a LANGE medical book

CW01665223

CURREN.
Diagnosis & Treatment Obstetrics & Gynecology

11TH EDITION

Alan H. DeCherney, MD
Chief, Reproductive Biology and Medicine Branch
National Institute of Child Health and Human Development
National Institutes of Health
Bethesda, Maryland

Lauren Nathan, MD
Associate Professor
Department of Osbstetrics and Gynecology
The David Geffen School of Medicine at UCLA
Los Angeles, California

Neri Laufer, MD
Professor and Chairman Department of Obstetrics and Gynecology
Hadassah University Hospital
Ein Kerem
Jerusalem, Israel

Ashley S. Roman, MD, MPH
Clinical Assistant Professor
Division of Maternal-Fetal Medicine
Department of Obstetrics and Gynecology
New York University School of Medicine
New York, New York

Mc Graw Hill Medical

New York Chicago San Francisco Lisbon London Madrid Mexico City
Milan New Delhi San Juan Seoul Singapore Sydney Toronto

The McGraw·Hill Companies

CURRENT Diagnosis & Treatment: Obstetrics & Gynecology, Eleventh Edition

1 2 3 4 5 6 7 8 9 0 DOC/DOC 17 16 15 14 13 12

ISBN 978-0-07-163856-2
MHID 0-07-163856-3
ISSN 0197-582X

Notice

Medicine is an ever-changing science. As new research and clinical experience broaden our knowledge, changes in treatment and drug therapy are required. The authors and the publisher of this work have checked with sources believed to be reliable in their efforts to provide information that is complete and generally in accord with the standards accepted at the time of publication. However, in view of the possibility of human error or changes in medical sciences, neither the authors nor the publisher nor any other party who has been involved in the preparation or publication of this work warrants that the information contained herein is in every respect accurate or complete, and they disclaim all responsibility for any errors or omissions or for the results obtained from use of the information contained in this work. Readers are encouraged to confirm the information contained herein with other sources. For example and in particular, readers are advised to check the product information sheet included in the package of each drug they plan to administer to be certain that the information contained in this work is accurate and that changes have not been made in the recommended dose or in the contraindications for administration. This recommendation is of particular importance in connection with new or infrequently used drugs.

This book was set in Minion Pro Regular by Cenveo Publisher Services.
The editors were Alyssa Fried and Harriet Lebowitz.
The production supervisor was Catherine Saggese.
Project management was provided by Sapna Rastogi, Cenveo Publisher Services.
RR Donnelly was printer and binder.

This book is printed on acid-free paper.

International Edition ISBN 978-0-07-174267-2; MHID 0-07-174267-0. Copyright © 2013. Exclusive rights by The McGraw-Hill Companies, Inc., for manufacture and export. This book cannot be re-exported from the country to which it is consigned by McGraw-Hill. The International Edition is not available in North America.

Contents

Section IV. Surgical & Medical Complications of Pregnancy

Section V. General Gynecology

Section VI. Gynecologic Oncology

Section VII. Reproductive Endocrinology & Infertility

Section VIII. Psychological & Social Issues

Authors

Paola Aghajanian, MD
Clinical Fellow in Maternal-Fetal Medicine
Department of Obstetrics and Gynecology
Los Angeles County–University of Southern California Medical Center
Los Angeles, California
Gestational Trophoblastic Diseases

Connie Alford, MD
Clinical Fellow
Eunice Kennedy Shriver, National Institute of Child Health and Human Development
National Institutes of Health
Bethesda, Maryland
Physiology of Reproduction in Women

Gayane Ambartsumyan, MD, PhD
Fellow Physician
Division of REI, Deptartment of Ob/Gyn
David Geffen School of Medicine at UCLA
Northridge, California
Infertility

Danielle D. Antosh, MD
Fellow
Department of Obstetrics and Gynecology
Washington Hospital Center
Washington, DC
Perioperative, Intraoperative, & Postoperative Complications in Gynecologic Surgery

Carol L. Archie, MD
Associate Clinical Professor Maternal-Fetal Medicine
Department of Obstetrics and Gynecology
David Geffen School of Medicine at UCLA
Los Angeles, California
Normal & Abnormal Labor & Delivery

Christina Arnett, MD
Department of Obstetrics & Gynecology
University of Southern California Medical Center
Los Angeles, California
Hematologic Disorders in Pregnancy

Gyamfi-Bannerman, MD
Associate Clinical Professor of Obstetrics and Gynecology
Division of Maternal-Fetal Medicine
Columbia University Medical Center
New York, New York
Thyroid & Other Endocrine Disorders During Pregnancy

Dvora Bauman, MD
Chaiman of Israeli PAG (Pediatric and Adolescent Gynecology) Society
Head of PAG Center
Department of Obstetrics and Gynecology
Bikur Holim Hospital
Jerusalem, Israel
Pediatric & Adolescent Gynecology

Shmuel Benenson, MD
Department of Clinical Microbiology and Infectious Diseases
Hadassah–Hebrew University Medical Center
Jerusalem, Israel
Antimicrobial Chemotherapy

Helene B. Bernstein, MD
Associate Professor
Reproductive Biology, Molecular Biology and Microbiology
Case Western Reserve University School of Medicine
Cleveland, Ohio
Normal Pregnancy

Jacob Bornstein MD, MPA
Professor and Associate Dean,
Faculty of Medicine in the Galilee,
Bar-Ilan University Chairman,
Department of Obstetrics and Gynecology
Western Galilee Hospital,
Nahariya, Israel President,
The International Society for the Study of Vulvovaginal Disease (ISSVD)
Benign Disorders of the Vulva & Vagina

Prof Amnon Brzezinski, MD
Professor
Department of Obstetrics and Gynecology
Hadassah Medical Center
Jerusalem, Israel
Contraception & Family Planning

Ronald T. Burkman, MD
Chair, Department of Obstetrics and Gynecology
Baystate Medical Center
Springfield, Massachusetts
Contraception & Family Planning

Melissa C. Bush, MD
Assistant Clinical Professor
Department of Obstetrics and Gynecology
University of California, Irvine
Orange, California
Multiple Gestation

Wendy Y. Chang, MD
Assistant Professor
Department of Obstetrics and Gynecology
David Geffen School of Medicine at UCLA
Los Angeles, California
Amenorrhea

Biing-Jaw Chen, MD
Anesthesiologist
Torrance, California
Obstetric Analgesia & Anesthesia

Alan H. DeCherney, MD
Chief, Reproductive Biology and Medicine Branch
National Institute of Child Health and Human Development
National Institutes of Health
Bethesda, Maryland
Imaging in Gynecology; Infertility; Amenorrhea; Assisted Reproductive Technologies: In Vivo Fertilization & Related Techniques; Antimicrobial Chemotherapy

Catherine M. DeUgarte, MD
Assistant Clinical Volunteer Faculty
Department of Obstetrics and Gynecology
UCLA
Los Angeles, California
Embryology of the Urogenital System & Congenital Abnormalities of the Genital Tract

Oliver Dorigo, MD, PhD
Assistant Professor
Department of Obstetrics and Gynecology
Division Gynecologic Oncology
David Geffen School of Medicine at UCLA
Los Angeles, California
Premalignant & Malignant Disorders of the Uterine Corpus; Radiation & Chemotherapy for Gynecologic Cancers

Samantha M. Dunham, MD
Clinical Assistant Professor
Department of Obstetrics and Gynecology
NYU School of Medicine
New York, New York
Early Pregnancy Risks

Wafic M. ElMasri, MD
Department of Obstetrics and Gynecology
Division Gynecologic Oncology
David Geffen School of Medicine at UCLA
Los Angeles, California
Radiation & Chemotherapy for Gynecologic Cancers

Nicole D. Fleming, MD
Fellow
Gynecologic Oncology
UCLA Medical Center
Los Angeles, California
Premalignant & Malignant Disorders of the Uterine Corpus

Amy A. Flick, MD
Fellow
Maternal-Fetal Medicine
UCLA
Los Angeles, California
Maternal Physiology During Pregnancy; Fetal & Early Neonatal Physiology

Michael D. Fox, MD
Department of Obstetrics and Gynecology
Division Chief, Reproductive Endocrinology and Infertility
University of Florida,
Jackonsonville, Florida
Endometriosis

Nathan S. Fox, MD
Associate Clinical Professor
Obstetrics, Gynecology, and Reproductive Science
Mount Sinai School of Medicine
New York, New York
Critical Care Obstetrics; Renal & Urinary Tract Disorders in Pregnancy

Shahin Ghadir, MD
Assistant Clinical Professor
Department of Obstetrics and Gynecology
David Geffen School of Medicine at UCLA
Los Angeles, California
Infertility

Johanna Weiss Goldberg, MD
Clinical Instructor
Department of Obstetrics and Gynecology
Joan and Sanford I Weill Medical College, Cornell University
New York, New York
Critical Care Obstetrics

T. Murphy Goodwin, MD
Professor of Obstetrics and Gynecology
Keck School of Medicine
University of Southern California
Los Angeles, California
Nervous System & Autoimmune Disorders in Pregnancy

Lisa Green, MD, MPH
Resident
Howard University Hospital
Washington DC
Antimicrobial Chemotherapy

Jeffrey S. Greenspoon, MD
Maternal-Fetal Medicine Specialist
Olive-View UCLA Medial Center
Los Angeles, California
Diabetes Mellitus in Pregnancy

Simi Gupta, MD
Maternal-Fetal Medicine Fellow
Department of Obstetrics and Gynecology
New York University
New York, New York
Imaging in Obstetrics

Vivian P. Halfin, MD
Associate Clinical Professor of Psychiatry and Obstetrics and Gynecology
Tufts University School of Medicine
Boston, Massachusetts
Domestic Violence & Sexual Assault

Afshan B. Hameed, MD
Associate Professor of Clinical Obstetrics & Gynecology
Associate Professor of Clinical Cardiology
Medical Director, Obstetrics
University of California, Irvine
Orange, California
Cardiac & Pulmonary Disorders in Pregnancy

Ryan J. Heitmann, DO
Clinical Fellow
Program in Reproductive and Adult Endocrinology
National Institutes of Health
Bethesda, Maryland
Anatomy of the Female Reproductive System

Micah J. Hill, DO
Clinical Fellow
Program in Reproductive and Adult Endocrinology
Eunice Kennedy Shriver National Institute of Child Health and Human Development
Bethesda, Maryland
Imaging in Gynecology

Prof Drorith Hochner-Celnikier, MD
Head, Department of Obstetrics and Gynecology
Hadassah Medical Organization
Mount Scopus, Jerusalem, Israel
Gynecologic History, Examination, & Diagnostic Procedures

Christine H. Holschneider, MD
Associate Professor
Department of Obstetrics and Gynecology
David Geffen School of Medicine at UCLA
Los Angeles, California
Surgical Diseases & Disorders in Pregnancy; remalignant & Malignant Disorders of the terine Cervix

Andy Huang, MD
Assistant Clinical Professor
Department of Obstetrics and Gynecology
UCLA
Los Angeles, California
Genetic Disorders & Sex Chromosome Abnormalities

Marc H. Incerpi, MD, PhD
Associate Professor
Department of Clinical Obstetrics and Gynecology, Division of Maternal-Fetal Medicine
Keck School of Medicine University of Southern California
Los Angeles, California
Operative Delivery

Carla Janzen, MD, PhD
Assistant Professor
Department of Obstetrics and Gynecology
UCLA
Los Angeles, California
Diabetes Mellitus in Pregnancy

Daniel A. Kahn, MD, PhD
Chief Resident Physician
Department of Obstetrics and Gynecology
David Geffen School of Medicine at UCLA
Los Angeles, California
Maternal Physiology During Pregnancy; Fetal & Early Neonatal Physiology

Laura Kalayjian, MD
Associate Professor of Neurology
Co-director, Comprehensive Epilepsy Center
University of Southern California Keck School of Medicine
Los Angeles, California
Nervous System & Autoimmune Disorders in Pregnancy

Amer Karam, MD
Assistant Clinical Professor
Department of Obstetrics and Gynecology
David Geffen School of Medicine at UCLA
Los Angeles, California
The Breast; Premalignant & Malignant Disorders of the Vulva & Vagina

Charles Kawada, MD
Department of Obstetrics, Gynecology, and Reproductive Biology
Harvard Medical School
Cambridge, Massachusetts
Gynecologic History, Examination, & Diagnostic Procedures

Lisa K. Kelly, MD
Assistant Professor of Pediatrics
Department of Pediatrics
Keck School of Medicine
Los Angeles, California
Normal Newborn Assessment & Care; Neonatal Resuscitation

Izabella Khachikyan, MD
Research Fellow
Department of PRAE
Eunice Kennedy Shriver National Institute of Child Health and Human Development
National Institutes of Health
Bethesda, Maryland
Benign Disorders of the Uterine Cervix

Karen Kish, MD
Clinical Assistant Professor
Department of Obstetrics & Gynecology
UT Southwestern Medical Center
Austin, Texas
Malpresentation & Cord Prolapse

Chad K. Klauser, MD
Clinical Assistant Professor
Division of Maternal Fetal Medicine
Department of Obstetrics and Gynecology
The Mount Sinai School of Medicine and NYU School of Medicine
New York, New York
Gastrointestinal Disorders in Pregnancy

Wing-Fai Kwan, MD
Anesthesiologist
Torrance, CA
Obstetric Analgesia & Anesthesia

Ofer Lavie, MD
Professor of Obstetrics and Gynecology
Department of Obstetrics and Gynecology
Faculty of Medicine of the Technion Israel Institute of Technology
Haifa, Israel
Benign Disorders of the Ovaries & Oviducts

Richard H. Lee, MD
Assistant Professor of Clinical Obstetrics and Gynecology
Associate Fellowship Director of Maternal-Fetal Medicine
Keck School of Medicine
University of Southern California
Los Angeles, California
Nervous System & Autoimmune Disorders in Pregnancy

Gary Levy, MD, MAJ, MC, USA
Clinical Fellow in Reproductive Endocrinology and Infertility
National Institutes of Health, Walter Reed National Military Medical Center
Clinical Instructor in Obstetrics and Gynecology
Uniformed Services University
Bethesda, Maryland
Premalignant & Malignant Disorders of the Ovaries & Oviducts

Jessica S. Lu, MPH
Medical Student
UCLA
Los Angeles, California
Domestic Violence & Sexual Assault

Michael C. Lu, MD, MPH
Associate Professor
Department of Obstetrics, Gynecology, and Public Health
UCLA Schools of Medicine and Public Health
Los Angeles, California
Domestic Violence & Sexual Assault

Gillian Mackay, MD
Assistant Professor
Department of Obstetrics and Gynecology
David Geffen School of Medicine at UCLA
Los Angeles, California
Sexually Transmitted Diseases & Pelvic Infections

Somjate Manipalviratn, MD
Department of Obstetric-Gynecology and Infertility
Superior A.R.T.
Bangkok, Thailand
Genetic Disorders & Sex Chromosome Abnormalities

John S. McDonald, MD
Professor
Department of Anesthesiology
Harbor-UCLA Medical Center
Torrance, California
Obstetric Analgesia & Anesthesia

Shobha H. Mehta, MD
Clinical Assistant Professor
Department of Obstetrics and Gynecology
Wayne State University
Detroit, Michigan
Assessment of At-Risk Pregnancy

Konstantinos G. Michalakis, MD
Department of Reproductive Endocrinology
National Institute of Health
Bethesda, Maryland
Assisted Reproductive Technologies: In Vivo Fertilization & Related Techniques

David A. Miller, MD
Professor of Obsterics, Gynecology and Pediatrics
Department of Obstetrics and Gynecology
Keck School of Medicine, University of Southern California
Los Angeles, California
Hypertension in Pregnancy

Martin N. Montoro, MD
Professor of Clinical Medicine and Obstetric Gynecology
Department of Maternal-Fetal Medicine
Keck School of Medicine/University of Southern California
Los Angeles, California
Cardiac & Pulmonary Disorders in Pregnancy

Aisling Murphy, MD
Clinical Fellow
Department of Obstetrics and Gynecology
David Geffen School of Medicine at UCLA
Los Angeles, California
Diabetes Mellitus in Pregnancy

Kenneth N. Muse, Jr., MD
Associate Professor & Director
Division of Reproductive Endocrinology
Department of Obstetrics & Gynecology
University of Kentucky
Lexington, Kentucky
Endometriosis

Lauren Nathan, MD
Associate Professor
Department of Obstetrics and Gynecology
David Geffen School of Medicine at UCLA
Los Angeles, California
Menopause & Postmenopause

Unzila Nayeri, MD
Fellow, Maternal-Fetal Medicine
Department of Obstetrics, Gynecology, and Reproductive Sciences
Yale University
New Haven, Connecticut
Congenital Fetal Infections

Sahadat K. Nurudeen, MD
Resident Physician
Department of Obstetrics and Gynecology
Georgetown University Hospital
Washington, DC
Physiology of Reproduction in Women

Sue M. Palmer, MD
Department of Obstetrics and Gynecology
University of Texas
Houston, Texas
Diabetes Mellitus in Pregnancy

Alan S. Penzias, MD
Surgical Director
Boston IVF
Boston, Massachusetts
Assisted Reproductive Technologies: In Vivo Fertilization & Related Techniques

Martin L. Pernoll, MD
Executive Dean
Kansas University School of Medicine
Kansas City, Kansas
Multiple Gestations

Caroline Pessel, MD
Maternal-Fetal Medicine Fellow
Department of Obstetrics and Gynecology
Columbia University Medical Center
New York, New York
The Normal Puerperium

Sarah B. H. Poggi, MD
Medical Director
The Brock Family Perinatal Diagnostic Center
Associate Professor
Department of Obstetrics and Gynecology
Inova Alexandria Hospital
Arlington, Virginia
Postpartum Hemorrhage & the Abnormal Puerperium

Karen Purcell, MD, PhD
Director
Department of Reproductive Services
Fertility for Family
San Jose, California
Premalignant & Malignant Disorders of the Ovaries & Oviducts

Elisabeth L. Raab, MD, MPH
Attending Neonatologist
Department of Neonatology
Childrens Hospital Los Angeles
Los Angeles, California
Normal Newborn Assessment & Care; Neonatal Resuscitation

Jeannine Rahimian, MD
Associate Clinical Professor
Department of Obstetrics and Gynecology
David Geffen School of Medicine at UCLA
Los Angeles, California
Disproportionate Fetal Growth

Andrei Rebarber, MD
Clinical Assistant Professor
Department of Obstetrics and Gynecology
Mount Sinai School of Medicine and NYU School of Medicine
New York, New York
Renal & Urinary Tract Disorders in Pregnancy

Ariel Revel, MD
Professor
Department of Obstetrics and Gynecology
Hadassah Medical Center and Hebrew University-Hadassah Medical School
Jerusalem, Israel
Hirsuitism

Ashley S. Roman, MD, MPH
Clinical Assistant Professor
Division of Maternal-Fetal Medicine
Department of Obstetrics and Gynecology
New York University School of Medicine
New York, New York
Normal & Abnormal Labor & Delivery; Imaging in Obstetrics; Late Pregnancy Complications; Hematologic Disorders in Pregnancy

Daniel H. Saltzman, MD
Clinical Professor
Department of Obstetrics and Gynecology
Division of Maternal Fetal Medicine
The Mount Sinai School of Medicine
New York, New York
Gastrointestinal Disorders in Pregnancy

Susan Sarajari, MD, PhD
Fellow
Division of Reproductive Endocrinology and Infertility
Department of Obstetrics and Gynecology
UCLA Medical Center and Cedars-Sinai Medical Center
Los Angeles, California
Endometriosis

Asher Shushan, MD
Associate Clinical Professor
Department of Obstetrics and Gynecology
Hebrew University
Jerusalem, Israel
Complications in Menstruation, Abnormal Uterine Bleeding

Alex Simon, MD
Director of IVF center
Department of Obstetrics and Gynecology
Hadassah University Hospital
Ein-Kerem, Jerusalem
Amenorrhea

Ramada S. Smith, MD
Director
Gaston Perinatal Center, Gaston Memorial Hospital
Gastonia, North Carolina
Critical Care Obstetrics

Robert J. Sokol, MD
Distinguished Professor of Obstetrics and Gynecology
Department of Obstetrics and Gynecology
Wayne State University School of Medicine
Detroit, Michigan
Assessment of At-Risk Pregnancy

Ella Speichinger, MD
Assistant Professor
Department of Obstetrics and Gynecology
David Geffen School of Medicine at UCLA
Los Angeles, California
Surgical Diseases & Disorders in Pregnancy

Pamela Stratton, MD
Head, Gynecology Consult Service
Program in Reproductive and Adult Endocrinology
Eunice Kennedy Shriver National Institute of Child Health and Human Development
Bethesda, Maryland
Benign Disorders of the Uterine Cervix

Stacy L. Strehlow, MD
Fellow, Maternal-Fetal Medicine
University of Southern California Women's and Children's Hospital
Los Angeles, California
Diabetes Mellitus in Pregnancy

Ann-Marie Surette, MD
Department of Obstetrics and Gynecology
NYU School of Medicine
New York, New York
Early Pregnancy Risks

Christopher M. Tarnay, MD
Associate Clinical Professor
Department of Obstetrics & Gynecology
David Geffen School of Medicine at UCLA
Los Angles, California
Urinary Incontinence & Pelvic Floor Disorders

Stephen Thung, MD, MSCI
Associate Professor
Department of Obstetrics and Gynecology
The Ohio State University
Columbus, Ohio
Congenital Fetal Infections

Bradley Trivax, MD
Fellow, Department of Reproductive Endocrinology and Infertility
UCLA Medial Center
Los Angeles, California
Genetic Disorders & Sex Chromosome Abnormalities

Ming C. Tsai, MD
Director
Department of Obstetrics and Gynecology
Bellevue Hospital Center
NYU School of Medicine
New York, New York
The Normal Puerperium

George VanBuren, MD
Associate Professor
Department of Reproductive Medicine
University Hospitals of Cleveland
Cleveland, Ohio
Normal Pregnancy

Sarah A. Wagner, MD
Assistant Professor
Department of Obstetrics and Gynecology
Loyola University Medical Center
Maywood, Illinois
Third-Trimester Vaginal Bleeding

Cecilia K. Wieslander, MD
Assistant Professor
Department of Obstetrics and Gynecology
David Geffen School of Medicine at UCLA
Los Angeles, California
Perioperative, Intraoperative, & Postoperative Complications in Gynecologic Surgery

Abigail Ford Winkel, MD
Assistant Professor
Department of Obstetrics & Gynecology
New York University School of Medicine
New York, New York
Dermatologic Disorders in Pregnancy

Keri S. Wong, MD
Department of Obstetrics and Gynecology
David Geffen School of Medicine at UCLA
757 Westwood Plaza, Suite B711
Los Angeles, California
Therapeutic Gynecologic Procedures

Preface

As in the previous editions, this text is a single-source reference for practitioners in both the inpatient and outpatient setting focusing on the practical aspects of clinical diagnosis and patient management.

Contained within the text is a thorough review of all of obstetrics and gynecology, including medical advances up to the time of publication. More than 1000 diseases and disorders are included.

A continued emphasis on disease prevention and evidence-based medicine remains paramount. In addition to diagnosis and treatment of disease, pathophysiology is a major area of focus. The concise format facilitates quick access.

A new and improved layout will certainly be appreciated, with more than 500 anatomic drawings, imaging studies, and diagrams as part of the basic text.

Medical students will find *Current Diagnosis & Treatment: Obstetrics & Gynecology* to be an authoritative introduction to the specialty and an excellent source for reference and review. House officers will welcome the concise practical information for commonly encountered health problems. Practicing obstetricians and gynecologists, family physicians, internists, nurse practitioners, nurse midwives, physician assistants, and other health care providers whose practice includes women's health can use the book to answer questions that arise in the daily practice of obstetrics and gynecology.

Medicine, including obstetrics and gynecology, is undergoing rapid change, and every attempt has been made to keep the Lange Series current. A great deal of effort has gone into checking the sources to make sure that this book presents standards of care and acceptable modes of treatment and diagnosis.

Everything that lies between the covers of the eleventh edition of *Current Diagnosis & Treatment: Obstetrics & Gynecology* has been updated, modified, and modernized from the tenth edition.

Alan H. DeCherney, MD
Lauren Nathan, MD
Neri Laufer, MD
Ashley S. Roman, MD, MPH

1 Anatomy of the Female Reproductive System

Ryan J. Heitmann, DO

Understanding human and pelvic anatomy is essential to the fundamental knowledge of an obstetrician/gynecologist. The basic facts and anatomic structures do not change, but our knowledge and understanding of relationships and function continues to increase. Advances in surgical techniques continue to place more importance on a physician's understanding of surgical landmarks. There can be significant variation in surgical anatomy, so the practitioner should be well versed in "normal" anatomy and prepared for the "nontextbook" cases.

ABDOMINAL WALL

Topographic Anatomy

The anterior abdominal wall is divided into sections for descriptive purposes and to allow the physician to outline relationships of the viscera in the abdominal cavity. The center point of reference is the sternoxiphoid process, which is in the same plane as the 10th thoracic vertebra. The upper 2 sections are formed by the subcostal angle; the lower extends from the lower ribs to the crest of the ilium and forward to the anterior superior iliac spines. The base is formed by the inguinal ligaments and the symphysis pubica.

The viscera are located by dividing the anterolateral abdominal wall into regions. One line is placed from the level of each ninth costal cartilage to the iliac crests. Two other lines are drawn from the middle of the inguinal ligaments to the cartilage of the eighth rib. The 9 regions formed (Fig. 1–1) are the epigastric, umbilical, hypogastric, and right and left hypochondriac, lumbar, and ilioinguinal.

Within the right hypochondriac zone are the right lobe of the liver, the gallbladder at the anterior inferior angle, part of the right kidney deep within the region, and, occasionally, the right colic flexure.

The epigastric zone contains the left lobe of the liver and part of the right lobe, the stomach, the proximal duodenum, the pancreas, the suprarenal glands, and the upper poles of both kidneys (Fig. 1–2).

The left hypochondriac region marks the situation of the spleen, the fundus of the stomach, the apex of the liver, and the left colic flexure.

Within the right lumbar region are the ascending colon, coils of intestine, and, frequently, the inferior border of the lateral portion of the right kidney.

The central umbilical region contains the transverse colon, the stomach, the greater omentum, the small intestine, the second and third portions of the duodenum, the head of the pancreas, and parts of the medial aspects of the kidneys.

Located in the left lumbar region are the descending colon, the left kidney, and the small intestine. Within the limits of the right ilioinguinal region are the cecum and appendix, part of the ascending colon, the small intestine, and, occasionally, the right border of the greater omentum.

The hypogastric region includes the greater omentum, loops of small intestine, the pelvic colon, and often part of the transverse colon.

The left ilioinguinal region encloses the sigmoid colon, part of the descending colon, loops of small intestine, and the left border of the greater omentum.

There is considerable variation in the position and size of individual organs due to differences in body size, conformation, and disease processes. Throughout life, variations in the positions of organs are dependent not only on gravity but also on the movements of the hollow viscera, which induce further changes in shape when filling and emptying. The need to recognize the relationships of the viscera to the abdominal regions becomes most apparent when taking into account the distortion that occurs during pregnancy. For example, the appendix lies in the right ilioinguinal region (right lower quadrant) until the 12th week of gestation. At 16 weeks, it is at the level of the right iliac crest. At 20 weeks, it is at the level of the umbilicus, where it will remain until after delivery. Because of this displacement, the symptoms of appendicitis will be different during the 3 trimesters. Similarly, displacement will also affect problems involving the bowel.

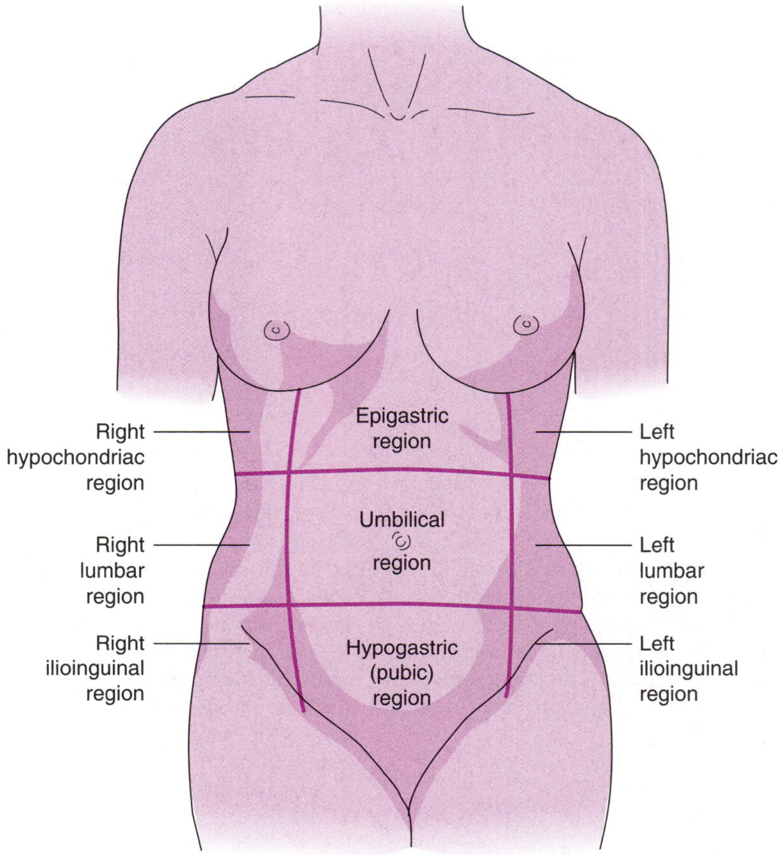

▲ **Figure 1–1.** Regions of the abdomen.

Skin, Subcutaneous Tissue, & Fascia

The abdominal skin is smooth, fine, and very elastic. It is loosely attached to underlying structures except at the umbilicus, where it is firmly adherent. Langer's lines are lines of tension based on the orientation of dermal fibers in the skin. On the anterior abdominal wall, these lines are arranged mostly in a transverse fashion. As a consequence, vertical incisions heal under more tension and therefore have a propensity to develop into wider scars. This is more noticeable in those patients who tend to form keloids. Conversely, transverse incisions, like a Pfannenstiel, heal with a much better cosmetic appearance.

Beneath the skin is the superficial fascia (tela subcutanea). This fatty protective fascia covers the entire abdomen. Below the navel, it consists principally of 2 layers: Camper's fascia, the more superficial layer containing most of the fat; and Scarpa's fascia (deep fascia), the fibroelastic membrane firmly attached to midline aponeuroses and to the fascia lata.

Arteries

Arteries of the Upper Abdomen

The lower 5 intercostal arteries (Fig. 1–3) and the subcostal artery accompany the thoracic nerves. Their finer, terminal branches enter the rectus sheath to anastomose with the superior and inferior epigastric arteries. The superior epigastric artery is the direct downward prolongation of the internal mammary artery. This artery descends between the posterior surface of the rectus muscle and its sheath to form an anastomosis with the inferior epigastric artery upon the muscle.

The inferior epigastric artery, a branch of the external iliac artery, usually arises just above the inguinal ligament and passes on the medial side of the round ligament to the abdominal inguinal ring. From there, it ascends in a slightly medial direction, passing above and lateral to the subcutaneous inguinal ring, which lies between the fascia transversalis

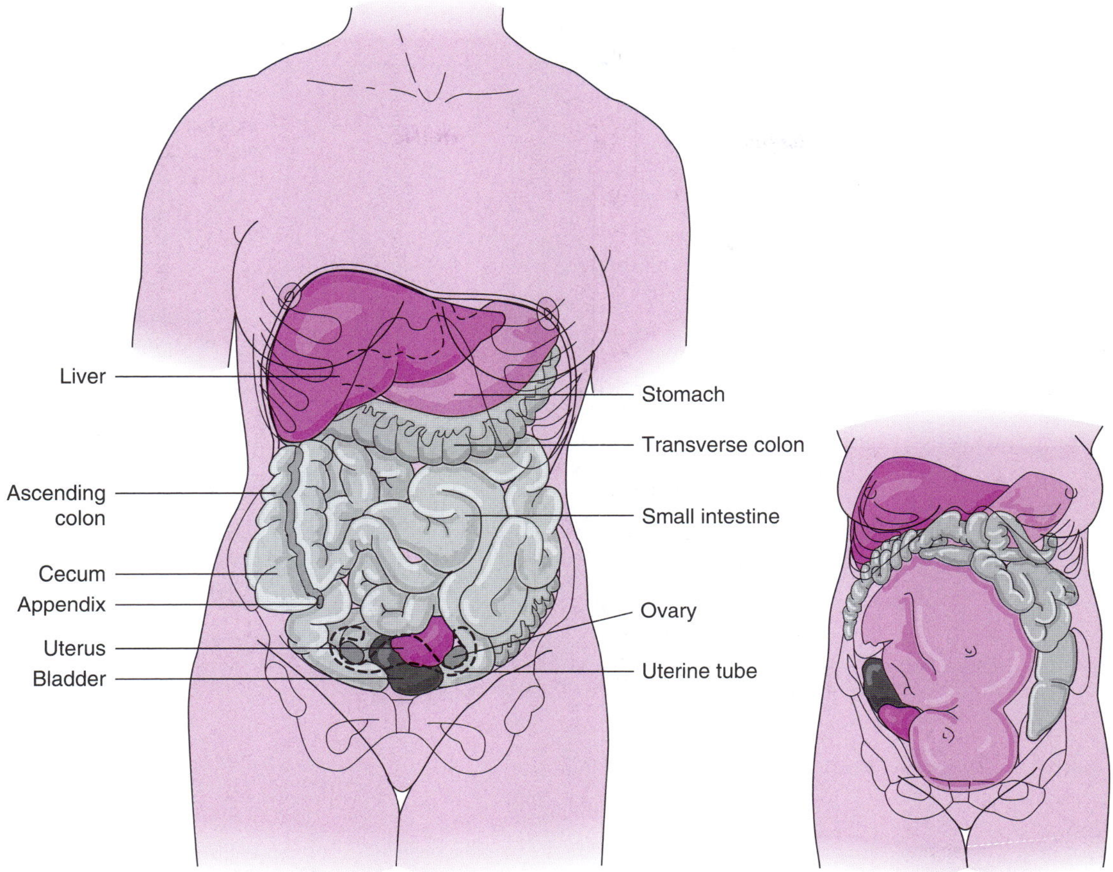

▲ **Figure 1–2.** Abdominal viscera in situ. Inset shows projection of fetus in situ.

and the peritoneum. Piercing the fascia transversalis, it passes in front of the linea semicircularis, turns upward between the rectus and its sheath, enters the substance of the rectus muscle, and meets the superior epigastric artery. The superior epigastric supplies the upper central abdominal wall, the inferior supplies the lower central part of the anterior abdominal wall, and the deep circumflex supplies the lower lateral part of the abdominal wall.

Arteries of the Lower Abdomen

The deep circumflex iliac artery is also a branch of the external iliac artery, arising from its side either opposite the epigastric artery or slightly below the origin of that vessel. It courses laterally behind the inguinal ligament lying between the fascia transversalis and the peritoneum. The deep circumflex artery perforates the transversus near the anterior superior spine of the ilium and continues between the transversus and internal oblique along and slightly above the crest of the ilium, finally running posteriorly to anastomose with the iliolumbar artery. A branch of the deep circumflex iliac artery is important to the surgeon because it forms anastomoses with branches of the inferior epigastric.

The various incisions on the abdomen encounter some muscle planes and vasculature of clinical significance. The McBurney incision requires separation of the external and internal oblique muscles and splitting of the transversus. The deep circumflex artery may be frequently encountered. The paramedian incision is made in the right or left rectus. Below the arcuate line, the fascia of the external and internal oblique, as well as the transversus muscles when present, goes over the rectus abdominis; above the arcuate line, the transversus and part of the internal oblique go under the rectus. The vasculature is primarily perforators and frequently the thoracoabdominal vein. Inferiorly, the superficial epigastric may be encountered.

In the Pfannenstiel or low transverse incision, the fascia of the external and internal oblique goes over the rectus muscle as well as the transversus muscle when present. After the fascia over the rectus is incised, the muscles can

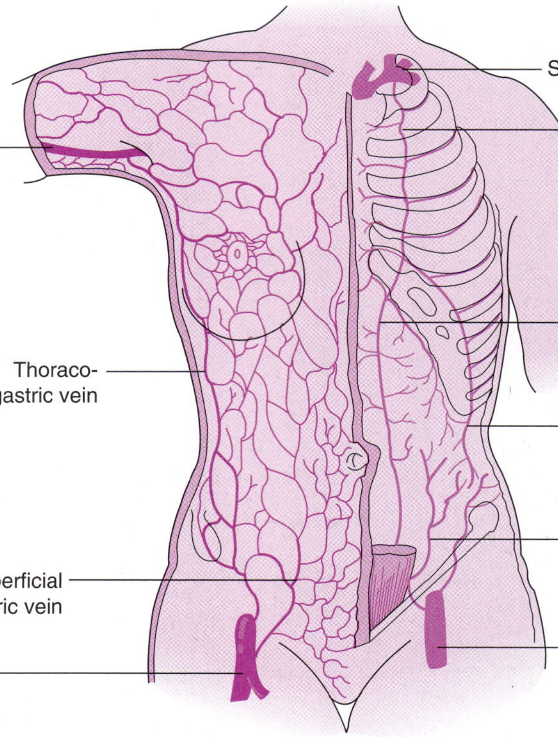

▲ **Figure 1–3.** Superficial veins and arteries of abdomen.

be separated. The superficial epigastric artery and vein are encountered in Camper's fascia. Laterally, the superficial and deep circumflex iliac arteries may be at the margin of the incision. Lying under the transversus muscle and entering the rectus approximately halfway to the umbilicus is the inferior epigastric artery.

In the Cherney incision, care should be taken to avoid the inferior epigastric artery, which is the primary blood supply to the rectus abdominis. Abdominal incisions are shown in Figure 1–4. The position of the muscles influences the type of incision to be made. The aim is to adequately expose the operative field, avoiding damage to parietal structures, blood vessels, and nerves. Low transverse incisions ideally do not extend past the lateral edges of the rectus muscles to avoid damage to the inferior epigastric vessels.

Veins

The superficial veins are more numerous than the arteries and form more extensive vascular networks. Above the level of the umbilicus, blood returns through the anterior cutaneous and the paired thoracoepigastric veins, the superficial epigastric veins, and the superficial circumflex iliac veins in the tela subcutanea. A cruciate anastomosis exists, therefore, between the femoral and axillary veins.

The deep veins correspond in name with the arteries they accompany. Below the umbilicus, these veins run caudally and medially to the external iliac vein; above that level, they run cephalad and laterally into the intercostal veins. Lymphatic drainage in the deeper regions of the abdominal wall follows the deep veins directly to the superficial inguinal nodes.

Lymphatics

The lymphatic drainage of the lower abdominal wall (Fig. 1–5) is primarily to the superficial inguinal nodes, 10–20 in number, which lie in the area of the inguinal ligament. These nodes may be identified by dividing the area into quadrants by intersecting horizontal and vertical lines that meet at the saphenofemoral junction. The lateral abdominal wall drainage follows the superficial circumflex iliac vein and drains to the lymph nodes in the upper lateral quadrant of the superficial inguinal nodes. The drainage of the medial aspect follows the superficial epigastric vein primarily to the lymph nodes in the upper medial quadrant of the superficial inguinal nodes. Of major clinical importance are the frequent anastomoses between the lymph vessels of the right and left sides of the abdomen.

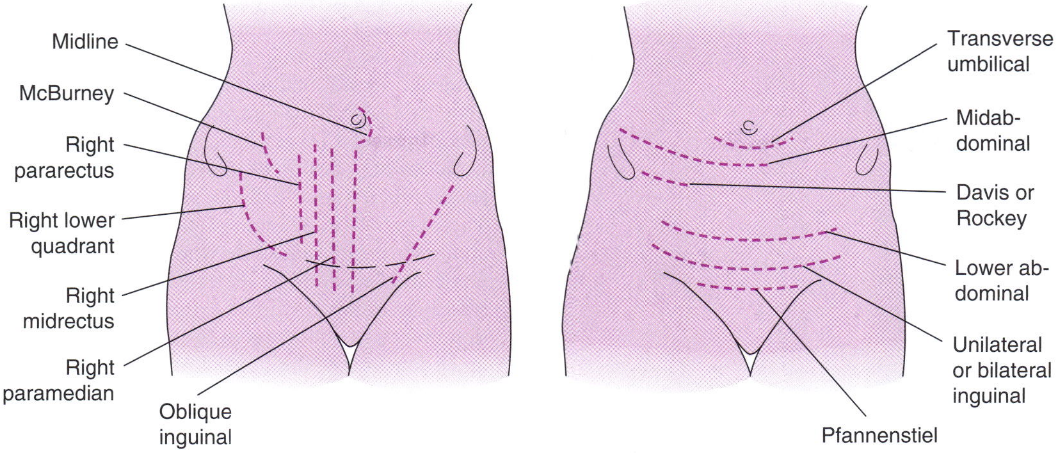

▲ **Figure 1–4.** Abdominal incisions. Transverse incisions are those in which rectus muscles are cut. A Cherney incision is one in which the rectus is taken off the pubic bone and then sewed back; the pyramidalis muscle is left on pubic tubercles.

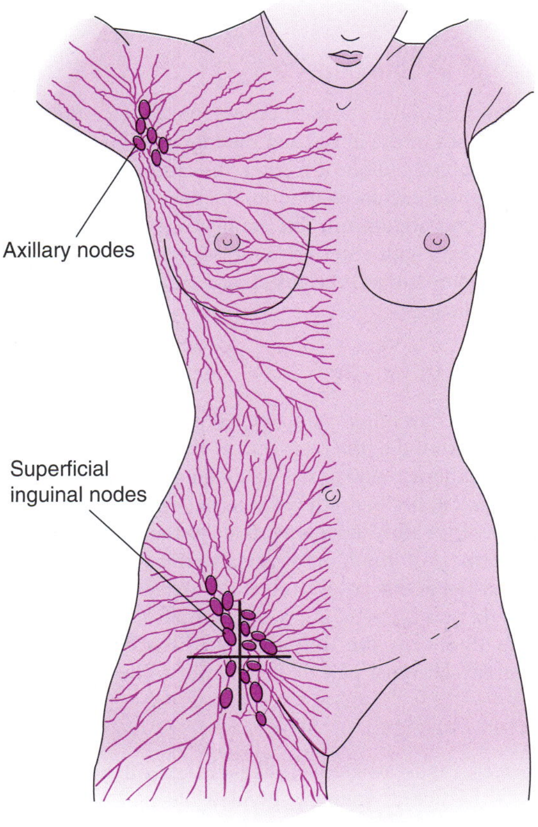

▲ **Figure 1–5.** Lymphatics of abdominal wall. Only one side is shown, but contralateral drainage occurs (ie, crosses midline to the opposite side).

Abdominal Nerves

The lower 6 thoracic nerves align with the ribs and give off lateral cutaneous branches (Fig. 1–6). The intercostal nerves pass deep to the upturned rib cartilages and enter the abdominal wall. The main trunks of these nerves run forward between the internal oblique and the transversus. The nerves then enter the rectus sheaths and the rectus muscles, and the terminating branches emerge as anterior cutaneous nerves.

The iliohypogastric nerve springs from the first lumbar nerve after the latter has been joined by the communicating branch from the last (12th) thoracic nerve. It pierces the lateral border of the psoas and crosses anterior to the quadratus lumborum muscle but posterior to the kidney and colon. At the lateral border of the quadratus lumborum, it pierces the aponeurosis of origin of the transversus abdominis and enters the areolar tissue between the transversus and the internal oblique muscle. Here, it frequently communicates with the last thoracic nerve and with the ilioinguinal nerve, which also originates from the first lumbar and last thoracic nerves.

The iliohypogastric divides into 2 branches. The iliac branch pierces the internal and external oblique muscles, emerging through the latter above the iliac crest and supplying the integument of the upper and lateral part of the thigh. The hypogastric branch, as it passes forward and downward, gives branches to both the transversus abdominis and internal oblique. It communicates with the ilioinguinal nerve and pierces the internal oblique muscle near the anterior superior spine. The hypogastric branch proceeds medially beneath the external oblique aponeurosis and pierces it just above the subcutaneous inguinal ring to supply the skin and symphysis pubica.

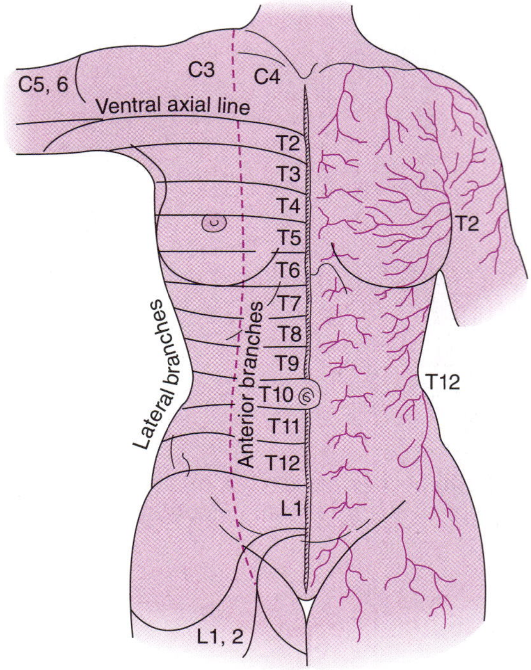

▲ **Figure 1–6.** Cutaneous innervation of the abdominal wall.

Similarly as with arteries and veins, care should be taken to avoid any nerve damage when performing surgery. With a low transverse incision, the iliohypogastric and ilioinguinal nerves are commonly encountered. Risk of damage or entrapment increases the more lateral an incision is made. When repairing the fascial layers, to help avoid entrapment of the iliohypogastric or ilioinguinal nerve, one should be careful not to place stitches lateral to the angle/apex of fascial incisions.

Abdominal Muscles & Fascia

The muscular wall that supports the abdominal viscera (Fig. 1–7) is composed of 4 pairs of muscles and their aponeuroses. The 3 paired lateral muscles are the external oblique, the internal oblique, and the transversus. Their aponeuroses interdigitate at the midline to connect opposing lateral muscles, forming a thickened band at this juncture, the linea alba, which extends from the xiphoid process to the pubic symphysis. Anteriorly, a pair of muscles—the rectus abdominis, with the paired pyramidalis muscles at its inferior border with its sheath—constitutes the abdominal wall.

Function of Abdominal Muscles

In general, the functions of the abdominal muscles are 3-fold: (1) support and compression of the abdominal viscera by the external oblique, internal oblique, and transversus muscles; (2) depression of the thorax in conjunction with the diaphragm by the rectus abdominis, external oblique, internal oblique, and transversus muscles, as evident in respiration, coughing, vomiting, defecation, and parturition; and (3) assistance in bending movements of the trunk through flexion of the vertebral column by the rectus abdominis, external oblique, and internal oblique muscles. There is partial assistance in rotation of the thorax and upper abdomen to the same side when the pelvis is fixed by the internal oblique and by the external oblique to the opposite side. In addition, the upper external oblique serves as a fixation muscle in abduction of the upper limb of the same side and adduction of the upper limb of the opposite side. The pyramidalis muscle secures the linea alba in the median line.

External Oblique Muscle

The external oblique muscle consists of 8 pointed digitations attached to the lower 8 ribs. The lowest fibers insert into the anterior half of the iliac crest and the inguinal ligament. At the linea alba, the muscle aponeurosis interdigitates with that of the opposite side and fuses with the underlying internal oblique.

Internal Oblique Muscle

The internal oblique muscle arises from thoracolumbar fascia, the crest of the ilium, and the inguinal ligament. Going in the opposite oblique direction, the muscle inserts into the lower 3 costal cartilages and into the linea alba on either side of the rectus abdominis. The aponeurosis helps to form the rectus sheath both anteriorly and posteriorly. The posterior layer extends from the rectus muscle rib insertions to below the umbilicus.

Transversus Muscle

The transversus muscle, the fibers of which run transversely and arise from the inner surfaces of the lower 6 costal cartilages, the thoracolumbar fascia, the iliac crest, and the inguinal ligament, lies beneath the internal oblique. By inserting into the linea alba, the aponeurosis of the transversus fuses to form the posterior layer of the posterior rectus sheath. The termination of this layer is called the arcuate line, and below it lies the transversalis fascia, preperitoneal fat, and peritoneum. Inferiorly, the thin aponeurosis of the transversus abdominis becomes part of the anterior rectus sheath.

Rectus Muscles

The rectus muscles are straplike and extend from the thorax to the pubis. They are divided by the linea alba and outlined laterally by the linea semilunaris. Three tendinous intersections cross the upper part of each rectus muscle, and a fourth may also be present below the umbilicus. The pyramidalis muscle, a vestigial muscle, is situated anterior to

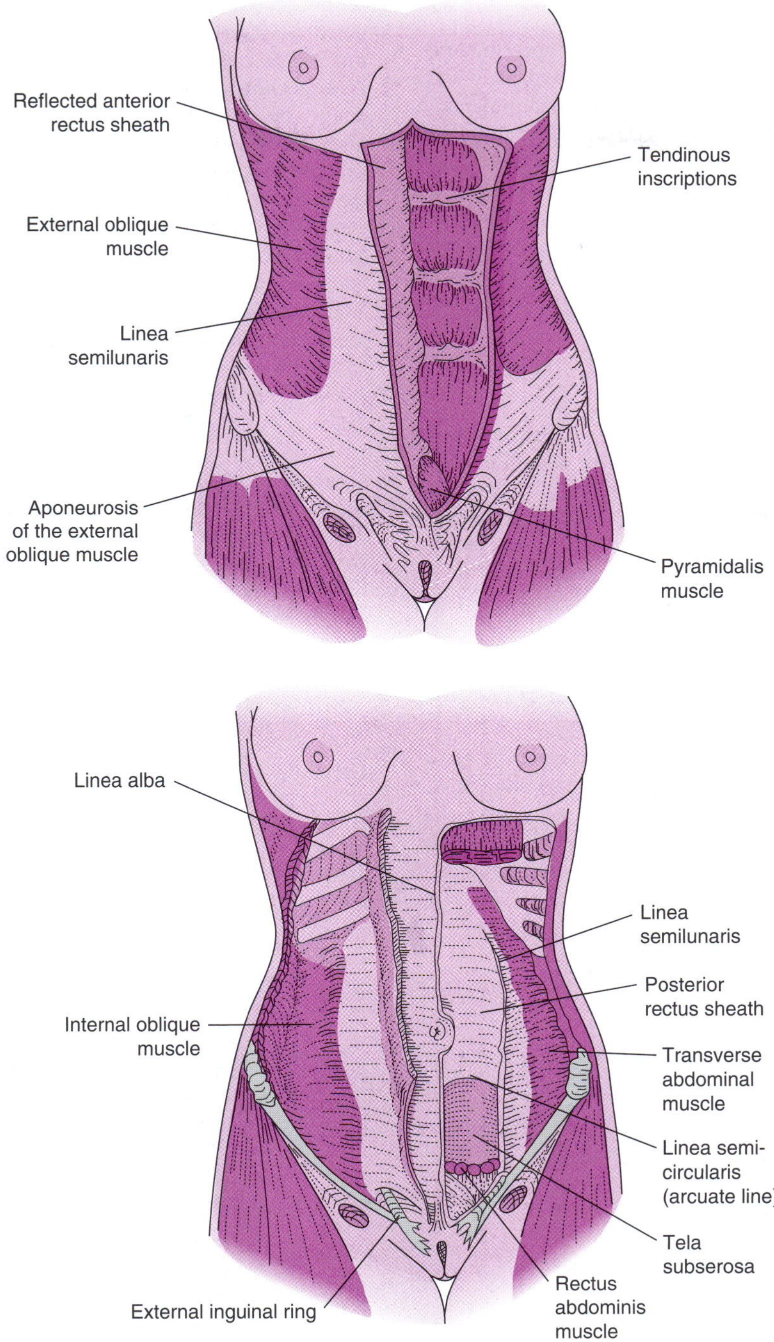

▲ **Figure 1–7.** Musculature of abdominal wall.

the lowermost part of the rectus muscle. It arises from and inserts into the pubic periosteum. Beneath the superficial fascia and overlying the muscles is the thin, semitransparent deep fascia. Its extensions enter and divide the lateral muscles into coarse bundles.

Special Structures

There are several special anatomic structures in the abdominal wall, including the umbilicus, linea alba, linea semilunaris, and rectus sheath.

Umbilicus

The umbilicus is positioned opposite the disk space between the third and fourth lumbar vertebrae, approximately 2 cm below the midpoint of a line drawn from the sternoxiphoid process to the top of the pubic symphysis. The umbilicus is a dense, wrinkled mass of fibrous tissue enclosed by and fused with a ring of circular aponeurotic fibers in the linea alba. Normally, it is the strongest part of the abdominal wall. It also represents the shortest distance between the skin and the abdominal cavity, and it is the most common place to enter the abdomen with the primary trochar when performing laparoscopic surgery.

Linea Alba

The linea alba, a fibrous band formed by the fusion of the aponeuroses of the muscles of the anterior abdominal wall, marks the medial side of the rectus abdominis; the linea semilunaris forms the lateral border, which courses from the tip of the ninth costal cartilage to the pubic tubercle. The linea alba extends from the xiphoid process to the pubic symphysis, represented above the umbilicus as a shallow median groove on the surface.

Rectus Sheath & Aponeurosis of the External Oblique

The rectus sheath serves to support and control the rectus muscles. It contains the rectus and pyramidalis muscles, the terminal branches of the lower 6 thoracic nerves and vessels, and the inferior and superior epigastric vessels. Cranially, where the sheath is widest, its anterior wall extends upward onto the thorax to the level of the fifth costal cartilage and is attached to the sternum. The deeper wall is attached to the xiphoid process and the lower borders of the seventh to ninth costal cartilages and does not extend upward onto the anterior thorax. Caudally, where the sheath narrows considerably, the anterior wall is attached to the crest and the symphysis pubica. Above the costal margin on the anterior chest wall, there is no complete rectus sheath (Fig. 1–8). Instead, the rectus muscle is covered only by the aponeurosis of the external oblique. In the region of the abdomen, the upper two-thirds of the internal oblique aponeurosis split at the lateral border of the rectus muscle into anterior and posterior lamellas. The anterior lamella passes in front of the external oblique and blends with the external oblique aponeurosis.

The posterior wall of the sheath is formed by the posterior lamella and the aponeurosis of the transversus muscle. The anterior and posterior sheaths join at the midline. The lower third of the internal oblique aponeurosis is undivided. Together with the aponeuroses of the external oblique and transversus muscles, it forms the anterior wall of the sheath. The posterior wall is occupied by transversalis fascia, which is spread over the interior surfaces of both the rectus and the transversus muscles, separating them from peritoneum and extending to the inguinal and lacunar ligaments. The transition from aponeurosis to fascia usually is fairly sharp, marked by a curved line called the arcuate line.

Variations of Abdominal Muscles

Variations have been noted in all of the abdominal muscles.

Rectus Muscle

The rectus abdominis muscle may differ in the number of its tendinous inscriptions and the extent of its thoracic

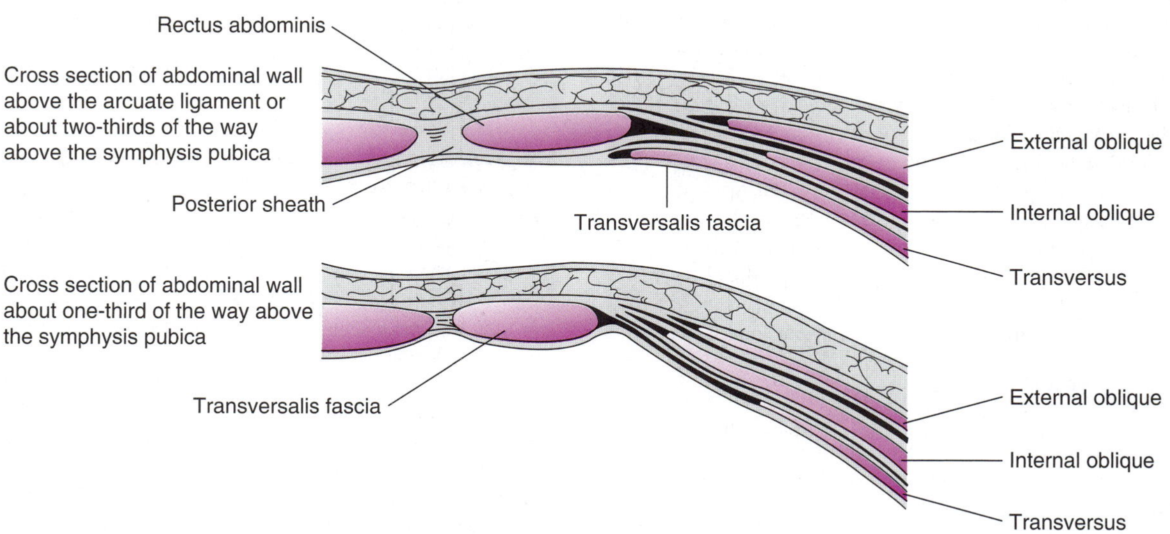

▲ **Figure 1–8.** Formation of rectus sheath.

attachment. Aponeurotic slips or slips of muscle on the upper part of the thorax are remnants of a more primitive state in which the muscle extended to the neck. Absence of part or all of the muscle has been noted. The pyramidalis muscle may be missing, only slightly developed, double, or extend upward to the umbilicus.

External Oblique Muscle

The external oblique muscle varies in the extent of its origin from the ribs. Broad fascicles may be separated by loose tissue from the main belly of the muscle, either on its deep or on its superficial surface. The supracostalis anterior is a rare fascicle occasionally found on the upper portion of the thoracic wall. Transverse tendinous inscriptions may also be found.

Internal Oblique Muscle

The internal oblique deviates at times, both in its attachments and in the extent of development of the fleshy part of the muscle. Occasionally, tendinous inscriptions are present, or the posterior division forms an extra muscle 7–7.5 cm wide and separated from the internal oblique by a branch of the iliohypogastric nerve and a branch of the deep circumflex iliac artery.

Transversus Muscle

The transversus muscle fluctuates widely in the extent of its development but is rarely absent. Rarely, it extends as far inferiorly as the ligamentum teres uteri (round ligament), and infrequently, it is situated superior to the anterior superior spine. However, it generally occupies an intermediate position.

BONY PELVIS

The pelvis (Fig. 1–9) is a basin-shaped ring of bones that marks the distal margin of the trunk. The pelvis rests on the lower extremities and supports the spinal column. It is composed of 2 innominate bones, one on each side, joined anteriorly and articulated with the sacrum posteriorly. The 2 major pelvic divisions are the pelvis major (upper or false pelvis) and the pelvis minor (lower or true pelvis). The pelvis major consists primarily of the space superior to the iliopectineal line, including the 2 iliac fossae and the region between them. The pelvis minor, located below the iliopectineal line, is bounded anteriorly by the pubic bones, posteriorly by the sacrum and coccyx, and laterally by the ischium and a small segment of the ilium.

Innominate Bone

The innominate bone is composed of 3 parts: ilium, ischium, and pubis.

Ilium

The ilium consists of a bladelike upper part or ala (wing) and a thicker, lower part called the body. The body forms the upper portion of the acetabulum and unites with the bodies of the ischium and pubis. The medial surface of the ilium presents as a large concave area: The anterior portion is the iliac fossa; the smaller posterior portion is composed of a rough upper part, the iliac tuberosity; and the lower part contains a large surface for articulation with the sacrum. At the inferior medial margin of the iliac fossa, a rounded ridge, the arcuate line, ends anteriorly in the iliopectineal eminence. Posteriorly, the arcuate line is continuous with the anterior margin of the ala of the sacrum across the anterior aspect of the sacroiliac joint. Anteriorly, it is continuous with the ridge or pecten on the superior ramus of the pubis.

The lateral surface or dorsum of the ilium is traversed by 3 ridges: the posterior, anterior, and inferior gluteal lines. The superior border is called the crest, and at its 2 extremities are the anterior and posterior superior iliac spines. The principal feature of the anterior border of the ilium is the heavy anterior inferior iliac spine. Important aspects of the posterior border are the posterior superior and the inferior iliac spines and, below the latter, the greater sciatic notch, the inferior part of which is bounded by the ischium. The inferior border of the ilium participates in the formation of the acetabulum.

The main vasculature (Fig. 1–10) of the innominate bone appears where the bone is thickest. Blood is supplied to the inner surface of the ilium through twigs of the iliolumbar, deep circumflex iliac, and obturator arteries by foramens on the crest, in the iliac fossa, and below the terminal line near the greater sciatic notch. The outer surface of the ilium is supplied mainly below the inferior gluteal line through nutrient vessels derived from the gluteal arteries. The inferior branch of the deep part of the superior gluteal artery forms the external nutrient artery of the ilium and continues in its course to anastomose with the lateral circumflex artery. Upon leaving the pelvis below the piriformis muscle, it divides into a number of branches, a group of which passes to the hip joint.

Ischium

The ischium is composed of a body, superior and inferior rami, and a tuberosity. The body is the heaviest part of the bone and is joined with the bodies of the ilium and pubis to form the acetabulum. It presents 3 surfaces. (1) The smooth internal surface is continuous above with the body of the ilium and below with the inner surface of the superior ramus of the ischium. Together, these parts form the posterior portion of the lateral wall of the pelvis minor. (2) The external surface of the ischium is the portion that enters into the formation of the acetabulum. (3) The posterior surface is the area between the acetabular rim and the posterior border. It is convex and is separated from the ischial tuberosity by a wide groove. The posterior border, with the ilium, forms the bony margin of the greater sciatic notch. The superior ramus of the ischium descends from the body of the bone to join the inferior ramus at an angle of approximately 90 degrees.

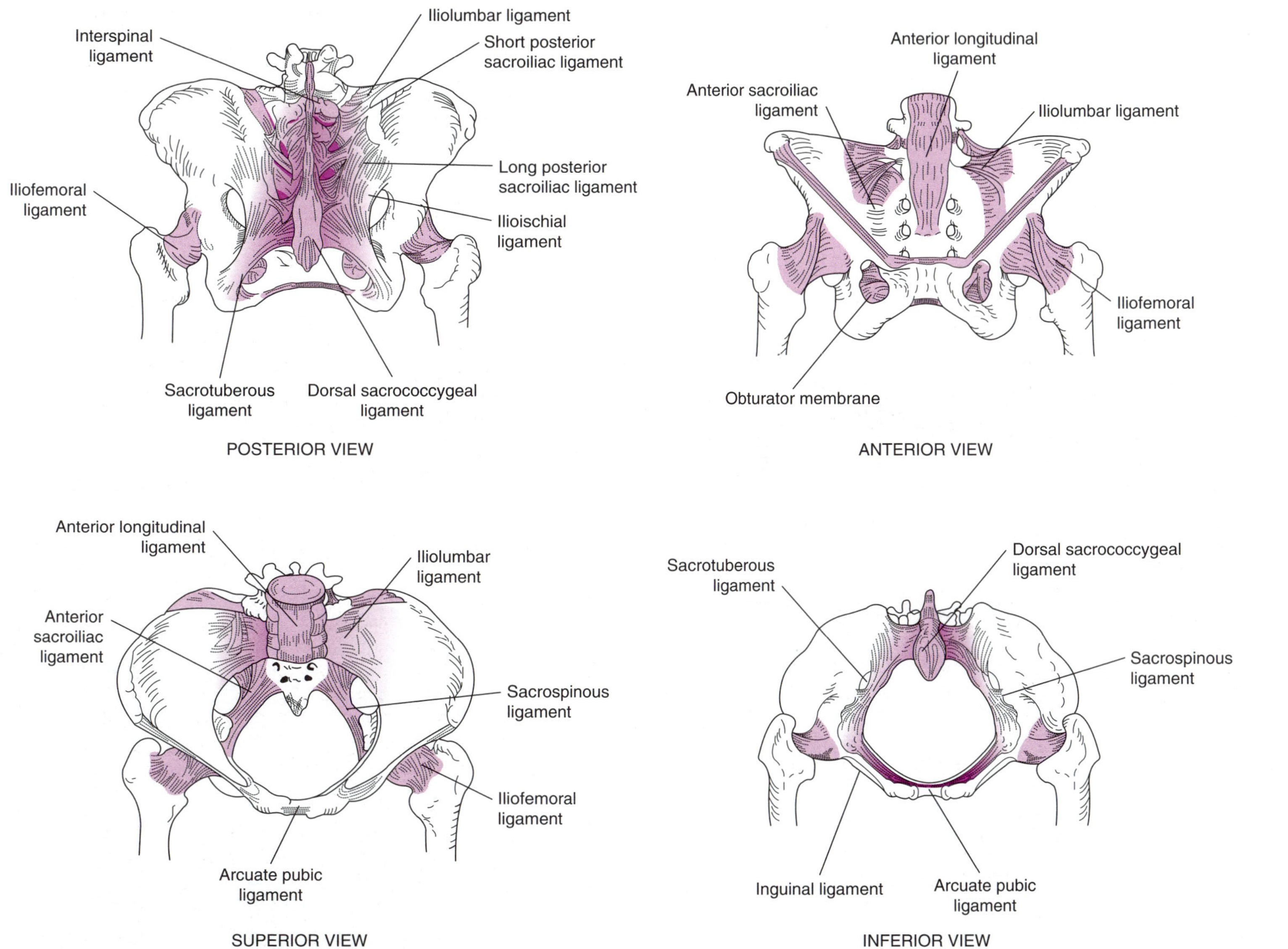

▲ **Figure 1–9.** The bony pelvis. (Reproduced, with permission, from Benson RC. *Handbook of Obstetrics & Gynecology*. 8th ed. Los Altos, CA: Lange; 1983.)

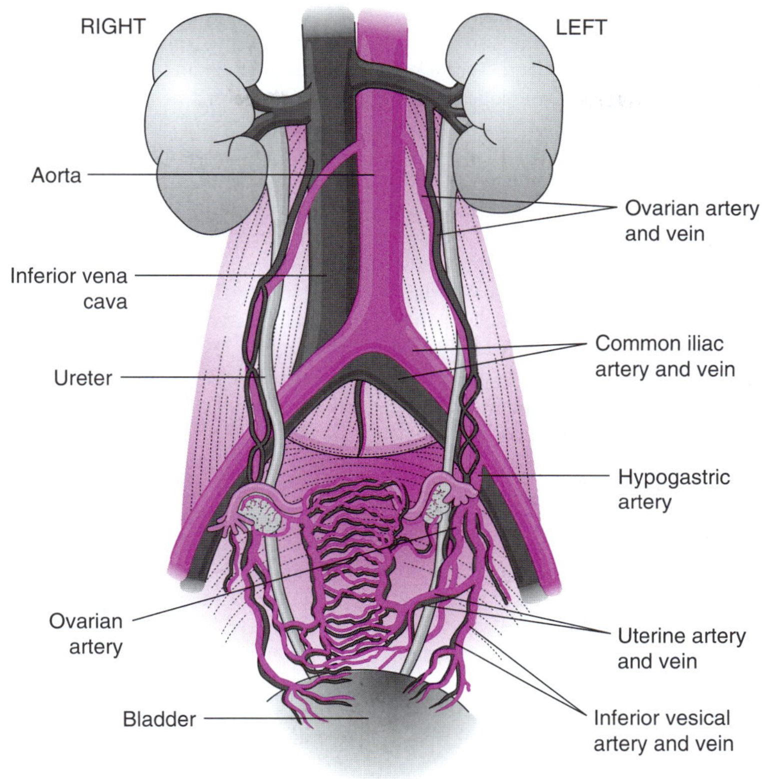

▲ **Figure 1–10.** Blood supply to pelvis.

The large ischial tuberosity and its inferior portion are situated on the convexity of this angle. The inferior portion of the tuberosity forms the point of support in the sitting position. The posterior surface is divided into 2 areas by an oblique line. The lesser sciatic notch occupies the posterior border of the superior ramus between the spine and the tuberosity. The inferior ramus, as it is traced forward, joins the inferior ramus of the pubis to form the arcus pubis (ischiopubic arch).

The ischium is supplied with blood from the obturator medial and lateral circumflex arteries. The largest vessels are situated between the acetabulum and the sciatic tubercle.

Pubis

The pubis is composed of a body and 2 rami, superior and inferior. The body contributes to the formation of the acetabulum, joining with the body of the ilium at the iliopectineal eminence and with the body of the ischium in the region of the acetabular notch. The superior ramus passes medially and forward from the body to meet the corresponding ramus of the opposite side at the symphysis pubica. The medial or fore portion of the superior ramus is broad and flattened anteroposteriorly. Formerly called "the body," it presents an outer and an inner surface, the symphyseal area, and an upper border or "crest."

Approximately 2 cm from the medial edge of the ramus and in line with the upper border is the prominent pubic tubercle, an important landmark. Below the crest are the anterior surface and the posterior or deep surface. The medial portion of the superior ramus is continuous below with the inferior ramus, and the lateral part presents a wide, smooth area anterosuperiorly, behind which is an irregular ridge, the pecten ossis pubis. The pecten pubis forms the anterior part of the linea terminalis. In front of and below the pectineal area is the obturator crest, passing from the tubercle to the acetabular notch. On the inferior aspect of the superior ramus is the obturator sulcus. The inferior ramus is continuous with the superior ramus and passes downward and backward to join the inferior ramus of the ischium, forming the "ischiopubic arch." The pubis receives blood from the pubic branches of the obturator artery and from branches of the medial and lateral circumflex arteries.

Pubic Symphysis

The pubic symphysis is a synarthrodial joint of the symphyseal surfaces of the pubic bones. The ligaments associated with it are (1) the interpubic fibrocartilage, (2) the superior pubic ligament, (3) the anterior pubic ligament, and (4) the arcuate ligament. The interpubic fibrocartilage is thicker in front than behind and projects beyond the edges of the bones, especially on the posterior aspect, blending intimately with the ligaments at its margins. Sometimes it is woven throughout, but often the interpubic fibrocartilage presents an elongated, narrow fissure with fluid in the interspace, partially dividing the cartilage into 2 plates.

The interpubic cartilage is intimately adherent to the layer of hyaline cartilage that covers the symphyseal surface of each pubic bone. The superior pubic ligament extends laterally along the crest of the pubis on each side to the pubic tubercle, blending in the middle line with the interpubic cartilage. The thick and strong anterior pubic ligament is closely connected with the fascial covering of the muscles arising from the conjoined rami of the pubis. It consists of several strata of thick, decussating fibers of different degrees of obliquity, the superficial being the most oblique and extending lowest over the joint. The arcuate ligament is a thick band of closely connected fibers that fills the angle between the pubic rami to form a smooth, rounded top to the pubic arch. Both on the anterior and posterior aspects of the joint, the ligament gives off decussating fibers that, interlacing with one another, strengthen the joint.

Sacrum

The sacrum is formed in the adult by the union of 5 or 6 sacral vertebrae; occasionally, the fifth lumbar vertebra is partly fused with it. The process of union is known as "sacralization" in the vertebral column. The sacrum constitutes the base of the vertebral column. As a single bone, it is considered to have a base, an apex, 2 surfaces (pelvic and dorsal), and 2 lateral portions. The base faces upward and is composed principally of a central part, formed by the upper surface of the body of the first sacral vertebra, and 2 lateral areas of alae. The body articulates by means of a fibrocartilage disk with the body of the fifth lumbar vertebra. The alae represent the heavy transverse processes of the first sacral vertebra that articulate with the 2 iliac bones. The anterior margin of the body is called the promontory and forms the sacrovertebral angle with the fifth lumbar vertebra. The rounded anterior margin of each ala constitutes the posterior part (pars sacralis) of the linea terminalis.

The pelvic surface of the sacrum is rough and convex. In the midline is the median sacral crest (fused spinal processes), and on either side is a flattened area formed by the fused laminae of the sacral vertebrae. The laminae of the fifth vertebra and, in many cases, those of the fourth and occasionally of the third are incomplete (the spines also are absent), thus leaving a wide opening to the dorsal wall of the sacral canal known as the sacral hiatus. Lateral to the laminae are the articular crests (right and left), which are in line with the paired superior articular processes above. The lateral processes articulate with the inferior articular processes of the fifth lumbar vertebra. The inferior extensions of the articular crests form the sacral cornua that bind the sacral hiatus laterally and are attached to the cornua of the coccyx. The cornua can be palpated in life and are important landmarks indicating the inferior opening of the sacral canal (for sacral-caudal anesthesia).

The lateral portions of the sacrum are formed by the fusion of the transverse processes of the sacral vertebrae. They form dorsally a line of elevations called the lateral sacral crests. The parts corresponding to the first 3 vertebrae are particularly massive and present a large area facing laterally called the articular surface, which articulates with the sacrum. Posterior to the articular area, the rough bone is called the sacral tuberosity. It faces the tuberosity of the ilium. The apex is the small area formed by the lower surface of the body of the fifth part of the sacrum. The coccyx is formed by 4 (occasionally 3 or 5) caudal or coccygeal vertebrae. The second, third, and fourth parts are frequently fused into a single bone that articulates with the first by means of a fibrocartilage. The entire coccyx may become ossified and fused with the sacrum (the sacrococcygeal joint).

The sacrum receives its blood supply from the middle sacral artery, which extends from the bifurcation of the aorta to the tip of the coccyx, and from the lateral sacral arteries that branch either as a single artery that immediately divides or as 2 distinct vessels from the hypogastric artery. The lowest lumbar branch of the middle sacral artery ramifies over the lateral parts of the sacrum, passing back between the last vertebra and the sacrum to anastomose with the lumbar arteries above and the superior gluteal artery below. The lateral sacral branches (usually 4) anastomose anteriorly to the coccyx with branches of the inferior lateral sacral artery that branch from the hypogastric artery. They give off small spinal branches that pass through the sacral foramens and supply the sacral canal and posterior portion of the sacrum.

Sacroiliac Joint

The sacroiliac joint is a diarthrodial joint with irregular surfaces. The articular surfaces are covered with a layer of cartilage, and the cavity of the joint is a narrow cleft. The cartilage on the sacrum is hyaline in its deeper parts but much thicker than that on the ilium. A joint capsule is attached to the margins of the articular surfaces, and the bones are held together by the anterior sacroiliac, long and short posterior sacroiliac, and interosseous ligaments. In addition, there are 3 ligaments (Fig. 1–11), classed as belonging to the pelvic girdle itself, which also serve as accessory ligaments to the sacroiliac joint: the iliolumbar, sacrotuberous, and sacrospinous ligaments.

The anterior sacroiliac ligaments unite the base and the lateral part of the sacrum to the ilium, blending with the periosteum of the pelvic surface and, on the ilium, reaching the arcuate line to attach in the paraglenoid grooves. The posterior sacroiliac ligament is extremely strong and consists essentially of 2 sets of fibers, deep and superficial,

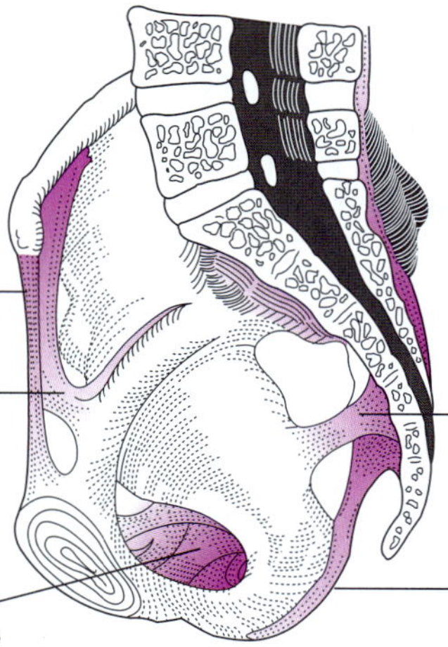

▲ **Figure 1–11.** Ligaments of the pelvis.

forming the short and long posterior sacroiliac ligaments, respectively. The short posterior sacroiliac ligament passes inferiorly and medially from the tuberosity of the ilium, behind the articular surface and posterior interior iliac spine, to the back of the lateral portion of the sacrum and to the upper sacral articular process, including the area between it and the first sacral foramen.

The long posterior sacroiliac ligament passes inferiorly from the posterior superior iliac spine to the second, third, and fourth articular tubercles on the back of the sacrum. It partly covers the short ligament and is continuous below with the sacrotuberous ligament. The interosseous ligaments are the strongest of all and consist of fibers of different lengths passing in various directions between the 2 bones. They extend from the rough surface of the sacral tuberosity to the corresponding surface on the lateral aspect of the sacrum, above and behind the articular surface.

Ligaments

The sacrotuberous ligament, in common with the long posterior sacroiliac ligament, is attached above to the crest of the ilium and posterior iliac spine and to the posterior aspect of the lower 3 sacral vertebrae. Below, it is attached chiefly to the medial border of the ischial tuberosity. Some of the fibers at the other end extend forward along the inner surface of the ischial ramus, forming the falciform process. Other posterior fibers continue into the tendons of the hamstrings.

The sacrospinous ligament is triangular and thin, extending from the lateral border of the sacrum and coccyx to the spine of the ischium. It passes medially (deep) to the sacrotuberous ligament and is partly blended with it along the lateral border of the sacrum.

The iliolumbar ligament connects the fourth and fifth lumbar vertebrae with the iliac crest. It originates from the transverse process of the fifth lumbar vertebra, where it is closely woven with the sacrolumbar ligament. Some of its fibers spread downward onto the body of the fifth vertebra, and others ascend to the disk above. It is attached to the inner lip of the crest of the ilium for approximately 5 cm. The sacrolumbar ligament is generally inseparable from the iliolumbar ligament and is regarded as part of it.

Foramens

Several foramens are present in the bony pelvis. The sacrospinous ligament separates the greater from the lesser sciatic foramen. These foramens are subdivisions of a large space intervening between the sacrotuberous ligament and the femur. The piriformis muscle passes out of the pelvis into the thigh by way of the greater sciatic foramen, accompanied by the gluteal vessels and nerves. The internal pudendal vessels, the pudendal nerve, and the nerve to the obturator internus muscle also leave the pelvis by this foramen, after which they enter the perineal region through the lesser sciatic foramen. The obturator internus muscle passes out of the pelvis by way of the lesser sciatic foramen.

The obturator foramen is situated between the ischium and the pubis. The obturator membrane occupies the obturator foramen and is attached continuously to the inner surface of the bony margin except above, where it bridges the obturator sulcus, converting the latter into the obturator canal, which provides passage for the obturator nerve and vessels.

On either side of the central part of the pelvic surface of the sacrum are 4 anterior sacral foramens that transmit the first 4 sacral nerves. Corresponding to these on the dorsal surface are the 4 posterior sacral foramens for transmission of the small posterior rami of the first 4 sacral nerves.

TYPES OF PELVES

Evaluation of the pelvis is best achieved by using the criteria set by Caldwell and Moloy, which are predicated upon 4 basic types of pelves: (1) the gynecoid type (from Greek *gyne* meaning woman); (2) the android type (from Greek *aner* meaning man); (3) the anthropoid type (from Greek *anthropos* meaning human); and (4) the platypelloid type (from Greek *platys* meaning broad and *pella* meaning bowl) (Fig. 1–12).

Gynecoid

In pure form, the gynecoid pelvis provides a rounded, slightly ovoid, or elliptical inlet with a well-rounded forepelvis (anterior segment). This type of pelvis has a well-rounded, spacious posterior segment, an adequate sacrosciatic notch, a hollow sacrum with a somewhat backward sacral inclination, and a Norman-type arch of the pubic rami. The gynecoid pelvis has straight side walls and wide interspinous and intertuberous diameters. The bones are primarily of medium weight and structure.

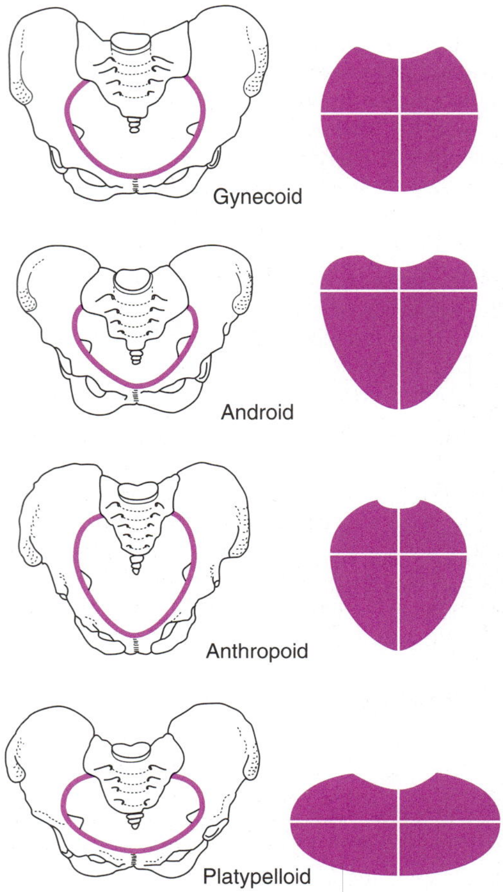

▲ **Figure 1–12.** Types of pelves. White lines in the diagrams at right (after Steele) show the greatest diameters of the pelves at left. (Reproduced, with permission, from Benson RC. *Handbook of Obstetrics & Gynecology*. 8th ed. Los Altos, CA: Lange; 1983.)

Android

The android pelvis has a wedge-shaped inlet, a narrow forepelvis, a flat posterior segment, and a narrow sacrosciatic notch, with the sacrum inclining forward. The side walls converge, and the bones are medium to heavy in structure.

Anthropoid

The anthropoid pelvis is characterized by a long, narrow, oval inlet; an extended and narrow anterior and posterior segment; a wide sacrosciatic notch; and a long, narrow sacrum, often with 6 sacral segments. The subpubic arch may be an angled Gothic type or rounded Norman type. Straight side walls are characteristic of the anthropoid pelvis, whose interspinous and intertuberous diameters are less than those of the average gynecoid pelvis. A medium bone structure is usual.

Platypelloid

The platypelloid pelvis has a distinct oval inlet with a very wide, rounded retropubic angle and a wider, flat posterior segment. The sacrosciatic notch is narrow and has a normal sacral inclination, although it is often short. The subpubic arch is very wide, and the side walls are straight, with wide interspinous and intertuberous diameters.

The pelvis in any individual case may be one of the 4 "pure" types or a combination of mixed types. When one discusses the intermediate pelvic forms, the posterior segment with its characteristics generally is described first and the anterior segment with its characteristics next (eg, anthropoid-gynecoid, android-anthropoid, or platypelloid-gynecoid). It is impossible to have a platypelloid-anthropoid pelvis or a platypelloid-android pelvis.

Pelvic Relationships

Several important relationships should be remembered, beginning with those at the inlet of the pelvis. The transverse diameter of the inlet is the widest diameter, where bone is present for a circumference of 360 degrees. This diameter stretches from pectineal line to pectineal line and denotes the separation of the posterior and anterior segments of the pelvis. In classic pelves (gynecoid), a vertical plane dropped from the transverse diameter of the inlet passes through the level of the interspinous diameter at the ischial spine.

These relationships may not hold true, however, in combination or intermediate (mixed type) pelves. The anterior transverse diameter of the inlet reaches from pectineal prominence to pectineal prominence; a vertical plane dropped from the anterior transverse passes through the ischial tuberosities. For good function of the pelvis, the anterior transverse diameter should never be more than 2 cm longer than the transverse diameter (Fig. 1–13).

Obstetric Conjugate

The obstetric conjugate differs from both the diagonal conjugate and the true conjugate. It is represented by a line

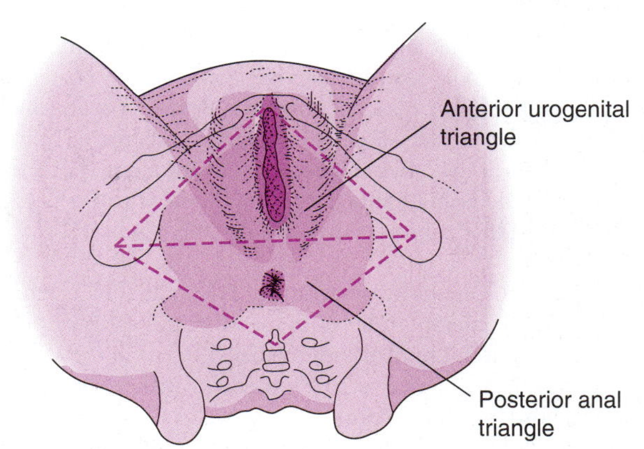

▲ **Figure 1–13.** Urogenital and anal triangles.

drawn from the posterior superior portion of the pubic symphysis (where bone exists for a circumference of 360 degrees) toward intersection with the sacrum. This point need not be at the promontory of the sacrum. The obstetric conjugate is divided into 2 segments: (1) the anterior sagittal, originating at the intersection of the obstetric conjugate with the transverse diameter of the inlet and terminating at the symphysis pubica; and (2) the posterior sagittal, originating at the transverse diameter of the inlet to the point of intersection with the sacrum.

Interspinous Diameter

A most significant diameter in the midpelvis is the interspinous diameter. It is represented by a plane passing from ischial spine to ischial spine. The posterior sagittal diameter of the midpelvis is a bisecting line drawn at a right angle from the middle of the interspinous diameter, in the same plane, to a point of intersection with the sacrum. This is the point of greatest importance in the midpelvis. It is sometimes said that the posterior sagittal diameter should be drawn from the posterior segment of the intersecting line of the interspinous diameter, in a plane from the inferior surface of the symphysis, through the interspinous diameter to the sacrum. However, this configuration often places the posterior sagittal diameter lower in the pelvis than the interspinous diameter. It is the interspinous diameter, together with the posterior sagittal diameter of the midpelvis, that determines whether or not there is adequate room for descent and extension of the head during labor.

Intertuberous Diameter

The intertuberous diameter of the outlet will reflect the length of the anterior transverse diameter of the inlet (ie, the former cannot be larger than the latter if convergent or straight side walls are present). Therefore, the intertuberous diameter determines the space available in the anterior segment of the pelvis at the inlet, and, similarly, the degree of convergence influences the length of the biparietal diameter at the outlet.

Posterior Sagittal Diameter

The posterior sagittal diameter of the outlet is an intersecting line drawn from the middle of the intertuberous diameter to the sacrococcygeal junction and reflects the inclination of the sacrum toward the outlet for accommodation of the head at delivery. It should be noted that intricate measurements of the pelvis are significant only at minimal levels. Evaluation of the pelvis for a given pregnancy, size of the fetus for a given pelvis, and conduct of labor engagement are far more important.

Outlets of the True Pelvis

The true pelvis is said to have an upper "inlet" and a lower "outlet." The pelvic inlet to the pelvis minor is bounded, beginning posteriorly, by (1) the promontory of the sacrum; (2) the linea terminalis, composed of the anterior margin of the ala sacralis, the arcuate line of the ilium, and the pecten ossis pubis; and (3) the upper border or crest of the pubis, ending medially at the symphysis. The conjugate or the anteroposterior diameter is drawn from the center of the promontory to the symphysis pubica, with 2 conjugates recognized: (1) the true conjugate, measured from the promontory to the top of the symphysis; and (2) the diagonal conjugate, measured from the promontory to the bottom of the symphysis.

The transverse diameter is measured through the greatest width of the pelvic inlet. The oblique diameter runs from the sacroiliac joint of one side to the iliopectineal eminence of the other. The pelvic outlet, which faces downward and slightly backward, is very irregular. Beginning anteriorly, it is bounded by (1) the arcuate ligament of the pubis (in the midline), (2) the ischiopubic arch, (3) the ischial tuberosity, (4) the sacrotuberous ligament, and (5) the coccyx (in midline). Its anteroposterior diameter is drawn from the lower border of the symphysis pubica to the tip of the coccyx. The transverse diameter passes between the medial surfaces of the ischial tuberosities.

INGUINAL REGION

The inguinal region of the abdominal wall is bounded by the rectus abdominis muscle medially, the line connecting the anterior superior iliac spines superiorly, and the inguinal ligament inferiorly. The region contains 8 layers of abdominal wall. These layers, from the most superficial inward, are (1) the skin, (2) the tela subcutanea (subcutaneous tissue), (3) the aponeurosis of the external oblique muscle, (4) the internal oblique muscle, (5) the transversus abdominis muscle (below the free border, the layer is incomplete), (6) the transversalis fascia, (7) the subperitoneal fat and connective tissue, and (8) the peritoneum. The tela subcutanea consists of the superficial fatty Camper's fascia, which is continuous with the tela subcutanea of the whole body, and the deeper membranous Scarpa's fascia, which covers the lower third of the abdominal wall and the medial side of the groin, both joining below the inguinal ligament to form the fascia lata of the thigh.

Subcutaneous (External) Inguinal Ring

A triangular evagination of the external oblique aponeurosis, the subcutaneous inguinal ring (external abdominal ring), is bounded by an aponeurosis at its edges and by the inguinal ligament inferiorly. The superior or medial crus is smaller and attaches to the symphysis pubica. The inferior or lateral crus is stronger and blends with the inguinal ligament as it passes to the pubic tubercle. The sharp margins of the ring are attributed to a sudden thinning of the aponeurosis. In the female, the ligamentum teres uteri (round ligament) pass through this ring. The subcutaneous inguinal ring is much smaller in the female than in the male, and the abdominal wall is relatively stronger in this region.

Abdominal (Internal) Inguinal Ring

The abdominal inguinal ring (internal abdominal ring) is the rounded mouth of a funnel-shaped expansion of transversalis fascia that lies approximately 2 cm above the inguinal ligament and midway between the anterior superior iliac spine and the symphysis pubica. Medially, it is bounded by the inferior epigastric vessels; the external iliac artery is situated below. The abdominal inguinal ring represents the area where the round ligament emerges from the abdomen. The triangular area medial to the inferior epigastric artery, bounded by the inguinal ligament below and the lateral border of the rectus sheath, is known as the trigonum inguinale (Hesselbach's triangle), the site of congenital direct hernias.

Inguinal Canal

The inguinal canal in the female is not well demarcated, but it normally gives passage to the round ligament of the uterus, a vein, an artery from the uterus that forms a cruciate anastomosis with the labial arteries, and extraperitoneal fat. The fetal ovary, like the testis, is an abdominal organ and possesses a gubernaculum that extends from its lower pole downward and forward to a point corresponding to the abdominal inguinal ring, through which it continues into the labia majora.

The processus vaginalis is an evagination of peritoneum at the level of the abdominal inguinal ring occurring during the third fetal month. In the male, the processus vaginalis descends with the testis. The processus vaginalis of the female is rudimentary, but occasionally a small diverticulum of peritoneum is found passing partway through the inguinal region; this diverticulum is termed the processus vaginalis peritonei (canal of Nuck). Instead of descending, as does the testis, the ovary moves medially, where it becomes adjacent to the uterus.

The intra-abdominal portion of the gubernaculum ovarii becomes attached to the lateral border of the developing uterus, evolving as the ligament of the ovary and the round ligament of the uterus. The extra-abdominal portion of the round ligament of the uterus becomes attenuated in the adult and may appear as a small fibrous band. The inguinal canal is an intermuscular passageway that extends from the abdominal ring downward, medially, and somewhat forward to the subcutaneous inguinal ring (about 3–4 cm). The canal is roughly triangular in shape, and its boundaries are largely artificial. The lacunar and inguinal ligaments form the base of the canal. The anterior or superficial wall is formed by the external oblique aponeurosis, and the lowermost fibers of the internal oblique muscle add additional strength in its lateral part. The posterior or deep wall of the canal is formed by transversalis fascia throughout and is strengthened medially by the falx inguinalis.

Abdominal Fossae

The abdominal fossae in the inguinal region consist of the foveae inguinalis lateralis and medialis. The fovea inguinalis lateralis lies lateral to a slight fold, the plica epigastrica, formed by the inferior epigastric vessels, and just medial to the abdominal inguinal ring, which slants medially and upward toward the rectus muscle. From the lateral margin of the tendinous insertion of the rectus muscle, upward toward the umbilicus, and over the obliterated artery extends a more accentuated fold, the plica umbilicalis lateralis. The fovea inguinalis medialis lies between the plica epigastrica and the plica umbilicalis lateralis, with the bottom of the fossa facing the trigonum inguinale (Hesselbach's triangle). This region is strengthened by the interfoveolar ligament at the medial side of the abdominal inguinal ring and the conjoined tendon lateral to the rectus muscle; however, these bands vary in width and thus are supportive.

Ligaments & Spaces

The falx inguinalis or conjoined tendon is formed by the aponeurosis of the transversus abdominis and internal oblique muscles. These fibers arise from the inguinal ligament and arch downward and forward to insert on the pubic crest and pecten ossis pubis, behind the inguinal and lacunar ligaments. The interfoveolar ligament is composed partly of fibrous bands from the aponeurosis of the transversalis muscle of the same and opposite sides. Curving medial to and below the internal abdominal ring, they attach to the lacunar ligament and pectineal fascia.

The inguinal ligament itself forms the inferior thickened border of the external oblique aponeurosis, extending from the anterior superior iliac spine to the pubic tubercle. Along its inferior border, it becomes continuous with the fascia lata of the thigh. From the medial portion of the inguinal ligament, a triangular band of fibers attaches separately to the pecten ossis pubis. This band is known as the lacunar (Gimbernat's) ligament. The reflex inguinal ligament (ligament of Colles or triangular fascia) is represented by a small band of fibers, often poorly developed, and derived from the superior crus of the subcutaneous inguinal ring and the lower part of the linea alba. These fibers cross to the opposite side to attach to the pecten ossis pubis. The inguinal ligament forms the roof of a large osseoligamentous space leading from the iliac fossa to the thigh. The floor of this space is formed by the superior ramus of the pubis medially and by the body of the ilium laterally.

The iliopectineal ligament extends from the inguinal ligament to the iliopectineal eminence, dividing this area into 2 parts. The lateral, larger division is called the muscular lacuna and is almost completely filled by the iliopsoas muscle, along with the femoral nerve medially and the lateral femoral cutaneous nerves laterally. The medial, smaller division is known as the vascular lacuna and is traversed by the external iliac (femoral) artery, vein, and lymphatic vessels, which do not completely fill the space. The anterior border of the vascular lacuna is formed by the inguinal ligament and the transversalis fascia. The posterior boundary is formed by the ligamentum pubicum superius (Cooper's ligament), a thickening of fascia along the public pecten where the pectineal fascia and iliopectineal ligament meet.

The transversalis fascia and iliac fascia are extended with the vessels, forming a funnel-shaped fibrous investment, the femoral sheath. The sheath is divided into 3 compartments: (1) the lateral compartment, containing the femoral artery; (2) the intermediate compartment, containing the femoral vein; and (3) the medial compartment or canal, containing a lymph node (nodi lymphatici inguinales profundi [node of Rosenmüller or Cloquet]) and the lymphatic vessels that drain most of the leg, groin, and perineum.

The femoral canal also contains areolar tissue, which frequently condenses to form the "femoral septum." Because of the greater spread of the pelvis in the female, the muscular and vascular lacunae are relatively large spaces. The upper or abdominal opening of the femoral canal is known as the femoral ring and is covered by the parietal peritoneum.

Arteries

In front of the femoral ring, the arterial branches of the external iliac artery are the inferior epigastric and the deep circumflex iliac. The inferior epigastric artery arises from the anterior surface of the external iliac, passing forward and upward on the anterior abdominal wall between peritoneum and transversalis fascia. It pierces the fascia just below the arcuate line, entering the rectus abdominis muscle or coursing along its inferior surface to anastomose with the superior epigastric from the internal thoracic. The inferior epigastric artery forms the lateral boundary of the trigonum inguinale (Hesselbach's triangle). At its origin, it frequently gives off a branch to the inguinal canal, as well as a branch to the pubis (pubic artery), which anastomoses with twigs of the obturator artery. The pubic branch of the inferior epigastric often becomes the obturator artery.

The deep circumflex iliac artery arises laterally and traverses the iliopsoas to the anterior superior iliac spine, where it pierces the transversus muscle to course between the transversus and the internal oblique, sending perforators to the surface. It often has anastomoses with penetrating branches of the inferior epigastric via its perforators through the rectus abdominis. The veins follow a similar course.

As the external iliac artery passes through the femoral canal, which underlies the inguinal ligament, it courses medial to the femoral vein and nerve, resting in what is termed the femoral triangle (Scarpa's triangle). The femoral sheath is a downward continuation of the inguinal ligament anterior to the femoral vessel and nerve.

The branches of the femoral artery supplying the groin are (1) the superficial epigastric, (2) the superficial circumflex iliac, (3) the superficial external pudendal, and (4) the deep external pudendal. The superficial epigastric artery passes upward through the femoral sheath over the inguinal ligament, to rest in Camper's fascia on the lower abdomen. The superficial circumflex iliac artery arises adjacent to the superior epigastric, piercing the fascia lata and running parallel to the inguinal ligament as far as the iliac crest. It then divides into branches that supply the integument of the groin, the superficial fascia, and the lymph glands, anastomosing with the deep circumflex iliac, the superior gluteal, and the lateral femoral circumflex arteries.

The superficial external pudendal artery arises from the medial side of the femoral artery, close to the preceding vessels. It pierces the femoral sheath and fascia cribrosa, coursing medially across the round ligament to the integument on the lower part of the abdomen and the labium majus, anastomosing with the internal pudendal. The deep external pudendal artery passes medially across the pectineus and adductor longus muscles, supplying the integument of the labium majus and forming, together with the external pudendal artery, a rete with the labial arteries.

Hernias

A hernia (Fig. 1–14) is a protrusion of any viscus from its normal enclosure, which may occur with any of the abdominal viscera, especially the jejunum, ileum, and greater omentum. A hernia may be due to increased pressure, such as that resulting from strenuous exercise, lifting heavy weights, tenesmus, or increased expiratory efforts, or it may result from decreased resistance of the abdominal wall (congenital

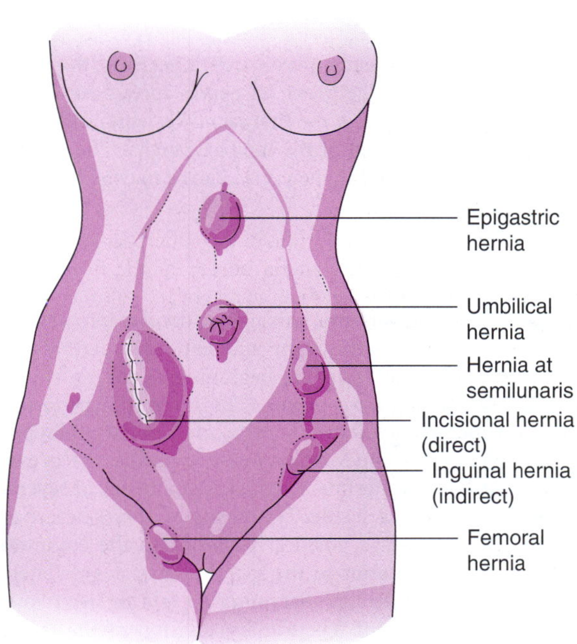

▲ **Figure 1–14.** Hernia sites.

or acquired), such as occurs with debilitating illness or old age, prolonged distention from ascites, tumors, pregnancy, corpulence, emaciation, injuries (including surgical incisions), congenital absence, or poor development. Hernias are likely to occur where the abdominal wall is structurally weakened by the passage of large vessels or nerves and developmental peculiarities. Ventral hernias occur through the linea semilunaris or the linea alba.

During early fetal development, portions of the mesentery and a loop of the intestine pass through the opening to occupy a part of the body cavity (the umbilical coelom) situated in the umbilical cord. Normally, the mesentery and intestine later return to the abdominal cavity. If they fail to do so, a congenital umbilical hernia results. Infantile umbilical hernias occur if the component parts fail to fuse completely in early postnatal stages. The unyielding nature of the fibrous tissue forming the margin of the ring predisposes to strangulation.

NERVES OF THE PELVIS

The pelvic autonomic system can be divided into the superior hypogastric plexus (the presacral plexus and the uterinus magnus), the middle hypogastric plexus, and the inferior hypogastric plexus. The superior hypogastric plexus begins just below the inferior mesenteric artery. It is composed of 1–3 intercommunicating nerve bundles connected with the inferior mesenteric ganglia, but no ganglia are an integral part of the plexus. The intermesenteric nerves receive branches from the lumbar sympathetic ganglia.

Superior Hypogastric Plexus

The superior hypogastric plexus continues into the midhypogastric plexus. The presacral nerves spread out into a latticework at the level of the first sacral vertebra, with connecting rami to the last of the lumbar ganglia. The greater part of the superior midhypogastric plexus may be found to the left of the midline.

Inferior Hypogastric Plexus

At the first sacral vertebra, this plexus divides into several branches that go to the right and left sides of the pelvis. These branches form the beginning of the right and left inferior hypogastric plexus. The inferior hypogastric plexus, which is the divided continuation of the midhypogastric plexus, the superior hypogastric plexus, the presacral nerve, and the uterinus magnus, is composed of several parallel nerves on each side. This group of nerves descends within the pelvis in a position posterior to the common iliac artery and anterior to the sacral plexus, curves laterally, and finally enters the sacrouterine fold or ligaments. The medial section of the primary division of the sacral nerves sends fibers (nervi erigentes) that enter the pelvic plexus in the sacrouterine folds. The plexus now appears to contain both sympathetic (inferior hypogastric plexus) and parasympathetic (nervi erigentes) components.

Nervi Erigentes

The sensory components, which are mostly visceral, are found in the nervi erigentes; however, if one takes into account the amount of spinal anesthetic necessary to eliminate uterine sensation, one must assume that there are a number of sensory fibers in the sympathetic component.

Common Iliac Nerves

The common iliac nerves originate separately from the superior hypogastric plexus and descend on the surface of the artery and vein, one part going through the femoral ring and the remainder following the internal iliac, finally rejoining the pelvic plexus.

Hypogastric Ganglion

On either side of the uterus, in the base of the broad ligament, is the large plexus described by Lee and Frankenhäuser, the so-called hypogastric ganglion. The plexus actually consists of ganglia and nerve ramifications of various sizes, as well as branches of the combined inferior hypogastric plexus and the nervi erigentes. It lies parallel to the lateral pelvic wall, its lateral surface superficial to the internal iliac and its branches; the ureter occupies a position superficial to the plexus. The middle vesical artery perforates and supplies the plexus, its medial branches supplying the rectal stalk. The greater part of the plexus terminates in large branches that enter the uterus in the region of the internal os, while another smaller component of the plexus supplies the vagina and the bladder. The branches of the plexus that supply the uterus enter the isthmus primarily through the sacrouterine fold or ligament. In the isthmus, just outside the entrance to the uterus, ascending rami pass out into the broad ligament to enter the body of the uterus at higher levels—besides supplying the uterine tubes. A part of the inferior hypogastric plexus may pass directly to the uterus without involvement in the pelvic plexus.

Ganglia are in close proximity to the uterine arteries and the ureters, in the adventitia of the bladder and vagina, and in the vesicovaginal septum. The nerve bundles entering the ganglia contain both myelinated and unmyelinated elements. Corpuscula lamellosa (Vater-Pacini corpuscles) may be found within the tissues and are often observed within nerve bundles, especially within those in the lower divisions of the plexus. Both myelinated and unmyelinated nerves are present within the uterus. The nerves enter along the blood vessels, the richest supply lying in the isthmic portion of the uterus. The fibers following the blood vessels gradually diminish in number in the direction of the fundus, where the sparsest distribution occurs. The fibers run parallel to the muscle bundles, and the nerves frequently branch to form a syncytium before terminating on the sarcoplasm as small free nerve endings.

Sensory Corpuscles

Vater-Pacini corpuscles (corpuscula lamellosa) are present outside the uterus. Dogiel and Krause corpuscles (corpuscula bulboidea) appear in the region of the endocervix. They may also be found in the broad ligament along with Vater-Pacini corpuscles and at the juncture of the uterine arteries with the uterus. These corpuscles may act to modulate the stretch response that reflexively stimulates uterine contractions during labor.

The innervation of the cervix shows occasional free endings entering papillae of the stratified squamous epithelium of the pars vaginalis. The endocervix contains a rich plexus of free endings that is most pronounced in the region of the internal os. The endocervix and the isthmic portion of the uterus in the nonpregnant state both contain the highest number of nerves and blood vessels of any part of the uterus. The presence here of a lamellar type of corpuscle has already been noted.

Nerves pass through the myometrium and enter the endometrium. A plexus with penetrating fibers involving the submucosal region is present in the basal third of the endometrium, with branches terminating in the stroma, in the basilar arterioles, and at the origin of the spiral arterioles. The outer two-thirds of the endometrium are devoid of nerves.

STRUCTURES LINING THE PELVIS

The walls of the pelvis minor are made up of the following layers: (1) the peritoneum, (2) the subperitoneal or extraperitoneal fibroareolar layer, (3) the fascial layer, and (4) the muscular layer. The anatomy of the floor of the pelvis is comparable to that of the walls except for the absence of an osseoligamentous layer.

Peritoneum

The peritoneum presents several distinct transverse folds that form corresponding fossae on each side. The most anterior is a variable fold, the transverse vesical, extending from the bladder laterally to the pelvic wall. It is not the superficial covering of any definitive structure. Behind it lies the broad ligament, which partially covers and aids in the support of the uterus and adnexa.

Ligaments

The broad ligament extends from the lateral border on either side of the uterus to the floor and side walls of the pelvis. It is composed of 2 layers, anterior and posterior, the anterior facing downward and the posterior facing upward, conforming to the position of the uterus. The inferior or "attached" border of the broad ligament is continuous with the parietal peritoneum on the floor and on the side walls of the pelvis. Along this border, the posterior layer continues laterally and posteriorly in an arc to the region of the sacrum, forming the uterosacral fold. Another fold—the rectouterine fold—frequently passes from the posterior surface of the cervix to the rectum in the midline.

The anterior layer of the broad ligament is continuous laterally along the inferior border with the peritoneum of the paravesical fossae and continuous medially with peritoneum on the upper surface of the bladder. Both layers of the attached border continue up the side walls of the pelvis to join with a triangular fold of peritoneum, reaching to the brim of the pelvis to form the suspensory ligament of the ovary or infundibular ligament. This ligament contains the ovarian vessels and nerves. The medial border of the broad ligament on either side is continuous with the peritoneal covering on both uterine surfaces. The 2 layers of the ligament separate to partially contain the uterus, and the superior or "free" border, which is laterally continuous with the suspensory ligament of the ovary, envelops the uterine tube.

The broad ligament can be divided into regions as follows: (1) a larger portion, the mesometrium, which is associated especially with the lateral border of the uterus; (2) the mesovarium, the fold that springs from the posterior layer of the ovary; and (3) the thin portion, the mesosalpinx, which is associated with the fallopian tube in the region of the free border. The superior lateral corner of the broad ligament has been referred to as the suspensory ligament of the ovary, or infundibulopelvic ligament, because it suspends the infundibulum as well as the ovary.

Fossae & Spaces

Corresponding to the peritoneal folds are the peritoneal fossae. The prevesical or retropubic space is a potential space that is crossed by the transverse vesical fold. It is situated in front of the bladder and behind the pubis. When the bladder is displaced posteriorly, it becomes an actual space, anteriorly continuous from side to side and posteriorly limited by a condensation of fatty areolar tissue extending from the base of the bladder to the side wall of the pelvis.

The vesicouterine pouch is a narrow cul-de-sac between the anterior surface of the body of the uterus and the upper surface of the bladder when the uterus is in normal anteflexed position. In the bottom of this pouch, the peritoneum is reflected from the bladder onto the uterus at the junction of the cervix and corpus. Therefore, the anterior surface of the cervix is below the level of the peritoneum and is connected with the base of the bladder by condensed areolar tissue.

The peritoneum on the posterior surface of the body of the uterus extends downward onto the cervix and onto the posterior fornix of the vagina. It is then reflected onto the anterior surface of the rectum to form a narrow cul-de-sac continuous with the pararectal fossa of either side. The entire space, bounded anteriorly by the cervix and by the fornix in the midline, the uterosacral folds laterally, and the rectum posteriorly, is the rectouterine pouch or cul-de-sac (pouch of Douglas).

Subperitoneal & Fascial Layers

The subperitoneal layer consists of loose, fatty areolar tissue underlying the peritoneum. External to the subperitoneal layer, a layer of fascia lines the wall of the pelvis, covering the muscles and, where these are lacking, blending with the periosteum of the pelvic bones. This layer is known as the parietal pelvic fascia and is subdivided into the obturator fascia, the fascia of the urogenital diaphragm, and the fascia of the piriformis.

The obturator fascia is of considerable thickness and covers the obturator internus muscle. Traced forward, it partially blends with the periosteum of the pubic bone and assists in the formation of the obturator canal. Traced upward, it is continuous at the arcuate line with the iliac fascia. Inferiorly, it extends nearly to the margin of the ischiopubic arch, where it is attached to the bone. In this lower region, it also becomes continuous with a double-layered triangular sheet of fascia, the fasciae of the urogenital diaphragm, passing across the anterior part of the pelvic outlet. A much thinner portion of the parietal pelvic fascia covers the piriformis and coccygeus muscles in the posterior pelvic wall. Medially, the piriformis fascia blends with the periosteum of the sacrum around the margins of the anterior sacral foramens and covers the roots and first branches of the sacral plexus.

Visceral pelvic fascia denotes the fascia in the bottom of the pelvic bowl, which invests the pelvic organs and forms a number of supports that suspend the organs from the pelvic walls. These supports arise in common from the obturator part of the parietal fascia, along or near the arcus tendineus. This arc or line extends from a point near the lower part of the symphysis pubica to the root of the spine of the ischium. From this common origin, the fascia spreads inward and backward, dividing into a number of parts classified as either investing (endopelvic) fascia or suspensory and diaphragmatic fascia.

Muscular Layer

The muscles of the greater pelvis are the psoas major and iliacus. Those of the lesser pelvis are the piriformis, obturator internus, coccygeus, and levator ani; they do not form a continuous layer.

Greater Pelvis

Psoas Major

The fusiform psoas major muscle originates from the 12th thoracic to the fifth lumbar vertebrae. Parallel fiber bundles descend nearly vertically along the side of the vertebral bodies and extend along the border of the minor pelvis, beneath the inguinal ligament, and on toward insertion in the thigh. The medial border inserts into the lesser trochanter, whereas the lateral border shares its tendon with the iliacus muscle. Together with the iliacus, it is the most powerful flexor of the thigh, acting as a lateral rotator of the femur when the foot is off the ground and free and as a medial rotator when the foot is on the ground and the tibia is fixed. The psoas component flexes the spine and the pelvis and abducts the lumbar region of the spine. The psoas, having longer fibers than the iliacus, gives a quicker but weaker pull.

Iliacus

The fan-shaped iliacus muscle originates from the iliac crest, the iliolumbar ligament, the greater part of the iliac fossa, the anterior sacroiliac ligaments, and frequently the ala of the sacrum. It also originates from the ventral border of the ilium between the 2 anterior spines. It is inserted in an oblique manner on the lateral surface of the tendon that emerges from the psoas above the inguinal ligament and directly on the femur immediately distal to the lesser trochanter. The lateral portion of the muscle arising from the ventral border of the ilium is adherent to the direct tendon of the rectus femoris and the capsule of the hip joint.

Lesser Pelvis

Piriformis

The piriformis has its origin from the lateral part of the ventral surface of the second, third, and fourth sacral vertebrae, from the posterior border of the greater sciatic notch, and from the deep surface of the sacrotuberous ligament near the sacrum. The fiber bundles pass through the greater sciatic foramen to insert upon the anterior and inner portion of the upper border of the greater trochanter. The piriformis acts as an abductor, lateral rotator, and weak extensor of the thigh.

Obturator Internus

The obturator internus arises from the pelvic surface of the pubic rami near the obturator foramen, the pelvic surface of the ischium between the foramen and the greater sciatic notch, the deep surface of the obturator internus fascia, the fibrous arch that bounds the canal for the obturator vessels and nerves, and the pelvic surface of the obturator membrane. The fiber bundles converge toward the lesser sciatic notch, where they curve laterally to insert into the trochanteric fossa of the femur. The obturator internus is a powerful lateral rotator of the thigh. When the thigh is bent at a right angle, the muscle serves as an abductor and extensor.

Coccygeus

The coccygeus muscle runs from the ischial spine and the neighboring margin of the greater sciatic notch to the fourth and fifth sacral vertebrae and the coccyx. A large part of the muscle is aponeurotic. It supports the pelvic and abdominal viscera and possibly flexes and abducts the coccyx.

Levator Ani

The levator ani muscle forms the floor of the pelvis and the roof of the perineum. It is divisible into 3 portions: (1) the iliococcygeus, (2) the pubococcygeus, and (3) the puborectalis.

1. Iliococcygeus—The iliococcygeus arises from the arcus tendineus, which extends from the ischial spine to the superior ramus of the pubis near the obturator canal and for a variable distance downward below the obturator canal. Its insertion is into the lateral aspect of the coccyx and the raphe that extends from the tip of the coccyx to the rectum. Many fiber bundles cross the median line.

2. Pubococcygeus—The pubococcygeus arises from the inner surface of the os pubis, the lower margin of the symphysis pubica to the obturator canal, and the arcus tendineus as far backward as the origin of the iliococcygeus. It passes backward, downward, and medially past the urogenital organs and the rectum, inserting into the anterior sacrococcygeal ligament, the deep part of the anococcygeal raphe, and each side of the rectum. The pubococcygeus lies to some extent on the pelvic surface of the insertion of the iliococcygeus.

3. Puborectalis—The puborectalis arises from the body and descending ramus of the pubis beneath the origin of the pubococcygeus, the neighboring part of the obturator fascia, and the fascia covering the pelvic surface of the urogenital diaphragm. Many of the fiber bundles interdigitate with those of the opposite side, and they form a thick band on each side of the rectum behind which those of each side are inserted into the anococcygeal raphe.

The levator ani serves to slightly flex the coccyx, raise the anus, and constrict the rectum and vagina. It resists the downward pressure that the thoracoabdominal diaphragm exerts on the viscera during inspiration.

Pelvic Diaphragm

The pelvic diaphragm (Fig. 1–15) extends from the upper part of the pelvic surface of the pubis and ischium to the rectum, which passes through it. The pelvic diaphragm is formed by the levator ani and coccygeus muscles and covering fasciae. The diaphragmatic fasciae cloaking the levator ani arise from the parietal pelvic fascia (obturator fascia), the muscular layer lying between the fasciae. As viewed from above, the superior fascia is the best developed and is reflected onto the rectum, forming the "rectal sheath." The coccygeus muscle forms the deeper portion of the posterolateral wall of the ischiorectal fossa, helping to bind the pelvic outlet. The diaphragm presents a hiatus anteriorly, occupied by the vagina and urethra. The pelvic diaphragm is the main support of the pelvic floor; it suspends the rectum and indirectly supports the uterus.

Arteries & Veins

The blood supply to the muscles lining the pelvis is primarily from branches of the hypogastric artery, accompanied by

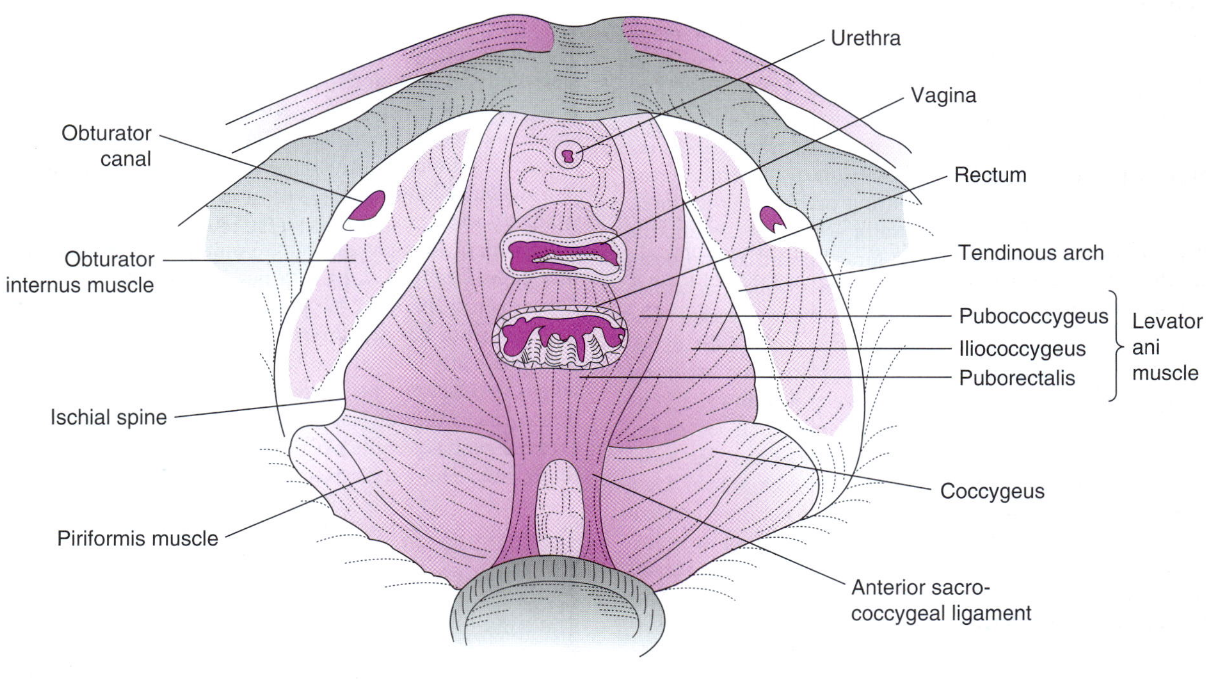

▲ **Figure 1–15.** Pelvic diaphragm from above.

contributions from the external iliac artery. The iliolumbar branch of the hypogastric artery runs upward and laterally beneath the common iliac artery, then beneath the psoas muscle to the superior aperture of the pelvis minor, where it divides into iliac and lumbar branches. The iliac supplies both the iliacus and psoas muscles. It passes laterally beneath the psoas and the femoral nerve and, perforating the iliacus, ramifies in the iliac fossa between the muscle and the bone. It supplies a nutrient artery to the bone and then divides into several branches that can be traced as follows: (1) upward toward the sacroiliac synchondrosis to anastomose with the last lumbar artery, (2) laterally toward the crest of the ilium to anastomose with the lateral circumflex and gluteal arteries, and (3) medially toward the pelvis minor to anastomose with the deep circumflex iliac from the external iliac. The lumbar branch ascends beneath the psoas and supplies that muscle along with the quadratus lumborum. It then anastomoses with the last lumbar artery.

Another branch of the hypogastric artery, the lateral sacral artery, may be represented as 2 distinct vessels. It passes medially in front of the sacrum and turns downward to run parallel with the sympathetic trunk. Crossing the slips of origin of the piriformis muscle, it sends branches to that muscle. On reaching the coccyx, it anastomoses in front of the bone with the middle sacral artery and with the inferior lateral sacral artery of the opposite side. The obturator artery usually arises from the hypogastric, but occasionally it may stem from the inferior epigastric or directly from the external iliac artery. It runs forward and downward slightly below the brim of the pelvis, lying between the peritoneum and endopelvic fascia. Passing through the obturator canal, it emerges and divides into anterior and posterior branches that curve around the margin of the obturator foramen beneath the obturator externus muscle.

When the obturator artery arises from the inferior epigastric or external iliac artery, its proximal relationships are profoundly altered, the vessel coursing near the femoral ring where it may be endangered during operative procedures. The anterior branch of the obturator artery runs around the medial margin of the obturator foramen and anastomoses with both of its posterior branch and the medial circumflex artery. It supplies branches to the obturator muscles. The internal pudendal artery is a terminal branch of the hypogastric artery that arises opposite the piriformis muscle and accompanies the inferior gluteal artery downward to the lower border of the greater sciatic foramen. It leaves the pelvis between the piriformis and coccygeus muscles, passing over the ischial spine to enter the ischiorectal fossa through the small sciatic foramen. Then, running forward through the canalis pudendalis (Alcock's canal) in the obturator fascia, it terminates by dividing into the perineal artery and the artery of the clitoris.

Within the pelvis, the artery lies anterior to the piriformis muscle and the sacral plexus of nerves, lateral to the inferior gluteal artery. Among the small branches that it sends to the gluteal region are those that accompany the nerve to the obturator internus. Another of its branches, the inferior hemorrhoidal artery, arises at the posterior part of the ischiorectal fossa. Upon perforating the obturator fascia, it immediately breaks up into several branches. Some of them run medially toward the rectum to supply the levator ani muscle. The superior gluteal artery originates as a short trunk from the lateral and back part of the hypogastric artery, associated in origin with the iliolumbar and lateral sacral and sometimes with the inferior gluteal or with the inferior gluteal and the internal pudendal. It leaves the pelvis through the greater sciatic foramen above the piriformis muscle, beneath its vein and in front of the superior gluteal nerve. Under cover of the gluteus maximus muscle, it breaks into a superficial and a deep division.

The deep portion further divides into superior and inferior branches. The inferior branch passes forward between the gluteus medius and minimus toward the greater trochanter, where it anastomoses with the ascending branch of the lateral circumflex. It supplies branches to the obturator internus, the piriformis, the levator ani, and the coccygeus muscles and to the hip joint. The deep circumflex iliac artery arises from the side of the external iliac artery either opposite the epigastric or a little below the origin of that vessel. It courses laterally behind the inguinal ligament, lying between the fascia transversalis and the peritoneum or in a fibrous canal formed by the union of the fascia transversalis with the iliac fascia. It sends off branches that supply the psoas and iliacus muscles, as well as a cutaneous branch that anastomoses with the superior gluteal artery.

VULVA

The vulva consists of the mons pubis, the labia majora, the labia minora, the clitoris, and the glandular structures that open into the vestibulum vaginae (Fig. 1–16). The size, shape, and coloration of the various structures, as well as the hair distribution, vary among individuals and racial groups. Normal pubic hair in the female is distributed in an inverted triangle, with the base centered over the mons pubis. Nevertheless, in approximately 25% of normal women, hair may extend upward along the linea alba. The type of hair is dependent, in part, on the pigmentation of the individual. It varies from heavy, coarse, crinkly hair in black women to sparse, fairly fine, lanugo-type hair in Asian women. The length and size of the various structures of the vulva are influenced by the pelvic architecture, as is the position of the external genitalia in the perineal area. The external genitalia of the female have their exact counterparts in the male.

Labia Majora

Superficial Anatomy

The labia majora are comprised of 2 rounded mounds of tissue, originating in the mons pubis and terminating in the perineum. They form the lateral boundaries of the vulva and are approximately 7–9 cm long and 2–4 cm wide, varying in

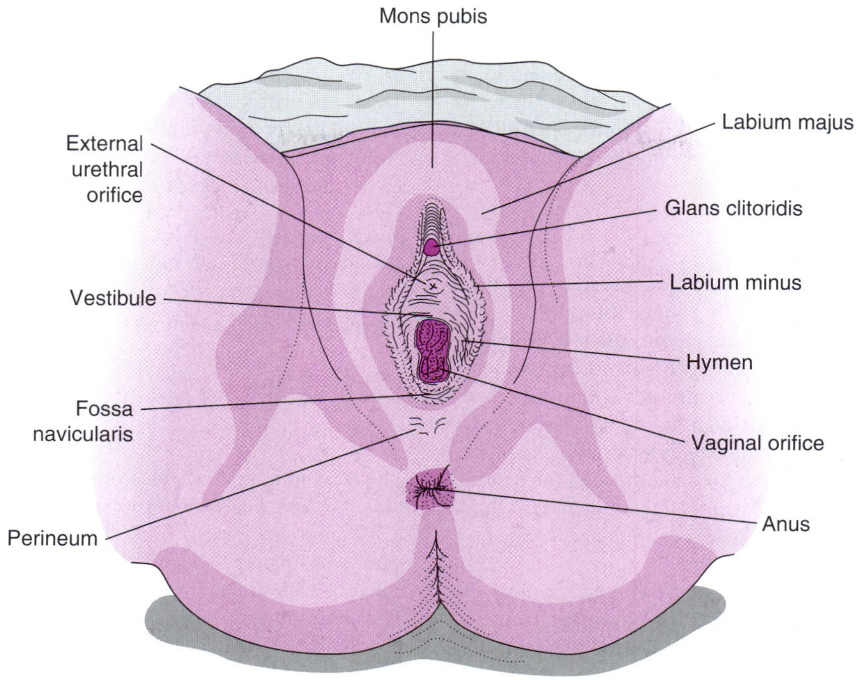

▲ **Figure 1–16.** External genitalia of adult female (parous).

size with height, weight, race, age, parity, and pelvic architecture. Embryologically, these permanent folds of skin are homologous to the scrotum of the male. Hair is distributed over their surfaces, extending superiorly in the area of the mons pubis from one side to the other. The lateral surfaces are adjacent to the medial surface of the thigh, forming a deep groove when the legs are together. The medial surfaces of the labia majora may oppose each other directly or may be separated by protrusion of the labia minora. The cleft that is formed by this opposition anteriorly is termed the anterior commissure. Posteriorly, the cleft is less clearly defined and termed the posterior commissure. The middle portion of the cleft between the 2 labia is the rima pudendi.

Deep Structures

Underlying the skin is a thin, poorly developed muscle layer called the tunica dartos labialis, the fibers of which course, for the most part, at right angles to the wrinkles of the surface, forming a crisscross pattern. Deep to the dartos layer is a thin layer of fascia, most readily recognizable in the old or the young because of the large amount of adipose and areolar tissue. Numerous sweat glands are found in the labia majora, with the greater number on the medial aspect. In the deeper substance of the labia majora are longitudinal bands of muscle that are continuous with the ligamentum teres uteri (round ligament) as it emerges from the inguinal canal. Occasionally, a persistent processus vaginalis peritonei (canal of Nuck) may be seen in the upper region of the labia. This can occasionally fill with fluid causing a cyst in the canal of Nuck to be present in the labia majora. Complete surgical obliteration of this persistent tract will solve this problem.

Arteries

The arterial supply into the labia majora comes from the internal and external pudendals, with extensive anastomoses. Within the labia majora is a circular arterial pattern originating inferiorly from a branch of the perineal artery, from the external pudendal artery in the anterior lateral aspect, and from a small artery of the ligamentum teres uteri superiorly. The inferior branch from the perineal artery, which originates from the internal pudendal as it emerges from the canalis pudendalis (Alcock's canal), forms the base of the rete with the external pudendal arteries. These arise from the medial side of the femoral and, occasionally, from the deep arteries just beneath the femoral ring, coursing medially over the pectineus and adductor muscles, to which they supply branches. They terminate in a circular rete within the labium majus, penetrating the fascia lata adjacent to the fossa ovalis and passing over the round ligament to send a branch to the clitoris.

Veins

The venous drainage is extensive and forms a plexus with numerous anastomoses. In addition, the veins communicate with the dorsal vein of the clitoris, the veins of the labia minora, and the perineal veins, as well as with the inferior hemorrhoidal plexus. On each side, the posterior labial veins connect with the external pudendal vein, terminating in the great saphenous vein (saphena magna) just prior to its entrance (saphenous opening) in the fossa ovalis. This large plexus is frequently manifested by the presence of large varicosities during pregnancy.

Lymphatics

The lymphatics of the labia majora are extensive and utilize 2 systems, one lying superficially (under the skin) and the other deeper, within the subcutaneous tissues. From the upper two-thirds of the left and right labia majora, superficial lymphatics pass toward the symphysis and turn laterally to join the medial superficial inguinal nodes. These nodes drain into the superficial inguinal nodes overlying the saphenous fossa. The drainage flows into and through the femoral ring (fossa ovalis) to the nodi lymphatici inguinales profundi (nodes of Rosenmüller or Cloquet; deep subinguinal nodes), connecting with the external iliac chain.

The superficial subinguinal nodes, situated over the femoral trigone, also accept superficial drainage from the lower extremity and the gluteal region. This drainage may include afferent lymphatics from the perineum. In the region of the symphysis pubica, the lymphatics anastomose in a plexus between the right and left nodes. Therefore, any lesion involving the labia majora allows direct involvement of the lymphatic structures of the contralateral inguinal area. The lower part of the labium majus has superficial and deep drainage that is shared with the perineal area. The drainage passes, in part, through afferent lymphatics to superficial subinguinal nodes; from the posterior medial aspects of the labia majora, it frequently enters the lymphatic plexus surrounding the rectum.

Nerves

The innervation of the external genitalia has been studied by many investigators. The iliohypogastric nerve originates from T12 and L1 and traverses laterally to the iliac crest between the transversus and internal oblique muscles, at which point it divides into 2 branches: (1) the anterior hypogastric nerve, which descends anteriorly through the skin over the symphysis, supplying the superior portion of the labia majora and the mons pubis; and (2) the posterior iliac, which passes to the gluteal area.

The ilioinguinal nerve originates from L1 and follows a course slightly inferior to the iliohypogastric nerve, with which it may frequently anastomose, branching into many small fibers that terminate in the upper medial aspect of the labium majus.

The genitofemoral nerve (L1–L2) emerges from the anterior surface of the psoas muscle to run obliquely downward over its surface, branching in the deeper substance of the labium majus to supply the dartos muscle and that vestige of the cremaster present within the labium majus. Its lumboinguinal branch continues downward onto the upper part of the thigh.

From the sacral plexus, the posterior femoral cutaneous nerve, originating from the posterior divisions of S1 and S2 and the anterior divisions of S2 and S3, divides into several rami that, in part, are called the perineal branches. They supply the medial aspect of the thigh and the labia majora. These branches of the posterior femoral cutaneous nerve are derived from the sacral plexus. The pudendal nerve, composed primarily of S2, S3, and S4, often with a fascicle of S1, sends a small number of fibers to the medial aspect of the labia majora. The pattern of nerve endings is illustrated in Table 1–1.

Labia Minora

Superficial Anatomy

The labia minora are 2 folds of skin that lie within the rima pudendi and measure approximately 5 cm in length and 0.5–1 cm in thickness. The width varies according to age and parity, measuring 2–3 cm at its narrowest diameter to 5–6 cm at its widest, with multiple corrugations over the surface. The labia minora begin at the base of the clitoris, where fusion of the labia is continuous with the prepuce, extending posteriorly and medially to the labia majora at the posterior commissure. On their medial aspects superiorly beneath the clitoris, they unite to form the frenulum adjacent to the urethra and vagina, terminating along the hymen on the right and left sides of the fossa navicularis and ending posteriorly in the frenulum of the labia pudendi, just superior to the posterior commissure. A deep cleft is formed on the lateral surface between the labium majus and the labium minus.

The skin on the labia minora is smooth, pigmented, and hairless. The color and distention vary, depending on the level of sexual excitement and the pigmentation of the individual. The glands of the labia are homologous to the glandulae preputiales (glands of Littre) of the penile portion of the male urethra.

Arteries

The main source of arterial supply (Fig. 1–17) occurs through anastomoses from the superficial perineal artery, branching from the dorsal artery of the clitoris, and from the medial aspect of the rete of the labia majora. Similarly, the venous pattern and plexus are extensive.

Veins

The venous drainage is to the medial vessels of the perineal and vaginal veins, directly to the veins of the labia majora, to the inferior hemorrhoidals posteriorly, and to the clitoral veins superiorly.

Lymphatics

The lymphatics medially may join those of the lower third of the vagina superiorly and the labia majora laterally, passing to

Table 1–1. Quantitative distribution of nerve endings in selected regions of the female genitalia.

	Touch			Pressure	Pain	Other Types	
	Meissner Corpuscles[1]	Merkel Tactile Disks[1]	Peritrichous Endings	Vater-Pacini Corpuscles[2]	Free Nerve Endings	Ruffini Corpuscles[2]	Dogiel and Krause Corpuscles[3]
Mons pubis	++++	++++	++++	+++	+++	++++	+
Labia majora	+++	++++	++++	+++	+++	+++	+
Clitoris	+	+	0	++++	+++	+++	+++
Labia minora	+	+	0	+	+	+	+++
Hymenal ring	0	+	0	0	+++	0	0
Vagina	0	0	0	0	+	0	0
					Occasionally		

[1]Also called corpuscula tactus.
[2]Also called corpuscula lamellosa.
[3]Also called corpuscula bulboidea.

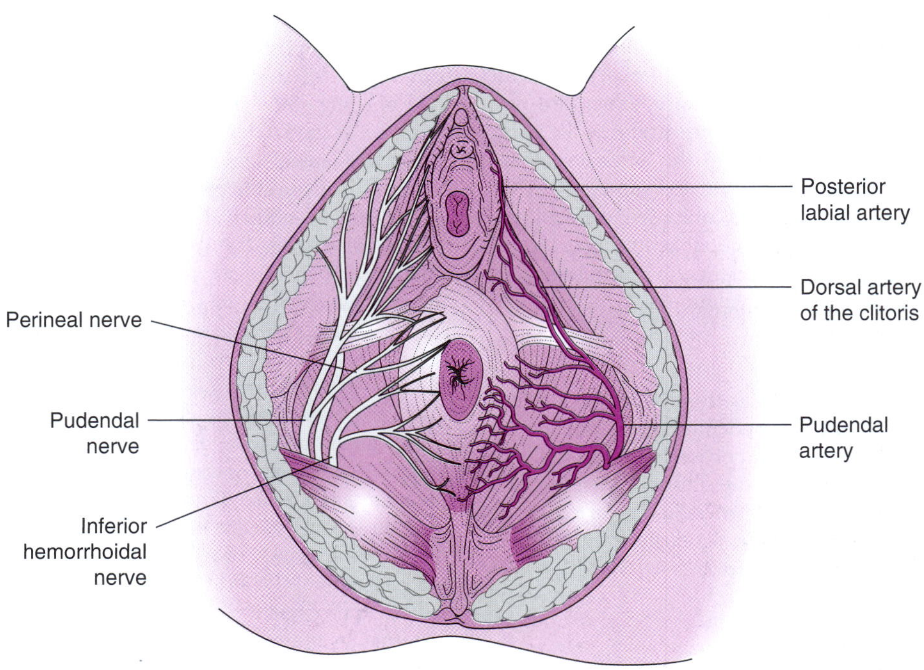

▲ **Figure 1–17.** Arteries and nerves of perineum.

the superficial subinguinal nodes and to the deep subinguinal nodes. In the midline, the lymphatic drainage coincides with that of the clitoris, communicating with that of the labia majora to drain to the opposite side.

Nerves

The innervation of the labia minora originates, in part, from fibers that supply the labia majora and from branches of the pudendal nerve as it emerges from the canalis pudendalis (Alcock's canal) (Fig. 1–17). These branches originate from the perineal nerve. The labia minora and the vestibule area are homologous to the skin of the male urethra and penis. The short membranous portion, approximately 0.5 cm of the male urethra, is homologous to the midportion of the vestibule of the female.

Clitoris

Superficial Anatomy

The clitoris is about 2 cm in length and is a homologue to the dorsal part of the penis. It consists of 2 small erectile cavernous bodies, terminating in a rudimentary glans clitoridis. The erectile body, the corpus clitoridis, consists of the 2 crura clitoridis and the glans clitoridis, with overlying skin and prepuce, a miniature homologue of the glans penis. The crura extend outward bilaterally to their position in the anterior portion of the vulva. The cavernous tissue, homologous to the corpus spongiosum penis of the male, appears in the vascular pattern of the labia minora in the female.

At the lower border of the pubic arch, a small triangular fibrous band extends onto the clitoris (suspensory ligament) to separate the 2 crura, which turn inward, downward, and laterally at this point, close to the inferior rami of the pubic symphysis. The crura lie inferior to the ischiocavernosus muscles and bodies. The glans is situated superiorly at the fused termination of the crura. It is composed of erectile tissue and contains an integument, hoodlike in shape, termed the prepuce. On its ventral surface, there is a frenulum clitoridis, the fused junction of the labia minora.

Arteries

The blood supply to the clitoris is from its dorsal artery, a terminal branch of the internal pudendal artery, which is the terminal division of the posterior portion of the internal iliac (hypogastric) artery. As it enters the clitoris, it divides into 2 branches, the deep and dorsal arteries. Just before entering the clitoris itself, a small branch passes posteriorly to supply the area of the external urethral meatus.

Veins

The venous drainage of the clitoris begins in a rich plexus around the corona of the glans, running along the anterior surface to join the deep vein and continuing downward to join the pudendal plexus from the labia minora, labia majora, and perineum, forming the pudendal vein.

Lymphatics

The lymphatic drainage of the clitoris coincides primarily with that of the labia minora, the right and left sides having access to contralateral nodes in the superficial inguinal chain. In addition, its extensive network provides further access downward and posteriorly to the external urethral meatus toward the anterior portion of the vestibule.

Nerves

The innervation of the clitoris is through the terminal branch of the pudendal nerve, which originates from the sacral plexus as previously discussed. It lies on the lateral side of the dorsal artery and terminates in branches within the glans, corona, and prepuce. The nerve endings in the clitoris vary from a total absence within the glans to a rich supply primarily located within the prepuce (Table 1–1). A total absence of endings within the clitoris itself takes on clinical significance when one considers the emphasis placed on the clitoris in discussing problems of sexual gratification in women.

Vestibule

Superficial Anatomy

The area of the vestibule is bordered by the labia minora laterally, by the frenulum labiorum pudendi (or posterior commissure) posteriorly, and by the urethra and clitoris anteriorly. Inferiorly, it is bordered by the hymenal ring. The opening of the vagina or junction of the vagina with the vestibule is limited by a membrane stretching from the posterior and lateral sides to the inferior surface of the external urethral orifice. This membrane is termed the hymen. Its shape and openings vary and depend on age, parity, and sexual experience. The form of the opening may be infantile, annular, semilunar, cribriform, septate, or vertical; the hymen may even be imperforate. In parous women and in the postcoital state, the tags of the hymenal integument are termed carunculae myrtiformes.

The external urethral orifice, which is approximately 2–3 cm posterior to the clitoris, on a slightly elevated and irregular surface with depressed areas on the sides, may appear to be stellate or crescentic in shape. It is characterized by many small mucosal folds around its opening. Bilaterally and on the surface are the orifices of the paraurethral and periurethral glands (ductus paraurethrales [ducts of Skene and Astruc]).

At approximately the 5 and 7 o'clock positions, just external to the hymenal rings, are 2 small papular elevations that represent the orifices of the ducts of the glandulae vestibulares majores or larger vestibular glands (Bartholin) of the female (bulbourethral gland of the male). The fossa navicularis lies between the frenulum labiorum pudendi and the hymenal ring. The skin surrounding the vestibule is stratified squamous in type, with a paucity of rete pegs and papillae.

Arteries

The blood supply to the vestibule is an extensive capillary plexus that has anastomoses with the superficial transverse perineal artery. A branch comes directly from the pudendal anastomosis with the inferior hemorrhoidal artery in the region of the fossa navicularis. The blood supply of the urethra anteriorly, a branch of the dorsal artery of the clitoris and the azygos artery of the anterior vaginal wall, also contributes.

Veins

Venous drainage is extensive, involving the same areas described for the arterial network.

Lymphatics

The lymphatic drainage has a distinct pattern. The anterior portion, including that of the external urethral meatus, drains upward and outward with that of the labia minora and the clitoris. The portion next to the urethral meatus may join that of the anterior urethra, which empties into the vestibular plexus to terminate in the superficial inguinal nodes, the superficial subinguinal nodes, the deep subinguinal nodes, and the external iliac chain. The lymphatics of the fossa navicularis and the hymen may join those of the posterior vaginal wall, intertwining with the intercalated lymph nodes along the rectum, which follow the inferior hemorrhoidal arteries. This pattern becomes significant with cancer. Drainage occurs through the pudendal and the hemorrhoidal chain and through the vestibular plexus onto the inguinal region.

Nerves

The innervation of the vestibular area is primarily from the sacral plexus through the perineal nerve. The absence of the usual modalities of touch is noteworthy. The vestibular portion of the hymenal ring contains an abundance of free nerve endings (pain).

Vestibular Glands

The glandulae vestibulares majores (larger vestibular glands or Bartholin glands) have a duct measuring approximately 5 mm in diameter. The gland itself lies just inferior and lateral to the bulbocavernosus muscle. The gland is tubular and alveolar in character, with a thin capsule and connective tissue septa dividing it into lobules in which occasional smooth muscle fibers are found. The epithelium is cuboid to columnar and pale in color, with the cytoplasm containing mucigen droplets and colloid spherules with acidophilic inclusions. The epithelium of the duct is simple in type, and its orifice is stratified squamous like the vestibule. The secretion is a clear, viscid, and stringy mucoid substance with an alkaline pH. Secretion is active during sexual activity.

The greater vestibular gland is homologous to the bulbourethral gland (also known as Cowper's glands, Duverney's glands, Tiedemann's glands, or the Bartholin glands of the male). If the opening to the gland becomes clogged, then a painful Bartholin's cyst can develop.

The arterial supply to the greater vestibular gland comes from a small branch of the artery on the bulbocavernosus muscle, penetrating deep into its substance. Venous drainage coincides with the drainage of the bulbocavernosus body. The lymphatics drain directly into the lymphatics of the vestibular plexus, having access to the posterior vaginal wall along the inferior hemorrhoidal channels. They also drain via the perineum into the inguinal area. Most of this minor drainage is along the pudendal vessels in the canalis pudendalis and explains, in part, the difficulty in dealing with cancer involving the gland. The innervation of the greater vestibular gland is from a small branch of the perineal nerve, which penetrates directly into its substance.

Muscles of External Genitalia

The muscles (Fig. 1–18) of the external genitalia and cavernous bodies in the female are homologous to those of the male, although they are less well developed.

Bulbocavernosus Muscle

The bulbocavernosus muscle and deeper bulbus vestibuli or cavernous tissues arise in the midline from the posterior part of the central tendon of the perineum, where each opposes the fibers from the opposite side. Each ascends around the vagina, enveloping the bulbus vestibuli (the corpus cavernosum bodies of the male) to terminate in 3 heads: (1) the fibrous tissue dorsal to the clitoris, (2) the tunica fibrosa of the corpus cavernosa overlying the crura of the clitoris, and (3) decussating fibers that join those of the ischiocavernosus to form the striated sphincter of the urethra at the junction of its middle and lower thirds.

The blood supply is derived from the perineal branch of the internal pudendal artery as it arises in the anterior part of the ischiorectal fossa. Deep to the fascia diaphragmatis urogenitalis inferior (Colles' fascia) and crossing between the ischiocavernosus and bulbocavernosus muscles, the pudendal artery sends 1–2 branches directly into the bulbocavernosus muscle and vestibular body, continuing anteriorly to terminate in the dorsal artery of the clitoris.

The venous drainage accompanies the pudendal plexus. In addition, it passes posteriorly with the inferior hemorrhoidal veins and laterally with the perineal vein, a branch of the internal pudendal vein. The lymphatics run primarily with those of the vestibular plexus, with drainage inferiorly toward the intercalated nodes of the rectum and anteriorly

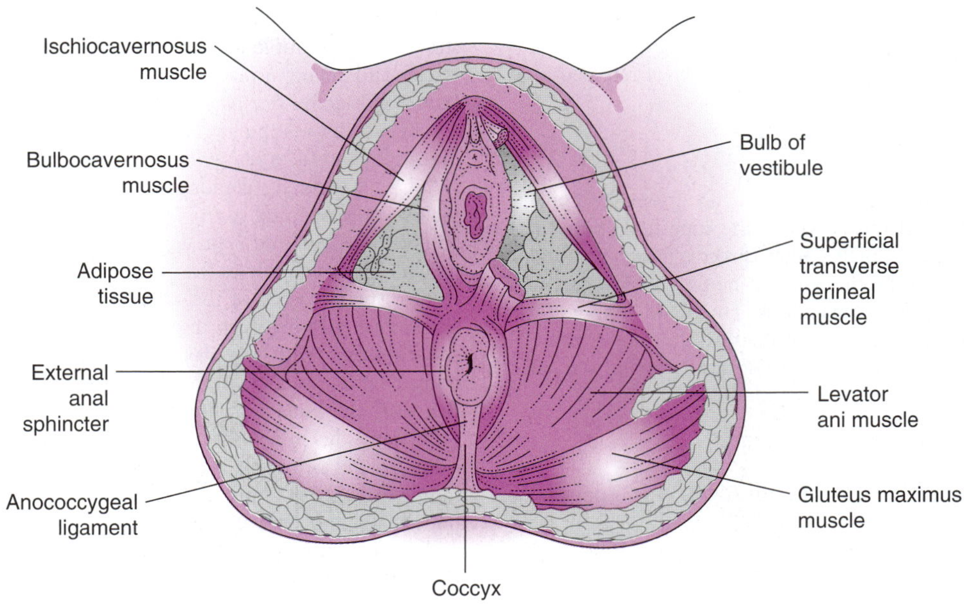

▲ **Figure 1–18.** Pelvic musculature (inferior view).

and laterally with the labia minora and majora to the superficial inguinal nodes. Contralateral drainage in the upper portion of the muscle and body is evident.

Ischiocavernosus Muscle

The ischiocavernosus muscle and its attendant cavernous tissue arise from the ischial tuberosity and inferior ramus to the ischium. It envelops the crus of its cavernous tissue in a thin layer of muscle ascending toward and over the medial and inferior surfaces of the symphysis pubica to terminate in the anterior surface of the symphysis at the base of the clitoris. It then sends decussating fibers to the region of the upper and middle thirds of the urethra, forming the greater part of the organ's voluntary sphincter. The blood supply is through perforating branches from the perineal artery as it ascends between the bulbocavernosus and ischiocavernosus muscles to terminate as the dorsal artery of the clitoris. The innervation stems from an ischiocavernosus branch of the perineal division of the pudendal nerve.

Transversus Muscle

The transversus perinei superficialis muscle arises from the inferior ramus of the ischium and from the ischial tuberosity. The fibers of the muscle extend across the perineum and are inserted into its central tendon, meeting those from the opposite side. Frequently, the muscle fibers from the bulbocavernosus, the puborectalis, the superficial transverse perinei, and occasionally the external anal sphincter will interdigitate. The blood supply is from a perforating branch of the perineal division of the internal pudendal artery, and the nerve supply is from the perineal division of the pudendal nerve.

Inferior Layer of Urogenital Diaphragm

The inferior layer of urogenital diaphragm is a potential space depending upon the size and development of the musculature, the parity of the female, and the pelvic architecture. It contains loose areolar connective tissue interspersed with fat. The bulbocavernosus muscles, with the support of the superficial transverse perinei muscles and the puborectalis muscles, act as a point of fixation on each side for support of the vulva, the external genitalia, and the vagina.

Surgical Considerations

A midline episiotomy is most effective to minimize trauma to vital supports of the vulva, bulbocavernosus, and superficial transverse perinei muscles. Overdistention of the vagina caused by the presenting part and body of the infant forms a temporary sacculation. If distention occurs too rapidly or if dilatation is beyond the resilient capacity of the vagina, rupture of the vaginal musculature may occur, often demonstrated by a cuneiform groove on the anterior wall and a tonguelike protrusion on the posterior wall of the vagina. Therefore, return of the vagina and vulva to the nonpregnant state is dependent upon the tonus of the muscle and the degree of distention of the vagina during parturition.

Special and deliberate consideration should be paid to the repair of the perineal body, the external anal sphincter, and the rectal mucosa. Whether created spontaneously or iatrogenically with episiotomy, lack of proper repair and

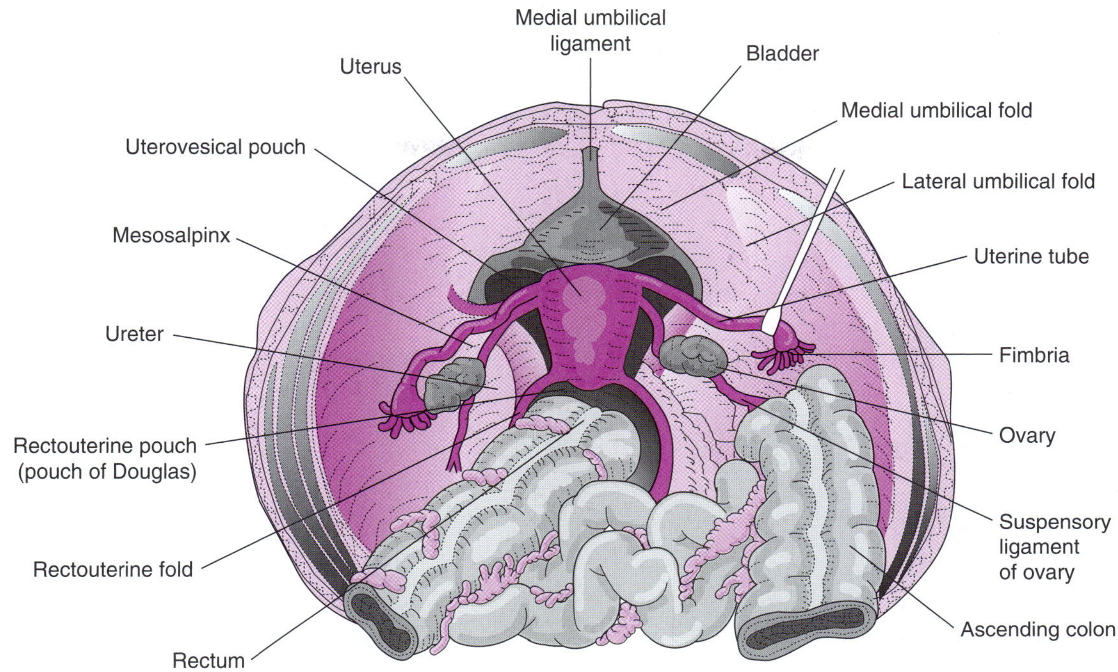

▲ **Figure 1–19.** Female pelvic contents from above.

attention to return of proper anatomic function will result in long-term morbidity with dyspareunia or anal incontinence.

CONTENTS OF THE PELVIC CAVITY

The organs that occupy the female pelvis (Figs. 1–19 to 1–21) are the bladder, the ureters, the urethra, the uterus, the uterine (fallopian) tubes or oviducts, the ovaries, the vagina, and the rectum.* With the exception of the inferior portion of the rectum and most of the vagina, all lie immediately beneath the peritoneum. The uterus, uterine tubes, and ovaries are almost completely covered with peritoneum and are suspended in peritoneal ligaments. The remainder are partially covered. These organs do not completely fill the cavity; the remaining space is occupied by ileum and sigmoid colon.

Bladder

Anatomy

The urinary bladder is a muscular, hollow organ that stores urine and lies posterior to the pubic bones and anterior to the uterus and broad ligament. Its form, size, and position vary with the amount of urine it contains. When empty, it takes the form of a somewhat rounded pyramid, having a base, a vertex (or apex), a superior surface, and a convex inferior surface that may be divided by a median ridge into 2 inferolateral surfaces.

Relationships

The superior surface of the bladder is covered with peritoneum that is continuous with the medial umbilical fold, forming the paravesical fossae laterally. Posteriorly, the peritoneum passes onto the uterus at the junction of the cervix and corpus, continuing upward on the anterior surface to form the vesicouterine pouch. When the bladder is empty, the normal uterus rests upon its superior surface. When the bladder is distended, coils of intestine may lie upon its superior surface. The base of the bladder rests below the peritoneum and is adjacent to the cervix and the anterior fornix of the vagina. It is separated from these structures by areolar tissue containing plexiform veins. The area over the vagina is extended as the bladder fills. The inferolateral surfaces are separated from the wall of the pelvis by the potential prevesical space, containing a small amount of areolar tissue but no large vessels. This surface is nonperitoneal and thus suitable for operative procedures. Posterolateral to the region facing the symphysis, each of the inferolateral surfaces is in relation to the fascia of the obturator internus, the obturator vessels and nerve, the obliterated umbilical artery above, and the fascia of the levator ani below. Posteriorly and medially, the inferior surface is separated from the base by an area called the urethrovesical junction, the most stationary portion of the bladder.

* The rectum is not described in this chapter.

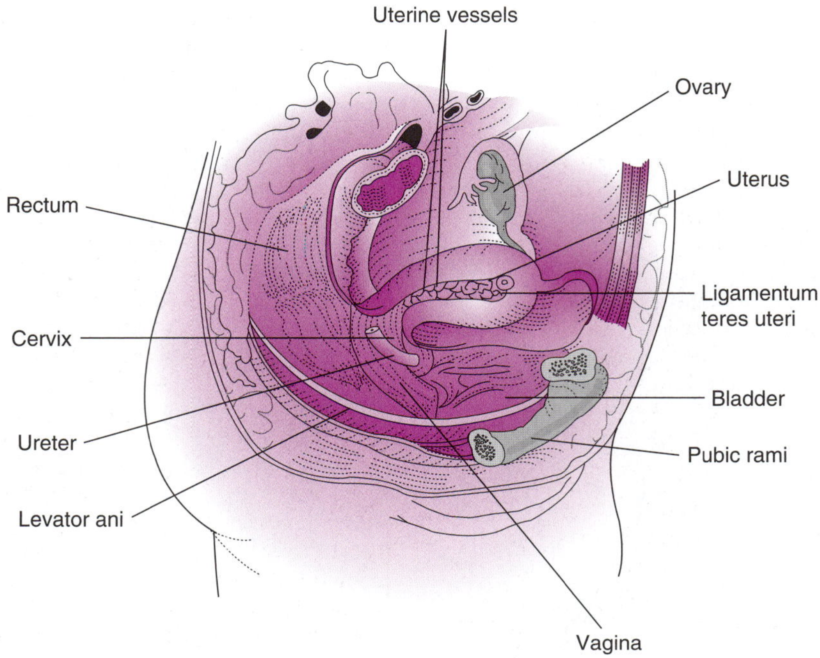

▲ **Figure 1–20.** Pelvic viscera (sagittal view).

Fascia, Ligaments, & Muscle

The bladder is enclosed by a thin layer of fascia, the vesical sheath. Two thickenings of the endopelvic fascia, the medial and lateral pubovesical or puboprostatic ligaments, extend at the vesicourethral junction abutting the levator ani muscle from the lower part of the anterior aspect of the bladder to the pubic bones. Similar fascial thickenings, the lateral true ligaments, extend from the sides of the lower part of the bladder to the lateral walls of the pelvis. Posteriorly, the vesicourethral junction of the bladder lies directly against the anterior wall of the vagina.

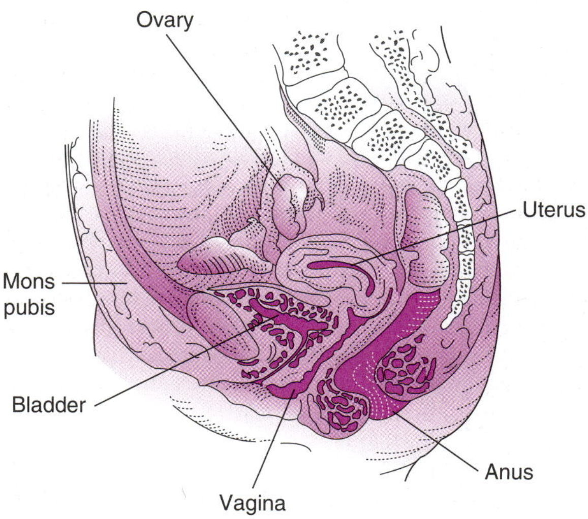

▲ **Figure 1–21.** Pelvic organs (midsagittal view). (Reproduced, with permission, from Benson RC. *Handbook of Obstetrics & Gynecology*. 8th ed. Los Altos, CA: Lange; 1983.)

A fibrous band, the urachus or medial umbilical ligament, extends from the apex of the bladder to the umbilicus. This band represents the remains of the embryonic allantois. The lateral umbilical ligaments are formed by the obliterated umbilical arteries and are represented by fibrous cords passing along the sides of the bladder and ascending toward the umbilicus. Frequently, the vessels will be patent, thus forming the superior vesical arteries. The peritoneal covering of the bladder is limited to the upper surface. The reflections of the peritoneum to the anterior abdominal wall and the corresponding walls of the pelvis are sometimes described as the superior, lateral, and posterior false ligaments. The muscle (smooth) of the bladder is represented by an interdigitated pattern continuous with and contiguous to the inner longitudinal and anterior circumferential muscles of the urethra. No distinct muscle layers are apparent.

Mucous Membrane

The mucous membrane is rose-colored and lies in irregular folds that become effaced by distention. The 3 angles of the vesical trigone are represented by the orifices of the 2 ureters and the internal urethral orifice. This area is redder in color and free from plication. It is bordered posteriorly by the plica interureterica, a curved transverse ridge extending between the orifices of the ureters. A median longitudinal elevation, the uvula vesicae, extends toward the urethral orifice. The internal urethral orifice is normally situated at the lowest point of the bladder, at the junction of the inferolateral and posterior surfaces. It is surrounded by a circular elevation, the urethral annulus, approximately level with the center of the symphysis pubica. The epithelial lining of the bladder is transitional in type. The mucous membrane rests on the submucous coat, composed of areolar tissue superficial to the muscular coat. There is no evidence of a specific smooth muscle sphincter in the vesical neck.

Arteries, Veins, & Lymphatics

The blood supply to the bladder comes from branches of the hypogastric artery. The umbilical artery, a terminal branch of the hypogastric artery, gives off the superior vesical artery prior to its obliterated portion. It approaches the bladder (along with the middle and inferior vesical arteries) through a condensation of fatty areolar tissue, limiting the prevesical "space" posterosuperiorly, to branch out over the upper surface of the bladder. It anastomoses with the arteries of the opposite side and the middle and inferior vesical arteries below. The middle vesical artery may arise from one of the superior vessels, or it may come from the umbilical artery, supplying the sides and base of the bladder. The inferior vesical artery usually arises directly from the hypogastric artery—in common with or as a branch of the uterine artery—and passes downward and medially, where it divides into branches that supply the lower part of the bladder. The fundus may also receive small branches from the middle hemorrhoidal, uterine, and vaginal arteries. The veins form an extensive plexus at the sides and base of the bladder from which stems pass to the hypogastric trunk.

The lymphatics, in part, accompany the veins and communicate with the hypogastric nodes. They also communicate laterally with the external iliac glands, and some of those from the fundus pass to nodes situated at the promontory of the sacrum. The lymphatics of the bladder dome are separate on the right and left sides and rarely cross, but extensive anastomoses are present among the lymphatics of the base, which also involve those of the cervix.

Nerves

The nerve supply to the bladder is derived partly from the hypogastric sympathetic plexus and partly from the second and third sacral nerves (the nervi erigentes).

Ureters

Anatomy & Relationships

The ureter is a slightly flattened tube that extends from the termination of the renal pelvis to the lower outer corner of the base of the bladder, a distance of 26–28 cm. It is partly abdominal and partly pelvic and lies entirely behind the peritoneum. Its diameter varies from 4–6 mm, depending on distention, and its size is uniform except for 3 slightly constricted portions.

The first of 3 constrictions is found at the junction of the ureter with the renal pelvis and is known as the upper isthmus. The second constriction—the lower isthmus—is at the point where the ureter crosses the brim of the pelvis minor. The third (intramural) constriction is at the terminal part of the ureter as it passes through the bladder wall.

The pelvic portion of the ureter begins as the ureter crosses the pelvic brim beneath the ovarian vessels and near the bifurcation of the common iliac artery. It conforms to the curvature of the lateral pelvic wall, inclining slightly laterally and posteriorly until it reaches the pelvic floor. The ureter then bends anteriorly and medially at about the level of the ischial spine to reach the bladder. In its upper portion, it is related posteriorly to the sacroiliac articulation; then, lying upon the obturator internus muscle and fascia, it crosses the root of the umbilical artery, the obturator vessels, and the obturator nerve.

In its anterior relationship, the ureter emerges from behind the ovary and under its vessels to pass behind the uterine and superior and middle vesical arteries. Coursing anteriorly, it comes into close relation with the lateral fornix of the vagina, passing 8–12 mm from the cervix and vaginal wall before reaching the bladder. When the ureters reach the bladder, they are about 5 cm apart. The ureters open into the bladder by 2 slitlike apertures, the urethral orifices, about 2.5 cm apart when the bladder is empty.

Wall of Ureter

The wall of the ureter is approximately 3 mm thick and is composed of 3 coats: connective tissue, muscle, and mucous membrane. The muscular coat has an external circular and an internal longitudinal layer throughout its course and an external longitudinal layer in its lower third. The mucous membrane is longitudinally plicated and covered by transitional epithelium. The intermittent peristaltic action of the ureteral musculature propels urine into the bladder in jets. The oblique passage of the ureter through the bladder wall tends to constitute a valvular arrangement, but no true valve is present. The circular fibers of the intramural portion of the ureter possess a sphincter like action. Still, under some conditions of overdistention of the bladder, urine may be forced back into the ureter.

Arteries, Veins, & Lymphatics

The pelvic portion of the ureter receives its blood supply from a direct branch of the hypogastric artery, anastomosing superiorly in its adventitia with branches from the iliolumbar and inferiorly with branches from the inferior vesical and middle hemorrhoidal arteries. Lymphatic drainage passes along the hypogastric vessels to the hypogastric and external iliac nodes, continuing up the ureters to their middle portion where drainage is directed to the periaortic and interaorticocaval nodes.

Nerves

The nerve supply is provided by the renal, ovarian, and hypogastric plexuses. The spinal level of the afferents is approximately the same as the kidney (T12, L1, L2). The lower third of the ureter receives sensory fibers and postganglionic parasympathetic fibers from the Frankenhäuser plexus and sympathetic fibers through this plexus as it supplies the base of the bladder. These fibers ascend the lower third of the ureter, accompanying the arterial supply. The middle segment appears to receive postganglions of sympathetic and parasympathetic fibers through and from the middle hypogastric plexus. The upper third is supplied by the same innervation as the kidney.

Urethra

Anatomy & Relationships

The female urethra is a canal 2.5–4 cm long. It extends downward and forward in a curve from the neck of the bladder (internal urethral orifice), which lies nearly opposite the symphysis pubica. Its termination, the external urethral orifice, is situated inferiorly and posteriorly from the lower border of the symphysis. Posteriorly, it is closely applied to the anterior wall of the vagina, especially in the lower two-thirds, where it actually is integrated with the wall, forming the urethral carina. Anteriorly, the upper end is separated from the prevesical "space" by the pubovesical (puboprostatic) ligaments, abutting against the levator ani and vagina and extending upward onto the pubic rami.

Anatomy of Walls

The walls of the urethra are very distensible, composed of spongy fibromuscular tissue containing cavernous veins and lined by submucous and mucous coats. The mucosa contains numerous longitudinal lines when undistended, the most prominent of which is located on the posterior wall and termed the crista urethralis. Also, there are numerous small glands (the homologue of the male prostate, paraurethral and periurethral glands of Astruc, ducts of Skene) that open into the urethra. The largest of these, the paraurethral glands of Skene, may open via a pair of ducts beside the external urethral orifice in the vestibule. The epithelium begins as transitional at the upper end and becomes squamous in the lower part.

External to the urethral lumen is a smooth muscle coat composed of an outer circular layer and an inner longitudinal layer in the lower two-thirds. In the upper third, the muscle bundles of the layers interdigitate in a basketlike weave to become continuous with and contiguous to those of the bladder. The entire urethral circular smooth muscle acts as the involuntary sphincter. In the region of the juncture of the middle and lower thirds of the urethra, decussating fibers (striated in type) form the middle heads of the bulbocavernosus and ischiocavernosus muscles and encircle the urethra to form the sphincter urethrae (voluntary sphincter).

Arteries & Veins

The arterial supply is intimately involved with that of the anterior vaginal wall, with cruciate anastomoses to the bladder. On each side of the vagina are the vaginal arteries, originating in part from the coronary artery of the cervix, the inferior vesical artery, or a direct branch of the uterine artery. In the midline of the anterior vaginal wall is the azygos artery, originating from the coronary or circular artery of the cervix. Approximately 5 branches traverse the anterior vaginal wall from the lateral vaginal arteries to the azygos in the midline, with small sprigs supplying the urethra. A rich anastomosis with the introitus involves the clitoral artery (urethral branches) as the artery divides into the dorsal and superficial arteries of the clitoris, a terminal branch of the internal pudendal artery. The venous drainage follows the arterial pattern, although it is less well defined. In the upper portion of the vagina, it forms an extensive network called the plexus of Santorini.

Nerves

The nerve supply is parasympathetic, sympathetic, and spinal. The parasympathetic and sympathetic nerves are derived from the hypogastric plexus; the spinal supply is via the pudendal nerve.

Uterus

Anatomy

The uterus is a pear-shaped, thick-walled, muscular organ, situated between the base of the bladder and the rectum. Covered on each side by the 2 layers of the broad ligament, it communicates above with the uterine tubes and below with the vagina. It is divided into 2 main portions, the larger portion or body above and the smaller cervix below, connected by a transverse constriction, the isthmus. The body is flattened so that the side-to-side dimension is greater than the anteroposterior dimension and larger in women who have borne children. The anterior or vesical surface is almost flat; the posterior surface is convex. The fallopian tubes join the uterus at the superior (lateral) angles. The round portion that extends above the plane passing through the points of attachment of the 2 tubes is termed the fundus. This portion is the region of greatest breadth.

The cavity of the body, when viewed from the front or back, is roughly triangular with the base up. The communication of the cavity below with the cavity of the cervix corresponds in position to the isthmus and forms the internal orifice (internal os uteri). The cervix, also called the portio vaginalis, is somewhat barrel-shaped and is 2–4 cm in length, its lower end joining the vagina at an angle varying from 45–90 degrees. It projects into the vagina and is divided into a supravaginal and a vaginal portion by the line of attachment. About one fourth of the anterior surface and half of the posterior surface of the cervix belong to the vaginal portion. At the extremity of the vaginal portion is the opening leading to the vagina, the external orifice (external os uteri), which is round or oval before parturition but takes the form of a transverse slit in women who have borne children. The cavity of the cervix is fusiform in shape, with longitudinal folds or furrows, and extends from the internal to the external orifice. The endocervical canal is composed of columnar, mucus-secreting cells, whereas the external cervix is lined by nonkeratinizing squamous epithelium. The junction between these 2 areas is called the squamocolumnar junction or transitional zone.

The size of the uterus varies, under normal conditions, at different ages and in different physiologic states. In the adult woman who has never borne children, it is approximately 7–8 cm long, 4–5 cm at its widest point, and 30–40 g in weight. In the prepubertal period, it is considerably smaller. In women who have borne children, it is larger. Its shape, size, and characteristics in the pregnant state become considerably modified depending on the stage of gestation.

Layers of Uterine Wall

The wall of the uterus is very thick and consists of 3 layers: serous, muscular, and mucous. The serous layer (perimetrium) is simply the peritoneal covering. It is thin and firmly adherent over the fundus and most of the body, and then thickens posteriorly and becomes separated from the muscle by the parametrium. The muscular layer (myometrium) is extremely thick at about 1.5–2.5 cm and continuous with that of the tubes and vagina. It also extends into the ovarian and round ligaments, into the cardinal ligaments at the cervix, and minimally into the uterosacral ligaments. Two principal layers of the muscular coat can be distinguished: (1) the outer layer, which is weaker and composed of longitudinal fibers; and (2) a stronger inner layer, the fibers of which are interlaced and run in various directions, having intermingled within them large venous plexuses. The muscle layer hypertrophies with the internal os to form a sphincter.

The cervix, from the internal os distally, progressively loses its smooth muscle, finally to be entirely devoid of smooth muscle and elastic in its distal half. It is, in fact, the "dead-end tendon" of the uterus, at which point, during the active component of labor, both the uterus and the vagina direct their efforts. The mucous layer (endometrium) is soft and spongy, composed of tissue resembling embryonic connective tissue. The surface consists of a single layer of ciliated columnar epithelium. The tissue is rather delicate and friable and contains many tubular glands that open into the cavity of the uterus.

Position & Axis Direction

The direction of the axis of the uterus varies greatly. Normally, the uterus forms a sharp angle with the vagina so that its anterior surface lies on the upper surface of the bladder and the body is in a horizontal plane when the woman is standing erect. There is a bend in the area of the isthmus, at which the cervix then faces downward. This position is the normal anteversion or angulation of the uterus, although it may be placed backward (retroversion), without angulation (military position), or to one side (lateral version). The forward flexion at the isthmus is referred to as anteflexion, or there may be a corresponding retroflexion or lateral flexion. There is no sharp line between the normal and pathologic state of anterior angulation.

Relationships

Anteriorly, the body of the uterus rests upon the upper and posterior surfaces of the bladder, separated by the uterovesical pouch of the peritoneum. The whole of the anterior wall of the cervix is below the floor of this pouch, and it is separated from the base of the bladder only by connective tissue. Posteriorly, the peritoneal covering extends down as far as the uppermost portion of the vagina; therefore, the entire posterior surface of the uterus is covered by peritoneum, and the convex posterior wall is separated from the rectum by the rectouterine pouch (cul-de-sac or pouch of Douglas). Coils of intestine may rest upon the posterior surface of the body of the uterus and may be present in the rectouterine pouch.

Laterally, the uterus is related to the various structures contained within the broad ligament: the uterine tubes, the round ligament and the ligament of the ovary, the uterine artery and veins, and the ureter. The relationships of the ureters and the uterine arteries are very important surgically. The ureters, as they pass to the bladder, run parallel with the cervix for a distance of 8–12 mm. The uterine artery crosses the ureter anterosuperiorly near the cervix, about 1.5 cm from the lateral fornix of the vagina. In effect, the ureter passes under the uterine artery "as water flows under a bridge."

Ligaments

Although the cervix of the uterus is fixed, the body is free to rise and fall with the filling and emptying of the bladder. The so-called ligaments supporting the uterus consist of the uterosacral ligaments, the transverse ligaments of the cervix (cardinal ligaments, cardinal supports, ligamentum transversum colli, ligaments of Mackenrodt), the round ligaments, and the broad ligaments. The cervix is embedded in tissue called the parametrium, containing various amounts of smooth muscle. There are 2 pairs of structures continuous with the parametrium and with the wall of the cervix: the uterosacral ligaments and the transverse (cardinal) ligament of the neck, the latter of which is the chief means of support and suspends the uterus from the lateral walls of the pelvis minor.

The uterosacral ligaments are, in fact, the inferior posterior folds of peritoneum from the broad ligament. They consist primarily of nerve bundles from the inferior hypogastric plexus and contain preganglionic and postganglionic fibers and C fibers of the sympathetic lumbar segments, parasympathetic in part from sacral components and in part from sensory or C fibers of the spinal segments.

The cardinal ligaments are composed of longitudinal smooth muscle fibers originating superiorly from the uterus and inferiorly from the vagina, fanning out toward the fascia visceralis to form, with the internal os of the cervix, the primary support of the uterus. There is a natural defect in the muscle at its sides (hilum of the uterus) and at the cervical isthmus (internal os), where the vasculature and nerve supply enter the uterus.

The round ligaments of the uterus, although forming no real support, may assist in maintaining the body of the uterus in its typical position over the bladder. They consist of fibrous cords containing smooth muscle (longitudinal) from the outer layer of the corpus. From a point of attachment to the uterus immediately below that of the ovarian ligament, each round ligament extends downward, laterally, and forward between the 2 layers of the mesometrium, toward the abdominal inguinal ring that it traverses and the inguinal canal, to terminate in a fanlike manner in the labia majora and become continuous with connective tissue. The round ligament is the gubernaculum (ligamentum teres uteri), vestigial in the female. It is accompanied by a funicular branch of the ovarian artery, by a branch from the ovarian venous plexus, and, in the lower part of its course, by a branch from the inferior epigastric artery (Sampson's artery), over which it passes as it enters the inguinal ring. Through the inguinal canal, it is accompanied by the ilioinguinal nerve and the external spermatic branch of the genitofemoral nerve.

The broad ligament, consisting of a transverse fold of peritoneum that arises from the floor of the pelvis between the rectum and the bladder, provides minimal support. In addition to the static support of these ligaments, the pelvic diaphragm (levator ani) provides an indirect and dynamic support. These muscles do not actually come in contact with the uterus, but they aid in supporting the vagina and maintain the entire pelvic floor in resisting downward pressure. The effectiveness of these muscles depends on an intact perineum (perineal body, bulbocavernosus muscle and body), for if it is lacerated or weakened the ligaments will gradually stretch and the uterus will descend. The uterus and its components and the vagina are, in fact, one continuous unit.

Arteries

The blood supply to the uterus is from the uterine and ovarian arteries. As a terminal branch of the hypogastric artery, the uterine artery runs downward and medially to cross the ureter near the cervix. It then ascends along the lateral border of the uterus in a tortuous course through the parametrium, giving off lateral branches to both uterine surfaces. Above, it anastomoses to join with the ovarian artery in the mesometrium, which creates the main accessory source of blood. The uterine arteries within the uterus form a series of arches over the fundus, creating cruciate anastomoses with the opposite side.

Branches of the arcuate arteries (radial) penetrate the myometrium at right angles to terminate in the basilar arterioles for the basilar portion of the endometrium and in the spinal arteries of the endometrium. The spinal arteries are tortuous in structure, not because of endometrial growth but because, ontogenically, an organ carries its arterial supply with it as it changes size and position. Therefore, the spiral arteries are able to maintain adequate arterial flow to the placenta while it is attached within the uterus.

On the other hand, the veins of the endometrium are a series of small sinusoids that connect to the larger sinusoids of the myometrium, the latter coalescing into the larger veins of the uterine complex. It is useful here to note the significance of the muscular role of the uterus in helping to control venous bleeding during parturition.

The arterial supply to the cervix is primarily through the cervical branches of the right and left uterine arteries, which form a rete around the cervix (coronary artery), creating the azygos artery in the midline anteriorly and posteriorly. Anastomoses between this artery and the vaginal artery on both sides afford cruciate flow on the anterior wall, whereas on the posterior wall of the vagina, anastomoses occur with the right and left middle hemorrhoidal arteries as they supply the wall and the rectum.

Veins

The veins form a plexus and drain through the uterine vein to the hypogastric vein. There are connections with the ovarian veins and the inferior epigastric by way of the vein accompanying the round ligament.

Lymphatics

Lymphatic drainage involves several chains of lymph nodes. From the subperitoneal plexus, the collecting trunks of the lower uterine segment may drain by way of the cervix to the external iliac chain or by way of the isthmus to the lateral sacral nodes. Drainage along the round ligament progresses to the superficial inguinal nodes, then to the femoral, and finally to the external iliac chain. Drainage laterally to the suspensory ligament of the ovary involves the lumbar pedicle and progresses in a retroperitoneal manner across and anteriorly to the ureter, to the lumbar nodes (interaorticocaval) that lie along the aorta, and inferiorly to the kidney.

Fallopian Tubes (Uterine Oviducts)

Anatomy

The fallopian tubes serve to convey the ova (eggs) to the uterus. They extend from the superior angles of the uterus to the region of the ovaries, running in the superior border of the broad ligament (mesosalpinx). The fallopian tubes and ovaries are collectively referred to as the adnexa. The course of each tube is nearly horizontal at first and slightly backward. Upon reaching the lower (uterine) pole of the ovary, the tube turns upward, parallel with the anterior (mesovarian) border, then arches backward over the upper pole and descends posteriorly to terminate in contact with the medial surface. Each tube is 7–12 cm long and may be divided into 4 parts: isthmus, ampulla, infundibulum, and interstitial.

The isthmus is the narrow and nearly straight portion immediately adjoining the uterus. It has a rather long intramural course, and its opening into the uterus, the uterine ostium, is approximately 1 mm in diameter. Following the isthmus is the wider, more tortuous ampulla. It terminates in a funnel-like dilatation, the infundibulum. The margins of the infundibulum are fringed by numerous diverging processes, the fimbriae, the longest of which, the fimbria ovarica, is attached to the ovary. The funnel-shaped mouth of the infundibulum, the abdominal ostium, is about 3 mm in diameter and actually leads into the peritoneal cavity, although it probably is closely applied to the surface of the ovary during ovulation. The interstitial is the portion of the tube that lies within the uterine wall. The innermost portion is seen from the uterine cavity as the tubal ostea.

Layers of Wall

The wall of the tube has 4 coats: serous (peritoneal), subserous or adventitial (fibrous and vascular), muscular, and mucous. Each tube is enclosed within a peritoneal covering except along a small strip on its lower surface, where the mesosalpinx is attached. At the margins of the infundibulum and the fimbriae, this peritoneal covering becomes directly continuous with the mucous membrane lining the interior of the tube. The subserous tissue is lax in the immediate vicinity of the tube. The blood and nerve supply is found within this layer. The muscular coat has an outer longitudinal and an inner circular layer of smooth muscle fibers, more prominent and continuous with that of the uterus at the uterine end of the tube. The mucous coat is ciliated columnar epithelium with coarse longitudinal folds, simple in the region of the isthmus but becoming higher and more complex in the ampulla. The epithelial lining extends outward into the fimbriae. The ciliary motion is directed toward the uterus.

Arteries & Veins

The blood supply to the tubes is derived from the ovarian and uterine arteries. The tubal branch of the uterine artery courses along the lower surface of the uterine tube as far as the fimbriated extremity and may also send a branch to the ligamentum teres. The ovarian branch of the uterine artery runs along the attached border of the ovary and gives off a tubal branch. Both branches form cruciate anastomoses in the mesosalpinx. The veins accompany the arteries.

Lymphatics

The lymphatic drainage occurs through trunks running retroperitoneally across and anterior to the ureter, into the lumbar nodes along the aorta, and inferior to the kidney.

Ovaries

Anatomy

The ovaries are paired organs situated close to the wall on either side of the pelvis minor, a little below the brim. Each measures 2.5–5 cm in length, 1.5–3 cm in breadth, and 0.7–1.5 cm in width, weighing about 4–8 g. The ovary has 2 surfaces, medial and lateral; 2 borders, anterior or mesovarian and posterior or free; and 2 poles, upper or tubal and lower or uterine. When the uterus and adnexa are in the normal position, the long axis of the ovary is nearly vertical, but it bends somewhat medially and forward at the lower end so that the lower pole tends to point toward the uterus. The medial surface is rounded and, posteriorly, may have numerous scars or elevations that mark the position of developing follicles and sites of ruptured ones.

Structure of Ovary

The ovary is covered by cuboid or low columnar epithelium and consists of a cortex and a medulla. The medulla is made up of connective tissue fibers, smooth muscle cells, and numerous blood vessels, nerves, lymphatic vessels, and supporting tissue. The cortex is composed of a fine areolar stroma, with many vessels and scattered follicles of epithelial cells within which are the definitive ova (oocytes) in various stages of maturity. The more mature follicles enlarge and project onto the free surface of the ovary, where they are visible to the naked eye. These are called graafian follicles. When fully mature, the follicle bursts, releasing the ovum and becoming transformed into a corpus luteum. The corpus luteum, in turn, is later replaced by scar tissue, forming a corpus albicans if pregnancy is not achieved that particular menstrual cycle.

Relationships

The upper portion of this surface is overhung by the fimbriated end of the uterine tube, and the remainder lies in relation to coils of intestine. The lateral surface is similar in shape and faces the pelvic wall, where it forms a distinct depression, the fossa ovarica. This fossa is lined by peritoneum and is bounded above by the external iliac vessels and below by the obturator vessels and nerve; its posterior boundary is formed by the ureter and uterine artery and vein, and the pelvic attachment of the broad ligament is located anteriorly.

The mesovarian or anterior border is fairly straight and provides attachment for the mesovarium, a peritoneal fold by which the ovary is attached to the posterosuperior layer of the broad ligament. Because the vessels, nerves, and lymphatics enter the ovary through this border, it is referred to as the hilum of the ovary.

Mesovarium

The ovary is suspended by means of the mesovarium, the suspensory ligament of the ovary (infundibulopelvic [IP] ligament), and the ovarian ligament. The mesovarium consists of 2 layers of peritoneum, continuous with both the epithelial coat of the ovary and the posterosuperior layer of the broad ligament. It is short and wide and contains branches of the ovarian and uterine arteries, with plexuses of nerves, the pampiniform plexus of veins, and the lateral end of the ovarian ligament. The suspensory ligament of the ovary is a triangular fold of peritoneum and is actually the upper lateral corner of the broad ligament, which becomes confluent with the parietal peritoneum at the pelvic brim. It attaches to the mesovarium as well as to the peritoneal coat of the infundibulum medially, thus suspending both the ovary and the tube. It contains the ovarian artery, veins, and nerves after they pass over the pelvic brim and before they enter the mesovarium.

The ovarian ligament is a band of connective tissue, with numerous small muscle fibers, that lies between the 2 layers of the broad ligament on the boundary line between the mesosalpinx and the mesometrium, connecting the lower (uterine) pole of the ovary with the lateral wall of the uterus. It is attached just below the uterine tube and above the attachment of the round ligament of the uterus and is continuous with the latter.

Arteries

The ovarian artery is the chief source of blood for the ovary. Though both arteries may originate as branches of the abdominal aorta, the left frequently originates from the left renal artery; the right, less frequently. The vessels diverge from each other as they descend. Upon reaching the level of the common iliac artery, they turn medially over that vessel and ureter to descend tortuously into the pelvis on each side between the folds of the suspensory ligament of the ovary into the mesovarium. An additional blood supply is formed from anastomosis with the ovarian branch of the uterine artery, which courses along the attached border of the ovary. Blood vessels that enter the hilum send out capillary branches centrifugally.

The veins follow the course of the arteries and, as they emerge from the hilum, form a well-developed plexus (the pampiniform plexus) between the layers of the mesovarium. Smooth muscle fibers occur in the meshes of the plexus, giving the whole structure the appearance of erectile tissue.

Lymphatics

Lymphatic channels drain retroperitoneally, together with those of the tubes and part of those from the uterus, to the lumbar nodes along the aorta inferior to the kidney. The distribution of lymph channels in the ovary is so extensive that it suggests the system may also provide additional fluid to the ovary during periods of preovulatory follicular swelling.

Nerves

The nerve supply of the ovaries arises from the lumbosacral sympathetic chain and passes to the gonad along with the ovarian artery.

Vagina

Anatomy

The vagina is a strong, hollow, fibromuscular canal approximately 7–9 cm long that extends from the uterus to the vestibule of the external genitalia, where it opens to the exterior. Its long axis is almost parallel with that of the lower part of the sacrum, and it meets the cervix of the uterus at an angle of 45–90 degrees. Because the cervix of the uterus projects into the upper portion, the anterior wall of the vagina is 1.5–2 cm shorter than the posterior wall. The circular cul-de-sac formed around the cervix is known as the fornix and is divided into 4 regions: the anterior fornix, the posterior fornix, and 2 lateral fornices. Toward its lower end, the vagina pierces the urogenital diaphragm and is surrounded by the 2 bulbocavernosus muscles and bodies, which act as a sphincter (sphincter vaginae).

Wall Structure

The vaginal wall is composed of a mucosal layer and a muscular layer. The smooth muscle fibers are indistinctly arranged in 3 layers: an outer longitudinal layer, circumferential layer, and a poorly differentiated inner longitudinal layer. In the lower third, the circumferential fibers envelop the urethra. The submucous area is abundantly supplied with a dense plexus of veins and lymphatics. The mucous layer shows many transverse and oblique rugae, which project inward to such an extent that the lumen in transverse section resembles an H-shaped slit. On the anterior and posterior walls, these ridges are more prominent, and the anterior column forms the urethral carina at its lower end, where the urethra slightly invaginates the anterior wall of the vagina. The mucosa of the vagina is lined throughout by nonkeratinized squamous epithelium. Even though the vagina has no true glands, there is a secretion present. It consists of cervical mucus, desquamated epithelium, and, with sexual stimulation, a direct transudate.

Relationships

Anteriorly, the vagina is in close relationship to the bladder, ureters, and urethra in succession. The posterior fornix is covered by the peritoneum of the rectovaginal pouch, which may contain coils of intestine. Below the pouch, the vagina rests almost directly on the rectum, separated from it by a thin layer of areolar connective tissue. Toward the lower end of the vagina, the rectum turns back sharply, and the distance between the vagina and rectum greatly increases. This space, filled with muscle fibers, connective tissue, and fat, is known as the perineal body. The lateral fornix lies just under the root of the broad ligament and is approximately 1 cm from the point where the uterine artery crosses the ureter.

The remaining lateral vaginal wall is related to the edges of the anterior portion of the levator ani. The vagina is supported at the introitus by the bulbocavernosus muscles and bodies, in the lower third by the levator ani (puborectalis), and superiorly by the transverse (cardinal) ligaments of the uterus. The ductus epoophori longitudinalis (duct of Gartner), the remains of the lower portion of the wolffian duct (mesonephric duct), may often be found on the sides of the vagina as a minute tube or fibrous cord. These vestigial structures often become cystic and appear as translucent areas.

Arteries & Veins

The chief blood supply to the vagina is through the vaginal branch of the uterine artery. After forming the coronary or circular artery of the cervix, it passes medially, behind the ureter, to send 5 main branches onto the anterior wall to the midline. These branches anastomose with the azygos artery (originating midline from the coronary artery of the cervix) and continue downward to supply the anterior vaginal wall and the lower two-thirds of the urethra. The uterine artery eventually anastomoses to the urethral branch of the clitoral artery. The posterior vaginal wall is supplied by branches of the middle and inferior hemorrhoidal arteries, traversing toward the midline to join the azygos artery from the coronary artery of the cervix. These branches then anastomose on the perineum to the superficial and deep transverse perineal arteries. The veins follow the course of the arteries.

Lymphatics

The lymphatics are numerous mucosal plexuses, anastomosing with the deeper muscular plexuses. The superior group of lymphatics joins those of the cervix and may follow the uterine artery to terminate in the external iliac nodes or form anastomoses with the uterine plexus. The middle group of lymphatics, which drain the greater part of the vagina, appears to follow the vaginal arteries to the hypogastric channels. In addition, there are lymph nodes in the rectovaginal septum that are primarily responsible for drainage of the rectum and part of the posterior vaginal wall. The inferior group of lymphatics forms frequent anastomoses between the right and left sides and either courses upward to anastomose with the middle group or enters the vulva and drains to the inguinal nodes.

Nerves

The innervation of the vagina contains both sympathetic and parasympathetic fibers. Only occasional free nerve endings are seen in the mucosa; no other types of nerve endings are noted.

SUMMARY

Even though the basic anatomy and structure of the human body is not changing, the evolution of surgical approaches and technologies is. This constantly ever-changing field requires the gynecologic surgeon to be well versed in female pelvic anatomy by constantly reviewing and studying its contents. Being knowledgeable and current with the female pelvis will allow even the most experienced, senior surgeon to adjust to situations where anatomy is altered secondary to disease processes, congenital malformation, or other unknown complications.

Berek J. *Berek and Novak's Gynecology*. 14th ed. Philadelphia, PA: Lippincott Williams & Wilkins; 2007.

Gabbe S, Niebyl JR, Simpson JL, et al (eds). *Obstetrics. Normal and Problem Pregnancies*. 5th ed. New York, NY: Churchill Livingston Elsevier; 2007.

Kass J, Chiou-Tan FY, Harrell JS, Zhang H, Taber KH. Sectional neuroanatomy of the pelvic floor. *J Comput Assist Tomogr* 2010;34:473–477. PMID: 19820518.

Rahn D, Phelan JL, Roshenraven SM, et al. Anterior abdominal wall nerve and vessel anatomy: clinical implications for gynecologic surgery. *Am J Obstet Gynecol* 2010;202:234.e1–e5. PMID: 20022582.

Schorge J, Schaffer J, Halvorson L, et al (eds). *Williams Gynecology*. New York, NY: McGraw-Hill; 2008.

2 Embryology of the Urogenital System & Congenital Anomalies of the Genital Tract

Catherine M. DeUgarte, MD

In the urogenital system, knowledge of the embryology is crucial in understanding the functions and interconnections between the reproductive and urologic systems. The adult genital and urinary systems are distinct in both function and anatomy, with the exception of the male urethra, where the 2 systems are interconnected. During development, these 2 systems are closely associated. The initial developmental overlap of these systems occurs 4–12 weeks after fertilization. The complexity of developmental events in these systems is evident by the incomplete separation of the 2 systems found in some congenital anomalies. For the sake of clarity, this chapter describes the embryology of each system separately, rather than following a strict developmental chronology.

In view of the complexity and duration of differentiation and development of the genital and urinary systems, it is not surprising that the incidence of malformations involving these systems is one of the highest (10%) of all body systems. Etiologies of congenital malformations are sometimes categorized on the basis of genetic, environmental, or genetic-plus-environmental (so-called polyfactorial inheritance) factors. Known genetic and inheritance factors reputedly account for about 20% of anomalies detected at birth, aberration of chromosomes for nearly 5%, and environmental factors for nearly 10%. The significance of these statistics must be viewed against reports that (1) an estimated one-third to one-half of human zygotes are lost during the first week of gestation and (2) the cause of possibly 70% of human anomalies is unknown. Even so, congenital malformations remain a matter of concern because they are detected in nearly 3% of infants, and 20% of perinatal deaths are purportedly due to congenital anomalies.

The inherent pattern of normal development of the genital system can be viewed as one directed toward somatic "femaleness," unless development is directed by factors for "maleness." The presence and expression of a Y chromosome (and its testis-determining genes) in a normal 46,XY karyotype of somatic cells directs differentiation toward a testis, and normal development of the testis makes available hormones for the selection and differentiation of the genital ducts. When male hormones are present, the mesonephric (wolffian) system persists; when male hormones are not present, the "female" paramesonephric (müllerian) ducts persist. Normal feminization or masculinization of the external genitalia is also a result of the respective timely absence or presence of androgen.

An infant usually is reared as female or male according to the appearance of the external genitalia. However, genital sex is not always immediately discernible, and the choice of sex of rearing can be an anxiety-provoking consideration. Unfortunately, even when genital sex is apparent, later clinical presentation may unmask disorders of sexual differentiation that can lead to problems in psychological adjustment. Whether a somatic disorder is detected at birth or later, investigative backtracking through the developmental process is necessary for proper diagnosis and treatment.

Overview of the First 4 Weeks of Development*

Transformation of the bilaminar embryonic disk into a trilaminar disk composed of **ectoderm, mesoderm,** and **endoderm** (the 3 embryonic germ layers) occurs during the third week by a process called **gastrulation** (Fig. 2–1). During this process, a specialized thickening of epiblast, the **primitive streak,** elongates through the midline of the disk. Some epiblastic cells become **mesoblastic cells,** which migrate peripherally between the epiblast and hypoblast, forming a middle layer of **embryonic mesoderm.** Other mesoblastic cells migrate into the hypoblastic layer and form **embryonic endoderm,** which displaces the hypoblastic cells. The remaining overlying epiblast becomes the **embryonic ectoderm.**

---

*Embryonic or fetal ages given in this chapter are relative to the time of fertilization and should be considered estimates rather than absolutes.

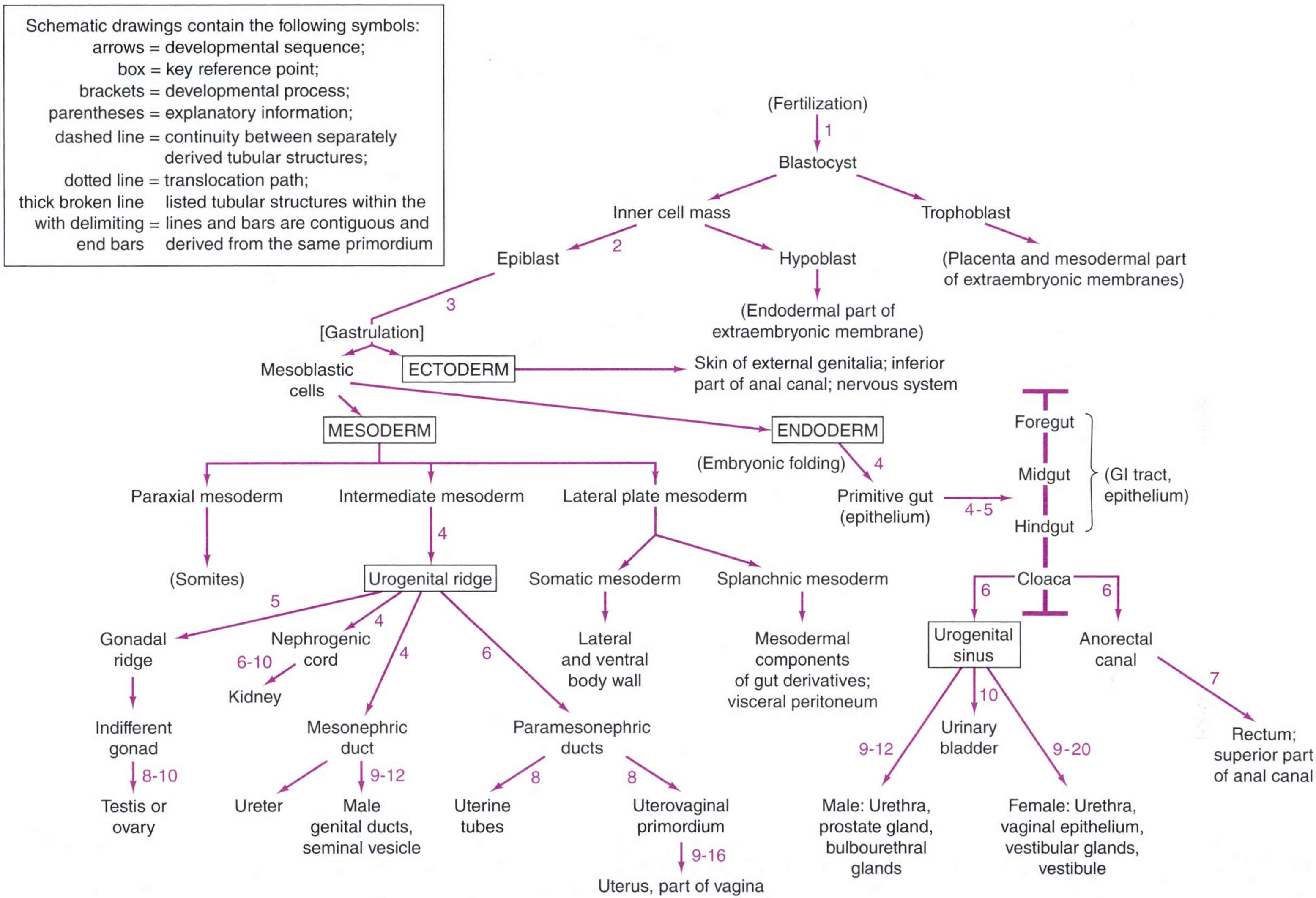

▲ **Figure 2–1.** Schematic overview of embryonic development of progenitory urinary and genital tissues and structures considered to be derivatives of embryonic ectoderm, mesoderm, or endoderm. Numbers indicate the weeks after fertilization when the indicated developmental change occurs. GI, gastrointestinal.

By the end of the third week, 3 clusters of mesoderm are organized on both sides of the midline neural tube. From medial to lateral, these clusters are **paraxial mesoderm,** which forms much of the axial skeleton; **intermediate mesoderm,** which is the origin of the **urogenital ridge** and, hence, much of the reproductive and excretory systems (Fig. 2–2); and **lateral plate mesoderm,** which splits and takes part in body cavity formation. The **intermediate mesoderm** is located between the paraxial and lateral plate mesoderm and is the origin of the **urogenital ridge** and, hence, much of the reproductive and excretory systems (Fig. 2–2). The primitive streak regresses after the fourth week. Rarely, degeneration of the streak is incomplete, and presumptive remnants form a teratoma in the sacrococcygeal region of the fetus (more common in females than in males).

Weeks 4 through 8 of development are called the **embryonic period** (the **fetal period** is from week 9 to term) because formation of all major internal and external structures, including the 2 primary forerunners of the urogenital system (urogenital ridge and urogenital sinus), begins during this time. During this period the embryo is most likely to develop major congenital or acquired morphologic anomalies in response to the effects of various agents. During the fourth week, the shape of the embryo changes from that of a trilaminar disk to that of a crescentic cylinder. The change results from "folding," or flexion, of the embryonic disk in a ventral direction through both its transverse and longitudinal planes. Flexion occurs as midline structures (neural tube and somites) develop and grow at a faster pace than more lateral tissues (ectoderm, 2 layers of lateral plate mesoderm enclosing the coelom between them, and endoderm). Thus, during transverse folding, the lateral tissues on each side of the embryo curl ventromedially and join the respective tissues from the other side, creating a midline ventral tube (the endoderm-lined **primitive gut**), a mesoderm-lined coelomic cavity (the **primitive abdominopelvic cavity**), and the incomplete ventral and lateral body wall. Concurrent longitudinal flexion ventrally of the caudal region of the disk establishes the pouchlike distal end, or **cloaca,** of the primitive gut as well as the distal attachment of the cloaca to the yolk sac through the allantois of the sac (Fig. 2–3).

A noteworthy point (see The Gonads) is that the primordial germ cells of the later-developing gonad initially are found close to the allantois and later migrate to the gonadal primordia. Subsequent partitioning of the cloaca during the sixth week results in formation of the anorectal canal and the **urogenital sinus,** the progenitor of the urinary bladder, urethra, vagina, and other genital structures (Fig. 2–1 and Table 2–1; see Subdivision of the Cloaca & Formation of the Urogenital Sinus).

Embryonic folding also moves the intermediate mesoderm—the forerunner of the **urogenital ridge**—to its characteristic developmental locations as bilateral longitudinal bulges in the dorsal wall of the new body cavity and lateral to the dorsal mesentery of the new gut tube. By the end of the fourth week of development, the principal structures (urogenital ridge and cloaca) and tissues that give rise to the urogenital system are present.

Tables 2–1 and 2–2 provide a general overview of urogenital development.

THE URINARY SYSTEM

Three excretory "systems" form successively, with temporal overlap, during the embryonic period. Each system has a different excretory "organ," but the 3 systems share anatomic continuity through development of their excretory ducts. The 3 systems are mesodermal derivatives of the urogenital ridge (Figs. 2–2 and 2–3), part of which becomes a longitudinal mass, the **nephrogenic cord.** The **pronephros,** or organ of the first system, exists rudimentarily, is nonfunctional, and regresses during the fourth week. However, the developing pronephric ducts continue to grow and become the mesonephric ducts of the subsequent kidney, the **mesonephros.** The paired mesonephroi exist during 4–8 weeks as simplified morphologic versions of the third, or permanent, set of kidneys, and they may have transient excretory function. Although the mesonephroi degenerate, some of their tubules, called **epigenital mesonephric tubules,** persist to participate in formation of the gonad and male ductuli efferentes (Fig. 2–4). The permanent kidney, the **metanephros,** begins to form in response to an inductive influence of a diverticulum of the mesonephric ducts during the fifth week and becomes functional at 10–13 weeks.

Differentiation of the caudal segment of the mesonephric ducts results in (1) incorporation of part of the ducts into the wall of the urogenital sinus (early vesicular trigone, see following text), and (2) formation of a ductal diverticulum, which plays an essential role in formation of the definitive kidney. If male sex differentiation occurs, the major portion of each duct becomes the epididymis, ductus deferens, and ejaculatory duct. Only small vestigial remnants of the duct sometimes persist in the female (**Gartner's duct; duct of the epoophoron**).

Metanephros (Definitive Kidney)

A. Collecting Ducts

By the end of the fifth week, a **ureteric bud,** or metanephric diverticulum, forms on the caudal part of the mesonephric duct close to the cloaca. The bud gives rise to the collecting tubules, calices, renal pelvis, and ureter (Fig. 2–2). The stalk of the elongating bud will become the **ureter** when the ductal segment between the stalk and the cloaca becomes incorporated into the wall of the urinary bladder (which is a derivative of the partitioned cloaca, see text that follows; Figs. 2–5 to 2–8). The expanded tip, or **ampulla,** of the bud grows into the adjacent metanephric mesoderm (**blastema**) and subdivides successively into 12–15 generations of buds, or eventual **collecting tubules.** From weeks 10–14, dilatation of the early generations of tubular branches successively produces the **renal pelvis,** the **major calices,** and the **minor calices,** while

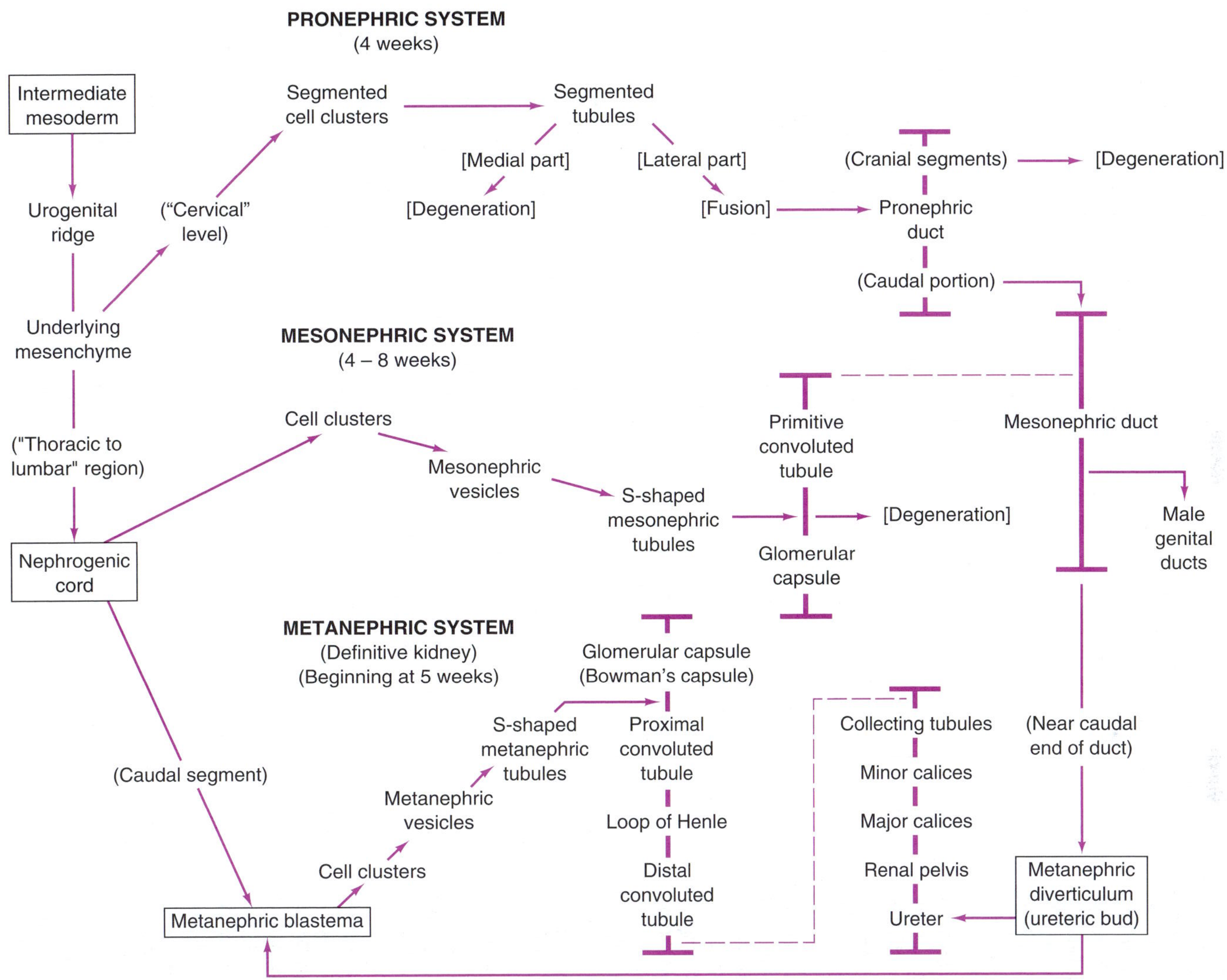

▲ **Figure 2–2.** Schematic drawing of formation of the definitive kidney and its collecting ducts. The pronephric duct is probably the only structure that participates in all 3 urinary systems, as its caudal portion continues to grow and is called the mesonephric duct when the mesonephric system develops. (Explanatory symbols are given in Fig. 2–1.)

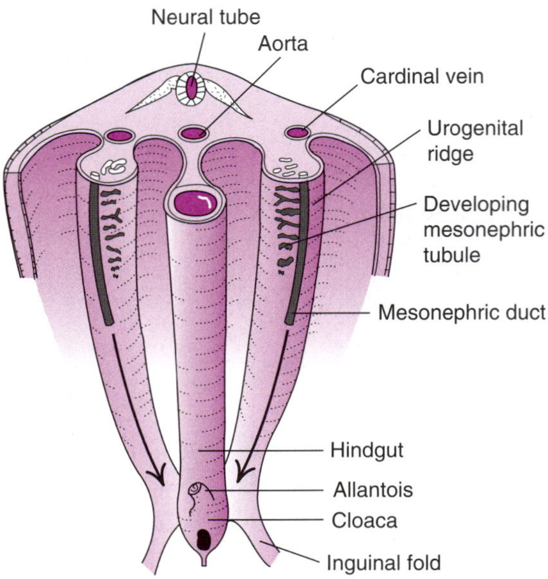

▲ **Figure 2–3.** Early stage in the formation of the mesonephric kidneys and their collecting ducts in the urogenital ridge. The central tissue of the ridge is the nephrogenic cord, in which the mesonephric tubules are forming. The mesonephric ducts grow toward (arrows) and will open into the cloaca. About 5 weeks' gestation.

the middle generations form the medullary collecting tubules. The last several generations of collecting tubules grow centrifugally into the cortical region of the kidney between weeks 24 and 36.

B. Nephrons

Continued maintenance of the intimate relationship of the metanephric blastema and ampulla is necessary for normal formation of the definitive excretory units (nephrons), which starts at about the eighth week. Formation of urine purportedly begins at about weeks 10–13, when an estimated 20% of the nephrons are morphologically mature.

The last month of gestation is marked by interstitial growth, hypertrophy of existing components of uriniferous tubules, and the disappearance of bud primordia for collecting tubules. Opinions differ about whether formation of nephrons ceases prenatally at about 28 or 32 weeks or postnatally during the first several months. If the ureteric bud fails to form, undergoes early degeneration, or fails to grow into the nephrogenic mesoderm, aberrations of nephrogenesis result. These may be nonthreatening (**unilateral renal agenesis**), severe, or even fatal (**bilateral renal agenesis, polycystic kidney**).

C. Positional Changes

Figure 2–9 illustrates relocation of the kidney to a deeper position within the posterior body wall, as well as the

Table 2–1. Adult derivatives and vestigial remains of embryonic urogenital structures.

Embryonic Structure	Male	Female
Indifferent gonad	*Testis*	*Ovary*
Cortex	*Seminiferous tubules*	*Ovarian follicles*
Medulla	*Rete testis*	*Medulla* Rete ovarii
Gubernaculum	Gubernaculum testis	*Ovarian ligament* *Round ligament of uterus*
Mesonephric tubules	*Ductus efferentes* Paradidymis	Epoophoron Paroophoron
Mesonephric duct	Appendix of epididymis *Ductus epididymidis* *Ductus deferens* *Ureter, pelvis, calices, and collecting tubules* *Ejaculatory duct and seminal vesicle*	Appendix vesiculosa Duct of epoophoron Duct of Gartner *Ureter, pelvis, calices, and collecting tubules*
Paramesonephric duct	Appendix of testis	Hydatid (of Morgagni) *Uterine tube* *Uterus* *Vagina (fibromuscular wall)*
Urogenital sinus	*Urinary bladder* *Urethra* (except glandular portion) Prostatic utricle *Prostate gland* *Bulbourethral glands*	*Urinary bladder* *Urethra* *Vagina* *Urethral and paraurethral glands* *Greater vestibular glands*
Müllerian tubercle	Seminal colliculus	Hymen
Genital tubercle	*Penis* *Glans penis* *Corpora cavernosa penis* *Corpus spongiosum*	*Clitoris* *Glans clitoridis* *Corpora cavernosa clitoridis* *Bulb of the vestibule*
Urogenital folds	*Ventral aspect of penis*	*Labia minora*
Labioscrotal swellings	*Scrotum*	*Labia majora*

Functional derivatives are in italics.

Modified and reproduced, with permission, from Moore KL, Persaud TVN. *The Developing Human: Clinically Oriented Embryology.* 5th ed. New York, NY: Saunders; 1993.

Table 2–2. Developmental chronology of the human urogenital system.

Age in Weeks[1]	Size (C-R) in mm	Urogenital System
2.5	1.5	Allantois present.
3.5	2.5	All pronephric tubules formed. Pronephric duct growing caudad as a blind tube. Cloaca and cloacal membrane present.
4	5	Primordial germ cells near allantois. Pronephros degenerated. Pronephric (mesonephric) duct reaches cloaca. Mesonephric tubules differentiating rapidly. Metanephric bud pushes into secretory primordium.
5	8	Mesonephros reaches its caudal limit. Ureteric and pelvic primordia distinct.
6	12	Cloaca subdividing into urogenital sinus and anorectal canal. Sexless gonad and genital tubercle prominent. Paramesonephric duct appearing. Metanephric collecting tubules begin branching.
7	17	Mesonephros at peak of differentiation. Urogenital sinus separated from anorectal canal (cloaca subdivided). Urogenital and anal membranes rupturing.
8	23	Earliest metanephric secretory tubules differentiating. Testis (8 weeks) and ovary (9–10 weeks) identifiable as such. Paramesonephric ducts, nearing urogenital sinus, are ready to unite a uterovaginal primordium. Genital ligaments indicated.
10	40	Kidney able to excrete urine. Bladder expands as sac. Genital duct of opposite sex degenerating. Bulbourethral and vestibular glands appearing. Vaginal bulbs forming.
12	56	Kidney in lumbar location. Early ovarian folliculogenesis begins. Uterine horns absorbed. External genitalia attain distinctive features. Mesonephros and rete tubules complete male duct. Prostate and seminal vesicle appearing. Hollow viscera gaining muscular walls.
16	112	Testis at deep inguinal ring. Uterus and vagina recognizable as such. Mesonephros involuted.
20–38 (5–9 months)	160–350	Female urogenital sinus becoming a shallow vestibule (5 months). Vagina regains lumen (5 months). Uterine glands begin to appear (5 months). Scrotum solid until sacs and testes descend (7–8 months). Kidney tubules cease forming at birth.

[1]After fertilization.
C–R, crown–rump length.
Modified and reproduced, with permission, from Arey LB. *Developmental Anatomy*. 7th ed. New York, NY: Saunders; 1965.

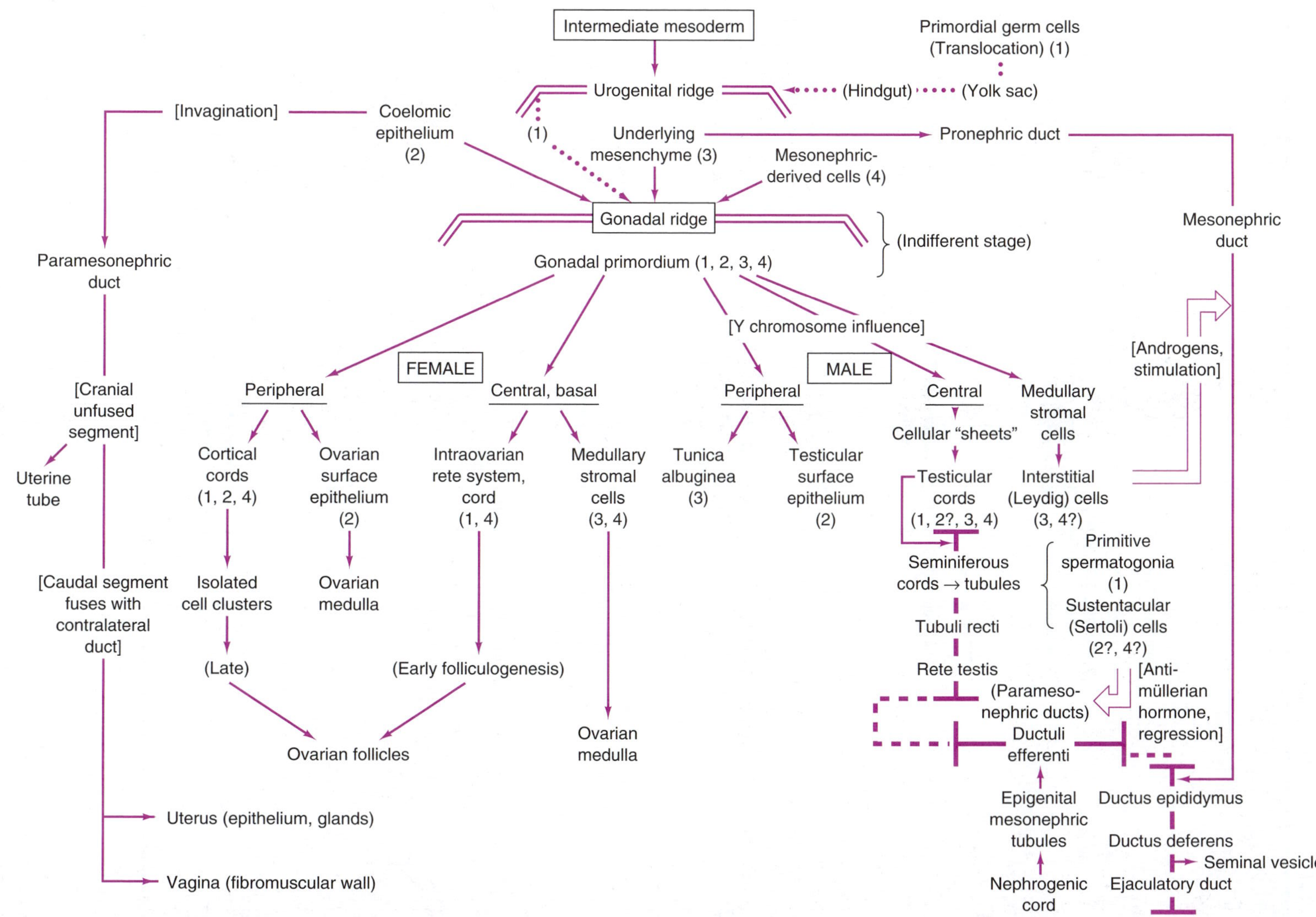

▲ **Figure 2–4.** Schematic drawing of the formation of the gonads and genital ducts.

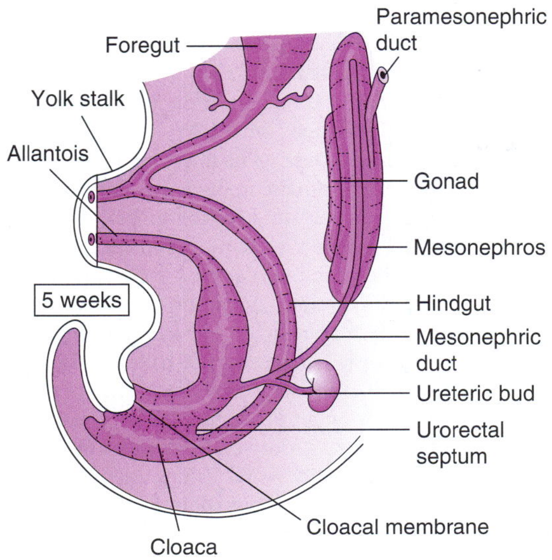

▲ **Figure 2–5.** Left-side view of urogenital system and cloacal region prior to subdivision of cloaca by urorectal septum (Tourneux and Rathke folds). Position of future paramesonephric duct is shown (begins in the sixth week). Gonad is in the indifferent stage (sexually undifferentiated).

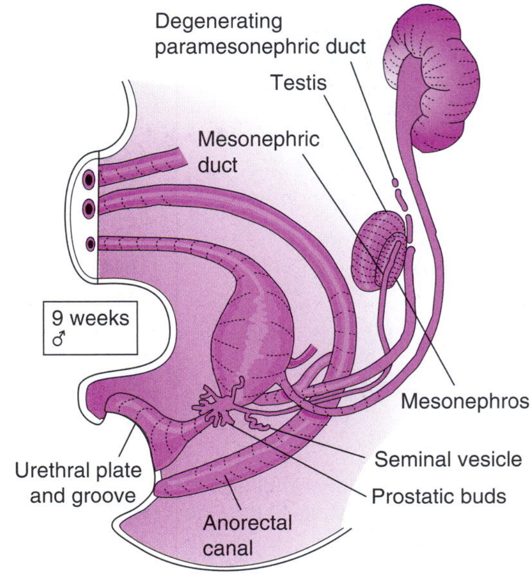

▲ **Figure 2–7.** Left-side view of urogenital system at an early stage of male sexual differentiation. Phallic part of urogenital sinus is proliferating anteriorly to form the urethral plate and groove. Seminal vesicles and prostatic buds are shown at a more advanced stage (about 12 weeks) for emphasis.

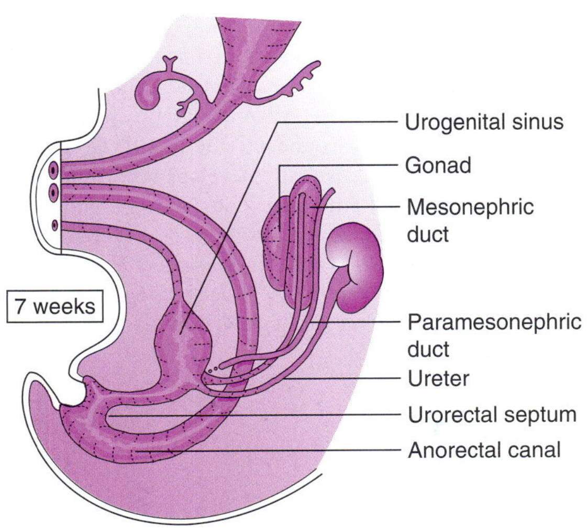

▲ **Figure 2–6.** Left-side view of urogenital system. Urorectal septum nearly subdivides the cloaca into the urogenital sinus and the anorectal canal. Paramesonephric ducts do not reach the sinus until the ninth week. Gonad is sexually undifferentiated. Note incorporation of caudal segment of mesonephric duct into urogenital sinus (compare with Fig. 2–5).

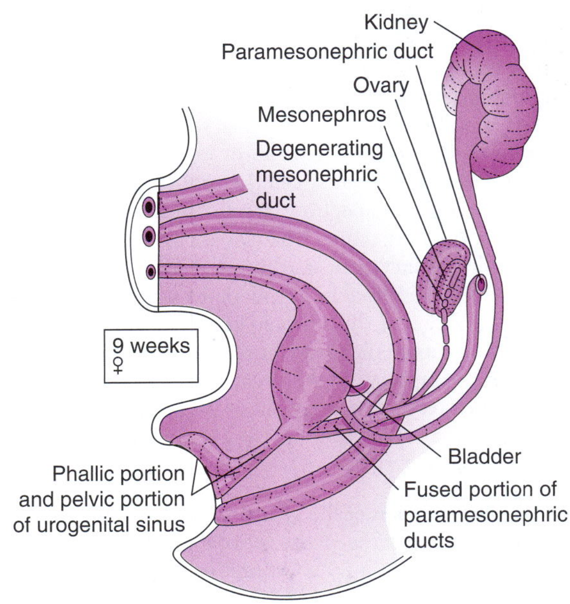

▲ **Figure 2–8.** Left-side view of urogenital system at an early stage of female sexual differentiation. Paramesonephric (müllerian) ducts have fused caudally (to form uterovaginal primordium) and contacted the pelvic part of the urogenital sinus.

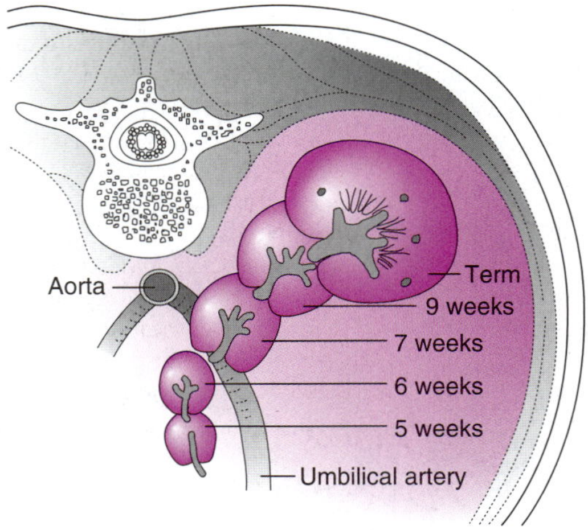

▲ **Figure 2–9.** Positional changes of the definitive kidney at 5 different stages but projected on one cross-sectional plane.

approximately 90-degree medial rotation of the organ on its longitudinal axis. Rotation and lateral positioning probably are facilitated by the growth of midline structures (axial skeleton and muscles). The "ascent" of the kidney between weeks 5 and 8 can be attributed largely to differential longitudinal growth of the rest of the lumbosacral area and to the reduction of the rather sharp curvature of the caudal region of the embryo. Some migration of the kidney may also occur. Straightening of the curvature also may be attributable to relative changes in growth, especially the development of the infraumbilical abdominal wall. As the kidney moves into its final position (lumbar 1–3 by the 12th week), its arterial supply shifts to successively higher aortic levels. Ectopic kidneys can result from abnormal "ascent." During the seventh week, the "ascending" metanephroi closely approach each other near the aortic bifurcation. The close approximation of the 2 developing kidneys can lead to fusion of the lower poles of the kidneys, resulting in formation of a single **horseshoe kidney,** the ascent of which would be arrested by the stem of the interior mesenteric artery. Infrequently, a **pelvic kidney** results from trapping of the organ beneath the umbilical artery, which restricts passage out of the pelvis.

THE GENITAL SYSTEM

Sexual differentiation of the genital system occurs in a basically sequential order: genetic, gonadal, ductal, and genital. **Genetic sex** is determined at fertilization by the complement of sex chromosomes (ie, XY specifies a genotypic male and XX a female). However, early morphologic indications of the sex of the developing embryo do not appear until about the eighth or ninth week after conception. Thus, there is a so-called **indifferent stage,** when morphologic identity of sex is not clear or when preferential differentiation for one sex has not been imposed on the sexless primordia. This is characteristic of early developmental stages for the gonads, genital ducts, and external genitalia. When the influence of genetic sex has been expressed on the indifferent gonad, **gonadal sex** is established. The **SRY** (**sex-determining region of the Y chromosome**) gene in the short arm of the Y chromosome of normal genetic males is considered the best candidate for the gene encoding for the **testis-determining factor** (**TDF**). TDF initiates a chain of events that results in differentiation of the gonad into a testis with its subsequent production of antimüllerian hormone and testosterone, which influences development of somatic "maleness" (see Testis). Normal genetic females do not have the SRY gene, and the early undifferentiated medullary region of their presumptive gonad does not produce the TDF (see Ovary).

The testis and ovary are derived from the same primordial tissue, but histologically visible differentiation toward a testis occurs sooner than that toward an ovary. An "ovary" is first recognized by the absence of testicular histogenesis (eg, thick tunica albuginea) or by the presence of germ cells entering meiotic prophase between the 8th and about the 11th week. The different primordia for male and female genital ducts exist in each embryo during overlapping periods, but establishment of male or female **ductal sex** depends on the presence or absence, respectively, of testicular products and the sensitivity of tissues to these products. The 2 primary testicular products are androgenic steroids (**testosterone** and nonsteroidal **antimüllerian hormone**) (see Testis). Stimulation by testosterone influences the persistence and differentiation of the "male" mesonephric ducts (**wolffian ducts**), whereas antimüllerian hormone influences regression of the "female" paramesonephric ducts (**müllerian ducts**). Absence of these hormones in a nonaberrant condition specifies persistence of müllerian ducts and regression of wolffian ducts (ie, initiation of development of the uterus and uterine tubes). **Genital sex** (external genitalia) subsequently develops according to the absence or presence of androgen. Thus, *the inherent pattern of differentiation of the genital system can be viewed as one directed toward somatic "femaleness" unless the system is dominated by certain factors for "maleness" (eg, gene expression of the Y chromosome, androgenic steroids, and antimüllerian hormone).*

THE GONADS

Indifferent (Sexless) Stage

Gonadogenesis temporally overlaps metanephrogenesis and interacts with tissues of the mesonephric system. Formation of the gonad is summarized schematically in Figure 2–4. Around the fifth week, the midportion of each urogenital ridge thickens as cellular condensation forms the **gonadal ridge.** For the next 2 weeks, this ridge is an undifferentiated cell mass, lacking either testicular or ovarian morphology.

As shown in Figure 2–4, the cell mass consists of (1) **primordial germ cells,** which translocate into the ridge, and a mixture of **somatic cells** derived by (2) proliferation of the coelomic epithelial cells, (3) condensation of the **underlying mesenchyme** of part of the urogenital ridge, and (4) ingrowth of **mesonephric-derived cells.**

The end of the gonadal indifferent stage in the male is near the middle of the seventh week, when a basal lamina delineates the coelomic epithelium and the developing tunica albuginea separates the coelomic epithelium from the developing testicular cords. The indifferent stage in the female ends around the ninth week, when the first oogonia enter meiotic prophase.

Primordial germ cells, presumptive progenitors of the gametes, become evident in the late third to early fourth week in the dorsocaudal wall of the yolk sac and the mesenchyme around the allantois. The **allantois** is a caudal diverticulum of the yolk sac that extends distally into the primitive umbilical stalk and, after embryonic flexion, is adjacent proximally to the cloacal hindgut. The primordial germ cells are translocated from the allantoic region (about the middle of the fourth week) to the urogenital ridge (between the middle of the fifth week and late in the sixth week). It is not known whether primordial germ cells must be present in the gonadal ridge for full differentiation of the gonad to occur. The initial stages of somatic development appear to occur independently of the germ cells. Later endocrine activity in the testis, but not in the ovary, is known to occur in the absence of germ cells. The germ cells appear to have some influence on gonadal differentiation at certain stages of development.

Testis

During early differentiation of the testis, there are condensations of germ cells and somatic cells, which have been described as platelike groups, or sheets. These groups are at first distributed throughout the gonad and then become more organized as primitive **testicular cords.** The cords begin to form centrally and are arranged somewhat perpendicular to the long axis of the gonad. In response to TDF, these cords differentiate into Sertoli cells. The first characteristic feature of male gonadal sex differentiation is evident around week 8, when the **tunica albuginea** begins to form in the mesenchymal tissue underlying the coelomic epithelium. Eventually, this thickened layer of tissue causes the developing testicular cords to be separated from the surface epithelium and placed deeper in the central region of the gonad. The surface epithelium reforms a basal lamina and later thins to a mesothelial covering of the gonad. The testicular cords coil peripherally and thicken as their cellular organization becomes more distinct. A basal lamina eventually develops in the testicular cords, although it is not known if the somatic cells, germ cells, or both are primary contributors to the lamina.

Throughout gonadal differentiation, the developing testicular cords appear to maintain a close relationship to the basal area of the mesonephric-derived cell mass. An interconnected network of cords, **rete cords,** develops in this cell mass and gives rise to the **rete testis.** The rete testis joins centrally with neighboring epigenital mesonephric tubules, which become the **efferent ductules** linking the rete testis with the epididymis, a derivative of the mesonephric duct. With gradual enlargement of the testis and regression of the mesonephros, a cleft forms between the 2 organs, slowly creating the mesentery of the testis, the **mesorchium.**

The differentiating testicular cords are made up of primordial germ cells (primitive spermatogonia) and somatic "supporting" cells (**sustentacular cells,** or **Sertoli cells**). Some precocious meiotic activity has been observed in the fetal testis. Meiosis in the germ cells usually does not begin until puberty; the cause of this delay is unknown. Besides serving as "supporting cells" for the primitive spermatogonia, Sertoli cells also produce the glycoprotein **antimüllerian hormone** (also called **müllerian-inhibiting substance**). Antimüllerian hormone causes regression of the paramesonephric (müllerian) ducts, apparently during a very discrete period of ductal sensitivity in male fetuses. At puberty, the seminiferous cords mature to become the seminiferous tubules, and the Sertoli cells and spermatogonia mature.

Shortly after the testicular cords form, the steroid-producing **interstitial (Leydig) cells** of the extracordal compartment of the testis differentiate from stromal mesenchymal cells, probably due to antimüllerian hormone. Mesonephric-derived cells may also be a primordial source of Leydig cells. Steroidogenic activity of Leydig cells begins near the 10th week. High levels of testosterone are produced during the period of differentiation of external genitalia (weeks 11–12) and maintained through weeks 16–18. Steroid levels then rise or fall somewhat in accordance with changes in the concentration of Leydig cells. Both the number of cells and the levels of testosterone decrease around the fifth month.

Ovary

A. Development

In the normal absence of the Y chromosome or the sex-determining region of the Y chromosome (SRY gene; see The Genital System), the somatic sex cords of the indifferent gonad do not produce TDF. In the absence of TDF, differentiation of the gonad into a testis and its subsequent production of antimüllerian hormone and testosterone do not occur (see Testis). The indifferent gonad becomes an ovary. Complete ovarian differentiation seems to require two X chromosomes (XO females exhibit ovarian dysgenesis, in which ovaries have precociously degenerated germ cells and no follicles and are present as gonadal "streaks"). The first recognition of a developing ovary around weeks 9–10 is based on the temporal absence of testicular-associated features (most prominently, the tunica albuginea) and on the presence of early meiotic activity in the germ cells.

Early differentiation toward an ovary involves mesonephric-derived cells "invading" the basal region (adjacent to mesonephros) and central region of the gonad (central and basal regions represent the primitive "medullary" region of the gonad). At the same time, clusters of germ cells are displaced somewhat peripherally into the "cortical" region of the gonad. Some of the central mesonephric cells give rise to the rete system that subsequently forms a network of cords (**intraovarian rete cords**) extending to the primitive cortical area. As these cords extend peripherally between germ clusters, several epithelial cell proliferations extend centrally, and some mixing of these somatic cells apparently takes place around the germ cell clusters. These early cordlike structures are more irregularly distributed than early cords in the testis and not distinctly outlined. The cords open into clusters of germ cells, but all germ cells are not confined to cords. The first oogonia that begin meiosis are located in the innermost part of the cortex and are the first germ cells to contact the intraovarian rete cords.

Folliculogenesis begins in the innermost part of the cortex when the central somatic cells of the cord contact and surround the germ cells while an intact basal lamina is laid down. These somatic cells are morphologically similar to the mesonephric cells that form the intraovarian rete cords associated with the oocytes and apparently differentiate into the presumptive granulosa cells of the early follicle. Folliculogenesis continues peripherally. Between weeks 12 and 20 of gestation, proliferative activity causes the surface epithelium to become a thickened, irregular multilayer of cells. In the absence of a basal lamina, the cells and apparent epithelial cell cords mix with underlying tissues. These latter cortical cords often retain a connection to and appear similar to the surface epithelium. The epithelial cells of these cords probably differentiate into granulosa cells and contribute to folliculogenesis, although this occurs after the process is well under way in the central region of the gonad. Follicles fail to form in the absence of oocytes or with precocious loss of germ cells, and oocytes not encompassed by follicular cells degenerate.

Stromal mesenchymal cells, connective tissue, and somatic cells of cords not participating in folliculogenesis form the **ovarian medulla** in the late fetal ovary. Individual **primordial follicles** containing diplotene oocytes populate the inner and outer cortex of this ovary. The rete ovarii may persist, along with a few vestiges of mesonephric tubules, as the vestigial epoophoron near the adult ovary. Finally, similar to the testicular mesorchium, the **mesovarium** eventually forms as a gonadal mesentery between the ovary and old urogenital ridge. Postnatally, the epithelial surface of the ovary consists of a single layer of cells continuous with peritoneal mesothelium at the ovarian hilum. A thin, fibrous connective tissue, the tunica albuginea, forms beneath the surface epithelium and separates it from the cortical follicles.

B. Anomalies of the Ovaries

Anomalies of the ovaries encompass a broad range of developmental errors from complete absence of the ovaries to supernumerary ovaries. The many variations of gonadal disorders usually are subcategorized within classifications of disorders of sex determination. Unfortunately, there is little consensus for a major classification, although most include pathogenetic consideration. Extensive summaries of the different classifications are offered in the references to this chapter.

Congenital absence of the ovary (no gonadal remnants found) is very rare. Two types have been considered, agenesis and agonadism. By definition, **agenesis** implies that the primordial gonad did not form in the urogenital ridge, whereas **agonadism** indicates the absence of gonads that may have formed initially and subsequently degenerated. It can be difficult to distinguish one type from the other on a practical basis. For example, a patient with female genital ducts and external genitalia and a 46,XY karyotype could represent either gonadal agenesis or agonadism. In the latter condition, the gonad may form but undergo early degeneration and resorption before any virilizing expression is made. *Whenever congenital absence of the ovaries is suspected, careful examination of the karyotype, the external genitalia, and the genital ducts must be performed.*

Descriptions of agonadism usually have indicated that the external genitalia are abnormal (variable degree of fusion of labioscrotal swellings) and that either very rudimentary ductal derivatives are present or there are no genital ducts. The cause of agonadism is unknown, although several explanations have been suggested, such as (1) failure of the primordial gonad to form, along with abnormal formation of ductal anlagen, and (2) partial differentiation and then regression and absorption of testes (accounting for suppression of müllerian ducts but lack of stimulation of mesonephric, or wolffian, ducts). Explanations that include teratogenic effects or genetic defects are more likely candidates in view of the associated incidence of nonsexual somatic anomalies with the disorder. The **streak gonad** is a product of primordial gonadal formation and subsequent failure of differentiation, which can occur at various stages. The gonad usually appears as a fibrouslike cord of mixed elements (lacking germ cells) located parallel to a uterine tube. Streak gonads are characteristic of **gonadal dysgenesis** and a 45,XO karyotype (**Turner's syndrome;** distinctions are drawn between Turner's syndrome and **Turner's stigmata** when consideration is given to the various associated somatic anomalies of gonadal dysgenesis). However, streak gonads may be consequent to genetic mutation or hereditary disease other than the anomalous karyotype.

Ectopic ovarian tissue occasionally can be found as **accessory ovarian tissue** or as **supernumerary ovaries.** The former may be a product of disaggregation of the embryonic ovary, and the latter may arise from the urogenital ridge as independent primordia.

SUBDIVISION OF THE CLOACA & FORMATION OF THE UROGENITAL SINUS

The endodermally lined urogenital sinus is derived by partitioning of the endodermal cloaca. It is the precursor of the urinary bladder in both sexes and the urinary and genital structures specific to each sex (Fig. 2–1). The cloaca is a pouchlike enlargement of the caudal end of the hindgut and is formed by the process of "folding" of the caudal region of the embryonic disk between 4 and 5 weeks' gestation (see Overview of the First 4 Weeks of Development; Figs. 2–1 and 2–3). During the "tail-fold" process, the posteriorly placed allantois, or allantoic diverticulum of the yolk sac, becomes an anterior extension of the cloaca (Figs. 2–3 and 2–5). Soon after the cloaca forms, it receives posterolaterally the caudal ends of the paired mesonephric ducts and hence becomes a junctional cistern for the allantois, the hindgut, and the ducts. A **cloacal membrane,** composed of ectoderm and endoderm, is the caudal limit of the primitive gut and temporarily separates the cloacal cavity from the extraembryonic confines of the amniotic cavity (Fig. 2–5).

Between weeks 5 and 7, 3 wedges of splanchnic mesoderm, collectively called the **urorectal septum,** proliferate in the coronal plane in the caudal region of the embryo to eventually subdivide the cloaca (Figs. 2–5 to 2–8). The superior wedge, called the **Tourneux fold,** is in the angle between the allantois and the primitive hindgut, and it proliferates caudally into the superior end of the cloaca (Fig. 2–5). The other 2 mesodermal wedges, called the **Rathke folds,** proliferate in the right and left walls of the cloaca. Beginning adjacent to the cloacal membrane, these laterally placed folds grow toward each other and the Tourneux fold. With fusion of the 3 folds creating a urorectal septum, the once single chamber is subdivided into the primitive **urogenital sinus** (ventrally) and the **anorectal canal** of the hindgut (dorsally; Figs. 2–6 to 2–8). The mesonephric ducts and allantois then open into the sinus. The uterovaginal primordium of the fused paramesonephric ducts will contact the sinusal wall between the mesonephric ducts early in the ninth week of development. However, it can be noted that the junctional point of fusion of the cloacal membrane and urorectal septum forms the **primitive perineum** (later differentiation creates the so-called perineal body of tissue) and subdivides the cloacal membrane into the **urogenital membrane** (anteriorly) and the **anal membrane** (posteriorly; Figs. 2–5, 2–8, and 2–10; see also Fig. 2–20).

THE GENITAL DUCTS

Indifferent (Sexless) Stage

Two pairs of genital ducts are initially present in both sexes: (1) the **mesonephric (wolffian) ducts,** which give rise to the male ducts and a derivative, the seminal vesicles; and (2) the **paramesonephric (müllerian) ducts,** which form the oviducts, uterus, and part of the vagina. When the adult structures are described as derivatives of embryonic ducts, this refers to the epithelial lining of the structures. Muscle and connective tissues of the differentiating structures originate from splanchnic mesoderm and mesenchyme adjacent to ducts. Mesonephric ducts are originally the excretory ducts of the mesonephric "kidneys" (see previous text), and they develop early in the embryonic period, about 2 weeks before development of paramesonephric ducts (weeks 6–10). The 2 pairs of genital ducts share a close anatomic relationship in their bilateral course through the urogenital ridge. At their caudal limit, both sets contact the part of the cloaca that is later separated as the urogenital sinus (Figs. 2–5, 2–6, and 2–10). *Determination of the ductal sex of the embryo (ie, which pair of ducts will continue differentiation rather than undergo regression) is established initially by the gonadal sex and later by the continuing influence of hormones.*

Formation of each paramesonephric duct begins early in the sixth week as an invagination of coelomic epithelium in the lateral wall of the cranial end of the urogenital ridge and adjacent to each mesonephric duct. The free edges of the invaginated epithelium join to form the duct except at the site of origin, which persists as a funnel-shaped opening, the future **ostium of the oviduct.** At first, each paramesonephric duct grows caudally through the mesenchyme of the urogenital ridge and laterally parallel to a mesonephric duct. More inferiorly, the paramesonephric duct has a caudomedial course, passing ventral to the mesonephric duct. As it follows the ventromedial bend of the caudal portion of the urogenital ridge, the paramesonephric duct then lies medial to the mesonephric duct, and its caudal tip lies in close apposition to its counterpart from the opposite side (Fig. 2–10). At approximately the eighth week, the caudal segments of the right and left ducts fuse medially and their lumens coalesce to form a single cavity. This conjoined portion of the Y-shaped paramesonephric ducts becomes the uterovaginal primordium, or canal.

Male: Genital Ducts

A. Mesonephric Ducts

The mesonephric ducts persist in the male and, under the stimulatory influence of testosterone, differentiate into the internal genital ducts (epididymis, ductus deferens, and ejaculatory ducts). Near the cranial end of the duct, some of the mesonephric tubules (epigenital mesonephric tubules) of the mesonephric kidney persist lateral to the developing testis. These tubules form a connecting link, the **ductuli efferentes,** between the duct and the rete testis (Fig. 2–10). The cranial portion of each duct becomes the convoluted **ductus epididymis.** The **ductus deferens** forms when smooth muscle from adjacent splanchnic mesoderm is added to the central segment of the mesonephric duct. The seminal vesicle develops as a lateral bud from each mesonephric duct just distal to the junction of the duct and the urogenital sinus (Fig. 2–7). The terminal segment of the duct between

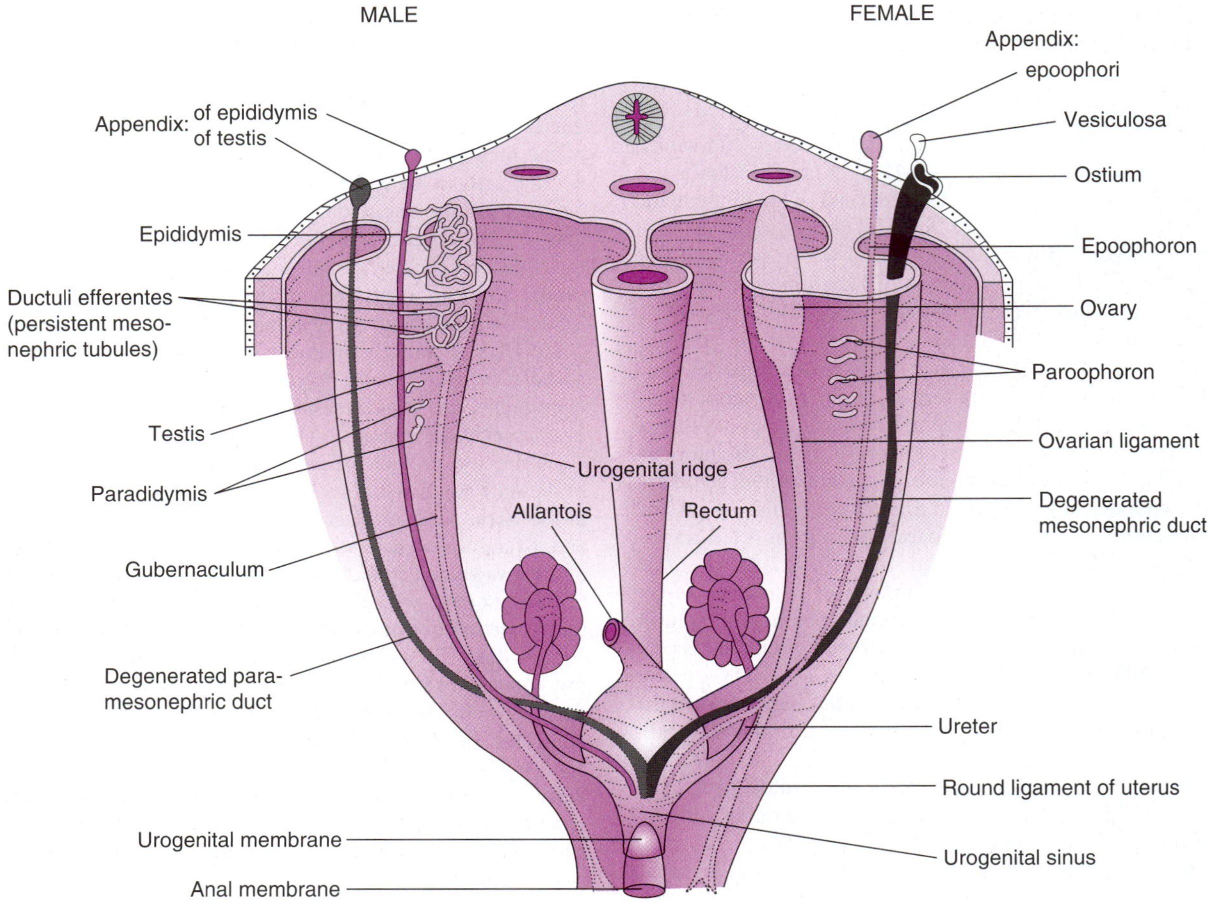

▲ **Figure 2–10.** Diagrammatic comparison between male and female differentiation of internal genitalia.

the sinus and seminal vesicle forms the **ejaculatory duct,** which becomes encased by the developing prostate gland early in the 12th week (see Differentiation of the Urogenital Sinus). A vestigial remnant of the duct may persist cranially near the head of the epididymis as the **appendix epididymis,** whereas remnants of mesonephric tubules near the inferior pole of the testis and tail of the epididymis may persist as the **paradidymis** (Fig. 2–10).

B. Paramesonephric Ducts

The paramesonephric ducts begin to undergo morphologic regression centrally (and progress cranially and caudally) about the time they meet the urogenital sinus caudally (approximately the start of the ninth week). Regression is effected by nonsteroidal antimüllerian hormone produced by the differentiating Sertoli cells slightly before androgen is produced by the Leydig cells (see Testis). Antimüllerian hormone is produced from the time of early testicular differentiation until birth (ie, not only during the period of regression of the paramesonephric duct). However, ductal sensitivity to antimüllerian hormone in the male seems to exist for only a short "critical" time preceding the first signs of ductal regression. Vestigial remnants of the cranial end of the ducts may persist as the **appendix testis** on the superior pole of the testis (Fig. 2–10). Caudally, a ductal remnant is considered to be part of the prostatic utricle of the seminal colliculus in the prostatic urethra.

C. Relocation of the Testes & Ducts

Around weeks 5–6, a bandlike condensation of mesenchymal tissue in the urogenital ridge forms near the caudal end of the mesonephros. Distally, this gubernacular precursor tissue grows into the area of the undifferentiated tissue of the anterior abdominal wall and toward the genital swellings. Proximally, the **gubernaculum** contacts the mesonephric duct when the mesonephros regresses and the gonad begins to form. By the start of the fetal period, the mesonephric duct begins differentiation and the gubernaculum adheres indirectly to the testis via the duct, which lies in the mesorchium of the testis. The external genitalia differentiate over the seventh to about the 19th week. By the 12th week, the testis is near the deep inguinal ring, and the gubernaculum is virtually at the inferior pole of the testis, proximally, and in the mesenchyme of the scrotal swellings, distally.

Although the testis in early development is near the last thoracic segment, it is still close to the area of the developing deep inguinal ring. With rapid growth of the lumbar region and "ascent" of the metanephric kidney, the testis remains relatively immobilized by the gubernaculum, although there is the appearance of a lengthy transabdominal "descent" from an upper abdominal position. The testis descends through the inguinal canal around the 28th week and into the scrotum about the 32nd week. Testicular blood vessels form when the testis is located on the dorsal body wall and retain their origin during the transabdominal and pelvic descent of the testis. The mesonephric duct follows the descent of the testis and hence passes anterior to the ureter, which follows the retroperitoneal ascent of the kidney (Fig. 2–10).

Hutson JM, Balic A, Nation T, Southwell B. Cryptorchidism. *Semin Pediatr Surg* 2010;19:215–224. PMID: 20610195.

Shaw CM, Stanczyk FZ, Egleston BL, et al. Serum antimüllerian hormone in healthy premenopausal women. *Fertil Steril* 2011;95:2718–2721. PMID: 21704216.

Turner ME, Ely D, Prokop J, Milsted A. Sry, more than testis determination? *Am J Physiol Regul Integr Comp Physiol* 2011;301:R561–R571. PMID: 21677270.

Vallerie AM, Breech LL. Update in Müllerian anomalies: diagnosis, management, and outcomes *Curr Opin Obstet Gynecol* 2010;22:381–387. PMID: 20724925.

Female: Uterus & Uterine Tubes

A. Mesonephric Ducts

Virtually all portions of these paired ducts degenerate in the female embryo, with the exception of the most caudal segment between the ureteric bud and the cloaca, which is later incorporated into the posterior wall of the urogenital sinus (Figs. 2–5 and 2–6) as the **trigone of the urinary bladder.** Regression begins just after gonadal sex differentiation and is finished near the onset of the third trimester. Cystlike or tubular vestiges of mesonephric duct (Fig. 2–11) may persist to variable degrees parallel with the vagina and uterus (**Gartner's cysts**). Other mesonephric remnants of the duct or tubules may persist in the broad ligament (**epoophoron**).

B. Paramesonephric Ducts

Differentiation of müllerian ducts in female embryos produces the uterine tubes, uterus, and probably the fibromuscular wall of the vagina. In contrast to the ductal/gonadal relationship in the male, ductal differentiation in the female

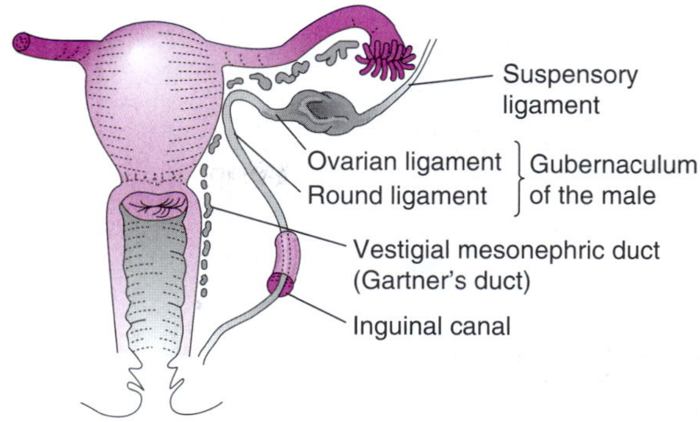

▲ **Figure 2–11.** Female genital tract. Gubernacular derivatives and mesonephric vestiges are shown.

does not require the presence of ovaries. Formation of the bilateral paramesonephric ducts during the second half of the embryonic period has been described [see Indifferent (Sexless) Stage]. By the onset of the fetal period, the 2 ducts are joined caudally in the midline, and the fused segment of the new Y-shaped ductal structure is the **uterovaginal primordium** (Fig. 2–8). The nonfused cranial part of each paramesonephric duct gives rise to the **uterine tubes** (oviducts), and the distal end of this segment remains open and will form the **ostium of the oviduct.**

Early in the ninth week, the uterovaginal primordium contacts medianly the dorsal wall of the urogenital sinus. This places the primordium at a median position between the bilateral openings of the mesonephric ducts, which joined the dorsal wall during the fifth week before subdivision of the urogenital sinus from the cloaca occurred (Figs. 2–8 and 2–9). A ventral protrusion of the dorsal wall of the urogenital sinus forms at the area of contact of the uterovaginal primordium with the wall and between the openings of the mesonephric ducts. In reference to its location, this protrusion is called the **sinusal tubercle** (**sinus tubercle, paramesonephric tubercle, müllerian tubercle**). This tubercle may consist of several types of epithelia derived from the different ducts as well as from the wall of the sinus.

Shortly after the sinusal tubercle forms, midline fusion of the middle and caudal portions of the paramesonephric ducts is complete, and the vertical septum (apposed walls of the fused ducts) within the newly established uterovaginal primordium degenerates, creating a single cavity or canal (Fig. 2–12). The solid tip of this primordium continues to grow caudally, while a mesenchymal thickening gradually surrounds the cervical region of the uterovaginal primordium. The primordium gives rise to the fundus, body, and isthmus of the uterus, specifically the endometrial epithelium and glands of the uterus. The endometrial stroma and smooth muscle of the myometrium are derived from adjacent splanchnic mesenchyme. The epithelium of the cervix forms from the lower aspect of the primordium. Development of the various components of the uterus covers

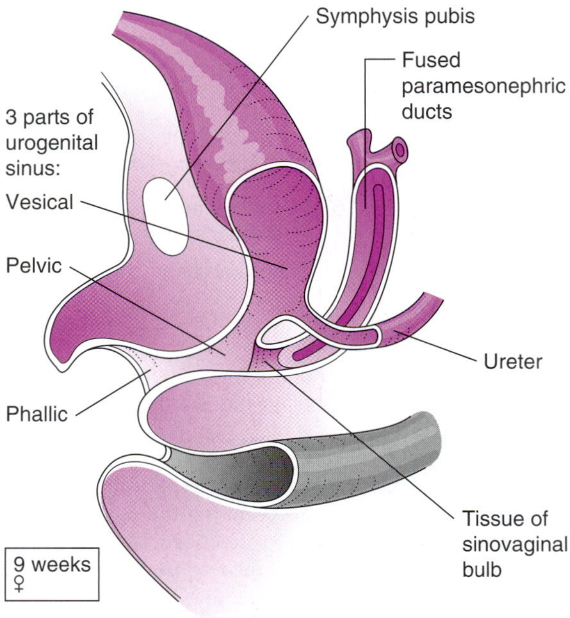

▲ **Figure 2–12.** Sagittal cutaway view of female urogenital sinus and uterovaginal primordium (fused paramesonephric ducts). Sinovaginal bulbs form in the 10th week.

the 3 trimesters of gestation. The basic structure is generated during the latter part of the first trimester. The initial formation of glands and muscular layer occurs near midgestation, whereas mucinous cells in the cervix appear during the third trimester.

The formation of the vagina is discussed in Differentiation of the Urogenital Sinus, even though the question of whether the vaginal epithelium is a sinusal or paramesonephric derivative (or both) has not been resolved. The fibromuscular wall of the vagina is generally considered to be derived from the uterovaginal primordium (Fig. 2–13).

C. Relocation of the Ovaries & Formation of Ligaments

Transabdominal "descent" of the ovary, unlike that of the testis, is restricted to a relatively short distance, presumably (at least partly) because of attachment of the gubernaculum to the paramesonephric duct. Hence, relocation of the ovary appears to involve both (1) a passive rotatory movement of the ovary as its mesentery is drawn by the twist of the developing ductal mesenteries and (2) extensive growth of the lumbosacral region of the fetus. The ovarian vessels (like the testicular vessels) originate or drain near the point of development of the gonad, the arteries from the aorta just inferior to the renal arteries and the veins to the left renal vein or to the vena cava from the right gonad.

Initial positioning of the ovary on the anteromedial aspect of the urogenital ridge is depicted in Figure 2–10, as is the relationship of the paramesonephric duct lateral to the degenerating mesonephros, the ovary, and the urogenital mesentery. The urogenital mesentery between the ridge and the dorsal body wall represents the first mesenteric support for structures developing in the ridge.

Alterations within the urogenital ridge eventually result in formation of contiguous double-layered mesenteries supporting the ovary and segments of the paramesonephric ducts. Enlargement of the ovary and degeneration of the adjacent mesonephric tissue bring previously separated layers of coelomic mesothelium into near apposition, establishing the mesentery of the ovary, the **mesovarium.** Likewise, mesonephric degeneration along the region of differentiation of the unfused cranial segment of the paramesonephric ducts establishes the **mesosalpinx.** Caudally, growth and fusion ventromedially of these bilateral ducts "sweep" the once medially attached mesenteries of the ducts toward the midline. These bilateral mesenteries merge over the fused uterovaginal primordium and extend laterally to the pelvic wall to form a continuous double-layered "drape," the **mesometrium of the broad ligament,** between the upper portion of the primordium and the posterolateral body wall. This central expanse of mesentery creates the rectouterine and vesicouterine pouches. The midline caudal fusion of the ducts also alters the previous longitudinal orientation of the upper free segments of the ducts (the oviducts) to a near transverse orientation. During this alteration, the attached mesovarium is drawn from a medial relationship into a posterior relationship with the paramesonephric mesentery of the mesosalpinx and the mesometrium.

The **suspensory ligament of the ovary,** through which the ovarian vessels, nerves, and lymphatics traverse, forms when cranial degeneration of the mesonephric tissue and regression of the urogenital ridge adjacent to the ovary reduce these tissues to a peritoneal fold.

The **round ligament of the uterus** and the **proper ovarian ligament** are both derivatives of the **gubernaculum,** which originates as a mesenchymal condensation at the caudal end of the mesonephros and extends over the initially short distance to the anterior abdominal wall (see Relocation of the Testes and Ducts). As the gonad enlarges and the mesonephric tissue degenerates, the cranial attachment of the gubernaculum appears to "shift" to the inferior aspect of the ovary. Distally, growth of the fibrous gubernaculum continues into the inguinal region. However, the midportion of the gubernaculum becomes attached, inexplicably, to the paramesonephric duct at the uterotubal junction. Formation of the uterovaginal primordium by caudal fusion of the paramesonephric ducts apparently carries the attached gubernaculum medially within the cover of the encompassing mesentery of the structures (ie, the parts of the developing broad ligament). This fibrous band of connective tissue eventually becomes 2 ligaments.

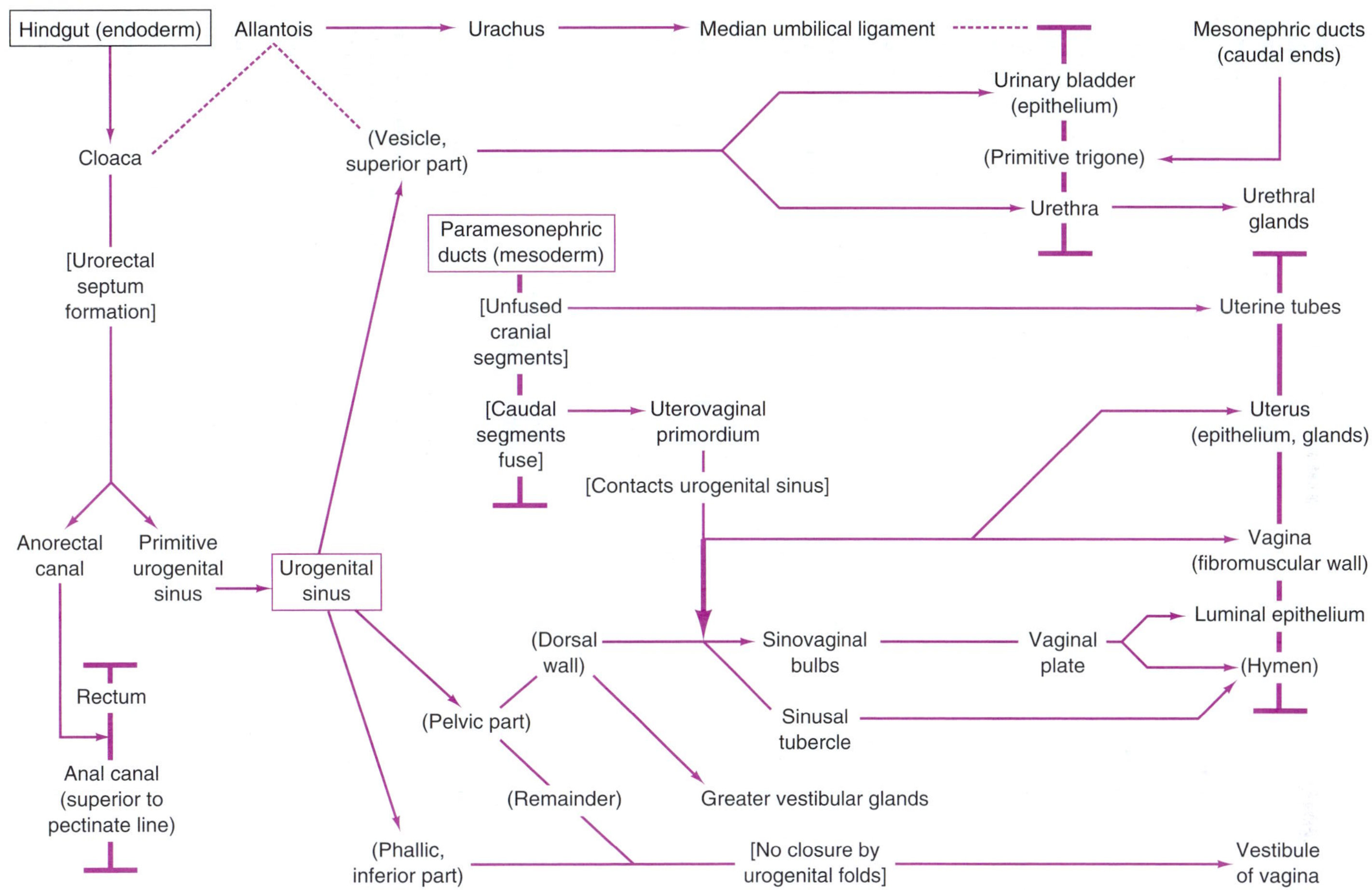

▲ **Figure 2–13.** Schematic drawing of differentiation of urogenital sinus and paramesonephric ducts in the female; formation of urinary bladder, urethra, uterine tubes, uterus, and vagina. (Explanatory symbols are given in Fig. 2–1.)

Cranially, the band is the proper ligament of the ovary, extending between the inferior pole of the ovary and the lateral wall of the uterus just inferior to the oviduct. Caudally, it continues as the uterine round ligament from a point just inferior to the proper ovarian ligament and extending through the inguinal canal to the labium majus.

D. Anomalies of the Uterine Tubes (Oviducts, Fallopian Tubes)

The uterine tubes are derivatives of the cranial segments of the paramesonephric (müllerian) ducts, which differentiate in the urogenital ridge between the sixth and ninth weeks (Fig. 2–10). Ductal formation begins with invagination of the coelomic epithelium in the lateral coelomic bay. The initial depression remains open to proliferate and differentiate into the ostium (Fig. 2–10). Variable degrees of **duplication of the ostium** sometimes occur; in such cases, the leading edges of the initial ductal groove presumably did not fuse completely or anomalous proliferation of epithelium around the opening occurred.

Absence of a uterine tube is very rare when otherwise normal ductal and genital derivatives are present. This anomaly has been associated with (1) ipsilateral absence of an ovary and (2) ipsilateral unicornuate uterus (and probable anomalous broad ligament). Bilateral absence of the uterine tubes is most frequently associated with lack of formation of the uterus and anomalies of the external genitalia. Interestingly, absence of the derivatives of the lower part of the müllerian ducts with persistence of the uterine tubes occurs more frequently than the reverse condition. This might be expected, as the müllerian ducts form in a craniocaudal direction.

Partial absence of a uterine tube (middle or caudal segment) also has been reported. The cause of partial absence is unknown, although several theories have been advanced. One theory holds that when the unilateral anomaly coincides with ipsilateral ovarian absence, a "vascular accident" might occur following differentiation of the ducts and ovaries. Obviously, various factors resulting in somewhat localized atresia could be proposed. From a different perspective, bilateral absence of the uterine tubes as an associated disorder in a female external phenotype is characteristic of **testicular feminization syndrome or androgen insensitivity syndrome** (nonpersistence of the rest of the paramesonephric ducts, anomalous external genitalia, hypoplastic male genital ducts, and testicular differentiation with usual ectopic location).

E. Anomalies of the Uterus

The epithelium of the uterus and cervix and the fibromuscular wall of the vagina are derived from the paramesonephric (müllerian) ducts, the caudal ends of which fuse medially to form the uterovaginal primordium. Most of the primordium gives rise to the uterus (Fig. 2–13). Subsequently, the caudal tip of the primordium contacts the pelvic part of the urogenital sinus, and the interaction of the sinus (sinovaginal bulbs) and primordium leads to differentiation of the vagina. Various steps in this sequential process can go awry, such as (1) complete or partial failure of one or both ducts to form (agenesis), (2) lack of or incomplete fusion of the caudal segments of the paired ducts (abnormal uterovaginal primordium), or (3) failure of development *after* successful formation (aplasia or hypoplasia). Many types of anomalies may occur because of the number of sites for potential error, the complex interactions necessary for the development of the müllerian derivatives, and the duration of the complete process.

Complete **agenesis of the uterus** is very rare, and associated vaginal anomalies are usually expected. Also, a high incidence of associated structural or positional abnormalities of the kidney has been reported; there has been speculation that the initial error in severe cases may be in the development of the urinary system and then in the formation of the paramesonephric ducts.

Aplasia of the paramesonephric ducts (**müllerian aplasia**) is more common than agenesis and could occur after formation and interaction of the primordium with the urogenital sinus. A rudimentary uterus or a vestigial uterus (ie, varying degrees of fibromuscular tissue present) is most frequently accompanied by partial or complete absence of the vagina. As in uterine agenesis, ectopic kidney or absence of a kidney is frequently associated with uterine aplasia (in about 40% of cases). **Uterine hypoplasia** variably yields a rudimentary or infantile uterus and is associated with normal or abnormal uterine tubes and ovaries. Unilateral agenesis or aplasia of the ducts gives rise to **uterus unicornis,** whereas unilateral hypoplasia may result in a rudimentary horn that may or may not be contiguous with the lumen of the "normal" horn (**uterus bicornis unicollis** with one unconnected rudimentary horn; Fig. 2–14). The status of the rudimentary horn must be considered for potential hematometra, or blood in the uterus that cannot exit, at puberty.

Anomalous **unification** caudally of the paramesonephric ducts results in many uterine malformations (Fig. 2–14). The incidence of defective fusion is estimated to be 0.1–3% of females. Furthermore, faulty unification of the ducts has been cited as the primary error responsible for most anomalies of the female genital tract. Partial or complete retention of the apposed walls of the paired ducts can produce slight (**uterus subseptus unicollis**) to complete (**uterus bicornis septus**) septal defects in the uterus. Complete failure of unification of the paramesonephric ducts can result in a double uterus (**uterus didelphys**) with either a single or double vagina.

F. Anomalies of the Cervix

Because the cervix forms as an integral part of the uterus, cervical anomalies are often the same as uterine anomalies. Thus, absence or hypoplasia of the cervix is rarely found

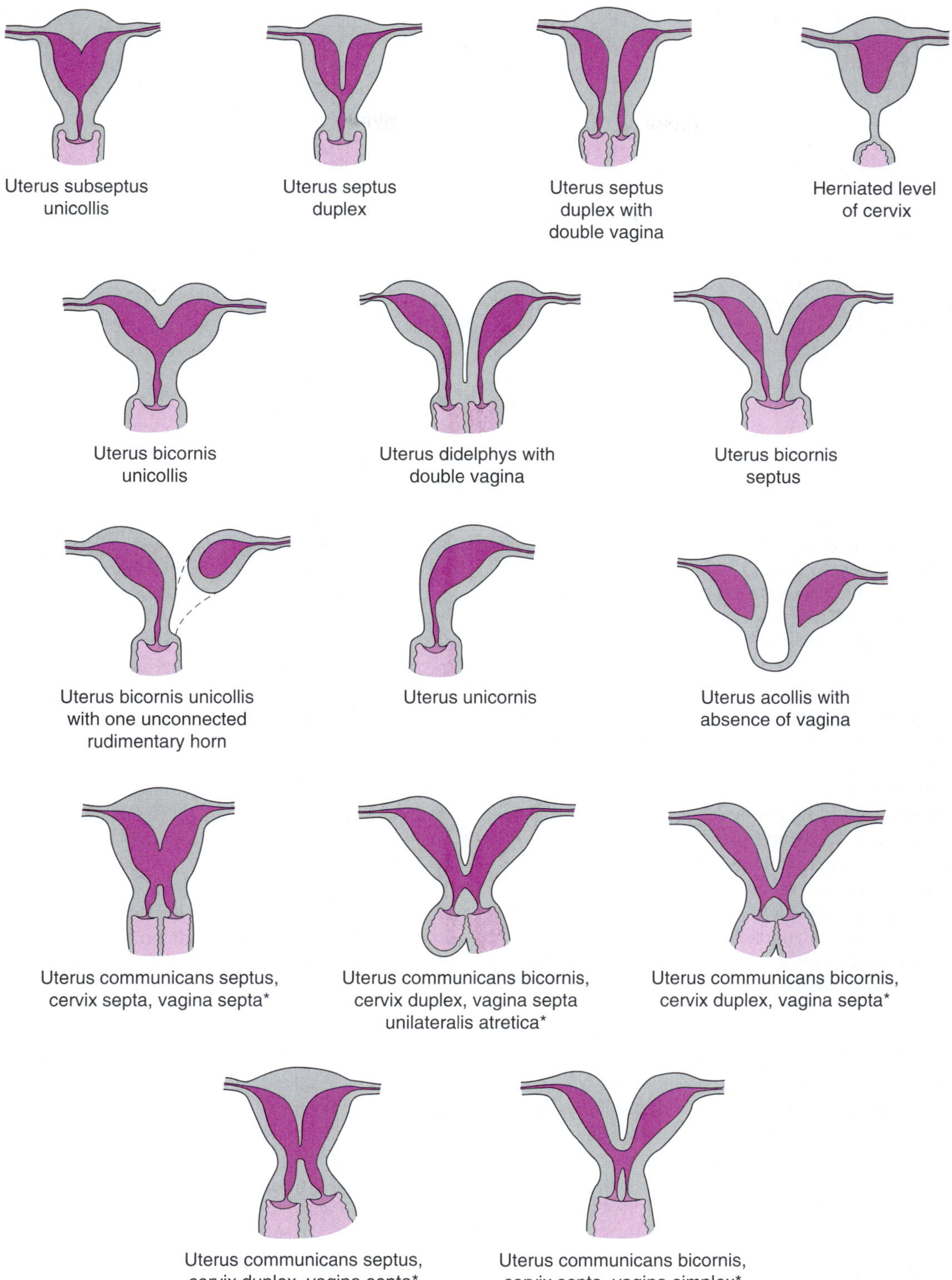

▲ **Figure 2–14.** Uterine anomalies. (*Redrawn and reproduced, with permission, from Toaff R. A major genital malformation: communicating uteri. *Obstet Gynecol* 1974;43:221.)

with a normal uterovaginal tract. The cervix appears as a fibrous juncture between the uterine corpus and the vagina.

Corbetta S, Muzza M, Avagliano L, et al. Gonadal structures in a fetus with complete androgen insensitivity syndrome and persistent Müllerian derivatives: comparison with normal fetal development. *Fertil Steril* 2011;95:1119.e9–e14. PMID: 20971460.

Dighe M, Moshiri M, Phillips G, Biyyam D, Dubinsky T. Fetal genitourinary anomalies—a pictorial review with postnatal correlation. *Ultrasound Q* 2011;27:7–21. PMID: 21343799.

Routh JC, Laufer MR, Cannon GM Jr, Diamond DA, Gargollo PC. Management strategies for Mayer-Rokitansky-Kuster-Hauser related vaginal agenesis: a cost-effectiveness analysis. *J Urol* 2010;184:2116–2121. PMID: 20850825.

DIFFERENTIATION OF THE UROGENITAL SINUS

Until differentiation of the genital ducts begins, the urogenital sinus appears similar in both sexes during the middle and late embryonic period. For purposes of describing the origin of sinusal derivatives, the sinus can be divided into 3 parts: (1) the **vesical part,** or the large dilated segment superior to the entrance of the mesonephric ducts; (2) the **pelvic part,** or the narrowed tubular segment between the level of the mesonephric ducts and the inferior segment; and (3) the **phallic part,** often referred to as the definitive urogenital sinus (the anteroposteriorly elongated, transversely flattened inferiormost segment) (Fig. 2–8). The **urogenital membrane** temporarily closes the inferior limit of the phallic part. The superior limit of the vesical part becomes delimited by conversion of the once tubular allantois to a thick fibrous cord, the **urachus,** by about 12 weeks. After differentiation of the vesical part of the sinus to form the epithelium of the **urinary bladder,** the urachus maintains its continuity between the apex of the bladder and the umbilical cord and is identified postnatally as the **median umbilical ligament.** Various anomalies of urachal formation can present as **urachal fistula, cyst,** or **sinus,** depending on the degree of patency that persists during obliteration of the allantois.

In both sexes, the caudal segments of each mesonephric duct between the urogenital sinus and the level of the ureter of the differentiating metanephric diverticulum (or ureteric bud) become incorporated into the posterocaudal wall of the vesical part (ie, urinary bladder) of the sinus (Figs. 2–5 and 2–6). As the dorsal wall of the bladder grows and "absorbs" these caudal segments, the ureters are gradually "drawn" closer to the bladder and eventually open directly and separately into it, dorsolateral to the mesonephric ducts (Figs. 2–6 and 2–7). The mesodermal segment of mesonephric duct incorporated into the bladder defines the epithelium of the **trigone of the bladder,** although this mesodermal epithelium is secondarily replaced by the endodermal epithelium of the sinusal bladder. After formation of the trigone, the remainder of each mesonephric duct (ie, the portion that was cranial to the metanephric diverticulum) is joined to the superior end of the pelvic part of the urogenital sinus. Thereafter, the ducts either degenerate (in females) or undergo differentiation (in males).

Male: Urinary Bladder, Urethra, & Penis (Fig. 2–15)

The urogenital sinus gives rise to the endodermal epithelium of the **urinary bladder,** the prostatic and membranous urethra, and most of the spongy (penile) urethra (except the glandular urethra). Outgrowths from its derivatives produce epithelial parts of the prostate and bulbourethral glands (Fig. 2–15). The **prostatic urethra** receives the ejaculatory ducts (derived from the mesonephric ducts) and arises from 2 parts of the urogenital sinus. The portion of this urethral segment superior to the ejaculatory ducts originates from the inferiormost area of the vesical part of the sinus. The lower portion of the prostatic urethra is derived from the pelvic part of the sinus near the entrance of the ducts and including the region of the sinusal tubercle—the latter apparently forming the seminal colliculus. Early in the 12th week, endodermal outgrowths of the prostatic urethra form the prostatic anlage, the **prostatic buds,** from which the glandular epithelium of the **prostate** will arise. Differentiation of splanchnic mesoderm contributes other components to the gland (smooth muscle and connective tissue), as is the case for mesodermal parts of the urinary bladder. The pelvic part of the sinus also gives rise to the epithelium of the **membranous urethra,** which later yields endodermal buds for the **bulbourethral glands.** The phallic, or inferior, part of the urogenital sinus proliferates anteriorly as the external genitalia form (during weeks 9–12) and results in incorporation of this phallic part as the endodermal epithelium of the **spongy (penile) urethra** (the distal glandular urethra is derived from ectoderm).

Early masculinization of the undifferentiated or indifferent genitalia takes place during the first 3 weeks of the fetal period (weeks 9–12) and is caused by androgenic stimulation. The phallus and urogenital folds gradually elongate to initiate development of the **penis.** The subjacent endodermal lining of the inferior part (phallic) of the urogenital sinus extends anteriorly along with the urogenital folds, creating an endodermal plate, the **urethral plate.** The plate deepens into a groove, the **urethral groove,** as the urogenital folds (now called **urethral folds**) thicken on each side of the plate. The urethral groove extends into the ventral aspect of the developing penis, and the bilateral urethral folds slowly fuse in a posterior to anterior direction over the urethral groove to form the **spongy (penile) urethra,** thereby closing the urogenital orifice (Fig. 2–15; see also Fig. 2–20). The line of fusion becomes the **penile raphe** on the ventral surface of the penis.

As closure of the urethral folds approaches the glans, the external urethral opening on this surface is eliminated.

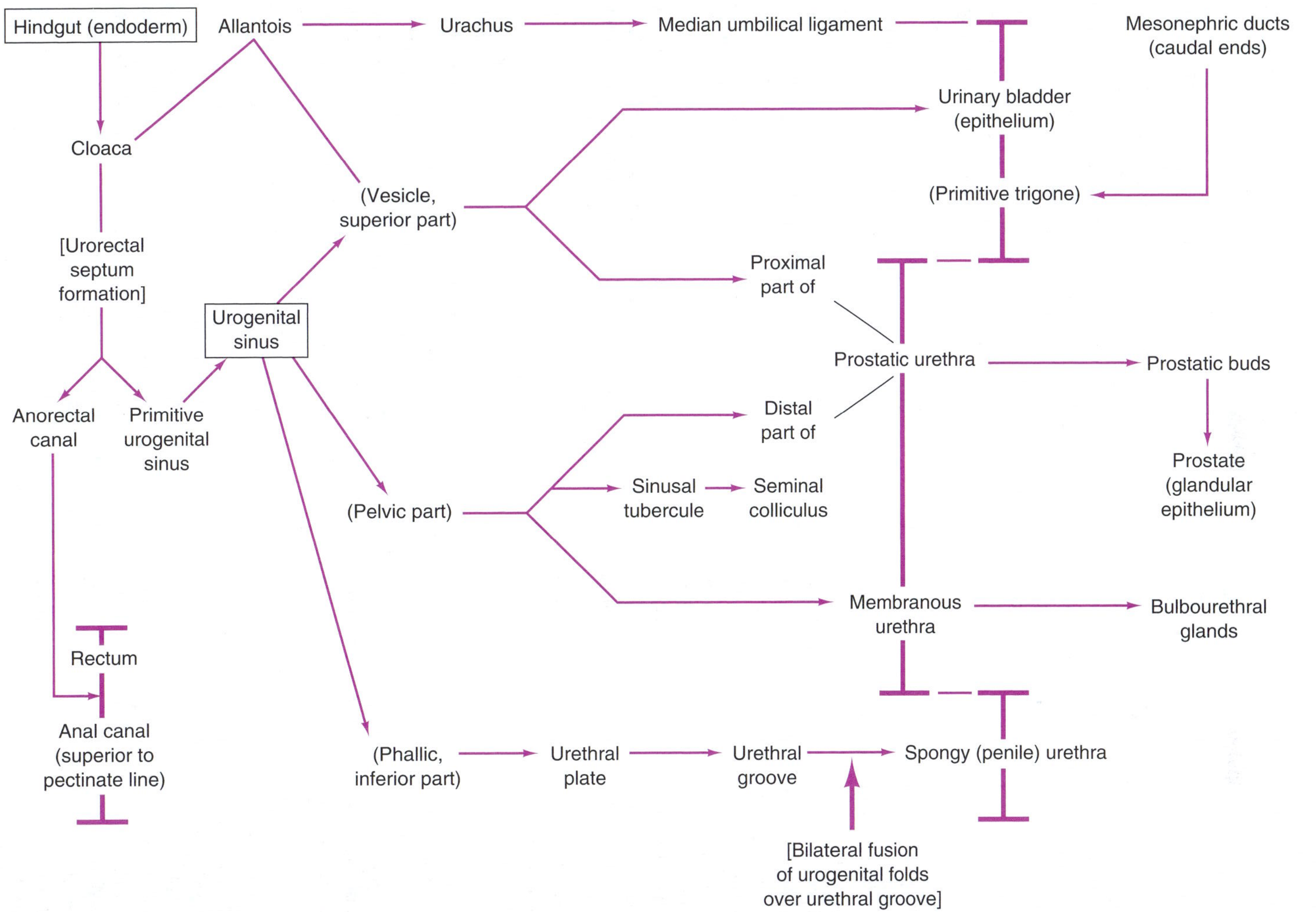

▲ **Figure 2–15.** Schematic drawing of male differentiation of the urogenital sinus; formation of urinary bladder and urethra. (Explanatory symbols are given in Fig. 2–1.)

Concurrently, an **ectodermal glandular plate** invaginates the tip of the penis. Canalization of the plate forms the distal end of the penile urethra, the **glandular urethra.** Thus, the external urethral meatus becomes located at the tip of the glans when closure of the urethral folds is completed (see Fig. 2–20). The **prepuce** is formed slightly later by a circular invagination of ectoderm at the tip of the **glans penis.** This cylindric ectodermal plate then cleaves to leave a double-layered fold of skin extending over the glans.

While the cloacal folds and phallic urogenital sinus were differentiating into the penis and the urethra, the **genital (labioscrotal)** swellings of the undifferentiated stage were enlarging lateral to the cloacal folds. Medial growth and fusion of the scrotal swellings to form the **scrotum** and **scrotal raphe** around the 12th week virtually complete the differentiation of the male external genitalia (see Figs. 2–20 and 2–22).

Female: Urinary Bladder, Urethra, & Vagina

A. Development

Differentiation of the female sinus is schematically presented in Figure 2–13 and illustrated in Figures 2–8, 2–12, 2–16, and 2–17. In contrast to sinusal differentiation in the male, the vesical part of the female urogenital sinus forms the epithelium of the **urinary bladder** and entire **urethra.** Derivatives of the pelvic part of the sinus include the epithelium of the **vagina,** the **greater vestibular glands,** and the **hymen.** Controversy exists about how the vagina is formed, mainly because of a lack of consensus about the origin and degree of inclusion of its precursory tissues (mesodermal paramesonephric duct, endodermal urogenital sinus, or even mesonephric duct). The most common theory is that 2 endodermal outgrowths, the **sinovaginal bulbs,** of the dorsal wall of the pelvic part of the urogenital sinus form bilateral to and join with the caudal tip of the uterovaginal primordium (fused paramesonephric ducts) in the area of the sinusal tubercle (Fig. 2–12). This cellular mass at the end of the primordium occludes the inferior aspect of the canal, creating an endodermal **vaginal plate** within the mesodermal wall of the uterovaginal primordium. Eventually, the vaginal segment grows, approaching the vestibule of the vagina. The process of growth has been described either as "downgrowth" of the vaginal segment away from the uterine canal and along the urogenital sinus or, more commonly, as "upgrowth" of the segment away from the sinus and toward the uterovaginal canal. In either case, the vaginal segment is extended between the paramesonephric-derived cervix and the sinus-derived vestibule (Figs. 2–12, 2–16, and 2–17). Near the fifth month, the breakdown of cells centrally in the vaginal plate creates the vaginal lumen, which is delimited peripherally by the remaining cells of the plate as the epithelial lining of the vagina. The solid vaginal fornices become hollow soon after canalization of the vaginal lumen is complete. The upper one-third to four-fifths of the vaginal epithelium has been proposed to arise from the uterovaginal primordium, whereas the lower two-thirds to one-fifth has been proposed as a contribution from the sinovaginal bulbs.

The fibromuscular wall of the vagina is derived from the uterovaginal primordium. The cavities of the vagina

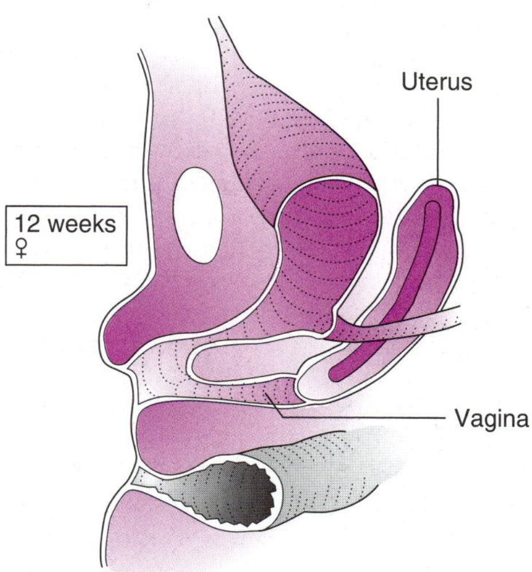

▲ **Figure 2–16.** Sagittal cutaway view of developing vagina and urethra.

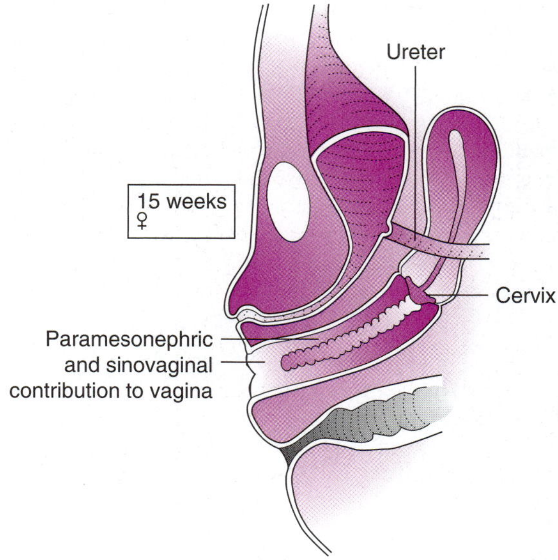

▲ **Figure 2–17.** Sagittal cutaway view of differentiated urogenital sinus and precanalization stage of vaginal development. The drawing depicts one of several theories about the relative contributions of paramesonephric ducts and sinovaginal bulbs to the vagina.

and urogenital sinus are temporarily separated by the thin **hymen,** which probably is a mixture of tissue derived from the vaginal plate and the remains of the sinusal tubercle. With concurrent differentiation of female external genitalia, inferior closure of the sinus does not occur during the 12th week of development, as it does in the male. Instead, the remainder of the pelvic part and all of the inferior phallic part of the urogenital sinus expand to form the **vestibule of the vagina.** Presumably, the junctional zone of pigmentation on the labia minora represents the distinction between endodermal derivation from the urogenital sinus (medially) and ectodermal skin (laterally).

B. Anomalies of the Vagina

The vagina is derived from interaction between the uterovaginal primordium and the pelvic part of the urogenital sinus (Fig. 2–13; see Development). The causes of vaginal anomalies are difficult to assess because integration of the uterovaginal primordium and the urogenital sinus in the *normal* differentiation of the vagina remains a controversial subject. Furthermore, an accurate breakdown of causes of certain anomalous vaginal presentations, as with many anomalies of the external genitalia, would have to include potential moderating factors of endocrine and genetic origin as well.

The incidence of absence of the vagina due to suspected **vaginal agenesis** is about 0.025%. Agenesis may be due to failure of the uterovaginal primordium to contact the urogenital sinus. The uterus is usually absent (Fig. 2–18). Ovarian agenesis is not usually associated with vaginal agenesis. The presence of greater vestibular glands has been reported with presumed vaginal agenesis; their presence emphasizes the complexity of differentiation of the urogenital sinus.

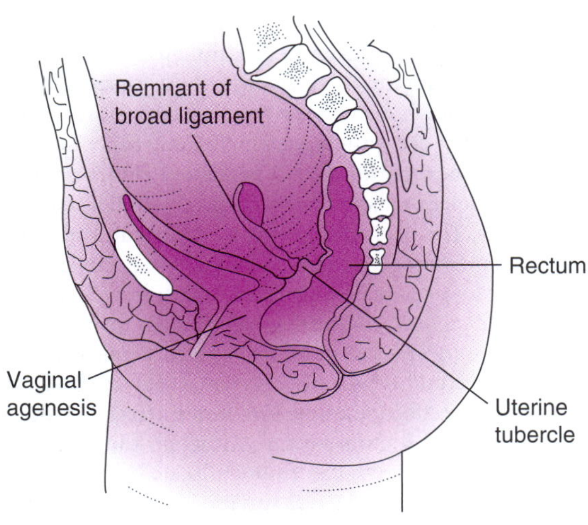

▲ **Figure 2–18.** Midsagittal view of vaginal agenesis and uterine agenesis with normal ovaries and oviducts.

Vaginal atresia, on the other hand, is considered when the lower portion of the vagina consists merely of fibrous tissue while the contiguous superior structures (the uterus, in particular) are well differentiated (perhaps because the primary defect is in the sinusal contribution to the vagina). In **müllerian aplasia** almost all of the vagina and most of the uterus are absent (Rokitansky-Küster-Hauser syndrome, with a rudimentary uterus of bilateral, solid muscular tissue, was considered virtually the same as this aplasia). Most women with absence of the vagina (and normal external genitalia) are considered to have müllerian aplasia rather than vaginal atresia.

Other somatic anomalies are sometimes associated with müllerian aplasia, suggesting multiple malformation syndrome. Associated vertebral anomalies are much more prevalent than middle ear anomalies, eg, müllerian aplasia associated with **Klippel-Feil syndrome** (fused cervical vertebrae) is more common than müllerian aplasia associated with Klippel-Feil syndrome plus middle ear anomalies ("conductive deafness"). **Winter's syndrome,** which is thought to be autosomal recessive, is evidenced by middle ear anomalies (somewhat similar to those in the triad above), renal agenesis or hypoplasia, and vaginal atresia (rather than aplasia of the paramesonephric ducts). **Dysgenesis** (partial absence) of the vagina and **hypoplasia** (reduced caliber of the lumen) have also been described.

Transverse vaginal septa (Fig. 2–19) are probably not the result of vaginal atresia but rather of incomplete canalization of the vaginal plate or discrete fusion of sinusal and primordial (ductal) derivatives. Alternative explanations are likely because the histologic composition of septa is not consistent. A rare genetic linkage has been demonstrated. A single septum or multiple septa can be present, and the location may vary in upper or lower segments of the lumen. **Longitudinal vaginal septa** can also occur. A variety of explanations have been advanced, including true duplication of vaginal primordial tissue, anomalous differentiation of the uterovaginal primordium, abnormal variation of the caudal fusion of the müllerian ducts, persistence of vaginal plate epithelium, and anomalous mesodermal proliferation. Septa may be imperforate or perforated. A transverse septum creates the potential for various occlusive manifestations (eg, hydrometrocolpos, hematometra, or hematocolpos), depending on the composition and location of the trapped fluid.

Abnormalities of the vagina are often associated with anomalies of the urinary system and the rectum because differentiation of the urogenital sinus is involved in formation of the bladder and urethra as well as the vagina and vestibule. Furthermore, if partitioning of the cloaca into the sinus and anorectal canal is faulty, then associated rectal defects can occur. Compound anomalies may affect the urinary tract or rectum. The urethra may open into the vaginal wall; even a single vesicovaginal cavity has been described. On the other hand, the vagina can open into a persistent urogenital sinus, as in

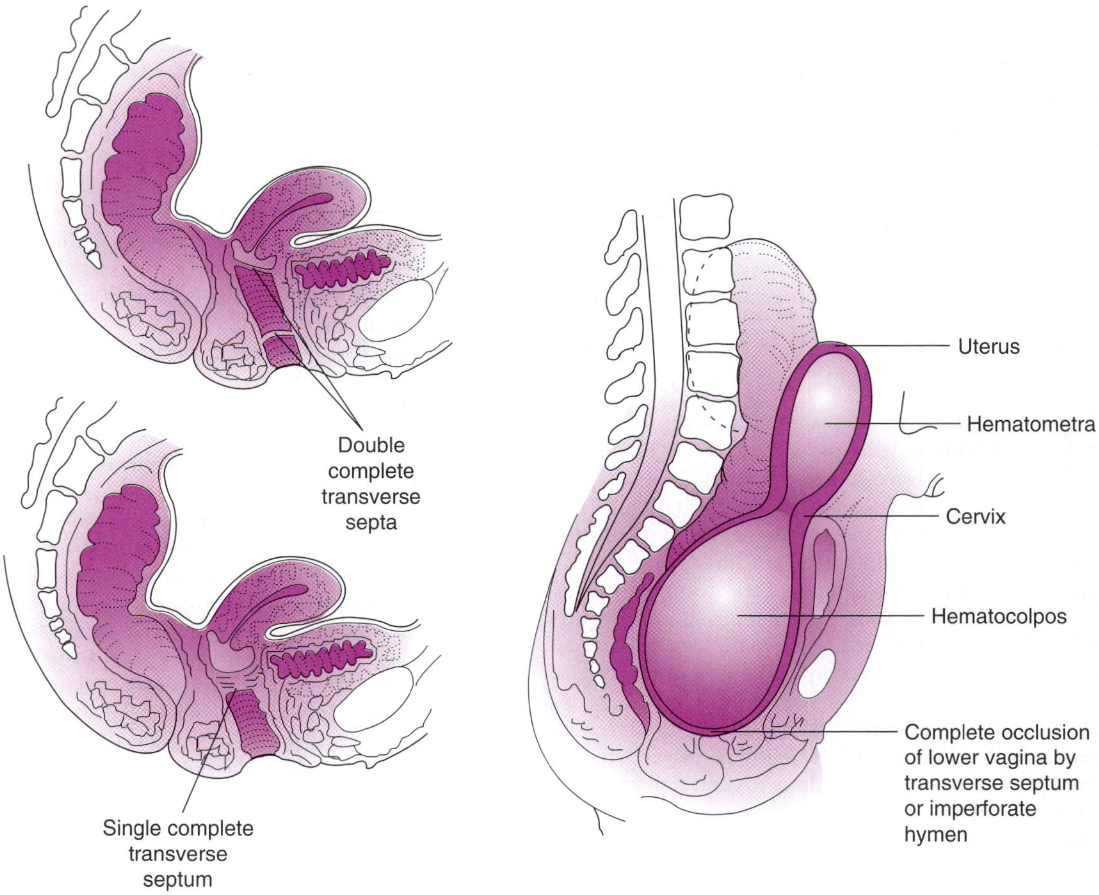

▲ **Figure 2–19.** Transverse vaginal septa.

certain forms of female pseudohermaphroditism. Associated rectal abnormalities include vaginorectal fistula, vulvovaginal anus, rectosigmoidal fistula, and vaginosigmoidal cloaca in the absence of the rectum (see Cloacal Dysgenesis).

C. Anomalies of the Hymen

The hymen is probably a mixture of tissue derived from remains of the sinusal tubercle and the vaginal plate. Usually, the hymen is patent, or perforate, by puberty, although an **imperforate hymen** is not rare. The imperforate condition can be the result of a congenital error of lack of central degeneration or the result of inflammatory occlusion after perforation. Obstruction of menstrual flow at puberty may be the first sign (Fig. 2–19).

D. Cloacal Dysgenesis (Including Persistence of the Urogenital Sinus)

Anomalous partitioning of the cloaca by abnormal development of the urorectal septum is rare, at least based on reported cases in the literature. As anticipated from a developmental standpoint, the incidence of associated genitourinary anomalies is high. Five types of cloacal or anorectal malformations are summarized in Table 2–3.

Rectocloacal fistula with a persistent cloaca provides a common canal or outlet for the urinary, genital, and intestinal tracts. The distinction between a canal and an outlet is one of depth (deep versus very shallow, respectively) of the persistent lower portion of the cloaca and, thus, the length of the individual urethral and vaginal canals emptying into the cloaca. The inverse relationship between depth (or length) of the cloaca and length of the vaginal and urethral canals is probably a reflection of the time when arrest of formation of the urorectal septum occurs. Although the bladder, the vagina, and the rectum can empty into a common cloaca as just described, other unusual variations of persistent cloaca can also occur.

For example, the vagina and rectum develop, but the urinary bladder does not develop as a separate entity from the cloaca. Instead, the vagina and rectum open separately into

Table 2–3. Cloacal malformations.

	Rectocloacal Fistula
Vestibule	Deformed; flanked by labia; clitoris in front, fourchette behind; anterior vestibule short, shallow, and moist; single external orifice in posterior half of vestibule (common conduit for urine, cervical mucus, and feces).
Bladder/urethra	Anterior; directed cranially and ventrally.
Vagina	Opens into the vault of cloaca.
Anus/rectum	Enters at highest and most posterior point; orifice is in midline and stenotic.
Disposition	Lengths of urethra and vagina are inversely proportionate to length of cloacal canal.
	Rectovaginal Fistula
Vestibule	Normal anatomy (2 orifices: urethral and vaginal).
Bladder/urethra	Normal.
Vagina	May be septate or normal.
Anus/rectum	Internal in the midposterior vaginal wall.
Disposition	Anus absent from perineum.
	Rectovestibular Fistula
Vestibule	Contains rectum, otherwise normal.
Urethra	Normal.
Vagina	Normal.
Anus/rectum	Small, sited at the fossa navicularis.
Disposition	Rectum is parallel with both vagina and urethra.
	Covered Anus
Vestibule	Normal.
Urethra	Normal.
Vagina	(Probably normal.)
Anus	At any point between the normal site and the fourchette; anocutaneous; anovulvar.
Disposition	Genital folds are abnormally fused anterior and posterior to common orifice and give rise to hypertrophied perineal raphe.
	Ectopic Anus
Vestibule	Normal.
Urethra	Normal.
Vagina	Normal.
Anus	Anterior to the normal site; normal function.
Disposition	Fault lies in the development of the perineum.

Modified and reproduced, with permission, from Okonkwo JEN, Crocker KM. Cloacal dysgenesis. *Obstet Gynecol* 1977;50:97–101.

a "urinary bladder," which has ureters entering posterolaterally to the vagina (vaginal orifice is in the "anatomic trigone" of the bladderlike structure). The external orifice from the base of this cloacal "bladder" is a single narrow canal. One explanation for this variant might be that arrest of formation of the urorectal septum occurs much earlier than does the separate development of distal portions of the 3 tracts (urethra, vagina, and anorectum) to a more advanced (but still incomplete) stage before urorectal septal formation ceases. The anomaly is probably rare.

With a **rectovaginal fistula,** the vestibule may appear anatomically normal, but the anus does not appear in the perineum. The defect probably results from anorectal agenesis due to incomplete subdivision of the cloaca (similar agenesis in the male could result in a rectourethral fistula). The development of the anterior aspect of the vagina completes the separation of the urethra from the vagina, so there is not a persistent urogenital sinus. **Anorectal agenesis** is reputedly the most common type of anorectal malformation, and usually a fistula occurs. Rectovaginal, anovestibular (or rectovestibular; Table 2–3), and anoperineal fistulas account for most anorectal malformations.

In the absence of the anorectal defect (normal anal presentation) but presence of a **persistent urogenital sinus** with a single external orifice, various irregularities of the urethra and genitalia can appear. The relative positions of urethral and vaginal orifices in the sinus can even change as the child grows. In the discussion of anomalies of the labia majora, there may be a persistent urogenital sinus in female pseudohermaphroditism due to congenital adrenal hyperplasia. The vagina opens into the persisting pelvic part of the sinus, which extends with the phallic part of the sinus to the external surface at the urogenital opening. The sinus can be deep and narrow in the neonate, approximating the size of a urethra, or it can be relatively shallow.

Urinary tract disorders associated with persistent urogenital sinus include duplication of the ureters, unilateral ureteral and renal agenesis or atresia, and lack of or abnormal ascent of the kidneys. Variations in the anomalies of derivatives of the urogenital sinus appear to be related in part to the time of arrest of normal differentiation and development of the urogenital sinus, as well as to the impact of other factors associated with abnormal sexual differentiation, such as the variable degrees of response to adrenal androgen in congenital adrenal hyperplasia.

THE EXTERNAL GENITALIA

Undifferentiated Stage

The external genitalia begin to form early in the embryonic period, shortly after development of the cloaca. The progenitory tissues of the genitalia are common to both sexes, and the early stage of development is virtually the same in females and males. Although differentiation of the genitalia can begin around the onset of the fetal period if testicular differentiation is initiated, definitive genital sex is usually not clearly apparent until the 12th week. Formation of external genitalia in the male involves the influence of androgen on the interaction of subepidermal mesoderm with the inferior parts of the endodermal urogenital sinus. In the female, this androgenic influence is absent.

The external genitalia form within the initially compact area bounded by the umbilical cord (anteriorly), the developing limb buds (laterally), the embryonic tail (posteriorly), and the cloacal membrane (centrally). Two of the primordia for the genitalia first appear bilaterally adjacent to the cloacal membrane (a medial pair of cloacal folds and a lateral pair of genital [labioscrotal] swellings). The **cloacal folds** are longitudinal proliferations of caudal mesenchyme located between the ectodermal epidermis and the underlying endoderm of the phallic part of the urogenital sinus. Proliferation and bilateral anterior fusion of these folds create the **genital tubercle,** which protrudes near the anterior edge of the cloacal membrane by the sixth week (Figs. 2–20 to 2–22). Extension of the tubercle forms the phallus, which at this stage is the same size in both sexes.

By the seventh week, the urorectal septum subdivides the bilayered (ectoderm and endoderm) cloacal membrane into the **urogenital membrane** (anteriorly) and the **anal membrane** (posteriorly). The area of fusion of the urorectal septum and the cloacal membrane becomes the **primitive perineum,** or **perineal body.** With formation of the perineum, the cloacal folds are divided transversely as **urogenital folds** adjacent to the urogenital membrane and **anal folds** around the anal membrane. As the mesoderm within the urogenital folds thickens and elongates between the perineum and the phallus, the urogenital membrane sinks deeper into the fissure between the folds. Within a week, this membrane ruptures, forming the **urogenital orifice** and, thus, opening the urogenital sinus to the exterior. Similar thickening of the anal folds creates a deep anal pit, in which the anal membrane breaks down to establish the **anal orifice** of the anal canal (Figs. 2–20 and 2–21).

Subsequent masculinization or feminization of the external genitalia is a consequence of the respective presence or absence of androgen and the androgenic sensitivity or insensitivity of the tissues. The significance of both of these factors (availability of hormone and sensitivity of target tissue) is exemplified by the rare condition (about 1 in 50,000 "females") of **testicular feminization,** wherein testes are present (usually ectopic) and produce testosterone and antimüllerian hormone. The antimüllerian hormone suppresses formation of the uterus and uterine tubes (from the paramesonephric ducts), whereas testosterone supports male differentiation of the mesonephric ducts to form the epididymis and ductus deferens. The anomalous feminization of the external genitalia is considered to be due to androgenic insensitivity of the precursor tissues consequent to an abnormal androgen receptor or postreceptor mechanism set by genetic inheritance.

Female

A. Development of External Genitalia

Feminization of the external genitalia proceeds in the absence of androgenic stimulation (or nonresponsiveness of the tissue). The 2 primary distinctions in the general process of feminization versus masculinization are (1) the lack of continued growth of the phallus and (2) the near absence of fusion of the urogenital folds and the labioscrotal swellings. Female derivatives of the indifferent sexual primordia for the external genitalia are virtually homologous counterparts of the male derivatives. Formation of the female genitalia is schematically presented in Figure 2–21.

The growth of the phallus slows relative to that of the urogenital folds and labioscrotal swellings and becomes the diminutive **clitoris.** The anterior extreme of the urogenital folds fuses superior and inferior to the clitoris, forming the **prepuce** and **frenulum of the clitoris,** respectively. The midportions of these folds do not fuse but give rise to the **labia minora.** Lack of closure of the folds leaves the urogenital orifice patent and results in formation of the **vestibule of the vagina** from the inferior portion of the pelvic part and the phallic part of the urogenital sinus at about the fifth month (Fig. 2–21). Derivatives of the vesical part of the sinus (the **urethra**) and the superior portion of the pelvic part of the sinus (**vagina** and **greater vestibular glands**) then open separately into the vestibule. The **frenulum of the labia minora** is formed by fusion of the posterior ends of the urogenital folds. The mesoderm of the labioscrotal swellings proliferates beneath the ectoderm and remains virtually unfused to create the **labia majora** lateral to the labia minora. The swellings blend together anteriorly to form the **anterior labial commissure** and the tissue of the **mons pubis,** while the swellings posteriorly less clearly define a **posterior labial commissure.** The distal fibers of the round ligament of the uterus project into the tissue of the labia majora.

B. Anomalies of the Labia Minora

In otherwise normal females, 2 somewhat common anomalies occur—labial fusion and labial hypertrophy. True labial fusion as an early developmental defect in the normally unfused midportions of the urogenital folds is purportedly less frequent than "fusion" due to inflammatory-type reactions. **Labial hypertrophy** can be unilateral or bilateral and may require surgical correction in extreme cases.

C. Anomalies of the Labia Majora

The labia majora are derived from the bilateral genital (labioscrotal) swellings, which appear early in the embryonic period and remain unfused centrally during subsequent sex differentiation in the fetal period. Anomalous conditions include **hypoplastic** and **hypertrophic labia** as well as different gradations of fusion of the labia majora.

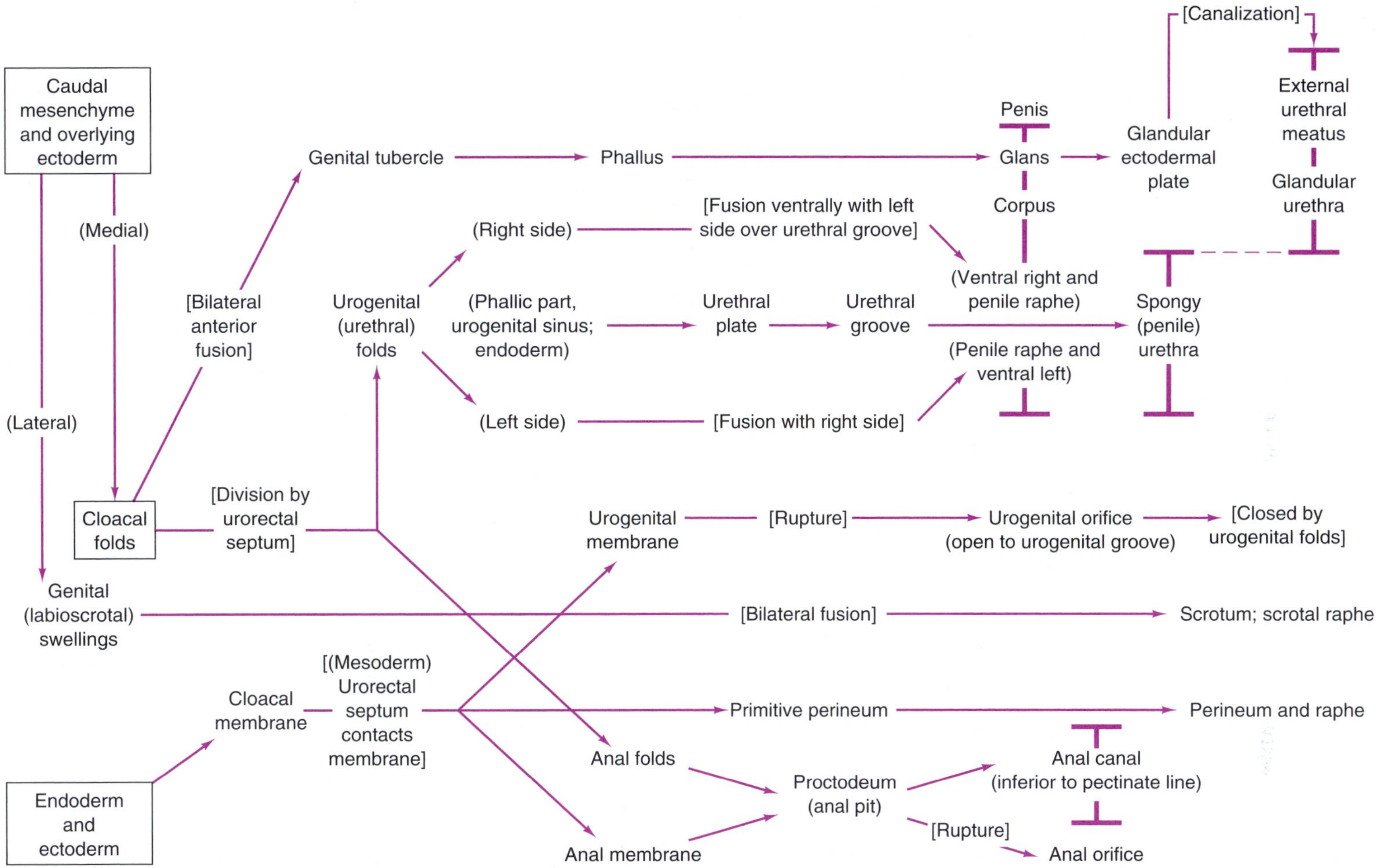

▲ **Figure 2–20.** Schematic drawing of formation of male external genitalia. (Explanatory symbols are given in Fig. 2–1.)

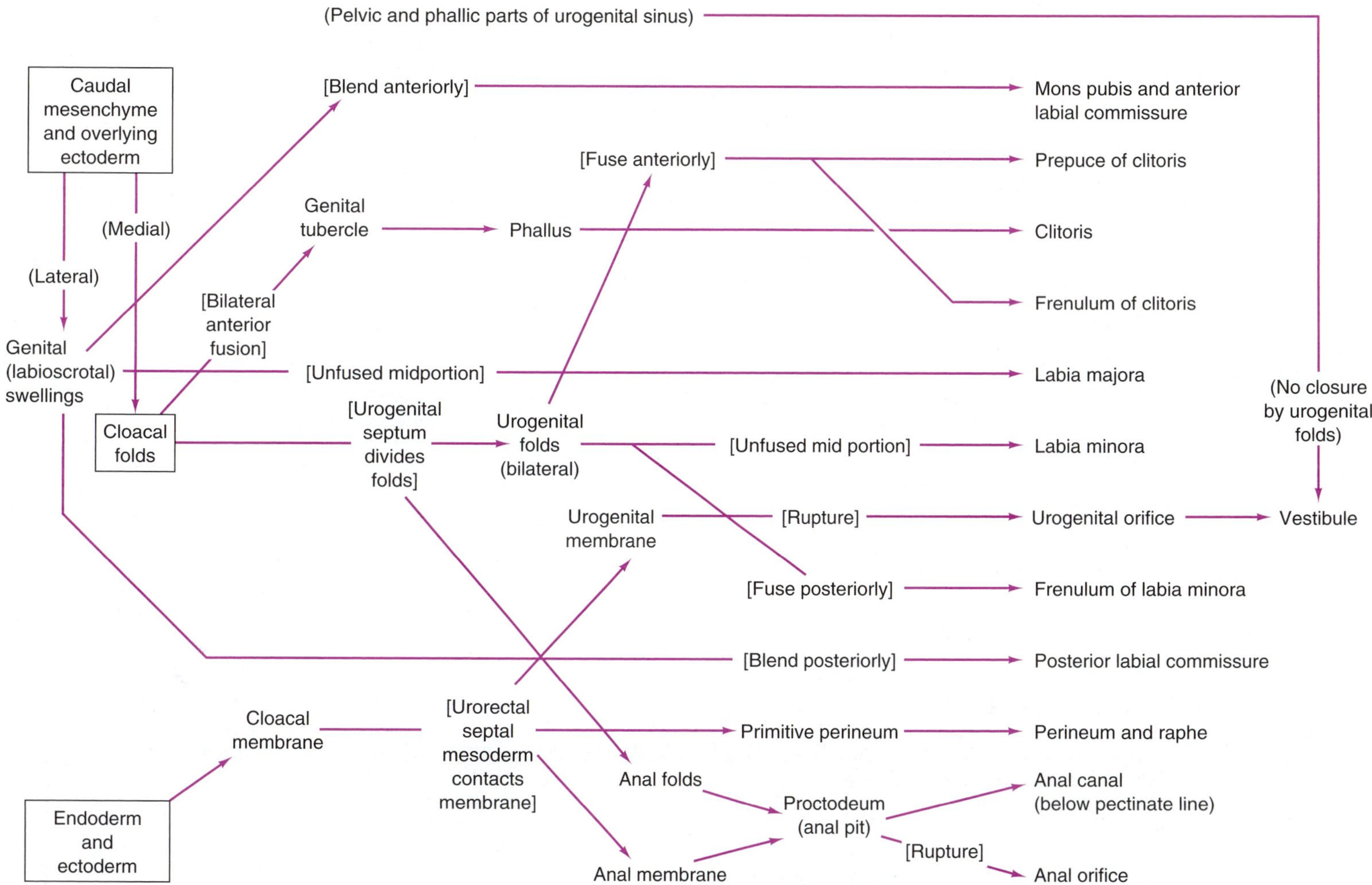

▲ **Figure 2–21.** Schematic drawing of formation of female external genitalia. (Explanatory symbols are given in Fig. 2–1.)

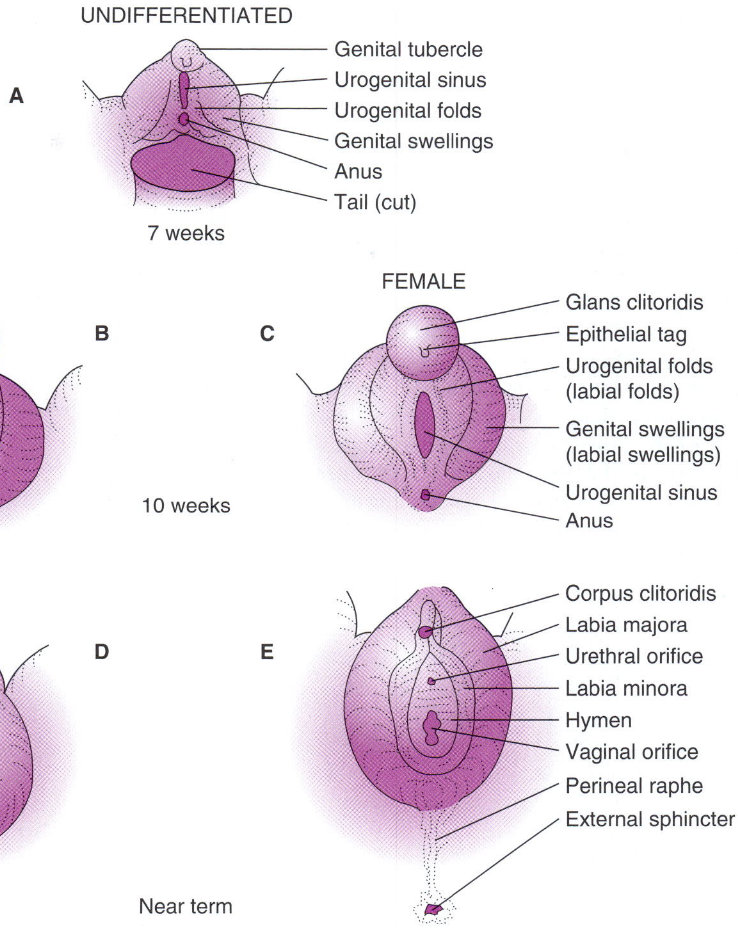

▲ **Figure 2–22.** Development of external genitalia. **A:** Before sexual differentiation and just after the urorectal septum divides the cloacal membrane. **B** and **D:** Male differentiation at about 10 weeks and near term, respectively. The urogenital folds fuse ventrally over the urethral groove to form the spongy urethra and close the inferior phallic part of the urogenital sinus. The glandular urethra forms by canalization of invaginated ectoderm from the tip of the glans. **C** and **E:** Female differentiation at about 10 weeks and near term, respectively. Until about 12 weeks, there is little difference in the appearance of female and male external genitalia. The urogenital folds fuse only at their anterior and posterior extremes, while the unfused remainder differentiates into the labia minor. (See also Figs. 2–20 and 2–21.)

Abnormal fusion (masculinization) of labioscrotal swellings in genetic females is most commonly associated with ambiguous genitalia of female pseudohermaphroditism consequent to **congenital adrenal hyperplasia (adrenogenital syndrome)**. Over 90% of females with congenital adrenal hyperplasia have a steroid 21-hydroxylase deficiency (autosomal recessive), resulting in excess adrenal androgen production. This enzyme deficiency has been reported to be "the most common cause of ambiguous genitalia in genetic females." Associated anomalies include clitoral hypertrophy and persistent urogenital sinus. Formation of a penile urethra is extremely rare.

D. Anomalies of the Clitoris

Clitoral agenesis is extremely rare and is due to lack of formation of the genital tubercle during the sixth week. Absence of the clitoris could also result from **atresia** of the genital tubercle. The tubercle forms by fusion of the anterior segments of the cloacal folds. Very rarely, these anterior segments fail to fuse, and a **bifid clitoris** forms. This anomaly also occurs when unification of the anterior parts of the folds is restricted by exstrophy of the cloaca or bladder. Duplication of the genital tubercle with consequent formation of a **double clitoris** is equally rare. **Clitoral hypertrophy**

alone is not common but may be associated with various intersex disorders.

E. Anomalies of the Perineum

The primitive perineum originates at the area of contact of the mesodermal urorectal septum and the endodermal dorsal surface of the cloacal membrane (at 7 weeks). During normal differentiation of the external genitalia in the fetal period, the primitive perineum maintains the separation of the urogenital folds and ruptured urogenital membrane from the anal folds and ruptured anal membrane, and later develops the perineal body. Malformations of the perineum are rare and usually associated with malformations of cloacal or anorectal development consequent to abnormal development of the urorectal septum. Imperforate anus has an incidence of about 0.02%. The simplest form (rare) is a thin membrane over the anal canal (the anal membrane failed to rupture at the end of the embryonic period). Anal stenosis can arise by posterior deviation of the urorectal septum as the septum approaches the cloacal membrane, causing the anal membrane to be smaller (with a relatively increased anogenital distance through the perineum). Anal agenesis with a fistula detected as an ectopic anus is considered to be a urorectal septal defect. The incidence of agenesis with a fistula is only slightly less than that without a fistula. In females, the fistula commonly may be located in the perineum (perineal fistula) or may open into the posterior aspect of the vestibule of the vagina (anovestibular fistula; see Cloacal Dysgenesis).

Lambert SM, Vilain EJ, Kolon TF. A practical approach to ambiguous genitalia in the newborn period. *Urol Clin North Am* 2010;37:195–205. PMID: 20569798.

Phillips TM. Spectrum of cloacal exstrophy. *Semin Pediatr Surg* 2011;20:113–118. PMID: 21453856.

Genetic Disorders & Sex Chromosome Abnormalities

3

Somjate Manipalviratn, MD
Bradley Trivax, MD
Andy Huang, MD

GENETIC DISORDERS

MENDELIAN LAWS OF INHERITANCE

1. Types of Inheritance

Autosomal Dominant

In autosomal dominant inheritance, it is assumed that a mutation has occurred in 1 gene of an allelic pair and that the presence of this new gene produces enough of the changed protein to give a different phenotypic effect. Environment must also be considered because the effect may vary under different environmental conditions. The following are characteristic of autosomal dominant inheritance:

1. The trait appears with equal frequency in both sexes.
2. For inheritance to take place, at least 1 parent must have the trait unless a new mutation has just occurred.
3. When a homozygous individual is mated to a normal individual, all offspring will carry the trait. When a heterozygous individual is mated to a normal individual, 50% of the offspring will show the trait.
4. If the trait is rare, most persons demonstrating it will be heterozygous (Table 3–1).

Autosomal Recessive

The mutant gene will not be capable of producing a new characteristic in the heterozygous state in this circumstance under customary environmental conditions—ie, with 50% of the genetic material producing the new protein, the phenotypic effect will not be different from that of the normal trait. When the environment is manipulated, the recessive trait occasionally becomes dominant. The characteristics of this form of inheritance are as follows:

1. The characteristic will occur with equal frequency in both sexes.
2. For the characteristic to be present, both parents must be carriers of the recessive trait.
3. If both parents are homozygous for the recessive trait, all offspring will have it.
4. If both parents are heterozygous for the recessive trait, 25% of the offspring will have it.
5. In pedigrees showing frequent occurrence of individuals with rare recessive characteristics, consanguinity is often present (Table 3–2).

X-Linked Recessive

This condition occurs when a gene on the X chromosome undergoes mutation and the new protein formed as a result of this mutation is incapable of producing a change in phenotype characteristic in the heterozygous state. Because the male has only 1 X chromosome, the presence of this mutant will allow for expression should it occur in the male. The following are characteristic of this form of inheritance:

1. The condition occurs more commonly in males than in females.
2. If both parents are normal and an affected male is produced, it must be assumed that the mother is a carrier of the trait.
3. If the father is affected and an affected male is produced, the mother must be at least heterozygous for the trait.
4. A female with the trait may be produced in 1 of 2 ways. (A) She may inherit a recessive gene from both her mother and her father; this suggests that the father is affected and the mother is heterozygous. (B) She may inherit a recessive gene from 1 of her parents and may express the recessive characteristic as a function of the

Table 3–1. Examples of autosomal dominant conditions and traits.

Achondroplasia
Acoustic neuroma
Aniridia
Cataracts, cortical and nuclear
Chin fissure
Color blindness, yellow-blue
Craniofacial dysostosis
Deafness (several forms)
Dupuytren's contracture
Ehlers-Danlos syndrome
Facial palsy, congenital
Huntington's chorea
Hyperchondroplasia
Intestinal polyposis
Keloid formation
Lipomas, familial
Marfan's syndrome
Mitral valve prolapse
Muscular dystrophy
Neurofibromatosis (Recklinghausen's disease)
Night blindness
Pectus excavatum
Adult polycystic renal disease
Tuberous sclerosis
von Willebrand's disease
Wolff-Parkinson-White syndrome (some cases)

Lyon hypothesis; this assumes that all females are mosaics for their functioning X chromosome. It is theorized that this occurs because at about the time of implantation, each cell in the developing female embryo selects 1 X chromosome as its functioning X and that all progeny cells thereafter use this X chromosome as their functioning X chromosome. The other X chromosome becomes inactive. Because this selection is done on a random basis, it is conceivable that some females will be produced

Table 3–2. Examples of autosomal recessive conditions and traits.

Acid maltase deficiency
Albinism
Alkaptonuria
Argininemia
Ataxia-telangiectasia
Bloom's syndrome
Cerebrohepatorenal syndrome
Chloride diarrhea, congenital
Chondrodystrophia myotonia
Color blindness, total
Coronary artery calcinosis
Cystic fibrosis
Cystinosis
Cystinuria
Deafness (several types)
Dubowitz's syndrome
Dysautonomia
Fructose-1,6-diphosphatase deficiency
Galactosemia
Gaucher's disease
Glaucoma, congenital
Histidinemia
Homocystinuria
Laron's dwarfism
Maple syrup urine disease
Mucolipidosis I, II, III
Mucopolysaccharidosis I-H, I-S, III, IV, VI, VII
Muscular dystrophy, autosomal recessive type
Niemann-Pick disease
Phenylketonuria
Sickle cell anemia
17α-Hydroxylase deficiency
18-Hydroxylase deficiency
21-Hydroxylase deficiency
Tay-Sachs disease
Wilson's disease
Xeroderma pigmentosum

Table 3–3. Examples of X-linked recessive conditions and traits.

Androgen insensitivity syndrome (complete and incomplete)
Color blindness, red-green
Diabetes insipidus (most cases)
Fabry's disease
Glucose-6-phosphate dehydrogenase deficiency
Gonadal dysgenesis (XY type)
Gout (certain types)
Hemophilia A (factor VIII deficiency)
Hemophilia B (factor IX deficiency)
Hypothyroidism, X-linked infantile
Hypophosphatemia
Immunodeficiency, X-linked
Lesch-Nyhan syndrome
Mucopolysaccharidosis II
Muscular dystrophy, adult and childhood types
Otopalatodigital syndrome
Reifenstein's syndrome

who will be using primarily the X chromosome bearing the recessive gene. Thus, a genotypically heterozygous individual may demonstrate a recessive characteristic phenotypically on this basis (Table 3–3).

X-Linked Dominant

In this situation, the mutation will produce a protein that, when present in the heterozygous state, is sufficient to cause a change in characteristic. The following are characteristic of this type of inheritance:

1. The characteristic occurs with the same frequency in males and females.
2. An affected male mated to a normal female will produce the characteristic in 50% of the offspring.
3. An affected homozygous female mated to a normal male will produce the affected characteristic in all offspring.
4. A heterozygous female mated to a normal male will produce the characteristic in 50% of the offspring.
5. Occasional heterozygous females may not show the dominant trait on the basis of the Lyon hypothesis (Table 3–4).

Table 3–4. Examples of X-linked dominant conditions and traits.

Acro-osteolysis, dominant type
Cervico-oculo-acoustic syndrome
Hyperammonemia
Orofaciodigital syndrome I

2. Applications of Mendelian Laws

Identification of Carriers

When a recessive characteristic is present in a population, carriers may be identified in a variety of ways. If the gene is responsible for the production of a protein (eg, an enzyme), the carrier often possesses 50% of the amount of the substance present in homozygous normal persons. Such a circumstance is found in galactosemia, where the carriers will have approximately half as much galactose-1-phosphate uridyltransferase activity in red cells as do noncarrier normal individuals.

At times, the level of the affected enzyme may be only slightly below normal, and a challenge with the substance to be acted upon may be required before the carrier can be identified. An example is seen in carriers of phenylketonuria, in whom the deficiency in phenylalanine hydroxylase is in the liver cells, and serum levels may not be much lower than normal. Nonetheless, when the individual is given an oral loading dose of phenylalanine, plasma phenylalanine levels may remain high because the enzyme is not present in sufficient quantities to act upon this substance properly.

In still other situations where the 2 alleles produce different proteins that can be measured, a carrier state will have 50% of the normal protein and 50% of the other protein. Such a situation is seen in sickle cell trait, where 1 gene is producing hemoglobin A and the other hemoglobin S. Thus, the individual has half the amount of hemoglobin A as a normal person and half the hemoglobin S of a person with sickle cell anemia. An interesting but important problem involves the detection of carriers of cystic fibrosis. This is the most common autosomal recessive disease in Caucasian populations of European background, occurring in 1 in 2500 births in such populations but found in the carrier state in 1 in 25 Americans. By 1990, over 230 alleles of the single gene responsible have been discovered. The gene is known as the cystic fibrosis transmembrane conductance regulator (CFTR), and the most common mutation, delta F508, accounts for about 70% of all mutations, with 5 specific point mutations accounting for over 85% of cases. Because so many alleles are present, population screening poses logistical problems that have yet to be worked out. Most programs screen for the most common mutations using DNA replication and amplification studies.

3. Polygenic Inheritance

Polygenic inheritance is defined as the inheritance of a single phenotypic feature as a result of the effects of many genes. Most physical features in humans are determined by polygenic inheritance. Many common malformations are determined in this way also. For example, cleft palate with or without cleft lip, clubfoot, anencephaly, meningomyelocele, dislocation of the hip, and pyloric stenosis each occur with a frequency of 0.5–2 per 1000 in white populations. Altogether, these anomalies account for slightly less than half of single primary defects noted in early infancy. They are present in siblings of affected infants—when both parents are normal—at a rate of 2–5%. They are also found more commonly among relatives than in the general population. The increase in incidence is not environmentally induced because the frequency of such abnormalities in monozygotic twins is 4–8 times that of dizygotic twins and other siblings. The higher incidence in monozygotic twins is called concordance.

Sex also plays a role. Certain conditions appear to be transmitted by polygenic inheritance and are passed on more frequently by the mother who is affected than by the father who is affected. Cleft lip occurs in 6% of the offspring of women with cleft lip, as opposed to 2.8% of offspring of men with cleft lip.

Many racial variations in diseases are believed to be transmitted by polygenic inheritance, making racial background a determinant of how prone an individual will be to a particular defect. In addition, as a general rule, the more severe a defect, the more likely it is to occur in subsequent siblings. Thus, siblings of children with bilateral cleft lip are more likely to have the defect than are those of children with unilateral cleft lip.

Environment undoubtedly plays a role in polygenic inheritance, because seasonal variations alter some defects and their occurrence rate from country to country in similar populations.

EPIGENETIC

Epigenetic is the regulation of gene expression not encoded in the nucleotide sequence of the gene. Gene expression can either be turned on or off by DNA methylation or histone modification (methylation, acetylation, phosphorylation, ubiquitination, or ADP-ribosylation). Epigenetic can subsequently be inherited by its descendants.

Genomic Imprinting

Genomic imprinting is an epigenetic process by which the male and female genomes are differently expressed. The imprinting mark on genes is either by DNA methylation or histone modification. The imprinting patterns are different according to the parental origin of the genes. Genomic imprints are erased in primordial germ cells and reestablished again during gametogenesis. The imprinting process is completed by the time of round spermatids formation in males and at ovulation of metaphase-II oocytes in females. The imprinted genes survive the global waves of DNA demethylation and remethylation during early embryonic development. In normal children, 1 set of chromosomes is derived from the father and the other from the mother. If both sets of chromosomes are from only 1 parent, the imprinted gene expression will be unbalanced. Prader-Willi syndrome and Angelman syndrome are examples of imprinting disorders. In Prader-Willi syndrome, both 15q13 regions are from the father, whereas in Angelman syndrome, both 15q13 regions are from the mother.

CYTOGENETICS

1. Identification of Chromosomes

In 1960, 1963, 1965, and 1971, international meetings were held in Denver, London, Chicago, and Paris, respectively, for the purpose of standardizing the nomenclature of human chromosomes. These meetings resulted in a decision that all autosomal pairs should be numbered in order of decreasing size from 1 to 22. Autosomes are divided into groups based on their morphology, and these groups are labeled by the letters A–G. Thus, the A group is comprised of pairs 1–3; the B group, pairs 4 and 5; the C group, pairs 6–12; the D group, pairs 13–15; the E group, pairs 16–18; the F group, pairs 19 and 20; and the G group, pairs 21 and 22. The sex chromosomes are labeled X and Y, the X chromosome being similar in size and morphology to the number 7 pair and thus frequently included in the C group (C-X) and the Y chromosome being similar in morphology and size to the G group (G-Y) (Fig. 3–1).

The short arm of a chromosome is labeled p and the long arm q. If a translocation occurs in which the short arm of a chromosome is added to another chromosome, it is written p+. If the short arm is lost, it is p−. The same can be said for the long arm (q+ and q−).

It has been impossible to separate several chromosome pairs from one another on a strictly morphologic basis because the morphologic variations have been too slight. However, there are other means of identifying each chromosome pair in the karyotype. The first of these is the incorporation of ^{3}H-thymidine, known as the autoradiographic technique. This procedure involves the incorporation of radioactive thymidine into growing cells in tissue culture just before they are harvested. Cells that are actively undergoing DNA replication will pick up the radioactive thymidine, and the chromosomes will demonstrate areas of activity. Each chromosome will incorporate thymidine in a different pattern, and several chromosomes can therefore be identified by their labeling pattern. Nonetheless, with this method it is not possible to identify each chromosome, although it is possible to identify chromosomes involved in pathologic conditions, eg, D_1 trisomy and Down syndrome.

Innovative staining techniques have made it possible to identify individual chromosomes in the karyotype and to identify small anomalies that might have evaded the observer using older methods. These involve identification

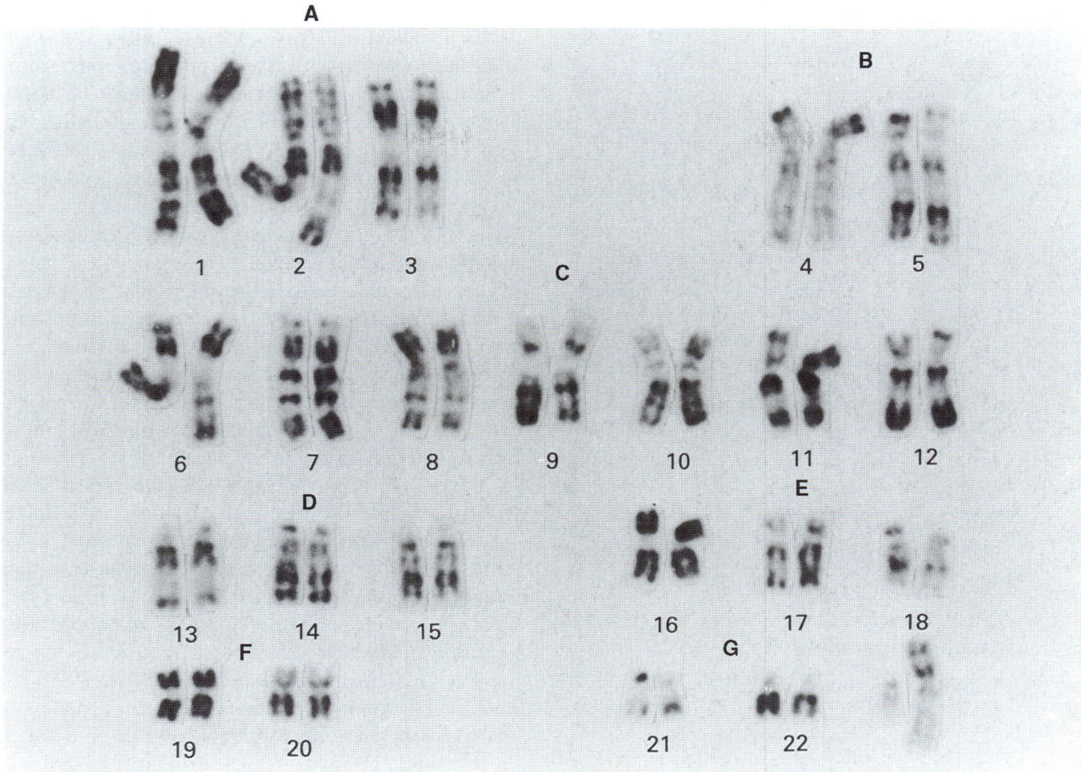

▲ **Figure 3–1.** Karyotype of a normal male demonstrating R banding.

of chromosome banding by a variety of staining techniques, at times with predigestion with proteolytic agents. Some of the more commonly used techniques are the following:

Q banding: Fixed chromosome spreads are stained without any pretreatment using quinacrine mustard, quinacrine, or other fluorescent dyes and observed with a fluorescence microscope.

G banding: Preparations are incubated in a variety of saline solutions using any 1 of several pretreatments and stained with Giemsa's stain.

R banding: Preparations are incubated in buffer solutions at high temperatures or at special pH and stained with Giemsa's stain. This process yields the reverse bands of G banding (Fig. 3–1).

C banding: Preparations are either heated in saline to temperatures just below boiling or treated with certain alkali solutions and then stained with Giemsa's stain. This process causes prominent bands to develop in the region of the centromeres.

2. Cell Division

Each body cell goes through successive stages in its life cycle. As a landmark, cell division can be considered as the beginning of a cycle. Following this, the first phase, which is quite long but depends on how rapidly the particular cell is multiplying, is called the G_1 stage. During this stage, the cell is primarily concerned with carrying out its function. Following this, the S stage, or period of DNA synthesis, takes place. Next there is a somewhat shorter stage, the G_2 stage, during which time DNA synthesis is completed and chromosome replication begins. Following this comes the M stage, when cell division occurs.

Somatic cells undergo division by a process known as **mitosis** (Fig. 3–2). This is divided into 4 periods. The first is **prophase**, during which the chromosome filaments shorten, thicken, and become visible. At this time they can be seen to be composed of 2 long parallel spiral strands lying adjacent to one another and containing a small clear structure known as the **centromere**. As prophase continues, the strands continue to unwind and may be recognized as chromatids. At the end of prophase, the nuclear membrane disappears and **metaphase** begins. This stage is heralded by the formation of a spindle and the lining up of the chromosomes in pairs on the spindle. Following this, **anaphase** occurs, at which time the centromere divides and each daughter chromatid goes to 1 of the poles of the spindle. **Telophase** then ensues, at which time the spindle breaks and cell cytoplasm divides. A nuclear membrane

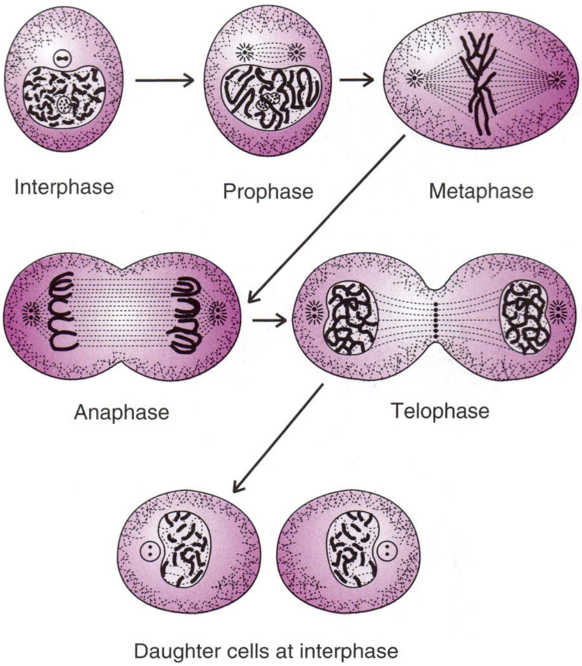

▲ **Figure 3–2.** Mitosis of a somatic cell.

now forms, and mitosis is complete. Each daughter cell has received chromosome material equal in amount and identical to that of the parent cell. Because each cell contains 2 chromosomes of each pair and a total of 46 chromosomes, a cell is considered to be **diploid**. Occasionally, an error takes place on the spindle, and instead of chromosomes dividing, with identical chromatids going to each daughter cell, an extra chromatid goes to 1 daughter cell and the other lacks that particular member. After completion of cell division, this leads to a trisomic state (an extra dose of that chromosome) in 1 daughter cell and a monosomic state (a missing dose of the chromosome) in the other daughter cell. Any chromosome in the karyotype may be involved in such a process, which is known as mitotic nondisjunction. If these cells thrive and produce their own progeny, a new cell line is established within the individual. The individual then has more than 1 cell line and is known as a **mosaic**. A variety of combinations and permutations have occurred in humans.

Germ cells undergo division for the production of eggs and sperm by a process known as **meiosis**. In the female it is known as oogenesis and in the male as spermatogenesis. The process that produces the egg and the sperm for fertilization essentially reduces the chromosome number from 46 to 23 and changes the normal diploid cell to an aneuploid cell, ie, a cell that has only 1 member of each chromosome pair. Following fertilization and the fusion of the 2 pronuclei, the diploid status is reestablished.

Meiosis can be divided into several stages (Fig. 3–3). The first is **prophase I**. Early prophase is known as the **leptotene stage**, during which chromatin condenses and becomes visible as a single elongated threadlike structure. This is followed by the **zygotene stage**, when the single threadlike chromosomes migrate toward the equatorial plate of the nucleus. At this stage, homologous chromosomes become arranged close to one another to form **bivalents** that exchange materials at several points known as **synapses**. In this way, genetic material located on 1 member of a pair is exchanged with similar material located on the other member of a pair. Next comes the **pachytene stage** in which the chromosomes contract to become shorter and thicker. During this stage, each chromosome splits longitudinally into 2 chromatids united at the centromere. Thus, the bivalent becomes a structure composed of 4 closely opposed chromatids known as a **tetrad**. The human cell in the pachytene stage demonstrates 23 tetrads. This stage is followed by the **diplotene stage**, in which the chromosomes of the bivalent are held together only at certain points called bridges or chiasms. It is at these points that crossover takes place. The sister chromatids are joined at the centromere so that crossover can only take place between chromatids of homologous chromosomes and not between identical sister chromatids. In the case of males, the X and Y chromosomes are not involved in crossover. This stage is followed by the last stage of prophase, known as **diakinesis**. Here the bivalents contract, and the chiasms move toward the end of the chromosome. The homologs pull apart, and the nuclear membrane disappears. This is the end of prophase I.

Metaphase I follows. At this time, the bivalents are now highly contracted and align themselves along the equatorial plate of the cell. Paternal and maternal chromosomes line up at random. This stage is then followed by **anaphase I** and **telophase I**, which are quite similar to the corresponding events in mitosis. However, the difference is that in meiosis the homologous chromosome of the bivalent pair separates and not the sister chromatids. The homologous bivalents pull apart, 1 going to each pole of the spindle, following which 2 daughter cells are formed at telophase I.

Metaphase, anaphase, and telophase of meiosis II take place next. A new spindle forms in metaphase, the chromosomes align along the equatorial plate, and, as anaphase occurs, the chromatids pull apart, 1 each going to a daughter cell. This represents a true division of the centromere. Telophase then supervenes, with reconstitution of the nuclear membrane and final cell division. At the end, a haploid number of chromosomes is present in each daughter cell (Fig. 3–3). In the case of spermatogenesis, both daughter cells are similar, forming 2 separate sperms. In the case of oogenesis, only 1 egg is produced, the nuclear material of the other daughter cell being present and intact but with very little cytoplasm, this being known as the **polar body**. A polar body is formed at the end of meiosis I and the end of

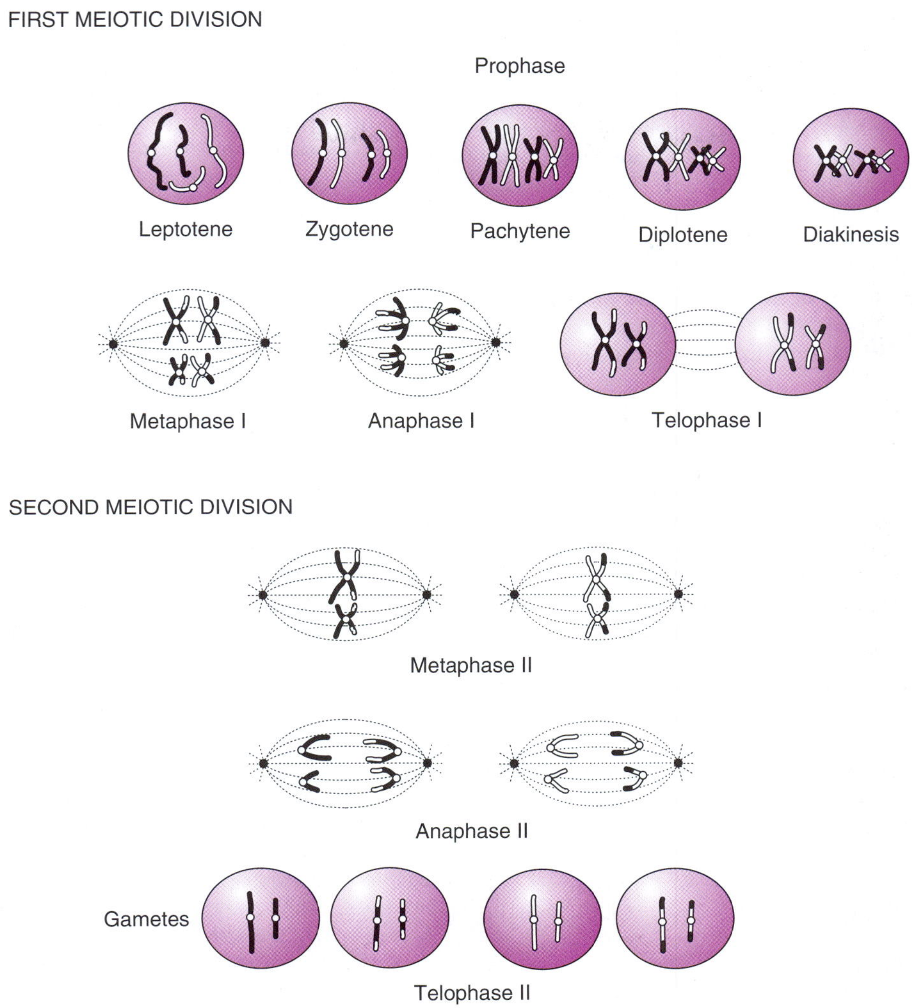

▲ **Figure 3–3.** Meiosis in the human.

meiosis II. Thus, each spermatogonium produces 4 sperms at the end of meiosis, whereas each oogonium produces 1 egg and 2 polar bodies.

Nondisjunction may also occur in meiosis. When it does, both members of the chromosome pair go to 1 daughter cell and none to the other. If the daughter cell that receives the entire pair is the egg, and fertilization ensues, a triple dose of the chromosome, or trisomy, will occur. If the daughter cell receiving no members of the pair is fertilized, a monosomic state will result. In the case of autosomes, this is lethal, and a very early abortion will follow. In the case of the sex chromosome, the condition may not be lethal, and examples of both trisomy and monosomy have been seen in humans. Any chromosome pair may be involved in trisomic or monosomic conditions.

3. Abnormalities in Chromosome Morphology & Number

As has been stated, nondisjunction may give rise to conditions of trisomy. In these cases, the morphology of the chromosome is not affected, but the chromosome number is. Be this as it may, breaks and rearrangements in chromosomes may have a variety of results. If 2 chromosomes undergo breaks and exchange chromatin material between them, the outcome is 2 morphologically new chromosomes known as **translocations**. If a break in a chromosome takes place and the fragment is lost, **deletion** has occurred. If the deletion is such that the cell cannot survive, the condition may be lethal. Nonetheless, several examples of deleted chromosomes in individuals who have survived have been identified. If a break takes place at either end of a chromosome and the chromosome heals by having the 2 ends fuse together, a ring chromosome is formed. Examples of these have been seen clinically in all of the chromosomes of the karyotype, and generally they exhibit a variety of phenotypic abnormalities.

At times a chromosome will divide by a horizontal rather than longitudinal split of the centromere. This leaves each daughter cell with a double dose of 1 of the arms of the chromosome. Thus, 1 daughter cell receives both long arms and the other both short arms of the chromosome. Such a chromosome is referred to as an **isochromosome**, the individual being essentially trisomic for 1 arm and monosomic for the other arm of the chromosome. Examples of this abnormality have been seen in humans.

Another anomaly that has been recognized is the occurrence of 2 breaks within the chromosome and rotation of the center fragment 180 degrees. Thus, the realignment allows for a change in morphology of the chromosome, although the original number of genes is preserved. This is called an **inversion**. At meiosis, however, the chromosome has difficulty in undergoing chiasm formation, and abnormal rearrangements of this chromosome, leading to partial duplications and partial losses of chromatin material, do take place. This situation may lead to several bizarre anomalies. If the centromere is involved in the inversion, the condition is called a **pericentric inversion**.

Breaks occasionally occur in 2 chromosomes, and a portion of 1 broken chromosome is inserted into the body of another, leading to a grossly abnormal chromosome. This is known as an **insertion** and generally leads to gross anomalies at meiosis.

4. Methods of Study

Sex Chromatin (X-Chromatin) Body (Barr Body)

The X-chromatin body was first seen in the nucleus of the nerve cell of a female cat in 1949 by Barr and Bertram. It has been found to be the constricted, nonfunctioning X chromosome. As a general rule, only 1 X chromosome functions in a cell at a given time. All other X chromosomes present in a cell may be seen as X-chromatin bodies in a resting nucleus. Thus, if one knows the number of X chromosomes, one can anticipate that the number of Barr bodies will be 1 less. If one counts the number of Barr bodies, the number of X chromosomes can be determined by adding 1.

Drumsticks on Polymorphonuclear Leukocytes

Small outpouchings of the lobes of nuclei in polymorphonuclear leukocytes of females have been demonstrated to be the X-chromatin body in this particular cell. Hence, leukocyte preparations may be used to detect X-chromatin bodies in much the same way as buccal cells are used.

Chromosome Count

In the karyotypic analysis of a patient, it is the usual practice to count 20–50 chromosome spreads for chromosome number. The purpose of this practice is to determine whether mosaicism exists because if a mosaic pattern does exist, there will be at least 2 cell lines of different counts. Photographs are made of representative spreads, and karyotypes are constructed so that the morphology of each chromosome can be studied.

Banding Techniques

As previously described, it is possible after appropriate pretreatment to stain metaphase spreads with special stains and construct a karyotype that demonstrates the banding patterns of each chromosome. In this way, it is possible to identify with certainty every chromosome in the karyotype. This is of value with problems such as translocations and trisomic conditions. Another use depends on the fact that most of the long arm of the Y chromosome is heterochromic and stains deeply with fluorescent stains. Thus, the Y chromosome can be identified at a glance, even in the resting nucleus.

APPLIED GENETICS & TERATOLOGY

1. Chromosomes & Spontaneous Abortion

An entirely new approach to reproductive biology problems became available with the advent of tissue culture and cytologic techniques that made it possible to culture cells from any tissue of the body and produce karyotypes that could be analyzed. In the early 1960s, investigators in a number of laboratories began to study chromosomes of spontaneous abortions and demonstrated that the earlier the spontaneous abortion occurred, the more likely it was due to a chromosomal abnormality. It is now known that in spontaneous abortions occurring in the first 8 weeks, the fetuses have about a 50% incidence of chromosome anomalies.

Of abortuses that are abnormal, approximately one-half are trisomic, suggesting an error of meiotic nondisjunction. One-third of abortuses with trisomy have trisomy 16. Although this abnormality does not occur in liveborn infants, it apparently is a frequent problem in abortuses. The karyotype 45,X occurs in nearly one-fourth of chromosomally abnormal abortuses. This karyotype occurs about 24 times more frequently in abortuses than in liveborn infants, a fact that emphasizes its lethal nature. Over 15% of chromosomally abnormal abortuses have polyploidy (triploidy or tetraploidy). These lethal conditions are seen only in abortuses except in extremely rare circumstances and are due to a variety of accidents, including double fertilization and a number of meiotic errors. Finally, a small number of chromosomally abnormal abortuses have unbalanced translocations and other anomalies.

Recurrent Pregnancy Loss

Couples who experience habitual abortion constitute about 0.5% of the population. The condition is defined as 2 or more spontaneous abortions. Several investigators have studied groups of these couples using banding techniques and have found that 10–25% of them have a chromosome anomaly in either the male or female partner. Those seen are 47,XXX, 47,XYY, and a variety of balanced translocation carriers. Those with sex chromosome abnormalities frequently demonstrate other nondisjunctional events. Chromosome anomalies are thus a major cause of habitual abortion, and the incorporation of genetic evaluation into such a work-up is potentially fruitful.

Lippman-Hand and Bekemans reviewed the world literature and studied the incidence of balanced translocation carriers among 177 couples who had 2 or more spontaneous abortions. These studies suggest that in 2–3% of couples experiencing early fetal loss, 1 partner will have balanced translocations. This percentage is not markedly increased when more than 2 abortions occur. Females had a somewhat higher incidence of balanced translocations than did males.

2. Chromosomal Disorders

This section is devoted to a brief discussion of various autosomal abnormalities. Table 3–5 summarizes some of the autosomal abnormalities that have been diagnosed. They are represented as syndromes, together with some of the signs typical of these conditions. In general, autosomal monosomy is so lethal that total loss of a chromosome is rarely seen in an individual born alive. Only a few cases of monosomy 21–22 have been reported to date, which attests to the rarity of this disorder. Trisomy may occur with any chromosome. The 3 most common trisomic conditions seen in living individuals are trisomies 13, 18, and 21. Trisomy of various C group chromosomes has been reported sporadically. The most frequently reported is trisomy 8. Generally, trisomy of other chromosomes must be assumed to be lethal, because they occur only in abortuses, not in living individuals. To date, trisomy of every autosome except chromosome 1 has been seen in abortuses.

Translocations can occur between any 2 chromosomes of the karyotype, and a variety of phenotypic expressions may be seen after mediocre arrangements. Three different translocation patterns have been identified in Down syndrome: 15/21, 21/21, and 21/22.

Deletions may also occur with respect to any chromosome in the karyotype and may be brought about by a translocation followed by a rearrangement in meiosis, which leads to the loss of chromatin material, or by a simple loss of the chromatin material following a chromosome break. Some of the more commonly seen deletion patterns are listed in Table 3–5.

The most frequent abnormality related to a chromosome abnormality is Down syndrome. Down syndrome serves as an interesting model for the discussion of autosomal diseases. The 21 trisomy type is the most common form and is responsible for approximately 95% of Down syndrome patients. There is a positive correlation between the frequency of Down syndrome and maternal age. Babies with Down syndrome are more often born to teenage mothers and even more frequently to mothers over 35. Although the reason for these findings is not entirely clear, it may be that, in older women at least, the egg has been present in prophase of the first meiotic division from the time of fetal life and that, as the egg ages, there is a greater tendency for nondisjunction to occur, leading to trisomy. A second theory is that coital habits are more erratic in both the very young and the older mothers, and this may lead to an increased incidence of fertilization of older eggs. This theory maintains that these eggs may be more likely to suffer nondisjunction or to accept abnormal sperm. Be this as it may, the incidence of Down syndrome in the general population is approximately 1 in 600 deliveries and at age 40 approximately 1 in 100 deliveries. At age 45, the incidence is approximately 1 in 40 deliveries (Table 3–6). The other 5% of Down syndrome patients are the result of translocations, the most common being the 15/21 translocation, but examples of 21/21 and 21/22 have been noted. In the case of 15/21, the chance of recurrence in a later pregnancy is theoretically 25%. In practice, a rate of 10% is observed if the mother is the carrier. When the father is the carrier, the odds are less because there may be a selection not favoring the sperm carrying both the 15/21 translocation and the normal 21 chromosome. In the case of 21/21 translocation, there is no chance for formation of a normal child because the carrier will contribute either both 21s or no 21 and, following fertilization, will produce either a monosomic 21 or trisomic 21. With regard to 21/22 translocation, the chance of producing a baby with Down syndrome is 1 in 2.

In general, other trisomic states occur with greater frequency in older women, and the larger the chromosome involved, the more severe the syndrome. Because trisomy 21 involves the smallest of the chromosomes, the phenotypic problems of Down syndrome are the least severe, and a moderate life expectancy may be anticipated. Even these individuals will be grossly abnormal, however, because of mental retardation and defects in other organ systems. The average life expectancy of patients with Down syndrome is much lower than for the general population.

3. Prenatal Diagnosis

Currently the most common use for applied genetics in obstetrics and gynecology is in prenatal counseling, screening, and diagnosis. Prenatal diagnosis first came into use in 1977 with the discovery of the significance of serum α fetoprotein (AFP). The United Kingdom Collaboration Study found that elevated AFP in maternal serum drawn between 16 and 18 weeks of gestation correlated with an increased incidence of neural tube defects (NTDs). Since that time,

Table 3–5. Autosomal disorders.

Type	Synonym	Signs
Monosomy		
Monosomy 21–22		Moderate mental retardation, antimongoloid slant of eyes, flared nostrils, small mouth, low-set ears, spade hands.
Trisomy		
Trisomy 13	Trisomy D: the "D_1" syndrome	Severe mental retardation, congenital heart disease (77%), polydactyly, cerebral malformations (especially aplasia of olfactory bulbs), eye defects, low-set ears, cleft lip and palate, low birth weight. Characteristic dermatoglyphic pattern.
Trisomy 18	Trisomy E: the "E" syndrome, Edward's syndrome	Severe mental retardation, long narrow skull with prominent occiput, congenital heart disease, flexion deformities of fingers, narrow palpebral fissures, low-set ears, harelip and cleft palate. Characteristic dermatoglyphics, low birth weight.
Trisomy 21	Down syndrome	Mental retardation, brachycephaly, prominent epicanthal folds. Brushfield spots, poor nasal bridge development, congenital heart disease, hypotonia, hypermobility of joints, characteristic dermatoglyphics.
Translocations		
15/21	Down syndrome	Same as trisomy 21.
21/21	Down syndrome	Same as trisomy 21.
21/22	Down syndrome	Same as trisomy 21.
Deletions		
Short arm chromosome 4 (4p–)	Wolf's syndrome	Severe growth and mental retardation, midline scalp defects, seizures, deformed iris, beak nose, hypospadias.
Short arm chromosome 5 (5p–)	Cri-du-chat syndrome	Microcephaly, catlike cry, hypertelorism with epicanthus, low-set ears, micrognathism, abnormal dermatoglyphics, low birth weight.
Long arm chromosome 13 (13q–)	. . .	Microcephaly, psychomotor retardation, eye and ear defects, hypoplastic or absent thumbs.
Short arm chromosome 18 (18p–)	. . .	Severe mental retardation, hypertelorism, low-set ears, flexion deformities of hands.
Long arm chromosome 18 (18q–)	. . .	Severe mental retardation, microcephaly, hypotonia, congenital heart disease; marked dimples at elbows, shoulders, and knees.
Long arm chromosome 21 (21q–)	. . .	Associated with chronic myelogenous leukemia.

much research effort has been aimed at perfecting the technique. We now can screen not only for NTDs but also for trisomy 21 and trisomy 18. In addition, cystic fibrosis, sickle cell disease, and Huntington's disease, as well as many inborn errors of metabolism and other genetic disorders, can now be identified prenatally.

Neural Tube Disease

Most neural tube diseases, eg, anencephaly, spina bifida, and meningomyelocele, are associated with a multifactorial inheritance pattern. The frequency of their occurrence varies in different populations (eg, rates as high as 10 per 1000 births in Ireland and as low as 0.8 per 1000 births in the western United States). Ninety percent are index cases, ie, they occur spontaneously without previous occurrence in a family. In general, if a couple has a child with such an anomaly, the chance of producing another affected child is 2–5%. If they have had 2 such children, the risk can be as high as 10%. However, other diagnostic possibilities involving different modes of inheritance should be considered. Siblings also run greater risks of having affected children, with the highest risk being to female offspring of sisters and the lowest to male offspring of brothers. Maternal serum screening is now available to all mothers between 16 and 20 weeks of gestation. If an elevation of 2.5 or more standard

Table 3–6. Estimates of rates per thousand of chromosome abnormalities in live births by single-year interval.

Maternal Age	Down Syndrome	Edward's Syndrome (Trisomy 18)	Patau's Syndrome (Trisomy 13)	XXY	XYY	Turner's Syndrome Genotype	Other Clinically Significant Abnormality[1]	Total[2]
< 15	1.0[3]	< 0.1[3]	< 0.1–0.1	0.4	0.5	< 0.1	0.2	2.2
15	1.0[3]	< 0.1[3]	< 0.1–0.1	0.4	0.5	< 0.1	0.2	2.1
16	0.9[3]	< 0.1[3]	< 0.1–0.1	0.4	0.5	< 0.1	0.2	
17	0.8[3]	< 0.1[3]	< 0.1–0.1	0.4	0.5	< 0.1	0.2	2.0
18	0.7[3]	< 0.1[3]	< 0.1–0.1	0.4	0.5	< 0.1	0.2	1.9
19	0.6[3]	< 0.1[3]	< 0.1–0.1	0.4	0.5	< 0.1	0.2	1.8
20	0.5–0.7	< 0.1–0.1	< 0.1–0.1	0.4	0.5	< 0.1	0.2	1.9
21	0.5–0.7	< 0.1–0.1	< 0.1–0.1	0.4	0.5	< 0.1	0.2	1.9
22	0.6–0.8	< 0.1–0.1	< 0.1–0.1	0.4	0.5	< 0.1	0.2	2.0
23	0.6–0.8	< 0.1–0.1	< 0.1–0.1	0.4	0.5	< 0.1	0.2	2.0
24	0.7–0.9	0.1–0.1	< 0.1–0.1	0.4	0.5	< 0.1	0.2	2.1
25	0.7–0.9	0.1–0.1	< 0.1–0.1	0.4	0.5	< 0.1	0.2	2.1
26	0.7–1.0	0.1–0.1	< 0.1–0.1	0.4	0.5	< 0.1	0.2	2.1
27	0.8–1.0	0.1–0.2	< 0.1–0.1	0.4	0.5	< 0.1	0.2	2.2
28	0.8–1.1	0.1–0.2	< 0.1–0.2	0.4	0.5	< 0.1	0.2	2.3
29	0.8–1.2	0.1–0.2	< 0.1–0.2	0.5	0.5	< 0.1	0.2	2.4
30	0.9–1.2	0.1–0.2	< 0.1–0.2	0.5	0.5	< 0.1	0.2	2.6
31	0.9–1.3	0.1–0.2	< 0.1–0.2	0.5	0.5	< 0.1	0.2	2.6
32	1.1–1.5	0.1–0.2	0.1–0.2	0.6	0.5	< 0.1	0.2	3.1
33	1.4–1.9	0.1–0.3	0.1–0.2	0.7	0.5	< 0.1	0.2	3.5
34	1.9–2.4	0.2–0.4	0.1–0.3	0.7	0.5	< 0.1	0.2	4.1
35	2.5–3.9	0.3–0.5	0.2–0.3	0.9	0.5	< 0.1	0.3	5.6
36	3.2–5.0	0.3–0.6	0.2–0.4	1.0	0.5	< 0.1	0.3	6.7
37	4.1–6.4	0.4–0.7	0.2–0.5	1.1	0.5	< 0.1	0.3	8.1
38	5.2–8.1	0.5–0.9	0.3–0.7	1.3	0.5	< 0.1	0.3	9.5
39	6.6–10.5	0.7–1.2	0.4–0.8	1.5	0.5	< 0.1	0.3	12.4
40	8.5–13.7	0.9–1.6	0.5–1.1	1.8	0.5	< 0.1	0.3	15.8
41	10.8–17.9	1.1–2.1	0.6–1.4	2.2	0.5	< 0.1	0.3	20.5
42	13.8–23.4	1.4–2.7	0.7–1.8	2.7	0.5	< 0.1	0.3	25.5
43	17.6–30.6	1.8–3.5	0.9–2.4	3.3	0.5	< 0.1	0.3	32.6
44	22.5–40.0	2.3–4.6	1.2–3.1	4.1	0.5	< 0.1	0.3	41.8

(continued)

Table 3–6. Estimates of rates per thousand of chromosome abnormalities in live births by single-year interval. *(Continued)*

Maternal Age	Down Syndrome	Edward's Syndrome (Trisomy 18)	Patau's Syndrome (Trisomy 13)	XXY	XYY	Turner's Syndrome Genotype	Other Clinically Significant Abnormality[1]	Total[2]
45	28.7-52.3	2.9-6.0	1.5-4.1	5.1	0.5	< 0.1	0.3	53.7
46	36.6-68.3	3.7-7.9	1.9-5.3	6.4	0.5	< 0.1	0.3	68.9
47	46.6-89.3	4.7-10.3	2.4-6.9	8.2	0.5	< 0.1	0.3	89.1
48	59.5-116.8	6.0-13.5	3.0-9.0	10.6	0.5	< 0.1	0.3	15.0
49	75.8-152.7	7.6-17.6	3.8-11.8	13.8	0.5	< 0.1	0.3	49.3

[1]XXX is excluded.
[2]Calculation of the total at each age assumes rate for autosomal aneuploidies is at the midpoints of the ranges given.
[3]No range may be constructed for those under 20 years by the same methods as for those 20 and over.
Reproduced, with permission, from Hook EB. Rates of chromosome abnormalities at different maternal ages. *Obstet Gynecol* 1981;58: 282–285.

deviations above the mean is noted, amniocentesis for AFP should be done along with a careful ultrasound study of the fetus for structural anomalies. Evidence for an NTD noted on ultrasound and suspected by amniotic fluid AFP elevation of 3.0 or more standard deviations indicates a diagnosis of an NTD and allows for appropriate counseling and decision making for the parents.

Maternal serum AFP screening detects about 85% of all open NTDs, thus allowing detection of 80% of all open NTDs and 90% of all anencephalic infants. Serum AFP screening does not detect skin-covered lesions or the closed form of NTDs. Thus, most encephaloceles may be missed.

Approximately 5–5.5% of women screened will have abnormally elevated values (≥ 2.5 times the mean). Most of these will be false-positive results (a repeat test should determine this) due to inaccurate dating of gestational age, multiple gestation, fetal demise or dying fetus, or a host of other structural abnormalities. In most cases, repeat AFP testing and ultrasound examination will identify the problem. If the serum AFP level remains elevated and ultrasound examination does not yield a specific diagnosis, amniotic fluid AFP levels should be measured as well as amniotic fluid acetylcholinesterase levels. Further testing and counseling may be necessary before a final diagnosis can be made. When the correct gestational age is used, the false-positive rate for second-trimester maternal screening is 3–4%.

Chromosomal Abnormalities

In 1984, maternal serum AFP levels were found to be lower in patients who delivered infants with Down syndrome. Using the AFP value with maternal age, 25–30% of fetuses with Down syndrome were detected prenatally. In 1988, 2 additional tests were added to the maternal AFP: human chorionic gonadotropin (hCG) and unconjugated estriol (uE_3). Using the "triple screen," a 60% detection rate for Down syndrome was accomplished. In addition, the use of uE_3 allowed for detection of trisomy 18.

Fetuses with Down syndrome have low maternal AFP, low uE_3, and high hCG. Fetuses with trisomy 18 have low values across all of the serum markers. The false-positive rate for women less than 35 years of age is 5%. Above this age cutoff, the false-positive rate is increased. The definitive diagnosis of a chromosomal abnormality must be confirmed with a fetal karyotype.

The risk of fetal trisomies increases with increasing maternal age. At age 35 the risk of a trisomy is approximately 1 in 200. At age 40 the risk is 1 in 20 (Table 3–6). Prior to the discovery of serum markers, advanced maternal age was used to guide which women received fetal karyotyping. Trisomies, however, are not the only abnormality increased in this population of women. Sex chromosome aneuploidies (47,XXY and 47,XXX) also occur at an increased rate in women 35 years of age and older. Despite the advances in serum screening, fetal karyotyping continues to be the gold standard for prenatal testing in this group of women. The use of maternal serum screening in this subset of women is hindered by a high false-positive rate, less than 100% detection rate for trisomy 18 and 21, and the lack of ability to screen for the sex chromosome aneuploidies.

Cystic Fibrosis

Cystic fibrosis affects 1 in 3300 individuals of European descent in the United States. The carrier frequency is 1 in 29 for North Americans of European descent and Ashkenazi Jewish descent and 1 in 60 for African Americans. A deletion of phenylalanine at position 508 of the CFTR gene on chromosome 7 leads to the disease. All individuals with a family history of cystic fibrosis or a high carrier frequency should be offered carrier testing. For couples who are both carriers of the defective allele, fetal testing may be provided.

Future Advances in Prenatal Screening

In the detection of certain trisomies, the triple-marker screen provides better sensitivity than any single marker alone. Nonetheless, the detection rate for trisomy 18 and trisomy 21 still remains quite low. According to the Serum Urine and Ultrasound Screening Study (SURUSS), integration of nuchal translucency measurement and pregnancy-associated plasma protein-A (PAPP-A) in the first trimester improves screening. This information in conjunction with early second-trimester measurement of AFP, uE_3, free β-hCG (or total hCG), and inhibin-A with maternal age provides the most effective method for screening of Down syndrome, with an 85% detection rate and 0.9% false-positive rate. As the field of prenatal diagnostics continues to evolve, higher detection rates with lower false-positive rates can be expected. With continued research and advancing technology, prenatal screening may move into the first trimester. It may involve new markers (proform of eosinophil major basic protein [proMBP], nasal bone) and may even involve markers taken in both the first and second trimesters.

Fetal Karyotyping

A. Amniocentesis

Amniocentesis for prenatal diagnosis of genetic diseases is an extremely useful tool in the following circumstances or classes of patients:

1. Maternal age 35 years or above
2. Previous chromosomally abnormal child
3. Three or more spontaneous abortions
4. Patient or husband with chromosome anomaly
5. Family history of chromosome anomaly
6. Possible female carrier of X-linked disease
7. Metabolic disease risk (because of previous experience or family history)
8. NTD risk (because of previous experience or family history)
9. Positive second-trimester maternal serum screen

Currently, so many metabolic diseases can be diagnosed prenatally by amniocentesis that when the history elicits the possible presence of a metabolic disease, it is prudent to check with a major center to ascertain the availability of a diagnostic method.

Amniocentesis generally is carried out at 15 to 17 weeks of gestation but can be offered earlier (12–14 weeks). The underlying risk of amniocentesis when performed at 15 weeks of gestation and beyond is increased risk of miscarriage. This risk is estimated at 1 in 200 (0.5%), which is approximately the risk of Down syndrome in a 35-year-old woman. When amniocentesis is performed prior to 15 weeks, the miscarriage rate is slightly increased. Table 3–7 lists some of the conditions that now can be diagnosed prenatally by biochemical means.

B. Chorionic Villus Sampling

Chorionic villus sampling (CVS) is a technique used in the first trimester to obtain villi for cytogenetic testing. Most commonly, it is performed transcervically; however, transabdominal routes may also be attempted. The value of CVS is that it can be performed earlier in the pregnancy, and thus the decision of pregnancy termination can be made earlier. The downfall of CVS, however, is a slightly higher miscarriage rate of 1–5% and an association with distal limb defects. These risks appear to be dependent on operator experience, and lower numbers have been reported when CVS is performed between 10 and 12 weeks of gestation.

Karyotyping & Fluorescence In Situ Hybridization Analysis

Once the fetal cells are obtained, they must be processed. Formal karyotyping should be performed on all specimens. This involves culturing the cells, replication, and eventually karyotyping. The entire process often takes 10–14 days until the final report becomes available. Fortunately, a quicker

Table 3–7. Examples of hereditary diseases diagnosable prenatally.

Lipidoses: Gaucher's, Tay-Sachs, Fabry's, etc.
Mucopolysaccharidoses: Hurler's, Hunter's, etc.
Aminoacidurias: Cystinosis, homocystinuria, maple syrup urine disease, etc.
Diseases of carbohydrate metabolism: Glucose-6-phosphate dehydrogenase deficiency, glycogen storage disease, etc.
Miscellaneous: Adrenogenital syndrome, Lesch-Nyhan syndrome, sickle cell disease, cystic fibrosis, Huntington's disease, etc.

analysis can be obtained for some of the most common chromosomal anomalies.

The fluorescence in situ hybridization (FISH) study is a rapid assay for the detection of specific chromosomal aneuploidies using fluorescent-labeled DNA probes. Currently, probes exist for chromosomes 13, 18, 21, and 22, as well as the X and Y sex chromosomes among others. The average time to obtain a result is 24 hours. However, certain chromosomal probes may return as quickly as 4 hours. The more rapid turnaround time can be attained because the probes are mixed with uncultured amniocytes obtained from amniotic fluid or cells from CVS. If a patient is late in gestation or if the ultrasound is highly suggestive of a certain chromosomal composite, FISH analysis may be an appropriate study. With the development of multicolor FISH, all human chromosomes are painted in 24 different colors, allowing identification of chromosome rearrangement.

Single Gene Defects

If 1 parent is affected and the condition is caused by an autosomal dominant disorder, the chances are 1 in 2 that a child will be affected. If both parents are carriers of an autosomal recessive condition, the chances are 1 in 4 that the child will be affected and 1 in 2 that the child will be a carrier. Carrier status of both parents can be assumed if an affected child has been produced or if a carrier testing program is available and such testing determines that both parents are carriers. Tay-Sachs disease and sickle cell disease detection programs are examples of the latter possibility.

When carrier testing is available and the couple is at risk, as with Tay-Sachs disease in Jewish couples and sickle cell disease in blacks, the physician should order these carrier tests before pregnancy is undertaken, or immediately if the patient is already pregnant. When parents are carriers and pregnancy has been diagnosed, prenatal diagnostic testing is indicated if a test is available. If a physician does not know whether or not a test exists or how to obtain the test, the local genetic counseling program, local chapter of the National Foundation/March of Dimes, or state health department should be called for consultation. These sources may be able to inform the physician about new research that may have produced a prenatal test. A new test may be likely because this area of research is very dynamic. If genetic counseling services are readily available, patients with specific problems should be referred to those agencies for consultation. It is impossible for a physician to keep track of all of the current developments in the myriad conditions caused by single gene defects.

X-linked traits are frequently amenable to prenatal diagnostic testing. When such tests are not available, the couple has the option of testing for the sex of the fetus. If a fetus is noted to be a female, the odds are overwhelming that it will not be affected, although a carrier state may be present. If the fetus is a male, the chances are 1 in 2 that it will be affected. With this information, the couple can decide whether or not to continue the pregnancy in the case of a male fetus. Again, checking with genetic counseling agencies may reveal a prenatal diagnostic test that has only recently been described or information such as gene linkage studies that may apply in the individual case.

All options should be presented in a nonjudgmental fashion with no attempt to persuade, based on the best information available at the time. The couple should be encouraged to decide on a course of action that suits their particular needs. If the decision is appropriate, it should be supported by the physician and the genetic counselor. Very rarely, the patient will make a decision the physician regards as unwise or unrealistic. Such a decision may be based on superstition, religious or mystical beliefs, simple naiveté, or even personality disorder. The physician should make every attempt to clarify the issues for the patient. Rarely, other resources such as family members or spiritual leaders may be consulted in strict confidence. The physician and the genetic counselor must clearly set forth the circumstances of the problem in the record, in case the patient undertakes a course of action that ends in tragedy and perhaps attempts to blame the professional counselors for not preventing it.

Genetic Counseling

Genetic counseling involves interaction between the physician, the family, and the genetic counselor. It is the physician's responsibility to utilize the services of the genetic consultant in the best interest of the patient. The genetic counselor will take a formal family history and construct a family tree (Fig. 3–4). The assessment of the underlying general population risk of a disease and the specific family risk should be provided. When a specific diagnosis is known in the proband

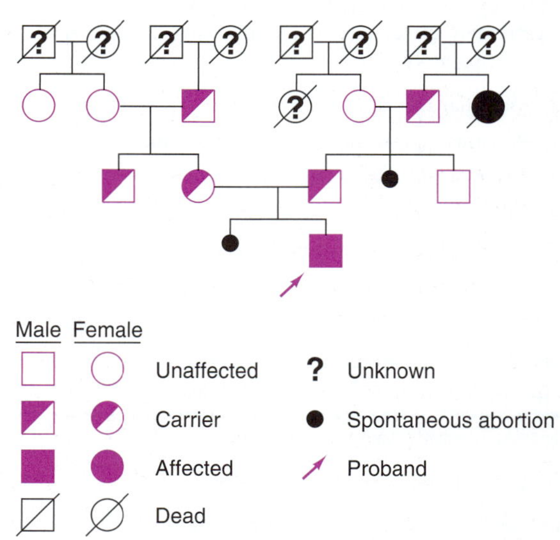

▲ Figure 3–4. Pedigree showing unaffected offspring, carrier offspring, and affected offspring in a family with an autosomal recessive trait (sickle cell anemia).

and the relatives are dead or otherwise not available, the counselor may ask to see photographs, which may show characteristics of the suspected condition. In many cases, when the pedigree is constructed, the inheritance pattern can be determined. If this can be done, the relative risks that future progeny will be affected can be estimated. This pedigree information is also useful in discussing the case with a genetic counselor.

GYNECOLOGIC CORRELATES

THE CHROMOSOMAL BASIS OF SEX DETERMINATION

Syngamy

The sex of the fetus normally is determined at fertilization. The cells of normal females contain 2 X chromosomes; those of normal males contain 1 X and 1 Y. During meiotic reduction, half of the male gametes receive a Y chromosome and the other half an X chromosome. Because the female has 2 X chromosomes, all female gametes contain an X chromosome. If a Y-bearing gamete fertilizes an ovum, the fetus is male; conversely, if an X-bearing gamete fertilizes an ovum, the fetus is female.

Arithmetically, the situation described previously should yield a male/female sex ratio of 100—the sex ratio being defined as 100 times the number of males divided by the number of females. However, for many years, the male/female sex ratio of the newborns in the white population has been approximately 105. Apparently the sex ratio at fertilization is even higher than at birth; most data on the sex of abortuses indicate a preponderance of males.

Abnormalities of Meiosis and Mitosis

The discussion in this section is limited to anomalies of meiosis and mitosis that result in some abnormality in the sex chromosome complement of the embryo.

Chromosome studies in connection with various clinical conditions suggest that errors in meiosis and mitosis do indeed occur. These errors result in any of the following principal effects: (1) an extra sex chromosome, (2) an absent sex chromosome, (3) 2 cell lines having different sex chromosomes and arising by mosaicism, (4) 2 cell lines having different sex chromosomes and arising by chimerism, (5) a structurally abnormal sex chromosome, and (6) a sex chromosome complement inconsistent with the phenotype.

By and large, an extra or a missing sex chromosome arises as the result of an error of disjunction in meiosis I or II in either the male or the female. In meiosis I, this means that instead of each of the paired homologous sex chromosomes going to the appropriate daughter cell, both go to 1 cell, leaving that cell with an extra sex chromosome and the daughter cell with none. Failure of disjunction in meiosis II simply means that the centromere fails to divide normally.

A variation of this process, known as anaphase lag, occurs when 1 of the chromosomes is delayed in arriving at the daughter cell and thus is lost. Theoretically, chromosomes may be lost by failure of association in prophase and by failure of replication, but these possibilities have not been demonstrated.

Persons who have been found to have 2 cell lines apparently have experienced problems in mitosis in the very early stage of embryogenesis. Thus, if there is nondisjunction or anaphase lag in an early (first, second, or immediately subsequent) cell division in the embryo, mosaicism may be said to exist. In this condition, there are 2 cell lines; 1 has a normal number of sex chromosomes, and the other is deficient in a sex chromosome or has an extra number of sex chromosomes. A similar situation exists in chimerism, except that there may be a difference in the sex chromosome: 1 may be an X and 1 may be a Y. This apparently arises by dispermy, by the fertilization of a double oocyte, or by the fusion, very early in embryogenesis, of 2 separately fertilized oocytes. Each of these conditions has been produced experimentally in animals.

Structural abnormalities of the sex chromosomes—deletion of the long or short arm or the formation of an isochromosome (2 short arms or 2 long arms)—result from injury to the chromosomes during meiosis. How such injuries occur is not known, but the results are noted more commonly in sex chromosomes than in autosomes—perhaps because serious injury to an autosome is much more likely to be lethal than injury to an X chromosome, and surviving injured X chromosomes would therefore be more common.

The situation in which there is a sex chromosome complement with an inappropriate genotype arises in special circumstances of true hermaphroditism and XX males (see later sections).

The X Chromosome in Humans

At about day 16 of embryonic life, there appears on the undersurface of the nuclear membrane of the somatic cells of human females a structure 1 μm in diameter known as the X-chromatin body. There is genetic as well as cytogenetic evidence that this is 1 of the X chromosomes (the only chromosome visible by ordinary light microscopy during interphase). In a sense, therefore, all females are hemizygous with respect to the X chromosome. However, there are genetic reasons for believing that the X chromosome is not entirely inactivated during the process of formation of the X-chromatin body. In normal females, inactivation of the X chromosome during interphase and its representation as the X-chromatin body are known as the Lyon phenomenon (for Mary Lyon, a British geneticist). This phenomenon may involve, at random, either the maternal or the paternal X chromosome. Furthermore, once the particular chromosome has been selected early in embryogenesis, it is always the same X chromosome that is inactivated in the progeny of that particular cell. Geneticists have found that the ratio of maternal to paternal X chromosomes inactivated is approximately 1:1.

The germ cells of an ovary are an exception to the X inactivation concept in that X inactivation does not characterize the meiotic process. Apparently, meiosis is impossible without 2 genetically active X chromosomes. Although random structural damage to 1 of the X chromosomes seems to cause meiotic arrest, oocyte loss, and therefore failure of ovarian development, an especially critical area necessary for oocyte development has been identified on the long arm of the X. This essential area involves almost all of the long arm and has been specifically located from Xq13 to Xq26. If this area is broken in 1 of the X chromosomes as in a deletion or translocation, oocyte development does not occur. However, a few exceptions to this rule have been described.

It is a curious biologic phenomenon that if 1 of the X chromosomes is abnormal, it is always this chromosome that is genetically inactivated and becomes the X-chromatin body, regardless of whether it is maternal or paternal in origin. Although this general rule seems to be an exception to the randomness of X inactivation, this is more apparent than real. Presumably, random inactivation does occur, but the disadvantaged cells—ie, those left with a damaged active X—do not survive. Consequently, the embryo develops only with cells with a normal active X chromosome (X-chromatin body) (Fig. 3–5).

If there are more than 2 X chromosomes, all X chromosomes except 1 are genetically inactivated and become X-chromatin bodies; thus, in this case, the number of X-chromatin bodies will be equal to the number of X chromosomes minus 1. This

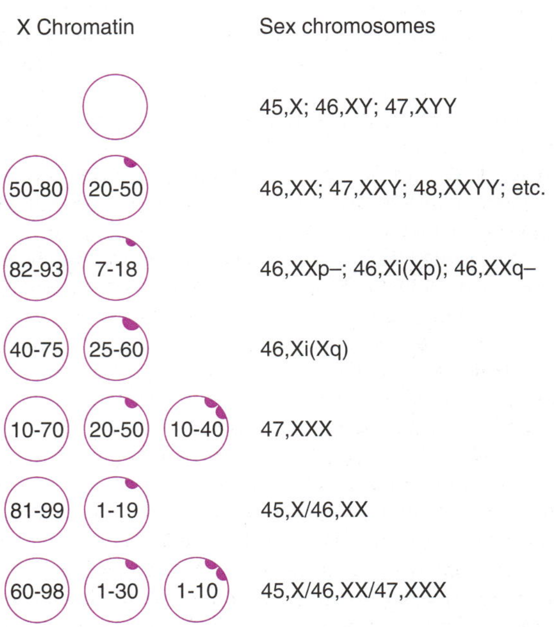

▲ **Figure 3–5.** Relation of X-chromatin body to the possible sex chromosome components.

type of inactivation applies to X chromosomes even when a Y chromosome is present, eg, in Klinefelter's syndrome.

Although the X chromosomes are primarily concerned with the determination of femininity, there is abundant genetic evidence that loci having to do with traits other than sex determination are present on the X chromosome. Thus, in the catalog of genetic disorders given in the 10th edition of *Mendelian Inheritance in Man*, 320 traits are listed as more or less definitely X-linked. Substantial evidence for X linkage has been found for about 160 of these traits; the rest are only suspected of having this relationship. Hemophilia, color blindness, childhood muscular dystrophy (Duchenne's dystrophy), Lesch-Nyhan syndrome, and glucose-6-phosphate dehydrogenase deficiency are among the better known conditions controlled by loci on the X chromosome. These entities probably arise from the expression of a recessive gene due to its hemizygous situation in males.

X-linked dominant traits are infrequent in humans. Vitamin D-resistant rickets is an example.

At least 1 disorder can be classified somewhere between a structural anomaly of the X chromosome and a single gene mutation. X-linked mental retardation in males is associated with a fragile site at q26, but a special culture medium is required for its demonstration. Furthermore, it has been shown that heterozygote female carriers for this fragile site have low IQ test scores.

The Y Chromosome in Humans

Just as the X chromosome is the only chromosome visible by ordinary light microscopy during interphase, the Y chromosome is the only chromosome visible in interphase, after exposure to quinacrine compounds, by fluorescence microscopy. This is a very useful diagnostic method.

In contrast to the X chromosome, few traits have been traced to the Y chromosome except those having to do with testicular formation and those at the very tip of the short arm, homologous with those at the tip of the short arm of the X. Possession of the Y chromosome alone, ie, without an X chromosome, apparently is lethal, because such a case has never been described.

Present on the Y chromosome is an area that produces a factor that allows for testicular development. This factor is termed testis-determining factor (TDF). Without the presence of TDF, normal female anatomy will develop. When TDF is present, testicular development occurs with subsequent differentiation of Sertoli cells. The Sertoli cells in turn produce a second factor central to male differentiation, müllerian-inhibiting factor (MIF), also termed antimüllerian factor (AMF). The presence of MIF causes the regression of the müllerian ducts and thereby allows for the development of normal internal male anatomy.

Y-Chromosome Microdeletion

In addition to sex determination function, human Y chromosome also has a role in spermatogenesis controlled by multiple genes along proximal Yq. The locus for spermatogenesis is on the euchromatic part of Yq (Yq11) called azoospermic factor (AZF). The AZF region is divided into three nonoverlapping regions AZFa, AZFb, and AZFc. The term "microdeletion" means that the size of the deleted segment is not visualized on karyotyping but must be discerned through molecular biology technique. There is no specific phenotype–genotype correlation between the degree of spermatogenic failure and type of Yq microdeletion. Complete deletion of AZFa and AZFb regions is associated with Sertoli cell-only syndrome and spermatogenic arrest, respectively. However, partial deletions of AZFa or AZFb or complete/partial deletions of AZFc are associated with a variable degree of spermatogenic failure ranging from oligozoospermia to Sertoli cell-only syndrome. There are reports of progressive impairment of spermatogenesis over time in patient with AZFc deletion. The fourth AZFd region, which was earlier proposed, does not exist based on the Y chromosome sequencing. There are many candidate genes within the deleted regions that are responsible for impaired spermatogenesis. The extensively studied genes are DAZ on AZFc region, RBMY1A1 on AZFb region, and USP9Y, DBY, and UTY on AZFa region. Because the deleted genes are expressed mainly in testes, men carrying the deletions have no abnormalities other than spermatogenic failure.

The incidence of Yq microdeletions in infertile men varies from 1–55% depending on study design. The most frequently deleted region is AZFc (~60%), whereas the deletion of the AZFa region is extremely rare (5%). The identification of Yq microdeletion has a prognostic value for the chance of successful testicular sperm retrieval. Men with complete deletion of AZFa and AZFb regions have almost no chance of having sperm recovered from surgical testicular sperm retrieval procedure, and no treatment is presently available for their fertility problem besides the use of donor sperm.

In the past, the majority of cases of Yq microdeletions have been de novo in infertile men during embryogenesis or from meiotic error in the germline of the fertile father. However, with the advent of assisted reproductive technologies, these infertile men can conceive genetic offspring with intracytoplasmic sperm injection (ICSI) technique, so Yq microdeletion can pass from generation to generation. A few studies show that when a Yq microdeletion is present in infertile men, ICSI-derived sons will inherit the same deletion. In view of genetic counseling, although Yq microdeletion is transmitted to the male offspring, the phenotype of male offspring regarding the degree of spermatogenesis is unpredictable due to the influence of the presence or absence of environmental factors that could affect spermatogenesis and the period of lifetime when spermatogenesis is assessed.

ABNORMAL DEVELOPMENT

1. Ovarian Agenesis–Dysgenesis

In 1938, Turner described 7 girls 15–23 years of age with sexual infantilism, webbing of the neck, cubitus valgus, and retardation of growth. A survey of the literature indicates that "Turner's syndrome" means different things to different writers. After the later discovery that ovarian streaks are characteristically associated with the clinical entity described by Turner, "ovarian agenesis" became a synonym for Turner's syndrome. After discovery of the absence of the X-chromatin body in such patients, the term ovarian agenesis gave way to "gonadal dysgenesis," "gonadal agenesis," or "gonadal aplasia."

Meanwhile, some patients with the genital characteristics mentioned previously were shown to have a normally positive X-chromatin count. Furthermore, a variety of sex chromosome complements have been found in connection with streak gonads. As if these contradictions were not perplexing enough, it has been noted that streaks are by no means confined to patients with Turner's original tetrad of infantilism, webbing of the neck, cubitus valgus, and retardation of growth but may be present in girls with sexual infantilism only. Since Turner's original description, a host of additional somatic anomalies (varying in frequency) have been associated with his original clinical picture; these include shield chest, overweight, high palate, micrognathia, epicanthal folds, low-set ears, hypoplasia of nails, osteoporosis, pigmented moles, hypertension, lymphedema, cutis laxa, keloids, coarctation of the aorta, mental retardation, intestinal telangiectasia, and deafness.

For our purposes, the eponym Turner's syndrome will be used to indicate sexual infantilism with ovarian streaks, short stature, and 2 or more of the somatic anomalies mentioned earlier. In this context, terms such as ovarian agenesis, gonadal agenesis, and gonadal dysgenesis lose their clinical significance and become merely descriptions of the gonadal development of the person. At least 21 sex chromosome complements have been associated with streak gonads (Fig. 3–6), but only about 9 sex chromosome complements have been associated with Turner's syndrome. However, approximately two-thirds of patients with Turner's syndrome have a 45,X chromosome complement, whereas only one-fourth of patients without Turner's syndrome but with streak ovaries have a 45,X chromosome complement.

Karyotype–phenotype correlations in the syndromes associated with ovarian agenesis are not completely satisfactory. Nonetheless, if gonadal development is considered as 1 problem and if the somatic difficulties associated with these syndromes are considered as a separate problem, one can make certain correlations.

With respect to failure of gonadal development, it is important to recall that diploid germ cells require 2 normal active X chromosomes. This is in contrast to the somatic cells, where only 1 sex chromosome is thought to be genetically active, at least after day 16 of embryonic life in the human, when the X-chromatin body first appears in the somatic cells. It is also important to recall that in 45,X persons no oocytes persist, and streak gonads are the rule. From these facts, it can be inferred that failure of gonadal development is not the result of a specific sex chromosome

45,X
46,XX
46,XY
46,XXp–
46,XXq–
46,Xi(Xp)
46,Xi(Xq)
46,XXq–?
45,X/46,XX
45,X/46,XY
45,X/46,Xi(Xq)
45,X/46,XXp–
45,X/46,XXq–
45,X/46,XXq–?
45,X/46,XX }
45,X/46,Xi(Xq) }
45,X/46,XX/47,XXX }
45,X/47,XXX }
45,X/46,XX/47,XXX }
45,X/46,Xi(Xq)/47,XXX }
45,X/46,XXr(X)
45,X/46,XX/46,XXr(X)
45,X/46,XXr(X)/47,XXr(X)r(X)
45,X/46,XX/47,XXX }
45,X/46,XXq– }

▲ **Figure 3–6.** The 21 sex chromosome complements that have been found in patients with streak gonads.

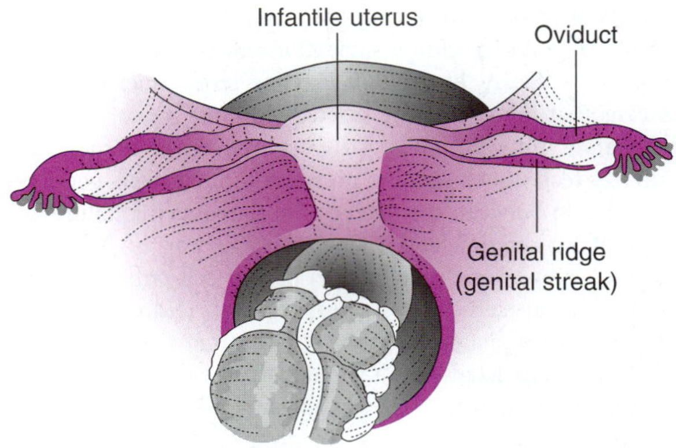

▲ **Figure 3–7.** Gonadal streaks in a patient with the phenotype of Turner's syndrome. (Redrawn and reproduced, with permission, from Jones HW Jr, Scott WW. *Hermaphroditism, Genital Anomalies and Related Endocrine Disorders.* 2nd ed. Philadelphia, PA: Williams & Wilkins; 1971.)

defect but rather of the absence of 2 X chromosomes with the necessary critical zones.

Karyotype–phenotype correlations with respect to somatic abnormalities are even sketchier than the correlations with regard to gonadal development. However, good evidence shows that monosomy for the short arm of the X chromosome is related to somatic difficulties, although some patients with long-arm deletions have somatic abnormalities.

History of Gonadal Agenesis

The histologic findings in these abnormal ovaries in patients with gonadal streaks are essentially the same regardless of the patient's cytogenetic background (Fig. 3–7).

Fibrous tissue is the major component of the streak. It is indistinguishable microscopically from that of the normal ovarian stroma. The so-called germinal epithelium, on the surface of the structure, is a layer of low cuboid cells; this layer appears to be completely inactive.

Tubules of the ovarian rete are invariably found in sections taken from about the midportion of the streak.

In all patients who have reached the age of normal puberty, hilar cells are also demonstrated. The number of hilar cells varies among patients. In those with some enlargement of the clitoris, hilar cells are present in large numbers. These developments may be causally related. Nevertheless, hilar cells are also found in many normal ovaries. The origin of hilar cells is not precisely known, but they are associated with development of the medullary portion of the gonad. Their presence lends further support to the concept that in ovarian agenesis the gonad develops along normal lines until just before the expected appearance of early oocytes. In all cases in which sections of the broad ligament have been available for study, it has been possible to identify the mesonephric duct and tubules—broad ligament structures found in normal females.

Clinical Findings

A. Symptoms & Signs

1. In newborn infants—The newborn with streak ovaries often shows edema of the hands and feet. Histologically, this edema is associated with large dilated vascular spaces. With such findings, it is obviously desirable to obtain a karyotype. However, some children with streak ovaries—particularly those who have few or no somatic abnormalities—cannot be recognized at birth.

2. In adolescents—The arresting and characteristic clinical finding in many of these patients is their short stature. Typical patients seldom attain a height of 1.5 m (5 ft) (Fig. 3–8). In addition, sexual infantilism is a striking finding. As mentioned earlier, a variety of somatic abnormalities may be present; by definition, if 2 or more of these are noted, the patient may be considered to have Turner's syndrome. Most of these patients have only 1 normal X chromosome, and two-thirds of them have no other sex chromosome. Patients of normal height without somatic abnormalities may also have gonadal streaks. Under these circumstances, there is likely to be a cell line with 2 normal sex chromosomes but

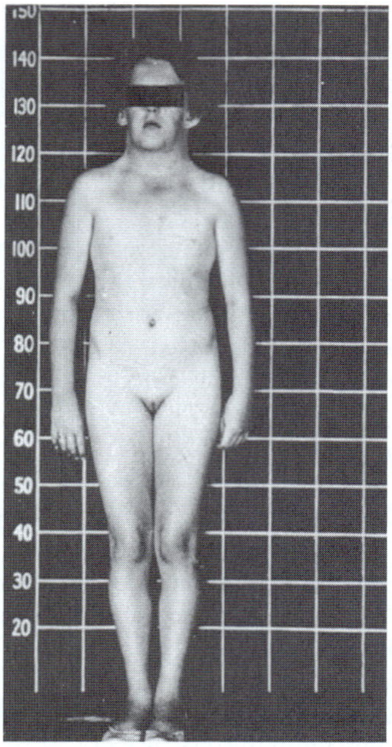

▲ **Figure 3–8.** Patient with Turner's syndrome. *(Reproduced, with permission, from Jones HW Jr, Scott WW. Hermaphroditism, Genital Anomalies and Related Endocrine Disorders.* 2nd ed. Philadelphia, PA: Williams & Wilkins; 1971.)

often a second line with a single X. The internal findings are exactly the same as in patients with classic Turner's syndrome, however.

B. Laboratory Findings

An important finding in patients of any age—but especially after expected puberty, ie, about 12 years—is elevation of total gonadotropin production. From a practical point of view, ovarian failure in patients over age 15 cannot be considered a diagnostic possibility unless the serum follicle-stimulating hormone level is more than 50 mIU/mL and luteinizing hormone level is more than 90 mIU/mL.

Nongonadal endocrine functions are normal. Urinary excretion of estrogens is low, and the maturation index and other vaginal smear indices are shifted well to the left.

▶ Treatment

Substitution therapy with estrogen is necessary for development of secondary characteristics.

Therapy with growth hormone will increase height. Whether ultimate height will be greater than it otherwise would be is uncertain, but current evidence suggests that it will be.

The incidence of malignant degeneration is increased in the gonadal streaks of patients with a Y chromosome, as compared with normal males. Surgical removal of streaks from all patients with a Y chromosome is recommended.

2. True Hermaphroditism

By classic definition, true hermaphroditism exists when both ovarian and testicular tissue can be demonstrated in 1 patient. In humans, the Y chromosome carries genetic material that normally is responsible for testicular development; this material is active even when multiple X chromosomes are present. Thus, in Klinefelter's syndrome, a testis develops with up to 4 Xs and only 1 Y. Conversely (with rare exceptions), a testis has not been observed to develop in the absence of the Y chromosome. The exceptions are found in true hermaphrodites and XX males, in whom testicular tissue has developed in association with an XX sex chromosome complement.

▶ Clinical Findings

A. Symptoms & Signs

No exclusive features clinically distinguish true hermaphroditism from other forms of intersexuality. Hence, the diagnosis must be entertained in an infant with any form of intersexuality, except only those with a continuing virilizing influence, eg, congenital adrenal hyperplasia. Firm diagnosis is possible after the onset of puberty, when certain clinical features become evident, but the diagnosis can and should be made in infancy.

In the past, most true hermaphrodites have been reared as males because they have rather masculine-appearing external genitalia (Fig. 3–9). Nevertheless, with early diagnosis, most should be reared as females.

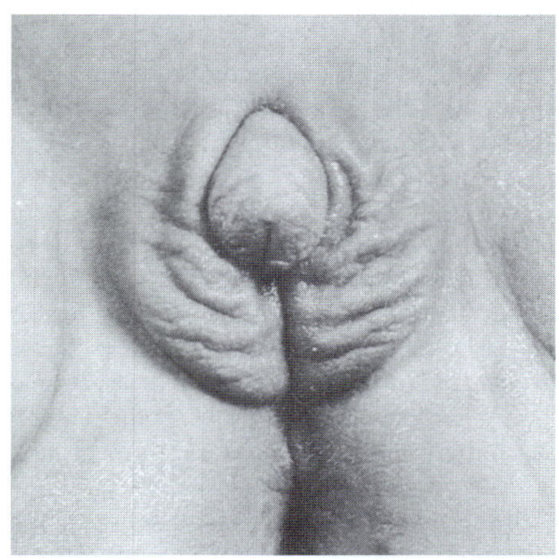

▲ **Figure 3–9.** External genitalia of a patient with true hermaphroditism. (Reproduced, with permission, from Jones HW Jr, Scott WW. *Hermaphroditism, Genital Anomalies and Related Endocrine Disorders.* 2nd ed. Philadelphia, PA: Williams & Wilkins; 1971.)

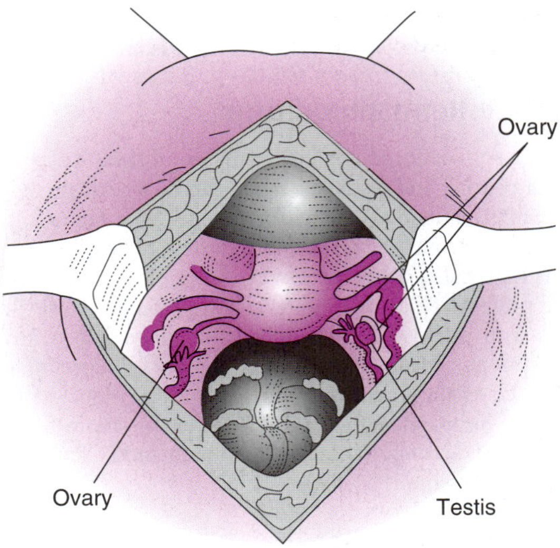

▲ **Figure 3–10.** Internal genitalia of a patient with true hermaphroditism. (Reproduced, with permission, from Jones HW Jr, Scott WW. *Hermaphroditism, Genital Anomalies and Related Endocrine Disorders.* 2nd ed. Philadelphia, PA: Williams & Wilkins; 1971.)

Almost all true hermaphrodites develop female-type breasts. This helps to distinguish male hermaphroditism from true hermaphroditism, because few male hermaphrodites other than those with familial feminizing hermaphroditism develop large breasts.

Many true hermaphrodites menstruate. The presence or absence of menstruation is partially determined by the development of the uterus; many true hermaphrodites have rudimentary or no development of the müllerian ducts (Fig. 3–10).

A few patients who had a uterus and menstruated after removal of testicular tissue have become pregnant and delivered normal children.

B. Sex Chromosome Complements

Most true hermaphrodites have X-chromatin bodies and karyotypes that are indistinguishable from those of normal females. In contrast to these, a few patients who cannot be distinguished clinically from other true hermaphrodites have been reported to have a variety of other karyotypes—eg, several chimeric persons with karyotypes of 46,XX/46,XY have been identified.

In true hermaphrodites, the testis is competent in its müllerian-suppressive functions, but an ovotestis may behave as an ovary insofar as its müllerian-suppressive function is concerned. The true hermaphroditic testis or ovotestis is as competent to masculinize the external genitalia as is the testis of a patient with the virilizing type of male hermaphroditism. This is unrelated to karyotype.

Deletion mapping by DNA hybridization has shown that most (but not all) XX true hermaphrodites have Y-specific sequences. Abnormal crossover of a portion of the Y chromosome to the X in meiosis may explain some cases. This latter statement is further supported by the finding of a positive H-Y antigen assay in some patients with 46,XX true hermaphroditism.

In general, the clinical picture of true hermaphroditism is not compatible with the clinical picture in other kinds of gross chromosomal anomalies. For example, very few true hermaphrodites have associated somatic anomalies, and mental retardation almost never occurs.

▶ Treatment

The principles of treatment of true hermaphroditism do not differ from those of the treatment of hermaphroditism in general. Therapy can be summarized by stating that surgical removal of contradictory organs is indicated, and the external genitalia should be reconstructed in keeping with the sex of rearing. The special problem in this group is how to establish with certainty the character of the gonad. This is particularly difficult in the presence of an ovotestis, because its recognition by gross characteristics is notoriously inaccurate, and one must not remove too much of the gonad for study. In some instances, the gonadal tissue of 1 sex is completely embedded within a gonadal structure primarily of the opposite sex.

3. Klinefelter's Syndrome

This condition, first described in 1942 by Klinefelter, Reifenstein, and Albright, occurs only in apparent males. As originally described, it is characterized by small testes, azoospermia, gynecomastia, relatively normal external genitalia, and otherwise average somatic development. High levels of gonadotropin in urine or serum are characteristic.

▶ Clinical Findings

A. Symptoms & Signs

By definition, this syndrome applies only to persons reared as males. The disease is not recognizable before puberty except by routine screening of newborn infants. Most patients come under observation at 16–40 years of age.

Somatic development during infancy and childhood may be normal. Growth and muscular development may also be within normal limits. Most patients have a normal general appearance and no complaints referable to this abnormality, which is often discovered during the course of a routine physical examination or an infertility study.

In the original publication by Klinefelter and coworkers, gynecomastia was considered an essential part of the syndrome. Since then, however, cases without gynecomastia have been reported.

The external genitalia are perfectly formed and in most patients are quite well developed. Erection and intercourse usually are satisfactory.

There is no history of delayed descent of the testes in typical cases, and the testes are in the scrotum. Neither is there any history of testicular trauma or disease. Although a history of mumps orchitis is occasionally elicited, this disease has not been correlated with the syndrome. However, the testes are often very small in contrast to the rest of the genitalia (about 1.5 × 1.5 cm).

Psychological symptoms are often present. Most studies of this syndrome have been performed in psychiatric institutions. The seriousness of the psychological disturbance seems to be partly related to the number of extra X chromosomes—eg, it is estimated that about one-fourth of XXY patients have some degree of mental retardation.

B. Laboratory Findings

One of the extremely important clinical features of Klinefelter's syndrome is the excessive amount of pituitary gonadotropin found in either urine or serum assay.

The urinary excretion of neutral 17-ketosteroids varies from relatively normal to definitely subnormal levels. There is a rough correlation between the degree of hypoleydigism as judged clinically and a low 17-ketosteroid excretion rate.

C. Histologic & Cytogenetic Findings

Klinefelter's syndrome may be regarded as a form of primary testicular failure.

Several authors have classified a variety of forms of testicular atrophy as subtypes of Klinefelter's syndrome. Be this as it may, Klinefelter believed that only those patients who have a chromosomal abnormality could be said to have this syndrome. Microscopic examination of the adult testis shows that the seminiferous tubules lack epithelium and are shrunken and hyalinized. They contain large amounts of elastic fibers, and Leydig cells are present in large numbers.

Males with positive X-chromatin bodies are likely to have Klinefelter's syndrome. The nuclear sex anomaly reflects a basic genetic abnormality in sex chromosome constitution. All cases studied have had at least 2 X chromosomes and 1 Y chromosome. The most common abnormality in the sex chromosome constitution is XXY, but the literature also records XXXY, XXYY, XXXXY, and XXXYY, and mosaics of XX/XXY, XY/XXY, XY/XXXY, and XXXY/XXXXY. In all examples except the XX/XXY mosaic, a Y chromosome is present in all cells. From these patterns, it is obvious that the Y chromosome has a very strong testis-forming impulse, which can operate in spite of the presence of as many as 4 X chromosomes.

Thus, patients with Klinefelter's syndrome will have not only a positive X-chromatin body but also a positive Y-chromatin body.

The abnormal sex chromosome constitution causes differentiation of an abnormal testis, leading to testicular failure in adulthood. At birth or before puberty, such testes show a marked deficiency or absence of germinal cells.

By means of nursery screening, the frequency of males with positive X-chromatin bodies has been estimated to be 2.65 per 1000 live male births.

Treatment

There is no treatment for the 2 principal complaints of these patients: infertility and gynecomastia. No pituitary preparation has been effective in the regeneration of the hyalinized tubular epithelium or the stimulation of gametogenesis. Furthermore, no hormone regimen is effective in treating the breast hypertrophy. When the breasts are a formidable psychological problem, surgical removal may be a satisfactory procedure. In patients who have clinical symptoms of hypoleydigism, substitution therapy with testosterone is an important physiologic and psychological aid. Donor sperm may be offered for treatment of infertility.

4. Double-X Males

A few cases of adult males with a slightly hypoplastic penis and very small testes but no other indication of abnormal sexual development have been reported. These males are sterile. Unlike those with Klinefelter's syndrome, they do not have abnormal breast development. They are clinically very similar to patients with Del Castillo's syndrome (testicular dysgenesis). Nevertheless, the XX males have a positive sex chromatin and a normal female karyotype. These may be extreme examples of the sex reversal that usually is partial in true hermaphroditism.

5. Multiple-X Syndromes

The finding of more than 1 X-chromatin body in a cell indicates the presence of more than 2 X chromosomes in that particular cell. In many patients, such a finding is associated with mosaicism, and the clinical picture is controlled by this fact—eg, if 1 of the strains of the mosaicism is 45,X, gonadal agenesis is likely to occur. There also are persons who do not seem to have mosaicism but do have an abnormal number of X chromosomes in all cells. In such persons, the most common complement is XXX (triplo-X syndrome), but XXXX (tetra-X syndrome) and XXXXX (penta-X syndrome) have been reported.

An additional X chromosome does not seem to have a consistent effect on sexual differentiation. The body proportions of these persons are normal, and the external genitalia are normally female. A number of such persons have been examined at laparotomy, and no consistent abnormality of the ovary has been found. In a few cases, the number of follicles appeared to be reduced, and in at least 1 case the ovaries were very small and the ovarian stroma poorly differentiated. About 20% of postpubertal patients with the triplo-X syndrome report various degrees of amenorrhea or some irregularity in menstruation. For the most part, however, these patients have a normal menstrual history and are of proved fertility.

Almost all patients known to have multiple-X syndromes have some degree of mental retardation. A few have mongoloid features. (The mothers of these patients tended to be older than the mothers of normal children, as is true with Down syndrome.) Perhaps these findings are in part circumstantial, as most of these patients were discovered during surveys in mental institutions. The important clinical point is that mentally retarded infants should have chromosomal study.

Uniformly, the offspring of triplo-X mothers have been normal. This is surprising, because theoretically in such cases meiosis should produce equal numbers of ova containing 1 or 2 X chromosomes, and fertilization of the abnormal XX ova should give rise to XXX and XXY individuals. Nevertheless, the triplo-X condition seems selective for normal ova and zygotes.

The diagnosis of this syndrome is made by identifying a high percentage of cells with double X-chromatin bodies in the buccal smear and by finding 47 chromosomes with a karyotype showing an extra X chromosome in all cells cultured from the peripheral blood. It should be noted that in the examination of the buccal smear, some cells have a single X-chromatin body. Hence, based on the chromatin examination, one might suspect XX/XXX mosaicism. Actually, in triplo-X patients, only a single type of cell can be demonstrated in cultures of cells from the peripheral blood. The absence of the second X-chromatin body in some of the somatic cells may result from the time of examination of the cell (during interphase) and from the spatial orientation, which could have prevented visualization of the 2 X-chromatin bodies (adjacent to the nuclear membrane). In this syndrome, the number of cells containing either 1 or 2 X-chromatin bodies is very high—at least 60–80%, as compared with an upper limit of about 40% in normal females.

6. Female Hermaphroditism due to Congenital Adrenal Hyperplasia

ESSENTIALS OF DIAGNOSIS

- Female pseudohermaphroditism, ambiguous genitalia with clitoral hypertrophy, and, occasionally, persistent urogenital sinus.
- Early appearance of sexual hair; hirsutism, dwarfism.
- Urinary 17-ketosteroids elevated; pregnanetriol may be increased.
- Elevated serum 17-hydroxyprogesterone level.
- Occasionally associated with water and electrolyte imbalance—particularly in the neonatal period.

General Considerations

Female hermaphroditism due to congenital adrenal hyperplasia is a clearly delineated clinical syndrome. The syndrome has been better understood since the discovery that cortisone may successfully arrest virilization. The problem usually is due to a deficiency of a gene required for 21-hydroxylation in the biosynthesis of cortisol.

If the diagnosis is not made in infancy, an unfortunate series of events ensues. Because the adrenals secrete an abnormally large amount of virilizing steroid even during embryonic life, these infants are born with abnormal genitalia (Fig. 3–11). In extreme cases, there is fusion of the scrotolabial folds and, in rare instances, even formation of a penile urethra. The clitoris is greatly enlarged so that it may be mistaken for a penis (Fig. 3–12). No gonads are palpable within the fused scrotolabial folds, and their absence has sometimes given rise to the mistaken impression of male cryptorchidism. Usually, there is a single urinary meatus at the base of the phallus, and the vagina enters the persistent urogenital sinus as noted in Figure 3–13.

During infancy, provided there are no serious electrolyte disturbances, these children grow more rapidly than normal. For a time, they greatly exceed the average in both height and weight. Unfortunately, epiphyseal closure occurs by about age 10, and as a result, these people are much shorter than normal as adults (Fig. 3–14).

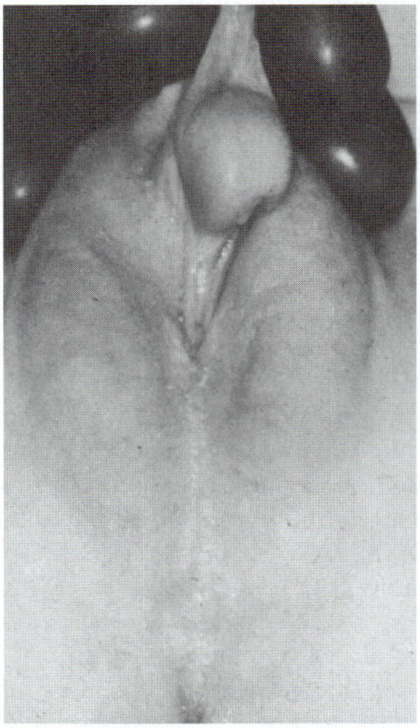

▲ **Figure 3–11.** External genitalia of a female patient with congenital virilizing adrenal hyperplasia. Compare with Figure 3–12. (Reproduced, with permission, from Jones HW Jr, Scott WW. *Hermaphroditism, Genital Anomalies and Related Endocrine Disorders.* 2nd ed. Philadelphia, PA: Williams & Wilkins; 1971.)

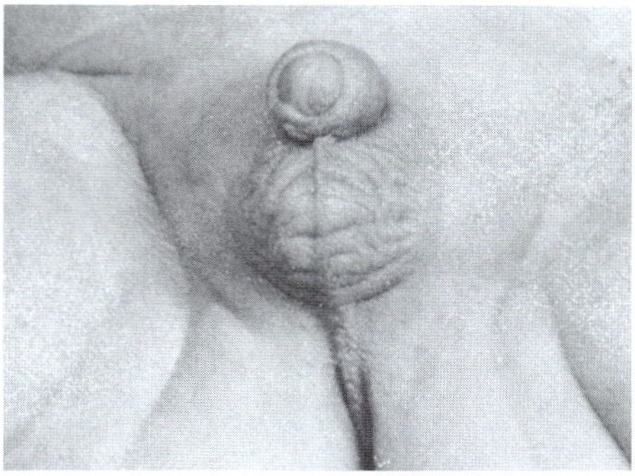

▲ **Figure 3–12.** External genitalia of a female patient with congenital virilizing adrenal hyperplasia. This is a more severe deformity than that shown in Figure 3–11.

The process of virilization begins at an early age. Pubic hair may appear as early as age 2 years but usually somewhat later. This is followed by growth of axillary hair and finally by the appearance of body hair and a beard, which may be so thick as to require daily shaving. Acne may develop early. Puberty never ensues. There is no breast development. Menstruation does not occur. During the entire process, serum adrenal androgens and 17-hydroxyprogesterone levels are abnormally high.

Although our principal concern here is with this abnormality in females, it must be mentioned that adrenal hyperplasia of the adrenogenital type may also occur in males, in whom it is called macrogenitosomia precox. Sexual development progresses rapidly, and the sex organs attain adult size at an early age. Just as in the female, sexual hair and acne develop unusually early, and the voice becomes deep. The testes are usually in the scrotum; however, in early childhood they remain small and immature, although the genitalia are of adult dimensions. In adulthood, the testes usually enlarge and spermatogenesis occurs, allowing impregnation rates similar to those of a control population. Somatic development in the male corresponds to that of the female; as a child, the male exceeds the average in height and strength, but (if untreated) as an adult he is stocky, muscular, and well below average height.

Both the male and the female with this disorder—but especially the male—may have the complicating problem of electrolyte imbalance. In infancy, it is manifested by vomiting, progressive weight loss, and dehydration and may be fatal unless recognized promptly. The characteristic findings are an exceedingly low serum sodium level, low CO_2-combining power level, and high potassium level. The condition is sometimes misdiagnosed as congenital pyloric stenosis.

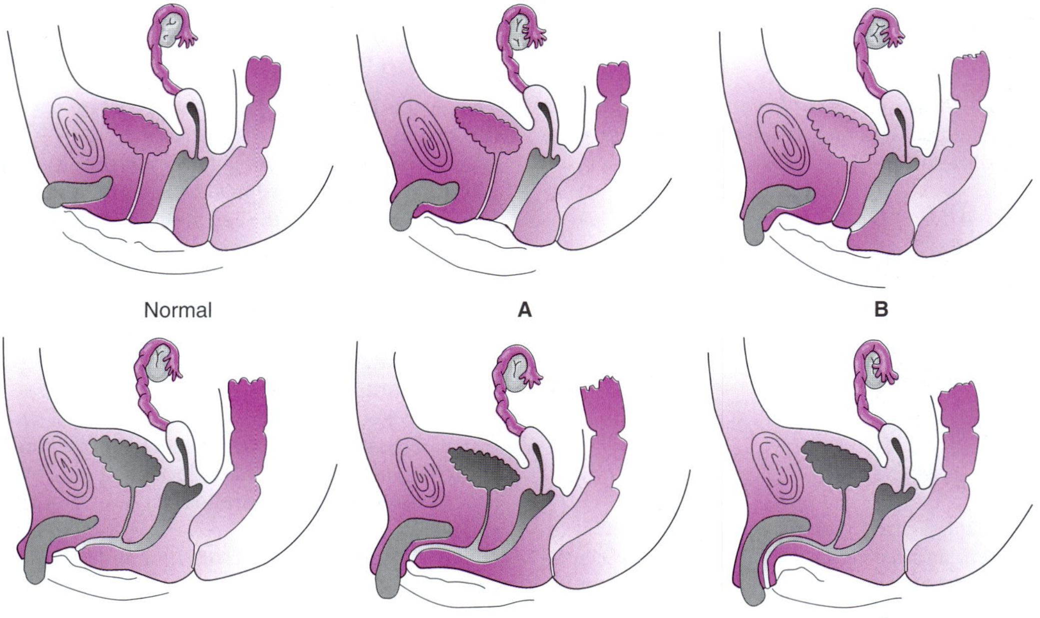

▲ **Figure 3–13.** Sagittal view of genital deformities of increasing severity **(A–E)** in congenital virilizing adrenal hyperplasia. (Redrawn and reproduced, with permission, from Verkauf BS, Jones HW Jr. Masculinization of the female genitalia in congenital adrenal hyperplasia. *South Med J* 1970;63:634–638.)

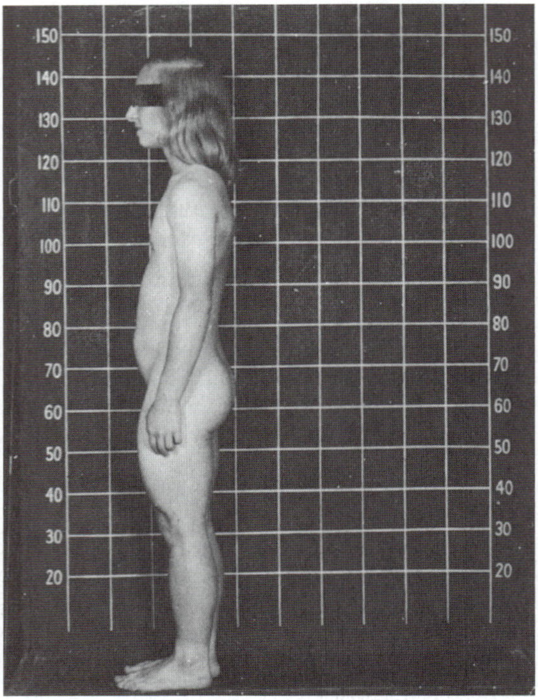

▲ **Figure 3–14.** Untreated adult with virilizing adrenal hyperplasia. Note the short stature and the relative shortness of the limbs. (Reproduced, with permission, from Jones HW Jr, Scott WW. *Hermaphroditism, Genital Anomalies and Related Endocrine Disorders.* 2nd ed. Philadelphia, PA: Williams & Wilkins; 1971.)

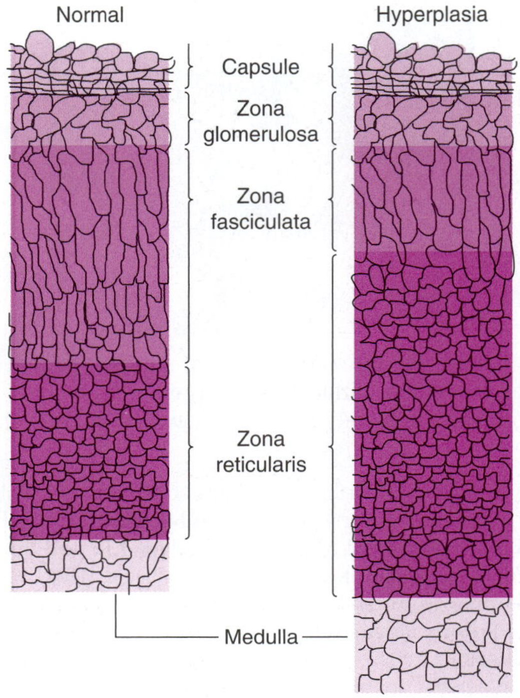

▲ **Figure 3–15.** Normal adrenal architecture and adrenal histology in congenital virilizing adrenal hyperplasia. Note the great relative increase in the zona reticularis.

A few of these patients have a deficiency in 11-hydroxylation that is associated with hypertension in addition to virilization.

Adrenal Histology

The adrenal changes center on a reticular hyperplasia, which becomes more marked as the patient grows older. In some instances, the glomerulosa may participate in the hyperplasia, but the fasciculata is greatly diminished in amount or entirely absent. Lipid studies show absence of fascicular and glomerular lipid but an abnormally strong lipid reaction in the reticularis (Fig. 3–15).

Ovarian Histology

The ovarian changes can be summarized by stating that in infants, children, and teenagers, there is normal follicular development to the antrum stage but no evidence of ovulation. With increasing age, less and less follicular activity occurs, and primordial follicles disappear. This disappearance must not be complete, however, because cortisone therapy, even in adults, usually results in ovulatory menstruation after 4–6 months of treatment.

Developmental Anomalies of the Genital Tubercle & Urogenital Sinus Derivatives

The phallus is composed of 2 lateral corpora cavernosa, but the corpus spongiosum is normally absent. The external urinary meatus is most often located at the base of the phallus (Fig. 3–11). An occasional case may be seen in which the urethra does extend to the end of the clitoris (Fig. 3–12). The glans penis and the prepuce are present and indistinguishable from these structures in the male. The scrotolabial folds are characteristically fused in the midline, giving a scrotum-like appearance with a median perineal raphe; however, they seldom enlarge to normal scrotal size. No gonads are palpable within the scrotolabial folds. When the anomaly is not severe (eg, in patients with postnatal virilization), fusion of the scrotolabial folds is not complete, and by gentle retraction it is often possible to locate not only the normally located external urinary meatus but also the orifice of the vagina.

An occasional patient has no communication between the urogenital sinus and the vagina. In no case does the vagina communicate with that portion of the urogenital sinus that gives rise to the female urethra or the prostatic urethra. Instead, the vaginal communication is via caudal urogenital sinus derivatives; thus, fortunately, the sphincter mechanism is not involved, and the anomalous communication is with

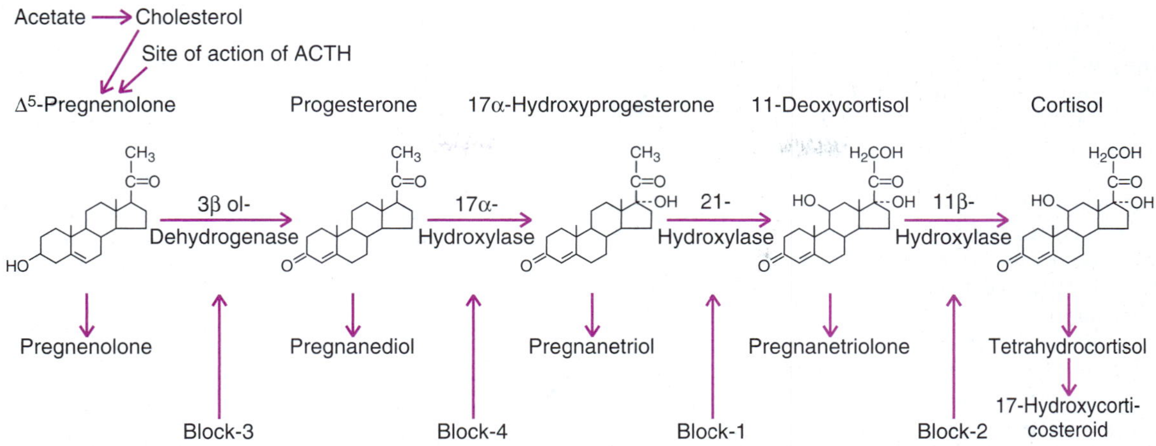

▲ **Figure 3–16.** Enzymatic steps in cortisol synthesis. Localization of defects in congenital adrenal hyperplasia.

that portion of the sinus that develops as the vaginal vestibule in the female and the membranous urethra in the male. From the gynecologist's point of view, it is much more meaningful to say that the vagina and (female) urethra enter a persistent urogenital sinus than to say that the vagina enters the (membranous [male]) urethra. This conclusion casts some doubt on the embryologic significance of the prostatic utricle, which is commonly said to represent the homologue of the vagina in the normal male.

Hormone Changes

Important and specific endocrine changes occur in congenital adrenal hyperplasia of the adrenogenital type. The ultimate diagnosis depends on demonstration of these abnormalities.

A. Urinary Estrogens

The progressive virilization of female hermaphrodites caused by adrenal hyperplasia would suggest that estrogen secretion in these patients is low, and this hypothesis is further supported by the atrophic condition of both the ovarian follicular apparatus and the estrogen target organs. Actually, the determination of urinary estrogens, both fluorometrically and biologically, indicates that it is elevated.

B. Serum Steroids

The development of satisfactory radioimmunoassay techniques for measuring steroids in blood serum has resulted in an increased tendency to measure serum steroids rather than urinary metabolites in diagnosing the condition and monitoring therapy. Serum steroid profiles of many patients with this disorder show that numerous defects in the biosynthesis of cortisol may occur. The most common defect is at the 21-hydroxylase step. Less frequent defects are at the 11-hydroxylase step and the 3β-ol-dehydrogenase step. Rarely, the defect is at the 17-hydroxylase step. In the most common form of the disorder—21-hydroxylase deficiency—the serum 17-hydroxyprogesterone level and, to a lesser extent, the serum progesterone level are elevated. This is easily understandable when it is recalled that 17-hydroxyprogesterone is the substrate for the 21-hydroxylation step (Fig. 3–16). Likewise, in the other enzyme defects, the levels of serum steroid substrates are greatly elevated.

Pathogenesis of Virilizing Adrenal Hyperplasia

The basic defects in congenital virilizing adrenal hyperplasia are 1 or more enzyme deficiencies in the biosynthesis of cortisol (Fig. 3–16). With the reduced production of cortisol, normal feedback to the hypothalamus fails, with the result that increased amounts of adrenocorticotropic hormone (ACTH) are produced. This excess production of ACTH stimulates the deficient adrenal gland to produce relatively normal amounts of cortisol—but also stimulates production of abnormally large amounts of estrogen and androgens by the zona reticularis. In this overproduction, a biologic preponderance of androgens causes virilization. These abnormal sex steroids suppress the gonadotropins so that untreated patients never reach puberty and do not menstruate.

Therefore, the treatment of this disorder consists in part of the administration of sufficient exogenous cortisol to suppress ACTH production to normal levels. This in turn should reduce overstimulation of the adrenal so that the adrenal will cease to produce abnormally large amounts of estrogen and androgen. The gonadotropins generally return to normal levels, with consequent feminization of the patient and achievement of menstruation.

The pathogenesis of the salt-losing type of adrenal hyperplasia involves a deficiency in aldosterone production.

Diagnosis

Hermaphroditism due to congenital adrenal hyperplasia must be suspected in any infant born with ambiguous or abnormal external genitalia. It is exceedingly important that the diagnosis be made at a very early age if undesirable disturbances of metabolism are to be prevented.

All patients with ambiguous external genitalia should have an appraisal of their chromosomal characteristics. In all instances of female pseudohermaphroditism due to congenital hyperplasia, the chromosomal composition is that of a normal female. A pelvic ultrasound in the newborn to determine the presence of a uterus is very helpful and, if positive, strongly suggests a female infant.

The critical determinations are those of the urinary 17-ketosteroid and serum 17-hydroxyprogesterone levels. If these are elevated, the diagnosis must be either congenital adrenal hyperplasia or tumor. In the newborn, the latter is very rare, but in older children and adults with elevated 17-ketosteroids, the possibility of tumor must be considered. One of the most satisfactory methods of making this different diagnosis is to attempt to suppress the excess androgens by administration of dexamethasone. In an adult or an older child, a suitable test dose of dexamethasone is 1.25 mg/45 kg (100 lb) body weight, given orally for 7 consecutive days. In congenital adrenal hyperplasia, there should be suppression of the urinary 17-ketosteroids on the seventh day of the test to less than 1 mg/24 h; in the presence of tumor, either there will be no effect or the 17-ketosteroid levels will rise.

Determination of urinary dehydroepiandrosterone (DHEA) or serum dehydroepiandrosterone sulfate (DHEAS) levels can also be helpful in differentiating congenital adrenal hyperplasia from an adrenal tumor. Levels in patients with congenital adrenal hyperplasia may be up to double the normal amount, whereas an adrenal tumor is usually associated with levels that are much higher than double the normal level.

Determination of the serum sodium and potassium levels and CO_2-combining power is also important to ascertain whether electrolyte balance is seriously disturbed.

Treatment

The treatment of female hermaphroditism due to congenital adrenal hyperplasia is partly medical and partly surgical. Originally, cortisone was administered; today, it is known that various cortisone derivatives are at least as effective. It is most satisfactory to begin treatment with relatively large doses of hydrocortisone divided in 3 doses orally for 7–10 days to obtain rapid suppression of adrenal activity. In young infants, the initial dose is about 25 mg/d; in older patients, 100 mg/d. After the output of 17-ketosteroids has decreased to a lower level, the dose should be reduced to the minimum amount required to maintain adequate suppression. This requires repeated measurements of plasma 17α-hydroxyprogesterone in order to individualize the dose.

It has been found that even with suppression of the urinary 17-ketosteroids to normal levels, the more sensitive serum 17-hydroxyprogesterone level may still be elevated. It seems difficult and perhaps undesirable to suppress the serum 17-hydroxyprogesterone values to normal because to do so may require doses of hydrocortisone that tend to cause cushingoid symptoms.

In the treatment of newborns with congenital adrenal hyperplasia who have a defect of electrolyte regulation, it is usually necessary to administer sodium chloride in amounts of 4–6 g/d, either orally or parenterally, in addition to cortisone. Furthermore, fludrocortisone acetate usually is required initially. The dose is entirely dependent on the levels of the serum electrolytes, which must be followed serially, but it is generally 0.05–0.1 mg/d.

In addition to the hormone treatment of this disorder, surgical correction of the external genitalia is usually necessary.

During acute illness or other stress, as well as during and after an operation, additional hydrocortisone is indicated to avoid the adrenal insufficiency of stress. Doubling the maintenance dose is usually adequate in such circumstances.

7. Female Hermaphroditism without Progressive Masculinization

Females with no adrenal abnormality may have fetal masculinization of the external genitalia with the same anatomic findings as in patients with congenital virilizing adrenal hyperplasia. Unlike patients with adrenogenital syndrome, patients without adrenal abnormality do not have elevated levels of serum steroids or urinary 17-ketosteroids, nor do they show precocious sexual development or the metabolic difficulties associated with adrenal hyperplasia as they grow older. At onset of puberty, normal feminization with menstruation and ovulation may be expected.

The diagnosis of female hermaphroditism not due to adrenal abnormality depends on the demonstration of a 46,XX karyotype and the finding of normal levels of serum steroids or normal levels of 17-ketosteroids in the urine. If fusion of the scrotolabial folds is complete, it is necessary to determine the exact relationship of the urogenital sinus to the urethra and vagina and to demonstrate the presence of a uterus by rectal examination or ultrasonography or endoscopic observation of the cervix. When there is a high degree of masculinization, the differential diagnosis between this condition and true hermaphroditism may be very difficult; an exploratory laparotomy may be required in some cases.

Classification

Patients with this problem may be seen because of a variety of conditions.

1. Exogenous androgen:
    a. Maternal ingestion of androgen
    b. Maternal androgenic tumor

c. Luteoma of pregnancy
d. Adrenal androgenic tumor

2. Idiopathic: No identifiable cause.
3. Special or nonspecific: The same as condition 2 except that it is associated with various somatic anomalies and with mental retardation.
4. Familial: A very rare anomaly.

8. Male Hermaphroditism

Persons with abnormal or ectopic testes may have external genitalia so ambiguous at birth that the true sex is not identifiable (Fig. 3–17). At puberty, these persons tend to become masculinized or feminized depending on factors to be discussed. Thus, the adult habitus of these persons may be typically male, ie, without breasts, or typically female, with good breast development. In some instances, the external genitalia may be indistinguishable from those of a normal female; in others, the clitoris may be enlarged; and in still other instances, there may be fusion of the labia in the midline, resulting in what seems to be a hypospadiac male. A deep or shallow vagina may be present. A cervix, a uterus, and uterine tubes may be developed to varying degrees; however, müllerian structures are often absent. Mesonephric structures may be grossly or microscopically visible. Body hair may be either typically feminine in its distribution and quantity or masculine in distribution and of sufficient quantity as to require plucking or shaving if the person is reared as a female. In a special group, axillary and pubic hair is congenitally absent. Although there is a well-developed uterus in some instances, all patients so far reported have been amenorrheic—in spite of the interesting theoretic possibility of uterine bleeding from endometrium stimulated by estrogen of testicular origin. There is no evidence of adrenal malfunction. In the feminized group, and less frequently in the nonfeminized group, there is a strong familial history of the disorder. Male hermaphrodites reared as females may marry and be well adjusted to their sex role. Others, especially when there has been equivocation regarding sex of rearing in infancy, may be less than attractive as women because of indecisive therapy. Psychiatric studies indicate that the best emotional adjustment comes from directing endocrine, surgical, and psychiatric measures toward improving the person's basic characteristics. Fortunately, this is consonant with the surgical and endocrine possibilities for those reared as females, because current operative techniques can produce more satisfactory feminine than masculine external genitalia. Furthermore, the testes of male hermaphrodites are nonfunctional as far as spermatogenesis is concerned. Only about one-third of male hermaphrodites are suitable for rearing as males.

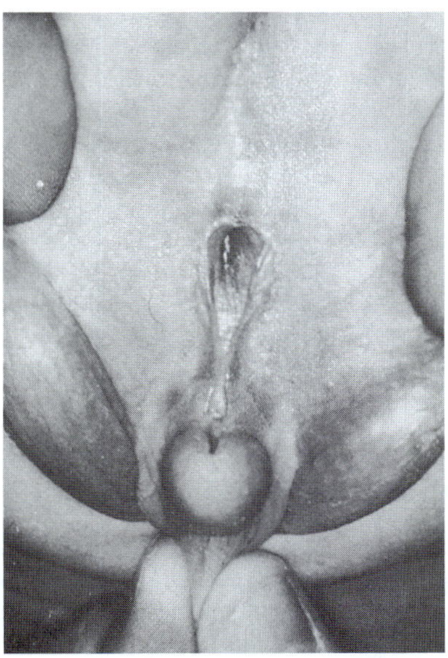

▲ **Figure 3–17.** External genitalia in male hermaphroditism. (Reproduced, with permission, from Jones HW Jr, Scott WW. *Hermaphroditism, Genital Anomalies and Related Endocrine Disorders.* 2nd ed. Philadelphia, PA: Williams & Wilkins; 1971.)

Classification

Since about 1970, considerable progress has been made in identifying specific metabolic defects that are etiologically important for the various forms of male hermaphroditism. Details are beyond the scope of this text. Nevertheless, it is important to point out that all cases of male hermaphroditism have a defect in either the biologic action of testosterone or the MIF of the testis. Furthermore, it now seems apparent that nearly all—if not all—of these defects have a genetic or cytogenetic background. The causes and pathogenetic mechanisms of these defects may vary, but the final common pathway is 1 of the 2 problems just mentioned; in the adult a study of the serum gonadotropins and serum steroids, including the intermediate metabolites of testosterone, can often pinpoint a defect in the biosynthesis of testosterone. In other cases, the end-organ action of testosterone may be defective. In children, the defect is sometimes more difficult to determine before gonadotropin levels rise at puberty, but one may suspect a problem by observing abnormally high levels of steroids that act as substrates in the metabolism of testosterone. A working classification of male hermaphroditism is as follows:

I. Male hermaphroditism due to a central nervous system defect
   A. Abnormal pituitary gonadotropin secretion
   B. No gonadotropin secretion
II. Male hermaphroditism due to a primary gonadal defect
   A. Identifiable defect in biosynthesis of testosterone

1. Pregnenolone synthesis defect (lipoid adrenal hyperplasia)
2. 3β-Hydroxysteroid dehydrogenase deficiency
3. 17α-Hydroxylase deficiency
4. 17,20-Desmolase deficiency
5. 17β-Ketosteroid reductase deficiency

B. Unidentified defect in androgen effect
C. Defect in duct regression (Figs. 3–18 and 3–19)
D. Familial gonadal destruction
E. Leydig cell agenesis
F. Bilateral testicular dysgenesis

III. Male hermaphroditism due to peripheral end-organ defect

A. Androgen insensitivity syndrome (Fig. 3–20)
1. Androgen-binding protein deficiency
2. Unknown deficiency

B. 5α-Reductase deficiency
C. Unidentified abnormality of peripheral androgen effect

IV. Male hermaphroditism due to Y chromosome defect

A. Y chromosome mosaicism (asymmetric gonadal differentiation) (Fig. 3–21)
B. Structurally abnormal Y chromosome
C. No identifiable Y chromosome

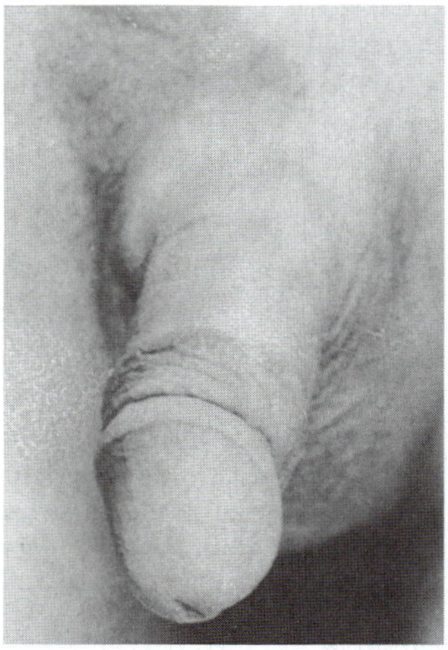

▲ **Figure 3–18.** External genitalia in male hermaphroditism. (Reproduced, with permission, from Jones HW Jr, Scott WW. *Hermaphroditism, Genital Anomalies and Related Endocrine Disorders.* 2nd ed. Philadelphia, PA: Williams & Wilkins; 1971.)

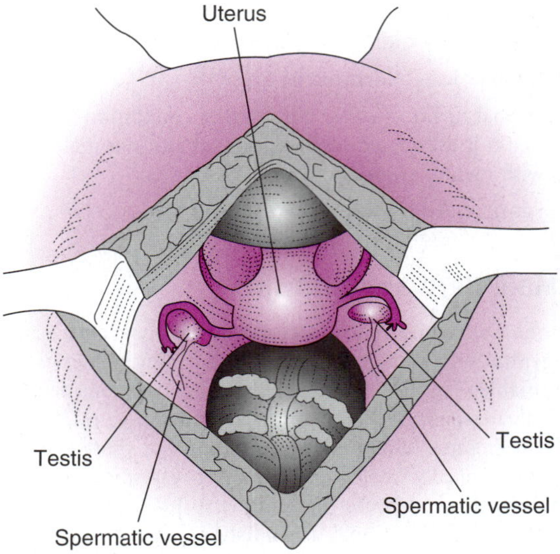

▲ **Figure 3–19.** Internal genitalia of the patient whose external genitalia are shown in Figure 3–18.

9. Differential Diagnosis in Infants with Ambiguous Genitalia

Accurate differential diagnosis is possible in most patients with ambiguous genitalia (Table 3–8). This requires a complex history of the mother's medication use, a complex sex chromosome study, rectal examination for the presence or absence of a uterus, measurement of serum steroid levels, pelvic ultrasonography, and information about other congenital anomalies. The following disorders, however, do not yield to differentiation by the parameters given in Table 3–8: (1) idiopathic masculinization, (2) the "special" forms of female hermaphroditism, (3) 46,XX true hermaphroditism, and, occasionally, (4) the precise type of male hermaphroditism. For these differentiations, laparotomy may be necessary for diagnosis and for therapy.

10. Treatment of Hermaphroditism

The sex of rearing is much more important than the obvious morphologic signs (external genitalia, hormone dominance, gonadal structure) in forming the gender role. Furthermore, serious psychological consequences may result from changing the sex of rearing after infancy. Therefore, it is seldom proper to advise a change of sex after infancy to conform to the gonadal structure of the external genitalia. Instead, the physician should exert efforts to complete the adjustment

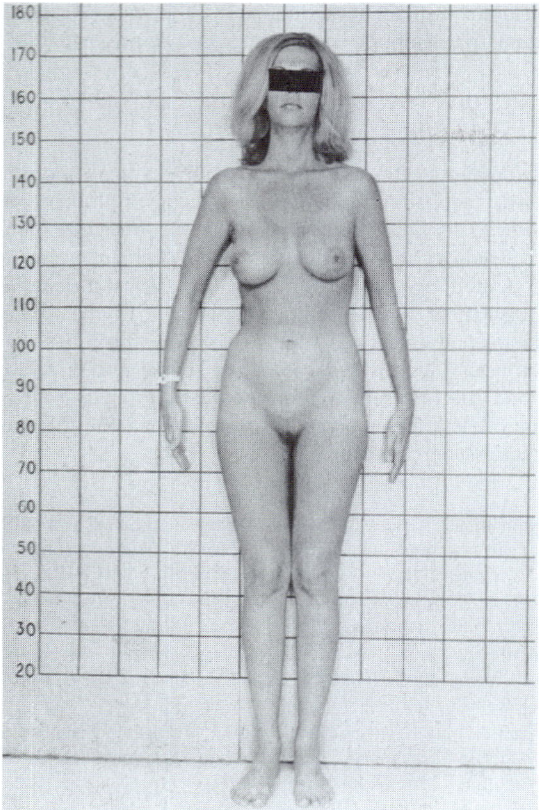

▲ **Figure 3–20.** Androgen insensitivity syndrome.

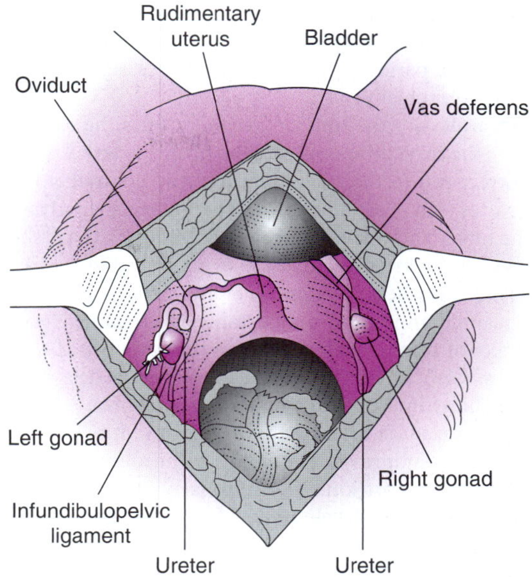

▲ **Figure 3–21.** Internal genitalia in asymmetric gonadal differentiation. (Reproduced, with permission, from Jones HW Jr, Scott WW. *Hermaphroditism, Genital Anomalies and Related Endocrine Disorders.* 2nd ed. Philadelphia, PA: Williams & Wilkins; 1971.)

Table 3–8. Differential diagnosis of ambiguous external genitalia.

Diagnosis	Karyotype	History	Uterus	Anomalies	17-KS	Sex Chromosomes
Adrenal hyperplasia	46,XX	+	+	–	E	XX
Maternal androgen	46,XX	+	+	–	N	XX
Idiopathic masculinization	46,XX	–	+	–	N	XX
Special or nonspecific	46,XX	–	+	–	N	XX
Female familial	46,XX	+	+	+	N	XX
True hermaphroditism	46,XX; 46,XY; etc	–	+ or –	–	N	XX or other
Male hermaphroditism	46,XY	+	+ or –	–	N	XY or other
Streak gonad	45,X; 46,XX; 46,XY; etc	–	+	+ or –	N	XO or other

+, positive; –, negative; N, normal; E, elevated; 17-KS, 17-ketosteroid level.

of the person to the sex role already assigned. Fortunately, most aberrations of sexual development are discovered in the newborn period or in infancy, when reassignment of sex causes few problems.

Regardless of the time of treatment (and the earlier the better), the surgeon should reconstruct the external genitalia to correspond to the sex of rearing. Any contradictory sex structures that may function to the patient's disadvantage in the future should be eradicated. Specifically, testes should always be removed from male hermaphrodites reared as females, regardless of hormone production. In cases of testicular feminization, orchiectomy is warranted because a variety of tumors may develop in these abnormal testes if they are retained, but the orchiectomy may be delayed until after puberty in this variety of hermaphroditism.

In virilized female hermaphroditism due to adrenal hyperplasia, suppression of adrenal androgen production by the use of cortisone from an early age will result in completely female development. It is no longer necessary to explore the abdomen and the internal genitalia in this well-delineated syndrome. The surgical effort should be confined to reconstruction of the external genitalia along female lines.

Patients with streak gonads or Turner's syndrome, who are invariably reared as females, should be given exogenous estrogen when puberty is expected. Those hermaphrodites reared as females who will not become feminized also require estrogen to promote the development of the female habitus, including the breasts. In patients with a well-developed system, cyclic uterine withdrawal bleeding can be produced even though reproduction is impossible. Estrogen should be started at about age 12 and may be given as conjugated estrogens, 1.5 mg/d orally (or its equivalent). In some patients, after a period of time, this dosage may have to be increased for additional breast development. In patients without ovaries who have uteri and in male hermaphrodites in the same condition, cyclic uterine bleeding can often be induced by the administration of estrogen for 3 weeks of each month. In other instances, this may be inadequate to produce a convincing "menstrual" period; if so, the 3 weeks of estrogen can be followed by 3–4 days of progestin (eg, medroxyprogesterone acetate) orally or a single injection of progesterone. Prolonged estrogen therapy increases the risk of subsequent development of adenocarcinoma of the corpus, so periodic endometrial sampling is mandatory in such patients.

Reconstruction of Female External Genitalia

The details of the operative reconstruction of abnormal external genitalia are beyond the scope of this chapter. However, it should be emphasized that the procedure should be carried out at the earliest age possible so as to enhance the desired psychological, social, and sexual orientation of the patient and to facilitate adjustment by the parents. Sometimes the reconstruction can be done during the neonatal period. In any case, operation should not be delayed beyond the first several months of life. From a technical point of view, early operation is possible in all but the most exceptional circumstances.

Briton-Jones C, Haines CJ. Microdeletions on the long arm of the Y chromosome and their association with male-factor infertility. *Hong Kong Med J* 2000;6:184–189. PMID: 10895412.

Eiben B, Glaubitz R. First-trimester screening: an overview. *J Histochem Cytochem* 2005;53:281–283. PMID: 15750002.

Horsthemke B, Ludwig M. Assisted reproduction: the epigenetic perspective. *Hum Reprod Update* 2005;11:473–482. PMID: 15994847.

Langer S, Kraus J, Jentsch I, Speicher MR. Multicolor chromosome painting in diagnostic and research application. *Chromosome Res* 2004;12:15–23. PMID: 14984098.

Lippman-Hand A, Bekemans M. Balanced translocations among couples with two or more spontaneous abortions: are males and females equally likely to be carriers? *Hum Genet* 1983;68:252–257. PMID: 6852821.

Rode L, Wφjdemann KR, Shalmi AC, et al. Combined first- and second-trimester screening for Down syndrome: an evaluation of proMBP as a marker. *Prenat Diagn* 2003;23:593–598. PMID: 12868091.

Sadeghi-Nejad H, Oates RD. The Y chromosome and male infertility. *Curr Opin Urol* 2008;18:628–632. PMID: 18832950.

Salozhin SV, Prokhorchuk EB, Georgiev GP. Methylation of DNA: one of the major epigenetic markers. *Biochemistry (Mosc)* 2005;70:525–532. PMID: 15948706.

Wald NJ, Rodeck C, Hackshaw AK, Rudnicka A. SURUSS in perspective. *Semin Perinatol* 2005;29:225–235. PMID: 16104673.

Physiology of Reproduction in Women

4

Connie Alford, MD
Sahadat Nurudeen, MD

This chapter is concerned with the function of the female reproductive system from birth, through puberty and adulthood, and finally to menopause.

After birth, the gonads are quiescent until they are activated by gonadotropins from the pituitary to bring about the final maturation of the reproductive system. This period of final maturation is known as adolescence. It is often called puberty, although strictly defined, puberty is the period when the endocrine and gametogenic functions of the gonads first develop to the point where reproduction is possible.

After sexual maturity, there are regular periodic changes of the adult female reproductive system, each in preparation for pregnancy. The cyclic changes are primarily divided into the ovarian and uterine cycle, though changes can also be seen in the uterine cervix, vagina, and breasts. Control of the cycle is exerted through the regulation of hypothalamic, pituitary, and ovarian hormones.

With advancing age, these cycles become irregular and eventually cease in the period known as menopause. The ovarian follicles are less responsive to central regulation, and there is an acute decrease in estrogen levels, which may lead to vasomotor symptoms, labile mood, and many changes in the female reproductive tract.

PUBERTY

The age at the time of puberty is variable. In Europe and the United States, it has been declining at the rate of 1–3 months per decade for more than 175 years. In the United States in recent years, puberty has generally been occurring between the ages of 8 and 13 in girls and 9 and 14 in boys depending on ethnic background.

Another event that occurs in humans at the time of puberty is an increase in the secretion of adrenal androgens (Fig. 4–1). The onset of this increase is called **adrenarche**. It typically happens in males and females before the onset of puberty occurring at age 8–10 years in girls and 10–12 years in boys. Dehydroepiandrosterone (DHEA) values peak at about 25 years of age and are slightly higher in boys. They then decline slowly to low values after the age of 60.

The increase in adrenal androgen secretion at adrenarche occurs without any changes in the secretion of cortisol or adrenocorticotropic hormone (ACTH). Adrenarche is probably due to a rise in the lyase activity of a 17α-hydroxylase. Thereafter, there is a gradual decline in this activity as plasma adrenal androgen secretion declines to low levels in old age.

In girls, the first event of puberty is **thelarche**, the development of breasts. The breasts develop under the influence of the ovarian hormones estradiol and progesterone, with estradiol primarily responsible for the growth of ducts and progesterone primarily responsible for the growth of lobules and alveoli. Thelarche is then followed by **pubarche**, the development of axillary and pubic hair. The adrenal androgens contribute significantly to the growth of axillary and pubic hair. Finally there is **menarche**, the first menstrual period. The initial periods are generally anovulatory with regular ovulation beginning about 1 year later.

The sequence of changes that occur at puberty in girls is summarized in Figure 4–2.

Control of the Onset of Puberty

In general, many factors can influence the timing of the initiation of puberty including general health, genetic influences, nutrition, and exercise. However, a neural mechanism is thought to be predominantly responsible for the onset of puberty. It depends on normal functioning of the hypothalamic-pituitary-gonadal axis. In children, the gonads can be stimulated by gonadotropins, the pituitary contains gonadotropins, and the hypothalamus contains gonadotropin-releasing hormone (GnRH). However, the gonadotropins are not secreted. In immature monkeys, normal menstrual cycles can be brought on by pulsatile injection of GnRH, and the cycles persist as long as the pulsatile injection is continued. In addition, GnRH is secreted in a pulsatile fashion in adults. Thus, it seems clear that during the period from birth

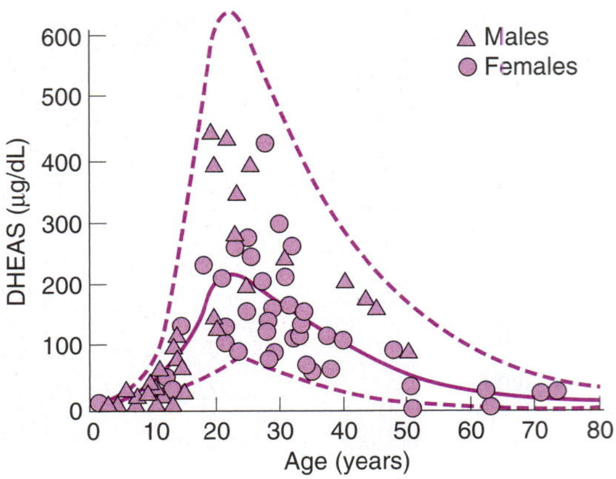

▲ Figure 4–1. Change in serum dehydroepiandrosterone sulfate (DHEAS) with age. The middle line is the mean, and the dashed lines identify ±1.96 standard deviations. (Reproduced with permission from Smith MR, Rudd BT, Shirley A, et al. A radioimmunoassay for the estimation of serum dehydroepiandrosterone sulfate in normal and pathological sera. *Clin Chim Acta* 1975;65:5.)

to puberty, a neural mechanism is operating to prevent the normal pulsatile release of GnRH. The nature of the mechanism inhibiting the GnRH pulse generator is unknown. Several theories have been suggested about this mechanism, including a recent study involving humans and mice, providing evidence that GPR54, a gene for a G protein–coupled receptor, is involved in the regulation of the processing or secretion of GnRH by the hypothalamus.

Relation to Leptin

It has been argued for some time that normally a critical body weight must be reached for puberty to occur. Thus, for example, young women who engage in strenuous athletics lose weight and stop menstruating. The same is seen in girls with anorexia nervosa. If these girls start to eat and gain weight, they menstruate again, ie, they "go back through puberty." It now appears that leptin, the satiety-producing hormone secreted by fat cells, may be the link between body weight and puberty. Leptin treatment has been shown to induce precocious puberty in immature female mice. However, more recent studies have suggested leptin to have a more permissive role for the onset of puberty rather than being a trigger. Observations of recombinant leptin administration in older, but not younger, children with leptin deficiency resulted in increased gonadotropin pulsatility. The role of leptin in the control of pubarche remains to be determined.

Sexual Precocity

Sexual precocity is pubertal development occurring before the age of 8 years in girls, and before the age of 9 years in boys. The major causes of precocious sexual development in humans are listed in Table 4–1. Early development of secondary sexual characteristics without gametogenesis is caused by abnormal exposure of immature males to androgen or females to estrogen. This syndrome should be called **precocious pseudopuberty** to distinguish it from true precocious puberty due to an early, but otherwise normal pubertal pattern of gonadotropin secretion from the pituitary (Fig. 4–3).

In 1 large series of cases, precocious puberty was the most frequent endocrine symptom of hypothalamic disease. It is interesting that in experimental animals and humans, lesions of the ventral hypothalamus near the infundibulum cause precocious puberty. The effect of the lesions may be due to an interruption of neural pathways that produce inhibition of the GnRH pulse generator or a local release of factors causing premature activation of the GnRH pulse generator. Pineal tumors are sometimes associated with precocious puberty, but there is evidence that these tumors are related only when there is secondary damage to the hypothalamus. Precocity due to this and other forms of hypothalamic damage probably occurs with equal frequency in both sexes, although the constitutional form of precocious puberty is more common in girls. In addition, it has now been proven that precocious gametogenesis and steroidogenesis can occur without the pubertal pattern of gonadotropin secretion (gonadotropin-independent precocity). At least in some cases of the condition, the sensitivity of luteinizing hormone (LH) receptors to gonadotropins is increased because of an activating mutation in the G protein that couples receptors to adenylyl cyclase.

Recent observational studies have proposed a link between low birth weight, increased weight gain during childhood, changes in insulin sensitivity, and subsequent hormonal changes, such as early pubarche. Although the association remains speculative, these studies suggest a programmed adaptation to improved postnatal nutritional status triggering a pathway of rapid growth and secondary sexual development.

Delayed or Absent Puberty

The normal variation in the age at which adolescent changes occur is so wide that puberty cannot be considered to be pathologically delayed until the absence of secondary sexual development by age 14 in girls or until the failure of menarche by the age of 17. Failure of maturation due to panhypopituitarism is associated with dwarfing and evidence of other endocrine abnormalities. Patients with the XO chromosomal pattern and gonadal dysgenesis are also dwarfed. In some individuals, puberty is delayed and menarche does not occur (primary amenorrhea), even though the gonads are present and other endocrine functions are normal.

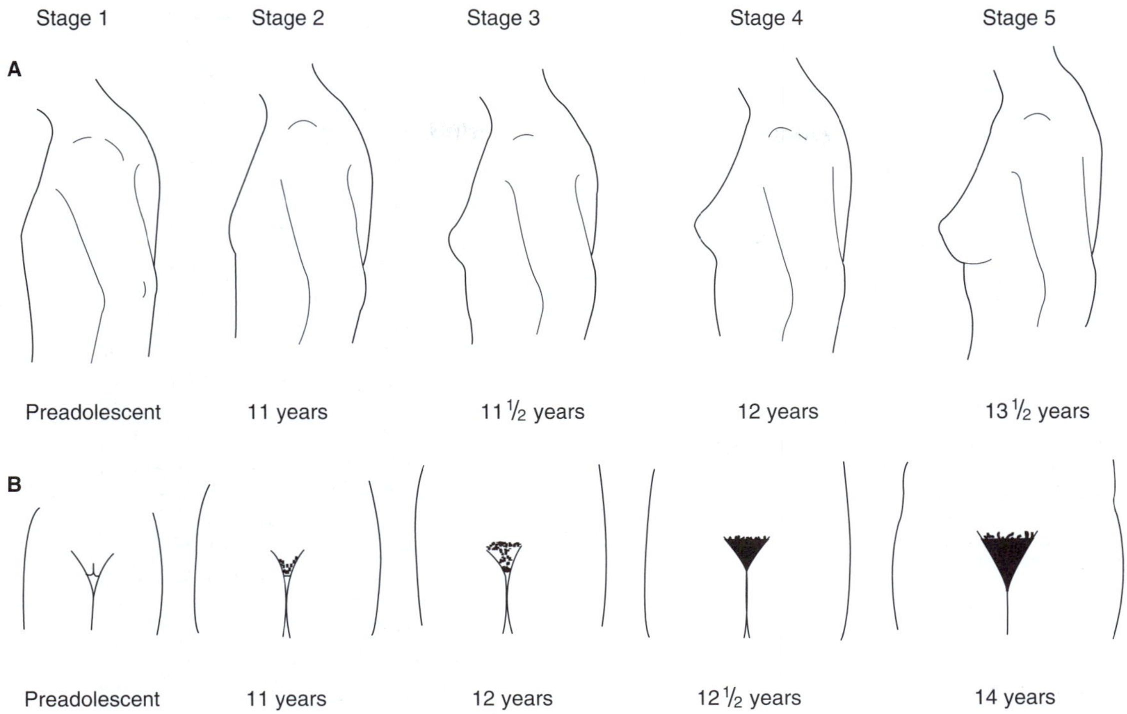

▲ **Figure 4–2.** Sequence of events at adolescence in girls. **A:** Stage 1: Preadolescent; elevation of breast papillae only. Stage 2: Breast bud stage (may occur between ages 8 and 13); elevation of breasts and papillae as small mounds, with enlargement of areolar diameter. Stage 3: Enlargement and elevation of breasts and areolas with no separation of contours. Stage 4: Areolas and papillae project from breast to form a secondary mound. Stage 5: Mature; projection of papillae only, with recession of areolas into general contour of breast. **B:** Stage 1: Preadolescent; no pubic hair. Stage 2: Sparse growth along labia of long, slightly pigmented, downy hair that is straight or slightly curled (may occur between ages 8 and 14). Stage 3: Darker, coarser, more curled hair growing sparsely over pubic area. Stage 4: Resembles adult in type but covers smaller area. Stage 5: Adult in quantity and type. (Redrawn, with permission, from Tanner JM. *Growth at Adolescence*. 2nd ed. New York, NY: Blackwell; 1962.)

REPRODUCTIVE FUNCTION AFTER SEXUAL MATURITY

Menstrual Cycle

The anatomy of the reproductive system of adult women is described in Chapter 1. Unlike the reproductive system of men, this system shows regular cyclic changes that teleologically may be regarded as periodic preparation for fertilization and pregnancy. In primates, the cycle is a **menstrual cycle**, and its most conspicuous feature is the cyclic vaginal bleeding that occurs with shedding of the uterine mucosa (**menstruation**). The length of the cycle is notoriously variable, but the average figure is 28 days from the start of one menstrual period to the start of the next. By common usage, the days of the cycle are identified by number, starting with the first day of menstruation.

Ovarian Cycle

From the time of birth, there are many **primordial follicles** under the ovarian capsule. Each contains an immature ovum (Fig. 4–4). At the start of each cycle, several of these follicles enlarge and a cavity forms around the ovum (antrum formation). This cavity is filled with follicular fluid. In humans, 1 of the follicles in 1 ovary starts to grow rapidly on about the sixth day and becomes the **dominant follicle**. The others regress, forming **atretic follicles**. It is not known how 1 follicle is singled out for development during this **follicular phase** of the menstrual cycle, but it seems to be related to the follicle's ability to produce estrogen, which is necessary for final maturation. The secretion of estrogen, in animal models, has been demonstrated even before the dominant follicle has emerged as morphologically dominant. Theoretically, depending on the position of the

Table 4–1. Classification of the causes of precocious sexual development in humans.

True precocious puberty
Constitutional
Cerebral: Disorders involving posterior hypothalamus
Tumors
Infections
Developmental abnormalities
Gonadotropin-independent precocity
Precocious pseudopuberty (no spermatogenesis or ovarian development)
Adrenal
Congenital virilizing adrenal hyperplasia (without treatment in males; following cortisone treatment in females)
Androgen-secreting tumors (in males)
Estrogen-secreting tumors (in females)
Gonadal
Interstitial cell tumors of testis
Granulosa cell tumors of ovary
Miscellaneous

Reproduced, with permission, from Barrett KE. *Ganong's Review of Medical Physiology*. 23rd ed. New York, NY: McGraw-Hill; 2010.

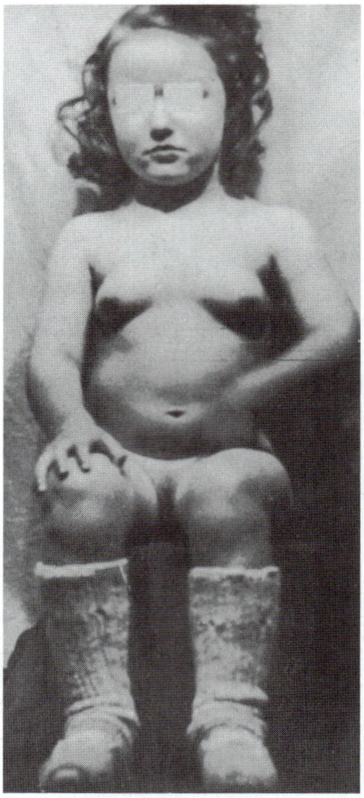

▲ **Figure 4–3.** Constitutional precocious puberty in a 3½-year-old girl. The patient developed pubic hair and started to menstruate at the age of 17 months.

follicle to the blood supply, there is a gradient of exposure to different amounts of hormones, growth factors, and other signaling molecules. Therefore, the follicle most responsive to follicle-stimulating hormone (FSH) is likely to be the first to produce estradiol.

The structure of a mature ovarian follicle (**graafian follicle**) is shown in Figure 4–4. The cells of the **theca interna** of the follicle are the primary source of circulating estrogens. The follicular fluid has a high estrogen content, and much of this estrogen comes from the **granulosa cells**.

At about the 14th day of the cycle, the distended follicle ruptures, and the ovum is extruded into the abdominal cavity. This is the process of **ovulation**. The ovum is picked up by the fimbriated ends of the uterine tubes (oviducts) and transported to the uterus. Unless fertilization occurs, the ovum degenerates or passes on through the uterus and out of the vagina.

The follicle that ruptures at the time of ovulation promptly fills with blood, forming what is sometimes called a **corpus hemorrhagicum**. Minor bleeding from the follicle into the abdominal cavity may cause peritoneal irritation and fleeting lower abdominal pain ("mittelschmerz"). The granulosa and theca cells of the follicle lining promptly begin to proliferate, and the clotted blood is rapidly replaced with yellowish, lipid-rich **luteal cells**, forming the **corpus luteum**. This is the **luteal phase** of the menstrual cycle, during which the luteal cells secrete estrogen and progesterone. Growth of the corpus luteum depends on its developing an adequate blood supply. There is evidence that vascular endothelial growth factor (VEGF) is essential for this process through regulation by the transcription factor, HIF-1α, under hypoxic conditions or by gonadotropin-stimulated conditions. If pregnancy occurs, the corpus luteum persists, and there are usually no more menstrual cycles until after delivery. If there is no pregnancy, the corpus luteum begins to degenerate about 4 days before the next menses (day 24 of the cycle) and is eventually replaced by fibrous tissue, forming a **corpus albicans**.

In humans, no new ova are formed after birth. During fetal development, the ovaries contain over 7 million germ cells; however, many undergo involution before birth, and others are lost after birth. At the time of birth, there are approximately 2 million primordial follicles containing ova, but approximately 50% of these are atretic. The remaining million ova undergo the first meiotic division at this time and arrest in prophase until adulthood. Atresia continues during development, and the number of ova in both the ovaries at the time of puberty is less than 300,000 (Fig. 4–5). Normally, only 1 of these ova per cycle (or about 400–500 in the course of a normal reproductive life) is stimulated to mature; the remainder degenerate. Just before ovulation, the first meiotic division is completed. One of the daughter cells, the **secondary oocyte**, receives most of the cytoplasm,

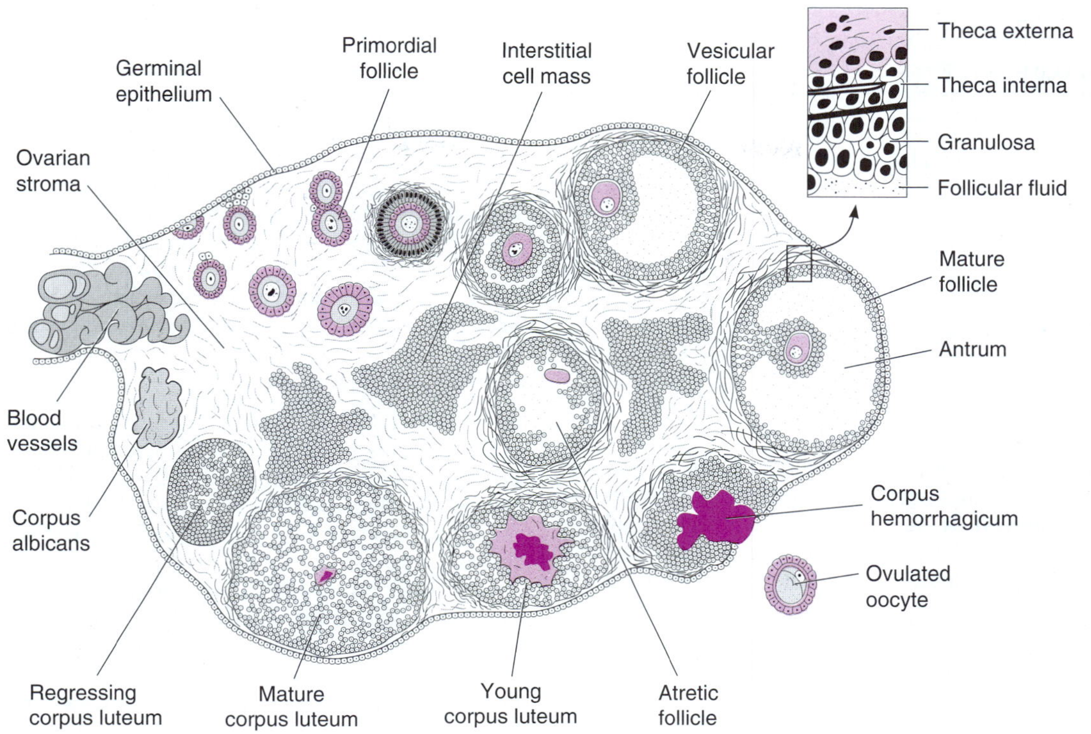

▲ **Figure 4–4.** Diagram of a mammalian ovary, showing the sequential development of a follicle, formation of a corpus luteum, and, in the center, follicular atresia. A section of the wall of a mature follicle is enlarged at the upper right. The interstitial cell mass is not prominent in primates.

while the other, the **first polar body**, fragments and disappears. The secondary oocyte immediately begins the second meiotic division, but this division stops at metaphase and is completed only when a sperm penetrates the oocyte. At that time, the **second polar body** is cast off, and the fertilized ovum proceeds to form a new individual.

Uterine Cycle

The events that occur in the uterus during the menstrual cycle terminate with the menstrual flow. By the end of each menstrual period, all but the deep layer of the endometrium has sloughed. Under the influence of estrogen secreted from the developing follicles, the endometrium regenerates from the deep layer and increases rapidly in thickness during the period from the fifth to 16th days of the menstrual cycle. As the thickness increases, the uterine glands are drawn out so that they lengthen (Fig. 4–6), but they do not become convoluted or secrete to any degree. These endometrial changes are called proliferative, and this part of the menstrual cycle is sometimes called the **proliferative phase**. It is also called the preovulatory or follicular phase of the cycle. After ovulation, the endometrium becomes more highly vascularized and slightly edematous under the influence of estrogen and progesterone from the corpus luteum. The glands become coiled and tortuous (Fig. 4–6), and they begin to secrete clear fluid. Consequently, this phase of the cycle is called the **secretory** or **luteal phase**. Late in the luteal phase, the endometrium, like the anterior pituitary, produces prolactin. The function of this endometrial prolactin has yet to be determined, though it has been suggested that prolactin may play a role in implantation.

The endometrium is supplied by 2 types of arteries. The superficial two-thirds of the endometrium, the stratum functionale, is shed during menstruation and is supplied by the long, coiled spiral arteries. The deep layer, which is not shed, is called the stratum basale and is supplied by short, straight basilar arteries.

When the corpus luteum regresses, hormonal support for the endometrium is withdrawn, causing vascular spasms in the spiral artery, ultimately leading to endometrial ischemia. The endometrium becomes thinner, which adds to the coiling of the spiral arteries. Leukocyte infiltration into the endometrial stroma initiates the breakdown of the extracellular matrix in the functionalis layer. Foci of necrosis appear in the endometrium and walls of the spiral arteries, which coalesce and lead to spotty hemorrhages that become confluent and ultimately produce menstrual flow.

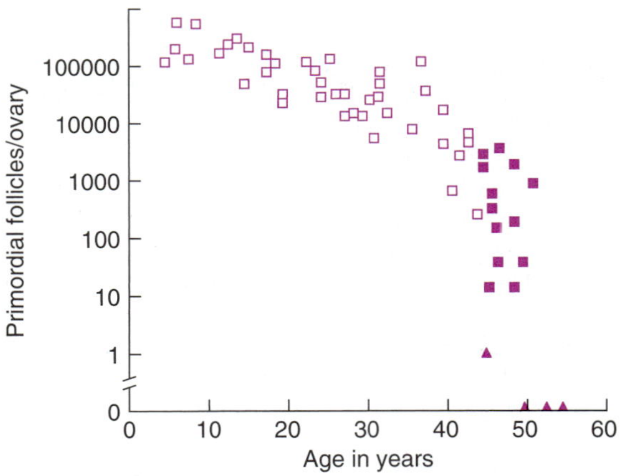

▲ **Figure 4–5.** Number of primordial follicles per ovary in women at various ages. □, premenopausal women (regular menses); ■, perimenopausal women (irregular menses for at least 1 year); ▲, postmenopausal women (no menses for at least 1 year). Note that the vertical scale is a log scale and that the values are from 1 rather than 2 ovaries. (Reproduced, with permission, from Richardson SJ, Senikas V, Nelson JF. Follicular depletion during the menopausal transition: evidence for accelerated loss and ultimate exhaustion. *J Clin Endocrinol Metab* 1987;65:1231.)

Spiral artery vasospasm serves to limit blood loss during menstruation and probably is produced by locally released prostaglandins. There are large quantities of prostaglandins in the secretory endometrium and in menstrual blood. Infusions of prostaglandin F_{2a} (PGF_{2a}) produce endometrial necrosis and bleeding. One theory of the onset of menstruation holds that in necrotic endometrial cells, lysosomal membranes break down and release proteolytic enzymes that foster the formation of prostaglandins from cellular phospholipids while promoting further local tissue destruction.

From the point of view of endometrial function, the proliferative phase of the menstrual cycle represents the restoration of the epithelium from the preceding menstruation, while the secretory phase represents the preparation of the uterus for implantation of the fertilized ovum. The length of the secretory phase is remarkably constant, about 14 days. The variations seen in the length of the menstrual cycle are mostly due to variations in the length of the proliferative phase. When fertilization fails to occur during the secretory phase, the endometrium is shed, and a new cycle begins.

Normal Menstruation

Menstrual blood is predominantly arterial, with only 25% of the blood being of venous origin. It contains tissue debris, prostaglandins, and relatively large amounts of fibrinolysin from the endometrial tissue. The fibrinolysin lyses clots, so menstrual blood does not normally contain clots unless the flow is excessive.

The usual duration of the menstrual cycle is 3–5 days, but flow as short as 1 day and as long as 8 days can occur in normal women. The average amount of blood loss is 30 mL but normally may range from slight spotting to 80 mL. Loss of more than 80 mL is abnormal. Obviously, the amount of flow can be affected by various factors, including not only the thickness of the endometrium, but also the medications and diseases that affect clotting mechanisms. After menstruation, the endometrium regenerates from the stratum basale.

Anovulatory Cycles

In some instances, ovulation fails to occur during the menstrual cycle. Such anovulatory cycles are common for the first 12–18 months after menarche and again before the onset of menopause. When ovulation does not occur, no corpus luteum is formed, and the effects of progesterone on the endometrium are absent. Estrogens continue to

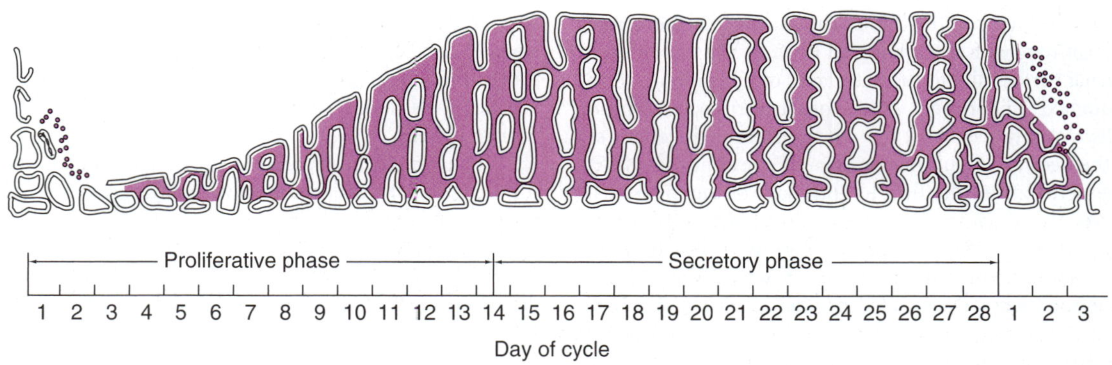

▲ **Figure 4–6.** Changes in the endometrium during the menstrual cycle. (Reproduced, with permission, from Ganong WF. *Review of Medical Physiology*. 22nd ed. New York, NY: McGraw-Hill; 2005.)

cause growth, however, and the proliferative endometrium becomes thick enough to break down and begin to slough. The time it takes for bleeding to occur is variable, but it usually occurs less than 28 days from the last menstrual period. The flow is also variable and ranges from scanty to relatively profuse.

Cyclic Changes in the Uterine Cervix

Although it is contiguous with the body of the uterus, the cervix of the uterus is different in a number of ways. The mucosa of the uterine cervix does not undergo cyclic desquamation, but there are regular changes in the cervical mucus. Estrogen makes the mucus much thinner and more alkaline, changes that promote the survival and transport of sperm. Progesterone makes it thick, tenacious, and cellular. The mucus is thinnest at the time of ovulation, and its elasticity, or **spinnbarkeit**, increases so that by midcycle a drop can be stretched into a long, thin thread that may be 8–12 cm or more in length. In addition, it dries in an arborizing, fern-like pattern when a thin layer is spread on a slide (Fig. 4–7). After ovulation and during pregnancy, it becomes thick and fails to form the fern pattern.

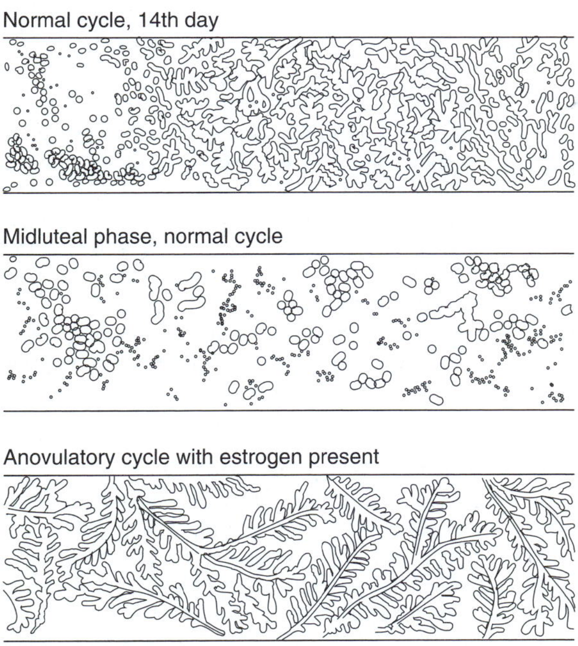

▲ Figure 4–7. Patterns formed when cervical mucus is smeared on a slide, permitted to dry, and examined under the microscope. Progesterone makes the mucus thick and cellular. In the smear from a patient who failed to ovulate (**bottom**), there is no progesterone to inhibit the estrogen-induced fern pattern. (Reproduced, with permission, from Barrett KE. *Ganong's Review of Medical Physiology*. 23rd ed. New York, NY: McGraw-Hill; 2010.)

Vaginal Cycle

Under the influence of estrogens, the vaginal epithelium becomes cornified, and these cornified epithelial cells can be identified in a vaginal smear. Under the influence of progesterone, a thick mucus is secreted, and the epithelium proliferates and becomes infiltrated with leukocytes. The cyclic changes in the vaginal smear in rats are particularly well known. The changes in humans and other species are similar but unfortunately not so clear-cut. However, the increase in cornified epithelial cells is apparent when a vaginal smear from an adult woman in the follicular phase of the menstrual cycle is compared, for example, with a smear taken from a prepubescent female.

Cyclic Changes in the Breasts

Although lactation normally does not occur until the end of pregnancy, there are cyclic changes in the breasts during the menstrual cycle. Estrogens cause proliferation of mammary ducts, whereas progesterone causes growth of lobules and alveoli (see Actions of Progesterone). The breast swelling, tenderness, and pain experienced by many women during the 10 days preceding menstruation probably are due to distention of the ducts, hyperemia, and edema of the interstitial tissue of the breasts. All of these changes regress, along with the symptoms, during menstruation.

Cyclic Changes in Other Body Functions

In addition to cyclic breast swelling and tenderness, there is usually a small increase in body temperature during the luteal phase of the menstrual cycle. This change in body temperature (see Indicators of Ovulation) probably is due to the thermogenic effect of progesterone.

Changes During Sexual Intercourse

During sexual excitation, the vaginal walls become moist as a result of transudation of fluid through the mucus membrane. A lubricating mucus is secreted by the vestibular glands. The upper part of the vagina is sensitive to stretch, while tactile stimulation from the labia minora and clitoris adds to the sexual excitement. The stimuli are reinforced by tactile stimuli from the breasts and, as in men, by visual, auditory, and olfactory stimuli. Eventually, the crescendo or climax known as orgasm may be reached. During orgasm, there are autonomically mediated rhythmic contractions of the vaginal wall. Impulses also travel via the pudendal nerves and produce rhythmic contractions of the bulbocavernosus and ischiocavernosus muscles. The vaginal contractions may aid in the transport of spermatozoa but are not essential for it, as fertilization of the ovum is not dependent on orgasm.

Indicators of Ovulation

Knowing when during the menstrual cycle ovulation occurs is important in increasing fertility or, conversely, in contraception. A convenient, but retrospective, indicator of the time of ovulation is a rise in the basal body temperature (Fig. 4–8). Accurate temperatures can be obtained by using a thermometer that is able to measure temperature precisely between 96 and 100°F. The woman should take her temperature orally, vaginally, or rectally in the morning before getting out of bed. The cause of temperature change at the time of ovulation is unknown but probably is due to the increase in progesterone secretion, as progesterone is thermogenic. A rise in urinary LH occurs during the rise in circulating LH that causes ovulation. This increase can be measured and used as another indicator of ovulation. Kits using dipsticks or simple color tests for detection of urinary LH are available for home use.

Ovulation normally occurs about 9 hours after the peak of the LH surge at midcycle (Fig. 4–8). The ovum lives approximately 72 hours after it is extruded from the follicle but probably is fertilizable for less than half this time. In a study of the relationship of isolated intercourse to pregnancy, 36% of women had a detected pregnancy following intercourse on the day of ovulation, but with intercourse on days after ovulation, the percentage was zero. Isolated intercourse of the first and second days before ovulation led to pregnancy in about 36% of the women. A few pregnancies resulted from isolated intercourse on day 3, 4, or 5 before ovulation, although the percentage was much lower, ie, 8% on day 5 before ovulation. Thus, some sperm can survive in the female genital tract and produce fertilization for up to 120 hours before ovulation, but the most fertile period is clearly the 48 hours before ovulation. However, for those interested in the "rhythm method" of contraception, if should be noted that there are rare but documented cases of pregnancy resulting from isolated coitus on every day of the cycle.

OVARIAN HORMONES

Chemistry, Biosynthesis, & Metabolism of Estrogens

The naturally occurring estrogens are **17β-estradiol**, **estrone**, and **estriol** (Fig. 4–9). They are C_{18} steroids, ie, they do not have an angular methyl group attached to the 10 position or a Δ^4-3-keto configuration in the A ring. They are secreted primarily by the granulosa and thecal cells of the ovarian follicles, the corpus luteum, and the placenta. The biosynthetic pathway involves their aromatization from androgens. Aromatase (CYP19) is the enzyme that catalyzes the conversion of androstenedione to estrone (Fig. 4–9). It also catalyzes the conversion of testosterone to estradiol.

Theca interna cells have many LH receptors, and LH acts on them via cyclic adenosine 3′,5′-monophosphate (cAMP) to increase conversion of cholesterol to androstenedione. Some of the androstenedione is converted to estradiol, which enters the circulation. The theca interna cells also supply androstenedione to granulosa cells. The granulosa cells only make estradiol when provided with androgens (Fig. 4–10), and they secrete the estradiol that they produce into the follicular fluid. They have many FSH receptors, and FSH facilitates the secretion of estradiol by acting via cAMP to increase the aromatase activity in these cells. Mature granulosa cells also acquire LH receptors, and LH stimulates estradiol production.

The stromal tissue of the ovary also has the potential to produce androgens and estrogens. However, it probably does so in insignificant amounts in normal premenopausal women. 17β-Estradiol, the major secreted estrogen, is in equilibrium in the circulation with estrone. Estrone is further metabolized to **estriol** (Fig. 4–9), probably mainly in the liver. Estradiol is the most potent estrogen of the three, and estriol is the least potent.

Two percent of the circulating estradiol is free. The remainder is bound to protein: 60% to albumin and 38% to the same gonadal steroid-binding globulin (GBG) that binds testosterone (Table 4–2).

In the liver, estrogens are oxidized or converted to glucuronide and sulfate conjugates. Appreciable amounts are secreted in the bile and reabsorbed in the bloodstream (enterohepatic circulation). There are at least 10 different metabolites of estradiol in human urine.

Secretion of Estrogens

The concentration of estradiol in plasma during the menstrual cycle is shown in Figure 4–8. Almost all of the estrogen comes from the ovary. There are 2 peaks of secretion: one just before ovulation and one during the midluteal phase. The estradiol secretion rate is 36 μg/d (133 nmol/d) in the early follicular phase, 380 μg/d just before ovulation, and 250 μg/d during the midluteal phase (Table 4–3). After menopause, estrogen secretion declines to low levels. For comparison, the estradiol production rate in men is about 50 μg/d (184 nmol/d).

Effects on Female Genitalia

Estrogens facilitate the growth of the ovarian follicles and increase the motility of the uterine tubes. Their role in the cyclic changes in the endometrium, cervix, and vagina is discussed earlier. They increase uterine blood flow and have important effects on the smooth muscle of the uterus. In immature and ovariectomized females, the uterus is small and the myometrium atrophic and inactive. Estrogens increase the amount of uterine muscle and its content of contractile proteins. Under the influence of estrogens, the myometrium becomes more active and excitable, and action potentials in the individual muscle fibers are increased. The "estrogen-dominated" uterus is also more sensitive to oxytocin.

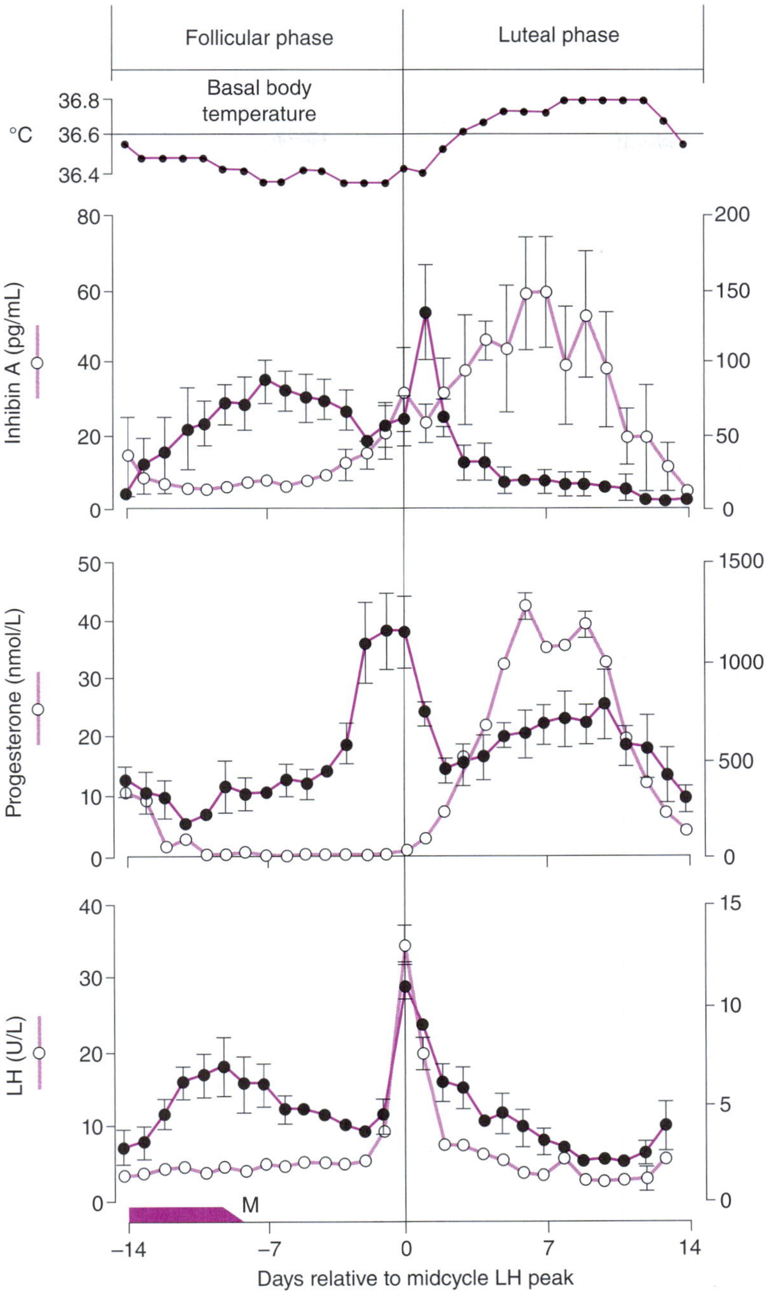

▲ Figure 4–8. Basal body temperature and plasma hormone concentrations (mean ± standard error) during the normal human menstrual cycle. Values are aligned with respect to the day of the midcycle luteinizing hormone (LH) peak. FSH, follicle-stimulating hormone. (Reproduced, with permission, from Barrett KE. *Ganong's Review of Medical Physiology*. 23rd ed. New York, NY: McGraw-Hill; 2010.)

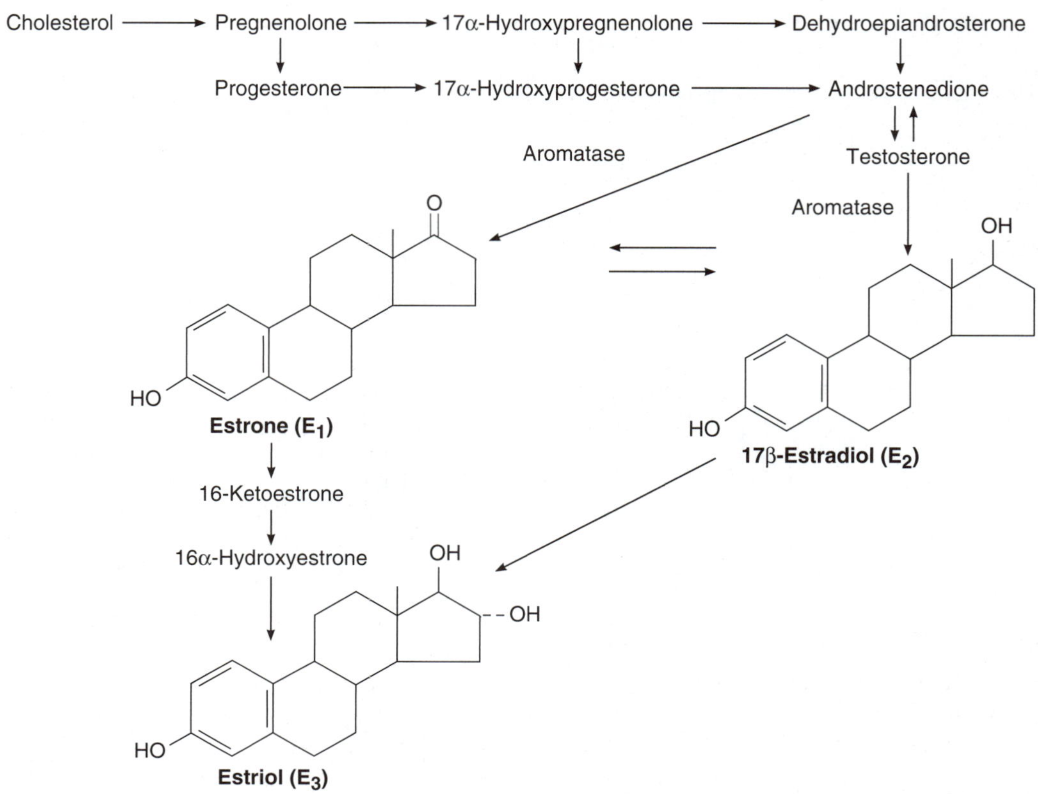

▲ **Figure 4–9.** Biosynthesis and metabolism of estrogens. (Reproduced, with permission, from Barrett KE. *Ganong's Review of Medical Physiology.* 23rd ed. New York, NY: McGraw-Hill; 2010.)

Prolonged treatment with estrogens causes endometrial hypertrophy. When estrogen therapy is discontinued, there is some sloughing and **withdrawal bleeding**. Some "breakthrough" bleeding may also occur during prolonged treatment with estrogens.

Effects on Endocrine Organs

Estrogens decrease FSH secretion. In some circumstances, estrogens inhibit LH secretion (negative feedback); in others, they increase LH secretion (positive feedback). Estrogens also increase the size of the pituitary. Women are sometimes given large doses of estrogens for 4–6 days to prevent conception during the fertile period (postcoital or "morning-after" contraception). In this instance, pregnancy probably is prevented by interference with implantation of the fertilized ovum rather than by changes in gonadotropin secretion.

Estrogens cause increased secretion of angiotensinogen and thyroid-binding globulin. They also cause epiphyseal closure in humans. In livestock, they exert an important

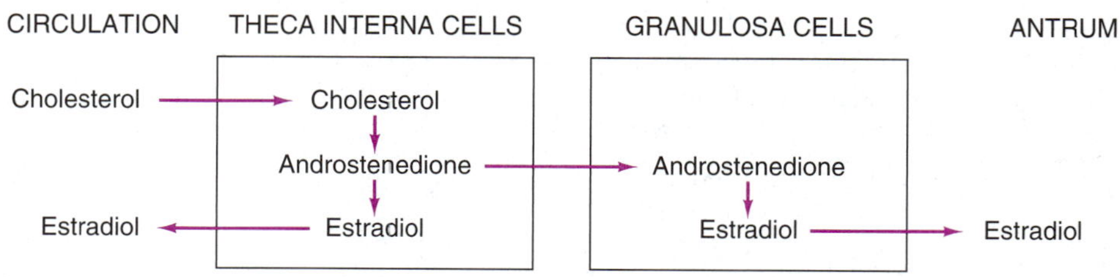

▲ **Figure 4–10.** Interactions between theca and granulosa cells in estradiol synthesis and secretion. (Reproduced, with permission, from Barrett KE. *Ganong's Review of Medical Physiology*. 23rd ed. New York, NY: McGraw-Hill; 2010.)

Table 4–2. Distribution of gonadal steroids and cortisol in plasma.

Steroid	% Free	% Bound to		
		CBG	GBG	Albumin
Testosterone	2	0	65	33
Androstenedione	7	0	8	85
Estradiol	2	0	38	60
Progesterone	2	18	0	80
Cortisol	4	90	0	6

CBG, corticosteroid-binding globulin; GBG, gonadal steroid-binding globulin.

protein anabolic effect, possibly by stimulating the secretion of androgens from the adrenal; estrogens have been used commercially to increase the weight of domestic animals.

Effects on the Central Nervous System

Estrogens are responsible for estrus behavior in animals, and they may increase libido in humans. They apparently exert this action by a direct effect on certain neurons in the hypothalamus (Fig. 4–11).

Estrogens increase the proliferation of dendrites on neurons and the number of synaptic knobs in rats. In humans, they have been reported to slow the progression of Alzheimer's disease, but this role of estrogen remains controversial.

Effects on the Breasts

Estrogens produce duct growth in the breasts and are largely responsible for breast enlargement at puberty

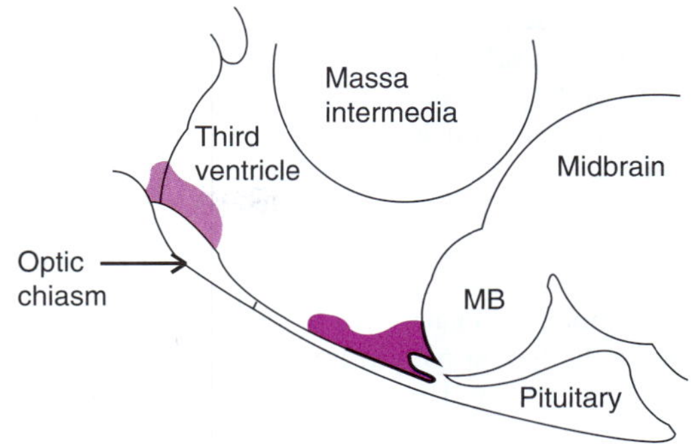

▲ **Figure 4–11.** Loci where implantations of estrogen in the hypothalamus affect ovarian weight and sexual behavior in rats, projected on a sagittal section of the hypothalamus. The implants that stimulate sex behavior are located in the suprachiasmatic area above the optic chiasm, whereas ovarian atrophy is produced by implants in the arcuate nucleus and surrounding ventral hypothalamus just above the pituitary stalk. MB, mamillary body. (Reproduced, with permission, from Barrett KE. *Ganong's Review of Medical Physiology*. 23rd ed. New York, NY: McGraw-Hill; 2010.)

in girls. Breast enlargement that occurs when estrogen-containing skin creams are applied locally is primarily due to systemic absorption of the estrogen, although a slight local effect is also produced. Estrogens are responsible for the pigmentation of the areolas. Pigmentation usually becomes more intense during the first pregnancy than it does at puberty.

Effects on Female Secondary Sex Characteristics

The body changes that develop in girls at puberty—in addition to enlargement of the breasts, uterus, and

Table 4–3. Twenty-four–hour production rates of sex steroids in women at different stages of the menstrual cycle.

Sex Steroids	Early Follicular	Preovulatory	Midluteal
Progesterone (mg)	1.0	4.0	25.0
17-Hydroxyprogesterone (mg)	0.5	4.0	4.0
Dehydroepiandrosterone (mg)	7.0	7.0	7.0
Androstenedione (mg)	2.6	4.7	3.4
Testosterone (μg)	144.0	171.0	126.0
Estrone (μg)	50.0	350.0	250.0
Estradiol (μg)	36.0	380.0	250.0

Modified and reproduced, with permission, from Yen SSC, Jaffe RB. *Reproductive Endocrinology*. 3rd ed. New York, NY: Saunders; 1991.

vagina—are due in part to estrogens, which are the "feminizing hormones," and in part simply to the absence of testicular androgens. Women have narrow shoulders, broad hips, thighs that converge, and arms that diverge (wide **carrying angle**). This body configuration, plus the female distribution of fat in the breasts and buttocks, is also seen in castrated males. In women, the larynx retains its prepubertal proportions, and the voice is high-pitched. There is less body hair and more scalp hair, and the pubic hair generally has a characteristic flattop pattern (**female escutcheon**). Growth of pubic and axillary hair in the female is due primarily to androgens rather than estrogens, although estrogen treatment may cause some hair growth. The androgens are produced by the adrenal cortex and, to a lesser extent, by the ovaries.

Other Actions of Estrogens

Normal women retain salt and water and gain weight just before menstruation. Estrogens can cause some degree of salt and water retention. However, aldosterone secretion is slightly elevated in the luteal phase, and this also contributes to premenstrual fluid retention.

Estrogens make sebaceous gland secretions more fluid and thus counter the effect of testosterone and inhibit formation of comedones ("blackheads") and acne. The liver palms, spider angiomas, and slight breast enlargement seen in advanced liver disease are due to increased circulating estrogens. The increase appears to be due to decreased hepatic metabolism of androstenedione, making more of this androgen available for conversion to estrogens.

Estrogens have a significant plasma cholesterol-lowering action. They produce vasodilatation and inhibit vascular smooth muscle proliferation, possibly by increasing the local production of nitric oxide (NO). Estrogen has also been shown to prevent expression of factors important in the initiation of atherosclerosis. These actions may account for the low incidence of myocardial infarction and other complications of atherosclerotic-vascular disease in premenopausal women. There is considerable evidence that small doses of estrogen may reduce the incidence of cardiovascular disease after menopause. However, some recently published data do not support this conclusion, and additional research is needed. Large doses of oral estrogen also promote thrombosis, apparently because the high concentrations of estrogen that reach the liver in the portal blood alter hepatic production of clotting factors.

Mechanism of Action

The 2 principal types of nuclear estrogen receptors are estrogen receptor-α (ER-α), which is encoded by a gene on chromosome 6, and estrogen receptor-β (ER-β), which is encoded by a gene on chromosome 14. Both are members of the nuclear receptor superfamily, which includes receptors for many different steroids. After binding estrogen, the nuclear receptors dimerize and bind to DNA, altering its transcription (Fig. 4–12). Some tissues contain one type or the other, but there is also overlap, with some tissues containing both ER-α and ER-β. ER-α is found primarily in the uterus, kidneys, liver, and heart; whereas ER-β is found primarily in the ovaries, prostate, lung, gastrointestinal tract, hemopoietic system, and central nervous system. The receptors also form heterodimers, with ER-α binding to ER-β. Male and female mice in which the gene for ER-α has been knocked out are sterile, develop osteoporosis, and continue to grow because their epiphyses do not close. ER-β female knockouts are infertile, but ER-β male knockouts are fertile even though they have hyperplastic prostates and loss of fat. Thus, the actions of the estrogen receptors are complex, multiple, and varied. However, this is not surprising because it is now known that both receptors exist in various isoforms and, like thyroid receptors, can bind to various activating and stimulating factors.

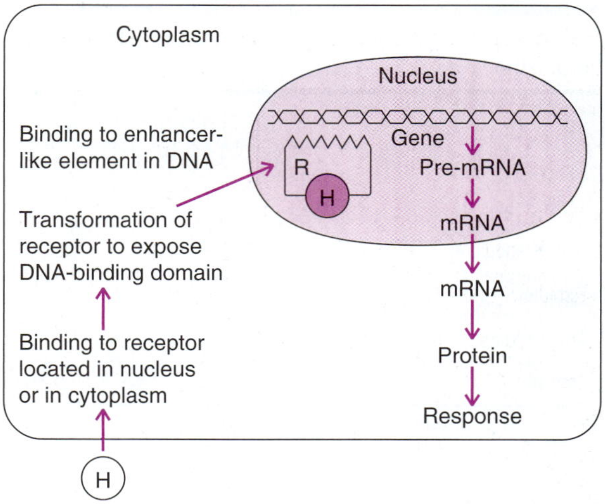

▲ **Figure 4–12.** Mechanism of action of steroid hormones. The estrogen, progestin, androgen, glucocorticoid, mineralocorticoid, and 1,25-dihydroxycholecalciferol receptors have different molecular weights, but all have a ligand-binding domain and a DNA-binding domain that is exposed when the ligand binds. The receptor–hormone complex then binds to DNA, producing increased or decreased transcription. H, hormone; R, receptor. (Reproduced, with permission, from Ganong WF. *Review of Medical Physiology*. 22nd ed. New York, NY: McGraw-Hill; 2005.)

Most of the actions of estrogens are genomic, ie, mediated by actions of the nucleus. However, some effects are so rapid that it is difficult to believe they are mediated via increased expression of mRNAs. These include effects on neuronal discharge in the brain and possibly feedback effects on gonadotropin secretion. Their existence has led to the hypothesis that, in addition to genomic actions, there are nongenomic effects of estrogens that are presumably mediated by membrane receptors. Similar rapid effects of progesterone, testosterone, and aldosterone may also be produced by membrane receptors.

Synthetic Estrogen

The ethinyl derivative of estradiol (Fig. 4–13) is a potent estrogen. Unlike naturally occurring estrogens, it is relatively active when given orally because it has an ethinyl group in position 17, which makes it resistant to hepatic metabolism. Naturally occurring hormones have low activity when given orally because the portal venous drainage of the intestine carries them to the liver, where they are largely inactivated before they can reach the general circulation. Some nonsteroidal substances and a few compounds found in plants have estrogenic activity. Plant estrogens rarely affect humans but may cause undesirable effects in farm animals. Diethylstilbestrol (Fig. 4–13) and a number of related compounds are strongly estrogenic, possible because they are converted to steroid-like ring structures in the body.

Estradiol reduces the hot flashes and other symptoms of the menopause, and it prevents the development of osteoporosis. It may reduce the initiation and progression of atherosclerosis and the incidence of myocardial infarctions. However, it also stimulates the growth of the endometrium and the breast, and it can lead to cancer of the uterus and possibly the breast. Therefore, there has been an active search for "tailor-made" estrogens that have the bone and cardiovascular effects of estradiol but lack its growth-stimulating effects on the uterus and the breast. Two of the selective estrogen receptor modulators (SERMs), **tamoxifen** and **raloxifene**, show promise in this regard. Neither combats the symptoms of menopause, but both have the bone-preserving effects of estradiol. They may also have cardioprotective effects, but the clinical relevance of these effects has not been established. In addition, tamoxifen does not stimulate the breast, and raloxifene does not stimulate the breast or uterus. The clinical uses of the 2 drugs are discussed elsewhere in this book.

Chemistry, Biosynthesis, & Metabolism of Progesterone

Progesterone (Fig. 4–14) is a C_{21} steroid secreted in large amounts by the corpus luteum and the placenta. It is an important intermediate in steroid biosynthesis in all tissues that secrete steroid hormones, and small amounts enter the

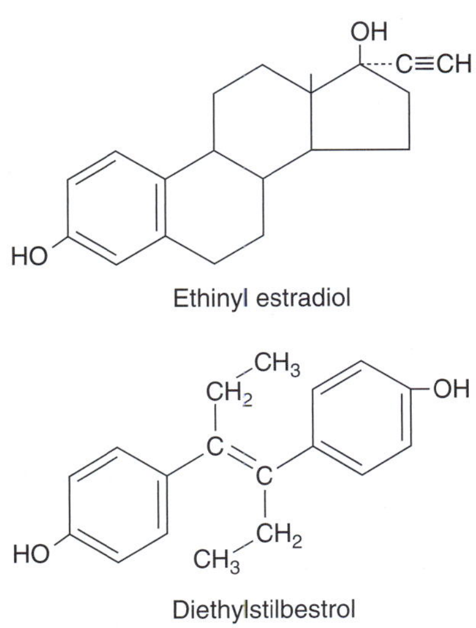

▲ **Figure 4–13.** Synthetic estrogens. (Reproduced, with permission, from Ganong WF. *Review of Medical Physiology*. 22nd ed. New York, NY: McGraw-Hill; 2005.)

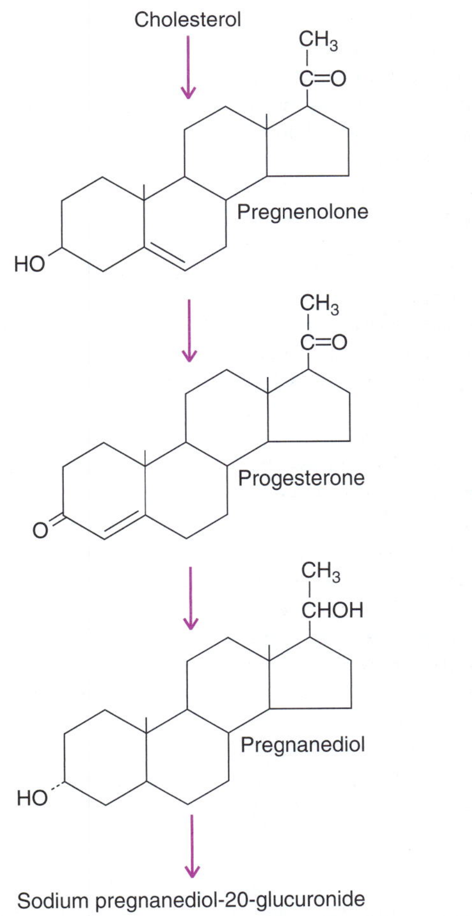

▲ **Figure 4–14.** Biosynthesis of progesterone and major pathway for its metabolism. Other metabolites are also formed. (Reproduced, with permission, from Barrett KE. *Ganong's Review of Medical Physiology*. 23rd ed. New York, NY: McGraw-Hill; 2010.)

circulation from the testes and adrenal cortex. The 20α- and 20β-hydroxy derivatives of progesterone are formed in the corpus luteum. About 2% of the progesterone in the circulation is free (Table 4–2), whereas 80% is bound to albumin and 18% is bound to corticosteroid-binding globulin. Progesterone has a short half-life and is converted in the liver to pregnanediol, which is conjugated to glucuronic acid and excreted in the urine (Fig. 4–14).

Secretion of Progesterone

The plasma progesterone level in women during the follicular phase of the menstrual cycle is approximately 0.9 ng/mL (3 nmol/L), whereas the level in men is approximately 0.3 ng/mL (1 nmol/L). The difference is due to secretion of small amounts of progesterone by cells in the ovarian follicle. During the luteal phase, the large amounts secreted by the corpus luteum cause ovarian secretion to increase about 20-fold. The result is an increase in plasma progesterone to a peak value of approximately 18 ng/mL (60 nmol/L) (Fig. 4–8).

The stimulating effect of LH on progesterone secretion by the corpus luteum is due to activation of adenylyl cyclase and involves a subsequent step that is dependent on protein synthesis.

Actions of Progesterone

The principal target organs of progesterone are the uterus, the breasts, and the brain. Progesterone is responsible for the progestational changes in the endometrium and the cyclic changes in the cervix and vagina described earlier. It has antiestrogenic effects on the myometrial cells, decreasing their excitability, their sensitivity to oxytocin, and their spontaneous electrical activity, while increasing their membrane potential. Progesterone decreases the number of estrogen receptors in the endometrium and increases the rate of conversion of 17β-estradiol to less active estrogens.

In the breast, progesterone stimulates the development of lobules and alveoli. It induces differentiation of estrogen-prepared ductal tissue and supports the secretory function of the breast during lactation.

The feedback effects of progesterone are complex and are exerted at both the hypothalamic and the pituitary level. Large doses of progesterone inhibit LH secretion and potentiate the inhibitory effects of estrogens, preventing ovulation.

Progesterone is thermogenic and probably is responsible for the rise in basal body temperature at the time of ovulation (Fig. 4–8). Progesterone stimulates respiration, and the fact that alveolar partial pressure of carbon dioxide (Pco_2) in women during the luteal phase of the menstrual cycle is lower than that in men is attributed to the action of secreted progesterone. In pregnancy, alveolar Pco_2 falls as progesterone secretion rises.

Large doses of progesterone produce natriuresis, probably by blocking the action of aldosterone on the kidney. The hormone does not have significant anabolic effect.

Mechanism of Action

The effects of progesterone, like those of other steroids, are brought about by an action on DNA to initiate synthesis of new mRNA. The progesterone receptor is bound to a heat shock protein in the absence of the steroid, and progesterone binding releases the heat shock protein, exposing the DNA-binding domain of the receptor. The synthetic steroid **mifepristone (RU-486)** binds to the receptor but does not release the heat shock protein, and it blocks the binding of progesterone. As the maintenance of early pregnancy depends on the stimulatory effect of progesterone on endometrial growth and its inhibition of uterine contractility, mifepristone causes absorption. In some countries, mifepristone combined with a prostaglandin is used to produce elective abortions.

Two isoforms of the progesterone receptor are produced by differential processing from a single gene on chromosome 11. Progesterone receptor A (PR_A) is a truncated form that when activated is capable of inhibiting some of the actions of progesterone receptor B (PR_B). A third isoform has been identified in humans, PR_C, which is thought to modulate the transcriptional activity of PR_A and PR_B. However, although the physiologic significance of the existence of the isoforms remains to be determined, it has been suggested that they have distinct tissue-specific responses to progesterone.

Substances that mimic the action of progesterone are sometimes called **progestational agents**, **gestagens**, or **progestins**. They are used along with synthetic estrogens as oral contraceptive agents.

RELAXIN

Relaxin is a polypeptide hormone that is secreted by the corpus luteum in women and by the prostate in men. During pregnancy, it relaxes the pubic symphysis and other pelvic joints while softening and dilating the uterine cervix, thus facilitating delivery. It also inhibits uterine contractions and may play a role in the development of the mammary glands. In nonpregnant women, relaxin is found in the corpus luteum and the endometrium during the secretory but not the proliferative phase of the menstrual cycle. Its function in nonpregnant women is unknown, but it is postulated that relaxin may play a role in follicular development, ovulation, and/or implantation. There is currently no evidence that endogenous relaxin contributes to reproductive processes in any species.

In most species, there is only 1 relaxin gene, but in humans there are 2 genes on chromosome 9 that code for 2 structurally different polypeptides with relaxin activity. However, only 1 of these genes is active in the ovary and the prostate. The structure of the polypeptide produced in these 2 tissues is shown in Figure 4–15.

INHIBINS & ACTIVINS

Both the ovaries and testes produce polypeptides called **inhibins** that inhibit FSH secretion. There are 2 inhibins,

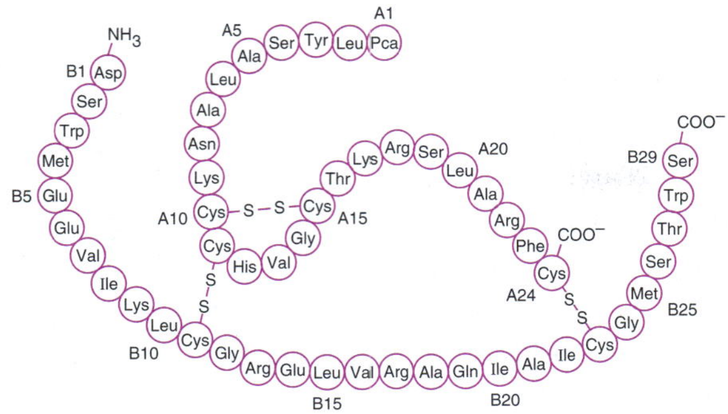

▲ **Figure 4–15.** Structure of human luteal and prostatic relaxin. Note the A and B chains are connected by disulfide bridges. Pca, pyroglutamic acid residue at N-terminal of A chain. (Modified and reproduced, with permission, from Winslow JW Shih A, Bourell JH, et al. Human seminal relaxin is a product of the same gene as human luteal relaxin. *Endocrinology* 1992;130:2660.)

and they are formed from 3 polypeptide subunits: a glycosylated α subunit with a molecular weight of 18,000, and 2 nonglycosylated β subunits, β_A and β_B, each with a molecular weight of 14,000. The subunits are formed from precursor proteins (Fig. 4–16). The α subunit combines with β_A to form a heterodimer and with β_B to form another heterodimer, with the subunits linked by disulfide bonds. Both $\alpha\beta_A$ (inhibin A) and $\alpha\beta_B$ (inhibin B) inhibit FSH secretion by a direct action on the pituitary, although it now appears that inhibin B is the FSH-regulating hormone in adults. Inhibins are produced by Sertoli cells in males and by granulosa cells in females.

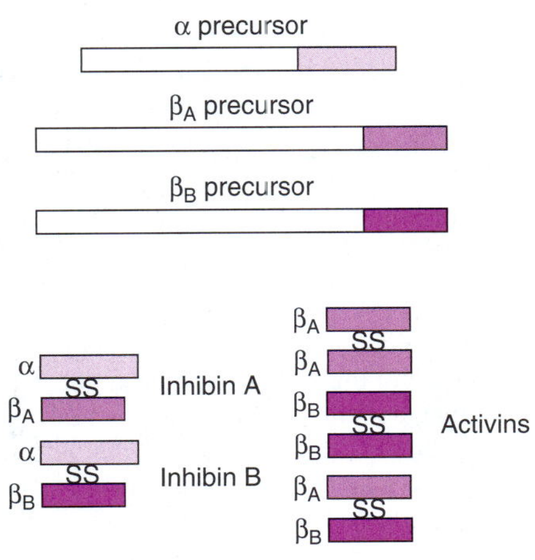

▲ **Figure 4–16.** Inhibin precursor proteins and the various inhibins and activins that are formed from them. SS, disulfide bonds. (Reproduced, with permission, from Ganong WF. *Review of Medical Physiology*. 22nd ed. New York, NY: McGraw-Hill; 2005.)

The heterodimer, $\beta_A\beta_B$, and the homodimers, $\beta_A\beta_A$ and $\beta_B\beta_B$, stimulate rather than inhibit FSH secretion and consequently are called **activins.** Their function in reproduction is unsettled. However, the inhibins and activins are members of the transforming growth factor-β superfamily of dimeric growth factors. Also included in this superfamily is the müllerian inhibitory substance (MIS), which is important in embryonic development of the gonads. Two **activin receptors** have been cloned, and both appear to be serine kinases. Inhibins and activins are found not only in the gonads, but also in the brain and many other tissues. In the bone marrow, activins are involved in the development of white blood cells. In embryonic life, activins are involved in the formation of mesoderm. All mice with a targeted deletion of the α-inhibin gene initially grew in a normal fashion but then developed gonadal stromal tumors, thus elucidating the role of the α-inhibin gene as a tumor suppressor gene.

In plasma, α_2-macroglobulin binds activins and inhibins. In tissues, activins bind to a family of 4 glycoproteins called **follistatins**. Binding of the activins inactivates their biologic activity, which may involve regulation of FSH production from gonadotropes in the anterior pituitary. However, the relation of follistatins to inhibin and their physiologic function remain unsettled.

PITUITARY HORMONES

Ovarian secretion depends on the action of hormones secreted by the anterior pituitary gland. The anterior pituitary gland secretes 6 established hormones: ACTH, growth hormone, thyroid-stimulating hormone (TSH), FSH, LH, and prolactin (Fig. 4–17). It also secretes 1 putative hormone: β-lipotrophic hormone (β-LPH).

The posterior pituitary differs from the anterior pituitary in that its hormones, oxytocin and arginine vasopressin, are secreted by neurons directly into the systemic circulation.

GONADOTROPINS

The gonadotropins, FSH and LH, act in concert to regulate the cyclic secretion of the ovarian hormones. They are glycoproteins made up of α and β subunits. The α subunits have the same amino acid composition as the α subunits in the glycoproteins, TSH and human chorionic gonadotropin (hCG). The specificity of these 4 glycoprotein hormones is imparted by the different structures of their β subunits. The carbohydrates in the gonadotropin molecules increase the potency of the hormones by markedly slowing their metabolism. The half-life of human FSH is about 170 minutes; the half-life of LH is about 60 minutes.

The receptors for FSH and LH are serpentine receptors coupled to adenylyl cyclase through G_S. In addition, each has an extended, glycosylated extracellular domain.

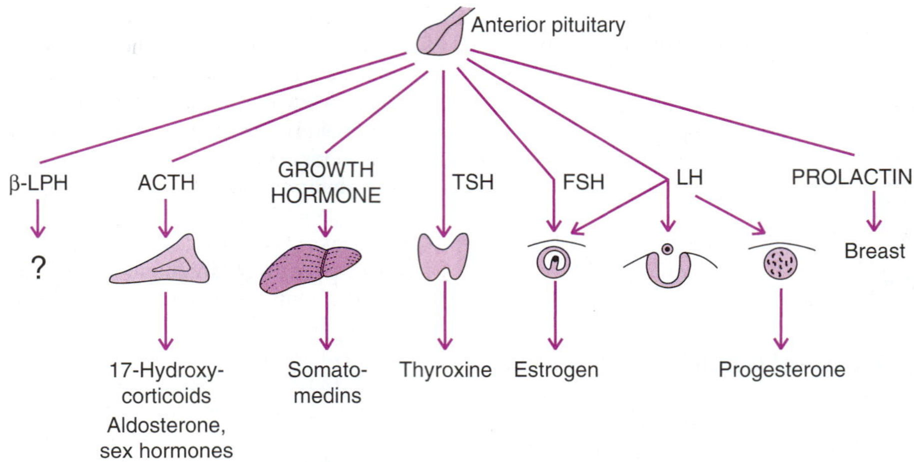

▲ **Figure 4–17.** Anterior pituitary hormones. In women, follicle-stimulating hormone (FSH) and luteinizing hormone (LH) act in sequence on the ovary to produce growth of the ovarian follicle, which secretes estrogen, then ovulation, followed by formation and maintenance of the corpus luteum, which secretes estrogen and progesterone. In men, FSH and LH control the functions of the testes. Prolactin stimulates lactation. β-LPH, β-lipotropic hormone; ACTH, adrenocorticotropic hormone; TSH, thyroid-stimulating hormone. (Reproduced, with permission, from Ganong WF. *Review of Medical Physiology*. 22nd ed. New York, NY: McGraw-Hill; 2005.)

HYPOTHALAMIC HORMONES

Secretion of the anterior pituitary hormones is regulated by the hypothalamic hypophysiotropic hormones. These substances are produced by neurons and enter the portal hypophysial vessels (Fig. 4–18), a special group of blood vessels that transmit substances directly from the hypothalamus to the anterior pituitary gland. The actions of these hormones are summarized in Figure 4–19. The structures of 6 established hypophysiotropic hormones are known (Fig. 4–20). No single prolactin-releasing hormone has been isolated and identified. However, several polypeptides that are found in the hypothalamus can increase prolactin secretion, and 1 or more of these may stimulate prolactin secretion under physiologic conditions.

The posterior pituitary hormones are produced in the cell bodies of neurons located in the supraoptic and paraventricular nuclei of the hypothalamus and transported down the axons of these neurons to their endings in the posterior lobe of the pituitary. The hormones are released from the endings into the circulation when action potentials pass down the axons and reach their endings. The structures of the hormones are shown in Figure 4–21.

CONTROL OF OVARIAN FUNCTION

FSH from the pituitary is responsible for the early maturation of the ovarian follicles, while FSH and LH together are responsible for the final maturation. A burst of LH secretion (Fig. 4–8) triggers ovulation and the initial formation of the corpus luteum. There is also a smaller midcycle burst of FSH secretion, the significance of which is uncertain. LH stimulates the secretion of estrogen and progesterone from the corpus luteum.

Hypothalamic Components

The hypothalamus occupies a key role in the control of gonadotropin secretion. Hypothalamic control is exerted by GnRH secreted into the portal hypophysial vessels. GnRH stimulates the secretion of both FSH and LH. It is unlikely that there is an additional separate follicle-stimulating hormone-releasing hormone (FRH).

GnRH is normally secreted in episodic bursts (**circhoral secretion**). These bursts are essential for normal secretion of gonadotropins, which are also exerted in a pulsatile fashion (Fig. 4–22). If GnRH is administered by constant infusion, the number of GnRH receptors in the anterior pituitary decreases (**downregulation**) and LH secretion falls to low levels. However, if GnRH is administered episodically at a rate of 1 pulse per hour, LH secretion is stimulated. This is true even when endogenous GnRH secretion has been prevented by a lesion of the ventral hypothalamus.

It is clear that, not only is this episodic nature of secretion of GnRH an important phenomenon, but that fluctuations in the frequency and amplitude of these GnRH bursts are also important in generating the other hormonal changes that are responsible for the menstrual cycle. Frequency is increased by estrogens and decreased by progesterone and testosterone. The frequency increases late in the follicular phase of the cycle, culminating in the LH surge. During the secretory phase, the frequency decreases as a result of the action of progesterone, but when estrogen and progesterone secretion decrease at the end of the cycle, frequency once again increases.

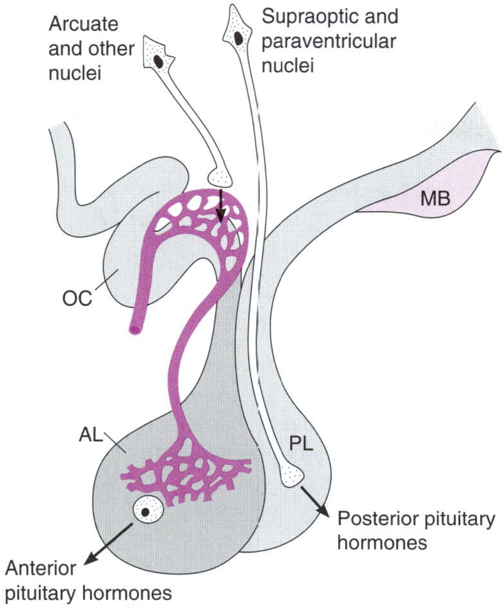

▲ **Figure 4–18.** Secretion of hypothalamic hormones. The hormones of the posterior lobe (PL) are released into the general circulation from the endings of supraoptic and paraventricular neurons, whereas hypophysiotropic hormones are secreted into the portal hypophysial circulation from the endings of arcuate and other hypothalamic neurons. AL, anterior lobe; MB, mamillary bodies; OC, optic chiasm. (Reproduced, with permission, from Ganong WF. *Review of Medical Physiology.* 22nd ed. New York, NY: McGraw-Hill; 2005.)

At the time of the midcycle LH surge, the sensitivity of the gonadotropes to GnRH is greatly increased because of their exposure to GnRH pulses of the frequency that exist at this time. This self-priming effect of GnRH is important in producing a maximum LH response.

The nature and the exact location of the GnRH pulse generator in the hypothalamus are still unsettled. However, it is known that norepinephrine and possibly epinephrine increase GnRH pulse frequencies. Conversely, opioid peptides, such as the enkephalins and β-endorphin, reduce the frequency of GnRH pulses.

The downregulation of pituitary receptors and the consequent decrease in LH secretion produced by constantly elevated levels of GnRH has led to the use of long-acting GnRH agonists to inhibit LH secretion in precocious puberty, endometriosis, leiomyomas, and cancer of the prostate.

Feedback Effects

Changes in plasma levels of LH, FSH, sex steroids, and inhibin B during the menstrual cycle are shown in Figure 4–8, and their feedback relations are diagrammed in Figure 4–23. At the start of the follicular phase, the inhibin B level is low and the FSH level is modestly elevated, fostering follicular growth. LH secretion is held in check by the negative feedback effect of the rising plasma estrogen level. At 36–48 hours before ovulation, the estrogen feedback effect becomes positive, which initiates the burst of LH secretion (LH surge) that produces ovulation. Ovulation occurs about 9 hours after the LH peak. FSH secretion also peaks, despite a small rise in inhibin B level, probably because of the strong stimulation of gonadotropes by GnRH. During the luteal phase, secretion of LH and FSH is low because of the elevated levels of estrogen, progesterone, and inhibin B.

It should be emphasized that a moderate, constant level of circulating estrogen exerts a negative feedback effect on LH secretion, whereas an elevated estrogen level exerts a positive feedback and stimulates LH secretion. It has been demonstrated in monkeys that there is also a minimum time that estrogen levels must be elevated to produce a positive feedback. When the circulating estrogen level was increased about 300% for 24 hours, only negative feedback was seen; but when it was increased about 300% for 36 hours or more, a brief decline in secretion was followed

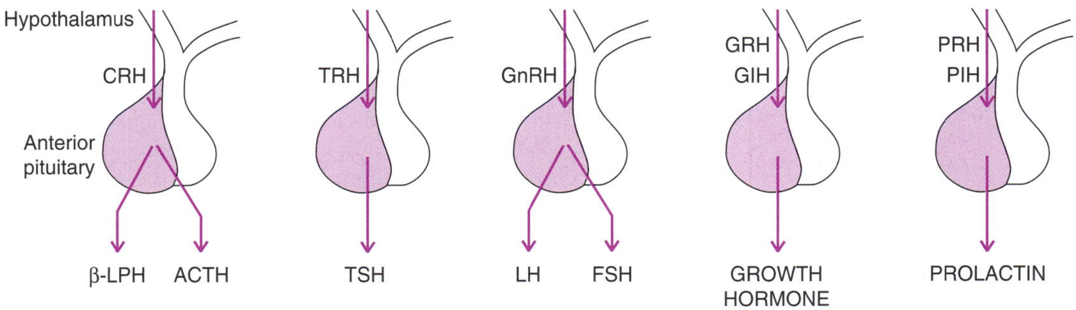

▲ **Figure 4–19.** Effects of hypophysiotropic hormones on the secretion of anterior pituitary hormones. β-LPH, β-lipotropic hormone; ACTH, adrenocorticotropic hormone; CRH, corticotropin-releasing hormone; FSH, follicle-stimulating hormone; GIH, growth-inhibiting hormone; GnRH, gonadotropin-releasing hormone; GRH, growth hormone-releasing hormone; LH, luteinizing hormone; PIH, prolactin-inhibiting hormone; PRH, prolactin-releasing hormone; TRH, thyroid-releasing hormone; TSH, thyroid-stimulating hormone. (Reproduced, with permission, from Ganong WF. *Review of Medical Physiology*. 22nd ed. New York, NY: McGraw-Hill; 2005.)

TRH	(pyro)Glu-His-Pro-NH_2
GnRH	(pyro)Glu-His-Trp-Ser-Tyr-Gly-Leu-Arg-Pro-Gly-NH_2
Somatostatin	Ala-Gly-Cys-Lys-Asn-Phe-Phe-Trp-Lys-Thr-Phe-Thr-Ser-Cys (S—S bridge between Cys residues)
CRH	Ser-Glu-Glu-Pro-Pro-Ile-Ser-Leu-Asp-Leu-Thr-Phe-His-Leu-Leu-Arg-Glu-Val-Leu-Glu-Met-Ala-Arg-Ala-Glu-Gln-Leu-Ala-Gln-Gln-Ala-His-Ser-Asn-Arg-Lys-Leu-Met-Glu-Ile-Ile-NH_2
GRH	Tyr-Ala-Asp-Ala-Ile-Phe-Thr-Asn-Ser-Tyr-Arg-Lys-Val-Leu-Gly-Gln-Leu-Ser-Ala-Arg-Lys-Leu-Leu-Gln-Asp-Ile-Met-Ser-Arg-Gln-Gln-Gly-Glu-Ser-Asn-Gln-Glu-Arg-Gly-Ala-Arg-Ala-Arg-Leu-NH_2
PIH	Dopamine

▲ **Figure 4–20.** Structures of hypophysiotropic hormones in humans. The structure of somatostatin shown is the tetradecapeptide (somatostatin 14). In addition, preprosomatostatin is the source of an N-terminal extended polypeptide containing 28 amino acid residues (somatostatin 28). Both forms are found in many tissues. CRH, corticotropin-releasing hormone; GnRH, gonadotropin-releasing hormone; GRH, growth hormone-releasing hormone; PIH, prolactin-inhibiting hormone; TRH, thyroid-releasing hormone. (Reproduced, with permission, from Ganong WF. *Review of Medical Physiology*. 22nd ed. New York, NY: McGraw-Hill; 2005.)

by a burst of LH secretion that resembled the midcycle surge. When circulating levels of progesterone were high, the positive feedback effect of estrogen was inhibited. There is evidence in primates that both the negative and the positive feedback effects of estrogen are exerted in the mediobasal hypothalamus via the ER-α receptors. The mechanism of the "switch" between negative and positive feedback remains unknown.

Control of Menstrual Cycle

In an important sense, regression of the corpus luteum (**luteolysis**) starting 3–4 days before menses is the key to the menstrual cycle. PGF_{2a} appears to be a physiologic luteolysin, but this prostaglandin is only active when endothelial cells producing endothelin-1 (ET-1) are present. Therefore, it appears that, at least in some species, luteolysis is produced by the combined action of PGF_{2a} and ET-1. In some domestic animals, oxytocin secreted by the corpus luteum appears to exert a local luteolytic effect, possibly by causing the release of prostaglandins. Once luteolysis begins, the estrogen and progesterone levels fall, followed by increased secretion of FSH and LH. A new crop of follicles develops, and then a single dominant follicle matures as a result of the action of FSH and LH. Near midcycle, there is a rise in estrogen secretion from the follicle. This rise augments the responsiveness of the pituitary to GnRH and triggers a burst of LH secretion. The resulting ovulation is followed by formation of a corpus luteum. There is a drop in estrogen secretion at first, but progesterone and estrogen levels then rise together, along with inhibin B. The elevated levels inhibit FSH and LH secretion for a while, but luteolysis again occurs and a new cycle begins.

Cys-Tyr-Phe-Gln-Asn-Cys-Pro-Arg-Gly-NH_2 (S—S bridge between Cys residues)

Arginine vasopressin

Cys-Tyr-Ile-Gln-Asn-Cys-Pro-Leu-Gly-NH_2 (S—S bridge between Cys residues)

Oxytocin

▲ **Figure 4–21.** Structures of arginine vasopressin and oxytocin. (Reproduced, with permission, from Ganong WF. *Review of Medical Physiology*. 22nd ed. New York, NY: McGraw-Hill; 2005.)

Reflex Ovulation

Female cats, rabbits, mink, and certain other animals have long periods of **estrus**, or heat, during which they ovulate only after copulation. Such **reflex ovulation** is brought about by afferent impulses from the genitalia and the eyes, ears, and nose that converge on the ventral hypothalamus and provoke an ovulation-inducing release of LH from the pituitary. In species such as rats, monkeys, and humans, ovulation is a spontaneous periodic phenomenon, but afferent impulses converging on the hypothalamus can also exert effects. Ovulation can be delayed for 24 hours in rats by administering pentobarbital or other neurally active drugs 12 hours before the expected time of follicle rupture. In women, menstrual cycles may be markedly influenced by emotional stimuli.

Contraception

Methods commonly used to prevent conception, along with their failure rates, are listed in Table 4–4. Contraception is

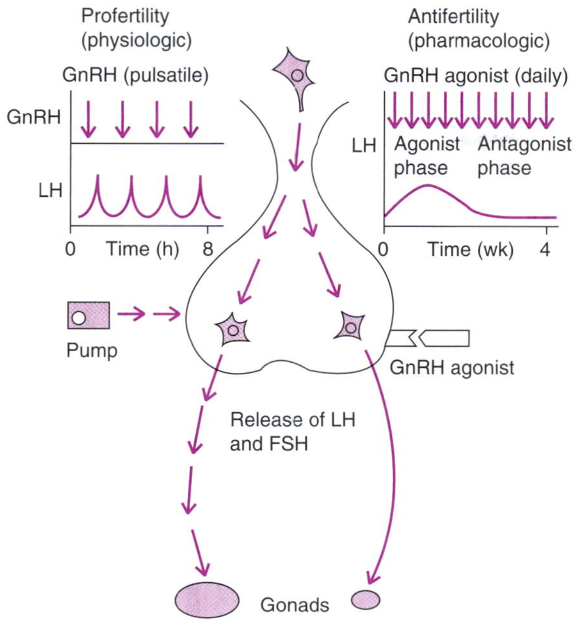

▲ **Figure 4–22.** Profertility and antifertility actions of gonadotropin-releasing hormone (GnRH) and its agonists. The normal secretion of GnRH is pulsatile, occurring at 30- to 60-minute intervals. This mode, which can be mimicked by timed injections, produces circhoral peaks of luteinizing hormone (LH) and follicle-stimulating hormone (FSH) secretion and promotes fertility. If GnRH is administered by continuous infusion or if 1 of its long-acting synthetic agonists is injected, there is initial stimulation of the pituitary receptors. However, this stimulation lasts for only a few days and is followed by receptor downregulation with inhibition of gonadotropin secretion (antifertility effect). (Reproduced, with permission, from Conn PM, Crowley WF Jr. Gonadotropin-releasing hormone and its analogues. *N Engl J Med* 1991;324:93.)

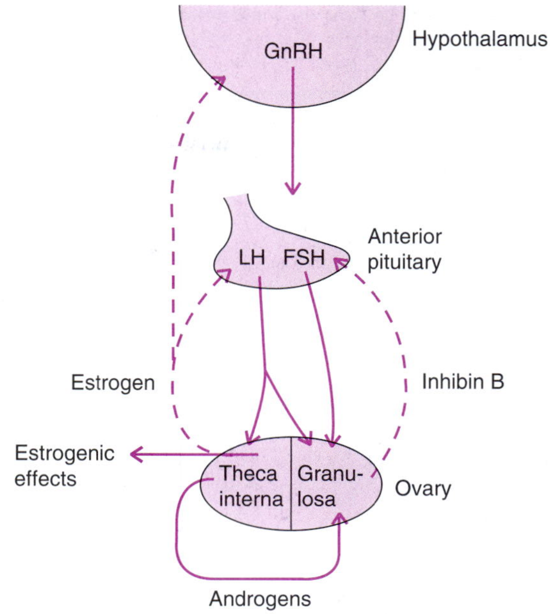

▲ **Figure 4–23.** Feedback regulation of ovarian function. The cells of the theca interna provide androgens to the granulosa cells, and the thecal cells produce the circulating estrogens, which inhibit the secretion of luteinizing hormone (LH), gonadotropin-releasing hormone (GnRH), and follicle-stimulating hormone (FSH). Inhibin B from the granulosa cells also inhibits FSH secretion. LH regulates thecal cells, whereas the granulosa cells are regulated by both LH and FSH. The dashed arrows indicate inhibition, and the solid arrows indicate stimulation. (Reproduced, with permission, from Ganong WF. *Review of Medical Physiology*. 22nd ed. New York, NY: McGraw-Hill; 2005.)

considered in detail in Chapter 58. It is briefly reviewed here because the techniques used are excellent examples of the practical application of the physiologic principles discussed in this chapter.

Among the most extensively used contraceptives are estrogens and/or progestins in varying doses and combinations. They interfere with gonadotropic secretion or implantation, and in some cases, inhibit the union of sperm with ova.

Once conception has occurred, abortion can be produced by progesterone antagonists such as mifepristone.

Implantation of foreign bodies in the uterus causes changes in the duration of the sexual cycle in a number of mammalian species. In humans, such foreign bodies do not alter the menstrual cycle, but they act as effective contraceptive devices. The 2 **intrauterine devices (IUDs)** available in the United States are T-shaped devices that contain copper or progestin. There is production of a local, sterile, inflammatory reaction secondary to the presence of the foreign body in the uterine cavity, which is thought to act as a spermicide inhibiting sperm capacitation, penetration, and survival. The progestin IUD thickens cervical mucus and may cause endometrial alterations that prevent implantation.

Implants made up primarily of progestins are now being increasingly used in some parts of the world. The implants are inserted under the skin and remain effective for 3 years. The 2 primary mechanisms of action include inhibition of ovulation and restriction of sperm penetration through cervical mucus. They often produce amenorrhea but otherwise appear to be well tolerated. Spontaneous breakthrough bleeding is, however, a common side effect.

PROLACTIN

Chemistry of Prolactin

Prolactin is another anterior pituitary hormone that has important functions in reproduction and pregnancy.

Table 4–4. Relative effectiveness of frequently used contraceptive methods.

Method	Failures per 100 Women-Years
Vasectomy	0.02
Tubal ligation and similar procedures	0.13
Oral contraceptive	
>50 μg estrogen and progestin	0.32
<50 μg estrogen and progestin	0.27
Progestin only	1.2
IUD	
Copper 7	1.5
Loop D	1.3
Diaphragm	1.9
Condom	3.6
Withdrawal	6.7
Spermicide	11.9
Rhythm	15.5

IUD, intrauterine device.

Data from Vessey M, Lawless M, Yeates D. Efficacy of different contraceptive methods. *Lancet* 1982;1:841. Reproduced with permission.

The human prolactin molecule contains 199 amino acid residues and 3 disulfide bridges (Fig. 4–24) and has considerable structural similarity to human growth hormone and human chorionic somatomammotropin (hCS). The half-life of prolactin, like that of growth hormone, is about 20 minutes. Structurally similar prolactins are secreted by the endometrium and by the placenta.

Receptors

The human prolactin receptor resembles the growth hormone receptor. It is one of the superfamily of receptors that includes the growth hormone receptor and receptors for many cytokines and hematopoietic growth factors. It dimerizes and activates the JAK-STAT and other intracellular enzymes cascades.

Actions

Prolactin causes milk secretion from the breast after estrogen and progesterone priming. Its effect on the breast causes increased production of casein and lactalbumin. However, the action of the hormone is not exerted on the cell nucleus and is prevented by inhibitors of microtubules. Prolactin also inhibits the effects of gonadotropins, possibly by an action at the level of the ovary. Consequently, it is a "natural contraceptive" that spaces pregnancies by preventing ovulation in lactating women. The function of prolactin in normal males is unsettled, but excess prolactin in normal males causes impotence. An action of prolactin that has been used in the past as the basis for a bioassay to assess this hormone is stimulation of the growth and "secretion" of the crop sacs in pigeons and other birds. The paired crop sacs are outpouchings of the esophagus that form, by desquamation of their inner cell layers, a nutritious material ("milk") that the birds feed to their young. However, prolactin, FSH, and LH are now regularly measured by radioimmunoassay.

Regulation of Prolactin Secretion

The normal plasma prolactin concentration is approximately 5 ng/mL in men and 8 ng/mL in women. Secretion is tonically inhibited by the hypothalamus, and a section of the pituitary stalk leads to an increase in circulating prolactin. Thus, the effect of the hypothalamic prolactin-inhibiting hormone (PIH), dopamine, is greater than the effect of the putative prolactin-releasing hormone. In humans, prolactin secretion is increased by stimulation of the nipple, exercise, and surgical or psychological stress (Table 4–5). The plasma prolactin level rises during sleep, with the rise starting after the onset of sleep and persisting throughout the sleep period. Secretion is increased during pregnancy, reaching a peak at the time of parturition. After delivery, the plasma concentration falls to nonpregnant levels in about 8 days. Suckling produces a prompt increase in secretion, but the magnitude of this rise gradually declines after a woman has been nursing for more than 3 months.

L-Dopa decreases prolactin secretion by increasing formation of dopamine. Bromocriptine and other dopamine agonists inhibit secretion because they stimulate dopamine receptors. Chlorpromazine and related drugs that block dopamine receptors increase prolactin secretion. Thyroid-releasing hormone (TRH) stimulates the secretion of prolactin in addition to TSH, plus there are additional prolactin-releasing polypeptides in hypothalamic tissue. Estrogens produce a slowly developing increase in prolactin secretion as a result of a direct action on the lactotropes.

It has not been established that prolactin facilitates the secretion of dopamine in the median eminence. Thus, prolactin acts in the hypothalamus in a negative feedback fashion to inhibit its own secretion.

Hyperprolactinemia

Up to 70% of patients with chromophobe adenomas of the anterior pituitary have elevated plasma prolactin levels. In some instances, the elevation may be due to damage to the pituitary stalk, but in most cases, the tumor cells are actually secreting the hormone. The hyperprolactinemia may cause galactorrhea, but in many individuals, there are no demonstrable abnormalities. Indeed, most women with galactorrhea have normal prolactin levels; definite elevations are found in less than one-third of patients with this condition.

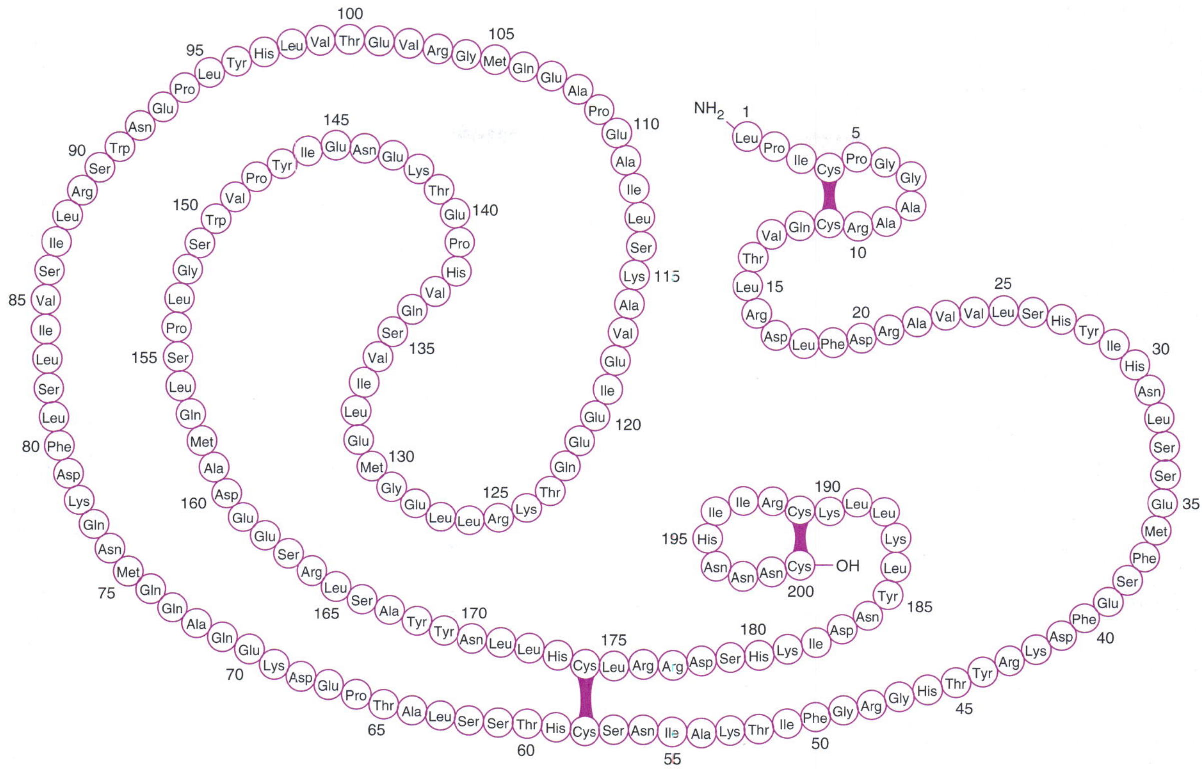

▲ **Figure 4–24.** Structure of human prolactin. (Reproduced, with permission, from Bondy PK, Rosenberg LE. *Metabolic Control and Disease.* 8th ed. New York, NY: Saunders; 1980.)

Another interesting observation is that 15–20% of women with secondary amenorrhea have elevated prolactin levels, and when prolactin secretion is reduced, normal menstrual cycles and fertility return. It appears that prolactin may produce amenorrhea by blocking the action of gonadotropins on the ovaries, but definitive proof of this hypothesis must await further research. The hypogonadism produced by prolactinomas is associated with osteoporosis due to estrogen deficiency.

Hyperprolactinemia in men is associated with impotence and hypogonadism that disappear when prolactin secretion is reduced.

MENOPAUSE

The human ovary gradually becomes unresponsive to gonadotropins with advancing age, and its function declines so that sexual cycles and menstruation disappear (menopause). This unresponsiveness is associated with and is probably caused by a decline in the number of primordial follicles (Fig. 4–5). The ovaries no longer secrete progesterone and 17β-estrodiol in appreciable quantities. Estrone is formed by aromatization of androstenedione in fat and other tissues, but the amounts are normally small. The uterus and vagina gradually become atrophic. As the negative feedback effect of the estrogens and progesterone is reduced, secretion of FSH and LH is increased, and plasma FSH and LH rise to high levels. Old female mice and rats have long periods of diestrus and increased levels of gonadotropin secretion, but a clear-cut "menopause" has apparently not been described in experimental animals.

In women, the menses usually become irregular and cease between the age of 45 and 55. The average age at onset of menopause has increased since the turn of the century and is currently about 51 years.

Sensation of warmth spreading from the trunk to the face ("hot flushes," also called hot flashes), night sweats, and various mood fluctuations are common after ovarian function has ceased. Hot flushes are said to occur in 75% of menopausal women and may last as long as 40 years. They are prevented by administration of estrogen. These vasomotor symptoms are not always specific to menopause; they also occur in premenopausal women and men whose gonads are removed surgically or destroyed by disease. Thus, the vasomotor symptoms result from acute estrogen withdrawal. However, it has been demonstrated that they coincide with surges of LH secretion. LH is secreted in episodic bursts at intervals of 30–60 minutes or more (circhoral secretion), and in the absence of gonadal hormones, these bursts are large. Each hot flush begins with the start of a burst. However, LH itself is not responsible for the symptoms, as they can continue after

Table 4–5. Factors affecting the secretion of human prolactin and growth hormone.

Factor	Prolactin	Growth Hormone
Sleep	I+	I+
Nursing	I++	N
Breast stimulation in nonlactating women	I	N
Stress	I+	I+
Hypoglycemia	I	I+
Strenuous exercise	I	I
Sexual intercourse in women	I	N
Pregnancy	I++	N
Estrogens	I	I
Hypothyroidism	I	N
TRH	I+	N
Phenothiazines, butyrophenones	I+	N
Opiates	I	I
Glucose	N	D
Somatostatin	N	D+
L-Dopa	D+	I+
Apomorphine	D+	I+
Bromocriptine and related ergot derivatives	D+	I

I, moderate increase; I+, marked increase; I++, very marked increase; N, no change; D, moderate decrease; D+, marked decrease.

Reproduced, with permission, from Barrett KE. *Ganong's Review of Medical Physiology*. 23rd ed. New York, NY: McGraw-Hill; 2010.

removal of the pituitary. Instead, it appears that some event in the hypothalamus initiates both the release of LH and the episode of flushing. Menopause and the clinical management of patients with menopausal symptoms are discussed in more detail in Chapter 59.

Bilezikjian LM, Blount AL, Leal AM, et al. Autocrine/paracrine regulation of pituitary function by activin, inhibin, and follistatin. *Mol Cell Endocrinol* 2004;225:29. PMID: 15451565.

Christian CA, Glidewell-Kenney C, Jameson JL, Moenter SM. Classical estrogen receptor α signaling mediates negative and positive feedback on gonadotropin-releasing hormone neuron firing. *Endocrinology* 2008;149:5328–5334. PMID: 18635656.

Duncan WC, van den Driesche S, Fraser HM. Inhibition of vascular endothelial growth factor in the primate ovary up-regulates hypoxia-inducible factor-1α in the follicle and corpus luteum. *Endocrinology* 2008;149:3313. PMID: 18388198.

Dunger DB, Ahmed ML, Ong KK. Early and late weight gain and the timing of puberty. *Mol Cell Endocrinol* 2006;254–255:140. PMID: 16824679.

Fortune JE, Rivera GM, Yang MY. Follicular development: the role of the follicular microenvironment is the selection of the dominant follicle. *Anim Reprod Sci* 2004;82–84:109. PMID: 15271447.

Ganong WF. *Review of Medical Physiology*. 22nd ed. New York, NY: McGraw-Hill; 2005.

Ibanez L, Valls C, Marcos MV, et al. Insulin sensitization for girls with precocious pubarche and with risk for polycystic ovary syndrome: effects of prepubertal initiation and postpubertal discontinuation of metaformin treatment. *J Clin Endocrinol Metab* 2004;89:4331. PMID: 15356029.

Jabbour HN, Critchley HOD. Potential roles of decidual prolactin in early pregnancy. *Reproduction* 2001;121:197. PMID: 11226044.

Jung H, Neumaier Probst E, Hauffa BP, et al. Association of morphological characteristics with precocious puberty and/or gelastic seizures in hypothalamic hamartoma. *J Clin Endocrinol Metab* 2003;88:4590. PMID: 14557427.

Kelley PA, Binart N, Lucas B, et al. Implications of multiple phenotypes observed in prolactin receptor knockout mice. *Front Neuroendocrinol* 2001;22:140. PMID: 11259135.

Knight PG, Glister C. TGF-β superfamily members and ovarian follicle development. *Reproduction* 2006;132:191. PMID: 16885529.

Knobil E, Neill JD (eds). *The Physiology of Reproduction*. 2nd ed, 2 vols. Philadelphia, PA: Raven Press; 1994.

Kronenberg HM, Melmed S, Polonsky K, et al (eds). *Williams Textbook of Endocrinology*. 11th ed. New York, NY: Saunders; 2008.

Larsen PR, Kronenberg HM, Melmed S, et al (eds). *Williams Textbook of Endocrinology*. 10th ed. New York, NY: Saunders; 2003.

Mani S. progestin receptor subtypes in the brain: the known and the unknown. *Endocrinology* 2008;149:2750. PMID: 18308838.

Mathews J, Gustattson J-A. Estrogen signaling: a subtle balance between ER and ER. *Mol Interv* 2003;3:281. PMID: 14993442.

Michala L, Creighton SM. Adolescent gynaecology. *Obstet Gynaecol Reprod Med* 2008;18:120–125.

Ness RB, Grisso JA, Vergona R, et al. Oral contraceptives, other methods of contraception and risk reduction for ovarian cancer. *Epidemiology* 2001;12:307. PMID: 11337604.

Palmer NR, Boepple PA. Variation in the onset of puberty: clinical spectrum and genetic investigation. *J Clin Endocrinol Metab* 2001;86:2364. PMID: 11397824.

Seminara SB, Messager S, Chatzidaki EE, et al. The GPR54 gene as a regulator of puberty. *N Engl J Med* 2003;349:1614. PMID: 14573733.

Sherwood OD. Relaxin's physiological roles and other diverse actions. *Endocr Rev* 2004;25:205. PMID: 15082520.

Welt CK, Chan JL, Bullen J, et al. Recombinant human leptin in women with hypothalamic amenorrhea. *N Engl J Med* 2004;351:987. PMID: 15342807.

The Breast

5

Amer Karam, MD

ANATOMY OF THE FEMALE BREAST

The breasts are secondary reproductive glands of ectodermal origin. They are frequently referred to as modified sweat glands. Each breast lies on the superior aspect of the chest wall. In women, the breasts are the organs of lactation, whereas in men, the breasts are normally functionless and undeveloped.

HISTOLOGY

The adult female breast contains glandular and ductal elements, stroma consisting of fibrous tissue that binds the individual lobes together and adipose tissue within and between the lobes.

Each breast consists of 12–20 conical lobes. The base of each lobe is in close proximity to the ribs. The apex, which contains the major excretory duct of the lobe, is deep to the areola and nipple. In turn, each lobe consists of a group of lobules. The lobules have several lactiferous ducts, which unite to form a major duct that drains the lobes as they course toward the nipple–areolar complex. Each of the major ducts widens to form an ampulla as they travel toward the areola and then narrow at its individual opening in the nipple. The lobules are held in place by a meshwork of loose, fatty areolar tissue. The fatty tissue increases toward the periphery of the lobule and gives the breast its bulk and hemispheric shape.

Approximately 80–85% of the normal breast is adipose tissue. The breast tissues are joined to the overlying skin and subcutaneous tissue by fibrous strands.

In the nonpregnant, nonlactating breast, the alveoli are small and tightly packed. During pregnancy, the alveoli hypertrophy, and their lining cells proliferate in number. During lactation, the alveolar cells secrete proteins and lipids, which comprise breast milk.

The deep surface of the breast lies on the fascia that covers the chest muscles. The fascial stroma, derived from the superficial fascia of the chest wall, is condensed into multiple bands that run from the breast into the subcutaneous tissues and the corium of the skin overlying the breast. These fascial bands—Cooper's ligaments—support the breast in its upright position on the chest wall. These bands may be distorted by a tumor, resulting in pathologic skin dimpling.

HISTOLOGIC CHANGES IN THE FEMALE BREAST DURING THE LIFE SPAN

In response to multiglandular stimulation during puberty, the female breast starts to enlarge and eventually assumes its conical or spherical shape. Growth is the result of an increase in acinar tissue, ductal size and branching, and deposits of adipose, the main factor in breast enlargement. Also during puberty, the nipple and areola enlarge. Smooth muscle fibers surround the base of the nipple, and the nipple becomes more sensitive to touch.

Once menses is established, the breast undergoes a periodic premenstrual phase during which the acinar cells increase in number and size, the ductal lumens widen, and breast size and turgor increase slightly. Many women have breast tenderness during this phase of the menstrual cycle. Menstrual bleeding is followed by a postmenstrual phase, characterized by a decrease in size and turgor, reduction in the number and size of the breast acini, and a decrease in diameter of the lactiferous ducts. Cyclic hormonal influences to the breast are quite variable.

In response to progesterone during pregnancy, breast size and turgidity increase considerably. These changes are accompanied by deepening pigmentation of the nipple–areolar complex, nipple enlargement, areolar widening, and an increase in the number and size of the lubricating glands in the areola. The breast ductal system branches markedly, and the individual ducts widen. The acini increase in number and size. In late pregnancy, the fatty tissues of the breasts are almost completely replaced by cellular breast parenchyma. After delivery with the rapid drop in progesterone and estrogen levels, the breasts, now fully mature, start to secrete milk. With cessation of nursing or administration of estrogens, which inhibit lactation, the breast rapidly returns to its prepregnancy state, with marked diminution of cellular elements and an increase in adipose deposits.

Following menopause, which typically occurs during the fifth decade of life, the breast undergoes a gradual process of atrophy and involution. There is a decrease in the number and size of acinar and ductal elements, so that the breast tissue regresses to an almost infantile state. Adipose tissue may or may not atrophy, with disappearance of the parenchymal elements.

GROSS ANATOMY (FIG. 5–1)

The adult female breast mound characteristically forms a near hemispheric contour on each side of the chest wall, usually extending from just below the level of the second rib inferiorly to the sixth or seventh rib. The breast mound is usually situated between the lateral sternal border and the anterior axillary fold. The breast tissue extends over a larger anatomic area than the more obvious breast mound. The superior portion of the breast tissue emerges gradually from the chest wall inferior to the clavicle, whereas the lateral and inferior borders are better defined. The major portion of the breast tissue is located superficial to the pectoralis major muscle and projects laterally and ventrally toward the tail of Spence. Smaller portions of breast tissue extend laterally and inferiorly to lie superficial to the serratus anterior and external oblique muscles and as far caudad as the rectus abdominis. The tail of Spence is a triangular tongue-shaped portion of breast tissue that extends superiorly and laterally toward the axilla, perforating the deep axillary fascia, and enters the axilla, where it terminates in close proximity to the axillary lymph nodes and vessels as well as the axillary blood vessels and nerves.

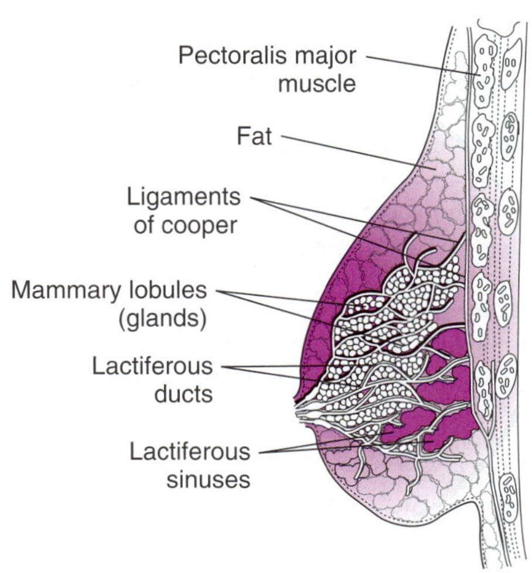

▲ **Figure 5–1.** Sagittal section of mammary gland.

The Nipple & Areola

The areola is a circular pigmented zone 2–6 cm in diameter at the tip of the breast. Its color varies from pale pink to deep brown depending on age, parity, and skin pigmentation. The skin of the areola contains multiple small, elevated nodules beneath which are located the sebaceous glands of Montgomery. The glands are responsible for lubrication of the nipple and help prevent cracks and fissures in the nipple–areolar complex that occur during breastfeeding. During the third trimester of pregnancy, the sebaceous glands of Montgomery markedly hypertrophy.

A circular smooth muscle band surrounds the base of the nipple. Longitudinal smooth muscle fibers branch out from this ring of circular smooth muscle to encircle the lactiferous ducts as they converge toward the nipple. The many small punctate openings at the superior aspect of the nipple represent the terminals of the major lactiferous ducts. As discussed earlier, the ampullae of the lactiferous ducts are deep to the nipple and the areola.

Blood Vessels, Lymphatics, & Nerves

A. Arteries (Fig. 5–2)

The breast has a rich blood supply with multiple arteries and veins. Perforating branches from the internal thoracic/mammary artery that penetrate the second to the fifth intercostal interspaces supply blood to the medial half of the breast. These arteries perforate the intercostal muscles and the anterior intercostal membrane to supply both the breast and the pectoralis major and minor muscles. During pregnancy, and not infrequently in advanced breast disease, the intercostal perforators may enlarge from engorgement. Small branches from the anterior intercostal arteries also supply the medial aspect of the breast. Laterally, the pectoral branch of the thoracoacromial branch of the axillary artery and the external mammary branch of the lateral thoracic artery, which also is a branch of the second segment of the axillary artery, supply the breast. The external mammary artery passes along the

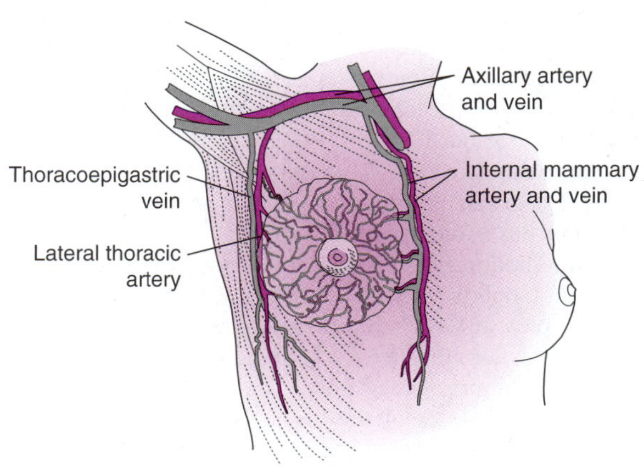

▲ **Figure 5–2.** Arteries and veins of the breast.

lateral free edge of the pectoralis major muscle to reach the lateral half of the breast. The artery usually is located medial to the long thoracic nerve.

The medial and lateral arteries, as they reach the breast, tend to arborize mainly in the supra-areolar area; consequently, the arterial supply to the upper half of the breast is almost twice that of the lower half.

B. Veins

Venous return from the breast closely follows the routes of the arterial system. Blood returns to the superior vena cava via the axillary and internal thoracic veins. It also returns via the vertebral venous plexuses, which are fed by the intercostal and azygos veins. Through the azygos veins, there is also some minor flow into the portal system. A rich anastomotic plexus of superficial breast veins is located in the subareolar region. In thin-skinned, fair individuals, these veins are normally visible, and they are almost always visible during pregnancy. Their presence makes for marked vascularity of sub- and para-areolar incisions. Venous return flow is greater in the superior quadrants than in the inferior quadrants of the breast.

C. Lymphatics (Fig. 5–3)

A thorough knowledge of the lymphatic drainage of the breast is of critical importance to the clinician. This is true because the lymphatic drainage has significant implications in several disease etiologies, including breast cancer. To a large extent, modern, less invasive surgical management techniques such as sentinel lymph node biopsy are based on a solid understanding of the pattern of lymphatic drainage in the breast.

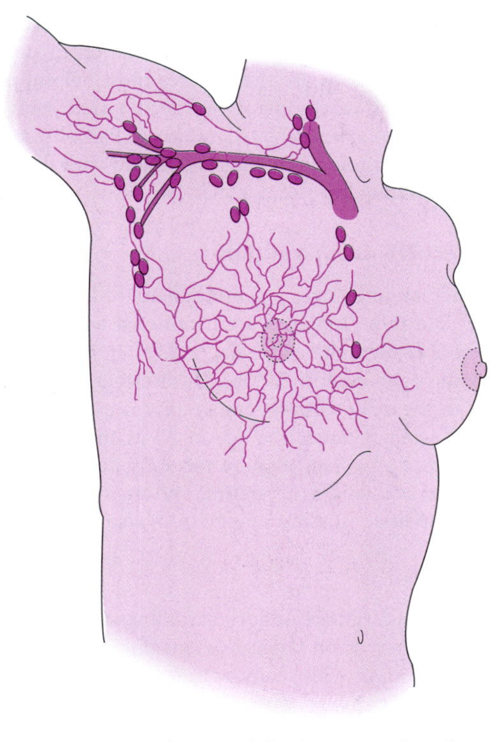

▲ **Figure 5–3.** Lymphatics of the breast and axilla.

Lymphatic drainage in the breast may be divided into 2 main categories: superficial (including cutaneous) drainage and deep parenchymatous drainage.

1. Superficial drainage—A large lymphatic plexus exists in the subcutaneous tissues of the breast deep to the nipple–areolar complex. This plexus drains the areola and nipple regions, including the cutaneous and subcutaneous tissues adjacent to the nipple–areolar complex. In addition, the superficial plexus drains the deep central parenchymatous region of the breast.

2. Deep parenchymatous drainage—The deep parenchymatous lymph vessels drain the remainder of the breast as well as some portion of the skin and subcutaneous tissues of the nipple–areolar complex not served by the superficial plexus. Small periductal and periacinal lymph vessels collect parenchymal lymph and deliver it to the larger interlobar lymphatics. Lymph from the cutaneous and nipple–areolar regions may drain either directly into the subareolar plexus or deeply into the parenchymatous lymph system. Once in the deep parenchymatous drainage, the lymph is delivered to the subareolar plexus for efferent transport.

The majority of lymphatic drainage from both the retroareolar and the deep interlobar lymphatics of the breast travel to the ipsilateral axillary lymph nodes. The route of drainage to the highest axillary node or nodes is not reproducible from patient to patient. In general, however, the drainage of the breast is to the anterior axillary or subpectoral nodes, which are located deep to the lateral border of the pectoralis major muscle, close to the lateral thoracic artery. From these nodes, lymph travels to nodes in close proximity to the lateral portion of the axillary vein. The lymph then passes superiorly, via the axillary chain of lymph vessels and nodes. Eventually, the drainage reaches the highest nodes of the axilla. Although this is the most regular pattern of lateral and superior breast lymphatic drainage, other paths are common, particularly when the lateral and superiorly directed channels are obstructed, for example, by tumor masses.

Surgeons usually classify the axillary lymph nodes in levels according to their relationship with the pectoralis minor muscle. Thus, lymph nodes located lateral or below the pectoralis minor muscle are classified as level I lymph nodes. Lymph nodes located deep to the pectoralis minor muscle constitute level II lymph nodes. Finally, lymph nodes located medially or superiorly to the upper margin of the pectoralis minor muscle constitute level III lymph nodes.

D. Nerves Encountered During Axillary Dissection

The lateral and anterior cutaneous branches of T4–6 supply the cutaneous tissues covering the breasts. Two major nerves and 2 smaller groups of nerves are in close proximity to the breast area and thus assume importance in breast surgery:

1. The **thoracodorsal nerve**, a branch of the posterior cord of the brachial plexus (C5–7), runs inferiorly along with the subscapular artery lying close to the posterior axillary wall and the ventral surface of the subscapular muscle. The nerve innervates the superior half of the latissimus dorsi muscle and is usually surrounded by a large venous plexus that drains into the subscapular veins.
2. The **long thoracic nerve** (nerve of Bell) arises from the anterior primary divisions of C5–7 at the level of the lower half of the anterior scalene muscle. In the neck, the nerve descends dorsal to the trunks of the brachial plexus on the inferior segment of the middle scalene muscle. Further descent places it dorsal to the clavicle and the axillary vessels. On the lateral thoracic wall, it descends on the external surface of the serratus anterior muscle along the anterior axillary line. The long thoracic nerve supplies filaments to each of the digitations of the serratus anterior muscle. Injury to this nerve results in a "winged" scapula.
3. The **intercostal brachial nerves** are 3 relatively minor cutaneous nerves that supply the skin of the medial surface of the upper arm. They transverse the lateral chest wall to the upper inner surface of the arm, passing across the base of the axilla.
4. The **medial and lateral pectoral nerves** supply the 2 pectoral muscles and pass from the axilla to the lateral chest wall. The lateral pectoral nerve, which arises from the lateral cord of the plexus, pierces the clavipectoral fascia membrane together with the thoracoacromial artery and supplies the pectoralis major muscle. The medial pectoral nerve, which arises from the medial cord of the brachial plexus but ends up being lateral to the lateral pectoral nerve, pierces the clavipectoral fascia and supplies the pectoralis minor muscle.

DISEASES OF THE BREAST

FIBROCYSTIC BREAST CHANGES

ESSENTIALS OF DIAGNOSIS

- Painful, often multiple, usually bilateral mobile masses in the breast.
- Rapid fluctuation in the size of the masses is common.
- Frequently, pain occurs or increases, as does size during the premenstrual phase of the cycle.
- Most common age is 30–50 years; occurrence is rare in postmenopausal women.

Pathogenesis

Fibrocystic breast changes, formerly known as fibrocystic disease, chronic cystic mastitis, or mammary dysplasia, are the most common cause of cyclic breast pain or mastalgia in reproductive age women. The term is imprecise and encompasses a wide spectrum of pathologic entities. The lesions are always associated with benign changes in the breast epithelium, some of which are found so frequently in normal breasts that they are probably variants of normal breast histology, but have, unfortunately, been termed a "disease." From a clinical standpoint, this entity is best described as nodular, sensitive breast.

Clinical Findings

Fibrocystic changes are common and affect more than 50% of women of reproductive age. These changes are thought to be the result of a hormonal imbalance that may produce asymptomatic breast lumps that are discovered by palpation. Cyclical breast pain or tenderness is often the presenting symptom and calls attention to the mass. The pain is caused by the proliferation of normal glandular breast tissue with estrogen stimulating the ductal elements and progesterone stimulating the stroma. There may be nonbloody, green or brown discharge from the nipple. In many cases, discomfort occurs or is increased during the premenstrual phase of the cycle. Fluctuations in size and rapid appearance or disappearance of a breast mass are common in cystic changes. In many women, caffeine seems to potentiate these symptoms. However, the role of caffeine as a direct cause of these symptoms has never been proven. Pain, fluctuation in size, and multiplicity of lesions are the features most helpful in differentiation from carcinoma. However, if a dominant mass is present, it should be evaluated by biopsy. Pathologists refer to a variety of histologic findings associated with fibrocystic changes including fibrosis, ductal hyperplasia, and adenosis.

Differential Diagnosis

Pain, fluctuation in size, and multiplicity of lesions help to differentiate these lesions from carcinoma and the benign entity of fibroadenoma. Final diagnosis often rests on biopsy and pathologic determination. Ultrasonography may be helpful in the diagnosis; mammography is usually not indicated for women under the age of 30 as the breast tissue in these young women may be too radiodense to allow a meaningful evaluation. Aspiration and/or sonography may be useful in differentiating a cystic from a solid mass.

Treatment

Once a benign diagnosis or normal findings have been established by biopsy or on clinical or imaging findings, simple reassurance will provide many patients with adequate relief.

For those patients who still seek treatment, symptomatic relief by avoiding trauma and by wearing a bra with adequate support can be very helpful. The role of caffeine consumption in the development and treatment of fibrocystic change has never been proven; however, many patients report relief of symptoms after abstinence from coffee, tea, and chocolate. Similarly, observational studies have suggested that low-fat diets can provide some relief. The data regarding the utility of vitamin E supplementation and evening primrose oil are controversial. Mild analgesics such as acetaminophen and nonsteroidal anti-inflammatory drugs (NSAIDs) can be used to relieve breast pain. For more symptomatic women, danazol and tamoxifen have been found to be effective, although their significant side effects have limited their acceptability and utility.

Prognosis

Exacerbations of pain, tenderness, and cyst formation may occur at any time until menopause, when symptoms subside. Patients should be reassured that single nonproliferative lesions like fibrocystic changes are not associated with an increased risk of breast cancer. On the other hand, the presence of multiple nonproliferative lesions or proliferative lesions (florid hyperplasia, sclerosing adenosis, and intraductal papillomas), particularly those with atypia (atypical lobular or ductal hyperplasia), is associated with an increased risk of subsequent breast cancer.

FIBROADENOMA OF THE BREAST

Pathogenesis

This common, benign neoplasm occurs most frequently in young women, usually within 20 years after puberty. It is somewhat more frequent and tends to occur at an earlier age in black women than in white women. The etiology of fibroadenomas is not known, but a hormonal relationship is likely since they can increase in size during pregnancy or with estrogen therapy and usually regress after menopause. Multiple tumors in 1 or both breasts are found in 10–15% of patients.

Clinical Findings

The typical fibroadenoma is a round, firm, discrete, relatively movable, nontender mass 1–5 cm in diameter. The tumor is usually discovered accidentally. Clinical diagnosis in young patients is generally not difficult. Fibroadenomas typically present as well-defined solid masses with benign imaging features on ultrasound and can be managed with core needle biopsy or short-term (3–6 months) follow-up with a repeat ultrasound and breast examination.

Differential Diagnosis

Definitive diagnosis can only be confirmed with a core biopsy or excision if the patient is symptomatic or wishes the mass to be excised. Cryoablation is an alternative to surgical excision of fibroadenomas, but should only be considered after a core biopsy diagnosis of fibroadenoma has been made.

Rapid growth sometimes raises the suspicion for a phyllodes tumor and can mandate an excision to confirm the diagnosis and rule out a malignancy.

Simple fibroadenomas do not raise the subsequent risk of breast cancer, although the presence of adjacent proliferative changes or a complex fibroadenoma is associated with a slightly increased risk.

Phyllodes tumors of the breast (previously called cystosarcoma phyllodes) are fibroepithelial tumors that tend to grow rapidly and may sometimes be confused with benign fibroadenomas. This tumor may reach a large size and, if inadequately excised, will recur locally. The lesion can be, but rarely is, malignant.

Treatment

Treatment is by local excision of the mass with a margin of surrounding normal breast tissue. The treatment of malignant phyllodes tumors is more controversial but generally involves wide local excision with appropriate margins. The role of radiation and chemotherapy is controversial. Breast conservation even for large tumors may not compromise cancer-specific survival.

NIPPLE DISCHARGE

Pathogenesis

Nipple discharge is usually characterized as normal lactation, galactorrhea or benign physiologic nipple discharge, and pathologic nipple discharge.

The most common causes of pathologic nipple discharge are intraductal papillomas and, less frequently, carcinoma and fibrocystic change with ectasia of the ducts. The discharge is usually unilateral, emanating from a single duct, and can be serous, bloody, or serosanguineous.

Clinical Findings

The important characteristics of the discharge and some other factors to be evaluated by history and physical examination are as follows:

1. Nature of discharge (serous, bloody, or other)
2. Association with or without a mass
3. Unilateral or bilateral
4. Single duct or multiple duct discharge
5. Discharge that is spontaneous, persistent or intermittent, or must be expressed
6. Discharge produced by pressure at a single site or by general pressure on the breast

7. Relation to menses
8. Premenopausal or postmenopausal
9. History of oral contraceptive use or estrogen replacement for postmenopausal symptoms

Differential Diagnosis

Galactorrhea or physiologic nipple discharge is frequently the result of hyperprolactinemia secondary to medications such as phenothiazines, endocrine tumors such as lactotroph adenomas, or endocrine abnormalities such as hypothyroidism and pituitary or hypothalamic disease (Table 5–1). Galactorrhea usually manifests as bilateral multiductal milky nipple discharge in the nonlactating breast. If the physical examination is otherwise normal, imaging is negative, and the discharge is multiductal and nonbloody, a pregnancy test, prolactin levels, renal and thyroid function tests, and appropriate endocrinologic follow-up may be necessary with appropriate treatment of the underlying cause.

Pathologic nipple discharge is usually unilateral, spontaneous serous or serosanguineous from a single duct and is usually caused by an intraductal papilloma or, more infrequently, by an intraductal malignancy. In either case, a palpable mass may not be present. The involved duct may be identified by pressure at different sites around the nipple at the margin of the areola. Bloody discharge is more suggestive of cancer but is usually caused by a benign papilloma in the duct. Cytologic examination is rarely helpful because negative findings do not rule out cancer, which is more likely in women older than age 50 years. Imaging modalities such as mammography and/or ultrasonography may reveal underlying abnormalities in the duct. Ductography can be used to delineate an intraductal filling defect, which may be causing the nipple discharge.

Table 5–1. Causes of galactorrhea.

Idiopathic
Drug induced
Phenothiazines, butyrophenones, reserpine, methyldopa, imipramine, amphetamine, metoclopramide, sulpiride, pimozide, oral contraceptive agents
Central nervous system (CNS) lesions
Pituitary adenoma, empty sella, hypothalamic tumor, head trauma
Medical conditions
Chronic renal failure, sarcoidosis, Schüller-Christian disease
Cushing's disease, hepatic cirrhosis, hypothyroidism
Chest wall lesions
Thoracotomy, herpes zoster

Reproduced, with permission, from Hindle WH. *Breast Disease for Gynecologists.* New York, NY: Appleton & Lange; 1990.

Treatment

In any case, surgical excision of the involved duct should be performed once the workup has ruled out additional breast findings that need to be addressed.

Purulent discharge can originate in a subareolar abscess and may require excision of the abscess and related lactiferous sinus.

FAT NECROSIS

Fat necrosis is a benign condition of the breast but is of clinical importance because it produces a mass, often accompanied by skin or nipple retraction, that is clinically indistinguishable from carcinoma. Trauma and surgery are the presumed etiology, although only about half of patients recall a history of injury to the breast. Ecchymosis is occasionally observed in conjunction with the mass. Tenderness may or may not be present. If untreated, the mass associated with fat necrosis gradually disappears. Should the mass not resolve after several weeks, a biopsy should be considered. Once the diagnosis is established, surgical excision is usually not necessary.

BREAST ABSCESS

During lactation and nursing, an area of redness, tenderness, and induration may develop in the breast. In its early stages, the infection can often be resolved while continuing nursing with the affected breast and administering an antibiotic. If the lesion progresses to form a palpable mass with local and systemic signs of infection, an abscess has developed and needs to be drained. Even in this setting breastfeeding or pumping can help in controlling the pain and discomfort associated with the infection as well as shorten the duration of the infection.

Less frequently, a subareolar abscess may develop in young or middle-age women who are not lactating. These infections tend to recur after simple incision and drainage unless the area is explored in a quiescent interval with excision of the involved lactiferous duct or ducts at the base of the nipple. Except for the subareolar type of abscess, infection in the breast is very rare unless the patient is lactating.

If a patient with a suspected breast infection does not respond to treatment, inflammatory breast cancer should be suspected especially when associated with axillary lymphadenopathy.

MALFORMATION OF THE BREAST

Many women consult their physicians for abnormalities in either the size or the symmetry of their breasts. Difference in size between the 2 breasts is common. If extreme, however, these differences may be corrected by cosmetic surgery, although the breast tissue in these individuals is otherwise normal.

Similarly, woman may complain of overly large breasts (macromastia). Studies fail to show any endocrinologic or pathologic abnormalities, and these patients may also be considered candidates for cosmetic surgery such as breast-reduction mammoplasty.

Less common malformations of the breast include amastia, complete absence of 1 or both breasts, or the presence of accessory nipples (polythelia) and breast tissue (polymastia) along the embryologic milk line, which occurs in 1–2% of whites.

PUERPERAL MASTITIS

See Chapter 10.

CARCINOMA OF THE FEMALE BREAST

ESSENTIALS OF DIAGNOSIS

- Early findings: Single, nontender, firm to hard mass with ill-defined margins; mammographic abnormalities and no palpable mass.
- Later findings: Skin or nipple retraction; axillary lymphadenopathy; breast enlargement, redness, edema, brawny induration, peau d'orange, pain, fixation of mass to skin or chest wall.
- Late findings: Ulceration; supraclavicular lymphadenopathy; edema of arm; bone, lung, liver, brain, or other distant metastases.

General Considerations

Cancer of the breast is the most common cancer in women, excluding nonmelanoma skin cancers. After lung cancer, it is the second most common cause of cancer death for women. The American Cancer Society estimates that over 210,000 new cases of cancer of the breast will be diagnosed in 2010, resulting in over 40,000 deaths. These figures include male breast cancer, which accounts for less than 1% of annual breast cancer incidence. The yearly breast cancer incidence has steadily decreased from 1999 to 2006. Similarly, the mortality from breast cancer has been decreasing since 1975, which is attributed to better screening and advances in treatment modalities. On average, the breast cancer death rate decreased by 2.3% per year from 1990 to 2001. The probability of developing the disease increases throughout life. The mean and median age of women with breast cancer is 60–61 years, and breast cancer is the main cause of death for women between the ages of 40 and 59.

At the present rate of incidence, a woman's risk of developing invasive breast cancer in her lifetime from *birth* to *death* is 1 in 8. This figure is from the Surveillance, Epidemiology, and End Results Program (SEER) of the National Cancer Institute (NCI) and is often cited but needs clarification. The data include all age groups in 5-year intervals with an open-ended interval at 85 years and above. When calculating risk, each age interval is weighted to account for the increasing risk of breast cancer with increasing age. A woman's risk of being diagnosed with invasive breast cancer by age is as follows:

- By age 30: 1 in 2000
- By age 40: 1 in 233
- By age 50: 1 in 53
- By age 60: 1 in 22
- By age 70: 1 in 13
- By age 80: 1 in 9
- In a lifetime: 1 in 8

In the United States, breast cancer is the most common cancer among women of all ethnic groups, although the incidence of the disease is highest among white patients. In general, rates reported from developing countries are lower than those reported from developed countries, with the notable exception of Japan. Some of the variability may be a result of underreporting, but lifestyle, sociodemographic, and environmental factors such as diet, exercise, parity, breastfeeding, and body weight are implicated as possible causes for this observed difference.

Women with a family history of breast cancer are more likely to develop the disease than controls. The risk of being diagnosed with breast cancer for a patient with 1 affected first-degree relative (mother or sister) is increased by almost 2-fold. With 2 affected first-degree relatives, the increased risk is almost 3-fold. The risk is even higher if those relatives were diagnosed at a young age. A family history of breast cancer is, however, only reported by 15–20% of patients with breast cancer. Inherited specific genetic mutations that predispose patients to breast cancer such as, BRCA1 and BRCA2 gene mutations, are rare, accounting for approximately 5% of all breast cancers. BRCA mutations place affected women at a significantly increased lifetime risk, up to a 70%, of being diagnosed with breast cancer.

Nulliparous women and women whose first full-term pregnancy was after age 30 years have a slightly higher incidence of breast cancer than multiparous women. Late menarche and artificial menopause are associated with a lower incidence of breast cancer, whereas early menarche (before age 12 years) and late natural menopause (after age 50 years) are associated with a slight increase in risk of developing breast cancer. The bulk of the currently available evidence supports a causal relationship between the use of postmenopausal combination hormone therapy and breast cancer, predominantly hormone receptor–positive breast cancer. On the other hand, a clear association has not been consistently established between oral contraceptive use and the risk of breast cancer.

Fibrocystic changes of the breast and other nonproliferative breast lesions are not associated with an increased risk of breast cancer. However, the presence of multiple nonproliferative lesions and the presence of proliferative changes, especially those associated with cytologic atypia, are associated with an increased incidence of cancer. Correspondingly, a personal history of breast cancer is the greatest risk factor for subsequent breast cancer events. In addition, a woman who has had cancer in 1 breast is at increased risk of not only a recurrence but also of a second primary in the ipsilateral breast, as well as in the contralateral breast. Women with cancer of the uterine corpus have a breast cancer risk significantly higher than that of the general population, and women with breast cancer have a comparably increased risk of endometrial cancer.

Women who are at greater-than-normal risk of developing breast cancer should be identified by their physicians and followed carefully. Screening programs involve periodic physical examination and screening mammography; screening magnetic resonance imaging of the breasts for those asymptomatic patients at highest risk may increase the detection rate of breast cancer and may improve the survival rate, although this has not yet been demonstrated. Unfortunately, more than 50% of women who develop breast cancer do not have significant identifiable risk factors.

Staging

The physical examination of the breast and additional preoperative studies are used to determine the clinical stage of a breast cancer. Clinical staging is based on the TNM (tumor, node, metastasis) system of the International Union Against Cancer. This classification considers tumor size, clinical assessment of axillary nodes, and the presence or absence of distant metastases. The assessment of the clinical stage is important in planning therapy. Histologic (or pathologic) staging is determined following surgery and along with clinical staging helps determine prognosis.

Clinical Findings

The majority of patients with breast cancer are diagnosed as a result of an abnormal mammogram and less often because of a palpable mass. The initial evaluation should include assessment of the local lesion, including a bilateral mammogram, if not previously performed, and breast ultrasound as indicated. The initial workup should include laboratory tests such as a complete blood count, liver function tests, and alkaline phosphatase. The search for distant spread should only be reserved for locally advanced breast cancers or if signs/symptoms of distant spread are present.

A. Symptoms

When the history is taken, special note should be made of the onset and duration of menarche, pregnancies, parity, artificial or natural menopause, date of last menstrual period, previous breast lesions and/or biopsies, hormonal supplementation, radiation exposure, and a family history of breast cancer. Back or other bone pain may be the result of osseous metastases. Systemic complaints or weight loss should raise the question of metastases, which may involve any organ but most frequently involve the bones, liver, and lungs. The more advanced the cancer in terms of aggressive histologic features, size of primary lesion, local invasion, and extent of regional node involvement, the higher is the incidence of metastatic spread to distant sites. Lymph node involvement is the single most significant prognostic feature and increases with increasing tumor size and aggressive histologic features such as pathologic grade.

Most patients with palpable breast cancers present with painless masses in the breast, most of which are discovered by the patient herself. Less frequent symptoms are breast pain; nipple discharge; erosion, retraction, enlargement, or itching of the nipple; and redness, generalized hardness, enlargement, or shrinking of the breast. Rarely, an axillary mass, swelling of the arm, or bone pain (from metastases) may be the first symptoms. Because of organized screening programs, fewer than 10% of breast cancers are detected solely on physical examination, and more than 90% are detected as a result of an abnormal mammogram

B. Signs

Inspection of the breast is the first step in physical examination and should be carried out with the patient sitting, arms at sides and then overhead. Abnormal variations in breast size and contour, minimal nipple retraction, and slight edema, redness, or retraction of the skin can be identified. Asymmetry of the breasts and retraction or dimpling of the skin can often be accentuated by having the patient raise her arms overhead or press her hands on her hips in order to contract the pectoralis muscles. Axillary and supraclavicular areas should be thoroughly palpated for enlarged nodes with the patient sitting (Fig. 5–4). Palpation of the breast for masses or other changes should be performed with the patient both seated and supine with the arm abducted (Fig. 5–5).

Breast cancer usually consists of a nontender, firm or hard lump with poorly delineated margins generally caused by local infiltration. Slight skin or nipple retraction is an important sign as it may affect staging. Minimal asymmetry of the breast may be noted. Very small (1–2-mm) erosions of the nipple epithelium may be the only manifestation of Paget's carcinoma. Watery, serous, or bloody discharge from the nipple is an occasional early sign but is more often associated with benign disease, as discussed earlier.

A lesion smaller than 1 cm in diameter may be difficult or impossible for a clinical examiner to feel and yet may be discovered by the patient's self-examination. During the premenstrual phase of the cycle, increased innocuous nodularity may suggest neoplasm or may obscure an underlying lesion. If there is any question regarding the nature of an

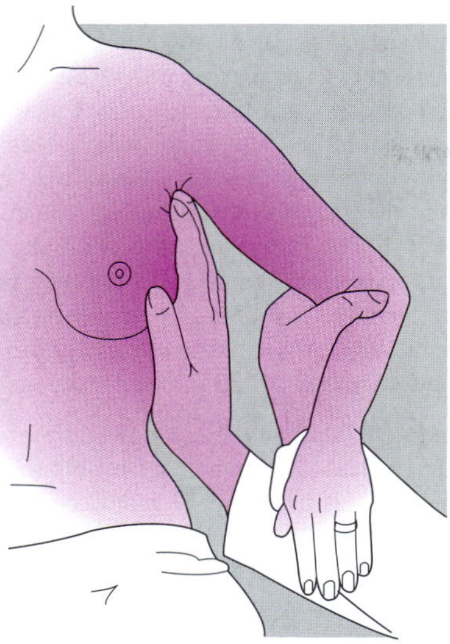

▲ **Figure 5–4.** Palpation of axillary region for enlarged lymph nodes.

abnormality under these circumstances, the patient should be asked to return after her period.

The following are characteristic of advanced carcinoma: edema, redness, nodularity, or ulceration of the skin; the presence of a large primary tumor (>5 cm); fixation to the chest wall; enlargement, shrinkage, or retraction of the breast; marked axillary lymphadenopathy; edema of the ipsilateral arm; supraclavicular lymphadenopathy; and distant metastases.

Most frequently, metastases initially tend to involve regional lymph nodes first, which may be clinically palpable, before spreading to distant sites. The axillary lymph nodes receive more than 85% of the lymphatic drainage from the breast. One or 2 movable, nontender, not particularly firm axillary lymph nodes 5 mm or less in diameter are frequently present and are generally of no clinical significance. Any firm or hard nodes larger than 5 mm in diameter are highly suspicious for nodal metastases. Axillary nodes that are matted or fixed to skin or deep structures indicate locally advanced disease (at least stage III). Histologic studies show that microscopic metastases are present in approximately 40% of patients with clinically negative nodes. Conversely, if the examiner believes that the axillary nodes are involved, this is confirmed in approximately 85% of cases on pathologic examination. The incidence of positive axillary nodes increases with the size of the primary tumor, the degree of local invasiveness of the neoplasm, and certain aggressive histologic features such as tumor grade.

Usually no nodes are palpable in the supraclavicular fossa. Firm or hard nodes of any size in this location or just beneath the clavicle (infraclavicular nodes) are indicative of locally advanced disease and suggest the strong possibility of distant metastatic sites of cancer. Biopsy or fine-needle aspiration to confirm nodal involvement in these areas is paramount. Ipsilateral supraclavicular nodes containing cancer indicate that the patient is in an advanced stage of the disease (stage IIIC). Edema of the ipsilateral arm, commonly caused by metastatic infiltration of regional lymphatics, is also a sign of advanced cancer.

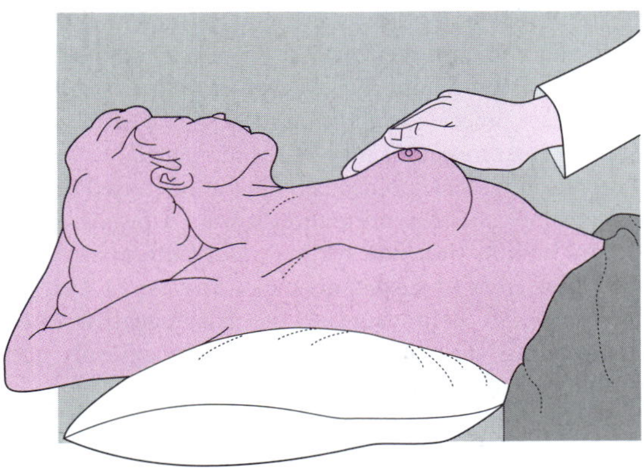

▲ **Figure 5–5.** Palpation of breasts. Palpation is performed with the patient supine and the arm abducted.

C. Special Clinical Forms of Breast Carcinoma

1. Paget's disease of the breast—Paget's disease of the breast refers to the eczematoid eruption and ulceration that arises from the nipple, can spread to the areola, and is associated with an underlying carcinoma. An underlying mass is palpable in about 50% of patients with Paget's disease. Of these masses, 95% are found to be an invasive cancer, mostly infiltrating ductal. For patients with Paget's disease and no underlying palpable mass, a noninvasive breast cancer or ductal carcinoma in situ is found in 75% of cases. Pain, itching, and/or burning are often the presenting symptoms, along with a superficial erosion or ulceration. Less frequently, a bloody discharge and nipple retraction are observed. The diagnosis is established most often by full-thickness biopsy of the lesion, which reveals the pathognomonic intraepithelial adenocarcinoma cells or Paget cells within the epidermis of the nipple. In 12–15% of patients with Paget's disease of the breast, no associated underlying intraparenchymal breast cancer is found.

Paget's disease is uncommon, accounting for approximately 1% of all breast cancers. It is frequently misdiagnosed and treated as dermatitis or bacterial infection, leading to an unfortunate delay in detection. Mastectomy has traditionally been the mainstay of therapy, although breast conservation followed by whole breast radiation can be attempted if nipple, areola, and wide local excision of the palpable mass or area of mammographic abnormality can be performed with an acceptable cosmetic result and negative margins. As for other forms of breast cancer, patients with only in situ disease need not have axillary evaluation, which is reserved for patients with an underlying palpable mass/invasive carcinoma or if a mastectomy is planned.

2. Inflammatory carcinoma—Inflammatory carcinoma is an aggressive form of breast cancer that is characterized by diffuse, brawny edema of the skin of the breast with an erysipeloid border, usually without an underlying palpable mass. Generally, this is a clinical diagnosis with pathologic confirmation of tumor embolization in the dermal lymphatics by biopsy of the overlying skin and should not be confused with noninflammatory locally advanced breast cancer. Inflammatory breast cancer is an aggressive but rare form of breast cancer representing less than 5% of cases. At presentation, nearly 35% of patients with inflammatory breast cancer have evidence of metastases. The inflammatory component, often mistaken for an infectious process, is caused by the blockage of dermal lymphatics by tumor emboli, which results in lymphedema and hyperemia. If a suspected skin infection does not rapidly respond (1–2 weeks) to a course of antibiotics, biopsy must be performed. Treatment usually consists of several cycles of neoadjuvant chemotherapy followed by surgery and/or radiotherapy depending on tumor response. A modified radical mastectomy is usually recommended for locoregional control as long as a complete resection of the tumor can be accomplished.

3. Occurrence during pregnancy or lactation—Pregnancy-associated breast cancer is defined as breast cancer that is diagnosed during pregnancy, in the first postpartum year, or anytime during lactation. The frequency of breast cancer during pregnancy or lactation ranges between 1:3000 and 1:10,000. The association of pregnancy and breast cancer presents a diagnostic and therapeutic dilemma for the patient and the physician. Women with breast cancer diagnosed during pregnancy or lactation tend to present at a later stage due in part to diagnostic delays. In the past, pregnancy-associated breast cancer was thought to lead to a worse outcome for the patient. More recent studies, however, have reported similar outcomes for women with breast cancer diagnosed during pregnancy and lactation when compared with nonpregnant breast cancer patients after controlling for stage, age, and other prognostic factors. Termination of the pregnancy, formerly performed routinely in the first two trimesters, has not been demonstrated to improve outcome. In most instances, modified radical mastectomy in pregnancy is the minimal treatment of choice, with the possible exception of the latter part of the third trimester, wherein breast-conservation therapy followed by postpartum radiotherapy may be considered. Most women with breast cancer diagnosed during pregnancy or lactation will be candidates for systemic chemotherapy. In general, the risk of fetal teratogenicity is highest during the first trimester and period of organogenesis. In the second or third trimester, chemotherapy is associated with a much lower risk or fetal toxicity but has been significantly linked to an increased risk of prematurity and growth retardation. In general, antimetabolites such as methotrexate, targeted antibodies such as trastuzumab, taxanes, and endocrine therapy should be avoided during pregnancy. Delivery of the infant should be delayed for a few weeks after the last dose of chemotherapy in order to minimize the risk of neutropenia in the fetus and infectious complication. The use of radiotherapy during pregnancy is contraindicated because of the potential for fetal damage. The decision to proceed with pregnancy termination should be individualized and based on the willingness of the patient to accept the potential teratogenic risk incurred by her breast cancer therapy.

4. Bilateral breast cancer—Clinically evident simultaneous bilateral breast cancer occurs in less than 1% of cases, but there is a 5–8% incidence of later occurrence of cancer in the second breast. Bilaterality occurs more often in women younger than age 50 years and is more frequently associated with a lobular carcinoma and in patients with hereditary breast cancer syndromes such as Li-Fraumeni syndrome. The incidence of second breast cancers increases directly with the length of time the patient is alive after her first cancer and is approximately 1.0% per year and is significantly higher in patients with hereditary breast cancer syndromes.

In patients with breast cancer, careful screening of the contralateral breast at the time of initial diagnosis and at regular intervals thereafter is warranted. Routine biopsy of the opposite breast is usually not indicated.

D. Mammography

Mammography is the breast imaging modality of choice and the only screening method that has been consistently found to decrease mortality of breast cancer. Some breast cancers can be identified by mammography as early as 2 years before reaching a size detectable by palpation.

Although false-positive and false-negative results are occasionally obtained with mammography, the experienced radiologist can interpret mammograms correctly in approximately 90% of cases. Ultrasound and magnetic resonance imaging (MRI) are not recommended for screening the general population, and their primary role is as adjuncts to an abnormal mammogram. For women at high risk for developing breast cancer, the addition of MRI and ultrasound to screening mammograms may be contemplated.

Because up to 15% of cancers that are detected on clinical exams are not seen on mammograms, a negative mammogram should preclude further intervention in patients with a dominant or suspicious mass. The use of a targeted ultrasound can help decrease the false-negative rate of mammograms and evaluate the mammographically occult palpable breast mass.

E. Cytology

Cytologic examination of nipple discharge or cyst fluid may be helpful on rare occasions. As a rule, mammography and breast biopsy are required when nipple discharge or cyst fluid is bloody or cytologically equivocal.

F. Biopsy

The diagnosis of breast cancer depends ultimately on examination of tissue removed by biopsy. Treatment should never be undertaken without an unequivocal histologic diagnosis of cancer. The safest course is biopsy examination of all suspicious masses found on physical examination and, in the absence of a mass, of suspicious lesions demonstrated by mammography. Approximately 30% of lesions thought to be definitely cancer prove on biopsy to be benign, and approximately 15% of lesions believed to be benign are found to be malignant. These findings demonstrate the fallibility of clinical judgment and the necessity for biopsy.

The simplest method is by fine-needle aspiration (FNA). This method is, however, limited by its inability to distinguish invasive from noninvasive breast cancers and the relatively high rate of nondiagnostic studies, especially for nonpalpable abnormalities and with less experienced practitioners.

In many centers, core needle biopsies, most often with image guidance, have replaced open surgical biopsies. Core needle biopsies offer the advantage of a more definitive histologic diagnosis, minimize the risk of inadequate samples, and allow the distinction between invasive and noninvasive breast cancers. Open surgical biopsies, often with wire localization, should be reserved for those lesions that are technically unattainable with core needle biopsies or in the event of core needle biopsy results that do not correlate with the imaging findings (discordant results).

In general, outpatient biopsy followed by definitive surgery at a later date gives patients time to adjust to the diagnosis of cancer, meet with members of the multidisciplinary team involved with managing breast cancer, and consider a second opinion as well as alternative forms of treatment. Studies show no adverse effects from the short (1–2 weeks) delay of the 2-step procedure, and this is the current recommendation of the NCI.

At the time of the initial biopsy of breast cancer, the specimen can also be analyzed with immunohistochemical staining for hormone and growth factor (eg, HER-2-Neu) receptors. Tumor analysis using reverse transcriptase polymerase chain reaction (RT-PCR) technology from pathologic specimens to assess the tumor recurrence risk is now available. Such tests can aid the patient and physician in the decision for further adjuvant therapy or not. At the time of pathologic confirmation of a breast cancer diagnosis, patients on hormone replacement therapy (HRT) should be instructed to stop hormone use until counseled by an oncologist.

G. Laboratory Findings

A complete blood cell count (CBC), chemistry panel including liver function tests (LFTs), and a β-human chorionic gonadotropin (β-hCG) in premenopausal patients should be obtained as part of the initial evaluation. An elevation in alkaline phosphatase or liver function may be an indication of distant metastatic disease and warrants further investigation. Hypercalcemia may be seen in advanced cases of metastatic cancer.

H. Imaging Studies

Most systematic reviews have concluded that the routine radiologic evaluation for metastatic disease is unnecessary in the majority of patients since the overall yield is low. In general, the prevalence of metastatic disease increases with the clinical stage of the disease. The Cancer Care Ontario Practice Guidelines Initiative recommends against routine staging for clinical stage I disease, whereas they recommend routine staging in patients with stage III disease and radionuclide bone scanning in patients with stage II disease. In general, imaging studies should be limited to patients with higher pretest probability of distant metastases, such as those with signs, symptoms, or laboratory abnormalities suggestive of distant metastases and those with locally advanced breast cancer.

The imaging modality of choice has not been standardized, although computed tomography (CT) scanning of chest, abdomen, and pelvis offers a more sensitive and attractive 1-visit option at the price of a higher risk of false-positive results, cost, and radiation exposure. In addition, evaluation for skeletal metastases with radionuclide bone scans would still be required.

The combination of positron emission tomography (PET) and CT scans is a promising tool in the staging and metastatic evaluation of breast cancer because it allows for the evaluation of visceral and bony metastases. However, data regarding its routine use in the metastatic workup of patients with breast cancer are lacking.

The American Society of Clinical Oncology has found that there is insufficient evidence to support the routine use of tumor markers such as CA 15-3, CA 27.29, and carcinoembryonic antigen (CEA). In general, assessment of myocardial function should be reserved for patients at high risk of cardiotoxicity (age >65 years or underlying heart disease) prior to initiating treatment with anthracyclines and in all patients scheduled to receive trastuzumab.

Early Detection

A. Screening Programs

Mammography remains the single best screening procedure for the early detection of breast cancer. The majority of breast cancers in the United States are detected as a result of an abnormal screening study. In general, depending on a woman's age and the density of her breasts, the sensitivity of mammography is 70–90%, and its specificity is greater than 90%. Yearly mammogram screening among women continues to increase, so that in 1997, roughly 85% of women had had a mammogram at least once previously. This was an increase of 15% from 1990 and of 47% from 1987. In 2008, the proportion of US women age 50–74 years who reported that they had a screening mammogram in the preceding 2 years was 81.1%. Lack of insurance coverage and lower socioeconomic status were associated with significantly lower prevalence of up-to-date mammography.

Despite a consensus on the importance of mammographic screening, mammography has still not been demonstrated unequivocally to decrease breast cancer mortality across all age groups. In women between 50 and 69 years of age, there is reasonable evidence, based largely on 8 randomized controlled trials, that screening mammography is beneficial. In elderly patients over the age of 70 years, however, the optimal frequency of screening is still unknown because they have not generally been included in most large cooperative screening trials and because of their limited life expectancy, which can affect gains in breast mortality. For younger women, the evidence is also not entirely clear. For women age 40–49 years, there appears to be a small benefit, which comes at the price of a higher number of patients in that age group who need to be screened. These results may be due to the lower prevalence of the disease and decreased sensitivity of mammograms in this age group as well as the possibility that younger women have faster growing tumors, which may be more readily missed at one screening and become clinically apparent before the subsequent screening. Nevertheless, in the Health Insurance Plan of Greater New York screening study from the United States, which with 18 years has the longest follow-up of any randomized mammography screening study, there was a 30% reduction in mortality in women older than 50 years of age. Despite academic debate and challenges and controversy in the news media, the consensus that screening mammography saves lives has been upheld.

Current screening recommendations from the American College of Radiology, the American Cancer Society, and the American Medical Association call for annual mammograms starting at age 40 years. The American College of Obstetricians and Gynecologists calls for screening mammography every 1–2 years for women age 40–49 and annually thereafter. There is no recommendation for a "baseline" examination prior to age 40 years, nor is there any evidence to support this practice in women younger than this age. Women with a genetic predisposition to breast cancer should be screened using a combination of screening mammography and MRI beginning at age 25 or based on the age of earliest onset breast cancer in the family. For women with a family history of breast cancer but without a genetic mutation, some authorities have suggested initiating screening with mammography before age 40, although data from randomized controlled trials on the efficacy of this approach is lacking.

B. Breast Examination

Even though several randomized controlled trials included clinical breast examination with mammography, the utility of clinical breast exams remains debatable. From these studies, it appears that mammography detected approximately 90% of breast cancers and clinical breast exams detected approximately 50% with significant but not total overlap. A recent review of the literature concluded that the effectiveness of clinical breast examination has yet to be proven. It also appears that sensitivity of clinical breast examination in the community setting is lower than that reported in the randomized trials due to a lack of standardization and procedural and examiner variability. Clinical breast examination remains an attractive and useful option in developing countries where screening mammography programs are prohibitively expensive, in the event of mammographically occult breast cancer, and in older women who are no longer being screened regularly.

The few randomized controlled trials that have examined breast self-examination have similarly failed to show a benefit in the rates of breast cancer diagnosis and mortality, suggesting that breast self-examination only be offered as an adjunct to regular screening and patients be educated about its limitations.

C. Genetic Testing

A positive family history of breast cancer is recognized as a risk factor for the subsequent development of breast cancer. With the discovery of 2 major breast cancer predisposition genes, BRCA1 (17q21) and BRCA2 (13q12-13), there has been increasing interest in genetic testing. Mutations in these 2 genes are associated with an elevated risk for breast cancer, as well as ovarian, colon, prostate, and pancreatic cancers. Of all women with breast cancer, approximately 5–10% may have mutations in BRCA1 or BRCA2. The estimated risk of a patient developing cancer with a BRCA1 or BRCA2 mutation is believed to be between 40% and 85%. Particular mutations may be more common in specific ethnic groups like the Ashkenazi Jewish population. Genetic testing is available and may be considered for members of high-risk families. The US Preventive Task Force, Kaiser Permanente, and the National Cancer Center Network have developed BRCA testing guidelines (Table 5–2). Because of the complexities of genetic testing, genetic counseling before and after testing is necessary.

Pathologic Types

Numerous pathologic subtypes of breast cancer can be identified histologically (Table 5–3). More than 95% of breast malignancies arise from the epithelial elements of the breast. These pathologic types are distinguished by the histologic appearance and growth pattern of the tumor. In general, breast cancer arises either from the epithelial lining of the

Table 5–2. Recommendations from the US Preventive Services Task Force on who should be offered genetic testing for BRCA mutations.

For non-Ashkenazi Jewish women:
Two first-degree relatives with breast cancer, 1 of whom was diagnosed at age 50 or younger
A combination of 3 or more first- or second-degree relatives with breast cancer regardless of age at diagnosis
A combination of both breast and ovarian cancer among first- and second-degree relatives
A first-degree relative with bilateral breast cancer
A combination of 2 or more first- or second-degree relatives with ovarian cancer, regardless of age at diagnosis
A first- or second-degree relative with both breast and ovarian cancer at any age
History of breast cancer in a male relative
For women of Ashkenazi Jewish descent:
Any first-degree relative (or 2 second-degree relatives on the same side of the family) with breast or ovarian cancer

large or intermediate-sized ducts (ductal) or from the epithelium of the terminal ducts of the lobules (lobular). The cancer may be invasive or in situ. Most breast cancers arise from the intermediate ducts and are invasive (invasive ductal or infiltrating ductal), and most histologic types are merely subtypes of invasive ductal cancer with unusual growth patterns (colloid, medullary, tubular, etc).

The histologic subtypes have only slight bearing on prognosis when outcomes are compared after accurate staging. Colloid (mucinous), medullary, papillary, adenoid cystic, and tubular histologies are generally believed to have a more favorable prognosis. Other histologic criteria have been studied in an attempt to substratify patients based on features such as tumor differentiation, lymphovascular space invasion, and tumor necrosis. Although these characteristics are important, stage is predominant and paramount in predicting outcome.

Table 5–3. Histologic types of breast cancer.

Type	Percent Occurrence
Invasive ductal (not otherwise specified)	80–85
Medullary	3–6
Colloid (mucinous)	3–6
Tubular	3–6
Papillary	3–6
Invasive lobular	4–10

The noninvasive cancers by definition lack the ability to spread. However, in patients whose biopsies show noninvasive intraductal cancer, associated invasive ductal cancers are present in 1–3% of cases. Lobular carcinoma in situ is considered by some to be a premalignant lesion that by itself is not a true cancer. It lacks the ability to spread but is associated with the subsequent development of invasive ductal cancer in 25–30% of cases within 15 years.

Hormone Receptor Sites

The presence or absence of estrogen and/or progesterone receptors in the nucleus of tumor cells is of critical importance in managing patients with initial, recurrent, and metastatic disease. Both estrogen receptors (ERs) and progesterone receptors (PRs) are nuclear hormone receptors. After binding their respective hormones in the cytoplasm of the target cell, the DNA-binding sites on the receptor are unmasked, and the activated complex migrates into the nucleus in order to bind to their respective hormone-responsive DNA elements. The responsiveness of breast cancer to hormonal therapy is best predicted by tumor expression of the ER and/or PR, and ER/PR-negative tumors are unlikely to benefit from endocrine therapy and would be better treated with systemic chemotherapy. Conversely, the magnitude of benefit from adjuvant endocrine therapy is directly related to the amount of ER.

ERs may be of prognostic significance, but current evidence is still unclear. For small node-negative tumors, the presence of ER is associated with lower likelihood of recurrence at 5 years when compared to ER-poor tumors. With longer follow-up, however, this initial advantage disappears primarily due to late recurrences. ER positivity is associated with a number of prognostic indicators, such as tumor grade and ploidy, but not with nodal metastases, and ER-positive tumors are more likely to metastasize to bone, soft tissue, and genital organs than are ER-negative tumors, which are more likely to spread to the liver, lung, and brain.

The Oxford Overview conducted by the Early Breast Cancer Trialists' Collaborative Group analyzed the data on each woman randomized to all trials of the treatment of operable breast cancer. In their last round of analysis published in 2005, the group showed that treatment with 5 years of tamoxifen when compared to no adjuvant endocrine therapy was associated with a 41% reduction in the annual risk of relapse and a 34% reduction in the annual death rate for women with ER-positive breast cancer.

It is advisable to obtain an ER assay for every breast cancer at the time of initial diagnosis. Receptor status may change after hormonal therapy, radiotherapy, or chemotherapy. The specimen requires special handling, and the laboratory should be prepared to process the specimen correctly.

HER2 & Response to Therapy

The HER2 gene encodes for a transmembrane glycoprotein that belongs to the epidermal growth factor receptor (EGFR) family of receptors, which play a key role in signal transduction controlling growth, differentiation, and possibly angiogenesis. Overexpression of the glycoprotein and/or amplification of its encoding gene is noted in 18–20% of breast cancer patients. HER2 overexpression/amplification is associated with an increased risk of recurrence and breast cancer death in the absence of systemic/targeted therapy and is also associated with resistance to endocrine therapy. However, HER2 overexpression/overamplification helps identify patients who benefit from the addition of agents that target the protein such as trastuzumab, a humanized monoclonal mouse antibody that binds the HER2 protein, and lapatinib, an oral tyrosine kinase inhibitor that blocks HER2. At least 4 large randomized controlled trials have shown that the addition of 1 year of trastuzumab to adjuvant therapy in patients with HER2-positive breast cancer significantly improves their disease-free and overall survival.

Curative Treatment

All oncologic treatment may be classified as curative or palliative. Curative treatment intent is advised for early-stage and locally advanced disease (clinical stages I to IIIC disease). Treatment intent is palliative for patients with stage IV disease and for previously treated patients who develop distant metastases or unresectable local recurrence.

A. Therapeutic Options

1. Radical mastectomy—Historically, Halsted is credited with performing the first modern radical mastectomy in 1882 in the United States. This surgical procedure was the en bloc removal of the breast, pectoral muscles, and axillary lymph nodes. It was the standard surgical procedure performed for breast cancer in the United States from the turn of the 20th century until the 1950s. During the 1950s, emerging information about lymph node drainage patterns prompted surgeons to undertake the extended radical mastectomy, which is a radical mastectomy and the removal of the internal mammary lymph nodes. It was postulated that a more extensive dissection of the draining lymphatics would improve control rates and translate into improved survival. A randomized trial, however, proved no benefit to the extended radical mastectomy versus the radical mastectomy, and the former was abandoned. Moreover, the failure of the extended radical mastectomy underscored the complications and morbidity of breast cancer surgery. This morbidity coupled with inadequate disease control led surgeons to explore less invasive and disfiguring techniques. Currently, radical mastectomy is rarely indicated or performed. Even in settings where radical resection may be entertained, such as invasion of the pectoralis muscles or large tumors, less invasive surgery coupled with neoadjuvant chemotherapy is preferred.

2. Modified radical mastectomy—Replacing radical mastectomy, the modified radical mastectomy (MRM) is the removal of the breast and underlying pectoralis major fascia, but not the muscle, and evaluation of selected axillary lymph nodes. Variations of this procedure include sacrificing the pectoralis minor muscle or not, and retracting, splitting, or transecting the pectoralis major to access the apex of the axilla for dissection. Because it is less invasive and less disfiguring, MRM provides a better cosmetic and functional result than radical mastectomy. Two prospective randomized trials, single-institution data, and several retrospective studies all demonstrate no difference in disease-free or overall survival rates between radical mastectomy and MRM for early-stage breast cancer. Until the early 1980s and the emergence of breast-conservation therapy (BCT), MRM was the standard treatment available to women for early-stage cancer. For locally advanced breast cancer and when the patient is not a candidate for BCT, or if the patient is not motivated for breast conservation, MRM remains a valid treatment option. A total mastectomy (simple mastectomy) is the removal of the whole breast, like an MRM, without the axillary dissection.

3. Breast-conservation therapy—BCT involves a surgical procedure such as a lumpectomy—an excision of the tumor mass with a negative surgical margin—an axillary evaluation, and postoperative irradiation. Several other operations, more limited in the scope of surgical dissection than MRM, such as segmental mastectomy, partial mastectomy, and quadrantectomy, are also used in conjunction with radiation and are part of the surgical component of BCT. As a result of 6 prospective randomized trials that showed no significant difference in local relapse, distant metastases, or overall survival between conservative surgery with radiation and mastectomy, BCT has gained increasing acceptance as a treatment option for stage I and II and selected stage III breast cancers.

B. Choice of Local Therapy

Breast cancer is a multidisciplinary disease in which surgeons, medical and radiation oncologists, radiologists, pathologists, nurses, and psychosocial support staff all play fundamental roles. Working with the patient, this team recommends the most appropriate treatment strategy. Clinical and pathologic stage, as well as biologic aggressiveness, are the principal determinants guiding local therapy, treatment strategy, and, ultimately, outcome. For early-stage breast cancer, including node-positive cases, much of the decision for initial local therapy rests with the patient. MRM is always a valid choice for addressing the local treatment of breast cancer. A patient's decision to undergo MRM does not necessarily obviate the role of radiation in the further management of breast cancer, and postmastectomy irradiation may still be recommended in approximately 20–25% of cases. To be a candidate for BCT, the patient must not be pregnant and cannot have multicentric breast cancer (evidence of cancer in >1 quadrant of the breast), locally advanced disease, diffuse microcalcifications on mammogram, or a prior history of ipsilateral breast irradiation. Relative contraindications are collagen-vascular disorders that could lead to a poor cosmetic outcome with irradiation and breast implants or psychiatric issues that would make close follow-up and surveillance difficult. These restrictions are only a portion of the decision-making process that must be completed before embarking on BCT.

Perhaps most importantly, the patient must be motivated and desire to maintain her breast in the face of a cancer diagnosis. This may entail some degree of physical, emotional, and psychological distress. For example, a patient may have to endure multiple re-excisions to obtain a negative surgical margin on the lumpectomy specimen. A patient may also experience resistance to BCT in areas where it is not commonly offered and where a multidisciplinary approach to breast cancer is not practiced. It has been shown that the surgical management of breast cancer differs considerably based on geographic location in the United States, independent of patient and tumor characteristics. Nevertheless, both physicians and patients pursue BCT because it allows the patient to preserve her breast without any decrement to survival, and the vast majority of women are pleased with the cosmetic result.

Because the treatment options for locally advanced and inflammatory breast cancers are in some ways less flexible than those for early-stage breast cancer, it is even more critical to engage the patient in the decision-making process for the choice of initial therapy. Many different strategies, which include mastectomy and less invasive surgeries, with or without neoadjuvant chemotherapy and adjuvant chemotherapy, radiation, and further maintenance interventions, are commonly used. In many settings, protocol therapy may be the most desirable treatment option.

Mastectomy

For about three-quarters of a century, radical mastectomy was considered standard therapy for breast cancer. The procedure was designed to remove the primary lesion, the breast in which it arose, the underlying muscle, and, by dissection in continuity, the axillary lymph nodes, which are most often the first site of regional spread beyond the breast. When radical mastectomy was introduced by Halsted, the average patient presented for treatment with locally advanced disease, and a relatively extensive procedure was often necessary just to remove all gross cancer. This is no longer the case. Patients now present with much smaller, less locally advanced lesions. Most of the patients in Halsted's original series would now be considered incurable by surgery alone, because they had extensive involvement of the chest wall, skin, and supraclavicular regions. Since the 1960s, MRM has supplanted the radical mastectomy because of its comparable disease control and a substantial decrease in morbidity and disfiguration.

In many cases, adjuvant therapy after MRM (eg, radiation) can even further reduce the incidence of local recurrence in certain patients with unfavorable tumor characteristics. In addition, 3 recent randomized trials of postmastectomy radiation, which confirmed a local control advantage, demonstrated an overall survival benefit in certain subsets of both pre- and postmenopausal women. For patients with ≥4 positive lymph nodes or large tumors ≥5 cm in diameter, postmastectomy radiation is strongly recommended. The role of postmastectomy radiation in patients with 1–3 positive nodes is more controversial. However, with increasing duration of follow-up, there is emerging evidence in favor of postmastectomy radiation for patients with 1–3 positive lymph nodes. Therefore, when deciding on initial local therapy, a patient must keep in mind that choosing MRM does not necessarily exclude a recommendation for adjuvant radiation.

Breast-Conservation Therapy

Because studies comparing radical mastectomy and MRM demonstrated no decrement in local control or survival, radical mastectomy has given way to MRM. In the 1980s, 6 prospective randomized trials were conducted worldwide that showed no significant difference in locoregional relapse or overall survival between breast-conserving surgery and radiation versus MRM for early-stage invasive breast cancer. In addition, an overview analysis showed equivalent survival with BCT as compared to mastectomy. Two of these studies included patients with node-positive breast cancer. With the addition of radiation to breast-conserving surgery techniques such as lumpectomy with an axillary evaluation, local failure is reduced to rates comparable to MRM with no compromise to overall survival.

There are a few absolute contraindications to BCT, which are mainly related to increased rates of in-breast recurrences or preclusion of use of radiation. These include persistently positive surgical margins, multicentric disease present in more than 1 quadrant of the breast, diffuse malignant-appearing calcifications throughout the breast precluding adequate resection, history of prior radiation therapy to the breast, and pregnancy. Other relative contraindications include a history of scleroderma due to an increased risk of skin toxicity associated with radiation and the large size of the tumor relative to the size of the breast, resulting in an unacceptable cosmetic outcome. Factors that are not contraindications to breast conservation include nodal metastases, tumor location, tumor subtype, and a family history of breast cancer.

Unfortunately, no subgroup of patient with breast cancer undergoing breast conservation has a low enough risk of recurrence to justify the elimination of adjuvant therapy. Some investigators are currently examining alternative strategies of delivering radiotherapy such partial breast irradiation and shortened courses of whole breast radiation in select patients with node-negative disease.

Axillary Evaluation

It is important to recognize that axillary evaluation is valuable both in planning therapy and in staging of the cancer. Axillary lymph node dissection has long been the mainstay for axillary staging in the treatment of patients with breast cancer. Although the removal of even occult cancer in axillary lymph nodes generally does not translate into an improvement in overall survival rates, regional failures will be lower. Axillary lymph node dissection is generally safe but may result in nerve damage and lymphedema, especially in patients receiving postoperative radiotherapy. Because of the potential for major morbidity associated with the procedure and questions regarding any survival advantage it would offer, some investigators examined the use of sentinel lymph node biopsy (SLNB) as an alternative to formal axillary dissection for the pathologic assessment of the clinically negative axilla. This procedure uses a tracer material that is injected into the tumor bed to map the tumor drainage to the primary or "sentinel" axillary lymph node(s). The sentinel lymph node is excised and pathologically examined. If the sentinel lymph node is found to harbor metastatic disease, a subsequent formal dissection is done. Conversely, if the sentinel lymph node is negative, no further surgical evaluation need be performed. Although this procedure relies heavily on the surgeon's expertise with a new technique and has some inherent limitations, when performed by an experienced team, a negative result carries a negative predictive value of 94–96%. Potential side effects and complications are minimized, and recovery is quick without sacrificing diagnostic or therapeutic results. A practical example of the benefits of SLNB is that, when used in conjunction with BCT, reported rates of lymphedema are lower than with axillary dissection.

Adjuvant Systemic Therapy

A. Hormonal Therapy

Adjuvant hormonal therapy or manipulation is recommended for all women whose breast cancer expresses hormone receptors. Even if the tumor does not express estrogen hormone receptor protein but only progesterone, hormonal therapy may be beneficial. This recommendation is made regardless of age, menopausal status, involvement or number of positive lymph nodes, or tumor size. The benefit of adjuvant hormonal therapy is seen across all subgroups of breast cancer patients, with both invasive and in situ lesions. Although the absolute decrease in recurrence, second primary breast cancer, and death may vary from group to group, there is a firmly established role for adjuvant hormonal intervention.

Until recently, 5 years of tamoxifen was considered to be the adjuvant hormonal therapy regimen of choice and remains a valuable option for both premenopausal and postmenopausal women with ER-positive tumors. Randomized trials support the 5-year duration, which is superior to shorter courses and does not expose the patient to the increased risk of adverse effects associated with longer use. Furthermore, use longer than 5 years does not appear to enhance the long-term benefit seen with just 5 years of use. Although tamoxifen carries an increased risk of endometrial cancer and venous thromboembolism, the benefits outweigh the risks for the vast number of patients. Surveillance screening procedures such as transvaginal ultrasound and endometrial biopsy are not necessary in asymptomatic patients on tamoxifen.

More recently, aromatase inhibitors (AI) such as anastrozole have been shown to be as effective if not more effective than tamoxifen in postmenopausal women with early-stage, invasive breast cancer. In fact, in at least 2 large trials, anastrozole and letrozole were found to be superior to tamoxifen in terms of disease-free survival, time to recurrence, and the incidence of contralateral breast cancer, although no significant difference in overall survival was seen. The toxicity profile of AIs is also different, making them useful for women who would like to avoid the tamoxifen-related side effects. Compared to tamoxifen, the use of AIs confers a smaller risk of endometrial cancer, venous thromboembolic events, and hot flashes. However, AIs are associated with a higher risk of musculoskeletal disorders, osteoporosis, and cardiac events when compared to tamoxifen. AIs are not typically used in premenopausal patients because the reduced estrogen feedback on the hypothalamus results in an increase in gonadotropin release, which paradoxically stimulates the ovary to produce more aromatase and androgen substrate.

B. Chemotherapy

Cytotoxic chemotherapy is commonly offered to women as adjuvant treatment for both early-stage and locally advanced breast cancer. The goal of adjuvant chemotherapy is to eliminate occult microscopic metastases that are often responsible for late recurrences. Cytotoxic chemotherapy offers benefits to the many early and the majority of locally advanced breast cancer patients, although the magnitude of benefit is more pronounced in premenopausal and node-positive patients. Cytotoxic chemotherapy is also considered by many to be the standard of care for patients with ER-negative tumors who are candidates for adjuvant systemic therapy because of adverse prognostic indicators such as tumor size >1 cm, positive lymph nodes, and high-grade disease.

The benefit of adding chemotherapy to endocrine therapy for patients with ER-positive tumors is more controversial, especially for patients with negative lymph nodes. The Oncotype DX 21-gene recurrence score assay is a potentially useful tool that could help predict patients with node-negative ER-positive tumors who have the lowest risk of distant recurrence, enough to justify elimination of chemotherapy.

Polychemotherapy (≥2 agents) is superior to single-agent chemotherapy. Duration for 3–6 months or 4–6 cycles appears to offer optimal benefit without subjecting the patient to undue toxicity associated with more prolonged treatment, which adds little benefit in terms of overall outcome. Cytotoxic chemotherapy with an anthracycline-based (doxorubicin or epirubicin) regimen is favored, because a small but statistically significant improvement in survival has been demonstrated compared with nonanthracycline-containing regimens. The cardiac toxicity caused by anthracyclines is not considered detrimental in women without significant cardiac disease but does occur in 1% of cases or less. Several trials have also demonstrated a survival advantage for regimens that include a taxane in addition to an anthracycline, particularly in node-positive tumors and other higher risk tumors. Alterations in dose schedule (eg, "dose-dense" regimens) also offer advantages over other combinations and administrations of chemotherapy for well-defined patient populations. As previously mentioned, several trials have shown that the addition of trastuzumab offers an overall and recurrence-free survival advantage in all but the most favorable HER2-positive tumors at the price of a small but significant increase in cardiac events, particularly for patients receiving an anthracycline-containing regimen. However, emerging data suggest the equivalence of taxane-based combinations with trastuzumab and those combinations containing anthracyclines with less cardiac toxicity. The choice of adjuvant chemotherapy is complex. The medical oncologist must consider multiple tumor and patient features and individualize treatment for breast cancer patients.

Several areas concerning chemotherapy have generated considerable interest but lack conclusive evidence. For instance, high-dose chemotherapy with bone marrow or stem cell rescue is not recommended. There is no evidence that high-dose regimens are superior to standard-dose polychemotherapy. Stem cell support or bone marrow transplant should be offered only on protocol. Further investigation is also needed to clarify the role of other biologic agents and dosing schedules. Trials need to enroll more patients older than age 70 years to assess the benefits and toxicities of adjuvant chemotherapy in this population. Finally, studies designed to measure quality of life need to be done to place the benefits versus toxicity question of adjuvant therapies into context.

The use of systemic therapy prior to surgery has become the mainstay of therapy for patients with locally advanced or inflammatory breast cancer but is increasingly being offered to patients with early-stage breast cancer to facilitate BCT instead of mastectomy.

Follow-Up Care

After primary treatment, breast cancer patients should be followed for life because of the long, insidious natural history of breast cancer. The goals of close breast cancer follow-up are to detect recurrences and second primaries after treatment in the ipsilateral breast and to detect new cancers in the contralateral breast. The risk of a second primary in the contralateral breast of a patient with a history of breast cancer is believed to be roughly 0.5–1% per year. Although there are no universally accepted guidelines, several consensus conferences have met to establish recommendations. After the completion of treatment, it is recommended that the patient undergo a physical examination every 4 months for the first 2 years, then every 6 months until year 5, and annually thereafter. A mammogram should be obtained annually for all patients and no less than 6 months after the completion of radiation therapy. For patients who received irradiation, a chest radiograph is also obtained yearly. Routine laboratory tests including CBC, chemistry profile, and LFTs can be ordered yearly, especially if the patient received chemotherapy, or else as needed. There is no role for routine bone scans or additional imaging unless the patient is symptomatic or there is clinical suspicion of an abnormality. Patients taking tamoxifen should have annual pelvic examinations and be counseled to report any irregular vaginal bleeding. Patients on AIs need periodic bone density studies and lipid panels to assess their cardiovascular risk factors.

A. Local Recurrence

The development of local recurrence correlates with stage and thus tumor size as well as the presence and number of positive axillary lymph nodes, margin status, nuclear grade, and histologic type. The median time to recurrence is roughly 4 years, with a 1–2% risk per year for the first 5 years and a 1% risk per year thereafter. Late failures occurring 15–20 years or more after treatment, however, do occur. The risk of local recurrence after BCT or MRM is generally <15%, 20 years after treatment. Positive axillary lymph nodes are prognostic for local failure at the chest wall after MRM, but they are not prognostic for a local failure after BCT.

The treatment of local recurrences depends on the initial local therapy. In the breast, failures after BCT can be treated with salvage mastectomy with salvage rates of approximately 50%. In general, there is no difference in overall survival for an isolated breast recurrence successfully treated with salvage mastectomy. Node failures are more ominous. Axillary failures have roughly a 50% 3- to 5-year disease-free survival, and supraclavicular failures have a 0–20% 3-year disease-free survival. All chest wall abnormalities should be biopsied to rule out recurrence and resected with a wide local excision if possible. Adjuvant salvage therapies such as radiation, cytotoxic chemotherapy, and hormonal therapy may also be instituted.

Local recurrence may signal the presence of widespread disease and is an indication for bone and liver scans, posteroanterior and lateral chest x-rays, and other examinations as needed to search for evidence of distant metastases. When there is no evidence of metastases beyond the chest wall and regional nodes, radical irradiation for cure and complete local excision can be attempted. Many patients with locally recurrent tumors will develop distant metastases within 2 years. For this reason, most physicians use systemic therapy for treatment of patients with local recurrence.

B. Edema of the Arm

Lymphedema of the arm is a significant and often dreaded complication of breast cancer treatment. Lymphedema occurs as a result of lymphatic disruption and insult caused primarily by local treatment modalities like surgery and radiation. Although each of these modalities carries its own risk with respect to arm edema, a combined-modality approach further increases this risk. With a typical level I/II axillary lymph node dissection and radiation, the risk of lymphedema is roughly <10%. This risk approached 30% when a more aggressive level III dissection was more commonly performed in the past. The rates of clinically significant lymphedema—that is, edema that affects function and is not merely detectable with sophisticated measurement tools—are generally considered to be much lower. With the advent of SLNB, lymphedema rates are expected to continue to improve.

Late or secondary edema of the arm may develop years after MRM, as a result of axillary recurrence or of infection in the hand or arm, with obliteration of lymphatic channels. Interestingly, there is frequently no obvious initiating event causing late arm swelling in a patient with a history of breast cancer treatment.

C. Breast Reconstruction

Breast reconstruction, with the implantation of a prosthesis or autologous tissue such as transverse rectus abdominis myocutaneous flap (TRAM), is now commonly offered following mastectomy and can be very frequently performed immediately after surgery. Therefore, reconstruction should be discussed with patients prior to mastectomy and is not an obstacle to the diagnosis of recurrent cancer.

Prognosis

The stage of breast cancer is the single most reliable indicator of prognosis. Patients with disease localized to the breast and no evidence of regional spread after microscopic examination of the lymph nodes have by far the most favorable prognosis. ERs and PRs appear to be an important prognostic variable because patients with hormone receptor–negative tumors and no evidence of metastases to the axillary lymph nodes have a much higher recurrence rate than do patients with hormone receptor–positive tumors and no regional metastases. The histologic subtype of breast cancer (eg, medullary, lobular, comedo) seems to have little significance in prognosis once these tumors are truly invasive.

Many patients who develop breast cancer will ultimately die of breast cancer. The mortality rate of breast cancer patients exceeds that of age-matched normal controls for nearly 20 years. Thereafter, the mortality rates are equal, although deaths that occur among the breast cancer patients are often directly the result of tumor. Five-year statistics do not accurately reflect the final outcome of therapy.

When cancer is localized to the breast, with no evidence of regional spread after pathologic examination, the clinical cure rate with most accepted methods of therapy is 75–80%. Exceptions to this may be related to the hormonal receptor content of the tumor, tumor size, host resistance, or associated illness. Patients with small ER- and PR-positive tumors and no evidence of axillary spread probably have a 5-year survival rate of nearly 90%. When the axillary lymph nodes are involved with the tumor, the survival rate drops to 50–60% at 5 years, and probably to less than 25% at 10 years. In general, breast cancer appears to be somewhat more aggressive in younger than in older women, which may be related to the fact that relatively fewer younger women have ER-positive tumors.

PALLIATIVE TREATMENT OF RECURRENT AND METASTATIC BREAST CANCER

This section discusses palliative therapy of disseminated disease incurable by surgery (stage IV).

Local Therapy

Patients with metastatic breast cancer are unlikely to be cured of their disease, and for many, the goals of care shift from cure to palliation, symptom control, and improved quality of life. In general, local therapy, such as palliative radiotherapy or surgery when technically feasible, should be reserved for patients in order to control their symptoms and minimize the risk of complications. As part of multimodality treatment, surgery for patients with metastatic breast cancer should be reserved for patients with a good performance status, minimal organ involvement, prolonged disease-free interval, or indolent disease growth when the likelihood of achieving complete resection of the tumor or metastasis is reasonable. A subset of these patients may achieve long-term survival as a result of surgery, although confirmatory data are still lacking. Palliative irradiation is also of value in the treatment of certain bone or soft tissue metastases to control pain or avoid pathologic fracture. Radiotherapy is especially useful in the treatment of the isolated bony metastasis and chest wall recurrences.

Hormonal Therapy

Disseminated disease may respond to prolonged endocrine therapy such as ovarian ablation or administration of drugs that block hormone receptor sites or that block hormone synthesis or production. Hormonal manipulation is usually more successful in postmenopausal women. A favorable response to hormonal manipulation occurs in about one-third of patients with metastatic breast cancer. In patients whose tumors contain ERs, the response is approximately 60%, and perhaps as high as 80% for patients whose tumors contain PRs as well. Tumors negative for both ERs and PRs have response rates to hormonal therapy that are 10% or less.

Because the quality of life during a remission induced by endocrine manipulation is usually superior to a remission after cytotoxic chemotherapy, it may be best to try endocrine manipulation as a first-line systemic treatment for tumor recurrence or palliation. However, it is better to forgo endocrine therapy in patients with rapidly growing visceral metastases in whom a period of ineffective therapy may lead to a significant decline in organ function and performance status. Thus, salvage endocrine therapy is best reserved for patients with minimal symptoms, no visceral involvement, and slow-growing tumors.

As a general rule, only 1 type of systemic therapy should be given at a time. The systemic modality may be given in combination with a local or regional treatment if symptomatic lesions develop. For instance, it may be necessary to irradiate a destructive lesion of weight-bearing bone while the patient is taking a hormonal agent or chemotherapy. The palliative systemic regimen should be changed only if the disease is clearly progressing but not if disease appears stable. This is especially important for patients with destructive bone metastases, because minor changes in the status of these lesions are difficult to determine radiographically. A plan of therapy that would simultaneously minimize toxicity and maximize benefits is often best achieved by hormonal manipulation.

The choice of endocrine therapy depends on the menopausal status of the patient. Women within 1 year of their last menstrual period are considered to be premenopausal, whereas women whose menstruation ceased more than 1 year ago are usually classified as postmenopausal. In the past, ovarian ablation, usually by bilateral surgical oophorectomy, or radiation was the standard method of hormone manipulation used in premenopausal women with advanced breast cancer. However, it has subsequently become clear that tamoxifen is equally effective and has none of the attendant risks of surgical ablation of the ovaries. Tamoxifen is recommended as the treatment of choice for hormonal therapy in the premenopausal woman with advanced breast cancer. For postmenopausal patients, AIs and tamoxifen are the initial therapy of choice for metastatic breast cancer amenable to endocrine manipulation, and a favorable response to initial hormonal therapy with tamoxifen is predictive of future responses to hormonal maneuvers.

The use of AIs, which work by blocking the conversion of testosterone to estradiol and androstenedione to estrogen both in the adrenal cortex and in peripheral tissue, including breast cancers themselves, is effective in postmenopausal patients.

Other hormonal agents have been found to be effective in premenopausal patients. Gonadotropin-releasing hormone (GnRH) agonists that act on the pituitary to eventually suppress follicle-stimulating hormone (FSH) and luteinizing hormone (LH) and the pituitary–ovarian axis, thereby decreasing estrogen production, have been used since the 1980s. They are an alternative to oophorectomy if used alone or can be combined with tamoxifen or AIs.

Progestins, megestrol acetate, and medroxyprogesterone acetate are alternative agents reserved mainly for cases resistant to tamoxifen and AIs.

Chemotherapy

Cytotoxic drugs should be considered for the treatment of metastatic breast cancer in the following instances: (1) if visceral metastases are present (especially brain or lymphangitic pulmonary spread), (2) if hormonal treatment is unsuccessful or the disease has progressed after an initial response to hormonal manipulation, or (3) if the tumor is ER and PR negative. With response rates of 35–55% in many series, the taxanes are quickly eclipsing the anthracyclines as the single most useful agents in the treatment of hormone-refractory metastatic breast cancer. Where once doxorubicin could achieve response rates of 40–50%, in some trials, the taxanes seem to offer a small overall survival advantage. In addition, they are generally well tolerated with an acceptable side effect profile. Questions about dosing, schedule of administration, and use with other agents, however, still have to be thoroughly answered.

Combination chemotherapy using multiple agents is appealing because, theoretically, the risk of drug resistance and cumulative toxicity is decreased. When compared to single-agent doxorubicin therapy, combination chemotherapy provides higher response rates and longer intervals until first progression. Nevertheless, the use of combination chemotherapy has never been shown to decrease drug resistance or toxicity in breast cancer. When combination chemotherapy has been compared to single-agent taxane therapy, although response rates were slightly lower, quality-of-life measurements were higher for the single agent. Thus, either a single-agent taxane or an anthracycline-containing combination regimen is frequently used as a first-line treatment. The use of cytotoxic chemotherapy or any other treatment modality should always be highly individualized, especially in the palliative setting.

Bisphosphonate Therapy

Bone is the most common site of metastatic disease at initial presentation and at the time of breast cancer recurrence. Bone metastases are often detected with a bone scan obtained in the staging of locally advanced cases or obtained because of clinical suspicion in the previously treated patient. Confirmation with plain radiographs, MRI, and/or CT is frequently needed because nearly 10% of lytic lesions may not be detected with a nuclear medicine scan. These other radiographic studies also help to delineate the extent of the metastatic disease. After bone metastases are confirmed, bisphosphonate therapy has been shown to diminish pain and decrease the rate of skeletal events and complications related to the bone metastases.

Bisphosphonate therapy should be administered with other palliative systemic treatments such as hormonal manipulation or chemotherapy. It is typically given intravenously every 3–4 weeks and continued indefinitely even though long-term studies are lacking. Regular dental exams, laboratory monitoring, and creatinine and renal function, as well as evaluation of calcium and vitamin D levels, are also recommended due to the risk of osteonecrosis of the jaw, renal insufficiency, and hypocalcemia associated with prolonged therapy.

Anderson GL, Limacher M, Assaf AR, et al. Effects of conjugated equine estrogen in postmenopausal women with hysterectomy: the Women's Health Initiative randomized controlled trial. *JAMA* 2004;291:1701–1712. PMID: 15082697.

Arisio R, Sapino A, Cassoni P, et al. What modifies the relation between tumour size and lymph node metastases in T1 breast carcinomas? *J Clin Pathol* 2000;53:846–850. PMID: 11127267.

Baum M, Buzdar A, Cuzick J, et al. Anastrozole alone or in combination with tamoxifen versus tamoxifen alone for adjuvant treatment of postmenopausal women with early-stage breast cancer: results of the ATAC (Arimidex, Tamoxifen Alone or in Combination) trial efficacy and safety update analyses. *Cancer.* 2003;98:1802–1810. PMID: 14584060.

Baxter N. Preventive health care, 2001 update: should women be routinely taught breast self-examination to screen for breast cancer? *CMAJ* 2001;164:1837–1846. PMID: 11450279.

Berry DA, Cronin KA, Plevritis SK, et al. Effect of screening and adjuvant therapy on mortality from breast cancer. *N Engl J Med* 2005;353:1784–1792. PMID: 16251534.

Bijker N, Rutgers EJ, Duchateau L, Peterse JL, Julien JP, Cataliotti L. Breast-conserving therapy for Paget disease of the nipple: a prospective European Organization for Research and Treatment of Cancer study of 61 patients. *Cancer* 2001;91: 472–477. PMID: 11169928.

Bristol IJ, Buchholz TA. Inflammatory breast cancer: current concepts in local management. *Breast Dis* 2005;22:75–83. PMID: 16761358.

Cardonick E, Iacobucci A. Use of chemotherapy during human pregnancy. *Lancet Oncol* 2004;5:283–291. PMID: 15120665.

Chen CY, Sun LM, Anderson BO. Paget disease of the breast: changing patterns of incidence, clinical presentation, and treatment in the U.S. *Cancer* 2006;107:1448–1458. PMID: 16933329.

Chu KC, Anderson WF, Fritz A, Ries LA, Brawley OW. Frequency distributions of breast cancer characteristics classified by estrogen receptor and progesterone receptor status for eight racial/ ethnic groups. *Cancer* 2001;92(1):37–45. PMID: 11443607.

Citron ML, Berry DA, Cirrincione C, et al. Randomized trial of dose-dense versus conventionally scheduled and sequential versus concurrent combination chemotherapy as postoperative adjuvant treatment of node-positive primary breast cancer: first report of Intergroup Trial C9741/Cancer and Leukemia Group B Trial 9741. J Clin Oncol 2003;21:1431–1439. PMID: 12668651.

Clarke M, Coates AS, Darby SC, et al. Adjuvant chemotherapy in oestrogen-receptor-poor breast cancer: patient-level meta-analysis of randomised trials. *Lancet* 2008;371:29–40. PMID: 18177773.

Clarke M, Collins R, Darby S, et al. Effects of radiotherapy and of differences in the extent of surgery for early breast cancer on local recurrence and 15-year survival: an overview of the randomised trials. *Lancet* 2005;366:2087–2106. PMID: 16360786.

Colditz GA, Rosner B. Cumulative risk of breast cancer to age 70 years according to risk factor status: data from the Nurses' Health Study. *Am J Epidemiol* 2000;152:950–964. PMID: 11092437.

Collaborative Group on Hormonal Factors in Breast Cancer. Breast cancer and breastfeeding: collaborative reanalysis of individual data from 47 epidemiological studies in 30 countries, including 50302 women with breast cancer and 96973 women without the disease. *Lancet* 2002;360:187–195. PMID: 12133652.

Dunstan CR, Felsenberg D, Seibel MJ. Therapy insight: the risks and benefits of bisphosphonates for the treatment of tumor-induced bone disease. Nat Clin Pract Oncol 2007;4:42–55. PMID: 17183355.

Early Breast Cancer Trialists' Collaborative Group. Effects of chemotherapy and hormonal therapy for early breast cancer on recurrence and 15-year survival: an overview of the randomised trials. *Lancet* 2005;365:1687–1717. PMID: 15894097.

Elmore JG, Armstrong K, Lehman CD, Fletcher SW. Screening for breast cancer. *JAMA* 2005;293:1245–1256. PMID: 15755947.

Elmore JG, Reisch LM, Barton MB, et al. Efficacy of breast cancer screening in the community according to risk level. *J Natl Cancer Inst* 2005;97:1035–1043. PMID: 16030301.

Erickson VS, Pearson ML, Ganz PA, Adams J, Kahn KL. Arm edema in breast cancer patients. *J Natl Cancer Inst* 2001;93: 96–111. PMID: 11208879.

Eubank WB, Mankoff DA. Evolving role of positron emission tomography in breast cancer imaging. Semin Nucl Med 2005;35(2):84–99. PMID: 15765372.

Familial breast cancer: collaborative reanalysis of individual data from 52 epidemiological studies including 58,209 women with breast cancer and 101,986 women without the disease. *Lancet* 2001;358:1389–1399. PMID: 11705483.

Fisher B, Anderson S, Bryant J, et al. Twenty-year follow-up of a randomized trial comparing total mastectomy, lumpectomy, and lumpectomy plus irradiation for the treatment of invasive breast cancer. *N Engl J Med.* 2002;347:1233–1241. PMID: 12393820.

Fisher B, Dignam J, Bryant J, Wolmark N. Five versus more than five years of tamoxifen for lymph node-negative breast cancer: updated findings from the National Surgical Adjuvant Breast and Bowel Project B-14 randomized trial. *J Natl Cancer Inst* 2001;93:684–690. PMID: 11333290.

Fisher ER, Anderson S, Tan-Chiu E, Fisher B, Eaton L, Wolmark N. Fifteen-year prognostic discriminants for invasive breast carcinoma: National Surgical Adjuvant Breast and Bowel Project Protocol-06. *Cancer* 2001;91(8 Suppl):1679–1687. PMID: 11309768.

Freedman DA, Petitti DB, Robins JM. On the efficacy of screening for breast cancer. *Int J Epidemiol* 2004;33:43–55. PMID: 15075144.

Freedman GM, Fowble BL. Local recurrence after mastectomy or breast-conserving surgery and radiation. *Oncology (Williston Park)*2000;14:1561–1581. PMID: 11125941.

Fyles AW, McCready DR, Manchul LA, et al. Tamoxifen with or without breast irradiation in women 50 years of age or older with early breast cancer. *N Engl J Med* 2004;351:963–970. PMID: 15342804.

Garber JE, Offit K. Hereditary cancer predisposition syndromes. *J Clin Oncol* 2005;23:276–292. PMID: 15637391.

Goldhirsch A, Ingle JN, Gelber RD, Coates AS, Thurlimann B, Senn HJ. Thresholds for therapies: highlights of the St Gallen International Expert Consensus on the primary therapy of early breast cancer 2009. *Ann Oncol* 2009;20:1319–1329. PMID: 19535820.

Guray M, Sahin AA. Benign breast diseases: classification, diagnosis, and management. *Oncologist* 2006;11:435–449. PMID: 16720843.

Harris L, Fritsche H, Mennel R, et al. American Society of Clinical Oncology 2007 update of recommendations for the use of tumor markers in breast cancer. *J Clin Oncol* 2007;25: 5287–5312. PMID: 17954709.

Hughes KS, Schnaper LA, Berry D, et al. Lumpectomy plus tamoxifen with or without irradiation in women 70 years of age or older with early breast cancer. *N Engl J Med* 2004;351:971–977. PMID: 15342805.

Humphrey LL, Helfand M, Chan BK, Woolf SH. Breast cancer screening: a summary of the evidence for the U.S. Preventive Services Task Force. *Ann Intern Med* 2002;137:347–360. PMID: 12204020.

Jahanfar S, Ng CJ, Teng CL. Antibiotics for mastitis in breastfeeding women. *Cochrane Database Syst Rev* 2009;1:CD005458. PMID: 19160225.

Jemal A, Siegel R, Xu J, Ward E. Cancer statistics, 2010. *CA Cancer J Clin* 2010;60:277–300. PMID: 20610543.

Khan QJ, O'Dea AP, Dusing R, et al. Integrated FDG-PET/CT for initial staging of breast cancer. *J Clin Oncol* 2007;25(18S):558. [Abstract]

Klauber-DeMore N, Tan LK, Liberman L, et al. Sentinel lymph node biopsy: is it indicated in patients with high-risk ductal carcinoma-in-situ and ductal carcinoma-in-situ with microinvasion? *Ann Surg Oncol* 2000;7:636–642. PMID: 11034239.

Kooistra BW, Wauters C, van de Ven S, Strobbe L. The diagnostic value of nipple discharge cytology in 618 consecutive patients. *Eur J Surg Oncol* 2009;35:573–577. PMID: 18986790.

Macdonald OK, Lee CM, Tward JD, Chappel CD, Gaffney DK. Malignant phyllodes tumor of the female breast: association of primary therapy with cause-specific survival from the Surveillance, Epidemiology, and End Results (SEER) program. *Cancer* 2006;107:2127–2133. PMID: 16998937.

Mansel RE, Fallowfield L, Kissin M, et al. Randomized multicenter trial of sentinel node biopsy versus standard axillary treatment in operable breast cancer: the ALMANAC Trial. *J Natl Cancer Inst* 2006;98:599–609. PMID: 16670385.

Morrogh M, Morris EA, Liberman L, Borgen PI, King TA. The predictive value of ductography and magnetic resonance imaging in the management of nipple discharge. *Ann Surg Oncol* 2007;14:3369–3377. PMID: 17896158.

Myers RE, Johnston M, Pritchard K, Levine M, Oliver T. Baseline staging tests in primary breast cancer: a practice guideline. *CMAJ* 2001;164:1439–1444. PMID: 11387916.

Nelson HD, Huffman LH, Fu R, Harris EL. Genetic risk assessment and BRCA mutation testing for breast and ovarian cancer susceptibility: systematic evidence review for the U.S. Preventive Services Task Force. *Ann Intern Med* 2005;143: 362–379. PMID: 16144895.

Nelson HD, Tyne K, Naik A, Bougatsos C, Chan BK, Humphrey L. Screening for breast cancer: an update for the U.S. Preventive Services Task Force. *Ann Intern Med* 2009;151:727–737, W237–742. PMID: 19920273.

Paik S, Shak S, Tang G, et al. A multigene assay to predict recurrence of tamoxifen-treated, node-negative breast cancer. *N Engl J Med* 2004;351:2817–2826. PMID: 15591335.

Parkin DM, Bray F, Ferlay J, Pisani P. Global cancer statistics, 2002. *CA Cancer J Clin* 2005;55:74–108. PMID: 15761078.

Pendas S, Dauway E, Giuliano R, Ku N, Cox CE, Reintgen DS. Sentinel node biopsy in ductal carcinoma in situ patients. *Ann Surg Oncol* 2000;7:15–20. PMID: 10674443.

Perazella MA, Markowitz GS. Bisphosphonate nephrotoxicity. *Kidney Int* 2008;74:1385–1393. PMID: 18685574.

Petrek JA, Pressman PI, Smith RA. Lymphedema: current issues in research and management. *CA Cancer J Clin* 2000;50:292–307. PMID: 11075239.

Piccart-Gebhart MJ, Procter M, Leyland-Jones B, et al. Trastuzumab after adjuvant chemotherapy in HER2-positive breast cancer. *N Engl J Med* 2005;353:1659–1672. PMID: 16236737.

Ragaz J, Olivotto IA, Spinelli JJ, et al. Locoregional radiation therapy in patients with high-risk breast cancer receiving adjuvant chemotherapy: 20-year results of the British Columbia randomized trial. *J Natl Cancer Inst* 2005;97:116–126. PMID: 15657341.

Randolph WM, Goodwin JS, Mahnken JD, Freeman JL. Regular mammography use is associated with elimination of age-related disparities in size and stage of breast cancer at diagnosis. *Ann Intern Med* 2002;137:783–790. PMID: 12435214.

Rastogi P, Anderson SJ, Bear HD, et al. Preoperative chemotherapy: updates of National Surgical Adjuvant Breast and Bowel Project Protocols B-18 and B-27. *J Clin Oncol* 2008;26:778–785. PMID: 18258986.

Romond EH, Perez EA, Bryant J, et al. Trastuzumab plus adjuvant chemotherapy for operable HER2-positive breast cancer. *N Engl J Med.* 2005;353:1673–1684. PMID: 16236738.

Sakorafas GH, Tsiotou AG. Selection criteria for breast conservation in breast cancer. *Eur J Surg* 2000;166:835–846. PMID: 11097148.

Saslow D, Boetes C, Burke W, et al. American Cancer Society guidelines for breast screening with MRI as an adjunct to mammography. *CA Cancer J Clin* 2007;57:75–89. PMID: 17392385.

Schnitt SJ. Benign breast disease and breast cancer risk: morphology and beyond. *Am J Surg Pathol* 2003;27:836–841. PMID: 12766590.

Schrenk P, Rieger R, Shamiyeh A, Wayand W. Morbidity following sentinel lymph node biopsy versus axillary lymph node dissection for patients with breast carcinoma. *Cancer* 2000;88:608–614. PMID: 10649254.

Singletary SE, Walsh G, Vauthey JN, et al. A role for curative surgery in the treatment of selected patients with metastatic breast cancer. *Oncologist* 2003;8:241–251. PMID: 12773746.

Smith I, Procter M, Gelber RD, et al. 2-year follow-up of trastuzumab after adjuvant chemotherapy in HER2-positive breast cancer: a randomised controlled trial. *Lancet* 2007;369:29–36. PMID: 17208639.

Srivastava A, Mansel RE, Arvind N, Prasad K, Dhar A, Chabra A. Evidence-based management of mastalgia: a meta-analysis of randomised trials. *Breast* 2007;16:503–512. PMID: 17509880.

Tatsumi M, Cohade C, Mourtzikos KA, Fishman EK, Wahl RL. Initial experience with FDG-PET/CT in the evaluation of breast cancer. *Eur J Nucl Med Mol Imaging* 2006;33:254–262. PMID: 16258765.

Thurlimann B, Keshaviah A, Coates AS, et al. A comparison of letrozole and tamoxifen in postmenopausal women with early breast cancer. *N Engl J Med* 2005;353:2747–2757. PMID: 16382061.

Velicer CM, Heckbert SR, Lampe JW, Potter JD, Robertson CA, Taplin SH. Antibiotic use in relation to the risk of breast cancer. *JAMA* 2004;291:827–835. PMID: 14970061.

Verkooijen HM. Diagnostic accuracy of stereotactic large-core needle biopsy for nonpalpable breast disease: results of a multicenter prospective study with 95% surgical confirmation. *Int J Cancer* 2002;99:853–859. PMID: 12115488.

Walter C, Al-Nawas B, du Bois A, Buch L, Harter P, Grotz KA. Incidence of bisphosphonate-associated osteonecrosis of the jaws in breast cancer patients. *Cancer* 2009;115:1631–1637. PMID: 19156913.

Normal Pregnancy and Prenatal Care

6

Helene B. Bernstein, MD, PhD
George VanBuren, MD

NORMAL PREGNANCY

Pregnancy (gestation) is the physiologic process of a developing fetus within the maternal body. Several terms are used to define the developmental stage of human conception and the duration of pregnancy. For obstetric purposes, the gestational age or menstrual age is the time elapsed since the first day of the last normal menstrual period (LNMP), which actually precedes the time of oocyte fertilization. The gestational age is expressed in completed weeks. The start of the gestation (based on the LNMP) is usually 2 weeks before ovulation, assuming a 28-day regular menstrual cycle. The developmental or fetal age is the age of the conception calculated from the time of implantation, which is 4 to 6 days after ovulation is completed. The menstrual gestational age of pregnancy is calculated at 280 days or 40 completed weeks. The estimated due date (EDD) may be estimated by adding 7 days to the first day of the last menstrual period and subtracting 3 months plus 1 year (Naegele's rule).

The period of gestation can be divided into units consisting of 3 calendar months each or 3 trimesters. The first trimester can be subdivided into the embryonic and fetal periods. The embryonic period starts at the time of fertilization (developmental age) or at 2 through 10 weeks' gestational age. The embryonic period is the stage at which organogenesis occurs and the time period during which the embryo is most sensitive to teratogens. The end of the embryonic period and the beginning of the fetal period occurs 8 weeks after fertilization (developmental age) or 10 weeks after the onset of the last menstrual period.

Definitions

The term **gravid** means "pregnant"; gravida is the total number of pregnancies that a women has had, regardless of the outcome. **Parity** is the number of births, both before and after 20 weeks' gestation, and comprises 4 components:

1. Full-term births
2. Preterm births: having given birth to an infant (alive or deceased) weighing 500 g or more, or at or beyond 20 completed weeks (based on the first day of the last menstrual period)
3. Abortions: pregnancies ending before 20 weeks, either induced or spontaneous
4. Living children

When gravidity and parity are calculated as part of the obstetric history, multiple births are designated as a single gravid event, and each infant is included as part of the parity total.

Live birth is the delivery of any infant (regardless of gestational age) that demonstrates evidence of life (eg, a heartbeat, umbilical cord pulsation, voluntary or involuntary movement), independent of whether the umbilical cord has been cut or the placenta detached. An **infant** is a live-born human from the moment of birth until the completion of 1 year of life (365 days).

A **preterm infant** is defined as one born between 20 weeks and 37 completed weeks of gestation (259 days). A **term infant** is one born between 37 0/7 and 40 0/7 weeks gestation (280 days). At term, a fetus usually weighs more than 2500 g. Depending on maternal factors such as obesity and diabetes, amniotic fluid volume, and genetic and racial factors, the baby may be larger or smaller than expected; therefore, the clinician must rely on objective data to determine fetal maturity. Fetal lung maturity is assumed after 39 weeks' gestation but can be verified at an earlier gestational age by analysis of amniotic fluid by amniocentesis.

A **postterm infant** is born after 42 weeks' gestation (294 days). A prolonged pregnancy may result in an excessive-size infant with diminished placental capacity. A postmature infant may exhibit characteristic cutaneous changes, including a loss of subcutaneous fat, wrinkled skin, and fine long hair on the arms. Predicting the end of a pregnancy is a difficult problem for prenatal care providers.

Prenatal mortality rates increase as gestation advances past the due date (EDD) and accelerates sharply after 42 weeks' gestation. It is not uncommon to offer induction of labor after 41 completed weeks, or 7 days past the due date. (See Chapter 14 on Late Pregnancy Complications.) Estimated gestational age can be determined by methods outlined later for ascertaining fetal age and EDD.

Increased morbidity and mortality may be associated with a **macrosomic infant** or a **large for gestational age** (LGA) fetus. This is defined as a fetus with an estimated fetal weight at or beyond the 90th percentile at any gestational age. At term, approximately 10% of newborn infants weigh more than 4000 g, and the weight of 1.5% of newborns is in excess of 4500 g. Excessive fetal size should be suspected in women with a previous macrosomic fetus or those with diabetes mellitus. A **low-birth-weight infant** is any live birth for which the infant's weight is less than or equal to 2500 g. An infant with fetal growth restriction is defined as one at or below the 10th percentile at any gestational age.

Using a system based on the duration of gestational age or fetal weight, an **abortion** is the expulsion or extraction of part (incomplete) or all (complete) of the placenta or membranes without an identified fetus or with a fetus (alive or deceased) weighing less than 500 g or with an estimated gestational age of less than 20 completed weeks or 139 days from the last menstrual period, if fetal weight is unknown.

A. Birth Rate & Fertility Rate

Birth rate is defined as the number of live births per 1000 population. The **fertility rate** is expressed as the number of live births per 1000 women ages 15–44 years (sexually active population group). The current birth rate is 13.83 per 1000 population in 2010, whereas the general fertility rate is 66.7 per 1000 women ages 15–44 years.

B. Neonatal & Perinatal Periods

The **neonatal** period is defined as birth until 28 days of life; during this interval, the infant is designated as a newborn or neonate. The **perinatal period** is the time from 28 weeks' gestation to the first 7 days of life; this also includes the late fetal and early neonatal period.

The **prenatal mortality rate** is the sum of late fetal deaths plus early neonatal deaths (death in the first 7 days of life). The **neonatal mortality rate** (NMR) is infant death from birth to within 28 days of life. The NMR is calculated as the number of neonatal deaths during a year, divided by the number of live births during the same year, expressed per 1000 live births.

American College of Obstetricians and Gynecologists. Fetal Macrosomia. ACOG Practice Bulletin No. 22. *Obstet Gynecol* 2000;96.

Centers for Disease Control and Prevention. National Center for Health Statistics. http://www.cdc.gov/nchs/data_access/Vitalstatsonline.htm#Downloadable. Accessed January 10, 2011.

ESSENTIALS OF DIAGNOSIS

- Diagnosis is made on the basis of amenorrhea and a positive pregnancy test.
- It is crucial to diagnose pregnancy as soon as possible in order to initiate appropriate prenatal care, avoid teratogen (an agent that can cause a deleterious fetal effect) exposure, and diagnose nonviable or ectopic pregnancies.

Clinical Findings

A. Symptoms & Signs

A number of clinical signs and symptoms may presumptively indicate pregnancy.

1. Amenorrhea—Cessation of menses is caused by hormones (estrogen and progesterone) produced by the corpus luteum. The abrupt cessation of menses in a healthy reproductive-aged female with predictable cycles is highly suggestive of pregnancy.

2. Nausea & vomiting—This is a common symptom (50% of pregnancies) that begins as early as 2 weeks' gestational age and customarily resolves at between 13 and 16 weeks' gestation. Hyperemesis gravidarum is an extreme form of nausea and vomiting and is characterized by dehydration, weight loss (up to 5%), and ketonuria. In extreme cases of hyperemesis gravidarum, hospitalization, intravenous therapy, antiemetics, and, if needed, parenteral nutrition are given. Uncomplicated nausea and vomiting is treated with frequent small meals, a dry diet, and emotional support. (See Chapter 29 on Gastrointestinal Disorders in Pregnancy for more discussion.)

3. Breast changes

A. MASTODYNIA—Breast tenderness may range from tingling to pain caused by hormonal changes affecting the mammary duct and alveolar system.

B. BREAST ENGORGEMENT—Breast engorgement and periareolar venous prominences are also seen early in pregnancy, especially in primiparous patients. **Montgomery's tubercles** are the portion of the areolar glands visible on the skin surface. These tubercles can be more pronounced during pregnancy secondary to hormonal changes occurring as early as 6–8 weeks' gestation.

C. COLOSTRUM SECRETION—Protein and antibody production may occur during pregnancy as early as 16 weeks' gestation. This secretion is not associated with preterm delivery.

D. Development of secondary breast tissue—Development of secondary breast tissue may occur across the nipple line. Hypertrophy of secondary breast tissue may occur in the axilla and cause a symptomatic mass.

4. Fetal movement—The initial perception of fetal movement occurs at 18–20 weeks' gestation in primiparous patients and as early as 14 weeks' gestation in multiparous patients. Maternal perception of movement is called **quickening**, but this is not a dependable sign of pregnancy.

5. Elevated basal body temperature—Progesterone produces a 0.5°F increase in the basal body temperature, which persists after the missed menses. The rise in temperature occurs within the luteal phase of the menstrual cycle.

6. Skin changes

A. Chloasma—The mask of pregnancy is skin darkening of the forehead, bridge of the nose, or cheek bones. This pregnancy-associated change is linked to genetic predisposition and usually occurs after 16 weeks' gestation. Chloasma is exacerbated by sunlight.

B. Linea nigra—Melanocyte-stimulating hormone increases, causing darkening of the nipples and the lower midline from the umbilicus to the pubis (linea nigra). This skin change is genetically based; skin lightens slightly after delivery of the fetus.

C. Striae—Striae marks of the breast and abdomen appear as irregular scars. The striae appear late in pregnancy and are caused by collagen separation.

D. Spider telangiectasia—These are common skin lesions of pregnancy that result from elevated plasma estrogen. Both the vascular stellate skin lesions as well as palmar erythema may be seen in pregnancy and also occur in patients with liver failure.

7. Pelvic organ changes

A. Chadwick's sign—Congestion of the pelvic vasculature causes bluish discoloration of the vagina and the cervix. This is a presumptive sign of pregnancy.

B. Hegar's sign—There is widening and softening of the body or isthmus of the uterus. This occurs at 6–8 weeks' menstrual age or gestational age. Estrogen and progesterone cause increased cervical softening and dilation at the external os.

C. Leukorrhea—There is an increase in vaginal discharge, containing epithelial cells and cervical mucous, secondary to hormonal changes.

D. Pelvic ligaments—There is relaxation of the sacroiliac and pubic symphysis during pregnancy. Relaxation is pronounced at the pelvic symphysis.

E. Abdominal enlargement—There is progressive abdominal enlargement with growth of uterus during pregnancy. From 18 to 34 weeks there is a good correlation between the uterine fundal measurement in centimeters and the gestational age in weeks.

F. Uterine contractions—Painless uterine contractions (**Braxton Hick's contractions**) are felt as tightening or pressure. They usually begin at approximately 28 weeks' gestation and increase in regularity with advancing gestational age. These contractions usually disappear with walking or exercise, whereas true labor contractions become more intense.

DIAGNOSIS

A. Fetal Heart Tones

Fetal heart tones (FHTs) are detectable by handheld Doppler (after 10 weeks' gestation) or by fetoscope (after 18–20 weeks' gestation). The normal heart rate is 110–160 beats per minute, with a higher fetal heart rate observed early in pregnancy.

B. Uterine Size/Fetal Palpation

Uterine size can be used to diagnose pregnancy secondary to uterine enlargement. Later in pregnancy, the fetus can be palpated through the maternal abdominal wall (after 22 weeks), and the position can be determined by Leopold's maneuvers.

C. Imaging Studies

Sonography is one of the most useful technical aids in diagnosing and monitoring pregnancy. Cardiac activity is discernible at 5–6 weeks via transvaginal sonogram, limb buds at 7–8 weeks, and finger and limb movements at 9–10 weeks. At the end of the embryonic period (10 weeks by LNMP), the embryo has a human appearance. The gestational age can be determined by the crown rump length between 6 and 13 weeks' gestation, with a margin of error of approximately 8% or 3–5 days.

D. Pregnancy Tests

Sensitive, early pregnancy tests measure changes in the level of human chorionic gonadotropin (hCG). There is a small degree of cross-reactivity between luteinizing hormone, follicle-stimulating hormone, and thyrotropin, which all share an α subunit with hCG. The β submit of hCG is produced by the syncytiotrophoblast 8 days after fertilization and may be detected in the maternal serum 8–11 days after conception or as early as 21–22 days after the LNMP. β-hCG levels peak at 10–12 weeks' gestation and decrease afterward. The half-life of hCG is 1.5 days. Generally, serum and urine levels return to normal (<5 mIU/mL), 21–24 days after delivery or after a fetal loss.

1. Home pregnancy test—hCG is a qualitative test that is performed on the first voided morning urine sample.

A positive test is usually indicated by a color change. Because the accuracy of the home pregnancy test depends on technique and interpretation, it should always be repeated in the office.

2. Urine pregnancy test—An antibody assay recognizing the β-hCG subunit is the initial lab test performed in the office to diagnose pregnancy. The test is reliable, rapid (1–5 minutes), and inexpensive, with a positive test threshold between 5 and 50 mIU/mL, characterized by a color change. This is the most common method to confirm pregnancy.

3. Serum pregnancy test—β-hCG can be detected within 7 days after conception or at a menstrual age of 21 days' gestation. The threshold for a positive test can be as low as 2–4 mIU/mL. Serial quantitative tests of β-hCG are be used to evaluate threatened abortion, ectopic pregnancy, or a molar pregnancy.

GESTATIONAL AGE DETERMINATION

The EDD (estimated date of delivery) and gestational age should be established based on the LNMP and Naegele's rule. Clinical parameters, discussed later, should be used as an adjunct to confirm or establish dating as needed.

Pregnancy Calendar or Calculator

Normally, human pregnancy lasts 280 days or 40 weeks (9 calendar months or 10 lunar months) from the LNMP. This may also be calculated as 266 days or 38 weeks from the last ovulation in a normal 28-day cycle. The easiest method of determining gestational age is with a pregnancy calendar or calculator. The EDD can be determined mathematically using Naegele's rule: subtract 3 months from the month of the LNMP and add 7 to the first day of the LNMP. Example: With an LNMP of July 14, the EDD is April 21.

CLINICAL PARAMETERS

Ultrasound

Ultrasound is used routinely to determine viability, estimate gestational age, screen for aneuploidy, and evaluate fetal anatomy and well-being. From 13 to 20 weeks, the most accurate parameter for gestational age assessment is the biparietal diameter, although this measurement is often used together with the head circumference, abdominal circumference, and femur length, with a margin of error (secondary to measurement) of 8% or approximately 7 days. After 24 weeks' gestation, the accuracy of ultrasound to estimate gestational age is diminished and is best used to assess growth or the estimated fetal weight.

Indications for ultrasound are as follows:

1. Dating.
2. Aneuploidy assessment—Discussed in Screening section (later).
3. Anatomical survey—A comprehensive anatomical survey can be performed as early as 16–18 weeks' gestation.
4. Cervical length assessment.
5. Fetal well-being can be monitored by ultrasound using the biophysical profile.

Uterine Size

An early first-trimester examination usually correlates well with the estimated gestational age. The uterus is palpable just at the pubic symphysis at 8 weeks. At 12 weeks, the uterus becomes an abdominal organ, and at 16 weeks, it is usually at the midpoint between the pubic symphysis and the umbilicus. Between 18 and 34 weeks' gestation, the uterus size or fundal height is measured in centimeters from the pubic symphysis to the upper edge of the uterine corpus, and the measurement correlates well with the gestational age in weeks (Fig. 6–1). The uterus is palpable at 20 weeks at the umbilicus. After 36 weeks, the fundal height may decrease as the fetal head descends into the pelvis.

Quickening

Maternal perception of fetal movement occurs between 18 and 20 weeks in the primiparous patient and at 14–18 weeks in the multigravida. The perceived fetal movement, or quickening, is often described as a butterfly-like movement rather than a kick.

Fetal Heart Tones

FHTs may be heard by a fetoscope at 18–20 weeks and by Doppler ultrasound as early as 10 weeks' gestation.

PREGNANCY FAILURE

Early

A. Diagnosis

The gold standard for diagnosis of early pregnancy failure is ultrasound. Definitive diagnosis requires recognition of a fetus in the absence of cardiac activity.

B. Laboratory Findings

In cases where ultrasound findings are equivocal, serial measurements of serum β-hCG levels with a failure to demonstrate an appropriate increase are helpful.

Late

C. Signs and Symptoms

In late pregnancy, the first sign of fetal demise is usually the absence of fetal movement as noted by the mother.

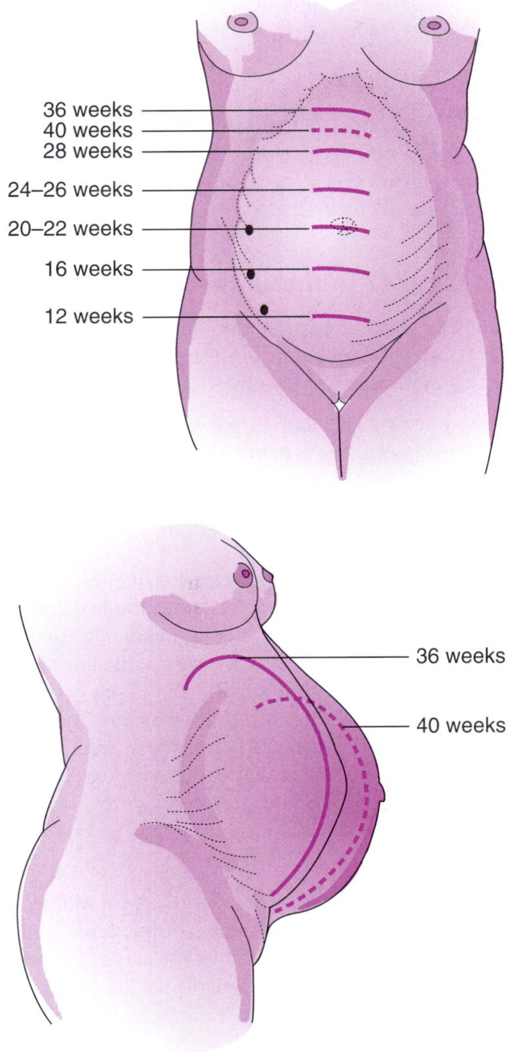

▲ **Figure 6–1.** Height of fundus at various times during pregnancy.

D. Diagnosis

If FHT cannot be appreciated, real-time ultrasonography is virtually 100% accurate in describing the absence of fetal heart motion.

E. Complications

Disseminated intravascular coagulopathy is a rare sequelae occurring after an intrauterine fetal demise (IUFD). Coagulation studies may be started 2 weeks after the demise of one twin, and delivery can be undertaken if serial serum fibrinogen levels fall below 200 mg/dL. In a singleton IUFD, coagulation studies including fibrinogen are done immediately after the diagnosis is made, and delivery is initiated promptly.

American College of Obstetricians and Gynecologists. Ultrasonography in Pregnancy. ACOG Practice Bulletin No. 101. *Obstet Gynecol* 2009;113:451–461. PMID: 19155920.

Owen J, Yost N, Berghella V, et al. Mid-trimester endovaginal sonography in women at high risk for spontaneous preterm birth. *JAMA* 2001;286:1340–1348. PMID: 11560539.

Wilcox AJ, Baird DD, Dunson D, McChesney R, Weinberg CR. Natural limits of pregnancy testing in relation to the expected menstrual period. *JAMA* 2001;286:1759–1761. PMID: 11594902.

PRENATAL CARE

Pregnancy is a normal physiologic process; however, complications that increase the mortality or morbidity to the mother and/or fetus occur in 5–20% of pregnancies. Our present system of prenatal care focuses on prevention.

Prenatal care providers must be familiar with the normal changes of pregnancy and the possible pathologic changes that may occur so that therapeutic measures can be initiated to reduce any risks to the mother or fetus. The purpose of prenatal care is to ensure a successful pregnancy outcome when possible, including the delivery of a live, healthy fetus. It's proven that mothers receiving prenatal care have a lower risk of complications, and one of the principal aims of prenatal care is the identification and special treatment of the high-risk patient—the one whose pregnancy, because of some factor in her medical history or an issue that develops during pregnancy, is likely to have a poor outcome.

Ideally, a woman planning pregnancy should have a medical evaluation before conception; this allows the physician to determine whether any risk factors will complicate a pregnancy in the context of a complete history and physical examination, along with prenatal laboratory studies. During the medical evaluation, the risks of cigarette smoking, alcohol and drug use, and exposure to known teratogens are discussed. Instructions on nutrition, exercise, and vitamins can be provided before pregnancy. For example, folic acid taken 3 months before conception may be beneficial in decreasing the incidence of open neural tube defects and cardiac anomalies.

Most women do not have a preconception evaluation, and the first prenatal visit may be scheduled well into the first and occasionally in the second or third trimester. Factors for delayed medical care should be reviewed with the patient, and any barriers—whether social, financial, or cultural—may be addressed for this and future pregnancies.

INITIAL OFFICE VISIT

The purpose of the first office visit is to identify any risk factors influencing the mother and/or fetus. A plan of care for a high-risk pregnancy may be established at the first prenatal visit, including pertinent consultations of subspecialists.

HISTORY

A. Obstetric History

The interview should include a discussion of current symptoms; this is also an ideal time to discuss any perceptions regarding childbearing (including potential birth plans) and the effect of the pregnancy on the patient's life.

Outcomes of all previous pregnancies provide important information for the current pregnancy; the following information should be obtained: length of gestation, birth weight, length of labor, type of delivery, fetal/neonatal outcome, anesthesia, and any complications occurring in previous pregnancies, including pregnancies ending before 20 weeks' gestation. If a caesarean section was performed, an operative report detailing the type of incision and any intraoperative complications should be obtained.

B. Medical History

Pregnancy may influence a number of maternal organ systems, and preexisting conditions may be exacerbated during pregnancy. Many cardiovascular, gastrointestinal, and endocrine disorders require careful evaluation and consultation regarding effects on the mother. For example, a prior blood transfusion may increase the risk of hemolytic disease of the newborn because of maternal antibodies produced secondary to a minor blood group mismatch. Medical conditions of particular relevance to pregnancy include diabetes and other endocrine diseases, hypertension, epilepsy, and autoimmune diseases.

C. Surgical History

A history of previous gynecologic, abdominal, or uterine surgery may necessitate a caesarean section. In addition, a history of cervical surgery, multiple induced abortions, or recurrent fetal losses may suggest cervical incompetence. Patients with a previous caesarean section may be candidates for vaginal delivery if they are adequately counseled and meet established guidelines.

D. Family History

A family history of diabetes mellitus should alert the clinician about an increased risk of gestational diabetes, especially if the patient has a history of a large infant or a previous birth defect, or an unexplained fetal demise. Glucose testing should be performed at the initial prenatal visit if there is a strong suspicion of undiagnosed pregestational diabetes rather than waiting until 24–28 weeks' gestation.

Awareness of familial disorders is also important in pregnancy management. Thus a brief, 3-generation pedigree is useful. Antenatal screening tests are available for many hereditary diseases. A history of twinning is important, because dizygotic twinning (polyovulation) may be a maternally inherited trait.

E. Social History

The prenatal history should include documentation of tobacco and alcohol use, any contact with intravenous drugs or drug users, or other drug use. Exposures (workplace and otherwise) should be evaluated.

Physical Examination

A complete physical examination should be performed at the first obstetric or prenatal visit; the pelvic examination is of special importance for the obstetrician, nurse, or midwife.

1. Bony pelvis—The configuration should be evaluated to determine whether the patient is at risk for cephalopelvic disproportion, which may lead to an operative delivery. Pelvimetry has been largely replaced, however, by clinical evaluation of the pelvis ("trial of labor").

A. PELVIC INLET—The anteroposterior diameter or diagonal conjugate may be estimated at the time of the initial pelvic examination. For this measurement, the index and middle finger are inserted into the vagina, the middle finger reaches the sacral promontory, and the tissue between the examiners' index and thumb is pushed against the patient's pubic symphysis. The distance between the tip of the examiner's finger and pubic symphysis pressure on the thumb measures the diagonal conjugate; the anterior diameter of the pelvic inlet is estimated by subtracting 1.5 cm from the measured diagonal conjugate (Fig. 6–2).

B. MIDPELVIS—The midpelvic space can be estimated by noting the prominence and closeness of the ischial spines. If the walls of the pelvis converge, and if the curve of the sacrum is straight/shallow, or if the sacrosciatic notches are narrowed, the midpelvis may be inadequate for a vaginal delivery.

C. PELVIC OUTLET—In contrast to the midpelvis, the pelvic outlet can be estimated by a physical examination. The shape of the outlet can be determined by palpation of the pubic rami from the symphysis to the ischial tuberosities with an estimation of the angle of the rami. A subpubic angle of less than 90 degrees suggests an inadequate pelvic outlet. A prominent coccyx decreases the anterior posterior diameter of the outlet and may further diminish the pelvic outlet.

2. Uterus—The uterus can be used to confirm gestational age in the first half of pregnancy. As the uterus enlarges, it becomes globular and often rotates to the right.

3. Cervical length—A nulliparous woman who has not undergone a vaginal delivery will have a closed external cervical os. A multiparous patient may have a greater opening or dilation of the external os. The average cervical length by bimanual examination in women averages between 3 and 4 cm. Women with a previous history of spontaneous preterm

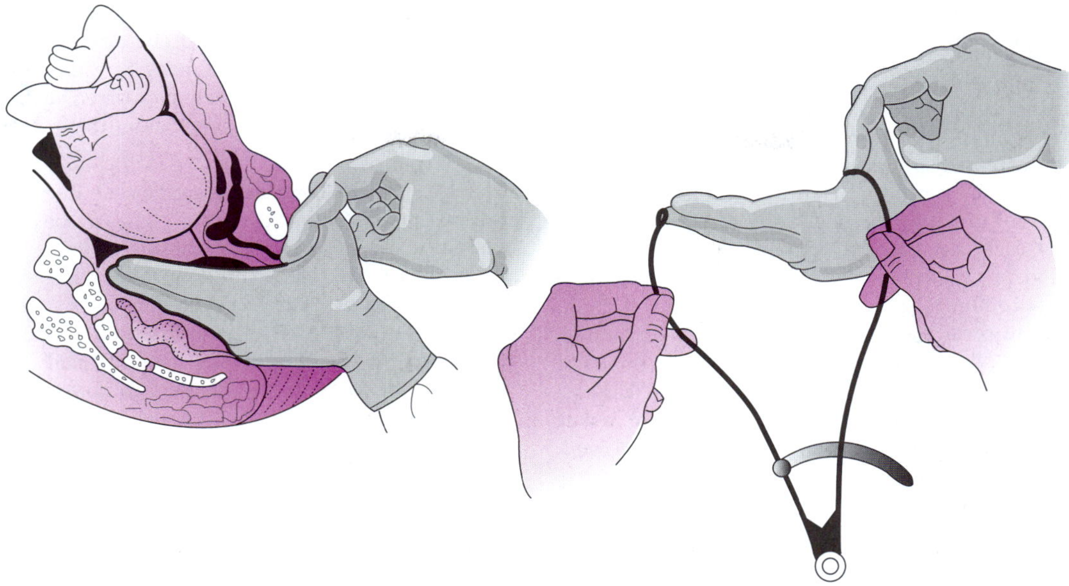

▲ **Figure 6–2.** Measurement of the diagonal conjugate (conjugata diagonalis). (Reproduced, with permission, from Benson RC. *Handbook of Obstetrics & Gynecology*. 8th ed. Los Altos, CA: Lange; 1983.)

birth may undergo a transvaginal sonogram (TVS) during the second trimester to evaluate her risk of recurrent preterm birth. Serial TVS exams may be necessary if there is any evidence of cervical dilation or cervical shortening on the initial sonogram.

4. Adnexal exam—During the pelvic exam, a bimanual examination is performed, and the cervical length and evaluation of both ovaries (the adnexa) can be performed.

Laboratory Tests

A. Initial Blood Tests

At the first prenatal visit, a number of screening tests are performed, including a complete blood count (hemoglobin, hematocrit, and platelets), blood group and Rh typing (ABO/Rh), screen for antibodies against blood group antigens, VDRL (Venereal Disease Research Laboratory) or RPR (rapid plasma reagent) for syphilis, hepatitis B surface antigen, and serology to detect antibodies against rubella and HIV. Women with a history of gestational diabetes are given a glucose challenge test (GCT) with oral ingestion of a solution containing 50 g of glucose. The venous glucose level is checked 1 hour after glucose ingestion.

B. Genetic Screening and Testing

1. Screening—First-trimester screening using a combination of a fetal nuchal translucency measurement and maternal serum analysis of pregnancy-associated plasma protein A (PAPP-A) and free or total β-hCG is used to screen for trisomy (21, 18, and 13). The detection rate of aneuploidy is between 85% and 87%, with a false-positive rate of less than 5%. With the use of first-trimester screening, maternal serum α fetoprotein (AFP) should be drawn at 15–18 weeks' gestation to screen for open neural tube defects.

For patients desiring aneuploidy assessment who did not receive first-trimester screening, a second trimester maternal serum quad screen is offered between 15 and 20 weeks' gestation (ideally at 16–18 weeks) to screen for neural tube defects and aneuploidy (chromosomal abnormalities). Analytes studied include serum β-hCG, unconjugated estriol, AFP, and inhibin. The detection rate of a quad screen is between 65% and 75% for trisomy 21, 18, and 13 and between 80% and 85% for open neural tube defects. The false-positive rate is approximately 5%.

Additional genetic testing includes hemoglobin electrophoresis to screen for hemoglobinopathies (including sickle cell disease risk) and cystic fibrosis screening, which has been added to prenatal screening at many institutions.

2. Invasive genetic testing—Invasive genetic testing must be offered to all women, especially those who will be 35 years of age or older at the time of delivery or who have a history of an abnormal pedigree or risk factors for inherited diseases. Chorionic villous sampling is performed between 9 and 13 weeks' gestation by either transabdominal or transvaginal technique. Amniocentesis is usually offered at between 15 and 20 weeks' gestation. The complication rate of these procedures is less than 1%, and the detection rate for aneuploidy is greater than 99%.

C. Urine Testing

At the initial prenatal visit, urinalysis and culture is performed. Approximately 2–12% of pregnant women have an asymptomatic urinary tract infection. If the bacterial count is greater than 10^5/mL, expressed as colony-forming units (CFU) on a voided specimen, then antibiotic sensitivity is performed.

Testing for urinary protein, glucose, and ketones is performed at each prenatal visit. Proteinuria of greater than or equal to 2+ on a standard dipstick (which correlates to greater than 300 mg/24 hours on a timed urine collection) may indicate renal disease or the onset of preeclampsia. The presence of glucosuria signifies that glucose transport to the kidney exceeds the transport capacity of the kidneys. This generally does not have clinical significance unless carbohydrate intolerance or gestational diabetes is present. During pregnancy in a known diabetic patient, the presence of urinary ketones usually indicates inadequate carbohydrate intake. In this case, the patient's diet should be reevaluated to ensure adequate carbohydrate intake.

D. Papanicolaou Smear (PAP)

Cervical cancer screening is performed at the initial prenatal visit unless there has been a normal exam within the past year.

E. Tuberculin Skin Test

A tuberculin skin test (**purified protein derivative**) is appropriate for high-risk patients.

E. Sexually Transmitted Diseases

1. Syphilis—Tests performed at the initial prenatal visit such as VDRL and the RPR screen in a sensitive, nonspecific manner for *Treponema pallidum*. A treponemal antibody test (FTA-ABS) is used to confirm syphilis infection after a positive VDRL or RPR screen in the absence of confirmed prior infection. Penicillin is the treatment of choice in pregnancy because of the ability of the agent to cross the placenta and treat the fetus as well as the mother. Erythromycin or ceftriaxone are alternative treatments outside of pregnancy, but penicillin is the treatment of choice for pregnant women. Because of the risk of treatment failure with secondary agents and congenital syphilis infection, penicillin desensitization is indicated in the setting of anaphylactic allergy. Monthly serologic tests (VDRL or RPR) are followed to assess treatment success of syphilis. These tests can remain positive after treatment; however, their titer should decrease substantially. The FTA-ABS will remain positive even after successful treatment.

2. Chlamydia—Screening consists of a DNA probe, which has a 90% specificity and sensitivity. An endocervical sample or urine sample can be used for diagnosis of chlamydia (CT). The agent of choice is azithromycin (1 g oral dose). Amoxicillin (500 mg oral dose three times a day for 7 days) is an alternative treatment. A test of cure is performed 2–3 weeks after completion of treatment. Screening for gonorrhea (GC) and CT are routinely performed at the time of PAP smear. In a high-risk population, these cultures are repeated at the third trimester (35–37 weeks' EGA).

3. Gonorrhea—GC can be detected by culture of the organism in Thayer-Morton agar or by a DNA probe as part of a combined GC/CT. GC may be transmitted to the infant and cause ophthalmic injury. Infection may be associated with preterm labor, preterm premature rupture of membranes, and intrapartum as well as postpartum infection. The drug of choice is ceftriaxone (125 mg intramuscularly [IM] one-time dose or 1 g intravenously every 24 hours for disseminated disease) secondary to prevalent penicillin-resistant strains. Patients with an allergy to penicillin are treated with a 2-g IM dose of spectinomycin.

4. Herpes simplex virus—Tissue culture or DNA polymerase chain reaction are used to detect active herpetic infections; serology can be used to assess a history of exposure. Oral acyclovir is used for primary and recurrent outbreaks. Prophylactic treatment at 36 weeks' gestation for women with documented genital herpes and recurrent outbreaks is recommended to reduce the chance of the patient having an active outbreak when she presents in labor. Regimens commonly used are acyclovir 400 mg twice daily or valacyclovir 1000 mg daily. When a patient is admitted for delivery, she should be asked about prodromal symptoms and examined for lesions of the cervix, vagina, and perineum. If no lesions or symptoms are present, vaginal delivery is permitted.

5. HIV—All obstetric patients should undergo HIV screening on an "opt out" basis at the first prenatal visit. The initial HIV screening test is an enzyme-linked immunosorbent assay (ELISA) followed by a confirmatory Western blot or immunofluorescence assay for patients with ELISA-positive tests.

If a woman has not had prenatal HIV testing (or care), a rapid HIV test is offered at the time of hospital admission. The goal of prenatal care and treatment of the HIV-positive pregnant patient is to appropriately treat the mother, reduce viral load, and minimize perinatal HIV transmission by providing antiretroviral prophylaxis intrapartum and to the infant. Treatment regimens should include prenatal highly active anti-retroviral therapy and intrapartum infusion of azidothymidine. Ongoing assessment of an HIV-infected pregnant woman involves serial measurements of the viral load and CD4 T-cell count. Cesarean delivery is recommended only for patients with high viral load (>1000 copies/mL); otherwise, mode of delivery is dictated by obstetric indications.

6. Other infections

A. Trichomonas—*Trichomonas vaginalis* can be identified in 20–30% of pregnant patients, but only 5–10%

of patients are symptomatic (itching, burning, or discharge). *T vaginalis* is a flagellated ovoid organism seen under magnification in warm normal saline solution. The discharge is described as foamy green and malodorous. Metronidazole has an efficacy of approximately 95% against *T vaginalis*. Metronidazole may be given as a single oral dose of 2 g, 500 mg twice daily for 7 days, or 250 mg 3 times daily for 7 days.

B. CANDIDIASIS—*Candida albicans* can be cultured from the vagina of many immunocompromised women (HIV, insulin-dependent diabetes mellitus, or pregnant). Symptoms of vaginal candidiasis include vaginal burning, itching, and a thick, white, curd-like discharge. Marked inflammation of the vagina and perineum may be noted, but fewer than 50% of women have symptoms.

The confirmatory test for candida is microscopic detection of hyphae or yeast buds on a KOH preparation. For uncomplicated candida yeast infections, topical therapy may be given for 3–7 days with agents such as miconazole, terconazole, clotrimazole, and butoconazole. In refractory cases, administration of systemic agents may be considered. Fluconazole (150-mg single oral dose) is the preferred agent in pregnancy.

C. BACTERIAL VAGINOSIS—Bacterial vaginosis (BV) is responsible for a large percentage of vaginitis during pregnancy. BV is a polymicrobial infection that is associated with many complications of pregnancy, including preterm labor, preterm premature rupture of membranes, chorioamnionitis, and endometritis.

SUBSEQUENT VISITS

The frequency of office visits is dependent on the gestational age, maternal condition, and any fetal complications. The standard schedule for prenatal office visits in uncomplicated patients is every 4 weeks from 0 to 32 weeks' gestation, every 2 weeks from 32 to 36 weeks' gestation, and weekly visits after 36 weeks' gestation.

At each visit, maternal weight, uterine fundal height, maternal blood pressure, and urinalysis by dipstick are documented. The FHTs should be documented. All findings should be recorded and compared with those from previous visits.

Maternal Weight Gain

The prepregnancy weight and the amount of weight gain during pregnancy are important. Maternal weight gain during pregnancy is due to a number of factors. The fetus (on average, 3500 g at term), the placenta (650 g) amniotic fluid (800 mg), breast enlargement (400 g) and uterus (970 g) are factors, as well as increased interstitial fluid and blood volume, which results in an additional 1200–1800 g of weight gain.

A woman who is 15% or more below ideal body weight or of short stature has a risk for a small for gestational age (SGA) infant and preterm delivery. A pregnant adolescent may have maternal compromise, as well as fetal jeopardy, if her diet is inadequate to meet her own growth requirements as well as that of the fetus. Inadequate maternal weight gain may reflect poor nutrition, inadequate nutrition absorption, or maternal illness, predisposing the mother to an inadequate volume expansion and the fetus to growth restriction. The American College of Obstetrics and Gynecology recommend a weight gain of 11.5–16 kg (25–35 lb) during a singleton pregnancy. Underweight women should gain more weight (12.5–18 kg or 28–40 lb), whereas obese women should gain less than 7–11.5 kg or 15–25 lbs.

Obese women (>30 body mass index [BMI]) and those with excessive maternal weight gain during pregnancy are more likely to have a macrosomic infant when compared with women with a normal BMI and appropriate weight gain during pregnancy.

Blood Pressure

The blood pressure tends to decrease 5–7 mm (both systolic and diastolic components) early in the second trimester, but the blood pressure measurement returns to normal levels in the third trimester. Blood pressure changes may provide a subtle sign of vascular compromise. Elevation of blood pressure may precede an increase in proteinuria seen with hypertension in pregnancy. Blood pressure is most accurately measured in a sitting position (with the arm at the level of the heart).

Fundal Height

There is a connection between the uterine size or fundal height (in centimeters) and the gestational age (in weeks) between 18 and 34 weeks. Measurement is made from the pubic symphysis to the top of the uterus (McDonald's technique). Fundal height is measured at each visit after 20 weeks' gestation. If the fundal height is discordant from the estimated gestational age by more than 2 (centimeters or weeks), further evaluation of fetal size and amniotic fluid via ultrasound is warranted.

Fetal Heart Tones

FHTs can be auscultated by 10–12 weeks' gestation using a handheld Doppler device; while in use, attention should be paid to the rate, rhythm, and presence of any irregularity of heart rate, as well as accelerations or decelerations. Abnormalities in rate or rhythm should be evaluated by ultrasound, electronic fetal heart rate monitoring, or even a fetal echocardiogram.

Edema

At each prenatal visit, findings should be noted, including transient episodes of general edema or swelling.

Lower extremity edema in late pregnancy is a natural consequence of hydrostatic changes in lower body circulation. Edema of the upper body (eg, face and hands), especially in association with relative or absolute increases in blood pressure, may be the first sign of preeclampsia, although edema is not part of the current diagnostic criteria. A moderate rise in blood pressure without excessive fluid retention may suggest a predisposition to chronic hypertension.

Fetal Size & Position

Manual assessment of fetal size and position is always indicated after approximately 26 weeks' gestation. The fetus may assume a number of positions before late gestation, but persistence of an abnormal lie into late pregnancy suggests abnormal placentation, uterine anomalies, or other problems that should be investigated by ultrasound. If an abnormal lie persists, consider external version after 37 weeks' gestation.

Laboratory Evaluations

A. Third-Trimester Laboratory Studies

1. Gestational diabetes screening—A 1-hour GCT, with a 50-g glucose load, is given between 24 and 28 weeks' gestation. If the 1-hour glucose test is abnormal, a 3-hour glucose tolerance test is performed. A 100-g glucose load is ingested after obtaining a fasting glucose level. Venous glucose levels are then measured at 1, 2, and 3 hours after the glucose load.

2. Complete blood count—This is normally repeated at the beginning of the third trimester to evaluate for anemia.

3. Group B streptococcus—The current recommendation is to perform routine screening for group B streptococcus (GBS) between 35 and 37 weeks' gestation. If the patient has a positive GBS culture at 35–37 weeks, or a positive urine culture for GBS anytime during the pregnancy, the patient is treated with penicillin (the drug of choice in the absence of allergy) at the time of admission in labor, decreasing the risk of early-onset group B streptococcal sepsis in the newborn.

COMMON COMPLAINTS

Ptyalism

Excessive salivation may be a complaint in a small percentage of pregnant women. The cause is unknown but may be associated with nausea and vomiting.

Pica

Pica is the ingestion of substances with no nutritive value; some common examples are ingestion of clay or laundry starch. Pica is harmful, as nutrition may be inadequate with the ingestion of nonnutritious bulk.

Urinary Frequency & Renal Function

Urinary frequency is a common complaint throughout pregnancy. Late in pregnancy, the enlarging uterus and fetus decrease bladder capacity, leading to frequency. The glomerular filtration rate increases 50% during pregnancy, and the serum creatinine decreases to a level of 0.4–0.6 mg/dL. Both the altered bladder and kidney function result from hormonal changes associated with pregnancy. Dysuria or hematuria may be a sign of infection. Approximately 2–12% of pregnant women have a urinary tract infection without symptoms. Diagnosis of a urinary tract infection will require a urinalysis as well as a urine culture with bacterial sensitivity.

Varicose Veins

Pressure by the enlarging uterus, which reduces venous return, as well as the relaxation of vascular smooth muscle by progesterone may result in enlargement of the peripheral veins in the lower extremities and development of varicosities. Specific therapy includes elevation of the lower extremities and the use of thigh-high compression stockings. These measures may reduce the degree of lower extremity edema and varicosity. Superficial varicosity is not evidence of deep venous thrombosis.

Joint & Back Pain

During pregnancy, relaxation may result in a small degree of separation or mobility at the pubic symphysis and sacroiliac articulations. The pregnant patient may experience an unstable pelvis, which results in pain. A pelvic girdle or maternity sling with bed rest may partially relieve the pelvic pain. The increasingly protuberant maternal abdomen results in lordosis. The patient may compensate the lordosis with backward thrust of the shoulders and forward thrust of the head. The corrective position may result in an exaggerated curvature of the maternal spine. A maternity girdle and low-heeled support shoes may reduce the back pain. Exercise and physical therapy may be helpful.

Leg Cramps/Numbness

Leg cramps are a common complaint with an unknown etiology. Theories for leg cramps include a reduced level of serum calcium or magnesium. Treatments include nutritional supplementation of calcium carbonate or calcium lactate. Magnesium citrate (300 mg per day) has also been used for leg cramps. Other therapies include local heat, massage, or flexion of the feet.

Breast Soreness

Physiologic breast engorgement may cause discomfort, especially during early and late pregnancy. A well-fitting brassiere worn 24 hours a day affords relief. Ice bags are temporarily effective. Hormone therapy is of no value.

Discomfort in the Hands

Acrodysesthesia of the hands consists of periodic numbness and tingling of the fingers (the feet are never involved). It affects at least 5% of pregnant women. In some cases it is thought to be a brachial plexus traction syndrome caused by drooping of the shoulders during pregnancy; carpal tunnel syndrome is a common cause of a similar symptom complex. The discomfort is most common at night and early in the morning. It may progress to partial anesthesia and impairment of manual proprioception. The condition is apparently not serious, but it may persist after delivery as a consequence of lifting and carrying the baby.

OTHER ISSUES RELATED TO PRENATAL CARE

Bathing

Bath water generally does not enter the vagina. Swimming and bathing are not contraindicated during pregnancy. However, in the third trimester, a patient may have impaired balance and is at risk for a fall.

Dental Care

There may be gum hypertrophy and gingival bleeding during pregnancy. Interdental papillae (epulis) may form in the upper gingiva and may have to be surgically removed. Normal dental procedures such as prophylaxis (cleaning), cavity restoration (filling), and periodontal restoration may be performed under local anesthesia. Antibiotics may be given for dental abscesses. Periodontal disease has been associated with an increased risk of preterm delivery in some studies.

Douching

Douching, which is seldom necessary, may be harmful during pregnancy and should be avoided.

Drugs, Nicotine, & Alcohol

1. Drugs—A **teratogen** is a toxin, drug, or a biologic agent that causes a harmful effect on a fetus. The US Food and Drug Administration has a classification system for drugs during pregnancy and lactation. The greatest effect of a drug is normally during the period of organogenesis (weeks 2–10 after LNMP). Drugs with the potential for addiction such as heroin, methadone, and benzodiazepines can cause major problems for the neonate, including withdrawal.

2. Nicotine & cigarette smoking—There is an increased risk of low-birth-weight infants with cigarette smoking by pregnant women. Smoking during pregnancy is associated with an increased risk of intrauterine growth restriction, placenta previa, placenta abruption, preterm birth, low birth weight, and perinatal mortality. Pregnant women should be urged not to smoke; but, if cessation is not possible, a reduction of the number of cigarettes smoked per day is encouraged. Pharmacologic agents may be offered to assist with smoking cessation.

3. Alcohol—The precise level of alcohol consumption that is safe during pregnancy cannot be determined. A fetal alcohol syndrome (FAS) after maternal ingestion (>2 oz daily) has been described, with an incidence from 1 in 600 to 1 in 1500 live births. The major features of FAS include pre- and postnatal growth restriction, cranial–facial dysmorphology (including microcephalus and microphthalmia), mental retardation, cardiac defects, and behavioral abnormalities. Infants whose mothers consume alcohol during pregnancy can have FAS or fetal alcohol effects (FAEs) or be normal. Pregnant women should be encouraged to avoid alcohol during pregnancy.

Exercise

Pregnant women should incorporate 30 minutes or more of moderate-intensity physical activity. Activities with risk of maternal injury, especially abdominal trauma, should be avoided. Aerobic and exercise classes have been designed for pregnant women. Pregnancy yoga classes are also available for women. Routines in yoga classes are designed for flexibility and joint protection.

Immunization

Killed virus, toxoid, or recombinant vaccines may be given during pregnancy. The American College of Obstetrics and Gynecology recommends that all pregnant women should receive the injectable influenza vaccine during the season (October–March). The "flu shot" is safe when given in any trimester. Furthermore, if administered during pregnancy, the vaccine appears to reduce the risk of infant respiratory disease within the first 6 months of life. Diphtheria and tetanus toxoid, hepatitis B vaccine series, and killed polio vaccine may be administered during pregnancy to women at risk.

Live attenuated vaccines (varicella, measles, mumps, polio, and rubella) should be given 3 months before pregnancy or postpartum. Live virus vaccines are contraindicated in pregnancy secondary to the potential risk of fetal infection. Viral shedding occurs in children receiving vaccination, but they do not transmit the virus; consequently, vaccination may be safely given to the children of pregnant women.

Secondary prophylaxis with immune globulin is recommended for pregnant women exposed to measles, hepatitis A, hepatitis B, tetanus, chicken pox, or rabies.

Intercourse

No adverse outcome can be directly attributed to sexual intercourse during pregnancy. If cramping, spotting, or bright red bleeding follows coitus, sexual activity should not occur until the patient is evaluated by her clinician. A patient with preterm labor or vaginal bleeding should not have coitus until evaluated by her clinician.

Nutritional Requirements

The mother's nutrition from the moment of conception is an important factor in the development of the infant's metabolic pathways and future well-being. The pregnant woman should be encouraged to eat a balanced diet and should be made aware of special needs for iron, folic acid, calcium, and zinc. The average woman weighing 58 kg (127 lb) has a normal dietary intake of 2300 kcal/d. An additional 300 kcal/d is needed during pregnancy, and an additional 500 kcal/d is needed during breastfeeding (Table 6–1). Consumption of fewer calories could result in inadequate intake of essential nutrients.

Table 6-1. Recommended daily dietary intake for nonpregnant, pregnant, and lactating women.

		Nonpregnant			Pregnant			Lactation		
	Units	14–18	19–30	31–50	14–18	19–30	31–50	14–18	19–30	31–50
Energy(kcal)	kcal/d	2000–2200	2000–2200	2000–2200	2300–2500	2300–2500	2300–2500	2500–2700	2500–2700	2500–2700
Protein	g/d	46	46	46	71	71	71	71	71	71
Carbohydrate	g/d	130	130	130	175	175	175	210	210	210
Water	L/d	2.7	2.7	2.7	3	3	3	3.8	3.8	3.8
Fiber	g/d	26	25	25	28	28	28	29	29	29
Vitamins										
A	μg/d	700	700	700	750	770	770	1300	1300	1300
B_6	mg/d	1.2	1.3	1.3	1.9	1.9	1.9	2	2	2
B_{12}	μg/d	2.4	2.4	2.4	2.6	2.6	2.6	2.8	2.8	2.8
C	mg/d	65	75	75	80	85	85	115	120	120
D	μg/d	5	5	5	5	5	5	5	5	5
E	mg/d	15	15	15	15	15	15	19	19	19
K	μg/d	75	90	90	75	90	90	75	90	90
Thiamin	mg/d	1	1.1	1.1	1.4	1.4	1.4	1.4	1.4	1.4
Riboflavin	mg/d	1	1.1	1.1	1.4	1.4	1.4	1.6	1.6	1.6
Niacin	mg/d	14	14	14	18	18	18	17	17	17
Folate	μg/d	400	400	400	500	500	500	600	600	600
Pantothenic acid	mg/d	5	5	5	6	6	6	7	7	7
Biotin	μg/d	25	30	30	30	30	30	35	35	35
Choline	mg/d	400	425	425	450	450	450	550	550	550
Elements										
Calcium	mg/d	1300	1000	1000	1300	1000	1000	1300	1000	1000
Iodine	μg/d	150	150	150	220	220	220	290	290	290
Iron	mg/d	15	18	18	27	27	27	10	9	9
Magnesium	mg/d	360	310	320	400	350	360	360	310	320
Phosphorus	mg/d	1250	700	700	1250	700	700	1250	700	700
Zinc	mg/d	9	8	8	12	11	11	13	12	12
Potassium	g/d	4.7	4.7	4.7	4.7	4.7	4.7	5.1	5.1	5.1

A. Protein

Protein needs in pregnancy are 1 g per kilogram per day plus 20 g per day in the second half of pregnancy (60–80 g per day for the average woman). Protein intake is crucial for embryonic development, and consumption of lean animal foods (chicken or fish), low-fat dairy products, and vegetable proteins such as legumes should be encouraged.

B. Calcium

Calcium intake should be 1200 mg per day during pregnancy and lactation. Calcium intake is of special concern for the pregnant adolescent and lactating woman. Low calcium intake is defined as less than 600 mg per day; should calcium intake be deficient during pregnancy, demineralization of the maternal skeleton may occur.

C. Iron

Every pregnant woman should have adequate iron intake for the increased red blood cell production that starts at approximately 6 weeks' gestation. In addition, women should have supplementation of 30 g per day of elemental iron during the second and third trimester. If iron deficiency anemia is diagnosed, the elemental iron dose may be increased to 60–120 mg per day.

D. Vitamins/Minerals

A well-balanced diet is critical to the nutrition of any pregnant woman. Folic acid has been shown to reduce the risk of neural tube defects (NTDs). A daily dose of 4 mg of folic acid is recommended for patients who have had a previous pregnancy affected by an NTD. Folic acid should be initiated a minimum of 1 month before conception and continued for the first 3 months after pregnancy. The recurrence risk of NTD is reduced by 70% with prenatal use of folic acid.

For all other women, a daily intake of at least 0.4 mg of folic acid before conception and through the first 3 months of pregnancy is recommended. Patients with insulin-dependent diabetes mellitus and those with seizure disorders treated with valproic acid and carbamazepine are at increased risk of an NTD (1%) and should receive at least 1 mg per day of folic acid. Vitamin B_{12} supplements are also desirable for strict vegetarian patients as well as those with megaloblastic anemia.

Travel

Travel (by automobile, train, or plane) does not adversely affect a pregnancy, but separation from the physician may be of concern.

Preparation for Labor

As term approaches, the patient must be instructed on the physiologic changes associated with labor. She is usually admitted to the hospital when contractions occur at 5- to 10-minute intervals. She should be told to seek medical advice for any of the following danger signals: (1) rupture of membranes, (2) vaginal bleeding, (3) decreased fetal movement, (4) evidence of preeclampsia (eg, marked swelling of the hands and face, blurring of vision, headache, epigastric pain, convulsions), (5) chills or fever, (6) severe or unusual abdominal or back pain, or (7) any other severe medical problems.

Abrams B, Altman SL, Pickett KE. Pregnancy weight gain: still controversial. *Am J Clin Nutr* 2000;71(Suppl):1233S. PMID: 1079939.

American College of Obstetricians and Gynecologists. ACOG Committee Opinion No. 267: Exercise during pregnancy and the postpartum period. *Obstet Gynecol* 2002;99:171–173. PMID: 11777528.

American College of Obstetricians and Gynecologists. ACOG Committee Opinion No. 438: Immunization during pregnancy. *Obstet Gynecol* 2009;114:398–400. PMID: 19623004.

American College of Obstetricians and Gynecologists. ACOG Committee Opinion No. 443: Air travel during pregnancy. *Obstet Gynecol* 2009;114:954–955. PMID: 19888065.

American College of Obstetricians and Gynecologists. ACOG Committee Opinion No. 468: Influenza vaccination during pregnancy. *Obstet Gynecol* 2010;116:1006–1007. PMID: 20859176.

American College of Obstetricians and Gynecologists. ACOG Committee Opinion No. 471: Smoking cessation during pregnancy. *Obstet Gynecol* 2010;116:1241–1244. PMID: 20966731.

American College of Obstetricians and Gynecologists. Screening for fetal chromosomal abnormalities. ACOG Practice Bulletin No. 77. *Obstet Gynecol* 2007;109:217–227. PMID: 17197615.

American College of Obstetricians and Gynecologists. Hemoglobinopathies in pregnancy. ACOG Practice Bulletin No. 78. *Obstet Gynecol* 2007;109:229–237. PMID: 17197616.

American College of Obstetricians and Gynecologists. Management of herpes in pregnancy. ACOG Practice Bulletin No. 82. *Obstet Gynecol* 2007;109:1489–1498. PMID: 17569194.

Koren G, Nulman I, Chudley AE, Loocke C. Fetal alcohol spectrum disorder. *CMAJ* 2003;169:1181–1185. PMID: 14638655.

AIDSinfo. Recommendations for Use of Antiretroviral Drugs in Pregnant HIV-1-Infected Women for Maternal Health and Interventions to Reduce Perinatal HIV Transmission in the United States: May 24, 2010. http://www.aidsinfo.nih.gov/Guidelines/GuidelineDetail.aspx?GuidelineID=9. Accessed January 11, 2011.

US Department of Agriculture Food and Nutrition Information Center. Dietary Reference Intakes. http://fnic.nal.usda.gov/nal_display/index.php?info_center=4&tax_level=3&tax_subject=256&topic_id=1342&level3_id=5140. Accessed January 19, 2011.

Verani JR, McGee L, Schrag SJ; Centers for Disease Control and Prevention (CDC). Prevention of perinatal group B streptococcal disease: revised guidelines from CDC, 2010. *MMWR Recomm Rep* 2010;59(RR-10):1–36. PMID: 21088663.

7 Normal & Abnormal Labor & Delivery

Carol L. Archie, MD
Ashley S. Roman, MD, MPH

LABOR AND DELIVERY

ESSENTIALS OF DIAGNOSIS

- Labor is a sequence of uterine contractions that results in effacement and dilatation of the cervix and voluntary bearing-down efforts, leading to the expulsion per vagina of the products of conception.
- Delivery is the mode of expulsion of the fetus and placenta.

Pathogenesis

Labor and delivery is a normal physiologic process that most women experience without complications. The goal of the management of this process is to foster a safe birth for mothers and their newborns. Additionally, the staff should attempt to make the patient and her support person(s) feel welcome, comfortable, and informed throughout the labor and delivery process. Physical contact between the newborn and the parents in the delivery room should be encouraged. Every effort should be made to foster family interaction and to support the desire of the family to be together. The role of the obstetrician/midwife and the labor and delivery staff is to anticipate and manage complications that may occur that could harm the mother or the fetus. When a decision is made to intervene, it must be considered carefully, because each intervention carries both potential benefits and potential risks. The best management in the majority of cases may be close observation and, when necessary, cautious intervention.

Physiologic Preparation for Labor

Before the onset of true labor, several preparatory physiologic changes commonly occur. The settling of the fetal head into the brim of the pelvis, known as **lightening**, usually occurs 2 or more weeks before labor in first pregnancies. In women who have had a previous delivery, lightening often does not occur until early labor. Clinically, the mother may notice a flattening of the upper abdomen and increased pressure in the pelvis. This descent of the fetus is often accompanied by a decrease in discomfort associated with crowding of the abdominal organs under the diaphragm (eg, heartburn, shortness of breath) and an increase in pelvic discomfort and frequency of urination.

During the last 4–8 weeks of pregnancy, irregular, generally painless uterine contractions occur with slowly increasing frequency. These contractions, known as **Braxton Hicks contractions**, may occur more frequently, sometimes every 10–20 minutes, and with greater intensity during the last weeks of pregnancy. When these contractions occur early in the third trimester, they must be distinguished from true preterm labor. Later, they are a common cause of "false labor," which is distinguished by the lack of cervical change in response to the contractions.

During the course of several days to several weeks before the onset of true labor, the cervix begins to soften, efface, and dilate. In many cases, when labor starts, the cervix is already dilated 1–3 cm in diameter. This is usually more pronounced in the multiparous patient, the cervix being relatively more firm and closed in nulliparous women. With cervical effacement, the mucus plug within the cervical canal may be released. When this occurs, the onset of labor is sometimes marked by the passage of a small amount of blood-tinged mucus from the vagina known as **bloody show**.

Mechanism of Labor

The mechanism of labor in the vertex position consists of engagement of the presenting part, flexion, descent, internal rotation, extension, external rotation, and expulsion (Table 7–1). The progress of labor is dictated by the pelvic dimensions and configuration, the size of the fetus, and the strength of the contractions. In essence, delivery proceeds along the line of least resistance, that is, by adaptation of the smallest achievable diameters of the presenting part to the most favorable dimensions and contours of the birth canal.

Table 7–1. Mechanisms of labor: vertex presentation.

Engagement	Flexion	Descent	Internal Rotation	Extension	External Rotation (Restitution)
Generally occurs in late pregnancy or at onset of labor. Mode of entry into superior strait depends on pelvic configuration.	Good flexion is noted in most cases. Flexion aids engagement and descent. (Extension occurs in brow and face presentations.)	Depends on pelvic architecture and cephalopelvic relationships. Descent is usually slowly progressive.	Takes place during descent. After engagement, vertex usually rotates to the transverse. It must next rotate to the anterior or posterior to pass the ischial spines, whereupon, when the vertex reaches the perineum, rotation from a posterior to an anterior position generally follows.	Follows distention of the perineum by the vertex. Head concomitantly stems beneath the symphysis. Extension is complete with delivery of the head.	After delivery, head normally rotates to the position it originally occupied at engagement. Next, the shoulders descend (in a path similar to that traced by the head). They rotate anteroposteriorly for delivery. Then the head swings back to its position at birth. The body of the baby is then delivered.

The sequence of events in vertex presentation is as follows:

A. Engagement

This usually occurs late in pregnancy in the primigravida, commonly in the last 2 weeks. In the multiparous patient, engagement usually occurs with the onset of labor. The head enters the superior strait in the occiput transverse position in 70% of women with a gynecoid pelvis (Figs. 7–1 and 7–2).

B. Flexion

In most cases, flexion is essential for both engagement and descent. This will vary, of course, if the head is small in relation to the pelvis or if the pelvis is unusually large.

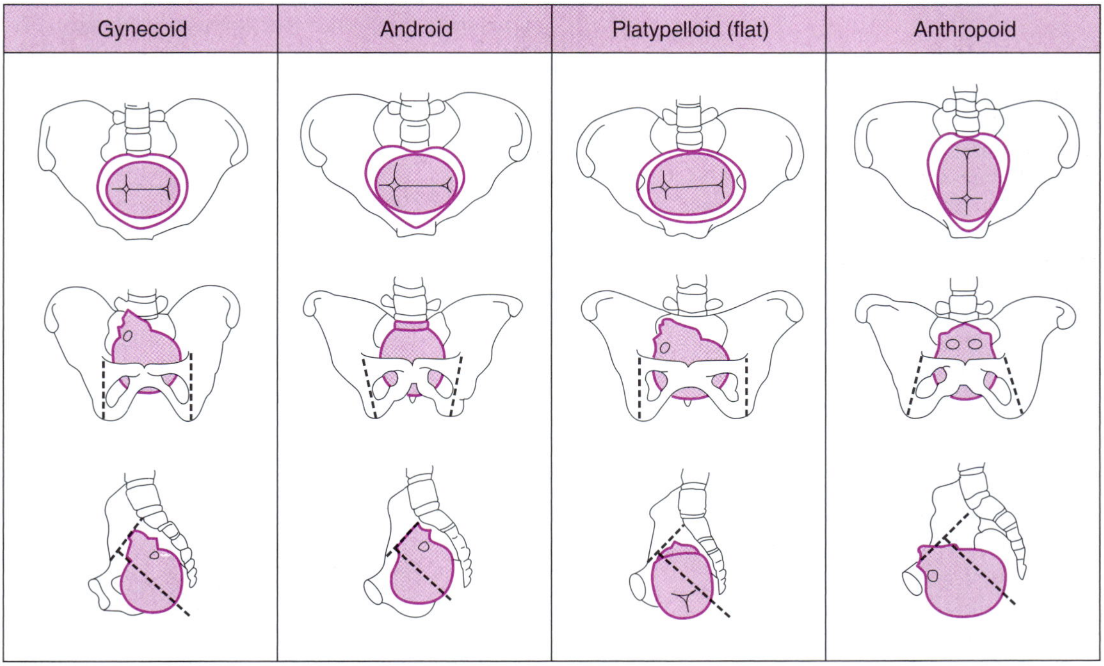

▲ **Figure 7–1.** Flexions of the fetal head in the 4 major pelvic types. (Reproduced, with permission, from Danforth DN, Ellis AH. Midforceps delivery: A vanishing art? *Am J Obstet Gynecol* 1963;86:29–37.)

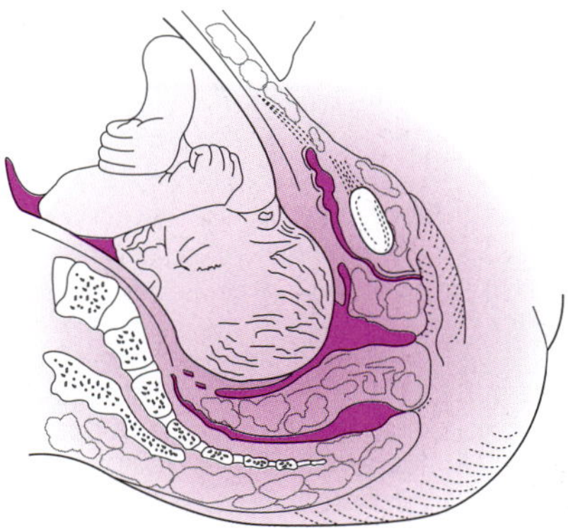

▲ **Figure 7–2.** Left occipitoanterior engagement.

When the head is improperly fixed—or if there is significant narrowing of the pelvic strait (as in the platypelloid type of pelvis)—there may be some degree of deflexion, if not actual extension. Such is the case with a brow (deflexion) or face (extension) presentation.

C. Descent

Descent is gradually progressive and is affected by the forces of labor and thinning of the lower uterine segment. Other factors also play a part (eg, pelvic configuration and the size and position of the presenting part). The greater the pelvic resistance or the poorer the contractions, the slower the descent. Descent continues progressively until the fetus is delivered; the other movements are superimposed on it (Fig. 7–3).

D. Internal rotation

With the descent of the head into the midpelvis, rotation occurs so that the sagittal suture occupies the anteroposterior diameter of the pelvis. Internal rotation normally begins with the presenting part at the level of the ischial spines. The levator ani muscles form a V-shaped sling that tends to rotate the vertex anteriorly. In cases of occipitoanterior vertex, the head has to rotate 45 degrees, and in occipitoposterior vertex, 135 degrees, to pass beneath the pubic arch (Fig. 7–4).

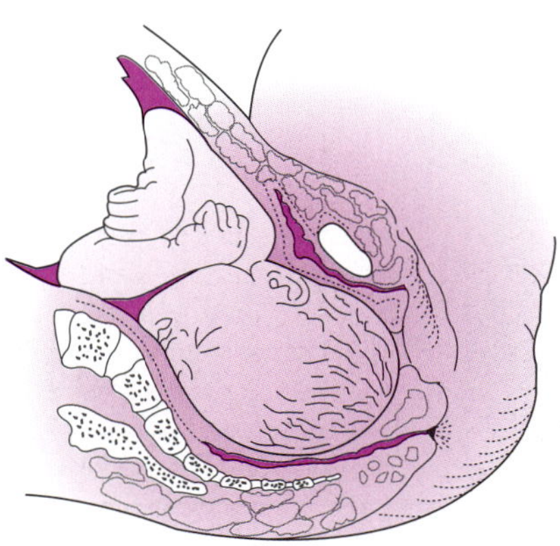

▲ **Figure 7–3.** Descent in left occipitoanterior position.

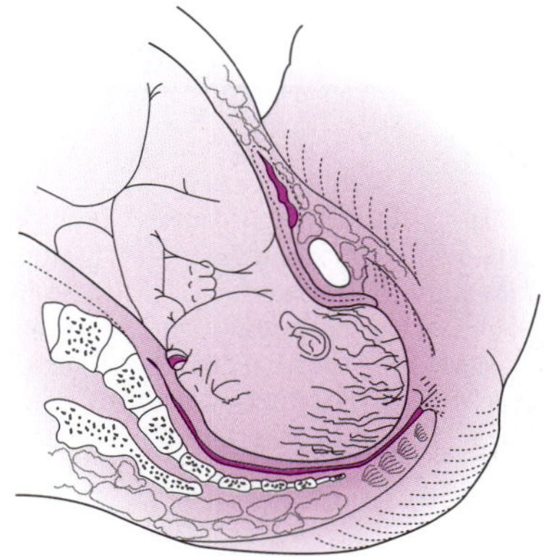

▲ **Figure 7–4.** Anterior rotation of head.

E. Extension

Because the vaginal outlet is directed upward and forward, extension must occur before the head can pass through it. As the head continues its descent, there is a bulging of the perineum, followed by crowning. Crowning occurs when the largest diameter of the fetal head is encircled by the vulvar ring (Fig. 7–5). At this time, spontaneous delivery is imminent.

F. External rotation

External rotation (restitution) follows delivery of the head when it rotates to the position it occupied at engagement. After this, the shoulders descend in a path similar to that traced by the head. The anterior shoulder rotates internally approximately 45 degrees to come under the pubic arch for delivery (Fig. 7–6). As this occurs, the head swings back to its position at birth.

▶ Clinical Findings

In true labor, the woman is usually aware of her contractions during the first stage. The intensity of pain depends

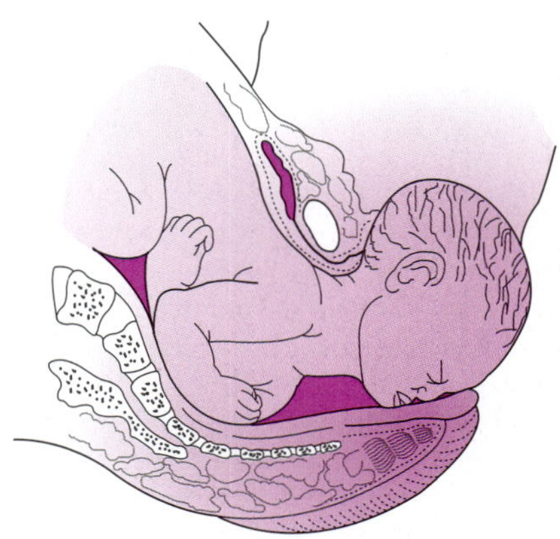

▲ **Figure 7–5.** Extension of the head.

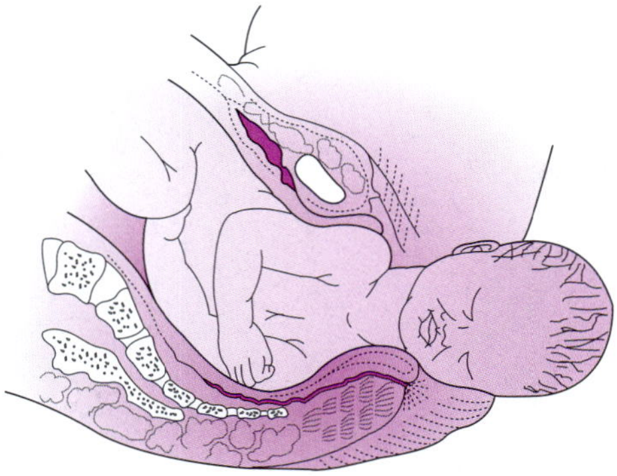

▲ **Figure 7–6.** External rotation of the head.

on the fetal/pelvic relationships, the quality and strength of uterine contractions, and the emotional and physical status of the patient. Few women experience no discomfort during the first stage of labor. Some women describe slight low back pain that radiates around to the lower abdomen. Each contraction starts with a gradual build-up of intensity, and dissipation of discomfort promptly follows the climax. Normally, the contraction will be at its height well before discomfort is reported. Dilatation of the lower birth canal and distention of the perineum during the second stage of labor will almost always cause discomfort.

Normal labor is a continuous process that has been divided into **three stages** for purposes of study, with the first stage further subdivided into two phases, the latent phase and the active phase.

- The first stage of labor is the interval between the onset of labor and full cervical dilatation.
- The second stage is the interval between full cervical dilatation and delivery of the infant.
- The third stage of labor is the period between the delivery of the infant and the delivery of the placenta.

In his classic studies of labor in 1967, Friedman presented data describing the process of spontaneous labor over time. The duration of the first stage of labor in primipara patients is noted to range from 6–18 hours, whereas in multiparous patients, the range is reported to be 2–10 hours. The lower limit of normal for the rate of cervical dilatation during the active phase is 1.2 cm per hour in first pregnancies and 1.5 cm per hour in subsequent pregnancies. The duration of the second stage in the primipara is 30 minutes to 3 hours and is 5–30 minutes for multiparas. For both, the duration of the third stage was reported to be 0–30 minutes for all pregnancies. These data, although extremely helpful as guidelines, should not be used as strict deadlines that trigger interventions if not met. Even if a numerical (statistical) approach is used to define "abnormal," the cutoff figure would not be the average range, but the 5th percentile numbers (eg, 25.8 hours for the first stage of labor in a primipara). The course that is more appropriate is to consider the overall clinical presentation and use the progress of labor to estimate the likelihood that successful vaginal delivery will occur.

The first stage of labor is evaluated by the rate of change of cervical effacement, cervical dilatation, and descent of the fetal head. The frequency and duration of uterine contractions alone is not an adequate measure of labor progress. The second stage of labor begins after full cervical dilatation. The progress of this stage is measured by the descent, flexion, and rotation of the presenting part.

Treatment

Women most likely to have a normal labor and delivery have had adequate prenatal care without significant maternal or fetal complications and are at 36 weeks' gestation or beyond. Whenever a pregnant woman is evaluated for labor, the following factors should be assessed and recorded:

- Time of onset and frequency of contractions, status of membranes, any history of bleeding, and any fetal movement.
- History of allergies, use of medication, and time, amount, and content of last oral intake.
- Prenatal records with special attention to prenatal laboratory results that impact intrapartum and immediate postpartum management (eg, HIV and hepatitis B status).
- Maternal vital signs, urinary protein and glucose, and uterine contraction pattern.
- Fetal heart rate, presentation, and clinical estimated fetal weight.
- Status of the membranes, cervical dilatation and effacement (unless contraindicated, eg, by placenta previa), and station of the presenting part.

If no complications are detected during the initial assessment and the patient is found to be in prodromal labor, admission for labor and delivery may be deferred. When a patient is admitted, a hematocrit or hemoglobin measurement should be obtained and a blood clot should be obtained in the event that a cross-match is needed. A blood group, Rh type, and antibody screen should also be done.

The First Stage of Labor

In the first stage of normal labor, the pregnant woman may be allowed to ambulate or sit in a comfortable chair as desired. When the patient is lying in bed, the supine position should be discouraged. Patients in active labor should avoid ingestion of solid food. Clear liquids, ice chips, or preparations for moistening the mouth and lips should be allowed. When significant amounts of fluids and calories are required because of long labor, they should be given intravenously.

Maternal pulse and blood pressure should be recorded at least every 2–4 hours in normal labor and more frequently if indicated. Maternal fluid balance (ie, urine output and intravenous and oral intake) should be monitored, and both dehydration and fluid overload should be avoided.

Management of discomfort and pain during labor and delivery is a necessary part of good obstetric practice. A patient's request is sufficient justification for providing pain relief during labor. Specific analgesic and anesthetic techniques are discussed in Chapter 24. Some patients tolerate the pain of labor by using techniques learned in childbirth preparation programs. Common methods of preparation include Lamaze, Bradley, Read, hypnotherapy, and prenatal yoga. Although specific techniques vary, these classes usually teach relief of pain through the application of principles of education, emotional support, touch, relaxation, paced breathing, and mental focus. The staff at the bedside should be knowledgeable about these pain-management techniques and should be supportive of the patient's decision to use them. When such methods fail to provide adequate pain relief, some patients will ask for medical assistance, and such requests should be respected. Indeed, the use of appropriate medical analgesic techniques should be explained to the patient and her labor partner and their use encouraged when medically indicated.

Reassurance of fetal well-being is sought through fetal monitoring. Fetal monitoring may be performed intermittently or continuously, depending on the presence or absence of risk factors for adverse perinatal outcome. In patients with no significant obstetric risk factors, either continuous or intermittent monitoring is acceptable. If the fetus is monitored intermittently, then the fetal heart rate should be auscultated or the electronic monitor tracing should be evaluated at least every 30 minutes in the active phase of the first stage of labor and at least every 15 minutes in the second stage of labor. In patients with obstetric risk factors such as hypertension, intrauterine fetal growth restriction, diabetes, or multiple gestations, continuous fetal monitoring is recommended.

Uterine contractions may be monitored by palpation, by tocodynamometer, or by internal pressure catheter. If monitored by palpation, the patient's abdomen should be palpated every 30 minutes to assess contraction frequency, duration, and intensity. For at-risk pregnancies, uterine contractions should be monitored continuously along with the fetal heart rate. This can be achieved by using either an external tocodynamometer or an internal pressure catheter in the amniotic cavity. The latter method is particularly useful when abnormal progression of labor is suspected or when the patient requires oxytocin for augmentation of labor.

The progress of labor is monitored by examination of the cervix. During the latent phase, especially when the membranes are ruptured, vaginal examinations should be done sparingly to decrease the risk of intrauterine infection. In the active phase, the cervix should be assessed approximately every 2 hours. The cervical effacement and dilatation and the station and position of the fetal head should be recorded (Fig. 7–7). Additional examinations to determine whether full dilation has occurred may be required if the patient reports the urge to push, or to search for prolapse of the umbilical cord or perform fetal scalp stimulation if a significant fetal heart rate deceleration is detected.

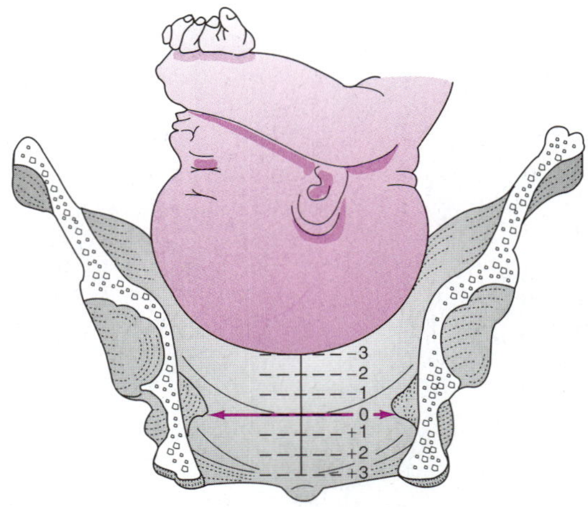

▲ **Figure 7–7.** Stations of the fetal head. (Reproduced, with permission, from Benson RC. *Handbook of Obstetrics & Gynecology*. 8th ed. Los Altos, CA: Lange; 1983.)

The therapeutic rupture of fetal membranes (amniotomy) has been largely discredited as a means of induction when used alone. Moreover, artificial rupture of the membranes increases the risk of chorioamnionitis and the need for antibiotics (especially if labor is prolonged), as well as the risk of cord prolapse if the presenting part is not engaged. Amniotomy may, however, provide information on the volume of amniotic fluid and the presence of meconium. In addition, rupture of the membranes may cause an increase in uterine contractility. Amniotomy should not be performed routinely. It should be used when internal fetal or uterine monitoring is required and may be helpful when enhancement of uterine contractility in the active phase of labor is indicated. Care should be taken to palpate for the umbilical cord and to avoid dislodging the fetal head. The fetal heart rate should be recorded before, during, and immediately after the procedure.

The Second Stage of Labor

At the beginning of the second stage of labor, the mother usually feels a desire to bear down with each contraction. This abdominal pressure, together with the force of the uterine contractions, expels the fetus. During the second stage of labor. the descent of the fetal head is measured to assess the progress of labor. The descent of the fetus is evaluated by measuring the relationship of the bony portion of the fetal head to the level of the maternal ischial spines (station) (Fig. 7–7). When the leading portion of the fetal skull is at the level of the ischial spines, the station is "0." The American College of Obstetricians and Gynecologists–endorsed method for describing station is to estimate the number of centimeters from the ischial spines. For instance, when the leading portion of the head is 2 cm above the ischial spines, this is reported as −2 station; when the leading portion of the skull is 3 cm below the ischial spines, this is reported as +3. Some practitioners find it useful to refer to station in estimated thirds of the maternal pelvis. An approximate correlation of these two methods would be as follows: 2 cm = +1, 4 cm = +2, and 6 cm = +3.

The second stage generally takes from 30 minutes to 3 hours in primigravid women and from 5–30 minutes in multigravid women. The median duration is 50 minutes in a primipara and 20 minutes in a multipara. These times may vary depending on the pushing efforts of the mother, the quality of the uterine contractions, and the type of analgesia.

Delivery

When the fetal head is noted to crown, delivery is imminent. Careful management by the practitioner with controlled efforts of the mother will minimize perineal trauma. Routine episiotomy is unnecessary and is associated with increased maternal blood loss, increased risk of disruption of the anal sphincter (third-degree extension) and rectal mucosa (fourth-degree extension), and delay in the patient's resumption of sexual activity. Further extension follows extrusion of the head beyond the introitus. Once the head is delivered, the airway is cleared of blood and amniotic fluid using a bulb suction device. The oral cavity is cleared initially, followed by clearing of the nares.

After the airway is cleared, an index finger is used to check whether the umbilical cord encircles the neck. If so, the cord can usually be slipped over the infant's head. If the cord is too tight, it can be cut between two clamps.

Delivery of the anterior shoulder is aided by gentle downward traction on the externally rotated head (Fig. 7–8).

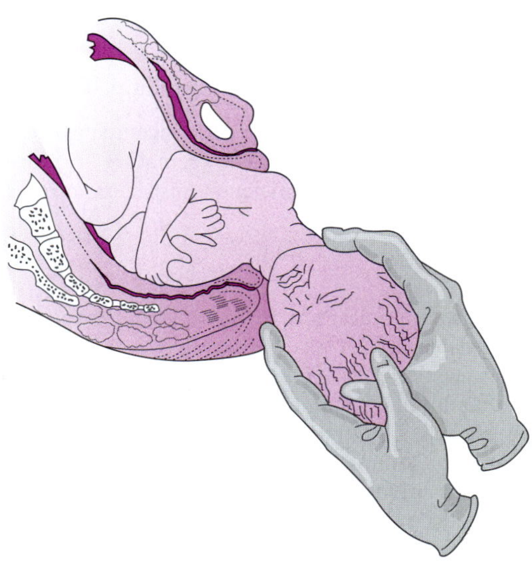

▲ **Figure 7–8.** Delivery of anterior shoulder.

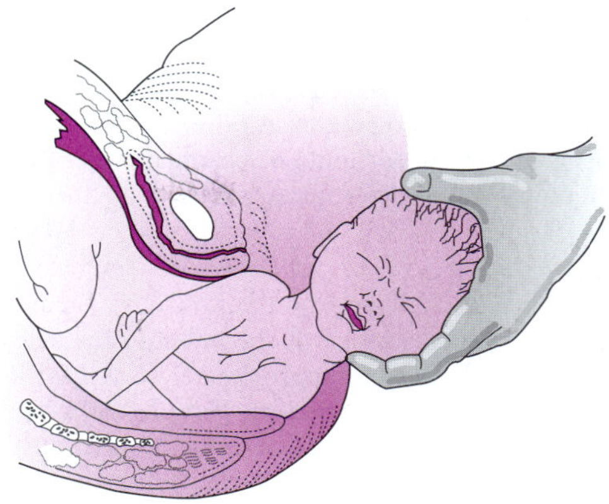

▲ **Figure 7–9.** Delivery of posterior shoulder.

The posterior shoulder is then delivered by gentle upward traction on the head (Fig. 7–9). The brachial plexus may be injured if excessive force is used. After these maneuvers, the body, legs, and feet are delivered with gentle traction on the shoulders.

After delivery, blood will be infused from the placenta into the newborn if the baby is held below the mother's introitus. Delayed cord clamping can result in neonatal hyperbilirubinemia as additional blood is transferred to the newborn infant. Generally, a vigorous newborn can be delivered directly from the introitus to the abdomen and waiting arms of a healthy, alert mother. Placing the child skin to skin (abdomen to abdomen) results in optimum warmth for the newborn. Then the cord, which has been doubly clamped, may be cut between the clamps by either the practitioner, the mother, or her partner.

Third Stage of Labor

Immediately after the baby is delivered, the cervix and vagina should be inspected for actively bleeding lacerations and surgical repair should be performed as needed. Repair of vaginal lacerations should be performed using absorbable suture material, either 2-0 or 3-0. The inspection and repair of the cervix, vagina, and perineum is often easier prior to the separation of the placenta before uterine bleeding obscures visualization.

Separation of the placenta generally occurs within 2–10 minutes of the end of the second stage, but it may take 30 minutes or more to spontaneously separate. Signs of placental separation are as follows: (1) a fresh show of blood appears from the vagina, (2) the umbilical cord lengthens outside the vagina, (3) the fundus of the uterus rises up, and (4) the uterus becomes firm and globular. When these signs appear, it is safe to place traction on the cord. The gentle traction, with or without counterpressure between the symphysis and fundus to prevent descent of the uterus, allows delivery of the placenta.

After the delivery of the placenta, attention is turned to prevention of excessive postpartum bleeding. Uterine contractions that reduce this bleeding may be enhanced with uterine massage and/or the infusion of a dilute solution of oxytocin. The placenta should be examined to ensure complete removal and to detect placental abnormalities.

Puerperium

The puerperium consists of the period after the delivery of the baby and placenta to approximately 6 weeks postpartum. The immediate postpartum period (within the first hour of delivery) is a critical time for both maternal and neonatal physiologic and emotional adjustment. During that hour, the maternal blood pressure, pulse rate, and uterine blood loss must be monitored closely. It is during this time that most postpartum hemorrhage usually occurs, largely as a result of uterine relaxation, retained placental fragments, or unrepaired lacerations. Occult bleeding (eg, vaginal wall hematoma formation) may manifest as increasing pelvic pain.

At the same time, maternal bonding to the newborn is evolving, and ideally breastfeeding is initiated. Early initiation of breastfeeding is beneficial to the health of both the mother and the newborn. Both benefit because babies are extremely alert and programmed to latch onto the breast during this period. Mother–infant pairs that begin breastfeeding early are most able to continue breastfeeding for longer periods of time. For the mother, nursing accelerates the involution of the uterus, thereby reducing blood loss by increasing uterine contractions. For the newborn, there are important immunologic advantages. For example, various maternal antibodies are present in breast milk, which provide the newborn with passive immunity against certain infections. Also immunoglobulin (Ig) A, a secretory immunoglobulin present in significant amounts in breast milk, protects the infant's gut by preventing attachment of harmful bacteria to cells of the gut mucosal surface. It is also believed that maternal lymphocytes pass through the infant's gut wall and initiate immunologic processes that are not yet fully understood. In addition to the immunologic benefits, breast milk is the ideal nutritional source for the newborn. Moreover, it is inexpensive and is usually in good supply. Given all the advantages (the preceding is only a partial list of the benefits), encouraging successful breastfeeding is an important health goal.

Induction and Augmentation of Labor

Induction of labor is the process of initiating labor by artificial means; augmentation is the artificial stimulation of labor that has begun spontaneously. Labor induction should be performed only after appropriate assessment of the mother and fetus. Additionally, the risks, benefits, and alternatives to induction in each case must be evaluated and explained to the patient. In the absence of medical indications for induction, fetal maturity must be confirmed by either exact pregnancy dating, first-trimester ultrasound measurements, and/or amniotic fluid analysis. Evaluation of the cervical status in terms of effacement and softening is important in predicting success of induction and is highly recommended before any elective induction (Table 7–2). Generally, induction should be done in response to specific indications and should not be done electively prior to 39 weeks gestational age.

Table 7–2. Bishop method of pelvic scoring for elective induction of labor.

Examination	Points		
	1	2	3
Cervical dilatation (cm)	1-2	3-4	5-6
Cervical effacement (%)	40-50	60-70	80
Station of presenting part	−1,−2	0	+1, 2
Consistency of cervix	Medium	Soft	. . .
Position of cervix	Middle	Anterior	. . .

Elective induction of labor may be performed safely when pelvic score is 9 or more.
(Modified and reproduced, with permission, from Bishop EH. Pelvic scoring for elective induction. *Obstet Gynecol* 1964;24:266.)

A. Indications

The following are common indications for induction of labor:

1. Maternal—Preeclampsia, diabetes mellitus, heart disease.

2. Fetal—Prolonged pregnancy, Rh incompatibility, fetal abnormality, chorioamnionitis, premature rupture of membranes, placental insufficiency, suspected intrauterine growth restriction.

B. Contraindications

Absolute contraindications to induction of labor include contracted pelvis; placenta previa; uterine scar because of previous classical caesarean section, myomectomy entering the endometrium, hysterotomy, or unification surgery; and transverse lie.

Labor induction should be carried out with caution in the following situations: breech presentation, oligohydramnios, multiple gestation, grand multiparity, previous caesarean section with transverse scar, prematurity, suspected fetal macrosomia.

Complications of Induction of Labor

A. For the mother

In many cases, induction of labor exposes the mother to more distress and discomfort than judicious delay and subsequent vaginal or caesarean delivery. The following hazards must be kept in mind: (1) failure of induction with increased risk of caesarean delivery; (2) uterine inertia and prolonged labor; (3) tumultuous labor and tetanic contractions of the uterus, causing premature separation of the placenta, rupture of the uterus, and laceration of the cervix; (4) intrauterine infection; and (5) postpartum hemorrhage.

B. For the fetus

An induced delivery exposes the infant to the risk of prematurity if the estimated date of conception has been inaccurately calculated. Precipitous delivery may result in physical injury. Prolapse of the cord may follow amniotomy. Injudicious administration of oxytocin or inadequate observation during induction could lead to fetal heart rate abnormalities or delivery of a baby with poor Apgar scores.

Methods of Cervical Ripening

Cervical ripening before induction of labor could facilitate the onset and progression of labor and increase the chance of vaginal delivery, particularly in primigravid patients.

A. Prostaglandin

Two forms of prostaglandins are commonly used for cervical ripening before induction at term: misoprostol (PGE_1) and dinoprostone (PGE_2). Although only dinoprostone, commercially available as prostaglandin gel, is currently Food and Drug Administration–approved for this use, off-label use of misoprostol for cervical ripening is widely practiced. Indeed, although both misoprostol and dinoprostone applied locally intravaginally can provide significant improvement in the Bishop score, a meta-analysis of randomized, controlled trials focusing on cervical ripening and induction of labor found the time to delivery was shorter and the rate of caesarean delivery was lower in the misoprostol group.

Dinoprostone comes prepackaged in a single-dose syringe containing 0.5 mg of PGE_2 in 2.5 mL of a viscous gel of colloidal silicon dioxide in triacetin. The syringe is attached to a soft-plastic catheter for intracervical administration, and the catheter is shielded to help prevent application above the internal cervical os. Misoprostol is manufactured in 100-μg unscored and 200-μg scored tablets that can be administered orally, vaginally, and rectally. PGE_2 should not be used in patients with a history of asthma, glaucoma, or myocardial infarction. Unexplained vaginal bleeding, chorioamnionitis, ruptured membranes, and previous caesarean section are relative contraindications to the use of prostaglandins for cervical ripening.

For cervical ripening and induction at term, misoprostol is given vaginally at a dose of 25 μg every 4–6 hours. With dinoprostone, usually 12 hours should be allowed for cervical ripening, after which oxytocin induction should be started. PGE_1 and PGE_2 have similar side-effect and risk profiles, including fetal heart rate deceleration, fetal distress, emergency caesarean section, uterine hypertonicity, nausea, vomiting, fever, and peripartum infection. However, a current literature review does not indicate any significant differences in reported side effects between control and treatment groups with prostaglandin cervical ripening.

B. Balloon catheter

A Foley catheter with a 25- to 50-mL balloon is passed into the endocervix above the internal os using tissue forceps. The balloon is then inflated with sterile saline, and the catheter is withdrawn gently to the level of internal cervical os. This method should induce cervical ripening over 8–12 hours. The cervix will be dilated 2–3 cm when the balloon falls out, which will make amniotomy possible, but effacement may be unchanged.

C. Hygroscopic dilators

Laminaria tents are made from desiccated stems of the cold-water seaweed *Laminaria digitata* or *L japonica*. When placed in the endocervix for 6–12 hours, the laminaria increases in diameter 3- to 4-fold by extracting water from cervical tissues, gradually swelling and expanding the cervical canal. Synthetic dilators like lamicel, a polyvinyl alcohol polymer sponge impregnated with 450 mg of magnesium sulfate, and dilapan, which is made from a stable nontoxic hydrophilic polymer of polyacrylonitrile, are also noted to be highly effective in mechanical cervical dilation.

Methods of Induction of Labor

A. Oxytocin

Intravenous administration of a very dilute solution of oxytocin is the most effective medical means of inducing labor. Oxytocin exaggerates the inherent rhythmic pattern of uterine motility, which often becomes clinically evident during the last trimester and increases as term is approached.

The dosage must be individualized. The administration of oxytocin is determined with a biologic assay: The smallest possible effective dose must be determined for each patient and then used to initiate and maintain labor. Constant observation by qualified attendants is required when this method is used.

In most cases it is sufficient to add 1 mL of oxytocin (10 units of oxytocin to 1 L of 5% dextrose in water [1 mU/mL]). One acceptable oxytocin infusion regimen is to begin induction or augmentation at 1 mU/min, preferably with an infusion pump or other accurate delivery system, and increase oxytocin in 2-mU increments at 15-minute intervals.

When contractions of 50–60 mm Hg (per the internal monitor pressure) or lasting 40–60 seconds (per the external monitor) occur at 2.5- to 4-minute intervals, the oxytocin dose should be increased no further. Oxytocin infusion is discontinued whenever hyperstimulation or fetal distress is identified, but can be restarted when reassuring fetal heart rate and uterine activity patterns are restored.

B. Amniotomy

Early and variable decelerations of the fetal heart rate are noted to be relatively common with amniotomy. Nonetheless, amniotomy may be an effective way to induce labor in carefully selected cases with high Bishop scores. Release of amniotic fluid shortens the muscle bundles of the myometrium; the strength and duration of the contractions are thereby increased, and a more rapid contraction sequence follows. The membranes should be ruptured with an amniohook. Make no effort to strip the membranes, and do not displace the head upward to drain off amniotic fluid. Because amniotomy has not been proven effective in augmenting labor uniformly, it is recommended that the active phase of labor be entered before performing amniotomy for augmentation. Amniotomy in selected cases, although slightly increasing the risk of infectious morbidity, could shorten the course of labor without increasing or reducing the incidence of operative delivery.

Bernal AL. Overview of current research in parturition. *Exp Physiol* 2000;86:213–222. PMID: 11429638.

Eason E, Labrecque M, Wells G, Feldman P. Preventing perineal trauma during childbirth: A systematic review. *Obstet Gynecol* 2000;95:464–471. PMID: 10711565.

el-Turkey M, Grant JM. Sweeping of the membrane is an effective method of induction of labor in prolonged pregnancy: A report of a randomized trial. *Br J Obstet Gynaecol* 1992;99:455–458. PMID: 1637758.

Forman A, Ulmsten U, Bányai J, Wingerup L, Uldbjerg N. Evidence for a local effect of intracervical prostaglandin E_2. *Am J Obstet Gynecol* 1982;143:756–60. PMID: 6954849.

Fraser WD, Sokol R. Amniotomy and maternal position in labor. *Clin Obstet Gynecol* 1992;35:535–545. PMID: 1521383.

Goldberg AB, Greenberg BS, Darney PD. Misoprostol and pregnancy. *N Engl J Med* 2001;344:38–41. PMID: 11136959.

Hansen AK, Wisborg K, Uldbjerg N, Henriksen TB. Elective caesarean section and respiratory morbidity in the term and near-term neonate. *Acta Obstet Gynecol Scand* 2007;86:389–94. PMID: 17486457.

Harbort GM Jr. Assessment of uterine contractility and activity. *Clin Obstet Gynecol* 1992;35:546–558. PMID: 1521384.

Kazzi GM, Bottoms SF, Rosen MG. Efficacy and safety of *Laminaria digitata* for preinduction ripening of the cervix. *Obstet Gynecol* 1982;60:440–443. PMID: 7121931.

Klein MC, Gauthier RJ, Robbins JM, et al. Relationship of episiotomy to perineal trauma and morbidity, sexual dysfunction, and pelvic floor relaxation. *Am J Obstet Gynecol* 1994;171:591–598. PMID: 8092203.

Lange AP, Secher NJ, Westergaard JG, Skovgård I. Prelabor evaluation of inducibility. *Obstet Gynecol* 1982;60:137–147. PMID: 7155472.

Martin JN Jr, Morrison JC, Wiser WL. Vaginal birth after cesarean section: The demise of routine repeat abdominal delivery. *Obstet Gynecol Clin North Am* 1988;15:719–736. PMID: 3226673.

McColgin SW, Hampton HL, McCaul JF, Howard PR, Andrew ME, Morrison JC. Stripping membranes at term: Can it safely reduce the incidence of postterm pregnancy? *Obstet Gynecol* 1990;76:678–680. PMID: 2216203.

Owen J, Hauth JC. Oxytocin for the induction or augmentation of labor. *Clin Obstet Gynecol* 1992;35:464–475. PMID: 1521376.

Renfrew MJ, Hannah W, Albers L, Floyd E. Practices that minimize trauma to the genital tract in childbirth: A systematic review of the literature. *Birth* 1998;25:143–160. PMID: 9767217.

Sheiner E, Segal D, Shoham-Vardi I, Ben-Tov J, Katz M, Mazor M. The impact of early amniotomy on mode of delivery and pregnancy outcome. *Arch Gynecol Obstet* 2000;264:63–67. PMID: 1104532.

Yamazaki H, Torigoe K, Numata O, et al. Neonatal clinical outcome after elective cesarean section before the onset of labor at the 37th and 38th week of gestation. *Pediatr Int* 2003;4:379–82. PMID: 12911470.

Maternal Physiology During Pregnancy & Fetal & Early Neonatal Physiology

8

Amy A. Flick, MD
Daniel A. Kahn, MD, PhD

Pregnancy involves a number changes in anatomy, physiology, and biochemistry, which can challenge maternal reserves. A basic knowledge of these adaptations is critical for understanding normal laboratory measurements, knowing the drugs likely to require dose adjustments, and recognizing women who are predisposed to medical complications during pregnancy.

CARDIOVASCULAR SYSTEM

Anatomic Changes

With uterine enlargement and diaphragmatic elevation, the heart rotates on its long axis in a left-upward displacement. As a result of these changes, the apical beat (point of maximum intensity) shifts laterally. Overall, the heart size increases by approximately 12%, which results from both an increase in myocardial mass and intracardiac volume (approximately 80 mL). Vascular changes include hypertrophy of smooth muscle and a reduction in collagen content.

Blood Volume

Blood volume expansion begins early in the first trimester, increases rapidly in the second trimester, and plateaus at about the 30th week (Fig. 8–1). The approximately 50% elevation in plasma volume, which accounts for most of the increment, results from a cascade of effects triggered by pregnancy hormones. For example, increased estrogen production by the placenta stimulates the renin–angiotensin system, which, in turn, leads to higher circulating levels of aldosterone. Aldosterone promotes renal Na^+ reabsorption and water retention. Progesterone also participates in plasma volume expansion through a poorly understood mechanism; increased venous capacitance is another important factor. Human chorionic somatomammotropin, progesterone, and perhaps other hormones promote erythropoiesis, resulting in the approximately 30% increase in red cell mass.

The magnitude of the increase in blood volume varies according to the size of the woman, the number of prior pregnancies, and the number of fetuses she is carrying. This hypervolemia of pregnancy compensates for maternal blood loss at delivery, which averages 500–600 mL for vaginal and 1000 mL for caesarean delivery.

Cardiac Output

Cardiac output increases approximately 40% during pregnancy, with maximum values achieved at 20–24 weeks' gestation. This rise in cardiac output is thought to result from the hormonal changes of pregnancy, as well as the arteriovenous-shunt effect of uteroplacental circulation.

Stroke volume increases 25–30% during pregnancy, reaching peak values at 12–24 weeks' gestation (Fig. 8–2). Thus elevations in cardiac output after 20 weeks of gestation depend critically on the rise in heart rate. Maximum cardiac output is associated with a 24% increase in stroke volume and a 15% rise in heart rate. Cardiac output increases in labor in association with painful contractions, which increase venous return and activate the sympathetic nervous system. Cardiac output is further increased, albeit transiently, at delivery.

Stroke volume is sensitive to maternal position. In lateral recumbency, stroke volume remains roughly the same from 20 weeks' gestation until term, but in the supine position stroke volume decreases after 20 weeks and can even decrease to nonpregnant levels by 40 weeks' gestation.

The resting maternal heart rate, which progressively increases over the course of gestation, averages at term approximately 15 beats/min more than the nonpregnant rate (Fig. 8–2). Of course, exercise, emotional stress, heat, drugs, and other factors can further increase heart rate.

Multiple gestations have even more profound effects on the maternal cardiovascular system. In twin pregnancies, cardiac output is approximately 20% greater than for singletons, because of greater stroke volume (15%) and heart rate (3.5%). Other differences include greater left ventricular end-diastolic dimensions and muscle mass.

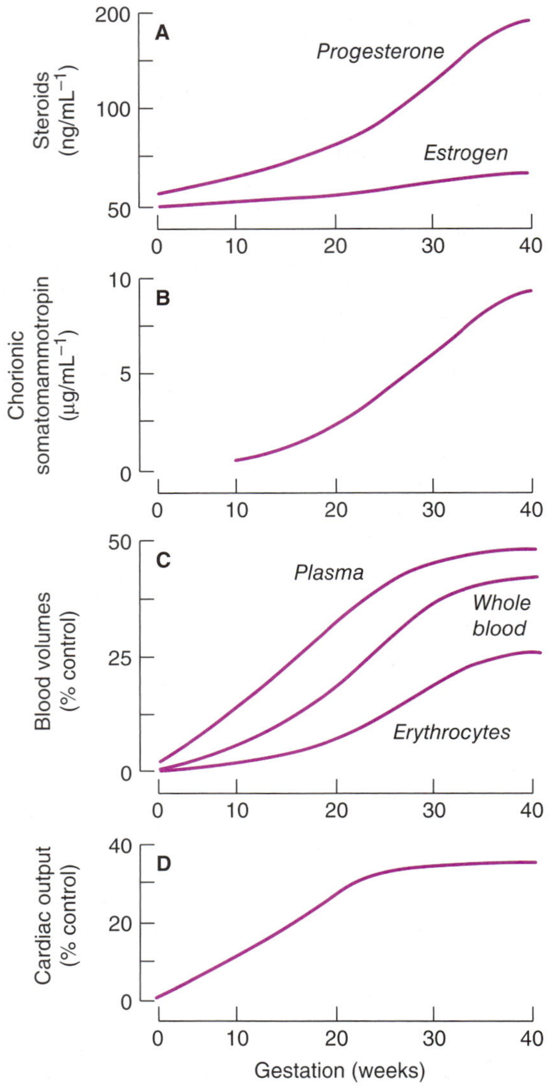

▲ **Figure 8–1.** Increases in maternal hormones (**A**, **B**), blood volume (**C**), and cardiac output (**D**) over gestation. % control represents the increment relative to nonpregnant values. (Modified, with permission, from Longo LD. Maternal blood volume and cardiac output during pregnancy: A hypothesis of endocrinologic control. *Am J Physiol* 1983;245:R720.)

Cardiac output is generally resistant to postural stress. For example, the decrease in cardiac output that develops immediately after standing does not occur in the middle of the third trimester, although some reduction can occur earlier in pregnancy. In the third trimester, the supine position can reduce cardiac output and arterial pressure caused by compression of the vena cava by the gravid uterus with an associated reduction in venous return to the heart.

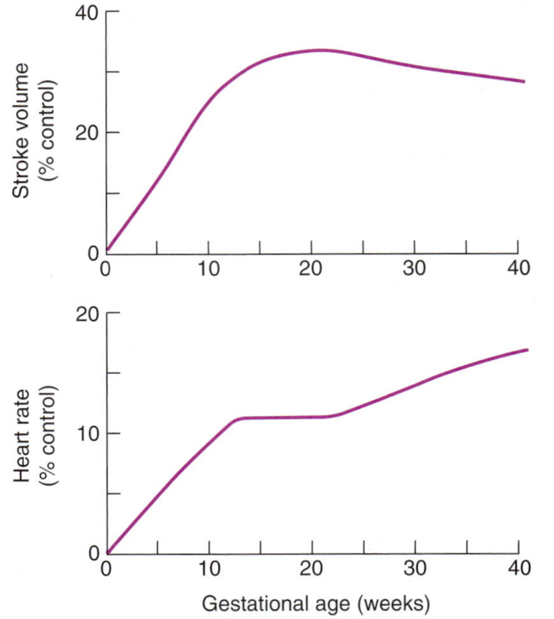

▲ **Figure 8–2.** Increases in maternal stroke volume and heart rate. The % control represents increment relative to measurements in patients who are not pregnant. (Reproduced, with permission, from Koos BJ. Management of uncorrected, palliated, and repaired cyanotic congenital heart disease in pregnancy. *Prog Ped Cardiol* 2004;19:250.)

Approximately 10% of gravidas will develop supine hypotensive syndrome, characterized by hypotension, bradycardia, and syncope. These women are particularly sensitive to caval compression because of reduced capacitance in venous collaterals. Shifting the gravida to a right or left lateral recumbent position will alleviate caval compression, increase blood return to the heart, and restore cardiac output and arterial pressure.

Blood Pressure

Systemic arterial pressure declines slightly during pregnancy, reaching a nadir at 24–28 weeks of gestation. Pulse pressure widens because the fall is greater for diastolic than for systolic pressures (Fig. 8–3). Systolic and diastolic pressures (and mean arterial pressure) increase to prepregnancy levels by approximately 36 weeks.

Venous pressure progressively increases in the lower extremities, particularly when the patient is supine, sitting, or standing. The rise in venous pressure, which can cause edema and varicosities, results from compression of the inferior vena cava by the gravid uterus and possibly from the pressure of the fetal presenting part on the common iliac veins. Lying in lateral recumbency minimizes changes in venous pressure. As expected, venous pressure in the lower extremities falls

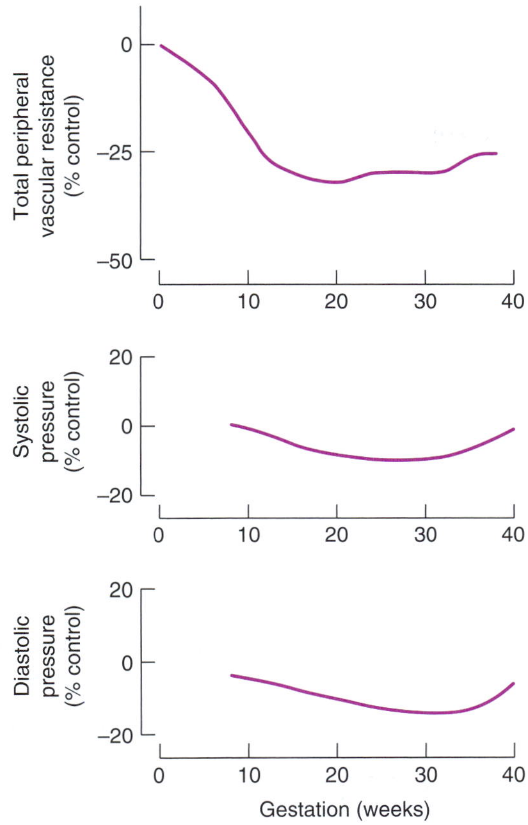

▲ **Figure 8–3.** Changes in maternal peripheral vascular resistance and arterial pressures over gestation. Pressures were measured in the left lateral recumbent position. The % control represents the relative change from nonpregnant values. (Modified, with permission, from Thornburg KL, Jacobson SL, Giraud GD, Morton MJ. Hemodynamic changes in pregnancy. *Semin Perinatol* 2000;24:11–14; Wilson M, Morganti AA, Zervoudakis I, et al. Blood pressure, the renin-aldosterone system and sex steroids throughout normal pregnancy. *Am J Med* 1980;68:97–104.)

immediately after delivery. Venous pressure in the upper extremities is unchanged by pregnancy.

Peripheral Vascular Resistance

Vascular resistance decreases in the first trimester, reaching a nadir of approximately 34% below nonpregnancy levels by 14 to 0 weeks of gestation with a slight increase toward term (Fig. 8–3). The hormonal changes of pregnancy likely trigger this fall in vascular resistance by enhancing local vasodilators, such as nitric oxide, prostacyclin, and possibly adenosine. Delivery is associated with nearly a 40% decrease in peripheral vascular resistance, although mean arterial pressure is generally maintained because of the associated rise in cardiac output.

Blood Flow Distribution

In absolute terms, blood flow increases to the uterus, kidneys, skin, breast, and possibly other maternal organs; the total augmented organ flow reflects virtually the entire increment in maternal cardiac output. However, when expressed as a percentage of cardiac output, blood flow in some of these organs may not be elevated compared with the nonpregnant state.

Blood flow to the uterus increases in a gestational age-dependent manner. Uterine blood flow can be as high as 800 mL/min, which is approximately 4 times the nonpregnant value. The increased flow during pregnancy results from the relatively low resistance in the uteroplacental circulation.

Renal blood flow increases approximately 400 mL/min above nonpregnant levels, and blood flow to the breasts increases approximately 200 mL/min. Blood flow to the skin also increases, particularly in the hands and feet. The increased skin blood flow helps dissipate heat produced by metabolism in the mother and fetus.

Strenuous exercise, which diverts blood flow to large muscles, has the potential to decrease uteroplacental perfusion and thus O_2 delivery to the fetus. Women who are already adapted to an exercise routine can generally continue the program in pregnancy; however, pregnant women should discuss their exercise plans with the physician managing the pregnancy.

HEART MURMURS & RHYTHM

The physiologic changes of pregnancy alter several clinical findings. For example, systolic ejection murmurs, which result from increased cardiac output and decreased blood viscosity, can be detected in 90% or more gravidas. Thus caution should be exercised in interpreting systolic murmurs in pregnant women.

The first heart sound may be split, with increased loudness of both portions, and the third heart sound may also be louder. Continuous murmurs or bruits may be heard at the left sternal edge, which arise from the internal thoracic (mammary) artery.

Pregnancy decreases the threshold for reentrant supraventricular tachycardia. Normal pregnancy can also be accompanied by sinus tachycardia, sinus bradycardia, and isolated atrial and ventricular premature contractions.

Electrocardiographic changes can include a 15- to 20-degree shift to the left in the electrical axis. Changes in ventricular repolarization can result in ST-segment depression or T-wave flattening. However, pregnancy does not alter the amplitude and duration of the P wave, QRS complex, or T wave.

PULMONARY SYSTEM

Anatomic Changes

Pregnancy alters the circulation of a number of tissues involved in respiration. For example, capillary dilatation leads to engorgement of the nasopharynx, larynx, trachea, and bronchi. Prominent pulmonary vascular markings observed on x-ray are consistent with increased pulmonary blood volume.

As the uterus enlarges, the diaphragm is elevated by as much as 4 cm. The rib cage is displaced upward, increasing the angle of the ribs with the spine. These changes increase the lower thoracic diameter by approximately 2 cm and the thoracic circumference by up to 6 cm. Elevation of the diaphragm does not impair its function. Abdominal muscles have less tone and activity during pregnancy, causing respiration to be more diaphragm dependent.

Lung Volumes and Capacities

Several lung volumes and capacities are altered by pregnancy (Table 8–1). Dead space volume increases because of relaxation of the musculature of conducting airways. Tidal volume and inspiratory capacity increase. Elevation of the diaphragm is associated with reduction in total lung capacity and functional residual capacity. The latter involves a decrease in both expiratory reserve and residual volumes.

Table 8–1. Effects of pregnancy on lung volumes and capacities.

	Definition	Change
I. Volumes		
Tidal	Volume inspired and expired with each normal respiratory cycle	↑ 35–50%
Inspiratory reserve	Maximum volume that can be inspired over normal end-tidal inspiration	↓
Expiratory reserve	Maximum volume that can be expired from resting end-tidal expiration	↓ 20%
Residual	Volume remaining in the lungs after maximum expiration	↓ 20%
II. Capacities		
Total lung	Total volume at the end of maximum inspiration	↓ 5%
Vital	Maximum volume expired after maximum inspiration	→
Inspiratory	Maximum volume inspired from end-tidal expiration	↑ 5–10%
Functional	Volume at end-tidal expiration that mixes with tidal air upon inspiration	↓ 20%

Respiration

Pregnancy has little effect on respiratory rate. Thus the increase in minute ventilation (approximately 50%) results from the rise in tidal volume. This increment in minute ventilation is disproportionately greater than the rise (approximately 20%) in total oxygen consumption in maternal muscle tissues (cardiac, respiratory, uterine, skeletal) and in the products of the fetal genome (placenta, fetus). This hyperventilation, which decreases maternal arterial PCO_2 to approximately 27–32 mm Hg, results in a mild respiratory alkalosis (blood pH of 7.4–7.5). The hyperventilation and hyperdynamic circulation slightly increase arterial PO_2.

Increased levels of progesterone appear to have a critical role in the hyperventilation of pregnancy, which develops early in the first trimester. As in the luteal phase of the menstrual cycle of nonpregnant women, the increased ventilation appears to be caused by the action of progesterone on central neurons involved in respiratory regulation. The overall respiratory effect appears to be a decrease in the threshold and an increase in the sensitivity of central chemoreflex responses to CO_2. Maternal hyperventilation may be protective in that that it prevents the fetus from being exposed to high CO_2 tensions, which might adversely affect the development of respiratory control and other critical regulatory mechanisms.

Functional measurement of ventilation can also change according to posture and duration of pregnancy. For example, the peak expiratory rate, which declines throughout gestation in the sitting and standing positions, is particularly compromised in the supine position.

RENAL SYSTEM

Anatomic Changes

During pregnancy, the length of the kidneys increases by 1–1.5 cm, with a proportional increase in weight. The renal calyces and pelves are dilated in pregnancy, with the volume of the renal pelvis increased up to 6-fold compared with the nonpregnant value of 10 mL. The ureters are dilated above the brim of the bony pelvis, with more prominent effects on the right. The ureters elongate, widen, and become more curved. The entire dilated collecting system may contain up to 200 mL of urine, which predisposes to ascending urinary infections. Urinary tract dilatation disappears in virtually all women by postpartum day 4.

Several factors likely contribute to the hydronephrosis and hydroureter of pregnancy: (1) Pregnancy hormones (eg, progesterone) may cause hypotonia of ureteral smooth muscle. Against this possibility is the observation that high progesterone levels in nonpregnant women do not cause hydroureter. (2) Enlargement of the ovarian vein complex in the infundibulopelvic ligament may compress the ureter at the brim of the bony pelvis. (3) Hyperplasia of smooth muscle in the distal one-third of the ureter may cause reduction in luminal size, leading to dilatation in the upper two-thirds. (4) The sigmoid colon and dextrorotation of the uterus likely reduce compression (and dilatation) of the left ureter relative to the right.

Renal Function

Renal plasma flow increases 50–85% above nonpregnant values during the first half of pregnancy, with a modest decrease in later gestation. The changes in renal plasma flow reflect decreases in renal vascular resistance, which achieves lowest values by the end of the first trimester. Elevated renal perfusion is the principal factor involved in rise in glomerular filtration rate (GFR), which is increased by approximately 25% in the second week after conception. GFR reaches a peak increment of 40–65% by the end of the first trimester and remains high until term (Fig. 8–4). The fraction of renal plasma flow that passes through the glomerular membrane (filtration fraction) decreases during the first 20 weeks of gestation, which subsequently rises toward term.

Hormones involved in these changes in renal vascular resistance may include progesterone and relaxin (via upregulation of vascular matrix metalloproteinase-2). Agents elaborated by the endothelium, such as endothelin (ET) (via activation of ET_B receptor subtype) and nitric oxide (via increased cyclic guanosine -3',5'-monophosphate), are likely to be critically involved in the reduction of renal vascular resistance. An additional factor is the increased cardiac output, which permits increased renal perfusion without depriving other organs of blood flow.

Urinary flow and sodium excretion rates in late pregnancy are increased 2-fold in lateral recumbency compared with the supine position. Thus measurements of urinary function must take into account maternal posture. Collection periods should be at least 12–24 hours to allow for errors caused by the large urinary dead space. However, reasonable estimates of urinary excretion of a particular substance over shorter time periods generally can be calculated by referencing the level to the creatinine concentration in the same sample of urine (substance/creatinine ratio) with the assumption that a pregnant woman excretes 1 g of creatinine per day. Creatinine production (0.7–1.0 g/day) by skeletal muscle is virtually unchanged by pregnancy.

Up to 80% of the glomerular filtrate is reabsorbed by the proximal tubules, a process that is independent of hormonal control. Aldosterone regulates sodium reabsorption in the distal tubules, whereas arginine vasopressin activity, which regulates free water clearance, determines the ultimate urine concentration. Pregnancy is associated with

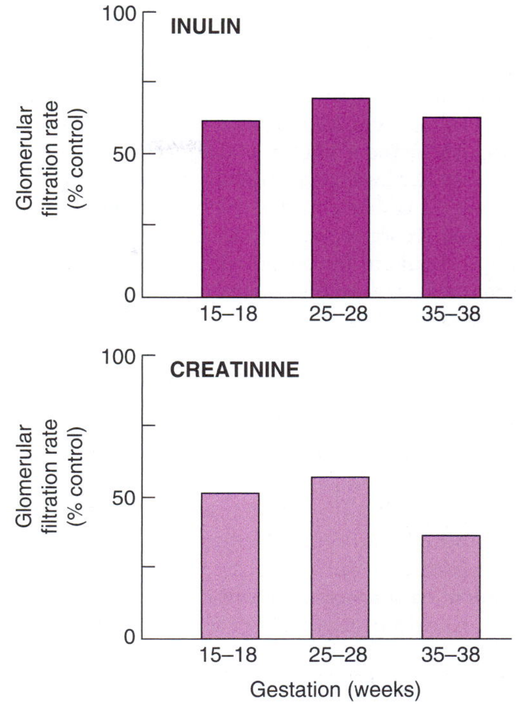

▲ **Figure 8–4.** Increases in glomerular filtration over gestation as reflected by changes in inulin and endogenous creatinine clearances. The % control represents relative change from postpartum values. (Data from Davison JM, Hytten FE. Glomerular filtration during and after pregnancy. *J Obstet Gynaecol Br Commonw* 1974;81:558.)

increased circulating concentrations of aldosterone. Even though the GFR increases dramatically during gestation, the volume of urine excreted per day is unchanged.

Renal clearance of creatinine increases as the GFR rises, with maximum clearances approximately 50% more than nonpregnant levels. The creatinine clearance decreases somewhat after approximately 30 weeks of gestation. The rise in GFR lowers mean serum creatinine concentrations (pregnant, 0.46 ± 0.13 mg/100 mL; nonpregnant, 0.67 ± 0.14 mg/100 mL) and blood urea nitrogen (pregnant, 8.17 ± 1.5 mg/100 mL; nonpregnant, 13 ± 3 mg/100 mL) concentrations.

Increased GFR with saturation of tubular resorption capacity for filtered glucose can result in glucosuria. In fact, more than 50% of women have glucosuria sometime during pregnancy. Increased urinary glucose levels contribute to increased susceptibility of pregnant women to urinary tract infection.

Urinary protein loss normally does not exceed 300 mg over 24 hours, which is similar to the nonpregnant state.

Thus proteinuria of more than 300 mg over 24 hours suggests a renal disorder.

Renin activity increases early in the first trimester and continues to rise until term. This enzyme is critically involved in the conversion of angiotensinogen to angiotensin I, which subsequently forms the potent vasoconstrictor angiotensin II. Angiotensin II levels also increase in pregnancy, but the vasoconstriction and hypertension that might be expected do not occur. In fact, normal pregnant women are very resistant to the pressor effects of elevated levels of angiotensin II and other vasopressors; this effect is likely mediated by increased vascular synthesis of nitric oxide and other vasodilators.

Angiotensin II is also a potent stimulus for adrenocortical secretion of aldosterone, which, in conjunction with arginine vasopressin, promotes salt and water retention in pregnancy. The net effect is a decrease in plasma sodium concentrations by approximately 5 mEq/L and a fall in plasma osmolality by nearly 10 mOsm/kg. These effects on electrolyte homeostasis likely involve a resetting of the pituitary osmostat. In pregnancy, the increased pituitary secretion of vasopressin is largely balanced by placental production of vasopressinase. Pregnant women who are unable to sufficiently augment vasopressin secretion can develop a diabetes insipidus–like condition characterized by massive diuresis and profound hypernatremia. Cases have been described with maternal sodium levels reaching 170 mEq/L.

Bladder

As the uterus enlarges, the urinary bladder is displaced upward and flattened in the anteroposterior diameter. One of the earliest symptoms of pregnancy is increased urinary frequency, which may be related to pregnancy hormones. In later gestation, mechanical effects of the enlarged uterus may contribute to the increased frequency. Bladder vascularity increases and muscle tone decreases, which increases bladder capacity up to 1500 mL.

GASTROINTESTINAL SYSTEM

Anatomic Changes

As the uterus grows, the stomach is pushed upward and the large and small bowels extend into more rostrolateral regions. Historically, it has been believed that the appendix is displaced superiorly in the right flank area. Recent literature has called this, and other common assumptions regarding pregnancy-associated changes, in to question. It is clear that organs return to their normal positions in the early puerperium.

Oral Cavity

Salivation appears to increase, although this may be caused in part by swallowing difficulty associated with nausea. Pregnancy does not predispose to tooth decay or to mobilization of bone calcium.

The gums may become hypertrophic and hyperemic; often, they are so spongy and friable that they bleed easily. This may be caused by increased systemic estrogen because similar problems sometimes occur with the use of oral contraceptives.

Esophagus & Stomach

Reflux symptoms (heartburn) affect 30–80% of pregnant women. Gastric production of hydrochloric acid is variable and sometimes exaggerated but more commonly reduced. Pregnancy is associated with greater production of gastrin, which increases stomach volume and acidity of gastric secretions. Gastric production of mucus also may be increased. Esophageal peristalsis is decreased. Most women first report symptoms of reflux in the first trimester (52% vs. 24% in the second trimester vs. 8.8% in the third trimester), although the symptoms can become more severe with advanced gestation.

The underlying predisposition to reflux in pregnancy is related to hormone-mediated relaxation of the lower esophageal sphincter (Fig. 8–5). With advancing gestation, the lower esophageal sphincter has decreased pressure as well as blunted responses to sphincter stimulation. Thus decreased motility, increased acidity of gastric secretions, and reduced function of the lower esophageal sphincter contribute to the increased gastric reflux. The increased prevalence of gastric reflux and delayed gastric emptying

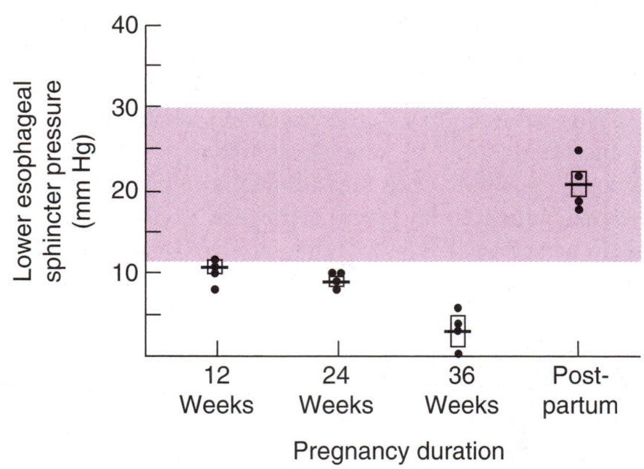

▲ **Figure 8–5.** Lower esophageal sphincter pressures for 3 periods of pregnancy and the postpartum state. The shaded area represents the normal range in nonpregnant women. The horizontal bars show the mean ± SE for measurements in 4 women. The rectangles show the mean ± SE for each gestational age. (Modified, with permission, from Van Theil DH, Gravaler JS, Joshi SN, et al. Heartburn in pregnancy. *Gastroenterology* 1977;72:666.)

of solid food make the gravida more vulnerable to regurgitation and aspiration with anesthesia. The rate of gastric emptying of solid foods is slowed in pregnancy, but the rate for liquids remains generally the same as in the nonpregnant state.

Intestines

Intestinal transit times are decreased in the second and third trimesters (Fig. 8–6), whereas first-trimester and postpartum transit times are similar. Transit times return to normal within 2–4 days postpartum.

The reduced gastrointestinal motility during pregnancy has been thought to be caused by increased circulating concentrations of progesterone. However, experimental evidence suggests that elevated estrogen concentrations are critically involved through an enhancement of nitric oxide release from the nonadrenergic, noncholinergic nerves that modulate gastrointestinal motility. Other factors may also be involved.

The slow transit time of food through the gastrointestinal tract potentially enhances water absorption, predisposing to constipation. However, diet and cultural expectations may be more important factors in this disorder.

Gallbladder

The emptying of the gallbladder is slowed in pregnancy and often incomplete. When visualized at caesarean delivery, the gallbladder commonly appears dilated and atonic. Bile stasis of pregnancy increases the risk for gallstone formation, although the chemical composition of bile is not appreciably altered.

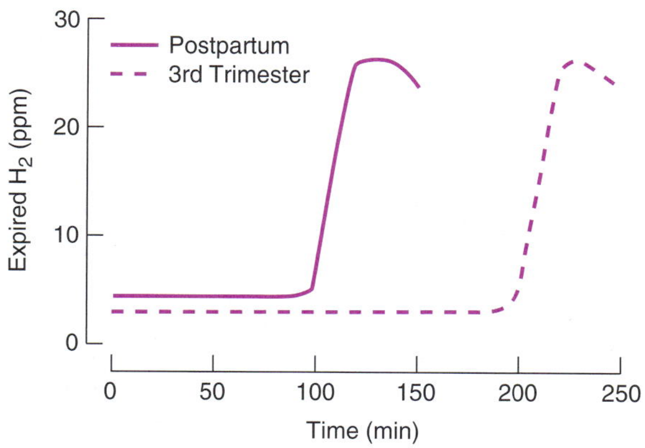

▲ **Figure 8–6.** Small-bowel transit times measured by the lactulose hydrogen breath method in a single woman in the third trimester and postpartum. Hydrogen concentrations in maternal breath were determined after administration of a lactulose meal. Hydrogen is released when bacteria in the colon break down lactulose. (Modified, with permission, from Wald A, Van Thiel DH, Hoeschstetter L, et al. Effect of pregnancy on gastrointestinal transit. *Dig Dis Sci* 1982;27:1015.)

Liver

Liver morphology does not change in normal pregnancy. Plasma albumin levels are reduced to a greater extent than the slight decrease in plasma globulins. This fall in the albumin/globulin ratio mimics liver disease in nonpregnant individuals. Serum alkaline phosphatase activity can double as the result of alkaline phosphatase isozymes produced by the placenta.

HEMATOLOGIC SYSTEM

Red Blood Cells

The red cell mass expands by approximately 33%, or by approximately 450 mL of erythrocytes for the average pregnant woman (Fig. 8–1). The increase is greater with iron supplementation. The greater increase in plasma volume accounts for the anemia of pregnancy. For example, maternal hemoglobin levels average 10.9 ± 0.8 (SD) g/dL in the second trimester and 12.4 ± 1.0 g/dL at term.

Iron

The enhanced erythropoiesis of pregnancy increases utilization of iron, which can reach 6–7 mg per day in the latter half of pregnancy. Many women begin pregnancy in an iron-deficient state, making them vulnerable to iron deficiency anemia. Thus supplemental iron is commonly given to pregnant women. Because the placenta actively transports iron from the mother to the fetus, the fetus generally is not anemic even when the mother is severely iron deficient.

White Blood Cells

The total blood leukocyte count increases during normal pregnancy from a prepregnancy level of 4300–4500/μL to 5000–12,000/μL in the last trimester, although counts as high as 16,000/μL have been observed in the last trimester. Counts in the 20,000–25,000/μL range can occur during labor. The cause of the rise in the leukocyte count, which primarily involves the polymorphonuclear forms, has not been established.

Polymorphonuclear leukocyte chemotaxis may be impaired in pregnancy, which appears to be a cell-associated defect. Reduced polymorphonuclear leukocyte adherence has been reported in the third trimester. These observations may predispose pregnant women to infection. Basophil counts decrease slightly as pregnancy advances. Eosinophil counts, although variable, remain largely unchanged.

Platelets

Some studies have reported increased production of platelets (thrombocytopoiesis) during pregnancy that is accompanied by progressive platelet consumption. Platelet counts fall below 150,000/μL in 6% of gravidas in the third trimester. This *pregnancy-associated thrombocytopenia*, which appears to be caused by increased peripheral consumption, resolves with delivery and is of no pathologic significance. Levels of prostacyclin (PGI_2), a platelet aggregation inhibitor, and thromboxane A_2, an inducer of platelet aggregation and a vasoconstrictor, increase during pregnancy.

Clotting Factors

Circulating levels of several coagulation factors increase in pregnancy. Fibrinogen (factor I) and factor VIII levels increase markedly, whereas factors VII, IX, X, and XII increase to a lesser extent.

Plasma fibrinogen concentrations begin to increase from nonpregnant levels (1.5–4.5 g/L) during the third month of pregnancy and progressively rise by nearly 2-fold by late pregnancy (4–6.5 g/L). The high estrogen levels of pregnancy may be involved in the increased fibrinogen synthesis by the liver.

Prothrombin (factor II) is only nominally affected by pregnancy. Factor V concentrations are mildly increased. Factor XI decreases slightly toward the end of pregnancy, and factor XIII (fibrin-stabilizing factor) is appreciably reduced, up to 50% at term. The free form of protein S declines in the first and second trimesters and remains low for the rest of gestation.

Fibrinolytic activity is depressed during pregnancy through a poorly understood mechanism. Plasminogen concentrations increase concomitantly with fibrinogen, but there is still a net procoagulant effect of pregnancy.

Coagulation and fibrinolytic systems undergo major alterations during pregnancy. Understanding these physiologic changes is critical for the management of some of the more serious pregnancy disorders, including hemorrhage and thromboembolic disease.

SKIN

Anatomic Changes

Hyperpigmentation is one of the well-recognized skin changes of pregnancy, which is manifested in the linea nigra and melasma, the *mask of pregnancy*. The latter, which is exacerbated by sun exposure, develops in up to 70% of pregnancies and is characterized by an uneven darkening of the skin in the centrofacial-malar area. The hyperpigmentation is probably because of the elevated concentrations of melanocyte-stimulating hormone and/or estrogen and progesterone effects on the skin. Similar hyperpigmentation of the face can be seen in nonpregnant women who are taking oral contraceptives.

Striae gravidarum consist of bands or lines of thickened, hyperemic skin. These "stretch marks" begin to appear in the second trimester on the abdomen, breasts, thighs, and buttocks. Decreased collagen adhesiveness and increased ground substance formation are characteristically seen in this skin condition. A genetic predisposition appears to be involved because not every gravida develops these skin changes. Effective treatment (preventive or therapeutic) has yet to be found.

Other common cutaneous changes include spider angiomas, palmar erythema, and cutis marmorata (mottled appearance of skin secondary to vasomotor instability). The development or worsening of varicosities accompanies nearly 40% of pregnancies. Compression of the vena cava by the gravid uterus increases venous pressures in the lower extremities, which dilates veins in the legs, anus (hemorrhoids), and vulva.

The nails and hair also undergo changes. Nails become brittle and can show horizontal grooves (Beau's lines). Thickening of the hair during pregnancy is caused by an increased number of follicles in anagen (growth) phase, and generalized hirsutism can worsen in women who already have hair that is thick or has a male pattern of distribution. The thickening of the hair ends 1–5 months postpartum with the onset of the telogen (resting) phase, which results in excessive shedding and thinning of hair. Normal hair growth returns within 12 months.

METABOLISM

Pregnancy increases nutritional requirements, and several maternal alterations occur to meet this demand. Pregnant women tend to rest more often, which conserves energy and thereby enhances fetal nutrition. The maternal appetite and food intake usually increase, although some have a decreased appetite or experience nausea and vomiting (see Chapter 6). In rare instances, women with pica may crave substances such as clay, cornstarch, soap, or even coal.

Pregnancy is associated with profound changes in structure and metabolism. The most obvious physical changes are weight gain and altered body shape. Weight gain results not only from the uterus and its contents, but also from increased breast tissue, blood volume, and water volume (approximately 6.8 L) in the form of extravascular and extracellular fluid. Deposition of fat and protein and increased cellular water are added to maternal stores. The average weight gain during pregnancy is 12.5 kg (27.5 lb).

Protein accretion accounts for approximately 1 kg of maternal weight gain, which is evenly divided between the mother (uterine contractile protein, breast glandular tissue, plasma protein, and hemoglobin) and the fetoplacental unit.

Total body fat increases during pregnancy, but the amount varies with the total weight gain. During the second half of pregnancy, plasma lipids increase (plasma cholesterol increases 50%, plasma triglyceride concentration may triple), but triglycerides, cholesterol, and lipoproteins decrease soon after delivery. The ratio of low-density lipoproteins to high-density lipoproteins increases during pregnancy. It has been suggested that most fat is stored centrally during midpregnancy and that as the fetus extracts more nutrition in the latter months, fat storage decreases.

Metabolism of carbohydrates and insulin during pregnancy is discussed in Chapter 31. Pregnancy is associated with insulin resistance, which can lead to hyperglycemia (gestational diabetes) in susceptible women. This metabolic disorder usually disappears after delivery, but may arise later in life as type 2 diabetes.

Maternal–Placental–Fetal Unit

Fetal genetics, physiology, anatomy, and biochemistry can now be studied with ultrasonography, fetoscopy, chorionic villus sampling, amniocentesis, and fetal cord and scalp blood sampling. Embryology and fetoplacental physiology must now be considered when providing direct patient care. Currently, some medical centers measure fetal pulse oximetry, fetal electroencephalograms, and fetal heart rate monitoring in determining the oxygenation status of the fetus. As the technology improves, we are reaching further into the early perinatal period to determine abnormal physiology and growth.

THE PLACENTA

A **placenta** may be defined as any intimate apposition or fusion of fetal organs to maternal tissues for physiologic exchange. The basic parenchyma of all placentas is the **trophoblast**; when this becomes a membrane penetrated by fetal **mesoderm**, it is called the **chorion**.

In the evolution of viviparous species, the yolk sac presumably is the most archaic type of placentation, having developed from the egg-laying ancestors of mammals. In higher mammals, the **allantoic sac** fuses with the chorion, forming the chorioallantoic placenta, which has mesodermal vascular villi. When the trophoblast actually invades the maternal endometrium (which in pregnancy is largely composed of decidua), a deciduate placenta results. In humans, maternal blood comes into direct contact with the fetal trophoblast.

DEVELOPMENT OF THE PLACENTA

Soon after ovulation, the endometrium develops its typical secretory pattern under the influence of progesterone from the corpus luteum. The peak of development occurs at approximately 1 week after ovulation, coinciding with the expected time for implantation of a fertilized ovum.

The first cleavage occurs during the next 36 hours after the cellular union of the egg and sperm. As the conceptus continues to divide and grow, the peristaltic activity of the uterine tube slowly transports it to the uterus, a journey that requires 6–7 days. Concomitantly, a series of divisions creates a hollow ball, the **blastocyst**, which then implants within the endometrium. Most cells in the wall of the blastocyst are trophoblastic; only a few are destined to become the embryo.

Within a few hours after implantation, the trophoblast invades the endometrium and begins to produce **human chorionic gonadotropin (hCG)**, which is thought to be important in converting the normal corpus luteum into the corpus luteum of pregnancy. As the cytotrophoblasts (**Langhans' cells**) divide and proliferate, they form transitional cells that are the likely source of hCG. Next, these transitional cells fuse, lose their individual membranes, and form the multinucleated **syncytiotrophoblast**. Mitotic division then ceases. Thus the syncytial layer becomes the front line of the invading fetal tissue. Maternal capillaries and venules are tapped by the invading fetal tissue to cause extravasation of maternal blood and the formation of small lakes (lacunae), the forerunners of the intervillous space. These lacunae fill with maternal blood by reflux from previously tapped veins. An occasional maternal artery then opens, and a sluggish circulation is established (hematotropic phase of the embryo).

The lacunar system is separated by trabeculae, many of which develop buds or extensions. Within these branching projections, the cytotrophoblast forms a mesenchymal core.

The proliferating trophoblast cells then branch to form secondary and tertiary villi. The **mesoblast**, or central stromal core, also formed from the original trophoblast, invades these columns to form a supportive structure within which capillaries are formed. The **embryonic body stalk** (later to become the umbilical cord) invades this stromal core to establish the fetoplacental circulation. If this last step does not occur, the embryo will die. Sensitive tests for hCG suggest that at this stage, more embryos die than live.

Where the placenta is attached, the branching villi resemble a leafy tree (the **chorion frondosum**), whereas the portion of the placenta covering the expanding conceptus is smoother (**chorion laeve**). When the latter is finally pushed against the opposite wall of the uterus, the villi atrophy, leaving the amnion and chorion to form the 2-layered sac of fetal membranes.

At approximately 40 days after conception, the trophoblast has invaded approximately 40–60 spiral arterioles, of which 12–15 may be called major arteries. The pulsatile arterial pressure of blood that spurts from each of these major vessels pushes the chorionic plate away from the decidua to form 12–15 "tents," or maternal **cotyledons**. The remaining 24–45 tapped arterioles form minor vascular units that become crowded between the larger units. As the chorionic plate is pushed away from the basal plate, the anchoring villi pull the maternal basal plate up into septa (columns of fibrous tissue that virtually surround the major cotyledons). Thus at the center of each maternal vascular unit there is 1 artery that terminates in a thin-walled sac, but there are numerous maternal veins that open through the basal plate at random. The human placenta has no peripheral venous collecting system. Within each maternal vascular unit is the fetal vascular "tree," with the tertiary free-floating villi (the major area for physiologic exchange) acting as thousands of baffles that disperse the maternal bloodstream in many directions.

FUNCTIONS OF THE MATERNAL–PLACENTAL–FETAL UNIT

The placenta is a complex organ of internal secretion, releasing numerous hormones and enzymes into the maternal bloodstream. In addition, it serves as the organ of transport for all fetal nutrients and metabolic products as well as for the exchange of oxygen and CO_2. Although fetal in origin, the placenta depends almost entirely on maternal blood for its nourishment.

The arterial pressure of maternal blood (60–70 mm Hg) causes it to pulsate toward the chorionic plate into the low-pressure (20 mm Hg) intervillous space. Venous blood in the placenta tends to flow along the basal plate and out through the venules directly into maternal veins. The pressure gradient within the fetal circulation changes slowly with the mother's posture, fetal movements, and physical stress. The pressure within the placental intervillous space is approximately 10 mm Hg when the pregnant woman is lying down. After a few minutes of standing, this pressure exceeds 30 mm Hg. In comparison, the fetal capillary pressure is 20–40 mm Hg.

Clinically, placental perfusion can be altered by many physiologic changes in the mother or fetus. When a precipitous fall in maternal blood pressure occurs, increased plasma volume improves placental perfusion. Increasing the maternal volume with saline infusion increases the fetal oxygen saturation. An increased rate of rhythmic uterine contractions benefits placental perfusion, but tetanic labor contractions are detrimental to placental and fetal circulation as they do not allow a resting period in which normal flow resumes to the fetus. An increased fetal heart rate tends to expand the villi during systole, but this is a minor aid in circulatory transfer.

Circulatory Function

A. Uteroplacental Circulation

The magnitude of the uteroplacental circulation is difficult to measure in humans. The consensus is that total uterine blood flow near term is 500–700 mL/min. Not all of this blood traverses the intervillous space. It is generally assumed that approximately 85% of the uterine blood flow goes to the cotyledons and the rest to the myometrium and endometrium. One may assume that blood flow in the placenta is 400–500 mL/min in a patient near term who is lying quietly on her side and is not in labor.

As the placenta matures, thrombosis decreases the number of arterial openings into the basal plate. At term, the ratio of veins to arteries is 2:1 (approximately the ratio found in other mature organs).

Near their entry into the intervillous spaces, the terminal maternal arterioles lose their elastic reticulum. Because the distal portions of these vessels are lost with the placenta, bleeding from their source can be controlled only by uterine contraction. Thus uterine atony causes postpartum hemorrhage.

B. Plasma Volume Expansion & Spiral Artery Changes

Structural alterations occur in the human uterine spiral arteries found in the decidual part of the placental bed. As a consequence of the action of cytotrophoblast on the spiral artery vessel wall, the normal musculoelastic tissue is replaced by a mixture of fibrinoid and fibrous tissue. The small spiral arteries are converted to large tortuous channels, creating low-resistance channels or arteriovenous shunts.

In early normal pregnancy, there is an early increase in plasma volume and resulting physiologic anemia as the red blood cell mass slowly expands. Immediately after delivery, with closure of the placental shunt, diuresis and natriuresis occur. When the spiral arteries fail to undergo these physiologic changes, fetal growth retardation often occurs with preeclampsia. "Evaluating uterine arteries, which serve the spiral arteries and the placenta in the pregnant women, offers an indirect method of monitoring the spiral arteries." Fleischer and colleagues (1986) reported that normal pregnancy is associated with a uterine artery Doppler velocimetry systolic/diastolic ratio of less than 2:6. With a higher ratio and a notch in the waveform, the pregnancy is usually complicated by stillbirth, premature birth, intrauterine growth retardation, or preeclampsia.

C. Fetoplacental Circulation

At term, a normal fetus has a total umbilical blood flow of 350–400 mL/min. Thus the maternoplacental and fetoplacental flows have a similar order of magnitude.

The villous system is best compared with an inverted tree. The branches pass obliquely downward and outward within the intervillous spaces. This arrangement probably permits preferential currents or gradients of flow and undoubtedly encourages intervillous fibrin deposition, commonly seen in the mature placenta.

Cotyledons (subdivisions of the placenta) can be identified early in placentation. Although they are separated by the placental septa, some communication occurs via the subchorionic lake in the roof of the intervillous spaces.

Before labor, placental filling occurs whenever the uterus contracts (*Braxton Hicks contractions*). At these times, the maternal venous exits are closed, but the thicker-walled arteries are only slightly narrowed. When the uterus relaxes, blood drains out through the maternal veins. Hence blood is not squeezed out of the placental lake with each contraction, nor does it enter the placental lake in appreciably greater amounts during relaxation.

During the height of an average first-stage contraction, most of the cotyledons are devoid of any flow and the remainder are only partially filled. Thus, intermittently—for periods of up to a minute—maternoplacental flow virtually ceases. Therefore, it should be evident that any extended prolongation of the contractile phase, as in uterine tetany, could lead to fetal hypoxia.

Endocrine Function

A. Secretions of the Maternal–Placental–Fetal Unit

The placenta and the maternal–placental–fetal unit produce increasing amounts of steroids late in the first trimester. Of greatest importance are the steroids required in fetal development from 7 weeks' gestation through parturition. Immediately after conception and until 12–13 weeks' gestation, the principal source of circulating gestational steroids (progesterone is the major one) is the corpus luteum of pregnancy.

After 42 days, the placenta assumes an increasingly important role in the production of several steroid hormones. Steroid production by the embryo occurs even before implantation is detectable in utero. Before implantation, production of progesterone by the embryo may assist ovum transport.

Once implantation occurs, trophoblastic hCG and other pregnancy-related peptides are secreted. A more sophisticated array of fetoplacental steroids is produced during organogenesis and with the development of a functioning hypothalamic–pituitary–adrenal axis. Adenohypophyseal basophilic cells first appear at approximately 8 weeks in the development of the fetus and indicate the presence of significant quantities of adrenocorticotropic hormone (ACTH). The first adrenal primordial structures are identified at approximately 4 weeks, and the fetal adrenal cortex develops in concert with the adenohypophysis.

The fetus and the placenta acting in concert are the principal sources of steroid hormones controlling intrauterine growth, maturation of vital organs, and parturition. The fetal adrenal cortex is much larger than its adult counterpart. From midtrimester until term, the large inner mass of the fetal adrenal gland (80% of the adrenal tissue) is known as the **fetal zone.** This tissue is supported by factors unique to the fetal status and regresses rapidly after birth. The outer zone ultimately becomes the bulk of the postnatal and adult cortex.

The trophoblastic mass increases exponentially through the seventh week, after which time the growth velocity gradually increases to an asymptote close to term. The fetal zone and placenta exchange steroid precursors to make possible the full complement of fetoplacental steroids. Formation and regulation of steroid hormones also take place within the fetus itself.

In addition to the steroids, another group of placental hormones unique to pregnancy are the polypeptide hormones, each of which has an analogue in the pituitary. These placental protein hormones include hCG and human chorionic somatomammotropin. The existence of placental human chorionic corticotropin also has been suggested.

A summary of the hormones produced by the maternal–placental–fetal unit is shown in Table 8–2.

B. Placental Secretions

1. Human chorionic gonadotropin—hCG was the first of the placental protein hormones to be described. It is a glycoprotein that has biologic and immunologic similarities to the luteinizing hormone (LH) from the pituitary. Recent evidence suggests that hCG is produced by the syncytiotrophoblast of the placenta. hCG is elaborated by all types of trophoblastic tissue, including that of hydatidiform moles, chorioadenoma destruens, and choriocarcinoma. As with all glycoprotein hormones (LH, follicle-stimulating hormone, thyroid-stimulating hormone [TSH]), hCG is composed of 2 subunits, α and β. The α subunit is common to all glycoproteins, and the β subunit confers unique specificity to the hormone.

Antibodies have been developed to the β subunit of hCG. This specific reaction allows for differentiation of hCG from pituitary LH. hCG is detectable 9 days after the midcycle LH peak, which occurs 8 days after ovulation and only 1 day after implantation. This measurement is useful because it can detect pregnancy in all patients on day 11 after fertilization. Concentrations of hCG rise exponentially until 9–10 weeks' gestation, with a doubling time of 1.3–2 days.

Concentrations peak at 60–90 days' gestation. Afterward, hCG levels decrease to a plateau that is maintained until delivery. The half-life of hCG is approximately 32–37 hours, in contrast to that of most protein and steroid hormones, which have half-lives measured in minutes. Structural characteristics of the hCG molecule allow it to interact with the human TSH receptor in activation of the membrane adenylate cyclase that regulates thyroid cell function. The finding of hCG-specific adenylate stimulation in the placenta may mean that hCG provides "order regulation" within the cell of the trophoblast.

2. Human chorionic somatomammotropin—Human chorionic somatomammotropin (hCS), previously referred to as designated **human placental lactogen**, is a protein hormone with immunologic and biologic similarities to the pituitary growth hormone. It is synthesized in the syncytiotrophoblastic layer of the placenta. It can be found

Table 8–2. Summary of maternal–placental–fetal endocrine-paracrine functions.

Peptides of exclusively placental origin
Human chorionic gonadotropin (hCG)
Human chorionic somatomammotropin (hCS)
Human chorionic corticotropin (hCC)
Pregnancy-associated plasma proteins (PAPP)
PAPP-A
PAPP-B
PAPP-C
PAPP-D (hCS)
Pregnancy-associated β_1 macroglobulin (β_1 PAM)
Pregnancy-associated α_2 macroglobulin (α_2 PAM)
Pregnancy-associated major basic protein (pMBP)
Placental proteins (PP) 1 through 21
Placental membrane proteins (MP) 1 through 7.
MP1 also known as placental alkaline phosphatase (PLAP)
Hypothalamic-like hormone (β-endorphin, ACTH-like)
Steroid of mainly placental origin
Progesterone
Hormones of maternal–placental–fetal origin
Estrone
Estradiol 50% from maternal androgens
Hormone of placental–fetal origin
Estriol
Hormone of corpus luteum of pregnancy
Relaxin
Fetal hormones
Thyroid hormone
Fetal adrenal zone hormones
α-Melanocyte-stimulating hormone
Corticotropin intermediate lobe peptide
Anterior pituitary hormone
Adrenocorticotropic hormone (ACTH)
Tropic hormones for fetal zone of placenta
β-Endorphin
β-Lipotropin

in maternal serum and urine in both normal and molar pregnancies. However, it disappears so rapidly from serum and urine after delivery of the placenta or evacuation of the uterus that it cannot be detected in the serum after the first postpartum day. The somatotropic activity of hCS is 3%, which is less than that of human growth hormone (hGH). In vitro, hCS stimulates thymidine incorporation into DNA and enhances the action of hGH and insulin. It is present in microgram-per-milliliter quantities in early pregnancy, but its concentration increases as pregnancy progresses, with peak levels reached during the last 4 weeks. Prolonged fasting at midgestation and insulin-induced hypoglycemia are reported to raise hCS concentrations. hCS may exert its major metabolic effect on the mother to ensure that the nutritional demands of the fetus are met.

It has been suggested that hCS is the "growth hormone" of pregnancy. The in vivo effects of hCS owing to its growth hormonelike and anti-insulin characteristics result in impaired glucose uptake and stimulation of free fatty acid release, with resultant decrease in insulin effect.

3. Placental proteins—A number of proteins thought to be specific to the pregnant state have been isolated. The most commonly known are the 4 pregnancy-associated plasma proteins (PAPPs) designated as PAPP-A, PAPP-B, PAPP-C, and PAPP-D. PAPP-D is the hormone hCS (described earlier). All these proteins are produced by the placenta and/or decidua. The physiologic role of these proteins, except for PAPP-D, are at present unclear. Numerous investigators have postulated various functions, ranging from facilitating fetal "allograft" survival and the regulation of coagulation and complement cascades to the maintenance of the placenta and the regulation of carbohydrate metabolism in pregnancy. In vitro studies of PAPP-A in knockout mouse models show it functioning as a regulator of local insulin-like growth factor bioavailability.

C. Fetoplacental Secretions

The placenta may be an incomplete steroid-producing organ that must rely on precursors reaching it from the fetal and maternal circulations (an integrated-maternal–placental–fetal unit). The adult steroid-producing glands can form progestins, androgens, and estrogens, but this is not true of the placenta. Estrogen production by the placenta is dependent on precursors reaching it from both the fetal and maternal compartments. Placental progesterone formation is accomplished in large part from circulating maternal cholesterol.

In the placenta, cholesterol is converted to pregnenolone and then rapidly and efficiently to progesterone. Production of progesterone approximates 250 mg per day by the end of pregnancy, at which time circulating levels are on the order of 130 mg/mL. To form estrogens, the placenta, which has an active aromatizing capacity, uses circulating androgens obtained primarily from the fetus but also from the mother.

The major androgenic precursor is **dehydroepiandrosterone sulfate (DHEAS)**. This compound comes from the fetal adrenal gland. Because the placenta has an abundance of sulfatase (sulfate-cleaving) enzyme, DHEAS is converted to free unconjugated DHEA when it reaches the placenta, then to androstenedione, testosterone, and finally estrone and 17β-estradiol.

The major estrogen formed in pregnancy is estriol; however, its functional value is not well understood. It appears to be effective in increasing uteroplacental blood flow, as it has a relatively weak estrogenic effect on other organ systems. Ninety percent of the estrogen in the urine of pregnant women is estriol.

Circulating progesterone and estriol are thought to be important during pregnancy because they are present in such large amounts. Progesterone may play a role in maintaining the myometrium in a state of relative quiescence during much of pregnancy. A high local (intrauterine) concentration of progesterone may block cellular immune responses to foreign antigens. Progesterone appears to be essential for maintaining pregnancy in almost all mammals examined. This suggests that progesterone may be instrumental in conferring immunologic privilege to the uterus.

Placental Transport

The placenta has a high rate of metabolism, with consumption of oxygen and glucose occurring at a faster rate than in the fetus. Presumably, this high metabolism requirement is caused by multiple transport and biosynthesis activities.

The primary function of the placenta is the transport of oxygen and nutrients to the fetus and the reverse transfer of CO_2, urea, and other catabolites back to the mother. In general, those compounds that are essential for the minute-by-minute homeostasis of the fetus (eg, oxygen, CO_2, water, sodium) are transported very rapidly by diffusion. Compounds required for the synthesis of new tissues (eg, amino acids, enzyme cofactors such as vitamins) are transported by an active process. Substances such as certain maternal hormones, which may modify fetal growth and are at the upper limits of admissible molecular size, may diffuse very slowly, whereas proteins such as IgG immunoglobulins probably reach the fetus by the process of pinocytosis. This transfer takes place by at least 5 mechanisms: simple diffusion, facilitated diffusion, active transport, pinocytosis, and leakage.

A. Mechanisms of Transport

1. Simple diffusion—Simple diffusion is the method by which gases and other simple molecules cross the placenta. The rate of transport depends on the chemical gradient, the diffusion constant of the compound in question, and the total area of the placenta available for transfer (Fick's law). The chemical gradient (ie, the differences in concentration in fetal and maternal plasma) is in turn affected by the rates of flow of uteroplacental and umbilical blood. Simple diffusion is also the method of transfer for exogenous compounds such as drugs.

2. Facilitated diffusion—The prime example of a substance transported by facilitated diffusion is glucose, the major source of energy for the fetus. Presumably, a carrier system operates *with* the chemical gradient (as opposed to active transport, which operates *against* the gradient) and may become saturated at high glucose concentrations. In the steady state, the glucose concentration in fetal plasma is approximately two-thirds that of the maternal concentration, reflecting the rapid rate of fetal utilization. Substances of low molecular weight, minimal electric charge, and high lipid solubility diffuse across the placenta with ease.

3. Active transport—Selective transport of specific essential nutrients and amnio acids are accomplished by enzymatic mechanisms.

4. Pinocytosis—Electron microscopy has shown pseudopodial projections of the syncytiotrophoblastic layer that reach out to surround minute amounts of maternal plasma. These particles are carried across the cell virtually intact to be released on the other side, whereupon they promptly gain access to the fetal circulation. Certain other proteins (eg, foreign antigens) may be immunologically rejected. This process may work both to and from the fetus, but the selectivity of the process has not been determined. Complex proteins, small amounts of fat, some immunoglobulins, and even viruses may traverse the placenta in this way. For the passage of complex proteins, highly selective processes involving special receptors are involved. For example, maternal antibodies of the IgG class are freely transferred, whereas other antibodies are not.

5. Leakage—Gross breaks in the placental membrane may occur, allowing the passage of intact cells. Despite the fact that the hydrostatic pressure gradient is normally from fetus to mother, tagged red cells and white cells have been found to travel in either direction. Such breaks probably occur most often during labor or with placental disruption (abruptio placentae, placenta previa, or trauma), caesarean section, or intrauterine fetal death. It is at these times that fetal red cells can most often be demonstrated in the maternal circulation. This is the mechanism by which the mother may become sensitized to fetal red cell antigens such as the D (Rh) antigen.

B. Placental Transport of Drugs

The placental membranes are often referred to as a "barrier" to fetal transfer, but there are few substances (eg, drugs) that will not cross the membranes at all. A few compounds, such as heparin and insulin, are of sufficiently large molecular size or charge that minimal transfer occurs. This lack of transfer is almost unique among drugs. Most medications are transferred from the maternal to the fetal circulation by simple diffusion, the rate of which is determined by the respective gradients of the drugs.

These diffusion gradients are influenced in turn by a number of serum factors, including the degree of drug-protein binding (eg, sex hormone binding globulin). Because serum albumin concentration is considerably lower during pregnancy, drugs that bind almost exclusively to plasma albumin (eg, warfarin, salicylates) may have relatively higher unbound concentrations and, therefore, an effectively higher placental gradient. By contrast, a compound such as carbon monoxide may attach itself so strongly to the increased total hemoglobin that there will be little left in the plasma for transport.

The placenta also acts as a lipoidal resistance factor to the transfer of water-soluble foreign organic chemicals; as a result, chemicals and drugs that are readily soluble in lipids are transferred much more easily across the placental barrier than are water-soluble drugs or molecules. Ionized drug molecules are highly water soluble and are therefore poorly transmitted across the placenta. Because ionization of chemicals depends in part on their pH-pK relationships, multiple factors determine this "simple diffusion" of drugs across the placenta. Obviously, drug transfer is not simple, and one must assume that some amount of almost any drug will cross the placenta.

ANATOMIC DISORDERS OF THE PLACENTA

Observation of structural alterations within the placenta may indicate fetal and maternal disease that otherwise might go undetected.

Twin-Twin Transfusion Syndrome

Nearly all monochorionic twin placentas show an anastomosis between the vessels of the 2 umbilical circulations, but differ in number, direction, and size of the anastomoses. These usually involve the major branches of the arteries and veins in the placental surface. Artery-to-artery communications are found in 75% of the monochorionic twin placentas. Less frequently found are vein-to-vein and artery-to-vein anastomoses. Of great pathologic significance are deep arteriovenous communications between the 2 circulations. This occurs when there are shared lobules supplied by an umbilical arterial branch from one fetus and drained by an umbilical vein branch of the other fetus. This is found in approximately half of all monochorionic twin placentas. Fortunately, one-way flow to the shared lobule may be compensated for by reverse flow through a superficial arterioarterial or venovenous anastomosis, if they coexist.

Twin-twin transfusion syndrome (TTS) arises when shared lobules causing blood flow from one twin to the other are not compensated for by the presence of superficial anastomosis or by shared lobules, causing flow in the opposite direction. This syndrome occurs in 15–20% of cases of monochorial placentation The twin receiving the transfusion is plethoric and polycythemic and may show cardiomegaly. The donor twin is pale and anemic and may have organ weights similar to those seen in the intrauterine malnutrition form of small for gestational age.

Placental Infarction

A placental infarct is an area of ischemic necrosis of placental villi resulting from obstruction of blood flow through the spiral arteries as a result of thrombosis. The lesions have a lobular distribution. However, the spiral arteries are not true end arteries, and if there is adequate flow through the arteries supplying adjacent lobules, sufficient circulation will be maintained to prevent necrosis. Thus ischemic necrosis of one placental lobule probably indicates not only that the spiral artery supplying the infarcted lobule is thrombosed, but that flow through adjacent spiral arteries is severely impaired. Placental infarction may serve as a mechanism allowing the fetus to redistribute blood flow to those placental lobules that are adequately supplied by the maternal circulation. Although often seen in mature placentas at low levels, the infarct must be extensive before the fetus is physiologically impaired.

Chorioangioma of the Placenta

A benign neoplasm occurring in approximately 1% of placentas and composed of fetoplacental capillaries may occur within the placenta. It is grossly visible as a purple-red, apparently encapsulated mass, variable in size, and occasionally multicentered. Placental hemangiomas, or "chorioangiomas," that measure 5 cm or more may be linked with maternal, fetal, and neonatal complications due to arteriovenous shunting of blood away from the fetus. Many placental tumors are accompanied by hydramnios, hemorrhage, preterm delivery, and fetal growth restriction.

Amniotic Bands

Close inspection of the fetal membranes, particularly near the umbilical cord insertion, may reveal band or stringlike membrane segments that are easily lifted above the placental surface. The origin of amniotic bands is unclear. Proposed mechanism include tearing in the amnion early in pregnancy as well as inherited developmental abnormality. They may cause constriction of the developing limbs or other digits. Amputation has been known to result. Syndactyly, clubfoot, and fusion deformities of the cranium and face may also be explained in certain instances on the basis of amniotic bands.

Placental Pathology

Any infant born with a complication may benefit from histologic evaluation of the placenta and umbilical cord.

Histopathologic features of a placenta with uteroplacental insufficiency include nonmarginal infarcts, shrunken placental villi, increased syncytial knots, increased perivillous fibrin, and multifocal and diffuse fibrin deposition. Similarly, if the ratio of nucleated red blood cells to leukocytes exceeds 2:3, this indicates fetal hypoxic stress. Chorangiosis is a pathologic change that indicates long-standing placental hypoperfusion or low-grade tissue hypoxia.

The presence of meconium and its location can also give insight into the possible time of the presumed insult. Under gross observation, meconium will stain the placenta and cord after 1–3 hours of exposure. Stained infant fingernails indicate meconium exposure for at least 6 hours. Stained vernix equates with exposure of meconium for 15 hours or longer.

Microscopic evaluation also sheds light on the timing of the release of meconium. Meconium-laden macrophages at the chorionic surface of the placenta can be seen when meconium has been present for 2–3 hours. When these macrophages are found deep within the extraplacental membranes, meconium has been present for at least 6–12 hours.

Lastly, when evaluation of the umbilical cord demonstrates necrobiotic and necrotic arterial media with surrounding meconium-laden macrophages, the release of meconium occurred more than 48 hours before delivery.

Abnormalities of Placental Implantation

Normally the placenta selects a location on the endometrium that benefits the growing fetus. However, there are numerous instances when the placental implantation site is not beneficial.

Placenta previa, or the implantation of the placenta over the cervical os, is the most common. The incidence at 12 weeks' gestation is approximately 6% because of the advancement of transvaginal imaging. Fortunately, most cases of placenta previa resolve by the time of delivery (reported incidence of 5/1000 births). A marginal placenta previa occurs when the edge of the placenta lies within 2–3 cm of the cervical os; the prevalence ranges from 10–45% when the less accurate abdominal ultra-sonogram is used.

Associated consequences of these abnormal placentation sites include increased risk for bleeding, both for the mother and the fetus, increased need for caesarean delivery, and possible risk of placenta accreta and increta or percreta, abruption, and growth restriction. Once the placental edge moves beyond 2–3 cm from the cervical os, these risks are minimized.

Placenta accreta is the most dangerous consequence of placenta previa. It involves abnormal trophoblastic invasion beyond the Nitabuch's layer. Placenta increta is the term used to describe invasion into the myometrium. Placenta percreta describes invasion through the serosa with possible invasion into surrounding tissues such as the bladder. Placenta accreta is associated with life-threatening postpartum hemorrhage and increased need for immediate hysterectomy.

The risk factors for placenta previa and placenta accreta are similar. Advanced maternal age, increased parity, and prior uterine surgery are common risk factors for both entities. The strongest correlation appears to exist with prior uterine surgeries. The prevalence of placenta previa after 1 prior caesarean delivery reaches 0.65% versus 0.26% in the unscarred uterus. However, after 4 or more caesarean deliveries the prevalence reaches 10%. Similarly, the frequency of accreta in the presence of placenta previa increases as the number of uterine surgeries increases. In patients with 1 prior uterine surgery, accreta occurs in 24% of placenta previas, whereas after 4 or more surgeries, the frequency of placenta accreta may be as high as 67%.

Placenta accreta may be suspected with certain ultrasound findings such as loss of the hypoechoic retroplacental myometrial zone, thinning or disruption of the hyperechoic uterine serosa-bladder interface, or with visualization of an exophytic mass. In all cases of placenta previa, and especially if placenta accreta is suspected, the patient must be counseled that hysterectomy may be needed to control excessive bleeding after delivery. Blood products must be available before delivery of the infant to ensure prompt replacement.

THE UMBILICAL CORD

Development

In the early stages, the embryo has a thick embryonic stalk containing 2 umbilical arteries, 1 large umbilical vein, the allantois, and the primary mesoderm. The arteries carry blood from the embryo to the chorionic villi, and the umbilical vein returns blood to the embryo. The umbilical vein and 2 arteries twist around one another.

In the fifth week of gestation, the amnion expands to fill the entire extraembryonic coelom. This process forces the yolk sac against the embryonic stalk and covers the entire contents with a tube of amniotic ectoderm, forming the umbilical cord. The cord is narrower in diameter than the embryonic stalk and rapidly increases in length. The connective tissue of the umbilical cord is called **Wharton's jelly** and is derived from the primary mesoderm. The umbilical cord can be found in loops around the baby's neck in approximately 23% of normal spontaneous vertex deliveries.

At birth, the mature cord is approximately 50–60 cm in length and 12 mm in diameter. A long cord is defined as more than 100 cm, and a short cord as less than 30 cm. There may be as many as 40 spiral twists in the cord, as well as false knots and true knots. When umbilical blood flow is interrupted at birth, the intra-abdominal sections of the umbilical arteries and vein gradually become fibrous cords. The course of the umbilical vein is discernible in the adult as a fibrous cord from the umbilicus to the liver (ligamentum teres) contained within the falciform ligament. The umbilical arteries are retained proximally as the internal iliac arteries and give off the superior vesicle arteries and the medial umbilical ligaments within the medial umbilical folds to the umbilicus. When the umbilical cord is cut and the end examined at the time of delivery, the vessels ordinarily are collapsed.

Analysis of the Umbilical Cord in Fetal Abnormalities

A segment of umbilical cord should be kept available as a source of umbilical cord blood for blood gas measurements at the time of delivery. Cord blood gases are a more objective measure of oxygenation than Apgar scores.

ABNORMALITIES OF THE UMBILICAL CORD

Velamentous Insertion

In velamentous insertion, the umbilical vessels divide to course through the membranes before reaching the chorionic plate. Velamentous insertion occurs in approximately 1% of placentas in singleton pregnancies, with multiple gestations having a 6–9 times higher incidence. When these vessels present themselves ahead of the fetus (vasa previa), they may rupture during labor or before to cause fetal exsanguination. When painless vaginal bleeding occurs, the blood may be tested to determine whether it is of fetal origin (Apt test). In practical terms, a high index of suspicion for vasa previa is needed because the time to fetal collapse with bleeding from vasa previa is often too rapid to allow test interpretation.

Short Umbilical Cord

It appears from indirect evidence in the human fetus that the length of the umbilical cord at term is determined by the amount of amniotic fluid present during the first and second trimesters and by the mobility of the fetus. If oligohydramnios, amniotic bands, or limitation of fetal motion occur for any reason, the umbilical cord will not develop to an average length. Amniocentesis performed to produce oligohydramnios in pregnant rats at 14–16 days results in significant reduction of umbilical cord length. The length of the umbilical cord does not vary with fetal weight, presentation, or placental size. Simple mechanical factors may determine the eventual length of the cord.

Knots in the Umbilical Cord

True knots occur in the cord in 1% of deliveries, leading to a perinatal loss of 6.1% in such cases. False knots are developmental variations with no clinical importance.

Loops of the Umbilical Cord

Twisting of the cord about the fetus may be the reason for excessive cord length. One loop of cord is present about the neck in 21% of deliveries, 2 loops in 2.5%, and 3 loops in 0.2%. The presence of loops increases as the amount of amniotic fluid increases, as the length of the umbilical cord increases and as fetal movement increases. When 3 loops are present, the cord is usually longer than 70 cm. One study of 1000 consecutive deliveries found 1 or more loops of cord around the neck in approximately 24% of cases. Retrospective studies suggest that neither single nor multiple loops are associated with adverse fetal outcomes.

Torsion of the Umbilical Cord

Torsion of the cord occurs counterclockwise in most cases. If twisting is extreme, fetal asphyxia may result.

Single Artery

A 2-vessel cord (absence of 1 umbilical artery) occurs in approximately 0.2–11% pregnancies, with risks depending on multiple gestation, ethnicity, maternal age, fetal sex, and smoking. The cause may be aplasia or atrophy of the missing vessel. The presence of single umbilical artery increases the risk for congenital and chromosomal anomalies. Associated malformations include neural tube defects, cardiac defects, genitourinary malformations, gastrointestinal malformations, and respiratory malformations. Acardiac twinning has also been documented. Level III ultrasound should be preformed.

Alfirevic Z, Stampalija T, Gyte GM. Fetal and umbilical Doppler ultrasound in normal pregnancy. *Cochrane Database Syst Rev* 2010;CD001450. PMID: 20687066.

Alkazaleh F, Chaddha V, Viero S, et al. Second-trimester prediction of severe placental complications in women with combined elevations in alpha-fetoprotein and human chorionic gonadotrophin. *Am J Obstet Gynecol* 2006;194:821–827. PMID: 16522419.

Ananth CV, Demissie K, Smulian JC, Vintzileos AM. Relationship among placenta previa, fetal growth restriction, and preterm delivery: A population-based study. *Obstet Gynecol* 2001;98:299–306. PMID: 11506849.

Anton L, Merrill DC, Neves LA, et al. The uterine placental bed Renin-Angiotensin system in normal and preeclamptic pregnancy. *Endocrinology* 2009;150:4316–4325. PMID: 19520788.

Brooks VL, Dampney RA, Heesch CM. Pregnancy and the endocrine regulation of the baroreceptor reflex. *Am J Physiol Regul Integr Comp Physiol* 2010;299:R439–R451. PMID: 20504907.

Cai LY, Izumi S, Koido S, et al. Abnormal placental cord insertion may induce intrauterine growth restriction in IVF-twin pregnancies. *Hum Reprod* 2006;21:1285–1290. PMID: 16497694.

Carlin A, Alfirevic Z. Physiological changes of pregnancy and monitoring. *Best Pract Res Clin Obstet Gynaecol* 2008;22:801–823. PMID: 18760680.

Conrad KP. Mechanisms of renal vasodilation and hyperfiltration during pregnancy. *J Soc Gynecol Investig* 2004;11:438–448. PMID: 15458740.

Derbyshire EJ, Davies J, Detmar P. Changes in bowel function: Pregnancy and the puerperium. *Dig Dis Sci* 2007;52:324–328. PMID: 17211700.

Desai DK, Moodley J, Naidoo DP. Echocardiographic assessment of cardiovascular hemodynamics in normal pregnancy. *Obstet Gynecol* 2004;104:20–29. PMID: 15228996.

Flo K, Wilsgaard T, Vårtun A, Acharya G. A longitudinal study of the relationship between maternal cardiac output measured by impedance cardiography and uterine artery blood flow in the second half of pregnancy. *BJOG* 2010;117(7):837–844. PMID: 20353457.

Flo K, Wilsgaard T, Acharya G. Relation between utero-placental and feto-placental circulations: A longitudinal study. *Acta Obstet Gynecol Scand* 2010;89:1270–1275. PMID: 20726828.

Granger JP. Maternal and fetal adaptations during pregnancy: Lessons in regulatory and integrative physiology. *Am J Physiol Regul Integr Comp Physiol* 2002;283:R1289–R1292. PMID: 12429557.

Harirah HM, Donia SE, Nasrallah FK, Saade GR, Belfort MA. Effect of gestational age and position on peak expiratory flow rate: A longitudinal study. *Obstet Gynecol* 2005;105:372–376. PMID: 15684167.

Jankowski M, Wang D, Mukaddam-Daher S, Gutkowska J. Pregnancy alters nitric oxide synthase and natriuretic peptide systems in the rat left ventricle. *J Endocrinol* 2005;184:209–217. PMID: 15642797.

Jensen D, Wolfe LA, Slatkovska L, Webb KA, Davies GA, O'Donnell DE. Effects of human pregnancy on the ventilatory chemoreflex response to carbon dioxide. *Am J Physiol Regul Integr Comp Physiol* 2005;288:R1369–R1375. PMID: 15677521.

Jeyabalan A, Lain KY. Anatomic and functional changes of the upper urinary tract during pregnancy. *Urol Clin North Am* 2007;34:1–6. PMID: 17145354.

Kirkegaard I, Uldbjerg N, Oxvig C. Biology of pregnancy-associated plasma protein-A in relation to prenatal diagnostics: An overview. *Acta Obstet Gynecol Scand* 2010;89:1118–1125. PMID: 20804336.

Lindheimer MD. Polyuria and pregnancy: Its cause, its danger. *Obstet Gynecol* 2005;105:1171–1172. PMID: 15863570.

Moertl MG, Ulrich D, Pickel KI, et al. Changes in haemodynamic and autonomous nervous system parameters measured non-invasively throughout normal pregnancy. *Eur J Obstet Gynecol Reprod Biol* 2009;144(Suppl 1):S179–S183. PMID: 19285779.

Muallem MM, Rubeiz NG. Physiological and biological skin changes in pregnancy. *Clin Dermatol* 2006:24:80–83. PMID: 16487877.

Robinson BK, Grobman WA. Effectiveness of timing strategies for delivery of individuals with placenta previa and accreta. *Obstet Gynecol* 2010;116:835–842. PMID: 20859146.

Sciscione AC, Hayes EJ; Society for Maternal-Fetal Medicine. Uterine artery Doppler flow studies in obstetric practice. *Am J Obstet Gynecol* 2009;201:121–126. PMID: 19646563.

Sheiner E, Abramowicz JS, Levy A, Silberstein T, Mazor M, Hershkovitz R. Nuchal cord is not associated with adverse perinatal outcome. *Arch Gynecol Obstet* 2006;274:81–83. PMID: 16374604.

Smith SD, Dunk CE, Aplin JD, Harris LK, Jones RL. Evidence for immune cell involvement in decidual spiral arteriole remodeling in early human pregnancy. *Am J Pathol* 2009;174:1959–1971. PMID: 19349361.

Stachenfeld NS, Taylor HS. Progesterone increases plasma volume independent of estradiol. *J Appl Physiol* 2005;98:1991–1997. PMID: 15718411.

Swansburg ML, Brown CA, Hains SM, Smith GN, Kisilevsky BS. Maternal cardiac autonomic function and fetal heart rate in preeclamptic compared to normotensive pregnancies. *Can J Cardiovasc Nurs* 2005:15:42–52. PMID: 16295797.

Taipale P, Hiilesmaa V, Ylostalo P. Diagnosis of placenta previa by transvaginal sonographic screening at 12–16 weeks in a non-selected population. *Obstet Gynecol* 1997;89:364–367. PMID: 9052586.

Toal M, Chan C, Fallah S, et al. Usefulness of a placental profile in high-risk pregnancies. *Am J Obstet Gynecol* 2007;196(4):363.e1–363.e7. PMID: 17403424.

Tihtonen K, Kööbi T, Yli-Hankala A, Uotila J. Maternal hemodynamics during cesarean delivery assessed by whole-body impedance cardiography. *Acta Obstet Gynecol Scand* 2005;84:355–361. PMID: 15762965.

Varga I, Rigó J Jr, Somos P, Joó JG, Nagy B. Analysis of maternal circulation and renal function in physiologic pregnancies; parallel examinations of the changes in the cardiac output and the glomerular filtration rate. *J Matern Fetal Med* 2000;9:97–104. PMID: 10902822.

Yagel S. The developmental role of natural killer cells at the fetal-maternal interface. *Am J Obstet Gynecol* 2009;201:344–350. PMID: 19788966.

Normal Newborn Assessment & Care

9

Elisabeth L. Raab, MD, MPH
Lisa K. Kelly, MD

A full-term newborn is a baby born at 37 weeks' or more gestation. Term newborns are evaluated in the delivery room immediately after birth to assure that they do not require respiratory or circulatory support, have no birth-related trauma or congenital anomalies requiring immediate intervention, and are transitioning as expected to extrauterine life. Approximately 97% of newborns are healthy and require only routine care in the nursery after birth. In the nursery, newborns receive a thorough evaluation to determine maturity, evaluate growth and development, and identify those with signs of acute illness or underlying congenital disease.

DELIVERY ROOM MANAGEMENT

At every delivery there should be at least 1 person whose primary responsibility is attending to the newborn. Although approximately 90% of the time no resuscitation will be required, the attendant must be able to recognize signs of distress in a newborn and carry out a skilled resuscitation.

After the umbilical cord is cut, newborns should be placed in a warm environment. They may be placed on the mother's chest, skin-to-skin, or they may be brought to a radiant warmer. Early skin-to-skin contact increases the likelihood and duration of breastfeeding, decreases infant crying, and facilitates bonding and is therefore encouraged when possible. However, it should only be done when the newborn is crying/breathing and has good tone and when there are no risk factors that increase the likelihood that resuscitation will be required (eg, prematurity). The infant is dried with prewarmed towels to prevent heat loss and the airway is positioned and cleared to ensure patency. The airway may be cleared by suctioning the mouth and nares with a bulb syringe or a suction catheter connected to mechanical suction. If the newborn is well-appearing and not at increased risk, the airway can be cleared simply by wiping the mouth and nose with a towel.

During this initial postpartum period, the newborn's respiratory effort, heart rate, color, and activity are evaluated to determine the need for intervention. If drying and suctioning do not provide adequate stimulus, it is appropriate to flick the soles or rub the back to stimulate breathing. It is important to note the presence of meconium in the amniotic fluid or on the newborn's skin. Although not contraindicated, it is no longer recommended that the obstetrician routinely suction the oropharynx of an infant born with meconium-stained amniotic fluid upon delivery of the head. If a newborn is in distress or has depressed respiratory effort after delivery and there is evidence that meconium was passed in utero, it is appropriate to intubate and suction the trachea before stimulating the baby in any way. Meconium can block the airway, preventing the newborn lungs from filling with oxygen, a vital step in normal transitioning. However, if the attempted intubation is prolonged or repeatedly unsuccessful, it may be appropriate to omit tracheal suctioning in favor of initiating positive pressure ventilation (PPV) in a depressed infant. Tracheal suctioning has not been shown to decrease the incidence of meconium aspiration syndrome or mortality rates in depressed infants born through meconium-stained fluid. An active, crying, well-appearing newborn does not require endotracheal intubation, regardless of the presence of meconium staining or the thickness of the meconium.

If a newborn remains apneic despite drying, suctioning, and stimulation, or if there are signs of distress such as grunting, central cyanosis, or bradycardia, resuscitation should quickly be initiated. PPV should be initiated in response to gasping, apnea and/or a heart rate below 100 beats/min and the decision to initiate PPV should ideally be made within the first 30–60 seconds after birth.

The Assignment of Apgar Scores

The Apgar score was introduced by Virginia Apgar in 1952 to quantitatively evaluate the newborn's condition after birth (Table 9–1). Scores between 0 and 2 in each of 5 different categories are assigned at 1 and 5 minutes of life. The score reflects the cardiorespiratory and neurologic status at those time points. If the score is <7 at 5 minutes, scores should be

Table 9–1. Apgar scoring.

Signs	Points Scored		
	0	1	2
Heartbeats per minute	Absent	Slow (<100)	>100
Respiratory effort	Absent	Slow, irregular	Good, crying
Muscle tone	Limp	Some flexion of extremities	Active motion
Reflex irritability	No response	Grimace	Cry or cough
Color	Blue or pale	Body pink, extremities blue	Completely pink

assigned every 5 minutes until the baby has a score of 7 or greater or has reached 20 minutes of life. The Apgar score is not what determines the need for resuscitation. Although scores are based on the same elements used to evaluate the newborn's status, the assessment of the need for intervention with PPV should ideally already have been made by the time the 1-minute Apgar score is assigned. Studies do not show a correlation between a low 1-minute Apgar score and outcome. However, the change between the scores at 1 and 5 minutes is a meaningful measure of the effectiveness of the resuscitation efforts, and a 5-minute score of 0–3 is associated with increased mortality in both preterm and full-term infants. It is important to know that factors such as prematurity, maternal medications, and congenital disease can adversely affect scores.

The Importance of the Prenatal & Intrapartum History

Knowledge of the prenatal and intrapartum history is essential for adequate care of the newborn. The history should be reviewed before delivery (if possible), as it may alter care in the immediate postpartum period. For example, information about the use of certain anesthetic drugs during labor and delivery alerts those attending the delivery to the possibility of newborn respiratory depression and allows them to anticipate a role for the use of naloxone in the resuscitation. Other important pieces of information are the presence of chronic disease in the mother (eg, diabetes mellitus, Grave's disease, or systemic lupus erythematosus), maternal illicit or prescription drug use, prenatal ultrasound findings, maternal screening laboratory test results, and the presence of risk factors for neonatal infection. All of these will affect how the newborn is monitored during the nursery admission and in the first few weeks of life, and adequate care is not possible without them.

A. The Initial Exam

Although a complete and detailed physical exam is delayed until the newborn is admitted to the nursery and has had time to transition to extrauterine life, a brief examination should be done shortly after delivery to rule out any problems that require immediate attention.

1. Airway—The airway should be evaluated for patency. A suction catheter may be passed through each naris if needed to remove secretions from the nasopharynx or if there is concern about the possibility of choanal atresia, but is not necessary if adequate clearance of secretions is achieved with a bulb syringe and the newborn is breathing comfortably. Although a suction catheter is an effective means of removing secretions, it should be used cautiously because it can induce bradycardia and cause trauma and edema to the mucous membranes.

2. Chest—The chest should be examined to determine the adequacy of the respiratory effort. One should assess chest wall movement, respiratory rate, and breathing pattern and look for signs of distress, such as retractions. Crackles are often audible initially, but should clear over time as fetal lung fluid is resorbed and the lungs inflate with air. Decreased or asymmetric breath sounds may result from pneumonia, atelectasis, a pneumothorax, mass, or effusion. Heart rate and rhythm should be evaluated, and the presence or absence of a murmur noted. The heart rate should be >100 beats/min.

3. Abdomen—The abdomen should be soft and nondistended. A distended, firm abdomen may indicate a bowel obstruction, pneumoperitoneum, or intra-abdominal mass. A scaphoid abdomen, when accompanied by respiratory distress, should raise the examiner's suspicion of a diaphragmatic hernia. The umbilical stump should be examined and the number of blood vessels noted. A single umbilical artery may be a clue to the presence of other anomalies, renal anomalies in particular.

4. Skin—The skin color should be evaluated. Although acrocyanosis, bluish discoloration of the hands and feet, may be seen in well newborns, central cyanosis of the trunk may be a sign that the newborn is not receiving sufficient oxygen. Cyanosis and pallor can result from a wide variety of causes such as sepsis, anemia, respiratory insufficiency with or without abnormally elevated cardiac vascular resistance, congenital heart disease, and hypoxic-ischemic injury with cardiac dysfunction; the pre- and intrapartum history is often useful in determining the etiology. Pulse oximetry is useful to help determine the oxygen saturation in the event of cyanosis. A cyanotic infant with a normal heart rate and respiratory effort may be given free-flow 100% oxygen by face mask or tubing held close to the nose and should be observed for improvement in skin coloring. If the skin does not become pink, the patient may require PPV to achieve improved oxygenation.

5. Genitalia—It is important to closely evaluate the genitalia before pronouncing the sex of the newborn. If there is ambiguity of the genitalia, the situation must be explained to the parents, and a full evaluation, including karyotyping and consultation with a pediatric endocrinologist and urologist, should be done before gender assignment.

5. General—Alertness, activity, tone, and movement of the extremities should be noted. The face and extremities should be evaluated for evidence of congenital anomalies or birth trauma. The most common birth-related injuries are nerve injuries (facial and brachial nerve palsies) and fractures (primarily clavicular). Unilateral peripheral facial nerve palsy should be suspected when the newborn has normal movement of the forehead, but difficulty closing the eye and flattening of the nasolabial folds on the affected side and an asymmetric facial expression with crying (the unaffected side will go down). Peripheral facial nerve injury is thought to result from compression of the nerve against the maternal sacrum during delivery and is not associated with the use of forceps in delivery. The risk of brachial plexus injury is increased when there is shoulder dystocia or the baby is large for gestational age (LGA). Erb's palsy (C5–C6 injury) manifests as an inability to externally rotate or abduct the shoulder; the affected arm is held adducted and internally rotated and is extended and pronated at the elbow ("waiter-tip" position). If the C5–T1 nerve roots are all affected, the function of the hand will be affected as well.

Casey BM, McIntire DD, Leveno KJ. The continuing value of the Apgar score for the assessment of newborn infants. *N Engl J Med* 2001;344:467. PMID: 11172187.

Dawson JA, Kamlin COF, Vento M, et al. Defining the reference range for oxygen saturation for infants after birth. *Pediatrics* 2010;125;e1340–e1347. PMID: 20439604.

Ehrenstein V. Association of Apgar scores with death and neurologic disability. *Clin Epidemiol* 2009;1:45–53. PMID: 20865086.

Roggensack A, Jefferies AL, Farine D, et al. Management of meconium at birth. *J Obstet Gynaecol Can* 2009;31:353–354. PMID: 19497156.

Weiner GM, Wyckoff M, Zaichkin J. 2010 American Heart Association guidelines for cardiopulmonary resuscitation and emergency cardiovascular care. *Circulation* 2010;122 (18 Suppl 3):S909–S919. PMID: 20956231.

CARE & OBSERVATION IN THE FIRST FEW HOURS OF LIFE

A single 1-mg intramuscular injection of vitamin K is recommended for all newborns to prevent bleeding as a result of vitamin K deficiency. Vitamin K prophylaxis has been standard of care since 1961, when it was first recommended by the American Academy of Pediatrics (AAP). Standard newborn care also includes applying either 0.5% erythromycin ointment, 1% silver nitrate solution, or 1% tetracycline ointment to the infant's eyes shortly after birth to prevent infectious neonatal conjunctivitis.

The well newborn may remain with the mother after birth and attempt an initial feed. There should be continued intermittent assessment to assure that there is no cardiorespiratory distress, temperature instability, altered level of activity, or other signs of distress. It is important that caregivers are aware that babies that require resuscitation after birth are at increased risk of difficulties with transitioning and must be monitored closely.

American Academy of Pediatrics, Committee on Fetus and Newborn. Controversies concerning vitamin K and the newborn policy statement. *Pediatrics* 2003;112:191. PMID: 12837888.

NEWBORN NURSERY CARE

Vital Signs

Vital signs should be recorded by the nursing staff for all newborns admitted to the nursery. Body temperature is typically measured in the axilla. Fever, defined as a temperature ≥38.0° Celsius (or 100.4° Fahrenheit), is often caused by excessive environmental heat or overbundling when it occurs shortly after birth. Hypothermia may result if newborns are left in the delivery room unbundled and off the radiant warmer. A newborn with hypothermia or hyperthermia whose temperature fails to normalize in response to appropriate environmental measures should be evaluated for possible sepsis and central nervous system pathology.

A normal respiratory rate for a newborn is typically between 40 and 60 breaths per minute. A normal heart rate for a newborn is generally 100–160 beats/min, but varies considerably with sleep and activity level. If measured, pulse oximetry should be >95% in the term infant. However, it is important to realize that oxygen saturations may remain low for several minutes after birth. Data indicate that it takes approximately 8 minutes on average for pulse oxygen saturations to rise above 90%. Neonatal resuscitation guidelines published by the AAP in 2010 target a preductal saturation of >80% by 5 minutes of life and 85–95% by 10 minutes of life in both term and preterm infants. Blood pressure varies with gestation and birth weight. There is still debate regarding what constitutes an abnormal blood pressure in a neonate, but hypotension in the first 12–24 hours of life is typically defined as a mean blood pressure less than the gestational age. Hypertension in the full-term newborn is defined as a systolic blood pressure >90 mm Hg and diastolic blood pressure >60 mm Hg and a mean blood pressure >70 mm Hg. Blood pressures should be measured in all 4 extremities if there is any suspicion of cardiac disease. Coarctation of the aorta is characterized by elevated blood pressure in the upper extremities and decreased pressure in the lower extremities.

Growth and Development

Weight, length, and head circumference should be measured and plotted on curves to assess intrauterine growth (Fig. 9–1). Newborns that are small for gestational age (SGA), historically defined as less than the 10th percentile on the growth curve, may warrant evaluation for congenital infections, chromosomal syndromes, or other causes if there is no identifiable cause for the growth retardation, such as multiple pregnancy or preeclampsia or other evidence of placental insufficiency. Infants that are SGA or LGA should be treated similarly to the infants of diabetic mothers and should be monitored for hypoglycemia in the first few hours of life.

Although gestational age is usually estimated before delivery by prenatal ultrasound (preferably early on in the pregnancy) or the mother's last menstrual period, information is sometimes unavailable or inaccurate, and maturity should be reassessed postnatally. There are measures, such as Ballard's modified version of the Dubowitz exam (Table 9–2), that incorporate multiple elements of the physical exam and may be useful at 12–24 hours of life to help determine gestational age.

Physical Exam

A physician should perform a complete physical exam of the newborn within the first 24 hours of life.

A. Skin

As on the initial brief examination, the color of the skin should be evaluated and the presence of cyanosis, pallor, or jaundice noted. The healthy newborn should be pink. Postterm infants often have dry, cracked skin. Clinical jaundice is rare in the first 24 hours of life and should trigger an evaluation. Plethora, often seen in infants of diabetic mothers, may indicate significant polycythemia. Practice varies, but most neonatologists consider a hematocrit >70% in an asymptomatic newborn and 65% in a symptomatic newborn grounds for a partial exchange transfusion. Symptoms of hyperviscosity include hypoxia, hypoglycemia, increased work of breathing, and seizures. Neurologic sequelae can be serious. Petechiae are often present over the face and upper torso, particularly when a nuchal cord is present. When present below the nipple line, petechiae should raise concern about the possibility of sepsis or platelet dysfunction. Bruising

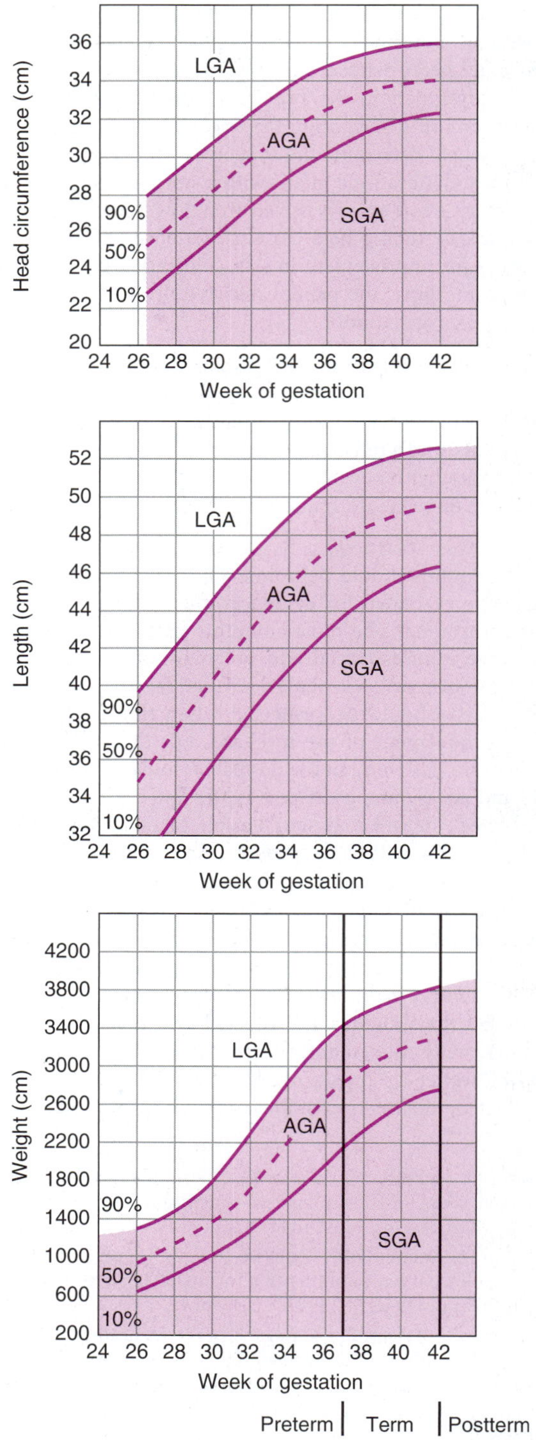

▲ **Figure 9–1.** Classification of newborns based on gestational age plotted against head circumference, length, and weight. AGA, appropriate for gestational age; LGA, large for gestational age; SGA, small for gestational age.

Table 9–2. Newborn maturity rating and classification.

	0	1	2	3	4	5
Neuromuscular maturity						
Posture 						
Square window (wrist) 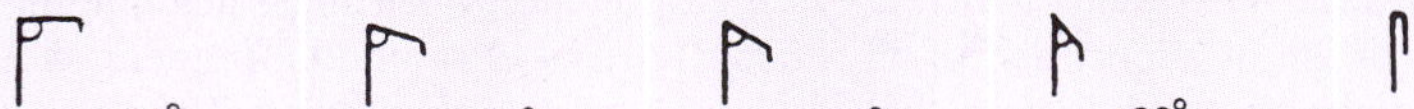	90°	60°	45°	30°	0°	
Arm recoil 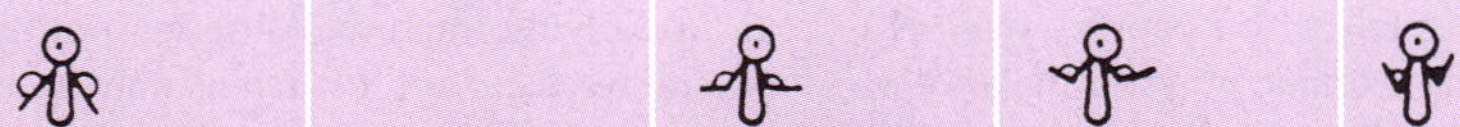	180°		100°–180°	90°–100°	< 90°	
Popliteal angle 	180°	160°	130°	110°	90°	< 90°
Scarf sign 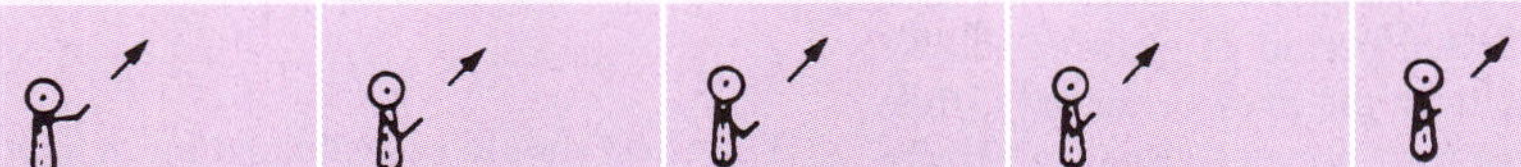						
Heel to ear 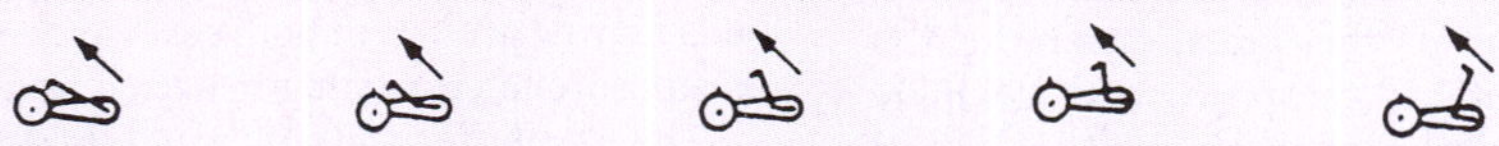						
Physical maturity						
Skin	Gelatinous, red, transparent	Smooth, pink; visible veins	Superficial peeling and/or rash; few veins	Cracking, pale area; rare veins	Parchment, deep cracking; no vessels	Leathery, cracked, wrinkled
Lanugo	None	Abundant	Thinning	Bald areas	Mostly bald	
Plantar creases	No crease	Faint red marks	Anterior transverse crease only	Creases anterior two-thirds	Creases cover entire sole	
Breast	Barely perceptible	Flat areola; no bud	Stippled areola; bud, 1-2 mm	Raised areola; bud, 3-4 mm	Full areola; bud, 5-10 mm	
Ear	Pinna flat; stays folded	Slightly curved pinna; soft; slow recoil	Well-curved pinna; soft; ready recoil	Formed and firm; instant recoil	Thick cartilage; ear stiff	
Genitalia (male)	Scrotum empty; no rugae		Testes descending; few rugae	Testes down; good rugae	Testes pendulous; deep rugae	
Genitalia (female)	Prominent clitoris and labia minora		Majora and minora equally prominent	Majora large; minora small	Clitoris and minora completely covered	

The following information should be recorded: Birth date and Apgar score at 1 and 5 minutes. Two separate examinations should be made within the first 24 hours to determine the estimated gestational age according to maturity rating. Each examination and the age of the infant at each examination should be noted. Maturity rating:

Score	5	10	15	20	25	30	35	40	45	50
Weeks	26	28	30	32	34	36	38	40	42	44

occurs frequently, especially with breech presentation, but should be noted because it may lead to excessive hemolysis and hyperbilirubinemia when extensive. Mongolian spots are dark purple-blue hyperpigmented areas usually over the back and buttocks that look like bruising, but are clusters of melanocytes deep within the dermis. They are present in a majority of black and Asian newborns and fade over time. Dermal sinuses, dimples, and cysts should be noted; they may indicate underlying defects or pose a risk for infection.

The most common newborn rash is erythema toxicum, which presents at 24–48 hours of life in almost half of all newborns as erythematous papular-pustular lesions that tend to spare the palms and soles. Other frequently seen benign rashes include milia, small white papules typically around the nares, and transient neonatal pustular melanosis, small vesicles or pustules present at birth that leave pigmented macules surrounded by scale when they disappear.

Hemangiomas and vascular malformations may be present at birth. Hemangiomas are benign tumors of vascular endothelium and are often not present at birth, but may be noted soon after. They eventually involute without therapy, but only after an initial period of growth, usually of 6–12 months. If present near the eyes or airways, they may require early intervention to prevent visual or airway compromise. In contrast, vascular malformations such as port-wine stains and salmon patches are always present at birth. Developmental anomalies composed of 1 or more types of vessels, they typically grow as the child grows and do not resolve spontaneously.

B. Head, Face, & Neck

The head should be evaluated for any asymmetry. The suture lines may be open or slightly overriding, but premature fusion requires intervention, as it presents a constraint to brain growth. The anterior fontanelle should be soft, not tense or bulging, when the newborn is calm. It is typically 1–4 cm in size and may be enlarged with hypothyroidism or increased intracranial pressure. The posterior fontanelle is typically <1 cm and may not be palpable.

Scalp edema (caput succedaneum) can most easily be differentiated from a cephalohematoma (a localized collection of blood under the dura mater) by noting whether or not the swelling crosses suture lines; cephalohematoma is typically confined by suture lines. A cephalohematoma should raise awareness of the possible development of hyperbilirubinemia as the collection of blood is broken down and resorbed. Skull fractures can occur, and the skull should be palpated carefully.

The face should be evaluated for dysmorphic features, malformations, and asymmetries. Micrognathia may cause significant airway compromise in the neonate and is associated with various syndromes. The palate should be palpated to ensure that it is not high-arched or clefted. A naris is patent if there is air movement through it (demonstrated by holding cotton in front of it) when the mouth and other naris are closed. Subconjunctival hemorrhages are a common finding as a result of the birth process. An absent red reflex should prompt an immediate ophthalmologic evaluation to rule out a congenital cataract, retinoblastoma, or glaucoma. Pupils should be equal and reactive. Abnormalities of the positioning or formation of the eyes, nose, or ears may suggest specific syndromes or chromosomal defects. Although preauricular tags and pits have been associated with renal malformations, there is no current evidence to suggest that their presence, when an isolated finding, is sufficient to warrant a renal ultrasound. The neck should be examined for masses, cysts, and webbing. The clavicles should be palpated for crepitus, swelling, and tenderness, which would suggest an underlying fracture. Although not usually detected until several weeks of age, torticollis may occur as a result of ischemia within, or hemorrhage into, the sternocleidomastoid muscle at birth. It manifests as a head tilt with or without a fibrous mass palpable in the muscle. Surgery is rarely necessary; the overwhelming majority of cases are managed with a home stretching regimen or physical therapy.

C. Chest

The chest should be evaluated for deformities such as widely spaced or accessory nipples and pectus excavatum. Breast buds may be present in both sexes and are normal, a product of exposure to circulating maternal hormones in utero.

The respiratory effort and rate should be evaluated, looking for signs of respiratory distress. Early on, tachypnea may be the only sign of pathologic processes as varied as pneumonia, amniotic fluid and/ or meconium aspiration syndrome, sepsis, or congenital heart disease (CHD). Breath sounds are auscultated, paying attention to the quality of the breath sounds, the air entry, and any asymmetry that is present across the lung fields. Asymmetry of the breath sounds may indicate an area of consolidation from atelectasis or infection, a pneumothorax, effusion, or mass. Upper airway sounds, such as congestion or stridor, are often mistaken for abnormal breath sounds on exam. The listener can usually distinguish noises of upper airway origin from those of intrathoracic origin by listening for the presence of the sounds over the patient's neck. Respiratory distress or an abnormal lung exam should be evaluated with a chest radiograph. In an emergency situation in which a pneumothorax is suspected, a transilluminator may be used. Transillumination is increased over the side of a pneumothorax, but it is sometimes difficult to assess accurately and should be confirmed by chest radiograph when possible before needle aspiration or chest tube placement.

A hyperdynamic precordium may indicate underlying heart disease with volume overload to one or both ventricles. The heart is auscultated to evaluate the heart rate and rhythm and characterize the heart sounds. A split-second heart sound can assure the examiner that both the aortic and pulmonary valves are present. A murmur should be described by where it is heard, what it sounds like, if it occurs in systole or diastole, and how loud it is. Murmurs are often audible in the newborn and are frequently innocent. Innocent murmurs are often attributed to a closing ductus arteriosus or foramen ovale, but the most commonly heard innocent murmur in the neonate is produced by peripheral pulmonic stenosis (PPS). PPS murmurs occur during systole and are best heard over the back or axillae.

Murmurs may or may not be present in newborns with CHD. Ventricular septal defects, the most common form of CHD, have a characteristic harsh, systolic murmur associated with them. However, the pressures in the newborn pulmonary system are still high (roughly equal to systemic pressures), and thus there is usually no flow gradient across a large ventricular defect to produce a murmur in the first few days of life. Complex CHD typically presents as cyanosis, tachypnea, or shock and will rarely present as an asymptomatic murmur. Signs may develop quickly with closure of the ductus arteriosus if the lesion has ductal-dependent pulmonary or systemic flow. The initial steps in evaluating a stable patient for suspected CHD include 4-extremity blood pressure measurements, measurement of pre- and postductal saturations, electrocardiogram, chest radiography, and a hyperoxia test. The diagnosis of CHD is usually established by echocardiogram.

D. Abdomen

The examiner should listen for bowel sounds and palpate the abdomen for masses, organomegaly, or abnormal musculature. The liver is easily palpable in the newborn and the inferior edge is usually 1–2 cm below the right costal margin. It is often possible to palpate the kidneys and spleen. Absence of the abdominal musculature may be associated with significant urinary tract abnormalities. The umbilical stump should be assessed for redness or induration that may suggest the presence of an infection. Umbilical hernias are common and typically require no intervention in infancy. Omphalocele and gastroschisis are major abdominal wall defects and require emergent surgical evaluation. Omphalocele is a midline abdominal wall defect. Bowel, and often liver, herniate through the defect, and the umbilicus is typically on the anterior aspect of the omphalocele. Unless ruptured, an omphalocele is covered by a membrane. Omphalocele is associated with aneuploidies, certain genetic syndromes such as pentalogy of Cantrell, and other congenital structural malformations. The defect in gastroschisis is typically to the right of the umbilicus on the abdominal wall, and the etiology of the defect is thought to be due to vascular interruption. The entire bowel may be externalized, but the liver typically remains internal. Unlike omphaloceles, the externalized bowel is not covered by a membrane. Other bowel abnormalities such as bowel atresias and malrotation of the bowel may be present in infants with gastroschisis. Fetuses with gastroschisis are also at increased risk of developing intrauterine growth restriction.

E. Genitalia

The penile length and clitoral size should be inspected to rule out ambiguous genitalia. The labia majora should cover the labia minora and clitoris in a term female. White mucouslike discharge from the vagina is often present and is physiologic.

The scrotum should be evaluated for hernias or masses and descent of the testicles. Transillumination of the scrotum will help to distinguish a hydrocele from an inguinal hernia. The position of the urethral meatus is important to note, as the presence of hypospadias should preclude routine circumcision to allow for optimal surgical correction of the hypospadias.

F. Anus

The rectum should be evaluated for patency and position. An anteriorly displaced rectum may be associated with a rectogenital fistula.

G. Musculoskeletal System

The extremities, spine, and hips are examined for signs of fracture, malformation, or deformation. Range of motion of the joints is assessed. Arthrogryposis, contractures of the joints, may be seen with neuromuscular disease or oligohydramnios as a result of decreased or limited movement in utero. Abnormalities of the extremities, such as polydactyly or syndactyly, are seen in different chromosomal abnormalities and syndromes and may help in making the diagnosis. Particular attention should be paid to the examination of the hips (despite the fact that a dislocation may not be detectable in the first weeks of life) because developmental dysplasia of the hip (DDH) can cause permanent damage if left undetected throughout the first year of life. Either the Barlow or Ortolani test may be used to determine whether a dislocation is present. The Barlow test involves positioning the patient on the back, bringing the knees together at midline, and then pushing down and out on the upper inner thighs. The Ortolani test involves pushing downward on the femurs while abducting the hips. With both maneuvers the dislocation is detected as a clunk as the femoral head is dislocated from the acetabulum (posteriorly with the Barlow, laterally with the Ortolani). Asymmetry of the gluteal folds and skin creases of the legs is another clue to the presence of DDH.

H. Neurologic System

Observing the activity level, alertness, and positioning of the newborn provides a tremendous amount of information about the overall state of health. A healthy, full-term newborn at rest should lie with the extremities flexed. Decreased tone may be a sign of neuromuscular or systemic illness such as sepsis. There should be spontaneous intermittent movement of all 4 limbs, and the baby should be alert during at least portions of the examination. Pupil size and symmetry should be noted. Primitive reflexes such as the Moro, grasp, suck, and tonic neck reflex should all be present at birth. To elicit the Moro reflex, the newborn is supported with a hand under the back and then rapidly dropped a few centimeters back toward the examination bed. The full Moro reflex consists of extension and then flexion and adduction of the arms ("embrace"), opening of the eyes, and a cry. Reflexes are elicited by tapping a finger over the appropriate tendon. Significant clonus may be a sign of central nervous system injury. A sacral dimple or tuft of hair over the sacral spine may indicate spina bifida occulta and should be evaluated with a spinal ultrasound; if the findings of the ultrasound are equivocal, a magnetic resonance imaging scan should be done at approximately 3 months of age.

Feeding

The benefits of breastfeeding on everything from the strength of the immune system to developmental outcomes and IQ have been well documented. Human milk is the most easily digested form of infant nutrition, and its caloric value is superior to formula. Mothers should be counseled prenatally about the benefits of breastfeeding and encouraged by their obstetric caregivers to consider breastfeeding. Contraindications to breastfeeding include HIV infection, active tuberculosis infection, and the use of certain medications. Maternal hepatitis C virus (HCV) infection is not a contraindication to breastfeeding. Transmission of HCV via breastmilk is not documented in the absence of coexisting maternal infection with HIV. Nevertheless, infected mothers should be informed that transmission via breastmilk is theoretically possible.

Breastfeeding may be difficult and frustrating for new mothers. It is important that the newborn nursery staff work to provide mothers with the support and knowledge they need to make breastfeeding a positive experience. It is also important that mothers of newborns who require bottle supplementation (eg, a dehydrated, jaundiced infant) are reassured that their efforts at breastfeeding will not be derailed by exposure to the bottle during a limited, medically necessary period, and that breastfeeding can still ultimately succeed.

Regardless of the overwhelming literature to support the value of breast milk, many mothers in the United States choose to bottle-feed their children. Selection of the formula given to the newborn is often based on what formula is available in the nursery or by the mother's preference. Standard-term infant formula contains iron supplementation and provides 20 kcal/oz. No one formula is better than another for healthy term infants. Mothers with a family history of lactose intolerance sometimes request soy formula, and standard soy formula will provide adequate nutrition for growth and development. Formulas such as Alimentum and Nutramigen are available for infants with more significant protein allergy. Premature infant formulas contain 24 kcal/oz and provide higher amounts of protein, medium-chain triglycerides, and vitamins and minerals (eg, calcium and phosphorous) than standard formulas. The AAP currently recommends formula for the first year of life.

Voiding and Stooling

Voiding should be monitored closely in the nursery. Changes in the baby's weight and the frequency of urination can be used to assess the hydration status and adequacy of intake in a breastfeeding baby. The time of the first void of urine and stool should be documented. Failure to void in the first 24 hours of life should prompt an evaluation of renal function and hydration status. Failure to pass stool in the first 48 hours of life should prompt an evaluation for possible bowel obstruction; 94% of normal term newborns will pass meconium in the first 24 hours of life. Obstruction can result from conditions such as bowel atresia or stenosis, Hirschsprung's disease, and meconium ileus.

American Academy of Pediatrics and American Heart Association. *Textbook of Neonatal Resuscitation*. 5th ed. Dallas, TX: American Academy of Pediatrics; 2006.

NEWBORN SCREENING & PROPHYLAXIS

The initial newborn exam may be normal despite the presence of serious occult illness. Signs of complex congenital heart disease, sepsis, gastrointestinal obstruction, significant jaundice, inborn errors of metabolism, and other illnesses may not be present until the second or third day of life at the earliest: shortly before, and at times after, the baby's discharge. Screening is done in the hopes of detecting disease before a patient becomes symptomatic and is usually reserved for processes that have a worse prognosis if not detected early and for which there is effective therapy. The maternal medical history, the obstetric and perinatal history, and state laws determine what screening is done on any given baby.

Standard newborn screening tests have traditionally screened for the following:

1. Phenylketonuria by Guthrie's test for phenylalanine level
2. Congenital hypothyroidism by thyroid function testing
3. Congenital syphilis by either rapid plasma reagent (RPR) or Venereal Disease Research Laboratory (VDRL) test (whichever test was performed on the mother)
4. ABO incompatibility using infant blood type and direct Coombs' test (standard if mother has O blood type, done at many institutions for all newborns)
5. Hearing loss (evaluated by auditory brainstem response or otoacoustic emissions)

Using tandem mass spectrometry, it is now possible to screen for as many as 50 congenital conditions from a single blood sample. Although it has been standard in many states for years now, expanded newborn screening was only adopted as a national standard in the United States in the spring of 2010.

Additional targeted screening often includes evaluation for infection, illicit drug exposure, hyperbilirubinemia, and hypoglycemia when there are risk factors that increase the yield of the testing. A history of rupture of amniotic membranes for >18 hours before delivery, maternal intrapartum fever, chorioamnionitis, and a positive maternal group B streptococcus culture without adequate treatment before delivery are all risk factors for newborn sepsis. A history of any of these risk factors warrants a screening evaluation of the asymptomatic newborn for laboratory evidence of infection. Screening is routinely done for hypoglycemia in infants of diabetic mothers as well as for SGA and LGA babies. At many institutions, infants of diabetic mothers are screened for polycythemia as well.

Information about maternal hepatitis B, HIV, herpes simplex virus (HSV), chlamydia, and syphilis status is essential to newborn care. Adequate prophylaxis for hepatitis B can prevent transmission in 95% of infants born to hepatitis B surface antigen–positive (HBsAg+) mothers. A baby born to a mother who is HBsAg+ should receive the hepatitis B vaccine and hepatitis B immune globulin (HBIG) within the first 12 hours of life to prevent hepatitis B virus transmission. If the mother's status is unknown, the newborn should receive the vaccine within 12 hours of birth, and every effort should be made to determine the mother's status. If the baby weighs more than 2 kg, HBIG can be given as late as 7 days of life if maternal status is positive or still unknown and still provide effective post-exposure prophylaxis. However, a baby who weighs <2 kg at birth should receive HBIG by 12 hours of postnatal life to receive adequate prophylaxis. Appropriate screening and treatment for infants born to mothers with a history of infection with HIV, chlamydia, HSV, or syphilis are detailed in the AAP's *Red Book*.

CIRCUMCISION

Routine circumcision is not currently recommended by the AAP. Although there is evidence that supports some medical benefits of circumcision (eg, decreased incidence of urinary tract infections during infancy, sexually transmitted disease, and penile cancer), the data are insufficient for the AAP to recommend the procedure for all newborn males, given concerns about the impossibility of informed consent in an infant and evidence of the pain and stress caused by the procedure. Parents should be provided with unbiased information about the procedure, and the decision to proceed should be left to them. If circumcision is performed, analgesia, either topical or by nerve block, should be given.

DISCHARGE PLANNING

The physician should complete another thorough examination on the day of discharge to reevaluate the overall health of the newborn. Anticipatory guidance should be given to parents to help them care for their newborns and recognize signs of illness and distress. Safety issues, such as the use of car seats, should be addressed. Parents should be alerted to problems such as fever, lethargy, and poor feeding that should prompt them to see a physician. They should be taught about expected newborn behavior, adequate feeding, monitoring of voiding and stooling, and umbilical cord care.

Anticipatory guidance is particularly important now that hospital stays after delivery are often only 36–48 hours. Criteria for newborn discharge at <48 hours of life are outlined in a 2004 AAP policy statement. Newborns discharged before 48 hours of life must be examined by a health care professional within 72 hours of the discharge, preferably within 48 hours. The plan for the newborn's first visit to the physician and any necessary follow-up laboratory testing or nursing visits to the home should be clearly established at the time of discharge, and parents should be able to demonstrate skill and comfort with feeding and tending to the baby's basic needs.

American Academy of Pediatrics. *AAP 2009 Red Book: Report of the Committee on Infectious Diseases*. 28th ed. Elk Grove Village, IL: American Academy of Pediatrics; 2009.

American Academy of Pediatrics, Committee on Fetus and Newborn. Policy statement: Hospital stay for healthy term newborns. *Pediatrics* 2010;125:405–409. PMID: 20100744.

10 The Normal Puerperium

Caroline Pessel, MD
Ming C. Tsai, MD

The puerperium, or postpartum period, generally lasts 6 weeks and is the period of adjustment after delivery when the anatomic and physiologic changes of pregnancy are reversed, and the body returns to the normal, nonpregnant state. The postpartum period has been arbitrarily divided into the immediate puerperium, or the first 24 hours after parturition, when acute postanesthetic or postdelivery complications may occur; the early puerperium, which extends until the first week postpartum; and the remote puerperium, which includes the period of time required for involution of the genital organs and return of menses, usually approximately 6 weeks.

ANATOMIC & PHYSIOLOGIC CHANGES DURING THE PUERPERIUM

Uterine Involution

The uterus increases markedly in size and weight during pregnancy (approximately 10 times the nonpregnant weight, reaching a crude weight of 1000 g) but involutes rapidly after delivery to the nonpregnant weight of 50–100 g. The gross anatomic and histologic characteristics of this process have been studied through autopsy, hysterectomy, and endometrial specimens. In addition, the decrease in size of the uterus and cervix has been demonstrated by magnetic resonance imaging, sonography, and computed tomography.

Immediately after delivery, the uterus weighs approximately 1 kg, and its size approximates that of a 20-week pregnancy (at the level of the umbilicus). At the end of the first postpartum week, it normally will have decreased to the size of a 12-week gestation and is palpable at the symphysis pubis (Fig. 10–1). In case of abnormal uterine involution, infection and retained products of conception should be ruled out.

Myometrial contractions, or **afterpains,** assist in involution. These contractions occur during the first 2–3 days of the puerperium and produce more discomfort in multiparas than in primiparas. Such pains are accentuated during nursing as a result of oxytocin release from the posterior pituitary. During the first 12 hours postpartum, uterine contractions are regular, strong, and coordinated (Fig. 10–2). The intensity, frequency, and regularity of contractions decrease after the first postpartum day as involutional changes proceed. Uterine involution is nearly complete by 6 weeks, at which time the organ weighs less than 100 g. The increase in the amount of connective tissue, elastin in the myometrium and blood vessels, and the increase in numbers of cells are permanent to some degree, so the uterus is slightly larger after pregnancy.

Changes in the Placental Implantation Site

After delivery of the placenta, there is immediate contraction of the placental site to a size less than half the diameter of the original placenta. This contraction, as well as arterial smooth muscle contractions, leads to hemostasis. Involution occurs by means of the extension and down growth of marginal endometrium and by endometrial regeneration from the glands and stroma in the decidua basalis.

By day 16, placental site, endometrial, and superficial myometrial infiltrates of granulocytes and mononuclear cells are seen. Regeneration of endometrial glands and endometrial stroma has also begun. Endometrial regeneration at the placental site is not complete until 6 weeks postpartum. In the disorder termed **subinvolution of the placental site,** complete obliteration of the vessels in the placental site fails to occur. Patients with this condition have persistent lochia and are subject to brisk hemorrhagic episodes. This condition usually can be treated with uterotonics. In the rare event that uterine curettage is performed, partly obliterated hyalinized vessels can be seen on the histologic specimen.

Normal postpartum discharge begins as **lochia rubra,** containing blood, shreds of tissue, and decidua. The amount of discharge rapidly tapers and changes to a reddish-brown

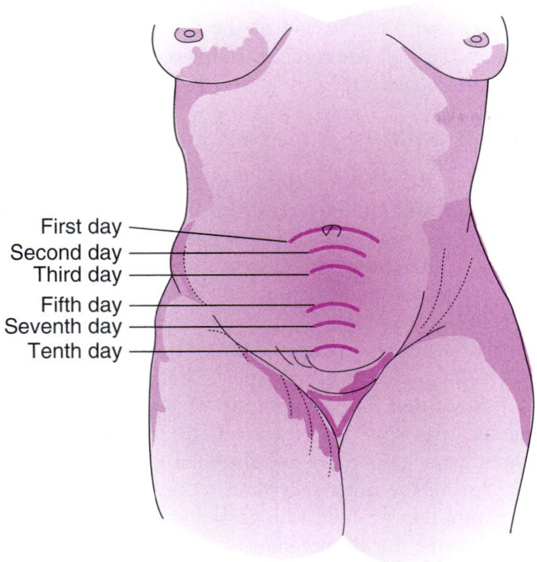

▲ **Figure 10–1.** Involutional changes in the height of the fundus and the size of the uterus during the first 10 days postpartum.

color over the next 3–4 days. It is termed **lochia serosa** when it becomes serous to mucopurulent, paler, and often malodorous. During the second or third postpartum week, the **lochia alba** becomes thicker, mucoid, and yellowish-white, coincident with a predominance of leukocytes and degenerated decidual cells. Typically during the fifth or sixth week postpartum, the lochial secretions cease as healing nears completion.

Changes in the Cervix, Vagina, & Muscular Walls of the Pelvic Organs

The cervix gradually closes during the puerperium; at the end of the first week, it is little more than 1 cm dilated. The external os is converted into a transverse slit, thus distinguishing the parous woman who delivered vaginally from the nulliparous woman or from one who delivered by caesarean section. Cervical lacerations heal in most uncomplicated cases, but the continuity of the cervix may not be restored, so the site of the tear may remain as a scarred notch.

After vaginal delivery, the overdistended and smooth-walled vagina gradually returns to its antepartum condition by about the third week. Thickening of the mucosa, cervical mucus production, and other estrogenic changes may be delayed in a lactating woman. The torn hymen heals in the form of fibrosed nodules of mucosa, the **carunculae myrtiformes**.

Two weeks after delivery, the fallopian tube reflects a hypoestrogenic state marked by atrophy of the epithelium. Fallopian tubes removed between postpartum days 5 and 15 demonstrate acute inflammatory changes that have not been correlated with subsequent puerperal fever or salpingitis. Normal changes in the pelvis after uncomplicated term vaginal delivery include widening of the symphysis and sacroiliac joints. Gas may be seen by ultrasonography

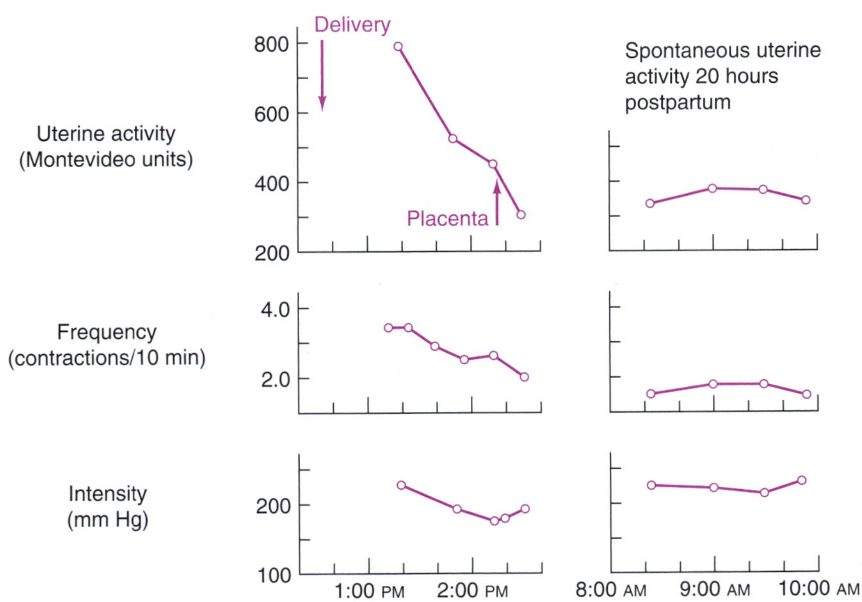

▲ **Figure 10–2.** Uterine activity during the immediate puerperium (**left**) and at 20 hours postpartum (**right**).

in the endometrial cavity a few days after an uncomplicated vaginal delivery. This sonographic observation is more often seen after caesarean section and after manual evacuation of placenta, and it does not necessarily indicate the presence of endometritis. Ovulation occurs as early as 27 days after delivery, with a mean time of 70–75 days in nonlactating women and 6 months in lactating women. In lactating women the duration of anovulation ultimately depends on the frequency of breastfeeding, duration of each feed, and proportion of supplementary feeds. Ovulation suppression is due to high prolactin levels, which remain elevated until approximately 3 weeks after delivery in nonlactating women and 6 weeks in lactating women. However, estrogen levels fall immediately after delivery in all mothers and remain suppressed in lactating mothers. Menstruation returns as soon as 7 weeks in 70% and by 12 weeks in all nonlactating mothers, and as late as 36 months in 70% of breastfeeding mothers.

The voluntary muscles of the pelvic floor and the pelvic supports gradually regain their tone during the puerperium. Tearing or overstretching of the musculature or fascia at the time of delivery predisposes to genital prolapse and genital hernias (cystocele, rectocele, and enterocele). Overdistention of the abdominal wall during pregnancy may result in rupture of the elastic fibers of the cutis, persistent striae, and diastasis of the rectus muscles. Involution of the abdominal musculature may require 6–7 weeks, and vigorous exercise is not recommended until after that time.

Urinary System

In the immediate postpartum period, the bladder mucosa is edematous as a result of labor and delivery. In addition, bladder capacity is increased. Overdistention and incomplete emptying of the bladder with the presence of residual urine are therefore common problems. The decreased bladder sensibility induced by intrapartum regional analgesia may lead to postpartum urinary retention; however, it is reversible and usually not detrimental to later urinary function. Nearly 50% of patients have a mild proteinuria for 1–2 days after delivery. Ultrasonographic examination demonstrates resolution of collecting system dilatation by 6 weeks postpartum in most women. Urinary stasis, however, may persist in more than 50% of women at 12 weeks postpartum. The incidence of urinary tract infection is generally higher in women with persistent dilatation. Significant renal enlargement may persist for many weeks postpartum.

Pregnancy is accompanied by an estimated increase of approximately 50% in the glomerular filtration rate. These values return to normal or less than normal during the eighth week of the puerperium. Endogenous creatinine clearance similarly returns to normal by 8 weeks. Renal plasma flow, which increased during pregnancy by 25% in the first trimester, falls in the third trimester and continues to fall to below normal levels for up to 24 months. Normal levels return slowly over 50–60 weeks. The glucosuria induced by pregnancy disappears. The blood urea nitrogen rises during the puerperium; at the end of the first week postpartum, values of 20 mg/dL are reached, compared with 15 mg/dL in the late third trimester.

Fluid Balance & Electrolytes

An average decrease in maternal weight of 10–13 lb occurs intrapartum and immediately postpartum due to the loss of amniotic fluid and blood as well as delivery of the infant and placenta. The average patient may lose an additional 4 kg (9 lb) during the puerperium and over the next 6 months as a result of excretion of the fluids and electrolytes accumulated during pregnancy. Contrary to widespread belief, breastfeeding has minimal effects on hastening weight loss postpartum. The magnitude of weight gain during pregnancy has impact on the postpartum weight retention. Women who gain more weight than the recommended range during the pregnancy tend to be heavier at 3 years postpartum than women who gained weight within recommended range during pregnancy, and this applies to both obese and nonobese patients.

There is an average net fluid loss of at least 2 L during the first week postpartum and an additional loss of approximately 1.5 L during the next 5 weeks. The water loss in the first week postpartum represents a loss of extracellular fluid. A negative balance must be expected of slightly more than 100 mEq of chloride per kilogram of body weight lost in the early puerperium. This negative balance probably is attributable to the discharge of maternal extracellular fluid. The puerperal losses of salt and water are generally larger in women with preeclampsia or eclampsia.

The changes occurring in serum electrolytes during the puerperium indicate a general increase in the numbers of cations and anions compared with antepartum values. Although total exchangeable sodium decreases during the puerperium, the relative decrease in body water exceeds the sodium loss. The diminished aldosterone antagonism due to falling plasma progesterone concentrations may partially explain the rapid rise in serum sodium. Cellular breakdown due to tissue involution may contribute to the rise in plasma potassium concentration noted postpartum. The mean increase in cations, chiefly sodium, amounts to 4.7 mEq/L, with an equal increase in anions. Consequently, the plasma osmolality rises by 7 mOsm/L at the end of the first week postpartum. In keeping with the chloride shift, there is a tendency for the serum chloride concentration to decrease slightly postpartum as serum bicarbonate concentration increases.

Metabolic & Chemical Changes

Total fatty acids and nonesterified fatty acids return to nonpregnant levels on about the second day of the puerperium. Both cholesterol and triglyceride concentrations decrease significantly within 24 hours after delivery, and this change is reflected in all lipoprotein fractions. Plasma triglycerides continue to fall and approach nonpregnant values 6–7 weeks postpartum. By comparison, the decrease in plasma cholesterol levels is slower; low-density lipoprotein cholesterol remains above nonpregnant levels for at least 7 weeks postpartum. Lactation does not influence lipid levels, but, in contrast to pregnancy, the postpartum hyperlipidemia is sensitive to dietary manipulation.

During the early puerperium, blood glucose concentrations (both fasting and postprandial) tend to fall below the values seen during pregnancy and delivery. This fall is most marked on the second and third postpartum days. Accordingly, the insulin requirements of diabetic patients are lower. Reliable indications of the insulin sensitivity and the blood glucose concentrations characteristic of the nonpregnant state can be demonstrated only after the first week postpartum. Thus a glucose tolerance test performed in the early puerperium may be interpreted erroneously if nonpuerperal standards are applied to the results.

The concentration of free plasma amino acids increases postpartum. Normal nonpregnant values are regained rapidly on the second or third postpartum day and are presumably a result of reduced utilization and an elevation in the renal threshold.

Cardiovascular Changes

A. Blood Coagulation

The production of both prostacyclin (prostaglandin I_2 [PGI_2]), an inhibitor of platelet aggregation, and thromboxane A_2, an inducer of platelet aggregation and a vasoconstrictor, is increased during pregnancy and the puerperium. Possibly, the balance between thromboxane A_2 and PGI_2 is shifted to the side of thromboxane A_2 dominance during the puerperium because platelet reactivity is increased at this time. Rapid and dramatic changes in the coagulation and fibrinolytic systems occur after delivery (Table 10–1). A decrease in the fibrinogen concentration begins during labor and reaches its lowest point during the first day postpartum. Thereafter, rising plasma fibrinogen levels reach prelabor values by the third or fifth day of the puerperium. This secondary peak in fibrinogen activity is maintained until the second postpartum week, after which the level of activity slowly returns to normal nonpregnant levels during the following 7–10 days. A similar pattern occurs with respect to factor VIII and plasminogen. Circulating levels of antithrombin III are decreased in the third trimester of pregnancy. Patients with a congenital deficiency of antithrombin III (an endogenous inhibitor of factor X) have recurrent venous thromboembolic disease, and a low level of this factor has been associated with a hypercoagulable state.

The fibrinolytic activity of maternal plasma is greatly reduced during the last months of pregnancy but increases rapidly after delivery. In the first few hours postpartum, an increase in tissue plasminogen activator (t-PA) activity develops, together with a slight prolongation of the thrombin time, a decrease in plasminogen activator inhibitors, and a significant increase in fibrin split products. Protein C is an important coagulation inhibitor that requires the nonenzymatic cofactor protein S (which exists as a free protein and as a complex) for its activity. The level of protein S, both total and free, increases on the first day after delivery

Table 10–1. Changes in blood coagulation and fibrinolysis during the puerperium.

	Time Postpartum				
	1 Hour	1 Day	3-5 Days	1st Week	2nd Week
Platelet count	↓	↑	↑↑	↑↑	↑
Platelet adhesiveness	↑	↑↑	↑↑↑	↑	0
Fibrinogen	↓	↓	↑	0	↓
Factor V		↑	↑↑	↑	0
Factor VIII	↓	↓	↑	↑	↓
Factors II, VII, X		↓	↓	↓↓	↓↓
Plasminogen	↓	↓↓	0	↓	↓
Plasminogen activator	↑↑↑	↑↑	0		
Fibrinolytic activity	↑	↑↑	↑↑	↑	
Fibrin split products	↑	↑↑	↑↑		

The arrows indicate the direction and relative magnitude of change compared with the late third trimester or antepartum values. Zero indicates a return to antepartum but not necessarily nonpregnant values.
(Data from Manning FA, et al. *Am J Obstet Gynecol* 1971;110:900; Bonnar J, et al. *Br Med J* 1970;2:200; Ygg J. *Am J Obstet Gynecol* 1969;104:2; and Shaper AG, et al. *J Obstet Gynaecol Br Commonw* 1968;75:433.)

and gradually returns to normal levels after the first week postpartum.

The increased concentration of clotting factors normally seen during pregnancy can be viewed as important reserve to compensate for the rapid consumption of these factors during delivery and in promoting hemostasis after parturition. Nonetheless, extensive activation of clotting factors, together with immobility, sepsis, or trauma during delivery, may set the stage for later thromboembolic complications (see Chapter 27). The secondary increase in fibrinogen, factor VIII, or platelets (which remain well above nonpregnant values in the first week postpartum) also predisposes to thrombosis during the puerperium. The abrupt return of normal fibrinolytic activity after delivery may be a protective mechanism to combat this hazard. A small percentage of puerperal women who show a diminished ability to activate the fibrinolytic system appear to be at high risk for the development of postpartum thromboembolic complications.

B. Blood Volume Changes

The total blood volume normally decreases from the antepartum value of 5–6 L to the nonpregnant value of 4 L by the third week after delivery. One-third of this reduction occurs during delivery and soon afterward, and a similar amount is lost by the end of the first postpartum week. Additional variation occurs with lactation. The volume expansion with increased water retention in the extracellular space during pregnancy may be viewed as a protective mechanism that allows most women to tolerate considerable blood loss during parturition. Normal vaginal delivery of a single fetus entails an average blood loss of approximately 400 mL, whereas caesarean section leads to a blood loss of nearly 1 L. If total hysterectomy is performed in addition to caesarean section delivery, the mean blood loss increases to approximately 1500 mL. Delivery of twins and triplets entails blood losses similar to those of operative delivery, but a compensatory increase in maternal plasma volume and red blood cell mass may be exacerbated in mothers carrying multiple gestations.

Dramatic and rapid readjustments occur in the maternal vasculature after delivery so that the response to blood loss during the early puerperium is different from that occurring in the nonpregnant woman. Delivery leads to obliteration of the low-resistance uteroplacental circulation and results in a 10–15% reduction in the size of the maternal vascular bed. Loss of placental endocrine function also removes a stimulus to vasodilatation.

A declining blood volume with a rise in hematocrit is usually seen 3–7 days after vaginal delivery (Fig. 10–3). In contrast, serial studies of patients after caesarean section indicate a more rapid decline in blood volume and hematocrit and a tendency for the hematocrit to stabilize or even decline in the early puerperium. Hemoconcentration occurs if the loss of red cells is less than the reduction in vascular capacity. Hemodilution takes place in patients who lose 20% or more

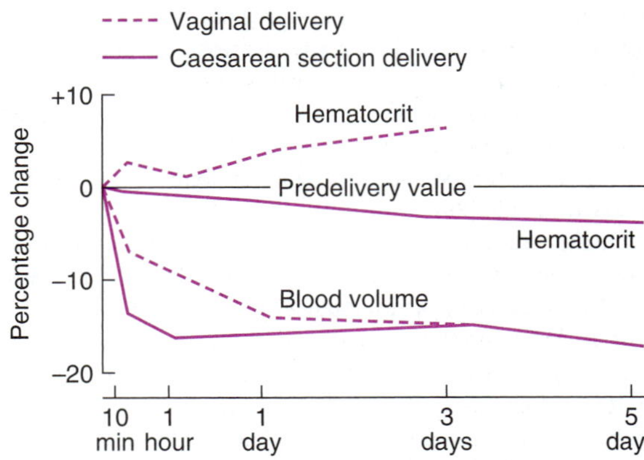

▲ **Figure 10–3.** Postpartum changes in hematocrit and blood volume in patients delivered vaginally and by caesarean section. Values are expressed as the percentage change from the predelivery hematocrit or blood volume. (Data from Ueland K, et al. Maternal cardiovascular dynamics. 1. Cesarean section under subarachnoid block anesthesia. *Am J Obstet Gynecol* 1968;100:42; PMID 5634434; and Ueland K, Hansen J. Maternal cardiovascular dynamics. 3. Labor and delivery under local and caudal analgesia. *Am J Obstet Gynecol* 1969;103: 8; PMID: 5761783.)

of their circulating blood volume at delivery. In patients with preeclampsia–eclampsia, resolution of peripheral vasoconstriction and mobilization of excess extracellular fluid may lead to significant expansion of vascular volume by the third postpartum day. Plasma atrial natriuretic peptide levels nearly double during the first days postpartum in response to atrial stretch caused by blood volume expansion and may have relevance for postpartum natriuresis and diuresis. Occasionally, a patient sustains minimal blood loss at delivery. In such a patient, marked hemoconcentration may occur in the puerperium, especially if there has been a preexisting polycythemia or a considerable increase in the red cell mass during pregnancy.

C. Hematopoiesis

The red cell mass increases by about 25% during pregnancy, whereas the average red cell loss at delivery is approximately 14%. Thus the mean postpartum red cell mass level should be about 15% above nonpregnant values. The sudden loss of blood at delivery, however, leads to a rapid and short-lived reticulocytosis (with a peak on the fourth postpartum day) and moderately elevated erythropoietin levels during the first week postpartum.

The bone marrow in pregnancy and in the early puerperium is hyperactive and capable of delivering a large number of young cells to the peripheral blood. Prolactin may play a minor role in bone marrow stimulation.

A striking leukocytosis occurs during labor and extends into the early puerperium. In the immediate puerperium, the white blood cell count may be as high as 25,000/mL, with an increased percentage of granulocytes. The stimulus for this leukocytosis is not known, but it probably represents a release of sequestered cells in response to the stress of labor.

The serum iron level is decreased and the plasma iron turnover is increased between the third and fifth days of the puerperium. Normal values are regained by the second week postpartum. The shorter duration of ferrokinetic changes in puerperal women compared with the duration of changes in nonpregnant women who have had phlebotomy is due to the increased erythroid marrow activity and the circulatory changes described previously.

Most women who sustain an average blood loss at delivery and who received iron supplementation during pregnancy show a relative erythrocytosis during the second week postpartum. Because there is no evidence of increased red cell destruction during the puerperium, any red cells gained during pregnancy will disappear gradually according to their normal life span. A moderate excess of red blood cells after delivery, therefore, may lead to an increase in iron stores. Iron supplementation is not necessary for normal postpartum women if the hematocrit or hemoglobin concentration 5–7 days after delivery is equal to or greater than a normal predelivery value. In the late puerperium, there is a gradual decrease in the red cell mass to nonpregnant levels as the rate of erythropoiesis returns to normal.

D. Hemodynamic Changes

The hemodynamic adjustments in the puerperium depend largely on the conduct of labor and delivery (eg, maternal position, method of delivery, mode of anesthesia or analgesia, and blood loss). Cardiac output increases progressively during labor in patients who have received only local anesthesia. The increase in cardiac output peaks immediately after delivery, at which time it is approximately 80% above the prelabor value. During a uterine contraction there is a rise in central venous pressure, arterial pressure, and stroke volume—and, in the absence of pain and anxiety, a reflex decrease in the pulse rate. These changes are magnified in the supine position. Only minimal changes occur in the lateral recumbent position because of unimpaired venous return and absence of aortoiliac compression by the contracting uterus (Poseiro's effect). Epidural anesthesia can interfere with the hemodynamic change by attenuating the progressive rise in cardiac output during labor and reduces the absolute increase observed immediately after delivery, probably by limiting pain, anxiety, and oxygen consumption.

Although major hemodynamic readjustments occur during the period immediately after delivery, there is a return to nonpregnant conditions in the early puerperium. A trend for normal women to increase their blood pressure slightly in the first 5 days postpartum reflects an increased uterine vascular resistance and a temporary surplus in plasma volume. A small percentage will have diastolic blood pressures of 100 mm Hg. Cardiac output (measured by Doppler and cross-sectional echocardiography) declines 28% within 2 weeks postpartum from peak values observed at 38 weeks' gestation. This change is associated with a 20% reduction in stroke volume and a smaller decrease in myocardial contractility indices. Postpartum resolution of pregnancy-induced ventricular hypertrophy takes longer than the functional postpartum changes (Fig. 10–4). In fact, limited data support a slow return of cardiac hemodynamics to prepregnancy levels

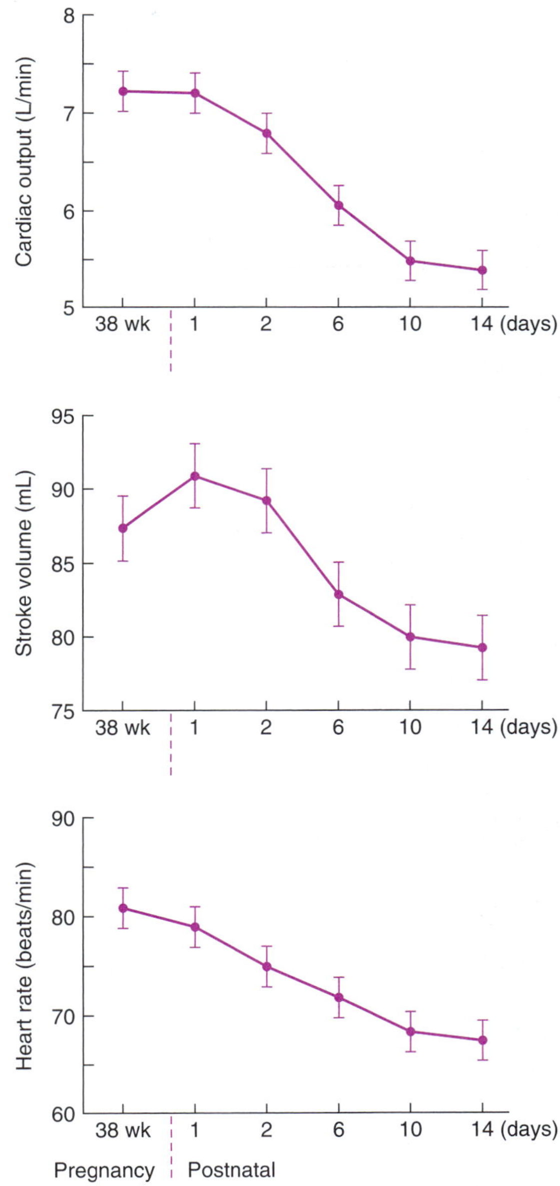

▲ **Figure 10–4.** Changes in cardiac output, stroke volume, and heart rate during the puerperium after normal delivery. (Reproduced, with permission, from Hunter S, Robson SC. Adaptation of the maternal heart in pregnancy. *Br Heart J* 1992;68:540.)

over a 1-year period. There are no hemodynamic differences between lactating and nonlactating mothers.

Respiratory Changes

The pulmonary functions that change most rapidly are those influenced by alterations in abdominal contents and thoracic cage capacity. Lung volumes change in the puerperium and gradually return to the nonpregnant states. The total lung capacity increases after delivery due to decreased intra-abdominal pressure on the diaphragm. An increase in resting ventilation and oxygen consumption and a less efficient response to exercise may persist during the early postpartum weeks. Comparisons of aerobic capacity before pregnancy and again postpartum indicate that lack of activity and weight gain contribute to a generalized detraining effect 4–8 weeks postpartum.

Changes in acid–base status generally parallel changes in respiratory function. The state of pregnancy is characterized by respiratory alkalosis and compensated metabolic acidosis, whereas labor represents a transitional period. A significant hypocapnia (<30 mm Hg), a rise in blood lactate, and a fall in pH are first noted at the end of the first stage of labor and extend into the puerperium. Within a few days, a rise toward the normal nonpregnant values of PCO_2 (35–40 mm Hg) occurs. Progesterone influences the rate of ventilation by means of a central effect, and rapidly decreasing levels of this hormone are largely responsible for the increased PCO_2 seen in the first week postpartum. An increase in base excess and plasma bicarbonate accompanies the relative postpartum hypercapnia. A gradual increase in pH and base excess occurs until normal levels are reached at approximately 3 weeks postpartum.

The resting arterial PO_2 and oxygen saturation during pregnancy are higher than those in nonpregnant women. During labor, the oxygen saturation may be depressed, especially in the supine position, probably as a result of a decrease in cardiac output and a relative increase in the amount of intrapulmonary shunting. However, a rise in the arterial oxygen saturation to 95% is noted during the first postpartum day. An apparent oxygen debt incurred during labor extends into the immediate puerperium and appears to depend on the length and severity of the second stage of labor. Many investigators have commented on the continued elevation of the basal metabolic rate for a period of 7–14 days after delivery. The increased resting oxygen consumption in the early puerperium has been attributed to mild anemia, lactation, and psychologic factors.

Pituitary–Ovarian Relationships

The plasma levels of placental hormones decline rapidly after delivery. Human placental lactogen has a half-life of 20 minutes and reaches undetectable levels in maternal plasma during the first day after delivery. Human chorionic gonadotropin (hCG) has a mean half-life of approximately 9 hours. The concentration of hCG in maternal plasma falls below 1000 mU/mL within 48–96 hours postpartum and falls below 100 mU/mL by the seventh day. Highly specific and sensitive radioimmunoassay for the subunit of hCG indicates virtual disappearance of hCG from maternal plasma between the 11th and 16th days after normal delivery. The regressive pattern of hCG activity is slower after first-trimester abortion than it is after term delivery and even more prolonged in patients who have undergone suction curettage for molar pregnancy.

Within 3 hours after removal of the placenta, the plasma concentration of 17β-estradiol falls to 10% of the antepartum value. The lowest levels are reached by the seventh postpartum day. Plasma estrogens do not reach follicular phase levels (>50 pg/mL) until 19–21 days postpartum in nonlactating women. The return to normal plasma levels of estrogens is delayed in lactating women. Lactating women who resume spontaneous menses achieve follicular-phase estradiol levels (>50 pg/mL) during the first 60–80 days postpartum. Lactating amenorrheic persons are markedly hypoestrogenic (plasma estradiol <10 pg/mL) during the first 180 days postpartum. The onset of breast engorgement on days 3–4 of the puerperium coincides with a significant fall in estrogen levels and supports the view that high estrogen levels suppress lactation.

The metabolic clearance rate of progesterone is high, and, as with estradiol, the half-life is calculated in minutes. By the third day of the puerperium, the plasma progesterone concentrations are below luteal phase levels (<1 ng/mL).

Prolactin levels in maternal blood rise throughout pregnancy to reach concentrations of 200 ng/mL or more. After delivery, prolactin declines in erratic fashion over a period of 2 weeks to the nongravid range in nonlactating women (Fig. 10–5). In women who are breastfeeding, basal concentrations of prolactin remain above the nongravid range and increase dramatically in response to suckling. As lactation progresses, the amount of prolactin released with each suckling episode declines. If breastfeeding occurs only 1–3 times each day, serum prolactin levels return to normal basal values within 6 months postpartum; if suckling takes place more than 6 times each day, high basal concentrations of prolactin will persist for more than 1 year. The diurnal rhythm of peripheral prolactin concentrations (a daytime nadir followed by a nighttime peak) is abolished during late pregnancy but is re-established within 1 week postpartum in non-nursing women.

Serum follicle-stimulating hormone (FSH) and luteinizing hormone (LH) concentrations are very low in all women during the first 10–12 days postpartum, whether or not they lactate. The levels increase over the subsequent days and reach follicular-phase concentrations during the third week postpartum (Fig. 10–5). At this time, marked LH pulse amplification occurs during sleep but disappears as normal ovulatory cycles are established. In this respect, the transition from postpartum amenorrhea to cyclic ovulation is reminiscent of

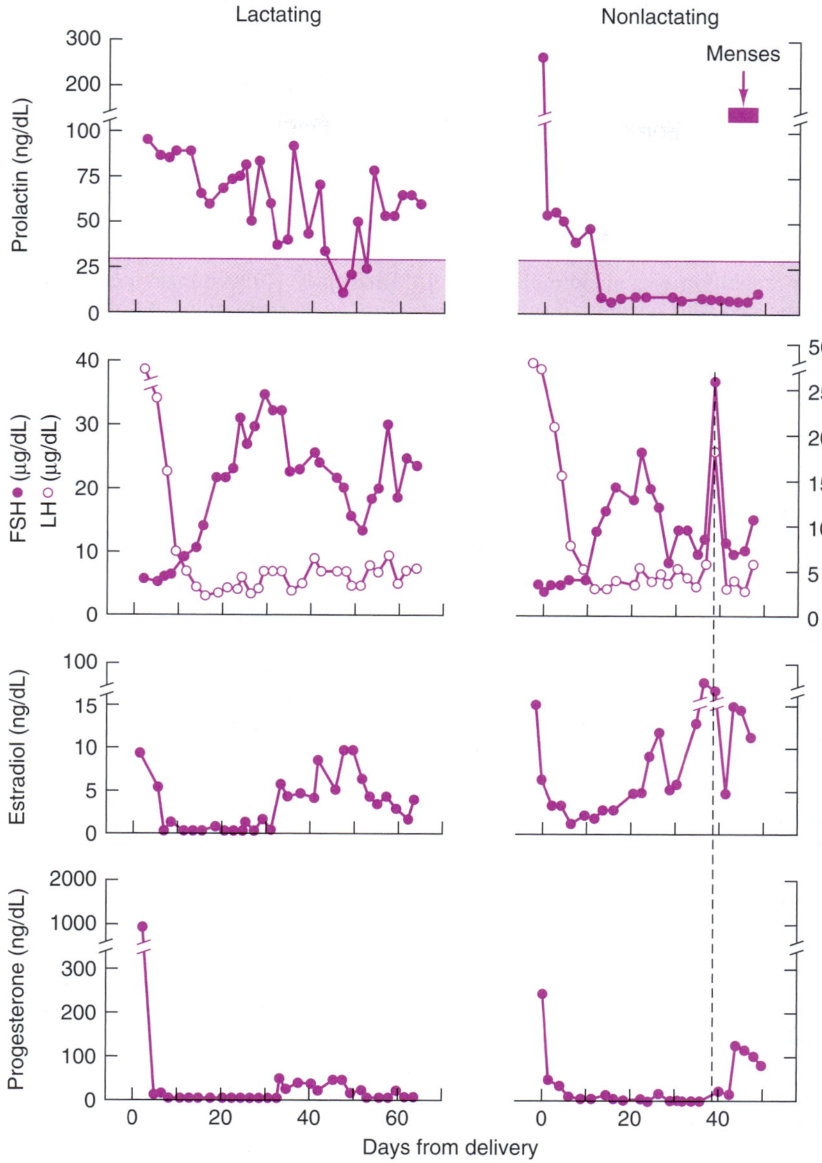

▲ **Figure 10–5.** Serum concentrations of prolactin, follicle-stimulating hormone (FSH), luteinizing hormone (LH), estradiol, and progesterone in a lactating and nonlactating woman during the puerperium. The hatched bars for the prolactin data represent the normal nongravid range. To convert the FSH and LH to milli-international units per milliliter, divide the FSH values by 2 and multiply the LH values by 4.5. (Reproduced, with permission, from Reyes FI, Winter JS, Faiman C. Pituitary-ovarian interrelationships during the puerperium. *Am J Obstet Gynecol* 1972;114:589.)

puberty, when gonadotropin secretion increases during sleep. There is a preferential release of FSH over LH postpartum during spontaneous recovery or after stimulation by exogenous gonadotropin-releasing hormone (GnRH). In the early puerperium, the pituitary is relatively refractory to GnRH, but 4–8 weeks postpartum, the response to GnRH is exaggerated. The low levels of FSH and LH postpartum are most likely related to insufficient endogenous GnRH secretion during pregnancy and the early puerperium, resulting in depletion of pituitary gonadotropin stores. The high estrogen and progesterone milieu of late pregnancy is associated with increased endogenous opioid activity, which may be responsible for suppression of GnRH activity in the puerperium. Resumption of FSH and LH secretion can be accelerated by administering a long-acting GnRH agonist during the first 10 days postpartum.

Because ovarian activity normally resumes upon weaning, either the suckling stimulus itself or the raised level of prolactin is responsible for suppression of pulsatile gonadotropin secretion. Hyperprolactinemia may not entirely account for the inhibition of gonadotropin secretion during lactation, as bromocriptine treatment abolishes the hyperprolactinemia of suckling but not the inhibition of gonadotropin secretion. Sensory inputs associated with suckling (if sufficiently intense), as well as oxytocin and endogenous opioids that are released during suckling, may affect the hypothalamic control of gonadotropin secretion, possibly by inhibiting the pulsatile secretion of GnRH. It appears that by 8 weeks after delivery, although ovarian activity still remains suppressed in fully breastfeeding women, pulsatile secretion of LH has resumed at a low and variable frequency in most women. However, the presence or absence of GnRH or LH pulses at 8 weeks does not predict the time of resumption of ovarian activity.

The time of appearance of the first ovulation is variable, and it is delayed by breastfeeding. Approximately 10–15% of non-nursing mothers ovulate by the time of the 6-week postpartum examination, and approximately 30% ovulate within 90 days postpartum. An abnormally short luteal phase is noted in 35% of first ovulatory cycles. The earliest reported time of ovulation as determined by endometrial biopsy is 33 days postpartum. Patients who have had a first-trimester abortion or ectopic pregnancy generally ovulate sooner after termination of pregnancy (as early as 14 days) than do women who deliver at term. Moreover, the majority of these women do ovulate before the first episode of postabortal bleeding—in contrast to women who have had a term pregnancy.

Endometrial biopsies in lactating women do not show a secretory pattern before the seventh postpartum week. Provided that nursing is in progress and that menstruation has not returned, ovulation before the tenth week postpartum is rare. In well-nourished women who breastfed for an extended period of time, fewer than 20% had ovulated by 6 months postpartum. Much of the variability in the resumption of menstruation and ovulation observed in lactating women may be due to individual differences in the strength of the suckling stimulus and to partial weaning (formula supplementation). This emphasizes the fact that suckling is not a reliable form of birth control. Because the period of lactational infertility is relatively short in Western societies, some form of contraception must be used if pregnancy is to be prevented. Among women who have unprotected intercourse only during lactational amenorrhea but adopt other contraceptive measures when they resume menstruation, only 2% will become pregnant during the first 6 months of amenorrhea. In underdeveloped countries, lactational amenorrhea and infertility may persist for 1–2 years owing to frequent suckling and poor maternal nutrition. When maternal dietary intake is improved, menstruation resumes at least 6 months earlier.

Other Endocrine Changes

Progressive enlargement of the pituitary gland occurs during pregnancy, with a 30–100% increase in weight achieved at term. Magnetic resonance imaging shows a linear gain in pituitary gland height of approximately 0.08 mm/wk during pregnancy. An additional increase in size occurs during the first week postpartum. Beyond the first week postpartum, however, the pituitary gland returns rapidly to its normal size in both lactating and nonlactating women.

The physiologic hypertrophy of the pituitary gland is associated with an increase in the number of pituitary lactotroph cells at the expense of the somatotropic cell types. Thus growth hormone secretion is depressed during the second half of pregnancy and the early puerperium. Because levels of circulating insulin-like growth factor (IGF)-1 increase throughout pregnancy, a placental growth hormone has been postulated and recently identified. Maternal levels of IGF-1 correlate highly with this distinct placental growth hormone variant, but not with placental lactogen during pregnancy and in the immediate puerperium.

Late pregnancy and the early puerperium are also characterized by pituitary somatotroph hyporesponsiveness to growth hormone-releasing hormone and to insulin stimulation. Whatever the inhibitory mechanism may be (possibly increased somatostatin secretion), it persists during the early postpartum period.

The rapid disappearance of placental lactogen and the low levels of growth hormone after delivery lead to a relative deficiency of anti-insulin factors in the early puerperium. It is not surprising, therefore, that low fasting plasma glucose levels are noted at this time and that the insulin requirements of diabetic patients usually drop after delivery. Glucose tolerance tests performed in women with gestational diabetes demonstrate that only 30% have abnormal test results 3–5 days after delivery, and 20% have abnormal glucose tolerance at 6 weeks postpartum. Because the early puerperium represents a transitional period in carbohydrate metabolism, the results of glucose tolerance tests may be difficult to interpret.

Evaluation of thyroid function is also difficult in the period immediately after birth because of rapid fluctuations in many indices. Characteristically, the plasma thyroxine level and other indices of thyroid function are highest at delivery and in the first 12 hours thereafter. A decrease to antepartum values is seen on the third or fourth day after delivery. Reduced available estrogens postpartum lead to a subsequent decrease in circulating thyroxine-binding globulin and a gradual diminution in bound thyroid hormones in serum. Serum concentrations of thyroid-stimulating hormone (TSH) are not significantly different postpartum from those of the pregnant or nonpregnant state. Administration of thyroid-releasing hormone in the puerperium results in a normal increase in both TSH and prolactin, and the response is similar in lactating and nonlactating patients. Because pregnancy is associated with some immunosuppressive effects, hyperthyroidism or hypothyroidism may recur postpartum in autoimmune thyroid disease. Failure of lactation and prolonged disability may be the result of hypothyroidism postpartum. In Sheehan's syndrome of pituitary infarction, postpartum cachexia and myxedema are seen secondary to anterior hypophyseal insufficiency.

Maternal concentrations of total and unbound (free) plasma cortisol, adrenocorticotropic hormone (ACTH), immunoreactive corticotropin-releasing hormone (CRH), and β-endorphin rise progressively during pregnancy and increase further during labor. Plasma 17-hydroxycorticosteroid levels increase from a concentration of 4–14 μg/dL at 40 weeks' gestation. A 2- to 3-fold increase is seen during labor. ACTH, CRH, and β-endorphin decrease rapidly after delivery and return to nonpregnant levels within 24 hours. Prelabor cortisol values are regained on the first day postpartum, but a return to normal, nonpregnant cortisol and 17-hydroxycorticosteroid levels is not reached until the end of the first week postpartum.

Much of the rise in total cortisol (but not in the unbound fraction) can be explained by the parallel increase in corticosteroid-binding globulin (CBG) during pregnancy. Displacement of cortisol from CBG by high concentrations of progesterone cannot account for the increased free cortisol levels because saliva progesterone levels (a measure of the unbound hormone) do not fluctuate, whereas a normal diurnal rhythm of saliva cortisol is maintained during pregnancy and postpartum. An extrapituitary source of ACTH, a progesterone-modulated decrease in the hypothalamic–pituitary sensitivity to glucocorticoid feedback inhibition, and an extrahypothalamic (eg, placental) source of CRH have been suggested as explanations for elevated plasma ACTH levels and the inability of dexamethasone to completely suppress ACTH in pregnant women.

In the third trimester, the placenta produces large amounts of CRH, which is released into the maternal circulation and may contribute to the hypercortisolemia of pregnancy. Present evidence suggests that it stimulates the maternal pituitary to produce ACTH while desensitizing the pituitary to further acute stimulation with CRH. Maternal hypothalamic control of ACTH production is retained (perhaps mediated by vasopressin secretion); this permits a normal response to stress and a persistent diurnal rhythm.

Overall, it is most likely that under the influence of rising estrogens and progesterone, there is a resetting of the hypothalamic–pituitary sensitivity to cortisol feedback during pregnancy, which persists for several days postpartum. Several studies have suggested a relationship between peripartum alterations in maternal levels of cortisol and β-endorphin and the development of postnatal mood disturbances.

The excretion of urinary 17-ketosteroids is elevated in late pregnancy as a result of an increase in androgenic precursors from the fetoplacental unit and the ovary. An additional increase of 50% in excretion occurs during labor. Excretion of 17-ketosteroids returns to antepartum levels on the first day after delivery and to the nonpregnant range by the end of the first week. The mean levels of testosterone during the third trimester of pregnancy range from 3 to 7 times the mean values for nonpregnant women. The elevated levels of testosterone decrease after parturition parallel with the gradual fall in sex hormone-binding globulin (SHBG). Androstenedione, which is poorly bound to SHBG, falls rapidly to nonpregnant values by the third day postpartum. Conversely, the postpartum plasma concentration of dehydroepiandrosterone sulfate remains lower than that of nonpregnant women, because its metabolic clearance rate continues to be elevated in the early puerperium. Persistently elevated levels of 17-ketosteroids or androgens during the puerperium are an indication for investigation of ovarian abnormalities. Plasma renin and angiotensin II levels fall during the first 2 hours postpartum to levels within the normal nonpregnant range. This suggests that an extrarenal source of renin has been lost with the expulsion of the fetus and placenta.

There is little direct information about the puerperal changes in numerous other hormones, including aldosterone, parathyroid hormone, and calcitonin. More research should be done on these important endocrine relationships in the puerperium.

De Santis M, Cavaliere AF, Straface G, Caruso A. Rubella infection in pregnancy. *Reprod Toxicol* 2006;21:390. PMID: 16580940.

Hellgren M. Hemostasis during normal pregnancy and pueperium. *Semin Thromb Hemost* 2003;29:125. PMID: 12709915.

Mulic-Lutvica A, Axelsson O. Postpartum ultrasound in women with postpartum endometritis, after cesarean section and after manual evacuation of the placenta. *Acta Obstet Gynecol Scand* 2007;86:210. PMID: 17364285.

Reader D, Franz MJ. Lactation, diabetes and nutrition recommendations. *Curr Diab Rep* 2004;4:370. PMID: 15461903.

Vesco KK, Dietz PM, Rizzo J, et al. Excessive gestational weight gain and postpartum weight retention among obese women. *Obstet Gynecol* 2009;114:1069. PMID 20168109.

CONDUCT AND MANAGEMENT OF THE PUERPERIUM

Most patients will benefit from 2–4 days of hospitalization after delivery. Only 3% of women with a vaginal delivery and 9% of women having a caesarean section have a childbirth-related complication requiring prolonged postpartum hospitalization or readmission. Although a significant amount of symptomatic morbidity may exist postpartum (painful perineum, breastfeeding difficulties, urinary infections, urinary and fecal incontinence, and headache), most women can return home safely 2 days after normal vaginal delivery if proper education and instructions are given, if confidence exists with infant care and feeding, and if adequate support exists at home. Earlier discharge is acceptable in select mothers and infants who have had uncomplicated labors and deliveries. Discharge criteria should be met and follow-up care provided. Optimal care includes home nursing visits through the fourth postpartum day.

Disadvantages of early discharge are the increased risks of rehospitalization of some neonates for hyperbilirubinemia and neonatal infection (eg, from group B streptococci).

Activities & Rest

The policy of early ambulation after delivery benefits the patient. Early ambulation provides a sense of well-being, hastens involution of the uterus, improves uterine drainage, and lessens the incidence of postpartum thromboembolic event. If the delivery has been uncomplicated, the patient may be out of bed as soon as tolerated. Early ambulation does not mean immediate return to normal activity or work. Commonly mothers complain of lethargy and fatigue. Therefore, rest is essential after delivery, and the demands on the mother should be limited to allow for adequate relaxation and adjustment to her new responsibilities. It is helpful to set aside a few hours each day for rest periods. Many mothers do not sleep well for several nights after delivery, and it is surprising how much of the day is occupied with the care of the newborn.

In uncomplicated deliveries, more vigorous activity, climbing stairs, lifting of heavy objects, riding in or driving a car, and performing muscle toning exercises may be resumed without delay. Specific recommendations should be individualized. Current American College of Obstetricians and Gynecologists committee opinions support gradual resumption of exercise routines as soon as medically and physically safe, as detraining may have occurred during pregnancy. No known maternal complications are associated with resumption of exercise, even in women who choose to resume an exercise routine within days. Exercise postpartum does not compromise lactation or neonatal weight gain. It may be beneficial in decreasing anxiety levels and decreasing the incidence of postpartum depression.

Diet

A regular diet is permissible as soon as the patient wishes in the absence of complication. Protein-rich foods, fruits, vegetables, milk products, and a high fluid intake are recommended, especially for nursing mothers. It is estimated that women will need approximately 500 kcal per day more than the recommended level for nonpregnant and nonlactating women. It may be advisable to continue the daily vitamin–mineral supplement during the early puerperium. Lactating women are advised to maintain calcium intake of 1000 mg per day and should be encouraged to drink plenty of fluids to maintain adequate hydration. After caesarean section, there is no evidence supporting compromised safety or comfort from the introduction of solid foods early and allowing the patient to decide when to eat postoperatively. In fact, early feeding as tolerated by the patient has been shown to be safe, to enhance patient satisfaction, to minimize hospital stay, and to facilitate a more rapid return to normal diet and bowel function.

Care of the Bladder

Most women empty the bladder during labor or have been catheterized at delivery. Even so, serious bladder distention may develop within 12 hours. A prolonged second stage of labor or operative delivery may traumatize the base of the bladder and interfere with normal voiding and is significantly associated with protracted urinary retention beyond the third postpartum day. In some cases, overdistention of the bladder may be related to pain or regional anesthesia. Mechanical bladder outlet obstruction may develop secondary to edema or local hematoma, functional obstruction may be secondary to pain, and detrusor underactivity may be due to bladder overdistention during labor. The marked polyuria noted for the first few days postpartum causes the bladder to fill in a relatively short time. Hence obstetric patients require catheterization more frequently than most surgical patients. The patient should be catheterized every 6 hours after delivery if she is unable to void or empty her bladder completely. Intermittent catheterization is preferable to an indwelling catheter because the incidence of urinary tract infection is lower. However, if the bladder fills to more than 1000 mL, 1–2 days of decompression by a retention catheter usually is required to establish voiding without significant residual urine. Postpartum voiding dysfunction is common but usually self-limited and spontaneously resolves within 3 days.

The incidence of true asymptomatic bacteriuria is approximately 5% in the early puerperium. Postpartum patients with a history of previous urinary tract infection, conduction anesthesia, and catheterization during delivery and operative delivery should have a bacterial culture of a midstream urine specimen. In cases of confirmed bacteriuria, antibiotic treatment should be given; otherwise, bacteriuria will persist in nearly 30% of patients. Three days of therapy is sufficient and avoids prolonged antibiotic exposure to the lactating mother.

Bowel Function

Pregnancy itself is associated with increased gastric emptying, but gastrointestinal motility is commonly delayed after labor and delivery. The mild ileus that follows delivery, together with perineal discomfort and postpartum fluid loss by other routes, predisposes to constipation during the puerperium. Milk of magnesia, 15–20 mL orally on the evening of the second postpartum day, usually stimulates a bowel movement by the next morning. If not, a rectal suppository, such as bisacodyl or a small tap water or oil retention enema, may be given. Less bowel stimulation will be needed if the diet contains sufficient roughage. Stool softeners, such as dioctyl sodium sulfosuccinate, may ease the discomfort of early bowel movements. Hemorrhoidal discomfort is a common complaint postpartum and usually responds to conservative treatment with compresses, suppositories containing corticosteroids, local anesthetic sprays or emollients, and sitz baths. Surgical treatment of hemorrhoids postpartum is rarely necessary unless thrombosis is extensive.

Operative vaginal delivery and lacerations involving the anal sphincter increase a woman's risk for anal incontinence. However, 5% of pregnant women overall have some degree of anal incontinence at 3 months postpartum. Complaints of fecal incontinence are often delayed because of embarrassment. Most cases are transient; however, cases persisting beyond 6 months require investigation and probable treatment.

Bathing

As soon as the patient is ambulatory, she may take a shower. Sitz or tub baths probably are safe if performed in a clean environment. Most patients prefer showers to tub baths because of the profuse flow of lochia immediately postpartum; however, sitz baths may be beneficial for perineal pain relief. Vaginal douching is contraindicated in the early puerperium. Tampons may be used whenever the patient is comfortable.

Care of the Perineum

Postpartum perineal care, even in the patient with an uncomplicated and satisfactorily repaired episiotomy or laceration, usually requires no more than routine cleansing with a bath or shower and analgesia.

Immediately after delivery, cold compresses (usually ice) applied to the perineum decrease traumatic edema and discomfort. The perineal area should be gently cleansed with plain soap at least once or twice per day and after voiding or defecation. If the perineum is kept clean, healing should occur rapidly. Cold or iced sitz baths, rather than hot sitz baths, may provide additional perineal pain relief for some patients. The patient should be put in a lukewarm tub to which ice cubes are added for 20–30 minutes. The cold promotes pain relief by decreasing the excitability of nerve endings and slowing nerve conduction, and by local vasoconstriction, which reduces edema, inhibits hematoma formation, and decreases muscle irritability and spasm. Episiotomy pain is easily controlled with nonsteroidal anti-inflammatory agents, which appear to be superior to acetaminophen or propoxyphene.

An episiotomy or repaired lacerations should be inspected daily. A patient with mediolateral episiotomy, a third- or fourth-degree laceration or extension, or extensive bruising or edema may experience severe perineal pain. In the case of persistent or unusual pain, a vaginal and/or rectal examination should be performed to identify a hematoma, perineal infection, or potentially fatal conditions, such as angioedema, necrotizing fasciitis, or perineal cellulitis. Episiotomy wounds rarely become infected, which is remarkable considering the difficulty of preventing contamination of the perineal area. In the event of infection, local heat and irrigation should cause the infection to subside. Appropriate antibiotics may be indicated if an immediate response to these measures is not observed. In rare instances, the wound should be opened widely and sutures removed for adequate drainage.

Uterotonic Agents

Prophylactic administration of oxytocin after the second stage of labor and/or after placental delivery is beneficial in preventing postpartum hemorrhage and the need for therapeutic uterotonics. The routine use of ergot preparations or prostaglandins may be as effective as oxytocin but has significantly more side effects. There appear to be no data supporting the prophylactic use of uterotonic agents beyond the immediate puerperium. These agents should be limited to patients with specific indications, such as postpartum hemorrhage or uterine atony.

Emotional Reactions

Several basic emotional responses occur in almost every woman who has given birth to a normal baby. A woman's first emotion is usually one of extreme relief, followed by a sense of happiness and gratitude that the new baby has arrived safely. A regular pattern of behavior occurs in the human mother immediately after birth of the infant. Touching, holding, and grooming of the infant under normal conditions rapidly strengthen maternal ties of affection. However, not all mothers react in this way, and some may even feel detached from the new baby. These reactions range from the common, physiologic, relatively mild, and transient "maternity blues," which affect some 50–70% of postpartum women, to more severe reactions including depression and rare puerperal psychosis.

Postpartum blues or maternity blues occur in up to 70% of postpartum women and appear to be a normal psychologic adjustment or response. It is generally characterized by tearfulness, anxiety, irritation, and restlessness. This symptomatology can be quite diverse and may include depression, feelings of inadequacy, elation, mood swings, confusion, difficulty concentrating, headache, forgetfulness, insomnia, depersonalization, and negative feelings toward the baby. These transient symptoms usually occur within the first few days after delivery and cease by postpartum day 10, although bouts of weeping may occur for weeks after delivery. The blues are self-limiting, but the distress can be diminished by physical comfort and reassurance. Evidence suggests that rooming-in during the hospital stay reduces maternal anxiety and results in more successful breastfeeding.

Prematurity or illness of the newborn delays early intimate maternal–infant contact and may have an adverse effect on the rapid and complete development of normal mothering responses. Stressful factors during the puerperium (eg, marital infidelity or loss of friends as a result of the necessary confinement and preoccupation with the new baby) may leave the mother feeling unsupported and may interfere with the formation of a maternal bond with the infant.

When a baby dies or is born with a congenital defect, the obstetrician should inform the mother and father about the problem together, if possible. The baby's normal, healthy features and potential for improvement should be emphasized, and positive statements should be made about the present availability of corrective treatment and the promises of ongoing research. In the event of a perinatal loss, parents should be assisted in the grieving process. They should be encouraged to see and touch the baby at birth or later, even if maceration or anomalies are present. Mementos such as footprints, locks of hair, or a photograph can be a solace to the parents after the infant has been buried. During the puerperium, the obstetrician has an important opportunity to help the mother whose infant has died work through her period of mourning or discouragement and to assess abnormal reactions of grief that suggest a need for psychiatric assistance. Pathologic grief is characterized by the inability to work through the sense of loss within 3–4 months, with subsequent feelings of low self-esteem.

Sexual Activity During the Postpartum Period

Establishment of normal prepregnancy sexual response patterns is delayed after delivery. However, it is safe to resume sexual activity when the woman's perineum is comfortable and bleeding is diminished. Although the median time for resumption of intercourse after delivery is 6 weeks and the normal sexual response returns at 12 weeks, sexual desire and activity vary tremendously among women. Sexual function significantly declines during the third trimester of pregnancy. This dysfunction peaks approximately 3 months postpartum and tends to improve within 6 months after delivery. During pregnancy women report lack of information and concerns about possible adverse outcomes for the pregnancy as reasons for their decreased sexual activity. Physical manifestations such as weight gain, breast tenderness, anxiety, and fatigue likely also contribute to avoidance of intercourse as the pregnancy progresses.

After delivery most women report low or absent sexual desire during the early puerperium and attribute this to fatigue, weakness, dyspareunia, vaginal dryness, urinary or fecal incontinence, irritative vaginal discharge, or fear of injury to the healing perineum. Early pelvic-floor muscle exercise appears to have positive effects on restoration of female sexual function. Significant predictors of dyspareunia at 6 months vary by study but have included breastfeeding, vacuum delivery, greater than first-degree lacerations, fecal incontinence, and history of previous dyspareunia. Approximately 90% of women restart sexual activity within 6 months after delivery, depending on the site and state of perineal or vaginal healing, return of libido, and vaginal atrophy resulting from breastfeeding. There is a gradual and steady recovery of sexual function postpartum, and by 12 months 80–85% of patients consider their sex lives unchanged and only 10–15% consider it worsened. The mode of delivery alone does not appear to have significant effect on sexual function 12–18 months after childbirth, as no difference in satisfaction or complications was found between women who delivered vaginally without episiotomy, heavy perineal laceration, or secondary operative interventions and women who underwent elective caesarean section.

Sexual counseling is indicated before the mother is discharged from the hospital. A discussion of the normal fluctuations of sexual interest during the puerperium is appropriate, as are suggestions for noncoital sexual options that enhance the expression of mutual pleasure and affection. The importance of sleep and rest and of the partner's emotional and physical support is emphasized. If milk ejection during sexual relations is a concern, nursing the baby before sexual intimacy can help. Sexual relations can generally be resumed by the third week postpartum, if desired. A water-soluble lubricant or vaginal estrogen cream is especially helpful in lactating amenorrheic mothers in whom vaginal atrophy occurs, usually because of low circulating estrogen levels. Patients should be informed that at least 50% of women engaging in sexual intercourse by 6 weeks will experience dyspareunia, which may persist up to 1 year. Dyspareunia also occurs in women with caesarean sections and in women using oral contraceptives who are not breastfeeding.

Postpartum Immunization

A. Prevention of Rh Isoimmunization

The postpartum injection of Rh_o (D) immunoglobulin* has been shown to prevent sensitization in the Rh-negative woman who has had fetal-to-maternal transfusion of Rh-positive fetal red cells. The risk of maternal sensitization rises with the volume of fetal transplacental hemorrhage. The usual amount of fetal blood that enters the maternal circulation is <0.5 mL. The usual dose of 300 μg of Rh_o (D) immunoglobulin is in excess of the dose generally required. Three hundred grams will neutralize approximately 30 mL of whole fetal blood (or 15 mL of Rh+ fetal red blood cells). If neonatal anemia or other clinical symptoms suggest the occurrence of a large transplacental hemorrhage, the amount of fetal blood in the maternal circulation can be estimated by the Kleihauer-Betke smear and the amounts of Rh_o (D) immunoglobulin to be administered adjusted accordingly.

* Trade names include Gamulin Rh, HypRho-D, and RhoGAM.

Rh_0 (D) immunoglobulin is administered after abortion without qualifications or after delivery to women who meet all of the following criteria: (1) The mother must be Rh_0 (D)-negative without Rh antibodies, (2) the baby must be Rh (D)+ or Rh (D)-/Du-positive, and (3) the cord blood must be Coombs-negative. If these criteria are met, a 1:1000 dilution of Rh_0 (D) immunoglobulin is cross-matched to the mother's red cells to ensure compatibility, and 1 mL (300 μg) is given intramuscularly to the mother within 72 hours after delivery. If the 72-hour interval has been exceeded, it is advisable to give the immunoglobulin rather than withhold it because it may still protect against sensitization 14–28 days after delivery, and the time required to mount a response varies among cases. The 72-hour time limit for administration of Rh immunoglobulin was a study limitation in a study in which patients in prison were allowed to be visited only every 3 days; thus the use of Rh immunoglobulin past the 3-day interval was never studied. Rh_0 (D) immunoglobulin should also be given after delivery or abortion when serologic tests of maternal sensitization to the Rh factor are questionable.

The average risk of maternal sensitization after abortion is approximately half the risk incurred by full-term pregnancy and delivery; the latter has been estimated at 11%. Women with pregnancy losses up to 12 weeks may receive a smaller dose of Rh immunoglobulin, as the 50-μg dose is sufficient to protect against 2.5 mL of Rh-positive fetal red blood cells. Even though mothers have received Rh_0 (D) immunoglobulin, they should be screened with each subsequent pregnancy because postpartum prophylaxis failures still exist. Failures are related to inadequate Rh_0 (D) immunoglobulin administration postpartum, an undetected very low titer in the previous pregnancy, and inexcusable oversights. Routine use of postpartum screening protocols to identify excess fetomaternal hemorrhage and strict adherence to recommended protocols for the management of unsensitized Rh-negative women will prevent most of these postpartum sensitizations.

B. Rubella Vaccination

A significant number of women of childbearing age estimated at 10–20% have never been immunized or exposed to rubella infection. The appropriate test for assessing rubella immunity is the immunoglobulin G serology. Women who are susceptible to rubella can be vaccinated safely and effectively with a live attenuated rubella virus vaccine (RA 27/3 strain) during the immediate puerperium. It is more immunogenic than earlier forms of the vaccine and is available in monovalent, bivalent (measles-rubella [MR]), and trivalent (measles-mumps-rubella [MMR]) forms. Seroconversion occurs in approximately 95% of women vaccinated postpartum. There is no contraindication to giving MMR vaccination while breastfeeding, and it is not associated with viral transmission to newborns. Women who receive rubella vaccinations are not contagious and cannot transmit infection to other susceptible children or adults. In addition, the serologic response against rubella is satisfactory when given concomitantly with other immunoglobulins such as Rh-immunoglobulin. Vaccinated patients should be informed that transient side effects can result from rubella vaccination. Mild symptoms such as low-grade fever and malaise may occur in fewer than 25% of patients and arthralgias and rash in fewer than 10%; rarely, overt arthritis may develop. Among adult women there is a 10–15% incidence of acute polyarthritis after immunization. In 2001, the US Centers for Disease Control and Prevention (CDC) changed the safe pregnancy interval after receiving the rubella vaccine from 3 months to 1 month. The receipt of vaccination during the pregnancy is not an indication for termination. The maximum theoretical risk of congenital rubella resulting from vaccination during early pregnancy is 1–2%.

C. Postpartum Tdap (Tetanus, Diphtheria, Pertussis) Vaccination

With the incidence of pertussis growing among adults and adolescents in the United States, there is a concomitant increased risk of transmission to susceptible populations, including infants. Infants do not have full immunity against pertussis until they have received at least 3 doses of pertussis-containing vaccine, making infants younger than 6 months the most susceptible. Pertussis is preventable through vaccination; however, immunity from childhood pertussis vaccines wanes after 5–10 years, making adolescent and adult populations again susceptible to pertussis. Infants under 12 months of age comprised 19% of cases and 92% of pertussis deaths in the United States from 2000–2004. Of those with pertussis, 63% required hospitalization, and 13% were diagnosed with pneumonia. The use of Tdap vaccine in the postpartum woman can provide protection to infants.

The Advisory Committee on Immunization Practices (ACIP) recommends routine postpartum Tdap for those pregnant women who previously have not received a dose of Tdap (including women who are breastfeeding) before discharge from the hospital or birthing center. If Tdap cannot be administered before discharge, it should be given as soon as it is feasible. The dose of Tdap replaces the next decennial dose of Td. Providers who choose to administer Tdap to pregnant women should discuss the lack of safety data with the pregnant patient.

D. Postpartum Influenza Vaccination

The ACIP recommends universal flu vaccination in the United States. Pregnant women are characterized by the CDC as a high-risk population because having the flu would place these women and their fetuses at increased risk of complications. The "flu shot" should thus be offered to these women as soon as flu season begins in September. This intramuscular form of the vaccine contains killed inactivated virus and is safe in pregnancy. The nasal-spray flu vaccine is not a safe option for pregnant women because it contains live albeit weakened flu viruses. If a pregnant woman does not receive the flu shot during pregnancy, then she should be given the vaccine in the immediate postpartum period. The ACIP strongly recommends that household contacts and caregivers of children younger than 6 months receive the flu shot, because children this young are at high risk for complications from the flu and are too young to be vaccinated themselves. Women in this postpartum period are eligible for either the flu shot or nasal-spray vaccine.

Contraception & Sterilization

The immediate puerperium has long been recognized as a convenient time for the discussion of family planning, although these discussions ideally should begin during prenatal care. Pregnancy prevention and birth control decisions should be made before discharge with a qualified nurse, physician, or physician's assistant or with the aid of educational tools. Anovulatory infertility lasts approximately 5 weeks in nonlactating women and >8 weeks in fully lactating women. The lactational pregnancy rate is approximately 1–2% at 1 year postpartum.

Tubal sterilization is the most common method of contraception used in the United States. It is the procedure of choice for women desiring permanent sterilization. It can be performed easily at the time of caesarean section or within 48 hours postpartum after vaginal delivery in uncomplicated patients without prolonging hospitalization or significantly increasing morbidity. Sterilization may not be advisable in women younger than 30 years, those of low parity, or when the neonatal outcome is in doubt and survival of the infant is not assured. Postponing tubal sterilization 6–8 weeks postpartum is desirable for many couples, as it allows time to ensure that the infant is healthy, to fully understand the implications of permanent sterilization, and, according to the US Collaborative Review on Sterilization, to decrease feelings of guilt and regret. It also allows for different surgical approaches to be discussed, including the hysteroscopic Essure device (Conceptus, Mountain View, CA), which has the benefit of avoiding abdominal incisions.

Appropriate counseling regarding risks of failure, permanence of the procedure, the medical risks, and the potential psychosocial reactions to the procedure should be discussed with the patient. Patient ambivalence at the last minute is not unusual, in which case it is advisable to defer the procedure until after the puerperium. The 10-year failure rate of postpartum sterilization ranges from 1–3% and varies with type of procedure performed. The risks of postpartum or interval tubal ligation are infrequent, and deaths from the procedure occur in 2–12 per 100,000 cases. Long-term complications, such as the posttubal syndrome (irregular menses and increased menstrual pain) have been reported in some 10–15% of women; however, well-controlled prospective studies have failed to confirm that these symptoms occur more frequently with sterilization than in controls.

Use of lactational amenorrhea for family planning in exclusively breastfeeding mothers provides 98% contraceptive protection for up to 6 months according to some studies; however, concurrent use of progestin-only pill is advisable to increase the contraceptive efficacy. When menses return, natural family planning may begin. This method, which has pregnancy rates comparable to those of barrier methods, uses detection of the periovulatory period by evaluating cervical mucus changes and/or basal body temperature changes. Patients should be aware that the natural method is not always reliable and can potentially increase the chance of pregnancy, especially in those women with irregular cycles.

Use of spermicides, a condom, or both may be prescribed until the postpartum examination; these methods carry a failure rate of 1.6–21 per 100 woman-years. Fitting of a diaphragm is not practical until involution of the reproductive organs has taken place and may be more difficult in lactating women with vaginal dryness. It should always be used in conjunction with a spermicidal lubricant containing nonoxynol-9. The failure rate for the diaphragm varies from 2.4–19.6 per 100 woman-years, with the lowest failure rates (comparable to the intrauterine device [IUD]) occurring in women who are older, motivated, experienced, or familiar with the technique.

Combined hormonal contraception, including the pill, patch, or ring, functions by suppressing ovulation, increasing cervical mucus viscosity, and lowering the receptivity of the endometrium to implantation. Oral contraception should be deferred until 6 weeks postpartum because of concerns about the postpartum hypercoagulable state. Of note, the vaginal ring produces the lowest estrogen levels of any combined hormonal contraceptive available. The typical use failure rate for combined hormonal contraception is 7–8% due primarily to missed pills or failure to resume therapy after the 7-day pill-free interval. Studies are inconclusive regarding estrogen's effect on milk letdown, and several studies have shown no deleterious effect of oral contraceptive pills on the breastfed infant. Progestin-only oral contraceptive (norethindrone 0.35 mg/d) has proven to be a safe option that does not suppress lactation and in fact may actually enhance lactation. Its contraceptive efficacy is maximum with exclusive breastfeeding, and additional or alternative contraceptive methods are advisable when breastfeeding frequency is decreased. The use of a long-acting progestin such as depot medroxyprogesterone acetate (Depo-Provera; Pfizer, New York, NY), 150 mg administered intramuscularly or 104 mg administered subcutaneously every 3 months, provides effective contraception (>99% contraceptive efficacy) for the lactating woman without increasing the risk of maternal thromboembolism or decreasing milk yield. However, concerns related to prolonged amenorrhea, prolonged return to fertility, the inconvenience of unscheduled bleeding, weight gain, skin changes, and reversible bone density reduction and lipid metabolism changes are potential reasons for discontinuation. On the other hand, the level of progestin in depot medroxyprogesterone acetate raises the seizure threshold and is the contraceptive of choice for women with seizure disorders.

Levonorgestrel implants placed after establishment of lactation (immediately postpartum or by 6 weeks) provide acceptable contraception with no effect on lactation or infant growth. They have gained little favor, probably because of irregular bleeding, high cost, and difficulty in insertion and removal.

Insertion of an IUD (copper-containing TCu 380 Ag) (Eurim-Pharm Vertriebs GmbH & Co KG, Austria) and ParaGard T380A (Duramed Pharmaceuticals Inc. Pomona, NY, USA), progesterone-releasing Progestasert (Janssen Pharmaceuticals Inc. Titusville, NJ, USA), or levonorgestrel-releasing Mirena (Bayer Healthcare Pharmaceuticals inc. Wayne, NJ, USA)) is highly effective in preventing pregnancy (<2–3 pregnancies per 100 woman-years) and is not considered an abortifacient. Ideally, an IUD should be placed at the first postpartum visit; however, it may be placed as early as immediately postpartum. In this latter case, the incidence of expulsion appears higher than with interval insertion. The main side effects include <1% risk of pelvic infection in the first 2 weeks after insertion, uterine perforation (<1%), expulsion (<3%), and abnormal uterine bleeding. The risk of ectopic pregnancy is lower among women with the Mirena or ParaGard compared with women using no contraception. The risk of uterine perforation during IUD insertion is higher in lactating women, probably because of the accelerated rate of uterine involution. Of note, the risk of expulsion is not increased in these lactating women. Uterine perforation is highest when insertion is performed in the first 1–8 weeks after delivery. The levonorgestrel IUD in particular has added noncontraceptive benefits, including an 80% rate of amenorrhea after 1 year, improvements in dysmenorrhea and endometriosis, and management of endometrial hyperplasia in poor surgical candidates.

Discharge Examination & Instructions

Before the patient's hospital discharge, the breasts and abdomen should be examined. The degree of uterine involution and tenderness should be noted. The calves and thighs should be palpated to rule out thrombophlebitis. The characteristics of the lochia are important and should be observed. The episiotomy wound should be inspected to see whether it is healing satisfactorily. A blood sample should be obtained for hematocrit or hemoglobin determination. Unless the patient has an unusual pelvic complaint, there is little need to perform a vaginal examination. The obstetrician should be certain that the patient is voiding normally, has normal bowel function, and is physically able to assume her new responsibilities at home.

The patient will require some advice on what she is allowed to do when she arrives home. Hygiene is essentially the same as practiced in the hospital, with a premium on cleanliness. Upon discharge from the hospital, the patient should be instructed to rest for at least 2 hours during the day, and her usual household activities should be curtailed. Activities, exercise, and return to work will be individualized. Accepted disability after delivery is 6 weeks. Various forms of social support are critical for mothers, especially those employed outside the home: available, high-quality day care; parental leave for both mothers and fathers; and support provided by the workplace such as flexible hours, the opportunity to breastfeed, on-site day care, and care for sick children. The patient who has had frequent prenatal visits to her obstetrician may feel cut off from the doctor during the interval between discharge and the first postpartum visit. She will feel reassured in this period if she receives thoughtful advice on what she is allowed to do and what she can expect when she arrives home. She should be instructed to notify the physician or nurse in the event of fever, vaginal bleeding, or back pain that does not resolve with over-the-counter pain medication. At the time of discharge, the patient should be informed that she will note persistent but decreasing amounts of vaginal lochia for approximately 3 weeks and possibly for a short period during the fourth or fifth week after delivery.

Postpartum Visit Examination

At the postpartum visit— 4–6 weeks after discharge from the hospital— the patient's weight and blood pressure should be recorded. Most patients retain approximately 60% of any weight in excess of 11 kg (24 lb) that was gained during pregnancy. A suitable diet may be prescribed if the patient has not returned to her approximate prepregnancy weight. If the patient was anemic upon discharge from the hospital or has been bleeding during the puerperium, a complete blood count should be determined. Persistence of uterine bleeding demands investigation and definitive treatment.

The breasts should be examined, and the adequacy of support, abnormalities of the nipples or lactation, and the presence of any masses should be noted. The patient should be instructed concerning self-examination of the breasts. A complete rectovaginal evaluation is required.

Nursing mothers may show a hypoestrogenic condition of the vaginal epithelium. Prescription of a vaginal estrogen cream to be applied at bedtime should relieve local dryness and coital discomfort without the side effects of systemic estrogen therapy. The cervix should be inspected and a Papanicolaou (Pap) smear obtained. Women whose prenatal smears are normal are still at risk for an abnormal Pap smear at their postpartum visit.

The episiotomy incision and repaired lacerations must be examined and the adequacy of pelvic and perineal support noted. Bimanual examination of the uterus and adnexa is indicated. At the time of the postpartum examination, most patients have some degree of retrodisplacement of the uterus, but this may soon correct itself. If marked uterine descensus is noted, or if the patient develops stress incontinence or symptomatic cystocele or rectocele, surgical correction should be considered if childbearing has been completed. Hysterectomy or vaginal repair is best postponed for at least 3 months after delivery to allow maximal restoration of the pelvic supporting structures.

The patient may resume full activity or employment if her course to this point has been uneventful. Once again, the patient should be advised regarding family planning and contraceptive practices. The postnatal visit is an important opportunity to consider general disorders such as backache and depression and to discuss infant feeding and immunization. Review of medical complications during the pregnancy and potential long-term impact of those pathologies should be discussed. Documentation of blood pressure should demonstrate normalization in women who experienced gestational hypertension or preeclampsia. Postpartum glucose tolerance testing and counseling of women with a history of gestational diabetes is also recommended. The rapport established between the obstetrician and the patient during the prenatal and postpartum periods provides a unique opportunity to establish a preventive health program in subsequent years.

Akman M, Tüzün S, Uzuner A, et al. The influence of prenatal counselling on postpartum contraceptive choice. *J Int Med Res* 2010;38:1243. PMID: 20925996.

American College of Obstetricians and Gynecologists. Exercise during pregnancy and the postpartum period. ACOG Committee Opinion No. 267, January 2002. PMID: 12053898.

American College of Obstetricians and Gynecologists. Rubella Vaccination. ACOG Committee Opinion No. 281, January 2002. PMID: 12800832.

American College of Obstetricians and Gynecologists. *Prevention of RhD Alloimmunization.* ACOG Practice Bulletin No. 75. Washington, DC: American College of Obstetricians and Gynecologists; 2006. PMID: 16880320.

American College of Obstetricians and Gynecologists. *Guideline for Perinatal Care/American Academy of Pediatrics and the American College of Obstetricians and Gynecologists.* 6th ed. Washington, DC: American College of Obstetricians and Gynecologists; 2007

Blumenthal P, Edelman A. Hormonal contraception. *Obstet Gynecol* 2008;112:670. PMID: 18757668.

Bonuck KA, Trombley M, Freeman K, et al. Randomized, controlled trial of a prenatal and postnatal lactation consultant intervention on duration and intensity of breastfeeding up to 12 months. *Pediatrics* 2005;116;1413. PMID: 16322166.

Chan LM, Westhoff CL. Tubal sterilization trends in the United States. *Fertil Steril* 2010;94:1. PMID: 20525387.

Citak N, Cam C, Arslan H, et al. Postpartum sexual function of women and the effects of early pelvic floor muscle exercises. *Acta Obstet Gynecol Scand* 2010;89:817. PMID: 20397759.

De Santis M, Cavaliere AF, Satraface G, Caruso A. Rubella infection in pregnancy. *Reprod Toxicol* 2006;21:390. PMID: 16580940.

Grimes DA, Lopez LM, Schulz KF, et al. Immediate post-partum insertion of intrauterine devices. *Cochrane Database Syst Rev* 2010;5:CD003036. PMID: 20464722.

Groutz A, Levin I, Gold R, et al. Protracted postpartum urinary retention: The importance of early diagnosis and timely intervention. *Neurourol Urodynam* 2010;10:1002–1006. PMID: 20860036.

Healy CM, Rench MA, Castagnini LA, Baker CJ. Pertussis immunization in a high-risk postpartum population. *Vaccine.* 2009;18;27:5599. PMID: 19647062.

Kapp N, Curtis KM. Combined oral contraceptive use among breastfeeding women: A systematic review. *Am J Med* 2010;123:863.e1. PMID: 20682139.

Kapp N, Curtis K, Nanda K. Progestogen-only contraceptive use among breastfeeding women: A systematic review. *Contraception* 2010;82:17. PMID: 20682140.

Klein K, Worda C, Leipold H, et al. Does the mode of delivery influence sexual function after childbirth? *J Womens Health (Larchmt)* 2009;18:1227. PMID: 19630552.

Liang CC, Chang SD, Wong SY, Chang YL, Cheng PJ. Effects of postoperative analgesia on postpartum urinary retention in women undergoing cesarean delivery. *J Obstet Gynaecol Res* 2010;36:991–995. PMID 20846254.

Lopez LM, Hiller JE, Grimes DA. Education for contraceptive use by women after childbirth. *Cochrane Database Syst Rev* 2010;CD001863. PMID: 20091524.

Mangesi L, Dowswell T. Treatments for breast engorgement during lactation. *Cochrane Database Syst Rev* 2010;9:CD006946. PMID: 20824853.

Serati M, Salvatore S, Siesto G, et al. Female sexual function during pregnancy and after childbirth. *J Sex Med* 2010;2782–2790. PMID: 20626601.

Tan TQ, Gerbie MV. Pertussis and patient safety: Implementing Tdap vaccine recommendations in hospitals. *Jt Comm J Qual Patient Saf* 2010;36:173. PMID: 20402374.

Van der Wijden C, Kleijnen J, Van den Berk T. Lactational amenorrhea for family planning. *Cochrane Database Syst Rev* 2003;CD001329. PMID: 14583931.

LACTATION

Physiology

The mammary glands are modified exocrine glands that undergo dramatic anatomic and physiologic changes during pregnancy and in the immediate puerperium. Their role is to provide nourishment for the newborn and to transfer antibodies from mother to infant.

During the first half of pregnancy, proliferation of alveolar epithelial cells, formation of new ducts, and development of lobular architecture occur. Later in pregnancy, proliferation declines, and the epithelium differentiates for secretory activity. At the end of gestation, each breast will have gained approximately 400 g. Factors contributing to increase in mammary size include hypertrophy of blood vessels, myoepithelial cells, and connective tissue; deposition of fat; and retention of water and electrolytes. Blood flow is almost double that of the nonpregnant state.

Lactation depends on a delicate balance of several hormones. An intact hypothalamic–pituitary axis is essential to the initiation and maintenance of lactation. Lactation can be divided into 3 stages: (1) mammogenesis, or mammary growth and development; (2) lactogenesis, or initiation of milk secretion; and (3) galactopoiesis, or maintenance of established milk secretion (Table 10–2).

Table 10–2. Multihormonal interaction in mammary growth and lactation.

Mammogenesis	Lactogenesis	Galactopoiesis
Estrogens	Prolactin	↓Gonadal hormones
Progesterone	↓Estrogens	Suckling (oxytocin, prolactin)
Prolactin	↓Progesterone	Growth hormone
Growth hormone	↓hPL(?)	Glucocorticoids
Glucocorticoids	Glucocorticoids	Insulin
Epithelial growth factor	Insulin	Thyroxinee and parathyroid hormone

Arrows signify that lower than normal levels of the hormone are necessary for the effect to occur. hPL, human placental lactogen.

Estrogen is responsible for the growth of ductal tissue and alveolar budding, whereas progesterone is required for optimal maturation of the alveolar glands. Glandular stem cells undergo differentiation into secretory and myoepithelial cells under the influence of prolactin, growth hormone, insulin, cortisol, and an epithelial growth factor. Although alveolar secretory cells actively synthesize milk fat and proteins from midpregnancy onward, only small amounts are released into the lumen. However, lactation is possible if pregnancy is interrupted during the second trimester.

Prolactin is a necessary hormone for milk production, but lactogenesis also requires a low-estrogen environment. Although prolactin levels continue to rise as pregnancy advances, placental sex steroids block prolactin-induced secretory activity of the glandular epithelium. It appears that sex steroids and prolactin are synergistic in mammogenesis but antagonistic in galactopoiesis. Therefore, lactation is not initiated until plasma estrogens, progesterone, and human placental lactogen levels fall after delivery. Progesterone inhibits the biosynthesis of lactose and α-lactalbumin; estrogens directly antagonize the lactogenic effect of prolactin on the mammary gland by inhibiting α-lactalbumin production. Human placental lactogen may also exert a prolactin-antagonist effect through competitive binding to alveolar prolactin receptors.

The maintenance of established milk secretion requires periodic suckling and the actual emptying of ducts and alveoli. Growth hormone, cortisol, thyroxine, and insulin exert a permissive effect. Prolactin is required for galactopoiesis, but high basal levels are not mandatory, because prolactin concentrations in the nursing mother decline gradually during the late puerperium and approach that of the nonpregnant state. However, if a woman does not breastfeed her baby, her serum prolactin concentration will return to nonpregnant values within 2–3 weeks. If the mother suckles twins simultaneously, the prolactin response is about double that when 1 baby is fed at a time, illustrating an apparent synergism between the number of nipples stimulated and the frequency of suckling. The mechanism by which suckling stimulates prolactin release probably involves the inhibition of dopamine, which is thought to be the hypothalamic prolactin-inhibiting factor.

Nipple stimulation by suckling or other physical stimuli evokes a reflex release of oxytocin from the neurohypophysis. Because retrograde blood flow can be demonstrated within the pituitary stalk, oxytocin may reach the adenohypophysis in very high concentrations and affect pituitary release of prolactin independently of any effect on dopamine. The release of oxytocin is mediated by afferent fibers of the fourth to sixth intercostal nerves via the dorsal roots of the spinal cord to the midbrain.

The paraventricular and supraoptic neurons of the hypothalamus make up the final afferent pathway of the milk ejection reflex. The central nervous system can modulate the release of oxytocin by either stimulating or inhibiting the hypothalamus to increase or decrease prolactin-inhibiting factor (dopamine) and thus the release of oxytocin from the posterior pituitary. Thus positive senses related to nursing and crying of infant and positive attitudes in pregnancy and toward breastfeeding can improve milk yield and the ultimate success of breastfeeding. Likewise, the expectation of nursing is sufficient to release oxytocin before milk letdown but is not effective in releasing prolactin in the absence of suckling. Contrarily, negative stimuli, such as pain, stress, fear, anxiety, insecurity, or negative attitudes, may inhibit the letdown reflex. Oxytocin levels may rise during orgasm, and sexual stimuli may trigger milk ejection.

Synthesis of Human Milk

Prolactin ultimately promotes milk production by inducing the synthesis of mRNAs for the production of milk enzymes and milk proteins at the membrane of mammary epithelial cells (alveolar cells). Milk synthesis and secretion are then initiated via four major transcellular and paracellular pathways. The substrates for milk production are primarily derived from the maternal gut or produced in the maternal liver. The availability of these substrates is aided by a 20–40% increased blood flow to the mammary gland, gastrointestinal tract, and liver, as well as increased cardiac output during breastfeeding. The principal carbohydrate in human milk is lactose. Glucose metabolism is a key function in human milk production, because lactose is derived from glucose and galactose; the latter originates from glucose-6-phosphate. A specific protein, α-lactalbumin, catalyzes lactose synthesis. This rate-limiting enzyme is inhibited by gonadal hormones during pregnancy. Prolactin and insulin, which enhance the uptake of glucose by mammary cells, also stimulate the formation of triglycerides. Fat synthesis takes place in the endoplasmic reticulum. Most proteins are synthesized de novo in the secretory cells from essential and nonessential plasma amino acids. The formation of milk protein and mammary enzymes is induced by prolactin and enhanced by cortisol and insulin.

Mature human milk contains 7% carbohydrate as lactose, 3–5% fat, 0.9% protein, and 0.2% mineral constituents expressed as ash. Its energy content is 60–75 kcal/dL. Approximately 25% of the total nitrogen of human milk represents nonprotein compounds (eg, urea, uric acid, creatinine, and free amino acids). The principal proteins of human milk are casein, α-lactalbumin, lactoferrin, immunoglobulin (Ig) A, lysozyme, and albumin. Milk also contains a variety of enzymes that may contribute to the infant's digestion of breast milk (eg, amylase, catalase, peroxidase, lipase, xanthine oxidase, and alkaline and acid phosphatase). The fatty acid composition of human milk is rich in palmitic and oleic acids and varies somewhat with the diet. The major ions and mineral constituents of human milk are Na^+, K^+, Ca^{2+}, Mg^{2+}, Cl^-, phosphorus, sulfate, and citrate. Calcium concentrations vary from 25–35 mg/dL and phosphorus concentrations from 13–16 mg/dL. Iron, copper, zinc, and trace metal contents vary considerably. All the vitamins except vitamin K are found in human milk in nutritionally adequate amounts. The composition of breast milk is not greatly affected by race, age, parity, normal diet variations, moderate postpartum dieting, weight loss, or aerobic exercise. Volume and caloric density may be reduced in extreme scenarios, such as developing countries where starvation or daily caloric intake is <1600 kcal/d. In addition, milk composition does not differ between the 2 breasts unless 1 breast is infected. However, the volume and concentration of constituents varies during the day. The volume per feed increases in the late afternoon and evening. Nitrogen peaks in the late afternoon. Fat concentrations peak in the morning and are lowest at night. Lactose levels remain fairly constant.

Colostrum, the premilk secretion, is a yellowish alkaline secretion that may be present in the last months of pregnancy and for the first 2–3 days after delivery. It has a higher specific gravity (1.040–1.060); a higher protein, vitamin A, immunoglobulin, and sodium and chloride content; and a lower carbohydrate, potassium, and fat content than mature breast milk. Colostrum has a normal laxative action and is an ideal natural starter food.

Ions and water pass the membrane of the alveolar cell in both directions. Human milk differs from the milk of many other species by having a lower concentration of monovalent ions and a higher concentration of lactose. The aqueous phase of milk is isosmotic with plasma; thus the higher the lactose, the lower the ion concentration. The ratio of potassium/sodium is 3:1 in both milk and mammary intracellular fluid. Because milk contains approximately 87% water and lactose is the major osmotically active solute, it follows that milk yield is largely determined by lactose production.

Immunologic Significance of Human Milk

The neonate's secretory immune system and cellular responses are immature. In particular, the IgM and IgA responses are poor, and cellular immunity is impaired for several months. Maternal transfer of immunoglobulins through breast milk provides support for the infant's developing immune system and thereby enhances neonatal defense against infection. All classes of immunoglobulins are found in milk, but IgA constitutes 90% of immunoglobulins in human colostrum and milk. The output of immunoglobulins by the breast is maximal in the first week of life and declines thereafter as the production of milk-specific proteins increases. Lacteal antibodies against enteric bacteria and their antigenic products are largely of the IgA class. IgG and IgA lacteal antibodies provide short-term systemic and long-term enteric humoral immunity to the breastfed neonate. IgA antipoliomyelitis virus activity present in breastfed infants indicates that at least some transfer of milk antibodies into serum does occur. However, maternal lacteal antibodies are absorbed systemically by human infants for only a very short time after birth. Long-term protection against pathogenic enteric bacteria is provided by the absorption of lacteal IgA to the intestinal mucosa. In addition to providing passive immunity, there is evidence that lacteal immunoglobulins can modulate the immunocompetence of the neonate, but the exact mechanisms have not been described. For instance, the secretion of IgA into the saliva of breastfed infants is enhanced in comparison with bottle-fed controls.

Breast milk is highly anti-infective, containing more than 4000 cells/mm^3, the majority of which are leukocytes. The total cell count is even higher in colostrum. In human milk, the leukocytes are predominantly mononuclear cells and macrophages. Both T and B lymphocytes are present. During maternal infection, antigen-specific lymphocytes can migrate to the breast mucosa or produce immunoglobulins, both of which are key in the fight against infection. Fully functional immunoglobulins are present, primarily as IgA, IgG, and IgM. Polymeric secretory IgA is easily transported across the mucous membrane of the breast, blocking the mucosal receptors of infectious agents.

Elements in breast milk other than immunoglobulins and cells have prophylactic value against infections. The marked difference between the intestinal flora of breastfed and bottle-fed infants is due to a dialyzable nitrogen-containing carbohydrate (bifidus factor) that supports the growth of *Lactobacillus bifidus* in breastfed infants. The stool of bottle-fed infants is more alkaline and contains predominantly coliform organisms and *Bacteroides* spp. *L bifidus* inhibits the growth of *Shigella* spp, *Escherichia coli,* and yeast. Human milk also contains a nonspecific antimicrobial factor, lysozyme (a thermostable, acid-stable enzyme that cleaves the peptidoglycans of bacteria), and a "resistance factor," which protect the infant against staphylococcal infection. Lactoferrin, an iron chelator, exerts a strong bacteriostatic effect on staphylococci and *E coli* by depriving the organisms of iron. Both C3 and C4 components of complement and antitoxins for neutralizing *Vibrio cholerae* are found in human milk. Unsaturated vitamin B_{12}–binding protein in milk renders the vitamin unavailable for utilization by *E coli* and *Bacteroides*. Finally, interferon in milk may provide yet another nonspecific anti-infection factor.

Human milk may also have prophylactic value in childhood food allergies. During the neonatal period, permeability of the small intestine to macromolecules is increased. Secretory IgA in colostrum and breast milk reduces the absorption of foreign macromolecules until the endogenous IgA secretory capacity of the newborn intestinal lamina propria and lymph nodes develops at 2–3 months of age. Protein of cow's milk can be highly allergenic in the infant predisposed by heredity. The introduction of cow's milk–free formulas has considerably reduced the incidence of milk allergy. Thus comparative studies on the incidence of allergy, bacterial and viral infections, severe diarrhea, necrotizing enterocolitis, tuberculosis, and neonatal meningitis in breastfed and bottle-fed infants support the concept that breast milk fulfills a protective function.

Advantages & Disadvantages of Breastfeeding

A. For the Mother

1. Advantages—Breastfeeding is convenient, economical, and emotionally satisfying to most women. It helps to contract the uterus and accelerates the process of uterine involution in the postpartum period, including decreased maternal blood loss. It promotes mother–infant bonding and self-confidence. Maternal gastrointestinal motility and absorption are enhanced. Ovulatory cycles are delayed with exclusive breastfeeding. According to epidemiologic studies, breastfeeding may help to protect against premenopausal cancer and ovarian cancer. American College of Obstetrics and Gynecologists recommends that exclusive breastfeeding be continued until the infant is at least 6 months old.

2. Disadvantages—Regular nursing restricts activities and may be perceived by some mothers as an inconvenience. Twins can be nursed successfully, but few women are prepared for the first weeks of almost continual feeding. Caesarean section may necessitate modifications of early breastfeeding routines. Difficulties such as nipple tenderness and mastitis may develop. Compared with nonlactating women, breastfeeding women have a significant decrease (mean 6.5%) in bone mineral content at 6 months postpartum, but there is "catch-up" remineralization after weaning.

There are few absolute contraindications to breastfeeding (see Disadvantages and Contraindications for the Infant).

A. For the Infant

1. Advantages—Breast milk is digestible, of ideal composition, available at the right temperature and the right time, and free of bacterial contamination. Infants of breastfed mothers have a decreased incidence of all of the following: diarrhea, lower respiratory tract infection, otitis media, pneumonia, urinary tract infections, necrotizing enterocolitis, invasive bacterial infection, and sudden infant death. Breastfed infants may have a decreased risk of developing insulin-dependent diabetes, Crohn's disease, ulcerative colitis, lymphoma, and allergic diseases later in life. Breastfed infants are less likely to become obese later in life. Suckling promotes infant–mother bonding. Cognitive development and intelligence may be improved.

2. Disadvantages and Contraindications—Absolute contraindications to breastfeeding include the use of street drugs or excess alcohol; human T-cell leukemia virus type 1; breast cancer; active herpes simplex infection of the breast; active pulmonary tuberculosis or human T-cell lymphotropic virus type I or II positive in the mother; galactosemia in the infant; and maternal intake of cancer chemotherapeutic agents, recent diagnostic or therapeutic radioactive isotopes, or recent exposure to radioactive materials. Specific precautions for individual medications should be reviewed when prescribing drugs to lactating women. HIV infection in the United States is also a contraindication to breastfeeding because it has been recognized as a mode of HIV transmission. Breastfeeding might pose an additional risk of vertical transmission (approximately 15%) above that present from the antepartum and intrapartum periods. The risk of HIV transmission through breast milk is substantially higher among women who become infected during the postpartum lactation period. Most mothers in developed countries who know of their seropositivity choose not to breastfeed; in underdeveloped countries where lactation is critical to infant survival, breastfeeding is recommended even among HIV-infected mothers.

Breastfeeding is not contraindicated for mothers who are hepatitis B surface antigen positive, or mothers who are infected with hepatitis C virus (positive hepatitis C virus antibody or virus-RNA–positive blood). The presence of fever or seropositivity for chronic exposure to cytomegalovirus (CMV) are also not contraindications to breastfeeding. Caution should be exercised in low-birth-weight babies where potential risk of transmission must be balanced against nutritional benefit. Freezing and pasteurization can decrease the CMV viral load in the mother's milk.

The milk of a nursing mother with cystic fibrosis is high in sodium and places the infant at risk for hypernatremia. A woman with clinically infectious varicella should be isolated from the infant and should neither breastfeed nor bottle-feed. Once the infant has received varicella zoster immune globulin and there are no skin lesions on the mother's breast, she may provide expressed milk for her infant. A small number of otherwise healthy breastfed infants develop unconjugated hyperbilirubinemia (sometimes exceeding 20 mg/dL) during the first few weeks of life because of the higher than normal glucuronyl transferase inhibitory activity of the breast milk. The inhibitor may be a pregnanediol, although increased milk lipase activity and free fatty acids are likely the critical factors.

Breastfeeding is not usually possible for weak, ill, or very premature infants or for infants with cleft palate, choanal atresia, or phenylketonuria. It is common practice in many nurseries to feed premature infants human milk collected fresh from their mothers or processed from donors. The effects of processing and storage on the persistence of viral agents are not well studied. CMV transmission through breast milk has been documented and may pose a significant hazard for preterm infants. It is recommended that seronegative preterm infants receive milk from seronegative donors only. Because maternal antibodies are present in breast milk, an otherwise healthy term infant may do better if breastfed.

Breastfeeding is not contraindicated in women who have undergone breast augmentation with saline implants. Many women with breast implants breastfeed successfully, but reduction mammoplasty involving nipple autotransplantation severs the lactiferous ducts and precludes nursing. The success rate of breastfeeding decreases approximately 25% and the need to supplement with formula increases 19% in women after augmentation. When nipple sensation is lost as a result of breast surgery, breastfeeding is not possible. Other postoperative factors, such as breast pain, capsular contracture, and pressure on the breast from the implant, may compromise a woman's ability to exclusively breastfeed. Finally, the psychologic concern that breastfeeding may compromise the results of a cosmetic surgery may interfere with breastfeeding attempts.

Principles & Techniques of Breastfeeding

In the absence of anatomic or medical complications, the timing of the first feeding and the frequency and duration of subsequent feedings largely determine the outcome of breastfeeding. Infants and mothers who are able to initiate breastfeeding within 1–2 hours of delivery are more successful than those whose initial interactions are delayed for several hours. Lactation is established most successfully if the baby remains with the mother and she can feed on demand for adequate intervals throughout the first 24-hour period. The initial feeding should last 5 minutes at each breast in order to condition the letdown reflex. At first, the frequency of feedings may be very irregular (8–10 times per day), but after 1–2 weeks a fairly regular 4- to 6-hour pattern will emerge.

When the milk "comes in" abruptly on the third or fourth postpartum day, there is an initial period of discomfort caused by vascular engorgement and edema of the breasts. The baby does not nurse so much by developing intermittent negative pressure as by a rhythmic grasping of the areola; the infant "works" the milk into its mouth. Little force is required in nursing because the breast reservoirs can be emptied and refilled without suction. Nursing mothers notice a sensation of drawing and tightening within the breast at the beginning of suckling after the initial breast engorgement disappears. They are thus conscious of the milk ejection reflex, which may even cause milk to spurt or run out.

Some women expend a great deal of emotion on the subject of breastfeeding, and a few are almost overwhelmed by fear of being unable to care for their babies in this way. If attendants are sympathetic and patient, however, a woman who wants to nurse usually can do so. Attendants must be certain that the baby "latches" on (actually over) the nipple and the areola so as to feed properly without causing pain for the mother.

The baby should nurse at both breasts at each feeding, because overfilling of the breasts is the main deterrent to the maintenance of milk secretion. Nursing at only 1 breast at each feeding inhibits the reflex that is provoked simultaneously in both breasts. Thus nursing at alternate breasts from 1 feeding to the next may increase discomfort due to engorgement and reduce milk output. It is helpful for the mother to be taught to empty the breasts after each feeding; a sleepy baby may not have accomplished this. The use of supplementary formula or other food during the first 6–8 weeks of breastfeeding can interfere with lactation and should be avoided except when absolutely necessary. The introduction of an artificial nipple, which requires a different sucking mechanism, will weaken the sucking reflex required for breastfeeding. Some groups, such as the La Leche League, recommend that other fluids be given by spoon or dropper rather than by bottle.

In preparing to nurse, the mother should (1) wash her hands with soap and water, (2) clean her nipples and breasts with water, and (3) assume a comfortable position, preferably in a rocking or upright chair with the infant and mother chest-to-chest. If the mother is unable to sit up to nurse her baby because of painful perineal sutures, she may feel more comfortable lying on her side. An alternative position is the football hold. A woman with large pendulous breasts may find it difficult to manage both the breasts and the baby. If the baby lies on a pillow, the mother will have both hands free to guide the nipple.

Each baby nurses differently; however, the following procedure is generally successful:

1. Allow the normal newborn to nurse at each breast on demand or approximately every 3–4 hours, for 5 minutes per breast per feeding the first day. Over the next few days, gradually increase feeding time to initiate the letdown reflex, but do not exceed 10–15 minutes per breast. Suckling for longer than 15 minutes may cause maceration and cracking of the nipples and thus lead to mastitis.

2. Stimulating the cheek or lateral angle of the baby's mouth should precipitate a reflex turn to the nipple and opening of the mouth. The infant is brought firmly to the breast, and the nipple and areola are placed into the mouth as far as the nipple–areola line. Slight negative pressure holds the teat in place, and milk is obtained with a peristaltic motion of the tongue. Compressing the periareolar area and expressing a small amount of colostrum or milk for the baby to taste may stimulate the baby to nurse.
3. Try to keep the baby awake by moving or patting, but do not snap its feet, work its jaw, push its head, or press its cheeks.
4. Before removing the infant from the breast, gently open its mouth by lifting the outer border of the upper lip to break the suction.

After nursing, gently wipe the nipples with water and dry them.

Milk Yield

The prodigious energy requirements for lactation are met by mobilization of elements from maternal tissues and from dietary intake. Physiologic fat stores laid down during pregnancy are mobilized during lactation, and the return to prepregnancy weight and figure is promoted. A variety of studies suggest that a lactating woman should increase her normal daily food intake by 500 kcal/d, but intakes of 2000–2300 calories are sufficient for lactating women. The recommended daily dietary increases for lactation are 20 g of protein; a 20% increase in all vitamins and minerals except folic acid, which should be increased by 50%; and a 33% increase in calcium, phosphorus, and magnesium. There is no evidence that increasing fluid intake will increase milk volume. Fluid restriction also has little effect because urine output will diminish in preference to milk output.

With nursing, average milk production on the second postpartum day is approximately 120 mL. The amount increases to about 180 mL on the third postpartum day and to as much as 240 mL on the fourth day. In time, milk production reaches approximately 300 mL/d.

A good rule of thumb for the calculation of milk production for a given day in the week after delivery is to multiply the number of the postpartum day by 60. This gives the approximate number of milliliters of milk secreted in that 24-hour period.

If all goes well, sustained production of milk will be achieved by most patients after 10–14 days. A yield of 120–180 mL per feeding is common by the end of the second week. When free secretion has been established, marked increases are possible.

Early diminution of milk production often is due to failure to empty the breasts because of weak efforts by the baby or ineffectual nursing procedures; emotional problems, such as aversion to nursing; or medical complications, such as mastitis, debilitating systemic disease, or Sheehan's syndrome. Late diminution of milk production results from too generous complementary feedings of formula, emotional or other illness, and pregnancy.

Adequate rest is essential for successful lactation. Sometimes it is difficult to ensure an adequate milk yield if the mother is working outside the home. If it is not possible to rearrange the nursing schedule to fit the work schedule or vice versa, it may be necessary to empty the breasts manually or by pump. Milk output can be estimated by weighing the infant before and after feeding. If there has been a bowel movement during feeding, the baby should be weighed before the diaper is changed.

It may be necessary to substitute bottle-feeding for breastfeeding if the mother's supply continues to be inadequate (<50% of the infant's needs) after 3 weeks of effort, if nipple or breast lesions are severe enough to prevent pumping, or if the mother is either pregnant or severely (physically or mentally) ill. Nourishment from the inadequately lactating breast can be augmented with the Lact-Aid Nursing Trainer (Lact-Aid International, Athens, TN), a device that provides a supplemental source of milk via a plastic capillary tube placed beside the breast and suckled simultaneously with the nipple. Disposable plastic bags serve as reservoirs, and the supplemental milk is warmed by hanging the bag next to the mother. The Lact-Aide supplementer has also been used to help nurse premature infants and to re-establish lactation after untimely weaning due to illness. The long-term success of breastfeeding is increased by a structured home support system of postnatal visits by allied health personnel or experienced volunteers.

Disorders of Lactation

A. Painful Nipples

Tenderness of the nipples, a common symptom during the first days of breastfeeding, generally begins when the baby starts to suck. As soon as milk begins to flow, nipple sensitivity usually subsides. If maternal tissues are unusually tender, dry heat may help between feedings. Nipple shields should be used only as a last resort because they interfere with normal sucking. Glass or plastic shields with rubber nursing nipples are preferable to shields made entirely of rubber.

Nipple fissures cause severe pain and prevent normal letdown of milk. Local infection around the fissure can lead to mastitis. The application of vitamin A and D ointment or hydrous lanolin, which does not have to be removed, is often effective. To expedite healing, the following steps are recommended. Apply dry heat for 20 minutes 4 times per day with a 60-watt bulb held 18 inches away from the nipple. Conduct prefeeding manual expression. Begin nursing on the side opposite the fissure with the other breast exposed to air to allow the initial letdown to occur atraumatically.

Apply expressed breast milk to nipples and let it dry in between feedings. If necessary, use a nipple shield while nursing, and take ibuprofen or acetaminophen with or without codeine just after nursing. On rare occasions, it may be necessary to stop nursing temporarily on the affected side and to empty the breast either manually or by gentle pumping. Commercially available hydrogel pad is another alternative to treat sore nipple. It is designed to be worn inside the bra to prevent and soothe painful, cracked, or bleeding nipples and contribute to the healing process. The hydrogel pad contains a low water/high glycerin content, which provides natural moisture to the area without causing skin maceration. Recent studies have shown that by retaining the internal natural moisture level of the skin, nipple trauma improves more quickly.

A cause of chronic severe sore nipples without remarkable physical findings is candidal infection. Prompt relief is provided by topical nystatin cream. Thrush or candidal diaper rash or maternal candidal vaginitis must be treated as well.

B. Engorgement

Engorgement of the breasts occurs in the first week postpartum and is due to vascular congestion and accumulation of milk. Vascularity and swelling increase on the second day after delivery, and the areola or breast may become engorged. Prepartum breast massage and around-the-clock demand feedings help to prevent engorgement in these patients. When the areola is engorged, the nipple is occluded and proper grasping of the areola by the infant is not possible. With moderately severe engorgement, the breasts become firm and warm, and the lobules may be palpable as tender, irregular masses. Considerable discomfort and often a slight fever can be expected.

Mild cases may be relieved by acetaminophen or other analgesics, cool compresses, and partial expression of the milk before nursing. In severe cases, the patient should empty the breasts manually or with an electric pump. Alternative treatments for breast engorgement include acupuncture, cabbage leaves, cold gel packs, pharmacologic treatments, and ultrasound, but none of them have proven to be superior for symptom relief.

C. Mastitis

Mastitis occurs most frequently in primiparous nursing patients and usually is caused by coagulase-positive *Staphylococcus aureus*. High fever should never be ascribed to simple breast engorgement alone. Inflammation of the breast seldom begins before the fifth day postpartum. Most frequently, symptoms of a painful erythematous lobule in an outer quadrant of the breast are noted during the second or third week of the puerperium. Inflammation may occur with weaning when the flow of milk is disrupted, or the nursing mother may acquire the infection during her hospital stay and then transmit it to the infant. Demonstration of antibody-coated bacteria in the milk indicates the presence of infectious mastitis. Many infants harbor an infection and, in turn, infect the mother's breast during nursing. Neonatal streptococcal infection should be suspected if mastitis is recurrent or bilateral.

Infection may be limited to the subareolar region but more frequently involves an obstructed lactiferous duct and the surrounding breast parenchyma. If cellulitis is not properly treated, a breast abscess may develop. When only mastitis is present, it is best to prevent milk stasis by continuing breastfeeding or by using a breast pump. Apply local heat, provide a well-fitted bra, and institute appropriate antibiotic treatment. Cephalosporins, methicillin sodium, and dicloxacillin sodium are the antibiotics of choice to combat penicillinase-producing bacteria.

The presence of pitting edema over the inflamed area and any degree of fluctuation suggest abscess formation. It is necessary to incise and open loculated areas and provide wide drainage. Although correct breastfeeding techniques and alternation of breast may decrease the formation of nipple crack and mastitis, there is currently insufficient evidence to show effectiveness of any of the interventions, including breastfeeding education, pharmacologic treatments, and alternative therapies, regarding the occurrence of mastitis.

D. Miscellaneous Complications

A galactocele, or milk-retention cyst, is caused by blockage of a milk duct. It usually will resolve with warm compresses and continuation of breastfeeding. Sometimes the infant will reject one or both breasts. Strong foods such as beans, cabbage, turnips, broccoli, onions, garlic, and rhubarb may cause aversion to milk or neonatal colic. A common cause of nursing problems is maternal fatigue.

Inhibition & Suppression of Lactation

Despite a recent upsurge in breastfeeding in Western countries, many women will not or cannot breastfeed, and others will fail in the attempt. Lactation inhibition is desirable in the event of fetal or neonatal death as well.

The oldest and simplest method of suppressing lactation is to stop nursing, to avoid nipple stimulation, to refrain from expressing or pumping the milk, and to wear a supportive bra. Analgesics are also helpful. Patients will complain of breast engorgement (45%), pain (45%), and leaking breasts (55%). Although the breasts will become considerably engorged and the patient may experience discomfort, the collection of milk in the duct system will suppress its production, and reabsorption will occur. After approximately 2–3 days, engorgement will begin to recede, and the patient will be comfortable again. Medical suppression of lactation with estrogens or bromocriptine is no longer recommended due to undesired side effect and medical complications.

American Academy of Pediatrics Committee on Pediatric AIDS. Human milk, breastfeeding, and transmission of human immunodeficiency virus in the United States (RE9542). *Pediatrics* 2003;112:1196. PMID: 14595069.

American Academy of Pediatrics Policy Statement. Breastfeeding and the use of human milk. *Pediatrics* 2005;115:496. PMID: 15687461.

American College of Obstetricians and Gynecologists. *Breastfeeding: Maternal and Infant Aspects.* ACOG Clinical Review Volume 12, issue 1. Washington, DC: American College of Obstetricians and Gynecologists; 2007.

American College of Obstetricians and Gynecologists. *Breastfeeding: Maternal and Infant Aspects.* ACOG Committee Opinion No. 361. Washington, DC: American College of Obstetricians and Gynecologists; 2007. PMID: 17267864.

Briggs GG, Freeman RK, Yaffe SJ (eds). *Drugs in Pregnancy and Lactation.* 7th ed. Philadelphia, PA: Lippincott Williams & Wilkins; 2005.

Crepinsek MA, Crowe L, Michener K, et al. Interventions for preventing mastitis after childbirth. *Cochrane Database Syst Rev* 2010;8:CD007239. PMID: 20687084.

Cruz N, Korchin L. Breastfeeding after augmentation mammoplasty with saline implants. *Ann Plastic Surg* 2010; 64: 530–533. PMID: 20354430.

Gartner LM, Morton J, Lawrence RA, et al. Breastfeeding and the use of human milk. *Pediatrics* 2005;115:496. PMID: 15687461.

Reshi P, Lone IM. Human immunodeficiency virus and pregnancy. *Arch Gynecol Obstet* 2010;281:781. PMID: 20035338.

11

Imaging in Obstetrics

Simi Gupta, MD
Ashley S. Roman, MD, MPH

Technology for imaging in obstetrics has advanced a great deal over the past decade, but the purpose remains the same: to evaluate the anatomy and well-being of the fetus and the mother. The primary imaging modality in obstetrics is the 2-dimensional (2D) ultrasound because it is safe and widely available. Three- and 4-dimensional (3D/4D) ultrasound and magnetic resonance imaging (MRI) are also being used in certain situations to enhance imaging techniques, but the cost of these modalities limits their widespread use. Finally, computed tomography (CT) scan has limited utility because of safety issues but may be necessary in evaluating certain maternal conditions.

ULTRASOUND IMAGING

Ultrasound evaluation uses sound waves at a frequency greater than that which the human ear can hear (>20,000 cycles per second or Hertz [Hz]) to obtain images. An ultrasound examination is performed in real time with images or video clips stored for review. Ultrasound probes contain a transducer that creates the ultrasound waves at different frequencies. Higher frequency transducers provide better resolution but have less tissue penetrations, whereas low-frequency transducers have lower resolution but better tissue penetration.

In obstetrics and gynecology, ultrasound imaging is generally performed 1 of 2 ways: either with a transvaginal probe or transabdominal probe. The choice of which probe to use generally depends on the structure of interest and its distance from the probe. For instance, imaging of the cervix or an early gestation is generally best achieved with a transvaginal probe, whereas evaluation of the fetus in the third trimester of pregnancy is best accomplished with transabdominal imaging.

Ultrasound during pregnancy when performed for medical indications is considered to be safe. There are no documented harmful effects to the fetus from diagnostic ultrasound. Ultrasound waves, however, are a form of energy and have been shown to raise tissue temperature with high energy output or prolonged exposure. To minimize this risk, it is recommended that energy output, as measured by the Mechanical Index, be kept less than 1.0 and that ultrasound be used for diagnostic purposes only (ie, not for entertainment purposes). Imaging of the fetus can be divided into ultrasound evaluations in the first trimester and evaluations in the second and third trimesters. In each trimester, the goals and the ability to evaluate the fetal anatomy differ.

First-Trimester Ultrasound Examination

There are a number of indications to perform first-trimester ultrasound. They include confirmation of an intrauterine pregnancy, assessment of pelvic pain and vaginal bleeding, estimation of gestational age, confirmation of viability, evaluation of number of gestations, genetic screening, evaluation of basic anatomy, and assessment of uterine and adnexal anomalies and pathology.

To begin with, a first-trimester ultrasound can be used to confirm an early pregnancy by documenting the location of a gestational sac and the presence or absence of a yolk sac and fetal pole. However, one should use caution in determining the location of a pregnancy based solely on the presence of a gestational sac because sometimes an intrauterine fluid collection could be a pseudogestational sac from an ectopic pregnancy and not a normal gestational sac. Please see Chapter 13 for a more thorough discussion of using ultrasound to evaluate for ectopic pregnancy.

An ultrasound in the first trimester can also be used to determine the gestational age and viability of a pregnancy by the presence or absence of cardiac activity. Gestational age should be determined by measuring the length of the fetal pole. If there is no fetal pole noted, the gestational age can be estimated by measuring the mean sac diameter of the gestational sac. To assess for viability, cardiac activity should be noted by transvaginal ultrasound when the fetal pole measures 4–5 mm, which corresponds to a gestational age of 6.0–6.5 weeks. Using transabdominal ultrasound, cardiac activity should be noted when the fetal pole corresponds

Table 11–1. Guidelines for evaluation of an abnormal pregnancy.

Type of Imaging	Findings Suggestive of Abnormal Pregnancy
Transabdominal ultrasound	1. Failure to detect a double decidual rim with an MSD of 10 mm or greater. 2. Failure to detect a yolk sac when the MSD is 20 mm or greater. 3. Failure to detect an embryo with cardiac activity when the MSD is 25 mm or greater.
Transvaginal ultrasound	1. Failure to detect a yolk sac when the MSD is 8 mm or greater. 2. Failure to detect cardiac activity when the MSD is 16 mm or greater.

MSD, mean sac diameter.

with a gestational age of 8 weeks. Table 11–1 includes some guidelines for evaluation of an abnormal pregnancy. However, there are exceptions to the guidelines, so a follow-up ultrasound may be considered in order not to terminate a normal pregnancy.

The first trimester is also the best time to determine the number of gestations and to evaluate the chorionicity and amnionicity of multifetal pregnancies. An ultrasound will be able to show the number of gestational sacs, number of yolk sacs, and the number of fetal poles with cardiac activity. In cases of multifetal pregnancies, an ultrasound will also show the location of the placenta or placentas, the number of yolk sacs, and the presence or absence of a dividing membrane or membranes. In monochorionic-monoamniotic twins, there will be no dividing membrane between the fetuses, and there will be a single yolk sac (Fig. 11–1).

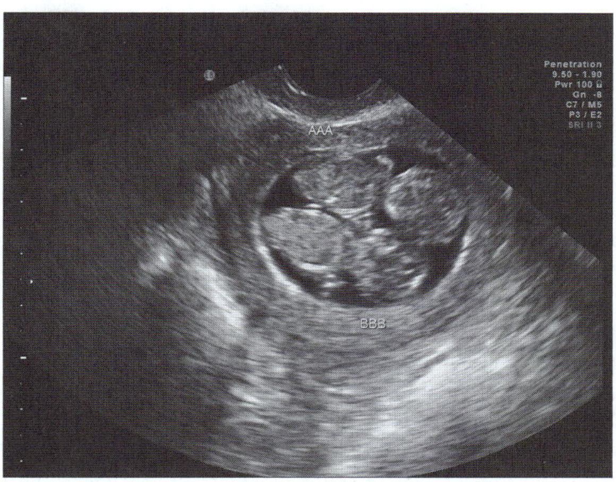

▲ **Figure 11–1.** Monochorionic monoamniotic twin gestation at 10 weeks' gestation. Note the lack of a dividing membrane and the close proximity of the fetuses. A single yolk sac was also noted.

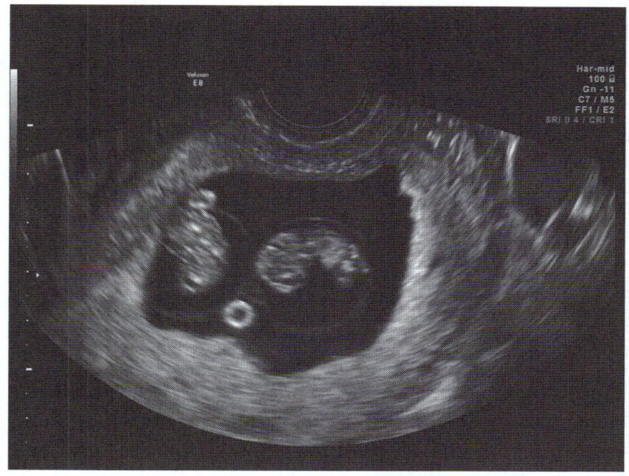

▲ **Figure 11–2.** Monochorionic diamniotic twin gestation at 9 weeks' gestation. Note the thin amnion surrounding each fetus and the 2 yolk sacs, both characteristic of the monochorionic diamniotic twin pregnancy at this early gestational age.

Monochorionic, diamniotic pregnancies in the early first trimester are characterized by a single chorion with 2 yolk sacs visualized. In many cases, the amnion may not be visible until approximately 8 weeks' gestation, at which time thin amniotic sacs may be seen surrounding each embryo (Fig. 11–2). By 10 weeks, monochorionic-diamniotic pregnancies are characterized by the T-sign on ultrasound, which represents a single placenta with 2 amnions. This is in contrast to dichorionic-diamniotic pregnancies, which will either show 2 separate placentas or show the classic lambda or twin-peak sign if there are fused placentas (Fig. 11–3). Conjoined twins can also be diagnosed during the first trimester based on ultrasound findings demonstrating a single

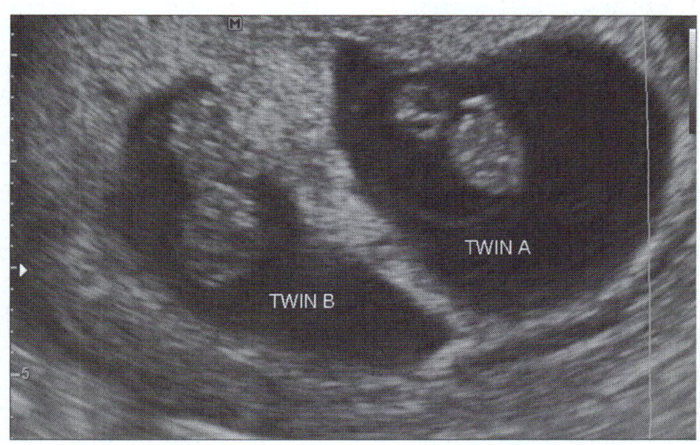

▲ **Figure 11–3.** Dichorionic diamniotic twin gestation at 8 weeks' gestation. Note the thick dividing membrane and wedge-shaped "lambda sign," the area at the top of the image, which represents the junction of the 2 placentas.

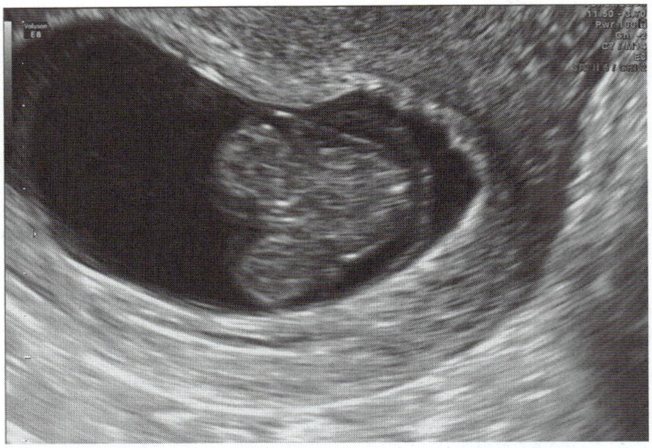

▲ **Figure 11–4.** Conjoined twin pregnancy at 9 weeks' gestation. Note the 2 fetal heads and apparent fusion at the thorax and abdomen. In this image, there is also a single amnion and chorion identified.

amnion, chorion, and yolk sac and 2 fetal poles that are fused (Fig. 11–4).

In the last 20 years, extensive research has shown that first-trimester ultrasound can also be used as a screening test for Down syndrome, trisomy 18, and trisomy 13. This is performed by measuring the nuchal translucency, or area of fluid that accumulates behind the fetal neck (Fig. 11–5). The combination of this measurement with maternal β human chorionic gonadotropin and pregnancy-associated plasma protein-A levels provides a patient-specific risk that the patient can use to determine whether she wants definitive testing for fetal chromosomal abnormalities with either chorionic villus sampling or an amniocentesis. More recently, research has shown that by incorporating the presence or absence of the nasal bone on ultrasound into the algorithm, the detection rate for Down syndrome in the first trimester is 94%, with a false-positive rate of 5%. Some institutions are also looking at impedance to flow in the ductus venosus and tricuspid regurgitation as markers of genetic abnormalities early in pregnancy.

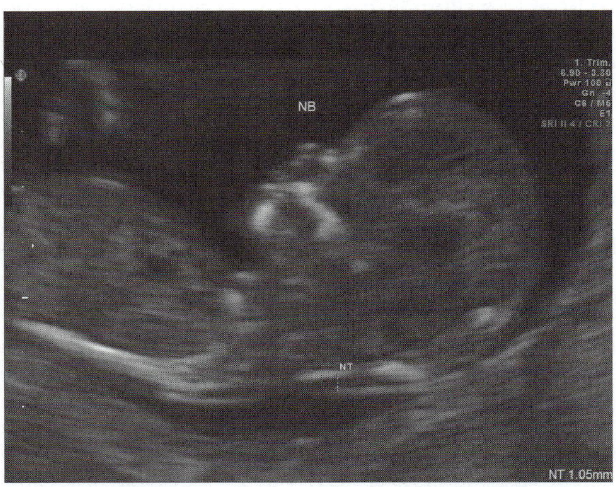

▲ **Figure 11–5.** Fetal nuchal translucency measurement at 12 weeks' gestation. The nuchal translucency refers to the echolucent space underneath the skin at the back of the neck. In this case, the nuchal translucency measurement was normal. In this figure, also note that the nasal bone is imaged. It is seen as a line underneath and parallel to the skin that is of equal or greater echogenicity than the skin.

Finally, with improvements in ultrasound technology and implementation of first-trimester screening for aneuploidy, more attention has been paid to the fetal anatomical survey in the first trimester. Although there are no official guidelines regarding what constitutes a fetal anatomical survey in the first trimester, it is possible to evaluate the fetal brain, spine, stomach, bladder, kidneys, abdominal cord insertion, and extremities during this period. Anatomical survey in the first trimester can currently detect a number of fetal anomalies, and surely as experience continues to grow, the number and type of anomalies detected will also increase. However, there are many structures that cannot be adequately evaluated in the first trimester, and there are many fetal anomalies that do not manifest on ultrasound until later in pregnancy. Therefore, an additional ultrasound is recommended in the second trimester.

Second- and Third-Trimester Ultrasound Examination

In the second and third trimesters, transvaginal and transabdominal ultrasound can be used for screening for chromosomal and nonchromosomal fetal anomalies, fetal growth, fetal well-being, fetal lie and presentation, placental anomalies, and cervical insufficiency. Additionally, it can be used for evaluating for gestational age, number of gestations, and viability if a first-trimester ultrasound was not performed.

A. Anatomy

The fetal anatomical evaluation recommended in current guidelines can be adequately assessed transabdominally after approximately 18 weeks of gestation and detects approximately 70% of major anatomical anomalies. However, the majority of the anatomy can be seen as early as 16 weeks transabdominally and even as early as 14 weeks transvaginally. If a patient is going to have a single second-trimester ultrasound to evaluate the basic fetal anatomy, it should be performed after 18 weeks' gestation. This is with the understanding that she may need to have a follow-up ultrasound after 20 weeks if further imaging of the brain and/or the heart is recommended. Some structures that are not required in current guidelines but that can be assessed (eg, the corpus callosum in the brain) cannot be reliably viewed until approximately 20 weeks' gestation. Therefore, some experts recommend 2 anatomy ultrasounds during pregnancy; the first can be performed at approximately 14–16 weeks' gestation to allow for early diagnosis of major structural

Table 11–2. AIUM guidelines for the fetal anatomical ultrasound.

Head, face, and neck	Cerebellum Choroid plexus Cisterna magna Lateral cerebral ventricles Midline falx Cavum septum pellucidi Upper lip Nuchal fold
Chest	Four-chamber view of the heart Outflow tracts of the heart if feasible
Abdomen	Stomach Kidneys Bladder Umbilical cord insertion (fetal abdomen) Umbilical cord vessel number
Spine	Cervical, thoracic, lumber, and sacral
Extremities	Legs and arms, presence or absence
Sex	Medically indicated only in multiple gestation

malformations and the second after 20 weeks' gestation to optimize evaluation of the heart and brain. Table 11–2 includes a guideline for fetal structures that should be assessed during a second-trimester anatomy ultrasound.

The second-trimester ultrasound can also be used as a genetic sonogram because major structural anomalies that can be seen are often associated with a chromosomal anomaly. Trisomy 13 and trisomy 18 fetuses have major structural anomalies that are identifiable by ultrasound in more than 80% of cases. However, fetuses with Down syndrome have major ultrasound-identifiable anomalies in only 25% of cases. These include certain cardiac anomalies, duodenal atresia, and ventriculomegaly. Ultrasound can also detect "soft" markers, which are variations in normal anatomy that are usually not clinically significant but can be associated with aneuploidy. Soft markers of Down syndrome include short femur or humerus length, renal pyelectasis, echogenic intracardiac foci, ventriculomegaly, or hyperechoic bowel. According to clinical studies, if the ultrasound does not reveal any soft markers, the risk of Down syndrome is reduced approximately 50–80%. A normal second-trimester genetic sonogram, however, does not eliminate the possibility of Down syndrome.

B. Growth

Ultrasound in the second and third trimester can also be used to evaluate fetal growth. Measurements of the biparietal diameter, head circumference, abdominal circumference or average abdominal diameter, and femoral diaphysis length can be calculated to determine an estimated fetal weight. This estimated fetal weight can be compared with the estimated fetal weights in published nomograms at each gestational age to evaluate the growth of the fetus. Indications for a fetal growth scan include measurement of fundal height less than expected based on gestational age, inability to measure fundal height because of fibroids or maternal obesity, multiple gestations, or maternal or fetal complications of pregnancy that are associated with fetal growth restriction.

The purpose of performing fetal growth scans is to identify fetal growth abnormalities (ie, fetal growth restriction and macrosomia). Intrauterine growth restriction is usually defined as an estimated gestational age less than the 10%. It can be associated with chromosomal and nonchromosomal anomalies, infection, and placental insufficiency. Identification of these fetuses is important because growth restriction is associated with fetal demise, and increased surveillance of the growth restricted fetuses may decrease this risk. Macrosomia can be defined as an estimated fetal weight greater than 4000 or 4500 g. Identification of these fetuses can be useful because of the association of macrosomia with postpartum hemorrhage, caesarean delivery, and shoulder dystocia. However, ultrasound is not a perfect estimate of fetal growth. The error rate can be as high as 15–20% depending on the gestational age and certain maternal characteristics such as body habitus and abdominal scar tissue. Also, if ultrasounds for growth are performed more often than every 2 weeks, the margin of error may be too great to determine whether appropriate growth has occurred. (See Chapter 16 on Disproportionate Fetal Growth for more detail.)

C. Evaluation of Fetal Well-Being

The purpose of using ultrasound for fetal surveillance is to identify fetuses that are at risk for intrauterine death or severe morbidity. Ideally, this will allow interventions such as early delivery in order to prevent these complications. Patients that may benefit from fetal surveillance include those with complaints such as decreased fetal movements, who carry fetuses with intrauterine growth restriction, or with medical or fetal complications that put them at risk for intrauterine death or severe morbidity. The 2 main methods of fetal surveillance are the biophysical profile or modified biophysical profile and Doppler ultrasound.

1. Biophysical profile—The biophysical profile (BPP) was first introduced in 1980. It consists of using 4 ultrasound parameters and a nonstress test to assign a score that gives a fetus's risk of hypoxia or intrauterine death. Table 11–3 shows the scoring of the fetal BPP. A score of 8 or 10 (of a possible score of 10) is considered normal. A score of 6 is considered equivocal, and a score of 4 or less is considered abnormal. Oligohydramnios, regardless of the composite score, warrants further evaluation.

The modified BPP consists of performing a nonstress test with only an evaluation of the amniotic fluid volume

Table 11–3. Parameters of the biophysical profile.

Variable	Two Points
Nonstress test	Reactive
Fetal breathing movements	One or more episodes of rhythmic breathing movements for 30 seconds or more
Fetal movement	Three or more discrete body or limb movement within 30 minutes
Fetal tone	One or more episodes of extension of a fetal extremity with return to flexion, or opening or closing of a hand
Amniotic fluid volume	A single maximum vertical pocket of 2 cm or more

Table 11–4. Interpretation of biophysical profile.

Score	Percent Risk of Umbilical Venous Blood pH <7.25	Risk of Fetal Death Within 1 Week (per 1000)
10/10	0	0.565
8/10 (normal AFV)	0	0.565
8/8 (NST not done)	0	0.565
8/10 (decreased AFV)	5–10	20–30
6/10 (normal AFV)	0	50
6/10 (decreased AFV)	>10	>50
4/10 (normal AFV)	36	115
4/10 (decreased AFV)	>36	>115
2/10 (normal AFV)	73	220
0	100	550

AFV, amniotic fluid volume; NST, nonstress test.
(Data from Manning FA. Fetal biophysical profile. *Obstet Gynecol Clin North Am* 1999;26:557–577.)

as measured by the amniotic fluid index (AFI). The AFI is calculated by dividing the uterus into 4 quadrants and measuring the maximum vertical pocket of amniotic fluid in each quadrant. The theory for this is based on the idea that the nonstress test is a measure of short-term fetal status, and the AFI is a measure of long-term fetal status. The AFI can measure long-term status because placental dysfunction can cause decreased renal perfusion, which can lead to oligohydramnios. If either the nonstress test is not reactive or the amniotic fluid index is less than 5 cm, the test is considered nonreactive. The stillbirth rate within a week of testing for a normal BPP or modified BPP is approximately 0.6–0.8 per 1000, giving a negative predictive value of greater than 99.9% for both tests. Risk of adverse pregnancy outcome as correlated with BPP score is shown in Table 11–4.

2. Fetal Doppler evaluation—Doppler ultrasound is emerging as a newer method to evaluate fetal well-being. Christian Doppler first described the Doppler effect in the 1800s as a way of describing the variation in the frequency of a light or sound wave as the source of that wave moves from a fixed point. In medicine, Doppler ultrasound is used as a measure of the speed at which blood is moving within a vessel. The 3 most common fetal arterial Dopplers are measured in the umbilical artery, middle cerebral artery, and uterine artery, whereas the most common fetal venous Doppler is measured in the ductus venosus. Umbilical artery Dopplers are a reflection of the placental circulation. As diseases begin to affect the placenta and increase resistance within the placenta, the end-diastolic flow in the umbilical artery begins to slow and eventually may become absent or even reversed.

Middle cerebral artery Dopplers work on a different principle (Fig. 11–6). In the presence of fetal hypoxemia, blood flow is redistributed to the brain, known as the brain-sparing effect. As a result, in worsening disease states, blood flow increases in the middle cerebral artery. This measurement can be used both for a general assessment of fetal well-being as well as an assessment for fetal anemia. Finally, ductus venosus Dopplers reflect cardiac compliance and cardiac afterload, which may increase with disease states that affect the placenta. Therefore, evaluation of the ductus venosus waveform can be used to assess fetal well-being.

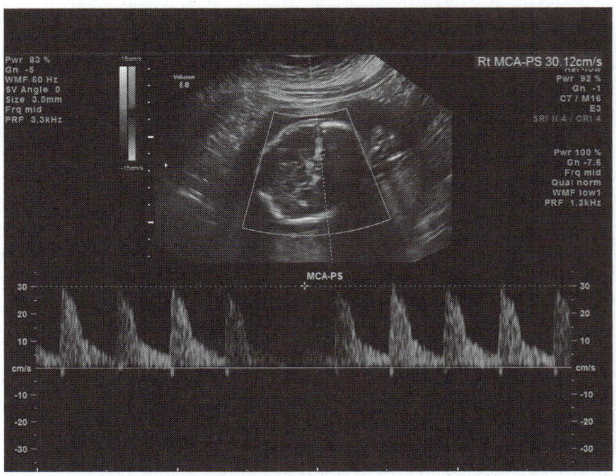

▲ **Figure 11–6.** Middle cerebral artery Dopplers to screen for fetal anemia. Color Doppler is used to identify the circle of Willis. The Doppler calipers are placed on the proximal third of the middle cerebral artery at a 0-degree angle (ie, dotted line overlaps the length of the middle cerebral artery). The peak systolic velocity is measured by measuring the peak of the waveforms.

D. Placental Location

In addition to the fetus, ultrasound in the second and third trimester can be used to evaluate the placenta for placental anomalies. It is standard to evaluate the placental location during the anatomy scan or third-trimester growth ultrasound, but if there is vaginal bleeding, one may also evaluate for placental abruption.

The placenta is usually described by its location, its relationship to the internal cervical os, and its appearance. Specifically, it is important to evaluate the placenta for any evidence of placenta previa. The distance of the lower edge of the placenta is measured in relation to the internal cervical os. Using ultrasound, the relationship of the placenta to the cervix can be described in 1 of 3 ways: complete previa, marginal previa, and no evidence of previa. If the placenta or placental edge covers the internal os, it is considered a complete placenta previa. A marginal placenta previa occurs when the placental edge is within 2 cm of the internal os but does not cover it. This is clinically significant because a placenta previa is associated with antenatal and intrapartum vaginal bleeding, and it is recommended that patients with a placenta previa have a caesarean section for delivery to decrease their risk of experiencing hemorrhage.

The placenta may also be evaluated for the presence of placenta accreta, which is most commonly associated with prior uterine surgery. A placenta accreta refers to trophoblastic villi that penetrate the decidua but not the myometrium and thus result in an abnormally adherent placenta. Other abnormalities of placental attachment include placenta increta, in which the trophoblastic villi penetrate the myometrium, and placenta percreta, in which the trophoblastic villi penetrate the myometrium and uterine serosa. On ultrasound, a placenta accreta can be suspected when there are placental lacunae, thinning of the myometrium over the placenta, and loss of the retroplacental hypoechoic space among other findings. Clinically, this is relevant because a placenta accreta can prevent separation of the placenta from the uterus after delivery of the fetus. Antenatal identification of placenta accreta can be used to ensure a planned delivery with the appropriate resources, which can reduce maternal morbidity and mortality.

Finally, ultrasound of the placenta can be used to evaluate for vaginal bleeding in the pregnant patient. The most concerning causes of third-trimester vaginal bleeding are placenta previa and placental abruption. Placenta previa may be suspected in the clinical scenario of painless vaginal bleeding and as noted before can be diagnosed by ultrasound. Placental abruption is often suspected when there is painful vaginal bleeding, but the sensitivity of ultrasound in diagnosing placental abruption is low. Ultrasound can only visualize hemorrhage in approximately 50% of cases of clinical placental abruption.

Maternal Evaluation

Ultrasound is also used in pregnancy to evaluate for maternal pathology, such as uterine fibroids and ovarian cysts or masses. However, imaging of certain maternal structures also has implications for obstetrical outcomes.

A. Cervical Evaluation

Ultrasound can be used to evaluate the cervix in the pregnant patient, as the shape and length of the cervix has been shown to correlate with preterm delivery. The best way to evaluate the cervix is by using transvaginal ultrasound. The most clinically applicable measurement is that of the cervical length. This is the distance of the closed cervix from the external os along the endocervical canal to the innermost closed portion of the cervix. It is also often standard to report the presence or absence of funneling or opening of the internal os. It is also important that approximately 3–5 minutes be spent evaluating the cervix because of the potential for dynamic changes. The shortest cervical length should be reported and used for clinical management.

The specific uses of cervical length measurements are rapidly evolving, but it is important to understand some basic principles for the use of these measurements. A normal cervical length measures between 25 and 50 mm from the mid-second trimester until the third trimester. A cervical length less than or equal to 25 mm at these gestational ages can be considered abnormal or "short." In the third trimester, there is physiologic shortening of the cervix, making the distinction between normal and abnormal more difficult. The earlier in gestation and the shorter the cervical length, the higher is the risk of preterm delivery. In Table 11–5, the risk of preterm birth by cervical length at 24 weeks is shown.

Cervical length measurements can be used in the second trimester in both low- and high-risk women to evaluate the risk for preterm birth. There are now many studies evaluating different treatment options, such as progesterone or cerclage, to help prevent preterm delivery based on the length of the cervix. In the late second and third trimester, cervical length can also be assessed in the symptomatic patient to help guide the need for hospitalization or the administration of steroids.

B. Maternal Doppler Evaluation

Uterine artery Dopplers are based on the theory that the spiral arterioles of the uterine arteries are meant to be maximally dilated to ensure adequate blood flow to the uterus. Worsening disease states are associated with a waveform notch and low end-diastolic velocity from high impedance circulation in the uterine artery. There have been a number of studies that have evaluated first- and second-trimester uterine artery Dopplers as a predictor of preeclampsia and intrauterine growth restriction. The studies have shown that in combination with abnormal maternal serum analytes, uterine artery Dopplers have a high sensitivity for prediction

Table 11–5. Sensitivity, specificity, and predictive value of cervical length at 24 weeks of gestation for preterm birth before 35 weeks of gestation.

	Cervical Length ≤ 20 mm	Cervical Length ≤ 25 mm	Cervical Length ≤ 30 mm
Sensitivity	23.0%	37.3%	54.0%
Specificity	97.0%	92.2%	76.3%
Positive predictive value	25.7%	17.8%	9.3%
Negative predictive value	96.5%	97.0%	97.4%

(Data modified from Iams J, Goldenberg R, Meis P. The length of the cervix and the risk of spontaneous premature delivery. *N Engl J Med* 1996;334:567–572.)

of these outcomes. Additional research is still being conducted to identify more accurately which patients to screen and with which combination of uterine artery Dopplers and serum analytes. Currently, besides close monitoring, aspirin is the only intervention that has been shown to decrease the risk of developing these adverse outcomes. Again, however, additional research is needed to determine which patients would benefit from this therapy.

American College of Obstetricians and Gynecologists. Practice bulletin 101: Ultrasonography in pregnancy. Washington, DC: ACOG; 2009.

American Institute of Ultrasound in Medicine. AIUM Practice Guideline for the Performance of Obstetrics Ultrasound Examinations. October 1, 2007. http://www.aium.org/publications/guidelines/obstetric.pdf. Accessed July 22, 2011.

Lovgren T, Dugoff L, Galan H. Uterine artery Doppler and prediction of preeclampsia. *Clin Obstet Gynecol* 2010;53:888–898. PMID: 21048456.

Manning FA. Fetal biophysical profile. *Obstet Gynecol Clin North Am* 1999;26:557–577. PMID: 10587955.

Nicolaides K. Screening for fetal aneuploidies at 11 to 13 weeks. *Prenat Diagn* 2011;31:7–15. PMID: 21210475.

Shipp T, Benacerraf B. Second trimester ultrasound screening for chromosomal abnormalities. *Prenat Diagn* 2002;22:296–307. PMID: 11981910.

Syngelaki A, Chelemen T, Dagklis T, et al. Challenges in the diagnosis of non-chromosomal abnormalities at 11–13 weeks. *Prenat Diagn* 2011;31:90–102. PMID: 21210483.

3D/4D ULTRASOUND

Up to this point, the discussion on imaging in obstetrics has been limited to 2D ultrasound. However, as technology is improving, the clinical uses of 3D and 4D ultrasound have started to be evaluated. The benefits of 3D ultrasound include improved evaluation of fetal anomalies, the ability to store information for reevaluation at a later time or by a different clinician, and improved maternal–fetal bonding. Specific fetal anomalies that have been studied with 3D include the fetal face, skeleton, neuroanatomy, and heart. 3D ultrasound not only helps to confirm a suspected anomaly seen in 2D ultrasound, but it also can help to explain findings to the parents. Figures 11–7 and 11–8 demonstrate 3D images of the fetal face. Figure 11–7 represents a normal fetal face, whereas Figure 11–8 demonstrates a fetus affected by unilateral cleft lip. Furthermore, 4D ultrasound can be used to evaluate fetal anomalies that may affect fetal movement.

American College of Obstetricians and Gynecologists. Practice bulletin 101: Ultrasonography in pregnancy. Washington, DC: ACOG; 2009.

American Institute of Ultrasound in Medicine. AIUM Practice Guideline for the Performance of Obstetrics Ultrasound Examinations. October 1, 2007. http://www.aium.org/publications/guidelines/obstetric.pdf. Accessed July 22, 2011.

Duckelmann A, Kalache K. Three-dimensional ultrasound in evaluating the fetus. *Prenat Diagn* 2010;30:631–638. PMID: 20572112.

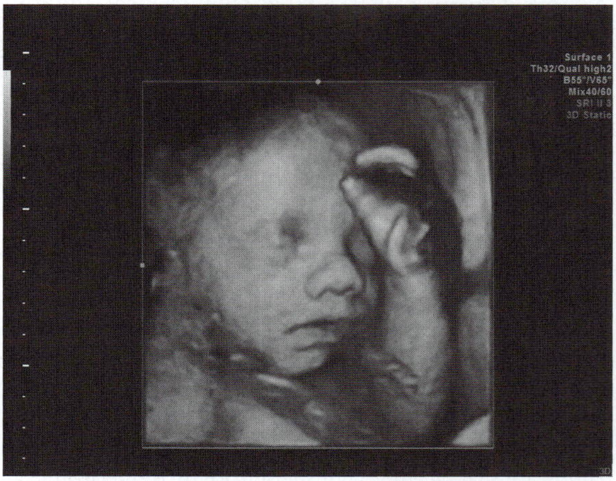

▲ **Figure 11–7.** 3D ultrasound image of normal fetal face at 29 weeks' gestation. Note the intact, smooth contour of the upper lip and symmetry of the nostrils.

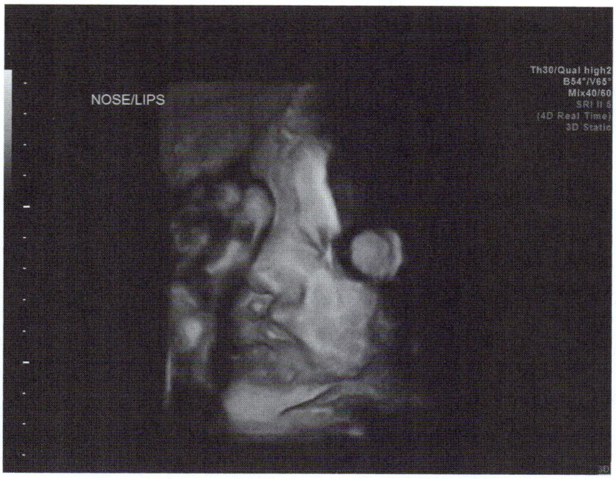

▲ **Figure 11–8.** 3D ultrasound image of fetal face affected by unilateral cleft lip at 35 weeks' gestation. Note the unilateral defect in the contour of the upper lip.

MAGNETIC RESONANCE IMAGING

Although ultrasound is the primary imaging modality used in obstetrics, MRI can be beneficial in certain cases. In the second trimester, obtaining or ascertaining a diagnosis is usually the purpose of the MRI, whereas in the third trimester, delivery planning is the goal. Abnormal fetal neuroanatomy, specifically ventriculomegaly, is the most common indication for a fetal MRI. MRI has been shown to alter the diagnosis or improve the accuracy of the diagnosis in up to 50% of studies performed for suspected fetal central nervous system anomalies. MRI can also be used to evaluate other fetal anomalies, such as genitourinary, gastrointestinal, cardiac, and musculoskeletal anomalies. For example, genitourinary anomalies are often associated with oligohydramnios, which can affect the imaging quality of ultrasound. MRI, on the other hand, is not dependent on the surrounding tissue, so it can be beneficial in these cases. In addition to fetal imaging, MRI has also been shown to be helpful in evaluating the placenta. In cases of suspected placenta accreta, increta, and percreta, where ultrasound findings are equivocal or a posterior placenta limits ultrasound evaluation, MRI can be used to more accurately diagnose the suspected abnormality.

Finally, although the safety of ultrasound in obstetrics has been well established, the safety of MRI is sometimes questioned. There have been no studies linking MRI to any teratogenic effects on the fetus. However, gadolinium use is not recommended during pregnancy. Although limited studies have not shown any adverse effect on the fetus, gadolinium has been shown to cross the placenta and may have a long half-life in the fetal compartment. For these reasons, it should not be used unless the potential benefit outweighs the potential risk of unknown fetal harm.

Bardo D, Ayetekin O. Magnetic resonance imaging for evaluation of the fetus and the placenta. *Amer J Perinatol* 2008;25:591–599. PMID: 18988323.

Chen M, Coakley F, Kaimal A, et al. Guidelines for computed tomography and magnetic resonance imaging use during pregnancy and lactation. *Obstet Gynecol* 2008;112(2, Part 1): 334–340. PMID: 18669732.

Assessment of At-Risk Pregnancy

12

Shobha H. Mehta, MD
Robert J. Sokol, MD

ESSENTIALS OF DIAGNOSIS

- A careful history to reveal specific risk factors
- A maternal physical examination organized to identify or exclude risk factors
- Routine maternal laboratory screening for common disorders
- Special maternal laboratory evaluations for disorders suggested by any evaluative process
- Comprehensive fetal assessment by an assortment of techniques over the entire course of the pregnancy

OVERVIEW

High-risk pregnancy is broadly defined as one in which the mother, fetus, or newborn is, or may possibly be, at increased risk of morbidity or mortality before, during, or after delivery. Factors that may lead to this increased risk include maternal health, obstetric abnormalities, and fetal disease. Table 12–1 provides an overview of some major categories that comprise a high-risk pregnancy.

The purpose of this chapter is to outline basic and essential aspects of diagnostic modalities available for determination of pregnancies at risk that can be used in practice in a rational manner.

The incidence of high-risk pregnancy varies according to the criteria used to define it. A great many factors are involved, and the effects of any given factor differ from patient to patient. Outcomes can include mortality of the mother and/or the fetus/neonate. Leading causes of maternal death include thromboembolic disease, hypertensive disease, hemorrhage, infection, and ectopic pregnancy. The leading causes of infant mortality (death from birth to 1 year of age) are congenital malformations and prematurity-related conditions. Although there is variation in definition depending on the resource, a perinatal death is one that occurs at any time after 28 weeks' gestation through the first 7 days after delivery. The perinatal mortality rate is the number of perinatal deaths per 1000 live births. Preterm birth is the leading cause of perinatal morbidity and neonatal mortality.

In assessing pregnancies to determine risk, several key concepts may offer tremendous insight. Human reproduction is a complex social, biochemical, and physiologic process that is not as successful as once thought. Approximately half of all conceptions are lost before pregnancy is even recognized. Another 15–20% are lost in the first trimester. Of this latter group, more than half have abnormal karyotypes and defy current methodologies for prevention of loss. However, many other causes of reproductive loss are amenable to diagnosis and treatment. In this chapter we discuss the indications and justifications for antepartum care and intrapartum management.

PRECONCEPTION CARE

Preconception evaluation and counseling of women of reproductive age has gained increasing acceptance as an important component of women's health. Care given in family planning and gynecology centers provides a potential opportunity to maximize maternal and fetal health benefits before conception. Issues of potential consequence to a pregnancy, such as medical problems, lifestyle (eg, substance abuse, weight, exercise), or genetic issues should be investigated and interventions devised before pregnancy. Specific recommendations include folic acid for the prevention of fetal neural tube defects (0.4 mg/d), strict blood sugar control in diabetic women, general management of any medical problems in the mother, avoidance of known teratogenic medications, and smoking cessation.

PRENATAL PERIOD

Initial Screening

The initial prenatal visit is important in evaluation and assessment of risk during the pregnancy and should take place as early in the pregnancy as possible, preferably in

Table 12–1. Major categories of high-risk pregnancies.

Fetal	
	Structural anomalies
	Chromosomal abnormalities
	Genetic syndromes
	Multiple gestations
	Infection
Maternal-fetal	
	Preterm labor
	Preterm premature rupture of membranes
	Cervical insufficiency
	Stillbirth
	Intrauterine growth restriction
	Abnormalities of placentation
	Preeclampsia
	Post-term
Maternal	
	Diabetes
	Chronic hypertension
	Cardiac
	Thyroid
	Infection

the first trimester. Information of vital importance includes maternal medical and obstetric history, physical examination, and key laboratory findings.

A. Maternal Age

Extremes of maternal age increase risks of maternal or fetal morbidity and mortality. Adolescents are at increased risk for preeclampsia–eclampsia, intrauterine growth restriction, and maternal malnutrition.

Women of increasing age at the time of delivery are at higher risk for preeclampsia, diabetes, and obesity, as well as other medical conditions. An increased risk of caesarean section, stillbirth, and placenta accreta are noted in women with advanced maternal age.

The risk of fetal aneuploidy increases with increasing age; the American College of Obstetricians and Gynecologists (ACOG), however, has recommended that maternal age of 35 years no longer be used as a cutoff to determine who is offered screening and who is offered invasive testing. Instead, patient counseling regarding options followed by maternal serum screening, ultrasound, and/or invasive testing, depending on patient's wishes, should occur.

B. Modality of Conception

It is important to differentiate spontaneous pregnancy from that resulting from assisted reproductive technologies (ART). Use of ART increases the risks of perinatal mortality (both stillbirths and early neonatal deaths), multifetal gestation, preterm birth (both singletons and multiples), congenital anomalies, and low birth weight.

C. Past Medical History

Many medical disorders can complicate the pregnancy course for the mother and thus the fetus. It is important that these diseases and their severity be addressed before conception if possible. During pregnancy, the patient may require aggressive management and additional visits and testing to follow the course of the disease, in addition to possible consultation or management of a high-risk specialist. Table 12–2 lists some of the most important disorders that may complicate pregnancy.

D. Family History

A detailed family history is helpful in determining any increased risk of heritable disease states (eg, Tay-Sachs, cystic fibrosis, sickle cell disease) that may affect the mother or fetus during the pregnancy or the fetus after delivery. Other relevant findings includes family history of thromboembolism, birth defects (particularly cardiac anomalies), and medical history of first-degree relatives (particularly diabetes).

E. Ethnic Background

Population screening for certain inheritable genetic diseases is not cost effective because of the relative rarity of those genes in the general population. However, many genetic diseases affect certain ethnicities in disproportionate amounts, allowing cost-effective screening of those particular groups. Table 12–3 lists several common inheritable genetic diseases for which screening is possible. It includes the group at risk as well as the method of screening.

Table 12–2. Some maternal diseases, disorders, and other complications of pregnancy.

Chronic hypertension
Diabetes mellitus
Thromboembolic disease
Thyroid disorders
Cardiac disease
Renal disease
Pulmonary disease (asthma, sarcoidosis)
Connective tissue disorders
Maternal cancer
Epilepsy
Blood disorders (anemia, coagulopathy, hemoglobinopathy)
Psychiatric disorders

Table 12–3. Common inheritable genetic diseases.

Disease	Population at Increased Risk	Method of Testing
Alpha thalassemia	Chinese, Southeast Asian, African	CBC Hemoglobin electrophoresis Mutation analysis
β thalassemia	Chinese, Southeast Asians, Mediterraneans, Pakistanis, Bangladeshis, Middle Easterners, African	CBC Hemoglobin electrophoresis
Bloom's syndrome	Ashkenazi Jews	Mutation analysis
Canavan's disease	Ashkenazi Jews	Mutation analysis
Cystic fibrosis	North American Caucasians of European ancestry, Ashkenazi Jews	Mutation analysis
Familial dysautonomia	Ashkenazi Jews	Mutation analysis
Fanconi's anemia	Ashkenazi Jews	Mutation analysis
Gaucher's disease	Ashkenazi Jews	Mutation analysis
Niemann-Pick disease	Ashkenazi Jews	Mutation analysis
Sickle cell disease and other structural hemoglobinopathies	African Americans, Africans, Hispanics, Mediterranean, Middle Easterners, Caribbean Indians	CBC Hemoglobin electrophoresis
Tay-Sachs	Ashkenazi Jews, French Canadians, Cajuns	Enzyme and mutation analysis

CBC, complete blood cell count.

F. Past Obstetric History

1. Recurrent abortion—A diagnosis of recurrent abortion is made after 3 or more consecutive spontaneous losses of a pregnancy before 20 weeks' gestation. Recurrent abortion is best investigated before another pregnancy occurs; workup can be initiated after 2 losses. If the patient is currently pregnant, however, as much of the workup as possible should be performed.

- Karyotype of abortus specimen
- Parental karyotype
- Survey for cervical and uterine anomalies
- Screening for hormonal abnormalities (ie, hypothyroidism)
- Infectious disease evaluation of the genital tract

The association between inherited thrombophilias and recurrent pregnancy loss is unclear; thus the testing for these is currently not recommended in the clinical setting. Screening for antiphospholipid antibodies (acquired thrombophilia) may be appropriate.

2. Previous stillbirth or neonatal death—A history of previous stillbirth or neonatal death should trigger an immediate investigation regarding the conditions or circumstances surrounding the event. If the demise was the result of a nonrecurring event, such as cord prolapse or traumatic injury, then the present pregnancy has a risk approaching the background risk. However, stillbirth or neonatal death may suggest a cytogenetic abnormality, structural malformation syndrome, or fetomaternal hemorrhage. Review of records, including autopsy, placental pathology, and karyotype if obtained, is vital. As with fetal loss, the association of unexplained stillbirth with inherited thrombophilias is unclear and testing is not recommended, although a maternal thrombophilia workup may be considered with stillbirth in the setting of severe placental thrombosis or infarcts, significant fetal growth restriction, or in the patient with a history of thrombosis.

3. Previous preterm delivery—A history of preterm birth confers an increased risk of early delivery in subsequent pregnancies. Furthermore, the risk of a subsequent preterm birth increases as the number of prior preterm births increases, and the risk decreases with each subsequent birth that is not preterm. The recurrence risk also rises as the gestational age of the previous preterm delivery decreases. Despite intense investigation, the incidence of preterm delivery has slightly increased in the United States, due in large measure to medical intervention producing indicated preterm deliveries. Eighty-five percent of preterm deliveries occur between 32 and 36 6/7 weeks, and they carry minimal fetal or neonatal morbidity. The remaining 15%

of preterm deliveries, however, account for nearly all of the perinatal morbidity and mortality. Common causes of perinatal morbidity in premature infants include respiratory distress syndrome, intraventricular hemorrhage, bronchopulmonary dysplasia, necrotizing enterocolitis, sepsis, apnea, retinopathy of prematurity, and hyperbilirubinemia. Preterm deliveries can be divided into 2 types: spontaneous and indicated, with indicated preterm deliveries caused by medical or obstetric disorders that place the mother and/or fetus at risk. The clinical risk factors most often associated with spontaneous preterm birth include history of previous preterm birth, genital tract infection, nonwhite race, multiple gestation, bleeding in the second trimester, and low prepregnancy weight. Recent multicenter trials have shown that progesterone in the form of 17α-hydroxyprogesterone caproate, given as weekly injections of 250 mg beginning in the second trimester, can decrease the risk of preterm delivery in patients with a history of prior spontaneous preterm delivery.

4. Rh alloimmunization or ABO incompatibility—All pregnant patients should undergo an antibody screen at the first prenatal visit. Those patients who are Rh (D)–negative with no evidence of anti-D alloimmunization should receive Rh (D) immunoglobulin (RhoGAM; Ortho-Clinical Diagnostics, Rochester, NY) 300 μg at 28 weeks of gestation. Patients who are Rh (D) sensitized can be followed with maternal titers and/or amniocentesis for fetal blood typing, followed by either serial amniocentesis for ΔOD_{450} or serial middle cerebral artery peak systolic velocity measurements, as well as fetal blood sampling via cordocentesis.

5. Previous preeclampsia–eclampsia—Previous preeclampsia–eclampsia increases the risk for hypertension in the current pregnancy, especially if underlying chronic hypertension or renal disease is present.

6. Previous infant with genetic disorder or congenital anomaly—A woman with a previous history of a fetus with a chromosomal abnormality is a frequent indication of cytogenetic testing, although this may be preceded by first- or second-trimester screening and anatomy ultrasound (US). The rate of recurrence depends on the abnormality.

7. Teratogen exposure—A teratogen is any substance, agent, or environmental factor that has an adverse effect on the developing fetus. Whereas malformations caused by teratogen exposure are relatively rare, knowledge of exposure can aid in the diagnosis and management.

A. DRUGS—Alcohol, antiseizure medications (phenytoin, valproic acid, etc.), lithium, mercury, thalidomide, diethylstilbestrol (DES), warfarin, isotretinoin, and so forth.

B. INFECTIOUS AGENTS—Cytomegalovirus, *Listeria*, rubella, toxoplasmosis, varicella, *Mycoplasma*, and so forth.

C. RADIATION—It is believed that medical diagnostic radiation delivering less than 0.05 Gy (5 rad) to the fetus has no teratogenic risk.

Physical Examination

Physical examination is important not only during the initial visit, but also throughout the pregnancy. Collection of maternal height and weight information allows for calculation of maternal body mass index, useful in risk assessment for many pregnancy abnormalities. In addition, weight gain is followed throughout the pregnancy, also a useful parameter for several risk factors in pregnancy. Vital sign abnormalities can lead to the diagnosis of many key obstetric complications. Fever, defined as a temperature of 100.4°F or greater, can be a sign of chorioamnionitis. Signs or symptoms of chorioamnionitis should be assessed, and, if chorioamnionitis is suspected, amniocentesis for microscopy and culture should be considered. Depending on clinical correlation, delivery may be necessary. Maternal tachycardia can be a sign of infection, anemia, or both. Isolated mild tachycardia (>100 beats/min) should be evaluated and followed up, as should maternal tachyarrhythmias. Maternal heart rate is noted to increase normally in pregnancy, however. The normal pattern of maternal blood pressure readings is a decrease from baseline during the first trimester, reaching its nadir in the second trimester, and slightly rising in the third trimester, although not as high as the baseline levels. Repeated blood pressure readings of 140/90 mm Hg taken 6 hours apart should be considered evidence of preeclampsia or gestational hypertension. Increases in systolic and diastolic blood pressure, although no longer part of the definition, may also be an indication of development of pregnancy-related hypertensive disease. The rest of the physical examination should be performed during the initial visit and focused examination during each visit. Fundal height measurements and fetal heart tone checks should also be performed.

Urinalysis

At the first prenatal visit, a clean-catch urine culture and sensitivity should be performed. Any growth should be treated with the appropriate antibiotics. At all subsequent visits, urine dipstick testing to screen for protein, glucose, leukocyte esterase, blood, or any combination of markers is useful in identifying patients with a change in baseline urinary composition.

Screening Tests

Screening tests during the initial visit include testing for rubella, rapid plasma reagin, hepatitis B, blood type, HIV, gonorrhea, and *Chlamydia*, and Pap smear.

American College of Obstetricians and Gynecologists. Inherited Thrombophilias in Pregnancy. ACOG Practice Bulletin No. 113. Washington, DC: American College of Obstetricians and Gynecologists; 2010.

American College of Obstetricians and Gynecologists. Screening for Fetal Chromosomal Anomalies. ACOG Practice Bulletin No. 77. Washington, DC: American College of Obstetricians and Gynecologists; 2007 (Reaffirmed 2008).

Branch DW, Gibson M, Silver RM. Clinical practice. Recurrent miscarriage. *N Engl J Med* 2010;363:1740–1747. PMID: 20979474.

Goldenberg RL, Culhane JF, Iams JD, Romero R. Epidemiology and causes of preterm birth. *Lancet* 2008;371:75–84. PMID: 18177778.

Mari G, Deter RL, Carpenter RL, et al. Noninvasive diagnosis by Doppler ultrasonography of fetal anemia due to maternal red cell alloimmunization. Collaborative group for Doppler assessment of the blood velocity in anemic fetuses. *N Engl J Med* 2000;342:9–14. PMID: 10620643.

Meis PJ, Klebanoff M, Thom E, et al. Prevention of recurrent preterm delivery by 17 alpha-hydroxyprogesterone caproate. *N Engl J Med* 2003;348:2479–2485. PMID: 12802023.

Mercer BM, Macpherson CA, Goldenberg RL, et al. Are women with recurrent spontaneous preterm births different from those without such history? *Am J Obstet Gynecol* 2006;194: 1176–1184. PMID: 16580328.

Reddy UM. Prediction and prevention of recurrent stillbirth. *Obstet Gynecol* 2007;110:1151–1164. PMID: 17978132.

Schieve LA, Ferre C, Peterson HB, Macaluso M, Reynolds MA, Wright VC. Perinatal outcome among singleton infants conceived through assisted reproductive technology in the United States. *Obstet Gynecol* 2004;103:1144–1153. PMID: 15172846.

ANTEPARTUM MANAGEMENT

Genetic Testing

A. First-Trimester Screening

Nuchal translucency, measured between 11(0/7) and 13(6/7) weeks, combined with maternal serum free β-human chorionic gonadotropin (β-hCG) and pregnancy-associated plasma protein-A levels, has been found to have 87.0% sensitivity for detection of trisomy 21, with a 5% false-positive rate. In the absence of chromosomal abnormalities, an increased nuchal translucency is associated with an increased risk of structural cardiac abnormalities and skeletal dysplasias, and so forth. Further US findings in the first trimester, including absence of nasal bone and abnormal ductus venosus Doppler findings, may further improve the detection rate for aneuploidy but require a high level of sonographic skill. Patients with an abnormal screening result can be offered invasive testing such as chorionic villus sampling for more accurate detection of fetal aneuploidy. The advantage of the first-trimester screen (as opposed to second-trimester maternal screening, discussed next) is that it allows for earlier detection of aneuploidy.

B. Second-Trimester Maternal Serum Screening

Frequently known as the "triple screen," this test includes maternal serum α-fetoprotein (MSAFP), β-hCG, and estriol. In some institutions, only the MSAFP is used, whereas in other institutions, a fourth test for inhibin is included, making it a "quad test." The usefulness of this screen is its ability to identify pregnancies at increased risk for open neural tube defects, as well as for certain chromosomal abnormalities, especially trisomy 21 (70% sensitivity for Down syndrome detection). This test is effective at 15–22 weeks' gestation and therefore can identify an at-risk pregnancy in time to pursue more definitive diagnosis, if desired. It is important to note, however, that maternal serum screening is not a definitive test and must be followed by invasive testing (discussed later) for karyotype determination.

The first- and second-trimester screen should not both be ordered independently during a pregnancy; this approach leads to unacceptably high false-positive rates for aneuploidy. Approaches have been developed, however, that allow for both tests to be used in combination to determine aneuploidy risk. One such approach is integrated aneuploidy screening, in which a single risk assessment is calculated using all 6 analytes after completion of both tests. Integrated screening has a Down syndrome detection rate of 95%, with a 5% false-positive rate. One major drawback is the withholding of information until the second trimester, precluding the benefits of early diagnosis and chorionic villus sampling. Another approach is stepwise sequential screening, which presents patients with risk-assessment results after completion of the first-trimester component and then again after the second-trimester blood draw. With this test, the detection rate for Down syndrome is 95%, with a 5% false-positive rate. Combined sequential screening is similar, but patients with a very low first-trimester risk do not have second-trimester analysis performed.

C. Screening for Carriers of Genetic Disease

Screening for sickle cell disease should be offered to individuals of African and African American descent and those from the Mediterranean basin, the Middle East, and India. Hemoglobin electrophoresis is the definitive test to determine the carrier status of sickle cell disease as well as other hemoglobinopathies.

Cystic fibrosis carrier screening should be discussed with all patients. Carrier rates, however, are highest in Caucasians, including parents of Eastern European Jewish (or Ashkenazi Jewish) descent. Furthermore, the detection rate of known mutations is highest in these groups and is lower in other groups. For instance, Asian Americans have a cystic fibrosis carrier rate of 1 in 94, and the detection rate of testing in this population is 49%. Current guidelines recommend offering information regarding testing to all groups but counseling lower-risk groups of the limitations of the testing.

Given the higher prevalence of other recessive genetic diseases among individuals of Ashkenazi Jewish descent, carrier screening should be offered for Tay-Sachs disease, Canavan's disease, and familial dysautonomia. Screening is also available for mucolipidosis IV, Niemann-Pick disease type A, Fanconi's anemia group C, Bloom's syndrome, and Gaucher's disease and may be considered in this population.

Preterm Labor Detection

Many patients present throughout pregnancy with signs and symptoms of preterm labor, specifically uterine contractions. Although the cost of missing true preterm labor is high, many patients are not in true labor, and the financial cost of aggressive management of these patients is also high. The accurate diagnosis of preterm labor may be aided by 2 screening tests: cervical length measurement and fetal fibronectin.

Gestational Diabetes Screening

Although recent consensus groups have recommended screening for gestational diabetes based on risk factors, many studies have shown this to be inadequate for detecting patients with gestational screening versus universal screening.

Routine screening consists of performing a glucose challenge test between 24 and 28 weeks. The test consists of a 50-g oral glucose load with a plasma glucose level drawn exactly 1 hour after. If the value is 140 mg/dL or over, a more specific glucose tolerance test (GTT) should be performed (the cutoff may be lowered to 130 mg/dL to improve sensitivity). The GTT involves obtaining a fasting plasma glucose level, giving a 100-g oral glucose load, then drawing plasma levels at 1 hour, 2 hours, and 3 hours after the glucose load. A test is considered positive for gestational diabetes if 2 of the 4 values are elevated. The thresholds proposed by Carpenter and Coustan are currently favored (fasting >95 mg/dL, 1 hour >180 mg/dL, 2 hour >155 mg/dL, 3 hour >140 mg/dL).

Group B Streptococcus

Group B streptococcus (GBS) asymptomatically colonizes between 10% and 30% of pregnant women, but perinatal transmission can result in a severe and potentially fatal neonatal infection. The current GBS testing protocol emphasizes the importance of culture screening and treatment over risk factor–based screening. For this reason, patients should be screened with a rectovaginal culture at 35–37 weeks. If the culture is positive, patients should be treated with intrapartum antibiotics. Intrapartum antibiotic prophylaxis has been shown to decrease the risk of perinatal GBS transmission. If the culture result is unknown, patients should be treated if in preterm labor, with rupture of membranes greater than or equal to 18 hours, or maternal fever greater than 100.4°F during labor. All patients with GBS bacteriuria during the pregnancy or a previous neonate with GBS sepsis should be treated with intrapartum antibiotics.

American College of Obstetricians and Gynecologists. Prevention of Early-Onset Group B Streptococcal Disease in Newborns. ACOG Committee Opinion No. 279. Washington, DC: American College of Obstetricians and Gynecologists; 2002.

American College of Obstetricians and Gynecologists. Screening for Fetal Chromosomal Anomalies. ACOG Practice Bulletin No. 77. Washington, DC: American College of Obstetricians and Gynecologists; 2007.

Gabbe SG, Graves CR. Management of diabetes mellitus complicating pregnancy. *Obstet Gynecol* 2003;102:857–868. PMID: 14551019.

Iams JD, Romero R, Culhane JF, Goldenberg RL. Primary, secondary, and tertiary interventions to reduce the morbidity and mortality of preterm birth. *Lancet* 2008; 371:164–175. PMID: 18191687.

Wapner RJ, Jenkins TM, Khalek N. Prenatal diagnosis of congenital disorders. In: Creasy RK, Resnik R (eds): *Maternal-Fetal Medicine: Principles and Practice*. Philadelphia, PA: Saunders Elsevier; 2009.

American College of Obstetricians and Gynecologists. Preconception and Prenatal Carrier Screening for Genetic Diseases in Individuals of Eastern European Jewish Descent. ACOG Committee Opinion No. 442. Washington, DC: American College of Obstetricians and Gynecologists; 2009.

FETAL ASSESSMENT

Performed during all trimesters, the techniques used are diverse, and the information obtained varies according to the quality of imaging, depth of investigation, and gestational age of pregnancy.

Ultrasound

Ultrasound (US) has evolved continuously over the last 30 years, with better equipment produced each year. Real-time sonography allows a 2-dimensional (2-D) image to demonstrate fetal anatomy, as well as characteristics such as fetal weight, movement, volume of amniotic fluid, and structural anomalies, such as myomas or placenta previa that may affect the pregnancy. Three-dimensional sonography allows volume to be ascertained, creating a 3-D–appearing image on the 2-D screen, which assists in identifying and clarifying certain anatomic anomalies. Most recently, 4-D machines have been developed, which produce 3-D video in real time. As the machines become more technically advanced and the computers that run them become faster, the images obtained will continue to improve and push the boundaries of sonographic prenatal diagnosis.

Diagnostic US is widely used in the assessment of the pregnancy and the fetus and offers a more than 80% detection rate of anomalies in experienced centers. The benefits and limitations of US should be discussed with all patients, and the decision to perform a US rests jointly with the physician and the patient.

A **standard** US examination should provide information such as fetal number, presentation, documentation of fetal viability, assessment of gestational age, amniotic fluid volume, placental location, fetal biometry, and an anatomic survey of the fetus(es). A **limited** US examination is a goal-directed search for a suspected problem or finding. A limited US can be used for guidance during procedures such as amniocentesis or external cephalic version, assessment of fetal well-being, or documentation of presentation or placental location intrapartum. A **specialized** US examination is performed when an anomaly is suspected based on history, biochemical abnormalities, or results of either the limited or standard scan. Other specialized examinations include fetal Doppler, biophysical profile (BPP), fetal echocardiogram, or additional biometric studies.

US evaluation of fetal anatomy may detect major structural anomalies. Gross malformations such as anencephaly and hydrocephaly are commonly diagnosed and rarely missed; however, more subtle anomalies such as facial clefts, diaphragmatic hernias, and cardiac defects are more commonly reported to have been missed by US. The basic fetal anatomy survey should include visualization of the cerebral ventricles, 4-chamber view of the heart, and examination of the spine, stomach, urinary bladder, umbilical cord insertion site, and renal region. Any indication of an anomaly should be followed by a more comprehensive sonogram. Typically, the fetal anatomic survey is performed at 17–20 weeks; however, there is controversy regarding the potential benefits of an earlier sonogram at 14–16 weeks using the transvaginal probe. The earlier scan allows earlier detection of anomalies that are almost always present by the second trimester, as well as allowing greater detailed viewing of the fetal anatomy by using the higher resolution vaginal transducers.

Aneuploidy Screening

Multiple second-trimester sonographic findings associated with aneuploidy or "markers" of aneuploidy have been identified. The presence of single or multiple markers adjusts the patient's age-related risk of aneuploidy based on the particular markers present. Such sonographic findings include, but are not limited to:

- Echogenic intracardiac focus
- Choroid plexus cysts
- Pyelectasis
- Echogenic bowel
- Short femur
- Increased nuchal fold

Chorionic Villus Sampling

Chorionic villus sampling (CVS) is an invasive test performed between 9 and 13 weeks' gestation and can be performed either transcervically or transabdominally. CVS is performed under sonographic guidance with the passing of a sterile catheter or needle into the placental site. Chorionic villi are aspirated and undergo cytogenetic analysis. The benefit of CVS over amniocentesis is its availability earlier in pregnancy. The overall pregnancy loss rate is higher than that of midtrimester amniocentesis, likely as a result of the increased background rate of spontaneous pregnancy loss between 9 and 16 weeks; limited data suggest that procedure-related loss rate for CVS appears to approach the rate of midtrimester amniocentesis. One disadvantage of CVS is that, unlike amniocentesis, it does not allow diagnosis of neural tube defects.

Amniocentesis

Amniocentesis is also performed under the guidance of ultrasonography. A needle is inserted transcutaneously through the maternal abdominal wall into the amniotic cavity, and fluid is removed. There are many uses for this amniotic fluid. In the early second trimester, these include AFP evaluation for neural tube defect assessment and the most common indication of cytogenetic analysis. In this case, amniocentesis is often performed between 15 and 20 weeks' gestation, and fetal cells from the amniotic fluid are obtained. Risks associated with the procedure are considered to be very low, with the risk of abortion as a result of amniocentesis considered to be between 1 in 200 to 1 in 450 amniocenteses.

Amniocentesis also provides a useful tool later in pregnancy, at low risk, for diagnosis of intra-amniotic inflammation and infection as a risk factor for preterm labor and adverse outcome, as well as documentation of fetal lung maturity.

Fetal Blood Sampling

Also referred to as cordocentesis or percutaneous umbilical blood sampling, fetal blood sampling is an option for chromosomal or metabolic analysis of the fetus. Benefits of the procedure include a rapid result turnaround and the ability to perform the procedure in the second and third trimesters. Intravascular access to the fetus is useful for assessment and treatment of certain fetal conditions such as Rh sensitization and alloimmune thrombocytopenia. However, there is a higher risk of fetal death compared with the other methods. Fetal loss rates are approximately 2%, but can vary depending on the fetal condition involved.

American College of Obstetricians and Gynecologists. Invasive Prenatal Testing for Aneuploidy. ACOG Practice Bulletin No. 88. Washington, DC: American College of Obstetricians and Gynecologists; 2007.

American College of Obstetricians and Gynecologists. Ultrasonography in Pregnancy. ACOG Practice Bulletin No. 101. Washington, DC: American College of Obstetricians and Gynecologists; 2009.

American Institute of Ultrasound in Medicine. AIUM practice guideline for the performance of an antepartum obstetric ultrasound examination. *J Ultrasound Med* 2010;29:157–166. PMID: 20040791.

Nicolaides KH. Nuchal translucency and other first-trimester sonographic markers of chromosomal abnormalities. *Am J Obstet Gynecol* 2004;191:45–67. PMID: 15295343.

Sonek JD, Cicero S, Neiger R, et al. Nasal bone assessment in prenatal screening for trisomy 21. *Am J Obstet Gynecol* 2006;195: 1219–1230. PMID: 16615922.

ANTEPARTUM FETAL TESTING

Fetal Movement Assessment

A decrease in maternal perception of fetal movement can precede fetal death, sometimes by several days. Perception of 10 distinct movements in a period of up to 2 hours is considered reassuring; if fewer, patients are often advised to undergo further testing.

Nonstress Test

Fetal movements associated with accelerations of fetal heart rate (FHR) provide reassurance that the fetus is not acidotic or neurologically depressed. A reactive and therefore reassuring nonstress test (NST) is defined as 2 or more FHR accelerations, at least 15 beats/min above the baseline and lasting at least 15 seconds within a 20-minute period. Vibroacoustic stimulation can elicit FHR accelerations that can reduce overall testing time without compromising detection of an acidotic fetus. In the case of a nonreassuring NST, further evaluation or delivery depends on the clinical context. In a patient at term, delivery is warranted. Pregnancy remote from term poses a more challenging dilemma to the clinician. If resuscitative efforts are not successful in restoring reactivity to the NST, then ancillary tests or testing techniques may prove useful in avoiding a premature iatrogenic delivery for nonreassuring FHR patterns, as the false-positive rate may be as high as 50–60%.

Biophysical Profile

The biophysical profile (BPP) is another way to assess fetal well-being. The BPP is composed of 5 components: NST, fetal breathing movements (30 seconds or more in 30 minutes), fetal movement (3 or more in 30 minutes), fetal tone (extension/flexion of an extremity), and amniotic fluid volume (vertical pocket of 2 cm or more). Each component is worth 2 points; a score of 8 or 10 is normal, 6 is equivocal, and 4 or less is abnormal. A BPP score of 10/10 or 8/10 with normal amniotic fluid volume is associated with a low risk of fetal asphyxia in the following week (approximately 1 per 1000).

Modified Biophysical Profile

Modified BPP combines NST, a short-term indicator of fetal acid–base status, with amniotic fluid index (AFI), a long-term indicator of placental function. AFI is measured by dividing the uterus into 4 equal quadrants and measuring the largest vertical pocket in each quadrant; the results are then summed and expressed in millimeters. The modified BPP has become a primary mode of antepartum fetal surveillance; a nonreactive NST or an AFI less than 50 mm (oligohydramnios) requires further fetal assessment or intervention.

Contraction Stress Test

The contraction stress test (CST) is based on the response of FHR to uterine contractions, with the premise that fetal oxygenation will be worsened during contractions. This can result in late decelerations in an already suboptimally oxygenated fetus. The test requires 3 contractions in 10 minutes to be adequate for interpretation. A positive or abnormal test is defined as late decelerations occurring with more than half of the contractions. A test is considered to be suspicious or equivocal if any late decelerations are seen (with fewer than 50% of contractions) and negative with no late decelerations. Contraindications to CST include any contraindications to labor, such as placenta previa or prior classic caesarean section. This test is now rarely used.

Growth Ultrasound

Growth US studies, performed every 3–4 weeks, are useful for assessment of fetuses that may be at risk for growth restriction secondary to medical conditions of pregnancy or fetal abnormalities.

Doppler Studies

Fetal Doppler studies initially were used to assess the placenta by evaluation of umbilical artery outflow. They have since evolved to a more comprehensive multivessel evaluation of fetal status. Doppler studies can be used to assess a compromised fetus (particularly the growth-restricted fetus) and may function as a diagnostic tool that alerts the clinician to the need for further intervention, including BPP, continuous fetal monitoring, or possibly delivery. In addition, the peak systolic velocity of the middle cerebral artery is used to assess fetal anemia in cases of alloimmunization and parvovirus infection.

Fetal Maturity Tests

A. Indications for Assessing Fetal Lung Maturity

ACOG has recommended that fetal pulmonary maturity should be confirmed before elective delivery before 39 weeks' gestation unless fetal maturity can be inferred from any of these criteria: fetal heart tones have been documented for 20 weeks by nonelectronic fetoscope or for 30 weeks by Doppler; 36 weeks have elapsed since a serum or urine hCG-based pregnancy test was reported to be positive; US measurement of crown–rump length at 6–11 weeks of gestation or measurements at 12–20 weeks support a

Table 12–4. Fetal maturity tests.

Test	Positive Discriminating Value	Positive Predictive Value	Relative Cost	Pros and Cons
TDx-FLM	>55	96–100%	Moderate	Minimal inter/intra-assay variability; simple test
L/S ratio	>2.0	95–100%	High	Large laboratory variation
PG	"Present"	95–100%	High	Not affected by blood, meconium; can use vaginal pooled sample
Lamellar body counts	30–40,000	97–98%	Low	Cutoff values still investigational
Optical density	OD 0.15	98%	Low	Simple technique
Foam stability index	>47	95%	Low	Affected by blood, meconium silicone tubes

FLM, fetal lung maturity; L/S, lecithin/sphingomyelin; PG, phosphatidylglycerol.

gestational age equal to or greater than 39 weeks. For those patients for whom delivery is mandated by fetal or maternal indications, testing of fetal lung maturity should not be performed, nor does a mature fetal lung maturity result before 39 weeks' gestation indicate delivery in the absence of appropriate clinical circumstances

1. Lecithin/sphingomyelin ratio—The lecithin/sphingomyelin (L/S) ratio for assessment of fetal pulmonary maturity was first introduced by Gluck and colleagues in 1971. The test depends on outward flow of pulmonary secretions from the lungs into the amniotic fluid, thereby changing the phospholipid composition of the latter and permitting measurement of the L/S ratio in a sample of amniotic fluid. In the absence of complications, the ratio of these 2 components reaches 2.0 at approximately 35 weeks. The presence of blood or meconium may interfere with test interpretation.

2. Phosphatidylglycerol—Phosphatidylglycerol (PG) is a minor constituent of surfactant. It begins to increase appreciably in amniotic fluid several weeks after the rise in lecithin. Its presence is more indicative of fetal lung maturity because PG enhances the spread of phospholipids on the alveoli.

3. Fluorescence polarization—The fluorescence polarization test, currently the most widely used test, uses polarized light to quantitate the competitive binding of a probe to both albumin and surfactant in amniotic fluid; thus it is a true direct measurement of surfactant concentration. It reflects the ratio of surfactant to albumin and is measured by an automatic analyzer, such as the TDx-FLM. An elevated ratio has been correlated with the presence of fetal lung maturity; the threshold for maturity is 55 mg of surfactant per gram of albumin.

Table 12–4 lists all fetal maturity tests available, discriminating levels, and specific characteristics of the tests.

American College of Obstetricians and Gynecologists. Antepartum Fetal Surveillance. ACOG Practice Bulletin No. 9. Washington, DC: American College of Obstetricians and Gynecologists; 1999 (Reaffirmed 2009).

American College of Obstetricians and Gynecologists. Fetal Lung Maturity. ACOG Practice Bulletin No. 97. Washington, DC: American College of Obstetricians and Gynecologists; 2008.

Baschat AA. Fetal growth restriction—from observation to intervention. *J Perinat Med* 2010;38:239–246. PMID: 20205623.

INTRAPARTUM MANAGEMENT

Fetal Heart Rate Monitoring

Use of electronic fetal monitoring (EFM) has been increasing over the last several decades, up to 85% in 2002. No randomized controlled trials have compared the benefits of EFM versus no form of monitoring during labor. Randomized clinical trials comparing EFM with intermittent auscultation showed an increase in caesarean section rate, caesarean section rate for fetal distress, and operative vaginal delivery rate, with no reduction in overall perinatal mortality, but possibly a decrease in perinatal mortality from fetal hypoxia. Given these findings, ACOG has stated that either EFM or intermittent auscultation is acceptable, given that guidelines for intermittent auscultation are met. Intermittent auscultation may not, however, be acceptable in high-risk patients.

Table 12–5. Three-tiered fetal heart rate interpretation system.

Category I Baseline rate: 110–160 beats/min Baseline FHR variability: moderate Late or variable decelerations: absent Early decelerations: present or absent Accelerations: present or absent
Category II All FHR tracings not categorized as category I or category III Examples include: Baseline rate Bradycardia not accompanied by absent baseline variability Tachycardia Baseline FHR variability Minimal or marked baseline variability Absent baseline variability with no recurrent decelerations Accelerations Absence of induced accelerations after fetal stimulation Periodic or episodic decelerations Recurrent variable decelerations accompanied by minimal or moderate baseline variability Prolonged deceleration more than 2 min but less than 10 min Recurrent late decelerations with moderate baseline variability
Category III Absent baseline FHR variability and any of the following: Recurrent late decelerations Recurrent variable decelerations Bradycardia Sinusoidal pattern

FHR, fetal heart rate.

Despite its widespread use, EFM suffers from poor interobserver and intraobserver reliability, uncertain efficacy, and a high false-positive rate. In 2008, a workshop sponsored by ACOG, the Eunice Kennedy Shriver National Institute of Child Health and Human Development (NICHD), and the Society of Maternal-Fetal Medicine recommended an EFM interpretive system based on a three-tiered approach (Table 12–5). Utility of this approach remains to be seen.

Fetal Heart Rate Definitions

The baseline is the mean FHR rounded to increments of 5 beats/min, at least 2 minutes in any 10-minute segment. Normal baseline is between 110 and 160 beats/min. Baseline FHR below 110 is defined as *bradycardia*; baseline FHR above 160 is defined as *tachycardia*. Either bradycardia (particularly when the new baseline is less than 80 beats/min) or tachycardia (particularly when associated with a decrease in variability or repetitive late or severe variable decelerations) suggests a nonreassuring fetal status. *Accelerations* (at 32 weeks or greater) are defined as elevations above the baseline of 15 beats/min lasting 15 seconds or longer; less than 32 weeks it is defined by elevations of 10 beats/min lasting at least 10 seconds. Two or more accelerations in a 20-minute interval are reassuring; this defines reactivity in an NST. *Variability* is defined by fluctuations in the FHR of 2 cycles per minute or greater and can range from absent to marked. Decelerations are categorized as early, late, and variable. *Early decelerations* generally mirror contractions in timing and shape and are generally not ominous, often representing head compression. *Late decelerations* are smooth falls in the FHR beginning after the contraction has started and ending after the contraction has ended. They are associated with fetal hypoxemia and a potential for perinatal morbidity and mortality. *Variable decelerations* are abrupt in decline and return to baseline, vary in timing with the contraction, and usually represent cord compression. These are most ominous when repetitive and severe (below 60 beats/min). A *prolonged deceleration* is a decrease of 15 beats/min below the baseline lasting between 2 and 10 minutes.

Ancillary Tests

A. Fetal Scalp Blood Sampling

In the presence of a nonreassuring FHR pattern, a scalp blood sample for determination of pH or lactate can be considered. Although the specificity is high (normal values rule out asphyxia), the sensitivity and positive predictive value of a low scalp pH in identifying a newborn with hypoxic–ischemic encephalopathy is low. For these reasons, in addition to the technical skill and expense of the procedure, fetal scalp pH is no longer used in many institutions.

B. Vibroacoustic Stimulation/Scalp Stimulation

The presence of an acceleration after a vaginal examination in which the examiner stimulates the fetal vertex with the examining finger or after vibroacoustic stimulation (as described earlier under "Nonstress Test") confirms the absence of acidosis (pH >7.2). Some clinicians prefer these methods over fetal scalp blood sampling because they are less invasive.

C. Fetal Pulse Oximetry

Fetal pulse oximetry, the measure of the fetus' oxygenation during labor, was developed with the goal of improving the specificity of FHR monitoring and decreasing the number of caesarean sections secondary to nonreassuring fetal status. It has not been demonstrated to be a clinically useful test in evaluating fetal status and is not recommended.

D. ST-Segment Analysis During Labor

ST-segment analysis via computerized real-time analysis of the ST-segment interval of the fetal electrocardiogram has been shown in initial studies to, in combination with intrapartum monitoring with EFM, increase the ability of obstetricians to identify compromised fetuses and to intervene more appropriately. A large multicenter randomized controlled trial is currently underway in the United States.

CONCLUSION

Assessing pregnancy to determine risk, as well as careful monitoring of pregnancies with a recognized risk, begins early in the gestation. Preconception counseling of patients with known medical or genetic disorders helps to optimize outcomes. Early and frequent prenatal care allows the care provider to screen his or her patient population to identify pregnancies at risk and act accordingly. Additionally, pregnancies identified as complicated by 1 or more issues can be followed by assortments of maternal and fetal surveillance techniques to maximize therapeutic treatment.

As technology advances and our ability to both diagnose and treat improve, the methods for assessment and care of the pregnancy at risk will be a constantly changing field.

American College of Obstetricians and Gynecologists. Intrapartum Fetal Heart Rate Monitoring: Nomenclature, Interpretation, and General Management Principles. ACOG Practice Bulletin No. 106. Washington, DC: American College of Obstetricians and Gynecologists; 2009.

American College of Obstetricians and Gynecologists. Management of Intrapartum Fetal Heart Rate Tracings. ACOG Practice Bulletin No.116. Washington, DC: American College of Obstetricians and Gynecologists; 2010.

Macones GA, Hankins GD, Spong CY, Hauth J, Moore T. The 2008 National Institute of Child Health and Human Development workshop report on electronic fetal monitoring: Update on definitions, interpretation, and research guidelines. *Obstet Gynecol* 2008;112:661–666. PMID: 18757666.

Mires G, Williams F, Howie P. Randomised controlled trial of cardiotocography versus Doppler auscultation of fetal heart at admission in labour in low risk obstetric population. *BMJ* 2001; 322:1457–1460. PMID: 11408301.

Neilson JP. Fetal electrocardiogram (ECG) for fetal monitoring during labour. *Cochrane Database Sys Rev* 2006; 3:CD000116. PMID: 16855950.

13 Early Pregnancy Risks

Ann-Marie Surette, MD
Samantha M. Dunham, MD

SPONTANEOUS ABORTION

ESSENTIALS OF DIAGNOSIS

- Suprapubic pain, uterine cramping, and/or back pain
- Vaginal bleeding
- Cervical dilation
- Passage of products of conception
- Quantitative β-human chorionic gonadotropin that is falling or not adequately rising
- Abnormal ultrasound findings (eg, empty gestational sac, lack of fetal growth or fetal cardiac activity)

General Considerations

Spontaneous abortion is the most common complication of pregnancy and is defined as the passing of a pregnancy at less than 20 weeks of gestation. It implies the spontaneous loss of an embryo or fetus weighing less than 500 g. **Threatened abortion** is bleeding arising from within the uterus that occurs before the 20th completed week in a viable pregnancy. The patient may or may not experience pain or cramping; however, there is no passage of products of conception and no cervical dilation. **Complete abortion** is the expulsion of all of the products of conception before the 20th completed week of gestation, whereas **incomplete abortion** is the expulsion of some, but not all, of the products of conception. **Inevitable abortion** refers to bleeding from within the uterus before the 20th week, with dilation of the cervix but without expulsion of the products of conception. The term **missed abortion** describes a nonviable pregnancy that has been retained in the uterus without cervical dilation and without the spontaneous passage of products of conception. In **septic abortion**, embryonic or fetal demise has occurred, and intrauterine infection has developed, which has the potential risk of spreading systemically.

Although the true incidence of spontaneous abortion is unknown, approximately 15% of clinically evident pregnancies and up to 50% of chemically evident pregnancies end in spontaneous abortion. Eighty percent of spontaneous abortions occur before 12 weeks' gestation.

The incidence of abortion is influenced by the age of the mother and by a number of pregnancy-related factors, including the number of previous spontaneous abortions, a previous intrauterine fetal demise, and a previous infant born with malformations or known genetic defects. Additionally, chromosomal abnormalities in either parent, such as balanced translocations, and medical comorbidities, such as thyroid disease and diabetes mellitus, may influence the rate of spontaneous abortion.

Pathogenesis

An abnormal karyotype is present in as many as 50% of spontaneous abortions occurring during the first trimester. The incidence decreases to 20–30% of second-trimester losses and to 5–10% of third-trimester losses. The majority of chromosome abnormalities are trisomies (56%), followed by polyploidy (20%) and monosomy X (18%).

Other suspected causes of spontaneous abortion are less common, and these include infection, anatomic defects, endocrine factors, immunologic factors, and exposure to toxic substances. In a significant percentage of spontaneous abortions, the etiology is unknown, even with genetic testing.

A. Genetic Abnormalities

Aneuploidy, an abnormal chromosomal number, is the most common genetic abnormality, accounting for up to 50% of clinical miscarriages. Monosomy X or Turner's syndrome is the single most common aneuploidy, comprising approximately 18% of these gestations. As a group, the autosomal trisomies account for more than half of aneuploid losses, with trisomy 16 being the most common. Autosomal trisomies have been noted for every chromosome except chromosome number 1. Most trisomic pregnancies end in miscarriage. The exceptions are trisomy 21, 18, and 13, which have survival to birth rates of 22%, 5%, and 3%, respectively.

Polyploidy, usually in the form of triploidy, is found in approximately 20% of all miscarriages. Polyploid conceptions typically result in an anembryonic gestation. Occasionally, these pregnancies will develop into partial hydatidiform moles.

The remaining half of early abortuses appear to have normal chromosomes. Of these, 20% have other genetic abnormalities that may account for the loss. Mendelian or polygenic factors resulting in anatomic defects may play a role. These factors tend to be more common in later fetal losses.

B. Maternal Factors

1. Systemic disease

A. Maternal infections—Organisms such as *Toxoplasma gondii,* herpes simplex virus, cytomegalovirus, and *Listeria monocytogenes* have been implicated in spontaneous abortion. Although these agents, as well as *Chlamydia trachomatis*, have been found in women with first-trimester losses, a causal relationship has not been established.

B. Other diseases—Endocrine disorders such as hypothyroidism, hyperthyroidism, hyperprolactinemia, and poorly controlled diabetes mellitus; cardiovascular disorders, such as hypertensive or renal disease; and autoimmune disorders, such as systemic lupus erythematosus and antiphospholipid syndrome, are associated with spontaneous abortion. At less than 10 weeks, the association between antiphospholipid syndrome and early pregnancy loss is controversial and less well established.

2. Uterine and cervical factors—Congenital anomalies that distort or reduce the size of the uterine cavity, such as unicornuate, bicornuate, or septate uterus, are associated with poor pregnancy outcomes (Fig. 13–1). There is an increased risk of miscarriage, as well as placental abruption, intrauterine growth restriction, and preterm labor. Of all uterine anomalies, septate uterus is the most common and can be removed by hysteroscopic resection, resulting in higher pregnancy and live birth rates (Fig. 13–2). Upper and lower genital tract structural changes have been observed in 25–33% of women whose mothers took diethylstilbestrol (DES) during pregnancy. Uterine anomalies, such as a T-shaped or hypoplastic uterus, carry an increased risk of miscarriage. DES was banned from use in pregnant women in 1971. As a result, pregnancy complications in DES daughters are less and less common, as these women are now 40 years and older. Acquired anomalies, such as fibroids (especially submucosal) and endometrial polyps, have been associated with spontaneous abortions as well.

The formation of scar tissue, or synechiae, within the uterine cavity that leads to problems such as infertility or recurrent miscarriage is known as Asherman's syndrome. These intrauterine adhesions or fibrosis are most commonly found after dilation and curettage (D&C) of the gravid uterus, either for spontaneous miscarriage, termination, or treatment of postpartum hemorrhage. Diagnosis is often confirmed with hysterosalpingogram, saline infusion sonogram, or hysteroscopy. Treatment is by resection of the adhesions using hysteroscopy.

Cervical insufficiency (previously known as cervical incompetence) is painless cervical shortening or dilation in the second or early third trimester, up to 28 weeks, resulting in preterm birth. Congenital uterine anomalies and DES anomalies are associated with cervical insufficiency. Procedures to treat dysplasia of the cervix such as cervical conization appear to increase the risk for cervical insufficiency.

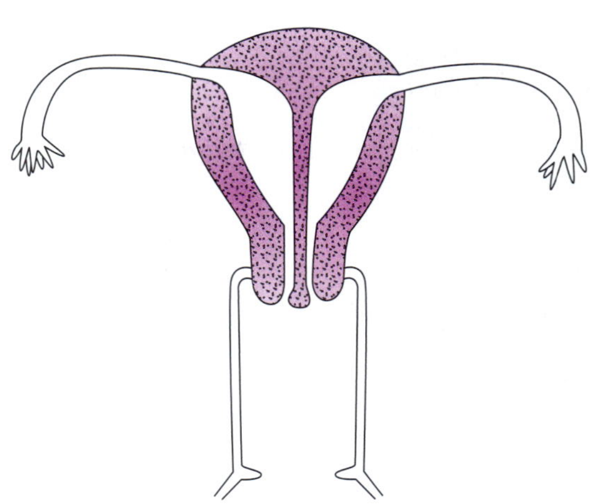

▲ **Figure 13–1.** Complete bicornuate uterus. (Reproduced, with permission, from Reichman DE, Laufer MR. Congenital uterine anomalies affecting reproduction. *Best Pract Res Clin Obstet Gynaecol* 2010;24:193. PMID: 19897423.)

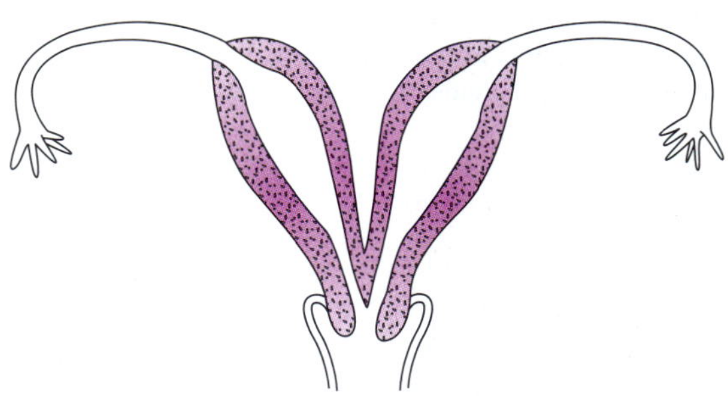

▲ **Figure 13–2.** Septate uterus. (Reproduced, with permission, from Reichman DE, Laufer MR. Congenital uterine anomalies affecting reproduction. *Best Pract Res Clin Obstet Gynaecol* 2010;24:193. PMID: 19897423.)

C. Toxic Factors

Exposure to antineoplastic drugs, anesthetic gases, alcohol, nicotine, or cocaine can result in spontaneous abortion. Other substances such as lead, ethylene oxide, and formaldehyde have also been associated with subsequent miscarriage.

D. Trauma

Direct trauma, such as a penetrating injury to the uterus, or indirect trauma, such as surgical removal of an ovary containing the corpus luteum, may result in spontaneous abortion. Amniocentesis or chorionic villus sampling are associated with a risk of pregnancy loss.

Pathology

In spontaneous abortion, hemorrhage into the decidua basalis often occurs. Necrosis and inflammation appear at the area of implantation. The pregnancy then becomes partially or entirely detached. Uterine contractions and dilation of the cervix result in expulsion of part or all of the products of conception.

Prevention

Some miscarriages can be prevented by early obstetric care and even preconception care, with adequate treatment of maternal comorbidities such as diabetes and hypertension, and by protection of pregnant women from environmental hazards and exposure to infectious diseases.

Clinical Findings

A. Threatened Abortion

Approximately 25% of pregnant women experience first-trimester bleeding. In most cases, this bleeding is caused by implantation into the endometrium. The cervix remains closed, and slight bleeding with or without cramping may be noted. Resolution of the bleeding and cramping carries a favorable prognosis; however, these women are at increased risk for subsequent miscarriage. First-trimester bleeding has also been associated with preterm premature rupture of membranes and preterm labor. Other causes, such as ectopic pregnancy and molar gestation, should also be considered.

B. Inevitable Abortion

Bleeding with cervical dilation, often with back or abdominal pain, indicate impending abortion. Unlike an incomplete abortion, the products of conception have not passed from the uterine cavity.

C. Incomplete Abortion

Incomplete abortion (Fig. 13–3) is defined as the passage of some but not all of the products of conception from the uterine cavity. Bleeding and cramping usually continue until all products of conception have been expelled. In general, severe pain and heavy bleeding occur and often require medical evaluation.

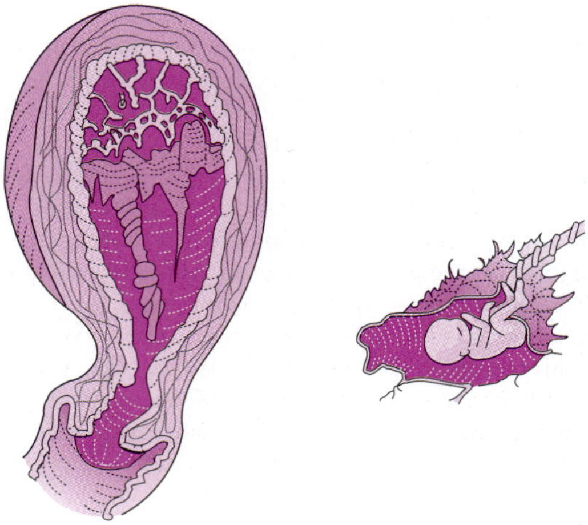

▲ **Figure 13–3.** Incomplete abortion. **Right:** Product of incomplete abortion. (Reproduced, with permission, from Benson RC. *Handbook of Obstetrics & Gynecology.* 8th ed. Los Altos, CA: Lange; 1983.)

D. Complete Abortion

In a complete abortion (Fig. 13–4), all of the products of conception have passed from the uterine cavity and the cervix is closed. Slight bleeding and mild cramping may continue for several weeks.

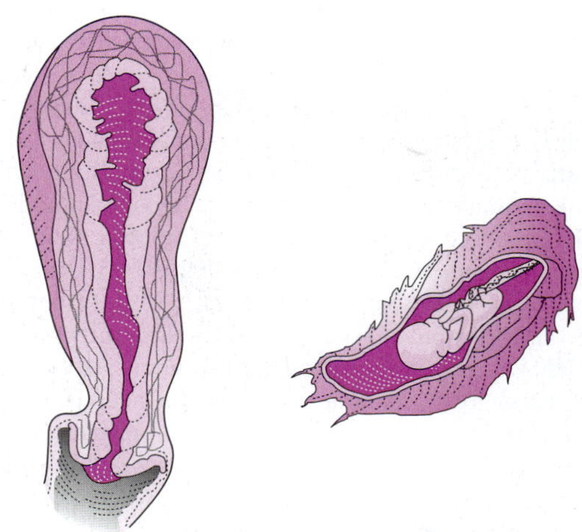

▲ **Figure 13–4.** Complete abortion. **Right:** Product of complete abortion. (Reproduced, with permission, from Benson RC . *Handbook of Obstetrics & Gynecology.* 8th ed. Los Altos, CA: Lange; 1983.)

E. Missed Abortion

Missed abortion is defined as a pregnancy that has been retained within the uterus after embryonic or fetal demise. Cramping or bleeding may be present, but often there are no symptoms. The cervix is closed, and the products of conception remain in situ.

F. Anembryonic Pregnancy

Anembryonic pregnancy (previously called *blighted ovum*) is an ultrasound diagnosis. It is a pregnancy in which the embryo fails to develop or is resorbed after loss of viability. On ultrasound, an empty gestational sac is seen without a fetal pole (Fig. 13–5). Clinical presentation is similar to that of a missed or threatened abortion: Mild pain or bleeding may be present; however, the cervix is closed, and the nonviable pregnancy is retained in the uterus.

Laboratory Findings

A. Complete Blood Count

If significant bleeding has occurred, the patient will be anemic. Both the white blood cell count and the sedimentation rate may be elevated, even without the presence of infection.

B. Pregnancy Tests

Falling or abnormally rising serum levels of β-human chorionic gonadotropin (hCG) are diagnostic of an abnormal pregnancy, either a failed intrauterine gestation or an ectopic pregnancy.

Ultrasound Findings

Transvaginal ultrasound is an essential diagnostic tool in diagnosing early normal and abnormal pregnancies. As early as 4–5 weeks of gestation, a gestational sac may be visualized in the uterus. In a normal intrauterine pregnancy, the sac is spherical and is eccentrically placed within the endometrium. At 5–6 weeks' gestation, a yolk sac will be present. In general, a gestational sac with a mean sac diameter (MSD) of ≥8 mm should contain a yolk sac. Similarly, a gestational sac with an MSD of >16 mm should also contain an embryo (Fig. 13–6). Pregnancies with a large gestational sac and no embryo are typically anembryonic gestations and are managed in a similar manner as a missed abortion (Fig. 13–5). Fetal heart motion is expected in embryos with a crown to rump length of >5 mm or at 6–7 weeks' gestation. If a repeat ultrasound in 1 week does not show embryonic cardiac activity, the diagnosis of embryonic demise is made.

In threatened abortion, ultrasound will reveal a normal gestational sac and a viable embryo. However, a large or irregular sac, an eccentric fetal pole, and/or a slow fetal heart rate (<85 beats/min) carry a poor prognosis. Miscarriage becomes increasingly less likely the further the gestation progresses. If a viable fetus of 6 weeks or less is seen on ultrasound, the risk of miscarriage is approximately 15–30%. The risk decreases to 5–10% at 7–9 weeks' gestation and to less than 5% after 9 weeks' gestation.

In an incomplete abortion, the gestational sac usually is irregularly shaped. Heterogenous, echogenic material representing retained products of conception is seen within the uterus. Endometrial thickness can be helpful in diagnosing an incomplete abortion; however, there is no consensus on a cutoff value to distinguish complete miscarriage from incomplete miscarriage. Color Doppler can be used to assess for flow within the tissue and can help differentiate retained products of conception that remain implanted within the uterus from tissue or blood that is in the process of expulsion. Thus, a combination of clinical and ultrasound findings must be used to determine management.

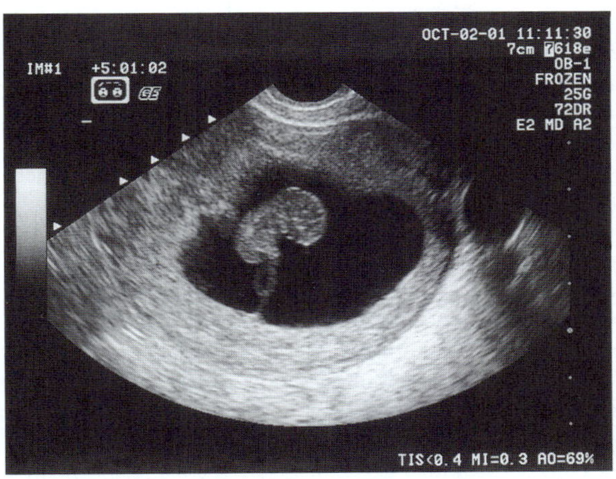

▲ **Figure 13–5.** Anembryonic pregnancy: large, irregular gestational sac without an embryo.

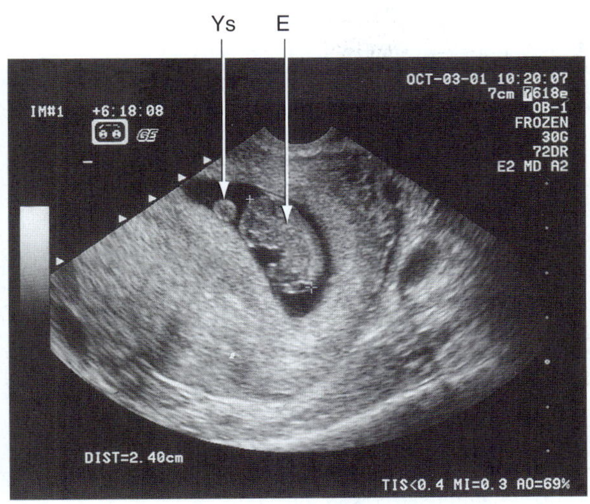

▲ **Figure 13–6.** Intrauterine pregnancy with gestational sac, yolk sac, and embryo.

The diagnosis of complete abortion is also based on clinical findings. On ultrasound, the endometrial lining appears thin, and no products of conception are visible within the cavity. Importantly, a complete abortion is only diagnosed with certainty if a previous intrauterine gestation was documented on ultrasound. Otherwise, hCG levels must be followed to confirm the absence of ectopic pregnancy.

Ectopic pregnancy may cause similar symptoms of miscarriage, such as bleeding and abdominal or pelvic pain. An adnexal mass may or may not be present. The presence of an ectopic pregnancy is exceedingly rare if an intrauterine pregnancy (gestational sac plus yolk sac) is seen on ultrasound. The chance of a simultaneous intrauterine and extrauterine pregnancy (heterotopic pregnancy) is approximately 1 in 3900, including spontaneous pregnancies and those conceived with assisted reproductive technology (ART).

Hydatidiform molar pregnancies usually end in miscarriage before the fifth month of gestation. Theca lutein cysts are present in 50% of cases and appear as bilateral, large, multiseptated ovarian cysts. These cysts are caused by excessive production of hCG by the abnormal trophoblastic tissue. The uterus may also be unusually large and contain a heterogenous endometrial mass classically described on ultrasound as a "swiss cheese" or "snowstorm" pattern. An early molar gestation may present simply as an anembryonic gestation or spontaneous abortion. Only partial molar gestations will contain fetal parts.

When findings on ultrasound are nonspecific, correlation with hCG levels can improve the ability to distinguish normal and abnormal pregnancies. In a normal pregnancy, the minimal rise in hCG is 53% over 48 hours. hCG values that rise slower than expected may be consistent with a failed intrauterine or ectopic pregnancy. Decreasing levels of hCG are also diagnostic of an abnormal pregnancy. In spontaneous abortion, the hCG values are expected to drop 21–35% in 2 days (depending on the initial hCG value). A slower decline is suggestive of an ectopic pregnancy.

Complications

Severe or persistent bleeding during or after spontaneous abortion may be life-threatening. The more advanced the gestation, the greater the likelihood of excessive blood loss. Infection, intrauterine adhesions (Asherman's syndrome), and infertility are other complications of abortion.

Perforation of the uterus may occur during procedures to remove retained products of conception, namely D&C. The rate of perforation during the first and second trimesters is approximately 0.5% for both induced and spontaneous abortions. Uterine perforation is more common during D&C performed in pregnancy because of the soft uterine wall and may be accompanied by injury to the bowel and bladder, hemorrhage, and infection. Surgical evacuation may also lead to cervical trauma and subsequent cervical insufficiency.

Treatment of Abortions

Successful management of spontaneous abortion depends on early diagnosis. Every patient should have a complete history taken and a physical examination performed. Laboratory studies include a complete blood count, blood type, and cervical cultures to determine pathogens in case of infection.

If the diagnosis of threatened abortion is made, pelvic rest can be recommended, although it has not been shown to prevent subsequent miscarriage. Prognosis is good when bleeding and/or cramping resolve.

If the diagnosis of a missed or incomplete abortion is made, options include surgical, medical, or expectant management. In the past, surgery was the standard of care because of concern that medical or expectant management would lead to higher rates of retained pregnancy tissue and subsequent infection. More recently, expectant or medical management are acceptable alternatives and have even shown lower rates of infection despite their higher rates of retained products of conception. These patients also avoid the risks of surgery, including uterine perforation, intrauterine adhesions, and cervical insufficiency. The advantages of performing a D&C include convenient timing and low rates of retained products of conception.

Expectant management allows the spontaneous passage of products of conception and avoids risks of surgery. Risks and side effects include unpredictable timing until the abortion is completed with the possibility of significant pain and bleeding, occasionally requiring emergent D&C. Expectant management also has the highest rates of retained pregnancy tissue, necessitating treatment with misoprostol (prostaglandin E1) or D&C.

Patients who choose medical management are given misoprostol, a drug that induces uterine contractions and expulsion of the products of conception. The risk of retained products is lower than with expectant management; however, repeat doses of medication may be needed to complete the abortion. As with expectant management, timing can be unpredictable, and symptoms of pain and/or bleeding may necessitate emergent D&C. Expectant or medical management of abortion assumes that prompt medical evaluation is available. Those options should not be considered if medical care is not easily accessible.

If the diagnosis of complete abortion is made, the patient should be observed for further bleeding. If bleeding is minimal, no further treatment is necessary. All products of conception should be examined and sent for pathologic examination to confirm an intrauterine pregnancy. If an intrauterine pregnancy was not previously seen on ultrasound and no pathology specimen is available, serial hCG levels are followed to confirm spontaneous abortion. If hCG levels decline more slowly than expected (eg, <21–35%), an ectopic pregnancy or retained products of conception must be considered. Molar gestation is also a possible diagnosis if hCG levels plateau or rise abnormally without an intrauterine pregnancy.

If a complete or partial hydatidiform molar pregnancy is diagnosed, surgical evacuation with suction D&C should be performed. As long as hCG levels are decreasing and remain undetectable after molar evacuation, there is no need for chemotherapy. However, if hCG levels start rising, plateau, or are persistent for more than 6 months, evaluation for malignant postmolar gestational trophoblastic disease is indicated.

Treatment of Complications

Uterine perforation may result in intraperitoneal bleeding, as well as injury to the bladder and/or bowel. In many cases, uterine perforation is asymptomatic and goes unrecognized. When perforation and bowel or bladder injury is suspected or when heavy bleeding is encountered, laparoscopy and/or laparotomy are indicated to determine the extent of the perforation and to evaluate for injury to other adjacent organs.

American College of Obstetricians and Gynecologists. *Diagnosis and Treatment of Gestational Trophoblastic Disease.* ACOG Practice Bulletin No. 53. Washington, DC: American College of Obstetricians and Gynecologists; 2004.

Chen B, Creinin M. Contemporary management of early pregnancy failure. *Clin Obstet Gynecol* 2007;67:88. PMID: 17304025.

Chung K, Allen R. The use of serial human chorionic gonadotropin levels to establish a viable or a nonviable pregnancy. *Semin Reprod Med* 2008;26:383. PMID: 18825606.

Dighe M, Cuevas C, Moshiri M, Dubinsky T, Dogra VS. Sonography in first trimester bleeding. *J Clin Ultrasound* 2008;36:352. PMID: 18335508.

Johns J, Jauniaux E. Threatened miscarriage as a predictor of obstetric outcome. *Obstet Gynecol* 2006;107:845. PMID: 16582121.

Nanda K, Peloggia A, Grimes D, Lopez L, Nanda G. Expectant care versus surgical treatment for miscarriage. *Cochrane Database Syst Rev* 2006;CD003518. PMID: 16625583.

Sawyer E, Jurkovic D. Ultrasonography in the diagnosis and management of abnormal early pregnancy. *Clin Obstet Gynecol* 2007;50:31. PMID: 17304023.

RECURRENT PREGNANCY LOSS

ESSENTIALS OF DIAGNOSIS

- Three or more consecutive pregnancy losses before 20 weeks of gestation

General Considerations

Recurrent miscarriage is defined as 3 or more consecutive pregnancy losses before 20 weeks of gestation, each with a fetus weighing less than 500 g. Recurrent pregnancy loss affects up to 5% of couples, often with no identifiable cause. The prognosis for a successful subsequent pregnancy correlates with the number of previous miscarriages. The risk of spontaneous abortion in a first pregnancy is approximately 15%, and this risk is at least doubled in women experiencing recurrent pregnancy loss.

Overall, the prognosis after repeated losses is good, with most couples having an approximately 60% chance of a viable pregnancy.

Pathogenesis & Treatment

Determining the etiology of recurrent miscarriage involves a comprehensive workup. This evaluation can be divided into 6 categories of possible causes: genetic, immunologic, endocrinologic, anatomic, microbiologic, and thrombophilic.

Table 13–1 summarizes a diagnostic workup and possible therapies for recurrent abortion.

A. Genetic Errors

Genetic errors associated with recurrent pregnancy loss include maternal and paternal karyotype abnormalities and recurrent aneuploidy.

A structural genetic factor is found in either partner in up to 8% of couples with recurrent miscarriage. Of these, balanced translocations are the most common and are found more frequently in the female partner. Less frequent findings include chromosome insertions, deletions, and inversions. When a karyotypic abnormality is found, genetic counseling should be provided because the likelihood of a subsequent healthy birth depends on the chromosome(s) involved and the type of rearrangement. Although couples affected by a structural genetic defect are more likely to have a miscarriage, the subsequent live birth rate can be as high as 70%. Despite the good prognosis, some patients opt for treatment with ART. If the defect is paternal, artificial insemination by a donor is available. For a maternal defect, a donor egg may be fertilized by the husband's sperm. Preimplantation genetic diagnosis is also available for parents who wish to use their own gametes.

In couples with normal karyotypes, recurrent fetal aneuploidy can be the cause of miscarriage. The most common aneuploidies found are the trisomies. Although miscarriages caused by trisomies are usually random events, the frequency of such events increases with advancing maternal age. In the general reproductive population, however, a trisomic miscarriage does not increase the risk of having a similar outcome in the next pregnancy. As a result, recurrent pregnancy loss with normal fetal chromosomes carries an overall higher recurrence risk, as this subset is presumably caused by maternal or paternal etiologies.

B. Uterine & Cervical Abnormalities

Anatomic abnormalities were the first described causes of recurrent miscarriage and account for up to 15% of recurrent

Table 13–1. Evaluation and management of recurrent early pregnancy loss.

Factor	Diagnostic Evaluation	Treatment
Genetic factors	Parental cytogenetics Three-generation pedigree	Genetic counseling Donor egg/sperm PGD
Anatomic factors	Ultrasound, hysterosalpingogram, hysteroscopy	Hysteroscopic metroplasty Lysis of adhesions Hysteroscopic myomectomy/polypectomy Cervical cerclage
Endocrine fctors	Midluteal progesterone level TSH level Prolactin level Fasting insulin and glucose, glucose tolerance test	Progesterone supplementation Synthroid Bromocriptine, cabergoline Metformin, insulin
Immunologic factors	Lupus anticoagulant Anticardiolipin IgG/IgM	ASA, heparin
Thrombophilic factors	Factor V Leiden Prothrombin gene mutation Fasting homocysteine Protein S/protein C activity Antithrombin activity	Heparin (insufficient data to routinely recommend)
Exogenous agents	Evaluate for tobacco, alcohol, drug use	Eliminate exposure

ASA, acetylsalicylic acid; Ig, immunoglobulin; PGD, preimplant genetic diagnosis; TSH, thyroid-stimulating hormone.
Data from Stephenson MD. Evaluation and management of recurrent early pregnancy loss. *Clin Obstet Gynecol* 2007;50:132.

pregnancy losses. Defects include congenital uterine anomalies, cervical insufficiency, submucosal leiomyomas and endometrial polyps, malformations from DES exposure in utero, and Asherman's syndrome.

The most common uterine malformation is a uterine septum. This anomaly is associated with first-trimester losses, presumably because of implantation failure on the relatively avascular septum. Other müllerian fusion abnormalities such as bicornuate and unicornuate uterus are less common and are more likely to cause second-trimester miscarriage or preterm delivery. Similarly, anomalies caused by DES exposure (eg, T-shaped uterus) can lead to second-trimester loss.

Structural defects such as submucosal leiomyomas and endometrial polyps likely interfere with implantation. In Asherman's syndrome, implantation is impeded by the presence of intrauterine adhesions and fibrosis. This scarring can also impair adequate blood supply to the endometrium. Diagnosis of uterine defects is usually accomplished with transvaginal ultrasound. A specific type of transvaginal ultrasound, in which saline is infused into the endometrial cavity (eg, saline infusion sonography), can help delineate defects such as leiomyomas, polyps, and intrauterine adhesions. Hysterosalpingogram or magnetic resonance imaging can detect uterine malformations. Treatment is primarily surgical, and minimally invasive procedures using hysteroscopy can be performed in many cases.

Cervical insufficiency classically presents in the second trimester with painless cervical dilation. Although no definite cause is found in many patients, cervical insufficiency has been associated with congenital uterine anomalies, trauma from procedures that dilate the cervix (eg, D&C), and excisional procedures such as a loop electrosurgical excision procedure or cold-knife conization.

If other causes of recurrent pregnancy loss are excluded and the presumed etiology is cervical insufficiency, a cervical cerclage is recommended between 13 and 16 weeks' gestation. Success rates with cerclage are 85–90%. Complications include bleeding, infection, rupture of membranes, and miscarriage. Contraindications to cerclage placement include bleeding of unknown etiology, infection, labor, ruptured membranes, and known fetal anomalies.

C. Endocrine Factors

Possible endocrine causes of recurrent miscarriage include thyroid disorders, hyperprolactinemia, poorly controlled diabetes mellitus, and luteal phase defect (eg, progesterone insufficiency).

Luteal phase defect (LPD) is thought to result from a deficiency in progesterone; however, the diagnosis remains controversial. Critics of this diagnosis note intraobserver and interobserver variations in biopsy results, the presence of LPD in normal women, and inconsistent results in women diagnosed with LPD. Furthermore, controlled studies demonstrating an improvement in pregnancy outcome with progesterone treatment are lacking. For these reasons, many experts are skeptical about the importance of LPD as an etiology of recurrent pregnancy loss.

The proposed mechanism in LPD is a relative lack of progesterone that causes a delay in endometrial development, preventing normal implantation. Inadequate hormonal support of the embryo may also be involved. In the past, the diagnosis of LPD was made by luteal phase endometrial biopsies that showed a lag in endometrial development when compared with the current day of the cycle. More recently, midluteal progesterone levels of <10 ng/mL have been used to diagnose an inadequate luteal phase. LPD is treated with supplemental progesterone.

Untreated hypothyroidism increases the risk of miscarriage. Hypothyroidism is diagnosed with a sensitive thyroid-stimulating hormone test, and patients should be euthyroid before attempting pregnancy. Hyperprolactinemia may be associated with recurrent pregnancy loss by competing with the hypothalamic–pituitary–ovarian axis, resulting in insufficient folliculogenesis, oocyte maturation, and/or a LPD. Treatment of hyperprolactinemia with a dopamine agonist may improve pregnancy outcomes. Patients with poorly controlled diabetes mellitus can similarly have an increased risk of miscarriage. These risks for recurrent pregnancy loss highlight the importance of diagnosing and treating underlying medical problems.

D. Infection

Infections such as *Toxoplasma gondii, Listeria monocytogenes,* herpes simplex, and cytomegalovirus have been implicated in spontaneous abortion, although a causal relationship has not been defined. No infectious agents have been clearly linked to recurrent pregnancy loss.

E. Immunologic Factors

Antiphospholipid syndrome is an autoimmune disorder defined by the presence of characteristic clinical features and antiphospholipid antibodies (lupus anticoagulant and/or anticardiolipin antibodies). The most common and serious complications of this disorder are venous and arterial thrombosis, in which the majority of thrombotic events are venous. The risk of thrombosis is significantly increased during pregnancy. Although the exact mechanism is unclear, the increased thrombotic potential in women with antiphospholipid syndrome is associated with recurrent pregnancy loss after 10 weeks' gestation. Therapy with aspirin with or without heparin has been shown to reduce pregnancy loss.

Women with systemic lupus erythematosus (SLE) have a higher rate of miscarriage and pregnancy loss in all trimesters. The prevalence of antiphospholipid antibodies in patients with SLE is estimated at 37%, and such antibodies are the most sensitive indicator of poor pregnancy outcomes.

Previously, the sharing of human leukocyte antigens between partners was thought to be associated with recurrent pregnancy loss. More recent studies, including a large, randomized controlled trial, do not support this theory. Despite the lack of diagnostic tests to identify an alloimmune factor associated with early pregnancy loss, there is evidence that there are immunologic interactions between the mother and her allogeneic pregnancy. Investigation is currently underway looking at the efficacy of active and passive immunotherapy in preventing recurrent miscarriage.

F. Thrombophilia

Certain inherited or acquired thrombophilic factors are associated with an increased risk of venous thromboembolism. These include a group of inherited gene mutations that predispose to arterial and/or venous thrombosis: factor V Leiden mutation, prothrombin gene mutation, hyperhomocysteinemia, methylenetetrahydrofolate reductase polymorphisms, and deficiencies in protein S, protein C, and antithrombin III. Despite the association between inherited thrombophilias and venous thromboembolism, a definitive causal link cannot be made between these diseases and uteroplacental thrombosis leading to adverse pregnancy outcomes.

Testing for maternal inherited thrombophilia may be considered when there is a personal history of thromboembolism in the absence of other risk factors such as surgery or prolonged immobilization. Testing is also indicated when a first-degree relative has a history of a high-risk thrombophilia or venous thromboembolism before age 50 years in the absence of risk factors. Currently, recurrent pregnancy loss is not an indication to screen for thrombophilias, with the exception of antiphospholipid antibodies. Likewise, there are insufficient data that treatment with heparin or other anticoagulant therapies improves pregnancy outcomes in women with inherited thrombophilia and recurrent pregnancy loss.

Allison JL, Schust DJ. Recurrent first trimester pregnancy loss: Revised definitions and novel causes. *Curr Opin Endocrinol Diabetes Obes* 2009;16:446. PMID: 19779333.

American College of Obstetricians and Gynecologists. *Inherited Thrombophilias in Pregnancy.* ACOG Technical Bulletin No. 113. Washington, DC: American College of Obstetricians and Gynecologists; 2010.

Reichman D, Laufer M. Congenital uterine anomalies affecting reproduction. *Best Pract Res Clin Obstet Gynaecol* 2010;24:193. PMID: 19897423.

Stephenson MD. Evaluation and management of recurrent early pregnancy loss. *Clin Obstet Gynecol* 2007;50:132. PMID: 17304030.

Yu D, Wong YM, Cheong Y, Xia E, Li TC. Asherman syndrome—one century later. *Fertil Steril* 2008;89:759. PMID: 18406834.

SEPTIC ABORTION

ESSENTIALS OF DIAGNOSIS

- Intrauterine infection involving the endometrium and products of conception

GENERAL CONSIDERATIONS

Mortality from abortion is rare in developed countries such as the United States, where induced abortions are legal. Abortion continues to be a leading cause of maternal death in countries where abortion remains illegal. These abortion-related deaths are primarily from sepsis as a result of unsterile instruments and poor surgical technique. Hemorrhage also accounts for a proportion of these deaths.

In septic abortion, infection usually begins as endometritis involving the endometrium and any retained products of conception. These patients present with fevers, chills, abdominal pain, vaginal bleeding, and malodorous vaginal discharge. Without treatment, endometritis may spread beyond the uterus, leading to peritonitis, bacteremia, and sepsis.

The 2 most common causes of septic abortion are retained products of conception and bacteria that have been introduced into the uterus via ascending infection. Pathogens that cause septic abortion are usually those seen in normal vaginal flora as well as sexually transmitted bacteria. Before performing D&C, screening for sexually transmitted infections is essential.

In evaluating septic abortion, a complete blood count, urinalysis, endocervical cultures, blood cultures, and abdominal x-ray to rule out uterine perforation should be obtained. Ultrasound should be performed to look for retained products of conception.

Treatment

Treatment of septic abortion involves hospitalization and intravenous antibiotic therapy. Selection of antibiotic agents should provide for both anaerobic and aerobic coverage. If retained products of conception are diagnosed, a D&C is indicated.

Griebel CP, Halvorsen J, Golemon TB, Day AAL. Management of spontaneous abortion. *Am Fam Physician* 2005;72:1243. PMID: 16225027.

ECTOPIC PREGNANCY

ESSENTIALS OF DIAGNOSIS

- Pregnancy implanted outside the endometrial cavity.
- The most common site of ectopic pregnancy is a fallopian tube.

Pathogenesis

In ectopic pregnancy, a fertilized ovum implants outside the endometrial cavity (Fig. 13–7). Nearly all ectopic pregnancies (>95%) occur in the fallopian tube (**tubal pregnancy**); however, an ectopic pregnancy may also be found implanted within the endocervical canal (**cervical pregnancy**), on or in the ovary (**ovarian pregnancy**), within a scar from a prior caesarean delivery (**caesarean scar pregnancy**), or within the peritoneal cavity (**abdominal pregnancy**).

Ectopic pregnancy occurs in approximately 1.5–2.0% of all pregnancies. The incidence has increased from 4.5 per 1000 in 1970 to 19.7 per 1000 in 1992, the last time data were reported by the US Centers for Disease Control and Prevention.

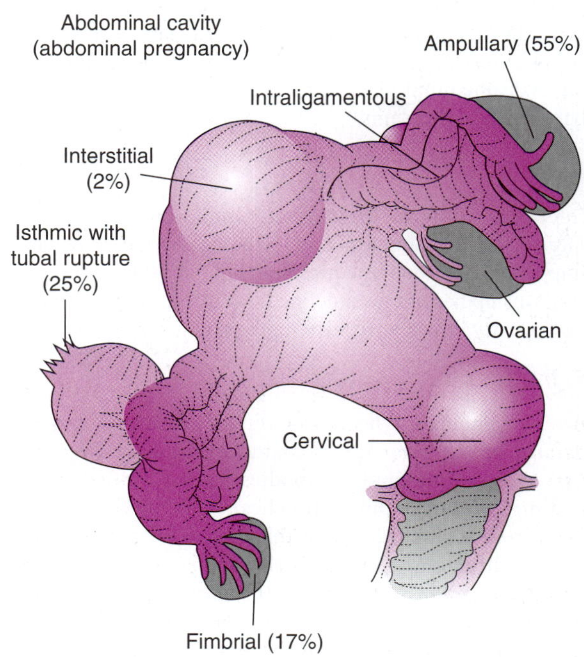

▲ Figure 13–7. Locations of ectopic pregnancies. (Reproduced, with permission, from: Benson RC. *Handbook of Obstetrics & Gynecology*. 8th ed. Los Altos, CA: Lange; 1983.)

This may be due, at least in part, to a higher incidence of pelvic inflammatory disease, use of assisted reproductive technology, and higher rates of tubal sterilization.

The morbidity and mortality associated with ectopic pregnancy has decreased dramatically, mainly because of earlier diagnosis with ultrasound and hCG levels and subsequent treatment before rupture. Nevertheless, ectopic pregnancy is the leading cause of pregnancy-related death in the first trimester and accounts for 4–10% of all pregnancy-related deaths.

Classification & Incidence

Ectopic pregnancy can be classified as follows (Fig. 13–7).

1. Tubal (>95%)—Includes ampullary (70%), isthmic (12%), fimbrial (11%), and interstitial (2%).

2. Other (<5%)—Includes cervical, ovarian, caesarean scar, and abdominal. Primary abdominal pregnancies have been reported, but most abdominal pregnancies result from tubal abortion or rupture with subsequent implantation in the bowel, omentum, or mesentery. Caesarean scar pregnancy is becoming an increasingly recognized clinical entity, with its incidence presumably paralleling the rise in caesarean section rates.

3. Heterotopic pregnancy—An ectopic pregnancy that occurs in combination with an intrauterine pregnancy. The risk of a heterotopic pregnancy is <1 in 30,000 of spontaneous pregnancies. The incidence ranges from 1 in 100 to 1 in 500 with assisted reproductive technologies.

There are many known risk factors for ectopic pregnancy, such as previous pelvic inflammatory disease, current and past smoking, and the presence of an intrauterine device (IUD). Despite our knowledge of these predisposing factors, up to one-third of ectopic pregnancies occur in women without any apparent risk factors.

A. Tubal Factors

Damage to the fallopian tube from a number of factors increases the risk of ectopic pregnancy. In pelvic inflammatory disease (PID), microorganisms ascend from the lower genital tract, infecting and causing inflammation of the uterus, fallopian tubes, and ovaries. Salpingitis can result in damage to fallopian tube cilia and blockage or closure of the tube. PID can also lead to adhesion formation among pelvic organs.

Other causes of distorted tubal anatomy leading to an increased risk of ectopic pregnancy include previous tubal surgery, endometriosis, uterine leiomyomas, and developmental abnormalities of the tube or abnormal tubal anatomy from in utero DES exposure. Up to one-third of pregnancies after tubal ligation and approximately 7% of pregnancies after sterilization reversal are ectopic. Additionally, one-third of pregnancies after an ectopic pregnancy are also ectopic implantations.

B. Assisted Reproductive Technology (ART)

The rate of ectopic pregnancy with ART ranges from 2.1% to as high as 8.6% of all clinical pregnancies. The etiology of ectopic pregnancy in patients undergoing ART and in vitro fertilization (IVF) is not completely understood, but several theories are currently under investigation.

Medications used to increase ovarian follicle production result in high levels of progesterone and estradiol that may affect tubal peristalsis and uterine relaxation. Women with tubal factor infertility undergoing IVF have even higher rates of ectopic pregnancy, and most physicians will recommend removal of diseased tubes before IVF. Ectopic pregnancy rates are associated with the number of transferred embryos as well as placement of the embryos.

C. Other Factors

Pregnancy is uncommon in women who use an IUD for contraception. However, approximately 5% of pregnancies that do occur in women using an IUD are ectopic pregnancies. Nevertheless, women with an IUD are overall less likely to develop an ectopic pregnancy than women who do not use contraception. Smoking also significantly increases the risk of ectopic pregnancy, likely because cigarette smoke affects cilia and smooth muscle function in the fallopian tube.

Timing of Rupture

Rupture of an ectopic pregnancy is usually spontaneous. Isthmic pregnancies tend to rupture earliest, at 6–8 weeks' gestation, because of the small diameter of this portion of the tube. Ampullary pregnancies rupture later, generally at 8–12 weeks. Interstitial pregnancies are the last to rupture, usually at 12–16 weeks, as the myometrium allows more room for the ectopic to grow. Interstitial rupture is quite dangerous because its proximity to uterine and ovarian vessels can result in massive hemorrhage.

Prevention

Prevention and early treatment of sexually transmitted diseases is important to prevent tubal damage and subsequent ectopic pregnancy. Smoking cessation can also help reduce the risk of ectopic pregnancy. Smoking decreases the motility of the fallopian tube cilia and makes a fertilized egg less likely to traverse the tube normally. Unfortunately, other known risk factors are more difficult to control, and up to one-third of ectopic pregnancies occur without any associated risk factors.

Clinical Findings

No specific symptoms or signs are pathognomonic for ectopic pregnancy, and many disorders can present similarly. Normal pregnancy, threatened or incomplete abortion, ovarian cyst rupture, ovarian torsion, gastroenteritis, and appendicitis can all be confused with ectopic pregnancy.

Because early diagnosis is crucial, a high index of suspicion should be maintained when any pregnant woman in the first trimester presents with bleeding and/or abdominal pain.

A. Symptoms

The following symptoms may assist in the diagnosis of ectopic pregnancy.

1. Pain—Pelvic or abdominal pain is present in almost 100% of cases. Pain can be unilateral or bilateral, localized or generalized. The presence of subdiaphragmatic or shoulder pain is suggestive of intra-abdominal bleeding. In tubal ectopic pregnancy, implantation typically occurs in the wall of the tube, in the connective tissue beneath the serosa. There may be little or no decidual reaction within the tube and minimal defense against the permeating trophoblast. The trophoblast invades blood vessels, causing local hemorrhage. A hematoma in the subserosal space enlarges as the pregnancy grows, and progressive distention of the tube eventually leads to pain and rupture.

2. Bleeding—Abnormal uterine bleeding occurs in roughly 75% of cases and represents decidual sloughing. Bleeding usually presents as intermittent, light spotting; however, bleeding may be heavier. A decidua cast is passed in 5–10% of ectopic pregnancies and may be mistaken for products of conception. Vaginal bleeding is of endometrial origin and results when the decidua breaks down from lack of progesterone support, a hallmark of an abnormal pregnancy. Occasionally the entire decidua may be shed in one or more large pieces as a decidual cast of the endometrial cavity. On pathologic examination, only decidua is seen, whereas chorionic villi are notably absent.

3. Amenorrhea—Secondary amenorrhea is variable. Approximately half of women with ectopic pregnancies have some bleeding at the time of their expected menses and may not realize they are pregnant.

4. Syncope—Dizziness, lightheadedness, and/or syncope may be part of the initial presentation and should raise suspicion for intra-abdominal bleeding from a ruptured ectopic pregnancy.

B. Signs

On examination, the following signs are important in the diagnosis of ectopic gestation.

1. Tenderness—Diffuse or localized abdominal tenderness is present in the majority of patients with ectopic pregnancies. Adnexal and/or cervical motion tenderness is also a common finding.

2. Adnexal Mass—A unilateral adnexal mass is palpated in one-third to one-half of patients. More often, unilateral adnexal fullness rather than a discrete mass is appreciated. Occasionally, a cul-de-sac mass is noted.

3. Uterine changes—The uterus may undergo the typical changes of pregnancy, including softening and a slight increase in size.

4. Hemodynamic instability—Vital signs will reflect the hemodynamic status of patients with tubal rupture and intra-abdominal bleeding.

C. Laboratory Findings

1. Hematocrit—The hematocrit is an important initial test that indirectly assesses the hemodynamic status of the patient and reflects the amount of intra-abdominal bleeding.

2. β-hCG—The qualitative serum or urine hCG assay is positive in virtually 100% of ectopic pregnancies. A positive result, however, does not help distinguish an intrauterine from ectopic pregnancy. More helpful is a quantitative hCG value that, in conjunction with transvaginal ultrasound, can often make the diagnosis. If ultrasound is nondiagnostic (eg, in an early ectopic, early normal pregnancy, or early failed pregnancy), serial hCG values can be followed. The hCG level should rise at a minimum of 53% over 48 hours in a normal pregnancy. An inappropriate rise in hCG has a sensitivity of 99% for an abnormal gestation. Of note, two-thirds of ectopic pregnancies have abnormally rising values, whereas the remaining third show a normal progression.

3. Progesterone—Serum progesterone levels may help confirm an ectopic pregnancy diagnosis. Serum progesterone values are independent of hCG levels. A serum progesterone level less than 5 ng/mL has a 100% specificity for identifying an abnormal pregnancy, but does not identify the location of the pregnancy. Progesterone levels greater than 20 ng/mL are associated with normal intrauterine pregnancies. All values in between 5 and 20 ng/mL are equivocal.

C. Diagnostic Tests

1. Ultrasound—Ultrasound is an essential part of the evaluation for an ectopic pregnancy. An initial transvaginal ultrasound can be used to visualize an intrauterine pregnancy or a definite ectopic gestation. If neither diagnosis is made, the patient is considered to have a "pregnancy of unknown location." Approximately 25–50% of women with an ectopic pregnancy initially present in this manner. An intrauterine pregnancy may not be visualized because the gestational sac has not yet developed or has collapsed. Likewise, an early ectopic pregnancy may be too small to be detected by ultrasound. When a diagnosis cannot be made, the patient is then followed with serial hCG levels and ultrasound until either an ectopic pregnancy, intrauterine gestation, or early pregnancy failure is confirmed.

In general, ultrasound should detect an intrauterine gestation when the hCG value falls within or surpasses the "discriminatory zone," defined as an hCG value between 1500 and 2000 mIU/mL. If the hCG level is higher than the discriminatory zone, and the transvaginal ultrasound is nondiagnostic, ectopic pregnancy or early abnormal pregnancy is likely. Caution should be used when interpreting hCG values because they may be falsely elevated in a pregnancy with multiple gestations.

A normal intrauterine sac appears regular and well defined on ultrasound. It has been described as an echolucent area having a "double ring" or "double decidual" sign, which represents the decidual lining and the chorion around the early gestational sac. In ectopic pregnancy, ultrasound may reveal only a thickened, decidualized endometrium. Decidual sloughing results in intracavitary fluid or blood and creates the so-called pseudogestational sac, a small and irregular structure that may be confused with an intrauterine gestational sac.

The presence of an adnexal mass with an empty uterus raises the suspicion for an ectopic pregnancy, especially if the hCG titers are above the discriminatory zone. Visualization of a gestational sac with a yolk sac or embryo within the adnexa confirms the diagnosis; however, it is more common to find a hyperechoic "tubal ring" or complex mass within the adnexae (Fig. 13–8). If rupture has occurred, anechoic or echogenic free fluid in the cul-de-sac may be visualized.

Ultrasound is increasingly being relied on to differentiate several less common types of ectopic pregnancies. Both interstitial tubal and caesarean section scar pregnancies can be difficult to distinguish from intrauterine gestations because of their proximity to the intrauterine cavity.

The most likely alternative diagnosis of an adnexal mass in early pregnancy is a corpus luteum cyst, which can also rupture and bleed, thus making its distinction from an ectopic pregnancy challenging.

2. Laparoscopy—In the past, laparoscopy was often used to diagnosis ectopic pregnancy. In current practice, however, transvaginal ultrasound has replaced laparoscopy as the preferred diagnostic tool. Compared with laparoscopy, ultrasound is equally effective in confirming the presence or absence of ectopic pregnancy. Ultrasound also has the advantages of being both cost-effective and noninvasive. In terms of surgical treatment for ectopic pregnancy, laparoscopy is the standard method, assuming the patient is hemodynamically stable.

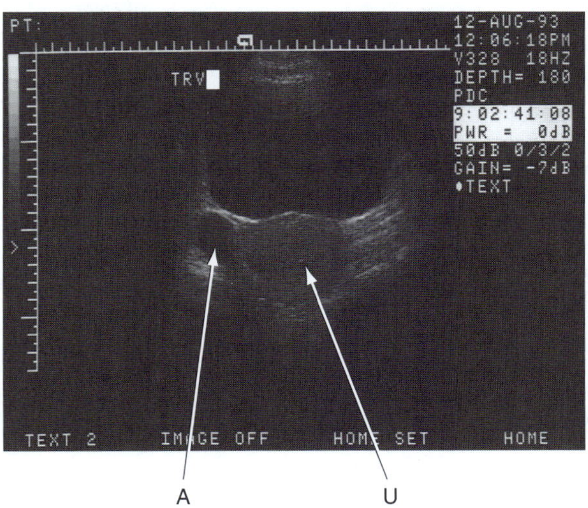

▲ **Figure 13–8.** Empty uterus (U) with an adnexal mass (A) suspicious for an ectopic pregnancy.

3. D&C—D&C can be performed to confirm or exclude intrauterine pregnancy. D&C is usually performed when an early ectopic or abnormal intrauterine gestation is suspected based on hCG levels and ultrasound. D&C should not be performed if a pregnancy is desired because it may remove a normal, early intrauterine gestation. If chorionic villi are seen on pathology examination of the D&C specimen, an intrauterine pregnancy is confirmed. On the other hand, if only decidua is obtained on D&C, ectopic pregnancy is highly likely.

4. Laparotomy—Immediate surgery is indicated in the hemodynamically unstable patient with a presumed ectopic pregnancy. Laparoscopy is generally the preferred surgical method for evaluation of suspected ectopic pregnancy in the stable patient; however, exploratory laparotomy can provide rapid access to control intra-abdominal hemorrhage. Laparotomy also may be performed if the laparoscopic approach does not allow adequate visualization or if scar tissue from previous surgeries makes the laparoscopic approach too difficult.

5. Culdocentesis—Culdocentesis, the vaginal passage of a needle into the posterior cul-de-sac, was once used to confirm the presence of hemoperitoneum. This technique has now been replaced by transvaginal ultrasound and is rarely performed in modern medicine.

6. Magnetic resonance imaging—Magnetic resonance imaging is a useful adjunct to ultrasound in cases in which an unusual ectopic location is suspected. The location of the ectopic pregnancy and recognition of cervical, caesarean scar, or interstitial pregnancy determines the options for treatment and management. In these types of ectopic pregnancy, conservative treatment with methotrexate is often preferred and usually attempted before surgery to avoid the potential catastrophic hemorrhage associated with surgical management in these cases.

Treatment

A. Expectant Management

Expectant management is appropriate and can be successful in a select population of patients. In general, these women should be asymptomatic, with lower starting hCG levels and evidence that the ectopic pregnancy is spontaneously resolving (eg, decreasing hCG levels). If the initial hCG level is less than 200 mU/mL, 88% of patients experience resolution with expectant management. These women should be educated about the potential risks of tubal rupture, intra-abdominal bleeding, and the need for emergent surgery.

B. Medical Management

Methotrexate (MTX) is a drug that inhibits the action of dihydrofolate reductase, thereby inhibiting DNA synthesis. MTX affects actively proliferating tissues such as bone marrow, intestinal mucosa, malignant cells, and trophoblastic tissue. This antimetabolite can be considered for women who are hemodynamically stable with a confirmed ectopic pregnancy or if clinical suspicion is high for an ectopic pregnancy. Although treatment of early ectopic pregnancy with MTX has significantly decreased the number of women who need surgery, there are several contraindications to its use.

Embryonic cardiac motion or the presence of a gestational sac larger than 3.5 cm are relative contraindications to MTX due to the higher rate of treatment failure in patients with either one of these findings. The level of hCG is also predictive of MTX success. With hCG values greater than 5000 mIU/mL, the failure rate is 14% with a single dose of MTX compared with 3.7% with a multiple-dose regimen. Because MTX affects rapidly dividing tissues within the body, it should not be given to women with blood dyscrasias or active gastrointestinal or respiratory disease. MTX is toxic to hepatocytes and is cleared by the kidneys; thus serum creatinine level and liver transaminases should be normal before administration. Patients must also be considered reliable for follow-up (Table 13–2).

There are three different regimens for giving MTX: single dose, two-dose, and a fixed multidose protocol. The single 50 mg/m^2 dose of MTX is most commonly used, given as an intramuscular injection. hCG levels are measured at 4 and 7 days posttreatment with an expected 15% decrease from day 4 to day 7. Weekly hCG levels are then checked until zero. If hCG levels do not drop appropriately, a second MTX dose or surgical intervention is advised. Overall, the fixed multidose regimen has been shown to be the most effective regimen, especially in treating more advanced gestations and those with embryonic cardiac activity. However, these patients may experience more side effects, and adherence to the treatment plan may be more difficult.

It is not unusual for women given MTX to have an increase in abdominal pain 2–3 days after administration, likely from the effect of the drug on trophoblast tissue and tubal distention or tubal abortion. Despite this common finding, monitoring for tubal rupture during MTX therapy is extremely important, and worsening pain should prompt immediate evaluation.

C. Surgical Treatment

Once the mainstay of therapy for ectopic pregnancy, surgical treatment is now mainly reserved for patients with contraindications to medical management and for those with evidence of tubal rupture. Despite declining rates of surgical management, surgery remains the most definitive treatment for ectopic pregnancies.

In a hemodynamically stable patient, laparoscopy is the standard approach for surgical management of a known or suspected ectopic pregnancy that is not amenable to medical treatment. In some instances, previous surgeries with subsequent intra-abdominal adhesions makes laparotomy the preferred approach. Tubal pregnancies can be treated with either linear salpingostomy or salpingectomy. The decision to perform either procedure depends on the patient's desire for future fertility as well as the appearance of the contralateral tube. If the contralateral tube appears abnormal and fertility is desired, a linear salpingostomy can be performed, and future fertility seems to be improved. In this technique, an incision is made along the fallopian tube, proximal to the ectopic pregnancy. The gestational tissue is gently removed from the tube with an effort to remove the ectopic in one piece.

Table 13–2. Contraindications to methotrexate in treatment of ectopic pregnancy.

Absolute contraindications
Breastfeeding
Overt or laboratory evidence of immunodeficiency
Alcoholism, alcoholic liver disease, or other chronic liver disease
Pre-existing blood dyscrasias, such as bone marrow hypoplasia, leukopenia, thrombocytopenia, or significant anemia
Known sensitivity to methotrexate
Active pulmonary disease
Peptic ulcer disease
Hepatic, renal, or hematologic dysfunction
Relative contraindications
Gestational sac larger than 3.5 cm
Embryonic cardiac motion

Data from American College of Obstetricians and Gynecologists. *Medical Management of Ectopic Pregnancy.* ACOG Practice Bulletin No. 3. Washington, DC: American College of Obstetricians and Gynecologists; 2008.

Patients who undergo linear salpingostomy are at risk for having persistent trophoblastic tissue and must be evaluated with weekly hCG levels until undetectable. hCG levels may remain elevated in up to 20% of patients who have undergone salpingostomy. In these cases, MTX is given, with high rates of resolution. Linear salpingostomy also increases the risk of a second ectopic pregnancy occurring in this tube, with rates up to 15%. In general, if the contralateral tube is normal, salpingectomy should be performed to reduce the risk of subsequent ectopic pregnancy.

Salpingectomy (removal of the fallopian tube) is preferred if the patient has completed child bearing, if the affected tube appears damaged, or if salpingostomy has already been performed on that tube. Salpingectomy is a simpler technique and carries minimal risk of retained trophoblastic tissue and postoperative tubal bleeding.

Interstitial pregnancies are uncommon, accounting for only 2–4% of all ectopic pregnancies. MTX and surgery can be offered to these patients. Expectant management is currently not recommended because it has not been well studied in these patients and the risks are considered greater than for tubal ectopics. Interstitial pregnancies implant into the vascular uterine cornua, and subsequent rupture can cause significant bleeding. MTX is a reasonable first-line therapy for the treatment of asymptomatic patients with an unruptured interstitial pregnancy, with reported success rates of >80%. Similar to MTX treatment of tubal pregnancies, close follow-up and patient education are necessary. Surgery is an option for patients who desire definitive management. Laparotomy was once the standard surgical approach; however, several laparoscopic techniques have now been described. Earlier diagnosis has allowed for management of interstitial pregnancies with less invasive surgical procedures.

D. Emergency Treatment

Immediate surgery is indicated when the diagnosis of a ruptured ectopic pregnancy is made. Blood products should be requested immediately because transfusion is often necessary. There is no place for conservative management in a patient with a ruptured ectopic. Even patients who initially present with normal vital signs can quickly become hemodynamically unstable. Rh_0 (D) immunoglobulin should be given to any Rh-negative mother with the diagnosis of ectopic pregnancy because sensitization may occur.

American College of Obstetricians and Gynecologists. *Medical Management of Ectopic Pregnancy.* ACOG Practice Bulletin No. 3. Washington, DC: American College of Obstetricians and Gynecologists; 2008.

Chang HJ, Suh CS. Ectopic pregnancy after assisted reproductive technology: What are the risk factors? *Curr Opin Obstet Gynecol* 2010;22:202. PMID: 20216415.

Ehrenberg-Buchner S, Sandadi S, Moawad N, Pinkerton J, Hurd W. Ectopic pregnancy: Role of laparoscopic treatment. *Clin Obstet Gynceol* 2009;52:372. PMID: 19661753.

Moawad NS, Mahajan ST, Moniz MH, Taylor SE, Hurd WW. Current diagnosis and treatment of interstitial pregnancy. *Am J Obstet Gyncol* 2010;202:15. PMID: 20096253.

Seeber BE, Barnhart KT. Suspected ectopic pregnancy. *Obstet Gynecol* 2006;107:399. PMID: 16449130.

EXPOSURE TO FETOTOXIC AGENTS

Many harmful agents are responsible for altering the biologic process of human development. Recognized teratogens include viruses (eg, rubella, cytomegalovirus, congenital lymphocytic choriomeningitis virus), environmental factors (eg, hyperthermia, irradiation), chemicals (eg, mercury, alcohol), and therapeutic drugs (eg, inhibitors of the renin–angiotensin system, thalidomide, isotretinoin, warfarin, valproic acid, carbamazepine).

Evaluation

When evaluating exposure to teratogens, it is important to consider gestational age at the time of exposure. Fetal development is most vulnerable during organogenesis (2–8 weeks postconception). Also important is the route of administration and dose of a particular medication, the length of exposure, and maternal and placental clearance. Passage into the placental circulation is necessary for a drug to cause a teratogenic effect. Table 13–3 lists some of the potential adverse effects related to the timing of exposure.

Table 13–3. Potential adverse effects of fetotoxic exposure at selected stages of development.

Timing	Potential Adverse Effect
Preimplantation (fertilization to implantation)	Miscarriage
Embryonic (2-9 weeks)	Miscarriage, structural malformations
Fetal (9–40 weeks)	Central nervous system abnormalities, growth restrictions, neurobehavioral abnormalities, reproductive effects, fetal demise

Data from Buhimschi CS, Weiner CP. Medications in pregnancy and lactation. *Obstet Gynecol* 2009;113:166. PMID: 19104374.

Table 13–4. Criteria used to define human teratogens.

Proven exposure at critical times during human development
Consistent dysmorphic findings in well-conducted epidemiologic studies
Specific defects or syndromes associated consistently with specific teratogens
Rare anatomic defects associated with environmental exposure
Proven teratogenicity in experimental animal models

Data from Buhimschi CS, Weiner CP. Medications in pregnancy and lactation. *Obstet Gynecol* 2009;113:166. PMID: 19104374.

Table 13–5. Common teratogens and their potential fetotoxic effects.

Teratogen	Potential Effects
Angiotensin-converting enzyme (ACE) inhibitors	**First-trimester exposure** Cardiovascular/CNS malformations **Second-trimester exposure** Oligohydramnios, anuria, renal failure, limb contractures, pulmonary hypoplasia
Selective serotonin reuptake inhibitors (SSRIs)	**Sertraline**: Increased risk of omphalocele, atrial, and ventricular septal defects **Paroxetine**: 1.5 to 2-fold increased risk of congenital cardiac malformations, anencephaly, omphalocele **All SSRIs**: Late exposure associated with transient neonatal respiratory distress
Anticonvulsants	**Valproic acid**: distinct craniofacial appearance, limb abnormalities, heart defects, CNS dysfunction **Carbamazepine**: facial dysmorphism, developmental delay, spina bifida, distal phalange, and fingernail hypoplasia **Phenytoin**: congenital heart defects, cleft palate
Anxiolytics (benzodiazepines)	Neonatal withdrawal, hypotonia, cyanosis, "floppy infant" syndrome
Alkylating agents	**Cyclophosphamide**: growth restriction, high-arched palate, microcephaly, flat nasal bridge, syndactyly, finger hypoplasia
Hormones/androgens	**Medroxyprogesterone acetate**: increased risk of hypospadias in male fetuses **Danazol**: androgenic effect on female fetuses
Antimetabolites (methotrexate)	Craniofacial, axial skeletal, cardiopulmonary, gastrointestinal malformations
Antithyroids	**Propylthiouracil**: fetal hypothyroidism, aplasia cutis **Methimazole**: fetal goiter, aplasia cutis, esophageal atresia, choanal atresia
Coumarin derivatives	**Warfarin**: nasal hypoplasia, microphthalmia, hypoplasia of the extremities, growth restriction, heart disease, scoliosis, deafness, CNS malformations, mental retardation
Lithium	Fetal and neonatal cardiac arrhythmias, hypoglycemia, nephrogenic diabetes insipidus, Ebstein's anomaly, polyhydramnios
Retinoids (isotretinoin)	Severe CNS, cardiovascular, endocrine malformations, mental retardation

Data from Buhimschi CS, Weiner CP. Medications in pregnancy and lactation. *Obstet Gynecol* 2009;113:166.

Table 13–6. Teratogenicity drug labeling required by the FDA.[1]

Category A: Well-controlled human studies have not disclosed any fetal risk.
Category B: Animal studies have not disclosed any fetal risk; or have suggested some risk not confirmed in controlled studies in women; or no adequate studies in women are available.
Category C: Animal studies have revealed adverse fetal effects; no adequate controlled studies in women are available.
Category D: Some fetal risk, but benefits may outweigh risk (eg, life-threatening illness, no safer effective drug).
Category X: Fetal abnormalities in animal and human studies; risk not outweighed by benefit. *Contraindicated in pregnancy*.

[1]The US Food and Drug Administration (FDA) has established 5 categories of drugs based on their potential for causing birth defects in infants born to women who use them during pregnancy. By law, the label must provide available information on teratogenicity.

Evaluation of studies examining toxic exposures is difficult because of the large number of possible fetotoxic agents and the complex interaction between these agents, the presence or absence of influences that may alter the effects of an agent, and the presence or absence of certain genotypes that might alter an individual's susceptibility. Therefore, specific criteria for recognizing teratogens in humans have been defined (Table 13–4). Table 13–5 lists common teratogens and their potential fetotoxic effects.

Counseling of parents should include review of the exposure history and discussion of the particular agent involved, as well as possible sequelae. In some cases, intervention may be possible. In other cases, if a pregnancy is found to develop abnormally, the parents may elect to abort an affected fetus. Effective counseling should provide the best information available to assist parents in what can be a very difficult decision.

The United States Food and Drug Administration standards for drug labeling with regard to teratogenicity are listed in Table 13–6.

Buhimschi CS, Weiner CP. Medications in pregnancy and lactation. *Obstet Gynecol* 2009;113:166. PMID: 19104374.

Van Gelder M, Van Rooij I, Miller R, Zielhius G, Jong-van den Berg L, Roeleveld N. Teratogenic mechanisms of medical drugs. *Hum Reprod Update* 2010;16:378. PMID: 20061329.

14 Late Pregnancy Complications

Ashley S. Roman, MD, MPH

PRETERM LABOR

ESSENTIALS OF DIAGNOSIS

- Estimated gestational age of greater than 20 0/7 weeks and less than 37 0/7 weeks
- Regular uterine contractions at frequent intervals
- Documented cervical change or appreciable cervical dilatation or effacement

Pathogenesis

Labor is the process of coordinated uterine contractions leading to progressive cervical effacement and dilatation by which the fetus and placenta are expelled. **Preterm labor** is defined as labor occurring after 20 weeks' but before 37 weeks' gestation. Although there is no strict definition in the literature regarding the amount of uterine contractions required for preterm labor, there is consensus that contractions need to be regular and at frequent intervals. Generally, more than 4 contractions per hour are needed to cause cervical change. The uterine contractions need not be painful to cause cervical change and may manifest themselves as abdominal tightening, lower back pain, or pelvic pressure. In addition, there must be demonstrated cervical effacement or dilatation to meet a diagnosis of preterm labor.

It is important to distinguish preterm labor from other similar clinical entities, such as cervical incompetence (cervical change in the absence of uterine contractions) and preterm uterine contractions (regular contractions in the absence of cervical change) because the treatment for these situations differs. Cervical incompetence may require cerclage placement, and preterm uterine contractions without cervical change is generally a self-limited phenomenon that resolves spontaneously and requires no intervention. If ruptured membranes accompany preterm labor, these cases are classified as preterm premature rupture of membranes (for discussion of diagnosis see Premature Rupture of Membranes).

Preterm birth complicates approximately 12% of all pregnancies in the United States. It is the number one cause of neonatal morbidity and mortality and causes 75% of neonatal deaths that are not due to congenital anomalies.

Thirteen percent of all infants are classified as low birth weight (<2500 g), of whom 25% are mature low-birth-weight infants and approximately 75% are truly premature. The latter group accounts for nearly two-thirds of infant deaths (approximately 25,000 annually in the United States). Approximately 30% of premature births are due to miscalculation of gestational age or to medical intervention required by the mother or fetus.

The care of premature infants is costly. Compared with term infants, those born prematurely suffer greatly increased morbidity and mortality (eg, functional disorders, abnormalities of growth and development). Thus every effort is made to prevent or inhibit preterm labor. If preterm labor cannot be inhibited or is best allowed to continue, it should be conducted with the least possible trauma to the mother and infant.

Many obstetric, medical, and anatomic disorders are associated with preterm labor. Some of the risk factors are listed in Table 14–1. Detailed discussions of these conditions are given in other chapters. The cause of preterm labor in 50% of pregnancies, however, is idiopathic. Although several prospective risk-scoring tools are in use, they have not been convincingly demonstrated to be of value.

Prevention

Unfortunately, there are few interventions known to prevent preterm labor. For women with a history of a prior spontaneous preterm birth, there is evidence indicating that progestin administered via either vaginal suppositories of progesterone or weekly intramuscular injections of 17-α hydroxyprogesterone caproate

Table 14–1. Risk factors associated with preterm labor.

Obstetric complications
In previous or current pregnancy
Severe hypertensive state of pregnancy
Anatomic disorders of the placenta (eg, abruptio placentae, placenta previa, circumvallate placenta)
Placental insufficiency
Premature rupture of membranes
Polyhydramnios or oligohydramnios
Previous premature or low-birth-weight infant
Low socioeconomic status
Maternal age <18 years or >40 years
Low prepregnancy weight
Nonwhite race
Multiple pregnancy
Short interval between pregnancies (<3 months)
Inadequate or excessive weight gain during pregnancy
Previous abortion
Previous laceration of cervix or uterus
Medical complications
Pulmonary or systemic hypertension
Renal disease
Heart disease
Infection: pyelonephritis, acute systemic infection, urinary tract infection, genital tract infection (eg, gonorrhea, herpes simplex, mycoplasmosis), fetotoxic infection (eg, cytomegalovirus infection, toxoplasmosis, listeriosis), maternal systemic infection (eg, pneumonia, influenza, malaria), maternal intra-abdominal sepsis (eg, appendicitis, cholecystitis, diverticulitis)
Heavy cigarette smoking
Alcoholism or drug addiction
Severe anemia
Malnutrition or obesity
Leaking benign cystic teratoma
Perforated gastric or duodenal ulcer
Adnexal torsion
Maternal trauma or burns
Surgical complications
Any intra-abdominal procedure
Conization of cervix
Previous incision in uterus or cervix (eg, caesarean delivery)
Genital tract anomalies
Bicornuate, subseptate, or unicornuate uterus
Congenital cervical incompetency

starting at 16–20 weeks until approximately 36–37 weeks reduces the risk of recurrent preterm birth by approximately 30%. Furthermore, vaginal progesterone may also reduce the risk of preterm birth in women found to have a short cervix on transvaginal ultrasound in the midtrimester. But, aside from these specific interventions, there is little we can do to prevent preterm labor.

Clinical Findings

A. Symptoms and Signs

1. Uterine contractions—Regular uterine contractions at frequent intervals as documented by tocometer or uterine palpation, generally more than 2 in one-half hour.

2. Dilation and effacement of cervix—This can be established by clinical examination or by transvaginal ultrasound. Documented cervical change in dilation or effacement of at least 1 cm or a cervix that is well effaced and dilated (at least 2 cm) on admission is considered diagnostic. On transvaginal ultrasound, a cervical length less than the 10th percentile (generally ≤2.5 cm) is also suggestive of cervical effacement.

3. Other signs—Many patients present with bloody mucous vaginal discharge, or "bloody show." More significant vaginal bleeding should be evaluated for abruptio placentae or placenta previa. Additionally, patients may report an increase in vaginal discharge or passage of their mucus plug.

B. Evaluation

Evaluation should include determination of the following:

1. Gestational age—Gestational age must be between 20 0/7 and 37 0/7 weeks' estimated gestational age (EGA), which should be calculated based on the patient's last menstrual period (LMP) or date of conception, if known, or the previous sonographic estimation if these dates are uncertain.

2. Fetal weight—Care must be taken to determine fetal size by ultrasonography.

3. Presenting part—The presenting part must be noted because abnormal presentation is more common in earlier stages of gestation.

4. Fetal monitoring—Continuous fetal monitoring should be performed to ascertain fetal well-being.

5. Tocodynamometry—Tocodynamometry should be performed to confirm the presence and frequency of contractions.

6. Physical examination—Physical examination should be performed to assess for cervical dilation, ruptured membranes (see section on Premature Rupture of Membranes), fundal tenderness, vaginal bleeding, and fever.

C. Laboratory Studies

1. Complete blood count with differential.
2. Urine obtained by catheter for urinalysis, culture, and sensitivity testing.
3. Ultrasound examination for fetal size, position, and placental location.
4. Amniocentesis may be useful to ascertain fetal lung maturity in instances in which EGA is uncertain, the size of the fetus is in conflict with the estimated

date of conception (too small, suggesting intrauterine growth restriction, or too large, suggesting more advanced EGA), or the fetus is more than 34 weeks' EGA. Specifically, the amniotic fluid can be tested for lecithin/sphingomyelin (L/S) ratio, the presence of phosphatidylglycerol, fluorescence polarization assay, or lamellar body count. Amniocentesis should also be performed in instances in which chorioamnionitis is suspected; the fluid should be tested for Gram's stain, bacterial culture, glucose levels, cell count, and, if available, interleukin-6 level.

5. Speculum examination should be performed. Cervical cultures should be sent for gonorrhea and chlamydia. A wet mount should be performed to look for signs of bacterial vaginosis. Group B streptococcus (GBS) cultures should be taken from the vaginal and rectal mucosa. A swab may also be used to test any fluid in the vaginal to see if it is amniotic fluid (see section on Premature Rupture of Membranes).
6. Hematologic workup in cases associated with vaginal bleeding (see Chapter 18).
7. Fetal fibronectin testing kits have been approved by the Food and Drug Administration (FDA) as a means to assess the risk of preterm birth in patients with preterm labor. A cervicovaginal swab is taken to look for the presence of fetal fibronectin. A negative test is effective at identifying women at low risk of imminent delivery (within 2 weeks). A positive test result, however, is less sensitive at predicting preterm birth. The test may be helpful in identifying patients at low risk of preterm birth who can be managed on an outpatient basis.

Differential Diagnosis

The differential diagnosis includes preterm contractions without labor (ie, without cervical change) and cervical insufficiency (ie, cervical dilation without uterine contractions). However, clinical examination and signs can help distinguish among these entities.

Complications

The primary complication of preterm labor is preterm birth and the resulting prematurity of the infant. Treatment is directed toward reducing the likelihood of preterm birth and reducing the risk of prematurity-related complications in the infant, such as respiratory distress syndrome and neurologic injury.

Treatment

Decisions regarding management are made based on EGA, estimated weight of the fetus, and existence of contraindications to suppressing preterm labor. Table 14–2 lists factors indicating that preterm labor should be allowed to continue. Once the patient is determined to not have any of these contraindications, the management of preterm labor depends on fetal gestational age. Generally, management falls into 1 of 2 categories: expectant management (observation) or intervention. For pregnancies between 24 0/7 and 34 0/7 weeks' EGA, intervention with corticosteroids has been shown to be of benefit in reducing neonatal morbidity and mortality rates. Although the efficacy of tocolysis has been much debated, it is generally accepted that a delay in delivery of 48 hours may be achieved at a minimum. Because this window can be used for corticosteroid administration, tocolysis is favored in many centers.

Table 14–2. Some cases in which preterm labor should not be suppressed.

Maternal factors
Severe hypertensive disease (eg, acute exacerbation of chronic hypertension, eclampsia, severe preeclampsia)
Pulmonary or cardiac disease (eg, pulmonary edema, adult respiratory distress syndrome, valvular disease, tachyarrhythmias)
Advanced cervical dilatation (>4 cm)
Maternal hemorrhage (eg, abruptio placentae, placenta previa, disseminated intravascular coagulation)
Fetal factors
Fetal death or lethal anomaly
Fetal distress
Intrauterine infection (chorioamnionitis)
Therapy adversely affecting the fetus (eg, fetal distress due to attempted suppression of labor)
Estimated fetal weight ≥2500 g
Erythroblastosis fetalis or fetal hydrops
Severe intrauterine growth retardation

Extremes of preterm gestational age pose special problems. Fetuses of very preterm pregnancies (20–23 weeks; EGA or estimated fetal weight [EFW] less than 550 g) are generally not considered to be viable. If these pregnancies can be continued for several more weeks, the fetuses will become viable, but have a high risk for significant morbidity if they are born in this periviable period and survive. Furthermore, intervention carries significant risks to the mother, including the risks of prolonged bed rest and side effects of tocolysis. Given these risks, expectant management is an acceptable and, in certain instances, preferable alternative to intervention. Mothers who choose intervention as opposed to expectant management should be extensively counseled by a multidisciplinary team, including the neonatologist, obstetrician, and social worker.

Conversely, once a pregnancy has continued beyond 34–37 weeks' EGA or EFW greater than 2500 g, the fetal survival rate is within 1% of the survival rate at 37 weeks. Fetal morbidity is less severe and is rarely a cause of long-term sequelae. Furthermore, corticosteroids have not been shown to be of benefit in fetuses of this age or size. Therefore, expectant management is usually the recommended course of action. Several factors should be considered when deciding between intervention and expectant management, including the certainty of the patient's dates, EFW, presence of maternal problems that could delay fetal lung maturity such as diabetes mellitus, and family history of late-onset respiratory distress syndrome (RDS).

There are other cases in which maternal or fetal factors indicate that preterm labor should be allowed to continue regardless of gestational age. Table 14–2 lists cases in detail.

The following is a protocol for management of pregnancies with preterm labor between 24 and 34 weeks' gestation.

A. Bed Rest

The role of bed rest in the management of preterm labor is controversial. Meta-analyses have failed to demonstrate prolongation of pregnancy. Bed rest is associated with an increased risk of maternal thromboembolism. At minimum, bed rest may be advised particularly during the initial evaluation of an episode of preterm labor to allow for close fetal and maternal monitoring.

B. Corticosteroids

The administration of corticosteroids to accelerate fetal lung maturity has become the standard of care in the United States for all women between 24 and 34 weeks' EGA at risk of preterm delivery within the following 7 days. It has been shown to decrease the incidence of neonatal respiratory distress, intraventricular hemorrhage, and neonatal mortality. Steroids can be given according to 1 of 2 protocols: (1) betamethasone 12 mg intramuscularly (IM) every 24 hours for a total of 2 doses; or (2) dexamethasone 6 mg IM every 12 hours for a total of 4 doses.

The optimal benefits of antenatal corticosteroids are seen 24 hours after administration, peak at 48 hours, and continue for at least 7 days. If therapy for preterm labor is successful and the pregnancy continues beyond 2 weeks, there are data suggesting that a single repeat course of steroids may be beneficial if the risk of preterm birth remains high and the patient is <33 weeks. More than 2 courses, however, may be associated with fetal growth abnormalities and delayed psychomotor development in the infant. In terms of safety of 1 or 2 courses of antenatal steroids, there does not appear to be an increased risk of infection or suppression of the fetal adrenal glands with steroid administration, and long-term follow-up of fetuses who received 1 or 2 courses of antenatal steroids shows no sequelae that can be attributed directly to steroid administration.

C. Tocolysis

If the patient continues to contract and falls into a high-risk group based on a history of preterm birth, positive fibronectin, short cervix on transvaginal sonography, or changing dilatation on cervical examination, tocolytic therapy may be initiated. When using tocolysis to treat preterm labor, it is important to keep the following goals in mind. The short-term goal is to continue the pregnancy for 48 hours after steroid administration, after which the maximum effect of the steroids can be achieved. The long-term goal is to continue the pregnancy beyond 34–36 weeks (depending on the institution), at which point fetal morbidity and mortality are dramatically reduced, and tocolysis can be discontinued.

Tocolytic therapy should be considered in the patient with cervical dilatation less than 5 cm. Successful tocolysis is generally considered fewer than 4–6 uterine contractions per hour without further cervical change.

The beta-mimetics and nifedipine are the most commonly used tocolytic agents. The decision to use a specific tocolytic should be carefully considered because of contraindications and side effects associated with each agent (Table 14–3).

1. Beta-mimetic adrenergic agents—Beta-mimetic adrenergic agents act directly on beta receptors (β_2) to relax the uterus. Their use is limited by dose-related cardiovascular side effects, including pulmonary edema, adult RDS, elevated systolic blood pressure and reduced diastolic blood pressure, and both maternal and fetal tachycardia. Other dose-related effects are decreased serum potassium level and increased blood glucose and plasma insulin levels and lactic acidosis. Maternal medical contraindications to the use of β-adrenergic agents include cardiac disease, hyperthyroidism, uncontrolled hypertension or pulmonary hypertension, asthma requiring sympathomimetic drugs or corticosteroids for relief, uncontrolled diabetes, and chronic hepatic or renal disease. Commonly observed effects during intravenous administration are palpitations, tremors, nervousness, and restlessness. The beta-mimetic in common use is terbutaline. Although it has been used in the past, ritodrine is no longer commercially available. Because of the side effects, beta-mimetic tocolysis in the United States is now limited almost exclusively to subcutaneous intermittent injections as a method of temporizing and triaging patients before definitive therapy with other agents.

Although not approved by the FDA for use as a tocolytic, terbutaline has been studied in the United States and is used widely as a tocolytic agent. For tocolysis, it is administered via subcutaneous boluses. Given the potential for maternal cardiac toxicity, terbutaline should only be used for a maximum of 48–72 hours and should only be used in an inpatient setting.

2. Magnesium sulfate—Although its exact mechanism of action is unknown, magnesium sulfate appears to inhibit calcium uptake into smooth muscle cells, reducing uterine contractility. The efficacy of magnesium is debated, but several small studies have shown an effect comparable to that of beta-mimetics, and it may be better tolerated than beta-mimetics. Magnesium sulfate may appear less likely to cause serious side effects than the beta-mimetics, but its therapeutic range is close to the range at which it will

Table 14–3. Side effects and complications of common tocolytics.

Tocolytic	Maternal Effects	Fetal/Neonatal Effects
Beta-mimetics (ritodrine, terbutaline)	Pulmonary edema Hypotension Tachycardia Nausea/vomiting Hyperglycemia Hypokalemia Cardiac arrhythmias	Tachycardia Hyperglycemia Hypoglycemia Ileus Possible increased risk for intraventricular hemorrhage
Magnesium sulfate	Flushing Nausea/vomiting Headache Generalized muscle weakness Shortness of breath Diplopia Pulmonary edema Chest pain Hypotension Tetany Respiratory depression	Lethargy Hypotonia Respiratory depression
Indomethacin	Gastrointestinal effects: Nausea/vomiting, heartburn, bleeding Coagulation disturbances Thrombocytopenia Renal failure Hepatitis Elevated blood pressure in hypertensive patients	Renal dysfunction Oligohydramnios Pulmonary hypertension Postpartum patent ductus arteriosus Premature constriction of ductus arteriosus in utero Increased risk for necrotizing enterocolitis and intraventricular hemorrhage
Nifedipine	Hypotension Tachycardia Headache Flushing Dizziness Nausea/vomiting	Tachycardia Hypotension

cause respiratory and cardiac depression. Therefore, patients receiving magnesium sulfate should be monitored closely for signs of toxicity, with frequent checks of deep tendon reflexes, pulmonary examinations, and strict calculations of the patient's fluid balance. These effects may be reversed by calcium gluconate (10 mL of a 10% solution given intravenously), and this antidote should be kept at the bedside when magnesium sulfate is used.

3. Calcium channel blockers—Calcium channel blockers such as nifedipine work as tocolytics by inhibiting calcium uptake into uterine smooth muscle cells via voltage-dependent channels, thereby reducing uterine contractility. Several studies have shown nifedipine to be equally or more efficacious than beta-mimetics in preterm labor. Other advantages are its low incidence of maternal side effects and ease of administration. Nifedipine can be given by mouth. A common regimen for tocolysis is nifedipine 20 mg by mouth, then 10–20 mg by mouth every 6 hours until contractions diminish sufficiently.

4. Prostaglandin synthase inhibitors—Prostaglandin synthase inhibitors such as indomethacin have been shown to be as effective as ritodrine for tocolysis, but their use has been limited by potentially serious fetal effects. Indomethacin works as a tocolytic by inhibiting prostaglandin synthesis, an important mediator in uterine smooth muscle contractility. The advantages of indomethacin are its ease of administration (it can be given by rectum or by mouth) and its potent tocolytic activity. However, it has been associated with oligohydramnios and premature closure of the ductus arteriosus. In preterm infants delivered before 30 weeks' EGA, some studies have demonstrated an increased risk of intracranial hemorrhage, necrotizing enterocolitis, and patent ductus arteriosus after birth. A common regimen for tocolysis is indomethacin 100 mg per rectum loading dose (or 50 mg by mouth), then 25–50 mg by mouth or rectum every 4–6 hours. Ultrasound should be performed every 48–72 hours to check for oligohydramnios. Because of the potentially serious fetal effects, many centers limit its use to infants less than 32 weeks' EGA and its duration of use to less than 48 hours.

5. Treatment with multiple tocolytics—All tocolytics have significant failure rates; therefore, if 1 tocolytic appears to be failing, that agent should be stopped and another agent should be tried. The use of multiple tocolytics at the same time appears to have an additive tocolytic effect, but also appears to increase the risk of serious side effects. For example, magnesium sulfate used in combination with nifedipine theoretically can cause serious maternal hypotension. Likewise, magnesium sulfate supplemented by 1–2 doses of subcutaneous terbutaline may be safe and effective, but sustained treatment with the 2 can increase the patient's risk of pulmonary edema. It should be remembered that the patient who is difficult to tocolyze may have an unrecognized chorioamnionitis or placental abruption, conditions that may be contraindications to use of any tocolysis at all.

6. Results of tocolytic therapy—With all tocolytics, a point may be reached where further therapy is not indicated. This may be due to adverse maternal or fetal response to the progress of labor. Thus, if cervical dilatation reaches 5 cm, the treatment should be considered a failure and abandoned. Conversely, if labor resumes after a period of quiescence, treatment should be carefully considered because the recrudescence of contractions may be a sign of intrauterine infection. In some cases, therapy may be reinstituted using the same or a different drug.

D. Antibiotics

Antibiotic therapy as a treatment of preterm labor and a means of prolonging pregnancy has been studied and has shown no benefit in delaying preterm birth in this population of patients. Patients with preterm labor should be started on antibiotics for prevention of neonatal GBS infection if the patient's GBS status is positive or unknown. Penicillin or ampicillin is used as first-line agents; cefazolin, clindamycin, erythromycin, or vancomycin can be used if the patient is allergic to penicillin. If the patient is successfully tocolyzed and there is no sign of imminent delivery or if the patient's most recent rectovaginal GBS culture (within 5 weeks) is negative, GBS prophylaxis can be discontinued.

E. Magnesium Sulfate for Fetal/Neonatal Neuroprotection

Several recent large trials have shown a reduced risk of cerebral palsy in fetuses exposed to magnesium sulfate in utero. The largest trial from the United States demonstrated a significant reduction in moderate to severe cerebral palsy in children at or beyond 2 years of age who received magnesium sulfate immediately before delivery. The optimal candidates for magnesium for this indication are not well defined, but it is reasonable to offer magnesium sulfate to any woman between 24 0/7 and 32 0/7 weeks of gestation immediately before delivery to reduce the risk of adverse neurologic outcomes (Table 14–4).

F. Conduct of Labor and Delivery

Premature infants younger than 34 weeks should be delivered in a hospital equipped for neonatal intensive care whenever possible, because inter-hospital transfer after birth is more hazardous. Although the route of delivery for very-low-birth-weight infants has been hotly debated, there is no conclusive evidence of a benefit to routine caesarean delivery. Indications for caesarean are the usual obstetrical indications, including nonreassuring fetal status, malpresentation, and history of prior caesarean.

Table 14–4. Protocol for use of magnesium sulfate for fetal neuroprotection.

Criteria for admission to protocol
Preterm birth anticipated within 2-24 hours. Gestational age of 24-31 6/7 weeks has been confirmed. Any specific contraindications to magnesium sulfate therapy have been ruled out.
Protocol
Begin intravenous infusion of magnesium sulfate loading dose, 6 g over 20-30 minutes, followed by a maintenance infusion of 2 g per hour. If delivery has not occurred after 12 hours and is no longer considered imminent, the infusion may be discontinued. If more than 6 hours has passed since discontinuation of magnesium sulfate and delivery is again believed to be imminent, another loading dose may be given followed by maintenance infusion.

Data from Rouse DJ, Hirtz DG, Thom E, et al. A randomized controlled trial of magnesium sulfate for the prevention of cerebral palsy. *N Engl J Med* 2008:359:895–905.

Table 14–5. Approximate neonatal survival of preterm infants.[1]

Gestation Age (weeks)	Birth Weight (g)	Survivors (%)	Intact[2] Survivors (%)
24–25	500–750	60	35
25–27	751–1000	75	60
28–29	1000–1250	90	80
30–31	1251–1500	96	90
32–33	1500–1750	99	98
>34	1751–2000	100	99

[1]Delivered in a tertiary care center.
[2]Intact defined as child without major disability such as blindness, deafness, or cerebral palsy.

If caesarean delivery is indicated, the decision to operate is based on maturity of the fetus and prognosis for survival. In borderline cases (23–24 weeks' gestation and 500–600 g EFW), the wishes of the parents with regard to intervention assume an important place. When performing a caesarean delivery, it is important to ascertain that the uterine incision is adequate for extraction of the fetus without delay or unnecessary trauma. This may require a vertical incision when the lower uterine segment is incompletely developed. Trauma to the newborn may be minimized by en caul delivery.

When birth follows the unsuccessful use of parenteral tocolytic agents, keep in mind the potential residual adverse effects of these drugs. β-Adrenergic agents may cause neonatal hypotension, hypoglycemia, hypocalcemia, and ileus. Magnesium sulfate may be responsible for respiratory and cardiac depression.

G. Cord pH & Blood Gases

Apgar scores are often low in low-birth-weight babies. This finding does not indicate asphyxia or compromised status but merely reflects the immaturity of the physiologic systems. Therefore, it is crucial to obtain cord pH and blood gas measurements for premature (and other high-risk) infants in order to document the status at birth. Cord pH and blood gas measurements may also be helpful in reconstructing intrapartum events, clarifying resuscitative measures, and determining the need for more intensive neonatal care.

Prognosis

Excellent neonatal care in the delivery room and nursery will do much to ensure a good prognosis for the preterm infant (see Chapter 22). Lower-birth-weight babies have a lesser chance of survival and a greater chance of permanent sequelae in direct relationship to size. Making generalizations regarding survival rates and sequelae is difficult because of the many causes of preterm delivery, the different levels of perinatal care, and the institutional differences in reported series. However, general figures for survival and morbidity have been reported and are helpful in counseling patients (Table 14–5).

Rouse DJ, Hirtz DG, Thom E, et al. A randomized controlled trial of magnesium sulfate for the prevention of cerebral palsy. *N Engl J Med* 2008:359:895–905. PMID: 18753646.

American College of Obstetricians and Gynecologists. *Assessment of Risk Factors for Preterm Birth. Clinical Management Guidelines for Obstetrician-Gynecologists.* ACOG Practice Bulletin No. 31. Washington, DC: American College of Obstetricians and Gynecologists; 2001.

American College of Obstetricians and Gynecologists. *Use of Progesterone to Reduce Preterm Birth.* ACOG Committee Opinion No. 419. Washington, DC: American College of Obstetricians and Gynecologists; 2008.

American College of Obstetricians and Gynecologists. *Magnesium Sulfate Before Anticipated Preterm Birth for Neuroprotection.* ACOG Committee Opinion No. 455. Washington, DC: American College of Obstetricians and Gynecologists; 2010.

American College of Obstetricians and Gynecologists. *Antenatal Corticosteroid Therapy for Fetal Maturation.* ACOG Committee Opinion No. 475. Washington, DC: American College of Obstetricians and Gynecologists; 2011.

Guinn DA, Atkinson MW, Sullivan L, et al. Single vs weekly courses of antenatal corticosteroids for women at risk of preterm delivery: A randomized controlled trial. *JAMA* 2001;286:1581–1587. PMID: 11585480.

Kenyon SL, Taylor DJ, Tarnow-Mordi W. ORACLE Collaborative Group. Broad-spectrum antibiotics for spontaneous preterm labour: The ORACLE II randomised trial. *Lancet* 2001;357:989–994. PMID: 11293641.

PREMATURE RUPTURE OF MEMBRANES

ESSENTIALS OF DIAGNOSIS

- History of a gush of fluid from the vagina or watery vaginal discharge
- Demonstration of amniotic fluid in the vagina on physical exam
- Absence of active labor

Pathogenesis

Rupture of the membranes may occur at any time during pregnancy. Premature rupture of the membranes (PROM) is defined as rupture of membranes before the onset of active labor. It becomes a particular problem if the fetus is preterm (preterm premature rupture of membranes [PPROM]) or, in the case of a term fetus, if the period of time between rupture of the membranes and the onset of labor is prolonged. If 24 hours elapse between rupture of the membranes and the onset of labor, the problem is one of prolonged PROM.

The exact cause of rupture is not known, although many conditions are associated with PROM (Table 14–6). PROM occurs in approximately 10.7% of all pregnancies. In approximately 94% of cases, this occurs at term or ≥37 weeks (approximately 20% of these are cases of prolonged rupture). Preterm fetuses (<37 weeks) account for approximately 5% of the total number of cases of PROM.

The pathophysiology of PROM is poorly understood. Risk factors include decidual hemorrhage, a history of spontaneous preterm birth in a prior pregnancy, bacterial colonization of the membranes, and invasive procedures such as amniocentesis. PROM is an important cause of preterm labor, prolapse of the cord, placental abruption, and intrauterine infection. Chorioamnionitis is an important sequela of PROM and may precede endomyometritis or sepsis of the newborn.

In extremely prolonged rupture of the membranes, the fetus may have an appearance similar to that of Potter's syndrome (ie, flattened facial features, wrinkling of the skin). If rupture of membranes with subsequent oligohydramnios occurs early in pregnancy at less than 26 weeks' EGA, it can cause pulmonary hypoplasia and limb positioning defects in the newborn.

Prevention

As with preterm labor, there are few interventions known to prevent PPROM. For women with a history of a prior spontaneous preterm birth, there is evidence indicating that progestin administered via either vaginal suppositories of progesterone or weekly intramuscular injections of 17-α hydroxyprogesterone caproate from 16 weeks until approximately 36–37 weeks reduces the risk of recurrent preterm birth by approximately 30%. Furthermore, vaginal progesterone may also reduce the risk of preterm birth in women found to have a short cervix on transvaginal ultrasound in the midtrimester. But, aside from these specific interventions, there is little we can do to prevent PPROM.

Clinical Findings

A. Symptoms

The diagnostic evaluation must be efficient and impeccably conducted to minimize the number of vaginal examinations and the risk of chorioamnionitis. Symptoms are the key to diagnosis; the patient usually reports a sudden gush of fluid or continued leakage. Additional symptoms that may be useful include the color and consistency of the fluid and the presence of flecks of vernix or meconium, reduced size of the uterus, and increased prominence of the fetus to palpation.

B. Sterile Speculum Examination

A most important step in accurate diagnosis is examination with a sterile speculum. This examination is the key to differentiating PROM from hydrorrhea gravidarum, vaginitis, increased vaginal secretions, and urinary incontinence. The examiner should look for the 3 hallmark confirmatory findings associated with PROM:

1. Pooling—the collection of amniotic fluid in the posterior fornix.
2. Nitrazine test—a sterile cotton-tipped swab should be used to collect fluid from the posterior fornix and apply

Table 14–6. Diseases and disorders associated with premature rupture of the membranes.

Maternal infection (eg, urinary tract infection, lower genital tract infection, sexually transmitted diseases)
Intrauterine infection
Cervical insufficiency
Multiple previous pregnancies
Hydramnios
Nutritional deficit
Decreased tensile strength of membranes
History of premature rupture of membranes or preterm birth in a prior pregnancy

it to Nitrazine (phenaphthazine) paper. In the presence of amniotic fluid, the Nitrazine paper turns blue, demonstrating an alkaline pH (7.0–7.25).

3. Ferning—Fluid from the posterior fornix is placed on a slide and allowed to air-dry. Amniotic fluid will form a fernlike pattern of crystallization.

Together, these 3 findings confirm ruptured membranes, although several factors may produce false-positive results. Alkaline pH on Nitrazine test can also be caused by vaginal infections or the presence of blood or semen in the sample. Cervical mucus can cause ferning, but usually patchy and less extensive than with PROM. During the speculum examination, the patient's cervix should be visually inspected to determine the degree of dilatation and effacement and the presence of cord prolapse. If vaginal pool is significant, the pool can be collected and sent for fetal lung maturity determination if the gestational age is greater than 32 weeks. Cervical secretions should also be sent for culture, and a wet mount should be performed.

If no free fluid is found, a dry pad should be placed under the patient's perineum and observed for leakage. Other confirmatory tests for PROM include observed loss of fluid from the cervical os when the patient coughs or performs a Valsalva maneuver during speculum examination and oligohydramnios on ultrasound examination. If the examiner still cannot confirm rupture of membranes and the patient's history is highly suspicious for PROM, it may be necessary to perform amniocentesis and inject a dilute solution of indigo carmine dye. This can be done after removal of amniotic fluid for pulmonary maturity testing, analysis for evidence of subacute intra-amniotic infection, and possible culture and sensitivity testing. After 15–30 minutes, examination of the patient's perineal pad will reveal blue dye if the membranes are ruptured.

C. Physical Examination

Once PROM is confirmed, a careful physical examination is necessary to search for other signs of infection. Given the risk of infection, there is no indication for digital cervical examination if the patient is in early labor. The sterile speculum examination is sufficient to distinguish between early and advanced labor.

D. Laboratory Studies

Initial laboratory studies should include a complete blood count with differential. In preterm pregnancies, evaluation should also include urine collected by catheterization for urinalysis, culture, and sensitivity testing and ultrasound examination for fetal size and amniotic fluid index. For patients between 32 and 34 weeks, a specimen of amniotic fluid collected from the vaginal pool or via amniocentesis can be sent for fetal lung maturity studies. Furthermore, many centers perform amniocentesis in all women with PPROM before 34 weeks to test for evidence of intra-amniotic infection.

E. Chorioamnionitis

In all cases of chorioamnionitis, it is safer for the fetus to be delivered than to be retained in utero. The most common organisms causing chorioamnionitis are those that ascend from the vagina (eg, *Escherichia coli*, *Bacteroides*, GBS, group D streptococcus, and other anaerobes). The most reliable signs of infection include the following: (1) Fever—the temperature should be checked every 4 hours. (2) Maternal leukocytosis—a daily leukocyte count and differential can be obtained. An increase in the white blood cell count or neutrophil count may indicate the presence of intra-amniotic infection. (3) Uterine tenderness—check every 4 hours. (4) Tachycardia—either maternal pulse >100 beats/min or fetal heart rate >160 beats/min—is suspicious. (5) Foul-smelling amniotic fluid.

A number of confounding factors may complicate the diagnosis of chorioamnionitis. For example, corticosteroid administration may cause mild leukocytosis (increase of 20–25%), and labor is associated with leukocytosis. If the diagnosis of chorioamnionitis is equivocal, amniocentesis can be performed to evaluate for evidence of infection, as described earlier in this chapter.

Differential Diagnosis

The differential diagnosis includes the increased physiologic vaginal discharge associated with pregnancy, vaginal infections such as bacterial vaginosis, and passage of a woman's mucus plug. Physical examination with testing of any vaginal discharge or pool can distinguish among these entities.

Complications

Complications associated with PROM are primarily associated with duration of membrane rupture and the development of chorioamnionitis. Treatment outlined below is directed toward expediting delivery and preventing chorioamnionitis and fetal/neonatal infection. Complications with PPROM are primarily related to prematurity and the risk of fetal/neonatal infection. As in patients with preterm labor, treatment is directed toward reducing the likelihood of preterm birth and reducing the risk of prematurity-related complications in the infant such as RDS and neurologic injury.

Treatment

The management of PROM depends on several factors, including gestational age and the presence or absence of chorioamnionitis.

A. Chorioamnionitis

If chorioamnionitis is present in the patient with PROM, the patient should be actively delivered *regardless of gestational age*. Broad-spectrum antibiotics should be started to treat the chorioamnionitis. If the patient is not in labor, labor should be induced to expedite delivery. Caesarean delivery should be reserved for the usual obstetric indications (eg, fetal malpresentation, nonreassuring fetal status).

B. Term Pregnancy Without Chorioamnionitis

The term pregnancy (EGA ≥37 weeks) with PROM in the absence of infection can be managed expectantly or actively. One large study found that starting induction of labor at presentation as opposed to expectant management reduced the time interval between PROM and delivery and the frequency of chorioamnionitis and postpartum febrile morbidity and neonatal antibiotic treatment. Therefore, active management with induction of labor at time of presentation for the woman with PROM at term is the preferred management strategy.

C. Preterm Pregnancy Without Chorioamnionitis

The principles of managing the preterm PROM patient are similar to those for managing the preterm labor patient. The key difference is the much increased risk of developing chorioamnionitis associated with preterm PROM. Pregnancies beyond 34 weeks' EGA can be managed as a term pregnancy with induction of labor or delivery via caesarean delivery (if indicated) because there is no evidence that antibiotics, corticosteroids, or tocolytics improve outcome in these patients.

Rupture of membranes before viability (ie, before 22–24 weeks of gestation) can be managed in one of several ways. One option is termination of pregnancy, given the high risk of adverse pregnancy outcome and prematurity. However, in the patient without evidence of chorioamnionitis, expectant management may be considered. Several case series have documented substantial survival rates (15–50%) with PPROM at 18–22 weeks. Although many patients may be unwilling to accept the risk of chorioamnionitis (30%) and even sepsis, they should be informed of the option of expectant management with antibiotic therapy.

For pregnancies with PROM between 24 and 34 weeks' EGA, several interventions have been shown to prolong pregnancy and improve outcome. After chorioamnionitis has been ruled out and a specimen of amniotic fluid from vaginal pool collection or amniocentesis sent for determination of fetal lung maturity, management should consist of the following interventions.

1. Antibiotics—Antibiotics have emerged as an important treatment for preterm PROM. In contrast to preterm labor, where antibiotics have shown no benefit in prolonging pregnancy, antibiotics appear to be effective in prolonging the latency period from rupture of membranes to delivery in patients with preterm PROM. They have also been shown to decrease the infection rate in these patients. A number of well-designed studies have shown improved neonatal outcomes with antibiotics alone and with antibiotics combined with corticosteroid therapy. Table 14–7 provides 1 recommended protocol for antibiotic use in preterm PROM.

2. Corticosteroids—The National Institutes of Health (NIH) consensus development panel recommends the use of steroids in PROM patients before 32 weeks' EGA in the absence of intra-amniotic infection. In this patient population, corticosteroids have been shown to decrease the rate of RDS, necrotizing enterocolitis, and intraventricular hemorrhage. The benefit of steroids at 32–33 weeks in women with PPROM is unclear. However, steroids may also be considered in patients with PPROM between 32 and 33 6/7 weeks, especially if pulmonary immaturity has been documented via testing of amniotic fluid.

3. Tocolytics—No study has shown that tocolytics alone improve fetal outcome in women with PPROM. In general, the use of tocolytics in the PPROM patient should be either avoided entirely or limited to 48 hours' duration to permit administration of corticosteroids and antibiotics.

4. Magnesium sulfate for fetal neuroprotection—As with the management of preterm labor, consideration should be given to administering magnesium sulfate for fetal neuroprotection if delivery is felt to be imminent in the PPROM patient between 24 and 32 weeks of gestation. See Table 14–4 for a suggested protocol.

Table 14–7. Antibiotic therapy for preterm premature rupture of membranes.

Once preterm PROM is confirmed, start:
Ampicillin 2 g IV every 6 hours plus
Erythromycin 250 mg IV every 6 hours
After 48 hours, if the patient is still undelivered, this regimen should be changed to:
Amoxicillin 250 mg by mouth every 8 hours plus
Erythromycin 333 mg by mouth every 8 hours
These antibiotics should be continued for 7 days if the patient remains undelivered. Women with GBS-positive cultures should receive prophylaxis intrapartum.

GBS, group B streptococcus; IV, intravenous; PROM, premature rupture of membranes.
Data from Mercer BM, Miodovnik M, Thurnau GR, et al. Antibiotic therapy for reduction of infant morbidity after preterm premature rupture of the membranes. *JAMA* 1997;278:989–995.

If after starting these interventions the fetal lung profile from testing of amniotic fluid returns as mature, the fetus should be delivered. Again, if at any time the patient shows signs of chorioamnionitis, the fetus should be delivered.

D. Role of Outpatient Management

In rare selected cases, patients who remain undelivered may be candidates for outpatient management. If leakage of fluid stops, the amniotic fluid volume normalizes, and the patient remains afebrile without evidence of increasing uterine irritability, she can be discharged home. These patients should be monitored very closely on an outpatient basis. They must be reliable and compliant with follow-up appointments. They also must take their temperature 4 times per day and be counseled on the warning signs of chorioamnionitis. These patients should also be monitored with frequent biophysical profiles; some sources recommend daily testing.

Seaward PG, Hannah ME, Myhr TL, et al. International multicentre term prelabor rupture of membranes study: evaluation of predictors of clinical chorioamnionitis and postpartum fever in patients with prelabor rupture of membranes at term. *Am J Obstet Gynecol* 1997;177:1024–1029. PMID: 9396886.

Mercer BM, Miodovnik M, Thurnau GR, et al. Antibiotic therapy for reduction of infant morbidity after preterm premature rupture of the membranes: A randomized controlled trial. *JAMA* 1997;278:989–995. PMID: 9307346.

Rouse DJ, Hirtz DG, Thom E, et al. A randomized controlled trial of magnesium sulfate for the prevention of cerebral palsy. *N Engl J Med* 2008:359:895–905. PMID: 18753646.

American College of Obstetricians and Gynecologists. *Premature Rupture of Membranes.* ACOG Practice Bulletin No. 80. Washington, DC: American College of Obstetricians and Gynecologists; 2007.

How HY, Cook CR, Cook VD, Miles DE, Spinnato JA. Preterm premature rupture of membranes: Aggressive tocolysis versus expectant management. *J Matern Fetal Med* 1998;7:8–12. PMID: 9502662.

Kenyon SL, Taylor DJ, Tarnow-Mordi W. ORACLE Collaborative Group. Broad-spectrum antibiotics for preterm, prelabour rupture of fetal membranes: The ORACLE I randomised trial. *Lancet* 2001;357:979–994. PMID: 11293641.

PROLONGED OR POSTTERM PREGNANCY

ESSENTIALS OF DIAGNOSIS

- Confirmation of gestational age greater than 42 completed weeks

Pathogenesis

The prolonged or postterm pregnancy is defined as pregnancy that has reached 42 weeks of gestation from the first day of the LMP or 40 weeks' gestation from the time of conception. Most fetuses will show effects of impaired nutritional supply (weight loss, reduced subcutaneous tissue, scaling, parchment-like skin). This condition is referred to as dysmaturity. The most common cause of prolonged pregnancy is incorrect dating due to variable length of the menstrual cycle. This has been reduced in recent years with widespread use of first-trimester ultrasound for dating. The cause of most cases of true prolonged pregnancy remains unknown. Experiments of nature, such as anencephalic fetuses and those with placental sulfatase deficiency, suggest that changes in placental steroid metabolism due to fetal hormonal signaling play a central role in the timing of delivery. At least 3% of infants are born after 42 completed weeks' gestation (in some series, as many as 12%). Because of the potential risks of dysmaturity, these infants deserve particular attention.

The maternal risks usually relate to large fetal size (ie, dysfunctional labor, arrested progress of labor, fetopelvic disproportion). Large fetal size may result in birth injury (eg, shoulder dystocia). Placental insufficiency is thought to be associated with aging of the placenta and is the basis for another group of fetal problems. Oligohydramnios, which is more common in postterm gestation, may lead to cord compromise.

Complications resulting from prolonged pregnancy result in a sharp rise in perinatal mortality and morbidity rates (2–3 times those of infants born at 37–42 weeks). Complications in the survivors increase the chance of neurologic sequelae.

Prevention

The most common cause of an apparent postterm pregnancy is an error in pregnancy dating. First-trimester ultrasound is an accurate way to confirm a patient's estimated date of delivery and has been shown to reduce the incidence of pregnancies diagnosed as postterm.

Clinical findings

The diagnosis of prolonged pregnancy is made by confirmation of the gestational age by referring to records of early pregnancy tests and ultrasound examinations, the exact time of conception (if known), and clinical parameters (eg, LMP, quickening, detection of fetal heart tones).

Differential Diagnosis

The most likely differential diagnosis of the suspected postterm pregnancy is incorrect pregnancy dating, which may be determined via a careful review of the patient's dating criteria. However, it may be difficult to ascertain the correct due date in a patient who presents for prenatal care late in pregnancy or has not had any early ultrasounds in pregnancy.

Treatment

The principal risk of labor induction has been thought to be an increased rate of caesarean birth. It has now been conclusively demonstrated, however, that induction of labor at 41 weeks does not increase the caesarean rate compared with expectant management with antepartum testing. Therefore, many authorities offer induction of labor at 41 completed weeks, reserving expectant management for those patients who refuse induction.

To adequately assess the risk of fetal compromise, the following is a useful protocol for pregnancies beyond 41 weeks' gestation:

1. Some form of fetal surveillance is advised, either with nonstress testing and measurement of amniotic fluid volume twice per week or with biophysical profiles twice per week.
2. Perform ultrasonic monitoring at least twice weekly to assess amniotic fluid volume (biophysical profiles may be obtained at the same time).
3. Have the mother count fetal movements each day.

The following additional precautions should be taken:

1. Decreased fetal movement warrants an immediate biophysical profile evaluation.
2. Abnormalities in the nonstress test mandate induction or a backup test such as the full biophysical profile.
3. An abnormal contraction stress test, decreased amniotic fluid volume, abnormal biophysical profile, or other signs of fetal distress require delivery.
4. A large or compromised fetus may require caesarean delivery (see discussion of macrosomia in Chapter 16).
5. In the absence of fetopelvic disproportion or fetal distress, labor can be induced. Fetal monitoring should be continuous.

American College of Obstetricians and Gynecologists. *Management of postterm pregnancy.* ACOG Practice Bulletin No. 55. Washington, DC: American College of Obstetricians and Gynecologists; 2004.

American College of Obstetricians and Gynecologists. *Assessment of Risk Factors for Preterm Birth. Clinical Management Guidelines for Obstetrician-Gynecologists.* ACOG Practice Bulletin No. 31. Washington, DC: American College of Obstetricians and Gynecologists; 2001.

American College of Obstetricians and Gynecologists. *Use of Progesterone to Reduce Preterm Birth.* ACOG Committee Opinion No. 419. Washington, DC: American College of Obstetricians and Gynecologists; 2008.

American College of Obstetricians and Gynecologists. *Magnesium Sulfate Before Anticipated Preterm Birth for Neuroprotection.* ACOG Committee Opinion No. 455. Washington, DC: American College of Obstetricians and Gynecologists; 2010.

American College of Obstetricians and Gynecologists. *Antenatal Corticosteroid Therapy for Fetal Maturation.* ACOG Committee Opinion No. 475. Washington, DC: American College of Obstetricians and Gynecologists; 2011.

RH ALLOIMMUNIZATION & OTHER BLOOD GROUP INCOMPATIBILITIES

ESSENTIALS OF DIAGNOSIS

- Maternal Rh-negativity and presence of antibody on indirect Coombs' test
- Rh or other antibody titer posing fetal risk
- May have a previous infant with hemolytic disease of the newborn
- Postnatal fetal cord blood findings of Rh-positivity and anemia (hemoglobin <10 g)

Pathogenesis

A fetus receives half of its genetic components from its mother and half from its father; therefore, the fetus may have red blood cell (RBC) antigens different from those of its mother. Some blood groups may act as antigens in individuals not possessing those blood groups. The antigens reside on red blood cells. If enough fetal cells cross into the maternal blood, a maternal antibody response may be provoked. If these maternal antibodies cross the placenta, they then can enter the fetal circulation and destroy the fetal erythrocytes, causing hemolytic anemia. This leads to fetal responses to meet the challenge of enhanced blood cell breakdown. These changes in the fetus and newborn are called erythroblastosis fetalis or fetal hydrops. Several blood groups are capable of producing fetal risk, but those in the Rh group have caused the overwhelming majority of cases of erythroblastosis fetalis, so the Rh group is used as the example.

The Rh blood group is the most complex human blood group. Rh antigens are lipoproteins that are confined to the red cell membrane. The Rh antigens are D, C, c, E, e, and G. The major antigen in this group, Rh (D), or Rh factor, is of particular concern. A woman who is lacking Rh(D) (otherwise known as Rh-negative) may carry an Rh-positive fetus if the fetus inherited the D antigen from the father. If fetal red blood cells pass into the mother's circulation in sufficient numbers, maternal IgG antibodies to the D antigen may develop and cross the placenta, causing hemolysis of fetal blood cells (Fig. 14–1). Hemolytic disease of the newborn may occur, and severe disease may cause fetal death.

In standard testing when the father is Rh-positive, 2 possibilities exist: he is either homozygous or heterozygous.

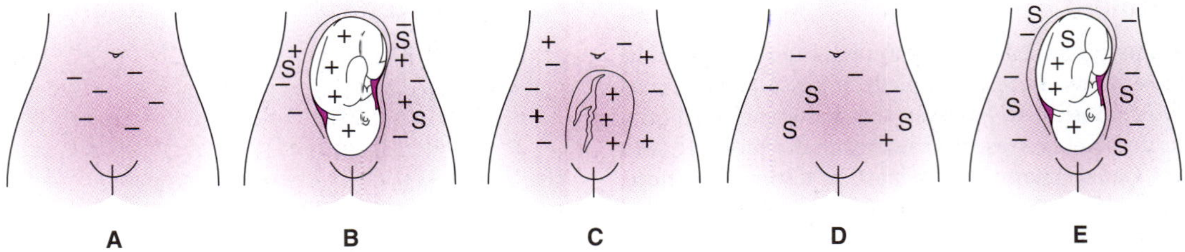

▲ **Figure 14–1.** **A:** Rh-negative woman before pregnancy. **B:** Pregnancy occurs. The fetus is Rh-positive. **C:** Separation of the placenta. **D:** After delivery, Rh alloimmunization occurs in the mother, and she develops antibodies (S) to the Rh-positive antigen. **E:** The next pregnancy with an Rh-positive fetus. Maternal antibodies cross the placenta, enter the fetal bloodstream, and attach to Rh-positive red cells, causing hemolysis.

Forty-five percent of Rh-positive persons are homozygous for D and 55% are heterozygous. If the father is homozygous, all of his children will be Rh-positive; if he is heterozygous, his children will have a 50% chance of being Rh-positive. By way of contrast, the Rh-negative individual is always homozygous.

Basque populations have the highest incidence of Rh negativity (30–35%). White populations in general have a higher incidence than other ethnic groups (15–16%). African Americans have a rate of 8%, African blacks 4%, Indoeurasians 2%, and North American Indians 1%.

In mothers who do not receive prophylaxis with anti-D immunoglobulin, the overall risk of alloimmunization for an Rh-positive ABO-compatible infant with an Rh-negative mother is approximately 16% after 2 deliveries of Rh-positive infants. Of these, 1.5–2% of reactions will occur antepartum and 7% within 6 months of delivery; the remainder (7%) manifest early in the second pregnancy, most likely as the result of an amnestic response. ABO incompatibility between an Rh-positive fetus and an Rh-negative mother provides some protection against Rh alloimmunization; in these cases the overall incidence is 1.5–2%. In mothers who receive prophylaxis with anti-D immunoglobulin administered both antepartum and postpartum, the risk of alloimmunization is reduced to 0.1%.

A. Maternal Rh Alloimmunization

Rh alloimmunization generally occurs by 1 of 2 mechanisms: (1) after incompatible blood transfusion or (2) after fetomaternal hemorrhage between a mother and an incompatible fetus. Fetomaternal hemorrhage may occur during pregnancy or at delivery. With no apparent predisposing factors, fetal red cells have been detected in maternal blood in 6.7% of women during the first trimester, 15.9% during the second trimester, and 28.9% during the third trimester. Predispositions to fetomaternal hemorrhage include spontaneous or induced abortion, amniocentesis, chorionic villus sampling, abdominal trauma (eg, due to motor vehicle accidents or external version), placenta previa, abruptio placentae, fetal death, multiple pregnancy, manual removal of the placenta, and caesarean section.

Although the exact number of Rh-positive cells necessary to cause alloimmunization of the Rh-negative pregnant woman is unknown, as little as 0.1 mL of Rh-positive cells can cause sensitization. Even with delivery, this amount occurs in less than half of cases.

Fortunately, there are other mitigating factors to Rh alloimmunization. A very important factor is that approximately 30% of Rh-negative persons never become sensitized (nonresponders) when given Rh-positive blood. ABO incompatibility also confers a protective effect (see Incidence).

The initial maternal immune response to Rh sensitization is low levels of immunoglobulin (Ig) M. Within 6 weeks to 6 months, IgG antibodies become detectable. In contrast to IgM, IgG is capable of crossing the placenta and destroying fetal Rh-positive cells.

B. Other Blood Group Alloimmunization

Of the other blood groups that may evoke an immunoglobulin capable of crossing the placenta (often called atypical or irregular immunizing antibodies), those that may cause severe fetal hemolysis (listed in descending order of occurrence) are Kell, Duffy, Kidd, MNSs, and Diego. P, Lutheran, and Xg groups may also cause fetal hemolysis, but it usually is less severe.

Prevention

Prevention of Rh (D) alloimmunization is possible by identifying women known to be negative for the Rh (D) antigen and administering anti-D immunoglobulin to prevent sensitization.

A. Prepregnancy or First Prenatal Visit

On the first prenatal visit, all pregnant women should be screened for the ABO blood group and the Rh(D) antigen. They should also undergo antibody screening (indirect Coombs' test). All Rh-negative mothers should receive prophylaxis according to the following protocol.

B. Visit at 28 Weeks

Antibody screening is performed. If negative, 300 μg of anti-D immunoglobulin (RhIgG) is given. If positive, the patient should be managed as Rh-sensitized.

C. Visit at 40 Weeks

If more than 12 weeks have elapsed since anti-D immunoglobulin administration, consideration should be given to administering 300 μg of anti-D immunoglobulin at 40 weeks of gestation.

D. Postpartum

If the infant is Rh(D)-positive, 300 μg of RhIgG is administered to the mother (provided maternal antibody screening is negative). Although RhIgG should generally be given within 72 hours after delivery, it has been shown to be effective in preventing alloimmunization if given up to 28 days after delivery. If the antibody screen is positive, the patient is managed as if she will be Rh-sensitized during the next pregnancy.

E. Special Fetomaternal Risk States

Several circumstances may occur during pregnancy that mandate administration of RhIgG to the unsensitized patient outside the management protocol described.

1. Abortion—Sensitization will occur in 2% of spontaneous abortions and 4–5% of induced abortions. In the first trimester, because of the small amount of fetal blood, 50 μg of RhIgG apparently is sufficient to prevent sensitization. However, because the cost of RhIgG has dropped, a full 300-μg dose is usually given. The same dose is recommended for exposure after the first trimester. The risk of Rh alloimmunization after threatened abortion is less well understood, but many experts agree that RhIgG should also be given to these patients.

2. Amniocentesis, Chorionic Villus Sampling, and Cord Blood Sampling—If the placenta is traversed by the needle, there is up to an 11% chance of sensitization. Therefore, administration of 300 μg of RhIgG is recommended when these procedures are performed in the unsensitized patient.

3. Antepartum Bleeding—In cases of antepartum vaginal bleeding or when there is evidence of a subchorionic hematoma or placenta abruption on ultrasound, administration of 300 μg of RhIgG is recommended. If the pregnancy is carried more than 12 weeks from the time of RhIgG administration, a repeat prophylactic dose is recommended.

4. External cephalic version—Fetomaternal hemorrhage occurs in 2–6% of patients who undergo external cephalic version, whether failed or successful; therefore, these patients should receive 300 μg of RhIgG.

F. Delivery With Fetomaternal Hemorrhage

Fetomaternal hemorrhage so extensive that it cannot be managed with 300 μg of RhIgG occurs in only approximately 0.4% of patients. The amount of hemorrhage can be quantified by the Kleihauer-Bethke test and additional doses of RhIgG given according to the amount of fetomaternal hemorrhage.

Clinical Findings

Hemolytic disease of the newborn occurs when the maternal antibodies cross the placenta and destroy the Rh-positive fetal red blood cells. Fetal anemia results, stimulating extramedullary erythropoietic sites to produce high levels of nucleated red cell elements. Immature erythrocytes are present in the fetal blood because of poor maturation control. Hemolysis produces heme, which is converted to bilirubin; both of these substances are neurotoxic. However, although the fetus is in utero, heme and bilirubin are effectively removed by the placenta and metabolized by the mother.

When fetal red blood cell destruction far exceeds production and severe anemia occurs, erythroblastosis fetalis may result. This is characterized by extramedullary hematopoiesis, heart failure, edema, ascites, and pericardial effusion. Tissue hypoxia and acidosis may result. Normal hepatic architecture and function may be disturbed by extensive liver erythropoiesis, which may lead to decreased protein production, portal hypertension, and ascites. On ultrasound, fetal hydrops may be visualized, which is defined as the presence of any 2 of the following: pleural effusion, ascites, pericardial effusion, increased skin thickness, polyhydramnios, or increased placental thickness.

In the immediate neonatal interval, the primary problem may relate to anemia and the sequelae mentioned previously. However, hyperbilirubinemia may also pose an immediate risk and certainly poses a risk as further red cell breakdown occurs. The immature (and often compromised) liver, with its low levels of glucuronyl transferase, is unable to conjugate the large amounts of bilirubin. This results in a high serum bilirubin level, with resultant kernicterus (bilirubin deposition in the basal ganglia).

Treatment

A. Management of the Unsensitized Rh-Negative Patient

Management of the pregnancy complicated by alloimmunization is guided by 2 factors: whether the patient has a history of an affected fetus in a previous pregnancy (ie, fetus with severe anemia or hydrops) and maternal antibody titers.

1. No history of previous fetus affected by rh alloimmunization—Once the antibody screen is positive for alloimmunization, these patients should be followed up with antibody titers at intake, 20 weeks' EGA, and then every 2–4 weeks. As long as antibody titers remain below the critical titer (<1:32 in our laboratory, but each laboratory must establish its own norms), there is no indication for further intervention. Once antibody titers reach 1:32, additional surveillance should be performed because a titer of 1:32 places the fetus at significant risk of hydrops and demise before 37 weeks. Ultrasound assessment of blood flow in the fetal middle cerebral artery (MCA) by Doppler has been shown to be a reliable and noninvasive screening tool for detecting moderate to severe fetal anemia. It is based on the concept that the fetus preserves oxygen delivery to the brain in the setting of anemia by increasing flow to the brain of the low viscosity blood. Ultrasound is performed to identify the circle of Willis, and blood flow in the proximal third of the MCA can be estimated using Doppler. High peak velocity blood flow in this area (>1.5 multiples of the median) correlates well with severe fetal anemia. This test can be performed at 2-week intervals in these patients, so more invasive diagnostic interventions can be avoided until evidence of severe anemia is observed.

In the past, amniocentesis has been used to determine amniotic fluid bilirubin levels and identify fetuses at risk of severe anemia; however, given the invasive nature of repeated amniocenteses, ultrasound for MCA Dopplers has widely replaced amniocentesis for this indication.

2. History of a prior fetus affected by rh alloimmunization—Antibody titers need not be followed in these pregnancies because amniocentesis is indicated by the history of prior affected fetus. Amniocentesis may be performed to determine the fetal genotype if the father of the fetus is determined to be heterozygous for D. If the fetus is determined to have the D antigen, that fetus is considered to be at risk of hemolytic disease and severe anemia regardless of maternal antibody titers. In general, after a first affected pregnancy, future pregnancies tend to manifest with more severe disease and at an earlier gestational age. For this reason, MCA Doppler surveillance should be initiated at 18 weeks and repeated every 1–2 weeks. Treatment of these patients is dictated by MCA Doppler.

3. Results of MCA Dopplers—Once it is determined that a patient should be followed with MCA Dopplers, the results of the MCA Dopplers will place the fetus into one of three categories:

A. UNAFFECTED OR MILDLY AFFECTED FETUS—The fetus that has normal MCA Doppler studies is considered to be unaffected or mildly affected. Testing should be repeated every 2–3 weeks, and delivery should be entertained at term or near term and after the fetus has achieved pulmonary maturity.

B. MODERATELY AFFECTED FETUS—The fetus that has MCA Doppler studies nearing 1.5 multiples of the median should be tested more frequently, every 1–2 weeks. Delivery may be required before term, and the fetus is delivered as soon as pulmonary maturity is reached. In some cases, enhancement of pulmonary maturity by use of corticosteroids may be necessary.

C. SEVERELY AFFECTED FETUS—The severely affected fetus has MCA Doppler studies >1.55 multiples of the median or has frank evidence of hydrops (eg, ascites, pleural or pericardial effusion, subcutaneous edema). Intervention usually is needed to allow the fetus to reach a gestational age at which delivery and neonatal risks are fewer than the risks of in utero therapy.

If the fetus is preterm, cordocentesis or percutaneous umbilical cord blood sampling is recommended at this stage to directly assess the fetal hematocrit. Intrauterine transfusions are generally performed between 18 and 35 weeks of gestation. Before 18 weeks, access to the umbilical vein is limited due to the small caliber of the vessel. After 35 weeks, the risk/benefit ratio favors delivery of a fetus with evidence of severe anemia. Once severe anemia is confirmed, intrauterine transfusion can be performed directly into the umbilical vein. The transfusion is performed using O-negative, cytomegalovirus-negative, washed, leukocyte-depleted, irradiated packed red cells. The intraperitoneal technique was used in years past but has largely been replaced by intravascular fetal transfusion secondary to its more predictable absorption.

After transfusion, repeat transfusions or delivery usually will be necessary, as production of fetal blood markedly decreases or ceases. Timing of these transfusions may be assisted by ultrasonic determination of MCA Doppler studies. Delivery should take place when the fetus has documented pulmonary maturity.

American College of Obstetricians and Gynecologists. *Prevention of Rh D Alloimmunization*. ACOG Practice Bulletin No. 4. Washington, DC: American College of Obstetricians and Gynecologists; 1999.

Mari G, Deter RL, Carpenter RL, et al. Noninvasive diagnosis by Doppler ultrasonography of fetal anemia due to maternal red-cell alloimmunization. Collaborative Group for Doppler Assessment of the Blood Velocity in Anemic Fetuses. *N Engl J Med* 2000;342:9–14. PMID: 10620643.

Saade GR. Noninvasive testing for fetal anemia. *N Engl J Med* 2000;342:52–53. PMID: 10620651.

STILLBIRTH

ESSENTIALS OF DIAGNOSIS

- Intrauterine fetal death at or beyond 20 weeks' gestation

Pathogenesis

Stillbirth affects <1% of pregnancies, with an incidence of approximately 6 per 1000 pregnancies in the United States.

Table 14–8. Risk factors and etiologies for stillbirth.

Maternal	Hypertensive disease Systemic lupus erythematosus Diabetes mellitus Thyroid disease Renal disease Intrahepatic cholestasis of pregnancy Obesity History of a prior stillbirth or fetus with intrauterine growth restriction Smoking/illicit drug use Advanced maternal age (≥35 years) Red cell or platelet alloimmunization
Fetal/placental	Multifetal gestation Congenital fetal infection (eg, parvovirus, listeria, syphilis, streptococcal infection) Intrauterine fetal growth restriction Fetal structural malformation Fetal aneuploidy Fetomaternal hemorrhage Placental abruption

There are a number of known risk factors for stillbirth, which are presented in Table 14–8.

In the past, cord accident was thought to be the cause of many stillbirths. However, more recent data suggest that a nuchal cord is found in approximately 30% of normal births and is most likely an incidental finding when a stillbirth is diagnosed. In order for a stillbirth to be attributed to cord accident, evidence of cord obstruction or compromise (ie, thrombosis) should be seen on pathologic examination, and other causes of stillbirth should be excluded.

In many cases, up to 50% of stillbirths, it is difficult to elucidate a cause of the stillbirth. In some cases, this may be attributable to incomplete workup. However, in many cases, the stillbirth may be unexplained despite a thorough evaluation.

Prevention

Compliance with prenatal care is an important strategy that may prevent stillbirth. The early diagnosis of fetal abnormalities and obstetrical complications such as preeclampsia may allow for the initiation of an appropriate surveillance strategy or timely delivery in order to avoid stillbirth.

Clinical Findings

Stillbirth is diagnosed with the absence of cardiac activity in a fetus at or beyond 20 weeks of gestational age on ultrasound or at birth. Some women with stillbirth may report decreased or absent fetal movement, vaginal bleeding, or abdominal pain.

However, in many cases, the patient may be asymptomatic for the stillbirth and may even report what she thought was normal fetal movement.

Treatment

Once a stillbirth is diagnosed, it is important to initiate an evaluation to determine the cause. A complete history and physical is the first step to look for findings suggestive of a possible cause. For instance, vaginal bleeding may be suggestive of placental abruption, and maternal fever and abdominal pain may indicate congenital fetal infection.

A. Evaluation

Ultrasound examination should be performed to confirm the fetal demise and the gestational age and to evaluate for any signs of fetal abnormality. Further testing can be divided into maternal and fetal testing (Table 14–9). The role of investigation for maternal inherited thrombophilia is controversial. Testing for maternal inherited thrombophilia should be considered if the fetus is severely growth restricted, if there is evidence of thrombosis on placental pathology, or if there is a personal or family history of deep venous thrombosis. Maternal toxicology screen should be considered if there is a suspicion for maternal drug abuse. Testing for diabetes should be performed if the patient was not screened during the pregnancy or if the fetus is large for gestational age. Placental pathology will test for evidence of abruption, thrombosis, or infarction. Additionally, placental pathology can evaluate for signs of viral or bacterial infection. Fetal autopsy is recommended for all stillbirths. However, the patient may decline, in which case external fetal evaluation and x-rays are recommended. Fetal karyotype may be obtained by testing amniotic fluid obtained via amniocentesis before delivery of the fetus or evaluation of fetal or placental tissue. One limitation to testing karyotype from any of these tissues is culture failure. Amniocentesis appears to have the highest yield in terms of success in determining fetal karyotype.

Table 14–9. Evaluation of stillbirth.

Maternal testing	Complete blood count Lupus anticoagulant Anticardiolipin antibodies Kleihauer Betke test Parvovirus IgG and IgM titer TSH RPR (syphilis testing) Type and screen
Fetal/placental testing	Placental pathology Fetal karyotype Fetal autopsy: if patient declines autopsy, external evaluation by pediatric geneticist and/or x-ray imaging of the fetus is recommended.

Ig, immunoglobulin; TSH, thyroid-stimulating hormone.

B. Delivery

Depending on the gestational age of the pregnancy, the pregnancy can be delivered by either induction of labor or dilation and evacuation. Some centers with expertise in late second-trimester dilation and evacuation may offer the procedure up to 26–28 weeks. With adequate cervical preparation before the procedure, an intact specimen can be obtained in many cases to allow for autopsy. Alternatively, labor induction can be performed regardless of gestational age. Hysterotomy or caesarean delivery is generally reserved for patients who fail induction of labor.

Prognosis

The prognosis for future pregnancies depends on the underlying cause of the stillbirth. For women in whom no etiology for stillbirth is found despite a thorough evaluation, the risk of recurrent stillbirth after 20 weeks is approximately 1–2%.

American College of Obstetricians and Gynecologists. *Management of Stillbirth*. ACOG Practice Bulletin No. 102. Washington, DC: American College of Obstetricians and Gynecologists; 2009.

Congenital Fetal Infections

15

Unzila Nayeri, MD
Stephen Thung, MD

PARVOVIRUS

ESSENTIALS OF DIAGNOSIS

- Caused by parvovirus B19, a single-stranded DNA virus
- Clinical manifestations: commonly asymptomatic, erythema infectiosum, systemic symptoms (fever, arthropathy, malaise), or aplastic crises
- Complications in pregnancy: fetal demise, fetal anemia, hydrops fetalis
- Diagnosis: serologic tests (immunoglobulin [Ig] G and IgM antibodies); serum viral DNA polymerase chain reaction
- Antenatal sonographic findings: fetal anemia, hydrops, elevated middle cerebral artery peak systolic velocity
- Fetal diagnosis: cordocentesis
- Fetal treatment: intrauterine blood transfusion

Pathogenesis

Parvovirus B19 infection, a common childhood infection, tends to be more frequent in late winter or early spring. The infection is caused by a single-stranded DNA virus, the B19 parvovirus, which is transmitted through respiratory secretions and hand-to-mouth contact. The virus has a predilection for rapidly dividing cells such as erythroid progenitor cells.

Prevalence of seropositivity increases with age, and about 50–60% of reproductive-aged women have documented antibodies to parvovirus B19 consistent with prior infection. Immunity is considered lifelong, although reinfection has been documented. The incidence of acute parvovirus infection during pregnancy is 3.3–3.8%. Schoolteachers, day care workers, and homemakers are most susceptible. Nonimmune individuals exposed in a classroom have a 20–30% risk of infection. The secondary attack rate for household members is up to 50%.

During pregnancy, the virus can cross the placenta and infect red cell progenitors in the fetal bone marrow. The virus suppresses erythropoiesis by attaching to the "P" antigen on red cell stem cells. This results in severe anemia and high-output congestive heart failure. In addition to the reduced survival of fetal red blood cells, anemia is further complicated by the increased demands of an expanding intravascular volume and the inability of the immature immune system to control the infection. Additionally, the virus can attack fetal myocardiocytes via the same "P" antigen and cause a cardiomyopathy, further exacerbating the congestive heart failure.

Prevention

Pregnant women who are susceptible to parvovirus B19 should avoid contact with known infected individuals. However, since 20% of infections are subclinical, exposure cannot be eliminated by identifying and excluding individuals with acute parvovirus B19 infection. Additionally, those with infection are infectious prior to the onset of symptoms. Therefore, a policy to routinely remove women from occupations considered high risk, such as day care attendants, is not recommended. On the other hand, patients should be counseled on careful hand washing and avoidance of sharing food and drink.

Clinical Findings

A. Symptoms & Signs (Table 15–1)

Parvovirus B19 causes the common childhood illness erythema infectiosum (also known as "fifth disease"). Erythema infectiosum is characterized by a low-grade fever, malaise, arthralgias, and a "slapped cheek" facial rash. Patients may also present with a "lace-like" erythematous rash on the trunk and extremities. The incubation period for parvovirus is 10–20 days. Although the typical rashes are more common

Table 15–1. Clinical manifestations of parvovirus.

Children	Adults	Fetal
"Slapped cheek" facial rash	No symptoms	Intrauterine fetal demise
Low-grade fever	Fever	Anemia
Malaise	Malaise	Hydrops fetalis
Arthralgias	Arthropathy	Thrombocytopenia
Erythematous rash on trunk and extremities	Erythematous rash on trunk and extremities	
	Aplastic crisis	

in children, adults may also present with dermatologic manifestations.

Systemic symptoms are noted 1–4 days prior to the onset of the rash. These symptoms include fever, malaise, and arthropathy, which is more common in adults. Patients with hemoglobinopathies such as sickle cell anemia are at risk for aplastic crises, which are usually self-limited. Patients infected with this virus are considered infectious 5–10 days following exposure up to the onset of symptoms. Once the rash presents, individuals are no longer infectious.

B. Laboratory Findings

Serologic testing is used to diagnose maternal parvovirus infection. Immunoglobulin (Ig) M antibody capture radioimmunoassay and enzyme-linked immunosorbent assay (ELISA) are commonly used, with sensitivities ranging from 80–90%. There are various possible combinations of serologic test results that indicate varying disease states (Table 15–2). IgM antibodies are detected 7–10 days after exposure, peak at 10–14 days, and remain positive for several months. Indicating prior infection, IgG antibodies present several days after IgM, plateau at 4 weeks, and persist for many years. When both IgM and IgG are positive, establishing the exact timing of infection is difficult.

Table 15–2. Possible serologic test results for parvovirus.

IgM	IgG	Interpretation
Negative	Negative	Susceptible
Negative	Positive	Prior immunity—protected against second infections
Positive	Negative	Acute infection—within previous 7 days
Positive	Positive	Subacute infection >7 days and <120 days

Reproduced, with permission, from Creasy RK, Resnik R, Iams J, et al (eds). *Creasy and Resnik's Maternal-Fetal Medicine: Principles and Practice.* 6th ed. Philadelphia, PA: Saunders Elsevier; 2009.

Polymerase chain reaction (PCR) assays may also be used to detect viral B19 DNA. In patients with a history of significant exposure and negative IgM serologies, PCR may be used to clarify the diagnosis because it is a sensitive method of detecting small amounts of viral DNA.

Fetal parvovirus infection is diagnosed using PCR analysis of viral B19 DNA in amniotic fluid obtained via amniocentesis. The more invasive method of percutaneous fetal blood sampling can also be used to directly test fetal blood for B19 IgM. This approach is rarely used because it is associated with a fetal loss rate of 1%.

Pregnant patients who have been exposed to parvovirus infection should undergo serologic testing for IgG and IgM antibodies. A woman with a positive IgG and a negative IgM antibody has had a prior infection and is therefore immunized. A positive IgM antibody indicates an acute or subacute parvovirus infection, depending on the IgG status. An infection that occurs during pregnancy and prior to 20 weeks increases the risk for fetal loss. On the other hand, infection after 20 weeks has a lower risk of fetal loss, yet infection remains associated with fetal anemia and hydrops. Patients should undergo serial ultrasound every 2 weeks for at least 10 weeks after the initial exposure to evaluate for evolving fetal hydrops from high-output cardiac failure. The ultrasound should also evaluate the fetus for severe fetal anemia by measuring the middle cerebral artery peak systolic flow (Fig. 15–1).

A pregnant woman who is negative for IgG and IgM is susceptible to infection. Therefore, in the case of a recent parvovirus exposure, additional testing with PCR of maternal blood for B19 DNA should be pursued given the possibility of false-negative serologies. The patient should also undergo repeat serologic testing in 3 weeks since IgM antibodies should eventually present in a true infection.

C. Imaging Studies

Ultrasound is a useful tool to screen for fetal anemia and hydrops. Sonographic signs of hydrops include fetal skin edema, ascites, or pleural or pericardial effusions. Doppler velocimetry of the fetal middle cerebral artery is considered an accurate tool to screen for severe fetal anemia (Fig. 15–2). Increases in the peak systolic velocity correlate with worsening fetal anemia. Suspected severe fetal anemia should be confirmed via cordocentesis, at which time therapeutic fetal blood transfusion may be performed.

Differential Diagnosis

Rubella
Enteroviruses
Arboviruses

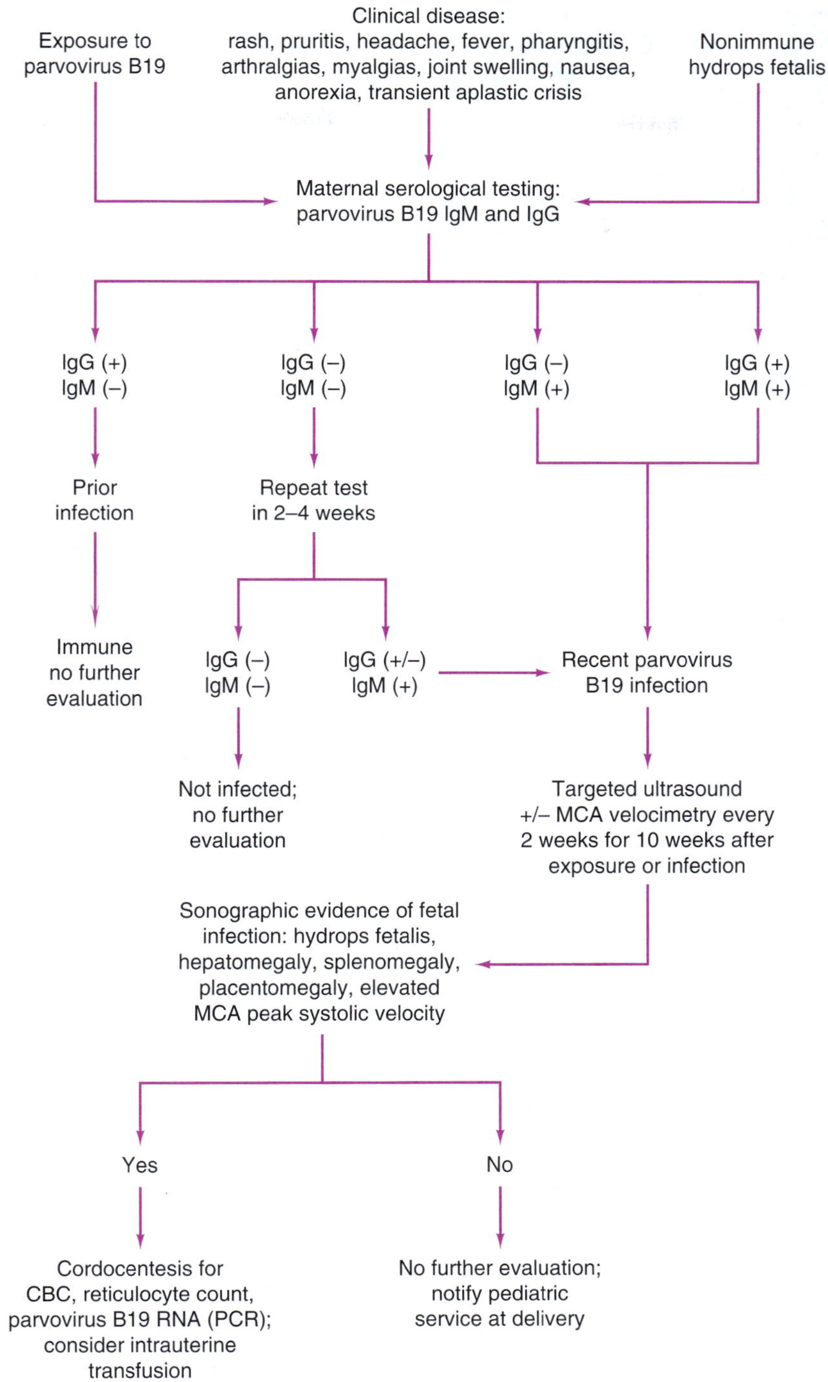

▲ **Figure 15–1.** Algorithm for evaluation and management of human parvovirus B19 infection in pregnancy. CBC, complete blood count; IgG, immunoglobulin G; IgM, immunoglobulin M; MCA, middle cerebral artery; PCR, polymerase chain reaction; RNA, ribonucleic acid. (Reproduced, with permission, from Cunningham FG, Leveno KJ, Bloom SL, Hauth JC, Rouse DJ, Spong CY. *Williams Obstetrics*. 23rd ed. http://www.accessmedicine.com. Copyright © The McGraw-Hill Companies, Inc. All rights reserved.)

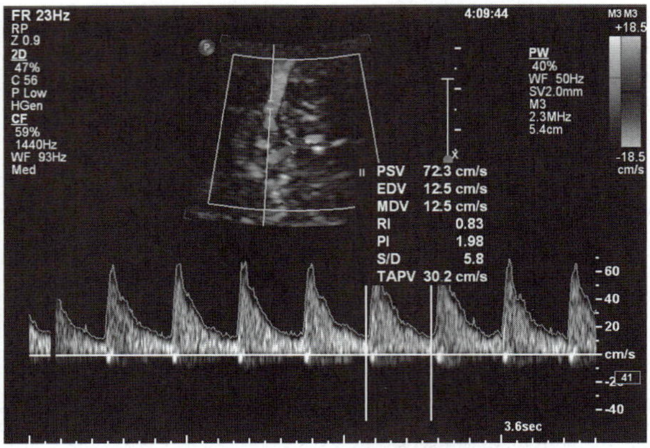

▲ **Figure 15–2.** Middle cerebral artery Doppler images showing elevated peak systolic velocity.

Streptococcal infection

Allergy

Drug reactions

In the setting of fetal hydrops:

Immune hydrops (Rh isoimmunization)

Nonimmune hydrops

Structural defects (cardiac tumors, neck masses, intracranial hemorrhage, etc)

Anemia (due to glucose-6-phosphate dehydrogenase deficiency, fetomaternal hemorrhage etc)

Infection (cytomegalovirus, syphilis, *Toxoplasma*, etc)

Genetic disorders

Placental disorders (chorangioma, chronic vein thrombosis)

Complications

Parvovirus infection in pregnancy has been linked to intrauterine fetal demise in the late second and third trimester. The risk of fetal loss in pregnancies infected prior to 20 weeks of gestation is 11%. The risk dramatically decreases to less than 1% if infection occurs after 20 weeks' gestation. Experts recommend that a workup for parvovirus be included in the evaluation of these intrauterine fetal demises.

In addition to causing fetal loss, the virus may lead to anemia and subsequent hydrops fetalis. The median interval between diagnosis of maternal infection and hydrops is 3 weeks. Fifty percent of cases occur within 2–5 weeks of maternal infection, and 93% of fetal manifestations occur within 8 weeks. The risk of anemia with hydrops depends on the gestational age at which maternal infection occurs. If infection occurs during the first 12 weeks of pregnancy, the risk of hydrops is 5–10%. This risk decreases to less than 5% if infection develops during weeks 13–20. After week 20 of gestation, the risk of hydrops is less than 1%. Hydropic fetuses with parvovirus are also at risk for severe thrombocytopenia. Despite studies linking parvovirus to teratogenicity in fetal animals and case reports of human infection and subsequent fetal malformations, most data suggest that parvovirus B19 is not a teratogen.

Treatment

Mild to moderate anemia is generally well tolerated by the fetus and resolves without sequelae. However, severe anemia can lead to hydrops fetalis and death. If severe anemia is suspected based on elevated Doppler middle cerebral artery peak systolic velocity or signs of hydrops, the fetal hematocrit should be assessed by percutaneous umbilical vein sampling (cordocentesis). Confirmed fetal anemia should be treated with intrauterine blood transfusion. The fetal platelet count should also be determined because the fetus is at risk for thrombocytopenia. Platelets should be available at the time of transfusion. Although there is a risk of fetal death after periumbilical blood sampling, multiple retrospective studies have demonstrated the benefit of such a procedure in hydropic fetuses with parvovirus infection. Usually, only 1 intrauterine transfusion is required because hematopoiesis recovers as the parvovirus infection is cleared.

The delivery of a neonate with hydrops should occur in a tertiary care setting to maximize pregnancy outcome. These infants generally require respiratory assistance with mechanical ventilation and may also require abdominal paracentesis and thoracocentesis of fetal ascites and pleural effusions to aid in resuscitation. Postnatal outcomes depend on gestational age, illness severity, and associated conditions.

Prognosis

Although parvovirus B19 infection during pregnancy is associated with fetal loss and hydrops fetalis, most intrauterine parvovirus infections have an excellent long-term prognosis. Historically, the mortality rate of fetal hydrops was close to 30%. With intrauterine transfusion therapy, over 90% of fetuses who require and survive these transfusions recover within 6–12 weeks with an overall mortality rate of less than 10%. Long-term neurologic and psychomotor outcomes of infants following intrauterine blood transfusion for hydrops have been reported. Most studies are reassuring and suggest no neurodevelopmental abnormalities, although the data are limited.

Borna S, Mirzaie F, Hanthoush-Zadeh S, Khazardoost S, Rahimi-Sharbaf F. Middle cerebral artery peak systolic velocity and ductus venosus velocity in the investigation of nonimmune hydrops. *J Clin Ultrasound* 2009;37:385–388. PMID: 19582828

Cunningham FG, Leveno KJ, Bloom SL, Hauth JC, Rouse DJ, Spong CY. Chapter 58: infectious diseases. In Cunningham FG, Leveno KJ, Bloom SL, Hauth JC, Rouse DJ, Spong CY (eds). *Williams Obstetrics*. 23rd ed. http://www.accessmedicine.com/content/aspx?aID=6048859. Accessed October 30, 2010.

de Haan TR, van den Akker ES, Porcelijn L, Oepkes D, Kroes AC, Walther FJ. Thrombocytopenia in hydropic fetuses with parvovirus B19 infection: incidence, treatment and correlation with fetal B19 viral load. *BJOG* 2008;115:76–81. PMID: 18053103.

de Jong EP, de Haan TR, Kroes AC, Beersma MF, Oepkes D, Walther FJ. Parvovirus B19 infection in pregnancy. *J Clin Virol* 2006;36:1–7. PMID: 16488187.

Duff P, Sweet R, Edwards R. Maternal and fetal infections. In Creasy RK, Resnik R, Iams J, et al (eds). *Creasy and Resnik's Maternal-Fetal Medicine: Principles and Practice.* 6th ed. Philadelphia, PA: Saunders Elsevier; 2009:775–776.

Enders M, Weidner A, Zoellner I, Searle K, Enders G. Fetal morbidity and mortality after acute human parvovirus B19 infection in pregnancy: prospective evaluation of 1018 cases. *Prenat Diagn.* 2004;24:513–518. PMID: 15300741.

Ergaz Z, Ornoy A. Parvovirus B19 in pregnancy. *Reprod Toxicol.* 2006;21:421–435. PMID: 16580942.

Matsuda H, Sakaguchi K, Shibasaki T, Takahashi H, Kawakami Y, Furuya K. Intrauterine therapy for parvovirus B19 infected symptomatic fetus using B19 IgG-rich high titer gammaglobulin. *J Perinat Med* 2005;33:561–563. PMID: 16318623.

Mendelson E, Aboudy Y, Smetana Z, Tepperberg M, Grossman Z. Laboratory assessment and diagnosis of congenital viral infections: rubella, cytomegalovirus (CMV), varicella-zoster virus (VZV), herpes simplex virus (HSV), parvovirus B19 and human immunodeficiency virus (HIV). *Reprod Toxicol* 2006;21:350–382. PMID: 16564672.

Nagel HT, de Haan TR, Vandenbussche FP, Oepkes D, Walther FJ. Long-term outcome after fetal transfusion for hydrops associated with parvovirus B19 infection. *Obstet Gynecol* 2007;109:42–47. PMID: 17197586.

Oepkes D, Seaward PG, Vandenbussche FP, et al. Doppler ultrasonography versus amniocentesis to predict fetal anemia. *N Engl J Med* 2006;355:156–164. PMID: 16837679.

Riley LE, Fernandez CJ. Parvovirus B19 infection in pregnancy. In: Hirsch MS, Edwards MS, Weisman LE, Lockwood CJ (eds). *UpToDate.* Waltham, MA: UpToDate; 2010. http://www.utdol.com. Accessed September 20, 2010.

Segata M, Chaoui R, Khalek N, Bahado-Singh R, Paidas MJ, Mari G. Fetal thrombocytopenia secondary to parvovirus infection. *Am J Obstet Gynecol* 2007;196:61.e1–61.e4. PMID: 17240236.

Servey JT, Reamy BV, Hodge J. Clinical presentations of parvovirus B19 infection. *Am Fam Physician* 2007;75:373–376. PMID: 17304879.

VARICELLA-ZOSTER VIRUS

ESSENTIALS OF DIAGNOSIS

- Caused by varicella-zoster virus (VZV), a single-stranded DNA virus
- Clinical manifestations: nonspecific prodromal symptoms and vesicular lesions
- Prevention: varicella vaccine; immunity following prior infection
- Diagnosis: usually clinical but can be confirmed by serologic tests for anti-VZV IgM
- Complications of maternal VZV in pregnancy: pneumonia, respiratory failure
- Congenital varicella infection: dermatomal scarring, chorioretinitis, limb hypoplasia, microcephaly, low birth weight
- Treatment of pregnant women: oral antivirals and, in the case of maternal complications such as pneumonia, intravenous antiviral therapy

Pathogenesis

The varicella-zoster virus (VZV) is a DNA virus that belongs to the herpesvirus family and causes varicella (chickenpox) and herpes zoster (shingles). Although a majority of infections occur in children, 2% of cases occur in adults. In children, the infection is often benign and self-limited, whereas in adults, it can be devastating. Adults over the age of 20 contribute to over half of varicella-related deaths.

The virus is transmitted by respiratory droplets and direct contact with vesicular lesions. Once droplets enter conjunctiva or nasal/oral mucosa, the virus replicates in regional lymph nodes and spreads to internal organs. Secondary viremia occurs as the virus is released into the bloodstream and attacks cutaneous tissue leading to VZV exanthem. Infectivity is present from 1–2 days prior to the onset of the rash up until the lesions crust over. VZV is highly infectious, with secondary attack rates approximating 90% in susceptible household contacts.

Following a primary VZV infection, the virus remains dormant in dorsal root ganglia. In the setting of impaired immunity, the virus may be reactivated to cause herpes zoster, a vesicular erythematous skin rash that presents along dermatomes. Although there are isolated case reports of reinfection, primary VZV is associated with lifelong immunity.

Prevention

To prevent the complications of VZV in pregnancy, all reproductive-aged women should be vaccinated for varicella if naturally acquired immunity is not present. Varivax, the varicella vaccine, is a live attenuated virus vaccine. The vaccine is contraindicated in pregnancy, immunocompromised states, systemic illnesses, and patients with allergies to neomycin (a component of the vaccine). One dose of the vaccine is sufficient in individuals ages 1–12, and 2 doses, administered 4–6 weeks apart, are required in those over the age of 12. Conception should be delayed until at least 1 month after the second dose. Pregnant patients known to be nonimmune to VZV should be counseled to avoid contact with individuals with varicella.

Clinical Findings

A. Symptoms & Signs (Table 15–3)

The incubation period is 10–21 days after the initial infection. The period of infectivity begins 48 hours prior to the

Table 15–3. Clinical manifestations of varicella infection.

Children	Adults	Fetal (Prenatal Ultrasound Findings)	Neonatal
Fever	Prodromal symptoms	Normal ultrasound findings	Low birth weight
Malaise	Vesicular rash	Spontaneous abortion	Disseminated vesicular rash
Myalgia	Pneumonia	Intrauterine fetal demise	Fever
Vesicular rash	Bacterial superinfection	Growth restriction	Dermatomal scarring
	Myocarditis	Limb hypoplasia	Pneumonia
	Death	Microcephaly	

onset of the rash and lasts until the vesicular lesions are crusted over. During this time period, patients experience prodromal symptoms such as fever, malaise, and myalgia. This is followed by a 6- to 10-day vesicular rash on the trunk, face, and scalp. The lesions usually occur in crops and evolve from vesicle to pustule to eventually a crusted over dry scab.

B. Laboratory Findings

Although the diagnosis of varicella is clinical, serologic tests can be performed to confirm the diagnosis in unclear cases. Using ELISA, anti-VZV IgM can be detected 3 days after the onset of symptoms and IgG can be detected 7 days after symptomatology. Immunofluorescence of vesicular lesions and viral cultures or viral DNA PCR of vesicular fluid can also establish the diagnosis.

Prenatal diagnosis of fetal varicella is possible by percutaneous umbilical vein blood sampling (cordocentesis) for identification of viral-specific antibody or DNA. The virus can also be identified by culture, antibody detection or viral DNA PCR in chorionic villi, or amniotic fluid. Although testing may be reassuring if test results are negative, positive test results do not correlate with severity of fetal infection. Invasive testing to make a fetal diagnosis is not routinely recommended.

C. Imaging Studies

Women with VZV who present with respiratory complaints should undergo imaging by chest x-ray. A diffuse or military infiltrative pattern usually distributed in the peribronchial region is suggestive of VZV pneumonia.

Although prenatal ultrasound can be used to look for markers of congenital VZV, the ultrasound is usually unremarkable. Ultrasound findings include hydrops, echogenic foci in liver and bowel, limb deformities, cardiac malformations, microcephaly, ventriculomegaly, and growth restriction.

Differential Diagnosis

Drug eruptions
Viral exanthems
Herpes simplex
Bullous pemphigoid
Dermatitis herpetiformis
Syphilis
Insect bites
Impetigo
Rickettsial disease

Complications

VZV infection occurs in 1–5 cases per 10,000 pregnancies. Pregnancies complicated by VZV infection are associated with maternal, fetal, and neonatal health risks.

Complications of primary VZV infection are more common in adults and include bacterial superinfection of vesicles, pneumonia, glomerulonephritis, myocarditis, adrenal insufficiency, and death. Patients may also experience benign cerebellar ataxia and Guillain-Barré syndrome.

VZV pneumonia occurs in up to 20% of adult cases of VZV and may be more severe in pregnant women. Symptoms include cough, shortness of breath, fever, and tachypnea and typically present within 1 week of the rash. VZV pneumonia is considered a medical emergency because pregnant patients are at risk for respiratory failure.

In terms of adverse effects on the pregnancy, acute VZV infection has been associated with spontaneous abortion, intrauterine fetal death, and congenital VZV syndrome. The risk of congenital VZV syndrome is low, close to 2%, and is limited to VZV exposure during the first 20 weeks of gestation.

Neonatal VZV is associated with up to a 25% mortality rate. Infants born to women who develop acute VZV from 5 days before delivery to 48 hours postpartum are at risk for serious consequences due to immaturity of the neonatal immune system and lack of maternal protective antibodies. Clinical manifestations of neonatal VZV include fever, disseminated vesicular rash, pneumonia, and encephalitis. Complications include dermatomal scarring, ocular abnormalities, chorioretinitis, limb hypoplasia, microcephaly, and low birth weight.

Treatment

At the first prenatal visit, all pregnant women should be questioned about prior VZV infection. About 70–90% of women who are uncertain about their prior history will actually have detectable antibodies and be immune. Patients with a well-defined history of infection should be reassured that second infections are extremely unlikely and that, in these cases, risks to the fetus are insignificant. It is unclear whether antenatal VZV screening of all pregnant women with negative or indeterminate VZV histories is cost effective.

If a susceptible pregnant patient is exposed to VZV, she should be treated within 72–96 hours (Fig. 15–3). Prophylactic intervention with varicella-zoster immune globulin (VZIG) in the incubation period can prevent or attenuate the manifestations of VZV, but it does not prevent fetal infection. Pregnant women who develop VZV despite immunoprophylaxis should be treated with oral acyclovir or valacyclovir for 1 week. Patients with pneumonia, encephalitis, or disseminated infection should have supportive care and be treated with intravenous acyclovir for 10 days.

Prognosis

Maternal VZV infection is associated with high maternal morbidity and mortality rates. Prognosis is improved with prompt medical attention, supportive care, and treatment of serious conditions such as pneumonia and encephalitis.

The risk of congenital VZV syndrome depends on the gestational age at which exposure occurs. Maternal infection after 20 weeks is not associated with congenital anomalies, and prognosis is favorable, as long as maternal health is optimized. Infection prior to 20 weeks is associated with a low risk of congenital VZV. Prenatal ultrasound diagnosis of fetal anomalies suggestive of congenital VZV syndrome carries a poorer prognosis.

Cunningham FG, Leveno KJ, Bloom SL, Hauth JC, Rouse DJ, Spong CY. Chapter 58: infectious diseases. In Cunningham FG, Leveno KJ, Bloom SL, Hauth JC, Rouse DJ, Spong CY (eds). *Williams Obstetrics*. 23rd ed. http://www.accessmedicine.com/content/aspx?aID=6048859. Accessed October 30, 2010.

Daley AJ, Thorpe S, Garland SM. Varicella and the pregnant woman: prevention and management. *Aust N Z J Obstet Gynaecol* 2008;48:26–33. PMID: 18275568.

Degani S. Sonographic findings in fetal viral infections: a systematic review. *Obstet Gynecol Surv* 2006;61:329–336. PMID: 16635273.

Duff P, Sweet R, Edwards R. Maternal and fetal infections. In Creasy RK, Resnik R, Iams J, et al (eds). *Creasy and Resnik's*

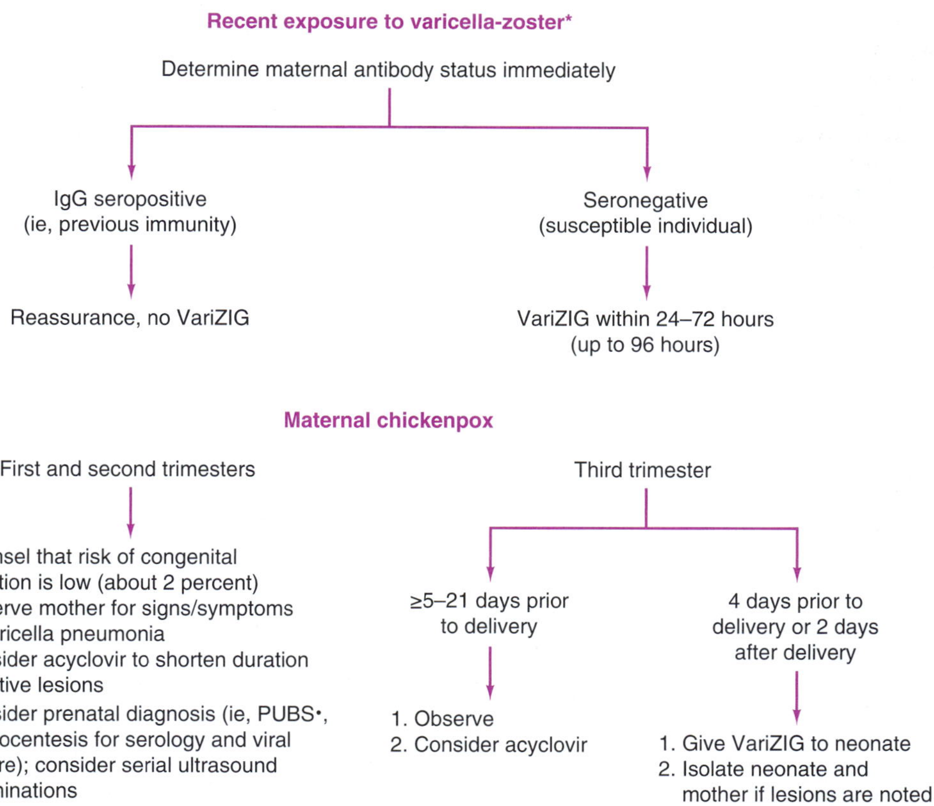

▲ Figure 15–3. Management of varicella-zoster infection in pregnancy. (*) If period of exposure is uncertain or diagnostic evaluation is delayed, consider immunoglobulin M (IgM) and serial immunoglobulin G (IgG) testing. Empiric use of VariZIG may be appropriate if susceptibility is suspected. (•) Percutaneous umbilical blood sampling. (Reproduced, with permission, from Riley LE. Varicella-zoster virus infection in pregnancy. In Hirsch MS, Lockwood CJ (eds). *UpToDate*. Waltham, MA: UpToDate; 2010. http://www.utdol.com.)

Maternal-Fetal Medicine: Principles and Practice. 6th ed. Philadelphia, PA: Saunders Elsevier; 2009:783–784.

Gardella C, Brown ZA. Managing varicella zoster infection in pregnancy. *Cleve Clin J Med* 2007;74:290–296. PMID: 17438678.

Koren G. Congenital varicella syndrome in the third trimester. *Lancet* 2005;366:1591–1592. PMID: 16271630.

Mendelson E, Aboudy Y, Smetana Z, Tepperberg M, Grossman Z. Laboratory assessment and diagnosis of congenital viral infections: rubella, cytomegalovirus (CMV), varicella-zoster virus (VZV), herpes simplex virus (HSV), parvovirus B19 and human immunodeficiency virus (HIV). *Reprod Toxicol* 2006;21:350–382. PMID: 16564672.

Riley LE. Varicella-zoster virus infection in pregnancy. In Hirsch MS, Lockwood CJ (eds). *UpToDate*. Waltham, MA: UpToDate; 2010. http://www.utdol.com. Accessed September 20, 2010.

Sauerbrei A, Wutzler P. Herpes simplex and varicella-zoster virus infections during pregnancy: current concepts of prevention, diagnosis and therapy. Part 2: varicella-zoster virus infections. *Med Microbiol Immunol* 2007;196:95–102. PMID: 17180380.

Tan MP, Koren G. Chickenpox in pregnancy: revisited. *Reprod Toxicol* 2006;21:410–420. PMID: 15979274.

RUBELLA

ESSENTIALS OF DIAGNOSIS

- Caused by an RNA virus transmitted via respiratory droplets
- Prevention: rubella vaccine
- Clinical manifestations: subclinical infection or mild, self-limited disease
- Diagnosis: serologic testing—rubella IgM and IgG antibodies
- Congenital rubella syndrome: deafness, ocular defects, central nervous system defects, and cardiac malformations

Pathogenesis

The rubella virus is part of the RNA togavirus family. Commonly referred to as the German measles, the virus is transmitted via respiratory droplets. From the respiratory tract, the virus replicates in lymph nodes and hematogenously disseminates throughout the body. Hematogenous spread of the virus across the placenta leads to fetal infection or congenital rubella syndrome (CRS). The virus causes cytopathic damage to vessels and ischemia in affected organs, leading to the various congenital defects.

Prevention

Primary prevention of rubella is possible through preconceptional vaccination. Since the introduction of the vaccine in 1969, the incidence of rubella in the United States has declined dramatically—from 0.45 per 100,000 in 1990 to 0.1 per 100,000 in 1999. The rubella vaccine consists of a live attenuated virus. Currently, the vaccine is recommended for all children from age 12–15 months and 4–6 years in conjunction with measles and mumps (MMR vaccine). Although it is recommended that women receiving the rubella vaccine delay conception for at least 1 month, there are no data to suggest an increase in complications if inadvertently given during pregnancy.

Reproductive-age women should be tested for immunity to rubella prior to pregnancy. If results indicate susceptibility, these patients should be vaccinated prior to conception. If patients are not seen before conception and instead present at the time of pregnancy, obstetricians should test for rubella at the first prenatal appointment. Susceptible women are counseled to avoid exposure to individuals with viral exanthems.

Pregnant women who are rubella nonimmune should be vaccinated immediately after delivery. Ninety-five percent of individuals receiving the vaccine will seroconvert. Vaccinated women can continue breastfeeding and will not transmit the virus to susceptible contacts. Postpartum vaccination programs have been shown to reduce rubella susceptibility in pregnant nonimmune women. A study in 2004 revealed that one-third of pregnant women are also susceptible to mumps. Therefore, the Centers for Disease Control and Prevention (CDC) recommends that rubella-susceptible women receive the MMR vaccine postpartum.

Clinical Findings

A. Symptoms & Signs (Table 15–4)

Acquired rubella may be subclinical or present as a mild, self-limited disease associated with an exanthem. Although 25–50% of individuals are asymptomatic, symptoms include low-grade fevers, conjunctivitis, cough, and malaise. The incubation period is 2–3 weeks. Symptoms usually last 1–5 days followed by the onset of the rash. The characteristic exanthem of rubella is a nonpruritic, erythematous, maculopapular rash. The rash typically starts on the face and then disseminates to the trunk and extremities lasting 1–3 days. Resolution of the rash follows the same pattern as dissemination. Patients may be contagious for 7–10 days as the virus is present in blood and nasopharyngeal secretions both prior to and following the onset of symptoms. Generalized tender lymphadenopathy, particularly postauricular adenopathy, may also be present. Female adolescents may present with rheumatologic sequelae, including morning stiffness and symmetric joint pain. Rare complications of rubella include thrombocytopenia, hemolytic anemia, and hepatitis.

B. Laboratory Findings

The diagnosis of rubella is usually established [CD1] by serologic testing of rubella-specific IgG and IgM, via

Table 15–4. Clinical manifestations of rubella.

Children	Adults	Fetal (Prenatal Ultrasound Findings)	Neonatal
Low-grade fever	Low-grade fever	Spontaneous abortion	Cataracts, retinopathy
Malaise	Malaise	Intrauterine fetal demise	Hearing impairment
Cough	Cough	Growth restriction	Microcephaly
Conjunctivitis	Conjunctivitis	Microcephaly	Hepatosplenomegaly
Nonpruritic maculopapular rash (face to trunk)	Nonpruritic maculopapular rash (face to trunk)	Hepatosplenomegaly	Hemolytic anemia, thrombocytopenia
Lymphadenopathy	Lymphadenopathy		Immune defects
	Rheumatologic symptoms		Panencephalitis

enzyme-linked immunoassays and other serologic tests. IgM antibody concentration reaches a peak 7–10 days after the onset of the infection and decreases over the next 4 weeks. The serum concentration of IgG rises slowly but remains positive over the lifetime of an individual. A rubella PCR or positive culture may also facilitate the diagnosis. The virus may be isolated from blood, nasal cavity, pharynx, or urine.

If rubella exposure occurs in a susceptible woman, serologic tests should be performed. If acute infection is documented with the presence of an IgM antibody, the patient should be counseled regarding the option for prenatal diagnosis. There are various methods to establish the prenatal diagnosis of rubella. Fetal blood via cordocentesis can be tested for rubella-specific IgM concentrations. This is limited in use because fetal immunoglobulins are unlikely to be present prior to 22–24 weeks. PCR can be performed on chorionic villi, fetal blood, and amniotic fluid. Although these tests can determine the presence of rubella in the fetal compartment, the results do not correlate with the level of fetal injury.

Differential Diagnosis

Rubeola

Roseola

Other viral exanthems

Drug reaction

Complications

Although the virus is usually self-limited in adults, rare complications of adult rubella have been reported. These serious complications include encephalitis, thrombocytopenia with hemorrhagic manifestations, neuritis, and conjunctivitis.

The virus can also adversely impact the developing fetus. Pregnant women infected with rubella are at higher risk for spontaneous abortion, fetal infection, growth restriction, and fetal demise. Due to the established rubella vaccination programs in the United States, the incidence of CRS has dramatically decreased, and there are now fewer than 50 cases of CRS each year. However, about 10–20% of reproductive-age women in the United States are not immune, and their fetuses are at risk for CRS. In developing countries without national guidelines for rubella vaccination, the burden of disease is higher, and CRS affects from 10–90 per 100,000 live births.

Rubella is considered one of the most teratogenic viruses during pregnancy. Congenital infection depends on the time of exposure to the virus. About 50–80% of neonates exposed to the virus prior to 12 weeks' gestation will manifest signs of congenital infection. The risk of CRS decreases with advancing gestational age. CRS is rare if infection occurs beyond 18 weeks' gestation.

Common anomalies associated with CRS include deafness (60–75%), eye defects such as cataracts or retinopathy (10–30%), central nervous system anomalies (10–25%), and cardiac malformations (10–20%). Other findings include microcephaly, growth retardation, hepatosplenomegaly, hemolytic anemia, and thrombocytopenia. Fetal infection is chronic and persistent after birth. Although most infants with CRS are asymptomatic at birth, they develop signs and symptoms over time. Because of the lack of clinical manifestations at birth and the risk for progression, timely diagnosis is important. Late manifestations of CRS include hearing loss, endocrine disorders, immune defects, and panencephalitis.

Treatment

Treatment for acute rubella infection in children and adults is supportive therapy. Glucocorticoids and platelet transfusion are considered in patients with complications such as thrombocytopenia or encephalopathy. Administration of immune globulin to susceptible women exposed to rubella during pregnancy is controversial.

The clinical benefit of immunoglobulins for postexposure prophylaxis of rubella and prevention of fetal infection has yet to be demonstrated.

Prognosis

Pregnant women with rubella have a favorable prognosis when it comes to their health. Unfortunately, the prognosis of CRS is potentially devastating because affected neonates commonly suffer serious sequelae and permanent damage.

Best JM. Rubella. *Semin Fetal Neonatal Med* 2007;12:182–192. PMID: 17337363.

Centers for Disease Control and Prevention (CDC). Progress toward elimination of rubella and congenital rubella syndrome–the Americas, 2003-2008. *MMWR Morb Mortal Wkly Rep* 2008;57:1176–1179. PMID: 18971920.

Cunningham FG, Leveno KJ, Bloom SL, Hauth JC, Rouse DJ, Spong CY. Chapter 58: infectious diseases. In Cunningham FG, Leveno KJ, Bloom SL, Hauth JC, Rouse DJ, Spong CY (eds). *Williams Obstetrics*. 23rd ed. http://www.accessmedicine.com/content/aspx?aID=6048859. Accessed October 30, 2010.

Degani S. Sonographic findings in fetal viral infections: a systematic review. *Obstet Gynecol Surv* 2006;61:329–336. PMID: 16635273.

De Santis M, Cavaliere AF, Straface G, Caruso A. Rubella infection in pregnancy. *Reprod Toxicol* 2006;21:390–398. PMID: 16580940.

Dontigny L, Arsenault MY, Martel MJ, et al. Rubella in pregnancy. *J Obstet Gynaecol Can* 2008;30:152–168. PMID: 18254998.

Duff P, Sweet R, Edwards R. Maternal and fetal infections. In Creasy RK, Resnik R, Iams J, et al (eds). *Creasy and Resnik's Maternal-Fetal Medicine: Principles and Practice*. 6th ed. Philadelphia, PA: Saunders Elsevier; 2009:775–776.

Duszak RS. Congenital rubella syndrome–major review. *Optometry* 2009;80:36–43. PMID: 19111256.

Elliman D, Sengupta N, El Bashir H, Bedford H. Measles, mumps, and rubella: prevention. *Clin Evid (Online)* 2007;2007:0316. PMID: 19454052.

Haas DM, Flowers CA, Congdon CL. Rubella, rubeola, and mumps in pregnant women: susceptibilities and strategies for testing and vaccinating. *Obstet Gynecol* 2005;106:295–300. PMID: 16055578.

Oster ME, Riehle-Colarusso T, Correa A. An update on cardiovascular malformations in congenital rubella syndrome. *Birth Defects Res A Clin Mol Teratol* 2010;88:1–8. PMID: 19697432.

Reef SE, Cochi SL. The evidence for the elimination of rubella and congenital rubella syndrome in the United States: a public health achievement. *Clin Infect Dis* 2006;43(Suppl 3):S123–S125. PMID: 16998770.

Reef SE, Redd SB, Abernathy E, Zimmerman L, Icenogle JP. The epidemiological profile of rubella and congenital rubella syndrome in the United States, 1998-2004: the evidence for absence of endemic transmission. *Clin Infect Dis* 2006;43(Suppl 3):S126–S132. PMID: 16998771.

Riley LE. Rubella in pregnancy. In Hirsch MS, Lockwood CJ (eds). *UpToDate*. Waltham, MA: UpToDate; 2010. http://www.utdol.com. Accessed September 20, 2010.

SYPHILIS

ESSENTIALS OF DIAGNOSIS

- Caused by the spirochete *Treponema pallidum*
- Stages:
  - Primary stage: defined by chancre
  - Secondary stage: systemic process involving a maculopapular rash, lymphadenopathy, flu-like symptoms, and condyloma lata
  - Latent stage: subclinical infection with positive serologic tests
    - Early latent syphilis: within 1 year of the initial infection
    - Late latent syphilis: infection 1 year after the primary infection
  - Tertiary stage: systemic disease with cardiovascular, neurologic, and cutaneous manifestations
- Diagnosis: direct visualization by dark field microscopy, serologic titers (VDRL and rapid plasma reagin, nonspecific treponemal tests; fluorescent treponemal antibody absorption test, treponemal-specific tests)
- Complications in pregnancy: spontaneous abortion, growth restriction, stillbirth, congenital anomalies, preterm delivery, fetal/neonatal infection, and neonatal death
- Treatment: penicillin

Pathogenesis

Syphilis is a chronic systemic infection caused by the motile spirochete *Treponema pallidum*. It is most commonly acquired through direct sexual contact. During pregnancy, infection can also occur via transplacental transmission. Exposure to open lesions containing the organisms facilitates transmission of the spirochete across mucous membranes or skin abrasions. The infection is acquired in 50–60% of partners after a single sexual exposure to an infected lesion. The tissue destruction observed in syphilis infections is a result of the immune response rather than a direct insult from the spirochete itself.

Although the incidence of syphilis steadily declined in the 1990s to early 2000s, there was a notable increase from 2003 to 2005. During this period, there was a parallel rise in the number of diagnosed cases of congenital syphilis (Fig. 15–4).

Prevention

Public health strategies, counseling, and education of patients on sexually transmitted infections can help reduce

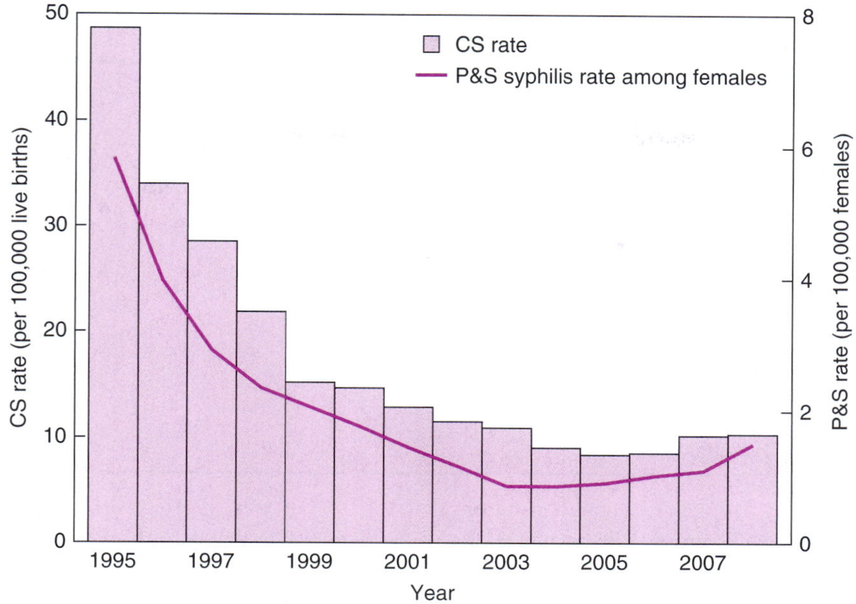

▲ **Figure 15–4.** Congenital syphilis (CS) rate among infants age <1 year and rate of primary and secondary (P&S) syphilis among females age ≥10 years. (Reproduced from Centers for Disease Control and Prevention. National Electronic Telecommunication System for Surveillance, United States, 1995–2008. http://www.cdc.gov/mmwr/preview/mmwrhtml/mm5914a1.htm.)

the risk of these infections. Although correct and consistent use of latex condoms may decrease the risk of syphilis transmission, sexual abstinence is the only guaranteed method to avoid transmission. Other risk factors associated with syphilis in pregnancy include poverty, sexual promiscuity, and illicit drug use. Avoiding activities leading to risky behavior, such as alcohol and drug use, may also help prevent transmission. The risk of syphilis can be further modified by early identification of infected patients, screening of high-risk populations, adequate treatment of patients and exposed individuals, and improved access to health care.

Congenital syphilis can be prevented by screening all pregnant women and treating those with evidence of infection. Patients should be encouraged to seek early prenatal care, and all pregnant women should undergo screening at the initial prenatal visit. High-risk patients should be rescreened in the third trimester, around 28 weeks of gestation, and in areas with high rates of congenital syphilis, rescreening upon admission in labor should be considered. Women with an intrauterine fetal demise after 20 weeks of gestation should also be evaluated for syphilis.

Clinical Findings

A. Symptoms & Signs

Syphilis is an infection that presents in different stages over a period of time if untreated. Early syphilis, which occurs within the first year after acquisition of the infection, includes primary and secondary syphilis. Latent syphilis refers to the absence of symptoms in the setting of positive serologies and often follows secondary syphilis. Tertiary or late syphilis, which involves the central nervous and cardiovascular systems, manifests years to decades after the initial infection. Table 15–5 summarizes the clinical manifestations of the various stages of syphilis.

The chancre, the characteristic lesion of primary syphilis, is a painless, nontender ulcer with an indurated base and raised border. The lesion is found at the site of inoculation. In women, it is most often found on the external genitalia, on the cervix, or in the vagina. Primary syphilis may also manifest with painless inguinal lymphadenopathy. The incubation period varies from 10–90 days, with a mean incubation time of 3 weeks. The primary chancre heals spontaneously in 3–6 weeks in the absence of treatment.

Secondary syphilis is a systemic process characterized by disseminated spread of the infection. This stage typically presents 6 weeks to 6 months after the onset of the primary chancre. Patients present with skin and mucous membrane lesions, along with flu-like symptoms (fever and myalgia) and generalized lymphadenopathy. The generalized maculopapular rash begins on the trunk and proximal extremities and spreads to the entire body, including the palms, soles, and scalp. Condyloma lata are wart-like lesions found in the genital area. The rash usually resolves spontaneously within 2–6 weeks. Patients then enter the latent stage of syphilis.

Table 15–5. Clinical manifestations of the various stages of syphilis.

Early		Latent		Late
Primary	Secondary	Early latent (<1 year from initial infection)	Late latent (>1 year from initial infection)	Tertiary
Chancre	Maculopapular rash (trunk to distal extremities), myalgia	No symptoms Positive serologies		Cardiovascular disease (aortic aneurysms, aortic insufficiency, coronary stenosis)
Inguinal lymphadenopathy	Fever, myalgias			Neurosyphilis (paralysis, tabes dorsalis, dementia)
	Generalized lymphadenopathy			Cutaneous lesions (gummas)
	Condyloma lata			

Patients with latent syphilis are usually asymptomatic with no findings on physical examination. Serologic tests continue to be positive during this time. Latent syphilis is further divided into early and late latent syphilis. If latent infection occurs within 1 year of the initial infection, it is defined as early latent syphilis. Late latent syphilis refers to infection that occurs 1 year after the time of initial infection. A patient can remain in the latent stage for many years.

About one-third of individuals with untreated syphilis will progress to the tertiary stage. Widespread tissue destruction in the tertiary stage results in cardiovascular disease, neurosyphilis, and cutaneous and osseous lesions. Obliterative endarteritis occurs as the spirochete develops a predilection for arterioles. Cardiovascular syphilis manifests with aortic aneurysms, aortic insufficiency, and coronary stenosis. Neurosyphilis is characterized by paralysis, paresthesias, tabes dorsalis, blindness, gait abnormalities, confusion, and dementia.

The Argyll-Robertson pupil (pupil that does not react to light but is able to accommodate) is pathognomonic for tertiary syphilis. Gummas are classic dermatologic manifestations. These gummas consist of necrosis surrounded by an inflammatory infiltrate encapsulated by proliferating connective tissue and form reddish-brown nodular lesions in the skin.

B. Laboratory Findings

Testing for syphilis can be performed either with direct visualization of the organism or by direct serologic testing. Using dark field microscopy, spirochetes can be identified in bodily fluid or lesions. More recently, direct fluorescent antibody stains have replaced dark field microscopy, but technicians still require a fluorescent microscope to visualize the organism. Serologic tests may initially return negative in the early stages of chancre formation. Therefore, these lesions should be sampled for detection of spirochetes and undergo dark field examination.

Serologic testing consists of a nonspecific screening test followed by a confirmatory treponemal antibody test. The nontreponemal screening tests include the Venereal Disease Research Laboratories (VDRL) test, rapid plasma reagin (RPR) test, or automated reagin test. Reported as a titer, these tests use cardiolipin antigens to detect circulating antibodies and can be used to follow response to treatment. In certain patients, however, a low titer may persist for a long period of time. Due to the nonspecific nature of these tests, false-positive results are not uncommon (0.2–3.2%) and may occur in a multitude of settings including various infections, malignancies, connective tissue diseases, and chronic liver disease.

The fluorescent treponemal antibody absorption test (FTA-ABS) is the most commonly used confirmatory test that detects antibodies specifically directed to treponemal cellular components. Because these tests remain positive even after treatment, they are not used to follow response to treatment. In pregnancy, seropositive women should be considered infected unless a treatment history is well documented and subsequent serologic antibody titers have declined.

Less than 10% of patients with untreated syphilis progress to symptomatic late neurosyphilis. In the absence of clinical signs or symptoms of neurologic involvement, the CDC does not recommend routine lumbar puncture in primary and secondary syphilis. However, in patients with latent syphilis, lumbar puncture should be performed if there are signs of neurologic involvement, evidence of active tertiary syphilis, treatment failure, or HIV infection. The diagnosis of neurosyphilis depends on a combination of tests including reactive serologies, abnormal cerebrospinal fluid (CSF) cell count, elevated protein, and/or reactive CSF VDRL.

Serial quantitative VDRL titers facilitate the diagnosis of reinfection or persistence of active syphilis. With adequate treatment, VDRL titers decrease and become negative within 6–12 months in early syphilis and within 12–24 months in late syphilis. Further diagnostic tests (such as lumbar puncture) and appropriate treatment are needed if titers continue to rise.

Congenital syphilis is diagnosed easily in the setting of a fetus with clinical manifestations of syphilis, placentomegaly, and positive laboratory studies confirming the infection. However, many neonates do not manifest signs and symptoms of congenital infection. Although cord blood may return positive for nonspecific tests for syphilis, the diagnosis is difficult due to the transplacental transfer of maternal nontreponemal and treponemal IgG antibodies to the fetus. In these complicated situations, treatment must be based on the diagnosis of syphilis in the mother, treatment status of the mother, comparison of maternal and infant nontreponemal serologic titers at the time of delivery, and presence of clinical findings of syphilis in the infant. Infants with positive VDRL tests results with no clinical evidence of syphilis should have monthly VDRL titers for at least 9 months; rising titers indicate the need for therapy.

Differential Diagnosis

Primary Syphilis

Granuloma inguinale
Lymphogranuloma venereum
Herpes simplex
Chancroid
Carcinoma
Trauma
Lichen planus
Psoriasis
Mycotic infections
Bowen's disease

Secondary Syphilis

Drug eruptions
Psoriasis
Lichen planus
Pityriasis rosea
Tinea versicolor
Parasitic infections
Viral exanthems
Rocky Mountain spotted fever

Complications

In addition to the aforementioned manifestations of the various stages of syphilis, complications of congenital syphilis result in significant neonatal morbidity. Although vertical transmission can occur at any time during pregnancy and at any stage of syphilis, the risk of congenital infection is greater in the earlier stages of the disease. Women with primary or secondary syphilis are more likely to transmit the disease to their fetuses than are women with latent disease. Maternal primary syphilis and secondary syphilis are associated with a 50% risk of congenital syphilis, whereas early latent syphilis carries a 40% risk of congenital syphilis. The risk of congenital syphilis is even lower, close to 10%, among patients with late latent syphilis. Although serious adverse outcomes are more likely to occur with transmission in the earlier stages, most pregnant women are in the latent stage of syphilis at the time of diagnosis and have had the infection for more than 1 year.

Although the spirochete can cross the placenta and infect the fetus as early as the sixth week of gestation, clinical manifestations do not appear until after the 16th week. By this time, the fetal immune system has matured and can respond to the spirochete. It is the immune reaction to the infection that is responsible for tissue destruction rather than direct injury by the spirochete. The risk of congenital syphilis is increased with infection late in pregnancy, treatment less than 30 days before delivery, inappropriate treatment of the mother, and the lack of prenatal serologic testing.

Untreated syphilis is associated with significant adverse effects on the pregnancy including spontaneous abortion, intrauterine growth restriction, fetal demise, congenital anomalies, preterm delivery, and neonatal death. Stillbirth rates range from 10–35%. Fetuses with congenital infections exhibit hepatosplenomegaly, ascites, polyhydramnios, placental thickening, and hydrops.

Congenital syphilis is divided into 2 clinical syndromes: early and late congenital syphilis (Table 15–6). Early congenital syphilis refers to the manifestations of syphilis within the first 2 years of life. These infants can present with a maculopapular rash, snuffles (flu-like syndrome associated with nasal discharge), mucous lesions, hepatosplenomegaly, jaundice, anemia, lymphadenopathy, chorioretinitis, and iritis. Late congenital syphilis presents after 2 years of age.

Table 15–6. Signs and symptoms of congenital syphilis.

Early (Symptoms within 2 Years of Life)	Late (Symptoms after 2 Years of Life)
Maculopapular rash	Frontal bossing
Snuffles	Short maxilla
Mucous lesions	Saddle nose
Hepatosplenomegaly	Saber shins
Jaundice	High palatal arch
Anemia	Hutchinson teeth
Lymphadenopathy	Interstitial keratitis
Chorioretinitis	Eighth nerve deafness

Findings consistent with late congenital syphilis include frontal bossing, short maxilla, saddle nose, saber shins, high palatal arch, Hutchinson teeth, interstitial keratitis, and eighth nerve deafness. Infants may also have other neurologic manifestations such as mental retardation, hydrocephalus, and optic nerve atrophy.

Treatment

Pregnant women with a history of sexual contact with a person with documented syphilis, positive dark field microscopic visualization of spirochetes, positive serologies via a specific treponemal test, or evidence of reinfection should be treated. Penicillin G is the treatment of choice for all stages of syphilis and is effective in treating maternal disease, preventing fetal transmission, and treating fetal disease (Table 15–7). Although alternatives to penicillin are available to treat nonpregnant penicillin-allergic patients, parenteral penicillin G is the only therapy with documented efficacy for syphilis during pregnancy because it crosses the placenta in adequate amounts, effectively treating the fetus. Therefore, it is recommended that patients with known penicillin allergy undergo desensitization followed by subsequent treatment with penicillin. Although erythromycin was previously used for treatment of syphilis in pregnancy, its efficacy for treatment of the fetus and prevention of transmission is inadequate. Doxycycline and tetracycline may be used to treat nonpregnant patients. The efficacy of antibiotics such as ceftriaxone and azithromycin is currently under investigation.

Desensitization can occur in an oral or intravenous manner. Regardless of the route, patients should undergo desensitization in a hospital setting due to potential serious IgE-mediated allergic reactions.

Early disease, with documentation that the initial infection occurred within the past year, is treated with a single dose of benzathine penicillin. Because of treatment failures even after adherence to recommended guidelines, some experts recommend additional therapy with a second dose of penicillin G 1 week after the initial dose. Despite adequate therapy, risk factors for treatment failure include high VDRL titers at the time of diagnosis, unknown duration of infection, treatment within 4 weeks of delivery, and ultrasound signs of fetal syphilis.

Late latent syphilis, latent syphilis of unknown duration, and tertiary syphilis should be treated with 3 doses of benzathine penicillin at weekly intervals. Neurosyphilis requires more intensive treatment with high doses of intravenous aqueous crystalline penicillin or intramuscular procaine penicillin for 10–14 days.

Patients may develop the Jarisch-Herxheimer reaction within several hours after treatment. Symptoms last for 12–24 hours and include fever, chills, myalgias, vasodilation, mild hypotension, and tachycardia. In addition to the symptoms present in nonpregnant individuals, women undergoing treatment in the second trimester are at risk for preterm contractions, preterm labor (highest risk 48 hours after treatment), decreased fetal movement, fetal distress, and fetal death. Patients improve with supportive therapy because the Jarisch-Herxheimer reaction is usually self-limited and resolves by 24–36 hours.

Response to therapy should be monitored with clinical and serologic examination at 1, 3, 6, 12, and 24 months after treatment. Titers usually decline at least 4-fold within 12–24 months of treatment. Patients with persistent clinical symptoms or with sustained 4-fold increases in the nontreponemal test titer have either failed therapy or become reinfected. These patients need retreatment, CSF analysis, and HIV testing. Pregnant women treated for syphilis need repeat serologic titers at 28–32 weeks of gestation and at delivery. Women at high risk for reinfection may have serologies checked monthly.

Table 15–7. CDC-recommended treatment of syphilis during pregnancy.

Diagnosis	Treatment
1. Primary, secondary, and early latent syphilis (<1 year)	Benzathine penicillin G, 2.4 MU IM in a single dose
2. Late latent syphilis (>1 year), latent syphilis of unknown duration, and tertiary syphilis	Benzathine penicillin G, 7.2 MU total, administered as 3 doses of 2.4 MU IM each at 1-week intervals
3. Neurosyphilis	Aqueous crystalline penicillin G, 18–24 MU per day administered as 3–4 MU IV every 4 hours or by continuous infusion for 10–14 days OR Procaine penicillin, 2.4 MU IM daily, plus probenecid 500 mg PO qid, both for 10–14 days
4. Penicillin-allergic	Pregnant women with a history of penicillin allergy should have allergy confirmed and then be desensitized

IM, intramuscular; IV, intravenous; MU, million units; PO, oral; qid, 4 times a day.
Modified, with permission, from Centers for Disease Control and Prevention. Sexually Transmitted Diseases Treatment Guidelines, 2006. *MMWR Recomm Rep* 2006;55:22–35.

After adequate treatment, nontreponemal serologic tests often become negative. The treponemal test results usually remain positive for life. Certain patients may have positive nontreponemal tests despite treatment. In these cases, titers are usually not higher than 1:8.

Prognosis

The number of cases of early syphilis has recently been rising, particularly among intravenous drug users and the HIV population. The syphilis rate among women increased from 1.1 cases per 100,000 females in 2007 to 1.5 cases per 100,000 females in 2008. Women of reproductive age make up 80% of the female population with syphilis. Therefore, syphilis is an important health concern. Serious sequelae for the fetus and neonate are due to the failure to diagnose or adequately treat maternal disease.

The efficacy of penicillin for treatment of syphilis in pregnancy ranges from 95–100%. Prognosis is usually favorable once the patient is adequately treated. However, pregnant patients require close follow-up because treatment failure may result in a congenitally infected fetus and neonate.

Centers for Disease Control and Prevention (CDC). Congenital syphilis – United States, 2003-2008. *MMWR Morb Mortal Wkly Rep* 2010;59:413–417. PMID: 20395934.

Centers for Disease Control and Prevention. Workowski KA, Berman SM. Sexually transmitted diseases treatment guidelines, 2006. *MMWR Recomm Rep* 2006;55:1–94. PMID: 16888612.

Chakraborty R, Luck S. Managing congenital syphilis again? The more things change.. . . *Curr Opin Infect Dis* 2007;20:247–252. PMID: 17471033.

Cheng JQ, Zhou H, Hong FC, et al. Syphilis screening and intervention in 500,000 pregnant women in Shenzhen, the People's Republic of China. *Sex Transm Infect* 2007;83:347–350. PMID: 176934449.

Coonrod DV, Jack BW, Stubblefield PG, et al. The clinical content of preconception care: infectious diseases in preconception care. *Am J Obstet Gynecol* 2008;199(6 Suppl 2):S296–S309. PMID: 19081424.

Cunningham FG, Leveno KJ, Bloom SL, Hauth JC, Rouse DJ, Spong CY. Chapter 58: infectious diseases. In Cunningham FG, Leveno KJ, Bloom SL, Hauth JC, Rouse DJ, Spong CY (eds). *Williams Obstetrics*. 23rd ed. http://www.accessmedicine.com/content/aspx?aID=6048859. Accessed October 30, 2010.

Doroshenko A, Sherrard J, Pollard AJ. Syphilis in pregnancy and the neonatal period. *Int J STD AIDS* 2006;17:221–227. PMID: 16595042.

Duff P, Sweet R, Edwards R. Maternal and fetal infections. In Creasy RK, Resnik R, Iams J, et al (eds). *Creasy and Resnik's Maternal-Fetal Medicine: Principles and Practice*. 6th ed. Philadelphia, PA: Saunders Elsevier; 2009:777–782.

Hollier LM. Syphilis. In Soper DE, Hollier LM, Eckert LO et al (eds). *Infectious Diseases in Obstetrics and Gynecology*. http://www.acog.org/publications/infectiousDiseases. Accessed September 20, 2010.

Hossain M, Broutet N, Hawkes S. The elimination of congenital syphilis: a comparison of the proposed World Health Organization action plan for the elimination of congenital syphilis with existing national maternal and congenital syphilis policies. *Sex Transm Dis* 2007;34(7 Suppl):S22–S30. PMID: 17592387.

Norwitz ER. Syphilis in pregnancy. In Lockwood CJ, Bartlett JG (eds). *UpToDate*. Waltham, MA: UpToDate; 2010. http://www.utdol.com. Accessed September 20, 2010.

Schmid GP, Stoner BP, Hawkes S, Broutet N. The need and plan for global elimination of congenital syphilis. *Sex Transm Dis* 2007;34(7 Suppl):S5–S10. PMID: 17592390.

Wolff T, Shelton E, Sessions C, Miller T. Screening for syphilis infection in pregnant women: evidence for the U.S. Preventive Services Task Force reaffirmation recommendation statement. *Ann Intern Med* 2009;150:710–716. PMID: 19451578.

Zhou P, Gu Z, Xu J, Wang X, Liao K. A study evaluating ceftriaxone as a treatment agent for primary and secondary syphilis in pregnancy. *Sex Transm Dis* 2005;32:495–498. PMID: 16041252.

CYTOMEGALOVIRUS

ESSENTIALS OF DIAGNOSIS

- Caused by double-stranded DNA herpes virus
- Prevention: strict personal hygiene
- Diagnosis: serologic testing in adults; amniotic fluid PCR for prenatal diagnosis
- Antenatal sonographic findings: microcephaly, ventriculomegaly, intracranial calcifications, hydrops, growth restriction, placentomegaly, and echogenic bowel

Pathogenesis

Cytomegalovirus (CMV) is a double-stranded DNA virus that belongs to the herpesvirus family. It has the ability to establish lifelong latency in the host after primary infection and can periodically reactivate with shedding of virus. CMV is the most common congenital infection. Birth prevalence estimates range from 0.2–2.5%.

Horizontal transmission of CMV results from transplantation of infected organs, blood transfusions, sexual contact, or contact with contaminated saliva or urine. Vertical transmission is due to transplacental infection, ingestion of genital tract secretions during delivery, or breastfeeding. Because the virus has the potential to remain latent in host cells after resolution of initial infection, CMV infections in pregnant women are either primary or recurrent. If the initial infection occurs during pregnancy, it is considered a primary infection. A recurrent infection refers to an infection in which maternal CMV antibodies are present prior to conception.

CMV seropositivity increases with age. In the United States, approximately 50–80% of adult women have serologic evidence of prior CMV infection. Although maternal pre-existing immunity decreases the risk of intrauterine transmission, the presence of antibodies is not absolutely protective against either reinfection or vertical transmission. The rate of seroconversion in pregnancy is about 1–4%.

Hematogenous spread of the virus across the placenta is responsible for congenital infection. Dissemination is more likely during primary infection. In the case of primary infection in pregnancy, there is a 50% risk of fetal infection. The rate of transmission increases as the pregnancy progresses, with the highest risk of transmission in the third trimester. However, the severity of fetal injury is greatest if maternal primary infection occurs in the first trimester. In the setting of recurrent infection, the risk of fetal transmission is overall lower, with a 5–10% risk.

Prevention

There is no vaccine to prevent CMV infection, and there is a lack of data to suggest that treatment of maternal infection prevents the risk of congenital CMV infection. For these reasons, routine prenatal screening for CMV is not recommended. Preventive measures, such as careful handwashing techniques, should be employed to decrease the risk of CMV infection during pregnancy. Susceptible individuals should avoid sharing food or drinks with young children. Seronegative pregnant women should also be transfused with CMV-negative blood products and counseled regarding safe sexual practices if not in a monogamous relationship.

Clinical Findings

A. Symptoms & Signs (Table 15–8)

Clinical manifestations of CMV depend on the integrity of the host immune system. Immunocompromised individuals are at risk for severe infection and may present with complications such as myocarditis, hepatitis, pneumonitis, retinitis, and/or meningoencephalitis. In pregnant women, CMV infections are either subclinical or consist of mild nonspecific symptoms. Fever, flu-like symptoms, or mild hepatitis are more likely to occur in individuals with primary infections rather than reinfection or reactivation. The incubation period for CMV is 1–2 months.

Table 15–8. Clinical manifestations of cytomegalovirus.

Immunocompetent Adults	Fetal (Prenatal Ultrasound Findings)	Neonatal
No symptoms	Ventriculomegaly	Hepatosplenomegaly
Low-grade fever	Intracranial calcifications	Chorioretinitis
Flu-like symptoms	Microcephaly	Hearing loss
Mild hepatitis	Growth restriction	Thrombocytopenia
	Fetal hydrops	Hepatitis
	Echogenic bowel	Liver dysfunction
	Meconium peritonitis	Disseminated intravascular coagulation

B. Laboratory Findings

Maternal infection during pregnancy is diagnosed by serologic testing. Primary infection is confirmed in the setting of seroconversion of CMV-specific IgG in paired acute and convalescent sera. Serum samples are collected 3–4 weeks apart and tested in parallel for anti-CMV IgG. Seroconversion from negative to positive or a significant increase in anti-CMV IgG titers is consistent with infection. IgM titers are not reliable in diagnosing CMV because the sensitivity of CMV IgM assays ranges from 50–90%. Additionally, IgM titers can remain positive for more than a year and revert from negative to positive in women with reactivation or reinfection with a different strain. Positive IgM titers decline over a period of 30–60 days. When CMV-specific IgG and IgM are both positive, CMV IgG avidity testing can be performed to confirm primary CMV infection. A low-avidity CMV IgG test is suggestive of CMV infection occurring in the preceding 6 months. Alternatively, a high-avidity test virtually excludes the possibility of a primary CMV infection occurring within the previous 4 months. Avidity testing is performed in the United States by Focus Diagnostics, a reference laboratory in California. Figure 15–5 depicts a management strategy for suspected maternal CMV infection.

The diagnosis of CMV can also be made by PCR antigen identification and viral culture. The highest concentrations of virus are found in urine, seminal fluid, saliva, and breast milk. Although viral cultures can be positive within 72–96 hours, a minimum of 21 days is required before the culture is reported as negative.

The preferred method for diagnosing congenital CMV is via PCR identification of CMV in amniotic fluid. Sensitivities of PCR range from 70–100%. Data suggest that sensitivities are higher if the testing is performed after 21 weeks' gestation and after a 6-week lag time between maternal infection and the procedure. This period allows sufficient time for the virus to infect the placenta and fetus with subsequent replication of the virus in the fetal kidney followed by excretion into the amniotic fluid. Therefore, if an amniocentesis is performed soon after infection and returns negative, the procedure should be repeated later in pregnancy. Identification of the virus or the viral load in the amniotic fluid does not correlate with the severity of fetal injury.

C. Imaging Studies

Prenatal ultrasound may help diagnose congenital CMV. Sonographic findings concerning for severe injury include

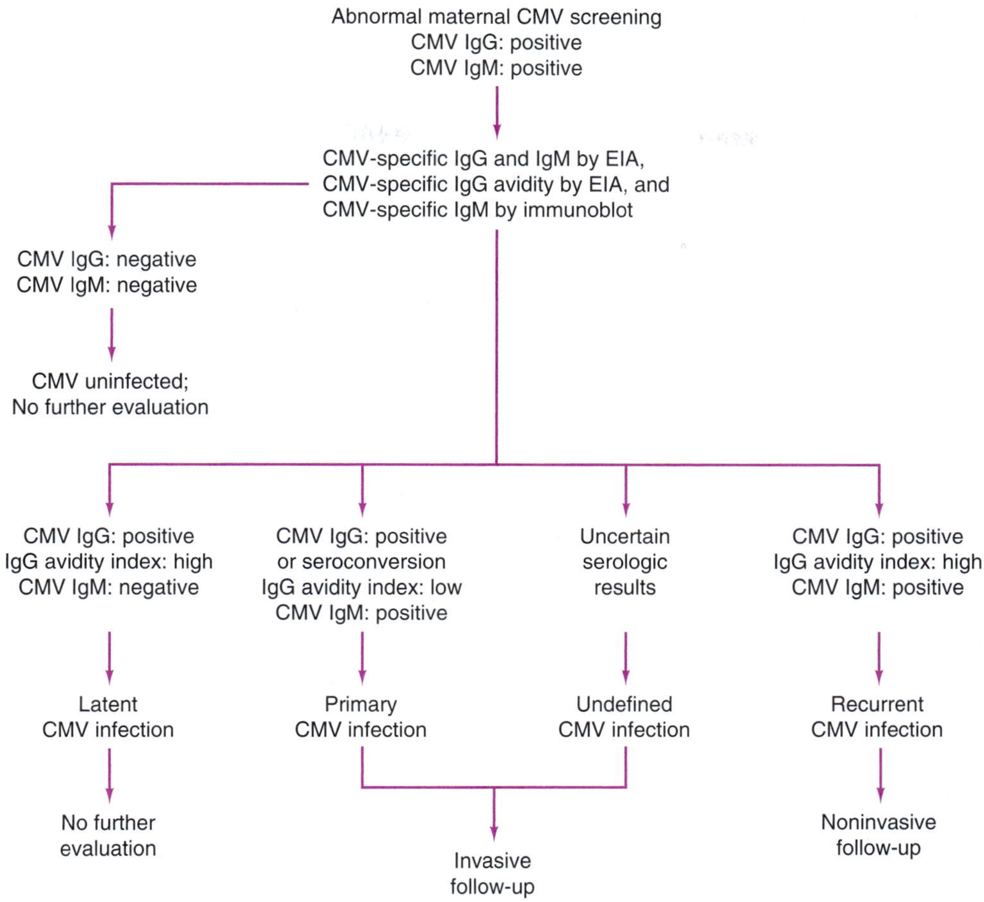

▲ **Figure 15–5.** Algorithm for evaluation of suspected maternal primary cytomegalovirus (CMV) infection in pregnancy. EIA, enzyme immunoassay; IgG, immunoglobulin G; IgM, immunoglobulin M. (Reproduced, with permission, from Cunningham FG, Leveno KJ, Bloom SL, Hauth JC, Rouse DJ, Spong CY. *Williams Obstetrics*, 23rd ed. http://www.accessmedicine.com. Copyright © The McGraw-Hill Companies, Inc. All rights reserved.)

microcephaly, ventriculomegaly, intracranial calcifications, hydrops, growth restriction, and oligohydramnios. Other ultrasound markers suggestive of infection include placentomegaly, echogenic bowel, meconium peritonitis, ascites, and pleural effusions. A normal ultrasound does not exclude the possibility of infection and sequelae.

Differential Diagnosis

Epstein-Barr virus
Acute hepatitis
Acute HIV
Human herpesvirus-6
Herpes simplex virus
Rubella
Enteroviral infections
Lymphocytic choriomeningitis virus
Toxoplasmosis

Complications

Congenital CMV is more likely in the setting of primary infection acquired earlier in the pregnancy. Approximately 5–15% of infants who develop congenital CMV are symptomatic at birth. Severe clinical manifestations include hepatosplenomegaly, intracranial calcifications, jaundice, growth restriction, microcephaly, chorioretinitis, hearing loss, thrombocytopenia, and hepatitis (Table 15–8). The most severely affected infants have a mortality rate of about 30%. Deaths are usually secondary to liver dysfunction, bleeding, disseminated intravascular coagulation, or secondary bacterial infections. Eighty percent of survivors have serious morbidity. Of the 85–90% of neonates who are asymptomatic at birth, 10–15% will develop hearing loss, chorioretinitis, or dental defects by the age of 2.

Treatment

Supportive therapy and symptomatic relief are recommended in infected immunocompetent pregnant women. Antiviral drugs, such as ganciclovir, should be used in immunocompromised patients with CMV because these medications decrease mortality and morbidity associated with serious CMV infections. Antiviral drugs have not been shown to decrease the risk of congenital CMV. Until recently, there has been no promising effective treatment for congenital CMV. More recent data suggest improved outcomes when using hyperimmune globulin as treatment and prophylaxis for congenital CMV infection. However, the study was limited in that it was neither randomized nor controlled, and therefore, its findings must be interpreted with caution.

Prognosis

Immunocompetent pregnant women with CMV have a favorable prognosis. However, congenital CMV poses a threat to infants and children and is, in fact, the most common congenital infection. It can be potentially devastating and is a major cause of permanent auditory, cognitive, and neurologic impairment.

Bodeus M, Kabamba-Mukadi B, Zech F, Hubinont C, Bernard P, Goubau P. Human cytomegalovirus in utero transmission: follow-up of 524 maternal seroconversions. *J Clin Virol* 2010;47:201–202. PMID: 20006542.

Cannon MJ. Congenital cytomegalovirus (CMV) epidemiology and awareness. *J Clin Virol* 2009;46(Suppl 4):S6–S10. PMID: 19800841.

Cannon MJ, Schmid DS, Hyde TB. Review of cytomegalovirus seroprevalence and demographic characteristics associated with infection. *Rev Med Virol* 2010;20:202–213. PMID: 20564615.

Cunningham FG, Leveno KJ, Bloom SL, Hauth JC, Rouse DJ, Spong CY. Chapter 58: infectious diseases. In Cunningham FG, Leveno KJ, Bloom SL, Hauth JC, Rouse DJ, Spong CY (eds). *Williams Obstetrics*. 23rd ed. http://www.accessmedicine.com/content/aspx?aID=6048859. Accessed October 30, 2010.

Duff P. Immunotherapy for congenital cytomegalovirus infection. *N Engl J Med* 2005;353:1402–1404. PMID: 16192488.

Duff P, Sweet R, Edwards R. Maternal and fetal infections. In Creasy RK, Resnik R, Iams J, et al (eds). *Creasy and Resnik's Maternal-Fetal Medicine: Principles and Practice*. 6th ed. Philadelphia, PA: Saunders Elsevier; 2009:764–766.

Focus Diagnostics Reference Laboratory Web Site. http://www.focusdx.com/focus/1-reference_laboratory/index.asp. Accessed November 18, 2010.

Guerra B, Simonazzi G, Banfi A, et al. Impact of diagnostic and confirmatory tests and prenatal counseling on the rate of pregnancy termination among women with positive cytomegalovirus immunoglobulin M antibody titers. *Am J Obstet Gynecol* 2007;196:221.e1–221.e6. PMID: 17346528.

Kanengisser-Pines B, Hazan Y, Pines G, Appelman Z. High cytomegalovirus IgG avidity is a reliable indicator of past infection in patients with positive IgM detected during the first trimester of pregnancy. *J Perinat Med* 2009;37:15–18. PMID: 18673093.

Kenneson A, Cannon MJ. Review and meta-analysis of the epidemiology of congenital cytomegalovirus (CMV) infection. *Rev Med Virol* 2007;17:253–276. PMID: 17579921.

Kylat RI, Kelly EN, Ford-Jones EL. Clinical findings and adverse outcome in neonates with symptomatic congenital cytomegalovirus (SCCMV) infection. *Eur J Pediatr* 2006;165:773–778. PMID: 16835757.

Malm G, Engman ML. Congenital cytomegalovirus infections. *Semin Fetal Neonatal Med* 2007;12:154–159. PMID: 17337260.

Nigro G, Adler SP, La Torre R, Best AM, Congenital Cytomegalovirus Collaborating Group. Passive immunization during pregnancy for congenital cytomegalovirus infection. *N Engl J Med* 2005;353:1350–1362. PMID: 16192480.

Ornoy A, Diav-Citrin O. Fetal effects of primary and secondary cytomegalovirus infection in pregnancy. *Reprod Toxicol* 2006;21:399–409. PMID: 16580941.

Sheffield JS, Boppana SB. Cytomegalovirus infection in pregnancy. In Wilkins-Haug L, Hirsch MS (eds). *UpToDate*. Waltham, MA: UpToDate; 2010. http://www.utdol.com. Accessed September 20, 2010.

TOXOPLASMOSIS

ESSENTIALS OF DIAGNOSIS

- Caused by an intracellular parasite
- Transmitted following consumption of undercooked meat or contact with oocysts from infected cat feces
- Clinical manifestations vary depending on the integrity of the immune system
- Diagnosis
  - Serologic testing in adults
  - DNA PCR of amniotic fluid for prenatal diagnosis
- Congenital toxoplasmosis: chorioretinitis, hydrocephalus, ventriculomegaly, and periventricular calcifications
- Treatment during pregnancy
  - Spiramycin therapy in women with documented acute toxoplasmosis
  - Therapy with pyrimethamine, sulfadiazine, and leucovorin if fetal diagnosis is confirmed

Pathogenesis

Toxoplasma gondii is an obligate intracellular parasite with 3 distinct life forms: trophozoite, cyst, and oocyst. Wild and domestic cats are the only known host for the oocyst. The oocyst is formed in the intestine and then shed in cat feces. The oocysts become infective 1–5 days later and may remain infectious for over a year. Other animals, such as cows, ingest the oocyst. The oocyst then becomes the invasive trophozoite, which then spreads throughout the body forming cysts in brain and muscle.

In developed countries, the prevalence of infection has declined over the last 30 years. Higher rates of infection are present in less developed countries and those with tropical climates where undercooked meats and unfiltered water are more prevalent. Ten to 50% of adults have evidence of previous infection. Maternal infection results from consumption of uncooked or undercooked meat or contact with oocysts from the feces of an infected cat. Following primary maternal infection, fetal infection occurs after transmission of parasites across the placenta. The trophozoite forms tissue cysts in the brain and muscle and can remain dormant for years.

About 50% of adults in the United States have developed immunity to *Toxoplasma*, and this immunity is generally lifelong, mediated by T lymphocytes, except in the case of immunocompromised patients. In the setting of primary infection, the overall rate of fetal infection is one-third. Although the risk of fetal infection increases with gestational age at seroconversion, severe infection is more likely with infection in the first trimester. The rate of vertical transmission increases from 10–15% in the first trimester, to 25% in the second trimester, and to more than 60% in the third trimester. Reinfection leading to congenital toxoplasmosis is exceedingly uncommon.

Prevention

Prevention of toxoplasmosis is extremely important in pregnancy. Pregnant women should avoid contact with cat litter. If cat litter is handled, gloves should be worn and hands should be thoroughly washed. Conscientious hand hygiene is also important following the preparation of meat. Fruits should be washed, and meat should be cooked thoroughly (to 152°F/66°C). Women should also avoid drinking unfiltered water and ingesting soil by observing strict hand hygiene after contact with soil.

Clinical Findings

A. Symptoms & Signs (Table 15–9)

Immunocompetent individuals with an acute infection may be either asymptomatic or present with vague nonspecific symptoms such as fatigue, fever, and myalgias. These patients may also present with lymphadenopathy. Immunocompromised patients, on the other hand, can have devastating consequences following infection. Neurologic dysfunction is not uncommon and includes encephalitis, meningoencephalitis, and intracerebral abscesses. Other manifestations include myocarditis and pneumonitis.

B. Laboratory Findings

Maternal diagnosis of toxoplasmosis is confirmed by serologic testing. Anti-*Toxoplasma* antibody can be detected using indirect fluorescent antibodies, indirect hemagglutination and agglutination tests, and ELISA. IgM-specific antibodies suggest acute infection. Diagnosis of an infection during pregnancy is most precise when 2 blood samples, greater than 2 weeks apart, document seroconversion from negative to positive *Toxoplasma*-specific IgM or IgG. In certain parts of Europe, women undergo serial testing with the goal of detecting early infection. However, the benefit of routine testing is controversial given the lack of data suggesting that treatment improves clinical outcomes. In the United States, diagnosis of a recent *Toxoplasma* infection is challenging in the setting of a single sample. IgM can remain positive for 10–13 months, and there is substantial variation among individuals. Twenty-five percent of women will have persistently positive IgM lasting years, and in certain patients, low IgG avidity will also remain positive for years. Rising IgG titers are also not useful due to the variation among laboratories. In the setting of a positive IgM and a negative IgG result with both tests positive 2 weeks later, recent infection is likely.

To confirm primary *Toxoplasma* infection, an avidity test for *Toxoplasma* IgG antibody is performed. In the

Table 15–9. Clinical manifestations of toxoplasmosis.

Immunocompetent Adults	Immunocompromised Adults	Fetal (Prenatal Ultrasound Findings)	Neonatal
No symptoms	Neurologic dysfunction: encephalitis, intracerebral abscesses	Ventriculomegaly	Hepatosplenomegaly
Fatigue	Myocarditis	Intracranial calcifications	Disseminated purpuric rash
Fever	Pneumonitis	Ascites	Chorioretinitis
Myalgia			Hearing loss
Lymphadenopathy			Neurologic dysfunction: seizures, mental retardation

setting of high-avidity IgG testing, infection within the previous 3–5 months is excluded. The functional avidity of IgG is low in the case of primary infection. In the United States, serologic diagnosis of an acute infection should be confirmed by the Palo Alto Medical Foundation Research Institute, a reference laboratory. The laboratory runs a panel of tests known as the Toxoplasma Serologic Profile, which includes the Sabin Feldman dye test, double-sandwich IgM ELISA, IgA and IgG ELISA, and a differential agglutination test.

The diagnosis of congenital toxoplasmosis is confirmed by identification of PCR toxoplasmic DNA in amniotic fluid. The sensitivity and specificity of real-time PCR are 92.2% and 100%, respectively. However, false-positive and false-negative tests do occur. Although the presence of *Toxoplasma*-specific IgM in fetal blood is extremely sensitive for diagnosis, due to the risk of fetal loss, cordocentesis is not widely used.

C. Imaging Studies

Ultrasonography is helpful in providing prognostic information. The most commonly noted abnormalities include intracranial calcifications and ventriculomegaly. These findings are usually seen after 21 weeks' gestation.

Differential Diagnosis

- CMV
- Disseminated tuberculosis
- Acute HIV
- Epstein-Barr virus (mononucleosis)
- Brain abscess
- Leukemia
- Lymphoma
- Pneumocystis pneumonia
- Progressive multifocal leukoencephalopathy
- Sarcoidosis
- Syphilis
- *Cryptococcus neoformans*
- *Aspergillus*

Complications

Although *Toxoplasma* infection is usually benign in immunocompetent pregnant women, infection in pregnancy can have serious consequences for the neonate. Approximately 3 per 1000 infants demonstrate evidence of congenital toxoplasmosis, with clinically significant infection present in 1 per 1000 pregnancies. Approximately 20% of neonates born to mothers with acute toxoplasmosis have clinical manifestations in infancy. These infants can present with hepatosplenomegaly, disseminated purpuric rash, ascites, and chorioretinitis. Central nervous system (CNS) manifestations include periventricular calcifications, ventriculomegaly, seizures, and mental retardation. The classic triad of congenital toxoplasmosis includes chorioretinitis, hydrocephalus, and periventricular calcifications.

Untreated asymptomatic infants at birth are at high risk for subsequently developing abnormalities. The most common delayed complication is chorioretinitis, which can result in vision loss. Additional sequelae that may manifest later in life include mental retardation, deafness, and seizures. Recent data do not suggest an association between congenital toxoplasmosis and reduced birth weight or small for gestational age infants.

Treatment

Toxoplasmosis infection in the immunocompetent adult is usually asymptomatic or self-limited and does not require treatment. Immunocompromised patients, on the other hand, should be treated with oral sulfadiazine and pyrimethamine.

Although there is no strong evidence demonstrating the efficacy of prenatal treatment, certain data suggest that prenatal therapy may reduce, but not eliminate, the risk of congenital infection. Therefore, therapy is usually offered to pregnant women diagnosed with acute infection. Treatment usually consists of spiramycin, a macrolide antibiotic that has the potential to concentrate in the placenta and, therefore, prevent fetal transmission. Because it does not cross the placenta, it is not used to treat fetal infection. Spiramycin is used commonly in Europe with favorable outcomes and is available in the United States through the CDC.

Pyrimethamine and sulfadiazine are folic acid antagonists that can be used to treat documented fetal infection. Pyrimethamine is teratogenic in animals, and both medications can cause bone marrow suppression. Due to the adverse effects of these medications, these drugs should only be used if fetal infection is confirmed. As of yet, there are no clinical trials to clearly demonstrate that the regimen is more effective than spiramycin. Leucovorin calcium (folinic acid) is added to the regimen to prevent bone marrow suppression. The efficacy and safety of other drugs such as azithromycin and clarithromycin in treating toxoplasmosis is currently under investigation.

Aggressive early treatment of neonates with congenital infection is recommended and includes therapy with pyrimethamine, sulfadiazine, and leucovorin for 1 year. Early therapy decreases the risk of late complications of toxoplasmosis.

Prognosis

Infection in immunocompetent women has a favorable prognosis. The prognosis of congenital toxoplasmosis is variable and depends on the clinical sequelae, which range from an asymptomatic state to severe neurologic morbidity.

Berrebi A, Assouline C, Bessieres MH, et al. Long-term outcome of children with congenital toxoplasmosis. *Am J Obstet Gynecol* 2010;203:552.e1–e6. PMID: 2063368.

Cortina-Borja M, Tan HK, Wallon M, et al. Prenatal treatment for serious neurological sequelae of congenital toxoplasmosis: an observational prospective cohort study. *PLoS Med* 2010;7(10):e1000351. PMID: 20967235.

Cunningham FG, Leveno KJ, Bloom SL, Hauth JC, Rouse DJ, Spong CY. Chapter 58: infectious diseases. In Cunningham FG, Leveno KJ, Bloom SL, Hauth JC, Rouse DJ, Spong CY (eds). *Williams Obstetrics*. 23rd ed. http://www.accessmedicine.com/content/aspx?aID=6048859. Accessed October 30, 2010.

Di Mario S, Basevi V, Gagliotti C, et al. Prenatal education for congenital toxoplasmosis. *Cochrane Database Syst Rev* 2009;1:CD006171. PMID: 19160267.

Duff P, Sweet R, Edwards R. Maternal and fetal infections. In Creasy RK, Resnik R, Iams J, et al (eds). *Creasy and Resnik's Maternal-Fetal Medicine: Principles and Practice*. 6th ed. Philadelphia, PA: Saunders Elsevier; 2009:782–783.

Feldman DM, Timms D, Borgida AF. Toxoplasmosis, parvovirus, and cytomegalovirus in pregnancy. *Clin Lab Med* 2010;30: 709–720. PMID: 20638583.

Galanakis E, Manoura A, Antoniou M, et al. Outcome of toxoplasmosis acquired during pregnancy following treatment in both pregnancy and early infancy. *Fetal Diagn Ther* 2007;22: 444–448. PMID: 17652934.

Gilbert R, Williams K. Toxoplasmosis and pregnancy. In Lockwood CJ, Weller PF (eds). *UpToDate*. Waltham, MA: UpToDate; 2010. http://www.utdol.com. Accessed September 20, 2010.

Gollub EL, Leroy V, Gilbert R, Chene G, Wallon M, European Toxoprevention Study Group (EUROTOXO). Effectiveness of health education on Toxoplasma-related knowledge, behaviour, and risk of seroconversion in pregnancy. *Eur J Obstet Gynecol Reprod Biol* 2008;136:137–145. PMID: 17977641.

Gras L, Wallon M, Pollak A, et al. Association between prenatal treatment and clinical manifestations of congenital toxoplasmosis in infancy: a cohort study in 13 European centres. *Acta Paediatr* 2005;94:1721–1731. PMID: 16420131.

Kodjikian L, Wallon M, Fleury J, et al. Ocular manifestations in congenital toxoplasmosis. *Graefes Arch Clin Exp Ophthalmol* 2006;244:14–21. PMID: 15906073.

Kravetz J. Congenital toxoplasmosis. *Clin Evid (Online)* 2008;2008:0906. PMID: 21418689.

Kur J, Holec-Gasior L, Hiszczynska-Sawicka E. Current status of toxoplasmosis vaccine development. *Expert Rev Vaccines* 2009;8:791–808. PMID: 19485758.

Lefevre-Pettazzoni M, Le Cam S, Wallon M, Peyron F. Delayed maturation of immunoglobulin G avidity: implication for the diagnosis of toxoplasmosis in pregnant women. *Eur J Clin Microbiol Infect Dis* 2006;25:687–693. PMID: 17024503.

Montoya JG, Remington JS. Management of Toxoplasma gondii infection during pregnancy. *Clin Infect Dis* 2008;47:554–566. PMID: 18624630.

Palo Alto Medical Foundation. Toxoplasma Serology Laboratory Web site. http://www.pamf.org/serology/clinicianguide.html. Accessed November 20, 2010.

Pappas G, Roussos N, Falagas ME. Toxoplasmosis snapshots: global status of Toxoplasma gondii seroprevalence and implications for pregnancy and congenital toxoplasmosis. *Int J Parasitol* 2009;39:1385–1394. PMID: 19433092.

SYROCOT (Systematic Review on Congenital Toxoplasmosis) Study Group, Thiebaut R, Leproust S, Chene G, Gilbert R. Effectiveness of prenatal treatment for congenital toxoplasmosis: a meta-analysis of individual patients' data. *Lancet* 2007;369:115–122. PMID: 17223474.

Thalib L, Gras L, Romand S, et al. Prediction of congenital toxoplasmosis by polymerase chain reaction analysis of amniotic fluid. *BJOG* 2005;112:567–574. PMID: 15842278.

Villena I, Ancelle T, Delmas C, et al. Congenital toxoplasmosis in France in 2007: first results from a national surveillance system. *Euro Surveill* 2010;15:19600. PMID: 20587361.

LISTERIA

ESSENTIALS OF DIAGNOSIS

- Caused by gram-positive motile *Bacillus*
- Preventive measures: thoroughly cooking raw meets, washing raw vegetables, avoiding unpasteurized foods
- Clinical manifestations in healthy pregnant women: asymptomatic, vague, flu-like symptoms including fever, chills, malaise, and myalgias
- Complications in pregnancy: fetal death, premature delivery, neonatal infection
- Diagnosis: cultures on blood, amniotic fluid, placenta
- Treatment: penicillin/ampicillin with or without gentamicin for synergistic effect

Pathogenesis

Listeria monocytogenes is a food-borne gram-positive motile **Bacillus** capable of causing life-threatening infections in humans. It is a facultative intracellular parasite that primarily inhabits soil and decaying vegetative matter. Animals carrying the organism contaminate foods of animal origin such as meat and dairy products. Although there are multiple species of *Listeria*, *L monocytogenes* is the only species that is considered pathogenic in humans. The organism's virulence is attributed to listeriolysin O, a pore-forming toxin, that enables the pathogen to suppress antigen-induced T-cell activation. Most *Listeria* infections in adults are due to oral ingestion followed by intestinal mucosal penetration and subsequent systemic infection.

Annually, there are approximately 1600 cases of listeriosis in the United States, with a 16% mortality rate. About 1 in 6 cases of listeriosis occurs during pregnancy. Recent data show that the overall incidence of listeriosis is decreasing, with a 26% decrease noted by the CDC from 1998 to 2009. Human listeriosis can occur as either a sporadic illness or an epidemic. The sporadic form occurs more commonly than the epidemic form (responsible for >95% of cases).

The epidemic form is due to widespread contamination of food products. High-risk foods include unpasteurized soft cheeses, processed/delicatessen meats, hot dogs, smoked seafood, and pâtés. Several outbreaks of listeriosis in the United States have been associated with Mexican-style soft cheeses made from unpasteurized milk.

Although *L monocytogenes* can be isolated from the feces of 1–5% of healthy adults, systemic infections usually occur in individuals with predisposing conditions such as pregnancy, old age, and immunocompromised states. Decreased cell-mediated immunity in pregnancy is believed to be the cause of increased susceptibility of pregnant women to listeriosis. Subsequent fetal and/or neonatal infection most likely occurs from hematogenous dissemination of the organism through the placenta, although ascending infection from cervical colonization with *L monocytogenes* may also play a role.

Prevention

Prevention of *Listeria* infections is important on a legislative as well as individual level. Government agencies such as the US Department of Agriculture (USDA) have instituted policy changes to reduce *L monocytogenes* contamination. Large-scale producers of ready-to-eat meat have been required to develop *L monocytogenes* control programs and institute various measures such as postpackaging pasteurization.

Individuals can prevent infection with *Listeria* by following certain recommendations. Recommendations include thoroughly cooking raw meats; carefully washing raw vegetables; avoiding unpasteurized milk or products made from unpasteurized milk; keeping uncooked meats and poultry separate from vegetables and from cooked foods and ready-to-eat foods; washing hands, knives, countertops, and cutting boards after handling and preparing uncooked foods; and consuming perishable and ready-to-eat foods as soon as possible. Pregnant women should also avoid soft cheeses such as feta, brie, and queso fresco and delicatessen meats.

Clinical Findings

A. Symptoms & Signs

In immunocompromised, elderly, and pregnant patients, *Listeria* can lead to invasive disease, such as meningitis and sepsis. In healthy adults, if ingested in high numbers, the organism can cause febrile gastroenteritis. The incubation period for *Listeria* is generally 6–90 days, but may be only 24 hours during widespread epidemics of gastroenteritis.

Listeriosis in pregnancy is most common in the third trimester. Although many pregnant infected women are asymptomatic, about two-thirds manifest nonspecific flu-like symptoms characterized by fever, chills, myalgias, malaise, and upper respiratory complaints. Infection is usually mild and self-limited, but pregnant women may present with signs and symptoms of sepsis. Listerial CNS infection in pregnancy is generally rare. Maternal listeriosis can lead to serious consequences such as fetal death, premature delivery, and neonatal infection.

B. Laboratory Findings

There are no specific clinical manifestations that help distinguish listeriosis from other infections that manifest with fever and nonspecific flu-like symptoms. Therefore, blood cultures are necessary in establishing the diagnosis. Routine cerebrospinal fluid analysis is limited because pregnant women do not usually present with CNS infections. Although routine stool cultures are not helpful in diagnosing systemic listeriosis, stool cultures using selective media may be valuable in patients with *Listeria* gastroenteritis. Amniocentesis may be performed to help diagnose fetal listerial infection. Additionally, cultures obtained from the uterus or placenta may also establish the diagnosis.

C. Imaging Studies

Magnetic resonance imaging (MRI) is superior to computed tomography scan for detecting *Listeria* lesions in the CNS. It is recommended that patients with *Listeria* meningitis or systemic listeriosis with CNS signs and symptoms undergo an MRI.

Differential Diagnosis

Maternal

Influenza

Urinary tract infection

Pyelonephritis

Meningitis

Fetal

Group B *Streptococcus*

Escherichia coli

Klebsiella pneumoniae

Complications

Maternal listeriosis is associated with fetal loss, premature delivery, neonatal infection, and neonatal death. In a review of 222 cases of maternal infection, the pregnancy was complicated by abortion or stillbirth in 20% of cases, while neonatal sepsis resulted in 68% of surviving neonates. Neonatal listeriosis has been divided into 2 distinct clinical and serologic entities: early-onset and late-onset disease. Early-onset disease occurs in infants infected in utero with signs of infection presenting soon after birth; it presents as diffuse sepsis with multiorgan involvement including liver, lungs, and CNS. Early-onset disease is associated with a high rate of fetal demise and neonatal mortality. Granulomatosis infantiseptica refers to a severe in utero infection in which disseminated abscesses and/or granulomas are present in multiple internal organs. Late-onset neonatal disease presents in term infants who present with signs and symptoms of infection days to weeks after delivery. These neonates usually present with meningitis and long-term neurologic sequelae such as mental retardation. Intrapartum transmission or nosocomial infection after delivery is usually responsible for late-onset disease. Both types of neonatal listeriosis are associated with a high neonatal mortality rate.

Treatment

Parenteral ampicillin or penicillin G is the recommended antibiotic regimen for treatment of listeriosis. Listerial microbial resistance to penicillins or derivatives of penicillins has not been described under natural conditions. Dose and duration of therapy depend on age and type of infection. Pregnant women are usually treated with ampicillin 2 g intravenously every 4–6 hours; this dose provides adequate transplacental penetration. Optimal duration of therapy in pregnancy has not been established and varies between 2 and 4 weeks. When complicated listerial infections are present—involving the CNS, endocarditis, or infections in neonates and immunocompromised adults—gentamicin may be added to ampicillin for a synergistic effect. Trimethoprim-sulfamethoxazole is effective in patients allergic to penicillins.

Prognosis

Although maternal prognosis after listerial infection is generally favorable, fetal and neonatal infection can be severe with perinatal case fatality rates ranging from 22–45%. Listeriosis carries a poorer prognosis for fetuses affected at earlier gestations. Prompt diagnosis and proper antibiotic therapy can significantly reduce the fetal and neonatal complications associated with maternal listeriosis.

Allerberger F, Wagner M. Listeriosis: a resurgent foodborne infection. *Clin Microbiol Infect* 2010;16:16–23. PMID: 20002687.

Bennion JR, Sorvillo F, Wise ME, Krishna S, Mascola L. Decreasing listeriosis mortality in the United States, 1990–2005. *Clin Infect Dis* 2008;47:867–874. PMID: 18752441.

Centers for Disease Control and Prevention (CDC). Preliminary FoodNet data on the incidence of infection with pathogens transmitted commonly through food–10 states, 2009. *MMWR Morb Mortal Wkly Rep* 2010;59:418–422. PMID: 20395935.

Cunningham FG, Leveno KJ, Bloom SL, Hauth JC, Rouse DJ, Spong CY. Chapter 58: infectious diseases. In Cunningham FG, Leveno KJ, Bloom SL, Hauth JC, Rouse DJ, Spong CY (eds). *Williams Obstetrics*. 23rd ed. http://www.accessmedicine.com/content/aspx?aID=6049068. Accessed June 1, 2010.

Duff P, Sweet R, Edwards R. Maternal and fetal infections. In Creasy RK, Resnik R, Iams J, et al (eds). *Creasy and Resnik's Maternal-Fetal Medicine: Principles and Practice*. 6th ed. Philadelphia, PA: Saunders Elsevier; 2009:773.

Gelfand M. Epidemiology and pathogenesis of Listeria monocytogenes infection. In Sexton DJ, Edwards MS (eds). *UpToDate*. Waltham, MA: UpToDate; 2011. http://www.utdol.com. Accessed June 1, 2011.

Gekara NO, Zietara N, Geffers R, Weiss S. Listeria monocytogenes induces T cell receptor unresponsiveness through pore-forming toxin listeriolysin O. *J Infect Dis* 2010;202:1698–1707. PMID: 20961225.

Gelfand M. Clinical manifestations and diagnosis of Listeria monocytogenes infection. In Sexton DJ, Kaplan MD (eds). *UpToDate*. Waltham, MA: UpToDate; 2011. http://www.utdol.com. Accessed June 1, 2011.

Gottlieb SL, Newbern EC, Griffin PM, et al. Multistate outbreak of listeriosis linked to turkey deli meat and subsequent changes in US regulatory policy. *Clin Infect Dis* 2006;42:29–36. PMID: 16323088.

Jackson KA, Iwamoto M, Swerdlow D. Pregnancy-associated listeriosis. *Epidemiol Infect* 2010;138:1503–1509. PMID: 20158931.

Janakiraman V. Listeriosis in pregnancy: diagnosis, treatment, and prevention. *Rev Obstet Gynecol* 2008;1:179–185. PMID: 19173022.

Lamont RF, Sobel J, Mazaki-Tovi, S, et al. Listeriosis in human pregnancy: a systematic review. *J Perinat Med* 2011;39:227–236. PMID: 21517700.

MacDonald PD, Whitwam RE, Boggs JD, et al. Outbreak of listeriosis among Mexican immigrants as a result of consumption of illicitly produced Mexican-style cheese. *Clin Infect Dis* 2005;40:677–682. PMID: 15714422.

Mylonakis E, Paliou M, Hohmann EL, Calderwood SB, Wing EJ. Listeriosis during pregnancy: a case series and review of 222 cases. *Medicine (Baltimore)* 2002;81:260–269. PMID: 12169881.

16 Disproportionate Fetal Growth

Jeannine Rahimian, MD, MBA

Weight at delivery once was considered evidence of prematurity (birthweight <2500 g) or postmaturity (macrosomia; birthweight >4500 g). These criteria later were revised upon the realization that birthweight can be reflective of other pathologic processes aside from prematurity. Abnormalities in fetal growth at each end of the spectrum—both large for gestational age fetuses and fetuses with suspected intrauterine growth restriction—are associated with an increased risk of adverse perinatal outcome. Normative standards applying to such ultrasound parameters as estimated fetal weight, abdominal circumference, and head circumference (HC) were developed.

Abnormal fetal growth or fetal size is most commonly defined on the basis of estimated fetal weight. Fetuses with an estimated fetal weight ≤ the 10th percentile are classified as having intrauterine growth restriction (IUGR), and those with a weight ≥ the 90th percentile are classified as large for gestational age (LGA). Both IUGR and LGA fetuses have increased risk for perinatal morbidity and mortality (Tables 16–1 and 16–2). The pathogenesis, differential diagnosis, and treatment are different for the 2 extremes of growth.

INTRAUTERINE GROWTH RESTRICTION

ESSENTIALS OF DIAGNOSIS

- Estimated fetal weight less than the 10th percentile for gestational age on ultrasound

Many terms have been used to describe fetuses with disproportionately small growth. **Intrauterine growth restriction** (IUGR) is used to designate a *fetus* that has not met its growth potential and is defined as estimated fetal weight (EFW) at or below the 10th percentile for gestational age. **Small for gestational age** (SGA) is a term that applies to the *infant* that is less than the 10th percentile at birth.

Pathogenesis

Approximately 70% of fetuses with EFW below the 10th percentile are simply constitutionally small; thus, the term IUGR is inaccurate for many fetuses. Distinguishing between normal and pathologic growth can be difficult, but a fetus with normal anatomy, normal amniotic fluid volume, and normal growth pattern over time will generally be constitutionally small rather than IUGR. Some nonpathologic factors that affect fetal birthweight are maternal height, paternal height, parity, ethnicity, and fetal sex.

A classification of IUGR pregnancy delineated by cause is given in Table 16–3. Any inference of suboptimal growth requires, by definition, serial observations. It cannot be emphasized too strongly that a pregnancy cannot be described as IUGR unless the gestational age is known with certainty.

Compared with an appropriate for gestational age (AGA) fetus, the IUGR fetus has altered body composition (including decreased body fat, total protein, whole body DNA and RNA, glycogen, and free fatty acids), altered distribution of weight among organs, and altered body proportions. Approximately 20% of IUGR infants are symmetrically small, with a relatively proportionate decrease in many organ weights. Eighty percent are asymmetrically small, with relative sparing of brain weight, especially when compared with that of the liver or thymus.

Numerous authors have differentiated between symmetric and asymmetric IUGR pregnancy in terms of cause and prognosis. *Symmetric IUGR* refers to infants in which all organs are decreased proportionally. Symmetric IUGR infants are more likely to have an endogenous defect that results in impairment of early fetal cellular hyperplasia. Symmetric IUGR infants have proportionately small brains, usually because of a decreased number of brain cells.

Table 16–1. Some complications associated with intrauterine growth restriction pregnancy.

Maternal Complications Complications due to underlying disease, preeclampsia, premature labor, caesarean delivery
Fetal Complications Stillbirth, hypoxia and acidosis, malformations
Neonatal Complications Hypoglycemia, hypocalcemia, hypoxia and acidosis, hypothermia, meconium aspiration syndrome, polycythemia, congenital malformations, sudden infant death syndrome
Long-Term Complications Lower IQ, learning and behavior problems, major neurologic handicaps (seizure disorders, cerebral palsy, mental retardation), hypertension

Although this may be the result of early, severe nutritional deprivation, the cause is more often a genetic disorder, infection, or other problem. Usually the thymus is small, with an average decrease of 25%. This decrease may explain in part the decreased cellular immunity seen in IUGR infants.

Asymmetric IUGR refers to infants in which organs are decreased disproportionately (abdominal circumference is affected to a greater degree than is HC). Asymmetric IUGR more likely is caused by intrauterine deprivation that results in redistribution of flow to the brain and heart at the expense of less important organs, such as the liver and kidneys. In asymmetric IUGR infants, brain weight is decreased only slightly compared with that of AGA controls, primarily as a result of decreased brain cell size and not because of decreased brain cell numbers. Cerebral abnormalities include decreased myelination, decreased utilization of metabolic substrates other than glucose, and altered protein synthesis. In experimental animals, these changes are more likely to produce adverse effects in the brain stem and cerebellum.

Table 16–2. Some complications of large for gestational age pregnancy.

Maternal Complications Caesarean section, postpartum hemorrhage, shoulder dystocia, perineal trauma, operative vaginal delivery
Fetal Complications Stillbirth, anomalies, shoulder dystocia
Neonatal Complications Low Apgar score, hypoglycemia, birth injury, hypocalcemia, polycythemia, jaundice, feeding difficulties
Long-Term Complications Obesity, type 2 diabetes, neurologic or behavioral problems

Table 16–3. Pathogenic classification of intrauterine growth restriction pregnancy.

A. Fetoplacental Causes
Genetic disorders
Autosomal: trisomy 13, 18, 21; ring chromosomes; chromosomal deletions; partial trisomies, partial deletions
Sex chromosomes: Turner's syndrome, multiple chromosomes (XXX, XYY)
Neural tube defects
Skeletal dysplasias: achondroplasia, chondrodystrophies, osteogenesis imperfecta
Abdominal wall defects
Other rare syndromes
Congenital infection
Viral: cytomegalovirus, rubella, herpes, varicella-zoster
Protozoan: toxoplasmosis, malaria
Bacterial: listeriosis
Placental disorders: placenta previa, placental infarction, chorionic villitis, chronic partial separation, placental malformations (circumvallate placenta, battledore placenta, placental hemangioma, twin-twin transfusion syndrome)
Multiple gestation
B. Maternal Factors
Coexistent maternal disease: hypertension, anemia (hemoglobinopathy, decreased normal hemoglobin [especially <12 g/dL]), renal disease (hypertension, protein loss), malnutrition (inflammatory bowel disease [ulcerative colitis, regional enteritis], pancreatitis, intestinal parasites), cyanotic cardiopulmonary disease
Substance abuse/drugs: alcohol, cigarette smoking, cocaine, heroin, warfarin, folic acid antagonists (methotrexate, aminopterin), anticonvulsants
Small maternal stature

This differential sparing is particularly prominent when deprivation occurs in the latter half of pregnancy. Deprivation early in pregnancy is associated with less cerebral sparing and diffusely slowed brain growth.

Although this classification is helpful in establishing a differential diagnosis and framework for discussion, it is not sufficiently precise to serve as a basis for decisions regarding intervention or viability.

A number of etiologies have been shown to have an association with IUGR, either symmetric or asymmetric.

A. Fetoplacental Causes

1. Congenital abnormalities—Genetic disorders account for approximately one-third of IUGR infants. The frequency of IUGR in chromosomally abnormal infants ranges from 20 to 60%, and the risk of an IUGR infant having a major congenital anomaly is 10%. An infant with an autosomal trisomy is more likely to be IUGR. The most common trisomy is **trisomy 21** (**Down syndrome**), with an incidence of 1.6 per 1000 live births. At term, such infants weigh an average of 350 g less than comparable normal infants and are 4 times more likely to be IUGR. This decrease is most apparent in the last 6 weeks of pregnancy. A similar decrease in birthweight occurs in translocation Down syndrome, whereas mosaic Down syndrome is associated with an intermediate decrease in birthweight.

The second most common autosomal trisomy is **trisomy 18** (**Edwards' syndrome**), which occurs in 1 in 6000–8000 live births. Eighty-four percent of these infants are IUGR. Ultrasound evaluation may reveal associated anomalies. The condition is associated with an increased likelihood of breech presentation, polyhydramnios, fetal neural tube defects, and visceral anomalies. The average birthweight of infants with trisomy 18 is almost 1000 g less than that of controls. In contrast to the placental weight in infants with trisomies 13 and 21, the placental weight in infants with trisomy 18 also is markedly reduced.

Trisomy 13 occurs in 1 in 5000–10,000 live births. More than 50% of affected infants have IUGR. Birthweights average 700–800 g less than those of controls.

Other more rare autosomal chromosome abnormalities, such as ring chromosomes, deletions, and partial trisomies, are associated with an increased likelihood of IUGR. Sex chromosome abnormalities may be associated with lower birthweight. Extra X chromosomes (>2) are associated with a 200-g to 300-g decrease in birthweight for each extra X. **Turner's syndrome** is associated with an average birthweight of approximately 400 g below average. Fetuses with mosaic Turner's syndrome are intermediately affected.

Growth impairment as a result of fetal chromosome abnormalities usually occurs earlier than impairment caused by placental abnormalities. However, there is considerable clinical overlap, so gestational age at the time of diagnosis is not always of clinical value.

Fetuses with neural tube defects frequently are IUGR, weighing approximately 250 g less than controls. Anencephalic fetuses are IUGR, even considering the absent brain and skull, with average third-trimester birthweights of approximately 1000 g less than matched controls. Certain dysmorphic syndromes are associated with an increased incidence of IUGR fetuses. **Achondroplasia** may be associated with low birthweight if either parent is affected but usually is associated with normal birthweight if a spontaneous mutation is the cause. **Osteogenesis imperfecta** consists of a spectrum of diseases, all of which result in IUGR fetuses.

Infants born with abdominal wall defects are characteristically IUGR, particularly those with **gastroschisis**.

Other autosomal recessive syndromes associated with IUGR include **Smith-Lemli-Opitz syndrome, Meckel's syndrome, Robert's syndrome, Donohue's syndrome,** and **Seckel's syndrome.** These conditions are rare and are most likely to be diagnosed antepartum in families with a previously affected child. Infants with renal anomalies such as renal agenesis (**Potter's syndrome**) or complete urinary tract outflow obstruction often have IUGR.

Other congenital anomalies associated with an increased incidence of IUGR outcome are **duodenal atresia** and **pancreatic agenesis**.

2. Congenital infections—(See also Chapter 15, Congenital Fetal Infections, for more discussion.) Chronic intrauterine infection is responsible for 5–10% of IUGR pregnancies (Table 16–3). The most commonly identified pathogen is cytomegalovirus (CMV). Although CMV can be isolated from 0.5 to 2% of all newborns in the United States, clinically obvious infection at the time of birth affects only 0.2–2 in 1000 live births. Active fetoplacental infection is characterized by cytolysis, followed by secondary inflammation, fibrosis, and calcification. Only infants with clinically apparent infection at birth are likely to be IUGR. Signs of congenital infection are nonspecific but include central nervous system involvement (eg, microcephaly), chorioretinitis, intracranial (periventricular) calcifications, pneumonitis, hepatosplenomegaly, and thrombocytopenia.

Congenital rubella infection increases the risk of IUGR. Infection in the first trimester results in the most severely affected fetuses, primarily as a result of microvascular endothelial damage. Such infants are likely to have structural cardiovascular and central nervous system defects such as microcephaly, deafness, glaucoma, and cataracts.

Other viruses implicated in causing IUGR are herpesvirus, varicella-zoster virus, influenza virus, and poliovirus, but the number of such cases is small. As expected by virtue of their chronic, indolent nature, protozoan infections are associated with IUGR. The most common protozoan, *Toxoplasma gondii,* usually is acquired by ingestion of raw meat. Only women with a primary infection are at risk for having an affected infant. The average incidence is 1 in 1000 live births in the United States, but the incidence varies widely among locations and social populations. Approximately 20% of newborns with congenital toxoplasmosis will have IUGR. Malaria is another protozoan infection associated with IUGR.

Although bacterial infections occur commonly in pregnancy and frequently are implicated in premature delivery, they are not commonly associated with IUGR. Chronic infection from *Listeria monocytogenes* is an exception. Infants usually are critically ill at the time of delivery and often have encephalitis, pneumonitis, myocarditis, hepatosplenomegaly, jaundice, and petechiae.

3. Placental factors—The placenta plays an important role in normal fetal growth. Placental weight has shown to be less with IUGR fetuses than with AGA fetuses, suggesting that appropriate fetal growth may depend on the size or weight of the placenta. Several placental abnormalities are associated with an increased likelihood of an IUGR fetus.

Placenta previa is associated with an increased incidence of IUGR, probably because of the unfavorable site of placental implantation. Complete placenta previa is associated with a higher incidence of IUGR than is partial placenta previa. Decreased functional exchange area as a result of **placental infarction** also is associated with an increased incidence of IUGR fetuses. **Premature placental separation** or varying degrees of placental abruption may occur at any time during pregnancy, with variable effects. When not associated with fetal death or premature labor, premature placental separation may increase the risk of IUGR. Malformations of the placenta or umbilical cord, such as **single umbilical artery (UA), velamentous umbilical cord insertion, circumvallate placenta, placental hemangioma, battledore placenta,** and **twin-twin transfusion syndrome,** also are associated with an increased risk of IUGR. **Chronic villitis,** chronic inflammation of placental villi, is seen with increased frequency when the placentas of IUGR pregnancies are examined histologically. Finally, **uterine anomalies** may be associated with impaired fetal growth, primarily because of suboptimal uterine blood flow.

4. Multiple gestation—Multiple gestation has long been associated with premature delivery. However, it also is associated with a 20–30% increased incidence of IUGR fetuses, most often as a result of placental insufficiency, twin-twin transfusion syndrome, preeclampsia, or anomalies. Fetal growth has a direct relationship to the number of fetuses present and the type of placentation (monochorionic vs. dichorionic). Serial ultrasound estimates of fetal weights should be considered in a multiple gestation pregnancy.

B. Maternal Factors

Numerous maternal diseases are associated with suboptimal fetal growth. Any woman who has borne 1 IUGR fetus is at increased risk for recurrence, with a 2-fold and 4-fold increased risk for IUGR birth after 1 or 2 IUGR births, respectively.

1. Hypertension—Hypertension is the most common maternal complication causing IUGR. Systemic hypertension results in decreased blood flow through the spiral arterioles and decreased delivery of oxygen and nutrients to the placenta and fetus. Hypertension may be associated with placental infarction.

2. Drugs—Both social drugs and prescribed medications can affect fetal growth. **Alcohol** use has long been known to be associated with impaired fetal growth. Virtually all infants with fetal alcohol syndrome exhibit signs of growth restriction.

Cigarette smoking is much more common among women of childbearing age in the United States than is alcoholism. Smoking causes one-third of IUGR cases and is the single most preventable cause of IUGR pregnancy in the United States today. Women who smoke have a 3-fold to 4-fold increase in IUGR infants. Birthweight is reduced by approximately 200 g, with the amount of growth restriction proportional to the number of cigarettes smoked per day. Women who quit smoking at 7 months' gestation have newborns with higher mean birthweights than do women who smoke throughout the entire pregnancy. Women who stop smoking before 16 weeks' gestation are not at increased risk for having an IUGR fetus.

Heroin and cocaine are also associated with an increased risk of IUGR, but confounding variables make determination of a direct cause-and-effect relationship difficult. Methadone use has not been shown to be associated with an increased incidence of IUGR.

Pharmacologic agents have been associated with an increased incidence of IUGR, primarily as a result of teratogenic effects. Warfarin has been associated with an increased incidence of IUGR, primarily as a result of the sequelae of intrauterine hemorrhage. Folic acid antagonists are associated with an increased risk of spontaneous abortion stillbirth, severe malformations, and IUGR.

IUGR fetuses are more common with maternally administered immunosuppressive drugs (eg, cyclosporine, azathioprine, corticosteroids), but when controlled for the underlying maternal disease, the medications per se probably have little effect on fetal growth. Furthermore, β-blockers are also associated with an increased risk of IUGR.

3. Malnutrition and malabsorption—Maternal weight at birth, prepregnancy weight, and weight gain during pregnancy account for 10% of the variance in fetal weight and increase the risk of delivering an infant <2500 g. Studies of infants borne by women who were pregnant during the Siege of Leningrad during World War II showed that daily intake must be reduced to <1500 kcal/d before a measurable effect on birthweight becomes evident. Maternal **malabsorption** may predispose to IUGR pregnancy. The most common clinical situations are inflammatory bowel disease (ulcerative colitis or regional enteritis), pancreatitis, and intestinal parasites. **Maternal eating disorders** such as bulimia and anorexia are also associated with IUGR.

4. Vascular disease and hypoxemia—Diseases that affect maternal microvascular perfusion can be associated with IUGR. These include collagen vascular disease, insulin-dependent diabetes mellitus associated with microvasculopathy, and preeclampsia. Also, chronic maternal hypoxemia due to pulmonary disease or cyanotic heart disease is associated with growth restriction.

5. Maternal features—A small woman may have a smaller-than-normal infant because of reduced growth potential. These mothers and infants are completely normal and healthy, but they are constitutionally small because of genetic variation. The ponderal index (PI) can be used to evaluate whether an infant is simply constitutionally small or is affected by IUGR. The PI is calculated using the following formula:

$$PI = [\text{Weight (in g)} \times 100]/[\text{length (in cm)}]^3$$

Infants affected by asymmetric IUGR will have a low PI (ie, they will be long, lightweight infants with a PI below the 10th percentile), whereas small normal infants will have a normal PI.

Women who were SGA at birth have a 2-fold increase in risk of IUGR in their offspring.

Maternal parity exerts a modest effect on birthweight. First-born infants tend to be smaller and more often categorized as IUGR. This effect decreases with successive deliveries and is not seen beyond the third birth.

6. Sex of fetus—At term, female fetuses are an average 5% (150 g) smaller and 2% (1 cm) shorter than male fetuses. Referring to separate norms for male and female fetuses may increase the power of biometry in assessing IUGR.

Prevention

Because many causes of IUGR are not preventable, few interventions have proved effective for prevention. Interventions that have shown benefit include smoking cessation, antimalarial chemoprophylaxis, and balanced protein and energy supplementation. Smoking is the single most common preventable cause of IUGR in infants born in the United States. As discussed in Maternal Factors, women who quit smoking at 7 months' gestation have newborns with higher mean birthweights than do women who smoke throughout the pregnancy. Women who quit smoking before 16 weeks' gestation are not at any increased risk for an IUGR infant. Limited data suggest that **balanced nutritional supplementation** improves mean birthweight. As expected, such supplementation more likely will benefit those with poor nutrition or adolescent pregnancies. Pregnant women should avoid close contact with individuals known to be infected or colonized with rubella virus or CMV. Nonpregnant women of reproductive age should be tested for immunity to rubella virus and, if susceptible, should be immunized prior to conception. Currently no vaccine exists for CMV.

Women of childbearing age should be tested for immunity to *T gondii* if this protozoan infection is clinically suspected. If the woman is immune, her risk of having an affected infant is remote. However, if she is susceptible, she should be cautioned to avoid cat feces and uncooked meat. If the screening immunoglobulin M (IgM) for *Toxoplasma* is positive, no action should be taken based on this result without confirmation by a regional reference laboratory with expertise in *Toxoplasma* testing.

Therapeutic medications are not a major cause of IUGR pregnancy, but benefits and risks should be weighed whenever medications are prescribed. Any woman of childbearing age should be questioned about the possibility of pregnancy before receiving therapeutic or diagnostic radiation to the pelvis.

Placental factors causing IUGR pregnancies are not generally preventable. It has been postulated that low-dose aspirin and dipyridamole may increase prostacyclin production in certain patients and thus prevent idiopathic uteroplacental insufficiency. The role of these agents in preventing IUGR resulting from placental insufficiency in at-risk populations is unclear at this time.

Preventive measures for the maternal diseases listed in Table 16–3 are beyond the scope of this chapter. Treatment of many of these conditions may decrease the likelihood of IUGR pregnancy. Treatment of hypertension has a positive effect on birthweight, at least in the third trimester. However, strict bed rest and hospitalization do not seem to have any beneficial effects for patients with a history of hypertension. Although a complex issue, protein supplements for patients with significant proteinuria may increase the amount of protein available for placental transfer. Correction of maternal anemia (of whatever cause) improves oxygen delivery to the fetus, thus improving fetal growth. However, routine supplements, such as with iron, have not been shown to be associated with any altered clinical outcomes.

Treatment of malabsorption syndrome (of whatever cause) can be expected to improve nutrient absorption and subsequent nutrient transfer to the fetus. Inflammatory bowel disease should be treated if required, but if possible, pregnancy should be deferred until the disease has been quiescent for approximately 6 months. Intestinal parasites should be appropriately treated and negative cultures confirmed prior to pregnancy.

Clinical Findings

A. Ultrasound Evaluation of Estimated Fetal Weight

The diagnosis of IUGR is made when biometric parameters on ultrasound indicate that the EFW is less than the 10th percentile for gestational age. In any pregnancy at risk for IUGR, baseline ultrasound studies should be obtained early in gestation. Careful attention should always be given to gestational dating (menstrual history, serial examinations, biochemical pregnancy testing, quickening, ultrasound). An IUGR outcome, however, may develop in pregnancies without identified risk factors. For some pregnancies, the first sign of IUGR may be a lagging fundal height on clinical examination. If the fundal height varies from the assigned gestational age by more than 2 cm, ultrasound is indicated to assess the EFW and amniotic fluid volume. Careful attention to fundal height measurement is associated with 46–86% sensitivity for detecting IUGR.

Ultrasound examination early in pregnancy is accurate in establishing the estimated date of confinement (EDC) and may sometimes identify genetic or congenital causes of IUGR pregnancy. Serial ultrasound examinations are important in documenting growth and excluding anomalies. An antenatal diagnosis of IUGR is not precise given that EFW cannot be measured directly and must be calculated from a combination of directly measured parameters. Overall prediction of weight via birthweight formulas can have a

10–20% error rate. Selection of the most useful biometric parameter depends on the timing of measurements. The crown–rump length is the best parameter for dating of pregnancy in the first trimester. The biparietal diameter (BPD) and HC are most accurate in the second trimester, with a margin of error of 7–11 days for BPD and 3–5 days for HC. HC is more useful in establishing gestational age in the third trimester because BPD loses its accuracy secondary to variations in shape. Abdominal circumference measurement is the single most sensitive measurement for evaluating fetal growth restriction. The fetal abdominal circumference reflects the volume of fetal subcutaneous fat and the size of the liver, which in turn correlates with the degree of fetal nutrition. Acidemia and hypoxemia are more common when the abdominal circumference is below the 5th percentile for gestational age.

The femur length is not helpful for identifying IUGR but can identify skeletal dysplasia. Because the definition of IUGR ultimately depends on birthweight and gestational age criteria, formulas that optimally predict birthweight in a given population will be the most important contributor to ultrasonographic criteria.

Fetuses from different populations show different growth patterns. The growth curves developed by Battaglia and Lubchenco in the 1960s do not reflect the variation in birthweight for various ethnic populations. The growth curves used today also do not reflect the median birthweight increase over the last 3 decades. Racial and ethnic anthropometric variations may suggest a need for specific charts for different communities.

Differential Diagnosis

If the fundal height on clinical examination is small, other diagnoses that should be entertained are oligohydramnios or a healthy pregnancy with the wrong due date (ie, the true gestational age is earlier than assigned). Ultrasound can help to differentiate among these diagnoses.

Complications

Numerous maternal and perinatal complications have been associated with IUGR pregnancies (Table 16–1). Underlying maternal disease is more likely to be present (Table 16–3), and these women require more intensive prenatal care. Premature labor or preeclampsia is more common. IUGR fetuses at any gestational age are less likely to tolerate labor well, and the need for operative delivery is increased.

Perinatal morbidity and mortality are significantly increased in low-birthweight infants, with an inverse relationship between neonatal weight and perinatal mortality. At any given gestational age, IUGR neonates have a higher mortality than do AGA neonates. However, at any given birthweight, outcomes are similar for IUGR and AGA neonates. Perinatal morbidity and mortality are especially increased in infants born at term with birthweights at or below the 3rd percentile. Increased risk of mortality is affected by the primary etiology of growth restriction and may be modified by the severity and progression of maternal factors (eg, hypertension control). With the advent of fetal surveillance, the perinatal mortality rate associated with IUGR has decreased to 2–3 times that of the AGA population. The past decade has witnessed increased attention to minimizing the perinatal complications of surviving IUGR neonates. With continued improvements in antenatal surveillance and neonatal care, the perinatal mortality rate for IUGR pregnancies in most centers now is 1.5–2 times that of the AGA population. Unfortunately, this rate likely will not reach that of the AGA population in the near future because of the persistent occurrence of lethal anomalies and severe congenital infections.

IUGR fetuses are at risk for in utero complications, including hypoxia and metabolic acidosis, which may occur at any time but are more likely to occur during labor. Up to 50% of growth-restricted fetuses exhibit abnormal fetal heart rate patterns, most often variable decelerations. Hypoxia is the result of increasing fetal oxygen requirements during pregnancy, with a rapid increase during the third trimester. If the fetus receives inadequate oxygen, hypoxia and subsequent metabolic acidosis will ensue. If undetected or untreated, this condition will lead to decreased glycogen and fat stores, ischemic end-organ damage, meconium-stained amniotic fluid, and oligohydramnios, eventually resulting in vital organ damage and intrauterine death.

IUGR infants are at increased risk for neonatal complications, including meconium aspiration syndrome, low Apgar scores, UA pH <7.0, need for intubation in the delivery room, seizures, sepsis, polycythemia, hypoglycemia, hypocalcemia, temperature instability, apneic episodes, and neonatal death. All IUGR infants require a thorough postnatal evaluation for congenital anomalies.

Treatment

The initial evaluation of the fetus suspected to be growth restricted involves:

- Evaluation for other evidence of fetal compromise. Depending on the gestational age, this may involve performing a biophysical profile and Doppler studies of umbilical and fetal vessels (see below for more details).
- Detailed fetal anatomic survey by ultrasound.
- Detailed maternal history for any evidence of recent infection, medication or drug exposure, any maternal medical disorders that are associated with IUGR such as hypertension, or any history of IUGR in a prior pregnancy.
- Physical examination and laboratory testing for any evidence of preeclampsia.
- Maternal serum testing for viral and parasitic infections if there is a history suggestive of recent infection.

The role of maternal evaluation for inherited and acquired thrombophilia is controversial in these patients. Studies have not demonstrated a consistent link between maternal thrombophilia and IUGR. If an association exists, it is likely a weak one.

Depending on the findings, consideration may be given to fetal karyotyping via genetic amniocentesis if IUGR presents prior to the third trimester and severe growth restriction is suspected (ie, EFW <3rd percentile). Amniocentesis should also be considered for karyotyping if any structural malformations are found or if there is polyhydramnios. Amniocentesis may also be performed to assess for pulmonary maturity for selected fetuses.

Treatment of IUGR pregnancy presupposes an accurate diagnosis. Even with the history, physical examination, and ultrasound examination, an accurate diagnosis remains difficult, and some IUGR pregnancies will not be detected. Conversely, some fetuses suspected to be growth restricted may have a normal birth weight or may be found to be constitutionally small.

All pregnant women who are smoking should be advised to discontinue cigarette smoking as well as use of alcohol and all recreational drugs. Although bed rest often is recommended, no evidence shows that bed rest results in improved outcome or increased fetal birthweight for fetuses with suspected IUGR. The increased uterine blood flow that occurs when the patient is in the lateral recumbent position theoretically may result in some benefit for fetuses with asymmetric IUGR. However, data do not support this theory.

Because IUGR fetuses are at risk for antepartum or intrapartum compromise, they should be followed carefully. The goal of fetal surveillance is to identify those fetuses at greatest risk of stillbirth and neonatal morbidity related to acidosis who may benefit from preterm delivery. The best method for monitoring a fetus with suspected IUGR is not well established; however, it typically involves ultrasound for biophysical profile and Doppler studies of umbilical and fetal vessels.

- **The biophysical profile (BPP)** is useful for assessing fetal well-being. With a normal BPP score, the risk of fetal asphyxia in the following week is low (approximately 1 in 1000). As part of the BPP, the amniotic fluid volume is assessed. Decreased amniotic fluid volume is clinically associated with IUGR. This finding is thought to result from decreased perfusion of the fetal kidneys, which leads to decreased urine production. **Oligohydramnios**, defined as a maximum vertical pocket of fluid <2 cm or amniotic fluid index of <5 cm, may be seen with IUGR infants, but the presence of a normal amniotic fluid index should not preclude the diagnosis of IUGR.
- **Umbilical artery (UA) Doppler velocimetry** can be used to estimate the likelihood of adverse perinatal outcome and is useful in determining the intensity of fetal surveillance. Placental circulatory insufficiency is associated with increased placental resistance, which is associated with decreased maternofetal oxygen transfer. This increase in placental resistance is manifested by a fall in forward blood flow through the UA due to increased downstream impedance. During the compensated stage, diastolic flow in the UA is reduced or absent. Reversal of diastolic flow in the UA is a sign of severe hypoxemia and acidemia. Although the use of UA Doppler studies for general population screening remains unproven, it is recommended as the primary method of surveillance for already identified IUGR fetuses. Doppler flow studies, in particular the systolic-to-diastolic ratio (S/D ratio), helps reduce unnecessary interventions and improve overall fetal outcome (including reducing the risk of perinatal death) in IUGR pregnancies. A recent study showed that of fetuses with suspected IUGR evaluated by Doppler studies, none of those with normal UA Doppler flow measurements were delivered with metabolic acidemia. This finding suggests that intense antenatal surveillance may be unnecessary in a fetus with a normal UA S/D ratio and normal amniotic fluid index. Abnormal UA flow is associated with an increased risk of caesarean or operative delivery.
- In fetuses with suspected IUGR, abnormal **middle cerebral artery (MCA) Doppler studies** and UA S/D ratios are strongly associated with low gestational age at delivery, low birthweight, and low UA pH. Also, mean birthweight, interval to delivery, need for emergent delivery, and occurrence of fetal distress all are related to the severity of abnormal Doppler findings after correction for gestational age. Abnormal Doppler cerebroplacental ratio (MCA pulsatile index divided by UA pulsatile index) also has been associated with a statistically significant increase in perinatal morbidity and mortality. Respiratory distress syndrome and intracranial hemorrhage are not associated with abnormal Doppler studies.
- Doppler studies of other fetal vessels such as the descending aorta, inferior vena cava, and ductus venosus have also been shown to correlate with fetal acidosis and risk of demise.

In addition to fetal kick counts, antepartum testing with BPP and UA Doppler are recommended once or twice per week for the fetus with suspected IUGR. The significance of abnormal UA Doppler results can be clarified by investigations of MCA circulation and Doppler studies of venous structures, including the ductus venosus.

Ultrasound examinations to assess adequacy of fetal growth should be performed at least every 3–4 weeks. Measurements should include BPD, HC, abdominal circumference, and femur length, especially in patients in whom an asymmetric IUGR fetus is suspected. Probably the most sensitive index of an asymmetric IUGR fetus is the abdominal circumference. The femur length/abdominal circumference ratio is a gestational age–independent ratio (normal 0.20–0.24). Asymmetric IUGR fetuses generally have a ratio >0.24.

Every IUGR pregnancy must be individually assessed for the optimal time of delivery (ie, the point at which the baby will do as well or better outside the uterus than inside). This would be whenever surveillance indicates fetal maturity, fetal compromise, or gestational age of 37–38 weeks (beyond which time there is no advantage to an IUGR fetus remaining in utero). Data are conflicting as to whether IUGR accelerates pulmonary maturity. Therefore, the current recommendation is to administer glucocorticoids to women likely to deliver before 34 weeks, as would be done with any other pregnancy.

IUGR pregnancies are at increased risk for intrapartum problems, so whenever possible, delivery should take place in a center where appropriate obstetric care, anesthesia, and neonatal care are readily available. Caesarean delivery may be necessary, and the presence of meconium-stained amniotic fluid or a compromised infant should be anticipated.

The mode of delivery must be individualized. Caesarean delivery is often indicated, especially when fetal monitoring reveals evidence of fetal compromise, malpresentation, or situations where traumatic vaginal delivery might be expected.

Continuous electronic fetal heart rate monitoring should be performed during labor in all cases, even if recent antepartum testing has been reassuring. Arteriovenous cord blood gas determinations also are useful; as many as 50% of IUGR infants have some degree of metabolic acidosis. Minimization of anesthesia is generally preferable, but controlled epidural anesthesia usually is safe. Maternal hypotension or hypovolemia must be avoided.

Prognosis

An IUGR pregnancy per se is not considered life-threatening for the mother. However, increased maternal morbidity and mortality may result from an underlying condition (eg, hypertension or renal disease). Most women who deliver IUGR infants can be expected to have long-term prognoses equivalent to those of women delivering AGA infants.

Infants with a low birthweight have a relatively high morbidity and mortality. Short-term morbidity includes impaired thermoregulation, hypoglycemia, polycythemia, and impaired immune function. Studies have shown that the rate of neonatal death, Apgar score at 5 minutes <3, UA pH <7.0, seizures during the first day of life, and incidence of intubation are significantly increased when the fetus is at or below the 3rd percentile for birthweight.

As for long-term prognosis for the infant, reports of national survey data show that IUGR infants appear to catch up in weight in the first 6 months of life. However, IUGR infants tend to remain physically small and are shorter, lighter, and have smaller HCs than do AGA infants.

Taken as a group, IUGR infants have more neurologic and intellectual deficits than do their AGA peers. IUGR infants have lower IQs as well as a higher incidence of learning and behavioral problems. Major neurologic handicaps, such as severe mental retardation, cerebral palsy, and seizures, are more common in IUGR infants. The incidence of sudden infant death syndrome (SIDS) is increased in IUGR infants, who account for 30% of all SIDS cases. Adults who were IUGR at birth are at higher risk for developing ischemic heart disease and related disorders, including hypertension, stroke, diabetes, and hypercholesterolemia.

Alfirevic Z, Stampalija T, Gyte GM. Fetal and umbilical Doppler ultrasound in high risk pregnancies. *Cochrane Database Syst Rev* 2010;1:CD007529. PMID: 20091637.

American College of Obstetricians and Gynecologists. *Clinical Management Guidelines: Intrauterine Growth Restriction. ACOG Practice Bulletin No. 12.* Washington, DC: American College of Obstetricians and Gynecologists; 2010.

Baschat AA, Galan HL, Bhide A, et al. Doppler and biophysical assessment in growth restricted fetuses: Distribution of test results. *Ultrasound Obstet Gynecol* 2006;27:41. PMID: 16323151.

Berghella V. Prevention of recurrent fetal growth restriction. *Obstet Gynecol* 2007;110:904. PMID: 17906027.

Lunde A, Melve KK, Gjessing HK, et al. Genetic and environmental influences on birth weight, birth length, head circumference, and gestational age by use of population based parent offspring date. *Am J Epidemiol* 2007;165:734. PMID: 17311798.

Zhang J, Merialdi M, Platt LD, et al. Defining normal and abnormal fetal growth: Promises and challenges. *Am J Obstet Gynecol* 2010;202:522. PMID: 20074690.

LARGE FOR GESTATIONAL AGE PREGNANCY

ESSENTIALS OF DIAGNOSIS

- EFW greater than the 90th percentile for gestational age on ultrasound.
- Macrosomia represents a subset of LGA fetuses weighing >4500 g.

Although the **large for gestational age (LGA)** fetus is defined according to the same concept as the IUGR fetus (LGA = heaviest 10% of newborns), LGA pregnancy has received substantially less attention since it is generally associated with fewer maternal and fetal complications than IUGR. *Large for gestational age* is defined as EFW above the 90th percentile for any specific gestational age. **Macrosomia** generally refers to fetuses with an EFW of at least 4500 g regardless of the gestational age; fetuses that are >4500 g are >95th percentile at any gestational age and therefore represent an extreme subset of LGA fetuses. The risk of morbidity is greater for infants born weighing between 4000 and 4500 g compared to the average population. However, the risk of infant morbidity is substantially increased at birthweights greater than 4500 g. Although there are numerous reports and studies regarding macrosomia, few data regarding LGA as defined here are available. Therefore, this section concentrates on fetal macrosomia, with additional comments regarding LGA pregnancies.

Pathogenesis

Numerous endocrinologic changes occur during pregnancy to ensure an adequate fetal glucose supply. In the second half of pregnancy, increased concentrations of human placental lactogen, free and total cortisol, and prolactin combine to produce modest maternal insulin resistance, which is countered by postprandial hyperinsulinemia. In those who are unable to mount this hyperinsulinemic response, relative hyperglycemia may develop (ie, gestational diabetes). Because glucose crosses the placenta by facilitated diffusion, fetal hyperglycemia ensues. This in turn produces fetal hyperinsulinemia with resultant intracellular transfer of glucose, leading to fetal macrosomia.

Factors that predispose to LGA pregnancy are listed in Table 16–4. As with IUGR pregnancy, diagnosis of LGA pregnancy depends on knowing with certainty the gestational age of the fetus.

A. Maternal Diabetes

Maternal diabetes, whether gestational, chemical, or insulin dependent, is the condition classically associated with fetal macrosomia. The "Pedersen hypothesis" was long assumed to account for fetal macrosomia, that is, the condition was the result of inadequate management of diabetes during pregnancy. Initial reports suggested that careful control of blood glucose level in insulin-dependent diabetic women would prevent fetal macrosomia, but recent studies have suggested that the problem is not so simple and that the incidence may correlate better with cord blood concentrations of maternally acquired anti-insulin immunoglobulin G (IgG) antibodies and/or increased serum levels of free fatty acids, triglycerides, and the amino acids alanine, serine, and isoleucine. Cord serum epidermal growth factor concentrations also have been found to be higher than normal in pregnancies complicated by prepregnancy diabetes and gestational diabetes.

A significant correlation exists between plasma leptin levels and neonatal birthweight, which suggests that leptin levels are directly related to the quantity of body fat tissue in fetal macrosomia.

Table 16–4. Factors that may predispose to fetal macrosomia or large for gestational age (LGA) pregnancy.

Maternal Factors
Diabetes (gestational, chemical, or insulin-dependent), obesity, postdatism, multiparity, advanced age, previous LGA infant, large stature
Fetal Factors
Genetic or congenital disorders, male gender

B. Maternal Obesity

Maternal obesity is associated with a 3- to 4-fold increased likelihood of fetal macrosomia. The increased risk of macrosomia associated with maternal obesity appears to be independent of comorbidities such as gestational or pregestational diabetes.

C. Postdatism

Prolonged pregnancy is more likely to result in a macrosomic fetus, presumably because of continued delivery of nutrients and oxygen to the fetus.

D. Genetic and Congenital Disorders

Several genetic and congenital syndromes are associated with an increased incidence of macrosomia. **Beckwith-Wiedemann syndrome** is frequently associated with fetal macrosomia, usually because of pancreatic islet cell hyperplasia (nesidioblastosis). Affected infants usually have hypoglycemia, macroglossia, and omphalocele. They also may have intestinal malrotation or visceromegaly. Although usually a sporadic event, other inheritance patterns have been suggested in a few families. Other rare syndromes include **Weaver's syndrome, Sotos' syndrome, Nevo's syndrome, Ruvalcaba-Myhre syndrome,** and **Marshall's syndrome. Carpenter's syndrome** and **fragile X syndrome** may be associated with an increased incidence of LGA infants.

E. Constitutionally Large Fetus

Fetuses who are suspected of being LGA may simply be large secondary to constitutional factors. **Large maternal stature** should be considered as contributing to macrosomia because birthweight tends to correlate more closely with maternal height than maternal weight. **Male fetuses** are more likely to be considered LGA because male fetuses are an average of 150 g heavier than appropriately matched female fetuses at each gestational week during late pregnancy. Series addressing fetal macrosomia generally report an increased incidence of male fetuses, usually approximately 60–65%. One recent study showed that male fetuses were twice as likely to be diagnosed with macrosomia as compared with female fetuses.

F. Maternal Weight Gain

Excessive maternal weight gain in pregnancy is associated with macrosomia. A weight gain of more than 40 lb significantly increased the incidence of macrosomia by an odds ratio of 3.3.

Prevention

Prevention of macrosomia and ensuing complications requires early detection of risk factors. Risk factors for having a macrosomic infant include multiparity, advanced maternal age, and previous delivery of a macrosomic infant. When controlled for gestational age and fetal gender, the average birthweight with successive pregnancies increases by 80–120 g up to the fifth pregnancy. Multiparity is also associated with other risk factors (eg, obesity, diabetes) and therefore may be a confounding variable. Advanced maternal age also contributes to increased birthweight. However, as with multiparity, it is also associated with obesity and diabetes.

Consideration should be given to evaluating patients with the risk factors noted in Table 16–4 for possible fetal macrosomia with an ultrasound estimate of fetal size and weight.

For patients with gestational or pregestational diabetes, adequate control of maternal glucose levels is thought to prevent the development of macrosomia, although neonatal complications despite excellent metabolic control have been reported. Prepregnancy weight and degree of weight gain are strong indicators for macrosomia regardless of glycemic control. However, the rates of macrosomia and complications are reduced overall when postprandial levels are monitored. Studies have shown that the risk of macrosomia is reduced to near normal in diabetic women who monitor 1-hour postprandial glucose levels and that 1-hour postprandial glucose levels are directly related to fetal abdominal circumference values. One study showed that when postprandial glucose levels were kept below 104 mg/dL, macrosomia rates of diabetic women were similar to those of nondiabetics. Chapter 31 reviews diabetes and pregnancy in more detail.

Infants of women who participate in regular aerobic exercise programs have lower average birthweights compared with infants in the general population but no demonstrable adverse effects. To date, no studies have evaluated the potential efficacy of exercise programs as a means of decreasing birthweight in women at risk for LGA pregnancy.

Clinical Findings

The first sign of macrosomia may be detected when the fundal height measurement on clinical examination exceeds the margin of error (>3 cm) for that gestational age. A diagnosis of macrosomia is made when the EFW on ultrasound (as determined by measurements of the HC, BPD, abdominal circumference, and femur length) exceeds 4500 g. Nonetheless, EFW by ultrasound is not very accurate. More than 30 different formulas for EFW calculation have been proposed, attesting to the inadequacy of each individual method. No single formula has been consistently better than the others. Even in skillful hands, the error of fetal weight estimates by ultrasound is 10–20%. One review of ultrasonographic diagnosis of macrosomia shows sensitivity ranging from 24 to 88% and specificity from 60 to 98%. The margin of error in estimating fetal weight means that the EFW by ultrasound must be at least 4750 g in order to predict a birthweight of 4000 g with a confidence interval of 90%. The best single measurement in evaluating macrosomia in diabetic mothers is abdominal circumference. An initial abdominal circumference above the 70th percentile is significantly associated with subsequent delivery of an LGA infant. Fetal body composition and fetal shoulder width cannot be accurately assessed by ultrasound.

Differential Diagnosis

If the fundal height on clinical examination is increased, the differential diagnosis includes polyhydramnios, fetal structural abnormality (such as sacrococcygeal teratoma), and undiagnosed multiple gestation in addition to macrosomia or LGA fetus. Ultrasound can differentiate among these diagnoses.

Complications

Macrosomic pregnancies are at increased risk for many fetal and maternal complications (Table 16–2). Macrosomic pregnancies are more likely to require **caesarean delivery**, usually because of failure to progress. In particular, primigravidas delivering a macrosomic infant are at increased risk for complications such **as prolonged labor, postpartum hemorrhage, operative vaginal delivery, and emergency caesarean section** as compared to delivering a normal weight infant. Primigravidas also have a higher risk of these complications compared with multiparous women delivering a macrosomic infant. Fetal distress, as determined by electronic fetal monitoring, is not more common in macrosomic pregnancies.

Shoulder dystocia occurs in 5–24% of vaginally delivered macrosomic fetuses. The incidence of shoulder dystocia correlates not only with increasing fetal weight but also with increasing chest circumference to HC. Shoulder dystocia of macrosomic infants also is related to maternal stature, but the association is not as clear. Approximately 10–15% of infants with shoulder dystocia experience brachial plexus injury; facial nerve injury and fractures of the humerus or clavicle also may be seen.

The risk of fetal **brachial plexus injury** in macrosomic infants delivered vaginally is 0.3–4%. Brachial plexus injury with shoulder dystocia is approximately 7% in infants whose birthweights exceed 4000 g but is 14% for mothers with gestational diabetes. The doubled risk may be secondary to increased fetal abdominal obesity in diabetic mothers. In diabetic patients, a correlation exists between the level of fetal truncal asymmetry (abdominal circumference/BPD ratio) as measured by ultrasound and the incidence and severity of shoulder dystocia. In addition to macrosomia, risk factors for shoulder dystocia include previous shoulder dystocia and maternal diabetes (3- to 4-fold increase compared to nondiabetic mothers). Lesser risk factors that are mediated through fetal size include previous delivery of a large fetus and excessive maternal weight gain during pregnancy. The risk of shoulder dystocia is similar in primigravidas and multigravidas delivering macrosomic infants.

Perineal trauma is more likely with a macrosomic pregnancy and is related to an increased incidence of shoulder dystocia and operative vaginal delivery. Vaginal delivery of a macrosomic infant increases by 5-fold the risk of third- or fourth-degree laceration.

Although gestational diabetes and postdatism predispose to fetal macrosomia, no evidence indicates that fetal macrosomia or an LGA fetus predisposes to gestational diabetes or postdatism.

The incidence of **stillbirth** remains higher in macrosomic fetuses than in controls of average weight. This problem has persisted even with the availability of fetal monitoring and presumably reflects the increased incidence of maternal diabetes and postdatism. Stillbirths are known to be increased in nonanomalous diabetic mothers, but the cause is not understood. Additionally, excessive prepregnancy weight is an independent risk factor for unexplained death. In fact, large fetal macrosomia is significantly associated with unexplained fetal death even after controlling for maternal age, diabetes, and hypertension.

Many of the neonatal complications of fetal macrosomia are the result of underlying maternal diabetes or birth trauma and include low Apgar scores, hypoglycemia, hypocalcemia, polycythemia, jaundice, and feeding difficulties. LGA infants have significantly higher absolute nucleated red blood cell counts, lymphocyte counts, and packed cell volumes. These hematologic abnormalities are the same for all LGA infants regardless of whether they are infants of nondiabetic mothers, insulin-dependent diabetic mothers, or non–insulin-dependent gestational diabetics. This situation is believed to reflect a compensatory increase in erythropoiesis as a result of chronic intrauterine hypoxia resulting from increased placental oxygen consumption and decreased fetal oxygen delivery.

LGA infants of diabetic mothers have an increased incidence of cardiac septal hypertrophy.

Treatment

Labor induction for suspected macrosomia has not been shown to reduce the risk of shoulder dystocia, and caesarean delivery reducing the incidence of fetal macrosomia and intrapartum complications remains an unproven hypothesis.

Several published reviews of fetal macrosomia suggest routine caesarean delivery for fetuses with estimated weights of 5000 g or more (or estimated weights ≥4500 g in diabetic pregnancies). This suggestion is based in part on the data given in Table 16–2 and in part on anthropometric studies suggesting that very macrosomic fetuses have bisacromial circumferences in excess of HCs. Because of current limitations in the sensitivity and specificity of ultrasound-derived fetal weight calculations, decisions regarding scheduled abdominal delivery must be partially based on clinical grounds. Such considerations are particularly warranted in women who are obese or are diabetic or in postdate pregnancies. Maternal age and maternal preference also should be considered when deciding on delivery method.

Intrapartum management considerations center on close observation of the patient's labor curve and avoidance of interventions that may be associated with an increased likelihood of traumatic vaginal delivery. Although data are conflicting, some studies have shown that patients with a protracted active phase of labor are more likely to experience shoulder dystocia. Close attention to a patient's progress during labor may help detect this risk factor for shoulder dystocia. Furthermore, vacuum-assisted vaginal delivery increases the risk of shoulder dystocia. If the estimate of fetal weight is greater than 4000 g, the vacuum should be avoided if the second stage is prolonged, and in general, the vacuum should be used with caution. Because of these factors, women at risk for macrosomic or LGA babies should deliver in facilities where adequate obstetric care, pediatric care, and anesthesia are available. Large-bore intravenous access must be established, and blood must be available. Delivery should occur in a setting where immediate operation can be accomplished.

Prognosis

Any woman who delivers an LGA baby should be informed that the risk of her having another LGA baby is increased by 2.5- to 4-fold. Such women should be screened for previously undiagnosed chemical or insulin-dependent diabetes and, even if screening is negative, should be followed carefully in any subsequent pregnancy to rule out gestational diabetes.

Obese women should be strongly encouraged to lose weight prior to becoming pregnant. Any woman who has delivered an LGA infant should be encouraged to seek early care for any subsequent pregnancy, if for no other reason than early confirmation of the EDC, which can minimize the likelihood of subsequent postdatism. Women who deliver an LGA infant with an underlying genetic or congenital disorder should receive genetic counseling regarding recurrence risks and the feasibility of antepartum diagnosis.

In addition to the many neonatal complications previously noted, infants of mothers with gestational or pregestational diabetes are at increased risk for subsequent obesity, type 2 diabetes, or both. Infants who suffer from neonatal complications are at increased risk for subsequent neurologic or behavioral problems.

American College of Obstetricians and Gynecologists. *Clinical Management Guidelines: Fetal Macrosomia. ACOG Practice Bulletin No. 22.* Washington, DC: American College of Obstetricians and Gynecologists; 2010.

Multiple Gestation

17

Melissa C. Bush, MD
Martin L. Pernoll, MD

ESSENTIALS OF DIAGNOSIS

- The incidence of multiple gestations has risen significantly over several decades, primarily due to increased use of fertility drugs for ovulation induction, superovulation, and assisted reproductive technologies (ART), such as in vitro fertilization (IVF).
- Compared with singleton pregnancies, twin pregnancies are more likely to be complicated by hypertensive disorders, gestational diabetes mellitus, anemia, preterm birth, ante- and postpartum hemorrhage, and maternal death.
- The perinatal mortality rate of twins is 3–4 times higher—and for triplets much higher still—than in singleton pregnancies as a result of chromosomal abnormalities, prematurity, structural anomalies, hypoxia, and trauma.
- This is particularly true of monozygotic twins, which are also uniquely susceptible to twin-twin transfusion syndrome.

Pathogenesis

In the United States, between 1980 and 2004, the twin rate climbed 101% with 68,339 twins born in 1980 and 137,085 twins born in 2006. Multiple gestations now comprise 3% of all pregnancies, and twins comprise 25–30% of deliveries resulting from assisted reproductive technologies (ART). Significant maternal and neonatal effects are felt from this increase in multiple births. The financial costs are also staggering, with combined costs of ART plus pregnancy care, delivery, and neonatal care reaching hundreds of thousands of dollars in some cases. Maternal morbidity and mortality rates are much higher in multiple pregnancy than in singleton pregnancy. Compared with singleton pregnancies, twin pregnancies are more likely to be complicated by hypertensive disorders, gestational diabetes mellitus, anemia, preterm birth, ante- and postpartum hemorrhage, and maternal death. Earlier and more precise sonography has revealed the incidence of multiple gestation to be 3.29–5.39% before 12 weeks. However, in over 20% of such cases, one or more of the pregnancies spontaneously disappears ("vanishing twin"). Although this event may be associated with vaginal bleeding, the prognosis remains good for the remaining twin.

Approximately two-thirds of twin pregnancies end in a singleton birth; the other embryo is lost from bleeding, is absorbed within the first 10 weeks of pregnancy, or is retained and becomes mummified (fetus papyraceous). Fetus papyraceous is a small, blighted, mummified fetus usually discovered at the delivery of a well-developed newborn. This occurs once in 17,000–20,000 pregnancies spontaneously and is also the result of multifetal reduction. The cause is thought to be death of one twin, amniotic fluid loss, or reabsorption and compression of the dead fetus by the surviving twin.

Twins can be monozygotic or dizygotic. Higher order multiples can result from either or both processes.

A. Monozygotic Multiple Gestation

Monozygotic twins ("identical twins") are the result of the division of a single fertilized ovum that subsequently divides into 2 separate individuals. Monozygotic twinning occurs in about 4–5 of 1000 pregnancies in all races. The rate is remarkably constant in all populations and is not influenced by heredity, age of the mother, or other factors. Monozygotic twins are always of the same sex. However, the twins may develop differently depending on the time of preimplantation division. Normally, monozygotic twins share the same physical characteristics (skin, hair and eye color, body build) and the same genetic features (blood characteristics: ABO, M, N, haptoglobin, serum group; histocompatible genes), and they are often mirror images of one another (one left-handed, the other right-handed, etc). However, their fingerprints differ.

The paradox of "identical" twins is that they may be the antithesis of identical. The very earliest splits are sometimes accompanied by a simultaneous chromosomal error, resulting in heterokaryotypic monozygotes, one with Down syndrome and the other normal. Furthermore, monozygotic twins may be discordant for fetal structural malformations.

Monozygotic triplets result from repeated twinning (also called supertwinning) of a single ovum. Conversely, trizygotic triplets develop by individual fertilization of 3 simultaneously expelled ova. Triplets may also be produced by the twinning of 2 ova and the elimination of 1 of the 4 resulting embryos. Similarly, quadruplets may be monozygotic, paired dizygotic, or quadrizygotic (ie, they may arise from 1 to 4 ova).

Monoamniotic twins are the rarest form of monozygotic twins, with an incidence of about 1:10,000 pregnancies (1–5% of monozygotic gestations). The perinatal mortality is much higher than that of other monozygotic twins (23%) mostly due to cord entanglement as a result of the absence of a dividing membrane.

1. Placenta & cord—The placenta and membranes of monozygotic twins vary (Fig. 17–1), depending on the time of initial division of the embryonic disk. Variations are noted below.

1. Division prior to the morula stage and differentiation of the trophoblast (day 3) results in separate or fused placentas, 2 chorions, and 2 amnions (dichorionic/diamniotic). (This process grossly resembles dizygotic twinning and accounts for almost one-third of monozygotic twinning.) This is clinically relevant since dichorionic twins have a much lower rate of complications.
2. Division after differentiation of the trophoblast but before the formation of the amnion (days 4–8) yields a single placenta, a common chorion, and 2 amnions (monochorionic/diamniotic). (This accounts for about two-thirds of monozygotic twinning.)

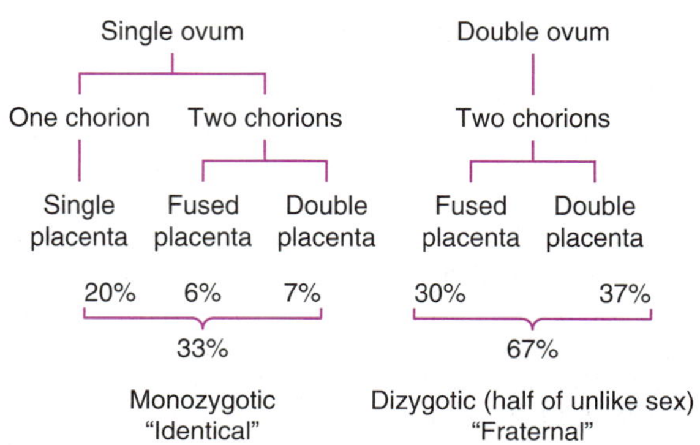

▲ **Figure 17–1.** Placental variations in twinning. (Reproduced, with permission, from Benson RC. *Handbook of Obstetrics & Gynecology*. 8th ed. Los Altos, CA: Lange; 1983.)

3. Division after differentiation of the amnion (days 8–13) results in a single placenta, 1 (common) chorion, and 1 (common) amnion (monochorionic/monoamniotic). This is rare.
4. Division later than day 15 may result in incomplete twinning. Just prior to that time (days 13–15), division may result in conjoined twins.

At delivery, the membranous T-shaped septum or dividing membrane of the placenta between the twins must be inspected and sectioned for evidence of the probable type of twinning (Fig. 17–2). Monochorionic, diamniotic twins most commonly have a transparent (<2 mm) septum made up of 2 amniotic membranes only (no chorion and no decidua). Dichorionic, diamniotic twins almost always have an opaque (thick) septum made up of 2 chorions, 2 amnions, and intervening decidua.

A monochorionic placenta can be identified by stripping away the amnion or amnions to reveal a single chorion over a common placenta. In virtually every case of monochorionic placenta, vascular communications between the 2 parts of the placenta can be identified by careful dissection or injection. In contrast, dichorionic placentas (of dizygotic twinning) only rarely have an anastomosis between the fetal blood vessels. All twin placentas are sent for pathologic examination to confirm chorionicity.

Placental and membrane examination is a certain indicator of zygosity in twins with monochorionic placentas because these are always monozygotic. Overall, approximately 1% of twins are monoamniotic, and these too are monozygotic. Determination of zygosity is clinically significant in case intertwin organ transplantation is needed later in life, as well as for assessing obstetrical risks. Monozygotic twins can rarely be discordant for phenotypic sex when one twin is phenotypically female due to Turner's syndrome (45,XO) and its sibling is male (46,XY).

Monochorionic placentation is associated with more disease processes as a result of placental vascular problems. Inequities of the placental circulation in one area (marginal insertion, partial infarction, or thinning) may lead to growth discordance between the twins. Due to vascular anastomoses in monochorionic placentation, standard multifetal reduction using intrathoracic potassium chloride can only be performed with dichorionic placentation.

The most serious problem with monochorionic placentas is local shunting of blood—also called **twin–twin transfusion syndrome.** This problem affects approximately 15% of monochorionic twin pregnancies and occurs because of vascular anastomoses to each twin that are established early in embryonic life. The possible communications are artery to artery, vein to vein, and combinations of these. Artery-to-vein communication is by far the most serious; it is most likely to cause twin–twin transfusion. In uncompensated cases, the twins, although genetically identical, differ greatly in size and appearance. The recipient twin is plethoric, edematous, and hypertensive. Ascites and kernicterus are likely. The heart,

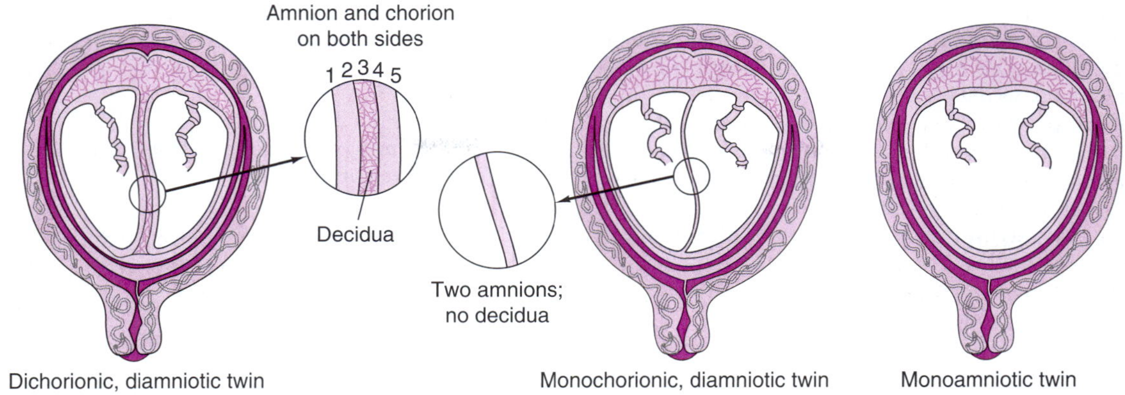

▲ **Figure 17–2.** Chorionic and amniotic membranes of twins. (Reproduced, with permission, from Benson RC. *Handbook of Obstetrics & Gynecology.* 8th ed. Los Altos, CA: Lange; 1983.)

liver, and kidneys are enlarged (glomerulotubal hypertrophy). Hydramnios follows fetal polyuria. Although ruddy and apparently healthy, the recipient twin with hypervolemia may die of heart failure during the first 24 hours after birth. The donor twin is small, pallid, and dehydrated (from growth restriction, malnutrition, and hypovolemia). Oligohydramnios may be present. Severe anemia, due to chronic blood loss to the other twin, may lead to hydrops and heart failure.

Velamentous insertion of the cord occurs in about 7% of twins but in only 1% of singletons. There is a corresponding increase in the potentially catastrophic vasa previa. The incidence of 2-vessel cord (single umbilical artery) is 4–5 times higher in monozygotic twins than in singletons.

Monochorionic, monoamniotic twins (1:100 sets of twins) have < a 90% likelihood of both surviving because of cord entanglement that compromises fetal-placental blood flow. Other common complications are congenital anomalies in 26% of monoamniotic twins and discordant birth weights, primarily due to twin–twin transfusion syndrome. Some authors advocate planned caesarean delivery at 32–34 weeks in an attempt to prevent in utero demise due to cord accidents, as well as continuous external fetal monitoring from about 27 weeks until delivery.

2. The fetus—There are several unusual fetal findings that may be seen in the setting of monozygotic twinning. Conjoined twins result from incomplete segmentation of a single fertilized ovum between the 13th and 14th days; if cleavage is further postponed, incomplete twinning (ie, 2 heads, 1 body) may occur. Lesser abnormalities are also noted, but these occur without regard to specific organ systems. Conjoined twins are described by site of union: pyopagus (at the sacrum); thoracopagus (at the chest); craniopagus (at the heads); and omphalopagus (at the abdominal wall). Curiously, conjoined twins usually are female. Numerous conjoined twins have survived separation.

An acardiac twin is a parasitic monozygotic fetus without a heart. It is thought to develop from reversed circulation, perfused by 1 arterial–arterial and 1 venous–venous anastomosis. This represents the twin reversed arterial perfusion (TRAP) syndrome. The otherwise normal donor twin is at risk for cardiac hypertrophy and failure and has a 35% mortality rate. Various methods of cord occlusion are being studied as in utero therapy.

B. Dizygotic Multiple Gestation

Dizygotic twins ("fraternal twins") are produced from separately fertilized ova. They bear only the resemblance of brothers or sisters and may or may not have the same blood type. Significant differences usually can be identified over time. Slightly more than 30% of twins are monozygotic; nearly 70% are dizygotic. Twins of different sexes are always dizygotic (fraternal). Twins of the same sex may be monozygotic or dizygotic. Although monozygotism is random—ie, it does not fit any discernible genetic pattern—dizygotism has hereditary determinants.

In North America, dizygotic twinning occurs about once in 83 conceptions and triplets occur about once in 8000 conceptions. A traditional approximation of the incidence of spontaneous multiple pregnancies is as follows:

Twins	1:80
Triplets	$1{:}80^2 = 1{:}6400$
Quadruplets (etc)	$1{:}80^3 = 1{:}512{,}000$

About 75% of dizygotic twins are the same sex. Many factors influence dizygotic twinning including age and ethnicity. Race is a factor, with multiple gestations most common in blacks, least common in Asians, and of intermediate occurrence in whites. The incidence of spontaneous dizygotic twinning varies from 1.3 in 1000 in Japan to 49 in 1000 in western Nigeria. The rate in the United States is about 12 in 1000. Spontaneous twinning increases with advancing maternal age. The widespread use of ART has increased the frequency of dizygotic twins with a minimal effect on the incidence of monozygotic twins.

Dizygotic twinning is more common among women who become pregnant soon after cessation of long-term oral contraception. This may be a reflection of high "rebound" gonadotropin secretion. Induction of ovulation in previously infertile patients has resulted in many multiple pregnancies—even the gestation of septuplets and octuplets. The estrogen analog clomiphene citrate increases the incidence of dizygotic pregnancy to about 5–10%.

Clinically, zygosity cannot be ascertained prenatally, so chorionicity seen on ultrasound is a useful surrogate marker for stratification of perinatal risk, with increased risks associated with monochorionicity.

Prevention

A. Multiple Gestations

Although ovulation induction agents result in fewer multiple pregnancies when used by experts, even in the best of hands, it is inevitable that some multiple pregnancies will occur. For example, clomiphene citrate induction of multiple ovulation increases the rate of dizygotic pregnancy above 5–10%.

With many forms of ART (eg, ovulation induction, in vitro fertilization), iatrogenic multiple pregnancies regularly occur in which the number of fetuses is so great that they may preclude any being carried to the point of viability. When this occurs, many authorities recommend multifetal pregnancy reduction by transabdominal intracardiac potassium chloride injection. Efforts are under way to recommend limiting the number of embryos transferred; legislation to this effect has been enacted in the United Kingdom. The American Society for Reproductive Medicine is now recommending single-embryo transfers in good-prognosis candidates.

Clinical Findings

With the ready availability of ultrasound, it is rare that multiple gestations go undiagnosed during pregnancy. Early diagnosis facilitates appropriate prenatal care.

A. Symptoms & Signs

All of the common annoyances of pregnancy are more troublesome in multiple gestations. The effects of multiple gestation on the patient include earlier and more severe pressure in the pelvis, nausea, backache, varicosities, constipation, hemorrhoids, abdominal distention, and difficulty in breathing. A "large pregnancy" may be indicative of twinning (distended uterus). Fetal activity is greater and more persistent in twinning than in singleton pregnancy.

Considering the possibility of multiple gestation is essential to early diagnosis. If one assumes that all pregnancies are multiple until proved otherwise, physical examination alone will identify most cases of twinning before the second trimester. Indeed, diagnosis of twinning is possible in over 75% of cases by physical examination. The following signs should alert the physician to the possibility or definite presence of multiple pregnancy:

1. Uterus larger than expected (>4 cm) for dates.
2. Excessive maternal weight gain that is not explained by edema or obesity.
3. Polyhydramnios, manifested by uterine size out of proportion to the calculated duration of gestation, is almost 10 times more common in multiple pregnancy.
4. History of assisted reproduction.
5. Elevated maternal serum α fetoprotein (MSAFP) values (see following section, Laboratory Findings).
6. Outline or ballottement of more than 1 fetus.
7. Multiplicity of small parts.
8. Simultaneous recording of different fetal heart rates, each asynchronous with the mother's pulse and with each other and varying by at least 8 beats/min. (The fetal heart rate may be accelerated by pressure or displacement.)
9. Palpation of 1 or more fetuses in the fundus after delivery of 1 infant.

Some of the common complications in early pregnancy may also occur as a result of multiple gestation. For example, maternal bleeding in the first trimester can indicate threatened or spontaneous abortion; however, the dead fetus may be 1 of twins, as demonstrated by real-time ultrasonography (1 anechoic or hypoechoic amniotic sac and 1 normal sac). In the second and third trimester, the demise of 1 fetus in a multiple gestation may rarely trigger disseminated intravascular coagulation (DIC), just as a singleton intrauterine demise might. This theoretical complication is so rare that DIC screening is no longer performed.

B. Laboratory Findings

The majority of multiple gestations are currently identified by using MSAFP screening or routine ultrasound. Indeed, identification of multiple gestation is so important for the institution of appropriate care that many authorities recommend routine ultrasonic scanning for early confirmation of gestational age and then again at 18–20 weeks. First-trimester ultrasonography is even more helpful for determining chorionicity and is becoming standard of care, especially since many patients undergo first-trimester ultrasound for nuchal translucency (NT) screening. Interestingly, NT measurements are similar for a given crown-rump length regardless if it is a singleton, twin, or higher order multiple gestation.

The maternal hematocrit and hemoglobin values and the red cell count usually are considerably reduced, in direct relationship to the increased blood volume. Indeed, maternal hypochromic normocytic anemia is almost universal because fetal demand for iron increases beyond the mother's ability to assimilate iron in the second trimester.

C. Ultrasound Findings

Ultrasonography is the preferred imaging modality for the diagnosis of multiple gestation and is potentially able to differentiate multiple gestation as early as 4–5 weeks (by endovaginal probe). Dichorionicity is suggested by fetuses of different genders, separate placentas, a thick (>2 mm) dividing membrane, or a "twin peak sign" in which the membrane inserts into 2 fused placentas. In the absence of these findings, monochorionicity is likely, particularly if the twins are spontaneously conceived. A first-trimester scan is highly recommended since definitive diagnosis of chorionicity may not be possible with second- and third-trimester scans. See the chapter on imaging in pregnancy (Chapter 11) for more details.

Differential Diagnosis

Multiple pregnancy must be distinguished from the following conditions.

A. Singleton Pregnancy

Inaccurate dates may give a false impression of the duration of the pregnancy, and the fetus may be larger than expected.

B. Polyhydramnios

Either single or multiple pregnancy may be associated with excessive accumulation of fluid.

C. Hydatidiform Mole

Although usually easily distinguished from multiple gestation, this complication must be considered in diagnosis early in pregnancy.

D. Abdominal Tumors Complicating Pregnancy

Fibroid tumors of the uterus, when present in great numbers, are readily identified. Ovarian tumors are generally single, discrete, and harder to diagnose. A distended bladder or full rectum may elevate the pregnant uterus.

E. Complicated Twin Pregnancy

If 1 dizygotic twin dies early in pregnancy and the other lives, the dead fetus may become flattened and mummified (fetus papyraceous; see earlier section on fetal pathologic factors). Its portion of a fused placenta will be pale and atrophic, but remnants of 2 sacs and 2 cords may be found. If 1 twin dies in late pregnancy, considerable enlargement of the uterus persists, although the findings on palpation may be unusual and only 1 fetal heartbeat will be heard. Ultrasonography can confirm the diagnosis.

Complications

A. Maternal

A gravida with a multiple pregnancy has about 5 times the likelihood of having a morbid (febrile, complicated) course as an average patient of the same parity with a single fetus.

Multiple gestations are associated with an increased incidence of maternal anemia, urinary tract infection, preeclampsia-eclampsia, hemorrhage (before, during, and after delivery), and uterine atony. Although blood volume is increased in multiple gestations, maternal anemia often develops because of greater demand for iron by the fetuses. However, prior anemia, poor diet, and malabsorption may precede or compound iron deficiency during multiple gestation. Hypochromic normocytic anemia is 2–3 times more common in multiple pregnancy than in singleton pregnancy. Urinary tract infection is at least twice as frequent in multiple pregnancy as in singleton pregnancy due to increased ureteral dilatation secondary to higher serum progesterone and uterine pressure on the ureters. Preeclampsia–eclampsia occurs about 3 times more often in multiple pregnancy than in a singleton pregnancy.

Additionally, respiratory tidal volume is increased, but the woman pregnant with twins often is "breathless" (possibly due to increased levels of progesterone). Marked uterine distention and increased pressure on the adjacent viscera and pelvic vasculature are typical of multiple gestation. Theca lutein cysts and even ascites may be seen as a result of abnormally high levels of chorionic gonadotropin in occasional multiple pregnancies. The maternal cardiovascular, respiratory, gastrointestinal, renal, and musculoskeletal systems are especially subject to stress in multiple pregnancy, combined with greater maternal–fetal nutritional requirements.

Placenta previa develops more frequently because of the large size of the placenta or placentas. Placenta previa may be responsible for antepartum bleeding, malpresentation, or unengagement of the first fetus. A large placenta (or placentas) and possibly fundal scarring or tumor may lead to low implantation of the placenta. Premature separation of the placenta may occur antepartum, perhaps in association with preeclampsia–eclampsia or with rupture of membranes of twin A and the initiation of strong uterine contractions, or after the delivery of the first twin. Careless traction on the first cord may encourage early partial separation of the placenta.

A thinned uterine wall, secondary to unusually large uterine contents, is associated with hypotonic uterine contractions and a longer latent stage of labor. However, prolonged labor is uncommon in multiple pregnancy because rupture of the membranes generally is followed by improvements in the uterine contraction pattern. Hemorrhage is about 5 times as frequent in multiple as in single pregnancies. Uterine atony often is accompanied by excessive loss of blood postpartum due to inability of the overdistended uterus to contract well and remain contracted after delivery.

Operative intervention is more likely in multiple pregnancy because of increased risk of obstetric problems such as malpresentation, prolapsed cord, and fetal distress.

Glucose tolerance tests demonstrate that rates of both gestational diabetes mellitus and gestational hypoglycemia are much higher in multiple gestation compared with findings in singleton pregnancy. This is not surprising given the placental origin of human placental lactogen, which causes insulin resistance.

B. Fetal

Perinatal mortality and morbidity rates are increased in multiple pregnancy, mainly because of preterm delivery and its complications (ie, trauma or asphyxia). The incidence of spontaneous abortion of at least 1 of several fetuses is increased in multiple pregnancy. Stillbirth occurs twice as often among twins as among singleton pregnancies. Common causes of fetal death are developmental anomalies, fetal growth restriction, cord compression, or placental disorders. In general, the higher the number of fetuses, the greater is the risk of fetal growth restriction.

Monochorionic twin pregnancies have a substantially increased risk of death as compared with their dichorionic counterparts because of the almost ever-present vascular anastomoses that may cause the twin–twin transfusion syndrome or acute feto-fetal hemorrhage after intrauterine demise of 1 twin. The greatest hazard from cord compression is cord entanglement of monozygotic twins with only 1 amniotic sac. Almost twice as many monozygotic as dizygotic twins die in the perinatal period. Attrition is even greater for triplets, quadruplets, and higher order pregnancies. Even so, preterm delivery and intrapartum complications are the most common causes of fetal loss and morbidity in multiple pregnancy.

Preterm premature rupture of the membranes and preterm labor and delivery, often with a long prodromal phase, are common occurrences in multiple pregnancy. The average gestational age at delivery is 36–37 weeks for twins, 33 weeks for triplets, and 31 weeks for quadruplets. Efforts to reduce the incidence of prematurity have thus far been largely unsuccessful. All too frequently, preterm delivery is occasioned by premature rupture of the membranes, which occurs in about 25% of twin, 50% of triplet, and 75% of quadruplet pregnancies. Delivery before the 36th week is twice as frequent in twin pregnancies as in singleton pregnancies. Intracranial injury is more common in premature infants, even those delivered spontaneously. An increased risk of cerebral palsy is found in twins, especially very low-birthweight babies, and also in liveborn co-twins of fetuses who died in utero.

Prolapse of the cord occurs 5 times more often in multiple than in singleton pregnancy. Premature separation of the placenta before delivery of the second twin may cause death of the second twin by hypoxia. When there are 2 separate placentas, 1 of them may deliver immediately after the first twin. Although the second twin may not be compromised, it is best to proceed with its delivery, both for its protection and to conserve maternal blood.

Major fetal structural malformations are present in approximately 2% of twin infants, compared with 1% of singletons, whereas minor malformations are found in 4% of twins compared with about 2.5% of singletons. Monozygotic twins are at higher risk than dizygotic twins.

Fetal malpresentation is more common in multiple gestations. Both twins present in cephalic presentation in almost 50% of cases. Twin A will be cephalic and twin B a breech in slightly more than 33% of cases (Fig. 17–3). Both fetuses will be breech presentations in 10% of cases, and almost that many will be single (or double) transverse presentations. Approximately 70% of first twins present by the vertex. Breech presentation occurs in slightly more than 25%. Overall, noncephalic presentation occurs 10 times more often in multiple pregnancy than in singleton pregnancy.

Treatment

A. Prenatal Diagnosis

The usual indications for prenatal diagnosis and counseling in a singleton pregnancy also apply to twin and higher order gestations. Because the incidence of twin gestation increases with maternal age, women with multiple gestations are often candidates for prenatal genetic diagnosis. Because the risk of aneuploidy is increased, some centers offer invasive testing to all patients carrying multiple gestations who will be over age 33 at delivery. Now that most patients have prenatal screening with ultrasound and/or maternal serum testing, the role of age is becoming less important for stratification of risk for aneuploidy. Genetic counseling should make clear

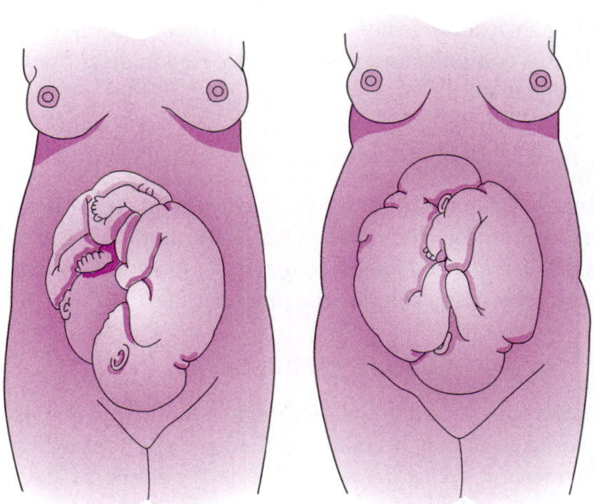

▲ **Figure 17–3.** **Left:** Both twins presenting by the vertex. **Right:** One cephalic and one breech presentation. (Reproduced, with permission, from Benson RC. *Handbook of Obstetrics & Gynecology*. 8th ed. Los Altos, CA: Lange; 1983.)

to the patient the need to obtain a sample from each fetus, the risk of a chromosomal abnormality, potential complications of the procedure, the possibility of discordant results, and the ethical and technical concerns when 1 fetus is found to be abnormal.

In twin pregnancies not accompanied by neural tube defects, the median MSAFP level will be 2.5-fold that of the median level for singleton pregnancies at 14–20 weeks' gestation. The levels in triplets and quadruplets are 3 and 4 times as high, respectively. A value greater than 4.5 times the median is considered abnormal for twin gestations and requires a targeted ultrasound and possible amniocentesis for the determination of amniotic fluid α fetoprotein and acetylcholinesterase. Serum screening is less effective in multiple gestations, with serum screening detecting only 47% of Down syndrome pregnancies. NT screening with first-trimester serum markers can detect about 70% of Down syndrome fetuses in twin pregnancies, with some added benefit to incorporating second-trimester markers.

Both amniocentesis and chorionic villus sampling can safely be performed in multiple gestations in experienced centers. Careful documentation of the location of the fetuses and the membrane separating the sacs is important in case there is discordance for aneuploidy. Selective termination of an aneuploid fetus can be performed via ultrasound-guided intracardiac injection of potassium chloride. The pregnancy can then continue carrying the normal twin only. Multifetal reduction may be performed to decrease the risk of serious perinatal morbidity and mortality associated with preterm delivery by reducing the number of fetuses from 3 or more to twins or even a singleton.

B. Antepartum Management

To prevent the complications of multiple gestation, it is imperative to make the diagnosis as early in pregnancy as possible. Later in pregnancy, ultrasonography is useful to monitor the growth of the fetuses and to detect structural anomalies. It is recommended to perform routine growth scans on twins every 4 weeks in the third trimester, or more frequently if growth restriction is detected. Antepartum testing is routinely performed in twins with suspected intrauterine growth restriction or growth discordance but is not universally performed in normally grown uncomplicated twins.

Enhanced antenatal care assists in improving outcome. The most commonly used techniques are iron and calcium supplementation, vitamin and folic acid administration (in an attempt to avoid anemia), a high-protein diet, and more weight gain than usual (ideal weight for height plus 35–45 lb). Supplementation with magnesium, zinc, and essential fatty acids has also been recommended.

There is not enough evidence to suggest a policy of routine hospitalization for bed rest in multiple pregnancy because no reduction in the risk of preterm birth or perinatal death is evident. There is also no evidence that prophylactic cerclage improves outcome. More frequent antenatal visits are scheduled, and several authorities recommend closely following cervical length by ultrasound. Early and prompt therapy for any complications (eg, vaginal infections, preeclampsia–eclampsia) should be instituted, bearing in mind that preeclampsia–eclampsia is a common complication of multiple pregnancy.

Tocolytic drugs may be used to suppress premature labor and extend gestation 48 hours so that the effects of steroids may be realized. There is no evidence that long-term oral or intravenous tocolysis improves outcome; however, this is still commonly practiced to a degree. Most authorities recommend starting with intravenous magnesium sulfate. If terbutaline is used, very close monitoring for pulmonary edema must be maintained, because this complication is much more likely with administration of β-mimetic agents in multiple gestation. Also, indomethacin is a very effective tocolytic in the second and early third trimesters, but it may influence fetal ductal constriction and decreased amniotic fluid volume, complications that appear to be gestational age dependent, so it should not be used after 32 weeks' gestation. Fetal fibronectin can be helpful, particularly when negative, to determine how aggressively to tocolyze.

Neonatal outcome is very much dependent on gestational age at delivery. In general, morbidity and mortality rates are similar for twins and singletons of equivalent gestational ages. Advances in neonatal intensive care have made survival possible even at 23 weeks' gestation, although usually with considerable morbidity, including but not limited to intraventricular hemorrhage, chronic lung disease, and necrotizing enterocolitis. Because intact survival is much more likely after 32–34 weeks, it is desirable to prolong gestation at least to this point when possible. The adage "1 day in utero saves 2 days in intensive care" applies to the economic as well as the emotional costs of caring for premature infants. For the dichorionic diamniotic twin pregnancy that is otherwise uncomplicated, recent studies have found that neonatal morbidity is reduced when delivery is at about 38 weeks, so routine delivery at that time is recommended, by either induction of labor or caesarean if indicated.

Optimal treatment of twin–twin transfusion syndrome in utero remains controversial. Laser therapy for ablation of anastomotic placental vessels is available in several centers around the United States and shows improved short-term survival as compared to expectant management and serial amnioreduction. Two-year neurodevelopmental outcomes are also improved in patients treated with laser. After delivery, therapy for twin–twin transfusion syndrome includes replacing blood in the donor twin to correct fluid and electrolyte imbalance. In the recipient twin, phlebotomy may be necessary until normal venous pressure is restored. Often, other therapy for cardiac failure (eg, digitalis) is necessary.

C. Labor & Delivery

All patients carrying a multiple gestation should be delivered in a well-equipped hospital by an experienced physician who has adequate assistance. It is desirable to have a pediatrician (or neonatologist) in attendance. Delivery must be done in the operating room in case an emergent caesarean section is needed for twin B. An early epidural is recommended; in case of emergent caesarean section, anesthesia is already established and general anesthesia can usually be avoided. Prematurity, trauma of manipulative delivery, and associated asphyxia are the major preventable causes of morbidity and mortality in twins, especially the second twin.

Admit the patient to the hospital at the first sign of suspected labor or preterm labor, if there is leakage of amniotic fluid, or if significant bleeding occurs. We instruct patients to come in for >4 contractions per hour at <34 weeks' gestation. An ultrasound evaluation should be performed to ascertain the presentation of each fetus and its estimated fetal weight. Routine, continuous electronic fetal heart rate monitoring is recommended. Labor should be conducted so that immediate caesarean section can be performed if required. A pediatric nurse team for each infant plus obstetric and anesthesiologic attendants should be present. Insert an intravenous line and send a specimen of blood for typing, antibody screening, and complete blood count.

If either twin shows signs of persistent compromise, proceed promptly to caesarean section delivery. Other indications for primary caesarean section include (but are not limited to) malpresentation, monoamniotic twins, gross disparity in fetal size, and placenta previa. In the United States, all higher order multiple gestations are delivered by caesarean delivery.

In a woman with a previous lower segment caesarean scar, limited literature suggests that delivery of twins does not mandate a repeat caesarean section in the absence of other complications. Concomitant with increasing rates of elective and nonelective caesarean section, caesarean by patient request is becoming more common. In addition, less resident training in vaginal breech delivery can decrease a clinician's comfort with breech extraction of a second twin.

Management of twins that are candidates for vaginal delivery may proceed as outlined below. Intrapartum twin presentations may be classified as follows: (1) twin A and twin B cephalic (slightly >40% of all twins); (2) twin A vertex and twin B noncephalic (almost 40%); and (3) twin A noncephalic and twin B cephalic, breech, or transverse (about 20%).

The current intrapartum management of twins is as follows. For cephalic–cephalic presentations in labor (category 1 above), vaginal delivery of both twins may be chosen in the absence of standard indications for caesarean section delivery. Of course, if either twin develops fetal distress, caesarean section delivery should be performed. Category 2 twins, each >32 weeks and weighing more than 1500–2000 g, can usually be managed successfully by vaginal delivery of both. This is generally accomplished by total breech extraction of twin B immediately after the delivery of twin A if the patient has been consented for this procedure. External cephalic version of twin B has also been described. While external version was previously recommended for conversion of twin B from breech to cephalic, now most operators deliver vaginal second twins by complete breech extraction. When either twin A or both twins are noncephalic (category 3), primary caesarean section should be performed. This is also sometimes recommended in cases of noncephalic twin B where the estimated fetal weight is much greater than that of twin A. The ultrasound machine should be in the operating room to confirm the presentation of twin B after the delivery of twin A. The amount of time between delivery of twin A and B is still a matter of controversy. If electronic fetal monitoring suggests fetal well-being, it is not necessary to deliver twin B within a prescribed amount of time such as 30 or 60 minutes. Difficult forceps operation or rapid extraction should be avoided, but forceps to protect the aftercoming premature head may be useful. The umbilical cord should be clamped promptly to prevent the second twin of a monozygotic twin pregnancy from exsanguinating into the first born.

Perform a vaginal examination immediately after delivery of twin A to note the presentation and station of the second twin, the presence of a second sac, an occult cord prolapse, or cord entanglement.

Cut the cord as far outside the vagina as possible so that it can hang loosely to permit vaginal examination or manipulation. This eliminates inadvertent cord traction on the placenta. Tag and label the cords (twin A and B) so that they may be associated with the proper placenta or placentas.

One twin may obstruct the delivery of both fetuses in locked twins. In this circumstance, twin A is always breech and twin B cephalic presentation, and the heads become impacted in the pelvis. Locked twins can be avoided by caesarean delivery in all cases in which it is known that twin A is not cephalic. However, if the obstetrician is presented with an emergent case of locked twins (Fig. 17–4), having an assistant support the twin already partially delivered as a breech while pushing both heads upward out of the pelvis with rotation of both fetuses may accomplish delivery of

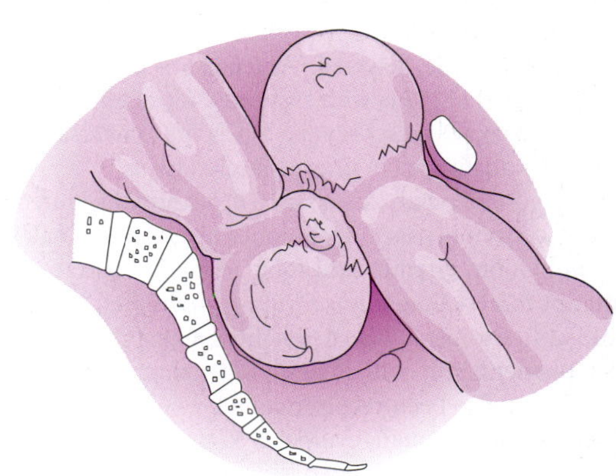

▲ **Figure 17–4.** Locked twins. (Reproduced, with permission, from Benson RC. *Handbook of Obstetrics & Gynecology*. 4th ed. Los Altos, CA: Lange; 1971.)

the first. This may require deep anesthesia. If this cannot be done, caesarean with abdominal delivery of both fetuses may be the safest route. An alternative while caesarean preparations are under way is to elevate the partially delivered twin, establish an airway, and protect the cord.

Postpartum hemorrhage is common in multiple pregnancy. Increased intravenous oxytocin, elevation, and massage of the fundus and an intravenous ergot or prostaglandin product (only after the last fetus is delivered) may be required. After delivery, if separation of the placenta is delayed or bleeding is brisk, manual extraction of the placenta may be necessary. Currently, we recommend prophylactic rectal misoprostol in the operating room followed by oral misoprostol every 6 hours for 24 hours after delivery for all multiple gestations.

Preeclampsia–eclampsia and premature labor and delivery are managed as outlined elsewhere in this book.

If it is desired to determine zygosity after delivery, concordance of placental examination, clinical comparisons, and hematologic and serologic tests provides presumptive evidence of monozygotic twinning. The total probability of diagnosis of zygosity is >95% using ABO, MNSs, Rh, Kell, Kidd, Duffy, and Lewis A and B antigens and approaches 100% using chromosomal analysis.

Prognosis

The US maternal mortality rate for women carrying a multiple gestation is only slightly higher than for singletons. With diligent care, many mothers and babies will do well. A history of previous dizygotic twins increases the likelihood of multiple gestation in a future pregnancy 10-fold.

Alexander JM, Leveno KJ, Rouse D, et al. Cesarean delivery for the second twin. *Obstet Gynecol* 2008;112:748–752. PMID: 18827115.

American College of Obstetricians and Gynecologists. *Multiple Gestation: Complicated Twin, Triplet and Higher-Order Multifetal Pregnancy. ACOG Practice Bulletin No. 56.* Washington, DC: American College of Obstetricians and Gynecologists; 2004.

Berghella V, Baxter JK, Hendrix NW. Cervical assessment by ultrasound for preventing preterm delivery. *Cochrane Database Syst Rev* 2009;3:CD007235. PMID: 19588421.

Blickstein I. Growth aberration in multiple pregnancy. *Obstet Gynecol Clin North Am* 2005;32:39–54. PMID: 15644288.

Bush MC, Malone FD. Down syndrome screening in twins. *Clin Perinatol.* 2005;32:373–836. PMID: 15922788.

Crowther CA, Han S. Hospitalisation and bed rest for multiple pregnancy. *Cochrane Database Syst Rev* 2010;7:CD000110. PMID: 20614420.

Dodd JM, Crowther CA. Elective delivery of women with a twin pregnancy from 37 weeks' gestation. *Cochrane Database Syst Rev* 2003;1:CD003582. PMID: 12535480.

Evans MI, Ciorica D, Britt DW, Fletcher JC. Update on selective reduction. *Prenat Diagn* 2005;9:807–813. PMID: 16170845.

Fox NS, Saltzman DH, Klauser CK, et al. Prediction of spontaneous preterm birth in asymptomatic twin pregnancies with the use of combined fetal fibronectin and cervical length. *Am J Obstet Gynecol* 2009;201:313.e1–e5. PMID: 19733285.

Fox NS, Silverstein M, Bender S, et al. Active second-stage management in twin pregnancies undergoing planned vaginal delivery in a U.S. population. *Obstet Gynecol* 2010;115:229–333. PMID: 20093893.

Hack KE, Derks JB, Elias SG, et al. Increased perinatal mortality and morbidity in monochorionic versus dichorionic twin pregnancies: Clinical implications of a large Dutch cohort study. *BJOG* 2008;115:58–67. PMID: 17999692.

Healy AJ, Gaddipati S. Intrapartum management of twins: Truths and controversies. *Clin Perinatol* 2005;32:455–473. PMID: 1592279.

Heyborne KD, Porreco RP, Garite TJ, Phair K, Abril D; Obstetrix/Pediatrix Research Study Group. Improved perinatal survival of monoamniotic twins with intensive inpatient monitoring. *Am J Obstet Gynecol* 2005;192:96–101. PMID: 15672009.

Lewi L, Gratacos E, Ortibus E, et al. Pregnancy and infant outcome of 80 consecutive cord coagulations in complicated monochorionic multiple pregnancies. *Am J Obstet Gynecol* 2006;194: 782–789. PMID: 16522413.

Luke B. Nutrition and multiple gestation. *Semin Perinatol* 2005;29:349–354. PMID: 16360494.

Moise KJ Jr, Johnson A, Moise KY, Nickeleit V. Radiofrequency ablation for selective reduction in the complicated monochorionic gestation. *Am J Obstet Gynecol* 2008;198:198.e1–e5. PMID: 18226623.

Murakoshi T, Ishii K, Matsushita M, et al. Monochorionic monoamniotic twin pregnancies with two yolk sacs may not be a rare finding: A report of two cases. *Ultrasound Obstet Gynecol* 2010;36:384–386. PMID: 20533442.

Oleszczuk JJ, Keith LG, Oleszczuk AK. The paradox of old maternal age in multiple pregnancies. *Obstet Gynecol Clin North Am* 2005;32:69–80. PMID: 15644290.

Ortibus E, Lopriore E, Deprest J, et al. The pregnancy and long-term neurodevelopmental outcome of monochorionic diamniotic twin gestations: A multicenter prospective cohort study from the first trimester onward. *Am J Obstet Gynecol* 2009;200:494.e1–e8. PMID: 19275567.

Peaceman AM, Kuo L, Feinglass J. Infant morbidity and mortality associated with vaginal delivery in twin gestations. *Am J Obstet Gynecol* 2009;200:462.e1–e6. PMID: 19318158.

Rustico MA, Baietti MG, Coviello D, Orlandi E, Nicolini U. Managing twins discordant for fetal anomaly. *Prenat Diagn* 2005;25:766–771. PMID: 16170860.

Shetty A, Smith AP. The sonographic diagnosis of chorionicity. *Prenat Diagn* 2005;25:735–739. PMID: 16170841.

Smith GC, Fleming KM, White IR. Birth order of twins and risk of perinatal death related to delivery in England, Northern Ireland, and Wales, 1994-2003: Retrospective cohort study. *BMJ* 2007;334(7593):576. PMID: 17337456.

Spadola AC, Simpson LL. Selective termination procedures in monochorionic pregnancies. *Semin Perinatol* 2005;29:330–337. PMID: 16360492.

Stone J, Ferrara L, Kamrath J, et al. Contemporary outcomes with the latest 1000 cases of multifetal pregnancy reduction (MPR). *Am J Obstet Gynecol* 2008;199(4):406.e1–e4. PMID: 19828991.

18 Third-Trimester Vaginal Bleeding

Sarah A. Wagner, MD

Vaginal bleeding in the third trimester can be very worrisome to a patient and clinician. When evaluating a patient with this problem, it is important to consider all the possible diagnoses in order to arrive at the appropriate conclusion and treatment. The most common causes of third-trimester vaginal bleeding are:

- Cervical bleeding associated with cervical change
- Abruptio placentae
- Placenta previa
- Vasa previa

Cervical bleeding associated with cervical change will be discussed in the section on the evaluation of preterm labor and labor at term.

ABRUPTIO PLACENTAE

Abruptio placentae (placental abruption) is defined as the premature separation of the normally implanted placenta from the uterine wall after 20 weeks of gestation but prior to the delivery of the infant. It is diagnosed retrospectively, evident only when the inspection of the placenta reveals a clot over the placental bed with disruption of the underlying placental tissue. The placental tissue may not show overt evidence of disruption if the abruption-to-delivery interval is short. One-third of all antepartum bleeding in the third trimester is due to placental abruption, and it will occur in 1 in 75–225 deliveries. About 1 in 830 abruptions end in fetal demise.

ESSENTIALS OF DIAGNOSIS

- Bleeding from the vagina
- Uterine activity
- Fetal heart rate abnormalities
- Changes in maternal hemodynamic status

Pathogenesis

Placental abruption may be the end of a chronic vascular pathologic process or may be due to a single inciting event. Bleeding due to vascular disruption accumulates and tracks along the decidua, separating the placenta from the remaining decidual layer. This may result in a partial abruption, referring to a self-limited hematoma that does not dissect the placental attachment further, or it may proceed to a complete abruption, leaving no decidual interface intact.

Abruption can be classified into 3 broad categories that allow for a description of the clinical and laboratory findings (Table 18–1).

- Grade 1: A small amount of vaginal bleeding and abnormal uterine activity or irritability are usually noted. The fetal heart rate tracing is within normal limits. Maternal hemodynamic status is normal, and all coagulation studies and laboratory values are within normal limits.
- Grade 2: A mild to moderate amount of vaginal bleeding is noted. Uterine activity may be tetanic or with frequent palpable and painful contractions. The fetal heart rate tracing may show decreased variability or late decelerations. Maternal hemodynamic status shows signs of compensation, including orthostatic hypotension and tachycardia, while maintaining overall blood pressure. Maternal fibrinogen may be decreased.
- Grade 3: External uterine bleeding may range from mild (likely concealed) to severe. The uterus is typically painful and tetanic. Fetal death has occurred. Maternal hemodynamic status is unstable, showing signs of severe volume depletion with hypotension and tachycardia. Thrombocytopenia and coagulation panel value abnormalities are present. Fibrinogen concentration level is typically <150 mg/dL.

The primary cause of placental abruption is unknown in most cases; however, it has been linked to several risk factors.

Table 18–1. Common causes of third-trimester bleeding.

Obstetric Causes	Nonobstetric Causes
Bloody show	Cervical cancer or dysplasia
Placenta previa	Cervicitis[1]
Abruptio placentae	Cervical polyps
Vasa previa	Cervical eversion
Disseminated intravascular coagulopathy (DIC)	Vaginal laceration
Uterine rupture	Vaginitis
Marginal sinus bleed[2]	

[1]Due to trichomoniasis, *Chlamydia trachomatis, Neisseria gonorrhoeae,* herpes simplex virus, etc.
[2]Marginal sinus bleed is a form of abruptio placentae.

Mechanical force or trauma is sometimes implicated, usually as a result of domestic violence or a motor vehicle accident. The clinical picture following a traumatic event can be severe in nature, and symptoms typically present within 24 hours. Blunt abdominal trauma can compress the placental interface, allowing for a shearing effect when decompression occurs. Rapid deceleration is the typical inciting event during a motor vehicle accident. Prolonged continuous fetal monitoring is critical in assuring the safety of the pregnancy. The mechanical force of rapid decompression of the uterus is an uncommon etiology. This can occur after the delivery of the first infant during the vaginal delivery of a twin gestation or after rupture of membranes in a patient with polyhydramnios.

Several factors can put a patient at risk for this disease. Maternal hypertension (>140/90 mm Hg) has been strongly associated with the occurrence of placental abruption. In fact, all hypertensive disorders of pregnancy have been implicated as risk factors. Forty to fifty percent of patients with grade 3 abruptions are found to have hypertensive disease of pregnancy.

Smoking is associated with a significant increase in the incidence of placental abruption, with a 2.5 relative risk of abruption severe enough to cause fetal death. Hypertension with concomitant cigarette smoking during pregnancy further increases the risk of abruption.

The relationship between age and the risk of placental abruption is not clear when other confounding factors, such as hypertension and multiparity, are corrected. Most authors feel that there is no direct correlation; however, a Norwegian study done over 15 years showed a strong relationship between placental abruption and maternal age among all levels of parity.

Increasing parity is a risk factor for placental abruption. The incidence in primigravidas is 1%, and this incidence increases to 2.5% in grand multiparas, correcting for confounding factors. This may be due to impaired decidualization after the implantation of multiple past placentas on the uterine wall.

Acquired or inherited thrombophilias may be associated with an increased risk of abruption. Factor V Leiden and prothrombin gene mutations have been implicated in multiple studies. Less common inherited thrombophilias, including protein C, protein S, and antithrombin deficiencies, may also be associated.

Approximately 2–5% of pregnancies that are complicated by preterm premature rupture of membranes will also be complicated by placental abruption. There is an even more substantial risk in patients who subsequently develop chorioamnionitis after rupturing membranes. It is difficult to ascertain whether the abruption is the cause or an effect of the ruptured membranes.

There is a well-known association between cocaine abuse and placental abruption, and up to 10% of women who use cocaine during pregnancy will incur this complications. It is likely due to acute vasoconstriction and disruption of vascular integrity directly as a result of cocaine use.

A history of placental abruption significantly predisposes a patient to another placental abruption. Five to 17% of all pregnancies complicated by abruption will recur in subsequent pregnancies. After 2 abruptions, the risk of recurrence increases to 25%. The reason for this association is unknown.

Clinical Findings

A. Symptoms & Signs

Most placental abruptions will present with the clinical triad, although many will not fill all 3 of the following categories:

- Fetal distress or fetal death: Fetal distress is typically the first clinical sign among patients who have continuous fetal monitoring during the abruption. A nonreassuring fetal heart rate tracing or poor biophysical profile score may indicate fetal compromise from a decrease in the placental exchange surface area or from severe maternal hypotension due to a large blood loss.
- Tetanic uterine activity (ie, contractions).
- Uterine bleeding, external or concealed.

Prompt evaluation is critical in caring for the patient with third-trimester uterine bleeding and possible placental abruption. All other common and potentially life-threatening causes of bleeding should be ruled out, including placenta previa, vasa previa, vaginal trauma, and vaginal or cervical malignancy. Once all other causes have been ruled out, placental abruption becomes the most likely diagnosis. Nearly 80% of patients with placental abruption will present with the complaint of vaginal bleeding. The 20% who do not exhibit this hallmark will commonly be diagnosed with labor or preterm labor. Patients occasionally complain of symptoms consistent with uterine tenderness and will be found to have increased uterine tone upon physical exam. Patients with these symptoms upon presentation will have a more severe abruption.

B. Laboratory Findings

Blood type and Rh status, hemoglobin, hematocrit, platelet count, coagulation studies, and fibrinogen level should be sent. A Kleihauer-Betke test should be sent for all women who are Rh negative.

C. Imaging Studies

Ultrasound has become important in the diagnosis and characterization of placental abruption. More than 50% of patients with confirmed abruption will have evidence of hemorrhage on ultrasound. Echogenicity, size, and location of the hemorrhage can be described, allowing the clinician to better understand the timing and severity of the abruption. If the ultrasound is performed during the early phases of the abruption, the area of hemorrhage will appear isoechoic or hyperechoic compared with the echogenicity of the placenta. The hematoma becomes hypoechoic within 1 week and sonolucent within 2 weeks of the initial hemorrhage.

The size and location of the hematoma are important in evaluating the severity of the abruption. A larger hematoma is associated with a worse prognosis than a smaller hematoma. A retroplacental hemorrhage has a worse prognosis than a subchorionic hemorrhage, which is defined as a collection of blood between the chorion and the decidua. A retroplacental hemorrhage that is >60 mL in volume has at least a 50% morality rate associated with it.

Prevention

Although no intervention has been shown to prevent placental abruption, known risk factors for placental abruption include poorly controlled maternal hypertension, smoking, and cocaine use. Counseling patients against smoking and cocaine use and helping them find appropriate cessation programs may reduce the risk of abruption, as may antihypertensive medication for women with poorly controlled hypertension.

Treatment

The hemodynamic status of the mother should be immediately evaluated and stabilization performed if necessary. Two large-bore intravenous lines should be placed, and the fetal heart rate should be monitored continuously. Crystalloid infusion should be started to rapidly correct the volume deficit, and packed red blood cells should be given if severe anemia is evident or if there is continued uterine bleeding. Urine output should be maintained above 30 mL/h. If no transfusion is required immediately, 4 units of packed red blood cells should be crossed and held nearby. Fresh frozen plasma should be administered for a fibrinogen level <100 mg/dL, and platelets should be given if the platelet count is <20,000 or <50,000 for a patient with severe continued hemorrhage or a requirement for emergent caesarean delivery. The clinician should not be falsely reassured by normal blood pressure and pulse, as the patient may have had hypertension previously and has had too rapid a volume loss to produce tachycardia.

Mode and timing of delivery depend greatly on the severity of the placental abruption and the gestational age of the pregnancy. If a grade 1 abruption has occurred and the gestational age is >37 weeks, the most appropriate course of action is induction or augmentation of labor with very close monitoring of the maternal and fetal status at all times. In the case of a preterm fetus with a grade 1 abruption, conservative management is indicated. Expectant management with short-term hospitalization has been shown to prolong the length of the pregnancy and has not been shown to increase morbidity or mortality of the fetus or the mother. If conservative management is pursued, administration of corticosteroids to promote fetal lung maturity is indicated if the gestational age is <34 weeks.

If the decision has been made to deliver the infant, close monitoring throughout labor and delivery is imperative. The hemodynamic status of the mother needs to be known at all times, and the fetal heart rate should be evaluated continuously. Serial coagulation studies and complete blood count should be obtained. If possible, an intrauterine pressure catheter should be use to evaluate uterine tone. If it appears that the patient's labor curve is progressing normally, a vaginal delivery is the preferable method of delivery.

An emergent caesarean section may be necessary at any point during labor. An increase in the resting tone of the myometrium may indicate a worsening of the abruption, and the possible compromise of blood flow to the fetus is an indication for emergent delivery. Other indications include a nonreassuring fetal heart rate tracing, severe hemorrhage, and disseminated intravascular coagulation. If an indication for emergent delivery has been identified, the maternal hemodynamic status should be quickly stabilized and correction of coagulopathy should be performed before proceeding. If the fetal status is reassuring and the caesarean is for maternal reasons, the correction of hypovolemia and coagulopathy can be done in a more controlled manner to avoid fluid overload prior to the surgery.

Prognosis

Outcome depends significantly on the gestational age of the fetus and the severity of the abruption. Prematurity, intrauterine growth restriction, caesarean delivery, and perinatal mortality are all increased in pregnancies that are complicated by placental abruption. In 1999, a review found that a pregnancy complicated by abruption, of any level of severity, had a 9-fold increase in the incidence of perinatal death, a 2-fold increase in the incidence of intrauterine growth restriction, and a 4-fold increase in the incidence of preterm birth.

Placental abruption is also associated with a substantial recurrence risk in future pregnancies of approximately 5–17%. After a history of 2 pregnancies affected by placental abruption, the risk of recurrence is approximately 25%. Unfortunately, there is no intervention that has been demonstrated to reduce the risk of recurrence. Preconception counseling should be targeted toward eliminating known risk factors such as smoking or cocaine use.

Ananth CV, Oyelese Y, Srinivas N, et al. Preterm premature rupture of membranes, intrauterine infection, and oligohydramnios: Risk factors for placental abruption. *Obstet Gynecol* 2004;104:71. PMID: 15229003.

PLACENTA PREVIA

When the placenta implants such that the placental tissue is located adjacent to or overlying the internal cervical os, it is called **placenta previa**. Placenta previa is the leading cause of third-trimester bleeding, complicating 4 in 1000 pregnancies over 20 weeks. The incidence is higher in early pregnancy prior to the development of the lower uterine segment, and most of these previas resolve as the pregnancy progresses.

There are 3 types of placenta previa (Fig. 18–1):

- Marginal placental previa: Characterized by the placenta being proximate to the margin of the internal os. It does not cover the os.
- Partial placenta previa: The placenta partially occludes the os, but does not completely cover it.
- Complete placenta previa: The internal os is fully covered by the placenta. This type is associated with the greatest risk of morbidity and mortality because it can cause the greatest amount of blood loss.

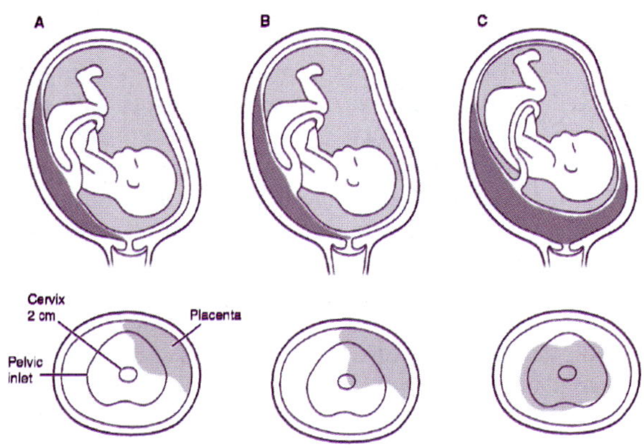

▲ **Figure 18–1.** **A:** Marginal placenta previa. **B:** Partial placenta previa. **C:** Complete placenta previa.

ESSENTIALS OF DIAGNOSIS

- Painless vaginal bleeding
- Ultrasonographic findings consistent with placenta previa

Pathogenesis

When a placenta implants in the lower part of the uterus, the pregnancy is at risk for placenta previa. There are several risk factors, including multiparity, increasing maternal age, history of prior caesarean section or uterine surgery, and multiple gestation.

Multiparas are at higher risk for placenta previa compared to nulliparas. The incidence of previa in nulliparas is 0.2%, whereas grand multiparas have an incidence of 5%. The theory behind this phenomenon is that once a placenta has implanted into a certain part of the uterine wall, it has permanently altered its constitution, making implantation at a different site more likely in subsequent pregnancies. Increasing maternal age has been a risk factor, and the cause of this association is unclear. The increased risk may be due to higher parity in older mothers, but it may also be an independent risk factor.

The risk of placenta previa increases directly with the number of uterine surgeries a patient has had in the past. This is mostly seen with increasing numbers of caesarean sections. The risk of placenta previa in second pregnancies after a first pregnancy delivered by caesarean section is 1–4%. The risk increases to nearly 10% in patients with 4 or more previous caesarean deliveries. Furthermore, it has been suggested that previas identified in the second trimester in patients with a previous caesarean delivery have a lower likelihood of resolving as the pregnancy progresses. Risk increases with previous curettage for spontaneous or induced abortion, thought to be due to a scarred active segment of the uterus.

Other risk factors for placenta previa include multiple gestation and smoking. This is due to the greater surface area of the placenta in these situations.

Placenta previa can be associated with several other conditions, including malpresentation, preterm premature rupture of membranes, and intrauterine growth restriction. There may also be an increased risk of congenital anomalies; however, there is no association with any specific anomaly.

Patients with placenta previa are at higher risk for developing placenta accreta, increta, or percreta.

- Placenta accreta: There is no decidua basalis, and the fibrinoid layer is incompletely developed.
- Placenta increta: The placenta invades the myometrium.
- Placenta percreta: The placenta penetrates the myometrium and may invade nearby viscera.

Previous uterine surgery is the risk factor most associated with placenta accreta. Patients with no prior uterine surgery and placenta previa will have accreta 4% of the time. Patients with 1 prior uterine surgery and placenta previa will have accreta 10–35% of the time. Multiple prior caesarean deliveries and placenta previa incurs a 60–65% risk of accreta. Two-thirds of patients with placenta accreta will require a caesarean-hysterectomy.

Clinical Findings

A. Symptoms & Signs

Placenta previa typically presents with painless vaginal bleeding, usually in the third trimester. Lack of pain with the presence of bleeding is what distinguishes placenta previa from placental abruption. The bleeding occurs in conjunction with the development of the lower uterine segment. As the myometrium becomes thinner, the placenta–decidua interface is disrupted, causing bleeding. The thinness of the lower uterine segment prevents it from contracting to minimize the bleeding from the uterine surface of the implantation site; however, sometimes the bleeding itself can irritate the myometrium and precipitate contractions.

The clinician should have a high index of suspicion for placenta previa in all patients who present with bleeding after 24 weeks. One-third of patients with placenta previa will present with bleeding before 30 weeks, one-third will present between 30 and 36 weeks, and one-third will present after 36 weeks. Ten percent of all women with previa will reach full term without an episode of bleeding. On average, a patient's first episode of bleeding will occur at 34 weeks, with delivery at 36 weeks. Risk of perinatal mortality and morbidity decreases linearly as gestational age increases.

B. Laboratory Findings

Baseline admission labs including blood type and Rh status, hemoglobin, hematocrit, and platelet count should be sent. Coagulation studies and fibrinogen concentration are not as important in patients with previa as in patients with abruption; however, if there is any doubt of the diagnosis, these should also be sent. A Kleihauer-Betke test should be sent for all women who are Rh negative.

C. Imaging Studies

Prior to the advent of routine second-trimester ultrasound, patients with placenta previa were diagnosed at the onset of bleeding. Currently, most cases are diagnosed by ultrasound in the second trimester, although most of these will resolve. Five to fifteen percent of all patients will have placenta previa at 17 weeks. Ninety percent of these will resolve by 37 weeks. This occurs because as the lower uterine segment develops, more distance is created between the placenta and the cervix. Complete previa and marginal or partial previa diagnosed in the second trimester will persist in 26% and 2.5% of patients, respectively. All patients who have placenta previa diagnosed before 24 weeks should have a sonogram between 28 and 32 weeks to reassess the position of the placenta.

Treatment

The initial management of a patient with a bleeding placenta previa is very similar to the initial management of a patient with placental abruption. Hemodynamic status of the mother should be immediately evaluated and stabilization performed if necessary. Large-bore intravenous lines should be placed, and the fetal heart rate should be monitored continuously.

Hemodynamic stabilization should be performed immediately. Crystalloid infusion should be started in order to rapidly correct a volume deficit, and packed red blood cells should be given if severe anemia is evident or if there is continued uterine bleeding. The goal hematocrit is at least 30% if the patient is bleeding. If no transfusion is required immediately, 4 units of packed red blood cells should be crossed and held nearby. The urine output should be maintained above 30 mL/h.

Subsequent management depends on gestational age, stability of the mother and fetus, the amount of bleeding, and presentation of the fetus. Delivery is always indicated if there is a nonreassuring fetal heart rate pattern despite resuscitation efforts, including maternal supplemental oxygen, left-side positioning, or intravascular volume replacement; if there is life-threatening maternal hemorrhage; or if the gestational age is >34 weeks and there is known fetal lung maturity. If the fetus is ≥37 weeks of gestational age and there is persistent bleeding or persistent uterine activity, delivery is also indicated. Digital cervical exams should be avoided.

Between 24 and 36 weeks, if maternal and fetal stability and well-being are assured, conservative expectant management may be indicated. About 75% of patients with symptomatic placenta previa are candidates for conservative management, and 50% of these patients can prolong their pregnancy by at least 4 weeks. Thirty percent of patients treated this way will progress to term without bleeding again. Seventy percent will have at least 1 more episode of bleeding, and 10% of these patients will have a third episode.

Conservative management, after stabilization has occurred and little or no uterine bleeding is noted, consists of several steps. Hydration and blood transfusion are given if necessary. Continuous fetal heart rate monitoring is required in cases where there is continued uterine bleeding, contractile activity, or intrauterine growth restriction. Tocolytic agents, if there is no suspicion for placental abruption, may be given if membranes have not been ruptured and there is contractile uterine activity. The patient should be restricted to bed rest with bathroom privileges. She should be given stool softeners, iron supplementation, and vitamin C. Steroids to promote fetal lung maturity should be administered if the gestational age is <34 weeks.

After steroids have been administered, if there is little or no uterine activity or bleeding, the patient may be a candidate for home therapy. To be considered for home therapy, the patient must be very reliable, have 24-hour contact via telephone, and have the ability to return quickly to the hospital at any time. She should remain on bed rest with bathroom privileges and should continue to take stool softeners and vitamin therapy. Strict instructions should be given regarding returning to the hospital if she experiences contractions or another episode of bleeding.

Fetal growth, amniotic fluid index, and placental location should be assessed by ultrasound every 3 weeks. Most experts agree that for the patient with complete placenta previa that is otherwise uncomplicated, delivery is recommended at 36–37 weeks.

If uterine bleeding is not excessive, patients with marginal previa may be delivered vaginally. Upon descent, the fetal head should tamponade bleeding. Abdominal delivery is indicated in most cases of placenta previa and in all cases of complete previa. If a caesarean section is performed, care should be taken not to disrupt the placenta upon fetal delivery. If possible, a uterine incision away from the placental bed should be used. For example, if there is an anterolateral placenta, a vertical incision in the lower uterine segment opposite the site of placental implantation should be used. A high transverse incision may be necessary for a low anterior placenta. In all cases, the operating room should be prepared for the possibility of the necessity to perform a hysterectomy.

As noted earlier, 66% of patients with placenta accreta will require a caesarean-hysterectomy. There are several surgical options if uterine preservation is important. The placenta can be removed and the uterine defect can be oversewn to abate the active focus of bleeding. The area of accreta can be resected and the uterus repaired. The last option includes leaving the placenta in situ. This is only acceptable in patients who are not actively bleeding. The cord should be ligated and cut close to its base. The patient should be treated with antibiotics and possibly methotrexate postpartum. In the rare case where bladder invasion is evident, the placenta should not be removed. These patients will likely require hysterectomy and partial cystectomy. (See Chapter 21.)

Prognosis

Neonatal outcomes have much improved in the last 20 years, secondary to conservative management, the liberal use of caesarean section, improved neonatal care, and earlier diagnosis. The perinatal mortality rate has fallen from 60% to 10% over the past several decades due to the ability to resuscitate and support infants who are increasingly more premature. Most mortality is due to prematurity. An earlier of episode of bleeding brings with it a higher risk of prematurity and thus a higher risk of mortality. The maternal mortality rate has decreased from 25% to <1% in patients with access to health care. Maternal mortality remains high in developing countries.

Ananth CV, Demissie K, Smulian JC, Vintzileos AM. Placenta previa in singleton and twin birth in the United States, 1989 through 1998: A comparison of risk factor profiles and associated conditions. *Am J Obstet Gynecol* 2003;188:275. PMID: 12548229.

Faiz AS, Ananth CV. Etiology and risk factors for placenta previa: An overview and meta-analysis of observational studies. *J Matern Fetal Neonatal Med* 2003;13:175. PMID: 12820840.

Laughon SK, Wolfe HM, Visco AG. Prior cesarean and the risk for placenta previa on second-trimester ultrasonography. *Obstet Gynecol* 2005;105(5 Pt 1):962–965. PMID: 15863531.

Sheiner E, Shoham-Vardi I, Hallak M, et al. Placenta previa: Obstetric risk factors and pregnancy outcome. *J Matern Fetal Med* 2001;10:414. PMID: 11798453.

Spong CY, Mercer BM, D'alton M, Kilpatrick S, Blackwell S, Saade G. Timing of indicated late-preterm and early-term birth. *Obstet Gynecol* 2011;118:323-33. PMID: 21775849.

Taipale P, Orden MR, Berg M, Manninen H, Alafuzoff I. Prenatal diagnosis of placenta accreta and percreta with ultrasonography, color Doppler, and magnetic resonance imaging. *Obstet Gynecol* 2004;104:537–540. PMID: 15339765.

VASA PREVIA

Vasa previa is a condition in which fetal vessels traverse the membranes in the lower uterine segment, crossing over the cervical os on front of the fetal head. This can occur with a velamentous insertion of the umbilical cord, where Wharton's jelly is not present to protect the fetal vessels, or in the case where a succenturiate lobe of the placenta has a vascular communication traversing the os. Rupture of these vessels can occur with or without rupturing membranes, and the result is fetal exsanguination. Vasa previa complicates approximately 1 in 1000 to 1 in 5000 pregnancies.

ESSENTIALS OF DIAGNOSIS

- Ultrasonographic evidence of vasa previa
- Painless vaginal bleeding upon rupture of membranes
- Fetal heart rate abnormalities
- Positive Apt, Ogita, or Loendersloot tests

Clinical Findings

A. Symptoms & Signs

The typical presentation of vasa previa is vaginal bleeding that occurs upon rupture of membranes with concomitant specific changes in the fetal heart rate tracing. With the onset of bleeding, the fetal heart responds to loss of intravascular volume with reflex tachycardia. Reflex tachycardia is usually followed by bradycardia accompanied by occasional accelerations. With severe fetal anemia, a sinusoidal fetal heart rate pattern may be seen. The clinician must have a high index of suspicion in order to make the correct diagnosis in enough time to prevent fetal death.

B. Laboratory Findings

Very rarely, the fetal heart rate does not show signs of acute volume loss, and the blood can be analyzed to determine its origin. The Apt, Ogita, and Loendersloot tests take between 5 and 10 minutes to perform and are available to identify fetal hemoglobin. They have varying sensitivities depending on the amount of dilution of the blood with amniotic fluid. However, these tests are primarily of historical interest. If a patient is bleeding from a diagnosed or strongly suspected vasa previa, caesarean delivery should be expedited.

C. Imaging Studies

With improvement in ultrasound technology and an increased awareness among providers about this disorder, many cases are now being diagnosed in the antepartum period via ultrasound. The ultrasound finding of either velamentous cord insertion or succenturiate lobe of the placenta should prompt providers to evaluate for vasa previa. The use of color Doppler during transvaginal ultrasound can clearly identify fetal vessels coursing through the fetal membranes and can establish the diagnosis. If the vessel is a fetal artery, pulsed Doppler can help confirm and measurement of the pulse rate can help to ascertain the diagnosis. Vasa previa can be distinguished from funic presentation (free loops of umbilical cord resting adjacent to the cervix) by mapping the fetal vessels from the placenta or cord insertion. Additionally, changes in maternal position may allow for free cord as in funic presentation to move, whereas vessels in a vasa previa will remain in place.

Treatment

If a patient presents with the previously mentioned classic findings, the appropriate course of action is to deliver immediately via caesarean section to prevent impending fetal demise. If the patient has been identified antenatally, it is recommended that the patient be monitored very closely for any evidence of vaginal bleeding and to administer corticosteroids to promote fetal lung maturity. Several experts recommend inpatient observation starting at 32 weeks. Inpatient observation allows for emergent caesarean in event of nonreassuring fetal testing, preterm labor, or preterm premature ruptured membranes. Empiric delivery at approximately 35 weeks of gestation without confirmation of lung maturity via amniocentesis is also recommended by several experts. Oyelese et al report that the mean gestational age at delivery in patients who are diagnosed antenatally is approximately 35 weeks, and almost 30% of these patients still require emergent delivery after membranes are ruptured. Because the rates of morbidity and mortality are so high after ruptured membranes in these patients, they recommend delivery at 35 weeks in order to avoid a catastrophic event and feel that it is justified even in the light of possible complications due to prematurity.

Prognosis

Fetal mortality has been reported as >50% in pregnancies complicated by vasa previa. Antenatal diagnosis increases the chance of fetal survival significantly. In one study, the rates of survival for fetuses and neonates with and without antenatal diagnosis were 97% and 44%, respectively.

Oyelese Y, Catanzarite V, Prefumo F, et al. Vasa previa: The impact of prenatal diagnosis on outcomes. *Obstet Gynecol* 2004;103:937. PMID: 15121568.

Malpresentation & Cord Prolapse

19

Karen Kish, MD

BREECH PRESENTATION

ESSENTIALS OF DIAGNOSIS

- Breech presentation occurs when the fetal pelvis or lower extremities engage the maternal pelvic inlet.
- Breech presentation may be suspected based on clinical examination, either by palpating fetal parts over the maternal abdomen or by pelvic examination.
- The diagnosis can be confirmed via ultrasound.

Breech presentation, which complicates 3–4% of all pregnancies, occurs when the fetal pelvis or lower extremities engage the maternal pelvic inlet. Three types of breech are distinguished, according to fetal **attitude** (Fig. 19–1). In **frank breech**, the hips are flexed with extended knees bilaterally. In **complete breech**, both hips and knees are flexed. In **footling breech**, 1 (single footling breech) or both (double footling breech) legs are extended below the level of the buttocks.

In singleton breech presentations in which the infant weighs less than 2500 g, 40% are frank breech, 10% complete breech, and 50% footling breech. With birth weights of more than 2500 g, 65% are frank breech, 10% complete breech, and 25% footling breech. The incidences of singleton breech presentations by birth weight and gestational age are listed in Table 19–1.

Fetal **position** in breech presentation is determined by using the fetal sacrum as the point of reference to the maternal pelvis. This is true for frank, complete, and footling breeches. Eight possible positions are recognized: sacrum anterior (SA), sacrum posterior (SP), left sacrum transverse (LST), right sacrum transverse (RST), left sacrum anterior (LSA), left sacrum posterior (LSP), right sacrum anterior (RSA), and right sacrum posterior (RSP). The **station** of the breech presenting part is the location of the fetal sacrum with regard to the maternal ischial spines.

Pathogenesis

Before 28 weeks, the fetus is small enough in relation to intrauterine volume to rotate from cephalic to breech presentation and back again with relative ease. As gestational age and fetal weight increase, the relative decrease in intrauterine volume makes such changes more difficult. In most cases, the fetus spontaneously assumes the cephalic presentation to better accommodate the bulkier breech pole in the roomier fundal portion of the uterus.

Breech presentation occurs when spontaneous version to cephalic presentation is prevented as term approaches or if labor and delivery occur prematurely before cephalic version has taken place. Some causes include oligohydramnios, polyhydramnios, uterine anomalies such as bicornuate or septate uterus, pelvic tumors obstructing the birth canal, abnormal placentation, advanced multiparity, and a contracted maternal pelvis.

In multiple gestations, each fetus may prevent the other from turning, with a 25% incidence of breech in the first twin, nearly 50% for the second twin, and higher percentages with additional fetuses. Additionally, 6% of breech presentations are found to have congenital malformations, which include congenital hip dislocation, hydrocephalus, anencephalus, familial dysautonomia, spina bifida, meningomyelocele, and chromosomal trisomies 13, 18, and 21. Thus, those conditions that alter fetal muscular tone and mobility increase the likelihood of breech presentation.

Clinical Findings

A. Palpation & Ballottement

Performance of Leopold's maneuvers and manual ballottement of the uterus through the maternal abdominal wall may confirm breech presentation. The softer, more ill-defined breech may be felt in the lower uterine segment above the pelvic inlet. Diagnostic error is common, however, if these maneuvers alone are used to determine presentation.

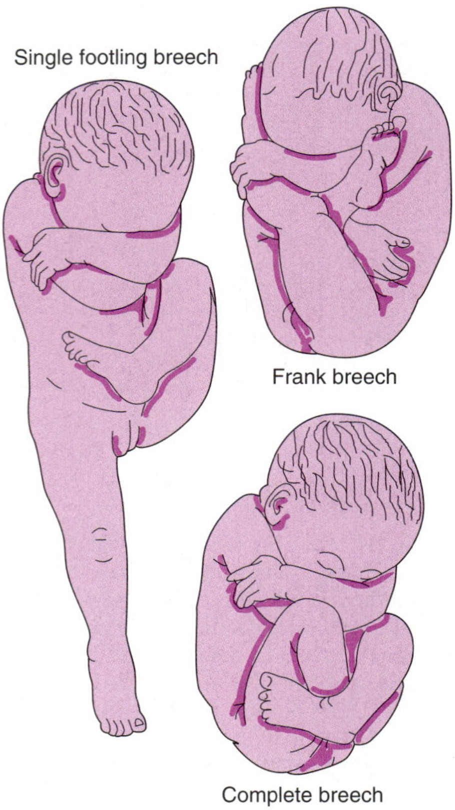

▲ **Figure 19–1.** Types of breech presentations. (Reproduced, with permission, from Pernoll ML. *Benson and Pernoll's Handbook of Obstetrics and Gynecology*. 10th ed. New York, NY: McGraw-Hill; 2001.)

B. Pelvic Examination

During vaginal examination, the round, firm, smooth head in cephalic presentation can easily be distinguished from the soft, irregular breech presentation if the presenting part is palpable. However, if no presenting part is discernible, further studies are necessary (ie, ultrasound).

C. Radiographic Studies

X-ray studies will differentiate breech from cephalic presentations and help determine the type of breech by locating the position of the lower extremities. X-ray studies can reveal multiple gestation and skeletal defects. Fetal attitude may be seen, but fetal size cannot readily be determined by x-ray film. Because of the risks of radiation exposure to the fetus with this technique, ultrasonography is now used instead of radiography to determine fetal presentation or malformations.

D. Ultrasound

Ultrasonographic scanning by an experienced examiner will document fetal presentation, attitude, and size; multiple gestation; location of the placenta; and amniotic fluid volume. Ultrasound also will reveal skeletal and soft tissue malformations of the fetus.

Complications

A. Birth Anoxia

Umbilical cord compression and prolapse may be associated with breech delivery, particularly in complete (5%) and footling (15%) presentations. This is due to the inability of the presenting part to fill the maternal pelvis, either because of prematurity or poor application of the presenting part to the cervix so that the umbilical cord is allowed to prolapse below the level of the breech (see below). Frank breech presentation offers a contoured presenting part, which is better accommodated to the maternal pelvis and is usually well applied to the cervix. The incidence of cord prolapse in frank breech is only 0.5% (the same as for cephalic presentations). Compression of the prolapsed cord may occur during uterine contractions, causing moderate to severe variable decelerations in the fetal heart rate and leading to fetal anoxia or death. If breech vaginal delivery is attempted, continuous electronic monitoring is mandatory during labor

Table 19–1. Incidence of singleton breech presentations by birthweight and gestational age.

Birthweight (g)	Gestational Age (weeks)	Incidence (%)
1000	28	35
1000–1499	28–32	25
1500–1999	32–34	20
2000–2499	34–36	8
2500	36	2–3
All weights		3–4

in these cases to detect ominous decelerations. If they occur, immediate caesarean delivery must be performed.

B. Birth Injury

The incidence of birth trauma during vaginal breech delivery is 6.7%, 13 times that of cephalic presentations (0.51%). Only high forceps and internal version and extraction procedures have higher rates of birth injury than do vaginal breech deliveries. The types of perinatal injuries reported in breech delivery include tears in the tentorium cerebellum, cephalohematomas, disruption of the spinal cord, brachial palsy, fracture of long bones, and rupture of the sternocleidomastoid muscles. Vaginal breech delivery is the main cause of injuries to the fetal adrenal glands, liver, anus, genitalia, spine, hip joint, sciatic nerve, and musculature of the arms, legs, and back.

Factors contributing to difficult vaginal breech delivery include a partially dilated cervix, unilateral or bilateral nuchal arms, and deflexion of the head. The type of procedure used may affect the neonatal outcome.

1. Partially dilated cervix—Delivery of a breech fetus may progress even though the cervix is only partially dilated because the bitrochanteric and bisacromial diameters are smaller than the biparietal diameter. This is true especially in prematurity. The hips and shoulders may negotiate the cervix, but the aftercoming head becomes entrapped, resulting in difficult delivery and birth injury.

2. Nuchal arms—During partial breech extraction and more often in total breech extraction, excessive downward traction on the body results in a single or double nuchal arm. This occurs because of the rapid descent of the body, leading to extension of 1 or both arms, which become lodged behind the neck. When delivery of the shoulder is difficult to accomplish, a nuchal arm should be suspected. To dislodge the arm, the operator rotates the body 180 degrees to bring the elbow toward the face. The humerus can then be identified and delivered by gentle downward traction. In cases of double nuchal arm, the fetus is rotated counterclockwise to dislodge and deliver the right arm and rotated clockwise to deliver the left arm. If this action is unsuccessful, the operator must insert a finger into the pelvis, identify the humerus, and possibly extract the arm, resulting in fracture of the humerus or clavicle. Nuchal arms cause a delay in delivery and increase the incidence of birth asphyxia.

3. Deflexion of the head—*Hyperextension of the head* is defined as deflexion or extension of the head posteriorly beyond the longitudinal axis of the fetus (5% of all breech deliveries). Causes of hyperextension include neck cysts, spasm of the neck musculature, and uterine anomalies, but over 75% have no known cause. Although deflexion may be documented by ultrasonographic or x-ray studies weeks before delivery, there is little apparent risk to the fetus until vaginal delivery is attempted. At that time, deflexion causes impaction of the occipital portion of the head behind the pubic symphysis, which may lead to fractures of the cervical vertebrae, lacerations of the spinal cord, epidural and medullary hemorrhages, and perinatal death. If head deflexion is diagnosed prior to delivery, caesarean section should be performed to avert injury. Caesarean section cannot prevent injuries such as minor meningeal hemorrhage or dislocation of the cervical vertebrae, which may develop in utero secondary to longstanding head deflexion.

4. Type of delivery—More complex delivery procedures have a higher rate of birth trauma. Whereas few infants are injured during spontaneous breech births, as many as 6% are injured during partial breech extraction and 20% during total breech extraction of singleton infants. Injuries associated with total breech extraction of singleton infants usually are extensive and severe, and this procedure should never be attempted unless fetal survival is in jeopardy and caesarean section cannot be immediately performed.

An additional important factor in breech injury and perinatal outcome is the experience of the operator. Inexperience may lead to hasty performance of obstetric maneuvers. Delay in delivery may result in birth asphyxia due to umbilical cord compression, but haste in the management of breech delivery results in application of excessive pressure on the fetal body, causing soft tissue damage and fracture of long bones. Too-rapid extraction of the body from the birth canal causes the arms to extend above the head, resulting in unilateral or bilateral nuchal arms and difficult delivery of the aftercoming head. All breech deliveries should be performed slowly and methodically by experienced obstetricians who execute the maneuvers with gentleness and skill—not speed.

Treatment

A. Antepartum Management

Following confirmation of breech presentation, the mother must be closely followed to evaluate for spontaneous version to cephalic presentation. If breech presentation persists beyond 36 weeks, external cephalic version should be considered (see below). Version is a procedure used to turn the fetal presenting part from breech to cephalic presentation (cephalic version) or from cephalic to breech presentation (podalic version). Because cephalic version is performed by manipulating the fetus through the abdominal wall, the maneuver is known as **external cephalic version.** Podalic version is performed by means of internal maneuvers and is known as **internal podalic version** (see below). External cephalic version is regaining popularity, whereas internal podalic version is rarely used.

In women considering a vaginal breech delivery of a singleton infant, radiographic pelvimetry using x-ray, computed tomography, or magnetic resonance imaging should be performed to rule out women with a borderline or contracted pelvis. Attempts at vaginal delivery with an inadequate pelvis are associated with a high rate of difficulty and significant trauma to mother and fetus. Difficult vaginal delivery may still occur in women with adequate pelvic measurements.

External cephalic version is used in the management of singleton breech presentations or in a nonvertex second twin. In carefully selected patients, it is safe for both mother and fetus. The goal is to increase the proportion of vertex presentations near term, thus increasing the chance for a vaginal delivery. In the past, external cephalic version was performed earlier in gestation but was accompanied by high reversion rates, making additional procedures necessary. Now it is performed in patients who have completed 36 weeks of gestation so that the risk of spontaneous reversion is decreased, and, if complications arise, delivery of a term infant can be accomplished. Current success rates for external cephalic version range from 35 to 85% (mean 60%).

Patients with unengaged singleton breech presentations of at least 36 weeks' gestation are candidates for external cephalic version. The procedure is more successful in multigravidas, those with a transverse or oblique lie, and those with a posterior placenta. Use of fetal heart rate monitoring and real-time ultrasonography is essential to document fetal well-being during the procedure. The use of tocolytics in external cephalic version is controversial. Recent evidence indicates that tocolytics offer an advantage in nulliparous women, but reports on which type of tocolytic confers the highest success rate are conflicting. Thus, these agents should be used at the discretion of the physician. Additionally, evidence regarding the use of regional anesthesia is inconsistent. Recent randomized controlled trials have shown an increased success rate in those with epidural anesthesia. However, the ultimate decision should be based on physician experience.

Contraindications to external cephalic version include engagement of the presenting part in the pelvis, marked oligohydramnios, placenta previa, uterine anomalies, presence of nuchal cord, multiple gestation, premature rupture of membranes, previous uterine surgery (including myomectomy or metroplasty), and suspected or documented congenital malformations or abnormalities (including intrauterine growth retardation).

Complications are rare, occurring in only 1–2% of all external cephalic versions. Complications include placental abruption, uterine rupture, rupture of membranes with resultant umbilical cord prolapse, amniotic fluid embolism, preterm labor, fetal distress, fetomaternal hemorrhage, and fetal demise. Thus, given the potential for catastrophic outcome, this procedure should be performed in a facility where immediate access to caesarean delivery is available. Patients require extensive counseling regarding the version procedure, with disclosure of all risks, benefits, and alternatives so that an informed medicolegal decision can be made.

1. Fetal heart rate abnormalities—These can be readily documented during external cephalic version by intermittent electronic fetal monitoring (EFM) or ultrasonographic surveillance. Fetal bradycardia occurs in 20% of cases, but normal cardiac activity usually will return if the procedure is stopped for a short time. If significant unremitting fetal cardiac alterations occur, the attempt at version should be discontinued and preparation for caesarean delivery undertaken immediately.

2. Fetomaternal transplacental hemorrhage (FMH)—This may occur during version and has been reported to occur in 6–28% of patients undergoing external cephalic version, although the amount of hemorrhage rarely results in clinically significant anemia. The **Kleihauer-Betke acid elution test** should be performed if this condition is suspected. In cases of an Rh-negative–unsensitized woman, Rh immune globulin (RhoGAM) should be administered after external cephalic version to cover the calculated amount of FMH.

3. Technique—External cephalic version is performed by first obtaining informed consent from the patient. An ultrasound examination is performed to verify presentation and to rule out fetal or uterine abnormalities. A nonstress test is done, and results must be reactive. If desired, a tocolytic is administered to prevent contractions or irritability. Anesthesia is also administered if desired. To perform the external cephalic version, both of the operator's hands are placed on the patient's abdomen, and a forward roll is attempted by lifting the breech upward while placing pressure on the head downward toward the pelvis. If this maneuver is unsuccessful, a backward roll can be attempted. Fetal well-being should be monitored intermittently with Doppler or real-time ultrasound scanning. The procedure should be abandoned in case of any significant fetal distress or patient discomfort or if multiple attempts are unsuccessful. Following the procedure, external fetal heart rate monitoring should be continued for 1 hour to ensure stability. If the patient is Rh negative, administer anti-D immune globulin. If the patient is stable, she can be sent home to await the onset of spontaneous labor if the version is successful. If unsuccessful, the patient can be scheduled for an elective caesarean section or a trial of labor with a breech vaginal delivery planned if the mother is a good candidate.

Recent studies have evaluated acupuncture and moxibustion (burning herbs to stimulate acupuncture points) to determine their role in facilitating spontaneous version of the breech fetus. To date, these trials have not found a consistent benefit to either mode.

B. Management during Labor

1. Examination—Patients with singleton breech presentations are admitted to the hospital with the onset of labor or when spontaneous rupture of membranes occurs because of the increased risk of umbilical cord complications. Upon admission, a repeat ultrasound is obtained to confirm the type of breech presentation and to ascertain head flexion. The fetus is again screened for lethal congenital malformations, such as anencephaly, which would preclude caesarean delivery for fetal indications. A thorough history is taken, and a physical examination is performed to evaluate the status of mother and fetus. Based on these findings, a decision must be made regarding the route of delivery (see below).

2. Electronic fetal monitoring—Continuous electronic fetal heart rate monitoring is essential during labor. If a fetal electrocardiographic electrode is needed, care should be taken to avoid injury to the fetal anus, perineum, and genitalia when attaching the electrode to the breech presenting part. An intrauterine pressure catheter can be used to assess the frequency, strength, and duration of uterine contractions. With the catheter in place, fetal distress or dysfunctional labor can easily be identified and the decision to proceed with a caesarean section made expeditiously to optimize fetal outcome.

3. Oxytocin—The use of oxytocin in the management of breech labor is controversial. Although some obstetricians condemn its use, others use oxytocin with benefit and without complications. Generally, oxytocin should be administered only if uterine contractions are insufficient to sustain normal progress in labor. Continuous fetal and uterine monitoring should be used whenever oxytocin is administered.

C. Delivery

The decision regarding route of delivery must be made carefully on an individual basis. Criteria for vaginal or caesarean delivery are outlined in Table 19–2.

Prior to 1975, virtually all viable singleton breech presentations were delivered vaginally. Caesarean section was reserved for specific fetal indications, such as unremitting distress or prolapsed umbilical cord, or maternal indications, such as placenta previa, abruptio placentae, or failure of progress in labor. However, breech infants delivered vaginally had a 5-fold higher mortality rate in comparison to cephalic presentations.

Recent studies have shown that planned caesarean delivery decreases perinatal and neonatal morbidity and mortality, with no difference in maternal morbidity and mortality versus planned vaginal breech delivery. Thus, caesarean delivery has now become much more common in breech presentation. Only obstetricians skilled in breech techniques should attempt any breech delivery, whether vaginal or caesarean. Nevertheless, broader familiarity with the technique is needed because unanticipated vaginal breech delivery is still encountered.

1. Caesarean delivery—The type of incision chosen is extremely important. If the lower uterine segment is well developed, as is usually the case in women at term in labor, a transverse "lower segment" incision is adequate for easy delivery. In premature gestations, in an unlabored uterus, or in many cases of malpresentation, the lower uterine segment may be quite narrow, and a low vertical incision is almost always required for atraumatic delivery.

2. Vaginal delivery—Obstetricians who contemplate performing a vaginal breech delivery should be experienced in the maneuver and should be assisted by 3 physicians: (1) an experienced obstetrician who will assist with delivery; (2) a pediatrician capable of providing total resuscitation of the newborn; and (3) an anesthesiologist, to ensure that the

Table 19–2. Criteria for vaginal or caesarean delivery in breech presentation.

Vaginal Delivery	Caesarean Delivery
Frank breech presentation	Estimated fetal weight of ≥3500 g or <1500 g
Gestational age of 34 weeks or more	Contracted or borderline maternal pelvic measurements
Estimated fetal weight of 2000–3500 g	Deflexed or hyperextended fetal head
Flexed fetal head	Prolonged rupture of membranes
Adequate maternal pelvis as determined by x-ray pelvimetry (pelvic inlet with transverse diameter of 11.5 cm and anteroposterior diameter of 10.5 cm; midpelvis with transverse diameter of 10 cm and anteroposterior diameter of 11.5 cm)	Unengaged presenting part Dysfunctional labor Elderly primigravida Mother with infertility problems or poor obstetric history Premature fetus (gestational age of 25–34 weeks)
No maternal or fetal indications for caesarean section Previable fetus (gestational age <25 weeks and weight <700 g)	Most cases of complete or footling breech over 25 weeks' gestation without detectable lethal congenital malformations (to prevent umbilical cord prolapse)
Documented lethal fetal congenital anomalies	Fetus with variable heart rate decelerations on electronic monitoring
Presentation of mother in advanced labor with no fetal or maternal distress, even if caesarean delivery was originally planned (a carefully performed, controlled vaginal delivery is safer in such cases than is a hastily executed caesarean section)	Footling presentation

mother is comfortable and cooperative during labor and delivery. The type of anesthesia required depends on the type of breech delivery. Multiparous women undergoing spontaneous breech delivery may require no anesthesia or only intravenous analgesia for pain relief during labor and a pudendal anesthetic during delivery. Epidural anesthesia may also be administered during labor or in anticipation of partial breech extraction, including application of Piper forceps to the aftercoming head. In emergency circumstances, complete relaxation of the perineum and uterus is essential for a successful outcome. This is accomplished by immediate induction of inhalation anesthesia or by administration of intravenous nitroglycerin.

A. Spontaneous vaginal delivery—During spontaneous delivery of an infant in the frank breech position, delivery occurs without assistance, and no obstetric maneuvers are applied to the body. The fetus negotiates the maternal pelvis as outlined below, while the operator simply supports the body as it delivers.

Engagement occurs when the bitrochanteric diameter of the fetus has passed the plane of the pelvic inlet. As the fetus descends into the pelvis (Fig. 19–2), the buttocks reach the levator ani muscles of the maternal pelvis. At this point, internal rotation occurs, whereby the anterior hip rotates beneath the pubic symphysis, resulting in a sacrum transverse position. The bitrochanteric diameter of the fetal pelvis is now in an anteroposterior position within the maternal pelvis. The breech then presents at the pelvic outlet and, upon emerging, rotates from sacrum transverse to sacrum anterior. Crowning occurs when the bitrochanteric diameter passes under the pubic symphysis. As this occurs, the shoulders enter the pelvic inlet with the bisacromial diameter in the transverse position. As descent occurs, the bisacromial diameter rotates to an oblique or anteroposterior diameter, until the anterior shoulder rests beneath the pubic symphysis. Delivery of the anterior shoulder occurs as it slips beneath the pubic symphysis. Upward flexion of the body allows for easy delivery of the posterior shoulder over the perineum.

As the shoulders descend, the head engages the pelvic inlet in a transverse or oblique position. Rotation of the head to the occiput anterior position occurs as it enters the midpelvis. The occiput then slips beneath the pubic symphysis, and the remainder of the head is delivered by flexion as the chin, mouth, nose, and forehead slip over the maternal perineum.

As delivery of the breech occurs, increasingly larger diameters (bitrochanteric, bisacromial, biparietal) of the body enter the pelvis, whereas in cephalic presentation, the largest diameter (biparietal diameter) enters the pelvis first. Particularly in preterm labors, the head is considerably larger than the body and provides a better "dilating wedge" as it passes through the cervix and into the pelvis. The smaller bitrochanteric and bisacromial diameters may descend into the pelvis through a partially dilated cervix, but the larger biparietal diameter may be trapped. Delivery in these cases is described in the following.

B. Partial breech extraction—Partial breech extraction (assisted breech extraction) is used when the operator discerns that spontaneous delivery will not occur or that expeditious delivery is indicated for fetal or maternal reasons. The body is allowed to deliver spontaneously up to the level of the umbilicus. The operator then assists in delivery of the legs, shoulders, arms, and head.

As the umbilicus appears at the maternal perineum, the operator places a finger medial to one thigh and then the other thigh, pressing laterally as the fetal pelvis is rotated away from that side by an assistant. Thus, the thigh is externally rotated at the hip and results in flexion of the knee and delivery of one, then the other, leg. The fetal trunk is then wrapped in a towel to support the body. When both scapulae are visible, the body is rotated counterclockwise. The operator locates the right humerus and laterally sweeps the arm across the chest and out the perineum (Fig. 19–3). In a similar fashion, the body is rotated clockwise to deliver the left arm. The head then spontaneously delivers by gently lifting the body upward and applying fundal pressure to maintain flexion of the fetal head (Fig. 19–4). During partial breech extraction, the anterior shoulder may be difficult to deliver if it is impacted behind the pubic symphysis. In this event, the body is gently lifted upward toward the pubic symphysis, and the operator inserts 1 hand along the hollow of the maternal pelvis and identifies the posterior humerus of the fetus. By gentle downward traction on the humerus, the posterior arm can be easily delivered, thus allowing for easier delivery of the anterior shoulder and arm.

The operator may elect to manually assist in delivery of the head by performing the **Mauriceau-Smellie-Veit maneuver** (Fig. 19–5). In this procedure, the index and middle fingers of 1 of the operator's hands are applied over the maxilla as the body rests on the palm and forearm of the operator. Two fingers of the operator's other hand are applied on either side of the neck with gentle downward traction. At the same time, the body is elevated toward the pubic symphysis, allowing for controlled delivery of the mouth, nose, and brow over the perineum. Likewise, Piper forceps may be used electively or when the Mauriceau-Smellie-Veit maneuver fails to deliver the aftercoming head. Piper forceps may only be used when the cervix is completely dilated and the head is engaged in the pelvis. Ideally, the head is in a direct occiput anterior position, but a left or right occiput anterior position is acceptable. Piper forceps should not be attempted in the occiput transverse positions because this may result in significant fetal and maternal injury. An assistant supports and slightly elevates the fetal trunk while the operator places each forceps blade alongside the fetal parietal bones (Fig. 19–6). After proper placement is confirmed, the forceps are locked, and gentle traction is applied to flex and

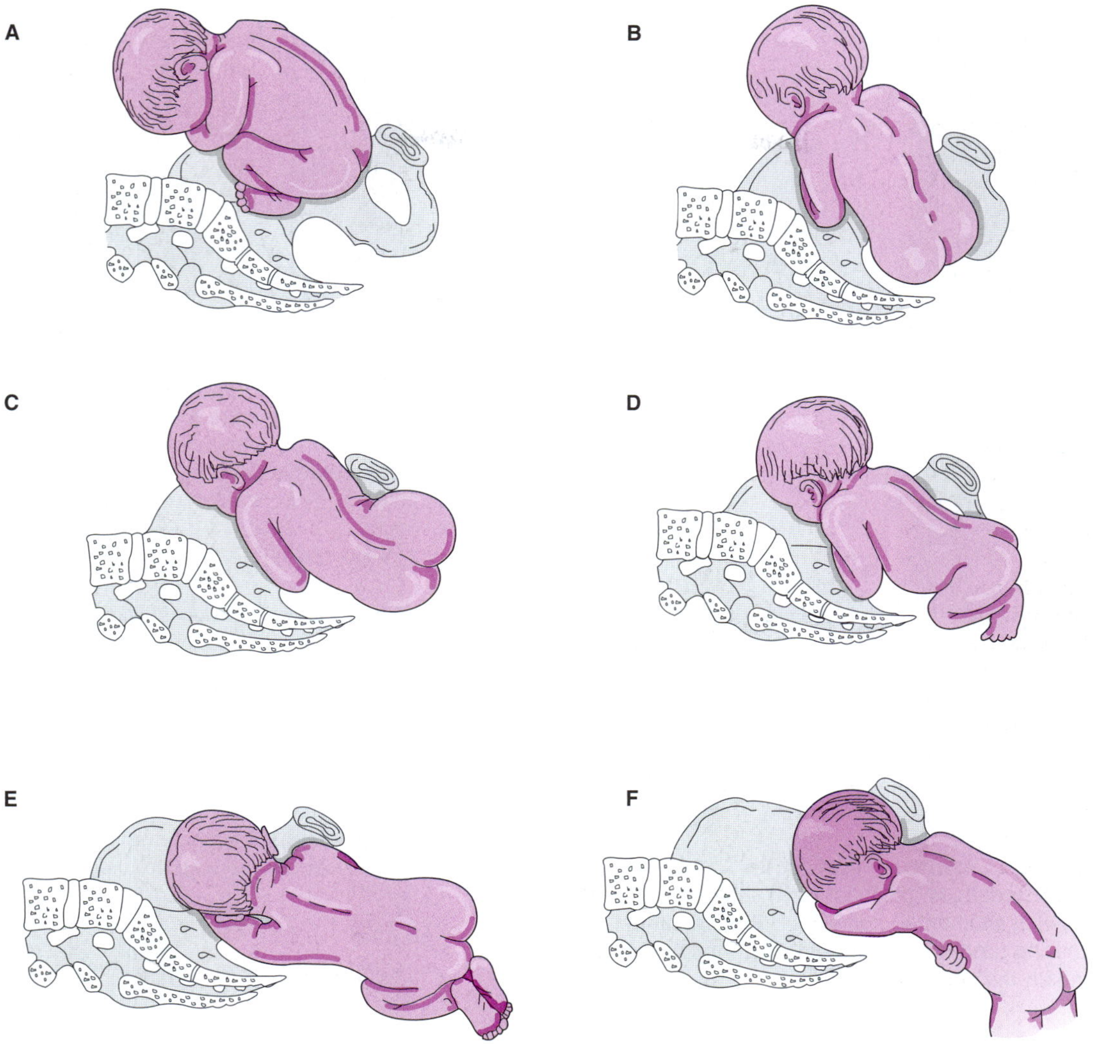

▲ **Figure 19–2.** Mechanism of labor in breech delivery. **A:** Mechanism of breech delivery. Right sacrum transverse at the onset of labor; engagement of the buttocks usually occurs in the oblique or transverse diameter of the pelvic brim. **B:** Early second stage. The buttocks have reached the pelvic floor, and internal rotation has occurred so that the bitrochanteric diameter lies in the anteroposterior diameter of the pelvic outlet. **C:** Late second stage. The anterior buttock appears at the vulva by lateral flexion of the trunk around the pubic symphysis. The shoulders have not yet engaged in the pelvis. **D:** The buttocks have been delivered, and the shoulders are adjusting to engage in the transverse diameter of the brim. This movement causes external rotation of the delivered buttocks so that the fetal back becomes uppermost. **E:** The shoulders have reached the pelvic floor and have undergone internal rotation so that the bisacromial diameter lies in the AP diameter of the pelvic outlet. Simultaneously, the buttocks rotate anteriorly through 90 degrees. This is called **restitution.** The head is engaging in the pelvic brim, and the sagittal suture is lying in the transverse diameter of the brim. **F:** The anterior shoulder is born from behind the pubic symphysis by lateral flexion of the delivered trunk.

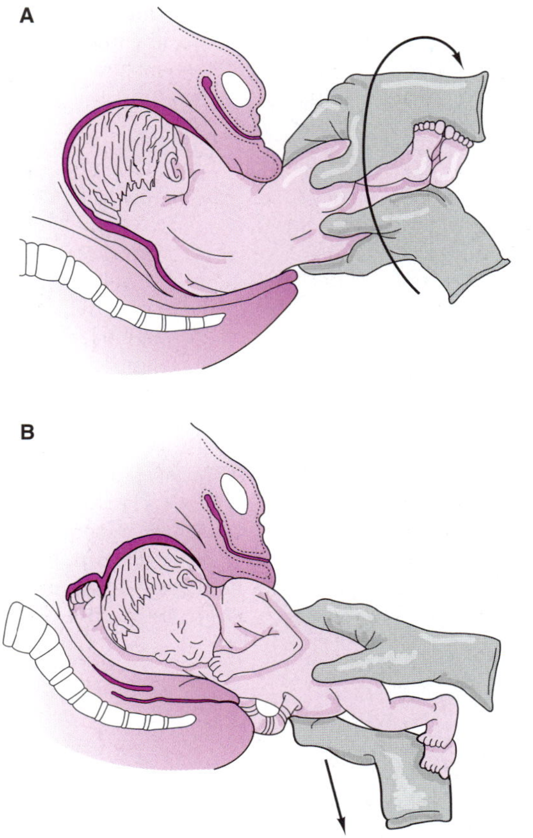

▲ **Figure 19–3.** Assisted delivery of the shoulders. **A:** Shoulders engaged, posterior (left) shoulder at lower level in pelvis than anterior shoulder. **B:** Rotation of trunk causing posterior shoulder to rotate to anterior and slip beneath the pubic symphysis.

deliver the head over the perineum. A midline episiotomy is often indicated to allow for easier application of the forceps and for delivery.

If, after delivery of the body, the spine remains in the posterior position and rotation is unsuccessful, extraction of the head in a persistent occiput posterior position may be accomplished by the **modified Prague maneuver.** One hand of the operator supports the shoulders from below, while the other hand gently elevates the body upward toward the maternal abdomen. This action flexes the head within the birth canal and results in delivery of the occiput over the perineum.

In premature breech presentations, the incompletely dilated cervix may allow delivery to the smaller body, but the relatively larger aftercoming head may be entrapped. Prompt delivery is mandatory because severe asphyxia leading to death may rapidly ensue. Gentle downward traction on the shoulders combined with fundal pressure applied by an assistant may effect delivery. If this fails, the anesthesiologist

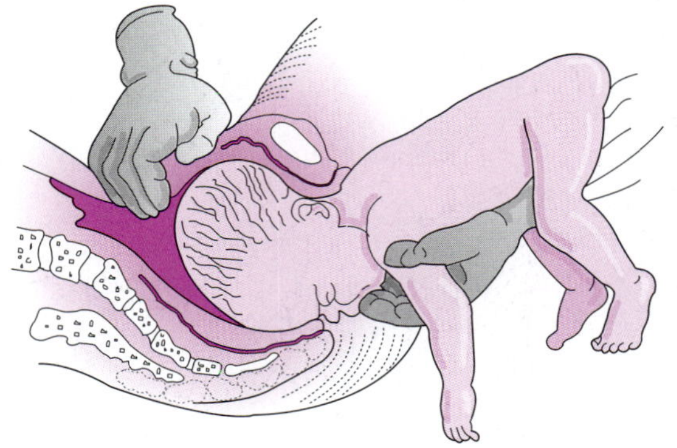

▲ **Figure 19–4.** Maneuver for delivery of the head. The fingers of the left hand are inserted into the infant's mouth or over the infant's mandible; the right hand exerts pressure on the head from above. (Modified and reproduced, with permission, from Pernoll ML. *Benson and Pernoll's Handbook of Obstetrics and Gynecology*. 10th ed. New York, NY: McGraw-Hill; 2001.)

should administer nitroglycerin or inhalation anesthesia to obtain complete relaxation of the lower uterine segment and pelvic floor with reattempt at delivery.

If delivery is still not accomplished, **Dührssen's incisions** must be considered to preserve fetal life. Incisions are made in the posterior cervix at the 6 o'clock position to loosen the entrapped head. Occasionally, additional incisions are necessary at the 2 and 10 o'clock positions. Dührssen's incisions invariably release the fetal head, but the maternal consequences may be severe with resultant hemorrhage.

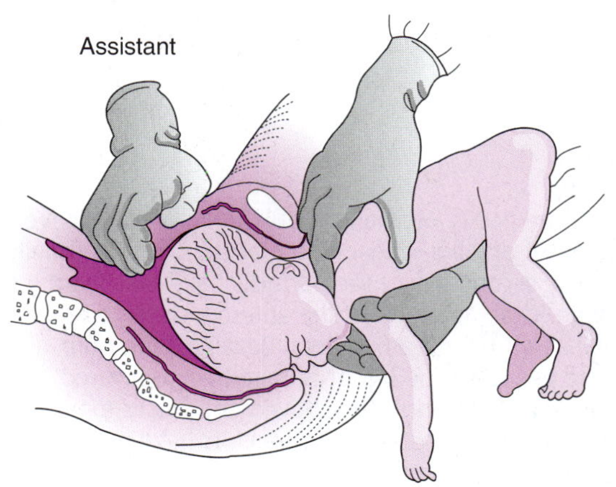

▲ **Figure 19–5.** Mauriceau-Smellie-Veit maneuver for delivery of the head. The fingers of the left hand are inserted into the infant's mouth or over the infant's mandible; the fingers of the right hand curve over the shoulders. An assistant exerts suprapubic pressure on the head. (Reproduced, with permission, from Pernoll ML. *Benson and Pernoll's Handbook of Obstetrics and Gynecology*. 10th ed. New York, NY: McGraw-Hill; 2001.)

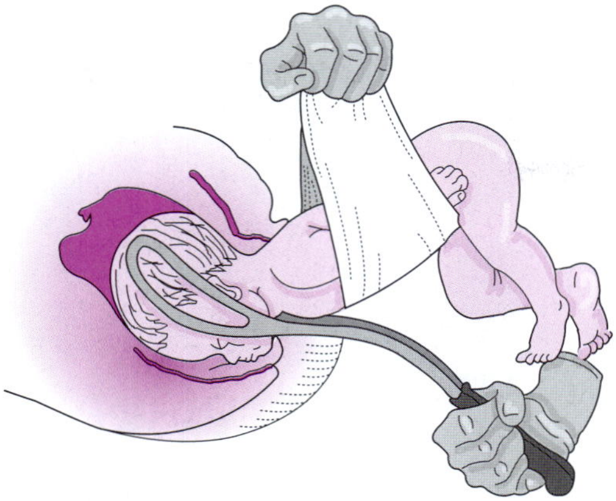

▲ **Figure 19–6.** Application of Piper forceps, using towel sling support. The forceps are introduced from below, left blade first, aiming directly at intended positions on sides of the head. (Reproduced, with permission, from Pernoll ML. *Benson and Pernoll's Handbook of Obstetrics and Gynecology*. 10th ed. New York, NY: McGraw-Hill; 2001.)

Thus, this procedure should be performed only in an emergent situation. Prevention of head entrapment can be accomplished by delivering viable premature breech gestations by caesarean section.

C. Total breech extraction—In total breech extraction (Fig. 19–7), the entire body is manually delivered. This procedure is used only occasionally when fetal distress is encountered and an expeditious delivery is indicated, and under certain conditions in the setting of delivery of a second twin in a nonvertex position following successful vaginal delivery of a first twin. Total breech extraction has been virtually replaced by caesarean delivery in modern obstetrics.

For complete or footling presentation, total breech extraction is accomplished by initially grasping both feet and applying gentle downward pressure until the buttocks are delivered (Fig. 19–8). A generous midline or mediolateral episiotomy is then performed. The operator gently grasps the fetal pelvis, with both thumbs placed directly on either side of the sacrum. The spine is rotated, if necessary, until it rests under the pubic symphysis. Gentle, firm downward pressure is applied to the body until both scapulas are visible. The shoulders, arms, and head are delivered as in partial breech extraction.

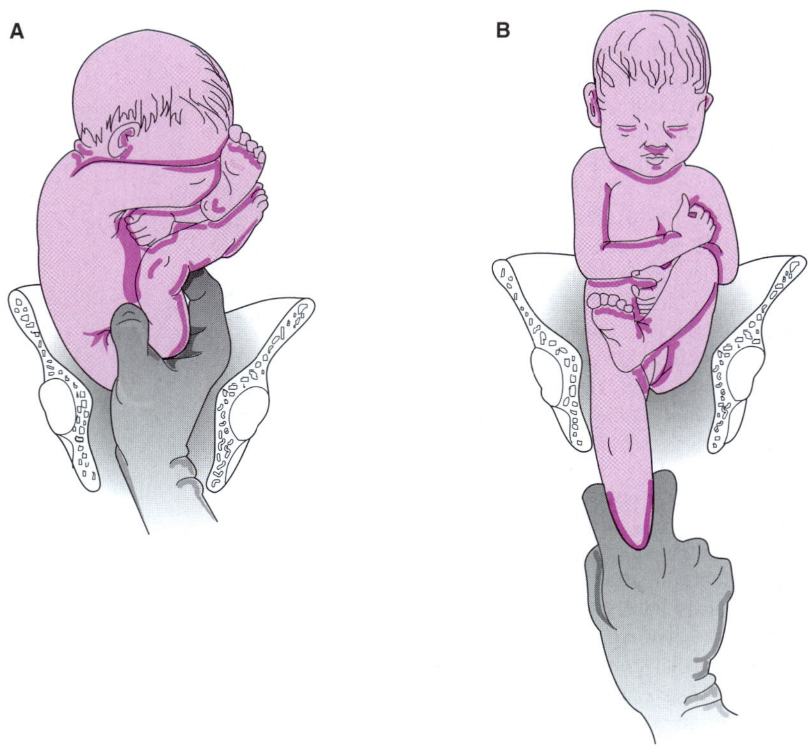

▲ **Figure 19–7.** Extraction of breech. **A:** Abduction of thigh and pressure in popliteal fossa cause the knee to flex and become accessible. **B:** Delivery of leg by traction on the foot.

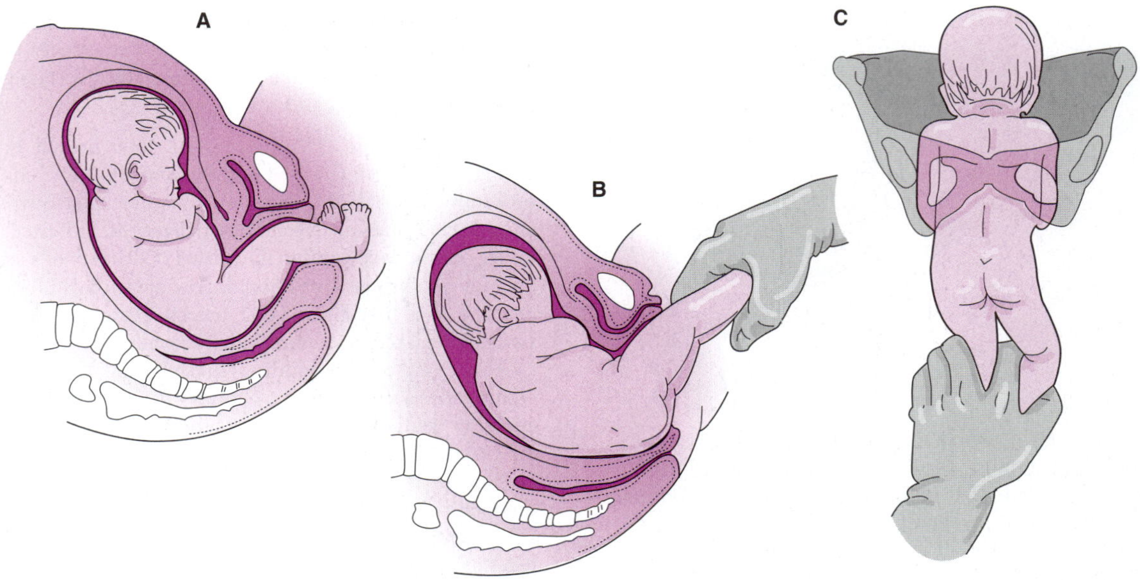

▲ **Figure 19–8.** Extraction of breech. **A:** Buttocks brought to hollow of sacrum. **B:** Traction on anterior leg causes buttocks to advance and rotate into direct anteroposterior diameter of pelvis. Continued downward traction causes the back to rotate anteriorly. **C:** Further downward traction causes the shoulders to engage in the transverse diameter of the inlet.

If the fetus is in frank breech presentation, the index finger of the right hand must initially be placed into the anterior groin of the fetus and gentle downward pressure applied (Fig. 19–9). As the fetus descends further into the birth canal, the left index finger is inserted into the posterior groin, and additional gentle downward traction is applied, until the buttocks are delivered through the vaginal introitus (Fig. 19–10). The fetus is gently rotated until the spine rests directly under the pubic symphysis. To deliver the extended legs from the birth canal, the operator places the index finger in the popliteal fossa of 1 leg and applies pressure upward and outward, causing the knee to flex. As the knee flexes, the foot is often seen or easily palpated. The lower leg is grasped firmly and gently delivered, and the opposite leg is then delivered. The rest of the body is extracted as previously described for footling presentation.

D. Internal podalic version—Internal podalic version is now rarely used because of the high fetal and maternal morbidity and mortality associated with the procedure. It is occasionally performed as a life-saving procedure or in cases of a noncephalic second twin (see Chapter 17 for delivery of a second twin). Internal podalic version is the only alternative to caesarean section for rapid delivery of the second twin in a noncephalic presentation if external cephalic version fails. Thus, when caesarean section is unavailable or when a life-threatening condition arises (maternal hemorrhage due to premature placental separation, fetal distress, prolapsed umbilical cord), internal version may be required.

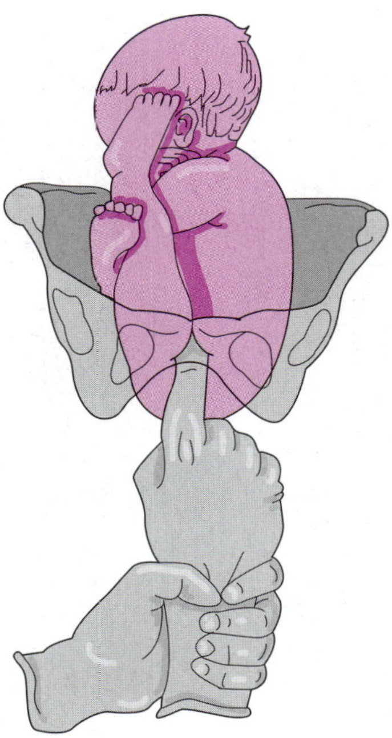

▲ **Figure 19–9.** Delivery of breech with 1 finger in the groin. The wrist is supported with the other hand. When the posterior groin is accessible, the index finger of the other hand is placed in the groin to complete delivery of the breech.

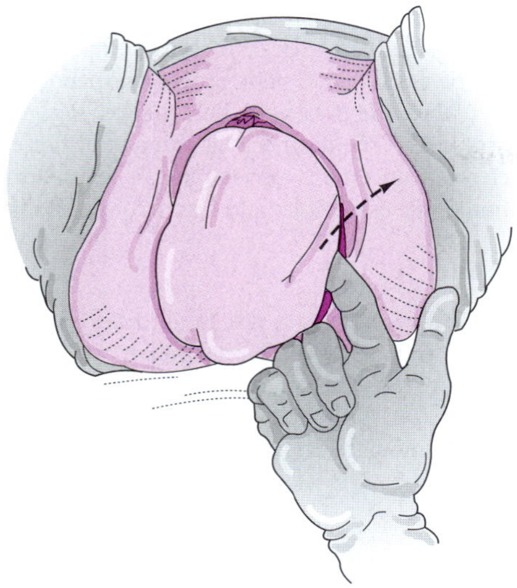

▲ **Figure 19–10.** Flexion and abduction of the thigh to deliver extended leg.

A life-threatening condition is the only indication for internal podalic version. The cervix must be completely dilated, and the membranes must be intact. A skilled operator is crucial for safe performance of this procedure. In several French studies, internal podalic version was found to be a reliable and effective technique with excellent long-term maternal and fetal prognoses.

Internal podalic version is contraindicated in cases in which the membranes are ruptured or oligohydramnios is present, precluding easy version. This procedure should not be performed through a partially dilated cervix or if the uterus is firmly contracted down on the fetal body. However, recent studies have indicated that intravenous nitroglycerin can be used to provide transient uterine relaxation without affecting maternal or fetal outcome.

Internal podalic version is associated with considerable risk of traumatic injury to both fetus and mother. Prior to 1950, when this procedure was performed much more frequently than it is today, associated uterine rupture and hemorrhage caused 5% of all maternal deaths. Perinatal mortality rates were 5–25% (primarily due to traumatic intracerebral hemorrhage and birth asphyxia). Considerable birth trauma, including long bone fractures, dislocations, epiphyseal separations, and central nervous system deficits, was also linked to this procedure. For these reasons, internal podalic version has been abandoned with rare exceptions in favor of caesarean section.

Internal podalic version is performed by first establishing an intravenous line for administration of parenteral fluids, including blood. Cross-matched blood should be available in the hospital blood bank. Anesthesia is then administered to relax the uterus. The patient is then placed in the dorsolithotomy position. The operator's hand is inserted through the fully dilated cervix along the fetal body until both feet are identified, and traction is applied to bring the feet into the pelvis and out the introitus. Then, both feet are firmly grasped. An amniotomy is then performed, and dorsal traction is applied on both lower extremities until both feet are delivered through the vagina. A total breech extraction for delivery of the body is then performed (Fig. 19–11).

Prognosis

The incidence of caesarean section for breech delivery has been steadily increasing, from approximately 30% in 1970 to 85% in 1999. A recent review of breech deliveries in California revealed an 88% caesarean section rate, with more vaginal deliveries performed in public teaching hospitals and far fewer in private facilities. A decreased number of practitioners currently are skilled in vaginal breech delivery,

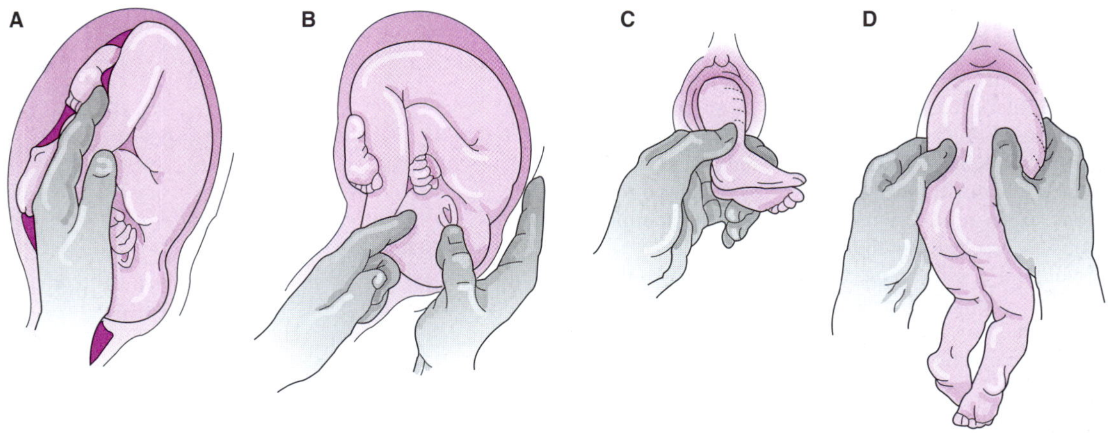

▲ **Figure 19–11.** Internal podalic version and extraction. **A:** Feet are grasped. **B:** Baby is turned; hand on abdomen pushes head toward uterine fundus. **C:** Feet are extracted. **D:** Torso is delivered. From this point onward, procedure is the same as for uncomplicated breech delivery.

and although academic faculty support its teaching, there are insufficient numbers of vaginal breech deliveries to properly teach this procedure at most institutions. It should be noted that caesarean section for the immature or malformed fetus does not improve chances for perinatal survival; vaginal delivery should be performed in these cases.

The Term Breech Trial Collaborative Group recently conducted a randomized controlled trial to compare planned caesarean section with vaginal birth for selected breech presentation pregnancies. They found that fetuses of women who underwent planned caesarean sections were less likely to die or to experience poor outcomes in the immediate neonatal period than were fetuses of women who underwent vaginal birth. There was no difference in the 2 groups in terms of maternal mortality or serious morbidity. They concluded that a policy of planned caesarean section will result in 7 caesarean births to avoid 1 infant death or serious morbidity. Because of the results of this trial, the American College of Obstetricians and Gynecologists recommends planned caesarean delivery for persistent breech presentations at term.

COMPOUND PRESENTATION

ESSENTIALS OF DIAGNOSIS

- *Compound presentation* is prolapse of a fetal extremity alongside the presenting part.
- Prolapse of the hand in cephalic presentation is most common, followed by prolapse of an upper extremity in breech presentation. Prolapse of a lower extremity in cephalic presentation is relatively rare.
- Compound presentations are uncommon, occurring in only 1 in 1000 pregnancies.

Pathogenesis

Obstetric factors that prevent descent of the presenting part into the pelvic inlet predispose to prolapse of an extremity alongside the presenting part (ie, prematurity, cephalopelvic disproportion, multiple gestation, grand multiparity, and hydramnios). Prematurity occurs in over 50% of compound presentations. In twin gestations, over 90% of compound presentations are associated with the second twin.

Because of poor application of the presenting part to the cervix found in compound presentations, umbilical cord prolapse is common (occurring in 11–20% of cases) and is a major contributor to fetal loss during labor.

Clinical Findings

The diagnosis of compound presentation is made by palpation of a fetal extremity adjacent to the presenting part on vaginal examination. The diagnosis is usually made during labor; as the cervix dilates, the prolapsed extremity is more easily palpated alongside the vertex or breech. Compound presentation may be suspected if poor progress in labor is noted, particularly when the presenting part fails to engage during the active phase. If the diagnosis of compound presentation is suspected but uncertain, ultrasound can be used to locate the position of the extremities and search for malformations.

Complications

Umbilical cord prolapse is a risk in all cases of compound presentation, and continuous fetal heart rate monitoring should be performed to detect fetal distress or changes in the fetal heart rate. Umbilical cord complications should be managed by immediate caesarean delivery (see below).

Treatment

Management of compound presentation depends on gestational age and type of presentation. Given that 50% of compound presentations are associated with prematurity, viability of the fetus should be documented prior to delivery. If the fetus is considered nonviable, labor should be permitted and vaginal delivery anticipated. The small size of the fetus makes dystocia or difficult vaginal delivery uncommon.

Labor can be allowed and vaginal delivery anticipated in viable cephalic presentations with a prolapsed hand. These cases generally pose no difficulty in labor or delivery because the hand moves upward into the lower uterine segment as the vertex descends into the birth canal. Therefore, expectant management (as opposed to manual reduction of the fetal hand into the uterus) is generally advised.

Prognosis

Compound presentations have been associated historically with perinatal mortality rates ranging from 9 to 19%. Contributing factors are prematurity, prolapsed umbilical cord, and traumatic vaginal delivery.

SHOULDER DYSTOCIA

ESSENTIALS OF DIAGNOSIS

- *Shoulder dystocia* is defined as an inability to deliver the shoulders after the head has delivered.
- Characteristically, after the head is delivered, the chin presses tightly against the perineum as the anterior shoulder becomes impacted behind the pubic symphysis.
- This condition is an acute obstetric emergency requiring prompt, skillful management in order to prevent significant fetal damage or death.
- The incidence of shoulder dystocia ranges from 0.15 to 1.7% of all vaginal deliveries.

Pathogenesis

Primary risk factors that can influence clinical management are fetal macrosomia, gestational or overt diabetes mellitus, a history of shoulder dystocia in a prior birth, a prolonged second stage of labor, and instrumental delivery, particularly a midpelvic delivery. Other risk factors, such as a history of a macrosomic infant, maternal obesity, multiparity, and postterm pregnancy, are mediated through the primary risk factors. However, most women who experience shoulder dystocia have no combination of risk factors that allows clinically useful identification.

Prevention

Efforts at prevention focus on patients with the clinically important risk factors: history of shoulder dystocia, macrosomia by estimated fetal weight (EFW), diabetes, prolonged second stage of labor, and instrumental delivery. Although no study has shown conclusively that offering caesarean delivery in the presence of various combinations of these risk factors is advisable from a risk–benefit analysis, most practitioners apply some or all of these in an attempt to reduce the risk of shoulder dystocia. An example of one approach follows.

1. Prior shoulder dystocia: Offer caesarean.
2. Prior brachial plexus injury: Strongly suggest caesarean.
3. Nondiabetic with macrosomia by EFW (varying thresholds applied between 4500 and 5000 g): Offer caesarean.
4. Diabetic with macrosomia (varying thresholds applied between 4000 and 4500 g): Offer caesarean.
5. Macrosomia by EFW: Avoid instrumental delivery.

It should be noted that labor induction in a nondiabetic woman due to suspected fetal macrosomia does not decrease the occurrence of shoulder dystocia nor does it decrease the rate of caesarean section.

Clinical Findings

Shoulder dystocia should be anticipated given any indications of macrosomia. The diagnosis is confirmed when gentle downward pressure on the head fails to deliver the anterior shoulder from behind the pubic symphysis. At this point, the fetus is at risk for asphyxiation as the fetus cannot expand its chest to breathe, and umbilical cord circulation is compressed within the birth canal. Confronted with this terrifying dilemma, the inexperienced operator often continues to apply downward pressure on the head in a vain attempt to deliver the anterior shoulder. Such action should be avoided, not only because it is ineffective but also because it can potentially damage the brachial plexus and result in permanent Erb's palsy. A number of maneuvers designed to alleviate shoulder dystocia without increasing traction have been described. No specific sequence of these maneuvers has be shown to be superior to any other, but a commonsense approach based on ease of performance and limitations of risk can be described. Initially, the operator places a hand in the birth canal to assess the posterior outlet. If inadequate, an episiotomy or a proctoepisiotomy is performed. At the same time, assistants including a pediatrician and an anesthesiologist are summoned to aid in the delivery.

Complications

Birth injuries related to shoulder dystocia include fracture of the humerus or clavicle and injury to the brachial plexus (**Erb's palsy**). Fractures of the humerus and clavicle generally heal without incident, and most injuries to the brachial plexus resolve with minimal or no neurologic deficit detectable during the neonatal period. However, approximately 10% of cases of Erb's palsies do not resolve. Studies attempting to distinguish the clinical course of patients with permanent injuries from those with transient injuries have found no clinically distinct characteristics. Some severe cases of shoulder dystocia may lead to hypoxic-ischemic encephalopathy and possible death. Maternal complications of shoulder dystocia include postpartum hemorrhage and lacerations involving the cervix, vagina, and perineum

Treatment

The **McRoberts' maneuver** should be used initially because it is simple and resolves shoulder dystocia in 42% of cases. The maternal legs are hyperflexed onto the maternal abdomen, resulting in flattening of the sacrum and cephalad rotation of the symphysis pubis. If the shoulders remain undelivered, suprapubic pressure is applied by an assistant to dislodge the anterior shoulder while gentle downward pressure on the head is applied. Suprapubic pressure and/or proctoepisiotomy increases success rates to between 54% and 58%. If these attempts are unsuccessful, the examiner can attempt to rotate the fetal shoulders into the oblique position by placing 2 fingers against the posterior shoulder and pushing it around toward the fetal chest (**Rubin maneuver**) or pushing the posterior shoulder around toward the fetal back (**Wood's maneuver**) in a corkscrew fashion.

If the maneuvers to this point fail, delivery of the posterior arm (Barnum maneuver) is indicated. The obstetrician's hand is inserted posteriorly into the hollow of the maternal sacrum, and the posterior arm of the fetus is identified. Gentle pressure by the examiner's forefinger on the fetal antecubital fossa will cause flexion of the arm. As the arm flexes across the chest, the forearm is gently grasped, and the hand and forearm are gently delivered from the birth canal. If not, the trunk can be rotated to bring the free arm anteriorly, resulting in delivery. Deliberate fracture of the clavicle also can be performed, preferably in a direction away from the fetal lungs. This action diminishes the size of the shoulder girdle and should facilitate delivery.

Finally, if all previous techniques fail, a **Zavanelli maneuver** can be performed in which the fetal head is replaced in anticipation of a caesarean delivery. A subcutaneous symphysiotomy also can be performed to allow disimpaction of the fetal shoulders. Both of these procedures can be very difficult, are associated with high maternal and fetal morbidity, and should be performed only when other conventional maneuvers have failed.

Prognosis

Women with a history of shoulder dystocia in a prior pregnancy are at increased risk of shoulder dystocia in future pregnancies. Retrospective data put this recurrence risk at 1–25%. It is reasonable to offer women with a history of shoulder dystocia caesarean delivery in future pregnancies.

UMBILICAL CORD PROLAPSE

ESSENTIALS OF DIAGNOSIS

- *Umbilical cord prolapse* is defined as descent of the umbilical cord into the lower uterine segment, where it may lie adjacent to the presenting part (occult cord prolapse) or below the presenting part (overt cord prolapse) (Fig. 19–12).
- In occult prolapse, the umbilical cord cannot be palpated during pelvic examination, whereas in funic presentation, which is characterized by prolapse of the umbilical cord below the level of the presenting part before the rupture of membranes occurs, the cord often can be easily palpated through the membranes.
- Overt cord prolapse is associated with rupture of the membranes and displacement of the umbilical cord into the vagina, often through the introitus.

Prolapse of the umbilical cord to a level at or below the presenting part exposes the cord to intermittent compression between the presenting part and the pelvic inlet, cervix, or vaginal canal. Compression of the umbilical cord compromises fetal circulation and, depending on the duration and intensity of compression, may lead to fetal hypoxia, brain damage, and death. In overt cord prolapse, exposure of the umbilical cord to air causes irritation and cooling of the cord, resulting in further vasospasm of the cord vessels. For these reasons, cord prolapse is considered to be an obstetric emergency.

The incidence of overt umbilical cord prolapse in cephalic presentations is 0.5%, frank breech 0.5%, complete breech 5%, footling breech 15%, and transverse lie 20%. The incidence of occult prolapse is unknown because it can be detected only by fetal heart rate changes characteristic of umbilical cord compression. However, some degree of occult prolapse appears to be common, given that as many as 50% of monitored labors demonstrate fetal heart rate changes compatible with umbilical cord compression. In most cases, the compression is transient and can be rectified simply by changing the patient's position.

Whether occult or overt, umbilical cord prolapse is associated with significant rates of perinatal morbidity and mortality because of intermittent compression of blood flow and resultant fetal hypoxia. The perinatal mortality rate associated with all cases of overt umbilical cord prolapse approaches 20%. Prematurity, itself a contributor to the incidence of umbilical cord prolapse, accounts for a considerable portion of this perinatal loss.

Pathogenesis

Any obstetric condition that predisposes to poor application of the fetal presenting part to the cervix can result in prolapse of the umbilical cord. Cord prolapse is associated with prematurity (<34 weeks' gestation), abnormal presentations (breech, brow, compound, face, transverse), occiput

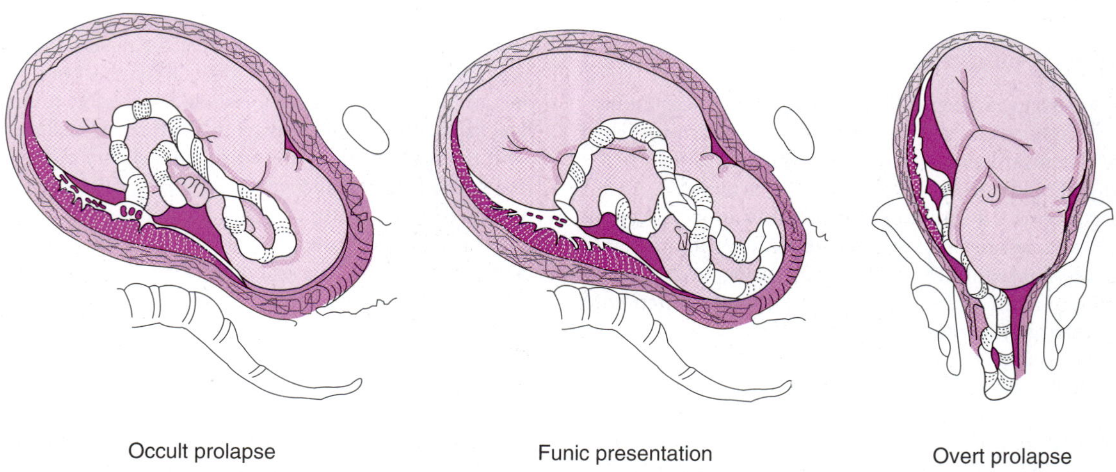

▲ **Figure 19–12.** Types of prolapsed cords.

posterior positions of the head, pelvic tumors, multiparity, placenta previa, low-lying placenta, and cephalopelvic disproportion. In addition, cord prolapse is possible with polyhydramnios, multiple gestation, or premature rupture of the membranes occurring before engagement of the presenting part. A recent study revealed that obstetric intervention contributes to nearly half of cases of umbilical cord prolapse. Examples cited include amniotomy, scalp electrode application, intrauterine pressure catheter insertion, attempted external cephalic version, and expectant management of preterm premature rupture of membranes.

Prevention

Patients at risk for umbilical cord prolapse should be treated as high-risk patients. Patients with fetal malpresentation or poorly applied cephalic presentations should be considered for ultrasonographic examination at the onset of labor to determine fetal lie and cord position within the uterine cavity. Because most prolapses occur during labor as the cervix dilates, patients at risk for cord prolapse should be continuously monitored to detect abnormalities of the fetal heart rate. Artificial rupture of membranes should be avoided until the presenting part is well applied to the cervix. At the time of spontaneous membrane rupture, a prompt, careful pelvic examination should be performed to rule out cord prolapse. Should amniotomy be required and the presenting part remains unengaged, careful needling of the membranes and slow release of the amniotic fluid can be performed until the presenting part settles against the cervix.

Clinical Findings

A. Overt Cord Prolapse

Overt cord prolapse can be diagnosed simply by visualizing the cord protruding from the introitus or by palpating loops of cord in the vaginal canal.

B. Funic Presentation

The diagnosis of funic presentation is made by pelvic examination if loops of cord are palpated through the membranes. Antepartum detection of funic presentation is discussed below.

C. Occult Prolapse

Occult prolapse is rarely palpated during pelvic examination. This condition can be inferred only if fetal heart rate changes (variable decelerations, bradycardia, or both) associated with intermittent compression of the umbilical cord are detected during monitoring.

Complications

A. Fetus

The fetus in good condition whose well-being is jeopardized by umbilical cord compression may exhibit violent activity readily apparent to the patient and the obstetrician. Variable fetal heart rate decelerations will occur during uterine contractions, with prompt return of the heart rate to normal as each contraction subsides. If cord compression is complete and prolonged, fetal bradycardia occurs. Persistent, severe, variable decelerations and bradycardia lead to development of hypoxia, metabolic acidosis, and eventual damage or death. As the fetal status deteriorates, activity lessens and eventually ceases. Meconium staining of the amniotic fluid may be noted at the time of membrane rupture.

B. Maternal

Caesarean section is a major operative procedure with known anesthetic, hemorrhagic, and operative complications. These risks must be weighed against the real risk to the fetus of continued hypoxia if labor were to continue.

Maternal risks encountered at vaginal delivery include laceration of the cervix, vagina, or perineum resulting from a hastily performed delivery.

C. Neonatal

The neonate at delivery may be hypoxic, acidotic, or moribund. A pediatric team should be present to effect immediate resuscitation of the newborn.

Treatment

A. Overt Cord Prolapse

The diagnosis of overt cord prolapse demands immediate action to preserve the life of the fetus. An immediate pelvic examination should be performed to determine cervical effacement and dilatation, station of the presenting part, and strength and frequency of pulsations within the cord vessels. If the fetus is viable, the patient should be placed in the knee–chest position, and the examiner should apply continuous upward pressure against the presenting part to lift and maintain the fetus away from the prolapsed cord until preparations for caesarean delivery are complete. Alternatively, 400–700 mL of saline can be instilled into the bladder in order to elevate the presenting part. Oxygen should be given to the mother until the anesthesiologist is prepared to administer a rapid-acting inhalation anesthetic for delivery. Successful reduction of the prolapsed umbilical cord has been described, but such an attempt may worsen fetal heart rate changes and should not delay preparation for caesarean delivery. Abdominal delivery should be accomplished as rapidly as possible through a generous midline abdominal incision, and a pediatric team should be on standby in the event immediate resuscitation of the newborn is necessary.

B. Occult Cord Prolapse

If cord compression patterns (variable decelerations) of the fetal heart rate are recognized during labor, an immediate pelvic examination should be performed to rule out overt cord prolapse. If occult cord prolapse is suspected, the patient should be placed in the lateral Sims or Trendelenburg position in an attempt to alleviate cord compression. If the fetal heart rate returns to normal, labor can be allowed to continue, provided no further fetal insult occurs. Oxygen should be administered to the mother, and the fetal heart rate should be continuously monitored electronically. Amnioinfusion can be performed via an intrauterine pressure catheter in order to instill fluid within the uterine cavity and possibly decrease the incidence of variable decelerations. If the cord compression pattern persists or recurs to the point of fetal jeopardy (moderate to severe variable decelerations or bradycardia), a rapid caesarean section should be accomplished.

C. Funic Presentation

The patient at term with funic presentation should be delivered by caesarean section prior to membrane rupture. However, there is no consensus on management if the fetus is premature. The most conservative approach is to hospitalize the patient on bed rest in the Sims or Trendelenburg position in an attempt to reposition the cord within the uterine cavity. Serial ultrasonographic examinations should be performed to ascertain cord position, presentation, and gestational age.

D. Route of Delivery

Vaginal delivery can be successfully accomplished in cases of overt or occult cord prolapse if, at the time of prolapse, the cervix is fully dilated, cephalopelvic disproportion is not anticipated, and an experienced physician determines that delivery is imminent. Internal podalic version, midforceps rotation, or any other operative technique is generally more hazardous to mother and fetus in this situation than is a judiciously performed caesarean delivery. Caesarean delivery is the preferred route of delivery in most cases. Vaginal delivery is the route of choice for the previable or dead fetus.

Prognosis

A. Maternal

Maternal complications include those related to anesthesia, blood loss, and infection following caesarean section or operative vaginal delivery. Maternal recovery is generally complete.

B. Neonatal

Although the prognosis for intrapartum cord prolapse is greatly improved, fetal mortality and morbidity rates still can be high, depending on the degree and duration of umbilical cord compression occurring before the diagnosis is made and neonatal resuscitation is started. If the diagnosis is made early and the duration of complete cord occlusion is <5 minutes, the prognosis is good. Gestational age and trauma at delivery also affect the final neonatal outcome. If complete cord occlusion has occurred for longer than 5 minutes or if intermittent partial cord occlusion has occurred over a prolonged period of time, fetal damage or death may occur.

Alouini S, et al. Management of umbilical cord prolapse and neonatal outcomes. *J Gynecol Obstet Biol Reprod* 2010;39:471–477. PMID: 20609529.

American College of Obstetricians and Gynecologists. Committee Opinion No. 340. Mode of term singleton breech delivery. *Obstet Gynecol* 2006;108:235–237. PMID: 16816088.

American College of Obstetricians and Gynecologists. *External Cephalic Version. ACOG Practice Bulletin No. 13.* Washington, DC: American College of Obstetricians and Gynecologists; 2000.

American College of Obstetricians and Gynecologists. *Shoulder Dystocia. ACOG Practice Bulletin No. 40.* Washington, DC: American College of Obstetricians and Gynecologists; 2002.

Athukorala C, et al. Intrapartum interventions for preventing shoulder dystocia. *Cochrane Database Syst Rev* 2006;4:CD005543. PMID: 17054263.

Bingham J, et al. Recurrent shoulder dystocia: A review. *Obstet Gynecol Surv* 2010;65:183–188. PMID: 20214833.

Boyle JJ, Katz VL. Umbilical cord prolapse in current obstetric practice. *J Reprod Med* 2005;50:303–306. PMID: 15971477.

Burgos J, et al. A prospective study of the factors associated with the success rate of external cephalic version for breech presentation at term. *Int J Gynaecol Obstet* 2011;112:48–51. PMID: 20870233.

Chauhan SP, et al. Shoulder dystocia with and without brachial plexus injury: Experience from three centers. *Am J Perinatol* 2007;24:365–371. PMID: 17566948.

Chinnock M, Robson S. Obstetric trainees' experience in vaginal breech delivery: Implications for future practice. *Obstet Gynecol* 2007;110:900–903. PMID: 17906026.

Collaris R, Tan PC. Oral nifedipine versus subcutaneous terbutaline tocolysis for external cephalic version: A double-blind randomized trial. *BJOG* 2009;116:74–80. PMID: 19087079.

Dilbaz B, et al. Risk factors and perinatal outcomes associated with umbilical cord prolapse. *Arch Gynecol Obstet* 2006;274: 104–107. PMID: 16538441.

Doumouchtsis SK, Arulkumaran S. Are all brachial plexus injuries caused by shoulder dystocia? *Obstet Gynecol Surv* 2009;64: 615–623. PMID: 19691859.

Doyle NM, et al. Outcomes of term vaginal breech delivery. *Am J Perinatol* 2005;22:325–328. PMID: 16118722.

Esakoff TF, et al. The association between birthweight 4000 g or greater and perinatal outcomes in patients with and without gestational diabetes mellitus. *Am J Obstet Gynecol* 2009;200:672.e1–4. PMID: 19376489.

Ford JB, et al. Recurrence of breech presentation in consecutive pregnancies. *BJOG* 2010;117:830–836. PMID: 20482538.

Gherman R, et al. Recurrent shoulder dystocia: A review. *Obstet Gynecol Surv* 2010;65:183–188. PMID: 20414833.

Guiltier MJ, et al. Moxibustion for breech version: A randomized controlled trial. *Obstet Gynecol* 2009;114:1034–1040. PMID: 20168104.

Gupta M, et al. Antenatal and intrapartum prediction of shoulder dystocia. *Eur J Obstet Gynecol Reprod Biol* 2010;151:134–139. PMID: 20427112.

Gurewitsch ED, Allen RH. Shoulder dystocia. *Clin Perinatol* 2007;34:365–385. PMID: 17765488.

Hannah M, et al. Planned cesarean section versus planned vaginal birth for breech presentation at term: A randomized multicentre trial. *Lancet* 2000;356:1375–1383. PMID: 11052579.

Hofmeyer GJ, Hannah ME. Planned cesarean section for term breech delivery. *Cochrane Database Syst Rev* 2003;3:CD000166. PMID: 12917886.

Hutton EK, Hofmeyer GJ. External cephalic version for breech presentation before term. *Cochrane Database Syst Rev* 2006;1:CD000084. PMID: 16437421.

Kayem G, et al. Early preterm breech delivery: Is a policy of planned vaginal delivery associated with increased risk of neonatal death? *Am J Obstet Gynecol* 2008;198:289.e1–6. PMID: 18241827.

Kok M, et al. Prediction of success of external cephalic version after 36 weeks. *Am J Perinatol* 2011;28:103–110. PMID: 20661845.

Kotaska A, et al. Vaginal delivery of breech presentation. *J Obstet Gynaecol Can* 2009;31:557–566, 567–578. PMID: 19646324.

Lewis DF, et al. Expectant management of preterm premature rupture of membranes and nonvertex presentation: What are the risks? *Am J Obstet Gynecol* 2007;196:566.e1–5. PMID: 17547897.

Lin MG. Umbilical cord prolapse. *Obstet Gynecol Surv* 2006;61:269–277. PMID: 16551378.

MacKenzie IZ, et al. Management of shoulder dystocia: Trends in incidence and maternal and neonatal morbidity. *Obstet Gynecol* 2007;110:1059–1068. PMID: 17978120.

Mahajan NN, et al. Internal podalic version for neglected shoulder presentation with fetal demise. *BJOG* 2009;116:180–184. PMID: 19656146.

Melendez J, et al. Severe shoulder dystocia leading to neonatal injury: A case control study. *Arch Gynecol Obstet* 2009;279:47–51. PMID: 18491119.

Menticoglou SM. A modified technique to deliver the posterior arm in severe shoulder dystocia. *Obstet Gynecol* 2006;108(3 Pt 2): 755–757. PMID: 17018492.

Nassar N, et al. Diagnostic accuracy of clinical examination for detection of non-cephalic presentation in late pregnancy: Cross sectional analytic study. *BMJ* 2006;333:578–580. PMID: 16891327.

Obeidat N, et al. Umbilical cord prolapse: A 10-year retrospective study in two civil hospitals, North Jordan. *J Obstet Gynaecol* 2010;30:257–260. PMID: 20373926.

Robilio PA, et al. Vaginal vs. cesarean delivery for preterm breech presentation of singleton infants in California: A population-based study. *J Reprod Med* 2007;52:473–479. PMID: 17694963.

Stitely ML, Gherman RB. Labor with abnormal presentation and position. *Obstet Gynecol Clin North Am* 2005;32:165–179. PMID: 15899353.

Traore Y, et al. Frequency of cord prolapse: Etiological factors and fetal prognosis in 47 cases in health center. *Mali Med* 2006;21:25–29. PMID: 17390525.

Yoshida M, et al. Effectiveness of epidural anesthesia of external cephalic version (ECV). *J Perinatol* 2010;30:580–583. PMID: 20485361.

20 Operative Delivery

Marc H. Incerpi, MD

An operative delivery refers to an obstetric procedure in which active measures are taken to accomplish delivery. Operative delivery can be divided into operative vaginal delivery and caesarean delivery. The last several years have seen a steady decline in the operative delivery with an increase in the caesarean section rate. In addition, vacuum-assisted vaginal delivery has become more common than forceps. Most recent data from births in the United States during 2005 indicate that the vacuum-to-forceps ratio is approximately 4:1. The success and safety of these procedures are based on operator skill, proper timing, and ensuring that proper indications are met while contraindications are avoided. This chapter explains how each procedure is performed, the indications and contraindications to the procedure, the potential complications, and how to minimize complications.

FORCEPS OPERATIONS

The obstetric forceps is an instrument designed to assist with delivery of the baby's head. The invention of the precursor to modern forceps is credited to Peter Chamberlin in the 1600s. It is used either to expedite delivery or to assist with certain abnormalities in the cephalopelvic relationship that interfere with advancement of the head during labor. The primary functions of the forceps are to assist with traction of the fetal head and/or to assist with rotation of the fetal head to a more desirable position.

Although forceps-assisted vaginal deliveries were once extremely popular, the most recent data demonstrate that only one-quarter of all operative vaginal deliveries are performed using forceps. The reverse was true approximately 10 years ago. In fact, many investigators are concerned that the use of forceps is becoming a lost art. The reasons often cited in contributing to the decline in the use of forceps are (1) medicolegal implications and fear of litigation, (2) reliance on caesarean section as a remedy for abnormal labor and suspected fetal jeopardy, (3) perception that the vacuum is easier to use and less risky to fetus and mother, and (4) decreased number of residency programs that actively train residents in the use of forceps. These factors have led to a cycle in which less teaching has led to a decrement in technical skills, an increased fear of litigation, and a resultant further decrease in the use of forceps.

THE OBSTETRIC FORCEPS

The obstetric forceps (Fig. 20–1) consists of 2 matched parts that articulate or "lock." Each part is composed of a blade, shank, lock, and handle. Each blade is designed so that it possesses 2 curves: the cephalic curve, which permits the instrument to be applied accurately to the sides of the baby's head, and the pelvic curve, which conforms to the curved axis of the maternal pelvis. The tip of each blade is called the toe. The front of the forceps is the concave side of the pelvic curve. The blades are referred to the left and right according to the side of the mother's pelvis on which they lie after application. During application, the handle of the left blade is held in the left hand, and the blade is applied to the left side of the mother's pelvis. Conversely, the handle of the right blade is held in the right hand and inserted so as to lie on the right side of the mother's pelvis. When the blades are inserted in this order, the right shank comes to lie atop the left so that the forceps articulate, or lock, as the handles are closed.

Physicians have been modifying 1 or more of the 4 basic parts since forceps were first invented. Although more than 600 kinds of forceps have been described, only a few are currently in use (Fig. 20–2). Although it is beyond the scope of this chapter to discuss all the different varieties of forceps and their indications, a brief comment on the more common types of forceps is appropriate. Simpson or Elliot forceps are most often used for outlet vaginal deliveries, whereas Kielland or Tucker-McLane forceps are used for rotational deliveries. Piper forceps are used in the United States for delivery of the aftercoming head in vaginal breech deliveries. The pelvic and cephalic curve, shank, blade, lock, and handle are different

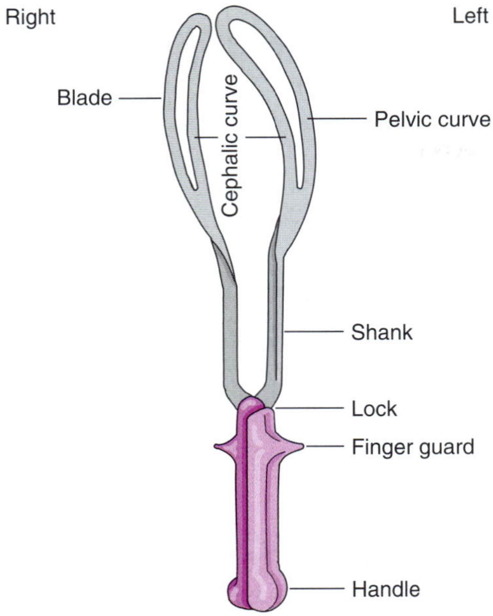

▲ **Figure 20–1.** DeLee modification of Simpson forceps. (Reproduced, with permission, from Benson RC. *Handbook of Obstetrics & Gynecology*. 8th ed. Los Altos, CA: Lange; 1983.)

for each type of forceps. These features determine the type of forceps that is best suited for the appropriate indication. For example, Piper forceps, which are specifically designed for breech deliveries, have a reverse pelvic curve compared to other forceps. Simpson forceps are suited for application to the molded fetal head, whereas Tucker-McLane forceps or Kielland forceps are more appropriate to the fetal head with little or no molding.

INDICATIONS & CONDITIONS FOR FORCEPS DELIVERY

In each of the following indications for forceps delivery, it must be emphasized that caesarean section is an alternative procedure that should be considered depending on the prevailing circumstances. Recognizing the inherent risks of both procedures, the obstetrician must decide which operation (vaginal delivery or caesarean section) will be safer for the mother and baby.

The indications for forceps delivery are as follows: (1) nonreassuring fetal heart rate pattern, (2) shortening of the second stage of labor for maternal reasons, (3) prolonged second stage of labor not due to dystocia, and (4) delivery of the aftercoming head in a breech presentation. A prolonged second stage of labor has been defined according to parity. In a nulliparous patient, a prolonged second stage is defined as more than 3 hours with a regional anesthetic or more than 2 hours without a regional anesthetic. In a multiparous patient, more than 2 hours with a regional anesthetic or more than 1 hour without a regional anesthetic constitutes a prolonged second stage of labor.

In order for the patient to be considered a candidate for forceps-assisted vaginal delivery with a cephalic presentation, *all* of the following prerequisites must be met: (1) complete cervical dilatation, (2) ruptured membranes, (3) fetal head engaged with the fetal head position known, (4) empty bladder, (5) no evidence of cephalopelvic disproportion, (6) adequate analgesia, (7) caesarean section capability, and (8) an experienced operator.

CLASSIFICATION OF FORCEPS DELIVERIES

In 1988 the American College of Obstetricians and Gynecologists redefined the classification of forceps. As discussed later, the same classification should be applied to vacuum delivery. This classification uses the leading bony point of the fetal skull and its relationship to the maternal ischial spines in centimeters as the point of reference. Each station of the fetal head refers to the relationship of the leading bony part of the fetal skull with respect to the ischial spines. The fetal head is said to be at 0 station when the head is at the level of the spines. When the head is above this level, the station is described as −1 through −5, corresponding to the number of centimeters above the level of the ischial spines. When the head is below this level, the station is described as +1 through +5, corresponding to the number of centimeters below the level of the ischial spines.

The classification of forceps is defined as follows:

1. **Outlet forceps** is the application of forceps when (a) the fetal scalp is visible at the introitus without separating the labia, (b) the fetal skull has reached the pelvic floor, (c) the sagittal suture is in the anteroposterior diameter or in the right or left occiput anterior or posterior position, and (d) the fetal head is at or on the perineum. According to this definition, rotation of the fetal head must be ≤45 degrees.
2. **Low forceps** is the application of forceps when the leading point of the fetal skull is at station +2 or greater and not on the pelvic floor. Low forceps have 2 subdivisions: (a) rotation ≤45 degrees and (b) rotation >45 degrees.
3. **Midforceps** is the application of forceps when the head is engaged but the leading point of the fetal skull is above station +2.

Only rarely should an attempt be made at forceps delivery above station +2. Under unusual circumstances, such as sudden onset of severe fetal or maternal compromise or transverse arrest, application of forceps above station +2 can be attempted while simultaneously initiating preparation for a caesarean delivery in case the forceps maneuver is unsuccessful. *Under no circumstances should forceps be applied to an unengaged head.*

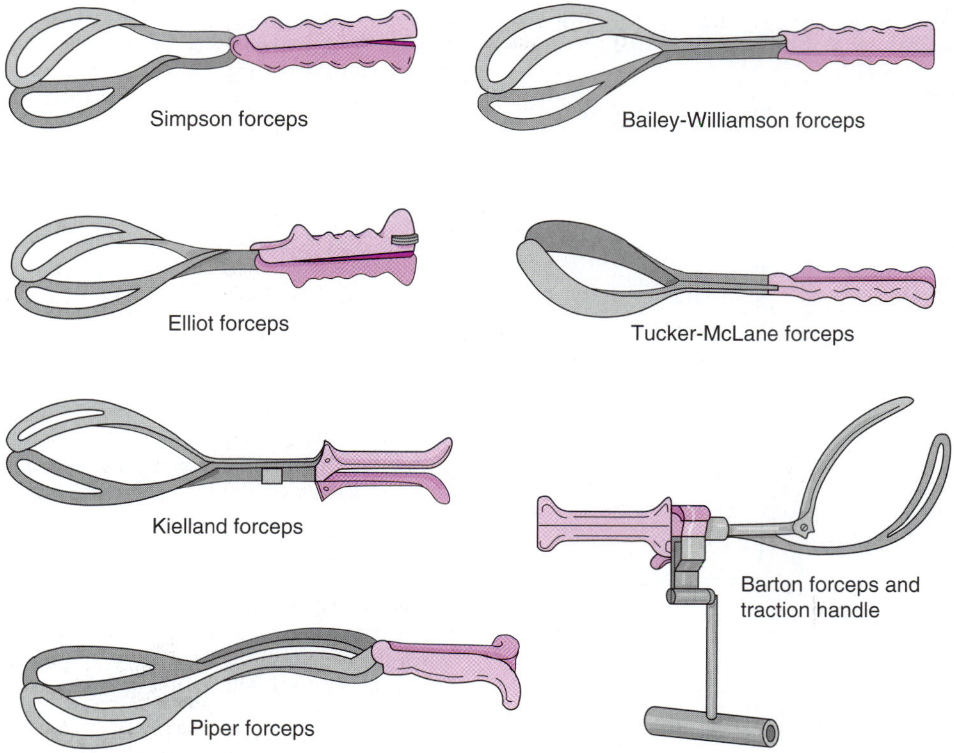

▲ **Figure 20–2.** Commonly used forceps. (Reproduced, with permission, from Benson RC. *Handbook of Obstetrics & Gynecology*. 8th ed. Los Altos, CA: Lange; 1983.)

PREPARATION OF THE PATIENT FOR FORCEPS DELIVERY

The patient must be placed in the dorsal lithotomy position and the bladder should be emptied. The legs should be comfortably placed in stirrups with the hips flexed and abducted. The abdomen and legs should be adequately draped, and the vagina and the perineum should be prepped in usual fashion. If conduction (spinal/epidural) anesthesia is to be used, it must be administered prior to the foregoing steps in delivery. If pudendal block or local infiltration is to be used, it should be administered after the preliminary examination has been performed and all is in readiness for delivery. An appropriate and effective anesthetic is essential to the performance of a forceps delivery.

The Preliminary Examination

Before the application of forceps, a careful examination if necessary to determine the following:

1. **The position of the fetal head**, which usually is easily determined by first locating the lambdoid sutures and then determining the direction of the sagittal suture. The posterior fontanelle is readily evident after the 3 sutures running into it are identified. If the most accessible fontanelle is found to have 4 sutures running into it, it is the anterior fontanelle and the position usually is occiput posterior. In the presence of marked edema of the scalp or caput succedaneum, both sutures and fontanelles may be masked, and the position can only be determined by feeling an ear and noting the direction of the pinna. It must be emphasized that if the position of the fetal head cannot be adequately determined, then forceps should not be applied.
2. **The station of the fetal head**, which is the relationship of the presenting part to the ischial spines, must be determined. In labor that proceeds swiftly without complications, such a determination usually is simple and accurate. However, when the first or especially the second stage of labor is prolonged and is further complicated by marked molding and a heavy caput, this relationship may suggest a false level of the head in the pelvis. If the head can be felt above the symphysis pubis, forceps should not be used.
3. **The adequacy of the pelvic diameters** of the midpelvis and outlet is determined by noting the following: (a) the prominence of the ischial spines, the degree to which

they shorten the transverse diameter of the midpelvis, and the amount of space between the spine and the side of the fetal head; (b) the contour of the accessible portion of the sacrum and the amount of space posterior to the head usually based on the length of the sacrospinous ligament; and (c) the width of the subpubic arch. This kind of appraisal is neither needed nor feasible for outlet forceps, but is essential for indicated low forceps or midforceps.

APPLICATION OF FORCEPS

A major concept to bear in mind is that the application of forceps should use finesse rather than force. Before the forceps are applied to the fetal head, a “phantom application” should be performed first. It is vital to inspect the forceps to ensure that they consist of a complete and matched set and that they articulate (lock) easily. Forceps should be applied in a delicate fashion in order to avoid potential injury to the vagina and perineum. The goal is for the blades to fit the fetal head as evenly and symmetrically as possible. The blades should lie evenly against the side of the head, covering the space between the orbits and ears (Fig. 20–3). It is important to emphasize that correct application prevents soft tissue and nerve injury, as well as bony injuries to the fetal head. After the forceps have been applied, they should articulate easily. If the forceps cannot be easily articulated, the forceps should be removed and a second attempt made. Once the forceps articulate, the following checks should be performed for delivery of an occiput anterior position before any traction is placed on the fetal head. (1) The sagittal suture should be perpendicular to the plane of the shanks. (2) The posterior fontanelle should be 1 fingerbreadth away from the shanks equidistant from the sides of the blades, and directly in front of the articulated forceps. (3) If fenestrated (open) blades are used, the amount of fenestration in front of the fetal head should admit no more than the tip of 1 finger. After these checks have been performed, then traction can safely be applied to the fetal head. Traction forces should be applied in the plane of least resistance and should follow the pelvic curve. This can best be accomplished by applying downward pressure on the shanks with outward pressure exerted upon the handle of the forceps. Once the fetal head begins to emerge out of the vagina, the forceps are disarticulated, and the head is delivered via a modified Ritgen maneuver. After delivery, it is important to ensure that no vaginal or perineal lacerations go unrecognized, paying particular attention to deep lateral vaginal sidewall (sulcal) lacerations. Lacerations, if present, should be repaired in customary fashion.

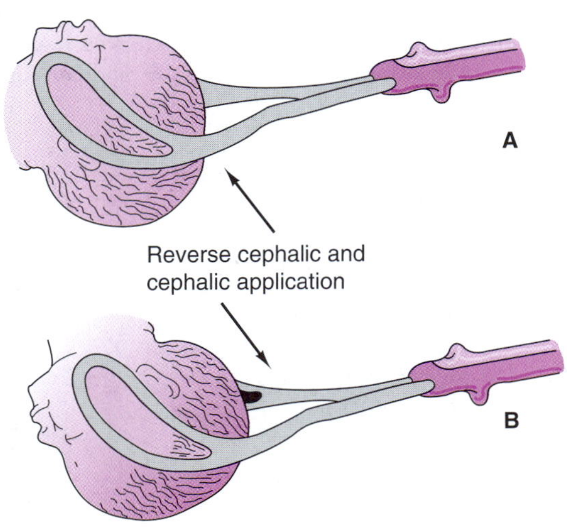

▲ **Figure 20–3.** Forceps correctly applied along occipitomental diameter of head in various positions of the occiput. **A:** Occiput posterior. **B:** Occiput anterior. (Reproduced, with permission, from Benson RC. *Handbook of Obstetrics & Gynecology*. 8th ed. Los Altos, CA: Lange; 1983.)

A more detailed step-by-step description of a forceps-assisted vaginal delivery in the occiput anterior position is as follows (Figs. 20–4 through 20–6). The left handle is held between the thumb and fingers of the left hand. Using 2 or 3 fingers of the right hand placed into the vagina, the blade is guided to its correct position on the left side of the fetal head (Fig. 20–4). This maneuver is repeated with the right hand and the right blade, using the fingers of the left hand placed into the vagina to guide the blade (Fig. 20–5). The handles are depressed slightly before locking, in order to place the blades properly along the optimal diameter of the fetal head (Fig. 20–6).

The forceps are designed such that they lock easily as the handles are closed if the application is accurate. If the handles are askew or if any force is needed to achieve precise articulation, the application is faulty and the position must be rechecked. If simple manipulation of the blades does not permit easy articulation, the forceps should be removed, the position verified (by feeling an ear, if necessary), and the blades reapplied correctly. After the 3 checks have been adequately performed, traction can be applied.

Obstetricians hold forceps for traction in different ways. One method is to grab the crossbar of the handle between the index and middle fingers of the left hand from underneath and to insert the middle and index fingers of the right hand in the crotch of the instrument from above. Another method is to grasp the handles with the fingers on the top of the handles or shanks and the thumbs on the bottom. Traction is made only in the axis of the pelvis along the curve of the birth canal. No more force is applied than can be exerted by the flexed forearms; the muscles of the back must be used, and the feet must not be braced. If a greater degree of traction is needed, the cause may be cephalopelvic disproportion, asynclitism of the fetal head, or an error in the evaluation of the pelvic diameters. The obstetrician then should reassess the possibility of successful vaginal delivery.

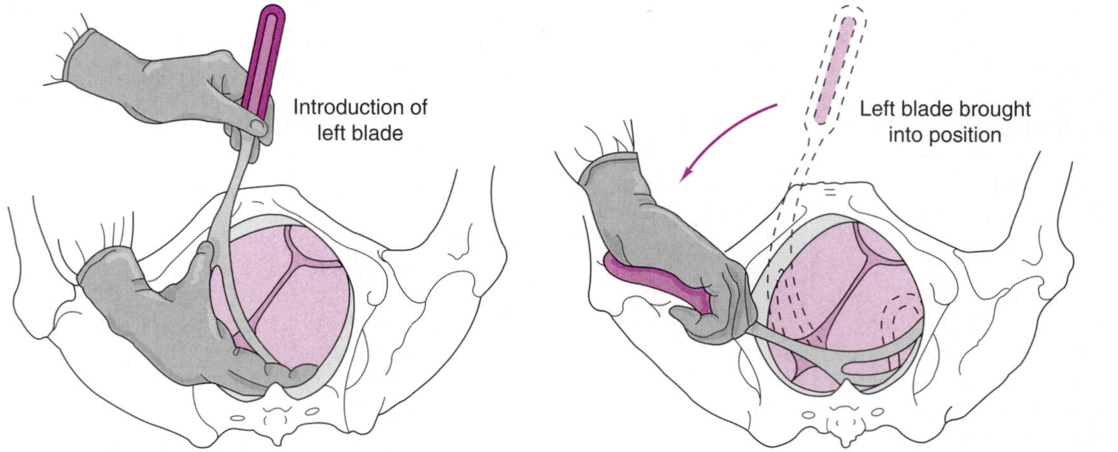

▲ **Figure 20–4.** Introduction of left blade (left blade, left hand, left side of pelvis). The handle is held with the fingers and thumb, not clenched in the hand. The handle is held vertically. The blade is guided with the fingers of the right hand. Placement of blade is completed by swinging the handle down to the horizontal plane.

As the head begins to distend the perineum, both the amount and direction of traction must be altered. The farther the head advances, the less the resistance offered by both the pelvis and soft parts; hence, only minimal traction should be applied as the head is about to be delivered. The head negotiates the final position of the pelvic curve by extension, and the physician should simulate this movement by elevating the handles of the forceps more and more as the head crowns (Fig. 20–7). If the forceps are allowed to remain in place throughout delivery of the fetal head, the handles will have passed the vertical plane as delivery of the head is completed. It is preferable to remove the forceps as the head crowns in the reverse order of their application by first disarticulating the forceps and raising the right handle until the blade is delivered. The left blade is then removed in similar fashion. Early removal of the forceps reduces the size of the mass that must pass through the introitus and thus reduces the likelihood of lacerations or extensions of episiotomies. After removal of the forceps, the head may recede; however, if the forceps have not been removed too soon, the head can be delivered by the use of the modified Ritgen

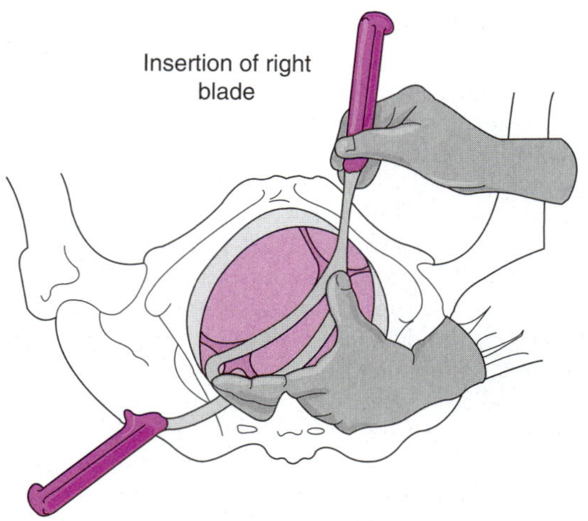

▲ **Figure 20–5.** Introduction of right blade (right blade, right hand, right side of pelvis). The left blade is already in place. The handle is grasped with the fingers and thumb, not gripped in the whole hand. The handle is held vertically. (Reproduced, with permission, from Benson RC. *Handbook of Obstetrics & Gynecology*. 8th ed. Los Altos, CA: Lange; 1983.)

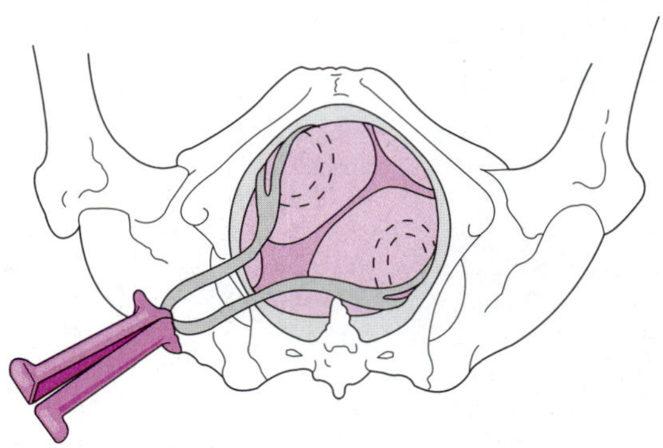

▲ **Figure 20–6.** Both blades introduced. The 2 handles are brought together and locked. If application is correct, the handles lock precisely, without the need for force. (Reproduced, with permission, from Benson RC. *Handbook of Obstetrics & Gynecology*. 8th ed. Los Altos, CA: Lange; 1983.)

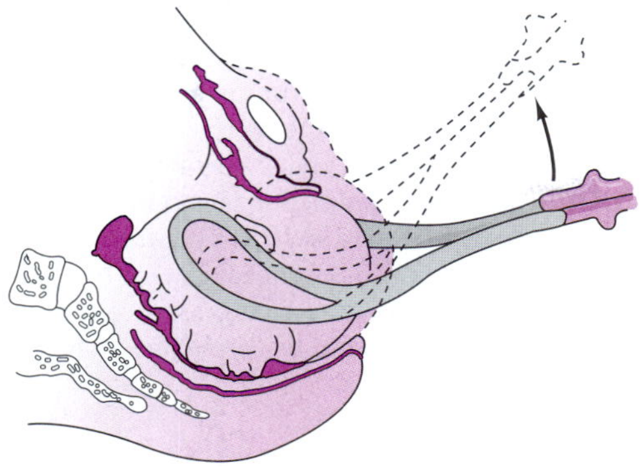

▲ **Figure 20–7.** Upward traction with low forceps. As the head extends, the handles are raised until they pass the vertical. Little force is needed. One hand suffices; the other hand may support the perineum. (Reproduced, with permission, from Benson RC. *Handbook of Obstetrics & Gynecology*. 8th ed. Los Altos, CA: Lange; 1983.)

maneuver during the next contraction. Because rotations with forceps and vaginal breech deliveries are now rarely, if ever performed, it is beyond the scope of this chapter to discuss these techniques.

DANGER & SAFETY OF FORCEPS

Although the use of forceps has fallen into disfavor over the last few years, few studies have prospectively evaluated the safety of forceps. A number of injuries to both mother and baby can result from the use of forceps, some serious and even fatal. Maternal complications include lacerations of the vagina and cervix, episiotomy extensions involving third- and fourth-degree lacerations, pelvic hematomas, urethral and bladder injuries, and uterine rupture. In addition, blood loss and the need for blood transfusion are increased in forceps deliveries. The baby may sustain minor facial lacerations, forceps marks, facial and brachial plexus palsies, cephalohematomas, skull fractures, intracranial hemorrhage, and seizures.

Many of these serious injuries and many of the minor ones inflicted by obstetric forceps result from errors in judgment rather than lack of technical skill. Such errors include failure to recognize the essential conditions for forceps delivery and lack of an appropriate indication for the operation as outlined earlier. The potential for injury increases in the following settings: (1) intervention occurs too early, before maximal molding and descent have been achieved by the patient's voluntary efforts, (2) continued traction is used in the presence of unrecognized cephalopelvic disproportion, (3) errors in diagnosis of the position of the fetal head, and (4) unwillingness to abandon the procedure and perform caesarean section. Most reports clearly demonstrate that maternal and/or fetal complications are more common with midforceps than with low or outlet forceps. The perception of increased fetal and maternal risk has served as one of the major driving forces contributing to the widespread decline in the use of forceps.

THE VACUUM EXTRACTOR

The idea of using a suction device applied to the fetal scalp to help facilitate deliver of the fetal head originated in the 1700s. The first vacuum cup was not designed until 1890. As one could well imagine, the first types of vacuum devices were crude, resembling a toilet plunger. In fact, the vacuum device did not gain much popularity until Malmström introduced a metal vacuum cup in 1954. The most common type of vacuum in use today is a pliable, Silastic cup with a handheld pump and gauge that allow delivery of the proper amount of suction pressure to the fetal head to effect delivery. Two models are shown in Figures 20–8 and 20–9. The vacuum extractor works by allowing the external traction forces applied to the fetal scalp to be transmitted to the fetal head. The traction on the vacuum apparatus increases the forces of delivery and facilitates passage of the fetus through the pelvis. In order for delivery to be accomplished, both traction on the fetal scalp and compression of the fetal head occur.

INDICATIONS & CONTRAINDICATIONS FOR VACUUM DELIVERY

With the exception of delivery of the aftercoming head in a breech presentation, the indications for vacuum use are similar to those of forceps: (1) nonreassuring fetal heart rate pattern, (2) shortening of the second stage of labor for maternal reasons, and (3) prolonged second stage of labor. In addition, as mentioned earlier, the classification of forceps deliveries is the same classification used for vacuum deliveries,

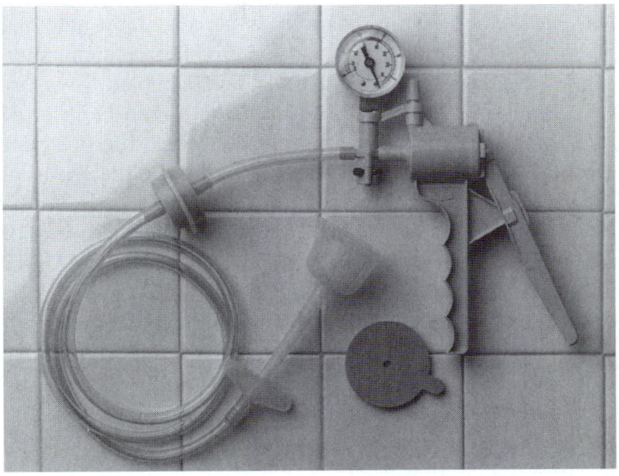

▲ **Figure 20–8.** Mityvac obstetrical vacuum delivery system includes extractor cup and pump. (Photograph reproduced with permission of CooperSurgical, Inc., Trumball, CT)

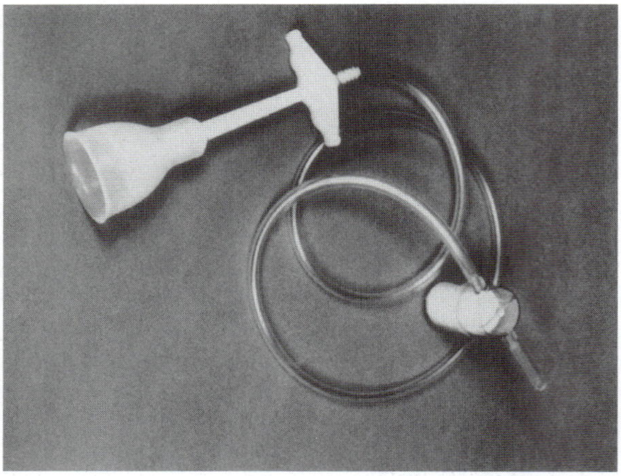

▲ **Figure 20–9.** CMI Tender Touch extractor cup. (Photograph reproduced with permission of Utah Medical Products.)

and the prerequisites are similar. Contraindications for vacuum delivery include the following: face presentation, breech presentation, true cephalopelvic disproportion, congenital anomalies of the fetal head (eg, hydrocephalus), gestational age <34 weeks, an unengaged fetal head, fetal demineralization disorder (eg, osteogenesis imperfecta), and known or suspected fetal bleeding diatheses (eg, hemophilia). In addition, caution must be exercised when the estimated fetal weight is >4000 g.

VACUUM APPLICATION

Before the vacuum is applied to the fetal head, the patient is prepared and the initial patient examination is performed as discussed earlier with regard to forceps deliveries. Application of the vacuum is perceived by many to be simpler than the use of the forceps. Before application occurs, the vacuum system should be assembled to ensure that no leaks are present. The cup should then be inserted into the vagina by directing pressure toward the posterior aspect of the vagina. The objective is to place the center of the cup directly over the sagittal suture at the *median flexion point* located approximately 3 cm anterior to the posterior fontanelle. This cup placement should allow for adequate maintenance of flexion of the fetal head during the entire procedure. The following checks should be performed prior to application of traction to the fetal head. (1) No maternal tissue should be included under the cup margin. (2) The cup should be placed in the midline over the sagittal suture and not off to the side of the head.

After the cup has been appropriately placed on the fetal scalp, an initial suction is applied, and the cup edges are reexamined to ensure that no maternal tissue is trapped underneath the vacuum cup. While the cup is held firmly against the fetal head, the pressure is increased to approximately 100–150 mm Hg to maintain the cup's position. The cup edges should be reexamined. If no maternal tissue is found under the cup edges, the pressure is increased to 500–600 mm Hg at the beginning of the uterine contraction. As the mother pushes, traction is applied downward along the pelvic axis. If more than 1 contraction is necessary, the vacuum pressure can be decreased to low levels between contractions. The axis of traction is then extended upward to a 45-degree angle to the floor as the head emerges. Once the head has completely delivered through the vagina, the suction is withdrawn and the cup removed.

EFFECTIVENESS & SAFETY OF VACUUM

Most reports demonstrate that the vacuum is effective, with a failure rate of approximately 10%. The following factors have been implicated in determining the effectiveness of vacuum delivery: cup design, shape, size, and traction site attachment, consistency and strength of vacuum, strength of maternal expulsive efforts and coordination with traction, fetal size and extent of cephalopelvic disproportion, station and deflection of the fetal head, and angle and technique of traction.

The safety of the vacuum has been called into question. In May 1998, the US Food and Drug Administration issued a Public Advisory Statement regarding fetal complications associated with vacuum delivery. The purpose of this statement was to advise practitioners that vacuum devices might cause serious or fetal complications when improperly used. As a result, the following recommendations were made. (1) The vacuum should be used only when a specific obstetric indication is present. (2) Persons using the vacuum should be experienced and aware of the indications, contraindications, and precautions. (3) Those who use the vacuum should read and understand the instructions for the particular instrument being used. (4) The neonatal care staff should be educated about the potential complications of vacuum. (5) Individuals responsible for the care of the neonate should be alerted that vacuum has been used. (6) All adverse reactions should be reported to the Food and Drug Administration.

Use of the vacuum has been associated with a variety of neonatal injuries ranging from benign superficial scalp markings to serious and potentially life-threatening intracranial hemorrhages. The most common neonatal complication is retinal hemorrhage, which may occur in as many as 50% of deliveries. Fortunately, the complication rarely has any clinical significance. Cephalohematoma involves bleeding beneath the periosteum and complicates approximately 6% of all vacuum deliveries. Because the bleeding is located under the periosteum, significant bleeding rarely results because of the inability of the blood to cross the sutures. Subgaleal hematoma, a more serious complication, occurs in 50 per 10,000 vacuum deliveries. The condition arises when bleeding occurs in the loose subaponeurotic tissues of the scalp. Because bleeding occurs above the periosteum, it is not contained by the sutures. Consequently, there is the potential for life-threatening hemorrhage. The subgaleal space actually extends from the orbits of the eyes to the nape of the neck. This potential space can accommodate over half of a newborn's blood volume. Intracranial hemorrhage occurs in approximately 0.35% of vacuum deliveries. It can be a catastrophic complication that includes subdural, subarachnoid, intraventricular, and/or intraparenchymal hemorrhage. These complications can be quite severe but fortunately are rare.

Most authorities agree that injury can be significantly decreased or eliminated if the following protocol is used. (1) Traction is applied only when the patient is actively pushing. (2) Applying torsion or twisting the cup in an attempt to rotate the head is prohibited. (3) The duration of time during which the cup is applied to the fetal head should not exceed 20 minutes. (4) The procedure should be abandoned after the cup has dislodged or "popped off" from the fetal head twice. It should not be applied a third time. (5) The procedure should be abandoned if there is no fetal descent after a single pull. (6) Neonatal staff should be present at the time of the vacuum delivery. (Note: This also applies to forceps deliveries.) (7) Under no circumstances should the operator switch from vacuum to forceps or vice versa. An excellent study examining neonatal injury associated with operative vaginal delivery clearly demonstrated that the greatest incidence of neonatal injury occurred in babies in whom both vacuum and forceps were used. The practitioner must be cognizant of the risk of shoulder dystocia, which is increased with instrumental delivery. Shoulder dystocia occurs more commonly with vacuum deliveries than with forceps deliveries. A simple ABC mnemonic for vacuum extraction is as follows:

A: **A**sk for help, **a**ddress the patient (obtain informed consent), **a**nesthesia

B: **B**ladder empty

C: **C**ervix fully dilated

D: **D**ownward traction, shoulder **d**ystocia

E: **E**xamine fetal head position

F: **F**lexion point

A detailed and complete delivery note should accompany each operative delivery. The medical record must document the indication for the procedure, the fetal station and head position at the time of the application(s) of forceps or vacuum, the type of device used, the total application time, the number of applications and "pop-offs" if vacuum was used, and if unsuccessful, the subsequent mode of delivery. It would also be prudent to include a comment in the medical record that the patient was informed of the potential complications of operative vaginal delivery.

Somewhat surprisingly, relatively few randomized, prospective studies have compared vacuum with forceps. In surveying the medical literature, the following conclusions can be drawn. On the whole, the vacuum extractor is less likely to achieve a successful vaginal delivery than is the forceps. The vacuum is significantly less likely to cause serious maternal injury than is the forceps. Although the vacuum is associated with a greater incidence of cephalohematoma, other facial/cranial injuries are more common with forceps. In comparing Apgar scores, the trend is toward more low 5-minute Apgar scores in the vacuum group than in the forceps group. Thus, an overall reduction in severe maternal injuries appears to be the most immediate benefit associated with the use of the vacuum. However, at this time, which instrument results in fewer major adverse neonatal effects remains to be determined.

Although both forceps and vacuum have proved to be useful in assisting with vaginal delivery, the vacuum is quickly becoming the preferred instrument of choice. Both forceps and vacuum extractors are acceptable and safe instruments for operative vaginal delivery. While candidates should be selected on an individualized basis and counseled accordingly, the skill of the operator should also influence the decision to attempt an operative delivery as well as the choice of instrument. Each instrument, however, has inherent risks. While the vacuum has been primarily associated with immediate neonatal morbidity, long-term data do not suggest any increased risk of neurodevelopmental delay in children delivered by either vacuum or forceps. In order to minimize both maternal and fetal risks, the operator must be familiar with the indications, contraindications, application, and use of the particular instrument. Guidelines similar to those discussed in this chapter should exist in order to facilitate a safe and effective delivery. While maternal morbidity may be slightly higher with forceps delivery, it is overall low in comparison with the morbidity that may be associated with delivery by caesarean section. In an era in which caesarean section rates are climbing, one must consider all of the available delivery modes and individualize them accordingly for each patient in order to ensure the most efficacious and safest delivery experience.

Caughey AB, Sandberg PL, Zlatnik MG, et al. Forceps compared with vacuum: Rates of neonatal and maternal morbidity. *Obstet Gynecol* 2005;106:908. PMID: 16260505.

Hook CD, Damos JR. Vacuum-assisted vaginal delivery. *Am Fam Physician* 2008;78:953. PMID: 18953972.

Johnson JH, Figueroa R, Garry D, Elimian A, Maulik D. Immediate maternal and neonatal effects of forceps and vacuum-assisted deliveries. *Obstet Gynecol* 2004;103:513. PMID: 14990415.

Miksovsky P, Watson WJ. Obstetric vacuum extraction: State of the art in a new millennium. *Obstet Gynecol Surv* 2001;56:736. PMID: 11719018.

CAESAREAN SECTION

Caesarean section or caesarean delivery refers to the delivery of a fetus, placenta, and membranes through an abdominal and uterine incision. The first documented caesarean section on a living person was performed in 1610. The patient died 25 days later. Since that time, numerous advances have made caesarean section a safe procedure. In the past 35 years, the rate of caesarean section has steadily increased from 5% to approximately 30%. Over this time, the maternal mortality ratio (maternal deaths per 100,000 births) has decreased from almost 300 to <10. The following factors are often cited as contributing to the increasing caesarean section rate: (1) lower operative vaginal delivery rates, (2) lower rates of vaginal births after caesarean section (VBAC), and (3) fewer vaginal breech deliveries. In order for the practitioner to perform this common operation safely, he or she must be aware of the indications, risks, operative technique, and potential complications of this procedure.

INDICATIONS

Caesarean section is used in cases where vaginal delivery either is not feasible or would impose undue risks to the mother or baby. Some of the indications for caesarean section are clear and straightforward, whereas others are relative. In some cases, fine judgment is necessary to determine whether caesarean section or vaginal delivery would be better. It is not practical to list all possible indications; however, hardly any obstetric complication has not been dealt with by caesarean section. The following indications are currently the most common.

Repeat Caesarean Section

A prior uterine incision from a myomectomy or previous caesarean section may weaken the uterine wall or predispose to rupture if labor is permitted. The initial dictum of "once a caesarean, always a caesarean" was held for many years. However, as multiple publications documenting the safety of VBAC began appearing in the literature, many physicians moved away from this long-held belief. In 2000, a national goal was set to lower the rate of repeat caesarean sections to 3% while increasing the VBAC rate to 35%. The major incentives that led to this change in philosophy were fewer delivery risks with vaginal delivery, less need for anesthesia, less postpartum morbidity, shorter hospital stay, lower costs, and the encouragement of earlier and often smoother interaction and bonding between mother and infant. As more and more VBACs were performed in less than ideal settings, more complications arose. There may be no greater obstetric catastrophe than a uterine rupture resulting in maternal and/or fetal death. In fact, there appears to be a trend back toward the belief of "once a caesarean, always a caesarean." Suffice it to say, "once a caesarean, always a controversy."

In general, patients who are the most suitable candidates for trial of labor after caesarean section (TOLAC) are those (1) with 1 prior low-transverse caesarean section, (2) who present in labor, (3) with nonrecurring conditions (eg, breech, abnormal fetal heart rate patterns, placenta previa in prior pregnancy), and (4) with a prior vaginal delivery. Patients who are not candidates for a TOLAC include women with a prior classical (vertical) uterine incision or prior myomectomy. If a trial of labor is to be conducted, the patient must be placed on continuous fetal heart rate and uterine activity monitoring, and a dedicated obstetrician and anesthesiologist must be immediately available to intervene in case uterine rupture is suspected. Prostaglandins for cervical ripening must be avoided, and oxytocin must be used in a judicious and conservative fashion, if at all. Current studies cite a maternal mortality rate of close to 1% in cases of uterine rupture and a perinatal mortality rate of approximately 50% in association with uterine rupture. Therefore, it is of utmost importance that equipment for both maternal and electronic fetal monitoring and appropriate obstetric and neonatal facilities are available. A large-bore intravenous catheter must be used, and blood for possible maternal transfusion must be available. Appropriate anesthesia, a fully equipped operating room, and obstetric and neonatal staff experienced in emergency care must all be immediately available.

Cephalopelvic Disproportion/Dystocia

Cases in which the fetal head is too large to traverse the pelvis should be managed by caesarean section. As discussed earlier, if the head does not engage during labor, operative vaginal delivery should not be attempted. Rather, caesarean section must be performed. Inlet disproportion should be suspected in the primigravida if the patient begins labor with the fetal head unengaged. In a significant number of these patients, the fetal head fails to engage, and caesarean section is indicated. Midpelvic disproportion may be suspected if the anteroposterior diameter is short, the ischial spines are prominent, the sacrospinous ligament is short, and the fetus is large. Outlet disproportion usually requires a trial of forceps or vacuum before a safe vaginal delivery is determined to be impossible.

Dystocia literally means "difficult labor." This occurs when a patient's labor progresses and then either stops completely (arrests) or becomes prolonged (protracted). When either of these situations occurs during labor, the patient warrants careful reassessment, including evaluation of the labor pattern, contraction pattern, estimated fetal weight and fetal presentation, and evaluation of the pelvis. In other words, the 3 P's (power, passenger, and pelvis) must be adequate in order for a vaginal delivery to occur.

Abnormal Fetal Lie & Malpresentation

Transverse lie and breech presentations are common indications for caesarean section. The trend toward caesarean delivery for breech deliveries has been hastened by a large randomized trial comparing breech infants born vaginally versus those born by caesarean section; better outcomes were achieved after caesarean section. Although some still consider vaginal breech delivery to be an acceptable option, experience with the technique is largely disappearing from practice. External cephalic version is a reasonable alternative for some patients and can be attempted to convert the fetus to cephalic presentation. However, this procedure is successful in allowing vaginal birth in only 50% of cases.

Fetal Heart Rate Tracing Abnormalities

Fetal monitoring before and during labor may disclose fetal problems that otherwise would not be evident. As a result of continuous fetal monitoring, the number of caesarean sections performed for a "nonreassuring fetal status" has increased. Best estimates demonstrate that approximately 10% of caesarean sections are performed for this indication.

Other Indications

In addition to the indications discussed earlier, other conditions that may lead to caesarean section are placenta previa, preeclampsia–eclampsia if remote from term, placental abruption, multiple gestations, fetal abnormalities (eg, hydrocephalus), cervical cancer, and active genital herpes infection. One other indication that is becoming more prevalent is patient choice. The idea of primary elective caesarean section continues to increase in popularity and generate controversy.

PREOPERATIVE PREPARATION FOR CAESAREAN SECTION

The following steps are generally taken before caesarean section is performed. The patient is made aware of the indications for the caesarean section, the alternatives, and the potential risks, benefits, and complications. She then signs a form indicating that she has received the appropriate information and consents to the procedure ("informed consent"). An intravenous 18-gauge needle should be in place with an appropriate intravenous solution running before the operation begins. The patient is given an antacid to minimize the likelihood of aspiration during anesthesia. A Foley catheter is placed to allow for continuous bladder drainage before, during, and after surgery. Anesthesia is administered, and the abdomen is prepped. The patient is covered with sterile drapes. Tilting the patient slightly to the left moves the uterus to the left of the midline and minimizes pressure on the inferior vena cava.

OPERATIVE PROCEDURE

Abdominal Incision

Opinions differ regarding the type of abdominal incision that should be performed. Most obstetricians use the transverse (Pfannenstiel) incision with or without transection of the rectus muscles because wound dehiscence is rare and because the cosmetic result is usually better. In cases in which the caesarean section must be performed urgently or emergently, especially in patients with prior abdominal surgery or marked obesity, the midline vertical suprapubic incision is preferred because it is much quicker and the exposure for expeditious delivery and resolving uterine bleeding (by hysterectomy, if needed) usually is better. In the presence of a prior lower abdominal scar, it is important to enter the peritoneal cavity at the upper end of the incision to avoid entering the bladder, which may have been pulled upward on the abdominal wall at the time of closure of the previous incision.

Uterine Incision

Before the uterine incision is made, laparotomy pads that have been soaked in warm saline and wrung out can be placed on either side of the uterus to catch the spill of amniotic fluid. The degree of dextrorotation should also be determined by noting the position of the round ligaments so that the uterine incision will be centered. Torsion should not be corrected; instead, access to the midline should be obtained by retracting the abdominal wall to the patient's right. The different types of uterine incisions will be discussed later.

Encountering the Placenta

If the placenta is encountered beneath the uterine incision, the operator should avoid cutting through it; otherwise serious fetal bleeding may result. If the placenta cannot be avoided, an incision can be made through it. However, the baby must be delivered as quickly as possible and the cord clamped immediately to prevent significant blood loss.

Delivery

The operator delivers the baby, and then the placenta delivers. Recent evidence has demonstrated that blood loss can be minimized by massaging the uterus to allow for spontaneous placental expulsion rather than by manually separating and extracting the placenta. After delivery of the placenta, the uterus should be massaged and oxytocin administered in a dilute intravenous solution at a rate sufficient to maintain a firm contraction. The uterine cavity is wiped clean with a sponge so as to remove any retained membranes. The uterus is exteriorized, and active bleeding sinuses are clamped with either Pennington clamps or ring forceps.

Closure of the Uterine Incision

The closure of the uterine incision is dependent on the type of incision that is made. In general, the entire thickness of the myometrium should be closed. In order to potentially decrease the likelihood of uterine rupture during a subsequent pregnancy, the uterine incision should be closed in 2 layers. The 2 types of uterine incisions used most often and discussed here are the classical uterine incision and the low-transverse uterine incision.

CLASSICAL CAESAREAN SECTION

This is the simplest to perform. However, it is associated with the greatest loss of blood and with a greater risk of uterine rupture with subsequent pregnancies when compared with low-transverse incisions. The currently accepted indications for classical caesarean section are placenta previa, transverse lie (especially back down), and preterm delivery in which the lower uterine segment is poorly developed. A classical caesarean section may be preferred if extremely rapid delivery is needed, because this type of incision may offer the fastest means of delivering the baby. Nonetheless, the hazards of this procedure must be weighed against the additional minute or so needed to dissect the bladder away from the lower uterine segment and make the transverse semilunar low-transverse uterine incision.

In performing a classical procedure, a vertical incision is made in the body of the uterus. A scalpel is used to enter the uterine activity, and the incision is enlarged with bandage scissors. The fetus is delivered through the incision. After the placenta and membranes are removed, the uterine defect is repaired with 3 layers of running, interlocking absorbable suture. Number 0 suture is recommended for the 2 deeper layers, and 2-0 suture is used for the superficial layer to reapproximate the serosal edges.

LOW-TRANSVERSE CAESAREAN SECTION

Because the low-transverse uterine incision (Figs. 20–10 through 20–17) is associated with less blood loss and the risk of subsequent uterine rupture is less than with a classical caesarean section, this type of caesarean delivery is performed more frequently. After the peritoneal cavity is opened and the uterus identified, the bladder fold of peritoneum is picked up with tissue forceps and incised transversely. The bladder is bluntly separated from the anterior aspect of the uterus inferiorly for a distance of 3–4 cm. The bladder is held away from this area by a specially designed bladder retractor. A transverse incision is made through the anterior uterine wall with the scalpel. Using either bandage scissors or fingers, the transverse incision is extended in a semilunar fashion and extended superiorly at the lateral edges in order to avoid the uterine vessels.

If the maneuver can be easily done, the fetal presenting part is elevated with the hand, making sure not to flex the wrist, thereby increasing the possibility of extension of the incision inferiorly toward the cervix. If the head is located deep in the pelvis, the head can safely be pushed up by an assistant inserting a hand into the vagina to elevate the fetal head for ease of delivery. After the baby and placenta are delivered, the uterus is exteriorized and clamps are placed on the cut edges of the uterus in areas of significant bleeding from the uterine sinuses. The uterine incision is generally closed in 2 layers using number 0 chromic catgut or other absorbable suture. After adequate hemostasis has been achieved, the bladder peritoneum either is reapproximated with suture or is left in place. Before the uterus is returned to the peritoneal cavity, the adnexa should be inspected for the presence of any pathology, such as ovarian cysts. Some practitioners prefer to close the anterior peritoneum with absorbable suture, whereas others prefer to leave it alone. The fascia, subcutaneous tissue, and skin are reapproximated in standard fashion.

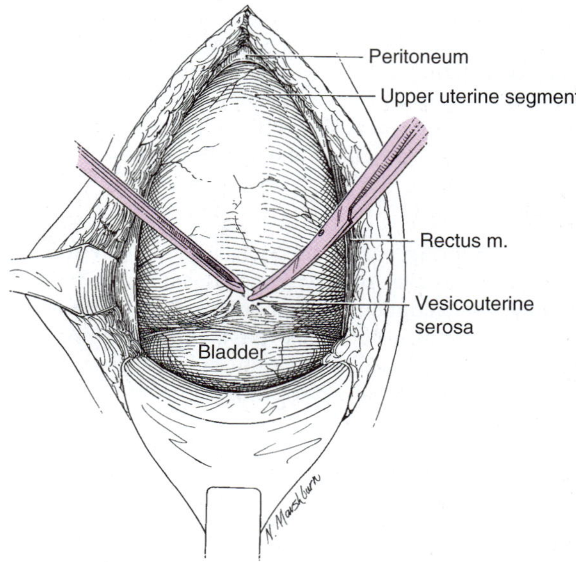

▲ **Figure 20–10.** The loose vesicouterine serosa is grasped with the forceps. The hemostat tip points to the upper margin of the bladder. The retractor is firmly positioned against the symphysis. m, muscle. (Reproduced, with permission, from Cunningham FG, Leveno KJ, Bloom SL, et al. *Williams Obstetrics*. 22nd ed. New York, NY: McGraw-Hill; 2005, p 594.)

COMPLICATIONS

The most common complications that result from caesarean section are postpartum hemorrhage, endometritis, and wound infection. Administering prophylactic antibiotics and ensuring hemostasis prior to closure of the abdomen have helped decrease the incidence of these complications. New data are emerging that demonstrate a lower risk of endometritis when antibiotics are given prior to the skin incision when compared to after clamping of the umbilical cord. The major factors affecting healing of the uterine incision are hemostasis, accuracy of apposition, quality and amount of suture material, and avoidance of infection and tissue strangulation. It can generally be stated that the longer the operative procedure, the greater is the likelihood of postoperative complications. Disasters following caesarean section are rare. Some clearly are not preventable. Others are the direct result of faulty surgical technique, especially lack of attention to hemostasis, inept or ill-chosen anesthesia, inadequate blood

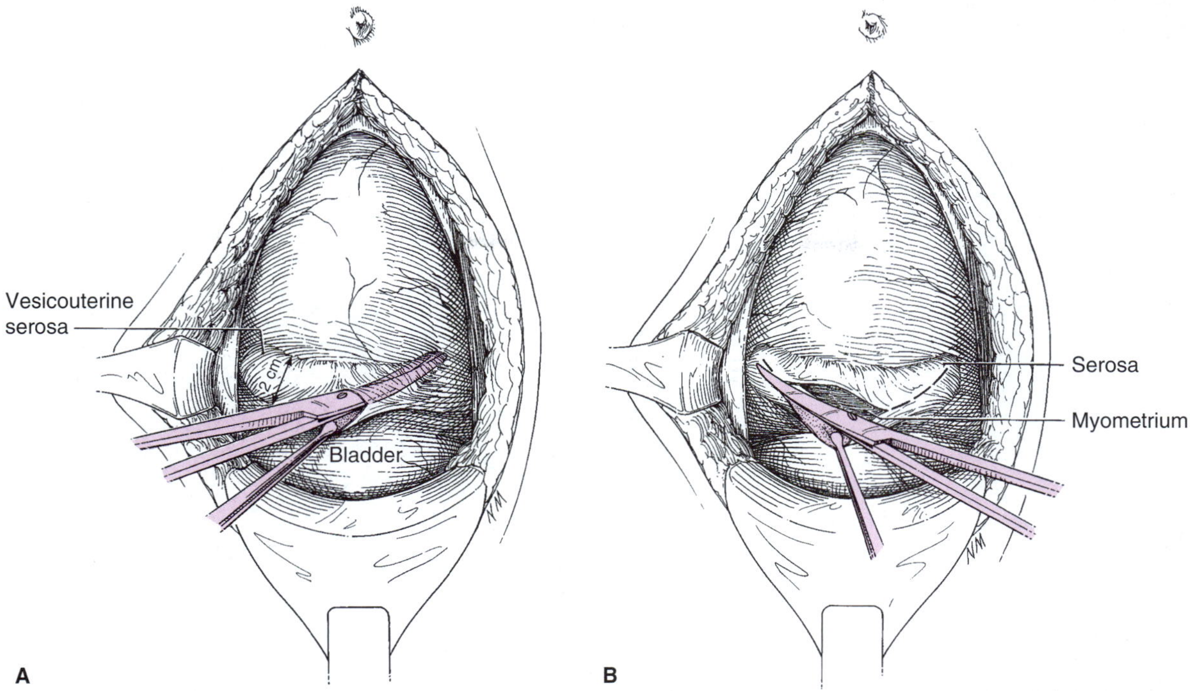

▲ **Figure 20–11.** The loose serosa above the upper margin of the bladder is elevated and incised laterally. (Reproduced, with permission, from Cunningham FG, Leveno KJ, Bloom SL, et al. *Williams Obstetrics*. 22nd ed. New York, NY: McGraw-Hill; 2005, p 594.)

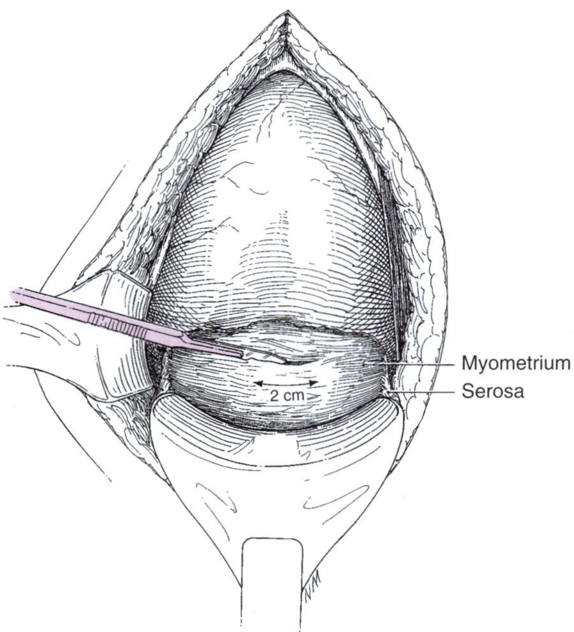

▲ **Figure 20–12.** The myometrium is incised carefully to avoid cutting the fetal head. (Reproduced, with permission, from Cunningham FG, Leveno KJ, Bloom SL, et al. *Williams Obstetrics*. 22nd ed. New York, NY: McGraw-Hill; 2005, p 595.)

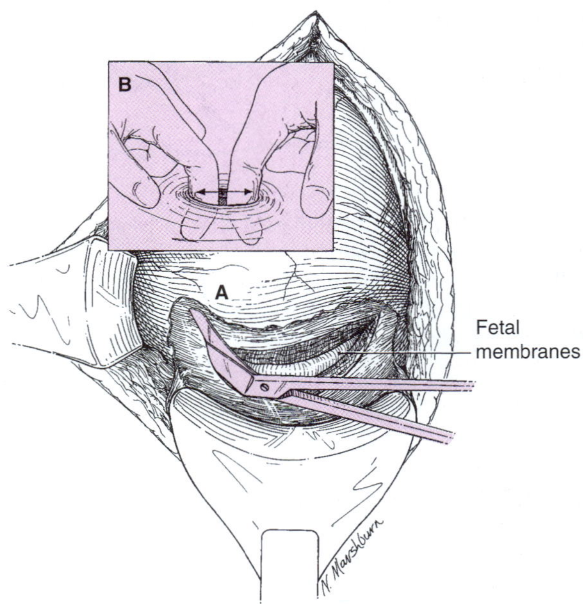

▲ **Figure 20–13.** After entering the uterine cavity, the incision is extended laterally with bandage scissors **(A)** or with fingers **(B)**. (Reproduced, with permission, from Cunningham FG, Leveno KJ, Bloom SL, et al. *Williams Obstetrics*. 22nd ed. New York, NY: McGraw-Hill; 2005, p 595.)

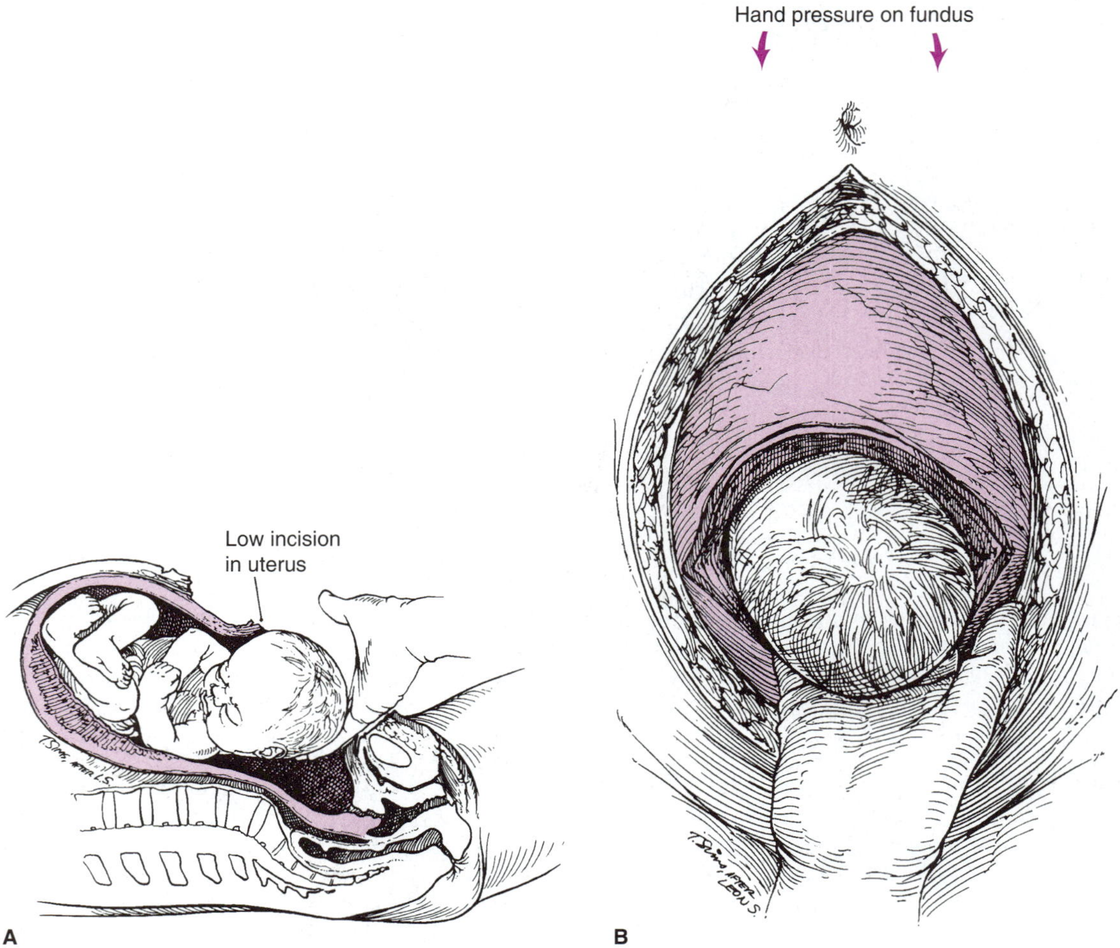

▲ **Figure 20–14. A:** Immediately after incising the uterus and rupturing the fetal membranes, the fingers are insinuated between the symphysis pubis and the fetal head until the posterior surface is reached. The head is lifted carefully anteriorly and, as necessary, superiorly to bring it from beneath the symphysis forward through the uterine and abdominal incisions. **B:** As the fetal head is lifted through the incision, pressure usually is applied to the uterine fundus through the abdominal wall to help expel the fetus. (Reproduced, with permission, from Cunningham FG, Leveno KJ, Bloom SL, et al. *Williams Obstetrics*. 22nd ed. New York, NY: McGraw-Hill; 2005, p 596.)

product replacement or transfusion of mismatched blood, and delayed diagnosis or mismanagement of infection.

Unfortunately, little information about the integrity of a particular scar in a subsequent pregnancy is gained by inquiry into the presence or absence of postoperative infection and location of the incision. In a later pregnancy, pain in the area of the scar may suggest dehiscence. Approximately 50% of all ruptures of classical uterine scars occur before the onset of labor. The incidence of uterine rupture is approximately 4–9% of classical scars and 0.7–1.5% of low-transverse scars. Rupture of a classical scar usually is catastrophic, occurring suddenly, totally, and with partial or total extrusion of the fetus into the abdominal cavity. Shock due to internal hemorrhage is a prominent sign. Rupture of the low-transverse scar usually is more subtle and almost always occurs during active labor. The most common presenting sign (present in more than 80% of cases) is a change in the fetal heart rate pattern. A newly recognized finding of variable or late decelerations should alert the obstetrician. Additional findings that might signal uterine rupture include vaginal bleeding, abdominal pain (especially over the prior incision site), and loss of fetal station. A scalp electrode to ensure a continuous fetal heart rate tracing should be utilized as soon as possible in

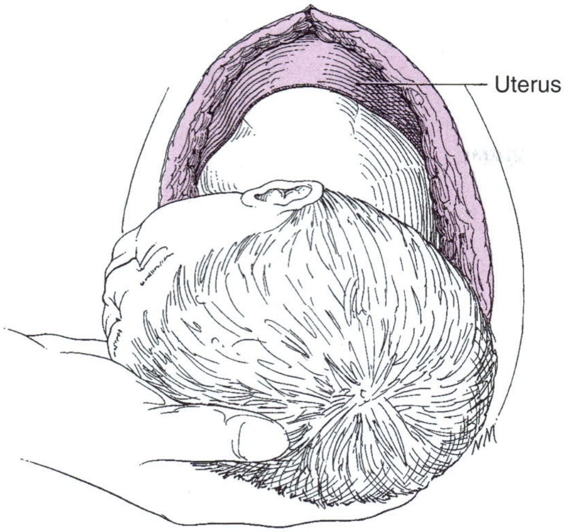

▲ **Figure 20–15.** The shoulders are delivered, and the oxytocin infusion is begun.

patients who are undergoing TOLAC. If uterine rupture is suspected, the patient must undergo surgery as soon as possible.

PERINATAL MORBIDITY & MORTALITY

Although it may appear on the surface that caesarean delivery is the safest for the baby, this may not be entirely true.

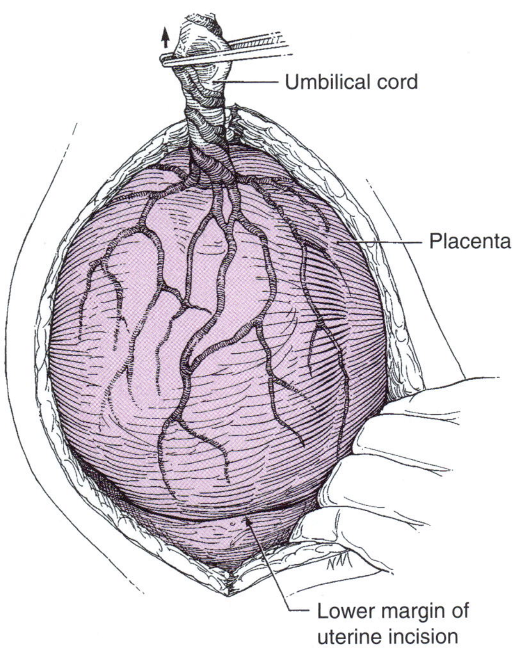

▲ **Figure 20–16.** Placenta bulging through the uterine incision as the uterus contracts.

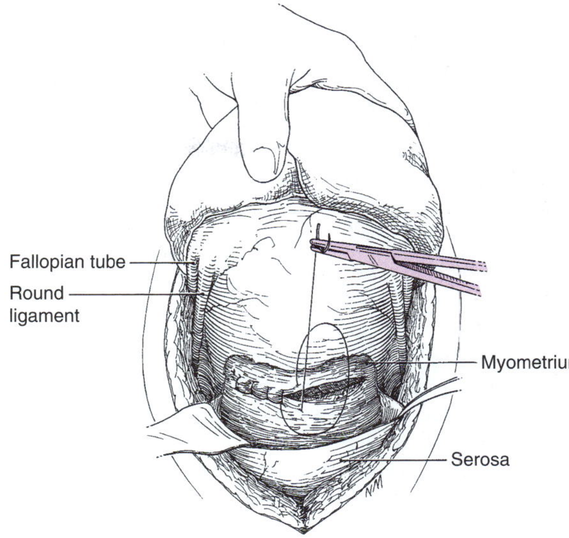

▲ **Figure 20–17.** The cut edges of the uterine incision are approximated with a running-lock suture.

Although usually benign, transient tachypnea of the newborn is more common with caesarean section than with vaginal delivery. The risk of fetal hemorrhage and hypoxia is present when the placenta is encountered below the uterine incision and is inadvertently or purposely transected. There is also the potential risk for laceration of the baby at the time that the uterine incision is made. Fetal laceration is reported to occur on an infrequent basis at a rate of approximately 0.2–0.4% of all caesarean sections. The usual site is on the face, in the area of the cheek, but it may also occur on the buttock, ear, head, or any other body site under the incision. Therefore, it is of great importance that care is taken when incising the layers of the uterus. This is especially true in a prolonged labor, in which the uterus may be very thin. Because of the potential complications to the baby inherent with each caesarean section, each infant should be examined by a trained professional as soon as possible after delivery.

American College of Obstetricians and Gynecologists. *Vaginal Birth after Previous Cesarean Delivery. Practice Bulletin No. 115.* Washington, DC: American College of Obstetricians and Gynecologists; 2010.

Goetzinger KR, Macones GA. Operative vaginal delivery: Current trends in obstetrics. *Womens Health* 2008;4:281. PMID: 19072477.

Gyamfi C, Juhasz G, Gyamfi P, Blumenfeld Y, Stone JL. Single-versus double-layer uterine incision closure and uterine rupture. *J Matern Fetal Neonatal Med* 2006;19:639. PMID: 17118738.

Kaimal AJ, Zlatnik MG, Cheng YW, et al. Effect of change in policy regarding the timing of prophylactic antibiotics on the rate of postcesarean delivery surgical-site infections. *Am J Obstet Gynecol* 2008;199:310.e1. PMID: 18771995.

Lydon-Rochelle M, Holt VL, Easterling TR, Martin DP. Risk of uterine rupture during labor among women with a prior cesarean delivery. *N Engl J Med* 2001;345:3. PMID: 11439945.

Nygaard I, Cruikshank DP. Should all women be offered elective cesarean delivery? *Obstet Gynecol* 2003;102:217. PMID: 12907089.

CAESAREAN HYSTERECTOMY

A major indication for caesarean hysterectomy is the inability to stop bleeding. The most common reason for performing caesarean hysterectomy is abnormal placental implantation, such as placenta accreta, increta, and percreta. As the caesarean section rate continues to escalate, these complications are becoming more common. Other indications for caesarean hysterectomy include intractable uterine atony, inability to repair a ruptured uterus, and large uterine myomas. Caesarean hysterectomy is a potentially morbid procedure because of increased blood loss and potential for injury to the bladder, ureter, or bowel.

The technical aspects of hysterectomy at the time of caesarean section are similar to those of hysterectomy in the nonpregnant patient except that all structures, cleavage planes, and pedicles are highly vascular. Therefore, there is significant risk for excessive blood loss and the need for the transfusion of blood products. In cases in which there is a suspicion that caesarean hysterectomy may need to be performed, the anesthesiologist and blood bank personnel should be informed. It is recommended that blood products (packed red blood cells and fresh frozen plasma) are available. Lastly, a vascular surgeon or gynecologic oncologist should be available to assist if needed. Studies have demonstrated that caesarean hysterectomy performed on a nonemergent basis is much safer than hysterectomy performed on an emergent basis. Specifically, injury to the bladder and ureter and the need for blood transfusions are more common when caesarean hysterectomy is performed emergently.

Oliphant SS, Jones KA, Wang L, Bunker CH, Lowder JL. Trends over time with commonly performed obstetric and gynecologic inpatient procedures. *Obstet Gynecol* 2010;116;926. PMID: 20859157.

Vacca A. Trials and tribulations of operative vaginal delivery. *BJOG* 2007;114:519. PMID: 17439561.

Yeomans ER. Operative vaginal delivery. *Obstet Gynecol* 2010;115:645. PMID: 20177298.

Postpartum Hemorrhage & the Abnormal Puerperium

21

Sarah B.H. Poggi, MD

POSTPARTUM HEMORRHAGE

ESSENTIALS OF DIAGNOSIS

- Postpartum hemorrhage denotes excessive bleeding (>500 mL in vaginal delivery) following delivery. Hemorrhage may occur before, during, or after delivery of the placenta. Actual measured blood loss during uncomplicated vaginal deliveries averages 700 mL, and blood loss often may be underestimated. Nevertheless, the criterion of a 500-mL loss is acceptable on historical grounds.
- Blood lost during the first 24 hours after delivery is *early postpartum hemorrhage*; blood lost between 24 hours and 6 weeks after delivery is *late postpartum hemorrhage*.

Pathogenesis

The incidence of excessive blood loss following vaginal delivery is 5–8%. Postpartum hemorrhage is the most common cause of excessive blood loss in pregnancy, and most transfusions in pregnant women are performed to replace blood lost after delivery. Hemorrhage is the third leading cause of maternal mortality in the United States and is directly responsible for approximately one-sixth of maternal deaths. In less developed countries, hemorrhage is among the leading obstetric causes of maternal death.

Causes of postpartum hemorrhage include uterine atony, obstetric lacerations, retained placental tissue, and coagulation defects.

A. Uterine Atony

Postpartum bleeding is physiologically controlled by constriction of interlacing myometrial fibers that surround the blood vessels supplying the placental implantation site. Uterine atony exists when the myometrium cannot contract.

Atony is the most common cause of postpartum hemorrhage (50% of cases). Predisposing causes include excessive manipulation of the uterus, general anesthesia (particularly with halogenated compounds), uterine overdistention (twins or polyhydramnios), prolonged labor, grand multiparity, uterine leiomyomas, operative delivery and intrauterine manipulation, oxytocin induction or augmentation of labor, previous hemorrhage in the third stage, uterine infection, extravasation of blood into the myometrium (Couvelaire uterus), and intrinsic myometrial dysfunction.

B. Obstetric Lacerations

Excessive bleeding from an episiotomy, lacerations, or both causes approximately 20% of postpartum hemorrhages. Lacerations can involve the uterus, cervix, vagina, or vulva. They usually result from precipitous or uncontrolled delivery or operative delivery of a large infant; however, they may occur after any delivery. Laceration of blood vessels underneath the vaginal or vulvar epithelium results in hematomas. Bleeding is concealed and can be particularly dangerous because it may go unrecognized for several hours and become apparent only when shock occurs.

Episiotomies may cause excessive bleeding if they involve arteries or large varicosities, if the episiotomy is large, or if a delay occurred between episiotomy and delivery or between delivery and repair of the episiotomy.

Persistent bleeding (especially bright red) and a well-contracted, firm uterus suggest bleeding from a laceration or from the episiotomy. When cervical or vaginal lacerations are identified as the source of postpartum hemorrhage, repair is best performed with adequate anesthesia.

Spontaneous rupture of the uterus is rare. Risk factors for this complication include grand multiparity, malpresentation, previous uterine surgery, and oxytocin induction of labor. Rupture of a previous caesarean section scar after vaginal delivery may be an increasingly important cause of postpartum hemorrhage.

C. Retained Placental Tissue

Retained placental tissue and membranes cause 5–10% of postpartum hemorrhages. Retention of placental tissue in the uterine cavity occurs in placenta accreta, which is an increasingly frequent diagnosis in this era of multiple caesarean deliveries. Retained placental tissue may also develop in cases managed by manual removal of the placenta, in mismanagement of the third stage of labor, and in unrecognized succenturiate placenta.

Ultrasonographic findings of an echogenic uterine mass strongly support a diagnosis of retained placental products. The technique probably is better used in cases of hemorrhage occurring a few hours after delivery or in late postpartum hemorrhage. Transvaginal duplex Doppler imaging also is effective in evaluating these patients. Some evidence indicates that sonohysterography may aid in the diagnosis of residual trophoblastic tissue. If the endometrial cavity appears empty, unnecessary dilatation and curettage may be avoided.

D. Coagulation Defects

Coagulopathies in pregnancy may be acquired coagulation defects seen in association with several obstetric disorders, including abruptio placentae, excess thromboplastin from a retained dead fetus, amniotic fluid embolism, severe preeclampsia, eclampsia, and sepsis. These coagulopathies may present as hypofibrinogenemia, thrombocytopenia, and disseminated intravascular coagulation. Transfusion of more than 8 U of blood in itself may induce a dilutional coagulopathy.

Von Willebrand's disease, autoimmune thrombocytopenia, and leukemia may occur in pregnant women.

Prevention

Prevention of hemorrhage is preferable to even the best treatment. All patients in labor should be evaluated for risk of postpartum hemorrhage. Risk factors include coagulopathy, hemorrhage, or blood transfusion during a previous pregnancy; anemia during labor; grand multiparity; multiple gestation; large infant; polyhydramnios; dysfunctional labor; oxytocin induction or augmentation of labor; rapid or tumultuous labor; severe preeclampsia or eclampsia; vaginal delivery after previous caesarean birth; general anesthesia for delivery; forceps delivery; and delay in placental delivery after vaginal delivery of the infant.

Complications

Although any woman may suffer excessive blood loss during delivery, women already compromised by anemia or intercurrent illness are more likely to demonstrate serious deterioration of condition, and anemia and excessive blood loss may predispose to subsequent puerperal infection. Major morbidity associated with transfusion therapy (eg, viral infection, transfusion reactions) is infrequent but is not insignificant. Moreover, other types of treatment for anemia may involve some risk.

Postpartum hypotension may lead to partial or total necrosis of the anterior pituitary gland and cause postpartum panhypopituitarism, or Sheehan's syndrome, which is characterized by failure to lactate, amenorrhea, decreased breast size, loss of pubic and axillary hair, hypothyroidism, and adrenal insufficiency. The condition is rare (<1 in 10,000 deliveries). A woman who has been hypotensive postpartum and who is actively lactating probably does not have Sheehan's syndrome. Hypotension also can lead to acute renal failure and other organ system injury. In extreme hemorrhage, sterility will result from hysterectomy performed to control intractable postpartum hemorrhage.

Treatment

A. Predelivery Preparation

All obstetric patients should have blood typed and screened on admission. Patients identified as being at risk for postpartum hemorrhage should have their blood typed and cross-matched immediately. The blood should be reserved in the blood bank for 24 hours after delivery. A large-bore intravenous catheter should be securely taped into place after insertion. Delivery room personnel should be alerted to the risk of hemorrhage. Severely anemic patients should be transfused as soon as cross-matched blood is ready.

With concerns associated with blood transfusion, autologous blood donation in obstetric patients at risk for postpartum hemorrhage has been advocated. Despite careful evaluation for risk factors, with the exception of cases of placenta previa, our ability to predict which patients will have hemorrhage and require blood transfusion remains poor; therefore, the cost of such an approach may not be justified.

B. Delivery

Following delivery of the infant, the uterus is massaged in a circular or back-and-forth motion until the myometrium becomes firm and well contracted. Excessive and vigorous massage of the uterus before, during, or after delivery of the placenta may interfere with normal contraction of the myometrium and, instead of hastening contraction, may lead to excessive postpartum blood loss.

C. Third Stage of Normal Labor; Placental Separation

The placenta typically separates from the uterus and is delivered within 5 minutes of delivery of the infant in 50% of cases and within 15 minutes in 90% of cases. Attempts to speed separation are of no benefit and may cause harm.

Spontaneous placental separation is impending if the uterus becomes round and firm, a sudden gush of blood comes from the vagina, the uterus seems to rise in the abdomen, and the umbilical cord moves down out of the vagina.

The placenta then can be removed from the vagina by gentle traction on the umbilical cord. Prior to placental separation, gentle steady traction on the cord combined with upward pressure on the lower uterine segment (Brandt-Andrews maneuver) ensures that the placenta can be removed as soon as separation occurs and provides a means of monitoring the consistency of the uterus. Adherent membranes can be removed by gentle traction with ring forceps. The placenta is inspected for completeness immediately after delivery.

Manual Removal of the Placenta

Opinion is divided about the timing of manual removal of the placenta. In the presence of hemorrhage, it is unreasonable to wait for spontaneous separation, and manual removal of the placenta should be undertaken without delay. Traditionally, in the absence of bleeding, many have advocated removal of the placenta 30 minutes after delivery of the infant. Newer evidence suggests that to prevent postpartum hemorrhage, a placenta that has not been delivered by 18 minutes should be removed.

Efforts to promote routine manual removal of the placenta were often made in the past. The rationale includes shortening the third stage of labor, decreasing blood loss, developing experience in manual removal as practice for dealing with placenta accreta, and providing a way to simultaneously explore the uterus. Evidence now indicates that manual removal of the placenta may be a risk factor for postpartum endometritis. These real or potential benefits must be weighed against the discomfort caused to the patient, the risk of infection, and the risk of causing more bleeding by interfering with normal mechanisms of placental separation.

Technique: The uterus is stabilized by grasping the fundus with a hand placed over the abdomen. The other hand traces the course of the umbilical cord through the vagina and cervix into the uterus to palpate the edge of the placenta. The membranes at the placental margin are perforated, and the hand is inserted between the placenta and the uterine wall, palmar side toward the placenta. The hand is then gently swept from side to side and up and down to peel the placenta from its attachments to the uterus. When the placenta has been completely separated from the uterus, it is grasped and pulled from the uterus.

The fetal and maternal sides of the placenta should be inspected to ensure that it has been removed in its entirety. On the fetal surface, incomplete placental removal is manifested as interruption of the vessels on the chorionic plate, usually shown by hemorrhage. On the maternal surface, it is possible to see where cotyledons have been detached. If evidence of incomplete removal is observed, the uterus must be re-explored and any small pieces of adherent placenta removed. The uterus should be massaged until a firm myometrial tone is achieved. Depending on the patient's other risk factors for postpartum endometritis, prophylactic antibiotics can be given at the time of manual removal of the placenta.

Immediate Postpartum Period

Uterotonic agents can be administered as soon as the infant's anterior shoulder is delivered. There is a significantly lowered incidence of postpartum hemorrhage in patients receiving oxytocin (either low-dose intravenous [IV] or intramuscular [IM]) at the time of delivery of the anterior shoulder and controlled cord traction compared to patients receiving IV oxytocin after placental delivery. There was no greater incidence of placental retention. However, populations without ultrasound screening for twins have a potential risk for entrapment of an undiagnosed second twin, and oxytocin should only be given after placental delivery. Routine administration of oxytocics during the third stage reduces the blood loss of delivery and decreases the chances of postpartum hemorrhage by 40%. Oxytocin, 10–20 U/L of isotonic saline, or other IV solution by slow IV infusion or 10 U IM can be used. Bolus administration should not be used because large doses (>5 U) can cause hypotension. Recently, sublingual misoprostol (800 μg) has been found to be clinically as effective as oxytocin (40 U/L) for treatment of postpartum hemorrhage. This information is particularly useful for low-resource areas because misoprostol does not have to be refrigerated or require specialized equipment for administration, but regardless of setting, misoprostol is a useful adjunct to treatment of postpartum hemorrhage. Ergot alkaloids (eg, methylergonovine maleate 0.2 mg IM) also can be routinely used, but they are not more effective than oxytocin and pose more risk because they rarely cause marked hypertension. This occurs most commonly with IV administration or when regional anesthesia is used. Ergot alkaloids should not be used in hypertensive women or in women with cardiac disease.

Repair of Lacerations

If bleeding is excessive before placental separation, manual removal of the placenta is indicated. Otherwise, excessive manipulation of the uterus should be avoided.

The vagina and cervix should be carefully inspected immediately after delivery of the placenta, with adequate lighting and assistants available. The episiotomy is quickly repaired after massage has produced a firm, tightly contracted uterus. A pack placed in the vagina above the episiotomy helps to keep the field dry; attaching the free end of the pack to the adjacent drapes reminds the operator to remove it after the repair is completed.

The tendency of bleeding vessels to retract from the laceration site is the reason for one of the cardinal principles of repair. Begin the repair above the highest extent of the laceration. The highest suture is also used to provide gentle traction to bring the laceration site closer to the introitus. Hemostatic ligatures are then placed in the usual manner, and the entire birth canal is carefully inspected to ensure that no additional bleeding sites are present. Extensive inspection also provides time to confirm that prior hemostatic efforts have been effective.

A cervical or vaginal laceration extending into the broad ligament should not be repaired vaginally. Laparotomy with evacuation of the resultant hematoma and hemostatic repair or hysterectomy are required.

Large or expanding hematomas of the vaginal walls require operative management for proper control. The vaginal wall is first exposed by an assistant. If a laceration accompanies the hematoma, the laceration is extended so that the hematoma can be completely evacuated and explored. When the bleeding site is identified, a large hemostatic ligature can be placed well above the site. This ensures hemostasis in the vessel, which is likely to retract when lacerated. The hematoma cavity should be left open to allow drainage of blood and ensure that bleeding will not be concealed if hemostasis cannot be achieved.

If no laceration is present on the vaginal side wall when a hematoma is identified, then an incision must be made over the hematoma to allow treatment to proceed as outlined.

Following delivery, recovery room attendants should frequently massage the uterus and check for vaginal bleeding.

Evaluation of Persistent Bleeding

If vaginal bleeding persists after delivery of the placenta, aggressive treatment should be initiated. It is not sufficient to perform perfunctory uterine massage, for instance, without searching for the cause of the bleeding and initiating definitive treatment. The following steps should be undertaken without delay:

1. Manually compress the uterus.
2. Obtain assistance.
3. If not already done, obtain blood for typing and crossmatching.
4. Observe blood for clotting to rule out coagulopathy.
5. Begin fluid or blood replacement.
6. Carefully explore the uterine cavity.
7. Completely inspect the cervix and vagina.
8. Insert a second IV catheter for administration of blood or fluids.

A. Measures to Control Bleeding

1. Manual exploration of the uterus—The uterus should be explored immediately in women with postpartum hemorrhage. Manual exploration also should be considered after delivery of the placenta in the following circumstances: (1) when vaginal delivery follows previous caesarean section; (2) when intrauterine manipulation, such as version and extraction, has been performed; (3) when malpresentation has occurred during labor and delivery; (4) when a premature infant has been delivered; (5) when an abnormal uterine contour has been noted prior to delivery; and (6) when there is a possibility of undiagnosed multiple pregnancy—to rule out twins.

Ensure that all placental parts have been delivered and that the uterus is intact. This should be done even in the case of a well-contracted uterus. Exploration performed for reasons other than evaluation of hemorrhage also should confirm that the uterine wall is intact and should attempt to identify any possible intrauterine structural abnormalities. Manual exploration of the uterus does not increase febrile morbidity or blood loss.

Technique: Place a fresh glove over the glove on the exploring hand. Form the hand into a cone and gently introduce it by firm pressure through the cervix while stabilizing the fundus with the other hand. Sweep the backs of the first and second fingers across the entire surface of the uterus, beginning at the fundus. In the lower uterine segment, palpate the walls with the palmar surface of 1 finger. Uterine lacerations will be felt as an obvious anatomic defect. All exploration should be gentle because the postpartum uterus is easily perforated.

Uterine rupture detected by manual exploration in the presence of postpartum hemorrhage requires immediate laparotomy. A decision to repair the defect or proceed with hysterectomy is made on the basis of the extent of the rupture, the patient's desire for future childbearing, and the degree of the patient's clinical deterioration.

2. Bimanual compression & massage—The most important step in controlling atonic postpartum hemorrhage is immediate bimanual uterine compression, which may have to be continued for 20–30 minutes or more. Fluid replacement should begin as soon as a secure IV line is in place. Typed and cross-matched blood is given when it is available. Manual compression of the uterus will control most cases of hemorrhage due to uterine atony, retained products of conception (once the products are removed), and coagulopathies.

Technique: Place a hand on the patient's abdomen and grasp the uterine fundus; bring it down over the symphysis pubis. Insert the other hand into the vagina, and place the first and second fingers on either side of the cervix and push it cephalad and anteriorly. The pulsating uterine arteries should be felt by the fingertips. Massage the uterus with both hands while maintaining compression. Prolonged compression (20–30 minutes) may be required but almost always is successful in controlling bleeding.

Insert a Foley catheter into the bladder during compression and massage because vigorous fluid and blood replacement will cause diuresis. A distended bladder will interfere with compression and massage, will contribute to the patient's discomfort, and may itself be a major contributor to uterine atony.

3. Curettage—Curettage of a large, soft postpartum uterus can be a formidable undertaking because the risk of perforation is high and the procedure commonly results in increased rather than decreased bleeding. The suction curette, even with a large cannula, covers only a small area of the postpartum uterus, and its size and shape increase the likelihood of perforation. A large blunt curette, the "banjo" curette, probably is the safest instrument for curettage of the postpartum uterus. It can be used when manual exploration fails to remove fragments of adherent placenta.

Curettage should be delayed unless bleeding cannot be controlled by compression and massage alone. Overly vigorous puerperal curettage can result in focal complete removal of the endometrium, particularly if the uterus is infected, with subsequent healing characterized by formation of adhesions and **Asherman's syndrome** (amenorrhea and secondary sterility due to intrauterine adhesions and uterine synechiae). If circumstances permit, ultrasonic evaluation of the postpartum uterus may distinguish those patients who will benefit from curettage from those who should be managed without it.

4. Uterine packing—Although once widely used for control of obstetric hemorrhage, uterine packing is no longer favored. The uterus may expand to considerable size after delivery of the placenta, thus accommodating both a large volume of packing material and a large volume of blood. The technique also demands considerable technical expertise because the uterus must be packed uniformly with 5 yards of 4-inch gauze, sometimes with the aid of special instrumentation (Torpin packer). However, this method has been used successfully, avoiding conversion to laparotomy in 9 reported cases. As a last resort, uterine packing may be particularly appropriate in centers where an interventional radiologist is not immediately available.

An alternative for uterine packing that relies on the same principle of uterine tamponade is the Bakri balloon. This device is an inflatable balloon that inflates up to 800 mL. Due to a double lumen port, drainage of blood can still occur so that concealed hemorrhage does not occur. The balloon can easily be moved after deflation vaginally. An advantage of the device is that it can be inserted at time of hemorrhage from a vaginal approach or at time of laparotomy; in either case, it can be removed vaginally. The success of the device has been described in case series.

5. Uterotonic agents—Oxytocin 20–40 U/L of crystalloid should be infused, if not already running, at a rate of 10–15 mL/min. Methylergonovine 0.2 mg can be given IM but is contraindicated if the patient is hypertensive. Intramyometrial injection of prostaglandin $F_{2\alpha}$ ($PGF_{2\alpha}$) to control bleeding was initially described in 1976. Intravaginal or rectal prostaglandin suppositories, intrauterine irrigation with prostaglandins, and intramyometrial injection of prostaglandins also have been reported to control hemorrhage from uterine atony. IM administration of 15-methylprostaglandin analogue was successful in treating 85% of patients with postpartum hemorrhage due to atony. Failures in these series occurred in women who had uterine infections or unrecognized placenta accreta. Side effects usually are minimal but may include transient oxygen desaturation, bronchospasm, and, rarely, significant hypertension. Transient fever and diarrhea may occur. Rectal misoprostol (800 μg), a prostaglandin E_1 analogue, has been found to be effective in the treatment of primary postpartum hemorrhage secondary to atony. As mentioned earlier, sublingual misoprostol (800 μg) has been found to be clinically as effective as oxytocin (40 U/L) for treatment of postpartum hemorrhage due to atony. This information is particularly useful for low-resource areas because misoprostol does not have to be refrigerated or require specialized equipment for administration.

6. Radiographic embolization of pelvic vessels—Embolization of pelvic and uterine vessels by angiographic techniques is increasingly common and has success rates that range from 85–95% in experienced hands. In institutions with trained interventional radiologists, the technique is worth considering in women of low parity as an alternative to hysterectomy. With the patient under local anesthesia, a catheter is placed in the aorta and fluoroscopy is used to identify the bleeding vessel. Pieces of absorbable gelatin sponge (Gelfoam) or coil are injected into the damaged vessel (most typically the uterine artery) or into the internal iliac vessels if no specific site of bleeding can be identified. If bleeding continues, further embolization can be performed. This technique has the advantage of being effective even when the cause of hemorrhage is extrauterine and in the presence or absence of uterine atony. Many authors recommend embolization before internal iliac ligation, because ligation obstructs the access route for angiography. Adequate recanalization can occur to maintain fertility, although at this point, there are only limited case series demonstrating maintenance of fertility with pelvic artery embolization in this setting (as opposed to use for uterine fibroids). Although pelvic artery embolization is clearly preferable to hysterectomy in a patient desiring fertility, it is important to remember that the procedure does have an inherent complication rate, about 3–5%, with reports in the medical literature of loss of circulation to the lower extremities, labial and buttock necrosis, and vesicovaginal fistula.

7. Operative management—The patient's wishes regarding further childbearing should be made clear as soon as laparotomy is contemplated for the management of postpartum hemorrhage. If the patient's wishes cannot be ascertained, the operator should assume that the childbearing function is to be retained. Whenever possible, the spouse or family members should also be consulted prior to laparotomy.

A. PRESSURE OCCLUSION OF THE AORTA—Immediate temporary control of pelvic bleeding may be obtained at laparotomy by pressure occlusion of the aorta, which will provide valuable time to treat hypotension, obtain experienced assistants, identify the source of bleeding, and plan the operative procedure. In the young and otherwise healthy patient, pressure occlusion can be maintained for several minutes without permanent sequelae.

B. Uterine artery ligation—During pregnancy, 90% of the blood flow to the uterus is supplied by the uterine arteries. Direct ligation of these easily accessible vessels can successfully control hemorrhage in 75–90% of cases, particularly when the bleeding is uterine in origin. Recanalization can occur, and subsequent pregnancies have been reported.

Technique: The uterus is lifted upward and away from the side to be ligated. Absorbable suture on a large needle is placed around the ascending uterine artery and vein on 1 side of the uterus, passing through the myometrium 2–4 cm medial to the vessels and through the avascular area of the broad ligament. The suture includes the myometrium to fix the suture and to avoid tearing the vessels. The same procedure is then performed on the opposite side. If the ligation is performed during caesarean section, the sutures can be placed just below the uterine incision under the bladder flap. It is not necessary to mobilize the bladder otherwise. Bilateral utero-ovarian artery ligation can also be performed in an attempt to reduce blood flow to the uterus. This technique should be performed with absorbable suture near the point of anastomoses between the ovarian artery and the ascending uterine artery at the utero-ovarian ligament.

C. B-Lynch brace suture—An alternative to the vessel ligation techniques is placement of a brace suture to compress the uterus in cases of diffuse bleeding from atony or percreta (Fig. 21–1). This technique, initially described in 1997, and in multiple small cases series since, has become increasing popular due to the simplicity of the procedure.

Technique: Laparotomy is made in the standard way for caesarean section, and a low-transverse uterine incision is made after the bladder is taken down. The uterus is exteriorized. To test the effectiveness of the method, the uterus is compressed manually, and another operator checks the vagina for decreased bleeding. Using no. 2 catgut, the uterus is punctured 3 cm from the right lower incision and 3 cm from the right lateral border. The suture is threaded to emerge 3 cm above the upper incision margin and 4 cm from the lateral border. The catgut is now visible anteriorly as it is passed over to compress the uterine fundus approximately 34 cm from the right cornual border. The suture is fed posteriorly and vertically to enter the posterior wall of the uterine cavity at the same level as the previous entry point. After manual compression, the suture is tightened and then passed posteriorly on the left side and passed around the uterine fundus again, this time on the left. The suture is brought

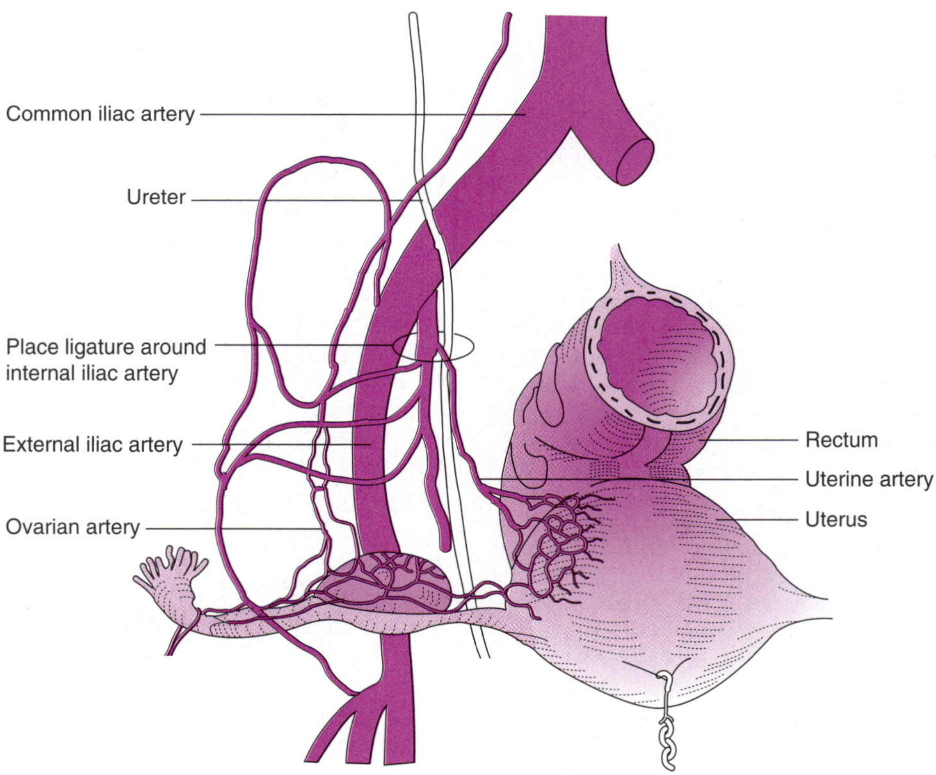

▲ **Figure 21–1.** B-Lynch brace suture

anteriorly to puncture the uterus at the upper part of the left uterine incision and then reemerge below the lower incision in a symmetric fashion. With 1 operator providing compression, the other throws the knot. The hysterotomy is closed in the standard fashion for a caesarean section.

D. Internal iliac artery ligation—Bilateral internal iliac (hypogastric) artery ligation is the surgical method most often used to control severe postpartum bleeding (Fig. 21–2). Exposure can be difficult, particularly in the presence of a large boggy uterus or hematoma. Failure rates of this technique can be as high as 57% but may be related to the skill of the operator, the cause of the hemorrhage, and the patient's condition before ligation is attempted.

Technique: The peritoneum lateral to the infundibulopelvic ligament is incised parallel with the ligament, or the round ligament is transected. In either case, the peritoneum to which the ureter will adhere is dissected medially, which removes the ureter from the operative field. The pararectal space is then enlarged by blunt dissection. The internal iliac artery on the lateral side of the space is isolated and doubly ligated (but not cut) with silk ligatures at its origin from the common iliac artery. The operator must be careful not to tear the adjacent thin veins. Blood flow distally to the uterus, cervix, and upper vagina is not occluded, but the pulse pressure is sufficiently diminished to allow hemostasis to occur by in situ thrombosis. Fertility is preserved, and subsequent pregnancies are not compromised.

E. Hysterectomy—Hysterectomy is the definitive method of controlling postpartum hemorrhage. Simple hemostatic

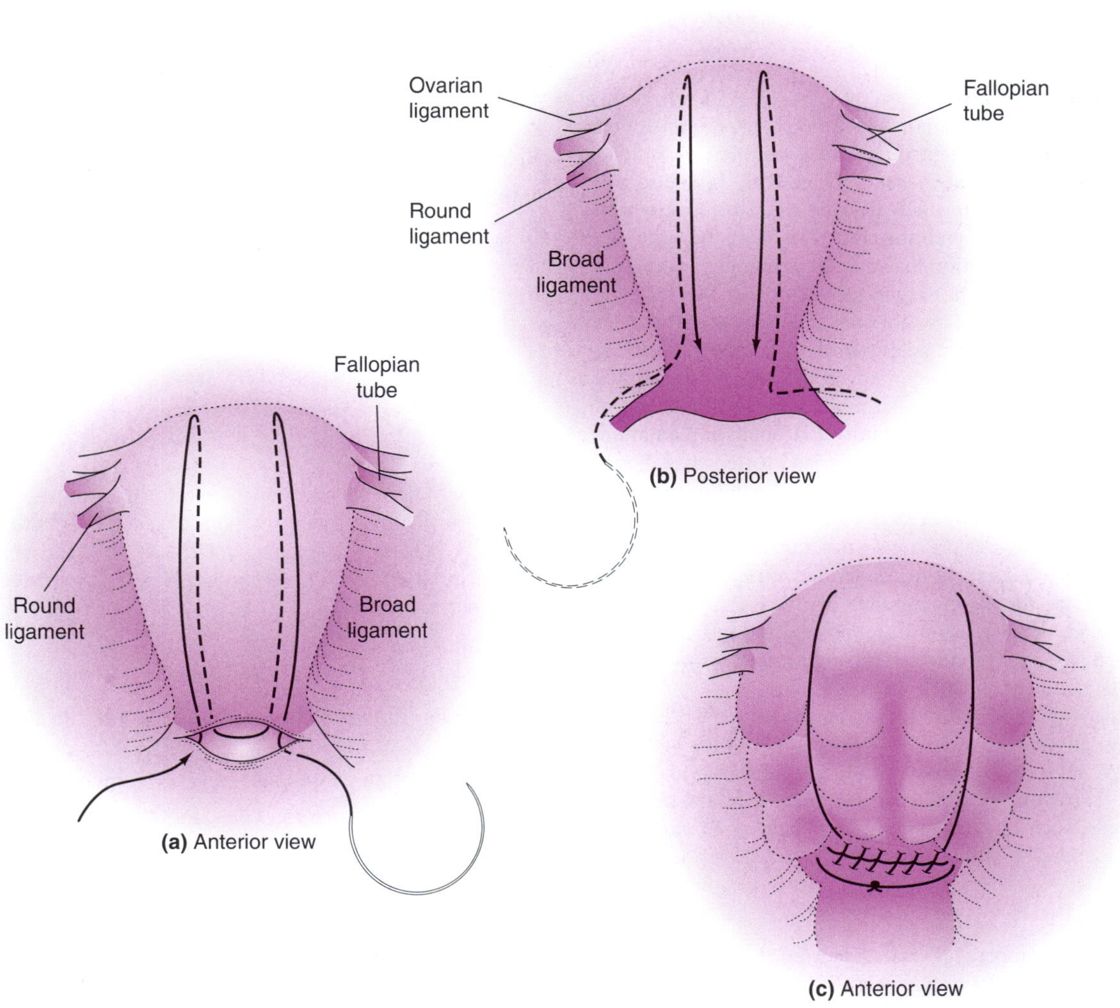

▲ **Figure 21–2.** Location of ligatures for right internal iliac (hypogastric) artery ligation.

repair of a ruptured uterus with or without tubal ligation in a woman of high parity or in poor condition for more extensive surgery may be preferred unless she has intercurrent uterine disease. The procedure is undoubtedly lifesaving.

8. Blood replacement—Blood and fluid replacement are required for successful management of postpartum hemorrhage. Massive transfusions may be necessary in patients with severe hemorrhage. Component therapy is advocated, with transfusion of packed cells, platelets, fresh-frozen plasma, and cryoprecipitate when indicated. Blood products should be obtained and given without delay when needed, because postponing transfusion may only contribute to the development of disseminated intravascular coagulation. In specialized settings, there may be a role for off-label use of recombinant activated factor VII, which was originally developed for hemophilia patients, but has been used successfully in several cases of fulminant postpartum hemorrhage.

B. Management of Delayed Postpartum Hemorrhage

Delayed postpartum hemorrhage (bleeding ≥2 weeks after delivery) is almost always due to subinvolution of the placental bed or retained placental fragments. Involution of the placental site is normally delayed when compared with that of the rest of the endometrium. However, for unknown reasons, in subinvolution the adjacent endometrium and the decidua basalis have not regenerated to cover the placental implantation site. The involutional processes of thrombosis and hyalinization have failed to occur in the underlying blood vessels, so bleeding may occur with only minimal trauma or other (unknown) stimuli. Although the cause of subinvolution is unknown, faulty placental implantation, implantation in the poorly vascularized lower uterine segment, and persistent infection at the implantation site have been suggested as possible factors. Uterine compression and bimanual massage, as previously described, control this type of bleeding, but it may be necessary to continue compression and massage for 30–45 minutes or longer. As previously mentioned, transvaginal ultrasound may aid in diagnosis of retained placental products. If imaging studies suggest intracavitary tissue, curettage is warranted.

Broad-spectrum antibiotics should be started when resuscitation allows. Oxytocin 10 U IM every 4 hours or 10–20 U/L IV solution by slow continuous infusion, 15-methyl $PGF_{2\alpha}$ (Prostin 15M) 0.25 mg IM every 2 hours, or ergot alkaloids, such as methylergonovine maleate 0.2 mg orally every 6 hours, should be administered for at least 48 hours.

▶ Prognosis

Postpartum hemorrhage has a recurrence rate of approximately 10% in future pregnancies. There are limited data on outcomes of pregnancies after uterine artery embolization or B-Lynch suture. It is unknown if these procedures put future pregnancies at increased risk of complications, although there are case reports and series of uneventful pregnancy outcomes after these procedures.

Blum J, Winikoff B, Raghavan S, et al. Treatment of post-partum haemorrhage with sublingual misoprostol versus oxytocin in women receiving prophylactic oxytocin: A double-blind randomized, non-inferiority trial. *Lancet* 2010;375:217–223. PMID: 20060162.

Clark SL, Belfort MA, Dildy GA, et al. Maternal death in the 21st century: Causes, prevention and relationship to cesarean delivery. *Am J Obstet Gynecol* 2008;199:36.e1–36.e5. PMID: 18455140.

Flood KM, Said S, Geary M, et al. Changing trends in peripartum hysterectomy over the last 4 decades. *Am J Obstet Gynecol* 2009;200:632.e1–632e6. PMID: 19306969.

Maassen MS, Lambers MD, Tutein Nolthenius RP, van der Valk PH, Elgersma OE. Complications and failure of uterine artery embolisation for intractable postpartum haemorrhage. *BJOG* 2009;116:55–61. PMID: 19016685.

Magann EF, Evans S, Chauhan SP, et al. The length of the third stage of labor and the risk of postpartum hemorrhage. *Obstet Gynecol* 2005;105:290–293. PMID: 15684154.

Sentilhes L, et al. B-Lynch suture for massive persistent post-partum hemorrhage following stepwise uterine devascularization. *Acta Obstet Gynecol Scand* 2008;87:1020–1026. PMID: 18927949.

Vitthala S, et al. Use of Bakri balloon in post-partum haemorrhage: A series of 15 cases. *Aust N Z J Obstet Gynaecol* 2009;49:191–194. PMID: 19432609.

PLACENTA ACCRETA

ESSENTIALS OF DIAGNOSIS

- A layer of decidua normally separates the placental villi and the myometrium at the site of placental implantation. A placenta that directly adheres to the myometrium without an intervening decidual layer is termed *placenta accreta.*
- Classification
  - A. By Degree of Adherence
    1. Placenta accreta vera—Villi adhere to the superficial myometrium.
    2. Placenta increta—Villi invade the myometrium.
    3. Placenta percreta—Villi penetrate the full thickness of the myometrium.
  - B. By Amount of Placental Involvement
    1. Focal adherence—A single cotyledon is involved.
    2. Partial adherence—One or several cotyledons are involved.
    3. Total adherence—The entire placenta is involved.

Pathogenesis

Estimates of the incidence of placenta accreta (all forms) vary from 1 in 2000 to 1 in 7000 deliveries. Placenta accreta vera accounts for approximately 80% of abnormally adherent placentas, placenta increta accounts for 15%, and placenta percreta accounts for 5%. The rate has risen over the last 2 decades, paralleling the increasing caesarean section rate. The condition has emerged as the major cause of peripartum hysterectomy in high-resource countries.

Both excessive penetrability of the trophoblast and defective or missing decidua basalis have been suggested as causes of placenta accreta. Histologic examination of the placental implantation site usually demonstrates the absence of the decidua and Nitabuch's layer. Cases of placenta accreta have been seen in the first trimester, suggesting that the process may occur at the time of implantation and not later in gestation.

Although the exact cause is unknown, several clinical situations are associated with placenta accreta, such as previous caesarean section, placenta previa, grand multiparity, previous uterine curettage, and previously treated Asherman's syndrome.

These conditions share a common possible defect in formation of the decidua basalis. The incidence of placenta accreta in the presence of placenta previa after 1 prior uterine incision is between 14% and 24%, after 2 is 23–48%, and after 3 is 35–50%. The incidence of placenta accreta after successful treatment of Asherman's syndrome may be as high as 15%.

Clinical Findings

Adverse effects from placenta accreta in pregnancy or during the course of labor and delivery are uncommon. Rarely, intra-abdominal hemorrhage or placental invasion of adjacent organs prior to labor has occurred, with the diagnosis made at laparotomy.

The diagnosis of placenta increta prior to delivery based on the lack of the sonolucent area normally seen beneath the implantation site during ultrasonographic examination is a finding confirmed in several reports. Sonographic antenatal diagnosis of the less invasive placental accreta also has been reported. Color Doppler imaging appears to be particularly helpful in diagnosis. Magnetic resonance imaging has also aided in the diagnosis of placenta accreta. The diagnosis is more often established when no plane of cleavage is found between the placenta or parts of the placenta and the myometrium in the presence of postpartum hemorrhage. Retained placental parts prevent the myometrium from contracting and thereby achieving hemostasis. Bleeding can be brisk. Inspection of the already separated placenta shows that portions are missing, and manual exploration may produce additional placental fragments.

Delayed spontaneous separation of the placenta is also an indication of an unusually adherent placenta. Focal or partial involvement may be manifested as difficulty in establishing a cleavage plane during manual removal of the placenta. Removal of a totally adherent placenta is difficult. Persistent efforts to manually remove a totally adherent placenta are futile and waste time, and they result in even more blood loss. Preparation for hysterectomy should begin as soon as the diagnosis is suspected.

Complications

The immediate morbidity associated with an abnormally adherent placenta is that associated with any type of postpartum hemorrhage. Massive blood loss and hypotension can occur. Intrauterine manipulation necessary to diagnose and treat placenta accreta may result in uterine perforation and infection. Sterility may occur as a result of hysterectomy performed to control bleeding. Perhaps due to diagnosis prior to delivery and preparation of the obstetric team, the condition is not a leading cause of mortality in the United States.

Recurrence may be common with lesser degrees of adherence.

Treatment

Fluid and blood replacement should begin as soon as excessive blood loss is diagnosed. Insertion of a second large-bore IV catheter may be necessary. Evaluation of puerperal hemorrhage should be performed as outlined earlier in Evaluation of Persistent Bleeding.

Conservative treatment of placenta accreta in women of low parity is increasingly attempted. A recent series described success in 131 of 167 women managed with serial IM methotrexate injections after pelvic artery embolization. The placenta (or portions of it) is left in situ if bleeding is minimal and will later slough off. Successful subsequent pregnancies have been reported, although the risk of recurrence of placenta accreta may be high.

Successful conservative treatment of placenta percreta is rare, but the conservative approach may be a reasonable option if only focal defects are present, blood loss is not excessive, and the patient wishes to preserve fertility. In anticipated cases of severe placenta accreta, preoperative balloon occlusion and embolization of the internal iliac arteries may minimize intraoperative blood losses. Successful embolization in unpredicted cases of placenta accreta has been reported. However, additional resection of adjacent organs, such as partial cystectomy, may be necessary in placenta percreta.

Prognosis

For women who were successfully treated with conservative management and uterine preservation, subsequent pregnancies have been reported, although the risk of recurrence of placenta accreta may be high.

Sentilhes L, Ambroselli C, Kayem G, et al. Maternal outcomes after conservative treatment for placenta accreta. *Obstet Gynecol* 2010;115:526–534. PMID: 20177283.

UTERINE INVERSION

ESSENTIALS OF DIAGNOSIS

- Uterine inversion is prolapse of the fundus to or through the cervix so that the uterus is in effect turned inside out.
- Almost all cases of uterine inversion occur after delivery and may be worsened by excess traction on the cord before placental separation.
- Nonpuerperal uterine inversion is rare and usually is associated with tumors (eg, polypoid leiomyomas).

Pathogenesis

In series reported within the past 30 years, the incidence of uterine inversion has varied from 1 in 4000 to 1 in 100,000 deliveries; an incidence of 1 in 20,000 is frequently cited. One worker reported no inversions in more than 10,000 personally conducted deliveries. More recent reviews indicate a greater incidence of uterine inversion, approximately 1 in 2000 to 1 in 2500 deliveries.

The exact cause of uterine inversion is unknown, and the condition is not always preventable. The cervix must be dilated, and the uterine fundus must be relaxed for inversion to occur. Rapid uterine emptying may contribute to uterine relaxation.

Conditions that may predispose women to uterine inversion include fundal implantation of the placenta, abnormal adherence of the placenta (partial placenta accreta), congenital or acquired weakness of the myometrium, uterine anomalies, protracted labor, previous uterine inversion, intrapartum therapy with magnesium sulfate, strong traction exerted on the umbilical cord, and fundal pressure.

Prevention

Many cases of uterine inversion result from mismanagement of the third stage of labor in women who already are at risk for developing uterine inversion. The following maneuvers are to be avoided: excessive traction on the umbilical cord, excessive fundal pressure, excessive intra-abdominal pressure, and excessively vigorous manual removal of the placenta.

Clinical Findings

The diagnosis of uterine inversion usually is obvious. Shock and hemorrhage are prominent, as is considerable pain. A dark red–blue bleeding mass is palpable and often visible at the cervix, in the vagina, or outside the vagina. A depression in the uterine fundus or even an absent fundus is noted on abdominal examination. Partial inversion in which the fundus stays within the vagina can escape immediate notice if the attendant is not aware of this complication.

If the uterus is inverted but does not protrude through the cervix, the inversion is *incomplete*. In *complete* inversion, the fundus has prolapsed through the cervix. Occasionally, the entire uterus may prolapse out of the vagina.

Puerperal inversion has also been classified on the basis of its duration. Acute inversion occurs immediately after delivery and before the cervix constricts. Once the cervix constricts, the inversion is termed *subacute*. Chronic inversion is noted more than 4 weeks after delivery. Today, nearly all cases of uterine inversion are of the acute variety and are recognized and treated immediately after delivery.

Differential Diagnosis

In some cases, a prolapsed fibroid may have clinical findings similar to uterine inversion; however, with a prolapsed fibroid, the uterine fundus should be palpable on abdominal examination.

Complications

The morbidity and mortality associated with uterine inversion correlate with the degree of hemorrhage, the rapidity of diagnosis, and the effectiveness of treatment.

The immediate morbidity is that associated with any postpartum hemorrhage; however, endomyometritis frequently follows uterine inversion. The intestines and uterine appendages may be injured if they are entrapped by the prolapsed uterine fundus. Death has occurred from uterine inversion, although with prompt recognition, definitive treatment, and vigorous resuscitation, the mortality rate in this condition should be quite low.

Treatment

Successful management of patients with uterine inversion depends on prompt recognition and treatment. If initial measures fail to relieve the condition, it may progress to the point at which operative treatment or even hysterectomy is necessary. Shock associated with uterine inversion typically is profound. Hemorrhage can be massive, and hypovolemia should be vigorously treated with fluid and blood replacement.

A. Manual Repositioning of the Uterus

Treatment should begin as soon as the diagnosis of uterine inversion is made. Assistance is vital. An initial attempt should be made to reposition the fundus. The inverted fundus, along with the placenta if it is still attached, is slowly and steadily pushed upward in the axis of the uterus (Fig. 21–3). If the placenta has not separated, do not remove it until an adequate IV infusion has been established.

If the initial attempt fails, induce general anesthesia, preferably with a halogenated agent (eg, halothane) to provide

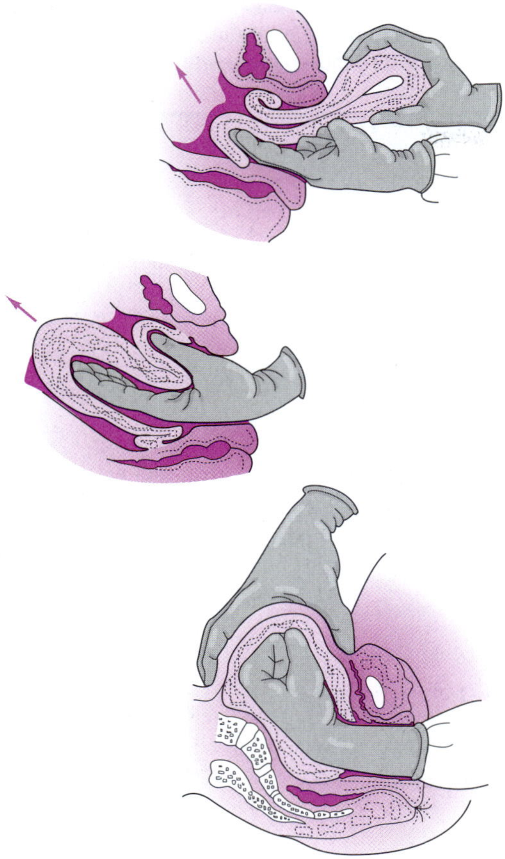

▲ **Figure 21–3.** Replacement of an inverted uterus.

uterine relaxation. Alternatively, 50 μg of IV nitroglycerin can be given as a bolus to relax the uterus and avoid intubation. The dose can be repeated at least once. While awaiting anesthesiology assistance, easily available tocolytics may be used effectively. Either IV magnesium sulfate or terbutaline 0.25 mg given as a bolus dose IV has been used successfully to achieve uterine relaxation in subacute inversion, and neither has been associated with bleeding.

Technique: The operator's fist is placed on the uterine fundus, and the fundus is gradually pushed back into the pelvis through the dilated cervix. The general anesthetic or uterine relaxant is discontinued. Infusion of oxytocin or ergot alkaloids is started and fluid and blood replacement continued. Alternatively, prostaglandins can be used to effect uterine contraction after repositioning. Bimanual uterine compression and massage are maintained until the uterus is well contracted and hemorrhage has ceased. The placenta can then be removed.

Antibiotics should be started as soon as is practical. Oxytocics or ergot alkaloids are continued for at least 24 hours. Frequent determinations of the hematocrit level should be made to ascertain the need for further blood replacement. Iron supplements should begin with resumption of oral intake.

B. Surgical Repositioning of the Uterus

Surgical repositioning of the uterus is rarely necessary in contemporary medical practice in the United States. However, when all other efforts have failed to reposition the everted uterus, operative intervention may be lifesaving. This is generally accomplished by a vertical incision through the lower uterine segment directly posterior. The uterus is repositioned by either pulling from above or, very rarely, pushing from below (using a sterile glove). The incision is then repaired as would be any uterine incision. Blood replacement, antibiotics, and careful monitoring are necessary for successful perioperative management.

Prognosis

It is not clear whether uterine inversion is at increased risk of recurrence in future pregnancies. The prognosis for women with uterine inversion in whom the uterus was successfully restored to its normal anatomic position is generally considered to be excellent.

POSTPARTUM & PUERPERAL INFECTIONS

General Considerations

Infections are among the most prominent puerperal complications. An improved understanding of the natural history of female genital infections and the availability of powerful antibiotics may have produced a complacent attitude toward puerperal infections that is unrealistic. Postpartum infections still are costly to both patients and society, and they are associated with an admittedly small but not negligible threat of serious disability and death.

Puerperal morbidity due to infection has occurred if the patient's temperature is higher than 38°C (100.4°F) on 2 separate occasions at least 24 hours apart following the first 24 hours after delivery. Overt infections can and do occur in the absence of these criteria, but fever of some degree remains the hallmark of puerperal infection, and the patient with fever can be assumed to have a genital infection until proved otherwise.

Incidence

Puerperal infectious morbidity affects 2–8% of pregnant women and is more common in those of low socioeconomic status, who have undergone operative delivery, with premature rupture of the membranes, with long labors, or who have multiple pelvic examinations.

Morbidity & Mortality

Postpartum infections are responsible for much of the morbidity associated with childbirth, and they either are directly responsible for or contribute to the death of approximately 7% of all pregnant women who die each year in the United States. The costs are considerable, not only in additional days of hospitalization and medications but also in time lost from work.

Sterility may result from the sequelae of postpartum infections, such as periadnexal adhesions. Hysterectomy occasionally is required in patients with serious postpartum or postoperative infection.

Pathogenesis

The flora of the birth canal of pregnant women is essentially the same as that of nonpregnant women, although variations in culture techniques and in the study populations have produced markedly different results. The vaginal flora typically includes aerobic and anaerobic organisms that are commonly considered pathogenic (Table 21–1). Several mechanisms appear to prevent overt infection in the genital tract, such as the acidity of the normal vagina; thick, tenacious cervical mucus; and maternal antibodies to most vaginal flora.

During labor and particularly after rupture of the membranes, some of the protective mechanisms are no longer present. Examinations and invasive monitoring apparatus probably facilitate the introduction of vaginal bacteria into the uterine cavity. Bacteria can be cultured from the amniotic fluid of most women undergoing intrauterine pressure monitoring, but overt postpartum infection is seen in fewer than 10% of these cases. Contractions during labor may spread bacteria present in the amniotic cavity to the adjacent uterine lymphatics and even into the bloodstream.

The postpartum uterus initially is devoid of mechanisms that keep it sterile, and bacteria may be recovered from the uterus in nearly all women in the postpartum period. Whether or not disease is clinically expressed depends on the presence of predisposing factors, the duration of uterine contamination, and the type and amount of microorganisms involved. The necrosis of decidua and other intrauterine contents (lochia) promotes an increase in the number of anaerobic bacteria, heretofore limited by lack of suitable nutrients and other factors necessary for growth.

Sterility of the endometrial cavity returns by the third or fourth postpartum week. Granulocytes that penetrate the endometrial cavity and the open drainage of lochia are effective in preventing infection in most patients.

Table 21–1. Percentage of organisms isolated from the vagina or cervix in normal pregnant and nonpregnant women.

Organism	Percentage Isolated
Aerobic bacteria	
Lactobacillus	17–97
Diphtheroids	14–83
Staphylococcus epidermidis	7–67
Staphylococcus aureus	0–12
α-Hemolytic streptococci	2–53
β-Hemolytic streptococci	0–93
Nonhemolytic streptococci	4–37
Group D streptococci	4–44
Escherichia coli	0–28
Gardnerella vaginalis	40–43
Neisseria gonorrhoeae	1–7
Mycoplasma	15–72
Ureaplasma	40–95
Anaerobic bacteria	
Lactobacillus	11–72
Bacteroides fragilis	0–20
Bacteroides species	0–50
Fusobacterium species	0–18
Peptococcus species	0–71
Peptostreptococcus species	12–40
Veillonella species	0–27
Clostridium species	0–17
Bifidobacterium species	0–32
Eubacterium species	0–36

Etiology

Almost all postpartum infections are caused by bacteria normally present in the genitalia of pregnant women. The lochia is an excellent culture medium for organisms ascending from the vagina. In women who have undergone caesarean section, more devitalized tissue and foreign bodies (sutures) are present, providing additional fertile ground for possible contamination and subsequent infection. Approximately 70% of puerperal soft tissue infections are mixed infections consisting of both aerobic and anaerobic organisms; infections occurring in women undergoing caesarean section are more likely to be serious.

General Evaluation

The source of infection should be identified, the likely cause determined, and the severity assessed. Most women with fever in the postpartum period have endometritis. Urinary tract infection is the next most common infection. Neglected or virulent endomyometritis may progress to more serious infection. Generalized sepsis, septic pelvic thrombophlebitis, or pelvic abscess may be the end result of an initial infection of the endometrial cavity.

1. Endometritis

ESSENTIALS OF DIAGNOSIS

- Infection of the endometrium
- Fever and a soft, tender uterus on physical examination

Pathogenesis

All of the following circumstances have led to higher than normal postpartum infection rates: prolonged rupture of the membranes (>24 hours), chorioamnionitis, an excessive number of digital vaginal examinations, prolonged labor (>12 hours), toxemia, intrauterine pressure catheters (>8 hours), fetal scalp electrode monitoring, preexisting vaginitis or cervicitis, operative vaginal deliveries, caesarean section, intrapartum and postpartum anemia, poor nutrition, obesity, low socioeconomic status, and coitus near term.

Caesarean section and low socioeconomic class are consistently associated with higher rates of postpartum infection, and caesarean section is easily the most common identifiable risk factor for development of puerperal infection. Some series report an infection rate of 40–80% following caesarean section delivery. Postpartum infection is more likely to be serious after caesarean section than after vaginal delivery. A history of bacterial vaginosis is associated with a higher risk of postcaesarean endometritis.

Clinical Findings

A. Symptoms & Signs

Fever and a soft, tender uterus are the most prominent signs of endometritis. The lochia may or may not have a foul odor. Leukocytosis is seen. In more severe disease, high fever, malaise, abdominal tenderness, ileus, hypotension, and generalized sepsis may be seen. Movement of the uterus causes increased pain.

1. Fever—Although the puerperium is a period of high metabolic activity, this factor should not raise the temperature above 37.2°C (99°F) and then only briefly in the first 24 hours postpartum. Modest temperature elevations may occur with dehydration. Any woman with a fever over 38°C (100.4°F) at any time in the puerperium should be evaluated.

Endometritis results in temperatures ranging from 38°C to over 40°C (100.4°F to >104°F), depending on the patient, the causative microorganism, and the extent of infection. The lower range of temperatures is more common. Endometritis usually develops on the second or third postpartum day. Early fever (within hours of delivery) and hypotension are almost pathognomonic for infection with β-hemolytic streptococci.

2. Uterine tenderness—The uterus is soft and exquisitely tender. Motion of the cervix and uterus may cause increased pain.

Abdominal tenderness is generally limited to the lower abdomen and does not lateralize. A carefully performed baseline examination should include an adnexal evaluation. Adnexal masses palpable on abdominal or pelvic examination are not seen in uncomplicated endometritis, but tubo-ovarian abscess may be a later complication of an infection originally confined to the uterus. Bowel sounds may be decreased and the abdomen distended and tympanitic.

Pelvic examination confirms the findings disclosed by abdominal examination.

B. Laboratory Findings

1. Hematologic findings—Leukocytosis is a normal finding during labor and the immediate puerperal period. White blood cell counts may be as high as 20,000/μL in the absence of infection, so higher counts can be anticipated in infection. Bacteremia is present in 5–10% of women with uncomplicated endometritis. *Mycoplasma* is frequently recovered from the blood of patients with postpartum fever. Infections with *Bacteroides* as the predominant organism are frequently associated with positive blood cultures.

2. Urinalysis—Urinalysis should be routinely performed in patients thought to have endometritis because urinary tract infections are often associated with a clinical picture similar to that of mild endometritis. If pyuria and bacteria are noted in a properly collected specimen, appropriate antibiotic therapy for urinary tract infections should be started and a portion of the specimen sent for culture.

3. Lochia cultures—Bacteria colonizing the cervical canal and ectocervix almost always can be recovered from lochia cultures, but they may not be the same organisms causing endometritis. Accurate cultures can be achieved only if specimens obtained transcervically are free from vaginal contamination. Material should be obtained using a speculum to allow direct visualization of the cervix and a gloved culture device (a swab that is covered while it is passed through a contaminated area, then uncovered to obtain a culture from the desired area). Transabdominal aspiration of uterine contents does secure an uncontaminated specimen, but routine use of this technique probably is not justified, and confirmation of placement within the uterine cavity may be difficult. Unless special means are taken to prevent cervical contamination and to ensure the recovery of anaerobic species, results of lochia cultures must be interpreted with great care.

4. Bacteriologic findings—Although the organisms responsible for puerperal infections vary considerably among hospitals, most puerperal infections are due to anaerobic streptococci, gram-negative coliforms, *Bacteroides* spp., and aerobic streptococci. *Chlamydia* and *Mycoplasma* are also implicated in many postpartum infections, but clinical isolates are rare because of the difficulty in culturing these organisms. Gonococci are recovered in varying degrees. The percentage of representative microorganisms recovered from women with endometritis is given in Table 21–2.

Patterns of bacterial isolates in puerperal infections in the patient's hospital are more important in guiding selection of appropriate antibiotics than are studies from the literature.

A. Aerobic bacteria—Group A streptococci are no longer a major cause of postpartum infection, but infection with these organisms still occurs occasionally, often associated with rapid progression of toxic shock syndrome. If more than an isolated instance of infection due to these streptococci occurs, immediate measures should be taken to halt a potential epidemic. Penicillin is highly effective.

Table 21–2. Percentage of organisms recovered from women with postpartum endomyometritis.

Organism	Percentage Isolated
Aerobic bacteria	
Group A streptococci	2-6
Group B streptococci	6-21
Group D streptococci	3-14
Enterococcus	12-21
Other streptococci	32
Staphylococcus epidermidis	28
Staphylococcus aureus	10
Escherichia coli	13-36
Gonococci	1-40
Gardnerella vaginalis	16
Anaerobic bacteria	
Bacteroides fragilis	19-75
Bacteroides species	17-100
Peptococcus	4-40
Peptostreptococcus	15-54
Veillonella species	10
Clostridium species	4-32

In as many as 30% of women with clinically recognized endometritis, group B streptococci are partly or wholly responsible for the infection. Classic presenting signs are high fever and hypotension shortly after delivery. However, group B streptococci are commonly recovered from the vaginas of pregnant women whether or not they have endometritis. Why some women with positive cultures develop serious illness whereas others do not undoubtedly depends on the presence of predisposing factors as well as other, as yet unknown, elements. It is interesting that positive cultures in women do not correlate well with the incidence of streptococcal infection in their newborns. Penicillin is the treatment of choice for patients with endometritis.

Group D streptococci, which include *Streptococcus faecalis*, are common isolates in endometritis. Ampicillin in high doses is the treatment of choice. Aminoglycosides are also effective against this group.

Staphylococcus aureus is not commonly seen in cultures from women with postpartum infections of the uterus. *Staphylococcus epidermidis* is frequently recovered from women with postpartum infections. These organisms are typically not seen in pure culture. When established staphylococcal infections require treatment, nafcillin, cloxacillin, or cephalosporins should be used.

Among the gram-negative aerobic organisms likely to be recovered in postpartum uterine infections, *Escherichia coli* is the most common. In postpartum uterine infections, *E coli* is more likely to be isolated from seriously ill patients, whereas in urinary tract infections, it is the most commonly isolated organism but is not necessarily found in the sickest patients. Hospital-acquired *E coli* is most susceptible to aminoglycosides and cephalosporins.

The incidence of *Neisseria gonorrhoeae* is 2–8% in pregnant women antepartum. Unless repeat screening examinations and treatment of patients with positive cultures are undertaken in women near term, the incidence of asymptomatic endocervical gonorrhea at delivery probably is only slightly less, and it is reasonable to believe that some cases of puerperal endometritis are gonococcal in origin.

Gardnerella vaginalis, a cause of vaginitis, is seen in isolates from women with postpartum infections, usually in those with a polymicrobial cause, although pure isolates have been reported.

Other gram-negative bacilli that are commonly encountered on medical and surgical wards (eg, *Klebsiella pneumoniae, Enterobacter, Proteus*, and *Pseudomonas* spp.) are uncommon causes of endometritis.

B. Anaerobic bacteria—Anaerobic bacteria are involved in puerperal infections of the uterus in at least 50% and perhaps as many as 95% of cases. They are much less commonly seen in urinary tract infections. Anaerobic peptostreptococci and peptococci are commonly recovered in specimens from women with postpartum infection, particularly with other anaerobic species. Clindamycin, chloramphenicol, and the newer cephalosporins are active against these organisms.

Bacteroides spp., particularly *Bacteroides fragilis*, are commonly found in mixed puerperal infections. These are likely to be the more serious infections (eg, puerperal pelvic abscess, caesarean section wound infections, and septic pelvic thrombophlebitis). When infection with this organism is suspected or confirmed, clindamycin, chloramphenicol, or third-generation cephalosporins should be used.

Gram-positive anaerobic organisms are represented only by *Clostridium perfringens*, which is not infrequently isolated from an infected uterus but which is a rare cause of puerperal infection.

c. Other organisms—*Mycoplasma* and *Ureaplasma* spp. are common genital pathogens that have been isolated from the genital tract and blood of postpartum women both with and without overt infection. These pathogens are frequently found in the presence of other bacteria. The role of these organisms in puerperal infections is unknown.

Chlamydia trachomatis is now thought to be the leading cause of pelvic inflammatory disease in some populations. Because the population most at risk for pelvic inflammatory disease is the same as that most likely to become pregnant, it is not surprising that *Chlamydia* is in some way involved in puerperal infections, but it is infrequently isolated as a cause of early postpartum endometritis. *Chlamydia* is more frequently associated with mild late-onset endometritis, so cultures for this organism should be obtained from patients with endometritis diagnosed several days after delivery. *Chlamydia* is difficult to culture, and it is possible that as more effective culture techniques become available, the place of this organism in the morbidity associated with postpartum infections will be clarified.

Differential Diagnosis

In the immediate postpartum period, involuntary chills are common and are not necessarily an indication of overt infection. Lower abdominal pain is common as the uterus undergoes involution with continuing contractions.

Extragenital infections are much less common than endometritis and urinary tract infections. Most of these infections can be effectively ruled out by history and examination alone. Patients should be asked, at a minimum, about coughing, chest pain, pain at the insertion site of IV catheters, breast tenderness, and leg pain. Examination of the breasts, chest, IV catheter insertion site, and leg veins should determine whether these areas might be the source of the postpartum fever. Chest x-ray films are rarely of benefit unless signs and symptoms point to a possible pulmonary cause of the fever.

Treatment

The choice of antibiotics for treatment of endometritis depends on the suspected causative organisms and the severity of the disease. If the illness is serious enough to require antibiotics, initial therapy should consist of IV antibiotics in high doses. Factors reinforcing the need for this approach include the large volume of the uterus, the expanded maternal blood volume, the brisk diuresis associated with the puerperium, and the difficulty in achieving adequate tissue concentrations of the antibiotic distal to the thrombosed myometrial blood vessels. Clindamycin plus an aminoglycoside is a standard first-line regimen. Good evidence now indicates that once-a-day dosing of gentamicin is as effective as the traditional thrice-daily regimen. Single-agent therapy with second- or third-generation cephalosporins is an acceptable alternative.

The response to therapy should be carefully monitored for 24–48 hours. Deterioration or failure to respond determined both clinically and by laboratory test results requires a complete reevaluation. Ampicillin is added when the patient has a less than adequate response to the usual regimen, particularly if *Enterococcus* spp. are suspected.

IV antibiotics are continued until the patient has been afebrile for 24–48 hours. Randomized and prospective trials have shown that additional treatment with oral antibiotics after IV therapy is unnecessary. Patients with documented concurrent bacteremia can be treated similarly, unless they have persistently positive blood cultures or a staphylococcal species cultured. If the patient remains febrile despite the standard antibiotic regimens, further evaluation should be initiated to look for abscess formation, hematomas, wound infection, and septic pelvic thrombophlebitis.

For patients known to be infected or at extremely high risk for infection at the time of delivery, initial therapy with 2- or 3-drug regimens in which 1 of the agents is clindamycin is prudent. Single-agent IV infusion of broad-spectrum agents such as piperacillin or cefoxitin appears to be equally effective.

Costantine MM, Rahman M, Ghulmiyah L, et al. Timing of perioperative antibiotics for cesarean delivery: A meta-analysis. *Am J Obstet Gynecol* 2008;301.e1–301.e6. PMID: 18771991.

Thurman AR. Post-cesarean delivery infectious morbidity: Focus on preoperative antibiotics and methicillin-resistant Staphylococcus aureus. *Am J Infect Control* 2010;38:612–616. PMID: 20627452.

2. Urinary Tract Infection

ESSENTIALS OF DIAGNOSIS

- Urine culture demonstrating the presence of bacteria in the urine in a patient symptomatic for urinary tract infection
- Pyelonephritis typically presents with symptoms of flank pain and/or systemic signs of fever, chills, and nausea/vomiting

Pathogenesis

Approximately 2–4% of women develop a urinary tract infection postpartum. After delivery, the bladder and lower urinary tract remain somewhat hypotonic, and residual urine and reflux result. This altered physiologic state, in conjunction with catheterization, birth trauma, conduction anesthesia, frequent pelvic examinations, and nearly continuous contamination of the perineum, is sufficient to explain the high incidence of lower urinary tract infections postpartum. In many women, preexisting asymptomatic bacteria, chronic urinary tract infections, and anatomic disorders of the bladder, urethra, and kidneys contribute to urinary tract infection postpartum.

Clinical Findings

A. Symptoms & Signs

Urinary tract infection usually presents with dysuria, frequency, urgency, and low-grade fever; however, an elevated temperature is occasionally the only symptom. White blood cells and bacteria are seen in a centrifuged sample of catheterized urine. A urine culture should be obtained. The history should be reviewed for evidence of chronic antepartum infections. If a woman had an antepartum urinary tract infection, then her postpartum infection likely is caused by the same organism. Repeated urinary tract infections call for careful postpartum evaluation. Urethral diverticulum, kidney stones, and upper urinary tract anomalies should be ruled out.

Urinary retention postpartum in the absence of regional anesthesia or well after its effects have worn off almost always indicates urinary tract infection.

Pyelonephritis may be accompanied by fever, chills, malaise, and nausea and vomiting. Characteristic signs of kidney involvement associated with pyelonephritis include costovertebral angle tenderness, dysuria, pyuria, and, in the case of hemorrhagic cystitis, hematuria.

B. Laboratory Findings

E coli is easily the most common organism isolated from infected urine in postpartum women (approximately 75% of cases). Other gram-negative bacilli are much less likely to be recovered. *E coli* is less likely to be the causative organism in women who had repeated urinary tract infections in the recent past.

Treatment

Antibiotics with specific activity against the causative organism are the cornerstone of therapy in uncomplicated cystitis. These drugs include sulfonamides, nitrofurantoin, trimethoprim-sulfamethoxazole, oral cephalosporins (cephalexin, cephradine), and ampicillin. Some hospitals report a high incidence of microbial resistance to ampicillin. The oral combination of amoxicillin-clavulanic acid provides a better spectrum of bacterial sensitivity. Sulfa antibiotics can be used safely in women who are breastfeeding if the infants are term without hyperbilirubinemia or suspected glucose-6-phosphate dehydrogenase deficiency. High fluid intake should be encouraged.

Pyelonephritis requires initial therapy with high doses of IV antibiotics, such as ampicillin 8–12 g/d or first-generation cephalosporins (cefazolin 3–6 g/d, cephalothin 4–8 g/d). An aminoglycoside can be added when resistant organisms are suspected or when the patient has clinical signs of sepsis. A long-acting third-generation cephalosporin, such as ceftriaxone 1–2 g every 12 hours, also can be used. The response to therapy may be rapid, but some women respond with gradual defervescence over 48 hours or longer. Urine cultures should be obtained to guide any necessary modifications in drug therapy if the patient's response is not prompt. Even with prompt resolution of fever, antibiotic therapy should be continued IV or orally for a total of 10 days. Urine for culture should be obtained at a postpartum visit after therapy has been completed.

3. Pneumonia

ESSENTIALS OF DIAGNOSIS

- Pneumonia typically presents with fever, chills, and productive cough.
- Women with obstructive lung disease, smokers, and those undergoing general anesthesia have an increased risk for developing pneumonia postpartum.

Clinical Findings

A. Symptoms & Signs

Symptoms and signs are the same as those of pneumonia in nonpregnant patients: productive cough, chest pain, fever, chills, rales, and infiltrates on chest x-ray film. In some cases, careful differentiation from pulmonary embolus is required.

B. X-Ray & Laboratory Findings

Chest x-ray film confirms the diagnosis of pneumonia. Gram-stained smears of sputum and material for culture should be obtained.

Streptococcus pneumoniae and *Mycoplasma pneumoniae* are the 2 most likely causative organisms. *S pneumoniae* can easily be identified on gram-stained smears. Infection with *M pneumoniae* can be suspected on clinical grounds.

Treatment

Appropriate antibiotics, oxygen (if the patient is hypoxic), IV hydration, and pulmonary toilet are the mainstays of therapy.

4. Caesarean Section Wound Infection

ESSENTIALS OF DIAGNOSIS

- Wound erythema and tenderness +/− drainage from the wound
- The patient may also demonstrate systemic signs of infection such as fever or malaise

Pathogenesis

Wound infection occurs in 4–12% of patients after caesarean section. The following risk factors predispose to subsequent wound infection in women undergoing caesarean section: obesity, diabetes, prolonged hospitalization before caesarean section, prolonged rupture of the membranes, chorioamnionitis, endomyometritis, prolonged labor, emergency rather than elective indications for caesarean section, and anemia.

Prevention

The high rate of infection (averaging 35–40%) after caesarean section is sufficient reason to consider prophylactic perioperative antibiotic administration. A major difference in practice in terms of prophylactic antibiotic administration prior to caesarean delivery has recently been advocated. While historically antimicrobial prophylaxis has been given after umbilical cord clamping, due to concerns regarding the masking of a neonatal infection, reductions in postcaesarean wound infection as great as 50% can be attributed to a single dose of cefazolin (1 g) given IV prior to skin incision.

Clinical Findings

A. Symptoms & Signs

Fever with no apparent cause that persists to the fourth or fifth postoperative day strongly suggests a wound infection. Wound erythema and tenderness may not be evident until several days after surgery. Occasionally, wound infections are manifested by spontaneous drainage, often accompanied by resolution of fever and relief of local tenderness. Rarely, a deep-seated wound infection becomes apparent when the skin overtly separates, usually after some strenuous activity by the patient.

B. Laboratory Findings

Gram-stained smears and culture of material from the wound may be helpful in guiding selection of the initial antibiotic. Blood cultures may be positive in the patient with systemic sepsis due to wound infection. The organisms responsible for most wound infections originate on the patient's skin. *S aureus* is the organism most commonly isolated. *Streptococcus* species, *E coli*, and other gram-negative organisms that may originally have colonized the amniotic cavity are also seen. Occasionally, *Bacteroides*, which comes only from the genital tract, is isolated from material taken from serious wound infections. In addition, methicillin-resistant *S aureus* (MRSA) is an emerging isolate from caesarean delivery wound infections. At this point, prophylactic antibiotic regimens have not addressed this particular organism.

Rarely, necrotizing fasciitis and the closely related synergistic bacterial gangrene can involve caesarean section incisions. They are recognized by their intense tissue destruction, lack of sensation in the involved tissues, and rapid extension. Radical debridement of necrotic and infected tissue is the cornerstone of treatment.

Treatment

A. Initial Evaluation

The incision should be opened along its entire length and the deeper portion of the wound gently explored to determine whether fascial separation has occurred. If the fascia is not intact, the wound is dissected to the fascial level, debrided, and repaired. Wound dehiscence has a high mortality rate and should be treated aggressively. Dehiscence is uncommon in healthy patients and with Pfannenstiel incisions. The skin can be left open to undergo delayed closure or to heal by primary intention.

If the fascia is intact, the wound infection can be treated by local measures.

B. Definitive Measures

Mechanical cleansing of the wound is the mainstay of therapy for caesarean wound infection. Opening the wound encourages drainage of infected material. The wound can be packed with saline-soaked gauze 2–3 times per day, which will remove necrotic debris each time the wound is unpacked. The wound can be left open to heal, or it can be closed secondarily when granulation tissue has begun to form.

Costantine MM, Rahman M, Ghulmiyah L, et al. Timing of perioperative antibiotics for cesarean delivery: A meta-analysis. *Am J Obstet Gynecol* 2008;301.e1–301.e6. PMID: 18771991.

Thurman AR. Post-cesarean delivery infectious morbidity: Focus on preoperative antibiotics and methicillin-resistant Staphylococcus aureus. *Am J Infect Control* 2010;38:612–616. PMID: 20627452.

5. Episiotomy Infection

ESSENTIALS OF DIAGNOSIS

- Pain at the episiotomy site
- Physical examination demonstrates disruption of the episiotomy wound

Pathogenesis

It is surprising that infected episiotomies do not occur more often than they do, because contamination at the time of delivery is universal. Subsequent contamination during the healing phase also should be common, yet infection and disruption of the wound are infrequent (0.5–3%). The excellent local blood supply is suggested as an explanation for this phenomenon.

In general, the more extensive the laceration or episiotomy, the greater are the chances for infection and breakdown of the wound. More tissue is devitalized in a large episiotomy, thereby providing greater opportunity for contamination. Women with infections elsewhere in the genital area probably are at greater risk for infection of the episiotomy.

Clinical Findings

A. Symptoms & Signs

Pain at the episiotomy site is the most common symptom. Spontaneous drainage is frequent, so a mass rarely forms. Incontinence of flatus and stool may be the presenting symptom of an episiotomy that breaks down and heals spontaneously.

Inspection of the episiotomy site shows disruption of the wound and gaping of the incision. A necrotic membrane may cover the wound and should be debrided if possible. A careful rectovaginal examination should be performed to determine whether a rectovaginal fistula has formed. The integrity of the anal sphincter should be evaluated.

B. Laboratory Findings

Infection with mixed aerobic and anaerobic organisms is common. *Staphylococcus* may be recovered from cultures of material from these infections. Culture results frequently are misleading because the area of the episiotomy typically is contaminated with a wide variety of pathogenic bacteria.

Treatment

Initial treatment should be directed toward opening and cleaning the wound and promoting the formation of granulation tissue. Warm sitz baths or Hubbard tank treatments help the debridement process. Attempts to close an infected, disrupted episiotomy are likely to fail and may make ultimate closure more difficult. Surgical closure by perineorrhaphy should be undertaken only after granulation tissue has thoroughly covered the wound site. There is an increasing trend toward early repair of episiotomy wound dehiscence, in contrast to conventional wisdom, which suggests a 3- to 4-month delay. Several large case series show excellent results once initial infection is treated.

6. Mastitis

ESSENTIALS OF DIAGNOSIS

- One or both breasts are tender, erythematous, and engorged on physical examination.
- With infectious mastitis or breast abscess, the patient commonly demonstrates fever and malaise.

Pathogenesis

Congestive mastitis, or breast engorgement, is more common in primigravidas than in multiparas. Infectious mastitis and breast abscesses also are more common in women pregnant for the first time and are seen almost exclusively in nursing mothers.

Infectious mastitis and breast abscesses are uncommon complications of breastfeeding. They almost certainly occur as a result of trauma to the nipple and the subsequent introduction of organisms from the infant's nostrils to the mother's breast. *S aureus* contracted by the infant while in the hospital nursery is the usual causative agent.

Clinical Findings

A. Symptoms & Signs

Breast engorgement usually occurs on the second or third postpartum day. The breasts are swollen, tender, tense, and warm. The patient's temperature may be mildly elevated. Axillary adenopathy can be seen.

Mastitis presents 1 week or more after delivery. Usually only 1 breast is affected and often only 1 quadrant or lobule. It is tender, reddened, swollen, and hot. There may be purulent drainage, and aspiration may produce pus. The patient is febrile and appears ill.

B. Laboratory Findings

The organism responsible for infectious mastitis and breast abscess almost always is *S aureus*. *Streptococcus* spp. and *E coli* are occasionally isolated. Leukocytosis is evident.

Treatment

A. Congestive Mastitis

The form of treatment depends on whether or not the patient plans to breastfeed. If she does not, tight breast binding, ice packs, restriction of breast stimulation, and analgesics help to relieve pain and suppress lactation. Medical suppression of lactation probably does not hasten involution of congested breasts unless the drug is taken very early after delivery. Bromocriptine 2.5 mg twice daily orally for 10 days is an effective regimen, although concerns about its side effect profile have curtailed its use. For the woman who is breastfeeding, manually emptying the breasts following infant feeding is all that is necessary to relieve discomfort.

B. Infectious Mastitis

Infectious mastitis is treated in the same way as congestive mastitis. Local heat and support of the breasts help to reduce pain. Cloxacillin, dicloxacillin, nafcillin, or a cephalosporin—antibiotic with activity against the commonly encountered causative organisms—should be administered. Infants tolerate the small amount of antibiotics in breast milk without difficulty. It may be prudent to check the infant for possible colonization with the same bacteria present in the mother's breast.

If an abscess is present, incision and drainage are necessary. The cavity should be packed open with gauze, which is then advanced toward the surface in stages daily. Most authorities recommend cessation of breastfeeding when an abscess develops. Antistaphylococcal antibiotics should be prescribed. Inhibition of lactation is also recommended.

POSTPARTUM DEPRESSION

ESSENTIALS OF DIAGNOSIS

- Depression that begins in the 12 months after delivery
- Criteria for diagnosis are the same as nonpregnancy-related depression
- Symptoms must be present nearly every day for at least 2 weeks

Pathogenesis

Considering the excitement, anticipation, and tension associated with imminent delivery, the marked hormonal alterations after delivery, and the substantial new burdens and responsibilities that result from childbirth, it is not surprising that some women experience depression after delivery. The incidence of postpartum depression is difficult to estimate, but the disorder is common. The pathogenesis is not well understood; genetic susceptibility combined with a major life event and hormonal changes in the puerperium appears to underlie many cases of postpartum depression. The greatest risk factor for depression is a history of depression prior to pregnancy. In women who suffered from depression before they became pregnant and in those without effective support mechanisms, the severity of depression may be more profound and the consequences far more serious. An openly psychotic state may develop within a few days after delivery and render the woman incapable of caring for herself or her newborn. In some cases, she may harm her infant and herself.

Clinical Findings

A. Symptoms & Signs

Symptoms of postpartum depression include derangements in sleep patterns, energy level, appetite, weight, and libido. Women often complain of depressed mood and/or anxiety. Other symptoms include irritability, anger, feelings of guilt, a sense of feeling overwhelmed, feelings of inadequacy, and inability to bond emotionally with the baby. To meet a diagnosis of postpartum depression, the symptoms must be present nearly every day for at least 2 weeks.

B. Laboratory Tests

Several screening tools are available for evaluating postpartum women for depression. The Edinburgh Postnatal Depression Scale is one such questionnaire that is able to identify most women with postpartum depression. Hypothyroidism is emerging as a cause of some cases of postpartum depression, and screening for this disorder should be considered if suggested by clinical presentation.

Differential Diagnosis

The main differential diagnosis of postpartum depression is postpartum blues. Postpartum blues, however, is characterized by transient symptoms of depression, whereas postpartum depression requires that the characteristic symptoms be present nearly every day for at least 2 weeks.

Complications

Complications of postpartum depression include poor bonding with the infant, which can impact child development. Additionally, women with postpartum depression are at increased risk of suicide and infanticide.

Treatment

The first step in managing women with postpartum depression is an evaluation to determine the severity of her depression and whether she is a threat to herself or others. Psychiatric consultation should be obtained for the postpartum woman who shows symptoms of severe depression or overt psychosis. Initial treatment options include psychosocial therapy and pharmacotherapy. Some antidepressant medications are compatible with breastfeeding, although all antidepressants are transferred through the breast milk in some amount. For women unresponsive to pharmacotherapy, electroconvulsive therapy has been used with success.

American College of Obstetricians and Gynecologists. *Use of Psychiatric Medications during Pregnancy and Lactation. ACOG Practice Bulletin No. 91*. Washington, DC: American College of Obstetricians and Gynecologists; 2008.

Brockington I. Postpartum psychiatric disorders. *Lancet* 2004;363:303–310. PMID: 14751705.

Hoffbrand S, Howard L, Crawley H. Antidepressant drug treatment for postnatal depression. *Cochrane Database Syst Rev* 2001;2:CD002018. PMID: 11406023.

Neonatal Resuscitation

22

Elisabeth L. Raab, MD, MPH
Lisa K. Kelly MD

Delivery of a high-risk fetus requires multidisciplinary prenatal decision making to ensure the best outcome for the newborn and mother. Obstetricians, neonatologists, and, in appropriate cases, pediatric medical and/or surgical subspecialists must work together to determine an appropriate plan of care for the fetus and delivery of the newborn and provide counseling for the family. Discovery of a significant complication during pregnancy often warrants referral of the mother to a perinatologist for further evaluation and possible treatment. When circumstances allow, the mother of a high-risk fetus should be transferred to a tertiary care center with experience in high-risk obstetric and neonatal care prior to delivery. Numerous studies have shown improved outcomes for low-birth-weight (LBW) infants (<2500 g) who are delivered at a center with a higher level of neonatal care.

Successful transition from fetal to ex utero life involves a complex series of hormonal and physiologic changes, many of which occur or begin before birth. Events such as cord compression, placental abruption, meconium aspiration, and premature delivery or the presence of infection or major congenital malformations may alter or prevent the essential postnatal transition. Any process that prevents or hinders the newborn from inflating the lungs with air and establishing effective ventilation, oxygenation, and/or circulation will result in a depressed newborn in need of resuscitation for survival.

RESUSCITATION OF THE HIGH-RISK INFANT

The American Academy of Pediatrics (AAP) guidelines mandate that at least 1 skilled person capable of carrying out resuscitation of a newborn be present at every delivery. When a delivery is identified as high risk, 2 or more skilled people may be required to provide adequate care. Often it is useful to assign roles to the resuscitation staff to ensure that the resuscitation flows as smoothly as possible. The equipment required for resuscitation, such as the bag and mask used for ventilation, the blender for oxygen and air delivery, the suction equipment, the radiant warmer, and the monitors, should be checked prior to the delivery. Communication between the obstetric and neonatal staff about the maternal medical and obstetric history as well as the prenatal history of the fetus is essential to ensure that the neonatal team can anticipate and interpret the problems the newborn may have in the delivery room.

Delivery Room Management

Although the expectations may be different and the need for resuscitation more common, the same principles apply to a high-risk delivery as to a routine delivery: The newborn should be kept warm and rapidly assessed to determine the need for intervention.

The initial evaluation and resuscitation may take place in the delivery room or, in centers with a high-risk delivery service, preferentially in an adjacent room specifically designed for high-risk resuscitations. Typically the newborn is brought immediately to a radiant warmer, although some institutions weigh extremely premature infants prior to transfer to the warmer bed in order to determine the birth weight if viability is in question. The infant is dried with prewarmed towels to prevent heat loss. At some centers, LBW newborns are put into polyurethane bags or wrapped with polyethylene occlusive wrap after delivery; these measures have been shown to significantly improve temperature stability during stabilization and transport to the neonatal intensive care unit (NICU). In addition, a knit hat is used to prevent heat loss from the head. Preterm infants are at increased risk for thermal instability given their greater body surface area to weight ratio, thinner skin, and relative paucity of subcutaneous fat compared to term infants. Hypothermia (body temperature <36°C) can occur rapidly in the preterm infant and may cause complications such as hypoglycemia and acidosis.

After rapidly drying the infant and removing the wet towels, the resuscitation team should position and clear the airway. The team then assesses the newborn's respiratory effort, heart rate, color, and activity to determine the need for intervention. Drying the patient and suctioning the airway

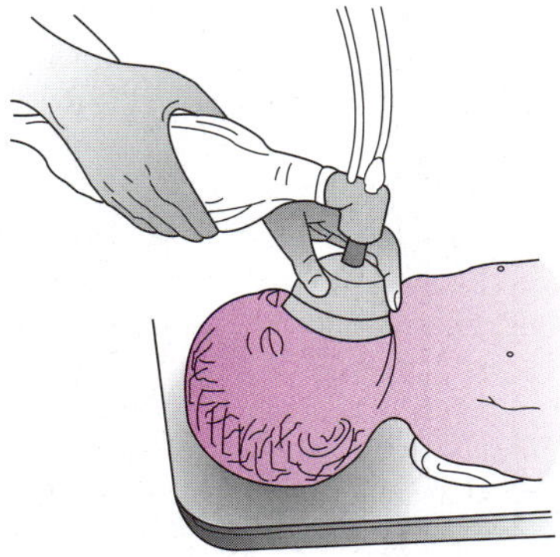

▲ **Figure 22–1.** Technique of bag and mask ventilation of the newborn. The neck should be slightly extended. An anesthesia bag should have a manometer attached; a self-inflating bag should have an oxygen reservoir attached.

usually provide adequate stimulation for the newborn to breathe. Rubbing the back or flicking the soles of the feet may be done to provide additional stimulus if initial respirations are irregular.

Positive-pressure ventilation (PPV) should be started if the newborn is apneic or has a heart rate less than 100 bpm. Figure 22–1 shows the correct positioning of the neck and placement of the mask. PPV will not be effective if the airway is not extended slightly and the mask is not applied to the face in the correct manner, with a tight seal around the nose and mouth. In addition, sufficient pressure must be given to produce adequate chest wall movement. A pressure manometer should be attached to the bag to monitor the amount of pressure that is being delivered. Overdistention of the lung causes significant trauma to the lung parenchyma and may cause complications such as a pneumothorax or lead to development of pulmonary interstitial emphysema (PIE), especially in the very-low-birth-weight (VLBW) neonate (birth weight <1500 g). Inability to move the chest wall with high pressures may indicate the lack of a good seal between the mask and the face, an airway obstruction, or significant pulmonary or extrapulmonary pathology compromising ventilation, such as pleural effusions, a congenital chest or abdominal mass, or a congenital diaphragmatic hernia (CDH). If the infant's respiration is markedly depressed, endotracheal intubation should be considered.

Chest compressions should be initiated if the heart rate is less than 60 bpm after 30 seconds of effective PPV. Figure 22–2 shows the acceptable methods for administering compressions to a neonate. Pressure should be applied to the sternum to depress it one-third of the anteroposterior diameter of the chest. Compressions should be coordinated with breaths: A single cycle should consist of 3 compressions followed by a single breath, and each cycle should last for

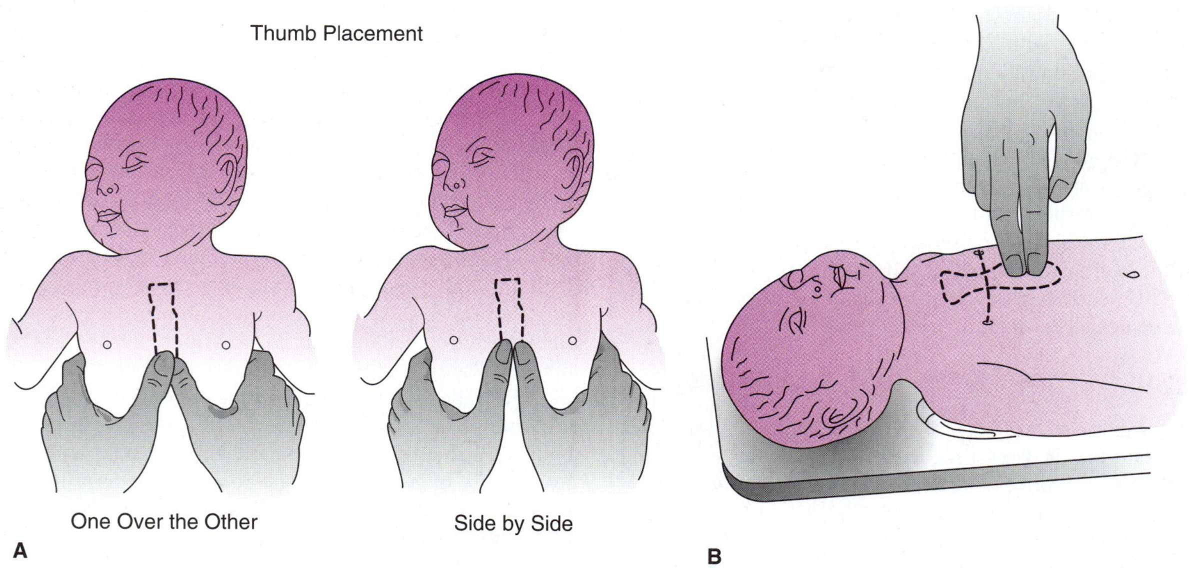

▲ **Figure 22–2.** **A:** Thumb technique for performing chest compressions on an infant. The two thumbs, placed either side by side or overlapping one another, are used to depress the lower third of the sternum, with the hands encircling the torso and the fingers supporting the back. **B:** Two-finger method for performing chest compressions on an infant. The tips of the middle finger and either the index finger or ring finger of one hand are used to compress the lower third of the sternum.

2 seconds. Compressions should be continued until the heart rate rises above 60 bpm. PPV should be continued until the heart rate is >100 bpm and the patient is showing adequate respiratory effort. If the heart rate remains <60 bpm after 30 seconds of compressions, administration of epinephrine is indicated. Failure to respond to PPV and chest compressions is a clear indication for endotracheal intubation; intubation should be attempted at this time if it has not already been performed. Figure 22–3 shows the landmarks used to guide placement of the endotracheal tube (ETT) between the vocal cords.

Epinephrine can be given via an ETT or an umbilical venous catheter. The standard dose of epinephrine in neonates is 0.01–0.03 mg/kg. The 2010 AAP guideline recommends giving epinephrine via the intravenous (IV) route and only giving endotracheal epinephrine if IV access cannot be obtained. If using the ETT, a dose of 0.05–0.1 mg/kg of the 1:10,000 concentration solution is recommended. The dose can be repeated every 3–5 minutes until the heart rate rises above 60 bpm.

When the infant's response to resuscitation is poor, other factors that may be complicating successful resuscitation of a newborn should be considered. Previous recommendations from the AAP have stated that the use of naloxone (Narcan) may be considered in cases of recent (<4 hours prior to delivery) administration of narcotics to the nonsubstance-using mother. However, the 2010 AAP recommendations do not recommend the use of naloxone under any circumstances and recommend only appropriate support of respiratory depression and oxygenation. Hypovolemia should be suspected if there is a perinatal history consistent with blood loss (eg, placental abruption, placenta previa) or sepsis and the baby is hypotensive and pale, with weak pulses and cool extremities. A 10 cc/kg IV infusion of normal saline, lactated Ringer's solution, or O-negative blood, if available and anemia is suspected, can be given to treat the suspected hypovolemia. The dose can be repeated if there is minimal improvement with the initial bolus. Metabolic acidosis may be present at birth if the baby was significantly distressed in utero or may develop after birth if oxygenation and/or perfusion are compromised. Although use of bicarbonate in resuscitation is not included in the AAP recommendations, significant acidosis will cause pulmonary vasoconstriction and poor myocardial contractility and should be treated. The umbilical artery can be catheterized to provide ongoing access to blood samples for determination of the extent of acidosis and the response to treatment during resuscitation. If bicarbonate is used, the dose is 2 mEq/kg IV of a 0.5 mEq/mL (4.2%) solution. Bicarbonate should be given slowly via an IV line and should be used only after ventilation is established so that the carbon dioxide (CO_2) produced with bicarbonate administration can be removed. Otherwise, bicarbonate administration may result in a significant increase in intracellular acidosis.

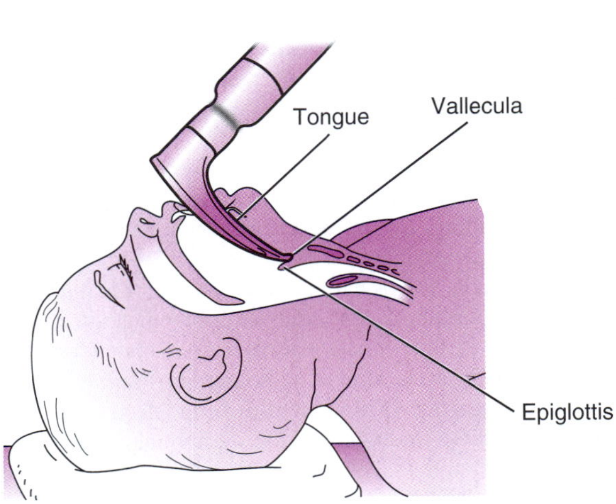

▲ **Figure 22–3.** Landmarks for placement of the laryngoscope.

Apgar scores are assigned at 1 and 5 minutes of life and continued at 5-minute intervals for up to 20 minutes as long as the score remains below 7. The Apgar score is a means of communicating the newborn's status during resuscitation; it should not be used to determine the need for resuscitation. The initial assessment of the newborn and assignment of the Apgar score are discussed in further detail in Chapter 9.

In the past, 100% oxygen has been the standard for neonatal resuscitation; however, 2 recent meta-analyses have demonstrated increased survival when resuscitation is initiated with air as compared to 100% oxygen. Therefore, the 2010 AAP recommendations now recommend beginning resuscitation with room air. There have been few studies looking at the use of blended oxygen and target oxygen saturations in either preterm or term infants. However, given the known toxicities of oxygen, the recent recommendations are to use blended oxygen when available and to target arterial saturations in the interquartile range for each gestational age (Fig. 22–4). If blended oxygen is not available and the baby remains bradycardic after 90 seconds of resuscitation, it is recommended to increase the oxygen to 100% until recovery of a normal heart rate.

Specific Considerations in the Delivery Room

A. Meconium

Meconium-stained fluid is present in 10–20% of deliveries. It is extremely rare if delivery takes place prior to 34 weeks' gestation. Passage of meconium in utero usually indicates fetal distress, and those personnel present at the delivery should be alerted by the presence of meconium to the possibility that the newborn may be depressed at birth.

It is no longer recommended by the AAP that all meconium-stained babies receive intrapartum suctioning.

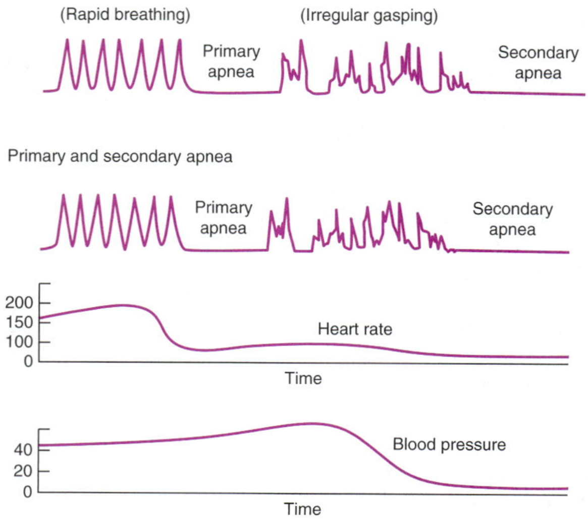

▲ **Figure 22–4.** Heart rate and blood pressure changes during apnea.

An active, crying, well-appearing infant does not require endotracheal intubation regardless of the presence of meconium staining or the thickness of the meconium. If the newborn is in distress or has depressed respiratory effort, the appropriate intervention is to intubate and suction the trachea before stimulating the baby in any way. If no meconium is suctioned from the airway, resuscitation should proceed according to the standard algorithm. If meconium is suctioned from the trachea, another attempt should be made to intubate the patient and suction the trachea again. However, if the patient has significant bradycardia, it may be appropriate to defer repeated suctioning and provide PPV.

The majority (94–97%) of infants born through meconium-stained fluid will not develop meconium aspiration syndrome, but when it does occur, infants are often critically ill. Meconium can block the airway and prevent the newborn's lungs from filling with air, a vital step in normal transitioning. Meconium aspiration into the lungs can cause obstruction of the small airways and consequently areas of atelectasis, gas trapping, and overdistention in addition to a chemical pneumonitis. The infant born through meconium may have pulmonary hypertension and inadequate oxygenation and requires close observation and early initiation of treatment when appropriate.

B. Asphyxia

Despite optimal prenatal care, some infants sustain injury prior to or during delivery that results in asphyxia. Perinatal asphyxia is characterized by the presence of hypoxemia, hypercapnia, and metabolic acidemia. It is the result of compromised oxygen delivery and blood flow to the fetus, either chronically or acutely, that stems from processes such as placental insufficiency, cord compression, trauma, and placental abruption.

If significant prepartum or peripartum hypoxic–ischemic injury has occurred, the infant likely will be depressed at birth and may not respond to initial interventions to establish respiration. The initial response in the newborn to hypoxemia is rapid breathing, followed shortly thereafter by a period of apnea, termed *primary apnea*. Drying the infant and rubbing the back or flicking the soles of the feet is sufficient to stimulate respiration during primary apnea. However, without intervention at this point, continued oxygen deprivation will lead to a series of gasps followed by a period of secondary apnea. It is important to recognize that an infant who does not respond to stimulation is likely exhibiting secondary apnea and requires further intervention. Respiration will not resume with stimulation if secondary apnea has begun, and positive pressure is necessary to reverse the process. Heart rate changes typically begin toward the end of primary apnea, whereas blood pressure typically is maintained until the period of secondary apnea.

Effective resuscitation of an asphyxiated newborn usually requires treatment of acidosis. Perinatal asphyxia may also be complicated by hypoglycemia and hypocalcemia. Myocardial dysfunction may be present, and fluid boluses and continuous infusion of inotrope may be required for adequate blood pressure support. However, in the presence of significant myocardial dysfunction, repeated volume boluses will worsen the cardiovascular status. In these cases, early administration of an inotrope (eg, dobutamine) with or without low to moderate doses of a vasopressor (eg, dopamine) is appropriate. In addition, seizures may occur in the newborn with perinatal asphyxia. Seizures usually are the result of hypoxic–ischemic injury to the cerebral cortex, but hypoglycemia and hypocalcemia also may cause seizure activity in the depressed neonate. In the newborn, phenobarbital (15–20 mg/kg IV) typically is given as the first-line treatment of seizures not caused by hypoglycemia or hypocalcemia. An additional 5–10 mg/kg bolus can be given to control status epilepticus. Asphyxiated infants are at increased risk for persistent pulmonary hypertension (discussed in detail later in the section Pathology & Care of the High-Risk Term Neonate).

The severity of the insult sustained by the newborn can be difficult to assess in the neonatal period. The presence of abnormal findings on the neurologic examination and the severity and persistence of those abnormalities are the most useful measures for assessing the degree of brain injury. Laboratory (umbilical cord and baby blood gases, serum creatinine level, liver function tests, blood lactate level, and cardiac enzyme levels) studies, radiographic (brain magnetic resonance imaging [MRI]) studies, and electroencephalographic (EEG) findings provide additional information to help predict the likelihood and anticipated extent of an adverse neurodevelopmental outcome. Early onset of seizure activity has been shown to increase the likelihood of a poor outcome. Infants with severe hypoxic–ischemic encephalopathy, which is characterized by absent reflexes, flaccid muscle tone, seizures, and a markedly altered level of consciousness, either die within several days of birth or have significant neurologic sequelae. It is a misconception that perinatal asphyxia is the cause of cerebral palsy. A minority of cases of cerebral palsy are actually attributable to intrapartum complications.

Several randomized, controlled studies have shown that induced hypothermia is protective in babies with mild-moderate asphyxia. Both selective hypothermia (ie, head cooling) and total body cooling have been shown to be effective. Devices are now available to regulate and safely cool neonates to a core temperature of 33.5–34.5°C. Therefore, it is now recommended that infants with moderate asphyxia should be cooled. Ideally the therapy should be initiated within 6 hours of the event (ie, birth). Timely transfer to a center that provides therapeutic hypothermia is of the utmost importance.

C. Shock

The newborn who fails to respond to initial attempts at resuscitation may be in circulatory shock. A number of different pathophysiologic processes can result in shock in the delivery room. Circulatory collapse can result from absolute (hemorrhage, capillary leak) or relative (vasodilatation) hypovolemia, cardiac dysfunction (asphyxia, congenital heart disease [CHD]), abnormal peripheral vasoregulation (prematurity, asphyxia, sepsis), or a combination of these factors. The peripartum history often helps elucidate the etiology. The presence of risk factors for sepsis (prolonged rupture of membranes, maternal fever, chorioamnionitis), hemorrhage (placenta previa, placental abruption, trauma), or perinatal asphyxia may be informative. Pallor or peripheral hyperemia, weak pulses with tachycardia, and cool or warm extremities are present on examination. Hypotension in the newborn immediately following delivery is commonly defined as a mean arterial pressure that is equal to or less than the gestational age. It is worth noting that blood pressure is normal in the early (compensated) phase of shock; hypotension may only develop as the process progresses.

As mentioned earlier in Delivery Room Management, a 10 cc/kg normal saline bolus typically is given to the newborn with hypotension. An additional 10–20 cc/kg is often given if the improvement in circulation is inadequate. Unmatched O-negative blood can be transfused in 10–15 cc/kg aliquots if severe anemia from blood loss is suspected. Volume should be administered slowly and judiciously to preterm infants who lack the mechanisms to autoregulate cerebral blood flow and protect the brain against reperfusion injury. Excessive volume may worsen the patient's status if cardiac dysfunction is the cause of hypotension. As discussed earlier, administration of sodium bicarbonate or THAM (tromethamine) may be indicated to treat metabolic acidosis in the newborn in shock. Vasopressor/inotrope infusions should be initiated in neonates who do not respond to volume resuscitation.

D. Cyanosis

Although acrocyanosis (cyanosis of the hands and feet) is often normal in the newborn, central cyanosis is not. Cyanosis is due to inadequate oxygen delivery to the tissue, either as a result of poor blood flow (peripheral vasoconstriction in acrocyanosis or low cardiac output in cardiogenic shock) or insufficiently oxygenated blood (pulmonary hypertension or severe parenchymal lung disease). Free-flow oxygen can be administered if a newborn has central cyanosis despite regular respirations. Free-flow oxygen can be delivered by holding a mask or oxygen tubing that is connected to a flowing source of 100% oxygen close to the baby's nose and mouth. Oxygen can be gradually withdrawn when the newborn turns pink. PPV is often indicated if the baby remains cyanotic despite free-flow oxygen. Lack of improvement of central cyanosis with administration of free-flow oxygen necessitates an evaluation of the cause of cyanosis. As discussed earlier, provision of 100% oxygen may have significant side effects if it is used for newborn resuscitation.

E. Prematurity

The delivery of a preterm infant requires a skilled multidisciplinary resuscitation team that has an understanding of the myriad problems associated with preterm delivery and has experience handling VLBW newborns. The presence at delivery of physicians, nurses, and a respiratory therapist trained in newborn resuscitation will optimize the early care of the newborn. Details of the delivery room care of the preterm infant are discussed in the section Delivery Room Management earlier in this chapter.

The neonatal team should meet with the family prior to delivery whenever possible. The parents should be informed about the prognosis for the fetus and need for intensive care admission if appropriate. It is critical that the family understand the plan for resuscitation in the delivery room and the anticipated short- and long-term problems the newborn may face. Often it is helpful to families to discuss the emotional impact of the admission and the possibility of a prolonged stay of their newborn in the intensive care unit. If the fetus is at the limits of viability, currently considered 23–24 weeks' gestation and/or weight <500 g, it is essential that the parents understand the considerable risk of death and the serious cognitive, motor, and pulmonary complications that may occur if the newborn does survive. The neonatal team must have a clear conversation with the parents about the possible options for postnatal management. Unfortunately, it often is difficult to make definitive plans given that the margin of error for prenatal determination of birth weight and gestational age is wide enough to have a significant impact on the viability of the fetus. Although many physicians have strong feelings of their own, it is vital that the course of resuscitation of a newborn at the limits of viability incorporates the family's wishes. Nevertheless, parents should understand that the fetus's viability will be reassessed after delivery, and that the maturity of the newborn, the newborn's condition at delivery, and the response to the resuscitative efforts made, in combination with available outcomes data, ultimately will determine the management in the delivery room.

F. Abdominal Wall Defects

Gastroschisis is the herniation of abdominal contents through an abdominal wall defect. The defect in gastroschisis usually is small and to the right of the umbilicus, and the intestines are unprotected by the peritoneal sac. *Omphalocele* also involves the herniation of abdominal contents through the abdominal wall, but the defect is in the umbilical portion of the abdominal wall, and the herniated viscera are covered by the peritoneal sac. Both defects require emergent care in the delivery room. Current delivery room recommendations suggest positioning the baby right side down to avoid kinking the mesenteric blood vessels and compromising blood flow to the intestines. The baby's lower body, including the defect and externalized organs, should be placed in a "bowel bag," which is then secured at the mid-thorax. This allows for direct visualization of the intestines while also limiting fluid losses. A nasogastric tube (at least 10 French) should be placed to allow for adequate decompression of the stomach and intestines.

Despite these measures, patients will still have increased heat and insensible fluid losses, and IV fluid should be started promptly at 1.5 times normal maintenance requirements to prevent dehydration and hypernatremia. Electrolytes and fluid status must be monitored closely. A surgical consultation should occur prenatally if the defect is diagnosed in utero. An urgent surgical evaluation should be obtained upon admission of the newborn to the NICU.

Kattwinkel J, Perlman JM, Aziz K, et al. Neonatal resuscitation: 2010 American Heart Association Guidelines for Cardiopulmonary Resuscitation and Emergency Cardiovascular Care. *Pediatrics* 2010;126:e1400–e1413. PMID: 20956432.

Paneth N. The evidence mounts against use of pure oxygen in newborn resuscitation. *J Pediatr* 2005;147:4–6. PMID: 16027683.

Saugstad OD. Oxygen for newborns: how much is too much? *J Perinatol* 2005;25(Suppl 2):S45. PMID: 15861173.

Spector LG, Klebanoff MA, Feusner JH, et al. Childhood cancer following neonatal oxygen supplementation. *J Pediatr* 2005;147:27–31. PMID: 16027689.

Tan A, Schulze A, O'Donnell CP, Davis PG. Air versus oxygen for resuscitation of infants at birth. *Cochrane Database Syst Rev* 2005;2:CD002273. PMID: 15846632.

PATHOLOGY & CARE OF THE PRETERM INFANT

In 2008, 12.3% of all births in the United States were preterm, a slight decrease from 12.8% in 2006. Advances in obstetric and neonatal care have markedly increased the survival of premature infants and improved outcomes. However, prematurity continues to account for a significant percentage of neonatal and infant mortality in the United States. As tinier and less mature infants survive, we face new ethical and medical challenges to continue improving the long-term and societal impact of the care provided in the NICU.

Respiratory Distress Syndrome

In 1959, Mary Ellen Avery and Jere Mead reported data showing that the severe respiratory disease seen in preterm infants, then known as hyaline membrane disease, was due in part to a deficiency of surfactant. Surfactant, a complex of phospholipids and protein secreted by type II pneumocytes, reduces surface tension in the alveoli of the lung. Its absence, or deficiency, results in diffuse microatelectasis and decreased functional residual capacity leading to the presentation of a "ground-glass" pattern and poor expansion of the lungs on chest radiograph (CXR). The lung disease of the preterm infant, now known as respiratory distress syndrome (RDS), also is a consequence of the immature architecture of the lung at the time of birth.

RDS presents as tachypnea and increased work of breathing that develops shortly after birth. Both oxygenation and ventilation are impaired, and blood gas analysis typically reveals hypoxia and a respiratory acidosis. Although most commonly seen in premature infants, RDS is associated with other conditions as well. Infants of diabetic mothers are at risk, even at term, because high levels of insulin in the fetus suppress lung maturation, including surfactant production. Without intervention, RDS typically worsens over the first few days of postnatal life. Historically, improvement was often heralded by a marked increase in urine output ("diuretic phase" of RDS).

The likelihood of RDS is inversely proportional to gestational age. It now is standard to give corticosteroids to mothers at risk of delivery before 32–34 weeks' gestation to hasten maturation of fetal organs, including the lungs, and to decrease the incidence and severity of RDS. Some larger preterm infants may require supplemental oxygen by nasal cannula or no respiratory assistance whatsoever. Babies with significant RDS typically require assisted ventilation. Ventilatory support can be given with continuous positive airway pressure (CPAP), a pressure- or volume-limited ventilator, or a high-frequency ventilator. A recent analysis concluded the data are not sufficient to recommend any mode of mechanical ventilation over the other as standard therapy for RDS. Provision of positive end-expiratory pressure (PEEP) (either as CPAP or PEEP) quickly after delivery is vital in order to prevent collapse of the lungs. If the lungs are allowed to collapse, oxygenation and ventilation will be compromised further and higher pressures will be required to reinflate the lungs, causing avoidable barotrauma and volutrauma to the lungs.

Exogenous surfactant administration has significantly reduced morbidity and mortality from RDS since its routine use began in the early 1990s. Prophylactic administration of surfactant to the preterm infant (ie, before 15 minutes of age) has been shown to reduce neonatal morbidity (pneumothorax and pulmonary interstitial edema) and mortality compared to rescue therapy (ie, waiting until after the diagnosis of RDS is made). Proposed explanations of this finding include a more homogeneous distribution of surfactant in the fluid-filled lung and the delivery of surfactant after a minimal period of PPV minimizing barotrauma and volutrauma to the lung. However, it is very important to ensure correct placement of the ETT prior to surfactant administration in the delivery room. If the ETT position cannot be determined, it may be better to delay surfactant until CXR has confirmed placement. If the degree of RDS is significant, an additional 2–4 doses of surfactant can be given every 6–12 hours depending on the surfactant preparation used. The newborn should be monitored closely after receiving surfactant because rapid changes in respiratory status usually occur, necessitating aggressive weaning of the ventilator settings. If the ventilator support is not weaned appropriately, the improving lung compliance will result in high tidal volume ventilation leading to volutrauma and hypocapnia. Complications such as obstruction of the ETT, pneumothorax, or pulmonary hemorrhagic edema may occur with surfactant. Pulmonary hemorrhagic edema likely is due to the surfactant administration-associated rapid decrease in pulmonary vascular resistance and the resulting pulmonary overcirculation through the ductus arteriosus. Blood gases should be checked frequently to prevent hypocapnia, which is associated with an increased incidence of periventricular leukomalacia (PVL) in the preterm neonate.

Despite the advances attributable to prenatal steroids, surfactant, and newer modes of ventilation, RDS continues to carry significant morbidity, including the risk of chronic lung disease, which is defined as the need for supplemental oxygen or ventilatory support at 36 weeks' postmenstrual age. New strategies have evolved over recent years to improve outcomes of newborns with RDS. Given the toxicities of oxygen, as discussed earlier, efforts are being made to limit exposure of preterm infants to hyperoxia. Many centers now aim to keep the oxygen saturation percent in the 80s or low 90s for preterm babies to prevent periods of hyperoxygenation and free-radical production. Although the data are scant and not well controlled, no current evidence suggests adverse neurologic effects of the lower saturations. However, it is recommended that saturations be kept in the high 90s once an infant's corrected gestational age reaches near-term. Future studies must be designed to investigate the potential side effects of lower saturations, including the development of pulmonary hypertension and subsequent cor pulmonale during infancy or early childhood.

Another recent change in neonatal practice has been the adoption of permissive hypercapnia. Permissive hypercapnia involves allowing CO_2 levels in the blood to rise above the normal value of 40 mm Hg in order to minimize the pressures required for ventilation and thereby reduce the lung injury caused by ventilator-induced barotrauma and volutrauma. This practice allows for infants to remain extubated who might have been reintubated in the past because of CO_2 retention. Although the procedure differs, CO_2 levels of 45–55 mm Hg are generally accepted, with some centers allowing higher CO_2 levels without a change in ventilatory management. The side effects of this approach are unknown, but hypercapnia may decrease the autoregulatory capacity of cerebral vessels, resulting in a more or less pressure-passive cerebral circulation. Therefore, the potential long-term neurodevelopmental effects of hypercapnia-associated pressure-passive cerebral circulation require investigation.

Encouraged by data from nonrandomized studies at Columbia University, many neonatologists are now trying to avoid intubation and/or mechanical ventilation, even in the tiniest babies. Using CPAP with nasal prongs for newborns with respiratory distress soon after birth (regardless of gestational age or birth weight) and a strategy of permissive hypercapnia, physicians at Columbia University reported a low incidence of bronchopulmonary dysplasia (BPD) compared to other tertiary care centers, without any significant increase in mortality. Because these findings require confirmation in appropriately designed randomized clinical trials, some centers have chosen an intermediate approach: VLBW infants are intubated for surfactant administration, but the ETT is removed shortly after and the period of mechanical ventilation is brief. Although approaches differ, early extubation is now a widely shared goal among neonatologists.

Dexamethasone was a key part of efforts to prevent and/or treat BPD for many years. However, a number of studies have shown a worse neurodevelopmental outcome in preterm infants who received dexamethasone treatment compared to controls with a similar degree of illness in the neonatal period. Many studies are still in progress, and data on long-term outcomes are not yet available, but the routine use of dexamethasone is no longer recommended. Dexamethasone is now reserved for those patients with the most severe lung disease, although, in general, no data support a better pulmonary outcome with its use. The available data suggest that there may be a window for dexamethasone use at 7–14 postnatal days, categorized as "moderately early" treatment, which has not been seen to cause any adverse outcomes. However, as mentioned earlier, a significant direct benefit associated with the use of dexamethasone is not available. Steroids also are now usually given in lower doses and shorter courses than in the past. The AAP currently recommends that neonatologists counsel parents about the risks and benefits of dexamethasone prior to initiating treatment. Future studies are needed to evaluate the effect, if any, of the newer treatment regimens on neurodevelopment outcome.

Nutrition

Providing optimal nutrition is an essential and challenging part of the care of the premature baby. Preterm infants are born with minimal nutrient stores and high metabolic demands, and growth failure is a frequent complication of prematurity. Supplying adequate nutrition for growth and development is complicated by the fact that many preterm newborns are too unstable to receive enteral nutrition in the first few days of postnatal life. There may be clear contraindications to enteral feeding, such as hypotension and vasopressor requirements, or factors can arise that can raise concerns about early initiation of enteral feeds, such as cocaine exposure in utero, indomethacin administration, the presence of a patent ductus arteriosus (PDA), or respiratory instability. Parenteral hyperalimentation is used to meet the newborn's initial fluid and nutritional requirements, but the ultimate goal is to meet those needs with enteral feedings given as early as safely possible.

An IV infusion of 10% glucose typically is started soon after birth to maintain glucose homeostasis. Extremely low-birth-weight (ELBW) babies (birth weight <1000 g) may require lower concentrations of dextrose because of higher total fluid requirements. Calcium supplementation in the dextrose infusion is standard for VLBW babies because transfer of calcium from mother to fetus primarily occurs during the third trimester, so VLBW babies are born with inadequate stores. The infusion rate of fluids typically is begun at 80–120 cc/kg/d depending on the immaturity and severity of illness of the neonate. Excessive fluids should be avoided because they have been associated with an increased risk for RDS, PDA, intraventricular hemorrhage (IVH), and necrotizing enterocolitis (NEC). Electrolytes and fluid status must be closely monitored over the first few days of life to determine appropriate fluid management. Depending on the level of immaturity, prenatal steroid exposure, and ambient humidity, ELBW infants may have enormous insensible losses and may develop hypernatremia if fluid needs are not met.

Protein breakdown can begin within the first postnatal days in preterm infants receiving only dextrose-containing fluids as nutrition. As a result, protein supplementation should be started as soon as possible to prevent a catabolic state. Parenteral hyperalimentation containing amino acids can be safely initiated immediately after delivery without development of acidosis, hyperammonemia, or uremia. The amino acid infusion should be started at 1.5–2.5 g/kg/d and advanced over several days to a goal of 3–4 g/kg/d.

Preterm newborns typically require a glucose infusion rate (GIR) of 6–8 mg/kg/min. The GIR is advanced in small increments to provide additional calories. Carbohydrate should account for approximately 40% of the 90–120 kcal/kg/d provided to the neonatal patient receiving parenteral nutrition. (Caloric requirements are higher with enteral feeding, typically 120–150 kcal/kg/d.) The need for GIR in excess of 15–18 mg/kg/min for adequate caloric support is rare. Glucose levels should be monitored and the dextrose infusion adjusted to maintain normoglycemia (ie, plasma glucose concentration 60–160 mg/dL). An insulin infusion can be started in the unusual event that hyperglycemia persists despite restricting the GIR to 4–6 mg/kg/min to continue to provide adequate calories for growth.

Intralipids provide the essential fatty acids required for multiple physiologic processes. Ideally, 40–50% of the daily caloric intake for a preterm infant receiving parenteral nutrition should come from fat. Usually a continuous 20% infusion at 0.5–1 g/kg/d is started on the first or second day of life, with the ultimate goal of providing 3 g/kg/d. Triglyceride and cholesterol levels must be monitored closely; elevated levels may require lower levels of lipid supplementation. Lipid infusion of 0.5–1 g/kg/d is required to prevent essential fatty acid deficiency.

In addition to providing protein, glucose, and fats, parenteral hyperalimentation provides electrolytes, vitamins, and minerals for the preterm infant unable to tolerate enteral feeds. Electrolyte levels must be monitored periodically to ensure appropriate levels. Particular attention must be paid to providing maximal amounts of calcium and phosphorous to VLBW infants who are at risk for developing osteopenia of prematurity.

It is important to begin enteral feeds as soon as possible in preterm infants. Delayed enteral feeding has adverse effects on the gut, such as mucosal atrophy, decreased digestive enzyme activity, and altered intestinal motility. In addition, long-term parenteral nutrition can cause cholestasis and presents an increased risk of infection because of the prolonged need for central venous access. Regimens for initiation of enteral feeding in VLBW infants vary but usually involve starting volumes of 10–20 mL/kg/d. Feeds are given via an orogastric or nasogastric tube for all but the most mature infants. The infant is monitored carefully for signs of feeding intolerance, such as abdominal distention, emesis, or large-volume gastric residuals while the feed volume is increased daily by 10–20 mL/kg. Some centers continue small-volume feeds for 5–10 days before advancing the volume toward the ultimate goal of 140–160 mL/kg/d.

Mothers of preterm infants should be encouraged to provide breast milk for their babies. Although infants are not typically developmentally ready to coordinate oral feeding until they reach 34 weeks' gestation and thus are unable to breastfeed initially, preterm infants can receive expressed breast milk via a gavage tube. The advantages of breastfeeding on everything from the appropriate function of the immune system to developmental outcomes and IQ are well documented. The caloric value of human milk clearly has proven to be superior to formula. Many NICUs now use pasteurized human breast milk banks to provide these benefits to infants whose mothers are unable to breastfeed. Human milk fortifiers are used to increase the protein, calories, calcium, phosphorous, vitamins, and minerals of mature human milk in order to meet the needs of the growing premature infant. Breast-fed infants should receive iron supplements once they reach the goal volume of enteral feeds.

Special formulas have been designed to better meet the nutritional needs of preterm infants receiving formula. Premature infant formulas contain 24 kcal/oz and provide higher amounts of protein, medium-chain triglycerides, vitamins, and minerals (eg, calcium and phosphorous) than standard formulas. If needed for adequate growth, the caloric content of preterm formula can be increased with any of a number of commercially available supplements, the majority of which provide additional calories as carbohydrate or fat. Although term infants gain an average of 30 g/d, 15–20 g/d is considered sufficient growth in the preterm infant.

Necrotizing Enterocolitis

NEC is a significant cause of morbidity and mortality in neonates. Although gastrointestinal in origin, NEC may lead to septic shock, respiratory failure, and death. Only 10% of cases occur in term newborns. The most premature and smallest infants are disproportionately affected; NEC occurs in 5–10% of all VLBW infants.

The presentation of NEC is highly variable. Signs and symptoms often are specific to the gastrointestinal tract, such as abdominal distention and/or erythema, emesis, bilious gastric residuals, and bloody stools; however, they may be nonspecific, such as apnea, temperature instability, and lethargy. Findings may be subtle initially, or the onset may be fulminant. Acidosis and thrombocytopenia are worrisome findings that may indicate necrotic bowel. Hyponatremia, due to upregulated sodium transport into the gut, and edema, due to increased capillary leak, often develop. Respiratory distress develops from abdominal competition due to inflammation and distention. The pathognomonic feature of NEC is the presence of intestinal pneumatosis on abdominal x-ray. Pneumatosis results from the production of hydrogen from bacteria in the bowel wall. Serial x-rays are obtained to follow disease progression. Air in the portal venous system or free air in the abdominal cavity indicates intestinal perforation, warranting surgical intervention for either an exploratory laparotomy to resect the necrotic bowel or placement of a right lower quadrant drain to decompress the abdomen if the patient is very small or unstable. Whether or not perforation has occurred, treatment of NEC typically includes 10–14 days of broad-spectrum antibiotics and discontinuation of enteral feeds. Many infants require fluid resuscitation and vasopressor/inotrope support. Seventy-five percent of infants with NEC survive, but half sustain long-term complications such as intestinal strictures and short gut syndrome.

Prematurity and enteral feeds have been clearly linked to NEC, but the pathogenesis of NEC is not well defined and is widely considered to be multifactorial. An infectious component is suggested by the association of certain organisms with outbreaks of NEC and the immature immune function of the preterm gastrointestinal tract. Mucosal injury as a result of altered intestinal and/or mucosal blood flow, either during periods of ischemia from hypotension or vascular spasm or during reperfusion and free-radical production, is believed to make the infant vulnerable. The presence of bacteria, ischemia and reperfusion, formula, and other unknown factors may all work together to trigger the inflammatory cascade responsible for the pathologic findings of NEC.

Risk factors for NEC include ELBW, polycythemia, umbilical catheters, enteral feeding, formula feeding, low Apgar scores, cyanotic heart disease, in utero cocaine exposure, and the presence of a PDA. Data on whether or not the rate of advancement of enteral feeds contributes to the development of NEC are conflicting. However, a recent study showed a decreased incidence of NEC in VLBW neonates who received small-volume feeds for 10 days before advancement compared to those who received daily 20 cc/kg advancement of feeds. The incidence of NEC has also been shown to decrease when standardized feeding regimens are instituted within a unit. The effect may be due to heightened awareness of signs and symptoms of feeding intolerance rather than to the actual specific regimen, but the effect has been reproduced and is dramatic.

NEC occurs less frequently in infants who receive breast milk. The protective effect of breast milk is speculated to result from the transfer of components of breast milk such as cytokines, immunoglobulins, growth factors, and probiotics to the infant. The protective effects of breast milk appear to occur even in those infants who are fed pasteurized donor breast milk. Other studies have shown a decreased incidence and severity of NEC in VLBW neonates who received supplementation with probiotic bacteria such as *Lactobacillus acidophilus*, *Bifidobacterium* spp., and *Streptococcus thermophilus*. However, further studies are needed to examine the safety of probiotics given recent reports of sepsis due to supplemented probiotic organisms. Antenatal steroids also have a protective effect against NEC, likely due to a demonstrated effect on gastrointestinal maturation and PDA closure.

Patent Ductus Arteriosus

During fetal life, close to 90% of the blood that leaves the right ventricle flows from the pulmonary artery to the aorta through the ductus arteriosus. After birth the pulmonary pressure falls, blood flow to the lungs increases, and the ductus arteriosus, primarily as a response to the increased oxygen tension in the blood and decreased circulating levels of prostaglandin E_2 (PGE_2), begins to close. Functional closure of the ductus arteriosus occurs within the first 1–2 days of postnatal life in the vast majority of term neonates, and definitive anatomic closure of the ductus usually is complete by the end of the first postnatal week. However, in neonates born prematurely, this process takes longer and may not always occur. In preterm neonates, failure of the ductus arteriosus to close is the result of several factors, including persistent hypoxia as a result of RDS and the continued presence of PGE_2. A PDA may be asymptomatic initially, but as the pulmonary pressure continues to fall, the left-to-right shunt of blood through the ductus arteriosus increases. Increasing left-to-right shunt produces pulmonary overcirculation (often with >50% of the left ventricular output shunting back into the lungs), worsening respiratory distress and gas exchange, an increasing oxygen requirement, and systemic hypotension. The presence of a PDA is suggested on physical examination by a hyperdynamic precordium (left ventricular overload), bounding palmar and brachial pulses, and a holosystolic precordial murmur. The pulse pressure usually is wide, and CXR typically demonstrates cardiomegaly and pulmonary congestion. Unless contraindications such as renal insufficiency, active bleeding, or thrombocytopenia are present, indomethacin, a nonselective inhibitor of the cyclooxygenase enzyme, is the first-line treatment of PDA because indomethacin effectively decreases prostaglandin synthesis. Indomethacin also has certain actions not directly related to inhibition of prostaglandin synthesis, such as a drug-induced decrease in global cerebral blood flow. This action may contribute to the indomethacin-induced decrease in severe IVH observed in ELBW neonates given indomethacin shortly after birth. However, there appears to be no significant long-term neurodevelopmental benefit of prophylactic indomethacin administration. In neonates with a PDA, fluids should be restricted to prevent worsening of pulmonary edema. Indomethacin may fail to achieve closure of the ductus, particularly in those who were born most prematurely or who received therapy later in postnatal life (beyond 10–14 days). Persistent patency of the ductus typically requires a repeat course of indomethacin followed by surgical ligation of the ductus, depending on the patient's age and clinical status. It should also be noted that the combination of indomethacin and postnatal steroid use has been shown to increase the likelihood of a spontaneous intestinal perforation. Therefore, care should be used when considering the use of those 2 drugs in combination.

Intraventricular Hemorrhage

IVH is one of the most feared complications of prematurity; severe IVH is a major risk for adverse long-term neurodevelopmental outcome. The incidence of IVH (approximately 20% in VLBW infants) is inversely proportional to gestational age. A number of factors combine to put the preterm neonate at risk. The blood vessels in the periventricular germinal matrix are abundant, immature, and fragile. These vessels may bleed when exposed to changes in blood flow. Sick newborns often experience periods of hypotension and hypertension, and they lack effective autoregulatory mechanisms to protect the brain during these variations in perfusion pressure. Changes in carbon dioxide levels in the blood also play an important role in regulating cerebral blood flow, and VLBW newborns may swing from hypocarbia to hypercarbia and back, particularly during the first few hours of life. In addition, bleeding may be aggravated by abnormal coagulation, particularly in the septic newborn.

Most IVH occurs during the first postnatal day; few cases occur after 5 days of life. Recent findings suggest that, at least in the VLBW neonate, IVH during the transitional period is caused by an ischemia–reperfusion cycle. Although IVH usually occurs without any clear outward signs that the process is occurring, a large bleed may cause a sudden change in mental status, a drop in hematocrit (Hct) level, and/or a full fontanelle. IVH is characterized as grade I when hemorrhage is confined to the region of the germinal matrix. Grade II IVH involves both the germinal matrix and the ventricles but does not fill or distend the ventricles. IVH grades I and II typically resolve and are not associated with a worse neurologic outcome than that expected for babies of the same gestational age without hemorrhages. Grade III IVH fills greater than 50% of the ventricles with blood and causes distention of the ventricles. Grade III IVH carries a significantly increased risk of mortality and adverse neurologic outcome because it more frequently evolves into ex vacuo or obstructive (fibrosis obstructs the ventricular system) hydrocephalus. IVH is classified as grade IV when the hemorrhage involves the brain parenchyma. This hemorrhage historically was considered to be an extension of IVH into the parenchyma but may more accurately represent a distinct process of venous infarction or severe ischemia followed by reperfusion in the periventricular white matter. Irrespective of the etiology, intraparenchymal hemorrhage results in tissue destruction and is associated with neurodevelopmental deficits in a marked majority of affected patients.

Although numerous preventative therapies have been evaluated (indomethacin, phenobarbital, vitamin E, morphine), none is currently recommended for routine prophylactic use. Every effort is made to keep blood pressure and carbon dioxide levels stable and within the normal range and to avoid unnecessary interventions, such as suctioning, which elevate intracranial pressure. Current guidelines recommend routine cranial ultrasound screening for infants less than 30 weeks' gestation between postnatal days 7 and 14 days and again when the infant reaches a corrected gestational age between 36 and 40 weeks. However, once IVH is detected, serial studies should be done to follow the bleed for progression and the ventricles for further dilation.

Performing an ultrasound study earlier than postnatal day 7 for newborns who are particularly unstable often is useful; the presence of a significant intraparenchymal bleed may help with decisions about direction of care for those whose viability is in question. Many centers advocate brain MRI prior to discharge to evaluate for white matter injury that may go undetected on cranial ultrasound and has been shown to be predictive of significant neurologic sequelae.

Retinopathy of Prematurity

Retinopathy of prematurity (ROP) is a disorder of retinal vascular proliferation that primarily affects premature infants. It is the second most common cause of blindness in children in the United States. Under normal conditions, the retina is completely vascularized by 36–40 weeks of gestation. The earlier in gestation delivery occurs, the larger the avascular region of the retina at birth and the greater the risk for ROP. The pathogenesis of ROP is not completely clear but seems to involve a period of vessel damage (from acidosis, hyperoxia, infection, etc) and cessation of vessel development followed by a period of abnormal proliferation. Hyperoxia and/or fluctuations in PaO_2 have been clearly shown to have an adverse effect on retinal development.

VLBW neonates, especially those who are critically ill and were born before 28 weeks' completed gestation, are at the highest risk for ROP. ROP tends to develop at 33 to 36 weeks' corrected gestation irrespective of the gestational age at birth. It may resolve spontaneously, as occurs in over 80–90% of cases, or, in rare cases, may progress to complete retinal detachment. Screening ophthalmologic examinations are recommended to monitor the progression of retinal vascularization in infants born at less than 31 weeks' gestation or weighing less than 1500 g. Screening should also be considered for infants weighing 1500–2000 g or born at 31 weeks' gestation or greater who have had an unstable course. The initial examination should be performed at 4 weeks of life or 30–31 weeks' corrected gestational age, whichever comes later. The frequency of repeat examinations is dictated by the findings, with the goal being early detection of ROP that meets criteria for surgical intervention.

American Academy of Pediatrics, Section on Ophthalmology. Screening examination of premature infants for retinopathy of prematurity. *Pediatrics* 2001;108:809. PMID: 11533356.

American Academy of Pediatrics, Subcommittee on Hyperbilirubinemia. Management of hyperbilirubinemia in the newborn infant 35 or more weeks of gestation. *Pediatrics* 2004;114:297. PMID: 15231951.

Askie LM, Henderson-Smart DJ, Irwig L, et al. Oxygen-saturation targets and outcomes in extremely preterm infants. *N Engl J Med* 2003;349:959–967. PMID: 12954744.

Halliday HL, Ehrenkranz RA, Doyle LW. Early postnatal (<96 hours) corticosteroids for preventing chronic lung disease in preterm infants. *Cochrane Database Syst Rev* 2003;1:CD001146. PMID: 12535402.

Halliday HL, Ehrenkranz RA, Doyle LW. Moderately early (7–14 days) postnatal corticosteroids for preventing chronic lung disease in preterm infants. *Cochrane Database Syst Rev* 2003;1:CD001144. PMID: 12535400.

Halliday HL, Ehrenkranz RA, Doyle LW. Delayed (>3 weeks) postnatal corticosteroids for preventing chronic lung disease in preterm infants. *Cochrane Database Syst Rev* 2009;1:CD001145. PMID: 19160189.

Kluckow M, Evans N. Low superior vena cava flow and intraventricular hemorrhage in preterm infants. *Arch Dis Child Fetal Neonatal Ed* 2000;82:F188–F194. PMID: 10794784.

Soll RF, Morley CJ. Prophylactic versus selective use of surfactant in preventing morbidity and mortality in preterm infants. *Cochrane Database Syst Rev* 2001;2:CD000510. PMID: 11405966.

Vohra S, Roberts RS, Zhang B, et al. Heat loss prevention (HeLP) in the delivery room: a randomized controlled trial of polyethylene occlusive skin wrapping in very preterm infants. *J Pediatr* 2004;145:750. PMID: 85580155.

PATHOLOGY & CARE OF THE HIGH-RISK TERM NEONATE

Persistent Pulmonary Hypertension

During fetal life, oxygenated blood is delivered to the fetus from the placenta. Pulmonary vascular resistance is elevated in utero; consequently minimal blood flow goes to the lungs. Instead, as noted in PDA, close to 90% of the output from the right ventricle passes from the pulmonary artery to the aorta through the ductus arteriosus. However, successful transition from fetal to extrauterine life requires a drop in pulmonary vascular resistance. The fall in pulmonary pressures results from a series of events that begins before birth but accelerates when a baby is born, the baby cries (filling the lungs with air), and the umbilical cord is cut (increasing the systemic resistance). A number of processes can interrupt this process, either by mechanically blocking the airways, thus preventing essential lung expansion and increase in the partial pressure of oxygen, or by preventing relaxation of the pulmonary vascular bed. Meconium aspiration syndrome, asphyxia, sepsis, pneumonia, and CDH are among the most common causes of persistently elevated pulmonary vascular resistance, termed *persistent pulmonary hypertension of the newborn* (PPHN).

PPHN results in severe hypoxia in the newborn. Blood continues to shunt away from the pulmonary circulation through the foramen ovale, ductus arteriosus, or both, bringing poorly saturated blood to the body. Treatment consists of interventions aimed at lowering the pulmonary vascular resistance. Acidosis and hypoxemia are potent pulmonary vasoconstrictors and are to be avoided. When possible, PaO_2 is maintained in the normal range (80–100 mm Hg). Supplemental oxygen is weaned cautiously because even relatively small changes can cause an acute decompensation. Every effort should be made to maintain left ventricular output and blood pressure (thus systemic perfusion) in the normal range and to keep the blood pH in the 7.3–7.4 range. Acidosis is a vasoconstrictor, but aggressive use of bicarbonate or THAM may not be beneficial. Although hyperventilation was used in the past to maintain an alkaline pH, concerns about ventilator-induced lung damage and the effect of hypocarbia on cerebral blood flow have altered this practice. In addition, studies have shown that it is the normalized pH, not the decreased CO_2, that improves pulmonary vasoconstriction. Most physicians adjust the ventilator support to target a $PaCO_2$ of 40–50. High-frequency ventilators are often used, allowing for higher mean airway pressures without increasing barotrauma and volutrauma to the lungs. Vasopressors, typically dopamine, are used to maintain systemic blood pressure. If there is evidence of myocardial dysfunction, an inotrope such as dobutamine typically is used, and vasopressor support is adjusted to prevent undesirable increases in systemic vascular resistance. Patients with PPHN are extremely sensitive to noise and tactile stimulation, so infusions of sedatives and analgesia are routinely used to minimize agitation. However, use of neuromuscular blockade is to be avoided because it does not appear to improve clinical outcome and is associated with significant side effects, including sensorineural hearing loss.

Nitric oxide is a selective pulmonary vasodilator. Inhaled nitric oxide (iNO) has been proven to improve oxygenation and decrease the need for extracorporeal membrane oxygenation (ECMO) in term infants with PPHN. iNO is routinely started at 20 ppm, although lower doses may be as effective. iNO is weaned as the patient stabilizes and the supplemental oxygen requirement falls. Despite the dramatic improvement in outcomes since the availability of iNO, a number of patients with PPHN will still require ECMO. Historically the criterion for ECMO has been a greater than 80% estimated risk of mortality with continued conventional medical management. General guidelines for the criteria for ECMO include an oxygenation index greater than 35–60 for between 0.5 and 6 hours, an alveolar–arterial oxygen difference greater than 605–620 (at sea level) for 4–12 hours, or a preductal PaO_2 less than 40 for more than 2 hours. ECMO is contraindicated in neonates less than 34 weeks' gestational age because of technical issues regarding catheter placement as well as the increased risk of intracranial bleeding in the preterm neonate. A preexisting grade II or higher IVH, signs of severe irreversible brain damage, lethal congenital anomalies, and nonreversible pulmonary disease are other contraindications to ECMO. Survival of patients with PPHN treated with ECMO varies depending on the underlying cause of PPHN. The survival rate of patients with meconium aspiration syndrome is greater than 90%, but the survival rate of patients with CDH is only 50%.

Congenital Diaphragmatic Hernia

CDH is a defect that results from incomplete development and closure of the diaphragm, usually at the foramen of Bochdalek at 8–10 weeks' gestation. The defect in the diaphragm allows the contents of the abdominal cavity to migrate into the chest, resulting in compression of the lungs and, in more severe cases, the heart. The compression leads to pulmonary hypoplasia, abnormal lung development, and potentially underdevelopment of 1 or both ventricles. Ninety percent of CDH involves the left hemidiaphragm. CDH is now generally prenatally diagnosed, but a number of cases still go undiagnosed, even with routine prenatal care.

A number of features should raise suspicion about the possibility of CDH in the newborn with cyanosis and respiratory distress. Breath sounds may be absent on the left side of the chest and the heart sounds shifted to the right. The abdomen tends to be scaphoid, as some of the abdominal organs typically have shifted into the thorax. It may be difficult to effectively ventilate and resuscitate the patient. If a CDH is suspected, mask and bag ventilation must be avoided. The patient should be intubated and a sump/replogle tube placed as soon as possible to prevent air from filling the stomach and bowel and thus compromising ventilation further. Many centers use sedation and sometimes paralysis to minimize activity and prevent competition from swallowed air. CXR observation of bowel loops in the chest confirms the diagnosis.

Surgical repair of the defect usually is delayed until the patient's condition stabilizes and the reactive component of the pulmonary hypertension has improved. Efforts are made to use the lowest ventilator settings tolerated to minimize ventilator-induced lung injury. Surfactant, iNO, high-frequency ventilation, and, if necessary, ECMO are often used to manage patients with CDH. However, surfactant administration has been shown to be of no benefit, and some studies suggest that it may be associated with an increased need for ECMO, so its routine use cannot be recommended. To date, the evidence also has not shown a clear benefit of iNO for patients with CDH. Additional studies are needed to evaluate the role of each of these interventions in the care of the patient with CDH.

Reported survival rates vary from approximately 35–80%, perhaps reflecting differences between centers and/or bias related to referral patterns. The prognosis depends on the severity of the underlying pulmonary hypoplasia and the degree of reactive pulmonary hypertension, as well as the presence of other anomalies or a chromosomal abnormality. Development of a pneumothorax has been shown to predict a poor outcome. Failure to achieve a preductal PaO_2 greater than 100 mm Hg or a $PaCO_2$ lower than 60 in the first 24 hours of life generally indicates a poor prognosis as well. Some physicians argue that infants in whom the $PaCO_2$ level never falls below 80 or who never achieve a preductal oxygen saturation of at least 85% for at least 1 hour have severe pulmonary hypoplasia and are not appropriate candidates for ECMO. However, the outcome of the individual patient is hard to predict, and every measure must be made to provide gentle ventilation and accept higher $PaCO_2$ and lower PaO_2 levels as long as systemic oxygen delivery is appropriate.

Transient Tachypnea of the Newborn

The differential diagnosis for the newborn with tachypnea in the first postnatal hours ranges from RDS to sepsis to CHD. One of the most common causes of tachypnea in the newborn is transient tachypnea of the newborn (TTN). TTN results when fetal lung fluid production fails to cease with the onset of labor. The incidence of TTN is significantly increased when the baby is delivered via caesarean section without labor especially if performed before 39 weeks of gestation.

The newborn presents with tachypnea, increased work of breathing, and cyanosis. Infants with TTN may require moderate supplemental oxygen; some may be sick enough to require intubation. CXR reveals interstitial and alveolar edema; fluid is characteristically seen in the right middle lobe fissure. Symptoms of TTN typically resolve over the first 24–48 hours (fetal lung fluid production ceases in response to stress), and CXR clears by the second or third day of life. However, TTN is a diagnosis of exclusion, and other causes of tachypnea and respiratory distress must be ruled out. An evaluation for sepsis (including initiation of antibiotic therapy pending culture results) as well as other causes of tachypnea is generally warranted.

Congenital Heart Disease

CHD occurs in approximately 1 in 100 live births, and approximately 3 in 1000 have CHD that requires surgical repair or results in death within the first year of life. CHD rarely presents in the delivery room. In fact, the majority of infants with prenatally diagnosed CHD initially appear well. Nevertheless, the newborn with cyanosis who fails to respond to 100% oxygen (hyperoxia test; see below) should be evaluated for structural heart disease. Complex CHD typically presents as cyanosis or congestive heart failure and circulatory shock and only rarely as an asymptomatic murmur in a newborn. Signs such as tachypnea, weak peripheral pulses, or cool extremities may develop quickly with closure of the ductus arteriosus if the lesion has ductal-dependent pulmonary or systemic flow. Right-sided obstructive lesions (eg, pulmonic atresia or stenosis), which are dependent on the ductus for pulmonary blood flow, tend to present with cyanosis due to diminished or absent pulmonary blood flow. Left-sided obstructive lesions (eg, coarctation of the aorta and hypoplastic left heart syndrome) typically present as shock and often are initially misdiagnosed as sepsis. However, statistically the term neonate who develops signs of shock after the first 24–48 hours of life is approximately 5 times more likely to have ductal-dependent CHD than bacterial sepsis.

The initial steps in evaluating a stable patient for suspected CHD include 4-extremity blood pressure measurements, measurement of preductal and postductal saturations, electrocardiogram, CXR, and hyperoxia test. If the PaO_2 level fails to increase above 100 after exposure to 100% fraction of inspired oxygen (FiO_2) for 15 minutes, cyanotic CHD is likely; if the PaO_2 level increases above 250, CHD is unlikely. CXR may reveal black lungs that signify diminished pulmonary blood flow (as occurs in right-sided obstructive lesions) or congestion (as occurs with obstructed pulmonary venous return). The diagnosis of CHD usually is established by echocardiogram, although cardiac catheterization is sometimes necessary to clarify the specifics of the abnormal anatomy in complex cases. Low-dose PGE infusion should be started when critical CHD is suspected in order to maintain or reestablish ductal patency. Once the diagnosis of cyanotic heart disease has been made, supplemental oxygen should be used sparingly but as necessary to keep oxygen saturations around 75–85% until surgical repair occurs. This supplementation should provide adequate oxygen delivery to prevent the development of metabolic acidosis without decreasing pulmonary vascular resistance and causing pulmonary overcirculation.

Esophageal Atresia/ Tracheoesophageal Fistula

Esophageal atresia occurs when there is an interruption in the separation of the foregut into the trachea and esophagus during the fourth week of gestation. In its most common form, there is a proximal esophageal pouch and a fistula between the trachea and the distal segment of the esophagus. The newborn with esophageal atresia typically presents in the first few hours after birth with copious secretions and coughing or gagging with the first feed. Respiratory distress may develop if secretions or feeds are aspirated. The prenatal istory often is remarkable for polyhydramnios due to the inability of the fetus to regulate amniotic fluid levels by swallowing. The diagnosis usually is apparent when a CXR reveals a nasogastric tube coiled in the proximal esophageal pouch. Absence of a gastric bubble on x-ray usually suggests that a distal fistula is not present. Emergent gastrostomy may be necessary to decompress the stomach. The feasibility of primary repair depends on the distance between the proximal and distal portions of the esophagus. If primary repair is not possible, initial surgery involves ligation of the fistula. Patients typically then undergo serial dilations of the proximal pouch and delayed anastomosis or may require colonic interposition if the gap remains too wide to close. Postoperative complications include leaking or stenosis at the anastomosis site, poor esophageal motility, and gastroesophageal reflux.

Polycythemia

Polycythemia, defined as a central venous Hct greater than 65%, results from either increased in utero erythropoiesis or from maternofetal or twin–twin transfusion. Increased in utero erythropoiesis occurs most often as a response to fetal hypoxia, usually from placental insufficiency. Erythropoiesis in the fetus is also increased with maternal diabetes, chromosomal abnormalities, and endocrine disorders such as congenital adrenal hyperplasia, thyroid disease, and Beckwith-Wiedemann syndrome. Maternofetal hemorrhage most commonly results from delayed cord clamping.

Polycythemia may cause congestive heart failure from volume overload, as in the case of the recipient twin in twin–twin transfusion syndrome. More commonly, the complications attributed to polycythemia arise from hyperviscosity rather than increased blood volume. Blood viscosity increases as the Hct level rises, placing the polycythemic infant at risk for complications from impaired blood flow and oxygen delivery. Polycythemia may present as hypoglycemia, poor feeding, respiratory distress, pulmonary hypertension, lethargy, jitteriness, or seizures. Infants are at increased risk for NEC, and thrombotic strokes may occur.

Although IV hydration may be useful, a symptomatic neonate with Hct level greater than 65% or an asymptomatic neonate with Hct level greater than 70% should undergo a partial exchange transfusion performed to decrease blood viscosity and ameliorate any symptoms. The volume of blood that should be removed and then replaced with isotonic saline (to lower the viscosity without causing hypovolemia) is determined by the following formula:

Volume to be exchanged = [Blood volume × (Observed hematocrit – Desired hematocrit)]/Observed hematocrit

Blood volume usually is estimated at 80–90 mL/kg in a term infant and 90–100 mL/kg in a preterm infant. The goal Hct usually is 55%. The hope is that partial exchange will prevent symptoms from worsening and further complications from developing, but long-term follow-up studies have failed to show any benefit.

Hyperbilirubinemia

Hyperbilirubinemia is a common problem in the neonatal period, affecting 60–70% of all infants born in the United States to some degree. In most instances, the level of the unconjugated form of bilirubin is elevated. Although the course usually is benign and an increase in serum bilirubin level occurs in all newborns during the first postnatal days, severe unconjugated hyperbilirubinemia can cause kernicterus and long-term neurologic damage.

Bilirubin is produced when heme-containing compounds such as hemoglobin are broken down. The initial unconjugated product is fat soluble but water insoluble, a form that can cross the blood–brain barrier and cause central nervous system toxicity but cannot be excreted. The blood carries bilirubin to the liver, where it is conjugated to a water-soluble and excretable form by the enzyme glucuronyl transferase. The immature hepatic enzyme function in the newborn impairs bilirubin conjugation and thus excretion. The shorter life span of red blood cells and increased red cell mass in neonates further predispose the newborn to elevated plasma concentrations of bilirubin, as does the increased reabsorption of bilirubin that occurs in the sterile newborn intestinal tract.

Hyperbilirubinemia may be severe when other coexisting factors increase hemolysis, decrease the rate of bilirubin conjugation, or impede excretion. Hemolysis is increased by abnormal red cell enzyme function (glucose-6-phosphate dehydrogenase [G6PD] deficiency, less frequently pyruvate kinase deficiency) or morphology (spherocytosis, elliptocytosis) and isoimmunization due to ABO, minor antigen, or Rh incompatibility. Sepsis can increase hemolysis. A number of inborn errors of metabolism and enzyme defects can impair conjugation. Conjugation is impaired when there is delayed maturation of the conjugating enzymes, as is thought to occur in cases of congenital hypothyroidism. Obstructed biliary flow, as in biliary atresia, and gastrointestinal obstruction cause decreased excretion. Many disease states are associated with hyperbilirubinemia.

Hyperbilirubinemia presents clinically as jaundice, a yellow-green discoloration of the skin and mucous membranes. A serum bilirubin level should be checked in all jaundiced newborns. It is standard policy in some nurseries to check a total serum bilirubin (TSB) level in all newborns prior to discharge. Most centers check a level within 24–48 hours of life in all VLBW infants as risk for sequelae from hyperbilirubinemia is believed to exist at lower serum bilirubin concentrations in preterm neonates. The etiology of the pathologic hyperbilirubinemia must be sought. A blood type, Coombs' test, Hct level, and reticulocyte count will provide important information, as will the parent's ethnicity, maternal blood type, and history of jaundice in siblings. It is important to determine whether it is the level of conjugated or unconjugated fraction of bilirubin that is elevated. The differential diagnosis, evaluation, and treatment are markedly different depending on whether or not the elevated portion is conjugated. A conjugated bilirubin level greater than 10% of the total value should prompt an investigation for biliary obstruction or causes of hepatocellular damage such as TORCH (toxoplasmosis, other agents, rubella, cytomegalovirus, herpes simplex) infection, galactosemia, and α_1-antitrypsin deficiency. A complete sepsis workup is indicated in the ill-appearing patient.

The AAP has established practice parameters to help direct the use of phototherapy and exchange transfusion for hyperbilirubinemia in infants of greater than 35 weeks' gestation. Phototherapy causes the photoisomerization of unconjugated bilirubin to a water-soluble form that can be excreted by the kidneys and gastrointestinal tract. Phototherapy is contraindicated for conjugated hyperbilirubinemia; it is ineffective and can cause a bronze staining of the skin. Figure 22–5 shows the current AAP recommendations for initiation of phototherapy. A patient should receive phototherapy if the TSB level lies above the line for the appropriate risk group for the patient. A newborn is considered to have risk factors if any of the following are present: isoimmune hemolytic disease, G6PD deficiency, asphyxia, significant lethargy, temperature instability, sepsis, acidosis, or albumin level less than 3.0 g/dL.

Insensible losses increase under phototherapy, and liberal IV fluids should be given in anticipation of increased daily fluid needs. Infants who appear well, are tolerating enteral feeds, and are not likely to require an exchange transfusion should continue feeding. Enteral nutrition will increase stooling and facilitate bilirubin excretion. IV fluid should be given in addition if oral intake is insufficient or if needed for adequate hydration.

Figure 22–6 shows the AAP guidelines for exchange transfusion. Exchange transfusion effectively removes anti-red blood cell antibodies circulating in the blood and may have an effect on removing circulating bilirubin. Twice the blood volume (estimated at 80–100 cc/kg) is slowly removed from the patient in aliquots of 5–10 cc, with each aliquot followed by transfusion of an equal volume of fresh type O-negative blood, reconstituted with plasma to a hematocrit of 45–50%. The guidelines shown in Figure 22–6 are intended to apply to the newborn who has a continuous rise in TSB level despite intensive phototherapy or to a neonate readmitted to the hospital after discharge who continues to have a TSB above the exchange level for 6 hours after initiation of phototherapy. Immediate exchange is recommended if the TSB is more than 5 mg/dL greater than the exchange threshold or if the patient has abnormal findings on neurologic examination that suggest acute bilirubin encephalopathy. Complications of exchange transfusion include hypocalcemia, hypoglycemia, hypothermia, coagulation abnormalities, apnea, and bradycardia. Many centers delay resuming oral feeds until 24–48 hours after exchange because of the increased risk of NEC after exchange.

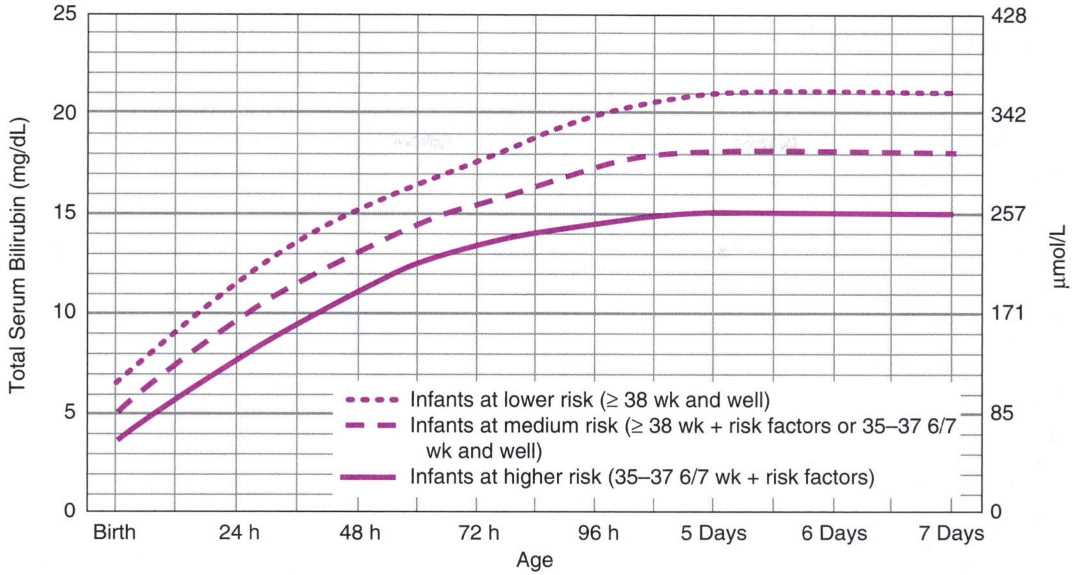

- Use total bilirubin. Do not subtract direct reacting or conjugated bilirubin.
- Risk factors = isoimmune hemolytic disease, G6PD deficiency, asphyxia, significant lethargy, temperature instability, sepsis, acidosis, or albumin < 3.0g/dL (if measured).
- For well infants 35–37 6/7 wk can adjust TSB levels for intervention around the medium risk line. It is an option to intervene at lower TSB levels for infants closer to 35 wks and at higher TSB levels for those closer to 37 6/7 wk.
- It is an option to provide conventional phototherapy in hospital or at home at TSB levels 2–3 mg/dL (35–50 mmol/L) below those shown but home phototherapy should not be used in any infant with risk factors.

▲ **Figure 22–5.** Guidelines for phototherapy in hospitalized infants of 35 or more weeks' gestation. G6PD, glucose-6-phosphate dehydrogenase; TSB, total serum bilirubin. (Data from the American Academy of Pediatrics, Subcommitte on hyperbilirubinemia: Management of hyperbilirubinemia in the newborn infant 35 or more weeks of gestation. *Pediatrics* 2004;114:297–316.)

Indications for phototherapy and exchange transfusion in preterm infants are not well established. A reasonable guideline is to begin phototherapy when the bilirubin concentration is equal to 0.5% of the birth weight (in grams) and to consider an exchange transfusion when the concentration reaches 1% of the birth weight. These numbers represent a very general guideline, however, and it is important that treatment decisions take into account the etiology of the jaundice and the patient's overall clinical status. The presence of significant bruising, hemolysis, sepsis, or acidosis should lower the physician's threshold for initiating treatment.

Infection

Infection is a significant cause of morbidity and mortality in the newborn. The immature newborn immune system places the neonate at increased risk for infection. The preterm infant, whose immune system is markedly immature and who has diminished levels of immunoglobulin compared to the term newborn, is at particularly high risk. Typically infection is acquired when organisms ascend into the uterine cavity and come into contact with the fetus, but infection can be acquired hematogenously, from the mother's blood, or at the time of delivery when the newborn passes through the vaginal canal.

A. Sepsis

Neonatal sepsis occurs in 1 in 1000 term infants and 1 in 4 preterm infants. Risk factors for neonatal sepsis include premature delivery, multiple pregnancy, prolonged rupture of amniotic membranes (>18 hours), maternal fever, maternal group B *Streptococcus* (GBS) colonization, and chorioamnionitis. The most common causes of early-onset (within the first week of life) sepsis are GBS and *Escherichia coli*. *Listeria monocytogenes*, enterococci, and several different gram-negative rod species are other identified causes of early-onset neonatal sepsis. Late-onset infection in hospitalized infants is more often due to *Staphylococcus* spp.

Signs and symptoms of sepsis in the newborn can be very subtle and nonspecific, such as temperature instability, hypoglycemia or hyperglycemia, apnea, poor feeding, or

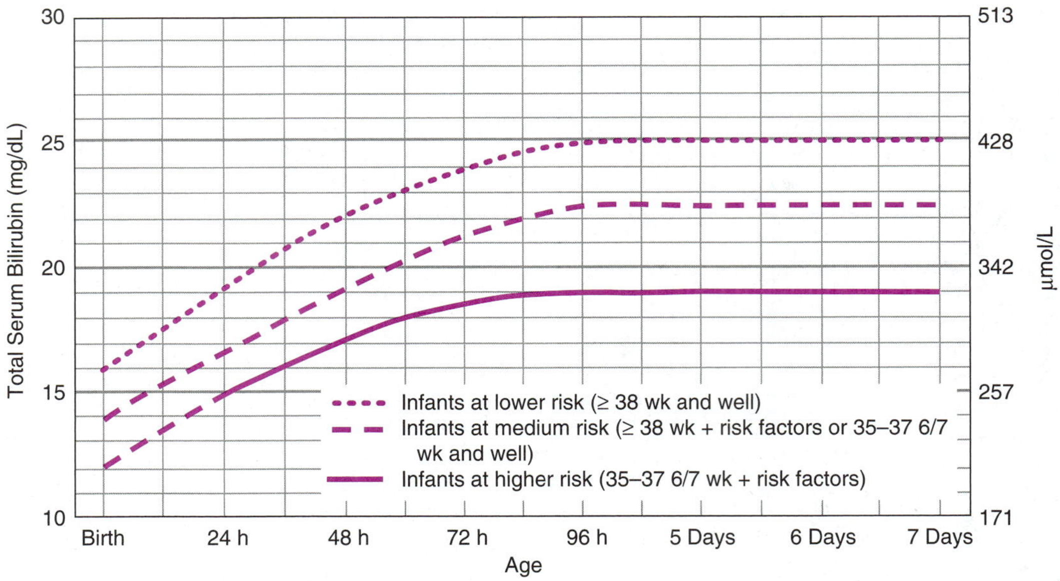

- The dashed lines for the first 24 hours indicate uncertainty due to a wide range of clinical circumstances and a range of responses to phototherapy.
- Immediate exchange transfusion is recommended if infant shows signs of acute bilirubin encephalopathy (hypertonia, arching, retrocolitis, opisthotonos, fever, high pitched cry) or if TSB is ≥5 mg/dL (85 µmol/L) above these lines.
- Risk factors—isoimmune hemolytic disease, G6PD deficiency, asphyxia, significant lethargy, temperature instability, sepsis, acidosis.
- Measure serum albumin and calculate B/A ratio.
- Use total bilirubin. Do not subtract direct reacting or conjugated bilirubin.
- If infant is well and 35–37 6/7 wk (median risk) can individualize TSB levels for exchange based on actual gestational age.

▲ **Figure 22–6.** Guidelines for exchange transfusion in infants of 35 or more weeks' gestation. G6PD, glucose-6-phosphate dehydrogenase; TSB, total serum bilirubin. (Data from the American Academy of Pediatrics, Subcommitte on hyperbilirubinemia: Management of hyperbilirubinemia in the newborn infant 35 or more weeks of gestation. *Pediatrics* 2004;114:297–316.)

tachypnea. In contrast, some neonates present in fulminant shock. A complete blood count and blood culture should be sent if sepsis is suspected and antibiotics should be started. A decreased or elevated white blood cell count, a predominance of immature white blood cell forms, and thrombocytopenia are suggestive of infection. Although nonspecific, an elevated C-reactive protein (CRP) level indicates the presence of an inflammatory or infectious process, and data support the negative predictive value of a CRP level in the evaluation for sepsis in the neonate. In addition, CXR is indicated to evaluate for pneumonia. Often differentiating an infiltrate from atelectasis, RDS, or retained lung fluid is difficult, but serial films may be useful in differentiating the various processes. There is debate about whether a culture of cerebrospinal fluid (CSF) is necessary in the newborn evaluated for early-onset sepsis. (A CSF culture is clearly warranted in suspected late-onset sepsis because the incidence of coexisting meningitis with late-onset bacteremia is very high.) Unless signs of meningitis (eg, seizure activity or altered mental status) or a documented positive blood culture is present, meningitis is unlikely in the immediate newborn period. However, studies have reported positive CSF cultures with concurrent negative blood cultures in asymptomatic neonates. The issue has been further complicated by the current widespread use of maternal intrapartum antibiotics. Consequently, given the ramifications of failure to diagnose or only partially treat a case of meningitis, CSF culture is a routine part of the newborn sepsis evaluation in many institutions, and if the infant is unable to have a lumbar puncture, meningitic doses of antibiotic should be used. Urine culture, a routine part of the sepsis evaluation for late-onset disease, is rarely useful in the first few days of life.

Antibiotics that provide broad-spectrum coverage, typically ampicillin and gentamicin in the first few days of life, should be continued for 48–72 hours pending the results of all cultures that were sent for analysis. Vancomycin and gentamicin are often used for nosocomial infections. If bacteremia is documented by a positive blood culture or highly suspected based on clinical status or laboratory findings, antibiotics should be continued for 7–10 days. IV antibiotics usually are continued for a minimum of 2 weeks for gram-positive meningitis and 3 weeks for gram-negative meningitis.

The Centers for Disease Control and Prevention (CDC) developed guidelines in 1996 that recommended screening for GBS colonization at 35–37 weeks' gestation. It was recommended that colonized women and those with other risk factors receive intrapartum antibiotic therapy beginning at least 4 hours prior to delivery. The incidence of early-onset GBS sepsis has been reduced by 65% in communities that have adopted the CDC GBS prevention guidelines. Currently, no evidence suggests an increased incidence of non-GBS early-onset sepsis with adoption of the guidelines, as had been feared.

B. Conjunctivitis

Infection of the conjunctiva may occur within the first few weeks of life. Prophylaxis with erythromycin 0.5% ophthalmic ointment immediately after delivery is now a standard part of newborn care. Conjunctivitis usually presents with injection of the conjunctiva and discharge from the eye, usually bilaterally, in the first week of life. Erythema of the conjunctiva helps differentiate conjunctivitis from lacrimal duct obstruction, a common cause of eye discharge in the neonate.

Chlamydia trachomatis and *Neisseria gonorrhoeae* are the most notable causes of neonatal conjunctivitis. Maternal treatment of either infection during pregnancy reduces the risk of infection in the neonate. Gonococcal conjunctivitis produces a purulent discharge and may cause serious complications, including blindness. A Gram stain and culture of the discharge should be performed if there is any suspicion of infection to determine appropriate therapy. It is important to recognize that the infant with *Chlamydia* conjunctivitis may have or may develop *Chlamydia* pneumonia. *Chlamydia* pneumonia commonly presents in the first 6 weeks of life with tachypnea and cough. The infant with gonococcal conjunctivitis should receive 7 days of IV or intramuscular treatment with a third-generation cephalosporin such as ceftriaxone. *Chlamydia* conjunctivitis is treated with oral erythromycin for 14 days.

C. Viral Infection

A number of viral infections can cause disease in the newborn. The infection may be acquired in utero or at the time of delivery. Antibody titers and cultures should be sent when congenital viral infection is suspected. A number of viruses (including cytomegalovirus [CMV], varicella, and parvovirus) and parasites such as *Toxoplasma gondii* are associated with congenital infection, and the presentation at birth varies significantly depending on the cause. Herpesvirus and enterovirus infections can present acutely with respiratory failure and/or shock. Hepatitis and coagulopathy are often seen in neonates with viral sepsis, even early in the disease process before end-organ damage is even suspected, and should raise suspicion about the possibility of a viral process. There is no maternal history of herpes simplex virus (HSV) in the majority of neonates diagnosed with HSV sepsis or encephalitis. Acyclovir is used to treat herpes viruses such as HSV and varicella.

Transmission from mother to infant at birth is one of the most efficient modes of hepatitis B virus (HBV). Between 80% and 90% of children born to mothers who are both hepatitis B surface antigen (HBsAg) and hepatitis B e antigen (HBeAg) positive will become infected, and 90% of those infants will become chronic HBV carriers. Transmission falls to less than 25% if HBeAg is negative and to 12% if anti-HBe is present. Babies born to HBsAg-positive mothers should receive hepatitis B immune globulin (HBIg) and the hepatitis B vaccine within 12 hours of delivery. If the mother's status is unknown at the time of delivery, the newborn should receive the vaccine within 12 hours of life. If the newborn weighs more than 2 kg, HBIg can be deferred for up to 7 days to allow determination of the mother's status according to the AAP *Red Book* guidelines. However, given the less reliable immune response to vaccine in the preterm host, HBIg should not be deferred in patients weighing less than 2 kg. Appropriate postexposure prophylaxis in the newborn has been shown to prevent transmission in 95% of exposures.

Perinatal infection with human immunodeficiency virus (HIV) now accounts for almost all new infections in preadolescents in the United States. The risk of perinatal transmission if an HIV-positive mother does not receive antiretroviral therapy during pregnancy is 13–39%. A trial of zidovudine during pregnancy and delivery, with continued treatment for the newborn for 6 weeks after delivery, showed a greater than 60% reduction in transmission. It is currently recommended that HIV-positive women receive zidovudine prophylaxis in addition to the standard current recommendations for antiretroviral therapy for all HIV-positive patients. Zidovudine prophylaxis/treatment of the newborn should be started and analysis for HIV DNA polymerase chain reaction sent when in utero exposure to HIV is recognized before 7 days of life.

Infant of the Diabetic Mother

From 50,000–100,000 infants are born to diabetic mothers every year in the United States. The infant of a diabetic mother (IDM) is at increased risk for congenital malformations, macrosomia, birth injury, and a number of postnatal complications, such as RDS, polycythemia, and hypoglycemia. With improved obstetric monitoring and neonatal care, perinatal mortality has decreased significantly over the past few decades. With decreased losses from stillbirths, perinatal asphyxia, and RDS, congenital malformations now represent the single most important cause of perinatal mortality and severe morbidity in IDMs.

Studies have shown that IDMs have a 2- to 8-fold higher risk of a structural malformation compared to infants born to nondiabetic mothers. The most common malformations in IDMs are neural tube defects, CHD, renal anomalies, and abnormalities of the genitourinary tract. The exact pathogenesis of the malformations is unclear, but various mechanisms, including altered levels of arachidonic acid and/or myoinositol, free-radical damage, and altered gene expression have been proposed. The risk of structural malformations has been clearly shown to correlate with poor glycemic control in the first trimester. Consequently, tight control of glucose levels must begin prior to conception in order to decrease the risk of structural malformations.

Metabolic alterations seen in IDMs are more closely associated with glycemic control later in pregnancy. Elevated maternal glucose levels result in elevated fetal glucose levels that produce hyperinsulinism in the fetus. Insulin is a growth factor, and abnormal exposure to insulin results in fetal macrosomia. After delivery, the hyperinsulinemic state persists, but there is no longer an ongoing supply of glucose coming across the placenta; the newborn is thus at risk for hypoglycemia. IDMs should be closely monitored after birth to ensure that glucose requirements are met. Severe and/or prolonged hypoglycemia can cause significant injury to the developing brain. Poor glucose control during the second and third trimesters is associated with an increased risk for macrosomia and neonatal hypoglycemia. Other metabolic derangements frequently seen in IDMs are hypocalcemia and hypomagnesemia.

IDMs are at increased risk for RDS. Surfactant production occurs later than normal in diabetic pregnancies. Polycythemia also occurs at a higher rate. The greater red cell volume, in turn, increases the risk of hyperbilirubinemia. Hyperglycemia and the resulting hyperinsulinemia in the fetus generate a catabolic state, causing oxygen consumption. Erythropoiesis is believed to occur as a response to fetal hypoxia.

Asymmetric hypertrophic cardiomyopathy is a frequent finding in IDMs. The cardiomyopathy may be asymptomatic, apparent only as cardiomegaly on CXR, or it may be clinically significant, usually as a result of left ventricular outflow tract obstruction and/or poor ventricular filling and cardiac output related to hypertrophy of the ventricular septum. The hypertrophy of the cardiac muscle resolves over time, and the only indicated treatment is supportive care.

Intrauterine Growth Restriction

Intrauterine growth restriction (IUGR) describes a pattern of aberrant and reduced fetal growth that is identified by prenatal ultrasound examinations. The growth restriction is classified as asymmetric if the head circumference, used as a marker for brain growth, is spared. IUGR refers to growth in utero, and IUGR newborns may or may not be small for gestational age (SGA). (The definition of SGA varies, but historically it has been defined as less than the 10th percentile for gestational age at birth.) IUGR can result from a range of processes that may originate with the fetus (chromosomal abnormalities, fetal gender, genetic inheritance, TORCH infection), the placenta (abnormal implantation or insertion of the cord, preeclampsia, placental insufficiency), or the mother (chronic disease such as diabetes, systemic lupus erythematosus, or cyanotic heart disease; smoking; abnormal uterine anatomy; low pregnancy weight gain). The etiology of IUGR in approximately 40% of patients is never determined. CMV and toxoplasmosis studies are sometimes sent for affected newborns to determine an infectious cause. However, given the number of idiopathic cases of IUGR, some have questioned the utility of sending these cultures for infants with no physical examination or imaging study findings suggestive of congenital infection. Prenatal management of the IUGR fetus is impacted by the increased risk of intrauterine demise and perinatal asphyxia with IUGR, but also requires consideration of the fact that gestational age at birth is still a major determinant of outcome in the premature growth-restricted infant. There is currently great interest in the connection between low birth weight and the development of type 2 diabetes, hypertension, and coronary artery disease in adulthood.

The Dysmorphic Infant

It is estimated that 2% of all newborns have a serious congenital malformation. Advances in prenatal care now allow for early diagnosis of many congenital birth defects or diseases, but many are still difficult or impossible to detect in utero. Dysmorphic features and structural abnormalities may be immediately apparent, or they may be subtle and identified only upon close inspection. Every newborn should undergo a thorough examination to identify features suggestive of underlying pathology, genetic abnormalities, or specific syndromes or disorders.

Transfer of the newborn to a referral center where an evaluation by a clinical geneticist or dysmorphologist can be conducted may be warranted if significant abnormalities are present. The remarkable progress in our understanding of human genetics over the past decade has dramatically increased our ability to identify the genetic defects responsible for countless diseases and syndromes. In addition, each year, more is understood about numerous multifactorial disorders, improving the odds that affected patients will be correctly diagnosed. A geneticist can help identify pertinent elements of the family, exposure, and prenatal history and direct a thorough but targeted radiologic and cytogenetic workup for the newborn. It is preferable to avoid making conclusions about the diagnosis (ie, a particular syndrome or sequence) until a complete evaluation has been performed. The emotional impact of an unsuspected defect or syndrome on the new parents should not be ignored, and misinformation can only hinder the process of acceptance (Table 22–1).

Table 22–1. Elements of counseling for developmental defects.

Description of the anomalies present
Cause of the condition (if known)
Indication of the prognosis
Discussion of immediate options
Therapeutic means that may be necessary
Potential for recurrence
Mode of inheritance (if known)
Late complications to be expected
In cases of death, the autopsy findings
Thorough answering of questions
Provisions for familial emotional support

Modified and reproduced, with permission, from Pernoll ML, King CR, Prescott GH. Genetics in obstetrics and gynecology. In: Wynn RM (ed). *Obstetrics and Gynecology Annual: 1980*. Vol 9. New York, NY: Appleton-Century-Crofts; 1980, p. 31.

Allan WC, Sobel DB. Neonatal intensive care neurology. *Semin Pediatr Neurol* 2004;11:119–128. PMID: 15259865.

American Academy of Pediatrics. *AAP 2003 Red Book: Report of the Committee on Infectious Diseases*. 26th ed. Elk Grove, IL: American Academy of Pediatrics; 2003.

Baltimore RS, Huie SM, Meek JI, et al. Early-onset neonatal sepsis in the era of group B streptococcal prevention. *Pediatrics* 2001;108:1094–1098. PMID: 11694686.

Berseth CL, Bisquera JA, Paje VU. Prolonging small feeding volumes early in life decreases the incidence of necrotizing enterocolitis in very low birth weight infants. *Pediatrics* 2003;111:529–534. PMID: 12613322.

Bin-Nun A, Bromiker R, Wilschanski M, et al. Oral probiotics prevent necrotizing enterocolitis in very low birth weight neonates. *J Pediatr* 2005;147:192–196. PMID: 16126048.

Boloker J, Bateman DA, Wung JT, et al. Congenital diaphragmatic hernia in 120 infants treated consecutively with permissive hypercapnia/spontaneous respiration/elective repair. *J Pediatr Surg* 2002;37:357–366. PMID: 11877648.

Centers for Disease Control and Prevention. National Center for Health Statistics. http://www.cdc.gov/nchs/. Accessed May 2010.

Cifuentes J, Bronstein J, Phibbs CS, et al. Mortality in low birth weight infants according to level of neonatal care at hospital of birth. *Pediatrics* 2002;109:745–751. PMID: 19986431.

Clark RH, Kueser TJ, Walker MW, et al. Low-dose nitric oxide therapy for persistent pulmonary hypertension of the newborn. *N Engl J Med* 2000;342:469. PMID: 10675427.

Dempsey EM, Barrington KJ. Short and long term outcomes following partial exchange transfusion in the polycythemic newborn: a systematic review. *Arch Dis Child Fetal Neonatal Ed* 2006;91:F2–F6. PMID: 16174666.

Hëller G, Richardson DK, Schnell R, et al. Are we regionalized enough? Early-neonatal deaths in low-risk births by the size of delivery units in Hesse, Germany 1990–1999. *Int J Epidemiol* 2002;31:1061. PMID: 12435785.

Khan N, Khazzi S. Yield and costs of screening growth-retarded infants for TORCH infections. *Am J Perinatol* 2000;17:131–135. PMID: 11012137.

Kunz AN, Noel JM, Fairchok MP. Two cases of Lactobacillus bacteremia during probiotic treatment of short gut syndrome. *J Pediatr Gastroenterol Nutr* 2004;38:457–458. PMID: 15085028.

Lin HC, Su BH, Chen AC, et al. Oral probiotics reduce the incidence and severity of necrotizing enterocolitis in very low birth weight infants. *Pediatrics* 2005;115:1–4. PMID: 15629973.

Martin JA, Kochanek KD, Strobino DM, et al. Annual summary of vital statistics—2003. *Pediatrics* 2005;115:619–634. PMID: 15741364.

Ment LR, Bada HS, Barnes P. Practice parameter: neuroimaging of the neonate: report of the Quality Standards Subcommittee of the American Academy of Neurology and the Practice Committee of the Child Neurology Society. *Neurology* 2002;58:1726–1738. PMID: 12084869.

Patole S. Prevention of necrotising enterocolitis: year 2004 and beyond. *J Matern Fetal Neonatal Med* 2005;17:69–80. PMID: 15804791.

Patole S, de Klerk N. Impact of standardized feeding regimens on incidence of neonatal necrotizing enterocolitis: a systematic review and meta-analysis of observational studies. *Arch Dis Child Fetal Neonatal Ed* 2005;90:F147-F151. PMID: 15724039.

Polin RA, Sahni R. Newer experience with CPAP. *Semin Neonatol* 2002;7:379–389. PMID: 12464500.

Schmidt B, Davis P, Moddemann D, et al. Trial of Indomethacin Prophylaxis in Preterms Investigators. Long-term effects of indomethacin prophylaxis in extremely-low-birth-weight infants. *N Engl J Med* 2001;344:1966–1972. PMID: 11430325.

Toby Study Group. Whole body hypothermia for the treatment of perinatal asphyxial encephalopathy: a randomized controlled trial. *BMC Pediatr* 2008;8:17. PMID: 18447921.

Tsao K, Lally KP. Surgical management of the newborn with congenital diaphragmatic hernia. *Fetal Diagn Ther* 2011;29:46–54. PMID: 20926849.

Van Meurs K. Is surfactant therapy beneficial in the treatment of the term newborn infant with congenital diaphragmatic hernia? *J Pediatr* 2004;145:312–316. PMID: 15343181.

Wunsch H, Mapstone J, Takala J. High-frequency ventilation versus conventional ventilation for the treatment of acute lung injury and acute respiratory distress syndrome: a systematic review and Cochrane analysis. *Anesth Analg* 2005;100: 1765–1771. PMID: 15920211.

23 Critical Care Obstetrics

Nathan S. Fox, MD
Johanna Weiss Goldberg, MD
Ramada S. Smith, MD

Critical care medicine has increasingly become an area of interest to the obstetrician–gynecologist. Pregnancy complications such as shock, thromboembolism, acute respiratory distress syndrome (ARDS), and coagulation disorders can lead to significant morbidity. Furthermore, the approach to these patients can be influenced by a variety of physiologic changes that are unique to pregnancy. This chapter provides a basic approach to some of the common clinical problems that often require complex multidisciplinary care and knowledge of invasive hemodynamic monitoring.

PULMONARY ARTERY CATHETERIZATION

The flow-directed pulmonary artery catheter has been a major addition to the clinician's armamentarium because of its applicability to a wide range of cardiorespiratory disorders. The catheter allows simultaneous measurement of central venous pressure (CVP), pulmonary artery pressure (PAP), pulmonary capillary wedge pressure (PCWP), cardiac output, and mixed venous oxygen saturation. The pulmonary artery catheter is a 7F triple-lumen polyvinyl chloride catheter with a balloon and thermodilution cardiac output sensor at the tip. The distal port is used to measure PAP when the balloon is deflated and PCWP when inflated. A proximal lumen is present 30 cm from the balloon tip; this can be used to monitor the CVP and to administer fluids and drugs. Both ports can be used to withdraw blood. Oximetric catheters also have 2 optical fibers that permit continuous measurement of mixed venous oxygen saturation by reflection spectrophotometry.

Insertion Technique

A 16-gauge catheter is used to gain access to the internal jugular or subclavian vein (Fig. 23–1). Pertinent anatomic landmarks for the internal jugular vein approach are shown in Figure 23–2. A guidewire is then introduced into the vein through the catheter, and the 16-gauge catheter sheath is removed. A pulmonary artery catheter is inserted over the guidewire, and the guidewire is removed. The central venous and pulmonary artery ports are connected to a pressure transducer, so that the characteristic waveforms of the various heart chambers can be identified as the catheter is advanced (Fig. 23–3). When the catheter is in the superior vena cava, the balloon is inflated with 1–1.5 mL of air, and the catheter is advanced forward into the main pulmonary artery. Table 23–1 shows the average distance in centimeters the catheter must be advanced from various insertion sites. From the main pulmonary artery, the flow of blood moves the catheter into a branch of the pulmonary artery, where it wedges and records the PCWP.

Criteria for verification of the true PCWP include (1) x-ray confirmation of catheter placement, (2) characteristic left atrial waveform configuration, (3) mean PCWP lower than mean PAP, (4) respiratory variation demonstrated by fluctuation of the PCWP waveform baseline with inspiration and expiration, and (5) blood samples showing higher oxygen tension and lower CO_2 tension than in arterial blood.

After deflation of the balloon, the pulmonary artery waveform should again be visualized. Fiberoptic catheters allow verification of PCWP by showing a sudden increase in mixed venous saturation to 95% or greater.

Indications for Invasive Monitoring

According to the American College of Obstetricians and Gynecologists, invasive hemodynamic monitoring may provide useful information for critical conditions during pregnancy such as:

- Shock (septic, hemorrhagic, cardiogenic, unexplained)
- Pulmonary edema (eg, severe pregnancy-induced hypertension [PIH], congestive heart failure [CHF], unexplained or refractory)
- Severe PIH with persistent oliguria unresponsive to fluid challenge
- ARDS
- Severe cardiac disease

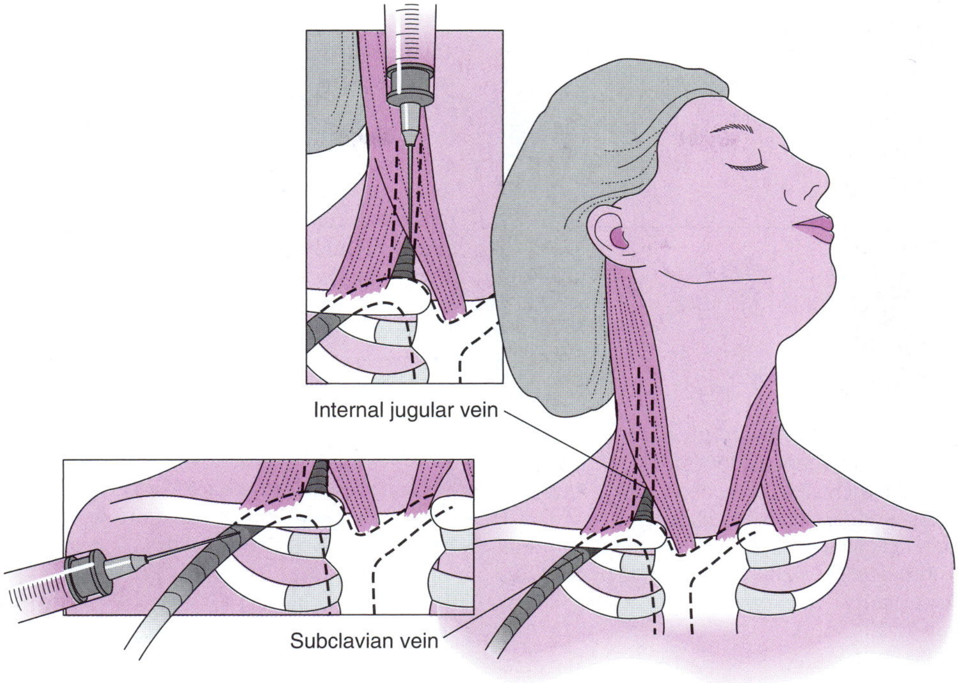

▲ **Figure 23–1.** Comparison of right internal jugular vein and subclavian vein vascular access sites for right heart catheterization.

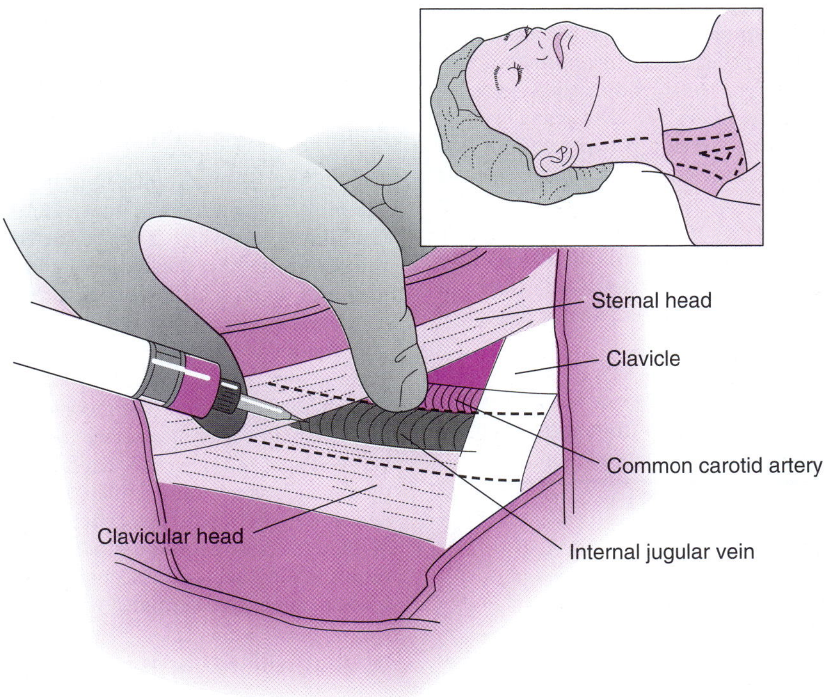

▲ **Figure 23–2.** Important anatomic landmarks associated with the internal jugular vein approach for right heart catheterization.

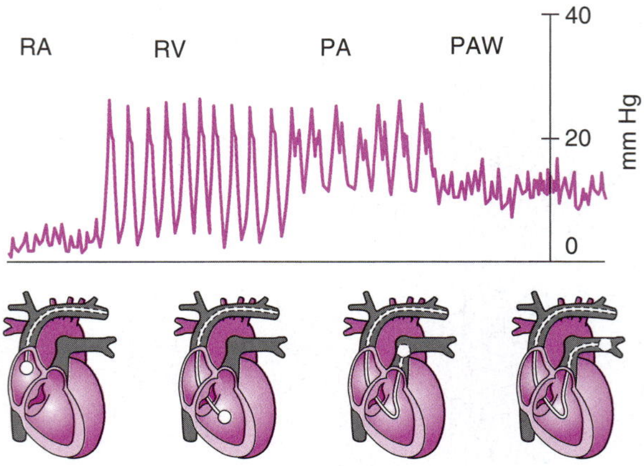

▲ **Figure 23–3.** Changes in waveforms observed during placement of a pulmonary artery catheter. RA, right atrium; RV, right ventricle; PA pulmonary artery; PAW, pulmonary artery wedge. (Reproduced, with permission, from Rosenthal MH. Intrapartum intensive care management of the cardiac patient. *Clin Obstet Gynecol* 1981;24:796.)

Hemodynamic Parameters Available With Pulmonary Artery Catheterization

During the diastolic period of the cardiac cycle, the left ventricle, left atrium, and pulmonary vascular bed essentially become a common chamber (Fig. 23–4). In a normal cardiovascular system, the left ventricular end-diastolic pressure (LVEDP), left atrial pressure, and PCWP are essentially interchangeable. A disparity may develop between PCWP and LVEDP when LVEDP is greater than 15 mm Hg; however, for clinical purposes, the PCWP provides a fairly accurate index of LVEDP, especially if the "a" wave (caused by retrograde transmission of the left atrial contraction) can be identified in the wedge tracing. The relationships described earlier can be substantially altered by mitral or aortic valvular disease.

Table 23–1. Distance to right atrium from various sites of insertion in pulmonary artery catheterization.

Vein	Distance to Right Atrium[1] (cm)
Internal jugular	15
Subclavian	15
Right antecubital	40
Left antecubital	50
Femoral	30

[1]Distance from right atrium to pulmonary artery is 8–15 cm.

A. Cardiac Output

The thermal sensing device in the tip of a pulmonary artery catheter allows for rapid determination of cardiac output by the thermodilution method. Five milliliters of 5% dextrose in water is injected through the central venous port at a constant distance from the thermistor tip. The use of this solution at room temperature can minimize sources of potential error associated with inaccurate temperature measurements and catheter warming. The change in pulmonary artery temperature is detected by the thermistor. The cardiac output is inversely proportional to the fall in temperature and is computed by planimetric or computerized methods. The average of 3 values within 10% of each other is typically utilized to calculate cardiac output.

B. Systemic Vascular Resistance

Systemic vascular resistance (SVR) represents the total resistance to forward flow of blood through the body's vascular tree. SVR is calculated as follows:

$$SVR = \frac{[(MAP - CVP)] \times 80}{CO}$$

During pregnancy, this parameter is usually in the range of 800–1200 dynes · s · cm^{-5}. Depending on the clinical condition, a reduction or increase in SVR may be desirable in the presence of normal blood pressure (eg, septic shock), in which a very low SVR may be seen despite normal or low blood pressure. In order to maintain vital organ perfusion, vasopressor therapy may be indicated to increase SVR.

C. Pulmonary Capillary Wedge Pressure

The PCWP provides important information on 2 basic parameters of cardiopulmonary function: (1) pulmonary venous pressure, which is a major determinant of pulmonary congestion; and (2) the left atrial and left ventricular filling pressures, from which ventricular function curves can be constructed.

Pulmonary capillary wedge pressure can be reliably assessed by CVP monitoring only in the absence of significant myocardial dysfunction. The measurement of PCWP has certain advantages over measurement of CVP alone. A disparity between right and left ventricular function may be seen in conditions such as myocardial infarction, valvular disease, sepsis, and severe PIH. Under these circumstances, the management of fluid therapy based on CVP alone could have adverse results. Additionally, cardiac output and mixed venous oxygen tension cannot be determined with a simple CVP catheter.

D. Ventricular Function Curves

Myocardial performance is best interpreted in terms of left ventricular function curves (ie, the Frank-Starling relationship). The cardiac output and PCWP are used to construct

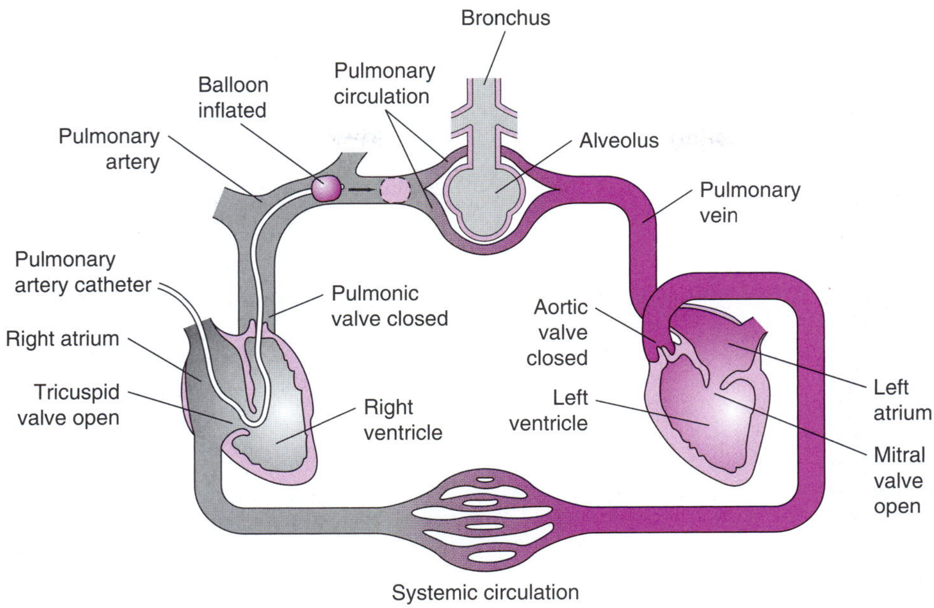

▲ **Figure 23–4.** Pulmonary capillary wedge pressure in diastole (ventricles relaxed).

the ventricular function curve by plotting the ventricular stroke work index against the mean atrial pressure or ventricular end-diastolic pressure (usually the PCWP). The left ventricular stroke work index is calculated by the following formula:

$$LVSWI = SVI \times (MAP - PCWP) \times 0.0136$$

(LVSWI = left ventricular stroke work index [g-m/m^2]; SVI = stroke volume index [mL/beat/m^2]; MAP = mean arterial pressure [mm Hg]; PCWP = pulmonary capillary wedge pressure [mm Hg]).

Ventricular function curves provide a useful index of cardiovascular status to guide inotropic and vasoactive drug therapy. Evaluation of myocardial contractility by ventricular function curves allows one to obtain optimal filling pressures and stroke volume index in critically ill patients. The effects of therapy (eg, diuretics, antihypertensive agents, or volume expanders) can be evaluated on the basis of performance. Under normal conditions, a small rise in filling pressure is accompanied by a rapid rise in stroke work. Unfavorable conditions such as hypoxia or myocardial depression produce a shift in the curve to the right and downward such that lower stroke work indices are seen at higher filling pressures.

E. Mixed Venous Oxygen Saturation

The mixed venous oxygen saturation (SvO_2) reflects the body's capacity to provide adequate tissue oxygenation. This parameter is affected by cardiac output, hemoglobin concentration, arterial oxygen saturation, and tissue oxygen consumption. An SvO_2 of 60–80% usually indicates normal oxygen delivery and demand with adequate tissue perfusion. An SvO_2 greater than 80% reflects increased oxygen delivery and decreased oxygen utilization. This situation may be seen in patients with hypothermia or sepsis who are receiving supplemental oxygen. A high SvO_2 may also provide confirmatory evidence that the pulmonary artery catheter is in the wedge position. Finally, a low SvO_2 (<60%) indicates increased oxygen demands with decreased oxygen delivery due to anemia, low cardiac output, or decreased arterial oxygen saturation.

Measurement of SvO_2 allows for continuous monitoring of cardiorespiratory reserve by providing an index of tissue oxygen delivery and utilization. Changes in SvO_2 will be apparent with infusion of vasoactive drugs, volume loading, or afterload reduction. Although many intensive care units rely on direct measurement of cardiac output alone, this parameter does not always accurately reflect tissue oxygenation. For instance, normal cardiac output might not be adequate to meet increased oxygen requirements in malignant hyperthermia or thyroid storm.

F. Maternal Oxygen Consumption

Mixed venous oxygen saturation results can be used with arterial blood gas analysis to provide useful information about the metabolic status of the critically ill obstetric patient. Resting maternal oxygen consumption progressively increases during pregnancy. Occasionally, one needs to pay particular attention to the metabolic status of critically ill women or those with ARDS. Factors such as tachycardia or fever that are associated with increased oxygen consumption should be minimized under these circumstances.

The Fick relationship:

$$CO = \frac{VO_2}{AvO_2 diff.} \times 100$$

provides a method for calculating oxygen consumption (VO_2), if the cardiac output (CO) and systemic arteriovenous oxygen (AvO_2) concentration difference is known. The AvO_2 difference can be calculated by subtracting the oxygen content of desaturated mixed venous blood from that of arterial blood that passes through the pulmonary artery catheter. For example, a patient with a cardiac output minus AvO_2 difference of 5 mL would have an oxygen consumption (VO_2) of 300 mL.

$$6000 \text{ mL min}^{-1} \times 5 \text{ mL per 100 mL blood}$$
$$VO_2 \ 100 = 300 \text{ mL min}^{-1}$$

An understanding of these relationships will allow the clinician to better understand how to use physiologic variables for interpreting the hemodynamic and pulmonary condition of critically ill patients.

G. Colloid Osmotic Pressure

The plasma colloid oncotic pressure (COP) is another measurement that can be useful in critical care (Table 23–2). Plasma COP is the pressure exerted by certain plasma proteins that hold fluid in the intravascular space. Albumin accounts for 75% of the oncotic pressure of plasma, with the rest coming from globulin and fibrinogen. It has been demonstrated in dogs that iatrogenic reduction in plasma proteins resulted in pulmonary edema with only minimal increases in left atrial pressure. Subsequent studies in humans identified cases of pulmonary edema in which normal or slightly elevated PCWP was present. From these studies, the important concept of a COP-PCWP gradient evolved. It appears that when the COP-PCWP gradient is less than 4 mm Hg, the likelihood of pulmonary edema is increased, although not all patients with a decreased gradient will develop pulmonary edema. The determination of COP and its relationship to the PCWP can play a crucial role in the detection of patients likely to develop pulmonary edema in the face of normal left-sided filling pressures.

Studies of pregnant women have demonstrated that patients with certain conditions in which the risk of pulmonary edema is markedly increased tend to have lowered COP (eg, hypovolemic shock, severe PIH, prolonged tocolytic therapy, and frank pulmonary edema).

Table 23–2. Serum colloid oncotic pressure during pregnancy.

	Normotensive (mm Hg)	Hypertensive (mm Hg)
Antepartum (term)	22.4 ± 0.5	17.9 ± 0.7
Postpartum (first 24 hours)	15.4 ± 2.1	13.7 ± 0.5

Complications

The most common complication associated with pulmonary artery catheter placement is dysrhythmia. More serious complications also include pulmonary infarction, thromboembolism, balloon rupture with air embolism, pulmonary artery or valve rupture, catheter knotting, infection, arterial puncture, thromboembolism, pneumothorax, and pulmonary hemorrhage. Table 23–3 summarizes the complication rates for pulmonary artery catheterization.

A. Dysrhythmia

Premature ventricular contractions may transiently occur as the catheter tip enters the right ventricle. However, they

Table 23–3. Complications of pulmonary artery catheterization.

Complication	Incidence (%)
Premature ventricular contractions	15–27
Arterial puncture	8
Superficial cellulitis	3
Thromboembolism	?
Pneumothorax	1–2
Balloon rupture	<1
Pulmonary infarction/ischemia	1–7
Pulmonary artery rupture	<1
Catheter knotting	<1
Catheter-related sepsis	1

(Reproduced, with permission, from Hankins GDV, Cunningham FG. Severe preeclampsia and eclampsia: Controversies in management. *Williams Obstetrics* 1991;18(suppl):11. Appleton & Lange.)

usually resolve after advancement of the catheter into the pulmonary artery. If the dysrhythmia is refractory to lidocaine, 50–100 mg given intravenously, the catheter should be withdrawn from the cardiac chambers.

B. Pulmonary Infarction

Pulmonary infarction may occur when the catheter migrates distally and wedges spontaneously for a prolonged period. This complication, as well as thromboembolism, may be avoided by monitoring the PCWP at regular intervals and by using a continuous heparinized flow system.

C. Balloon Rupture

Balloon rupture can be avoided by limiting the number of balloon inflations and by inflating only to the smallest necessary volume. Inflation of the balloon beyond 2 mL of air is unnecessary and may be harmful. To avoid rupture of a pulmonary artery branch, inflation of the balloon should be stopped immediately when the wedge tracing is seen.

D. Catheter Knotting

Catheter knotting is usually the result of advancing the catheter 10–15 cm farther than is necessary to reach the right ventricle or pulmonary artery. Withdrawing the catheter while the balloon is still inflated may cause tricuspid rupture or chordae tendineae tears.

E. Infection and Phlebitis

Infection and phlebitis can be minimized by using aseptic technique. The risk of associated sepsis is related to excessive catheter manipulation and the duration of catheterization.

NONINVASIVE MONITORING FOR CRITICALLY ILL PATIENTS

Pulse oximetry is a simple tool that can be used with invasive monitoring for patients with cardiovascular or respiratory compromise. The correlation between pulse oximetry and direct blood oxygen saturation is excellent when oxygen saturation is greater than 60%. Factors adversely affecting the accuracy of pulse oximetry include movement, peripheral vasoconstriction, hypotension, anemia, hypothermia, intravascular dye, and possibly nail polish.

OBSTETRIC SHOCK

Shock may be defined as an imbalance between oxygen supply and demand. The basic underlying defect is a significant reduction in the supply of oxygenated blood to various tissues due to inadequate perfusion. In obstetrics, this reduction often results from hemorrhage, sepsis, or pump failure. The physiologic compensation common to all shock states involves tachycardia and peripheral vasoconstriction to maximize cerebral and cardiac perfusion by way of the sympathetic nervous system. Failure of these compensatory mechanisms will lead to a predominance of anaerobic metabolism and lactic acidosis, which can be potentially devastating to the patient and fetus. Cardiogenic shock may be seen in pregnant women with cardiac dysrhythmias, congenital heart disease, peripartum cardiomyopathy, and congestive heart failure. The following discussion will focus on 2 of the more common shock syndromes complicating pregnancy—those related to hemorrhage and sepsis.

HYPOVOLEMIC SHOCK

ESSENTIALS OF DIAGNOSIS

- Recent history of acute blood loss or excessive diuresis
- Hypotension, tachycardia, tachypnea, and oliguria with progression to altered mental status
- Precipitous drop in hematocrit (if from hemorrhage)

Pathogenesis

Hypovolemic shock is a leading cause of maternal mortality in the United States and is most commonly associated with obstetric hemorrhage. Bleeding severe enough to cause hemorrhagic shock may result from a wide variety of conditions, including ruptured ectopic pregnancy; abruptio placentae; placenta previa; placenta accreta; rupture, atony, or inversion of the uterus; surgical procedures; obstetric lacerations; or retained products of conception.

During normal pregnancy, the blood volume expands by approximately 1500 mL. This hypervolemia results from hormonal alterations and may be considered protective against peripartum bleeding. During acute hemorrhage, the body responds to volume loss by hemodynamic, volume-altering, and hormonal mechanisms.

Hemodynamic adjustments result from activation of the sympathetic nervous system. These changes include vasoconstriction of arteriolar resistance vessels, constriction of venous capacitance vessels, and redistribution of blood flow away from peripheral organs to preserve adequate cerebral and cardiac blood flow.

Volume adjustments occur from extravascular fluid shifts into the intravascular compartment. The rate of plasma refill depends on the magnitude of volume depletion.

If these mechanisms are insufficient to restore circulatory function, other compensatory effects, such as secretion of antidiuretic hormone (ADH), cortisol, aldosterone, and catecholamines will occur. Epinephrine, in addition to causing peripheral vasoconstriction, will have inotropic and chronotropic effects on the heart. ADH, cortisol, and aldosterone will help conserve water and salt, which may then result in reduced blood flow to the kidneys and decreased urine output.

These homeostatic mechanisms serve to maintain adequate tissue perfusion until approximately 25–30% of the circulating blood volume is lost. Inadequate tissue perfusion and oxygenation will then lead to anaerobic metabolism and lactic acidosis. Over a prolonged period of vasoconstriction, there may be decompensation of the peripheral vasculature leading to damaged or leaky capillaries. Observations of blood flow regulation during pregnancy suggest that uterine arteries have limited capacity to autoregulate fetoplacental perfusion. Thus uteroplacental blood flow is critically dependent on systemic maternal cardiac output.

Clinical Findings

The clinical manifestations of hemorrhagic shock depend on the quantity and rate of volume depletion. Orthostatic signs and symptoms may be masked by the hypervolemia of pregnancy, especially if a source of bleeding is not evident. Additionally, because pregnant women usually are young and healthy, their ability to tolerate significant blood loss is greater than a typical medical patient. Therefore, they may experience significant blood loss before showing some of the signs or symptoms of shock. Obvious hypotension and tachycardia in the presence of external bleeding should alert the clinician to the possibility of shock. A careful physical examination will identify decreased tissue perfusion in several different organ systems, including the heart, brain, kidneys, lungs, and skin. Altered mental status, dizziness, diaphoresis, and cold, clammy extremities, as well as a fast, "thready" pulse are common findings in significant hemorrhagic shock. Oliguria (<30 mL/h), CVP of less than 5 cm H_2O, and PCWP of less than 5 mm Hg are all consistent with significant volume depletion. Fetal heart monitoring may reveal bradycardia or late decelerations.

Differential Diagnosis

Hypovolemic shock should be differentiated from other shock syndromes resulting from sepsis or heart failure. Usually, there is a history of profound bleeding. Because shock may affect several organ systems, it is essential that its underlying cause be identified. Patients with septic shock will tend to be febrile, with associated abnormal white blood cell counts and clinical evidence of infection. Cardiogenic shock may be associated with clinical and radiographic evidence of pulmonary congestion or a previous history of heart disease.

Complications

Electrolyte imbalance, acidosis, acute tubular necrosis, stress-induced gastric ulceration, pulmonary edema, and ARDS are common complications associated with hemorrhagic shock. Myocardial infarction is a rare complication in the obstetric population.

Treatment

The treatment of hemorrhagic shock should be directed toward replacing blood volume and optimizing cardiac performance. The source of bleeding should be controlled. Uterine atony that is unresponsive to massage and oxytocin may benefit from methylergonovine (0.2 mg intramuscularly), 15-methyl prostaglandin $F_{2\alpha}$ (0.25 mg intramuscularly), or misoprostol (1000 mcg rectally). Persistent bleeding may require uterine artery ligation, hypogastric artery ligation, or even caesarean hysterectomy. Decisions regarding blood and fluid replacement should be guided by central pressures and urine output, although pulmonary artery catheterization is rarely necessary. A military antishock trousers suit will mobilize blood pooled in the lower body and return it to the central circulation, improving systemic cardiac output and organ perfusion. Supplemental oxygen will minimize tissue hypoxia and fetal acidosis.

Initial rapid volume replacement with crystalloid solution given through a large-bore intravenous site is a temporizing measure until blood replacement is possible. Typically, 1–2 L of lactated Ringer's solution can be administered as rapidly as possible. Compared with normal saline, the electrolyte composition of lactated Ringer's solution more closely approximates plasma, and the metabolism of lactate to bicarbonate provides some buffering capacity for acidosis.

Guidelines for perioperative transfusion of red blood cells have been defined by the National Institutes of Health. Initial treatment of hemorrhagic shock should involve volume replacement by crystalloid or colloid solutions that do not carry risks for disease transmission or transfusion reaction. The use of perioperative red blood cell transfusion should not rely solely on the dogma of "transfusing to a hematocrit above 30%" as the sole criterion because there is poor evidence supporting its usefulness. The decision of whether to transfuse red cells should also take into account other factors such as patient age, hemodynamic status, anticipated bleeding, and medical or obstetrical complications. If it is necessary to transfuse large amounts of blood, it is important to note and correct the presence of electrolyte imbalances, acid–base abnormalities, hypothermia, and the dilution of platelets and coagulation factors, which may require the transfusion of other blood products.

The risk of posttransfusion hepatitis has been dramatically decreased by testing blood products with a commercially available hepatitis C assay. The test is a qualitative, enzyme-linked immunosorbent assay (ELISA) for the detection of antibody to hepatitis C virus (anti-HCV) in human serum or plasma. The ELISA test has a specificity of 99.84% in a low prevalence population. A supplemental assay, the recombinant immunoblot assay, can be performed on blood that has a repeat reactive anti-HCV.

Fluid balance from intravenous infusions or urine output should be meticulously recorded with daily weights. Oliguria refractory to volume loading may be improved by the addition of intravenous dopamine in low doses (2–5 μg/kg/min) to improve renal perfusion. A diuretic such as bumetanide 0.5–1 mg administered intravenously (IV), not to exceed 10 mg/day, should be considered for patients with prolonged oliguria despite normal or elevated pulmonary capillary wedge pressures.

Blood tests should include complete blood count, serum electrolytes, creatinine, arterial blood gas analysis, and coagulation profile. Urinalysis is also important. A baseline chest radiograph and electrocardiogram are desirable. Typed and cross-matched transfusion products should be available from the blood bank. One to 2 ampules of sodium bicarbonate (50–100 mEq) can be administered intravenously to correct acidosis (pH <7.20). Frequent serial hematocrits may provide an index of acute blood loss. A baseline hematologic profile (prothrombin time [PT], partial thromboplastin time [PTT], fibrinogen, platelets) is necessary to evaluate the possibility of coagulopathy.

Prognosis

Maternal and fetal survival rates are directly related to the magnitude of volume depletion and length of time the patient remains in shock. If the hemorrhage is controlled and intravascular volume is restored within a reasonable interval, the prognosis is generally good in the absence of associated complications. However, the return of fetal blood flow may lag behind correction of maternal flow.

American College of Obstetricians and Gynecologists. *Postpartum Hemorrhage.* ACOG Practice Bulletin No. 76. Washington, DC: ACOG; October 2006.

SEPTIC SHOCK

ESSENTIALS OF DIAGNOSIS

- History of recent hospitalization or surgery
- Pelvic or abdominal infection with positive confirmatory cultures
- Temperature instability, confusion, hypotension, oliguria, cardiopulmonary failure

Pathogenesis

Septic shock is a life-threatening disorder secondary to bacteremia. The American College of Obstetricians and Gynecologists defines septic shock as sepsis with hypotension despite adequate fluid resuscitation, with the presence of perfusion abnormalities including (but not limited to) lactic acidosis and oliguria. The incidence of bacteremia in obstetric patients has been estimated to be between 0.7% and 10%. Although gram-negative bacteria are usually responsible for most of these infections, septic shock may also result from infection with other bacteria, fungi, protozoa, or viruses. The most common cause of obstetric septic shock is postoperative endometritis (85%). Other commonly associated conditions include antepartum pyelonephritis, septic abortion, and chorioamnionitis.

Sepsis may lead to a systemic inflammatory response that can be triggered not only by infections, but also by noninfectious disorders, such as trauma and pancreatitis. However, there is strong evidence to support the concept that endotoxin is responsible for the pathogenesis of gram-negative septic shock. *Escherichia coli* has been implicated in 25–50% of cases of septic hypotension, but a variety of other organisms may be causative, including *Klebsiella, Enterobacter, Serratia, Proteus, Pseudomonas, Streptococcus, Peptostreptococcus, Staphylococcus, Fusobacterium, Clostridium*, and *Bacteroides*. The gram-negative endotoxin theory does not explain gram-positive shock, although an understanding of the proposed mechanisms will serve to exemplify the multisystemic effects of this disorder.

Endotoxin is a complex lipopolysaccharide present in the cell walls of gram-negative bacteria. The active component of endotoxin, lipid A, is responsible for initiating activation of the coagulation, fibrinolysis, complement, prostaglandin, and kinin systems. Activation of the coagulation and fibrinolysis systems may lead to consumptive coagulopathy. Complement activation leads to the release by leukocytes of mediators that are responsible for damage to vascular endothelium, platelet aggregation, intensification of the coagulation cascade, and degranulation of mast cells with histamine release. Histamine will cause increased capillary permeability, decreased plasma volume, vasodilatation, and hypotension. Release of bradykinin and β-endorphins also contributes to systemic hypotension. Early stages of septic shock involve low SVR and high cardiac output with a relative decrease in intravascular volume. Late or cold shock subsequently involves an endogenous myocardial depressant factor that has not been isolated. This factor is associated with decreased cardiac output and continued low SVR in the absence of pressor agents. Recent studies suggest that tumor necrosis factor (TNF) may lead to depressed myocardial function during septic shock. Monocytes and macrophages incubated with endotoxin produce this 17-kDa polypeptide within 40 minutes. Direct injection of TNF into animals leads to many of the changes seen in endotoxic shock. Other possible factors include interleukin (IL)-1, IL-6, IL-8, interferon gamma, and granulocyte stimulating factor.

Clinical Findings

A. Symptoms and Signs

Septic shock can be divided into 3 stages: preshock, early shock (warm shock), and late (or cold) shock. In preshock, patients present with tachypnea and respiratory alkalosis (above the mild respiratory alkalosis seen in normal pregnancy). Their condition is best described as a moderate hyperdynamic state, with elevated cardiac output, decreasing SVR, and normal blood pressures. Response to therapy will be greatest at this stage. Early shock is a more hyperdynamic state. Blood pressure drops (systolic blood pressure < 60 mm Hg), and SVR decreases dramatically (< 400 dynes · s · cm^{-5}). Altered mental status, temperature instability, and sinusoidal fluctuations in arterial blood pressure may be seen at this stage. As this condition progresses into late shock, activation of the sympathetic nervous system with release of catecholamines will lead to intense vasoconstriction, which serves to shunt blood from the peripheral tissues to the heart and brain (cold shock). The compensatory vasoconstriction results in increased cardiac work. Lactic acidosis, poor coronary perfusion, and the influence of myocardial depressant factor may also contribute to poor cardiac performance (Fig. 23–5). The fetus is more resistant to the effects of endotoxin than the mother; however, alterations in uteroplacental flow can lead to hypoxia, acidosis, placental abruption, intracranial hemorrhage, and fetal demise.

The clinical manifestations of septic shock depend on the target organs affected. The most common cause of death in patients with this condition is respiratory insufficiency secondary to ARDS.

B. Laboratory Findings

Complete blood cell count, serum electrolytes, urinalysis, baseline arterial blood gases, chest radiograph, and a coagulation profile are laboratory studies important in the management of these patients. Hematologic findings may include significant anemia, thrombocytopenia, and leukocytosis. Serum electrolytes are often abnormal because of acidosis, fluid shifts, or decreased renal perfusion. Urinalysis permits evaluation of renal involvement. In addition to urine cultures, aerobic and anaerobic blood cultures may be helpful to confirm the diagnosis and guide antibiotic therapy.

Arterial blood gas measurements and a chest radiograph will facilitate clinical assessment of the ventilatory and oxygenation status. Early stages of septic shock will be associated with respiratory alkalosis, which later progresses to metabolic acidosis.

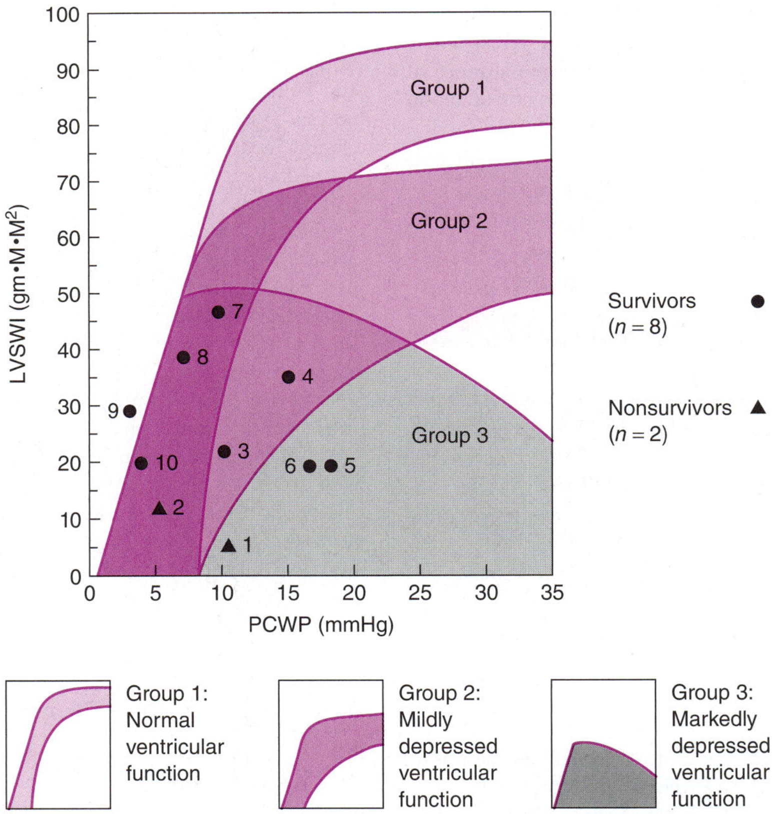

▲ **Figure 23–5.** Presenting left ventricular function of 10 pregnant women with septic hypotension. LVSWI, left ventricular stroke work index; PCWP, pulmonary capillary wedge pressure. (Reproduced, with permission, from Lee W, Clark SL, Cotton DB, et al. Septic shock during pregnancy. *Am J Obstet Gynecol* 1988;159:410.)

A baseline electrocardiogram (ECG) should be performed to rule out myocardial infarction or cardiac dysrhythmia. Abdominal radiographic studies may be useful to rule out other intrapelvic or intra-abdominal sources of obstetric sepsis (eg, bowel perforation, uterine perforation, tubo-ovarian abscess). Significant disseminated intravascular coagulation (DIC) will be identified by abnormal PT, PTT, or fibrinogen levels.

Differential Diagnosis

The differential diagnosis should include other hypovolemic and cardiogenic shock syndromes. Additional causes of acute cardiopulmonary compromise include amniotic fluid embolism, pulmonary thromboembolism, cardiac tamponade, aortic dissection, and diabetic ketoacidosis. The history, physical examination, and laboratory studies will usually be sufficient to distinguish between these diagnoses.

Complications

Numerous complications may occur with septic shock, depending on the target organs involved. Aside from ARDS, some of the more serious complications include congestive heart failure and cardiac dysrhythmias. Systemic hypotension and ischemic end-organ damage can lead to hepatic failure or renal insufficiency. Fetal or maternal demise are the most dire outcomes.

Treatment

Successful management of obstetric septic shock depends on early identification and aggressive treatment focused on stabilization of the patient, removal of underlying causes of sepsis, broad-spectrum antibiotic coverage, and treatment of associated complications. Febrile patients with mild hypotension who respond rapidly to volume infusion alone do not require invasive monitoring. In other cases, the pulmonary artery catheter should be used to guide specific therapeutic maneuvers for optimizing myocardial performance and maintaining systemic cardiac output and blood pressure. A hemodynamic approach for stabilizing pregnant women with septic shock should include (1) volume repletion and hemostasis, (2) inotropic therapy with dopamine on the basis of left ventricular function curves, and (3) addition of peripheral vasoconstrictors (phenylephrine first, then norepinephrine) to maintain afterload (Fig. 23–6).

A. General Measures

Septic shock during pregnancy should be treated with a broad-spectrum antibiotic regimen such as ampicillin, gentamicin, and clindamycin. Aminoglycoside maintenance doses should be titrated in relation to serum peak and trough levels, or a 24-hour dosing regimen may be used. Newer antibiotics such as imipenem, cilastatin, vancomycin, and the extended spectrum penicillins (eg, ticarcillin) are also proving to be effective therapies. There must be a careful search for infected or necrotic foci that can result in persistent bacteremia, and surgical intervention may be necessary. In one study, 40% of septic obstetric patients required surgical removal of infected products of conception, and all survived. If chorioamnionitis is present in the septic obstetric patient, prompt delivery is necessary. However, if the pregnancy is not the cause of infection, immediate delivery is usually not required. Supportive care should also include control of fever with antipyretics, hypothermic cooling blankets, or both. Correction of maternal acidosis, hypoxemia, and systemic hypotension will usually improve any abnormalities in the fetal heart tracing.

B. Cardiovascular Support

Aggressive treatment of obstetric septic shock must rapidly and effectively reverse organ hypoperfusion, improve oxygen delivery, and correct acidosis. Priority should be given to cardiopulmonary support with the additional understanding that other major organ systems can also be severely affected.

A sequential hemodynamic approach for stabilizing obstetric septic shock with volume repletion, inotropic therapy, and peripheral vasoconstrictors is recommended. Volume therapy initially begins with 1–2 L of lactated Ringer's solution infused over approximately 15 minutes. However, it is important that volume infusion not be withheld in a hypotensive patient pending placement of a pulmonary artery catheter. The total amount of crystalloid administered should be guided by the presence or absence of maternal hypoxemia secondary to pulmonary edema and left ventricular filling pressures, as estimated by PCWP.

In general, myocardial performance will be optimized according to the Starling mechanism at a PCWP of 14–16 mm Hg. Such preload optimization is mandatory before the initiation of inotropic therapy. Blood component therapy can also be an important adjunctive measure if the patient has experienced significant hemorrhage and has developed an associated coagulopathy.

If the shock state persists despite volume replacement and adequate hemostasis, efforts should be directed toward improving myocardial performance and vascular tone. Inotropic agents such as dopamine, dobutamine, or isoproterenol are excellent choices for improving myocardial contractility in an obstetric patient with a failing heart (Table 23–4). We recommend dopamine as the first-line drug of choice for treating septic hypotension when inotropic therapy is indicated. This substance is a chemical precursor of norepinephrine that has alpha-adrenergic, beta-adrenergic, and dopaminergic receptor stimulating actions. The dopamine infusion is initiated at 2–5 μg/kg/min and titrated against its effect on improving cardiac output and blood pressure in patients with obstetric septic shock. At low doses (0.5–5.0 μg/kg/min), this sympathomimetic amine acts primarily on the dopaminergic receptors, leading to vasodilation and improved perfusion of the renal and mesenteric vascular beds.

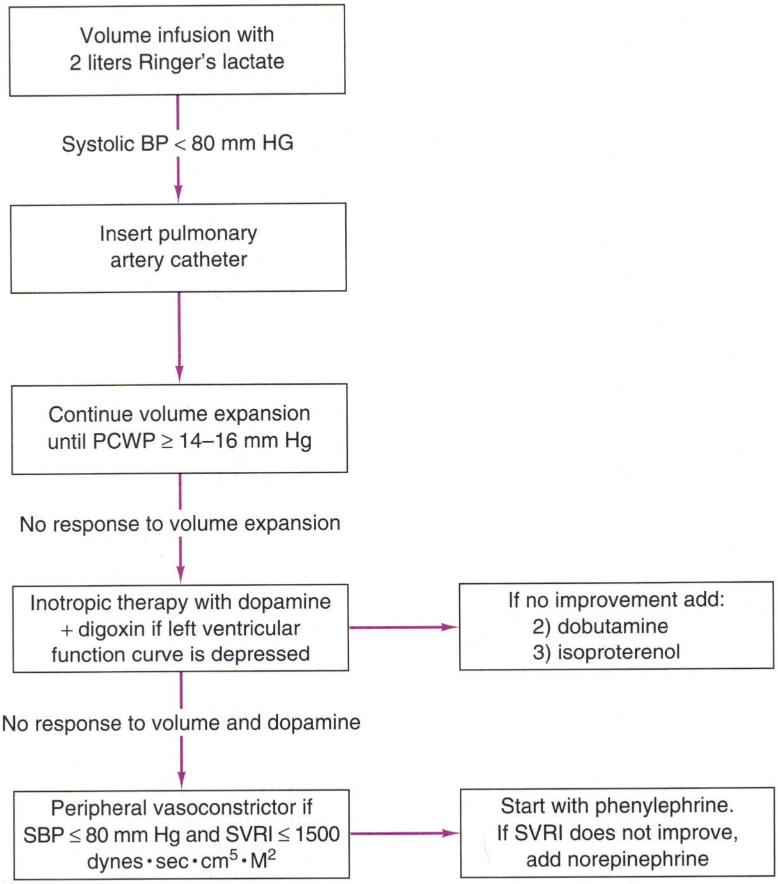

▲ **Figure 23–6.** Hemodynamic algorithm for treatment of obstetric septic shock. SVRI, systemic vascular resistance index; PCWP, pulmonary capillary wedge pressure; SBP, systolic blood pressure. (Reproduced, with permission, from Lee W, Clark SL, Cotton DB, et al. Septic shock during pregnancy. *Am J Obstet Gynecol* 1988;159:410.)

Table 23–4. Sympathomimetic and vasopressor drugs useful for therapy of obstetric septic shock.

Agent	Maintenance Dose Range[1]	Therapeutic Goals
Inotropic		
Dopamine	2-10 μg/kg/min	Cardiac index ≥ 3 L/min/m^2 SBP ≥ 80 mm Hg
Dobutamine	2-10 μg/kg/min	Optimize left ventricular function curves
Isoproterenol	1-20 μg/min	
Vasopressors		
Phenylephrine	1–5 μg/min	SVRI ≥ 1500 dynes · 5 · cm^{-5}· Cm^{-2}
Norepinephrine	1-4 μg/min	

SBP, systolic blood pressure; SVRI, systemic vascular resistance index.
[1]Drug dosages that are administered by μg/kg/min can be prepared by the following method:
1.5 mg × body weight (kg) = total mg in 250 mL 5% dextrose in water
10 mL/h = 1 μg/kg/min
20 mL/h = 2 μg/kg/min

Higher dopamine doses (5.0–15.0 μg/kg/min) are associated with predominant effects on the β receptors of the heart. The beta-adrenergic effects are responsible for improved myocardial contractility, stroke volume, and cardiac output. Much higher dopamine dosages (15–20 μg/kg/min) will elicit an alpha-adrenergic effect, similar to a norepinephrine infusion, and result in generalized vasoconstriction. Vasoconstrictive action associated with high doses of infused dopamine can actually be detrimental to organ perfusion and will rarely be useful under these clinical circumstances. Although myocardial performance after dopamine therapy is best evaluated by ventricular function curves, it is reasonable to maintain a systemic cardiac index above 3 L/min/m^2.

If satisfactory ventricular function is not achieved with dopamine, a second inotropic agent such as dobutamine (2–20 μg/kg) should be added to the dopamine regimen. Dobutamine is a direct myocardial β_1 stimulant that increases cardiac output with only minimal tachycardia. Isoproterenol should be considered a third-line agent, which can be titrated at 1–20 μg/min. This drug acts primarily on beta-adrenergic receptors to increase contractility and heart rate. However, potential side effects may include ventricular ectopy, excessive tachycardia, and undesired vasodilatation. Digoxin is commonly added to the previously described regimen to improve the force and velocity of myocardial contraction. This agent is given in a loading dose of 0.5 mg IV, followed by 0.25 mg every 4 hours for a total dose of 1.0 mg. IV digoxin should be given under continuous ECG monitoring with special attention to serum potassium levels. The usual maintenance dosage during pregnancy is 0.25–0.37 mg/dL depending on plasma drug levels.

A peripheral vasoconstrictor may be initiated if there is a reduced systemic vascular resistance index (SVRI; less than 1500 dynes · s · cm^{-5}) accompanied by a systolic blood pressure of less than 80 mm Hg despite inotropic therapy. It should be emphasized that maintenance of afterload appears to be a major hemodynamic determinant associated with maternal survival. Because of its pure alpha-adrenergic activity (which increases SVR), phenylephrine (1–5 μg/kg/min) is the initial drug of choice. Norepinephrine is only indicated for septic shock patients with decreased afterload who do not respond to volume loading, inotropic therapy, and phenylephrine. This drug is a mixed adrenergic agonist with a primary effect on the alpha receptors, which leads to generalized vasoconstriction and increased SVR. Although the therapy of septic shock should focus primarily on stabilization of maternal factors, vasopressor agents should be administered cautiously during pregnancy because they have been reported to decrease uterine blood flow in animals with experimentally induced spinal hypotension.

Some investigators have advocated large doses of corticosteroids for the acute management of septic shock, but human clinical trials have failed to demonstrate any conclusive benefit.

Newer investigational agents include corticosteroids and antiendotoxin therapy. Multicenter trials of endotoxin antibodies have suggested a possible improvement in mortality rate and organ failure in some subgroups of nonpregnant septic patients.

Prognosis

Despite all medical and surgical therapeutic options, the overall maternal mortality rate in septic shock is approximately 50%. The prognosis is worsened by the presence of ARDS or preexisting medical problems.

AMNIOTIC FLUID EMBOLISM

ESSENTIALS OF DIAGNOSIS

- Sudden, unexplained peripartum respiratory distress, cardiovascular collapse, and coagulopathy
- Bleeding secondary to coagulopathy or uterine atony (common)
- Amniotic fluid debris in right side of the heart on autopsy

Pathogenesis

Amniotic fluid embolism is a rare but potentially devastating complication of pregnancy that often results in poor obstetric outcome. Most of the information about amniotic fluid embolism has been derived from clinical reports, because the rarity of the disorder does not allow for clinical trials, and no suitable animal model exists. The first major review of the literature regarding this condition was by Morgan in 1979. This evaluated 272 cases. Since that time, a national registry was initiated by Clark. The incidence of amniotic fluid embolism is difficult to estimate and may be anywhere from 1 in 8000 to 1 in 30,000.

The basic mechanism of disease is related to the effects of amniotic fluid on the respiratory, cardiovascular, and coagulation systems. One of the classic theories hypothesized that the following 3 primary acute events occur: (1) pulmonary vascular obstruction, leading to sudden decreases in left ventricular filling pressures and cardiac output; (2) pulmonary hypertension with acute cor pulmonale; and (3) ventilation-perfusion inequality of lung tissue, leading to arterial hypoxemia and its metabolic consequences.

Only a small volume of amniotic fluid (1–2 mL) is transferred to the maternal circulation during normal labor. Thus enhanced communication between the amniotic fluid sac and the maternal venous system is necessary for amniotic fluid embolism to occur. Sites of entry may include endocervical veins lacerated during normal labor, a disrupted placental implantation site, and traumatized uterine veins.

Squamous cells and trophoblastic tissue are often found in the maternal pulmonary vasculature of patients who underwent pulmonary artery catheterization. However, one must see more specific material such as mucin, fetal debris, vernix, lanugo, and squamous cells coated with white blood cells and granular debris to confirm the diagnosis. If meconium is present, a more dramatic response is seen. Fetal demise has also been shown to worsen this condition. Once amniotic debris enters the venous system, it travels rapidly to the cardiopulmonary circulation, leading to shock and arterial hypoxemia. Myocardial dysfunction may result from ischemic injury or right ventricular dilatation. Some experimental evidence suggests that amniotic fluid may have a direct myocardial depressant effect. Endothelin, a vasoconstrictive peptide found in vascular endothelial cells, has been implicated. Other factors that may play a role include proteolytic enzymes, histamine, prostaglandins, complement, and biogenic amines (eg, serotonin). These mediators are seen in other shock states such as sepsis and anaphylaxis, leading Clark to suggest that amniotic fluid embolism be termed "anaphylactoid syndrome of pregnancy." The effects of systemic hypotension and hypoxemia may lead to cardiopulmonary collapse, renal insufficiency, hepatic failure, seizures, and coma.

Amniotic fluid embolism is almost always associated with some form of DIC. The etiology of coagulopathy associated with amniotic fluid embolism is incompletely understood, but it is known that amniotic fluid has potent total thromboplastin and antifibrinolytic activity, both of which increase with advancing gestational age. Once clotting is triggered in the pulmonary vasculature, local thrombin generation can cause vasoconstriction and microvascular thrombosis.

Limited hemodynamic observations with pulmonary artery catheterization suggest that in humans with amniotic fluid embolism, left ventricular dysfunction is the only significant hemodynamic alteration that is consistently documented. The response to amniotic fluid embolus in humans may be biphasic, initially resulting in intense vasospasm, severe pulmonary hypertension, and hypoxia. The transient period of right heart failure with hypoxia is later followed by a secondary phase of left heart failure, as reflected by elevated pulmonary artery pressure with subsequent return of right heart function. This biphasic theory may account for the extremely high maternal mortality rate within the first hour (25–34%) and explains why pulmonary hypertension can be difficult to document in patients with this disorder.

Clinical Findings

A. Symptoms and Signs

In his classic review of 272 patients with amniotic fluid embolus, Morgan characterized the main presenting clinical features: 51% presented with respiratory distress and cyanosis, 27% with hypotension, and only 10% with seizures. The Clark national registry noted 30% of patients presented with seizures or seizure-like activity, 27% with dyspnea, 17% with fetal bradycardia, and 13% with hypotension. Between 37% and 54% of patients exhibited an associated bleeding diathesis. Risk factors identified in the Morgan study included multiparity, tumultuous labor, or tetanic uterine contractions. Other studies have noted risk factors including advanced maternal age, use of uterine stimulants, caesarean section, uterine rupture, high cervical lacerations, premature separation of the placenta, and intrauterine fetal demise. Clark, however, was unable to identify any notable risk factors. Other presenting signs that have been described include tachypnea, peripheral cyanosis, bronchospasm, and chest pain.

B. Laboratory Findings

Arterial blood oxygen tension typically indicates severe maternal hypoxemia. This hypoxemia may result from ventilation-perfusion inequality with atelectasis and associated pulmonary edema. The diagnosis of significant coagulopathy is manifested by the presence of microangiopathic hemolysis, hypofibrinogenemia, prolonged clotting times, prolonged bleeding time, and elevated fibrin split products. The chest radiograph is nonspecific, although pulmonary edema is often noted. The ECG typically reveals unexplained tachycardia, nonspecific ST- and T-wave changes, and a right ventricular strain pattern. Lung scans occasionally identify perfusion defects resulting from amniotic fluid embolism even though chest radiographic findings are normal.

Differential Diagnosis

Many conditions may mimic the effects of amniotic fluid embolism on the respiratory, cardiovascular, and coagulation systems. Pulmonary thromboembolism can result in severe hypoxemia with pulmonary edema. In contrast to amniotic fluid embolism, chest pain is a relatively common finding. Congestive heart failure due to fluid overload or preexisting heart disease may mimic the cardiorespiratory compromise observed during amniotic fluid embolism. Hypotension may result from several disorders, including septic chorioamnionitis or postpartum hemorrhage. Pulmonary aspiration (Mendelson's syndrome) is associated with tachycardia, shock, respiratory distress, and production of a frothy pink sputum, but is usually also associated with bronchospasm and wheezing. Other conditions in the differential diagnosis include air embolism, myocardial infarction, anaphylaxis, placental abruption, eclampsia, uterine rupture, transfusion reaction, and local anesthesia toxicity.

Treatment

Amniotic fluid embolism remains one of the most devastating and unpreventable conditions complicating pregnancy. Therapeutic measures are supportive and should be directed toward minimizing hypoxemia with supplemental oxygen, maintaining blood pressure, and managing associated coagulopathies. Patients with poor oxygenation often require intubation and positive end-expiratory pressure. Adequate oxygenation will minimize related cerebral and myocardial ischemia and acidosis-induced pulmonary artery vasospasm. Pulmonary artery catheterization should be considered in the absence of coagulopathy to guide inotropic therapy with dopamine. If invasive hemodynamic monitoring is not available, rapid digitalization should be considered. Finally, the development of consumptive coagulopathy may require replacement of depleted hemostatic components in cases with significant uncontrollable bleeding or abnormal clotting parameters.

Prognosis

Maternal mortality rates range from 60–80%; however, a recent study quoted a 26.4% mortality rate. Of those patients who do not survive, 25% die within the first hour, and 80% within the first 9 hours. Correspondingly high perinatal morbidity and mortality rates would be expected.

PULMONARY THROMBOEMBOLISM

ESSENTIALS OF DIAGNOSIS

- Unexplained chest pain and dyspnea (most frequent presenting symptoms)
- History of pulmonary embolism, deep venous thrombosis, prolonged immobilization, or recent surgery
- Physical examination: usually nonspecific, depending on extent of cardiopulmonary involvement, but may include tachycardia, wheezing, pleural friction rub, and pulmonary rales
- Laboratory evaluation: decreased arterial blood oxygen tension to less than 90 mm Hg in the sitting position
- Diagnostic studies: pulmonary radionuclide ventilation-perfusion scanning, spiral computed tomography, and angiography

Pathogenesis

Pulmonary thromboembolism is a rare complication of pregnancy (0.09%) but is a significant cause of maternal morbidity and mortality. Mortality has been documented as 12.8% if untreated and 0.7% if therapy is instituted. The diagnosis of deep venous thrombosis (DVT) occurs in the antepartum period approximately half the time and is evenly distributed throughout each trimester. Pulmonary embolism has a higher incidence in the postpartum period. Predisposing factors commonly include advanced maternal age, obesity, traumatic delivery, abdominal delivery, thrombophlebitis, and endometritis. Patients with underlying thrombophilias or previous thrombotic events are at greater risk for this condition.

More than 100 years ago, Virchow postulated that the basic mechanism of thrombus formation is related to a combination of vessel injury, vascular stasis, and alterations in blood coagulability. Venous thrombi consist of fibrin deposits and red blood cells with varying amounts of platelet and white blood cell components. In most cases, lower extremity and pelvic thrombi are responsible for the pathologic sequelae.

Ordinarily, the vascular endothelium does not react with either platelets or the blood coagulation system unless it is disrupted by vessel injury. Such injury exposes subendothelial cells to blood elements responsible for activation of the extrinsic coagulation cascade. Disruption of the vascular endothelium may occur during traumatic vaginal delivery or caesarean section.

Pregnancy is associated with venous stasis, especially in the lower extremities, because the enlarging uterus reduces blood return to the inferior vena cava by direct mechanical effects. Hormonal factors may also contribute to vasodilatation and stasis during pregnancy. Stasis prevents the hepatic clearance of activated coagulation factors and minimizes mixing of these factors with their serum inhibitors. In this manner, venous stasis becomes another predisposing factor for the formation of thrombi. Stasis secondary to prolonged bedrest for medical or obstetric complications will predispose a pregnant woman to increased venous stasis and formation of vascular thrombi. The period of greatest risk for thrombosis and embolism appears to be the immediate postpartum, especially after caesarean delivery.

The maternal circulation becomes hypercoagulable from alterations in the coagulation and fibrinolytic systems. Serum concentrations of most coagulation proteins, such as fibrinogen and factors II, VII, VIII, IX, and X, increase during pregnancy. These changes are also associated with decreased fibrinolytic activity, which is responsible for the conversion of plasminogen to the active proteolytic enzyme plasmin.

Women with congenital or acquired thrombophilias are at increased risk for thrombosis; in fact, up to half of women who have these events in pregnancy may have an underlying disorder. The most commonly recognized thrombophilia in the white population is factor V Leiden mutation (5%). Other less common but significant disorders include prothrombin gene mutation G20210A (2–4%), antithrombin III deficiency (0.02–0.2%), protein C deficiency (0.2–0.5%), protein S deficiency (0.08%), and hyperhomocysteinemia (1%). The antiphospholipid antibody syndrome also significantly increases maternal risk of thromboembolism and other pregnancy complications.

Once a venous thrombus is formed, it may dislodge from its peripheral vascular origin and enter the central maternal circulation. Propagation of the original venous clot or recurrent pulmonary emboli are possible. DVTs limited to the calf rarely embolize, but approximately 20% extend to the proximal lower extremity.

Clinical Findings

A. Symptoms and Signs

The subsequent cardiopulmonary effects of pulmonary embolus will depend on the location and size of thrombi in the lung. A patient with a large embolus affecting the central pulmonary circulation may present with acute syncope, respiratory distress, and shock. Smaller emboli may not have significant clinical sequelae.

No single symptom or combination of symptoms is sensitive or specific for the diagnosis of pulmonary embolus. Classic triads (hemoptysis, chest pain, and dyspnea; or dyspnea, chest pain, and apprehension) are rarely seen (Table 23–5). Chest pain and dyspnea were the most common symptoms in patients with angiographically documented pulmonary emboli (more than 80%). Physical findings include tachycardia, tachypnea (rate >16/min), pulmonary rales, wheezing, and pleural friction rub.

Table 23–5. Symptoms and signs in 327 patients with pulmonary embolus confirmed by angiography.

Symptom or Sign	Frequency (%)
Chest pain	88
Pleuritic	74
Nonpleuritic	14
Dyspnea	84
Apprehension	59
Cough	53
Hemoptysis	30
Sweating	27
Syncope	13
Respiration more than 16/min	92
Pulmonary rales	58
Pulse more than 100/min	44
Fever (>37.8 °C [99.7 °F])	43
Phlebitis	32
Heart gallop	34
Diaphoresis	36
Edema	24
Heart murmur	23
Cyanosis	19

(Adapted and reproduced, with permission, from Bell WR, Simon TL, DeMets DL. The clinical features of submassive and massive pulmonary emboli. *Am J Med* 1977;62:355.)

B. Laboratory Findings

There are no specific routine laboratory findings associated with the diagnosis of pulmonary embolus, although arterial blood gas measurements will often reveal significant hypoxemia. In the upright position, almost all healthy young pregnant women will have an arterial blood oxygen tension greater than 90 mm Hg. An alveolar-atrial (A-a) gradient of greater than 20 is suspicious for pulmonary embolus. The ECG may reveal unexplained tachycardia associated with cor pulmonale (right axis deviation, S wave in lead I, Q wave plus T wave inversion in lead III). A chest roentgenogram may be normal or may show infiltrates, atelectasis, or effusions. Thirty percent of patients with a pulmonary embolus will have a normal chest x-ray.

It is generally accepted that a normal radionuclide perfusion study can effectively rule out pulmonary embolus. Perfusion studies are occasionally equivocal, and ventilation scanning may be required to clarify the diagnosis. Ventilation scanning will improve the specificity of the perfusion study, because this will rule out airway disorders that may be responsible for reduced pulmonary perfusion. The radiation exposure is minimal (<0.1 rad). Unfortunately, a V/Q scan can only confirm a diagnosis if it is normal or indicates high probability of embolus. Therefore, 40–60% of patients will require further testing.

Spiral computed tomography (CT) is a newer form of imaging that has a sensitivity and specificity of 94% in the nonpregnant patient. Spiral CT may also be helpful in detecting other abnormalities causing pulmonary symptoms (eg, pleural effusions, consolidation, emphysema, pulmonary masses). However, this study may miss emboli below the segmental level. Magnetic resonance imaging has limited value in diagnosing pulmonary embolism in pregnancy because it has not been well studied.

If the previously mentioned studies are equivocal, pulmonary angiography should be considered. Subsequent exposure of the fetus to the relatively low levels of ionizing radiation from angiography can be minimized with appropriate pelvic shielding and selective angiography on the basis of prior radionuclide scanning.

Noninvasive Doppler should be considered as an initial diagnostic test for suspected DVT involving the lower extremities. Compression ultrasound uses firm compression with the transducer probe to detect intraluminal filling defects. Imaging is most useful for the distal iliac, femoral, and popliteal veins. Doppler is also useful for the proximal iliac veins. Sensitivity is 95%, with a 96% specificity. Impedance plethysmography measures impedance flow with pneumatic cuff inflation. Sensitivity and specificity are 83% and 92%, respectively. Compression of the inferior vena cava by the gravid second- or third-trimester uterus may cause false-positive results.

If the above noninvasive tests are inconclusive, it may be helpful to confirm the extent of the original thrombotic event by venography with pelvic shielding. The soleal calf sinuses and the valves involving the popliteal and femoral veins are the sources of most deep venous thrombi. Venography is associated with induced phlebitis in approximately 3–5% of procedures performed. Radiofibrinogen methods to detect thrombus formation will result in placental transfer of radioactive iodine and are contraindicated in pregnant or nursing women.

Differential Diagnosis

Any condition potentially related to cardiopulmonary compromise during pregnancy should be included in the differential diagnosis. This includes amniotic fluid and air emboli, spontaneous pneumothorax, septic shock, and preexisting heart disease.

Treatment

A. Preventive Treatment

Once predisposing risk factors to pulmonary embolus are identified, it is important to minimize the possibility of further complications. In patients at higher risk for DVT, prophylactic measures should be directed toward preventing venous stasis that leads to clot formation. Mechanical maneuvers such as raising the lower extremities 15 degrees above the horizontal, keeping the legs straight rather than bent at the knees when sitting, or performing calf flexion exercises may be useful, as may external pneumatic compression. One method used to prevent perioperative thrombophlebitis includes minidose heparin prophylaxis, 5000 U subcutaneously 2 hours before surgery and every 12 hours until routine ambulation is achieved. Minidose heparin prophylaxis significantly decreases not only the incidence of DVT but also the incidence of fatal pulmonary emboli. Subcutaneous minidose heparin may be reinstituted approximately 6 hours after delivery. Postpartum or postoperative ambulation is important in minimizing thromboembolic complications during this high-risk period. Some women may require therapeutic anticoagulation during pregnancy to prevent a thromboembolic event. Included in this category are women with artificial heart valves, antithrombin III deficiency, antiphospholipid antibody syndrome, history of rheumatic heart disease and atrial fibrillation, homozygosity for factor V Leiden or prothrombin gene mutation, and recurrent thromboembolic disease. Therapeutic anticoagulation can be achieved by using subcutaneous heparin 2–3 times a day, adjusting for a PTT of 2.0–3.0 times normal. Low molecular weight heparin (LMWH) can also be used. LMWH does not cross the placenta, and it has been shown to be relatively safe in pregnancy. In addition, complications of heparin therapy (osteoporosis, thrombocytopenia) are less common with this medication, and dosing in pregnancy usually may require fewer adjustments. The PTT does not need to be followed; instead, peak antifactor Xa levels can be checked every 4–6 weeks. It is controversial whether other disorders, such as protein C or S deficiency, or a family history of thrombophilias, require anticoagulation therapy. These patients may benefit from minidose heparin prophylaxis. LMWH can also be used for prophylaxis. The typical dose is either weight-based or empiric.

B. Treatment of Documented Pulmonary Embolism

Once pulmonary embolism is documented, therapeutic intervention should be directed to correction of arterial hypoxemia and any associated hypotension. Other measures should prevent clot propagation or recurrent emboli. Supplemental oxygen should be given to achieve an arterial oxygen tension of at least 70 mm Hg. A loading dose of 5000–10,000 U of heparin should be given intravenously by continuous infusion, followed by a maintenance dose of approximately 1000 U/h. The PTT should be maintained at 1.5–2.5 times control values. Other investigators recommend the use of heparin levels for monitoring anticoagulation therapy. Heparin levels may be measured on the third or fourth day and should be approximately 0.2 μg/mL, not to exceed 0.4 μg/mL. Alternatively, LMWH can also be used for therapeutic anticoagulation. Leg elevation, bedrest, and local heat will be beneficial to patients who have associated DVT. Intravenous morphine may be helpful in alleviating anxiety and ameliorating chest pain.

Intrapartum care of pulmonary embolus is complicated, and individual treatment approaches may vary. Selected patients with recent pulmonary thromboembolism, ileofemoral DVT, or heart valve prosthesis should probably continue full anticoagulation with high-dose heparin during labor or surgical procedures. Under these circumstances, the risk for potential bleeding complications from anticoagulant needs to be balanced against the risk of thromboembolism. Although there is a higher incidence of wound hematomas associated with peripartum anticoagulation, there is no clear evidence that this regimen is associated with excessive postpartum hemorrhage after normal vaginal delivery.

Postpartum patients receiving heparin may be switched over to warfarin once oral intake is tolerated. Warfarin is considered safe during breastfeeding. Heparin should be continued for the first 5–7 days of warfarin therapy. By the time heparin is discontinued, the international normalized ratio should be 2.0–3.0 times the normal value. Alternatively, it may be desirable to continue moderate doses of subcutaneous heparin (10,000 U twice daily) or LMWH. Postpartum anticoagulation should be continued for at least 3 months if the patient developed pulmonary embolus in the third trimester.

C. Complications of Treatment

The major complication of anticoagulant therapy is maternal or fetal hemorrhage. Heparin does not cross the placenta due to its large molecular weight, but it has been associated with maternal thrombocytopenia and osteoporosis. These effects can be reduced with LMWH. Warfarin is known to cross the placental barrier, and its use in the first trimester has been associated with embryopathy (nasal hypoplasia and stippled epiphyses) in approximately 5–8% of fetuses. Fetal nervous system abnormalities (eg, hydrocephalus) have also been noted with the use of warfarin during pregnancy.

A small percentage of patients will experience recurrent pulmonary emboli despite full anticoagulation. These patients may be candidates for vena caval ligation by a transabdominal approach under general or regional anesthesia. If the pelvis is suspected as the source of embolus, the right ovarian vein should also be ligated. It has been estimated that approximately 95% of patients with pulmonary embolism massive enough to cause hypotension eventually die. In this context, pulmonary artery embolectomy may be life-saving.

Placement of a vena caval umbrella via the internal jugular vein is an option for unstable patients with recurrent emboli who would not be prime surgical candidates. Although abdominal radiography is required for this procedure, placement of the umbrella filter does not require general anesthesia. This strategy will prevent larger emboli from reaching the pulmonary circulation.

Prognosis

Pulmonary embolus, with a mortality rate of 12–15% if left untreated, will develop in approximately one-fourth of untreated patients with antenatal DVT. In a review of pregnancies complicated by DVT treated with anticoagulant therapy, the incidence of pulmonary embolus was 4.5% of patients, with a maternal mortality rate of less than 1%.

American College of Obstetricians and Gynecologists. *Thromboembolism in Pregnancy*. ACOG Practice Bulletin No. 19. Washington, DC: ACOG; August 2000.

DISSEMINATED INTRAVASCULAR COAGULATION

ESSENTIALS OF DIAGNOSIS

- History of recent bleeding diathesis, especially concurrent with placental abruption, amniotic fluid embolism, fetal demise, sepsis, preeclampsia–eclampsia, or saline abortion.
- Clinical evidence of multiple bleeding points associated with purpura and petechiae on physical examination.
- Laboratory findings classically include thrombocytopenia, hypofibrinogenemia, and elevated PT, elevated D-dimer, and fibrin split products that do not easily correct with replacement.

Pathogenesis

DIC is a pathologic condition associated with inappropriate activation of coagulation and fibrinolytic systems. It should be considered a secondary phenomenon resulting from an underlying disease state. The most common obstetric conditions associated with DIC are intrauterine fetal death, amniotic fluid embolism, pre-eclampsia-eclampsia, HELLP (hemolysis, elevated liver enzymes, and low platelet count syndrome), placenta previa, and placental abruption. Saline-induced abortion is also a cause. It is a separate condition from dilutional coagulopathy, which often follows hemorrhage and volume replacement with crystalloid and red blood cells. Dilutional coagulopathy represents a diminished amount of factors and can be easily corrected b replacing these factors. DIC, however, represents a cascade of events leading to the activation of the coagulation cascade and continued consumption of the clotting factors.

The most widely accepted theory of blood coagulation entails a "cascade theory" (Fig. 23–7). Basically, the coagulation system is divided into intrinsic and extrinsic systems. The intrinsic system contains all the intravascular components required to activate thrombin by sequential activation of factors XII, XI, IX, X, V, and II (prothrombin). The extrinsic system is initially activated by tissue thromboplastin, leading to sequential activation of factors VII, X, V, and prothrombin. Both the intrinsic and extrinsic pathways converge to activate factor X, which subsequently reacts with activated factor V in the presence of calcium and phospholipid to convert prothrombin to thrombin.

Thrombin is a proteolytic enzyme responsible for splitting fibrinogen chains into fibrinopeptides, leading to the formation of fibrin monomer. This central enzyme is capable of activating factor XIII to stabilize the newly formed fibrin clot and will enhance the activity of factors V and VIII.

Activation of the coagulation system also stimulates the conversion of plasminogen to plasmin as a protective mechanism against intravascular thrombosis. Plasmin is an enzyme that inactivates factors V and VIII and is capable of lysing fibrin and fibrinogen to form degradation products. Thus the normal physiologic hemostatic mechanism represents a delicate and complex balance between the coagulation and fibrinolytic systems.

Pregnancy is considered to represent a hypercoagulable state. With the exception of factors XI and XIII, there is an overall increase in the activity of coagulation factors. Fibrinogen rises as early as 12 weeks' gestation and reaches a peak level of 400–650 mg/dL in late pregnancy. The fibrinolytic system is depressed during pregnancy and labor but returns to normal levels within 1 hour of placental delivery. The early puerperium is accompanied by a secondary rise in fibrinogen, factors VIII, IX, X, and anti-thrombin III; a return to nonpregnant levels occurs by 3–4 weeks postpartum.

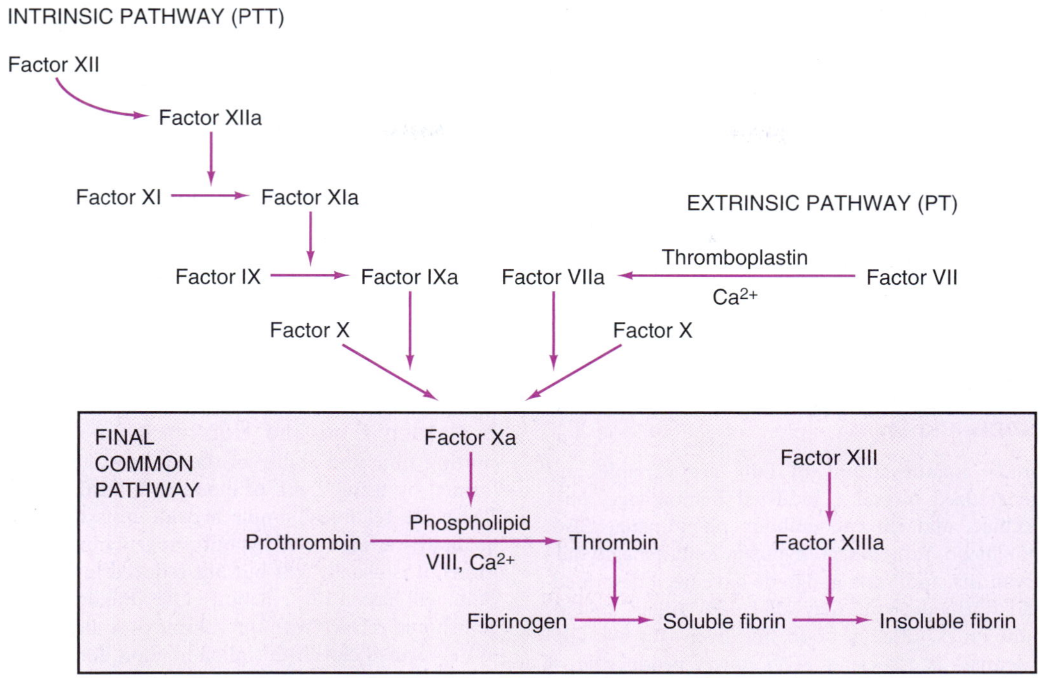

▲ **Figure 23–7.** Coagulation cascade mechanism.

The complex pathophysiology of DIC is characterized by (1) procoagulant system activation, (2) fibrinolytic system activation, (3) inhibitor consumption, (4) cytokine release, (5) cellular activation, and (6) resultant end-organ damage. DIC occurs as a secondary event in a wide variety of illnesses associated with excess production of circulating thrombin. The pathophysiologic factors responsible for inappropriate activation of the clotting mechanism include endothelial cell injury, liberation of thromboplastin from injured tissue, and release of phospholipid from red cell or platelet injury. All these mechanisms may contribute to development of a bleeding diathesis resulting from increased thrombin activity. Additionally, widespread DIC will cause increased platelet aggregation, consumption of coagulation factors, secondary activation of the fibrinolytic system, and deposition of fibrin into multiple organ sites, which can result in ischemic tissue damage. The associated thrombocytopenia and presence of fibrin split products will impair hemostasis.

Specific obstetric conditions associated with DIC include the following.

A. Placental Abruption

DIC may occur in placental abruption involving liberation of tissue thromboplastin or possible intrauterine consumption of fibrinogen and coagulation factors during the formation of retroplacental clot. This leads to activation of the extrinsic coagulation mechanism. Placental abruption is one of the most common obstetric causes of DIC.

B. Retained Dead Fetus Syndrome

Another cause of DIC is retained dead fetus syndrome involving liberation of tissue thromboplastin from nonviable tissue. This cause is less common in recent years due to advanced ultrasound technology and the earlier detection of this condition.

C. Amniotic Fluid Embolism

This involves not only the release of tissue thromboplastin, but also the intrinsic procoagulant properties of amniotic fluid itself. It is likely that the associated hypotension, hypoxemia, and tissue acidosis will encourage the activation of coagulation factors.

D. Preeclampsia-Eclampsia

This condition is associated with chronic coagulation abnormalities that may lead to thrombocytopenia and elevation of fibrin degradation products. It is uncertain whether endothelial damage activates procoagulant proteins and platelets or the reverse, although the former is more likely. Eclampsia is associated with DIC 11% of the time; with HELLP syndrome this increases to 15%. Preeclampsia together with placental abruption also significantly increases this association.

E. Saline or Septic Abortion

Saline-induced abortion has been associated with subclinical DIC. Severe cases of DIC have occurred in 1 in 400 to 1 in 1000 cases. Disease may be related to the release of tissue thromboplastin from the placenta. Septic abortion may also cause release of tissue thromboplastin or release of bacterial endotoxin (phospholipids).

F. Other

Other triggers of DIC include septicemia, viremias (eg, HIV, varicella, cytomegalovirus, hepatitis), drugs, and acidosis.

Clinical Findings

A. Symptoms and Signs

Acute clinical manifestations of DIC are variable and include generalized bleeding, localized hemorrhage, purpura, petechiae, and thromboembolic phenomena. Also, fever, hypotension, proteinuria, hypoxia, hemorrhagic bullae, acral cyanosis, and frank gangrene have been described. Widespread fibrin deposits may affect any organ system, including the lungs, kidneys, brain, and liver. Chronic DIC (eg, fetal demise) is associated with slower production of thrombin and may be associated with minimal or absent clinical signs and symptoms.

B. Laboratory Findings

Although histologic diagnosis of fibrin deposits is the only definitive manner by which DIC may be confirmed, there are a host of indirect tests suitable for the clinical evaluation of coagulopathy.

1. Platelets—Platelets are decreased (<100,000/μL) in more than 90% of cases. In the absence of other causes, spontaneous purpura usually does not occur when platelet counts are greater than 30,000/μL.

2. Prothrombin time—PT measures the time required for clotting by the extrinsic pathway and is dependent on the ultimate conversion of fibrinogen to fibrin. It is prolonged in only 50–75% of patients with DIC. The explanations for the normal PTs are, first, the presence of circulating activated clotting factors such as thrombin or factor Xa, that accelerate the formation of fibrin; and second, the presence of early degradation products, which are rapidly clottable by thrombin; these may cause the test to register a normal or fast PT.

3. Partial thromboplastin time—PTT is frequently normal in DIC (40–50% of the time) and is not as helpful for establishing the diagnosis. This test measures the function of the intrinsic and final common pathways of the coagulation cascade.

4. Thrombin time (TT)—TT is elevated in 80% of patients with DIC. It is affected only by the amount of circulating fibrinogen or the presence of thrombin inhibitors such as fibrin degradation products and heparin. This test specifically measures the time necessary for conversion of fibrinogen to fibrin.

5. Fibrinogen—Fibrinogen is often decreased, with approximately 70% of patients with DIC having a serum level less than 150 mg/dL. The normal physiologic increase of serum fibrinogen levels during pregnancy may mask a pathologic decrease in this parameter.

6. Fibrin split products—Values greater than 40 μg/mL are suggestive of DIC. These are elevated in 85–100% of patients with DIC. These degradation products are diagnostic of the plasmin biodegradation of fibrinogen or fibrin, so indicate only the presence of plasmin.

7. Clotting time and clot retraction—Observation of clotting time and ability of the clot to retract can be performed by using 2 mL of blood in a 5-mL glass test tube. These are relatively simple bedside tests that can provide qualitative evidence of hypofibrinogenemia. When the clot forms, it is usually soft but not reduced in volume (adding celite will hasten this reaction). Over the next half hour, the clot should retract, with the volume of serum exceeding that of the formed clot. If this phenomenon does not occur, low serum fibrinogen levels can be suspected.

8. Peripheral blood smear—A peripheral blood smear reveals schistocytes in approximately 40% of patients with DIC.

9. Bleeding time—The time required for hemostasis after skin puncture will become progressively prolonged as the platelet count falls below 100,000/μL. Spontaneous continuous bleeding from puncture sites may develop if the platelet count falls below 30,000/μL.

10. Newer tests—Several of these laboratory findings are more reliable than the classic studies.

A. D-DIMER—This is a neoantigen formed as a result of plasmin digestion of cross-linked fibrin when thrombin initiates the transition of fibrinogen to fibrin and activates factor XIII to cross-link the fibrin formed. The test is specific for fibrin (not fibrinogen) degradation products and is abnormal in 90% of cases.

B. ANTITHROMBIN III LEVEL—This is abnormal in 89% of cases.

C. FIBRINOPEPTIDE A—This is abnormal 75% of the time.

Differential Diagnosis

Most acute episodes of generalized bleeding in obstetric patients will be related to pregnancy, but other rare causes of congenital or acquired coagulopathies need to be considered. These include idiopathic thrombocytopenic purpura, hemophilia, and von Willebrand's disease. Placental abruption is often associated with uterine tenderness, fetal bradycardia, and uterine bleeding. DIC associated with fetal demise usually does not become apparent until at least 5 weeks after the absence of heart tones has been documented. Amniotic fluid embolus is typically associated with acute onset of respiratory distress and shock. Preeclampsia is characterized by hypertension and proteinuria, which may lead to eclamptic seizures.

Complications

In addition to the potential complications of uncontrolled hemorrhage previously discussed, widespread fibrin deposition may affect any major organ system. This may include the liver (hepatic failure), kidneys (tubular necrosis), and lungs (hypoxemia).

Treatment

Although individual measures will be dictated by the specific obstetric condition, the primary, most important treatment of pregnancy-related DIC is correction of the underlying cause. In most cases, prompt termination of the pregnancy is required. Moderate or low-grade DIC may not be associated with clinical evidence of excessive bleeding and often will require close observation but no further therapy.

Supportive therapy should be directed to the correction of shock, acidosis, and tissue ischemia. Cardiopulmonary support, including inotropic therapy, blood replacement, and assisted ventilation, should be implemented with the patient in close proximity to a delivery suite. Fetal monitoring, careful recording of maternal fluid balance, and serial evaluation of coagulation parameters are extremely important. If sepsis is suspected, antibiotics should be employed. Central monitoring with a pulmonary artery catheter is relatively contraindicated due to potential bleeding complications. Vaginal delivery, without episiotomy if possible, is preferable to caesarean section. Failure of improvement in the coagulopathy within several hours after delivery suggests sepsis, liver disease, retained products of conception, or a congenital coagulation defect.

Blood component therapy should be initiated on the basis of transfusion guidelines reported by the National Institutes of Health. Criteria for red cell transfusions were discussed earlier (see Hypovolemic Shock). Fresh-frozen plasma has only limited and specific indications, which include massive hemorrhage, isolated factor deficiencies, reversal of warfarin, antithrombin II deficiency, immunodeficiencies, and thrombocytopenic purpura. Although most cases of severe obstetric hemorrhage will lead to laboratory evidence of coagulation abnormalities, transfusion of fresh-frozen plasma may not always benefit these patients; the amount transfused is usually insufficient for replacing coagulation factors lost by dilution or clot formation. Even with massive obstetric hemorrhage, most procoagulant levels are above 30% of normal values, which is sufficient for maintaining clinical hemostasis in most patients. Specific replacement of fibrinogen should be accomplished by cryoprecipitate. Each unit of cryoprecipitate carries approximately 250 mg of fibrinogen. Platelets should only be administered in the face of active bleeding with a platelet count < 50,000/μL or prophylactically with platelet count 20–30,000/μL or less or after massive transfusion (>2 times blood volume). Platelets should be transfused on the basis of 1 U/10 kg body weight to raise the cell count above 50,000/μL. However, it should be noted that clotting factors containing fibrinogen may be associated with enhanced hemorrhage and also with thrombosis when given to patients with DIC. For this reason, they should be administered with extreme caution. Obstetricians should remember that Rh immune globulin should be given to Rh-negative recipients of platelets from Rh-positive donors.

Subcutaneous low-dose heparin or LMWH may be effective in treating the intravascular clotting process of DIC. Heparin acts as an anticoagulant by activating antithrombin III but has little effect on activated coagulation factors. Anticoagulation is contraindicated in patients with fulminant DIC and central nervous system insults, fulminant liver failure, or obstetric accidents. The one instance, however, in which heparin has been demonstrated to benefit pregnancy-related DIC is in the case of the retained dead fetus with an intact vascular system, in which case heparin may be administered to interrupt the coagulation process and thrombocytopenia for several days until safe delivery may be implemented.

Prognosis

Most cases of obstetric DIC will improve with delivery of the fetus or evacuation of the uterus. The maternal and fetal prognosis will be more closely related to the associated obstetric condition than to the coagulopathy.

Bick RL. Syndromes of disseminated intravascular coagulation in obstetrics, pregnancy, and gynecology. *Hematol Oncol Clin North Am* 2000;13:999–1044. PMID: 11005032.

Ginsberg JS, Greer I, Hirsh J. Use of antithrombotic agents during pregnancy. *Chest* 2001;119:122S. PMID: 11157646.

ACUTE RESPIRATORY DISTRESS SYNDROME (ARDS)

ESSENTIALS OF DIAGNOSIS

- History of gastric aspiration, infection/sepsis, preeclampsia-eclampsia, seizures, hemorrhage, coagulopathy, or amniotic fluid embolism
- Progressive respiratory distress with decreased lung compliance
- Severe hypoxemia refractory to oxygen therapy

- Diffuse infiltrates on chest roentgenogram
- Normal PCWP, with absence of radiographic evidence of congestive heart failure

Pathogenesis

ARDS is a severe form of lung disease with acute onset, characterized by bilateral infiltrates on chest x-ray, no evidence of intravascular volume overload (PCWP no greater than 18 mm Hg), and severely impaired oxygenation, demonstrated by a ratio of arterial oxygen tension (PaO_2) to the fraction of inspired oxygen (FIO_2) of less than 200 mm Hg. ARDS appears to occur more commonly in obstetric patients than in the general population. Its incidence in the nonpregnant population is 1.5 per 100,000, but it has been estimated to occur in between 1 in 3000 and 1 in 10,000 pregnant patients. ARDS has many causes, including gastric aspiration, amniotic fluid embolism, sepsis, coagulopathy, massive blood transfusion, and shock. It can be easily confused with cardiogenic pulmonary edema secondary to alterations in preload, myocardial contractility, or afterload. A basic understanding of the differences between cardiogenic and noncardiogenic pulmonary edema is essential before rational therapeutic intervention may be implemented.

The basic underlying pathologic change responsible for ARDS is lung injury that results in damage to the pulmonary epithelium and endothelial tissue. This, in turn, leads to enhanced vascular permeability. Factors determining the net flux of lung fluid between the capillary lumen and interstitial space are quantitatively related by the Starling equation:

$$\text{Net fluid flux} = \kappa[(\text{Pcap} - \text{Pis}) - (\pi\text{cap} - \pi\text{is})]$$

(κ = filtration coefficient, Pcap = pulmonary capillary hydrostatic pressure, Pis = interstitial space hydrostatic pressure, πcap = pulmonary capillary serum colloid osmotic pressure, $\pi$is = interstitial space fluid colloid osmotic pressure)

Normally, fluid flows from the capillary system to the interstitial space and is returned to the systemic circulation by the pulmonary lymphatic system. An increase in left atrial pressure is observed when the left ventricle is unable to pump all the returning blood into the left atrium. Accordingly, the pulmonary capillary hydrostatic pressure increases, facilitating net movement of lung fluid into the interstitial space. When capillary fluid efflux into the interstitial space exceeds lymphatic resorption, the clinical presentation of pulmonary edema will occur. Although colloid osmotic pressure in the interstitial space and serum also plays a role in pulmonary edema, the most common factor is increased capillary hydrostatic pressure secondary to increased preload (fluid overload), afterload (severe hypertension), and decreased myocardial contractility (postpartum cardiomyopathy).

Capillary membrane permeability plays a much larger role in the genesis of noncardiogenic pulmonary edema (ARDS). Such injury due to hypoxic ischemia, vasoactive substances, chemical irritation, or microthrombi facilitates further efflux of capillary fluid and plasma proteins into the interstitium. This increase in permeability acutely produces atelectasis and diminished compliance of the lung, and damage is usually nonuniform. As the functional capability of atelectatic bronchioles diminishes, shunting and hypoxemia develop.

Maternal physiologic changes can contribute to the severity of ARDS. It has been suggested that decreased extrathoracic compliance, decreased functional residual capacity, higher oxygen deficit, limited cardiac output increases, and anemia may adversely affect the clinical presentation and course of ARDS during pregnancy.

Clinical Findings

A. Symptoms and Signs

Classic signs of respiratory distress are tachypnea, intercostal retractions, and even cyanosis, depending on the degree of hypoxemia. Fetal tachycardia or late decelerations may reflect maternal hypoxemia and uteroplacental insufficiency. Pulmonary rales in noncardiogenic pulmonary edema will be indistinguishable from those of cardiogenic pulmonary edema, but physical findings consistent with the cardiogenic disorder (ventricular gallop, jugular venous distention, and peripheral edema) are not typical features of ARDS. Unfortunately, the physiologic changes of pregnancy may mask the significance of these physical findings during the more subtle stages of respiratory distress.

B. Laboratory Findings

Arterial blood gas determinations will reveal a progressive moderate to severe hypoxemia despite oxygen therapy. Depending on the obstetric cause of ARDS, other laboratory findings will be variable or nonspecific. The initial chest roentgenogram will often be normal, even in the presence of clinically significant respiratory distress. Within the next 24–48 hours, patchy or diffuse infiltrates will progress to prominent alveolar infiltrates (Fig. 23–8). Unlike in cardiogenic pulmonary edema, the heart will most likely be of normal size in a patient with ARDS. PCWP measured by right heart catheterization is the procedure most helpful in differentiating ARDS and pulmonary edema. The PCWP is elevated (>20 mm Hg) in cardiogenic pulmonary edema but is often normal in ARDS.

Measurement of endobronchial fluid COP has also been used to differentiate capillary permeability-induced pulmonary edema from hydrostatic or cardiogenic pulmonary edema. In pulmonary edema secondary to capillary permeability, the COP of endobronchial fluid obtained from endotracheal tube suctioning is usually greater than 75% of the simultaneously obtained plasma COP. In cardiogenic pulmonary edema, the COP of the endobronchial fluid is usually less than 60% that of plasma.

Histopathologically, idiopathic pulmonary fibrosis and ARDS are remarkably similar. Both show evidence of acute alveolar injury, which is characterized by interstitial inflammation, hemorrhage, and edema. This is followed by

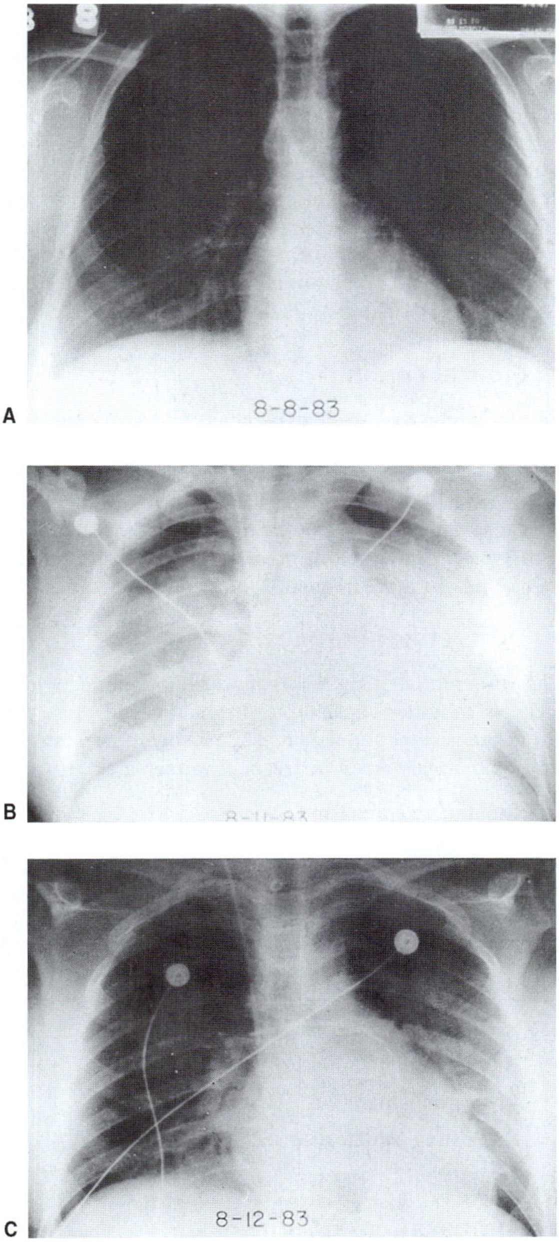

▲ **Figure 23–8.** Sequence of chest radiographs from a 21-year-old woman during her first pregnancy with antepartum pyelonephritis and acute respiratory distress syndrome (ARDS). **A:** Normal chest film. **B:** Bilateral patchy pulmonary densities have developed, consistent with the diagnosis of ARDS. Much of the apparent increase in heart size is related to shallow inspiration and supine technique. **C:** ARDS has improved dramatically, with only minimal residual pulmonary densities.

a hypercellular phase, loss of alveolar structure, and pulmonary fibrosis.

Differential Diagnosis

ARDS should be differentiated from infectious pneumonitis and cardiogenic causes of pulmonary edema. Cardiogenic pulmonary edema will usually respond more rapidly to diuretic therapy than will ARDS, in which abnormalities in capillary membrane permeability are not quickly resolved by such intervention.

Treatment

Therapy should be directed toward the prevention of hypoxemia, correcting acid–base abnormalities, removal of inciting factors, and hemodynamic support appropriate for the specific cause (eg, amniotic fluid embolus, DIC). Cardiogenic pulmonary edema is usually treated with a combination of diuretics, inotropic therapy, and afterload reduction. If a hemodynamic profile is not immediately available by pulmonary artery catheter, the clinician may elect to begin oxygen and furosemide (20 mg IV) for the presumptive diagnosis of cardiogenic pulmonary edema. By contrast, it should be apparent that the basic therapy for ARDS is supportive. Endotracheal intubation with mechanical ventilation is almost always required. The pulmonary artery catheter will be helpful in guiding fluid management and optimizing cardiac performance. Additionally, mixed venous oxygen saturation from the distal port of the pulmonary artery catheter will provide an index of oxygen utilization.

In obstetric patients, reasonable therapeutic goals for cardiorespiratory support include a mechanical ventilator tidal volume of less than 10 mL/kg, PCWP 8–12 mm Hg, arterial blood oxygen tension greater than 60 mm Hg, and mixed venous oxygen tension greater than 30 mm Hg. If unable to maintain PaO_2 of at least 60 mm Hg on 50% or less inspired oxygen, positive end-expiratory pressure (PEEP) in amounts of up to 15 cm H_2O may be helpful. However, it is important to avoid barotrauma to the remaining functional alveolar units, so high tidal volumes and pressures should be avoided. If the mixed venous tension is low, transfusion of red blood cells or inotropic therapy may improve oxygen transport and delivery.

Since the presence of capillary membrane abnormalities in ARDS is associated with rapid equilibration of proteinaceous material between the capillaries and interstitial spaces, intravenous colloid replacement should be discouraged in lieu of crystalloid resuscitation. A policy of relative fluid restriction should be followed, but only if the following criteria are met: stable fetus, no evidence of metabolic acidosis, normal renal function, and no need for vasopressor therapy or PEEP. Sedation and pain relief should be used liberally and may help to decrease oxygen consumption. Nutritional support for patients on prolonged mechanical ventilation must be considered; enteral feeding is preferred, as it may reduce the translocation of gut bacteria into the body. Prospective controlled studies have not demonstrated the benefit of steroid therapy for ARDS. Once therapy for cardiopulmonary support has been implemented, a thorough search for predisposing factors to ARDS must be identified for specific intervention.

Potential future therapies for ARDS include high-frequency ventilation, extracorporeal membrane oxygenation, intravenous oxygen, inhaled nitric oxide, surfactant replacement, oxygen-free radical scavengers, arachidonic acid metabolite inhibitors, antiprotease agents, antiendotoxin antibodies, anti-tumor necrosis factor antibodies, and other immunologic therapies for sepsis.

The timing of delivery in these patients is unclear from the literature. Based on the high rates of fetal death, preterm labor, fetal heart rate abnormalities, and perinatal asphyxia, most authorities recommend delivery after a gestational age of 28 weeks. In one review, only 10 of 39 patients with antepartum ARDS were discharged undelivered, and all had pyelonephritis or *Varicella*. Caesarean section should be reserved for standard obstetrical indications.

Prognosis

Older series suggested a mortality rate as high as 50–60% for patients with ARDS. More recent reviews show rates of 39–44%. One study of 41 patients demonstrated a 24.4% mortality rate; this has been attributed to possible differences in patient population as well as improvements in critical care. Many affected patients developed pulmonary complications that included barotrauma and pneumothorax. Fortunately, survivors of ARDS usually do not demonstrate permanent long-term pulmonary dysfunction.

Catanzarite V, Willms D, Wong D, et al. Acute respiratory distress syndrome in pregnancy and the puerperium: Causes, courses, and outcome. *Obstet Gynecol* 2001;97:760. PMID: 11339930.

CARDIOPULMONARY ARREST

ESSENTIALS OF DIAGNOSIS

- Cardiopulmonary arrest can be caused by a number of conditions during pregnancy.
- Without treatment, mortality is high for both the patient and the fetus.
- Treatment should follow standard basic and advanced cardiac life support algorithms, with some minor modifications due to pregnancy.
- Perimortem caesarean delivery may assist resuscitation by relieving aortocaval compression and increasing venous return to the heart. If necessary, it should be performed within 5 minutes of arrest for maximal effect.

Pathogenesis

Many of the critical conditions discussed in this chapter can lead to cardiopulmonary arrest. Cardiopulmonary arrest during pregnancy poses a unique challenge in that both the patient and the fetus are acutely at risk of severe morbidity and mortality. The prevalence ranges from 1 in 20,000 to 1 in 50,000 pregnancies, but this prevalence is likely increasing due to the increased prevalence of advanced maternal age and obesity in pregnancy, as well as women with other chronic medical problems becoming pregnant with the assistance of assisted reproductive technologies.

Clinical Findings

Cardiopulmonary arrest in pregnancy presents similar to nonpregnant women, beginning with symptoms such as chest pain, weakness, shortness of breath, and diaphoresis, and eventually leading to cardiac arrest. However, due to the vague nature of some of the early symptoms and overlap with typical symptoms of pregnancy, early warning signs may be missed more frequently in pregnant women.

Differential Diagnosis

The differential diagnosis of cardiopulmonary arrest includes conditions specific to pregnancy, and those present in the general population. The most common causes of cardiopulmonary arrest in pregnant women are:

1. Pulmonary embolism
2. Hemorrhage
3. Sepsis
4. Peripartum cardiomyopathy
5. Stroke
6. Preeclampsia–eclampsia
7. Anesthesia-related complications
8. Amniotic fluid embolism
9. Myocardial infarction
10. Preexisting cardiac disease
11. Trauma

Complications

Mortality is very high for pregnant women with cardiopulmonary arrest. Fetal demise is also very common. Due to this, treatment should be initiated immediately with the goal to maximize maternal cardiac output and ventilation.

Treatment

Due to the high mortality associated with cardiopulmonary arrest during pregnancy, resuscitation should follow standard algorithms of basic and advanced cardiac life support, with some modifications for the pregnancy. It is not proper to defer potential life-saving treatment for the patient due to a fear of exposing the fetus to medications and therapies. The most effective interventions for saving the fetus are those that save the mother's life. Therefore, medications used in resuscitation protocols should be used without hesitation.

It may be difficult to perform cardiac compressions due to a large uterus and engorged breasts. Compressions should not be performed in the supine position, as the gravid uterus may cause aortocaval compression, diminished venous return, and subsequent decreased cardiac output. Patients should be positioned with a left lateral tilt before compressions are applied. This can be accomplished using a moving table or a wedge or with manual displacement of the uterus. Defibrillation and cardioversion have been successfully used during pregnancy without disturbance of the fetal cardiac conduction system. It is important, however, to remove fetal monitors to prevent arcing.

The decision to perform a perimortem caesarean section should be made rapidly, within 4–5 minutes of cardiac arrest, to optimize both maternal and neonatal survival. This extreme measure can maximize maternal survival by relieving aortocaval compression and increasing blood flow back to the heart. Although the minimum gestational age for perimortem caesarean delivery is controversial, aortocaval compression begins as early as 20 weeks; therefore, hysterotomy should be considered as part of resuscitative measures in pregnancies of at least 20–22 weeks or greater.

Prognosis

Unfortunately, prognosis is poor, but it depends on the etiology of the cardiopulmonary arrest, coexisting morbidities, and the ability to begin resuscitation expeditiously and effectively.

American College of Obstetricians and Gynecologists. *Critical Care in Pregnancy*. ACOG Practice Bulletin No. 100. Washington, DC: ACOG; February 2009.

24 Obstetric Analgesia & Anesthesia

John S. McDonald, MD
Biing-Jaw Chen, MD
Wing-Fai Kwan, MD

Analgesia is the loss or modulation of pain perception. It can be (1) local and affect only a small area of the body, (2) regional and affect a larger portion of the body, or (3) systemic. Analgesia is achieved by the use of hypnosis (suggestion), systemic medication, regional agents, or inhalational agents.

Anesthesia is the total loss of sensory perception and may include loss of consciousness. It is induced by various agents and techniques. In obstetrics, **regional anesthesia** is accomplished with local anesthetic techniques (epidural, spinal) and **general anesthesia** with systemic medication and endotracheal intubation.

The terms *analgesia* and *anesthesia* are sometimes confused in common usage. Analgesia denotes those states in which only modulation of pain perception is involved. Anesthesia denotes those states in which mental awareness and perception of other sensations are lost. Attempts have been made to divide anesthesia into various components, including analgesia, amnesia, relaxation, and loss of reflex response to pain. Analgesia can be regarded as a component of anesthesia if viewed in this way.

The use of techniques and medications to provide pain relief in obstetrics requires an expert understanding of their effects to ensure the safety of both mother and fetus.

ANATOMY OF PAIN

It may be academic to argue that pain should be defined as the parturient's response to the stimuli of labor, because agreement on a definition of pain has eluded scholars for centuries.

Nevertheless, it should be appreciated that the "pain response" is a response of the total personality and cannot be dissected systematically and scientifically. Physicians are obligated to provide a comfortable or at least a tolerable labor and delivery. Many patients are tense and apprehensive at the onset of labor, although they may have little or no discomfort. The physician must be knowledgeable of the options for pain relief and respond to the patient's needs and wishes.

The evolution of pain in the first stage of labor originally was described as involving spinal segments T11 and T12. Subsequent research has determined that segments T10–L1 are involved. Discomfort is associated with ischemia of the uterus during contraction as well as dilatation and effacement of the cervix. Sensory pathways that convey nociceptive impulses of the first stage of labor include the uterine plexus, the inferior hypogastric plexus, the middle hypogastric plexus, the superior hypogastric plexus, the lumbar and lower thoracic sympathetic chain, and the T10–L1 spinal segments.

Pain in the second stage of labor also is produced by distention of the vagina and perineum. Sensory pathways from these areas are conveyed by branches of the pudendal nerve via the dorsal nerve of the clitoris, the labial nerves, and the inferior hemorrhoidal nerves. These are the major sensory branches to the perineum and are conveyed along nerve roots S2, S3, and S4. Nevertheless, other nerves, such as the ilioinguinal nerves, the genital branches of the genitofemoral nerves, and the perineal branches of the posterior femoral cutaneous nerves, may play a role in perineal innervation.

Although the major portion of the perineum is innervated by the 3 major branches of the pudendal nerve, innervation by the other nerves mentioned may be important in some patients. The type of pain reported may be an ache in the back or loins (referred pain, perhaps from the cervix), a cramp in the uterus (due to fundal contraction), or a "bursting" or "splitting" sensation in the lower vaginal canal or pudendum (due to dilatation of the cervix and vagina).

Dystocia, which usually is painful, may be due to fetopelvic disproportion; tetanic, prolonged, or dysrhythmic uterine contractions; intrapartum infection; or many other causes.

SAFETY OF OBSTETRIC ANESTHESIA

Substantial advances in the quality and safety of obstetric anesthesia have been made in the past 3 decades. Outdated techniques, such as "twilight sleep" and mask anesthesia, have been recognized as ineffective or unsafe and have been replaced by epidural infusion of narcotic/local anesthesia mixtures and patient-controlled analgesia during labor and postoperatively. When required, general anesthesia is provided using short-acting drugs with well-known fetal effects, and careful attention is focused on airway management.

Maternal mortality relating to anesthesia has been reduced 10-fold since the 1950s, largely because of an enhanced appreciation of special maternal risks associated with anesthesia. The overall anesthesia-related death rate in the United States now is as low as 1.0 per million live births, a 5-fold decline in the last decade. Regional anesthesia now is more commonly performed for caesarean delivery, fewer births occur in hospitals performing fewer than 500 deliveries per year, and having both in-house anesthesia and obstetric physician coverage is more common. Historically, women have a higher chance of dying under general anesthesia than regional anesthesia during caesarean deliveries. During the 1970s and 1980s, the case fatality rate for general anesthesia during caesarean delivery was 32.3 per million and the rate for regional anesthesia was 1.9 per million. Thus 17 women died under general anesthesia for every 1 who died from regional anesthesia. By the 1990s, that ratio dropped to 6 to 1. In the 2000s, the case fatality rate for general anesthesia during caesarean delivery has decreased to 6.5 per million and case fatality rate for regional anesthesia has slightly increased to 3.8. The relative risk of general compared with regional anesthesia fell to 1.7. General anesthesia now seems just as safe as a spinal or epidural for caesarean delivery. The decline in deaths under general anesthesia could be attributed to better anesthetic monitoring, better management of difficult airway-failed intubation, and expertise with laryngeal airway mask and other airways devices. Difficulty with intubation, aspiration, and hypoxemia leading to cardiopulmonary arrest are the leading causes of anesthesia-related maternal death under general anesthesia. And the leading causes of anesthesia-related maternal death from regional anesthesia are high spinal or epidural block, respiratory failure, and drug reaction.

Another point of concern is that the overall maternal mortality (not related specifically to anesthesia) has increased in the United States since 1985. This increase in maternal mortality is most pronounced in older parturients (older than 35 years), particularly in black parturients. Cardiomyopathy, hypertension, obesity, and hemorrhage are the principal etiologies associated with these rising mortality rates and are important factors for the anesthesiologist to consider.

TECHNIQUES OF ANALGESIA WITHOUT THE USE OF DRUGS

Psychophysical Methods

Three distinct psychologic techniques have been developed as a means of facilitating the birth process and making it a positive emotional experience: "natural childbirth," psychoprophylaxis, and hypnosis. So-called *natural childbirth* was developed by Grantly Dick-Read in the early 1930s and popularized in his book *Childbirth Without Fear*. Dick-Read's approach emphasized the reduction of tension to induce relaxation. The psychoprophylactic technique was developed by Velvovski, who published the results of his work from Russia in 1950. In Russia in the mid-1950s, it became evident that obstetric psychoprophylaxis was a useful substitute for poorly administered or dangerously conducted anesthesia for labor and delivery. This method was later introduced in France by Lamaze. Hypnosis for pain relief has achieved periodic spurts of popularity since the early 1800s and depends on the power of suggestion.

Many obstetricians argue that psychoprophylaxis can largely eliminate the pain of childbirth by diminishing cortical appreciation of pain impulses rather than by depressing cortical function, as occurs with drug-induced analgesia. Relaxation, suggestion, concentration, and motivation are factors that overlap other methods of preparation for childbirth. Some of them are closely related to hypnosis.

These techniques can significantly reduce anxiety, tension, and fear. They provide the parturient with a valuable understanding of the physiologic changes that occur during labor and delivery. In addition, they provide an opportunity for closer understanding and communication between the patient and her mate, who may be an important source of comfort to her during the stressful process of childbirth. If psychophysical techniques do no more than this, they deserve the obstetrician's support.

Studies undertaken to assess the effectiveness of psychophysical techniques have reported widely divergent results, with effectiveness ranging from as low as 10–20% to as high as 70–80%. The overall benefit is best judged by the parturient herself, with validation by the observations of attendants. As is no doubt true in other aspects of medical practice in which emotional overlay and subjective reporting play a role in the evaluation of specific types of therapy, the personality and level of enthusiasm of the doctor can strongly influence the patient's reactions to a given therapy. Practitioners who are skeptical of psychophysical techniques cannot expect to accomplish very much using them.

None of these psychophysical techniques should be forced on a patient, even by a skillful provider. The patient must not be made to feel that she will fail if she does not choose to complete her labor and delivery without analgesic medication. It must be made clear to the patient from the outset that she is expected to ask for help if she feels she wants or needs it. All things considered, psychophysical techniques should be viewed as adjuncts to other analgesic methods rather than substitutes for them.

The effectiveness of hypnosis is partially due to the well-known, although incompletely understood, mechanisms by which emotional and other central processes can influence a person's overall responses to the pain experience. Verbal suggestion and somatosensory stimulation may help to alleviate discomfort associated with the first stage of labor. In addition, hypnotic states may provide apparent analgesia and amnesia for distressing, anxiety-provoking experiences. Finally, hypnotic techniques may substantially improve the parturient's outlook and behavior by reducing fear and apprehension. However, certain practical points with regard to hypnosis must be considered because the time needed to establish a suitable relationship between physician and patient often is more than can be made available in the course of a busy medical practice.

ANALGESIC, AMNESTIC, & ANESTHETIC AGENTS

General Comments & Precautions

1. If the patient is prepared psychologically for her experience, she will require less medication. Anticipate and dispel her fears during the antenatal period and in early labor. Never promise a painless labor.
2. Individualize the treatment of every patient, because each one reacts differently. Unfavorable reactions to any drug can occur.
3. Know the drug you intend to administer. Be familiar with its limitations, dangers, and contraindications as well as its advantages.
4. All analgesics given to the mother will cross the placenta. Systemic medications produce higher maternal and fetal blood levels than regionally administered drugs. Many drugs have central nervous system depressant effects. Although they may have the desired effect on the mother, they also may exert a mild to severe depressant effect on the fetus or newborn.

The ideal drug will have an optimal beneficial effect on the mother and a minimal depressant effect on the offspring. None of the presently available narcotic and sedative medications used in obstetrics has selective maternal effects. The regional administration of local anesthetics accomplished this goal to a large extent because the low maternal serum levels that are produced expose the fetus to insignificant quantities of drugs.

Pharmacologic Aspects

A. Route of Administration

Systemic techniques of analgesia and anesthesia include both oral and parenteral routes of administration. Parenteral administration includes subcutaneous, intramuscular, and intravenous injection. Sedatives, tranquilizers, and analgesics usually are given by intramuscular injection. In some cases, the intravenous route is preferred.

The advantages of intravenous administration are (1) avoidance of variable rates of uptake due to poor vascular supply in fat or muscle; (2) prompt onset of effect; (3) titration of effect, avoiding the "peak effect" of an intramuscular bolus; and (4) smaller effective doses because of earlier onset of action.

The disadvantages of intravenous injection are inadvertent arterial injection and the depressant effect of overdosage, but the advantage of smaller dosage outweighs the disadvantages.

Always administer the lowest concentration and the smallest dose to obtain the desired effect.

B. Physical and Chemical Factors

Anesthetics penetrate body cells by passing through the lipid membrane boundary. This membrane is not permeable to charged (ionized) drugs but is permeable to unionized forms of drugs. Much of the total drug transfer is dependent on the degree of lipid solubility, so local anesthetics are characterized by aromatic rings that are lipophilic, and all are lipid-soluble. The intermediate amine radical of a local anesthetic is a weak base that in aqueous solutions exists partly as undissociated free base and partly as dissociated cation. Figure 24–1 shows the equilibrium for such an existence and the Henderson-Hasselbalch equation, with which the proportion of the anesthetic in the charged and uncharged forms can be determined. The ratio of the cation to the base form of the drug is important, because the base form is responsible for penetration and tissue diffusion of the local anesthetic, whereas the cation form is responsible for local analgesia when the drug contacts the site of action within the sodium channel on the axolemma.

The pK_a of a drug is the pH at which equal proportions of the free base and cation form occur. Most local anesthetics used in obstetric analgesia have pK_a values ranging from 7.7–9.1 (Table 24–1). Because the pH of maternal blood is equal to or greater than 7.4, the pK_a of local anesthetics is so close that significant changes in maternal and fetal acid–base balance may result in fluxes in the base versus the

$$\underset{\text{Cation}}{R{:}NH^{+}} + OH^{-} \rightleftharpoons \underset{\text{Base}}{R{:}N} + HOH$$

$$pH = pK_a + \log \frac{\text{Base}}{\text{Cation}}$$

▲ **Figure 24–1.** Local anesthetics are weak bases coexisting as undissociated free base and dissociated cation. Their proportion can be calculated by means of the Henderson-Hasselbalch equation.

Table 24–1. pKa values of the more commonly used local anesthetics.

Drug	Brand Name	pKa
Bupivacaine	Marcaine	8.1
Chloroprocaine	Nesacaine	8.7
Etidocaine	Duranest	7.7
Lidocaine	Xylocaine	7.9
Ropivacaine	Naropin	8.0
Tetracaine	Pontocaine	8.5

cation forms of the drug. For example, a rising pH shifts a given amount of local anesthetic cation to the base form; conversely, a fall in pH generates more of the cationic form.

Physical factors are important in drug transfer. Drugs with a molecular weight (MW) under 600 cross the placenta without difficulty, whereas those with MW over 1000 do not. A molecule such as digoxin (MW 780.95) crosses the ovine placenta very poorly. Molecular weights of most local anesthetics are in the 200–300 range. From the physical aspect, most local anesthetics cross the maternal–fetal barrier by simple diffusion according to the principles of Fick's law (Fig. 24–2), which states that the rate of diffusion of a drug depends on the concentration gradient of the drug between the maternal and fetal compartments and the relationship of the thickness and total surface available for transfer.

C. Placental Transfer

Factors other than the physical or chemical properties of a drug may affect its transfer across the placenta. These factors include the rate and route of drug administration and the distribution, metabolism, and excretion of the drug by the mother and fetus. Fick's law may appear to be a simple method of determining drug transfer, but other complexities exist: differential blood flow on either side of the placenta, volume of maternal and fetal blood, and various shunts in the intervillous space that are important determinants of the final amount of drug a fetus may receive. Certain maternal disorders, such as hypertensive cardiovascular disease, diabetes, and preeclampsia-eclampsia, may alter placental blood flow and in some way affect the extent of drug distribution.

$$Q/T = K\left[\frac{A(C_M - C_F)}{D}\right]$$

▲ **Figure 24–2.** Fick's law. A, surface area available for drug transfer; C_M, maternal drug concentration; C_F, fetal drug concentration; D, membrane thickness; K, diffusion constant of the drug; Q/T, rate of diffusion.

As the placenta matures, the thickness of the epithelial trophoblastic layer progressively decreases. This reduction may cause the thickness of the tissue layers between the maternal and fetal compartments to decrease 10-fold (from as much as 25 μm in early gestation to 2 μm at term in some species). As gestation progresses, the surface area of the placenta also increases. At term, these changes in physical structure tend to favor improved transfer of drugs across the placenta.

Placental transfer is affected by the pH of the blood on both sides of the placenta. The pH of the blood on the fetal side of the placenta normally is 0.1–0.2 U lower than that on the maternal side. Therefore, passage of drug to the fetal unit results in a tendency for more of the drug to exist in the ionized state. Because the maternal–fetal equilibrium is established only between the unionized fraction of the drug on either side of the barrier, this physiologic differential will expedite maternal–fetal transfer of drug. With more drug in the ionized form in the fetal unit, the new equilibrium that arises results in a greater total (ionized plus unionized) drug load in the fetus. Because the pK_a values of commonly used local anesthetics are closer to the maternal blood pH, these agents tend to accumulate on the fetal side of the placenta. This also is true of other basic drugs such as morphine, meperidine, and propranolol. Further decreases in the fetal pH lead to additional drug entrapment in the fetus. For acidic drugs (eg, thiopental) the shift in total drug concentration is in the opposite direction, that is, toward the maternal side of the placenta.

In summary, the rate of transfer of a drug is governed mainly by (1) lipid solubility, (2) degree of drug ionization, (3) placental blood flow, (4) molecular weight, (5) placental metabolism, and (6) protein binding.

D. Fetal Distribution

After a drug deposited in the maternal compartment passes through the maternal–fetal barrier, the drug must reach the fetus and undergo distribution (Fig. 24–3). The response of the fetus and newborn depends on drug concentration in vessel-rich organs, such as the brain, heart, and liver. Drugs transferred from the maternal to the fetal compartment of the placenta are then diluted before distribution to the various fetal vital organs. Approximately 85% of the blood in the umbilical vein, which passes from the placenta to the fetus, passes through the fetal liver and then into the inferior vena cava. The remainder bypasses the liver and enters the vena cava primarily via the ductus venosus. An admixture of blood coming from the lower extremities, the abdominal viscera, the upper extremities, and the thorax further reduces the drug concentration. Blood from the right atrium shunts from right to left through the foramen ovale into the left atrium, resulting in a final concentration on the left side of the heart that is only slightly lower than that in the vena cava.

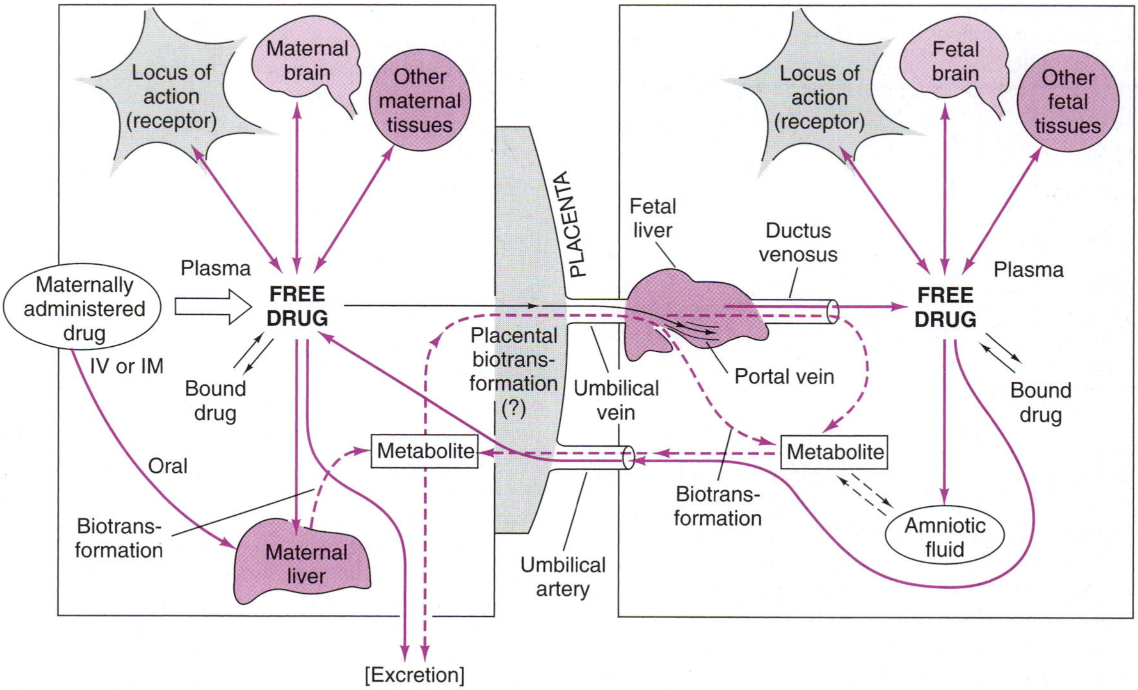

▲ **Figure 24–3.** Relationship between maternal and fetal compartments and distribution of drugs between them. Drug is passed from the maternal compartment, via the placenta (a partial barrier), to the fetal compartment, where the principles of drug dynamics (ie, distribution, biotransformation, and excretion) determine the eventual specific organ tissue levels. One purely mechanical barrier exists between the maternal and fetal compartments, which attains importance in the late first and second stages of labor—the umbilical cord, which is susceptible to partial and total occlusion.

The amount of drug ultimately reaching a vital organ is related to that organ's blood supply. Because the central nervous system is the most highly vascularized fetal organ, it receives the greatest amount of drug. Once the drug reaches the fetal liver, it may either be bound to protein or metabolized.

The uptake of drug by fetal tissues can be very rapid after either intravenous or epidural administration. Measurable concentrations of local anesthetics have been found in fetal tissues as early as 1–2 minutes after injection. Lipid solubility of a drug is important in developing concentrations in certain organs with high lipid content, such as the adrenal, ovary, liver, and brain.

Drug metabolism and excretion are the final features of the fetal distribution picture. The fetal liver is able to metabolize drugs and numerous substrates as early as the second trimester, an ability that improves to term. Narcotics and sedatives are metabolized much more slowly by the fetal liver, producing a prolonged effect of these drugs in the newborn who is exposed in utero. Finally, the ability of the fetus to excrete drugs is also reduced by reduced renal function.

Systemic Analgesics & Anesthetics

A. Sedatives (Hypnotics)

The principal use of sedative–hypnotic drugs is to produce drowsiness. For many years, these drugs were the only ones available to reduce anxiety and induce drowsiness. The latent phase of the first stage of labor can be managed by either psychologic support alone or utilization of sedative–hypnotic compounds. Psychologic support may be complemented by the use of sedatives. When properly used, these drugs induce tranquility and an enhanced feeling of well-being. They are poor analgesics and do not raise the pain threshold appreciably in conscious subjects. Amnesia does not occur. Labor may be slowed by large doses of sedatives, especially when given too early in the first stage.

The use of barbiturates alone for obstetric analgesia is not common practice and should be discouraged. The required dosage is dangerous to the fetus, which is extremely sensitive to central nervous system depression by these drugs. Periodic apnea and even abolition of all movements outlast the effects of the barbiturates on the mother.

B. Tranquilizers & Amnestics

These drugs are used principally to relieve apprehension and anxiety and to produce a calm state. Additionally, they may potentiate the effects of other sedatives. An analgesic-potentiating effect is often claimed for this group of agents but has not been definitely demonstrated. Hydroxyzine and diazepam are popular tranquilizer–amnestics. Scopolamine, which was widely popular in obstetrics in the past, produces no analgesia but has a mild sedative and marked amnestic effect. Scopolamine is no longer used because the amnesia produced is excessive and prolonged. Diazepam should be avoided during labor because it has a long chemical half-life, which is even more prolonged in the neonate. Diazepam readily crosses the placenta and is found in significant concentrations in fetal plasma. At present, diazepam is not recommended if the neonate is premature because of the threat of kernicterus. Other potential side effects related to the use of diazepam are fetal hypotonia, hypothermia, and a loss of beat-to-beat variability in the fetal heart rate.

One of the controversies over diazepam concerns the content of sodium benzoate and benzoic acid buffers. Both compounds are potent uncouplers of the bilirubin–albumin complex, and some investigators have suggested that the neonate may be more susceptible to kernicterus because of an increase level of free circulating bilirubin. However, because injectable diazepam is effective in the treatment of human newborn seizure disorders, opiate withdrawal, and tetanus and because it is regarded as a useful adjunct in obstetric analgesia, a study was undertaken in animals in which comparable quantities of sodium benzoate were injected to determine whether significant amounts of bilirubin would be made available to the circulation. Midazolam, a short-acting water-soluble benzodiazepine, appears to be devoid of the neonatal effects seen with diazepam and is more rapidly cleared. In small doses it could conceivably become a useful anxiolytic for the laboring patient. Midazolam is 3–4 times more potent than diazepam, and there is a brief delay in the onset of its sedative effect after intravenous injection. Doses should be kept below 0.075 mg/kg to avoid excessive anterograde amnesia.

C. Narcotic Analgesics

Systemic analgesic drugs (including narcotics) are commonly used in the first stage of labor because they produce both a state of analgesia and mood elevation. The favored drugs are codeine 60 mg intramuscularly or meperidine 50–100 mg intramuscularly or 25–50 mg (titrated) intravenously. The combination of morphine and scopolamine was once popular for its "twilight sleep" effect but is rarely used now. Common undesirable effects of this combination of drugs are nausea and vomiting, cough suppression, intestinal stasis, and diminution in frequency, intensity, and duration of uterine contractions in the early first stage of labor. Also, amnesia is excessive for these patients.

Morphine is not used in active laboring patients because of the excessive respiratory depression seen in the neonate compared with equipotent doses of other narcotics. Fetuses who are of young gestational age, are small for dates, or have undergone trauma or long labor are more susceptible to narcosis.

Fentanyl is a popular synthetic narcotic that has been used in obstetrics in both the systemic and epidural compartments. Its use in the epidural compartment has met with good success when combined with small quantities and low concentrations of bupivacaine. Data supporting its use come from both Europe and the United States.

Sufentanil is a derivative of fentanyl with increased potency and lipophilicity. It is widely used for intrathecal and epidural analgesia during labor. Potential adverse effects of sufentanil include possible placental deposition and neonatal respiratory depression. Adding intrathecal or epidural sufentanil to bupivacaine improves labor analgesia with faster onset and longer duration compared with bupivacaine alone. The usual dose is 3–5 μg intrathecally and 10–15 μg epidurally.

Remifentanil is a newer ultra short-acting synthetic opioid with rapid onset (approximately 1 minute) after intravenous administration. It is rapidly metabolized by nonspecific blood and tissue esterases, not depending on renal or hepatic function, and hence it does not accumulate in the fetus. This rapid onset and elimination facilitate its effective and safe use during labor. Remifentanil has been administered as intravenous analgesia for labor using a variety of methods, including baseline infusion, PCA boluses (with or without baseline infusion), and target-controlled infusions.

Butorphanol (Stadol) is a synthetic parenteral analgesic that has agonist and antagonist of opioid properties. It is 5 times as potent as morphine and 40 times as potent as meperidine. The typical doses are 1–2 mg intravenously or intramuscularly every 3–4 hours. Onset of analgesia is within a few minutes after intravenous injection. There is less respiratory depression compared with an equivalent dose of morphine due to ceiling effect from its agonist-antagonist properties. This property makes butorphanol particularly useful for labor analgesia, when respiratory depression of the fetus/neonate is a concern.

Nalbuphine (Nubain) is a mixed agonist/antagonist opioid similar to butorphanol commonly used for parenteral labor analgesia. Its potency is equivalent to that of morphine on a milligram basis. The onset of action after intravenous injection is 2–3 minutes with duration of 5–6 hours. The usual dose is 10–20 mg intravenously every 4–6 hours. It is metabolized predominantly by the liver and excreted by the kidney.

D. Thiobarbiturate

Intravenous anesthetics such as thiopental and thiamylal are widely used in general surgery. However, less than 4 minutes after a thiobarbiturate is injected into the mother's vein, the concentrations of the drug in the fetal and maternal blood will be equal. The mother will lose consciousness and airway protective reflexes with a thiopental dose of 1.5–2 mg/kg; therefore, it should be used only in association with general endotracheal anesthesia. Thiopental doses of 3–4 mg/kg are used for induction of general anesthesia.

E. Propofol

Propofol is a newer induction agent that was introduced into practice in the United States in the early 1990s. As an induction agent, it is similar to the barbiturates in mild cardiac depression and loss of peripheral vasomotor tone. It offers the advantages of rapid clearance, short duration of action, antiemetic properties, and reduced risk of airway reactivity. It is an ideal agent for induction of general anesthesia at a dose of 2 mg/kg in parturients. It also can be used in 10- to 20-mg increments during surgery under regional block to treat nausea and vomiting. Neonatal Apgar scores and umbilical gases are similar after induction with propofol or barbiturates.

F. Etomidate

Etomidate is an intravenous induction agent that has been used in obstetric anesthesia since 1979. It produces a rapid onset of anesthesia with minimal cardiorespiratory effects. This property makes it ideal for parturients who are hemodynamically unstable or who would not tolerate hemodynamic aberrations well. With an induction dose of 0.2–0.3 mg/kg, etomidate undergoes a rapid hydrolysis that leads to quick recovery. Etomidate crosses the placenta rapidly; however, large variations in the UV/MV (umbilical vein : maternal vein) ratio (0.04–0.5) have been reported. Etomidate may cause pain at the injection site and involuntary muscle movements in some patients.

G. Ketamine

The phencyclidine derivative ketamine produces anesthesia by a dissociative interruption of afferent pathways from cortical perception. It has become a useful and widely used adjunctive agent in obstetrics because maternal cardiovascular status and uterine blood flow are well maintained. Effective maternal analgesia results from low doses of 0.25–0.5 mg/kg but without loss of consciousness or protective reflexes. The margin of safety is narrow, however, so it should be used only by physicians able to easily secure and protect the airway if loss of consciousness occurs. For caesarean delivery, general anesthetic induction can be produced with 1–2 mg/kg intravenously. Ketamine stimulates the cardiovascular system to maintain heart rate, blood pressure, and cardiac output. It is useful in the setting of major blood loss, when rapid induction of general anesthesia is required. However, it has significant hallucinogenic effects that limit its utility in obstetrics.

H. Inhalation Anesthetics

Inhaled anesthetics are administered as a component of general anesthesia. In the past, inhaled anesthetics were given during labor in subanesthetic concentrations to treat contraction pain, but they are no longer used for this indication. The mask administration of these gases to the conscious laboring patient can result in airway obstruction, aspiration, and hypoxia. Also, the vaporized gases would unacceptably contaminate the labor room environment because effectively scavenging of exhaust gases from the room is not possible. Finally, of all the presently used volatile anesthetics, only nitrous oxide has analgesic properties at subanesthetic concentrations.

The most commonly used inhaled anesthetics in pregnancy are nitrous oxide, sevoflurane, desflurane, and isoflurane. These drugs all readily cross the placenta and produce significant blood concentrations in the fetus. During the brief exposure to maternally administered anesthetic gases, the fetus is not adversely affected. Fetal cardiac output is slightly reduced by these drugs, but critical organ blood flow is unaffected, and fetal acid–base status is unchanged. Exposure to minimum alveolar concentrations of anesthetic gases for more than 15 minutes is associated with reduced Apgar scores, but other parameters of fetal and newborn well-being are unimpaired.

The term parturient is more sensitive to the anesthetic effects of all inhaled anesthetics, presumably as a result of elevated progesterone levels. This increased sensitivity of 20–30% compared with nonpregnant subjects places the patient at increased risk for obtundation and aspiration; therefore, these drugs should not be administered without preparation for endotracheal intubation. Volatile agents except N_2O produce uterine relaxation, and high concentrations should be avoided during delivery to prevent uterine atony and postpartum hemorrhage. At low concentrations (<1%), they produce amnesia, and their tocolytic effects are easily counteracted by standard infusions of oxytocin (Pitocin).

REGIONAL ANESTHESIA

Regional anesthesia is achieved by injection of a local anesthetic (Table 24–2) around the nerves that pass from spinal segments to the peripheral nerves responsible for sensory innervation of a portion of the body. More recently, narcotics have been added to local anesthetics to improve analgesia and reduce some side effects of local anesthetics. Regional nerve blocks used in obstetrics include the following: (1) lumbar epidural and caudal epidural block, (2) subarachnoid (spinal) block, (3) combined spinal epidural block, and (4) pudendal block.

Infiltration of a local anesthetic drug and pudendal block analgesia carry minimal risks. The hazards increase with the amount of drug used. The safety and suitability of regional anesthesia depend on proper selection of the drug and the patient and the obstetrician–gynecologist's knowledge,

Table 24–2. Drugs used for local anesthesia.

	Tetracaine (Pontocaine)	Lidocaine (Xylocaine)	Bupivacaine (Marcaine)	Chloroprocaine (Nesacaine)	Ropivacaine (Naropin)
Potency*	10	2-3	9-12	3	9-12
Toxicity*	10	1-1.5	4-6	1	3-4
Stability	Stable	Stable	Stable	Stable	Stable
Total maximal dose	50-100 mg	350-500 mg	175-200 mg	800-1000 mg	200-250 mg
Infiltration					
Concentration	0.05-0.1%	0.5-1%	0.25%	1-2%	0.2-0.5%
Onset	10-20 min	3-5 min	5-10 min	3-5 min	5-10 min
Duration	1½-3 h	1-2 h	1½-4 h	30-60 min	1½-4 h
Nerve block					
Concentration	0.25-0.5%	1-2%	0.25-0.5%	2%	0.5-1%
Onset	20-30 min	10-20 min	20-30 min	10-20 min	20-30 min
Duration	3-10 h	2-4 h	4-12 h	30-60 min	5-8 h
Epidural					
Concentration	—	1-2%	0.06-0.5%	2-3%	0.05-1%
Onset	—	5-15 min	15-20 min	5-10 min	15-20 min
Duration		1-2 h	2-5 h	30-60 min	2-4 h
Subarachnoid					
Concentration	0.25-1%	2-5%	0.5-0.75%	2%	0.5-1%
Dose	5-20 mg	40-100 mg	0.75-15 mg	35-50 mg	15-22.5 mg
Onset	Fast	Fast	Fast	Fast	Fast
Duration	90-200 min	45-90 min	75-150 min	30-45min	75-150 min

*Compared with procaine.

experience, and expertise in the diagnosis and treatment of possible complications. Major conductive anesthesia and general anesthesia in obstetrics require specialized knowledge and expertise in conjunction with close maternal and fetal monitoring. This field of expertise has developed as a subspecialty within anesthesia, reflecting the need for specialized understanding of the obstetric patient and her response and of the fetal responses to anesthesia.

Patient Selection

Regional anesthesia is appropriate for labor analgesia, caesarean delivery, and other obstetric operative procedures (eg, postpartum tubal ligation, cervical cerclage). Most patients prefer to remain awake; however, occasionally a choice is made to provide general anesthesia.

The anesthesiologist will assess the patient to determine the relative risks of general versus regional anesthesia. For example, some forms of valvular heart disease may contraindicate regional block, and general anesthesia may be considered more appropriate. Other contraindications to regional anesthesia include infection, coagulopathy, hypovolemia, progressive neurologic disease, and patient refusal.

Patient Preparation

The woman who is well informed and has a good rapport with her physician generally is a calm and cooperative candidate for regional or general anesthesia. The patient and her partner should be well informed early in her pregnancy of the options for labor anesthesia as well as for caesarean section if that circumstance arises. The anesthesiologist can be involved early in pregnancy if the patient has special concerns about anesthesia (family history of anesthetic risk, previous back surgery, coagulation problems). Some hospitals have obstetric anesthesia preassessment clinics that deal with these patient concerns.

Local Anesthetic Agents

A local anesthetic drug blocks the action potential of nerves when their axons are exposed to the medication. Local anesthetic agents act by modifying the ionic permeability of the cell membrane to stabilize its resting potential. The smaller the nerve fiber, the more sensitive it is to local anesthetics because the susceptibility of individual nerve fibers is inversely proportional to the cross-sectional diameter of the fibers. Hence, with regional anesthesia, the patient's perception of light touch, pain, and temperature and her capacity for vasomotor control are obtunded sooner and with a smaller concentration of the drug than is the perception of pressure or the function of motor nerves to striated muscles. The exception to this rule is the sensitivity of autonomic nerve fibers that are blocked by the lowest concentration of local anesthetic despite their being larger than some sensory nerves.

Only anesthetic drugs that are completely reversible and nonirritating and cause minimal toxicity are clinically acceptable. Other desirable properties of regional anesthetic agents include rapidity of onset, predictability of duration, and ease of sterilization. Table 24–2 summarizes the local anesthetics commonly used in obstetrics and gynecology together with their uses and doses.

All local anesthetics have certain undesirable dose-related side effects when absorbed systemically. All these drugs are capable of stimulating the central nervous system and may cause bradycardia, hypertension, or respiratory stimulation at the medullary level. Moreover, they may produce anxiety, excitement, or convulsions at the cortical or subcortical level. This response stimulates grand mal seizures because it is followed by depression, loss of vasomotor control, hypotension, respiratory depression, and coma. Such an episode of indirect cardiovascular depression often is accentuated by a direct vasodilatory and myocardial depressant effect. The latter is comparable to the action of quinidine. This effect explains why lidocaine is useful for treatment of certain cardiac arrhythmias.

Chloroprocaine is an ester derivative that was popular in 1970s primarily because of its rapid onset and short duration of action and its low toxicity to the fetus. It is metabolized by plasma cholinesterase and therefore does not demand liver enzyme degradation, as do the more complex and longer acting amide derivatives. Chloroprocaine has a half-life of 21 seconds in adult blood and 43 seconds in neonatal blood. Direct toxic effects on the fetus are minimized because fewer drugs are available for transfer in the maternal compartment.

The potency of chloroprocaine is comparable to that of lidocaine and mepivacaine, and the drug is 3 times more potent than procaine. Its average onset of action ranges from 6–12 minutes and persists for 30–60 minutes, depending on the amount used. Chloroprocaine is often used for urgent caesarean delivery when epidural catheter is already placed to avoid general anesthesia.

Bupivacaine, the amide local anesthetic, is related to lidocaine and mepivacaine but has some very different physicochemical properties. It has a much higher lipid solubility, a higher degree of binding to maternal plasma protein, and a much longer duration of action. More than with other local anesthetics, the concentration of bupivacaine can be reduced to produce sensory block with minimal motor block. Because injection of bupivacaine for labor pain relief now is mostly in the form of continuous small-volume and minimal concentration administration via a pump mechanism, the complications previously of concern, such as hypotension and convulsions, are now rare.

A word of caution is needed regarding the administration of bupivacaine for caesarean delivery. This drug has been implicated in certain cardiovascular catastrophes associated with initial drug injection, such as cardiac arrests that were refractory to full and appropriate resuscitative attempts. Although these catastrophes are rare, the practitioner is well advised to inject no more than 5 mL of the drug at any one time, to wait 4–5 minutes, then to repeat the procedure until the desired volume has been delivered. The maximum concentration of bupivacaine now allowed by the Food and Drug Administration (FDA) for obstetric epidural anesthesia is 0.5%. The dose of more than 3 mg/kg is considered a toxic dose now. The safety of bupivacaine can be enhanced by giving it in fractional doses (eg, 5 mL every 5 minutes).

Ropivacaine is a newer amide local anesthetic introduced into the United States in the mid-1990s. It is less lipid-soluble than bupivacaine, and initial studies suggested that it produced less motor blockade and was less cardiotoxic than its homologue bupivacaine. Later studies have been less convincing in documenting improved efficacy and safety, but ropivacaine has replaced bupivacaine in some institutions. There is ongoing study of the safety and efficacy of levobupivacaine, the levorotatory isomer of bupivacaine, which may also prove less cardiotoxic than its racemic parent molecule. Both of these newer amide local anesthetics are used in doses and concentrations similar to those of bupivacaine.

Local Infiltration Analgesia

Local tissue infiltration of dilute solutions of anesthetic drugs generally yields satisfactory results because the target is the fine nerve fibers. Nevertheless, one must keep in mind the dangers of systemic toxicity when large areas are anesthetized or when reinjection is required. It is good practice, therefore, to calculate in advance the milligrams of drug and volume of solution that may be required to keep the total dosage below the accepted toxic dose.

Infiltration in or near an area of inflammation is contraindicated. Injections into these zones may be followed by rapid systemic absorption of the drug as a result of increased vascularity of the inflamed tissues. Moreover, the injection may introduce or aggravate infection.

Regional Analgesia Techniques

A. Lumbar Epidural Block

This analgesic technique is well suited to obstetric anesthesia. Either bolus injections or continuous infusion of local anesthetics is used for labor, vaginal delivery, or caesarean surgery. Narcotics are added to supplement the quality of the block.

After the patient is evaluated, an epidural block can be placed once labor is established. Drug dosages can be adjusted as circumstances change. The catheter can be used for surgery and postoperative analgesia if necessary. The second stage of labor is prolonged by epidural anesthesia; however, the duration of the first stage is unaffected. The use of outlet forceps is increased, but fetal outcome is not adversely affected by epidural block.

The epidural block technique must be exact, and inadvertent massive (high) spinal anesthesia occasionally occurs. Other undesirable reactions include the rapid absorption syndrome (hypotension, bradycardia, hallucinations, and convulsions), postpartum backache, and paresthesias. Epidural block should eradicate pain between T10 and L1 for the first stage of labor and between T10 and S5 for the second stage of labor.

The procedure is as follows. Inject 3 mL of a 1.5% aqueous solution of lidocaine or similar agent into the catheter as a test dose. If spinal anesthesia does not result after 5–10 minutes, inject an additional 5 mL. Inject 10 mL of the anesthetic solution in total to slowly accomplish an adequate degree and suitable level of anesthesia. Once the block is established, a continuous infusion of 10–12 mL/h will maintain the block for labor. Bupivacaine 0.125–0.25% is most often used for an epidural block, with fentanyl 2–5 µg/mL in the epidural mixture.

The mother is nursed in a wedged or lateral position to prevent aortocaval compression. The sympathectomy produced by the block predisposes the patient to venous pooling and reduced venous return. Maternal blood pressure must be measured frequently when the epidural is in effect.

B. Caudal Block

Caudal anesthesia (Fig. 24–4) is an epidural block approached through the caudal space. It can provide selective sacral block for the second stage of labor; however, it is rarely used now because of complications specific to the obstetric patient. The descent of the fetal head against the perineum, in addition to the sacral edema at term, obscures the landmarks of the sacral hiatus. This makes the caudal procedure technically challenging, and reports of transfixing the rectum and fetal skull puncture with the epidural needle have led many anesthesiologists to avoid this technique. Lumbar epidural anesthesia is considered a safer alternative.

C. Spinal Anesthesia

Spinal anesthesia currently is the anesthetic of choice for caesarean delivery. Spinal anesthesia can be performed

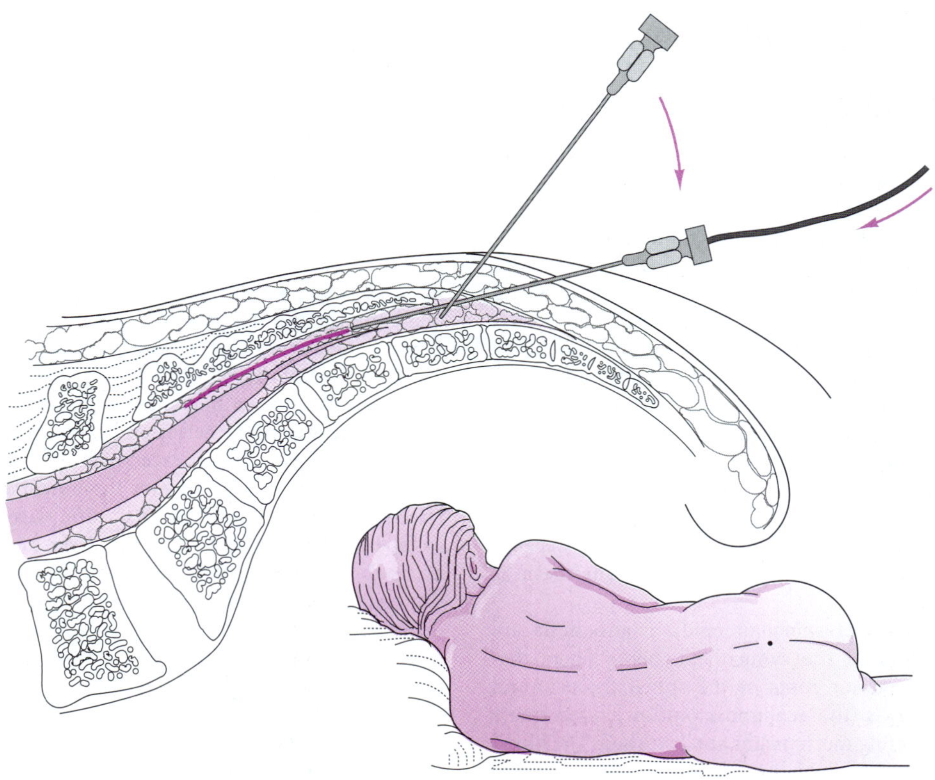

▲ **Figure 24–4.** Caudal catheter in place for continuous caudal anesthesia.

more quickly than epidural anesthesia and provides ideal operating conditions, including dense sensory and motor block. The onset of sympathectomy is more abrupt than with epidural block, so care must be taken to ensure that the patient is adequately preloaded with 1.5–2 L of saline solution before performing the technique. Spinal anesthesia is used less commonly these days to alleviate the pain of delivery and the third stage of labor. The advantages of spinal anesthesia are that the mother remains conscious to witness delivery, no inhalation anesthetics or analgesic drugs are required, the technique is not difficult, and good relaxation of the pelvic floor and lower birth canal is achieved. Prompt anesthesia is achieved within 5–10 minutes. The dosage of spinal anesthetic is small. Complications are rare and easy to treat. However, spinal headache occurs in 1–2% of patients.

D. Combined Spinal–Epidural Analgesia

The use of combined spinal–epidural anesthesia (CSE) became popular in the mid 1990s as an alternative to epidural anesthesia for labor. A small dose of local anesthetic and narcotic (2.5 mg bupivacaine and 25 μg fentanyl) is injected through a spinal needle, which is introduced through the epidural needle and advanced into the intrathecal space. The spinal needle is withdrawn and the epidural catheter placed for later use. The spinal medication produces immediate pain relief and minimal motor block and may allow ambulation. Later in labor, the epidural catheter is used for continuous infusion of epidural solution, similar to that described for standard epidural anesthesia in labor.

Detractors of CSE argue that the technique may increase the incidence of post–lumbar puncture headache and that ambulation even after low-dose spinal injection is unsafe for both mother and baby. Finally, because the technique is technically cumbersome, it may be associated with higher complication rates, although the studies did not support this statement.

The most serious consequence of spinal or epidural anesthesia is maternal mortality. Maternal deaths associated with use of 0.75% bupivacaine for caesarean delivery and labor were reported in the late 1980s, prompting the FDA to outlaw the use of this drug in obstetrics. These deaths were attributed to venous uptake of the drug and immediate and lasting myocardial depression from the local anesthetic, which did not respond to appropriate cardiac resuscitative efforts. Today maternal mortality associated with regional anesthesia is lower, primarily because bolus dosing of high concentrations of local anesthesia is no longer performed.

Most side effects of spinal or epidural anesthesia are secondary to block of the sympathetic nerve fibers that accompany the anterior roots of the spinal thoracic and upper lumbar nerves (thoracolumbar outflow). Thus many physiologic regulating mechanisms are disturbed. The blood pressure falls as a result of loss of arterial resistance and venous pooling—assuming no compensation is made by change of the patient's position (eg, Trendelenburg position). If high thoracic dermatomes (T1–T5) are blocked, alteration of the cardiac sympathetic innervation slows the heart rate and reduces cardiac contractility. Epinephrine secretion by the adrenal medulla is depressed. Concomitantly, the unopposed parasympathetic effect of cardiac slowing alters vagal stimulations. As a result of these and related changes, shock follows promptly, especially in hypotensive or hypovolemic patients. Moreover, a precipitous fall in the blood pressure of the arteriosclerotic hypertensive patient is inevitable.

Fluids, oxygen therapy for adequate tissue perfusion, shock position to encourage venous return, and pressor drugs given intravenously are recommended.

In the past, postdural puncture headache (PDPH) due to leakage of cerebrospinal fluid through the needle hole in the dura was an early postoperative complication in up to 15% of patients. Small-caliber needles (25F) decrease the incidence of headache to 8–10%. With the introduction of pencil-point Whitaker and Sprotte spinal needles, the incidence of PDPH has been reduced to 1–2%. Therapy for PDPH includes recumbent position, hydration, sedation, and, in severe cases, epidural injection of 10–20 mL of the patient's fresh blood to "seal" the defect.

Rarely, spinal or epidural anesthesia caused nerve injury and transient or permanent hypesthesia or paresthesia. Excessive drug concentration, sensitivity, or infection may have been responsible for some of these complications. The incidence of serious complications of spinal or epidural anesthesia is considerably lower than that of cardiac arrest during general anesthesia.

E. Paracervical Block

Paracervical block is no longer considered a safe technique for the obstetric patient. In the past, paracervical anesthesia was used to relieve the pain of the first stage of labor. Pudendal block was required for pain during the second stage of labor. Sensory nerve fibers from the uterus fuse bilaterally at the 4–6 o'clock and 6–8 o'clock positions around the cervix in the region of the cervical–vaginal junction. Ordinarily, when 5–10 mL of 1% lidocaine or its equivalent is injected into these areas, interruption of the sensory input from the cervix and uterus promptly follows.

Many now consider paracervical block to be contraindicated in obstetrics because of the potential adverse fetal effects. Many reports in the literature place the incidence of fetal bradycardia at 8–18%. However, recent work with accurate fetal heart rate monitoring associated with continuous uterine contraction patterns suggests that the incidence is closer to 20–25%. Some researchers have attempted to investigate the significance of the bradycardia. One explanation is that an acid–base disturbance in the fetus does not occur unless the bradycardia lasts longer than 10 minutes and that neonatal depression is rare unless associated with delivery during the period of bradycardia. There seems to be little difference in the incidence and severity of fetal bradycardia by paracervical block between complicated and uncomplicated patients. Other disadvantages of paracervical block include maternal trauma and bleeding, fetal trauma and direct injection, inadvertent intravascular injection with convulsions, and short duration of the block.

F. Pudendal Nerve Block

Pudendal block has been one of the most popular of all nerve block techniques in obstetrics. The infant is not depressed, and blood loss is minimal. The technique is simplified by the fact that the pudendal nerve approaches the spine of the ischium on its course to innervate the perineum. Injection of 10 mL of 1% lidocaine on each side will achieve analgesia for 30–45 minutes approximately 50% of the time.

Both the transvaginal and transcutaneous methods are useful for administering a pudendal block. The transvaginal technique has important practical advantages over the transcutaneous technique. The "Iowa trumpet" needle guide can be used, and the operator's finger should be placed at the end of the needle guide to palpate the sacrospinous ligament, which runs in the same direction and is just anterior to the pudendal nerve and artery. Appreciating the sensation of the needle puncturing the ligament usually is difficult. This facet of the technique (no definite end point) may make it difficult for the inexperienced clinician to perform. Aspiration of the syringe for possible inadvertent entry into the pudendal artery should be accomplished, and, if no blood is returned, 10 mL of local anesthetic solution should be injected in a fanlike fashion on the right and left sides. The successful performance of the pudendal block requires injection of the drug at least 10–12 minutes before episiotomy. Often in clinical practice, pudendal block is performed within 4–5 minutes of episiotomy, so the local anesthetic may not have adequate time to take effect.

1. Advantages and disadvantages—Advantages of pudendal nerve block are its safety, ease of administration, and rapidity of onset of effect. Disadvantages include maternal trauma, bleeding, and infection; rare maternal convulsions due to drug sensitivity; occasional complete or partial failure; and regional discomfort during administration.

The pudendal perineal block, like any other nerve block, demands some technical experience and knowledge of the innervation of the lower birth canal. Nevertheless, in spite of a well-placed bilateral block, skip areas of perineal analgesia may be noted. The possible reason is that although the pudendal nerve of S2–S4 derivation does contribute to the majority of fibers for sensory innervation to the perineum, other sensory fibers also are involved. For example, the inferior hemorrhoidal nerve may have an origin independent from that of the sacral nerve and therefore will not be a component branch of the pudendal nerve. In this case, it must be infiltrated separately. In addition, the posterior femoral cutaneous nerve (S1–S3) origin may contribute an important perineal branch to the anterior fourchette bilaterally. In instances in which this nerve plays a major role in innervation, it must be blocked separately by local skin infiltration.

Two other nerves contribute to the sensory innervation of the perineum: the ilioinguinal nerve, of L1 origin, and the genital branch of the genitofemoral nerve, of L1 and L2 origin. Both of these nerves sweep superficially over the mons pubis to innervate the skin over the symphysis of the mons pubis and the labium majus. Occasionally, these nerves must also be separately infiltrated to provide optimal perineal analgesic effect. Thus it should be apparent that a simple bilateral pudendal nerve block may not be effective in many cases. For maximum analgesic effectiveness, in addition to a bilateral pudendal block, superficial infiltration of the skin from the symphysis medially to a point halfway between the ischial spines may be necessary. Thus a true perineal block may be regarded as a regional technique.

Either lumbar epidural or caudal epidural block should eradicate pain between the T10 and S5 levels for the second stage. All of these nerves are denervated because they all are derived from L1–S5 segments.

2. Procedure (Fig. 24–5)

1. Palpate the ischial spines vaginally. Slowly advance the needle guide toward each spine. After placement is achieved, the needle is advanced through the guide to penetrate approximately 0.5 cm. Aspirate, and if the needle is not in a vessel, deposit 5 mL below each spine. This blocks the right and left pudendal nerves. Refill the syringe when necessary, and proceed in a similar manner to anesthetize the other areas specified. Keep the needle moving while injecting and avoid the sensitive vaginal mucosa and periosteum.
2. Withdraw the needle and guide approximately 2 cm and redirect toward an ischial tuberosity. Inject 3 mL near the center of each tuberosity to anesthetize the inferior hemorrhoidal and lateral femoral cutaneous nerves.
3. Withdraw the needle and guide almost entirely and then slowly advance toward the symphysis pubica almost to the clitoris, keeping approximately 2 cm lateral to the labial fold and approximately 1–2 cm beneath the skin. Injection of 5 mL of lidocaine on each side beneath the symphysis will block the ilioinguinal and genitocrural nerves.

If the procedure explained is carefully and skillfully done, only slight discomfort will be felt during the injections. Prompt flaccid relaxation and good anesthesia for 30–60 minutes can be expected. A summary of anesthetic approaches in labor is shown in Figure 24–6.

Prevention & Treatment of Local Anesthetic Overdosage

The correct dose of any local anesthetic is the smallest quantity of drug in the greatest dilution that will provide adequate

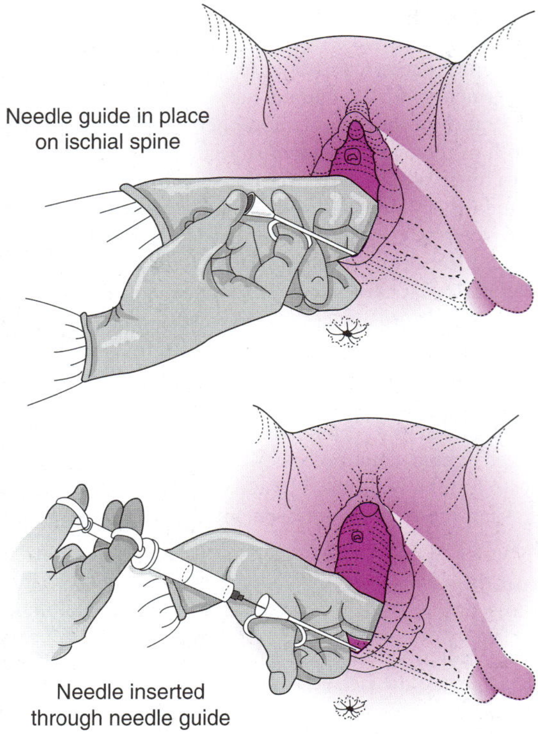

▲ **Figure 24–5.** Use of needle guide ("Iowa trumpet") in pudendal anesthetic block. (Reproduced, with permission, from Benson RC. *Handbook of Obstetrics & Gynecology*. 8th ed. Los Altos, CA: Lange; 1983.)

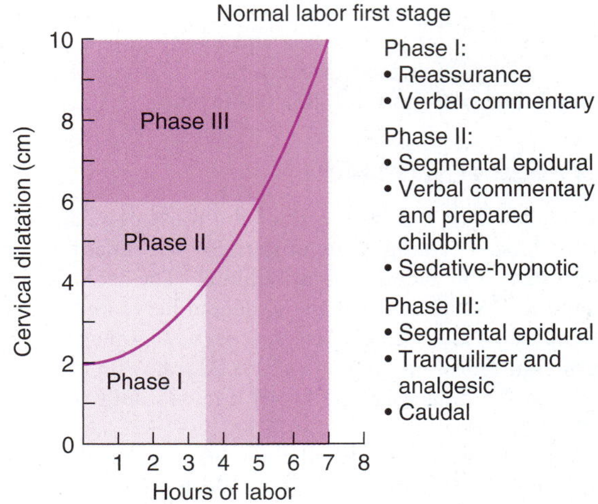

▲ **Figure 24–6.** First-stage management in a primipara can be divided into 3 phases. Phase I (early labor) should be managed by simple reassurance and verbal commentary if the patient has received adequate antepartum education. An epidural may be performed once labor is well established. Phase II can be handled by a segmental epidural block, continued reassurance, a sedative-hypnotic drug, a narcotic, or a tranquilizer. Phase III, the accentuated phase of labor, can be handled by segmental epidural block, a combination tranquilizer and analgesic, or a caudal epidural block. However, use of reassurance and verbal commentary in conjunction with prepared childbirth methods may be adequate for some patients to tolerate the discomfort of phase III labor.

analgesia. The pregnant patient is more likely to have an intravascular drug injection because of venous distention in the epidural space and may be more susceptible to the toxic effects of local anesthetics (Table 24–3). Injection of the drug into a highly vascularized area will result in more rapid systemic absorption than, for example, injection into the skin. To prevent too-rapid absorption, the operator can add epinephrine to produce local vasoconstriction and prolong the anesthetic. A final concentration of 1:200,000 is desirable, especially when a toxic amount is approached. Epinephrine is contraindicated in patients with increased cardiac irritability of medical or drug origin.

Treatment of local anesthetic overdosage manifested by central nervous system toxicity (a convulsion) is generally achieved effectively and without incident. However, the clinician must be aware of certain basic principles. These include the recognition of prodromal signs of a central nervous system toxic reaction and immediate treatment as required. A toxic central nervous system reaction to local anesthetics consists of ringing in the ears, diplopia, perioral numbness, and deep, slurred speech. An adequate airway must be maintained, and the patient should receive 100% oxygen, with respiratory assistance if necessary. Protection of

Table 24–3. Toxic doses of local anesthetics commonly used in obstetrics.

Drug	Toxic Dose
Lidocaine	5 mg/kg, plain 7 mg/kg with epinephrine
Bupivacaine[1]	2.5 mg/kg, plain 3.5 mg/kg with epinephrine
Chloroprocaine	11 mg/kg, plain 14 mg/kg with epinephrine
Tetracaine	1.5 mg/kg, plain
Ropivacaine	3 mg/kg, plain 3.5 mg/kg with epinephrine

[1] Dose as low as 90 mg have produced cardiac arrest.
All epinephrine concentrations 1:200,000.

the patient's airway and immediate injection of thiopental 50 mg or midazolam 1–2 mg usually stop the convulsion immediately. Succinylcholine was recommended in the past, but it is a potent neuromuscular relaxant that requires placement of an endotracheal tube with positive-pressure ventilation. Studies have indicated that cellular metabolism is greatly increased during convulsive episodes so that a definite increase in cellular oxygenation occurs—hence the use of a depressant selective for the hypothalamus and thalamus because these sites are the foci of irritation.

Local anesthetics-induced cardiotoxicity, especially by bupivacaine, is serious consequence when local anesthetic overdosage happens. The treatment of this complication is usually difficult, and the patient may suffer from arrhythmias (ventricular tachycardia) to even cardiac arrest. Intralipid intravenous infusion is recommended for bupivacaine-induced cardiotoxicity. Current guidelines suggest that 20% lipid emulsion initially be administered as a bolus of 1.5 mL/kg over 1 minute. After completion of the bolus, a continuous infusion of 0.25 mL/kg/min should be started. If the patient does not respond to the initial bolus, 1 to 2 additional boluses may be administered. The rate of the infusion may be increased to 0.5 mL/kg if there is persistent hypotension. The infusion should be continued until 10 min after the patient regains hemodynamic stability. An upper limit of 10 mL/kg is the recommended upper limit for administration in 30 minutes. Any patient that has had local anesthetic toxicity should be monitored for 12 hours after the event, as recurrence of cardiovascular instability has been shown to occur even after lipid administration.

ANESTHESIA FOR CAESAREAN DELIVERY

With few exceptions, all caesarean deliveries in the United States are performed with spinal, epidural, or general anesthesia. Maternal and neonatal outcomes are good when these techniques are performed effectively. In 1982, more than half of the caesarean births in the United States were performed under general anesthesia. By 1998, the rate had dropped to less than 10% of all caesarean births. Spinal anesthesia has become more common than epidural anesthesia for caesarean delivery in the past few years, primarily as a result of the introduction of newer spinal needles that prevent post–lumbar puncture headaches. Although the majority of anesthesia-related maternal mortality is associated with caesarean birth, the rate has continued to decline dramatically over the last few decades and now is less than 1.5 anesthesia-related deaths per million live births in the United States.

Regional Analgesia

A. Lumbar Epidural Block

Lumbar epidural blockade can be used for caesarean analgesia and adequate analgesia for operative delivery. As mentioned in the discussion of regional anesthesia, the major hazard of the regional analgesic technique is blockade of sympathetic fibers and a decrease in vascular resistance, along with venous pooling and hypotension. However, this can be greatly alleviated by elevating the patient's right hip to prevent compression of the vena cava by the gravid uterus when the patient is lying on the operating table. In addition, the anesthesiologist can rotate the operating table 15–20 degrees to the left to rotate the uterus away from the vena cava.

An epidural catheter can be placed immediately before surgery, or a catheter used to provide pain relief for labor can be reinjected for the surgery. After the catheter is suitably placed and taped in position, the patient should be rotated slightly out of the supine position to remove the hazard of vena cava occlusion when local anesthetic is injected as a test dose. Lidocaine 2% with epinephrine 1:200,000 can be used, or lidocaine 2% without epinephrine can be used if cardiovascular instability is present. Bupivacaine 0.5% or mepivacaine 1.5% with or without epinephrine (as described for lidocaine) also can be used. The total dosage for the therapeutic test is approximately 3 mL, which is an adequate amount to ascertain whether or not inadvertent subarachnoid injection of the drug has occurred. Incremental injections of 5 mL are then titrated to produce a T4–T6 sensory level. Usually a total volume of 18–20 mL of local anesthetic is required.

The blood pressure is monitored every 5 minutes and the dermatome levels examined every 5 minutes for the first 20 minutes to ascertain the height and density of the analgesic block. Usually a waiting period of only 15–20 minutes is needed for adequate analgesic block for incision. During this time, the patient's abdomen is surgically scrubbed and prepared and the patient draped for caesarean delivery. If a brief episode of hypotension occurs, the patient is given a rapid infusion of lactated Ringer's solution. In addition, the uterus must be shifted away from the vena cava. If these measures are not sufficient to relieve a brief episode of hypotension, 5–10 mg of ephedrine or 50–100 μg of phenylephrine can be administered intravenously for a mild vasopressor effect.

B. Subarachnoid Block

Spinal block is now the most common anesthesia used for elective caesarean delivery in the United States. The advantages are immediate onset of analgesia, so no waiting period is needed for the block to become effective, and the absence of drug transmission from the maternal to the fetal compartment because the anesthetic is deposited in the subarachnoid space in such small quantities. In addition, subarachnoid block may be a simpler technique to perform because the end point is definite—the identification of fluid from the subarachnoid space. The disadvantages are a more profound and rapid onset of hypotension and more frequent nausea and vomiting due either to unopposed parasympathetic stimulation of the gastrointestinal tract or to hypotension. Subarachnoid block usually is achieved via the paramedian or midline technique, details of which are beyond the scope of this text. The agents most commonly used for subarachnoid analgesia are lidocaine 5% (50–75 mg) and bupivacaine 10–12.5 mg. As with the lumbar epidural technique, the patient is prehydrated with 500–1000 mL of lactated Ringer's solution.

After the technical aspects of the procedure have been completed, the patient is placed in the supine position with the uterus displaced to the left as described. If hypotension occurs, the uterus should be pushed farther to the left to improve return of blood from the lower extremities into the circulation and increase right atrial pressure and thus cardiac output, and a bolus of Ringer's lactate should be given. If these measures are not successful, the patient should receive ephedrine 5–10 mg or phenylephrine 50–100 μg intravenously to sustain a mild vasopressor effect. During a period of hypotension, the mother should receive oxygen by mask to increase oxygen delivery to the uteroplacental bed. Newer spinal needles are associated with a low incidence (1–2%) of spinal headache (PDPH). As a result, spinal anesthesia is becoming more popular for elective caesarean surgery.

C. Combined Spinal-Epidural Anesthesia

The combination of spinal and epidural technique (CSE) has increased in popularity and may provide rapid and effective anesthesia for caesarean delivery. Advantages of CSE include the rapid onset of surgical anesthesia with a smaller spinal dose and ability to extend the duration by activation of epidural anesthesia. The use of smaller local anesthetic dose may decrease the incidence of maternal hypotension, which can be significantly detrimental both to the mother and the fetus.

General Anesthesia

General anesthesia is indicated for caesarean delivery when regional techniques cannot be used because of coagulopathy, infection, hypovolemia, or urgency. Some patients prefer to be "put to sleep" and refuse regional techniques.

Ideally, general anesthesia for caesarean delivery should cause the mother to be unconscious, feel no pain, and have no unpleasant memories of the procedure; the fetus should not be jeopardized, with minimal depression and intact reflex irritability.

General anesthesia for caesarean delivery is substantially modified from the typical nonobstetric technique. A rapid sequence technique is used with cricoid pressure to prevent aspiration, with recognition that the risks for the term obstetric patient include (1) full stomach (and aspiration), (2) difficulty with laryngoscopy and intubation, and (3) rapid desaturation if intubation is unsuccessful.

A. Patient Preparation

Preoperative medication usually is not required when the patient is brought to the caesarean section room. Alert the patient preoperatively that she may have a lucid "window" during the operative procedure when she experiences pain or hears voices. Explain that the condition results from the need to maintain a light analgesic state in order to protect the fetus from large doses of drugs. The patient should be prepared with 30 mL of nonparticulate antacid to offset gastric acidity. The patient is given 100% oxygen with a close-fitting mask for 3 minutes before induction.

B. Procedure

When the surgeon is ready to make the incision, thiopental 2.5 mg/kg should be injected intravenously and cricoid pressure exerted by an assistant. Immediately, succinylcholine 120–140 mg intravenously should be administered, and intubation and inflation of the cuff performed. Intubation is confirmed by auscultation and monitoring end-tidal CO_2 before the cricoid pressure is released and the incision made. After 6–8 breaths of 100% oxygen, the patient should be given nitrous oxide 50% with oxygen 50% until delivery of the fetus. Low concentrations of halothane or isoflurane (0.5%) will reduce the incidence of awareness. Intermediate-acting muscle relaxants maintain paralysis. An attempt must be made to keep the induction-to-delivery time under 10 minutes. Five minutes is required for redistribution of barbiturate back across the placenta into the maternal compartment. After delivery of the fetus, the nitrous oxide concentration can be increased to 70% if oxygen saturation is more than 98% and intravenous narcotics and benzodiazepines injected for supplemental anesthesia.

The patient should be fully awakened and on her side before extubation. Postoperative analgesia can be provided by patient-controlled administration of morphine or meperidine.

With this approach, good neonatal outcomes are anticipated if induction-to-delivery times and uterine entry-to-delivery times are kept to a minimum.

Local Anesthesia

Local infiltration anesthesia as a primary technique for caesarean delivery is very rarely used. When used, local anesthesia is performed to provide supplemental anesthesia in patients with inadequate epidural or spinal blockade. However, there may be situations when regional or general anesthesia is not immediately available, and caesarean delivery under local anesthesia may be necessary for fetal indications (eg, prolonged fetal bradycardia during the first stage of labor). The general nerve supply of the abdominal wall is composed of 6 of the lowest thoracic nerves, the ilioinguinal and the iliohypogastric nerves bilaterally. The 3 primary nerves that make up the sensory input from the abdomen all end as anterior cutaneous nerves in the abdominal wall. For emergent caesarean delivery, one can use 1% lidocaine in a 10-mL syringe with a 3.5-inch 25-gauge spinal needle injected just under the skin from the umbilicus to near symphysis pubis. If the knife follows this line during incision, the patient will not feel pain. Then, the subcutaneous, muscle and rectal sheath layers are injected as the abdomen is opened. This is the most rapid method for analgesia and delivery by caesarean section and may be a choice in cases in which anesthesia is not available or possible for a period of time. The major disadvantages of local infiltration are the potential for systemic toxicity and technical difficulties in providing adequate anesthesia for surgery, but it can be life-saving for the fetus when immediate delivery is needed for fetal indications.

ANESTHESIA FOR SPECIAL OBSTETRICAL CIRCUMSTANCES

Multiple Gestations

A. Psychoanalgesia

The psychoprophylactic technique helps to prepare the patient for the intrapartum experience. When the labor progresses normally, psychoanalgesia can effectively reduce apprehension and enhance the pleasurable aspects of childbirth. It also may prepare the patient for an understanding of some of the complications of multiple gestations (uterine inertia in the first stage of labor, uterine atony in the third stage, and possible need for caesarean delivery) and reduce the total amount of drugs required for analgesia.

B. Pudendal Nerve Block

Pudendal nerve block usually is reserved for cases in which epidural block is not available. Analgesia is more limited and does not provide as effective analgesia should version or breech extractions of the second twin be required.

C. Epidural Block

This technique is useful as a first-stage analgesic method, but only a segmental type should be used (T10–L2) to prevent the increased hazard of hypotension secondary to a combined large-segment sympathetic block and vena cava occlusion. Ideal management entails the use of lumbar epidural block for the first stage of labor and low caudal block for the late second stage of labor. Epidural anesthesia does not affect fetal outcome with twin delivery but has the advantage of enabling the obstetrician to intervene more easily if the second twin presents abnormally. The need for a general anesthetic can be avoided if an epidural is in place and a caesarean section is required urgently for delivery of the second twin.

D. Spinal Block

The low subarachnoid block is rarely used at the end of the second stage for crowning, delivery, and episiotomy. A low spinal block does not provide a sufficiently high block for caesarean section should it be required urgently (eg, in malpresentation or cord prolapse of the second twin). Therefore, an epidural anesthetic is always preferable for the labor and delivery of multiple births.

E. Inhalation Analgesics

Nitrous oxide is the only inhalation anesthetic that is analgesic at low concentrations. Experience is needed to use nitrous oxide safely because the pregnant patient is sensitive to the drug's anesthetic effects and she can easily become obtunded. Loss of airway reflexes and aspiration are causes of maternal mortality.

General endotracheal anesthesia can be used for caesarean delivery of twins. Neonatal depression is more likely if the induction-to-delivery time is long (>8 minutes), especially if the uterine incision-to-delivery time also is prolonged (>3 minutes).

Midforceps Delivery

Midforceps delivery is rarely used in current practice given the limited number of practitioners skilled in the technique. Midforceps delivery generally involves both rotation and traction. Therefore, the anesthetic regimen must provide relaxation as well as analgesia for the perineum, lower vagina, and upper birth canal. In order for the obstetrician to perform the procedures necessary for delivery, optimal conditions must be provided so that maternal and fetal trauma can be minimized. Regional analgesia with a lumbar, caudal, epidural, or subarachnoid block is preferred because these blocks provide analgesia and optimal relaxation.

The Trapped Head

On the rare occasion when breech delivery is complicated by a trapped head, the application of forceps or other manipulations may be required urgently. If an epidural block is in place, no further analgesia will be required; however, if one is not in place, immediate anesthesia and pelvic relaxation will be required to facilitate rapid delivery and minimize trauma. The best technique for this purpose is general anesthesia with halothane after suitable protection of the patient from the hazards of aspiration. Protection should include use of antacid 30 mL orally and adequate oxygenation, followed by thiopental 200 mg intravenously, succinylcholine 80–100 mg intravenously, and rapid intubation with cricoid pressure. Another approach described in the literature is administration of 50–100 μg intravenous nitroglycerin to relax the lower uterine segment.

Preeclampsia–Eclampsia

This syndrome is classically described as the proteinuric hypertension. However, it can affect multiple organ systems and be associated with other variants, the most notable being HELLP syndrome, the constellation of hemolysis, elevated liver enzymes and low platelet count. Preeclampsia–eclampsia accounts for approximately 20% of maternal deaths per year in the United States. The primary pathologic characteristic of this disease process is generalized arterial spasm and endothelial dysfunction. As gestation lengthens, there is a tendency toward a fluid shift from the vascular to the extravascular compartment with resultant hypovolemia—in spite of an expanded extracellular fluid space.

It is estimated that nearly 50% of eclamptic patients who die have myocardial hemorrhages or areas of focal necrosis. Major disorders of central nervous system function probably are caused by cerebral vasospasm. Optimal anesthetic management of these patients during the intrapartum period must include a careful preanesthetic evaluation of the cardiovascular and central nervous systems.

The physiologic changes of severe preeclampsia–eclampsia are exaggerated by regional block as a result of restricted intravascular volume, which may lead to considerable depression of blood pressure. Small subgroups of these patients suffer from reduced cardiac output (compared with normal pregnancy), decreased intravascular fluid space, and marked increases in SVR. Patients with severe hemodynamic changes may require direct monitoring of pulmonary artery and wedge pressures to manage labor and the effects of epidural anesthesia. Uterine blood flow is increased with epidural block because of the favorable reduction of SVR, as long as central filling pressures and mean arterial pressure are well maintained.

Regional and general anesthesia is used in the management of preeclamptic patients. Contraindications to regional anesthesia include coagulopathy and urgency for delivery in the setting of nonreassuring fetal testing. The latter may mitigate against taking excessive time for placing a spinal or epidural if the baby requires immediate delivery.

Epidural anesthesia may be preferred to spinal anesthesia in cases of severe hypertension. The more graduated onset of sympathetic block with this technique is thought to produce less hypotension than would occur with spinal block. However, recent evidence suggests that adequate volume preloading of these patients, who by definition are depleted intravascularly, results in similar hemodynamic responses to both regional techniques. More study is required to confirm these findings. However, spinal and epidural anesthesia now usually is encouraged for the management of preeclamptic patients. Obstetricians have become aware that epidural anesthesia is a valuable adjunct in the management of hypertension as a result of the pain relief as well as the vasodilation produced by epidural block. In the past, epidural anesthesia was avoided because of an exaggerated concern over hypotension; now epidural anesthesia is encouraged if the patient's volume status is well managed and if coagulopathy does not complicate the clinical picture.

Hemorrhage and Shock

Intrapartum obstetric emergencies demand immediate diagnosis and therapy for a favorable outcome for the mother and fetus. Placenta previa and abruptio placentae can be accompanied by serious maternal hemorrhage. Aggressive obstetric management may be indicated, but superior anesthetic management will play a major role in reducing maternal and fetal morbidity and mortality rates. The primary threat to the mother is blood loss, which reduces her effective circulating blood volume and her oxygenation potential. Similarly, the chief hazard to the fetus is diminished uteroplacental perfusion secondary to maternal hypovolemia and hypotension. The perinatal mortality rate associated with placenta previa and abruptio placentae ranges from 15–20% in some studies and up to 50–100% in other studies. The overall morbidity and mortality rates for both the fetus and the mother depend on the gestational age and health of the fetus, the extent of the hemorrhage, and the therapy given.

Good anesthetic management demands early consultation. Reliable intravenous lines should be established early. In addition, recommendations for treatment and control of shock must be formulated. Prompt caesarean delivery often is indicated. Ketamine can support blood pressure for induction. A modified nitrous oxide–oxygen relaxant method of general anesthesia will provide improved oxygenation for both the mother and the fetus and will have a minimal effect on maternal blood pressure. As surgery progresses, it may be necessary to administer large volumes of warm blood, intravenous fluids, or even vasopressors when imperative. Regional block is contraindicated in the presence of hypovolemia.

Umbilical Cord Prolapse

Umbilical cord prolapse is an acute obstetric emergency that is a critical threat to the fetus. Often, because of confusion, irrational behavior by the medical staff may threaten the mother's life. For example, a haphazard rapid induction of anesthesia without attention to many of the essential safety details may be attempted. Naturally, prolapse of the umbilical cord is incompatible with fetal survival unless the fetal presenting part is elevated at once and maintained in that position to avoid compression of the cord. There then should be adequate time for methodical, safe induction of anesthesia. General anesthesia is induced as soon as the abdomen is prepped and draped. In the rush of the emergency situation, the anesthesiologist must remain meticulous in his or her assessment and management of the mother's airway. A failed intubation and its consequent cardiorespiratory arrest constitute the leading cause of anesthetic maternal mortality.

Breech Delivery

Epidural anesthesia can be used for the labor patient with a breech presentation. The need for breech extraction is not increased by the use of epidural anesthesia, and a functioning epidural may prevent the need for general anesthesia should an emergency arise at delivery.

If an epidural block is not in place at the time of delivery, the anesthesiologist must be prepared to proceed with an immediate endotracheal general anesthesia if the after-coming fetal head becomes trapped. Drugs, monitors, and anesthetic equipment must be prepared in anticipation of such an event.

Because vaginal breech delivery is associated with an increased risk of perinatal mortality in singleton pregnancies, excellent communication and cooperation between the obstetrician and the anesthesiologist is greatly needed to succeed in an atraumatic delivery. Instead of vaginal delivery, most obstetricians perform caesarean delivery for singleton fetuses in breech presentation now.

Emergency Caesarean Section

General anesthesia is the technique most suitable for the urgent cesarean delivery. It entails placement of an endotracheal tube with an inflated cuff to protect the patient from aspiration of gastric contents into the lung after administration of adequate barbiturate and a muscle relaxant to facilitate endotracheal intubation. Several safety measures must be taken. (1) Give 30 mL of a nonparticulate antacid (sodium citrate) within 15 minutes of induction. (2) Accomplish denitrogenation with 100% oxygen by tight-fitting mask. (3) Inject thiopental 2.5 mg/kg intravenously. (4) Apply cricoid pressure. (5) Give succinylcholine 100–120 mg intravenously. (6) Intubate the trachea and inflate the cuff. (7) Give 6–8 deep breaths of 100% oxygen. (8) Continue to administer nitrous oxide 50% with oxygen 50%, half minimum alveolar concentration (MAC) of volatile agents, and maintain relaxation with muscle relaxants. (9) Supplement with short-acting narcotics and midazolam after the baby is delivered.

These steps should be instituted rapidly and with effective communication between the anesthesiologist and the obstetrician, who should be scrubbed and prepared to make the incision. With this technique, anesthesia can be induced and the fetus delivered within 30 minutes from the time caesarean section is ordered. To prevent vena cava occlusion from the gravid uterus, a wedge should be placed under the patient's right hip or the operating table rotated slightly to the left.

ANESTHESIA FOR NONOBSTETRIC COMPLICATIONS

Anesthesiologists use the following classification system developed by the American Society of Anesthesiologists (ASA). It is used in both emergency and nonemergent situations to record physical status and to ascertain that proper materials are available for the anticipated procedure.

Class 1: No organic, physiologic, biochemical, or psychiatric disturbance

Class 2: Mild to moderate systemic disturbance that may or may not be related to the reason for surgery, eg, heart disease that only slightly limits physical activity, essential hypertension, anemia, extremes of age, obesity, chronic bronchitis)

Class 3: Severe systemic disturbance that may or may not be related to the reason for surgery (eg, heart disease that limits activity, poorly controlled hypertension, diabetes mellitus with vascular complications, chronic pulmonary disease that limits activity)

Class 4: Severe systemic disturbance that is life-threatening with or without surgery (eg, congestive heart failure, crescendo angina pectoris, advanced pulmonary, renal, and hepatic dysfunction)

Class 5: Moribund patient who has little chance of survival but is submitted to surgery as a last resort (resuscitative effort) (eg, uncontrolled hemorrhage as from a ruptured abdominal aneurysm, cerebral trauma, pulmonary embolus)

Emergency operation (E): Any patient in whom an emergency operation is required (eg, otherwise healthy 30-year-old woman who requires dilatation and curettage for moderate but persistent hemorrhage [ASA class 1E])

Hypertension

Pre-existing hypertensive cardiovascular disease in a pregnant woman should be differentiated from preeclampsia–eclampsia. Unlike the latter, the manifestations of hypertensive disease usually are present before week 20 of pregnancy and persist after delivery. The untreated disease by itself presents a serious challenge to the obstetrician and increases maternal and fetal risk. Chronic hypertension does not specifically contraindicate any of the anesthetic options, but the anesthesiologist must assess and manage abnormalities of volume and vascular resistance to prevent hypotension. Systemic analgesia with sedatives and tranquilizers may be selected for first-stage pain relief, but a hazard still remains.

Heart Disease

Pregnancy superimposed on heart disease presents serious problems in anesthetic management. Patients with functional class I or II rheumatic or congenital heart disease usually fare well throughout pregnancy. Except for patients with fixed cardiac output (moderate to severe aortic stenosis or mitral stenosis), regional analgesia epidural block provides ideal management of first- and second-stage pain relief. This avoids undesirable intrapartum problems such as anxiety, tachycardia, increased cardiac output, and the Valsalva maneuver. The lumbar epidural catheter can be activated for first-stage analgesia with sensory levels of T10 through L2 segments. With the restricted epidural technique, wide variations in blood pressure usually will be avoided and adequate analgesia provided.

Patients with valvular heart disease must be thoroughly assessed before onset of labor so that the anesthesiologist can determine the risks of regional block, tolerance to volume loading, and sympathectomy and determine the need for invasive monitoring. These patients require thorough physical examination, electrocardiography, echocardiography, and Doppler assessment of valve areas and left ventricular function.

Patients with stenotic lesions may not tolerate fluid loading or sympathetic block. Epidural narcotic anesthesia does not provide complete analgesia for labor but may be an appropriate choice if the patient does not tolerate the autonomic effects of local anesthetics. Patients with regurgitant valve lesions generally do well with this afterload reduction of epidural local anesthesia. Central monitoring of preload is indicated with severe lesions.

Marfan's syndrome and ischemic heart disease require early and aggressive management of labor pain to prevent hypertension and tachycardia. Early lumbar epidural anesthesia with narcotic/local anesthetic mixtures is recommended.

Diabetes Mellitus

Diabetes presents unique problems in anesthetic management because of the hazard to the fetus. The patient with diabetes requires a detailed regimen of antepartum care that extends through the intrapartum and the neonatal period. Moreover, hypotension presents an anesthetic hazard in situations of reduced fetal reserve common to diabetes. The latent phase of labor is best managed with psychological support, mild sedatives, or tranquilizers. The latter part of the first stage can be managed with small intravenous doses of narcotics or epidural block. If labor continues without signs of fetal distress and analgesia for the second stage is desired, either local or pudendal block or epidural or saddle block is appropriate. If a patient is allowed to undergo the stress of labor but fetal decompensation is evident, operative delivery must be performed at once, with emphasis on preventing hypotension. Careful regional block can be used if time permits. If time does not permit placement of a regional block, emergency general endotracheal anesthesia is indicated. Blood glucose levels should be measured intraoperatively because the unconscious patient cannot report hypoglycemia.

Gastrointestinal Difficulties

Gastrointestinal nonstriated muscle has diminished tone and motility during pregnancy. Some medical gastrointestinal difficulties present special problems in management during the intrapartum period. Peptic ulcer often improves during pregnancy, but in some cases the disease worsens in the last trimester and causes serious problems during labor and the immediate postpartum period. Ulcer perforation and hematemesis are rare in labor. Nonetheless, good management of analgesia during delivery is necessary to decrease anxiety and apprehension.

Ulcerative colitis may worsen during pregnancy. Perinatal and maternal mortality rates are not increased because symptomatic management usually is adequate. Regional ileitis may become more severe during pregnancy.

Chronic pancreatitis may be reactivated during pregnancy. Acute pancreatitis occasionally occurs in the third trimester. The significant laboratory values are elevated serum amylase and reduced serum calcium levels, along with typical symptoms of epigastric pain and nausea and vomiting.

Sympathetic blocking techniques are not contraindicated for anesthetic management of the first and second stages of labor in these gastrointestinal disorders that may coincide with pregnancy. It is clinically desirable to alleviate anxiety and apprehension in the first stage of labor because tension may exacerbate the disease process. Therefore, a tranquilizer–narcotic combination early in the first stage of labor should be considered and then lumbar epidural block for first- and second-stage management. Subarachnoid block can be administered to manage the second stage of labor successfully, with use of a true saddle block obtunding chiefly the sacral fibers.

Psychiatric Disorders

Most patients approaching delivery look on the experience as one of the happiest times of their lives. However, some patients undergo severe emotional stress during the third trimester and as delivery nears.

The obstetrician and the anesthesiologist should talk openly with a psychiatric patient about the problems of labor and delivery management and offer suggestions for management of discomfort so that she will have minimal emotional stress. The ideal technique is the combined use of lumbar epidural block for the first stage and lumbar or caudal epidural block for the second stage. It is best to carefully point out to the patient the reasons for choosing the technique and to review the technical points of the procedure so that she will not be alarmed when the block is attempted. These techniques are preferred because they afford early and continuous analgesia during labor and delivery.

TREATMENT OF COMPLICATIONS OF ANESTHETICS

Resuscitation of the Mother

Anesthesia is responsible for 10% of maternal mortality. The most common cause of maternal death is failure to intubate the trachea at induction of general anesthesia. Less frequently, maternal death results from inadvertent intravascular injection of local anesthetic (toxic reaction) or inadvertent intrathecal injection of anesthetic (total spinal).

When faced with maternal cardiovascular collapse, full cardiopulmonary resuscitation (CPR) is indicated:

1. Establish a patent airway.
2. Aspirate mucus, blood, and vomitus with a tracheal suction apparatus. Use a laryngoscope for direct visualization of air passages and intubate the trachea.

3. Administer oxygen by artificial respiration if respirations are absent or weak. If high spinal anesthesia has occurred, continue to ventilate the patient until paralysis of the diaphragm has dissipated.
4. Give vasopressors intravenously (ephedrine 10–20 mg). Place the patient in the wedged supine position with the feet elevated and give transfusions of plasma, plasma expanders, and blood for traumatic or hemorrhagic shock.
5. Specifically treat cardiac arrhythmias in accordance with advanced cardiac life support (ACLS) recommendations.
6. Provide external cardiac massage in the absence of adequate rhythm and blood pressure.
7. Consider immediate caesarean delivery to salvage fetus and improve venous return if the patient does not immediately respond to efforts.

Full cardiopulmonary arrest can be averted if the prodromal symptoms are recognized and treated immediately. A total spinal block is recognized by excessive and dense sensory and motor block to a test injection of local anesthesia through the epidural catheter. Further injections are avoided, and the patient's blood pressure is supported with fluid, positioning, and vasopressors.

An intravascular injection of local anesthetic is recognized early by symptoms of drowsiness, agitation, tinnitus, perioral tingling, bradycardia, and mild hypotension. The patient should be immediately given 100% oxygen and a small dose of diazepam (5 mg), midazolam (1 mg), or thiopental (50 mg). Further treatment may not be needed. The patient must be watched closely and the epidural catheter removed.

Aya AGM, Mangin R, Vialles N, Ferrer JM, Robert C, Ripart J, de La Coussaye JE. Patients with severe preeclampsia experience less hypotension during spinal anesthesia for elective cesarean delivery than healthy parturients: A prospective cohort comparison. *Anesth Analg* 2003;97:867–872. PMID: 12933418.

Bucklin BA, Hawkins JL, Anderson JR, et al. Obstetric anesthesia workforce survey: Twenty-year update. *Anesthesiology* 2005;103:645–653. PMID: 16129992.

Hawkins JL, Chang J, Palmer SK, Charles P, Callaghan WM. Anesthesia-related maternal mortality in the United States: 1979–2002. *Obstet Gynecol* 2011;117:69–74. PMID: 21173646.

MacKay AP, Berg CJ, Atrash HK. Pregnancy-related mortality from preeclampsia and eclampsia. *Obstet Gynecol* 2001;97:533–538. PMID: 11275024.

Mhyre JM. What's new in obstetric anesthesia in 2009? An update on maternal patient safety. *Anesth Analg* 2010;111:1480–1487. PMID: 20861422.

Practice guidelines for obstetric anesthesia: An updated report by the American Society of Anesthesiologists Task Force on Obstetric Anesthesia. *Anesthesiology* 2007;106:843–863. PMID: 17413923.

Toledo P. The role of lipid emulsion during advanced cardiac life support for local anesthetic toxicity. *Int J Obest Anesth* 2011;20:60–63. PMID: 21112763.

Visalyaputra S, Rodanant O, Somboonviboon W, Tantivitayatan K, Thienthong S, Saengchote W. Spinal versus epidural anesthesia for cesarean delivery in severe preeclampsia: A prospective randomized, multicenter study. *Anesth Analg* 2005;101:862–868. PMID: 16116005.

Weinberg GL. Lipid infusion therapy: Translation to clinical practice. *Anesth Analg* 2008;106:1340–1342. PMID: 18420841.

Wong CA, Scavone BM, Peaceman AM, et al. The risk of cesarean delivery with neuraxial analgesia given early versus late in labor. *N Engl J Med* 2005;352:655–665. PMID: 15716559.

Surgical Disorders in Pregnancy

25

Ella Speichinger, MD
Christine H. Holschneider, MD

The incidence of surgical disease is the same in pregnant and nonpregnant patients. A total of 1.5–2% of all pregnancies undergo nonobstetric surgical intervention. Presenting symptoms of surgical diseases are often similar in pregnant and nonpregnant patients. The most common surgical disorders in pregnancy are appendicitis, cholecystitis, intestinal obstruction, adnexal torsion, trauma, and cervical and breast disease. Limited imaging can be performed during pregnancy if results would significantly alter management. The second trimester is the preferred time for nonurgent surgery. Surgery should not be delayed in any trimester if systemic infection or severe disease is suspected, as this is associated with higher risk to mother and fetus. Whenever possible, regional anesthesia should be performed. Pregnancy does not change prognosis, which depends largely on the extent of disease at diagnosis. A multidisciplinary approach with maternal–fetal medicine, surgery, anesthesia, and neonatology during treatment planning is invaluable to ensure optimal outcomes for both the mother and fetus.

Surgical interventions other than caesarean section are performed in 1.5–2.0% of all pregnancies. Altered anatomy and physiology and potential risks to the mother and fetus make diagnosis and management of surgical disorders more difficult during pregnancy. The interests of mother and fetus are best served by the obstetrician's active participation with the anesthesiologist, neonatologist, and general surgeon throughout the mother's diagnosis and management of a nonobstetric surgical disorder. It is imperative that the obstetrician be well informed about the ways in which surgical disorders influence pregnancy and vice versa, the risks of diagnostic and therapeutic procedures to the fetus, and appropriate management of preterm labor in the immediate postoperative period.

Surgical disorders can be either incidental to or directly related to the pregnancy. Diagnostic evaluation requires gentle, sensitive elicitation of physical signs, at times without sophisticated diagnostic aids that involve risk to the developing fetus. Good judgment regarding the timing, methods, and extent of treatment is important. In the absence of peritonitis, visceral perforation, or hemorrhage, surgical disorders during gestation generally have little effect on placental function and fetal development.

MATERNAL CONSIDERATIONS

Pregnancy is accompanied by physiologic and anatomic changes that alter the evaluation and management of the surgical patient. The 30–50% increase in plasma volume during pregnancy affects cardiac output and may alter drug distribution and laboratory test results. Red cell mass increases but not as much as the plasma volume, resulting in a slight physiologic anemia. Colloid osmotic pressure is decreased during pregnancy. Increased interstitial fluid is seen as mild edema, particularly in the lower extremities. Systemic vascular resistance decreases during pregnancy. Systolic and diastolic blood pressures characteristically drop during the early second trimester, with a gradual return to baseline by term. Functional pulmonary residual capacity decreases due to limitation of diaphragmatic excursion. Minute ventilation increases due to increased tidal volume and respiratory rate. A compensated mild respiratory alkalosis exists. Increased renal blood flow is evidenced by increased glomerular filtration rate and decreased serum creatinine and blood urea nitrogen values. Gastrointestinal motility is diminished, resulting in delayed gastric emptying and constipation. The enlarging uterus may alter the anatomic relation among the different organs. When the patient is in the supine position, the enlarged uterus may compress the inferior vena cava and result in the hypotensive vena cava compression syndrome.

ACOG Committee Opinion No. 284: Nonobstetric surgery in pregnancy. *Obstet Gynecol* 2003;102:431. PMID: 12907126.

Price LC, Slack A, Nelson-Piercy C. Aims of obstetric critical care management. *Best Pract Res Clin Obstet Gynaecol* 2008;22:775–799. PMID: 18693071.

FETAL CONSIDERATIONS

Optimal care of the pregnant surgical patient requires that potential hazards to the fetus be minimized. This includes risks associated with the maternal disease, diagnostic radiologic procedures, therapeutic drugs, anesthesia, and surgery. Assessment of the risks and benefits to the mother is relatively easy but less so for the fetus because of its relative inaccessibility.

A number of imaging modalities are available for diagnosis during pregnancy, including ultrasound (US), magnetic resonance imaging (MRI), computed tomography (CT), and x-ray.

Radiation Exposure

Although no definite harmful effects from the diagnostic use of US and MRI during pregnancy are reported, exposure to radiation is associated with fetal risks. Limited diagnostic CT or x-ray procedures can be undertaken with care in the pregnant patient. The fetus should be shielded whenever possible. The risk of adverse fetal effects associated with radiation exposure changes with gestational age and is related to the radiation dose to the fetus. These risks fall principally into 2 categories: teratogenicity and carcinogenicity. For example, within 2 weeks of fertilization, the embryo is most susceptible to implantation failure. If implantation was not affected, teratogenicity is extremely unlikely. Before 8 weeks, the fetus is at risk for radiation-induced growth restriction. At 8–15 weeks, the embryo is the most susceptible to mental retardation, with an approximately 4% risk on exposure at 10 cGy and 60% at 150 cGy. Teratogenic effects are unlikely in embryos older than 20 weeks. The most common fetal defects seen with direct fetal irradiation of 10 cGy or more are microcephaly, mental retardation, intrauterine growth restriction, and eye abnormalities. Current evidence suggests no increased structural or developmental fetal risk with radiation doses less than 5 cGy. The second set of concerns exists regarding in utero radiation exposure and its association with an increase in childhood neoplasms. The risk appears to be dose-related. Natural background fetal radiation exposure is estimated at 0.1 cGy. Fetal exposure to 2–5 cGy is estimated to translate into a relative risk of 1.5–2.0 for fatal childhood cancer, recognizing that the absolute risk is still very low (2 in 2000). Table 25–1 outlines estimates of fetal radiation exposure with various diagnostic procedures.

Table 25–1. Estimated fetal radiation exposure from common diagnostic radiologic procedures.

Procedure	Fetal Exposure cGy (rad)
Chest x-ray (2 views)	$2\text{-}7 \times 10^{-5}$
Mammogram (4 views)	$7\text{-}20 \times 10^{-3}$
Abdominal x-ray (1 view)	0.1–0.3
Hip x-ray (1 view)	$1\text{-}2 \times 10^{-3}$
Ventilation-perfusion scan	0.01–0.04
Helical CT chest	$1\text{-}10 \times 10^{-3}$
CT abdomen	1.7–3.5
CT pelvis	1.0–4.6

Note. Gray (Gy) is the International System unit for the radiation absorbed dose rad, which is the old but still frequently used unit (1 Gy = 100 rad; 1cGy = 1 rad). Radiographic exposure from a single diagnostic procedure to less than 5 cGy (5 rad) has not been associated with an increase in fetal abnormalities or pregnancy loss. Although concerns about exposure in the range from 5–10 cGy (5–10 rad) have been raised, serious developmental risk to the fetus is not known until the absorbed dose reaches 10 cGy (10 rad).

Exposure to Contrast

Traditionally, it has been recommended that use of iodine contrast be avoided during pregnancy. Although in vivo animal studies have not documented teratogenesis, ionic contrast when instilled directly into the amniotic sac during amniofetography has provoked neonatal hypothyroidism. Intravenous use of nonionic contrast media has been reported to have no effect on neonatal thyroid function. Given the existing data, the American College of Radiology states that definitive conclusions regarding the safety of intravascular iodinated contrast use cannot be made and recommends its use in pregnancy only if necessary. Before administration, it is important to weigh information that will be obtained by the addition of iodine contrast and to obtain informed consent. It is essential that infants whose mothers have received iodine contrast have thyroid function tested postnatally.

Gadolinium crosses the placenta and is thought to be excreted by the fetal kidneys into the amniotic fluid. There is a theoretical concern for toxicity related to persistence of free gadolinium. The American College of Radiology discourages its use in pregnancy, stating it should be used only if absolutely essential and following informed consent. However, the US Food and Drug Administration classifies gadolinium as a class C drug, and the European Society of Radiology states that based on available evidence, the use of gadolinium in pregnancy appears to be safe.

In summary, routine preoperative radiologic procedures are not justified. However, if clinical management of the pregnant patient would be significantly altered based on the findings of a judiciously performed radiologic procedure, the limited fetal exposure risk is generally warranted. Gadolinium should be considered only if the diagnostic information gained from the study is essential for the health of the mother. When multiple diagnostic images are required, consultation with a dosimetry expert may be helpful in calculating estimated fetal dose.

Surgical and Anesthesia Risks

Fortunately, most women who require surgery during pregnancy are otherwise relatively healthy and undergo an uneventful postoperative course. Generally, the safety of nonobstetric surgery in pregnancy and general anesthesia has been well established. Nevertheless, some increased risks are associated with surgery and anesthesia during pregnancy, and purely elective surgical procedures should be postponed until after pregnancy. Individual studies have suggested a possible increase in neural tube defects; other registries have documented adverse effects including low birth weight, prematurity, intrauterine growth restriction, and early neonatal death, but they are thought to correlate with the underlying condition that necessitates the surgical procedure. A review of 54 articles documenting pregnancy outcomes of nonobstetric surgical procedures between 1966 and 2002 found a low rate of miscarriage, congenital abnormalities, and preterm birth, but firm conclusions cannot be made, as no suitable control group existed. Thus, despite the general safety of anesthetic agents in pregnancy, some concern remains regarding teratogenicity in early gestation, and all but truly emergent surgery should be postponed until the second trimester. The second trimester is the preferred surgery time over the third trimester, as the risk of preterm labor and spontaneous abortion is lowest at that time. Whenever possible, regional anesthesia should be performed. No known reproductive toxicity is associated with currently used local anesthetic agents at recommended dose ranges. Short-term postoperative use of narcotic analgesic agents, frequently in combination with acetaminophen or nonsteroidal anti-inflammatory drugs before 32 weeks, generally appears to produce no adverse fetal effects.

Because intrauterine asphyxia is a major risk to the fetus consequent to maternal surgery, monitoring and maintaining maternal oxygen-carrying capacity, oxygen affinity, arterial PO_2, and placental blood flow throughout the preoperative, operative, and postoperative periods are important. For gestations greater than 18 weeks, attention should be given to providing uterine displacement to prevent venocaval compression when the patient is in the supine position. Supplemental oxygen administration and maintenance of circulating volume also assist fetal oxygenation. A reduction in maternal blood pressure can lead directly to fetal hypoxia. Greater reductions in uteroplacental perfusion by direct vascular constriction and an increase in uterine tonus are noted in association with the use of vasopressors, especially those with predominantly α-adrenergic activity. Ephedrine, with its peripheral beta-adrenergic effect, produces much less vasospasm and has traditionally been the vasopressor of choice in the pregnant patient, especially for treating hypotensive complications of regional anesthesia. More recent data find phenylephrine a good alternative with no untoward fetal effects.

To ensure fetal well-being, continuous electronic fetal heart rate monitoring should be used when maternal surgery is performed after 24 weeks as long as the monitoring device can function outside the sterile surgical field. In some cases, intraoperative electronic fetal monitoring may be considered in previable pregnancies to facilitate maternal positioning and oxygenation. At minimum, if the fetus is considered to be viable, electronic fetal and contraction monitoring is advised both before and after the procedure to assess fetal well-being and to evaluate for signs of preterm labor.

The severity of the inflammatory response associated with the disease requiring surgery appears to be more important in determining pregnancy outcome than is the use of anesthesia or the surgical procedure itself. Premature labor does not appear to be a common result of procedures such as exploratory laparotomy unless visceral perforation and peritonitis are encountered or a low pelvic procedure is performed with significant uterine manipulation. Prophylactic use of tocolytics in this setting is controversial. Often, a single dose of a beta-adrenergic agent such as terbutaline is sufficient to arrest contractions. Use of indomethacin may be preferred if significant inflammation is present; however, patency of fetal ductus arteriosus and amniotic fluid index should be monitored if used for more than 48 hours. If possible, uterine activity should be monitored after surgery to detect preterm labor and allow for early intervention. There are no studies to guide the decision to administer prophylactic glucocorticoids at the time of nonobstetric surgery. In the absence of systemic maternal infection, glucocorticoids should be considered if the gestation is between 24 and 34 weeks to reduce perinatal morbidity and mortality if preterm delivery occurs. Additionally, there is no literature to support progesterone supplementation perioperatively unless the corpus luteum is removed before 12 weeks of gestation.

Chen MM, Coakley FV, Kaimal A, Laros RK. Guidelines for computed tomography and magnetic resonance imaging use during pregnancy and lactation. *Obstet Gynecol* 2008;112:333–340. PMID: 18669732.

Cohen-Kerem R, Railton C, Oren D, et al. Pregnancy outcome following nonobstetric surgical intervention. *Am J Surg* 2005;190:467–473. PMID: 16105538.

McCollough CH, Schueler BA, Atwell TD, et al. Radiation exposure and pregnancy: When should we be concerned? *Radiographics* 2007;27:909–917.

The American College of Obstetricians and Gynecologists. Committee Opinion: Nonobstetric surgery during pregnancy. *Obstet Gynecol* 2011;117:420–421. PMID: 21252774.

DIAGNOSTIC CONSIDERATIONS

History

Clues to the cause of surgical disorders in pregnancy are often found in a careful review of the medical history. The stage and status of pregnancy are also relevant.

Pain

Pain is the most prominent symptom encountered with acute abdominal conditions complicating pregnancy. Generalized abdominal pain, guarding, and rebound strongly suggest peritonitis secondary to bleeding, exudation, or leakage of intestinal contents. Peritoneal signs can be less obvious in pregnancy as the uterus may displace the infected organ from contact with the parietal peritoneum. Cramping with lower central abdominal pain suggests a uterine disorder. Lower abdominal pain on either side suggests torsion, rupture, or hemorrhage of an ovarian cyst or tumor. Right lower or midabdominal pain suggests appendicitis. Disorders of the descending and sigmoid colon with left lower quadrant pain are infrequently encountered because of the relatively young age of obstetric patients. Midabdominal pain early in gestation suggests an intestinal origin. Upper abdominal pain is often related to the liver, spleen, gallbladder, stomach, duodenum, or pancreas. Constipation is a common problem but is rarely associated with other symptoms.

Other Symptoms

Abdominal pain associated with nausea and vomiting after the first trimester usually suggests a gastrointestinal disorder. Nausea and vomiting associated with the inability to pass gas or stool points to an intestinal obstruction. Diarrhea is seldom encountered in association with acute surgical problems except as a symptom of recurrent ulcerative colitis.

Syncope associated with pain and signs of peritoneal irritation usually indicate an acute abdominal emergency with rupture of a viscus, ischemia, or hemorrhage. A temperature of 38 °C (100.4 °F) or greater suggests infection, which may be localized by other clinical findings. Fever can also be associated with later stages of visceral necrosis in the cases of torsion or intestinal ischemia. Vaginal bleeding usually points to an intrauterine or cervical problem. Urinary tract infection is often accompanied by urinary frequency and urgency.

Physical Examination

The patient with an acute abdomen should undergo careful assessment of the reproductive organs, and her vital signs and general condition should be noted as well as the presence or absence of bowel sounds, abdominal rigidity or rebound tenderness, and the presence or absence of a mass. The fewest possible number of abdominal examinations should be gently performed without haste and with adequate explanation, using the flat part of the hand and starting in an asymptomatic area.

Laboratory Studies

Several laboratory studies routinely used in the evaluation of surgical disease have altered normal values during pregnancy; they are discussed where appropriate for the specific disease entity. The white blood cell count is considered elevated if the value is above 16,000/μL in any trimester. An interval of several hours usually passes between onset of hemorrhage and detection of lowered hematocrit values.

ANESTHESIA

The type of anesthesia is determined primarily by the planned surgical procedure. All general anesthetic agents cross the placenta but are not thought to be teratogenic. Regional anesthesia minimizes fetal exposure but may either not be appropriate for the surgical procedure or the maternal condition. If general anesthesia is anticipated, it is important to consider the physiologic changes in pregnancy, such as increased oropharyngeal swelling and decreased glottic opening, which can complicate intubation and ventilation. Obesity and preeclampsia can exacerbate these difficulties, leading to aspiration, failed intubation, and subsequent maternal and fetal hypoxia. Despite this, successful general anesthesia optimizes maternal and fetal oxygenation and reduces intraoperative uterine irritability. During either regional or general anesthesia, liberal oxygen supplementation should be employed to avoid maternal and fetal hypoxia.

Cheek TG, Baird E. Anesthesia for nonobstetric surgery: Maternal and fetal considerations. *Clin Obstet Gynecol* 2009;52:535–545. PMID: 20393407.

Lynch J, Scholz S. Anaesthetic-related complications of caesarean section. *Zentralbl Gynakol* 2005;127:91–95. PMID: 15800840.

PRINCIPLES OF SURGICAL MANAGEMENT

Delay in diagnosis and performance of surgery is the factor primarily responsible for increased maternal morbidity rates and perinatal loss, especially with maternal abdominal trauma. Immediate surgical exploration is generally indicated in the presence of unmistakable signs of peritoneal irritation, evidence of strangulating intestinal obstruction with possible gangrene, or intra-abdominal hemorrhage. In subacute conditions, care should be used in deciding to proceed with surgery. Surgery that is not urgent and can be delayed is best deferred until the second trimester or puerperium. Surgical techniques usually are not altered because of the pregnancy. Essentials of good preoperative care include adequate hydration, availability of blood for transfusion, and appropriate preoperative medication that will not decrease oxygenation for mother and fetus. Gestational age, uterine size, the specific surgical disorder, and the anticipated type of surgery to be performed are important factors in the selection of the abdominal incision. At operation, the least extensive procedure necessary should be performed with as little manipulation of the uterus as possible. Unless an obstetric indication is present or the uterus interferes with performance of a procedure, it usually is best not to perform a caesarean delivery during an abdominal operation.

Postoperative care depends on the gestational age and the operation performed. For patients whose gestation has reached viability, electronic monitoring of fetal heart rate and uterine activity should be continued in the immediate postoperative period, with staff capable of performing an emergent caesarean section readily available. Oversedation and fluid or electrolyte imbalance are to be avoided. Encouragement of early maternal activity and resumption of normal food intake are generally recommended.

THROMBOPROPHYLAXIS

Both pregnancy and surgery increase the risk of venous thromboembolism (VTE). Beginning in early pregnancy, vitamin K coagulation factors and type-1 plasminogen activator inhibitor increase, whereas protein S levels decrease. Surgery increases venous stasis and causes endothelial damage. Both mechanical and pharmacologic thromboprophylaxis reduce the incidence of symptomatic VTE. Pneumatic compression devices have few contraindications and should be considered for all pregnant women undergoing surgery. Pharmacologic thromboprophylaxis should be weighed against the patient's risk of thrombosis versus perioperative bleeding. Pregnant women who have an inherited or acquired thrombophilia, prolonged immobilization, past history of VTE, malignancy, age older than 35 years, multiple gestation, systemic illness, or obesity are at increased risk for VTE.

Bates SM, Greer IA, Pabinger I, et al. Venous thromboembolism, thrombophilia, antithrombotic therapy, and pregnancy: American College of Chest Physicians Evidence-Based Clinical Practice Guidelines (8th Ed.). *Chest* 2008;133:844S–886S. PMID: 18574280.

Dargaud Y, Rugeri L, Vergnes MC, et al. A risk score for the management of pregnant women with increased risk of venous thromboembolism: A multicentre prospective study. *Br J Haematol* 2009;145:825–835. PMID: 19388925.

LAPAROSCOPY IN PREGNANCY

Over the past 2 decades, laparoscopy has been increasingly used during pregnancy in the management of a variety of surgical disorders, most commonly for the exploration and treatment of adnexal masses, for appendectomy, and for cholecystectomy, but also for more technical surgical procedures such as nephrectomy, splenectomy, or retroperitoneal lymphadenectomy. The major advantages are decreased postoperative morbidity, less pain, shorter hospital stay, and postoperative recovery time. There may also be benefits specific to pregnancy, such as less uterine manipulation and better visualization around the enlarged uterus. Possible drawbacks are the risk of injury to the pregnant uterus, technical difficulty with exposure because of the enlarged uterus, increased carbon dioxide absorption, and decreased uterine blood flow secondary to excessive intra-abdominal pressure. Knowledge of the short- and long-term effects of laparoscopy on the human fetus is limited. Laparoscopy has been performed during all trimesters. During the first half of pregnancy, the risks inherent to the laparoscopic procedure do not appear to be substantially increased compared with the risks in nonpregnant patients. The largest population-based study of 2181 laparoscopies and 1522 laparotomies before 20 weeks' gestation did not find any differential impact of laparoscopy versus laparotomy on perinatal outcome. Fetal loss appears to be associated with maternal disease severity rather than with operative technique. Risks of uterine injury can be mitigated by placing a supraumbilical port 6 cm above the fundus using the open (Hasson's) technique; others recommend inserting the Veres needle in the left upper quadrant. Trocar placement under ultrasound guidance has also been described. Because there is uncertainty regarding the possible adverse effects of pneumoperitoneum and potential for fetal acidosis, attempts should be made to keep intra-abdominal pressure between 8 and 12 mm Hg and not to exceed 15 mm Hg. Intraoperative CO_2 monitoring should be used to maintain end-tidal CO_2 between 32 and 34 mm Hg.

Corneille MG, Gallup TM, Bening T, et al. The use of laparoscopic surgery in pregnancy: Evaluation of safety and efficacy. *Am J Surg* 2010;200:363–367. PMID: 20800715.

Guidelines Committee of SAGES. Guidelines for diagnosis, treatment, and use of laparoscopy for surgical problems during pregnancy. *Surg Endosc* 2008;22:849–861. PMID: 18288533.

GASTROINTESTINGAL DISEASES & DISORDERS

Early accurate diagnosis of serious abdominal surgical disease during pregnancy is more difficult for the following reasons: (1) altered anatomic relationships, (2) impaired palpation and detection of nonuterine masses, (3) depressed symptoms, (4) symptoms that mimic the normal discomforts of pregnancy, and (5) difficulty in differentiating surgical and obstetric disorders. In general, elective surgery should be avoided during pregnancy, but operation should be performed promptly for definite or probable acute disorders. The approach to surgical problems in pregnant or puerperal patients should be the same as in nonpregnant patients, with prompt surgical intervention when indicated. The risk of inducing labor with diagnostic laparoscopy or laparotomy is low, provided unnecessary manipulation of the uterus and adnexa is avoided. Spontaneous abortion is most likely to occur if surgery is performed before 14 weeks' gestation or when peritonitis is present.

APPENDICITIS

ESSENTIALS OF DIAGNOSIS

- Symptoms include abdominal pain, usually localized to right lower or mid quadrant, with nausea, vomiting, and/or anorexia.
- Patients may have an elevated white blood cell count with a left shift.
- Ultrasound or CT scan demonstrates enlargement or inflammation of the appendix.

Clinical Findings

Acute appendicitis is the most common extrauterine complication of pregnancy for which surgery is performed. Suspected appendicitis accounts for nearly two-thirds of all nonobstetric exploratory celiotomies performed during pregnancy; most cases occur in the second and third trimesters.

Appendicitis occurs in 0.1–1.4 per 1000 pregnancies. Although the incidence of disease is not increased during gestation, rupture of the appendix occurs 2–3 times more often during pregnancy secondary to delays in diagnosis and operation. Maternal and perinatal morbidity and mortality rates are greatly increased when appendicitis is complicated by peritonitis.

A. Symptoms & Signs

The diagnosis of appendicitis in pregnancy is challenging. Signs and symptoms often are atypical and not dramatic. Right lower quadrant or middle quadrant pain almost always is present when acute appendicitis occurs in pregnancy but may be ascribed to so-called round ligament pain or urinary tract infection. In nonpregnant women, the appendix is located in the right lower quadrant (65%), in the pelvis (30%), or retrocecally (5%). Traditionally it was taught that pregnancy displaces the appendix upwardly. However, some retrospective studies suggest that there is only minimal appendiceal migration throughout pregnancy.

The most consistent clinical symptom encountered in pregnant women with appendicitis is vague pain on the right side of the abdomen, although atypical pain patterns abound. Muscle guarding and rebound tenderness are much less demonstrable as gestation progresses. If pain changes from localized tenderness to a more diffuse nature, appendiceal perforation should be suspected. Rectal and vaginal tenderness are present in 80% of patients, particularly in early pregnancy. Nausea, vomiting, and anorexia usually are present, as in the nonpregnant patient. During early appendicitis, the temperature and pulse rate are relatively normal. High fever is not characteristic of the disease, and 25% of pregnant women with appendicitis are afebrile.

B. Laboratory Findings

The relative leukocytosis of pregnancy (normal 6000–16,000/μL) clouds interpretation of infection. Although not all patients with appendicitis have white blood cell counts above 16,000/μL, at least 75% show a left shift in the differential. Urinalysis may reveal significant pyuria (20%) as well as microscopic hematuria. This is particularly true in the latter half of pregnancy, when the appendix migrates closer to the retroperitoneal ureter.

C. Imaging

In the nonpregnant patient, CT of the abdomen with and without contrast has become an important tool aiding in the diagnosis of appendicitis. To avoid the risk of radiation to the fetus, US has a distinct role as the first-line imaging modality in pregnancy (Fig. 25–1). Graded compression ultrasonography has been found to have a high positive predictive value but average sensitivity in diagnosing appendicitis. MRI is helpful in further aiding the diagnosis in patients for whom sonographic findings are nondiagnostic. If US is nondiagnostic and MRI is not available, CT may be appropriate. A noncompressible appendix on ultrasound is abnormal, whereas MRI or CT may demonstrate an enlarged, fluid-filled appendix with or without a fecalith. An appendix measuring > 6 mm should be considered abnormal.

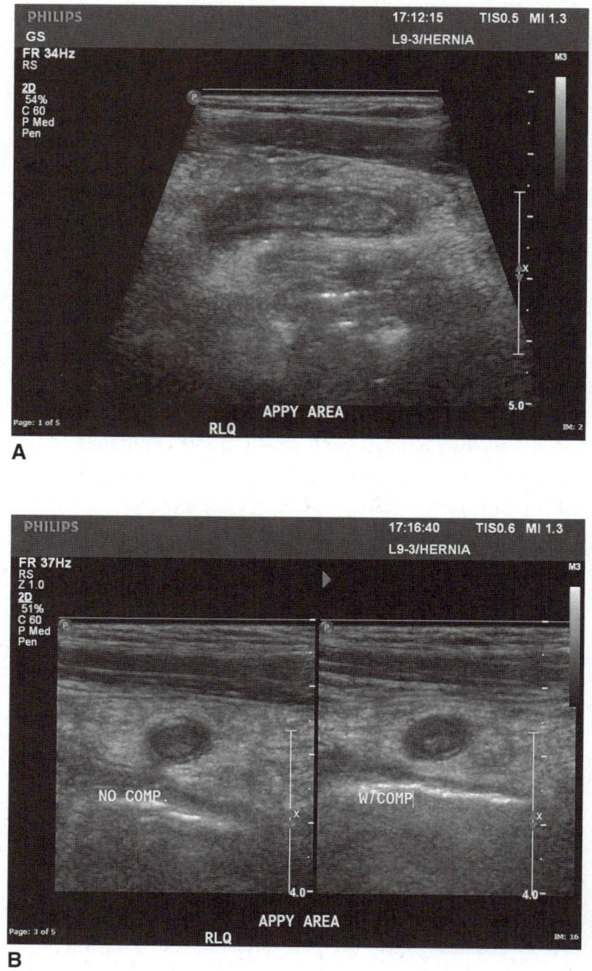

▲ **Figure 25–1.** Acute appendicitis diagnosed by graded compression ultrasonography. **A:** Longitudinal image of the right lower quadrant demonstrates the appendix as a blind-ending, thick-walled tubular structure. **B:** Transverse images with and without compression demonstrate this structure remains at least 6 mm thick with compression. (Images used, with permission, from Dr. Maitraya Patel, Olive View-UCLA Medical Center, Sylmar, CA.)

Differential Diagnosis

Pyelonephritis is the most common misdiagnosis in patients with acute appendicitis in pregnancy. The differential diagnosis of appendicitis includes gastrointestinal disorders such as gastroenteritis, small bowel obstruction, diverticulitis, pancreatitis, mesenteric adenitis, diverticulitis, and neoplasm; also possible are gynecologic and obstetric disorders such as ruptured corpus luteum cyst, adnexal torsion, ectopic pregnancy, placental abruption, early labor, round ligament syndrome, chorioamnionitis, degenerating myoma, or salpingitis.

Complications

Postoperative preterm labor has been reported to occur in 25% of second-trimester and as high as 50% of third-trimester patients. Most preterm deliveries occur within the first postoperative week. Perinatal loss may occur in association with preterm labor and delivery or with generalized peritonitis and sepsis, occurring in 0–1.5% of uncomplicated appendicitis cases. Twenty-five percent of pregnant women with appendicitis will progress to perforation; this risk is greatest when surgery is delayed more than 24 hours. With appendiceal rupture, fetal loss rates are reportedly as high as 30%, and maternal mortality rates as high as 4% are reported. This is of particular concern because appendiceal rupture occurs most frequently in the third trimester.

Treatment

Immediate surgical intervention is indicated once the diagnosis of appendicitis is made. In the setting of active labor, the surgery should be performed immediately postpartum. Delaying treatment increases the risk of perforation, which in turn increases the risk of fetal loss. Under appropriate conditions, laparoscopic appendectomy may be as safe as open appendectomy. A systematic review of 637 cases of laparoscopic appendectomy showed a significantly higher rate of fetal loss (6% vs. 3.1%), though equal or lesser rates of preterm delivery compared with open appendectomy. Large series report a negative surgical exploration rate between 13% and as high as 55%, likely due to the many processes that may mimic appendicitis in pregnancy. When the appendix appears normal at laparotomy, careful exploration for other nonobstetric and obstetric conditions is important.

Treatment of nonperforated acute appendicitis complicating pregnancy is appendectomy. A single dose of preoperative prophylactic antibiotics should be routinely given. In the setting of perforation, peritonitis, or abscess formation, broad-spectrum intravenous antibiotics should be continued until culture and sensitivities can narrow antibiotic choice. If drainage is necessary for generalized peritonitis, drains should be placed transabdominally and not transvaginally. During the first trimester, a transverse incision at McBurney's point or over the area of maximal tenderness is generally considered appropriate. If the diagnosis is not certain, a vertical midline incision can be made. Laparoscopy is an alternate surgical approach used with increasing frequency, especially in the first half of pregnancy. In the late second or third trimester, a muscle-splitting incision centered over the point of maximal tenderness usually provides optimal appendiceal exposure. As a rule, appendiceal disease is managed and the pregnancy is left alone. A Smead-Jones combined mass and fascial closure with secondary wound closure 72 hours later may be advisable when the appendix is gangrenous or perforated or in the presence of peritonitis or abscess formation.

Induced abortion is rarely indicated. Depending on the gestational age and expert neonatal care available, abdominal delivery occasionally is performed when peritonitis, sepsis, or a large appendiceal or cul-de-sac abscess occurs. Data are limited, so making definitive recommendations regarding the use of prophylactic tocolytics is difficult. It appears unnecessary in uncomplicated appendicitis but may be appropriate with advanced disease. Caution is indicated because of reports that tocolytics are associated with an increased risk of pulmonary edema in women with sepsis. Labor that follows shortly after surgery in the late third trimester should be allowed to progress because it is not associated with a significant risk of wound dehiscence. At times, the large uterus may help wall off an infection, which after delivery may become disrupted, leading to an acute abdomen within hours postpartum.

Prognosis

Better fluid and nutritional support, use of antibiotics, safer anesthesia, prompt surgical intervention, and improved surgical technique have been important elements in the significant reduction of maternal mortality from appendicitis during pregnancy. Similarly, the fetal mortality rate has significantly improved over the past 50 years. Perinatal loss is low and maternal mortality negligible in cases of uncomplicated appendicitis, but increase significantly in the setting of peritonitis or appendiceal rupture. Thus it is imperative to avoid surgical delay. A higher negative laparotomy or laparoscopy rate may be an acceptable trade-off for a lower fetal mortality rate.

Oto A, Ernst RD, Shah R, et al. Right-lower-quadrant pain and suspected appendicitis in pregnant women: Evaluation with MR imaging–initial experience. *Radiology* 2005;234:445–451. PMID: 15591434.

Pates JA, Avendanio TC, Zaretsky MV, McIntire DD, Twickler DM. The appendix in pregnancy: Confirming historical observations with a contemporary modality. *Obstet Gynecol* 2009;114:805–808. PMID: 19888038.

Walsh CA, Tang T, Walsh SR. Laparoscopic versus open appendectomy in pregnancy: A systematic review. *Int J Surg* 2008;6:339–344. PMID: 18342590.

CHOLECYSTITIS & CHOLELITHIASIS

ESSENTIALS OF DIAGNOSIS

- Patients usually present with abdominal pain in the right upper quadrant or epigastric region.
- Serum laboratories may demonstrate an elevation in the white blood cell count and/or elevated liver enzymes.
- Ultrasound of the right upper quadrant of the abdomen is usually diagnostic in these cases.

Clinical Findings

Gallbladder disease is one of the most common medical conditions and the second most common surgical disorder during pregnancy. Gallstones are responsible for 90% of cholecystitis in Western countries; parasitic infections are a less common cause. Acute cholecystitis occurs in 1 in 1600 to 1 in 10,000 pregnancies. Well-described risk factors for cholelithiasis are age, female sex, fertility, obesity, and family history. It has been estimated that at least 3.5% of pregnant women harbor gallstones. Multiparas are at increased risk of gallbladder disease. Both progesterone and estrogen increase bile lithogenicity; progesterone decreases gallbladder contractility. These changes are seen by the end of the first trimester of pregnancy.

A. Symptoms and Signs

Signs and symptoms are similar to those seen in the nonpregnant state and include anorexia, nausea, vomiting, dyspepsia, and intolerance of fatty foods. Biliary tract disease may cause right upper quadrant, epigastric, right scapular, shoulder, and even left upper quadrant or left lower quadrant pain that tends to be episodic. Biliary colic attacks often are of acute onset, seemingly are triggered by meals, and may last from a few minutes to several hours. Fever, right upper quadrant pain, and tenderness under the liver with deep inspiration (Murphy's sign) are often present in patients with acute cholecystitis. In severe cases the patient may have mild jaundice or appear septic.

B. Laboratory Findings

An elevated white blood cell count with an increase in immature forms is seen with acute cholecystitis. Aspartate transaminase (AST) and alanine transaminase (ALT) levels are often increased. Modest increases in the alkaline phosphatase and bilirubin levels are anticipated very early in cholecystitis or common duct obstruction. However, a more characteristic pattern of relatively normal AST and ALT levels with elevated alkaline phosphatase and bilirubin levels is generally found after the first day of the attack. These changes are not diagnostic and do not signify common bile duct stone or obstruction alone, but when present they serve to support the diagnosis. Elevated lipase and amylase support the diagnosis of an associated pancreatitis.

C. Imaging

US findings of gallbladder stones, a thickened gallbladder wall, fluid collection around the gallbladder, a dilated common bile duct, or even swelling in the pancreas are suggestive of cholelithiasis and cholecystitis. The diagnostic accuracy of US for detecting gallstones in pregnancy is 95%, making it the diagnostic test of choice.

Differential Diagnosis

The major diagnostic difficulty imposed by pregnancy is differentiating between cholecystitis and appendicitis. In addition to its association with gallstones, cholecystitis can be infectious secondary to *Salmonella typhi* or parasites. A number of other lesions of the biliary tract occur rarely during gestation, including choledochal cysts, which are seen as a spherical dilatation of the common bile duct with a very narrow or obstructed distal end. Associated pancreatitis may be present. Severe preeclampsia with associated right upper quadrant abdominal pain and abnormal liver function tests; hemolysis, elevated liver enzymes, and low platelet count (HELLP) syndrome; acute fatty liver of pregnancy; and acute viral hepatitis are in the differential diagnosis. The presence of proteinuria, nondependent edema, hypertension, and sustained increases in AST and ALT levels compared with alkaline phosphatase level are clinical and laboratory features usually associated with preeclampsia. Peptic ulcer disease, myocardial infarction, and herpes zoster also have overlapping symptoms.

Complications

Secondary infection with enteric flora such as *Escherichia coli*, *Klebsiella*, or *Streptococcus faecalis* complicates one-fifth of cases. Pancreatitis may frequently accompany cholecystitis during pregnancy. Removal of the gallbladder and gallstones may be preferred over conservative medical therapy when pancreatitis is concurrent, as it is associated with fetal loss in 3–20% of pregnant patients. Other uncommon complications of cholecystitis during gestation are retained intraductal stones, gangrenous cholecystitis, galbladder perforation with biliary peritonitis, cholecystoenteric fistulas, and ascending cholangitis.

Treatment

The initial management of symptomatic cholelithiasis and cholecystitis in pregnancy is nonoperative with bowel rest, intravenous hydration, correction of electrolyte imbalances, and analgesics. If antibiotics are not routinely given, they should be administered if no improvement is seen in 12–24 hours or if systemic symptoms are noted. This therapy results in resolution of acute symptoms in most patients. Surgical intervention is indicated if symptoms fail to improve with medical management, for recurrent episodes of biliary colic, and for complications such as recurrent cholecystitis, choledocholithiasis, and gallstone pancreatitis. Because recurrence rates for symptomatic biliary disease during pregnancy may be as high as 60–92%, active surgical management, especially in the second trimester, has been advocated in recent years. Recent literature has demonstrated the safety of open and laparoscopic cholecystectomy during pregnancy. Endoscopic retrograde cholangiopancreatography (ERCP) with endoscopic sphincterotomy may be an alternative for selected patients with common bile duct stones. Operative therapy for uncomplicated cholecystitis performed during the second and third trimesters does not appear to be associated with an appreciable increase in morbidity and mortality rates or fetal loss.

Prognosis

The outcomes for mother and fetus after uncomplicated gallbladder surgery are excellent. Morbidity and mortality rates increase with maternal age and extent of disease.

Andriulli A, Loperfido S, Napolitano G, et al. Incidence rates of post-ERCP complications: A systematic survey of prospective studies. *Am J Gastroenterol* 2007;102:1781–1788. PMID: 17509029.

Date RS, Kaushal M, Ramesh A. A review of the management of gallstone disease and its complications in pregnancy. *Am J Surg* 2008;196:599–608. PMID: 18614143.

Jackson H, Granger S, Price R, et al. Diagnosis and laparoscopic treatment of surgical diseases during pregnancy: An evidence-based review. *Surg Endosc* 2008;22:1917–1927. PMID: 18553201.

ACUTE PANCREATITIS

ESSENTIALS OF DIAGNOSIS

- Patients usually present with epigastric pain that may radiate to the back.
- Serum amylase and lipase levels are elevated, findings diagnostic of pancreatitis.
- Ultrasound may demonstrate an enlarged pancreas and fluid within the peritoneal cavity.

Clinical Findings

The incidence of acute pancreatitis in pregnancy reportedly ranges from 1 in 1000 to 1 in 5000 deliveries. Pancreatitis occurs most frequently in the third trimester and puerperium. The mortality rate associated with acute pancreatitis may be higher during pregnancy because of delayed diagnosis. The ultimate cause of pancreatitis is the presence of activated digestive enzymes within the pancreas. Many cases of pancreatitis are idiopathic. As in the nonpregnant state, cholelithiasis is the most commonly identified cause, followed by alcoholism, lipidemia, viral and drug-induced pancreatitis, familial pancreatitis, structural abnormalities of the pancreas or duodenum, severe abdominal trauma, vascular disease, and preeclampsia-associated pancreatitis.

A. Symptoms & Signs

Gravidas with pancreatitis usually present with severe, steady epigastric pain that often radiates to the back in general approximation of the retroperitoneal location of the pancreas. Often exacerbated by food intake, its onset may be gradual or acute and is frequently accompanied by nausea and vomiting. During gestation, patients may present primarily with vomiting with little or no abdominal pain. Although physical examination is rarely diagnostic, several findings of note may be present, including a low-grade fever, tachycardia, and orthostatic hypotension. The latter finding may be present with hemorrhagic pancreatitis in addition to Cullen's sign (periumbilical ecchymosis) and Turner's sign (flank ecchymosis). Epigastric tenderness and ileus also may be present.

B. Laboratory Findings

The cornerstone of diagnosis is the determination of serum amylase and lipase levels. Interpretation of serum amylase levels in pregnancy is difficult at times because of the physiologic, up to 2-fold rise in serum amylase level during pregnancy. A laboratory serum amylase level that is more than 2 times above the upper limit of normal suggests pancreatitis. However, an elevated serum amylase level is not specific for pancreatitis because cholecystitis, bowel obstruction, hepatic trauma, or a perforated duodenal ulcer can cause similar serum amylase level elevations. Serum amylase levels usually return to normal within a few days of an attack of uncomplicated acute pancreatitis. Serum lipase level is a pancreas-specific enzyme and lipase elevation can guide the differential diagnosis toward pancreatitis. In severe pancreatitis, hypocalcemia develops as calcium is complexed by fatty acids liberated by lipase.

C. Imaging

Sonographic examination may demonstrate an enlarged pancreas with a blunted contour, peritoneal or peripancreatic fluid, and abscess or pseudocyst formation. Ultrasonography allows for the diagnosis of cholelithiasis, which may be etiologic for pancreatitis. The mere presence of gallstones, however, does not demonstrate etiologic relevance. US is also helpful for evaluating other differential diagnostic considerations.

Differential Diagnosis

Especially pertinent in the differential diagnosis of pancreatitis in pregnancy are hyperemesis gravidarum, preeclampsia, ruptured ectopic pregnancy (often with elevated serum amylase levels), perforated peptic ulcer, intestinal obstruction or ischemia, acute cholecystitis, ruptured spleen, liver abscess, and perinephric abscess.

Complications

Although all of the usual complications of pancreatitis can occur in parturients, there is no special predisposition to complications during pregnancy. Acute complications include hemorrhagic pancreatitis with severe hypotension and hypocalcemia, acute respiratory distress syndrome, pleural effusions, pancreatic ascites, abscess formation, and liponecrosis.

Treatment

Treatment of acute pancreatitis is aimed at correcting any underlying predisposing factors and treating the pancreatic inflammation. In pregnancy, acute pancreatitis is managed as it is in the nonpregnant state, except that nutritional supplementation is considered at an earlier point in treatment to protect the fetus, either via nasojejunal tube feeding of an elemental formula or total parenteral nutrition. Treatment is primarily medical and supportive, including bowel rest with or without nasogastric suction, intravenous fluid and electrolyte replacement, and parenteral analgesics. Antibiotics are reserved for cases with evidence of an acute infection. In patients with gallstone pancreatitis, consideration is given to early cholecystectomy or ERCP after the acute inflammation subsides. In pancreatitis not caused by gallstones, surgical exploration is reserved for patients with pancreatic abscess, ruptured pseudocyst, severe hemorrhagic pancreatitis, or pancreatitis secondary to a lesion that is amenable to surgery. Pregnancy does not influence the course of pancreatitis.

Prognosis

Maternal mortality rates as high as 37% were reported before the era of modern medical and surgical management. Respiratory failure, shock, need for massive fluid replacement, and severe hypocalcemia are predictive of disease severity. Most recent single-institution series reflect a reduced maternal mortality rate of less than 1%; perinatal death ranges from 3–20%, depending on severity of disease. Preterm labor appears to occur in a high proportion of patients with acute pancreatitis in later gestation.

Eddy JJ, Gideonsen MD, Song JY, Grobman WA, O'Halloran P. Pancreatitis in pregnancy. *Obstet Gynecol* 2008;112:1075–1081. PMID: 18978108.

Luminita CS, Steidl ET, Rivera-Alsina ME. Acute hyperlipidemic pancreatitis in pregnancy. *Am J Obstet Gynecol* 2008;98:e57. PMID: 18359475.

PEPTIC ULCER DISEASE

ESSENTIALS OF DIAGNOSIS

- Patients typically present with epigastric discomfort.
- Endoscopy is diagnostic of peptic ulcer disease.
- Pathogenesis

Pathogenesis

Pregnancy appears to be somewhat protective against the development of gastrointestinal ulcers, as gastric secretion and motility are reduced and mucus secretion is increased. Close to 90% of women with known peptic ulcer disease experience significant improvement during pregnancy, but more than half will have recurrence of symptoms within 3 months postpartum. Thus peptic ulcer disease occurring as a complication of pregnancy or diagnosed during gestation is encountered infrequently, although the exact incidence is unknown. Infection with *Helicobacter pylori* is associated with the development of peptic ulcer disease.

Clinical Findings

Signs and symptoms of peptic ulcer disease in pregnancy can be mistakenly dismissed as being a normal part of the gravid state. Dyspepsia is the major symptom of ulcers during gestation, although reflux symptoms and nausea are also common. Epigastric discomfort that is temporally unrelated to meals is often reported. Abdominal pain might suggest a perforated ulcer, especially in the presence of peritoneal signs and systemic shock. Endoscopy is the diagnostic method of choice for these patients if empiric clinical therapy, including lifestyle and diet modifications, antacids, antisecretory agents, and treatment for *H pylori* when positive, fail to improve symptoms.

Differential Diagnosis

Gastroesophageal reflux disease and functional or nonulcer dyspepsia are common occurrences in pregnancy and may result in symptoms very similar to those of peptic ulcer disease. Biliary colic, chronic pancreatitis, Mallory-Weiss tears, and irritable bowel syndrome must also be considered. In recent years the diagnosis of persistent hyperemesis gravidarum has been linked to *H pylori* infection. Women with jaundice, persistent symptoms of dysphagia or odynophagia, weight loss, occult gastrointestinal bleeding, a family history of gastrointestinal cancers or unexplained anemia postpartum should be assessed for malignancy. A history of prior gastric surgery should prompt an evaluation for surgical complications. Ulcer perforation should be suspected in the setting of sudden, severe, diffuse abdominal pain followed by tachycardia and peritoneal signs.

Complications

Fewer than 100 parturients with complications of peptic ulcer disease, such as perforation, bleeding, and obstruction, have been reported. Most of these cases have occurred in the third trimester of pregnancy. Gastric perforation during pregnancy has an exceedingly high mortality rate, partly because of the difficulty in establishing the proper diagnosis. Other causes of upper gastrointestinal bleeding in pregnancy are reflux esophagitis and Mallory-Weiss tears. Surgical intervention is indicated for significant bleeding ulcerations. In patients requiring surgery for complicated peptic ulcers late in the third trimester, concurrent caesarean delivery may be indicated to enhance operative exposure of the upper abdomen and to prevent potential fetal death or damage from maternal hypotension and hypoxemia.

Treatment

Dyspepsia during pregnancy first should be treated with dietary and lifestyle changes, supplemented with antacids or sucralfate. When symptoms persist, H_2-receptor antagonists or, in severe cases, proton pump inhibitors can be used. Administration of triple-drug therapy for *H pylori* during pregnancy is controversial; because complications from peptic ulcer disease during pregnancy are low and there are theoretical concerns of teratogenicity from treatment, it is often deferred until postpartum. Empiric treatment of *H pylori* without testing is not recommended.

Chen YH, Lin HC, Lou HY. Increased risk of low birthweight, infants small for gestational age, and preterm delivery for women with peptic ulcer. *Am J Obstet Gynecol* 2010;202:164.e1–164.e8. PMID: 20113692.

Engemise S, Oshowo A, Kyei-Mensah A. Perforated duodenal ulcer in the puerperium. *Arch Gynecol Obstet* 2009;279:407–410. PMID: 18642012.

Talley N, Vakil N. Guidelines for the management of dyspepsia. Practice Parameters Committee of the American College of Gastroenterology. *Am J Gastroenterol* 2005;100:2324–2337. PMID: 16181387.

ACUTE INTESTINAL OBSTRUCTION

ESSENTIALS OF DIAGNOSIS

- Patients typically present with the classic triad of abdominal pain, vomiting, and obstipation.
- The diagnosis is confirmed with abdominal x-ray series.

Pathogenesis

Intestinal obstruction is an infrequently encountered complication of pregnancy that is estimated to occur in approximately 1–3 of every 10,000 pregnancies. However, it is the third most common nonobstetric reason for laparotomy during pregnancy (following appendicitis and biliary tract disease). It occurs most commonly in the third trimester. The most common causes of mechanical obstruction are adhesions (60%) and volvulus (25%), followed by intussusception, hernia, and neoplasm. Volvulus is much more prevalent during pregnancy; the risk is greatest when uterine size rapidly changes (eg, second trimester and immediately postpartum).

Clinical Findings

The same classic triad of abdominal pain, vomiting, and obstipation is observed in pregnant and nonpregnant women with intestinal obstruction. Pain may be diffuse, constant, or periodic, occurring every 4–5 minutes with small-bowel obstruction or every 10–15 minutes with large-bowel obstruction. Bowel sounds are of little value in making an early diagnosis of obstruction, and tenderness to palpation typically is absent with early obstruction. Vomiting occurs early with small-bowel obstruction. Guarding and rebound tenderness are observed in association with strangulation or perforation. Late in the course of disease, fever, oliguria, and shock occur as manifestations of massive fluid loss into the bowel, acidosis, and infection. The classic findings of bowel ischemia include fever, tachycardia, localized abdominal pain, marked leukocytosis, and metabolic acidosis. Unfortunately, most laboratory abnormalities arise once bowel ischemia has progressed to bowel necrosis.

The diagnosis usually is confirmed by radiologic studies, which should be obtained when intestinal obstruction is suspected. A single abdominal series (upright and supine abdominal film) is nondiagnostic in up to 50% of early cases, but serial films usually reveal progressive changes that confirm the diagnosis. Volvulus should be suspected when a single, grossly dilated loop of bowel is seen. A volvulus primarily occurs at the cecum but may also be seen at the sigmoid colon. Occasionally, more extensive radiologic imaging is indicated, given the high risk of fetal death with delayed treatment.

Differential Diagnosis

The diagnosis of hyperemesis gravidarum in the second and third trimesters should be viewed with caution and made only after gastrointestinal causes of the symptoms including pancreatitis have been excluded. Mesenteric ischemia, adynamic ileus of the colon, and acute colonic pseudo-obstruction (Ogilvie's syndrome) are included in the differential diagnosis but are rarely seen during pregnancy.

Prognosis

Intestinal obstruction in pregnancy is associated with a maternal mortality rate of 6%, often secondary to infection and irreversible shock. Early diagnosis and treatment are essential for an improved outcome. Perinatal mortality is approximately 20% and usually results from maternal hypotension and resultant fetal hypoxia and acidosis.

Treatment

The management of bowel obstruction in pregnancy is essentially no different from treatment of nonpregnant patients. The cornerstones of therapy are bowel decompression, intravenous hydration, correction of electrolyte imbalances, and timely surgery when indicated. The patient's condition must be rapidly stabilized. The amount of fluid loss often is underestimated and may be 1–6 L by the time obstruction is identified on a scout film. Aggressive hydration is needed to support both the mother and the fetus. A nasogastric tube should be placed. Colonoscopy has been used successfully in the reduction of volvulus averting laparotomy. Ogilvie's syndrome can be managed with bowel rest, rehydration, and a rectal tube for large bowel decompression. Surgery is mandatory if perforation or gangrenous bowel is suspected or when the patient's symptoms do not resolve with medical management. A vertical midline incision on the abdomen provides the best operative exposure and can be extended as needed. Surgical principles for intraoperative management apply similarly to pregnant and nonpregnant patients. Caesarean delivery is performed first if the large uterus prevents adequate exposure of the bowel in term pregnancies or if indicated obstetrically. The entire bowel should be examined carefully because there may be more than 1 area of obstruction or limited bowel viability.

Dietrich CS 3rd, Hill CC, Hueman M. Surgical diseases presenting in pregnancy. *Surg Clin North Am* 2008;88:403–419. PMID: 18381120.

Parangi S, Levine D, Henry A, Isakovich N, Pories S. Surgical gastrointestinal disorders during pregnancy. *Am J Surg* 2007;193:223–232. PMID: 17236852.

INFLAMMATORY BOWEL DISEASE

(See Chapter 29, Gastrointestinal Disorders in Pregnancy, for more details.)

ESSENTIALS OF DIAGNOSIS

- Crohn's disease is one subcategory, characterized by insidious onset; episodes of low-grade fever, diarrhea, and right lower quadrant pain; and perianal disease with abscess and fistulas formed. Radiographic evidence of ulceration, structuring, or fistulas of the small intestine or colon. May involve any segment of the gastrointestinal tract from the mouth to the anus.
- Ulcerative colitis is the other subcategory of inflammatory bowel disease, manifesting with bloody diarrhea, lower abdominal cramps, fecal urgency, anemia, and low serum albumin. It is diagnosed with sigmoidoscopy and only involves the colon.

Clinical Findings

Inflammatory bowel disease (IBD) (Crohn's disease and ulcerative colitis) often affects women in their childbearing years; however, initial presentation of IBD during pregnancy is rare. IBD presents with crampy abdominal pain and diarrhea stained with blood or mucus. More rarely the patient has weight loss and fevers.

Differential Diagnosis

Because some of the early IBD symptoms are found in normal pregnancies, diagnosis can be delayed, leading to poorer outcome. Initial evaluation should begin with ultrasound, which can also evaluate gallbladder, pancreas, and adnexa. Bowel wall thickening or abscess formations may be seen. Gold standard for diagnosis is endoscopy with biopsy, which can be safely performed during pregnancy.

Treatment

Initial management includes dietary modifications or bulking agents. Other medications that have been safely used in pregnancy are sulfasalazine, prednisone, and occasionally antibiotics. Patients receiving sulfasalazine should be given folate supplementation because sulfasalazine inhibits its absorption. Patients taking corticosteroids should receive stress-dose steroids during delivery or in surgery. Safety data of immunosuppressant use such as cyclosporine and anti–tumor necrosis factor-α in pregnancy are limited, but these agents have been used for persistent flares. Surgery during pregnancy is indicated for intestinal obstruction, megacolon, perforation, hemorrhage, abscess formation, and failed medical management. Delivery route should be based on obstetric indications except for patients who have active perianal disease; those with an ileal pouch and anastomosis may consider caesarean section to prevent injury to the anal sphincter.

Prognosis

The impact of IBD on pregnancy outcomes is controversial, though in general maternal and fetal outcomes are improved if IBD is in remission before conception. Postpartum flare is more common in Crohn's disease than ulcerative colitis.

Ilnyckyj A. Surgical treatment of inflammatory bowel diseases and pregnancy. *Best Pract Res Clin Gastroenterol* 2007;21:819–834. PMID: 17889810.

Reddy D, Murphy SJ, Kane SV, et al. Relapses of inflammatory bowel disease during pregnancy: In-hospital management and birth outcomes. *Am J Gastroenterol* 2008;103:1203–1209. PMID: 18422816.

HEMORRHOIDS

ESSENTIALS OF DIAGNOSIS

- Patients with hemorrhoids typically present with complaints of painless bleeding, prolapse, pain, pruritus, and/or fecal soilage.
- Hemorrhoids are visible on physical examination or anoscopy.

Pathogenesis

Pregnancy is the most common cause of symptomatic hemorrhoids. Approximately 9–35% of pregnant and postpartum women suffer from hemorrhoids. Higher incidences of constipation, increased blood volume, and venous congestion secondary to the enlarging uterus contribute to hemorrhoid formation.

Clinical Findings

Patients with hemorrhoids typically present with complaints of painless bleeding, prolapse, pain, pruritus, and/or fecal soilage. On physical examination, hemorrhoids are visualized as a protrusion into or out of the anal canal. Internal hemorrhoids may require anoscopy for visualization.

Treatment

The current management approach to hemorrhoid disease is conservative, with simple outpatient treatment preferred, particularly during pregnancy and the puerperium. Medical therapy with dietary changes, avoidance of excessive straining, fiber supplementation, stool softeners, and hemorrhoidal analgesics often is the only requirement for nonthrombosed hemorrhoids. Often 6 weeks or longer are needed to perceive improvement. If conservative treatments fail, rubber-band ligation, infrared coagulation, or sclerotherapy appear to be safe during pregnancy. Hemorrhoidectomy is the best means of definitive therapy for hemorrhoidal disease but is rarely necessary during pregnancy. It should be considered postpartum if the patient continues to fail to respond to conservative measures, if hemorrhoids are severely prolapsed and require manual reduction, or if associated pathology such as ulceration, severe bleeding, fissure, or fistula is present. Thrombosis or clots in the vein lead to severe symptoms. If thrombosed external hemorrhoids remain tender and persist despite conservative treatment, surgical excision under local anesthesia is preferred over clot extraction, as this results in a high rate of clot recurrence.

Longo SA, Moore RC, Canzoneri BJ, Robichaux A. Gastrointestinal conditions during pregnancy. *Clin Colon Rectal Surg* 2010; 23:80–89. PMID: 21629625.

SPONTANEOUS HEPATIC & SPLENIC RUPTURE

ESSENTIALS OF DIAGNOSIS

- Patients with spontaneous hepatic or splenic rupture typically present with severe abdominal pain and the rapid onset of shock.

Pathogenesis

Intra-abdominal hemorrhage during pregnancy has diverse causes, including trauma, preexisting splenic disease, and preeclampsia–eclampsia. Often, the exact cause cannot be determined preoperatively. Spontaneous hepatic rupture may be associated with severe preeclampsia–eclampsia. (See Chapter 26, Hypertension in Pregnancy, for more details on preeclampsia–eclampsia.)

Clinical Findings

Spontaneous hepatic or splenic rupture is usually manifested by severe abdominal pain and shock, with thrombocytopenia and low fibrinogen levels.

Treatment

Exploratory celiotomy in conjunction with aggressive transfusion of blood products including packed red blood cells, fresh-frozen plasma, and platelets should be undertaken immediately, as this has been associated with improved survival rates.

Bleeding from a lacerated or ruptured spleen does not cease spontaneously and requires immediate surgical attention. Evidence of a hemoperitoneum on imaging studies or a hemorrhagic peritoneal lavage in association with a falling hematocrit level and abdominal pain establish the presence of a hemoperitoneum.

RUPTURED SPLENIC ARTERY ANEURYSM

ESSENTIALS OF DIAGNOSIS

- Women with ruptured splenic artery aneurysm typically present with epigastric, left upper quadrant, or left shoulder pain.
- The diagnosis is usually confirmed by abdominal radiography or ultrasound.

Pathogenesis

Autopsy data suggest that splenic artery aneurysm occurs in 0.1% of adults and appear to be more common in women. It is estimated that 6–10% of lesions will rupture, with portal hypertension and pregnancy being the main risk factors. Twenty-five to 40% of ruptures occur during gestation, especially in the last trimester, and are a major cause of intraperitoneal hemorrhage. Pregnant women who develop ruptured splenic artery aneurysm have a 75% mortality rate, with an even higher fetal mortality rate of up to 95%. Most patients with this condition are thought preoperatively to have placental abruption or uterine rupture.

Clinical Findings

Before rupture, the presenting symptoms may be completely absent or vague. The most common symptom is vague epigastric, left upper quadrant, or left shoulder pain. In approximately 25% of patients a 2-stage rupture is seen, with a smaller primary hemorrhage into the lesser sac, which may allow for temporary tamponade of the bleeding until complete rupture into the peritoneal cavity occurs, causing hemorrhagic shock. A bruit may be audible. A highly diagnostic finding on flat x-ray film of the abdomen is demonstration in the upper left quadrant of an oval calcification with a central lucent area. In stable clinical situations, angiography can provide positive confirmation and is the gold standard for diagnosis. In pregnancy, however, ultrasonography and pulsed-wave Doppler studies are preferred in order to minimize fetal radiation exposure.

Treatment

A splenic artery aneurysm in a woman of childbearing age should be treated in a timely manner, even during pregnancy, because of the increased risk of rupture and associated mortality. The elective operative mortality rate reportedly ranges between 0.5% and 1.3%.

He MX, Zheng JM, Zhang S, et al. Rupture of splenic artery aneurysm in pregnancy: A review of the literature and report of two cases. *Am J Forensic Med Pathol* 2010;31:92–94. PMID: 20032776.

Parangi S, Levine D, Henry A, Isakovich N, Pories S. Surgical gastrointestinal disorders during pregnancy. *Am J Surg* 2007;193:223–232. PMID: 17236852.

PELVIC DISEASES & DISORDERS

OVARIAN MASSES

ESSENTIALS OF DIAGNOSIS

- Most ovarian masses during pregnancy present as an incidental finding on routine obstetrical ultrasound to evaluate the fetus.
- Some women may experience pelvic pain or discomfort due to the mass.

Pathogenesis

The incidental finding of an adnexal mass in pregnancy has become more common with the routine use of ultrasonography. As many as 1–4% of pregnant women are diagnosed with an adnexal mass. The majority of the masses are functional or corpus luteum cysts and spontaneously resolve by 16 weeks' gestation. More than 90% of unilateral, noncomplex masses less than 5 cm in diameter that are noticed in the first trimester are functional and resolve spontaneously. Patients who undergo assisted reproduction present a special subgroup, as their ovaries frequently have ovarian cysts in the first trimester due to ovarian hyperstimulation. Pathologic ovarian neoplasms tend not to resolve. The most common pathologic ovarian neoplasms during pregnancy are benign cystic teratoma, serous or mucinous cystadenoma, and cystic corpus luteum. Of the adnexal masses that persist, 1–10% will be malignant.

Clinical Findings

Most adnexal masses discovered during pregnancy are found as incidental findings at time of ultrasound performed for evaluation of the fetus. Thus most women are asymptomatic for the ovarian mass. However, some women may experience pelvic pain or discomfort related to the mass.

Differential Diagnosis

Ovarian masses must be differentiated from lesions of the colon, pedunculated leiomyomas, pelvic kidneys, and congenital abnormalities of the uterus. If ultrasound cannot distinguish between leiomyoma and ovarian neoplasm, MRI can improve diagnostic precision.

Treatment

The 3 main reasons for advising surgery for an adnexal mass in pregnancy are the risks of rupture, torsion, and malignancy. Determination of the actual risk of rupture or torsion of a benign-appearing adnexal mass in pregnancy remains an unsettled issue. It is estimated that only approximately 2% of such masses will rupture during gestation, and the incidence of torsion in recent published series ranges from 0–15%. The challenge to the clinician is to weigh for each individual patient these risks against the risks of abdominal surgery during pregnancy, including miscarriage, rupture of membranes, and preterm labor. If adnexal masses diagnosed in the first trimester require surgery in pregnancy, it is generally advisable to perform the operation via laparotomy or laparoscopy in the second trimester unless signs or symptoms suggestive of torsion or highly aggressive malignancy indicate the need for more immediate intervention. Similarly, asymptomatic ovarian masses that are initially noted in the third trimester of pregnancy can be followed until the time of delivery or postpartum because the size of the uterus may present access problems and because preterm labor may be inadvertently induced.

The risk of malignancy can be largely gauged by the ultrasonographic characteristics of the mass. Ultrasonography usually facilitates delineation of the size and morphology of adnexal masses. If the mass is unilateral, mobile, and cystic, anaplastic elements are less likely and operation can be deferred.

Any adnexal lesion that is present after 14 weeks' gestation, is growing in size on serial ultrasonographic evaluations, contains solid and complex components or internal papillae, is fixed, is surrounded by abdominal ascites, or is symptomatic warrants surgical exploration and pathologic diagnosis.

Marret H, Lhomme C, Lecuru F, et al. Guidelines for the management of ovarian cancer during pregnancy. *Eur J Obstet Gynecol Reprod Biol* 2010;149:18–21. PMID: 20042265.

Schmeler KM, Mayo-Smith WW, Peipert JF, Weitzen S, Manuel MD, Gordinier ME. Adnexal masses in pregnancy: Surgery compared with observation. *Obstet Gynecol* 2005;105:1098–1103. PMID: 15863550.

Schwartz N, Timor-Tritsch IE, Wang E. Adnexal masses in pregnancy. *Clin Obstet Gynecol* 2009;52:570–585. PMID: 20393410.

Yen CF, Lin SL, Murk W, et al. Risk analysis of torsion and malignancy for adnexal masses during pregnancy. *Fertil Steril* 2009;91:1895–1902. PMID: 18359024.

TORSION OF THE ADNEXA

ESSENTIALS OF DIAGNOSIS

- Adnexal torsion may be suspected in the woman with an adnexal mass who experiences the sudden onset of pelvic pain, usually severe in nature.
- Ultrasound is useful in confirming the presence of an adnexal mass.
- Laparoscopy or laparotomy is diagnostic for confirming the presence of torsion.

Pathogenesis

Torsion of the adnexa can involve the ovary, tube, and ancillary structures, either separately or together. The most common time for occurrence of adnexal torsion is between 6 and 14 weeks and in the immediate puerperium. Although torsion of normal adnexa has been described, it commonly is associated with a cystic neoplasm.

Clinical Findings

Symptoms include abdominal pain and tenderness that usually are sudden in onset and result from occlusion of the vascular supply to the twisted organ. Shock and peritonitis may ensue. Ultrasonography frequently demonstrates an adnexal mass and altered blood flow on Doppler studies. The diagnosis of torsion is ultimately made at surgery.

Treatment

Prompt operation is necessary to prevent tissue necrosis, preterm labor, and potential perinatal death. Laparoscopy appears to be as safe as laparotomy for mother and fetus. The right ovary is involved more frequently than is the left ovary. Benign cystic teratomas and cystadenomas are the most common histologic findings in ovaries that have undergone torsion. Traditional thinking has been that ovarian cysts that have undergone torsion must not be untwisted before pedicle clamping because of the concern for potential fatal thromboembolic complications. However, recent series on both nonpregnant and pregnant patients demonstrate that adnexa that had undergone torsion can safely be untwisted, followed by the appropriate removal of the mass (eg, cystectomy). Oophoropexy may be performed to prevent future re-occurrence of the torsion. These adnexa are capable of recovering and being functional. Salpingo-oophorectomy can be reserved for the management of active bleeding or suspicious neoplasms. If cystectomy includes corpus luteum before 12 weeks' gestation, progesterone supplementation should be initiated.

CARCINOMA OF THE OVARY

(See also Chapter 50, Premalignant and Malignant Disorders of the Ovaries and Oviducts.)

ESSENTIALS OF DIAGNOSIS

- Symptoms of ovarian cancer are often vague and mimic some of the common symptoms associated with pregnancy.
- Certain ultrasound findings, although not diagnostic of malignancy, can be suggestive of malignancy.
- The diagnosis is confirmed on pathologic examination of surgically excised tissue.

Pathogenesis

Carcinoma of the ovary occurs in less than 0.1% of all gestations and has been encountered in all trimesters. Between 1% and 10% of all ovarian tumors complicating pregnancy are malignant. Consistent with the young age of the pregnant population, most malignant neoplasms are germ cell tumors (dysgerminoma, endodermal sinus tumor, malignant teratoma, embryonal carcinoma, and choriocarcinoma) and tumors of low malignant potential, but cystadenocarcinomas do occur. The majority of ovarian malignancies diagnosed in pregnancy are early-stage disease.

Clinical Findings

Symptoms of ovarian cancer are often vague and include bloating, increasing abdominal girth, and urinary frequency, findings that are common during pregnancy. Most cases of ovarian cancer diagnosed during pregnancy are found when an adnexal mass is seen during routine ultrasound to evaluate the fetus. Ultrasound findings suggestive of ovarian malignancy are a mass with a solid component or thick septations, evidence of flow within the solid component on color Doppler interrogation, and the presence of other masses in the pelvis suggestive of enlarged nodes.

Treatment

Solid and complex ovarian tumors with significant solid components discovered during pregnancy generally should be treated surgically because of the low but significant incidence of cancer (1–10%). The treatment of gestational ovarian cancer follows the same principles as that for the nonpregnant patient. If the adnexal mass is complex, laparoscopy may be considered if intact removal in an endoscopic bag is feasible. If an open approach is taken, the incision needs to be of sufficient size not only to remove the tumor intact, but also to properly explore the abdomen and to reduce uterine manipulation until the definitive surgical course of management is determined. Upon abdominal entry, peritoneal washings should be obtained and the contralateral ovary examined. If abnormal in appearance, biopsy should be performed; otherwise, routine biopsy is unnecessary. Adequate tissue should be obtained for histologic diagnosis on frozen section. If the tumor is benign, residual ovarian tissue should be conserved if possible.

If malignant, staging is performed. Conservative surgery is appropriate for an encapsulated tumor if no evidence of uterine or contralateral ovarian involvement is seen. In more advanced stages, the extent of surgery, including tumor debulking, will depend on gestational age and the patient's wishes with regard to the pregnancy. Early termination of pregnancy does not improve outcome of ovarian cancer. In some cases, optimal surgical cytoreduction of the tumor to <1cm residual disease can be accomplished with the uterus and pregnancy left in situ. Neoadjuvant chemotherapy may offer an interim treatment for selected patients diagnosed at midgestation to allow for fetal maturity before extensive surgical cytoreduction. Elevated tumor markers, such as α-fetoprotein, lactate dehydrogenase, β-human chorionic gonadotropin, and cancer antigen-125, during the preoperative workup of an adnexal mass must be interpreted with caution because pregnancy itself may cause an increase in these values.

LEIOMYOMAS

ESSENTIALS OF DIAGNOSIS

- The diagnosis of leiomyomas in pregnancy is made based on ultrasound

Clinical Findings

Uterine leiomyomas are found in 0.1–3.9% of pregnancies. Most women with fibroids during pregnancy are asymptomatic. A degenerating leiomyoma or one undergoing torsion is characterized by acute abdominal pain with point tenderness over the site of the leiomyoma. Ultrasonography is of great value to document the location, size, and consistency of leiomyomas in a pregnant uterus. Cystic changes in leiomyomas are often visualized when clinical signs of degeneration are present.

Complications

A large cohort study of obstetric outcomes of women diagnosed ultrasonographically with uterine leiomyomas in pregnancy found an increased risk of caesarean delivery (mostly before labor onset), breech presentation, malposition, preterm delivery, placenta previa, and severe postpartum hemorrhage. Uterine leiomyomas may further complicate pregnancy by undergoing degeneration or torsion, or by causing mechanical obstruction of labor.

Treatment

Conservative treatment with analgesia, reassurance, and supportive therapy almost always is adequate. Occasionally, surgery during pregnancy is indicated for torsion of an isolated, pedunculated leiomyoma. With the exception of a pedunculated leiomyoma on a narrow stalk, myomectomy should not be performed during pregnancy because of the risk of uncontrollable hemorrhage.

Qidwai GI, Caughey AB, Jacoby AF. Obstetric outcomes in women with sonographically identified uterine leiomyomata. *Obstet Gynecol* 2006;107:376–382. PMID: 16449127.

Vergani P, Locatelli A, Ghidini A, et al. Large uterine leiomyomata and risk of cesarean delivery. *Obstet Gynecol* 2007;109:410–414. PMID: 17267843.

CANCER IN PREGNANCY

The incidence of cancer in pregnancy is approximately 1 in 1000. The most common malignancies diagnosed during pregnancy are cervical cancer (26%; see also Chapter 48, Premalignant and Malignant Disorders of the Uterine Cervix), breast cancer (26%), leukemias (15%), lymphomas (10%; see also Chapter 34, Hematologic Disorders in Pregnancy), and malignant melanomas (8%). Once cancer is diagnosed during pregnancy, a multidisciplinary team of maternal–fetal medicine specialists, oncologists, surgeons, and radiation oncologists can assist the patient in making difficult decisions regarding treatment timing and continued pregnancy.

CERVICAL CANCER

(See also Chapter 48, Premalignant and Malignant Disorders of the Uterine Cervix.)

ESSENTIALS OF DIAGNOSIS

- The diagnosis of cervical cancer during pregnancy is usually made on the basis of cervical biopsy after abnormal pap smear or detection of cervical mass.
- Pregnancy should not limit evaluation of abnormal cervical cytology or evaluation of a cervical mass.

Pathogenesis

Invasive cervical cancer complicates approximately 0.05% of pregnancies. Diagnosis during pregnancy occurs more frequently in areas in which routine prenatal cytologic examination is done. Significantly abnormal cervical cytology in pregnancy calls for colposcopic evaluation.

Clinical Findings

As is the case with nonpregnant patients, cervical cancer in pregnancy primarily presents with bleeding, but the diagnosis is frequently missed because the bleeding is assumed to be pregnancy-related rather than due to cancer. The possibility of cancer must be kept in mind, and if a cervical lesion or mass is seen during prenatal care, it must be biopsied.

Treatment

The diagnosis and management of invasive cervical cancer during pregnancy presents the patient and the physician with many challenges. Management is determined by the stage of the cancer, the gestational age, and the patient's desires regarding the pregnancy. Pregnancy does not appear to affect the prognosis for women with cervical cancer and the fetus is not affected by the maternal disease, but may suffer morbidity from its treatment (eg, preterm delivery).

If the pregnancy is early and the disease is stage I–IIA, radical hysterectomy and therapeutic lymphadenectomy can be performed with the fetus left in situ, unless the patient is unwilling to terminate the pregnancy. Women at a gestational age closer to fetal viability or who decline termination may decide to continue the pregnancy after careful discussion regarding the maternal risks. Delivery in patients with cervical dysplasia and carcinoma in situ may be via the vaginal route. Patients with invasive cervical cancer should be delivered by caesarean section to avoid potential cervical hemorrhage and dissemination of tumor cells during vaginal delivery. A caesarean radical hysterectomy with therapeutic lymphadenectomy is the procedure of choice for patients with stage IA2–IIA2 disease once fetal maturity is established. As in the nonpregnant patient, radiation with concomitant chemotherapy is used for the treatment of more advanced disease. In the first trimester, irradiation may be carried out with the expectation of spontaneous abortion. In the second trimester, interruption of the pregnancy by hysterotomy before radiation therapy should be considered, although some experts advocate proceeding with immediate radiation treatment, again awaiting spontaneous evacuation of the uterus. In selected cases with locally advanced disease in which the patient declines pregnancy termination, consideration may be given to neoadjuvant chemotherapy in an effort to prevent disease progression during the time needed to achieve fetal maturity. Delivery should be by caesarean section. A lymphadenectomy can be performed at the same time. Postpartum the patient should receive chemoradiation following guidelines established for the nonpregnant patient.

BREAST CANCER

ESSENTIALS OF DIAGNOSIS

- Women with breast cancer during pregnancy usually present with a breast mass or thickening.
- The diagnosis is confirmed with biopsy.
- Pregnancy should not limit a thorough evaluation of a breast mass.

Breast cancer is the most common cancer diagnosed in women in the United States. One of every 5 cases occurs in women younger than 45 years, and 2–5% of women with breast cancer are pregnant when the diagnosis is made. In the United States, the incidence of breast cancer in pregnancy is 3 per 10,000 live births. For this reason, careful breast examination should be performed during prenatal and postnatal care, and a family history should be obtained.

Clinical Findings

Pregnancy- and lactation-related changes in the breast increase the frequency and range of breast problems and make the diagnosis of breast cancer more difficult. A painless lump is the most common presentation of gestational breast cancer. Bloody nipple discharge may be a presenting symptom and requires workup. Any mass found by the patient or by the obstetrician should be fully evaluated without undue delay.

Differential Diagnosis

The differential diagnosis is broad and includes lactating adenoma, galactocele, milk-filled cyst, fibroadenoma, abscess, and cancer.

Complications

Management of the pregnant woman with breast carcinoma is difficult because it requires careful consideration of both mother and fetus. The general approach to treatment of breast cancer in pregnancy should be similar to that in nonpregnant patients and should not be delayed because of pregnancy.

Treatment

Initial management of the pregnant patient with a breast mass does not differ significantly from that for nonpregnant women. When a localized lesion is present, breast ultrasonography is the preferred first imaging modality during pregnancy. It is safe and helpful in distinguishing between cystic and solid masses. Although the sensitivity of mammography is diminished by the breast changes in pregnancy, the study still may be helpful for selected patients with inconclusive ultrasound examinations. With low-dose mammography and appropriate shielding, fetal radiation exposure is minimal. Nonetheless, it is generally recommended that the procedure be avoided during the first trimester. Gadolinium-enhanced breast MRI is an imaging technique that may be indicated in selected patients, although there is a paucity of data on MRI features of pregnancy-associated breast cancer. Cystic lesions should be aspirated and the fluid, if bloody, examined cytologically. Malignant cells are rarely found in nonbloody fluid. Fine-needle aspiration, core biopsy, or incisional biopsy can be used in some cases, but surgical excisional biopsy may be most appropriate for clinically suspicious or cytologically equivocal lesions. The increased vascularity of the breasts is associated with a higher rate of bleeding, and the lactating breast is prone to infectious complications, but neither pregnancy nor lactation appears to interfere with excisional biopsy in an outpatient setting.

Breast cancer is classified according to the tumor-node metastasis (TNM) staging system. If a pregnant woman has clinically positive nodes or suspicious symptoms, she should undergo radiographic staging of lung, liver, and bone; asymptomatic women with clinically node-negative early-stage breast cancer do not. This can be done with plain films with abdominal shielding, abdominal ultrasound, MRI, and radionuclide bone scans, which are thought to be safe in pregnancy.

Termination of pregnancy has not been shown to improve survival rates. Modified radical mastectomy is the preferred local management of pregnant patients with breast cancer, with the goal of avoiding the need for adjuvant radiation therapy. Radical mastectomy is well tolerated during pregnancy. Breast-conserving surgery, which must be combined with adjuvant radiation, is limited primarily to patients presenting in the late second and third trimester, for whom surgery is performed during pregnancy and radiation treatment postponed until after delivery. For a patient who desires breast-conserving surgery outside the third trimester, a detailed discussion is imperative. For management of the lymph nodes, axillary dissection has been the traditional treatment of choice. Sentinel lymph node biopsy can be safely performed during pregnancy using colloid, but outcomes data are limited.

Adjuvant chemotherapy is frequently recommended for premenopausal women with breast cancer. The recommendation of chemotherapy for a pregnant woman with breast cancer is a complex decision, but the indications for adjuvant chemotherapy for gestational breast cancer are generally the same as for the nonpregnant patient. Chemotherapy during the first trimester is contraindicated as it is associated with miscarriage and major malformations. The chemotherapeutic agents used in gestational breast cancer are generally the same as those used in nonpregnant patients; cyclophosphamide, doxorubicin, and fluorouracil have been given successfully during the second and third trimesters, with no measurable increase in congenital malformations but an increased incidence of prematurity and intrauterine growth restriction. Neoadjuvant chemotherapy may be a treatment option in select patients with locally advanced or metastatic gestational breast cancer. Chemotherapy should be stopped after 35 weeks to decrease the risk of neonatal neutropenia. Use of radiation and endocrine therapy should be avoided during pregnancy. Breastfeeding should be avoided during chemotherapy, hormone therapy, or radiation. There is no contraindication to breastfeeding after completion of therapy for breast cancer.

The results of treatment are much the same stage for stage as they are in nonpregnant patients, but pregnancy-associated breast cancers tend to be more advanced at diagnosis (larger tumor size, more frequently involved lymph nodes), resulting in an overall worse prognosis for this group of patients as a whole. Diagnostic delay is blamed for more advanced disease at diagnosis.

Prognosis

Subsequent pregnancies need not necessarily be discouraged after a suitable period of recuperation and observation, as subsequent pregnancy does not increase the risk of recurrence or death from breast cancer. For women who are breast cancer antigen (BRCA)-1 or BRCA-2 mutation carriers, there is no evidence that pregnancy decreases their breast cancer risk. With respect to fetal outcomes, there appears to be an increase in preterm birth among women receiving chemotherapy during pregnancy. There are no reported cases of metastatic disease to the fetus.

Amant F, Deckers S, Van Calsteren K, et al. Breast cancer in pregnancy: Recommendations of an international consensus meeting. *Eur J Cancer* 2010;46:3158–3168. PMID: 20932740.

Azim HA Jr, Pavldis N, Peccatori F. Treatment of the pregnant mother with cancer: A systematic review on the use of cytotoxic, endocrine, targeted agents and immunotherapy during pregnancy. Part II: Hematological tumors. *Cancer Treat Rev* 2010;36:110–121. PMID: 20018452.

Loibl S, Von Minckwitz G, Gwyn K, et al. Breast carcinoma during pregnancy: International recommendations from an expert meeting. *Cancer* 2006;106:237–246. PMID: 16342247.

Pereg D, Koren G, Lischner M. Cancer in pregnancy: Gaps, challenges and solutions. *Cancer Treat Rev* 2008;34:302–312. PMID: 18291591.

O'Meara AT, Cress R, Xing G, et al. Malignant melanoma in pregnancy: A population-based evaluation. *Cancer* 2005;103: 1217–1226. PMID: 15712209.

LYMPHOMAS AND LEUKEMIAS

(See also Chapter 34, Hematologic Disorders in Pregnancy.)

ESSENTIALS OF DIAGNOSIS

- Most women diagnosed with Hodgkin's lymphoma during pregnancy present with painless lymphadenopathy.
- Biopsy is necessary to make a diagnosis of Hodgkin's lymphoma.
- Patients with leukemia may experience symptoms related to pancytopenia.
- Leukemia may be suspected on the basis of circulating blasts on peripheral blood smear.
- The diagnosis of leukemia is made on the basis of bone marrow biopsy.

Clinical Findings

The incidence of Hodgkin's lymphoma in pregnancy is estimated to be 1 in 1000 to 1 in 6000 pregnancies, with non-Hodgkin's lymphomas being significantly less frequent.

The typical presentation is painless adenopathy, and adequate biopsy is essential for diagnosis. Hodgkin's lymphoma is curable even in advanced stages, and prognosis and stage distribution in pregnancy is comparable to those in the nonpregnant patient.

The incidence of leukemia in pregnancy is estimated at 1 in 100,000. The acute leukemias are more frequent. The diagnosis is made by examination of bone marrow samples, which can be safely performed during pregnancy. Acute leukemia places pregnant patients at very high risk for bleeding and infection complications.

Treatment

Approximately 70% of patients present with early-stage disease and can be treated with either single-agent chemotherapy or, in selected cases, modified supradiaphragmatic radiation.

Patients in early pregnancy presenting with extensive infradiaphragmatic disease, for which radiation therapy would be a significant component of curative therapy, should consider termination of pregnancy because of the associated significant teratogenic risks. Standard chemotherapy regimens appear moderately safe to use in the second and third trimester.

Treatment of acute leukemia should be started immediately after diagnosis for an attempt at cure. Depending on the gestational age, the management during pregnancy poses many challenges to the patient, her family, and the treating physicians. Chronic myelogenous leukemia can be treated with interferon throughout pregnancy. There are rare reports of lymphoma and leukemia metastases to the fetus.

MALIGNANT MELANOMA

ESSENTIALS OF DIAGNOSIS

- Patients with melanoma usually present with a suspicious skin lesion.
- The diagnosis is made by biopsy or excision of the lesion.

Approximately 30–35% of women diagnosed with melanoma are of childbearing age, and approximately 0.1–1% of female melanoma patients are pregnant.

Clinical Findings

Most present with stage I disease. Clinical signs of melanoma are the same in pregnant and nonpregnant women. Suspicious lesions are those that have changed in size, color, or shape; bleed; or are ulcerated. The diagnosis is made by excision, allowing for microstaging. Tumor thickness, tumor site, and presence of metastases are the most important prognostic factors.

Treatment/Prognosis

There has been long-standing controversy regarding the prognosis of pregnancy-associated melanoma, but more recent evidence suggests that patients with early primary lesions and wide surgical excision with appropriate margins have a prognosis comparable to that of their nonpregnant counterparts. Moreover, pregnancy termination has not been shown to improve survival. Data on higher stage melanoma diagnosed in pregnancy are limited. Malignant melanoma is the tumor that most frequently metastasizes to the placenta or fetus, accounting for more than half of all tumors with fetal involvement. Postpartum the placenta should be sent for pathologic evaluation.

CARDIAC DISEASE

ESSENTIALS OF DIAGNOSIS

- Cardiac disease complicates 1–4% of all pregnancies in the United States.
- Rheumatic and congenital heart disease constitute the majority of cases.

Treatment

Patients requiring cardiac surgery should undergo the procedure before becoming pregnant. Nevertheless, the rare patient will require cardiac surgery during pregnancy. Most available reports on cardiac surgery during pregnancy involve closed and open mitral valvuloplasties and mitral or aortic valve replacement.

Cardiac surgery can be performed with good results in pregnancy, although there is maternal and fetal risk. Operations should generally be performed early in the second trimester when organogenesis is complete and there is comparatively less hemodynamic burden and less risk of preterm labor than later in gestation.

Prognosis

Maternal mortality rates average 1–9%, related to the specific procedure performed and the patient's preoperative cardiovascular status. Percutaneous balloon valvuloplasty should be considered the preferred technique to treat valvular disease during pregnancy. Perinatal mortality is expected in 2–10% of percutaneous balloon valvuloplasties. Perinatal loss is thought to be greater after open valvular or bypass surgery due largely to the nonpulsatile blood flow and hypotension associated with cardiopulmonary bypass. Close fetal surveillance by electronic heart rate and uterine contraction monitoring is essential during any cardiac surgical procedure, whether or not cardiopulmonary bypass is used. During bypass, blood flow to the uterus can be assessed indirectly by changes in the fetal heart rate, and alterations in flow can be made accordingly.

Weiss BM. Managing severe mitral valve stenosis in pregnant patients—Percutaneous balloon valvuloplasty, not surgery, is the treatment of choice. *J Cardiothorac Vasc Anesth* 2005;19:277–278. PMID: 15868549.

NEUROLOGIC DISEASE

(See also Chapter 33, Nervous System and Autoimmune Disorders in Pregnancy.)

ESSENTIALS OF DIAGNOSIS

- The most common neurosurgical emergency to complicate pregnancy is intracranial hemorrhage.
- Symptoms and signs of subarachnoid hemorrhage include headache, nausea and vomiting, stiff neck, photophobia, seizures, and a decreasing level of consciousness.

Pathogenesis

Intracranial hemorrhage during pregnancy is rare (1–5 per 10,000 pregnancies) but is associated with significant maternal and fetal mortality and serious neurologic morbidity in survivors. Cerebral aneurysm rupture is responsible for approximately 70% of intracranial hemorrhage; arteriovenous malformations (AVM) cause 25%, and the remaining cases are due to eclampsia, coagulopathy, trauma, and intracranial tumors. During pregnancy the risk of bleeding from an AVM that had not bled previously is 3.5%, which is close to the annual bleeding rate in the nonpregnant patient. However, mortality due to a bleeding AVM in pregnancy is higher (30%) than in the nonpregnant state (10%). The risk of rebleeding from an AVM in the same pregnancy is 27%. Intracranial hemorrhage with associated neurologic damage during pregnancy (limited capacity for decision making, persistent vegetative state, brain death) poses significant medical and ethical challenges in caring for the mother and fetus.

Most commonly, bleeding from an aneurysm occurs in the subarachnoid space, whereas bleeding from an AVM is located within the brain parenchyma.

Clinical Findings

Symptoms and signs of subarachnoid hemorrhage include headache, nausea and vomiting, stiff neck, photophobia, seizures, and a decreasing level of consciousness. The headache usually is very sudden in onset, whereas the headache associated with intraparenchymal bleeding usually is somewhat less severe and is slower in onset. Focal neurologic deficits may be absent in up to 40% of patients. CT or MRI confirm the diagnosis of an intracranial bleed. Cerebral angiography may be needed to identify and characterize an aneurysm or AVM.

Treatment

Early surgical or endovascular intervention after aneurysmal hemorrhage during pregnancy is associated with reduced maternal and fetal mortality. Neurosurgical centers with significant experience in cerebral aneurysm procedures have better outcomes than lower volume centers. For patients with AVM, the decision to treat the lesion during pregnancy is less clear but should follow the same guidelines that apply to nonpregnant patients.

Prognosis

Once the intracranial hemorrhage has been effectively treated, vaginal delivery can proceed according to obstetric indications. For women who have not received definitive treatment, delivery route is controversial. Maternal and fetal mortality appear the same with elective caesarean delivery or instrumental vaginal delivery under regional anesthesia. Aneurysm rupture has been reported during elective caesarean delivery, which is not considered protective. Regardless of delivery route, blood pressure control is imperative.

Qaiser R, Black P. Neurosurgery in pregnancy. *Semin Neurol* 2007; 27:476–481. PMID: 17940927.

TRAUMA

ESSENTIALS OF DIAGNOSIS

- Automobile accidents are the most common nonobstetric cause of death during pregnancy.
- The most common cause of fetal death is death of the mother.
- Initial treatment focuses on immediate stabilization of the mother followed by evaluation of the fetus.

Pathogenesis

Approximately 7% of pregnancies are complicated by trauma, such as motor vehicle accidents (40%), falls (30%), direct assaults to the maternal abdomen (20%), and other causes (10%). Automobile accidents are the most common nonobstetric cause of death during pregnancy. The most common cause of fetal death is death of the mother. The second most common cause of fetal death is placental abruption. Pregnant women with traumatic injuries may be victims of physical abuse. Suicide also contributes to injury-related death. A pregnancy may increase family stress; therefore, the practitioner should be alert for signs of abuse and/or depression.

Treatment

The primary initial goal in treating a pregnant trauma victim is to stabilize the mother's condition. Rapid hemorrhage can occur because approximately 600 mL of blood flow is directed to the uterus each minute. To optimize maternal and fetal outcome, an organized team approach to the pregnant trauma patient is essential. Maternal assessment and management are similar to those for the nonpregnant patient, keeping in mind the goal of protecting the fetus from unnecessary drug and radiation exposure. The fetus should be evaluated early during trauma assessment, and after fetal viability is reached, continuous fetal heart rate and uterine activity monitoring should be instituted, as long as it does not interfere with maternal resuscitative efforts. This information becomes critical when making management decisions for mother and fetus. Emergent caesarean section should be initiated if cardiopulmonary resuscitation has been unsuccessful after 4 minutes; this may provide the fetus with a greater chance for intact survival and allow for a successful maternal resuscitation. Caesarean delivery is also indicated if there is a nonreassuring fetal heart rate tracing in the setting of a stable mother, or if the enlarged uterus does not allow for repair of maternal injuries.

After immediate stabilization, the fetal heart rate and uterine contractions should be monitored for posttraumatic placental abruption. This usually occurs quite soon after the injury but rarely manifests as late as 5 days after trauma. Monitoring should continue for at least 4 hours after the trauma unless suspicious findings, including uterine contractions, vaginal bleeding, abdominal or uterine tenderness, postural hypotension, and fetal heart rate abnormalities, are noted. If any of these signs occur or if the trauma was severe, monitoring should be extended to 24–48 hours. Nonreassuring fetal heart rate patterns and fetal death can occur despite mild maternal trauma or pain. Ultrasound is helpful if abruption is visualized, but many are not. There is little evidence that the Kleihauer-Betke test reliably predicts significant fetomaternal hemorrhage, but it is recommended to determine if additional doses of Rh_o (D) immunoglobulin are needed for Rh-negative patients. Routine coagulation profiles are not clinically helpful in the setting of a stable mother.

Brown HL. Trauma in pregnancy. *Obstet Gynecol* 2009;114: 147–160. PMID: 19546773.

Katz V, Balderston K, Defreest M. Perimortem cesarean delivery: Were our assumptions correct? *Am J Obstet Gynecol* 2005;192:1916–1920. PMID: 15970850.

Muench MV, Canterino JC. Trauma in pregnancy. *Obstet Gynecol Clin North Am* 2007;34:555–583. PMID: 17921015.

26 Hypertension in Pregnancy

David A. Miller, MD

Hypertension is a common medical disorder that affects 20–30% of adults in the United States and complicates as many as 5–8% of all pregnancies. Hypertensive disorders of pregnancy rank among the leading causes of maternal morbidity and mortality. Approximately 15% of maternal deaths are attributable to hypertension, making it the second leading cause of maternal mortality in the United States. Severe hypertension increases the mother's risk of heart attack, cardiac failure, cerebral vascular accidents, and renal failure. The fetus and neonate also are at increased risk from complications such as poor placental transfer of oxygen, fetal growth restriction, preterm birth, placental abruption, stillbirth, and neonatal death.

Hypertension is defined as a sustained blood pressure higher than 140/90 mm Hg. In the nonpregnant patient, essential hypertension accounts for more than 90% of cases; however, many other conditions must be considered (Table 26–1). In the pregnant patient, hypertension may be attributable to any of the conditions summarized in Table 26–1. In addition, unique forms of hypertension, gestational hypertension and preeclampsia, occur only during pregnancy. Gestational hypertension is characterized by elevated blood pressure diagnosed for the first time during pregnancy in patients without evidence of proteinuria. Preeclampsia is characterized by the onset of hypertension and proteinuria, usually during the third trimester of pregnancy. The National High Blood Pressure Education Program Working Group stated that edema occurs too frequently in normal pregnant women to be a useful marker in the diagnosis of preeclampsia. Therefore, edema is no longer recommended as a diagnostic criterion for preeclampsia. Management of preeclampsia differs from the management of other forms of hypertension during pregnancy. Therefore, it is important to distinguish preeclampsia from other forms of hypertension that may complicate pregnancy.

Classification of hypertension during pregnancy can be viewed as a continuum. On one end of the spectrum is the patient with hypertension that was present before pregnancy (or was recognized during the first half of pregnancy), does not worsen appreciably during pregnancy, and persists after delivery. This condition would be classified as chronic hypertension. On the other end of the spectrum is the patient with no evidence of chronic hypertension who experiences the abrupt onset of hypertension and proteinuria late in pregnancy followed by complete resolution postpartum. In this case, the hypertension observed during pregnancy may be the result of factors related entirely to pregnancy and not to an underlying medical cause. This condition would be classified as preeclampsia. Between these 2 extremes are gestational hypertension and cases in which varying degrees of preeclampsia are superimposed upon varying degrees of chronic hypertension. These broad categories have some value in estimating risk. Isolated mild to moderate chronic hypertension may have little effect on pregnancy outcome. On the other hand, severe hypertension of any cause may increase the risk to mother and fetus. The highest risks are associated with preeclampsia or eclampsia. The classification system of hypertension in pregnancy proposed by the National High Blood Pressure Education Program Working Group is summarized in Table 26–2.

CHRONIC HYPERTENSION

ESSENTIALS OF DIAGNOSIS

- Hypertension with onset before pregnancy or before 20th week of gestation
- Persistence of hypertension beyond 12 weeks postpartum
- Blood pressure ≥140 mm Hg systolic or ≥90 mm Hg diastolic

Table 26–1. Causes of chronic hypertension.

Idiopathic Essential hypertension
Vascular disorders Renovascular hypertension Aortic coarctation
Endocrine disorders Diabetes mellitus Hyperthyroidism Pheochromocytoma Primary hyperaldosteronism Hyperparathyroidism Cushing's syndrome
Renal disorders Diabetic nephropathy Chronic renal failure Acute renal failure Tubular necrosis Cortical necrosis Pyelonephritis Chronic glomerulonephritis Nephrotic syndrome Polycystic kidney
Connective tissue disorders Systemic lupus erythematosus

Pathogenesis

Chronic hypertension complicates as many as 5% of pregnancies. It is characterized by a history of high blood pressure before pregnancy, elevation of blood pressure during the first half of pregnancy, or high blood pressure that lasts for longer than 12 weeks after delivery. The pathogenesis of chronic hypertension or essential hypertension is poorly understood. Factors that may contribute to the development of chronic hypertension are derangements in sympathetic neural activity or angiotensin II activity. There appears to be a genetic component in that hypertension is more common in individuals with a family history of hypertension. Other risk factors that predispose one to develop chronic hypertension during a person's lifetime are African American race, obesity, dyslipidemia, and physical inactivity.

Clinical Findings

Chronic hypertension is defined as women who have a blood pressure of ≥140 mmHg systolic or ≥90 mmHg diastolic before pregnancy, during the first 20 weeks of pregnancy, or >12 weeks after pregnancy. During the first trimester of pregnancy, women with a history of chronic hypertension will likely manifest blood pressure elevations. However, during normal pregnancy, maternal blood volume increases by 40–60%. Cardiac output and renal blood flow increase significantly. Blood pressure normally decreases throughout the first half of pregnancy under the influence of progesterone, reaching a nadir in midpregnancy and returning to prepregnancy levels by the end of the third trimester. For this reason, blood pressure may normalize during the second trimester in women with underlying chronic hypertension.

Evaluation of the patient with chronic hypertension is directed at end organs and systems most likely to be

Table 26–2. Classification of hypertension in pregnancy.

Definition of hypertension	
Mild:	Systolic blood pressure ≥140 mm Hg or Diastolic blood pressure ≥90 mm Hg
Severe:	Systolic blood pressure ≥160 mm Hg or Diastolic blood pressure ≥110 mm Hg
Chronic hypertension	
Hypertension with onset before pregnancy or before 20th week of gestation Use of antihypertensive medications before pregnancy Persistence of hypertension beyond 12 weeks postpartum	
Preeclampsia	
Hypertension that occurs after 20 weeks of gestation in a woman with previously normal blood pressure. Systolic blood pressure ≥140 mm Hg or diastolic blood pressure ≥90 mm Hg on 2 occasions at least 6 hours apart. Proteinuria, defined as urinary excretion of ≥0.3 g protein in a 24-hour urine specimen. This finding usually correlates with a finding of 1+ or greater on dipstick. Note edema is no longer a diagnostic criterion. Note a systolic rise of 30 mm Hg or a diastolic rise of 15 mm Hg is no longer a diagnostic criterion.	
Eclampsia	
New-onset grand mal seizures in a woman with preeclampsia that cannot be attributed to other causes	
Superimposed preeclampsia–eclampsia	
Preeclampsia or eclampsia that occurs in a woman with a preexisting chronic hypertension	
Gestational hypertension	
Hypertension detected for the first time after midpregnancy Distinguished from preeclampsia by the absence of proteinuria Working diagnosis only during pregnancy	
Transient hypertension of pregnancy	
Gestational hypertension that resolves by 12 weeks postpartum. If proteinuria develops in a patient with gestational hypertension, the diagnosis is preeclampsia. If gestational hypertension does not resolve by 12 weeks postpartum, the diagnosis is chronic hypertension.	

affected by hypertension, including the eyes, heart, kidneys, uteroplacental circulation, and the fetus. Laboratory tests include a complete blood count, glucose screen, electrolyte panel, serum creatinine, urinalysis, and urine culture. In some cases, additional tests may be needed. In patients with possible renal disease (serum creatinine ≥0.8 mg/dL, urine protein >1+ on dipstick), a 24-hour urine collection for creatinine clearance and total protein will provide baseline information that may be helpful in diagnosing the onset of preeclampsia later in pregnancy. An electrocardiogram may reveal left ventricular hypertrophy in the patient with long-standing hypertension. Chest radiography with abdominal shielding or echocardiogram may reveal cardiomegaly.

Differential Diagnosis

In women with hypertension, underlying disorders must be excluded (Table 26–1). The search for an underlying cause should include a complete history and physical examination, taking into account the normal changes that accompany pregnancy. Blood pressure should be measured in both arms with the patient in a sitting position and the arm at the level of the heart, and multiple measurements should be obtained on different occasions. If possible, measurements should be obtained outside of the office setting. The fifth Korotkoff sound should be used to determine diastolic pressure. Auscultation of the flanks may reveal a renal artery bruit. Funduscopic examination may reveal typical findings associated with long-standing hypertension or possibly diabetes. An enlarged thyroid gland may indicate thyroid disease. Absent peripheral pulses suggest coarctation of the aorta. Heart, skin, and joints should be evaluated thoroughly. Antinuclear antibody may help suggest a diagnosis of collagen vascular disease. A suppressed thyroid-stimulating hormone level suggests hyperthyroidism. Rarely, elevated urinary catecholamine levels may point to pheochromocytoma.

Complications

Complications related to chronic hypertension include superimposed preeclampsia, fetal growth restriction, preterm birth, and placental abruption. The risk of developing one of these complications correlates with the degree of maternal blood pressure elevation; the higher the blood pressure, the greater the risk of one of these complications. Unfortunately, the benefit of maternal blood pressure control appears to be limited to preventing maternal morbidities and does not appear to extend to reducing the risk of these obstetric complications.

Treatment

Management of the chronic hypertensive patient during pregnancy is targeted to 2 goals: (1) maternal blood pressure control to minimize the risk of maternal complications related to blood pressure elevations such as stroke and myocardial infarction, and (2) early detection of any obstetrical or fetal complications related to chronic hypertension.

A number of antihypertensives have been shown to be safe and effective during pregnancy in controlling maternal blood pressure. Treatment of elevated blood pressure with antihypertensives reduces the risk of maternal morbidities related to hypertension but does not reduce the risk of fetal complications such as intrauterine growth restriction, preeclampsia, and placental abruption.

A. Treatment of Mild Chronic Hypertension

In pregnant women with mild hypertension and no evidence of renal disease, serious medical complications are rare. Moreover, there is no consensus that antihypertensive medication can reduce the risk of fetal death, growth restriction, placental abruption, preeclampsia, or eclampsia in these women. Therefore, antihypertensive medication is not usually necessary. Avoidance of alcohol and tobacco is encouraged. Sodium restriction may be considered (2–3 g/d). Rigorous activity should be avoided, as should weight reduction. Despite the lack of evidence supporting the benefit of antihypertensive therapy in women with blood pressure <180/110 mm Hg, many clinicians are reluctant to withhold medication when the blood pressure remains ≥150/100 mm Hg despite lifestyle modifications. A practical management algorithm using a blood pressure of 150/100 mm Hg as the threshold for initiation of antihypertensive therapy in women without evidence of end-organ involvement and 140/90 mm Hg as the threshold in women with evidence of renal involvement is summarized in Figure 26–1. Prenatal visits are scheduled every 2–4 weeks until 34–36 weeks and weekly thereafter. At each visit, blood pressure, urine protein, and fundal height are evaluated. Patients are questioned regarding signs and symptoms of preeclampsia, including headache, abdominal pain, blurred vision, scotomata, rapid weight gain, or marked swelling of the hands and/or face. Antepartum fetal monitoring usually is started around 32–34 weeks, and, in most cases, delivery is accomplished by 39–40 weeks' gestation.

B. Treatment of Severe Chronic Hypertension

Women with sustained blood pressure ≥180/110 mm Hg or those with evidence of renal disease may be at higher risk for serious complications, such as heart attack, stroke, or progression of renal disease, and are candidates for antihypertensive medication. As summarized in Figure 26–1, many clinicians would use a lower threshold of 150/100 mm Hg for instituting antihypertensive therapy during pregnancy.

Frequent prenatal visits may be needed to check the effectiveness of the medication. Fetal growth, blood pressure, and proteinuria are assessed at each visit, and evidence

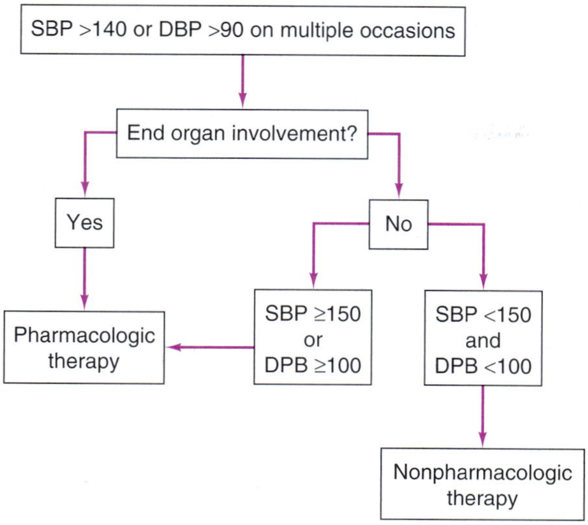

▲ **Figure 26–1.** Management algorithm for chronic hypertension in pregnancy. DBP, diastolic blood pressure; SBP, systolic blood pressure.

of superimposed preeclampsia is aggressively sought. Management of preeclampsia is described later in this chapter. In women with evidence of renal disease, some clinicians measure creatinine clearance and 24-hour urinary protein excretion each trimester. Sonographic assessment of fetal growth is performed every 2–4 weeks, antepartum testing is initiated by 32–34 weeks, and delivery is accomplished after 38 weeks or when fetal lung maturity is demonstrated. In some cases, hypertension worsens significantly during pregnancy without the development of overt preeclampsia. If exacerbation of chronic hypertension necessitates preterm delivery, corticosteroids should be considered in attempt to accelerate fetal maturity.

C. Antihypertensive Therapy in Chronic Hypertension

Several choices for initial antihypertensive therapy during pregnancy are available. Methyldopa has been studied extensively and is recommended by many as the first-line antihypertensive agent in pregnancy. It is a centrally acting alpha-adrenergic agonist that appears to inhibit vasoconstricting impulses from the medullary vasoregulatory center. The total daily dosage of 500 mg to 2 g is administered in 2–4 divided doses. Peak plasma levels occur 2–3 hours after administration, and the maximum effect occurs 4–6 hours after an oral dose. The agent is excreted primarily by the kidney. Sedation and postural hypotension are the most common side effects. A positive direct Coombs' test may be seen, usually after 6–12 months of therapy. Hemolytic anemia may occur in these patients and is an indication to stop the medication. Fever, liver function abnormalities, granulocytopenia, and thrombocytopenia are rare side effects.

Labetalol is an alpha$_1$-adrenergic blocker and a nonselective beta-adrenergic blocker. The beta-blockade/alpha-blockade ratio is 7:1. A large body of clinical evidence suggests that use of labetalol is safe during pregnancy. It appears to lack teratogenicity and crosses the placenta in small amounts. One randomized study showed no advantages of labetalol over methyldopa. Another study reported a higher incidence of small for gestational age newborns in patients treated with labetalol. The usual starting dose is 100 mg twice per day (BID), and the dose can be increased weekly to a maximum of 2400 mg daily. Titration increments should not exceed 200 mg BID.

Nifedipine is a calcium channel blocker that has been used during pregnancy for tocolysis and treatment of hypertension. Several reports suggest that nifedipine use is safe during pregnancy; however, the cumulative experience with this agent is not as extensive as with methyldopa and labetalol. When nifedipine is used for treatment of chronic hypertension during pregnancy, the long-acting formulation (Procardia XL, Adalat CC) may improve patient compliance. The principal benefit of this agent is once-daily dosing. The usual starting dose is 30 mg daily. If necessary, the dose may be increased to 60–90 mg daily. The neuromuscular-blocking action of magnesium may be potentiated by simultaneous calcium channel blockade; therefore, nifedipine should be used with caution in patients receiving magnesium sulfate. The sublingual route of administration is associated with unpredictable blood levels and should be avoided.

Other antihypertensive medications used in pregnancy include atenolol, metoprolol, prazosin, minoxidil, hydralazine, thiazide diuretics, and clonidine. Published experience with these agents is limited, and they should not supplant methyldopa, labetalol, or nifedipine as first-line agents in pregnancy.

Use of angiotensin-converting enzyme inhibitors (enalapril, captopril) during pregnancy is associated with fetal hypocalvaria, renal defects, anuria, and fetal and neonatal death. These agents are contraindicated in pregnancy. With few exceptions, diuretics (furosemide, hydrochlorothiazide) should be avoided during pregnancy. Fetal bradycardia, growth retardation, and neonatal hypoglycemia have been reported in patients treated with blockers.

D. Fetal Assessment in Chronic Hypertension

Pregnancies complicated by chronic hypertension, regardless of the cause, are at increased risk for poor fetal growth. An initial ultrasound examination should be performed as early as possible to confirm the due date and to ensure that no obvious fetal anomalies are present. Thereafter, fetal growth may be assessed by ultrasound as needed, usually no more frequently than every 2–4 weeks. Antepartum fetal monitoring usually is started by 32–34 weeks. If the nonstress test is used as the method of surveillance, it should be accompanied by assessment of amniotic fluid volume. Doppler velocimetry of the umbilical, uterine, and middle cerebral arteries are helpful in optimizing the timing of delivery, particularly in cases of suspected fetal growth restriction.

Prognosis

Pregnancy outcome usually is good in patients with mild chronic hypertension and no other serious medical conditions. Fetal growth restriction, superimposed preeclampsia, placental abruption, and preterm delivery are the most common complications. The outlook is less favorable in women with severe hypertension early in pregnancy and in those with evidence of end-organ compromise, such as renal insufficiency and/or cardiovascular disease. By necessity, management is individualized. Close monitoring for development of fetal growth restriction and superimposed preeclampsia is indicated.

American College of Obstetricians and Gynecologists. Chronic hypertension in pregnancy. ACOG Practice Bulletin No. 29. *Obstet Gynecol* 2001;98:177. PMID 11508256.

Report of the National High Blood Pressure Education Program Working Group on high blood pressure in pregnancy. *Am J Obstet Gynecol* 2000;183:S1. PMID 10920346.

GESTATIONAL HYPERTENSION

ESSENTIALS OF DIAGNOSIS

- Maternal blood pressure elevation of ≥140 mm Hg systolic or ≥90 mm Hg diastolic on 2 occasions 6 hours apart in a previously normotensive woman ≥20 weeks' gestation
- No evidence of proteinuria

Pathogenesis

Gestational hypertension appears to affect approximately 6% of pregnancies. The pathogenesis of gestational hypertension is unclear, and it is equally unclear whether gestational hypertension represents an early stage of preeclampsia or whether it is an entirely separate disease entity. Gestational hypertension is considered to be a provisional diagnosis as many women with gestational hypertension will go on to be diagnosed with either preeclampsia or chronic hypertension. If preeclampsia has not developed and the maternal blood pressure has returned to normal by 12 weeks postpartum, then a diagnosis of transient hypertension of pregnancy is made.

Clinical Findings

A diagnosis of gestational hypertension is made when (1) maternal blood pressure is elevated to ≥140 mm Hg systolic or ≥90 mm Hg diastolic on 2 occasions 6 hours apart in a previously normotensive woman ≥20 weeks' gestation, and (2) there is no evidence of proteinuria. Gestational hypertension is classified as mild or severe based on the degree of blood pressure elevation. It is considered to be severe when the systolic blood pressure is persistently ≥160 mm Hg or the diastolic blood pressure is persistently ≥110 mm Hg.

Complications

Approximately 15–25% of women diagnosed with gestational hypertension go on to develop preeclampsia. Women with mild gestational hypertension do not appear to be at increased risk of preterm birth, intrauterine growth restriction, abruption, or stillbirth. Women with severe gestational hypertension, however, are at increased risk of adverse outcomes, including preterm birth, intrauterine growth restriction, and placental abruption.

Treatment

Given the 15–25% risk of progression to preeclampsia, treatment includes close surveillance for signs and symptoms of preeclampsia. Patient education regarding symptoms of preeclampsia (headache, visual changes, epigastric or abdominal pain) is recommended. Initial evaluation includes 24-hour urine collection to confirm the absence of significant proteinuria and serum laboratory evaluation to evaluate hepatic transaminases, creatinine, hematocrit, platelets, and lactic acid dehydrogenase. Derangements in any of these serum laboratories would be indicative of a diagnosis of preeclampsia as opposed to gestational hypertension.

For the patient with mild gestational hypertension, fetal surveillance with ultrasound for fetal growth approximately once per month and weekly biophysical profiles can assess fetal well-being. Antihypertensives are not recommended in women with mild gestational hypertension, as they have not been shown to improve outcomes. Delivery is recommended at 39–40 weeks' gestation.

Because severe gestational hypertension is associated with an increased risk of adverse outcomes at a rate similar to that of severe preeclampsia, women with severe gestational hypertension are generally managed the same way as women with severe preeclampsia (see Treatment section under Preeclampsia, later).

Prognosis

Most women experience normalization of their blood pressure within 2 weeks after delivery. Approximately 15% of women diagnosed with gestational hypertension will have persistently elevated blood pressure >12 weeks after delivery and will meet a diagnosis of chronic hypertension. The recurrence rate of gestational hypertension in future pregnancies is approximately 25%.

PREECLAMPSIA

ESSENTIALS OF DIAGNOSIS

- Maternal blood pressure elevation of ≥140 mm Hg systolic or ≥90 mm Hg diastolic on 2 occasions 6 hours apart
- Proteinuria ≥300 mg in a 24-hour urine specimen

Pathogenesis

Preeclampsia complicates 5–7% of all pregnancies. Preeclampsia occurs with increased frequency among young, nulliparous women. However, the frequency distribution is bimodal, with a second peak occurring in multiparous women greater than 35 years of age. Among daughters of preeclamptic women, the risk of preeclampsia is significantly higher than the population risk. Other predisposing factors for preeclampsia are listed in Table 26–3.

Normal pregnancy is associated with decreased maternal sensitivity to endogenous vasopressors. Apparent early in gestation, this effect leads to expansion of the maternal intravascular space and a decline in blood pressure throughout the first half of pregnancy, with a nadir at midgestation. Thereafter, continued expansion of intravascular volume leads to a gradual rise in the blood pressure to prepregnancy levels by term. Women destined to develop preeclampsia do not exhibit normal refractoriness to endogenous vasopressors. As a result, normal expansion of the intravascular space does not occur, and the normal decline in blood pressure during the first half of pregnancy may be absent or attenuated. Despite normal to elevated blood pressure, intravascular volume is reduced.

Table 26–3. Risk factors for preeclampsia.

Age <20 years or >35 years
Nulliparity
Multiple gestation
Hydatidiform mole
Diabetes mellitus
Thyroid disease
Chronic hypertension
Renal disease
Collagen vascular disease
Antiphospholipid syndrome
Family history of preeclampsia

The etiology of preeclampsia is not known; however, a growing body of evidence suggests that maternal vascular endothelial injury plays a central role in the disorder. Some reports suggest that endothelial damage in preeclampsia results in decreased endothelial production of prostaglandin I_2 (prostacyclin), a potent vasodilator and inhibitor of platelet aggregation. Endothelial cell injury exposes subendothelial collagen and can trigger platelet aggregation, activation, and release of platelet-derived thromboxane A_2 (TXA_2), a potent vasoconstrictor and stimulator of platelet aggregation. Decreased prostacyclin production by dysfunctional endothelial cells and increased TXA_2 release by activated platelets and trophoblast may be responsible for reversal of the normal ratio of prostacyclin and TXA_2 observed in preeclampsia. The predominance of TXA_2 may contribute to the vasoconstriction and hypertension that are central features of the disorder. Elevated intravascular pressure combined with damaged vascular endothelium results in movement of fluid from the intravascular to the extravascular spaces, leading to edema in the brain, retinae, lungs, liver, and subcutaneous tissues. Hypertension and glomerular endothelial damage lead to proteinuria. The resultant decrease in intravascular colloid oncotic pressure contributes to further loss of intravascular fluid. Hemoconcentration is reflected in a rising hematocrit. Consumption of platelets and activation of the clotting cascade at the sites of endothelial damage may lead to thrombocytopenia and disseminated intravascular coagulation (DIC). Soluble fibrin monomers produced by the coagulation cascade may precipitate in the microvasculature, leading to microangiopathic hemolysis and elevation of the serum lactate dehydrogenase level. Cerebral edema, vasoconstriction, and capillary endothelial damage may lead to hyperreflexia, clonus, convulsions, or hemorrhage. Hepatic edema and/or ischemia may lead to hepatocellular injury and elevation of serum transaminases and lactate dehydrogenase levels. The right upper quadrant or epigastric pain observed in severe preeclampsia is thought to be caused by stretching of Glisson's capsule by hepatic edema or hemorrhage. Intravascular fluid loss across damaged capillary endothelium in the lungs may result in pulmonary edema. In the retinae, vasoconstriction and/or edema may lead to visual disturbances, retinal detachment, or blindness. Movement of fluid from the intravascular space into the subcutaneous tissues produces the characteristic nondependent edema of preeclampsia.

Endothelial damage appears to be capable of triggering a cascade of events culminating in the multiorgan system dysfunction observed in preeclampsia. However, the mechanism of endothelial injury remains speculative. In one theory, decreased placental oxygenation triggers the placenta to release an unknown factor into the maternal circulation. This circulating factor is capable of damaging or altering the function of maternal endothelial cells and triggering the cascade of events described. In support of this theory, cultured trophoblasts exposed to a hypoxic environment release a variety of potentially vasoactive factors, including thromboxane, interleukin-1, and tumor necrosis factor. Moreover, serum from preeclamptic women, when applied to human endothelial cell cultures, alters the release of a variety of procoagulant, vasoactive, and mitogenic factors, including endothelin, nitric oxide, and prostacyclin. Serum from the same woman 6 weeks after delivery does not produce this effect. Likewise, serum from a nonpreeclamptic woman at the same gestational age fails to trigger these endothelial changes. In many cases, reduced placental oxygenation may be explained by maternal vasculopathy (chronic hypertension, renal disease, collagen vascular disease) and in others by abnormal placental mass (multiple gestation, diabetes, hydatidiform mole). In another subset of patients, reduced placental oxygenation late in pregnancy may be the result of abnormal endovascular trophoblast invasion early in pregnancy. In the first trimester of a normal pregnancy, proliferating trophoblast invades the decidual segments of the maternal spiral arteries, replacing endothelium and destroying the medial elastic and muscular tissue of the arterial wall. The arterial wall is replaced by fibrinoid material. During the second trimester, a second wave of endovascular trophoblastic invasion extends down the lumen of the spiral arteries deeper in the myometrium. The endothelium and musculoelastic architecture of the spiral arteries are destroyed, resulting in dilated, thin-walled, funnel-shaped vessels that are passive conduits of the increased uteroplacental blood flow of pregnancy. In some women destined to develop preeclampsia, the first wave of endovascular trophoblastic invasion may be incomplete, and the second wave does not occur. As a result, the deeper segments of the spiral arteries are not remodeled but instead retain their musculoelastic architecture and their ability to respond to endogenous vasoconstrictors, reducing maternal perfusion of the placenta and predisposing to relative placental hypoxia later in pregnancy. In addition, myometrial portions of the spiral arteries exhibit a unique abnormality characterized by vessel wall damage, fibrinoid necrosis, lipid deposition, and macrophage and mononuclear cell infiltration of vessel walls and surrounding tissues. These changes, histologically similar to those observed in atherosclerosis, are referred to as acute atherosis and may lead to vascular lumen obliteration and placental infarction. Importantly, these changes are attributed to abnormal endovascular trophoblastic invasion during the second trimester of pregnancy, predisposing the fetus to suboptimal placental perfusion early in gestation. Interestingly, the clinical manifestations are observed most often in the third trimester, possibly due to increasing fetal and placental oxygen demands with advancing gestation.

The reason that endovascular trophoblastic invasion progresses normally in most pregnancies but abnormally in others is unclear. One theory maintains that maternal antibodies directed against paternal antigens on invading trophoblasts are necessary to shield those antigens from recognition by decidual natural killer cells, protecting the invading trophoblast from attack and rejection by the cellular arm of the maternal immune system. Supporting this theory is the observation that preeclampsia appears to be associated with primi-paternity and the presumed lack of previous maternal exposure and sensitization to paternal trophoblast antigens in a previous pregnancy. Additional support for this theory is provided by the observation that preeclampsia is more common among women using barrier contraception than among those using nonbarrier forms of contraception before pregnancy. This suggests that maternal exposure (and presumably sensitization) to paternal antigens on sperm is protective against preeclampsia. The observed inverse relationship between duration of cohabitation before pregnancy and the incidence of preeclampsia provides further evidence that maternal sensitization to paternal antigens is protective against preeclampsia. The interplay between immunology and genetics is underscored by the observation that preeclampsia may be more common in pregnancies in which the father was the product of a preeclamptic pregnancy. Applied to the theory under discussion, this suggests that some genetically determined paternal antigens are less antigenic than others and therefore less likely to provoke an antibody response in an exposed mother, decreasing maternal production of "blocking" antibodies and increasing the likelihood of abnormal placental invasion and preeclampsia. Alternatively, paternally inherited genes may code for altered fetal production of insulin-like growth factor-2, an insulin homologue related to placental invasion. Other genes that may be inherited from the father and play a role in the development of preeclampsia include genes coding for angiotensinogen, methylenetetrahydrofolate reductase, and the factor V Leiden mutation.

Some studies have demonstrated that invading trophoblastic cells in normal pregnancy undergo an "antigenic shift" to resemble vascular endothelial antigens, masking them from recognition and rejection by decidual natural killer cells. Invading trophoblasts in preeclamptic pregnancies may fail to make this antigenic shift, exposing them to recognition by natural killer cells and halting normal invasion.

Recent work has demonstrated that soluble fms-like tyrosine kinase-1 (sFlt-1) is increased in the placenta and serum of women with preeclampsia. This protein adheres to placental growth factor and vascular endothelial growth factor (VEGF), preventing their interaction with endothelial receptors and causing endothelial dysfunction. Interrupted angiogenesis may contribute to faulty placental invasion early in pregnancy and subsequent risk for placental hypoxia–ischemia and preeclampsia. Unbound placental growth factor and VEGF have been found in decreased concentration during and even before the development of clinical preeclampsia.

Genetic, immunologic, and other factors govern the complex interaction between the maternal host and the invading trophoblast. Detailed discussion of these and other possible etiologies of the entity of preeclampsia are beyond the scope of this chapter. Regardless of the etiology, thorough familiarity with the clinical aspects of the disorder can help guide thoughtful and coherent management.

Preeclampsia exerts an effect on many different maternal organ systems:

A. Brain

Pathologic findings in preeclampsia-induced cerebral injury include fibrinoid necrosis, thrombosis, microinfarcts, and petechial hemorrhages, primarily in the cerebral cortex. Cerebral edema may be observed. Head computed tomographic findings include focal white matter hypodensities in the posterior cerebral hemispheres, temporal lobes, and brain stem, possibly reflecting petechial hemorrhage with resultant local edema. Magnetic resonance imaging may reveal occipital and parietal abnormalities in the watershed distribution of the major cerebral arteries, as well as lesions in the brain stem and basal ganglia. Subarachnoid or intraventricular hemorrhage may occur in severe cases.

B. Heart

Preeclampsia is characterized by the absence of normal intravascular volume expansion, a reduction in normal circulating blood volume, and a loss of normal refractoriness to endogenous vasopressors, including angiotensin II. Invasive hemodynamic monitoring in preeclamptic patients has yielded conflicting information. Depending on disease severity, effects of previous therapy, and other factors, preeclampsia has been described variously as a state of abnormally high cardiac output and low systemic vascular resistance, a state of abnormally low cardiac output and high systemic vascular resistance, or a state of high cardiac output and high systemic vascular resistance. These divergent observations underscore the complexity of the disorder.

C. Lungs

Alterations in colloid oncotic pressure, capillary endothelial integrity, and intravascular hydrostatic pressure in preeclampsia predispose to noncardiogenic pulmonary edema. In women with preeclampsia superimposed on chronic hypertension, preexisting hypertensive cardiac disease may exacerbate the situation, superimposing cardiogenic pulmonary edema on noncardiogenic, preeclampsia-related pulmonary edema. Excessive administration of intravenous (IV) fluid and postpartum mobilization of accumulated extravascular fluid also increase the risk of pulmonary edema. In eclampsia, pulmonary injury may result from aspiration of gastric contents, leading to pneumonia, pneumonitis, or adult respiratory distress syndrome.

D. Liver

Histologic lesions in the liver are characterized by sinusoidal fibrin deposition in the periportal areas with surrounding hemorrhage and portal capillary thrombi. Centrilobular necrosis may result from reduced perfusion. Inflammation is not characteristic. Subcapsular hematomas may develop. In severe cases involving hepatocellular necrosis and DIC, intrahepatic hematomas may progress to liver rupture. Right upper quadrant pain or epigastric pain are classic symptoms attributed to stretching of Glisson's capsule. Elevation of serum transaminases is a hallmark of HELLP (hemolysis, elevated liver enzymes, and low platelets) syndrome.

E. Kidneys

Distinct histologic changes have been described in the kidneys of women with preeclampsia. The classic renal lesion of preeclampsia, glomeruloendotheliosis, is characterized by swelling and enlargement of glomerular capillary endothelial cells, leading to narrowing of the capillary lumen. There is an increased amount of cytoplasm containing lipid-filled vacuoles. Mesangial cells may be swollen as well. Immunoglobulins, complement, fibrin, and fibrin degradation products have been observed in the glomeruli, but their presence is variable.

F. Eyes

Retinal vasospasm, retinal edema, serous retinal detachment, and cortical blindness may occur in the setting of preeclampsia. Blindness is uncommon and usually transient, resolving within hours to days of delivery.

Prevention

The observed alteration in the ratio of vasoconstrictive and vasodilatory prostaglandins in preeclampsia led investigators to study the effectiveness of prostaglandin synthesis inhibitors in preventing the disorder. Several small trials of low-dose aspirin reported significant reductions in the incidence of preeclampsia in high-risk populations. However, in 1994 the Collaborative Low-Dose Aspirin Study in Pregnancy (CLASP) Collaborative Group reported a large randomized trial comparing low-dose aspirin with placebo in more than 9300 high-risk patients. Low-dose aspirin did not reduce the incidence of preeclampsia in this high-risk population. Because the risks of the regimen are few, some physicians may reasonably choose to use it.

Calcium is essential in the synthesis of nitric oxide, a potent vasodilator believed to contribute to the maintenance of reduced vascular tone in pregnancy. Calcium supplementation during pregnancy has been proposed as a means to prevent preeclampsia. Although individual studies have demonstrated mixed results regarding the efficacy of calcium supplementation, a meta-analysis concluded that calcium supplementation of at least 1 gram daily during pregnancy appears to reduce the risk of preeclampsia by approximately 50%.

Clinical Findings

A diagnosis of preeclampsia is made based on 2 criteria: (1) elevated maternal blood pressure of ≥140 mm Hg systolic or ≥90 mm Hg diastolic on 2 occasions 6 hours apart, and (2) proteinuria ≥300 mg in a 24-hour urine specimen. In the past, the classic diagnostic triad included hypertension, proteinuria, and edema. Recently, the National High Blood Pressure Education Working Group recommended eliminating edema as a diagnostic criterion because it is too frequent an observation during normal pregnancy to be useful in diagnosing preeclampsia. In addition to the classic findings of hypertension and proteinuria, women with preeclampsia may complain of scotomata, blurred vision, or pain in the epigastrium or right upper quadrant. Examination often reveals brisk patellar reflexes and clonus. Laboratory abnormalities include elevated levels of hematocrit, lactate dehydrogenase, serum transaminases and uric acid, and thrombocytopenia. Although biochemical evidence of DIC may be detected with increased fibrin degradation products, hypofibrinogenemia and prolongation of the prothrombin time and activated partial thromboplastin time usually are seen only in cases complicated by abruption or multiple organ failure.

Preeclampsia is classified into mild or severe based on the degree of hypertension and proteinuria and the presence of other findings (Table 26–4). The HELLP syndrome is a variant of preeclampsia that is characterized by hemolysis, elevated liver enzymes, and low platelets. It complicates 10% of cases of severe preeclampsia and up to 50% of cases of eclampsia. Right upper quadrant pain, nausea, vomiting, and malaise are common. Hypertension and proteinuria are variable. The hallmark of the disorder is microangiopathic hemolysis leading to elevation of serum lactate dehydrogenase level and fragmented red blood cells on peripheral smear. Transaminase levels are elevated, thrombocytopenia is present, and DIC may be evident. Management is similar to that of severe preeclampsia. (See Chapter 29, Gastrointestinal Disorders in Pregnancy, for a more extensive review of HELLP syndrome.)

Complications

Complications related to preeclampsia include preterm birth, intrauterine fetal growth restriction, placental abruption, maternal pulmonary edema, and eclampsia. The estimated incidence of eclampsia is 1–3 per 1000 preeclamptic patients. Eclampsia is defined as one or more generalized convulsions in the setting of preeclampsia.

Table 26–4. Classification of preeclampsia.

Mild Preeclampsia	Severe Preeclampsia
Blood pressure ≥140 mm Hg systolic or ≥90 mm Hg diastolic but <160/110 mm Hg	Blood pressure ≥160 mm Hg systolic or ≥110 mm Hg diastolic on 2 occasions at least 6 hours apart while the patient is on bed rest
Proteinuria ≥300 mg/24 h but <5 g/24 h	Proteinuria of 5 g or higher in 24-hour urine specimen or 3+ or greater on 2 random urine samples collected at least 4 hours apart
Asymptomatic	Oliguria <500 mL in 24 hours Cerebral or visual disturbances Pulmonary edema or cyanosis Epigastric or right upper quadrant pain Impaired liver function Thrombocytopenia Fetal growth restriction

Treatment

In the management of preeclampsia, with few exceptions, maternal interests are best served by immediate delivery. However, this approach may not be in the best interest of the fetus. In the case of extreme prematurity, for example, the fetus may benefit from a period of expectant management during which corticosteroids are administered to accelerate fetal maturation. The decision to proceed with immediate delivery versus expectant management is based on several factors, including disease severity, fetal maturity, maternal and fetal condition, and cervical status.

A. Mild Preeclampsia

Women with mild preeclampsia are hospitalized for further evaluation and, if indicated, delivery. If mild preeclampsia is confirmed and the gestational age is 40 weeks or greater, delivery is indicated. At gestational ages of 37–40 weeks, cervical status is assessed and, if favorable, induction is initiated. If the cervical status is unfavorable, preinduction cervical ripening agents are used as needed. Occasionally, women with very unfavorable cervical examinations between 37 and 40 weeks may be managed expectantly for a limited time with bed rest, antepartum fetal surveillance, and close monitoring of maternal condition, including blood pressure measurement every 4–6 hours and daily assessment of patellar reflexes, weight gain, proteinuria, and symptoms. A complete blood count and levels of serum transaminases, lactate dehydrogenase, and uric acid should be checked weekly to twice weekly. Delivery is indicated if the cervical status becomes favorable, antepartum testing is abnormal, the gestational age reaches 40 weeks, or evidence of worsening preeclampsia is seen. If expectant management is undertaken after 37 weeks, the patient should understand that the only known benefit is a possible reduction in the rate of caesarean birth.

Women with mild preeclampsia before 37 weeks' gestation are managed expectantly with bed rest, twice-weekly antepartum testing, and maternal evaluation as described. Corticosteroids are administered if the gestational age is <34 weeks; amniocentesis is performed as needed to assess fetal pulmonary maturity. When extended expectant management is undertaken, fetal growth is assessed with ultrasound every 3–4 weeks. Occasionally, outpatient management is reasonable in carefully selected, reliable, asymptomatic patients with minimal proteinuria and normal laboratory test results. This approach includes bed rest at home, daily fetal movement counts, twice-weekly antepartum testing, serial evaluation of fetal growth, and frequent assessment, often by a visiting nurse, of blood pressure, proteinuria, weight gain, patellar reflexes, and symptoms. Any evidence of disease progression constitutes an indication for hospitalization and consideration of delivery. The benefit of prophylactic intrapartum magnesium sulfate in preventing convulsions in patients with mild preeclampsia has not been demonstrated conclusively in the literature.

B. Severe Preeclampsia

Severe preeclampsia mandates hospitalization. Delivery is indicated if the gestational age is 34 weeks or greater, fetal pulmonary maturity is confirmed, or evidence of deteriorating maternal or fetal status is seen. Acute blood pressure control may be achieved with hydralazine, labetalol, or nifedipine. The goal of antihypertensive therapy is to achieve a systolic blood pressure <160 mm Hg and a diastolic blood pressure <105 mm Hg. Overly aggressive control of the blood pressure may compromise maternal perfusion of the intervillous space and adversely affect fetal oxygenation. Hydralazine is a peripheral vasodilator that can be given in doses of 5–10 mg administered intravenously (IV). The onset of action is 10–20 minutes, and the dose can be repeated in 20–30 minutes if necessary. Labetalol can be administered in doses of 5–20 mg by slow IV push. The dose can be repeated in 10–20 minutes. Nifedipine is a calcium channel blocker that can be used in doses of 5–10 mg orally. The sublingual route of administration should not be used. The dose can be repeated in 20–30 minutes, as needed.

Management of severe preeclampsia before 34 weeks is controversial. In some institutions, delivery is accomplished regardless of fetal maturity. In others, delivery is delayed for a limited period of time to permit the administration of corticosteroids. Four large randomized controlled trials comparing magnesium sulfate with other methods of treatment to prevent convulsions in women with severe preeclampsia have demonstrated that magnesium sulfate is associated with a significantly lower rate of eclampsia than either no treatment or nimodipine. Lucas and colleagues reported no seizures among 1049 preeclamptic women receiving magnesium sulfate prophylaxis. Nonetheless, tonic–clonic convulsions may occur despite magnesium sulfate therapy. Magnesium sulfate is initiated, fetal status is monitored continuously, and antihypertensive agents are used as needed to maintain a systolic blood pressure <160 mm Hg and a diastolic blood pressure <105 mm Hg. Between 33 and 35 weeks, consideration should be given to amniocentesis for pulmonary maturity studies. If mature, immediate delivery is indicated. If immature, corticosteroids are administered and, if possible, delivery is delayed 24–48 hours. Between 24 and 32 weeks, antihypertensive therapy is instituted as indicated, corticosteroids are administered, and extensive maternal counseling is undertaken to clarify the risks and benefits of pregnancy prolongation. Neonatology consultation is helpful to delineate the neonatal risks specific to gestational age and estimated fetal weight. The duration of expectant management is determined on an individual basis, taking into account maternal wishes, estimated fetal weight, gestational age, and maternal and fetal status. Expectant management is contraindicated in the presence of fetal compromise, uncontrollable hypertension, eclampsia, DIC, HELLP syndrome, cerebral edema, pulmonary edema, or evidence of cerebral or hepatic hemorrhage. When severe preeclampsia is diagnosed before 24 weeks of gestation, the likelihood of a favorable outcome is low. Thorough counseling should address realistically the risks and anticipated benefits of expectant management and should include the option of pregnancy termination. If an appropriately informed patient declines the option of pregnancy termination, expectant management should proceed as outlined previously.

C. Intrapartum Management of Preeclampsia

In women with preeclampsia without contraindications to labor, vaginal delivery is the preferred approach. Cervical ripening agents and oxytocin are used as needed. If magnesium sulfate is used for seizure prophylaxis, it is administered as an IV loading dose of 4–6 g over 20–60 minutes, followed by a maintenance dose of 1–2 g/h. Urine output and serum creatinine level are monitored, and the magnesium dose is adjusted accordingly to prevent hypermagnesemia. Patellar reflexes and respiratory rate should be assessed frequently. In the presence of patellar reflexes, serum magnesium levels usually are unnecessary. Therapeutic magnesium levels range from 4–8 mg/dL. Loss of patellar reflexes is observed at magnesium levels of 10 mg/dL or higher, respiratory paralysis may occur at levels of 15 mg/dL or above, and cardiac arrest is possible with levels in excess of 25 mg/dL. Calcium gluconate (10 mL of 10% solution) should be available in the event of hypermagnesemia. To avoid pulmonary edema, total IV fluids should not exceed 100 mL/h. Pain control is achieved with regional anesthesia or with intramuscular or IV narcotic analgesics. Invasive hemodynamic monitoring is reserved for refractory pulmonary edema, adult respiratory distress syndrome, or oliguria unresponsive to fluid challenge. If caesarean section is required, platelets should be available for possible transfusion for patients with platelet counts <50,000/mm^3. Use of other blood products is guided by clinical and laboratory findings.

D. Management of Eclampsia

In most cases eclamptic seizures are self-limited, lasting 1–2 minutes. The first priorities are to ensure that the airway is clear and to prevent injury and aspiration of gastric contents. Diazepam or lorazepam should be used only if seizures are sustained. Nearly all tonic–clonic seizures are accompanied by a prolonged fetal heart rate deceleration that resolves after the seizure has ended. Once the patient has been stabilized, delivery is indicated. If possible, a 10- to 20-minute period of in utero resuscitation should be permitted before delivery. Convulsions alone do not constitute an indication for caesarean section. However, if vaginal birth is not possible within a reasonable period of time, caesarean delivery is performed in most cases. A number of studies suggest that magnesium sulfate is superior to phenytoin, diazepam, and a lytic cocktail at preventing recurrent seizures in women with eclampsia.

Altman D, Carroli G, Duley L, et al. Magpie Trial Collaboration Group: Do women with preeclampsia, and their babies, benefit from magnesium sulfate? The Magpie Trial: A randomized placebo-controlled trial. *Lancet* 2002;359:1877–1890. PMID 12057549.

American College of Obstetricians and Gynecologists. Diagnosis and management of preeclampsia and eclampsia. ACOG Practice Bulletin No. 33. *Obstet Gynecol* 2002;99:159. PMID 16175681.

Belfort M, Anthony J, Saade G. The Nimodipine Study Group: A comparison of magnesium sulfate and nimodipine for the prevention of preeclampsia. *N Engl J Med* 2003;348:304–311. PMID 12540643.

Caritis S, Sibai B, Hauth J, et al. Low-dose aspirin to prevent preeclampsia in women at high risk. National Institute of Child Health and Human Development Network of Maternal-Fetal Units. *N Engl J Med* 1998;338:701–705. PMID: 9494145.

CLASP (Collaborative Low-dose Aspirin Study in Pregnancy) Collaborative Group. CLASP: A randomized trial of low-dose aspirin for the prevention and treatment of pre-eclampsia among 9364 pregnant women. *Lancet* 1994;343:619–629. PMID: 7906809.

Chambers JC, Fusi L, Malik IS, et al. Association of maternal endothelial dysfunction with preeclampsia. *JAMA* 2001;285:1607. PMID 11268269.

Duley L. Pre-eclampsia and hypertension. *Clin Evid* 2002;7:1296. PMID 12230748.

Duley L, Gulmezoglu AM, Henderson-Smart DJ. Magnesium sulphate and other anticonvulsants for women with pre-eclampsia. *Cochrane Database Syst Rev* 2003;CD000025. PMID 12804383.

Duley L, Henderson-Smart DJ, Knight M, King JF. Antiplatelet agents for preventing pre-eclampsia and its complications. *Cochrane Database Syst Rev* 2004:CD004659. PMID 14974075.

Esplin MS, Fausett MB, Fraser A, et al. Paternal and maternal components of the predisposition to preeclampsia. *N Engl J Med* 2001;344:867. PMID 11259719.

Hofmeyr GJ, Lawrie TA, Atallah AN, Duley L. Calcium supplementation during pregnancy for preventing hypertensive disorders and related problems. *Cochrane Database Syst Rev* 2010;CD001059. PMID: 20687064.

Isler CM, Barrilleaux PS, Magann EF, Bass JD, Martin JN Jr. A prospective, randomized trial comparing the efficacy of dexamethasone and betamethasone for the treatment of antepartum HELLP (hemolysis, elevated liver enzymes, and low platelet count) syndrome. *Am J Obstet Gynecol* 2001;184:1332. PMID 11408849.

Lain KY, Roberts JM. Contemporary concepts in the pathogenesis and management of preeclampsia. *JAMA* 2002;287:3183. PMID 12076198.

Levine RJ, Maynard SE, Qian C, et al. Circulating angiogenic factors and the risk of preeclampsia. *N Engl J Med* 2004;350:672. PMID 14764923.

Livingston JC, Livingston LW, Ramsey R, Mabie BC, Sibai BM. Magnesium sulfate in women with mild preeclampsia: A randomized controlled trial. *Obstet Gynecol* 2003;101:217–220. PMID 12576241.

Lucas MF, Leveno KJ, Cunningham FG. A comparison of magnesium sulfate with phenytoin for the prevention of eclampsia. *N Engl J Med* 1995;333:201–205. PMID: 7791836.

O'Brien JM, Milligan DA, Barton JR. Impact of high-dose corticosteroid therapy for patients with HELLP (hemolysis, elevated liver enzymes, and low platelet count) syndrome. *Am J Obstet Gynecol* 2000;183:921. PMID 11035338.

Sibai BM, Caritis SN, Thom E, et al. Prevention of preeclampsia with low-dose aspirin in health, nulliparous pregnant women. The National Institute of Child Health and Human Development Network of Maternal-Fetal Units. *N Engl J Med* 1993;329:1213–1218. PMID: 8413387.

CONCLUSION

Hypertensive disorders of pregnancy remain among the most common causes of adverse maternal and perinatal outcome. These disorders can be regarded as a spectrum of disease, ranging from isolated chronic hypertension to pure preeclampsia–eclampsia. Isolated mild or moderate chronic hypertension appears to have little effect on pregnancy outcome. Morbidity and mortality are highest among patients with severe preeclampsia or eclampsia.

Appropriate management of newly diagnosed chronic hypertension entails a thorough search for an underlying cause. Close maternal and fetal surveillance is necessary, and a high index of suspicion must be maintained for the development of superimposed preeclampsia.

The management of preeclampsia is influenced by many factors, including disease severity, gestational age, and fetal condition. Optimal management requires an appreciation of the complexity of the disease process and familiarity with its manifestations in multiple organ systems. Maternal and fetal risks and benefits must be assessed thoroughly. Individualized treatment plans should be formulated and discussed with the patient, and she should be encouraged to participate in major decisions regarding her care. In atypical cases, alternative diagnoses must be considered.

Cardiac & Pulmonary Disorders in Pregnancy

27

Afshan B. Hameed, MD, FACC
Martin N. Montoro, MD

CARDIAC DISORDERS IN PREGNANCY

CARDIOVASCULAR CHANGES IN NORMAL PREGNANCY

Hemodynamic adaptations of pregnancy are geared to augment blood flow to the developing fetoplacental unit. These alterations may stress the maternal cardiovascular system, leading to signs and symptoms similar to those seen in heart disease. Women with preexisting cardiovascular disease are particularly at risk, as they may exhibit marked clinical deterioration during the course of pregnancy.

Blood volume begins to increase as early as 6 weeks of gestation and continues to rise until midpregnancy. The hormonally mediated increase in plasma volume is disproportionately higher than the red cell mass, resulting in the so-called physiologic anemia of pregnancy. Cardiac output (CO) is increased by 50% above the nonpregnant state as a product of increased stroke volume, along with an increased heart rate by 10–20 beats/min. CO peaks in the mid-second trimester and plateaus thereafter. Myocardial contractility improves, left atrial and left ventricular chamber sizes increase, and peripheral vascular resistance falls (effects of progesterone, circulating prostaglandins, atrial natriuretic peptides, endothelial nitric oxide, and the low-resistance vascular bed of the placenta). The systemic arterial pressure falls during the first trimester, remains stable during the second trimester, and returns to pregestational levels before term. The reduction in diastolic pressure is more pronounced than the reduction in systolic pressure, leading to a wide pulse pressure. Supine hypotensive or uterocaval syndrome may occur in 0.5–11% of pregnancies and is related to the acute occlusion of inferior vena cava by the gravid uterus in the supine position; it is characterized by significant decreases in blood pressure and heart rate. This contrasts with the tachycardia seen with hypotension in the nonpregnant state. Patients usually complain of lightheadedness, nausea, dizziness, and syncope in extreme cases. Symptoms are alleviated by changing to a left lateral recumbent position.

Hemodynamic changes during labor and delivery are in part related to the fear, anxiety, and pain experienced by the patient at that stage. Additionally, uterine contractions displace 300–500 mL of blood with each contraction, further augmenting CO. Oxygen consumption increases 3-fold. These changes in CO are less pronounced if the patient remains in the supine position with leftward tilt and receives adequate analgesia. Immediately after delivery, relief of caval compression coupled with autotransfusion from the contracting uterus produces a further increase in CO. This may lead to acute cardiac decompensation in the immediate postpartum period. Most of these physiologic changes revert to prepregnancy levels by 2 weeks postpartum.

HEART DISEASE

Heart disease is surpassing other causes of maternal mortality in recent years. Cardiac disease complicates approximately 1% of all pregnancies. Pregnant patients with significant symptoms on exertion, such as patients in New York Heart Association (NYHA) functional classes III and IV (Table 27–1), have high event rates and may succumb to complications of heart disease, such as heart failure, arrhythmias, and stroke. Patients with stenotic lesions (eg, mitral or aortic stenosis) and minimal baseline symptoms (NYHA class I or II) may deteriorate rapidly.

As a greater proportion of the pediatric population is surviving surgical correction of congenital anomalies, many children are reaching adulthood and subsequently becoming pregnant. Pregnant women with congenital heart disease now outnumber those with rheumatic heart disease in most developing countries. Acquired conditions such as ischemic heart disease are also not uncommon today as women are delaying childbearing to the third and fourth decades of life. As the general population becomes more susceptible to diabetes mellitus, morbid obesity, and hypertension, more frequent encounters with ischemic heart disease in pregnant patients are expected.

Table 27–1. New York Heart Association functional classification of heart disease.

Class I	No signs or symptoms (chest pain or shortness of breath)
Class II	No symptoms at rest, slight limitation with mild to moderate activity (walking >2 blocks)
Class III	No symptoms at rest, marked limitation with less than ordinary activity (walking <2 blocks)
Class IV	Symptoms at rest

CARDIOVASCULAR EVALUATION DURING PREGNANCY

Most women with heart disease have successful pregnancies, but complacency in the diagnosis and management of pregnant patients can have direct consequences for both the mother and the fetus. Therefore, it is essential to evaluate every pregnant woman with heart disease for her risk of adverse outcomes during pregnancy, labor, delivery, and postpartum. In general, all such women should be referred to a tertiary care center for a multidisciplinary management by an obstetrician, cardiologist, clinical geneticist, and neonatologist.

Preconception Counseling

Care of women with cardiac disease should ideally begin with preconception counseling. Certain conditions may need treatment before attempting pregnancy. Cardiac conditions associated with high maternal mortality include pulmonary hypertension (primary and secondary), peripartum and other cardiomyopathies with reduced ejection fraction, Marfan's syndrome with aortic root enlargement, and complicated coarctation of aorta (Table 27–2). These patients should be advised against pregnancy and offered termination of pregnancy at an appropriate gestational age. In general, valve stenoses are problematic in pregnancy, and regurgitant lesions are relatively well tolerated. Management principles in pregnant women are similar to those in the nonpregnant state. Preconception counseling allows for optimal timing for conception, completion of all diagnostic procedures beforehand (especially those involving radiation exposure), discontinuation of teratogenic drugs, and scheduling of corrective/palliative surgery before pregnancy.

The initial evaluation should include a careful medical history, comprehensive physical examination, and noninvasive diagnostic testing. Common findings in normal pregnancy are listed in Table 27–3. Siu et al identified the

Table 27–2. High-risk pregnancy in women with heart disease.

Etiology	Disease
Pump failure	Severe cardiomyopathy
Symptomatic valve narrowing	MS, AS, PS
Cyanotic heart disease	Tetralogy of Fallot, transposition of great arteries
Aortic rupture	Marfan's syndrome with dilated aorta
Artificial prosthesis	Mechanical heart valves
Elevated pulmonary artery pressures	Eisenmenger's syndrome, primary pulmonary hypertension, pulmonary vascular disease

AS, aortic stenosis; MS, mitral stenosis; PS, pulmonary stenosis.

Table 27–3. Common findings in normal pregnancy.

Symptoms	Fatigue, decreased exercise capacity
	Lightheadedness, syncope
	Palpitations
	Dyspnea, orthopnea
Physical examination	Distended neck veins
	Increased intensity of S_1, exaggerated splitting
	Exaggerated splitting of S_2
	Midsystolic, soft, ejection-type murmurs (lower left sternal border or over the pulmonary area)
	Third heart sound
	Continuous murmurs (cervical venous hum, mammary soufflé)
	Brisk, diffused, displaced left ventricular impulse
	Palpable right ventricular impulse
Electrocardiogram	QRS axis deviation
	Small Q and inverted P in lead III (abolished by inspiration)
	Sinus tachycardia, higher incidence of arrhythmias
Chest radiograph	Horizontal position of heart
	Increased lung markings
Echocardiography	Slightly increased systolic and diastolic left ventricular dimensions
	Moderate increase in size of right atrium, right ventricle, and left atrium
	Functional pulmonary, tricuspid, and mitral regurgitation

following prognostic indicators to predict cardiac events in pregnancy (ie, heart failure, arrhythmia, stroke, death):

1. **N**ew York Heart Association (NYHA) functional class ≥II (or cyanosis)
2. **O**utlet obstruction of the left heart
3. **P**rior cardiac event (heart failure, arrhythmia, stroke)
4. **E**jection fraction <40%

The risk of a cardiac event with 0, 1, and >1 prognostic indicators were estimated to be 5%, 27%, and 75%, respectively.

Most pregnant patients experience reduced exercise tolerance and easy fatigability. This may be aggravated by the weight gained during gestation and physiologic anemia of pregnancy. Syncopal episodes or lightheadedness may occur due to mechanical compression of the inferior vena cava by the gravid uterus leading to poor venous return to the heart, especially in the third trimester. Other frequent complaints include hyperventilation and orthopnea (from mechanical pressure of the enlarged uterus on the diaphragm). Palpitations are common and probably are related to the hyperdynamic circulation of pregnancy rather than arrhythmias in most cases. Signs and symptoms of cardiovascular disease are listed in Table 27–4.

Hyperventilation is a common phenomenon in pregnancy and is likely related to the effect of progesterone on the respiratory center. It is important to differentiate hyperventilation from dyspnea, which is a common finding in congestive heart failure. Bibasilar crackles are commonly heard in normal pregnancy and result from atelectasis that develops from basal compression of the lungs due to uterine enlargement and the subsequent increase in intra-abdominal pressure.

The physical examination should focus on facial, digital, or skeletal abnormalities that suggest the presence of congenital anomalies. One should observe for clubbing, cyanosis, or pallor. The first heart sound usually is widely split (which can be misinterpreted as a fourth heart sound). A loud first heart sound suggests mitral stenosis (MS), whereas a low-intensity first heart sound indicates first-degree heart block. A widely split second heart sound goes along with atrial septal defect (ASD), whereas a paradoxically split sound occurs in severe left ventricular hypertrophy or left bundle branch block. A third heart sound is normal in pregnancy. A fourth heart sound, ejection click, opening snap, or mid to late systolic click suggests heart disease. Functional systolic murmurs can be heard in most pregnant women and can result from the hyperkinetic circulation of pregnancy. These murmurs are midsystolic and are heard best at the lower left sternal border and over the pulmonic area. Continuous benign murmurs, such as the cervical venous hum and mammary soufflé, also result from increased flow secondary to the hemodynamic changes of pregnancy. The venous hum is best heard over the right supraclavicular fossa, and the mammary soufflé is best auscultated over the breast in late gestation. Diastolic murmurs heard during pregnancy require further investigation by echocardiography and Doppler ultrasound.

Table 27–4. Signs and symptoms indicative of significant cardiovascular disease.

Symptoms	Progressively worsening shortness of breath
	Cough with frothy pink sputum
	Paroxysmal nocturnal dyspnea
	Chest pain with exertion
	Syncope preceded by palpitations or exertion
	Hemoptysis
Physical examination	Abnormal venous pulsations
	Rarely audible S_1
	Single S_2 or paradoxically split S_2
	Loud systolic murmurs, any diastolic murmur
	Ejection clicks, late systolic clicks, opening snaps
	Friction rub
	Sustained right or left ventricular heave
	Cyanosis or clubbing
Electrocardiogram	Significant arrhythmias
	Heart blocks
Chest radiograph	Cardiomegaly
	Pulmonary edema

Diagnostic Tests

A. Electrocardiography

The QRS axis in normal pregnancy usually is within normal limits but can shift to the extreme right or left of that range. A small Q wave and an inverted P wave in lead III are abolished by deep inspiration. Greater R-wave amplitude can be seen in leads V_1 and V_2. The incidences of sinus tachycardia and premature atrial/ventricular beats, as well as the susceptibility to paroxysmal supraventricular and ventricular arrhythmias, are increased.

B. Chest Radiograph

The radiation exposure from a routine chest radiograph is minimal; however, chest x-ray films still should not be taken casually in pregnancy. Chest x-ray may be performed for appropriate indications with abdominopelvic protective lead shielding. The findings on chest films may mimic abnormal disease conditions. Straightening of the left heart border due to enlargement of the main pulmonary artery can be seen. The heart is more horizontal, and the lung markings are more prominent due to redistribution secondary to increased pulmonary venous pressure.

C. Echocardiography

Small pericardial effusions are common in normal pregnant women late in pregnancy. Dilation of mitral, tricuspid, and pulmonary annuli and enlargement of all the cardiac chambers are seen. Mild physiologic regurgitation of these valves is observed. Transthoracic echocardiography can be used safely on both the mother and the fetus to rule out congenital heart disease, ventricular dilatation, and aortic root disease. Doppler ultrasound can evaluate the significance of valvular lesions, estimate pulmonary pressures, and rule out intracardiac shunts. Transesophageal echocardiography can improve visualization of posteriorly situated cardiac structures, such as the left atrium and mitral valve.

D. Exercise Stress Testing

Stress testing usually is indicated for preconception workup for estimation of myocardial reserve to determine whether a woman can safely carry a pregnancy to term. Some low-level exercise protocols have been developed for implementation during pregnancy to evaluate for ischemic heart disease. These protocols allow the heart rate to go up to only 70% of age-predicted heart rate and are considered safe in the first half of pregnancy.

E. Cardiac Catheterization

Pulmonary artery catheterization without fluoroscopy, at the bedside, is a relatively safe procedure and allows for hemodynamic monitoring during labor and delivery in select patients. Left or right heart catheterization under fluoroscopy should be undertaken only when absolutely essential (eg, for percutaneous coronary intervention or balloon valvuloplasty). Every effort should be taken to shield the abdominal and pelvic areas and to avoid radiation exposure of the fetus.

VALVULAR HEART DISEASE

1. Mitral Stenosis

ESSENTIALS OF DIAGNOSIS

- Mitral stenosis (MS) is the most common valve lesion seen in pregnancy.
- It is characterized by narrowing of the opening within the mitral valve.

Pathogenesis

Mitral stenosis may be congenital or due to rheumatic heart disease, Libman-Sacks endocarditis in lupus, or Lutembacher's syndrome (MS in association with an atrial septal defect). Rheumatic heart disease develops after a group A β-hemolytic streptococcal infection of the upper airway. Even though its incidence in developing countries has declined as a result of the prevalent use of antibiotics, rheumatic valvular disease still afflicts a large majority of women of childbearing age in Asia, Central America, and South America.

Clinical Findings

The characteristic findings include a right ventricular lift, a loud first heart sound (S_1), an accentuated pulmonic component of the second heart sound (P_2), an opening snap, and a low-frequency diastolic rumble at the apex with presystolic accentuation (if the patient is in sinus rhythm). The murmur is best heard with the bell of the stethoscope in the left lateral decubitus position. The electrocardiogram often is normal but may indicate left atrial enlargement, right-axis deviation, or even right ventricular hypertrophy. Echocardiogram is diagnostic.

Complications

The increased left atrial pressure may predispose the patient to atrial arrhythmias (ie, atrial fibrillation). This new-onset atrial fibrillation can precipitate acute decompensation even in the setting of mild to moderate MS due to acceleration of ventricular rate that decreases the diastolic filling period and thus increases pulmonary venous pressure. The pregnant cardiac patient also is at risk for developing thromboembolic complications in a setting of existing hypercoagulable state as well as venous stasis in the legs.

Treatment

The goals are to prevent/treat tachycardia and atrial fibrillation, prevent fluid overload, and alleviate pain and anxiety. Beta blockers, diuretics, and occasionally digitalis and anticoagulants may be necessary to treat congestive failure and atrial arrhythmias. Patients with chronic atrial fibrillation should be anticoagulated with subcutaneous heparin. Anemia, infection, and thyrotoxicosis should be corrected. Large fluctuations in hemodynamics due to venous pooling in the legs should be prevented by the use of elastic support hose, especially late in pregnancy. Medical management remains the first-line therapy in patients with MS. In patients with severe MS, mitral valvotomy may be performed for symptom relief before pregnancy. Balloon valvuloplasty has become a preferred, less invasive procedure, especially for patients with a noncalcified, pliable valve with excellent results. Mitral valve placement is considered as a last resort due to high maternal morbidity and fetal loss rates and should be deferred until after the pregnancy if possible.

Patients with MS should be delivered vaginally at term unless caesarean section is indicated for obstetric reasons.

Narcotic-epidural anesthesia is the preferred option for delivery. Other considerations include maintenance of meticulous fluid balance, oxygen administration, and left lateral decubitus position during labor. The second stage of labor may be shortened with use of outlet forceps. Careful hemodynamic monitoring during labor and delivery is indicated in patients with compromised circulation. Postpartum uterotonics should be given cautiously and blood loss carefully monitored. Redistribution of fluid from the interstitial to the intravascular space immediately postpartum may precipitate pulmonary edema in these patients.

Prognosis

The risk of developing heart failure increases progressively throughout pregnancy and in the peripartum period. Labor imposes an additional load, and congestive failure may develop for the first time during labor in a previously well-controlled patient with MS. The overall mortality rate in women with rheumatic mitral valve disease is 1% overall and reaches 3–4% in women with class III and IV severity.

2. Mitral Regurgitation

ESSENTIALS OF DIAGNOSIS

- Mitral regurgitation is characterized by a mitral valve that does not close properly during systole, leading to leakage of blood from the left ventricle into the left atrium.

Pathogenesis

Mitral regurgitation (MR) is one of the most common valvular lesions seen in adulthood. The most common cause of MR is mitral valve prolapse, which is seen in approximately 50% of cases of MR. With mitral valve prolapse, there is myxomatous degeneration of the valve, which causes stretching out of the valve and chordae tendineae. MR can also be caused by ischemic heart disease, rheumatic fever, and Marfan's syndrome.

Clinical Findings

Mitral regurgitation is generally well tolerated in pregnancy. The characteristic finding on physical examination is a long systolic murmur that ends with the second heart sound and is best heard at the apex with radiation into the axilla. An associated third heart sound is often present, and an opening snap may be present with associated mitral valve stenosis.

Complications

Severe MR may lead to left atrial enlargement, atrial fibrillation, and/or congestive heart failure (CHF).

Treatment

No treatment is indicated in an asymptomatic patient. Symptoms are usually related to CHF and respond well to digitalis, diuretics, and vasodilators. Anticoagulation should be used for atrial fibrillation.

3. Mitral Valve Prolapse

ESSENTIALS OF DIAGNOSIS

- Prolapse of one or both mitral valve leaflets into the left atrium during systole

Pathogenesis

Mitral valve prolapse (MVP) is a common congenital cardiac lesion in the general population. However, only 2–4% of the affected individuals have significant MR. It can be inherited as an autosomal dominant disorder with incomplete penetrance. MVP may be an idiopathic finding; it may also be seen in conjunction with other disorders such as Marfan's syndrome, autosomal dominant polycystic kidney disease, and Ehlers-Danlos syndrome.

Clinical Findings

On physical examination, patients with MVP may have a midsystolic click and/or a midsystolic or late systolic murmur at the apex of the left ventricle. Echocardiogram confirms the findings and can also evaluate for MR.

Treatment

All patients with a history of MVP should undergo comprehensive prepregnancy clinical evaluation and echocardiography.

Prognosis

MVP is generally well tolerated in pregnancy unless associated with severe MR, left atrial enlargement, left ventricular dysfunction, or atrial fibrillation. Severe MR can worsen during pregnancy, and patients may develop progressive atrial enlargement, atrial fibrillation, and clinical decline. Select patients should be referred for mitral valve repair before pregnancy.

4. Aortic Stenosis

ESSENTIALS OF DIAGNOSIS

- Narrowing of the area within the aortic valve

Pathogenesis

In reproductive years, the most common cause of aortic stenosis (AS) is bicuspid aortic valve followed by rheumatic heart disease. Bicuspid aortic valve may be associated with aortic root enlargement and is important in the preconception evaluation and counseling.

Clinical Findings

Common symptoms include chest pain due to decreased coronary perfusion, syncope due to decreased cerebral perfusion, and congestive heart failure due to increased left atrial pressure. Physical examination is significant for diminished and delayed carotid pulse. Left ventricular apical impulse is usually displaced and sustained with a harsh systolic ejection murmur that can be heard in the second right intercostal space. Electrocardiogram may demonstrate left ventricular hypertrophy and left atrial enlargement.

Complications

Pregnancy is contraindicated if the patient has severe AS without symptoms, history of symptomatic AS, or history of heart failure, syncope, or cardiac arrest. AS causes a fixed CO, decreased coronary and cerebral perfusion, and an increase in the left atrial pressure. Hemodynamic changes of pregnancy put these patients at an elevated risk.

Treatment

Patients with mild to moderate AS who are asymptomatic should be advised to restrict their physical activity and can be managed expectantly during pregnancy. Patients with severe AS should strongly be considered for mechanical relief of their obstruction. Aortic balloon valvuloplasty can be performed before pregnancy *or* after 20 weeks of gestation if the valve anatomy is favorable. Aortic valve replacement is considered a last resort and is associated with significant fetal loss and maternal morbidity.

OTHER CARDIAC VALVULAR LESIONS

1. Aortic Regurgitation

Patients with aortic insufficiency tolerate pregnancy well because the fall in peripheral resistances favors forward blood flow and decreases the regurgitant fraction.

2. Pulmonary Stenosis

Isolated pulmonary stenosis is well tolerated in pregnancy. Favorable maternal and fetal outcomes have been reported in the absence of right ventricular failure. Transvalvular pressure gradients of >60 mm Hg may warrant relief of obstruction. Right ventricular failure or arrhythmias may be seen.

CONGENITAL CARDIAC LESIONS

ESSENTIALS OF DIAGNOSIS

- Congenital cardiac lesions are structural malformations of the heart present at birth that developed during fetal life or perinatal transition.
- With improvements in cardiac care, more children who were born with cardiac malformations are reaching reproductive age.
- Congenital cardiac lesions are associated with an increased risk of fetal and maternal complications.

Pathogenesis

With advances in the care of children born with cardiac structural malformations during the 20th century, more women with congenital heart defects—repaired or unrepaired—are reaching reproductive age. Congenital cardiac defects may be classified as cyanotic or acyanotic. The most common acyanotic congenital cardiac lesion is bicuspid aortic valve. The presence of congenital cyanotic heart disease is not an absolute contraindication to pregnancy but does increase the risk of fetal loss. Heart failure occurs in 47% patients with cyanotic heart disease versus 13% with acyanotic lesions, and maternal mortality approaches 4–16% in uncorrected lesions.

Women with congenital heart defects in general are at increased risk of maternal and fetal complications during pregnancy. The absolute risk of each complication varies according to the underlying lesion. The maternal complications associated with congenital heart defects in pregnant women include heart failure, arrhythmias, thromboembolism, endocarditis, and pulmonary hypertension.

Fetal complications related to maternal cardiac disease are an increased risk of miscarriage, stillbirth, intrauterine growth restriction and prematurity, and in many cases iatrogenic preterm birth for maternal indications. Fetuses of women with congenital heart disease are also at increased risk of congenital heart defect. The recurrence risk depends on the specific type of defect, but in general, the risk is approximately 5–10%.

Clinical Findings, Treatment, and Prognosis

Clinical findings, treatment, and prognosis vary according to underlying heart lesion. General tenets of management of women with congenital heart disease during the antepartum period are close surveillance for maternal symptoms of decompensation during pregnancy, fetal surveillance for evidence of pregnancy loss or intrauterine growth restriction, and fetal echocardiogram (usually performed at 20 weeks) to assess for recurrent congenital heart defect.

In terms of labor management, women with repaired or unrepaired defects with normal cardiac function may be allowed to labor and deliver normally. In many cases, however, women may require a more controlled labor and delivery with planned induction of labor and assisted second stage with vacuum or forceps. Caesarean delivery is usually reserved for obstetrical indications due to the increased blood loss and increased risk of postdelivery infection when compared with vaginal birth. The management of pregnancies in women with specific cardiac defects is discussed next.

A. Coarctation of Aorta

The most common site of coarctation is distal to the left subclavian artery. Unoperated coarctation of aorta is rarely encountered in pregnancy. Postrepair coarctation patients require careful prepregnancy evaluation to exclude important cardiovascular residua or sequelae. It is a rare cause of secondary hypertension and may be associated with ASD and ventricular septal defect (VSD), bicuspid aortic valve, Berry aneurysm of the circle of Willis, and hypertension. A gradient of <20 mm Hg across the coarctation is associated with favorable maternal and fetal outcomes. Patients with coarctation are at risk for aortic aneurysm, dissection and rupture, CHF, cerebrovascular accident due to uncontrolled hypertension or rupture of intracranial aneurysm, and bacterial endocarditis. The key is to avoid hypotension and excessive blood loss at the time of delivery.

B. Atrial Septal Defect

Atrial septal defect (ASD) is one of the most common congenital heart defects seen in adults. Secundum ASD is the most commonly seen during pregnancy, and the majority of these patients have uncomplicated pregnancies. Primum ASDs may be associated with cleft mitral valve. Partial anomalous pulmonary venous connection is characteristically associated with sinus venosus ASD. There is an additional risk for pulmonary hypertension and arrhythmias. Physical examination includes systolic ejection murmur at the left sternal border and wide fixed split second heart sound. Electrocardiogram may reveal a partial right bundle branch block, right axis deviation, right ventricular hypertrophy, or left axis deviation in patients with ostium primum defects.

Patients with large defects are prone to CHF, atrial fibrillation, and paradoxical embolism. Consider prophylactic anticoagulation and meticulous leg care in the peripartum period (compression stockings, leg squeezers) in patients with large ASDs to prevent embolization. Systemic hypertension may lead to an increase in left to right shunt, which may lead to pulmonary volume overload. The key is to avoid volume overload.

C. Ventricular Septal Defect

Most ventricular septal defects (VSD) encountered during pregnancy have either been repaired or are clinically insignificant. VSD is generally well tolerated during pregnancy. Patients with large defects are at risk for CHF, arrhythmias, and pulmonary hypertension. Systemic hypertension may lead to an increase in left to right shunt, which may lead to pulmonary volume overload similar to an ASD.

D. Patent Ductus Arteriosus

Patent ductus arteriosus (PDA) is an uncommon lesion encountered in pregnancy. Most patients with small PDA tolerate pregnancy well. Symptoms are primarily fatigue and dyspnea. Physical examination findings include widened pulse pressure and a continuous murmur in the pulmonic area. Moderate-size PDA may cause left atrial and left ventricular enlargement with associated left ventricular volume overload and heart failure. These patients are at risk for pulmonary hypertension and reversal of shunt (right to left) secondary to elevated pulmonary pressures (Eisenmenger's syndrome). Systemic hypertension may lead to an increase in left to right shunt, which may lead to pulmonary volume overload/CHF similar to that seen in ASD and VSD physiology.

E. Eisenmenger's Syndrome

Eisenmenger's syndrome is the reversal of a left to right shunt (ASD, VSD, PDA) due to progressive pulmonary hypertension. Right to left shunting leads to systemic arterial oxygen desaturation and central cyanosis. The degree of cyanosis is determined by the extent of pulmonary vascular obstructive disease. Maternal mortality approaches 30–50% and fetal loss may be as high as 75%. It is one of the few conditions in which pregnancy is contraindicated. If the patient is seen for the first time early in pregnancy, she should strongly be advised to terminate pregnancy. Various pulmonary vasodilators have been successfully used in pregnancy to lower the pulmonary pressures, but the overall prognosis remains grim. In these patients, the pulmonary pressures may reach systemic levels, and therefore, a minimal lowering of systemic blood pressure may cause massive right to left shunting. This may lead to worsening hypoxia, setting up a vicious cycle of further pulmonary vasoconstriction, and may result in rapid hemodynamic deterioration. Therefore, continuous pulse oximetry and oxygen administration to keep oxygen saturations above 90% is beneficial. Narcotic epidural or general endotracheal anesthesia should be used to avoid risk of systemic hypotension. Although these patients are at high risk for thromboembolism due to hypercoagulability of pregnancy and polycythemia, the benefit of anticoagulation has not been confirmed. Patients may undergo assisted vaginal delivery if they are stable, and caesarean section is reserved for obstetrical indications and/or for unstable patients. Patients with Eisenmenger's syndrome may have serious complications in the postpartum period, and therefore, prolonged hospitalization is recommended.

F. Tetralogy of Fallot

Patients with conotruncal abnormalities, including tetralogy of Fallot (TOF), complex pulmonary atresia, or truncus arteriosus, have an increased prevalence of 22q11.2 microdeletion. All adult patients considering pregnancy or reproduction should be screened for 22q11.2 microdeletion, as this has an important impact on the chance of congenital heart disease in the offspring, and be offered prepregnancy genetic counseling. Most patients with TOF have had prior intracardiac repair, but they remain at increased risk of maternal and fetal complications. Poor prognostic indicators in patients with TOF are hematocrit >65%, history of syncope, CHF, cardiomegaly, right ventricular hypertrophy, and oxygen saturations <90%.

G. Marfan's Syndrome

Marfan's syndrome is an autosomal dominant condition that causes cystic medial necrosis of the aorta and may lead to dissecting aneurysm in pregnancy. There is an increased risk of rupture, dissection, and cardiovascular complications if aortic root diameter is more than 4 cm. Patients with aortic root dilatation ≥4 cm should be advised against pregnancy and offered termination if pregnant. Prophylactic beta-blockers should be considered to retard the progression of aortic root dilatation in pregnancy. In addition to the more ominous cardiovascular complications, obstetrical morbidities, including uterine inversion, postpartum hemorrhage, and rectovaginal perforation, have been reported.

PERIPARTUM CARDIOMYOPATHY

ESSENTIALS OF DIAGNOSIS

- Peripartum cardiomyopathy is a dilated cardiomyopathy of unknown cause.
- It usually is diagnosed during late pregnancy or in the 4–5 months after delivery.
- It is diagnosed with the finding of left ventricular systolic dysfunction in a woman with no history of cardiac disease.

Pathogenesis

At present, the etiology of peripartum cardiomyopathy is unclear. A number of pathophysiologic mechanisms have been proposed, including inflammation, myocarditis, an abnormal maternal immunologic response to fetal antigens, and other environmental factors. A single clear cause, however, has not been identified.

Clinical Findings

Patients usually present with dyspnea, cough, chest discomfort, or fatigue. The diagnosis is based on the following criteria:

- Presentation with heart failure during the last month of pregnancy or within 5 months postpartum
- Absence of an underlying cause for the heart failure
- No history of heart disease before presentation
- Evidence of left ventricular systolic dysfunction by an ejection fraction <45% or reduced shortening fraction

Echocardiogram typically reveals a reduction in cardiac contractility and dilation of the left ventricle without hypertrophy. Serial B-type natriuretic peptide levels may be a useful marker to follow through the pregnancy.

Complications

Patients with ejection fraction of <35% are at risk or thromboembolism; therefore, prophylactic anticoagulation during pregnancy and full anticoagulation for 7–10 days after delivery should be considered.

Treatment

Patients with a diagnosis of peripartum cardiomyopathy should be delivered after stabilization of the mother. Principles of therapy are similar to that in the nonpregnant state, including supportive care (consisting of bed rest and fluid and salt restriction) and medical therapy. Medical therapy includes diuretics, vasodilators, and digitalis with or without beta-blockers. The use of angiotensin-converting enzyme inhibitors is contraindicated during pregnancy.

Prognosis

Cardiac function normalizes within 6 months of delivery in approximately half of patients with peripartum cardiomyopathy. Long-term outcomes of patients with previous history of peripartum cardiomyopathy is related to recovery of left ventricular ejection fraction (LVEF). Patients with recovered LVEF have a 20% risk of developing heart failure during future pregnancy. On the other hand, patients with persistent left ventricular dysfunction have a 30% risk of congestive heart failure and 17% risk of maternal mortality in their subsequent pregnancy. There is considerable controversy regarding the safety of subsequent pregnancy in patients with a history of peripartum cardiomyopathy and normalization of left ventricular function. It is recognized that left ventricular systolic function may decline with the subsequent pregnancy, even in patients who had normalization after the prior pregnancy. Careful prepregnancy counseling and discussion about the risks, including the potential for life-threatening complications, should be outlined with the patient and partner before proceeding with a subsequent pregnancy.

PREGNANCY AFTER PROSTHETIC HEART VALVE REPLACEMENT

ESSENTIALS OF DIAGNOSIS

- Patients with prosthetic heart valve are particularly at risk during pregnancy due to difficulties in maintaining adequate and consistent levels of anticoagulation.

Pathogenesis

Many women with a history of valvular heart disease may have undergone prosthetic valve replacement before pregnancy, either with mechanical or bioprosthetic valves. The use of bioprosthetic/tissue valve obviates the need for anticoagulants, but the life span of bioprosthetic valves is only 8–10 years, and anticoagulation may still be required if the patient is in atrial fibrillation. Compared with mechanical valves, the high rate of bioprosthetic valve deterioration is primarily determined by the younger age group (ie, childbearing years ([29% vs. 82%]). Recent studies report no impact of pregnancy on the overall bioprosthetic valve longevity. The majority of pregnant women have mechanical prosthesis in place these days.

Complications

Women with prosthetic valves during pregnancy are at risk of a number of complications, including valve failure, heart failure, thromboembolism, bleeding related to anticoagulation, and infection.

Treatment

Management of women with mechanical valves involves careful therapeutic anticoagulation. The options include oral anticoagulation with warfarin, unfractionated heparin, and low-molecular-weight heparin. Use of warfarin in the first trimester of pregnancy carries the risk of teratogenicity, as it crosses the placental barrier and can affect fetal cartilage and bone development. Warfarin in doses <5 mg/day has significantly lower risk of fetal complications. As warfarin crosses the placental barrier, it may cause fetal anticoagulation with risk of intracranial bleeding at the time of delivery. Therefore, warfarin is not a preferred agent toward the end of pregnancy, and patients are generally switched to a heparin preparation at 36 weeks of gestation. Unfractionated heparin and low-molecular-weight heparin do not cross the placental barrier and have no teratogenic threat to the fetus. Three regimens for anticoagulation during pregnancy are heparin throughout the pregnancy, warfarin throughout the pregnancy, or a combination of both drugs using heparin during the first trimester to minimize the possible teratogenic effect of warfarin, switching to warfarin in the late first trimester, then switching back to heparin in the late third trimester in anticipation of delivery in order to minimize fetal anticoagulation. There is considerable controversy regarding the best approach to the patient who requires anticoagulation for a mechanical heart valve during pregnancy. The risk to the mother versus the risk to the fetus must be discussed and carefully reviewed. It should be emphasized that regardless of the anticoagulation regimen used, meticulous monitoring and follow-up are mandatory.

SUMMARY

Most pregnant patients with cardiac disease have successful outcomes with careful follow-up. Valvular stenotic lesions pose a high risk to the mother and the fetus, whereas regurgitant lesions are tolerated well by pregnant women. Extremely high-risk patients should be advised against pregnancy and be offered termination if they become pregnant. A team of high-risk obstetrician, cardiologist, and anesthesiologist is recommended to optimize maternal and fetal outcome.

Abbas AE, Lester SJ, Connolly H. Pregnancy and the cardiovascular system. *Int J Cardiol* 2005;98:179–189. PMID: 15686766.

Bonow RO, Carabello B, de Leon AC, et al. ACC/AHA Guidelines for the Management of Patients with Valvular Heart Disease. Executive Summary. A report of the American College of Cardiology/American Heart Association Task Force on Practice Guidelines (Committee on Management of Patients with Valvular Heart Disease). *J Heart Valve Dis* 1998;7: 672–707. PMID: 9870202.

Campuzano K, Roqué H, Bolnick A, Leo MV, Campbell WA. Bacterial endocarditis complicating pregnancy: Case report and systematic review of the literature. *Arch Gynecol Obstet* 2003;268:251–255. PMID: 12728325.

Hameed AB, Chan K, Ghamsary M, Elkayam U. Longitudinal changes in the B-type natriuretic peptide levels in normal pregnancy and postpartum. *Clin Cardiol* 2009; 32:E60–E62. PMID: 19455566.

Friedrich E, Hameed A. Fluctuations in the anti-factor Xa levels with therapeutic enoxaparin anticoagulation in pregnancy. *J Perinatol* 2010;30:253–257. PMID: 19829297.

Hameed AB, Mehra A, Rahimtoola SH. The role of catheter balloon commisurotomy for severe mitral stenosis in pregnancy. *Obstet Gynecol* 2009;114:1336–1340. PMID: 19935039.

Elkayam U, Tummala PP, Rao K, et al. Maternal and fetal outcomes of subsequent pregnancies in women with peripartum cardiomyopathy. *N Engl J Med* 2001;344:1567–1571. PMID: 11372007.

Elkayam U, Bitar F. Valvular heart disease and pregnancy: Part II: Prosthetic valves. *J Am Coll Cardiol* 2005;46:403–410. PMID: 16053950.

Elkayam U, Bitar F. Valvular heart disease and pregnancy: Part I: Native valves. *J Am Coll Cardiol* 2005;46:223–230. PMID: 16022946.

Hameed A, Karaalp IS, Tummala PP, et al. The effect of valvular heart disease on maternal and fetal outcome of pregnancy. *J Am Coll Cardiol* 2001;37:893–899. PMID: 11693767.

Hung L, Rahimtoola SH. Prosthetic heart valves and pregnancy. *Circulation* 2003;107:1240–1246. PMID: 12628941.

Reimold SC, Rutherford JD. Clinical practice. Valvular heart disease in pregnancy. *N Engl J Med* 2003;349:52–59. PMID: 12840093.

Siu SC, Sermer M, Colman JM, et al. Prospective multicenter study of pregnancy outcomes in women with heart disease. *Circulation* 2001;104:515–521. PMID: 11479246.

Sutton SW, Duncan MA, Chase VA, Marce RJ, Meyers TP, Wood RE. Cardiopulmonary bypass and mitral valve replacement during pregnancy. *Perfusion* 2005;20:359–368. PMID: 16363322.

PULMONARY DISORDERS IN PREGNANCY

ASPIRATION PNEUMONITIS

ESSENTIALS OF DIAGNOSIS

- Aspiration of gastric contents can occur during pregnancy, most commonly during labor or after delivery.
- Aspiration can lead to pneumonitis that may be life-threatening.

Pathogenesis

A number of factors in pregnancy contribute to an increased risk of aspiration and aspiration pneumonitis. The risk of aspiration of gastric contents is increased during pregnancy due to elevated intra-abdominal pressure, decreased gastroesophageal sphincter tone, delayed gastric emptying, and diminished laryngeal reflexes. Aspiration may be the result of passive regurgitation or active vomiting. Aspiration was reported to account for 30–50% of maternal deaths related to anesthetic complications, and if bacterial infection after aspiration occurred, usually after 24–72 hours, the mortality rate could be even higher. Due to advances in obstetric— and particularly anesthetic—management, the incidence of aspiration pneumonitis and its complications has been considerably reduced. Aspiration pneumonitis has also been called Mendelson's syndrome, named after the physician who described a large series of women with this complication in association with aspiration at time of operative intervention.

Prevention

Given the high risk associated with aspiration pneumonitis, including the possibility of maternal death, every effort should be made to prevent this potentially catastrophic condition. General anesthesia is the main risk factor related to aspiration, and expert airway management during induction and intubation is extremely important.

Oral intake during labor is not generally recommended. Women undergoing elective caesarean delivery should not be given anything by mouth for at least 6–8 hours before the procedure. All anesthetized obstetric patients should be intubated. Laryngeal reflexes will generally prevent aspiration while patients are awake, but the reflexes will be altered in patients who are given excessive sedation, in patients who are under anesthesia, or in patients with seizures. Pain, anxiety, narcotics, and labor itself may cause delayed gastric emptying and increased intragastric pressure. Lowering the volume of gastric contents to <25 mL and raising the gastric pH to >2.5 will reduce the risk of pulmonary injury if aspiration occurs. Clear, nonparticulate systemic alkalizers (eg, sodium citrate-Bacitra, or Alka-Seltzer) must be used instead of particulate oral antacids (eg, magnesium trisilicate, Maalox, Riopan). Thirty milliliters of a clear antacid should be routinely given to all women 30 minutes before induction of anesthesia.

Gastric acidity may also be reduced by histamine-2 (H_2) receptor blockers. Cimetidine and ranitidine have been reported to be safe for use during pregnancy. Metoclopramide may increase lower esophageal sphincter tone and enhance gastric emptying. However, antacids are preferred, particularly in emergency situations, because they are reliable and fast acting. H_2 blockers and metoclopramide are not recommended for routine use.

Clinical Findings

The pathologic mechanism, clinical manifestations, and outcome depend on the volume (≥25 mL), acidity (pH ≤2.5), and composition (presence or absence of solid particles) of the aspirate. Small volumes of a very acidic aspirate will be highly toxic, whereas relatively large volumes of a buffered aspirate can be relatively well tolerated. Aspiration of large, solid particulate matter may occlude portions of the larger bronchi, resulting in hypoxia, pulmonary hypertension, and even death. With smaller particles, bronchial obstruction occurs more distally, resulting in atelectasis, hypoxia, and inflammation of the bronchial mucosal and respiratory distress. Symptoms immediately after aspiration include dyspnea, bronchospasm, cyanosis, tachycardia, and even respiratory arrest. The patient will be hypoxic, hypercapnic, and acidotic. If infection supervenes, fever and leukocytosis will occur 48–72 hours later. The localization of the chest X Ray abnormalities will depend on the patient's position when the aspiration occurred: a) at the lung bases if she was upright, b) in the upper lobes or in the superior segment of the lower lobes if she was supine. A picture of diffuse interstitial pulmonary edema ("white out") may be seen after aspiration of large amounts of very acidic material.

Treatment

If aspiration occurs during anesthesia, immediate intubation and suction should be performed, followed by ventilation and adequate oxygenation. Positive end-expiratory pressure may help to better expand areas of fluid-filled collapsed lung. Bronchoscopic suction should be performed as soon as possible if the aspirate contains solid particles. A chest x-ray film should be taken and serial blood gas determinations made. These patients should be managed in the intensive care unit.

If the gastric fluid pH is >3.0 and the patient appears to be well oxygenated, she can be followed closely with periodic chest x-ray films and blood gas determinations. The picture usually resolves without antibiotics in 48–72 hours, except when infection occurs. Therefore, antibiotics should not be given routinely or empirically; they should be administered when clinical evidence and cultures indicate the presence of a superimposed bacterial infection. The bacterial flora is often polymicrobial but anaerobes from the mouth usually predominate, and therefore penicillin or clindamycin are the antibiotics more often recommended. The use of corticosteroids is not universally agreed upon.

Calthorpe N, Lewis M. Acid aspiration prophylaxis in labour: Survey of UK obstetric units. *Int J Obstet Anesth* 2005;14: 300–304. PMID: 16154737.

De Souza DG, Doar LH, Metha SH, et al. Aspiration prophylaxis and rapid sequence induction for elective cesarean delivery: Time to reassess old dogma? *Anesth Analg* 2010;110: 1503–1505. PMID: 20418311.

Hawkins JL, Chang J, Palmer SK, et al. Anesthesia-related maternal mortality in the United States: 1979-2002. *Obstet Gynecol* 2011;117:69–74. PMID: 21173646.

Mitka M. Experts, organizations debate whether women in labor can safely eat and drink. *JAMA* 2010;303:927–978. PMID: 20215600.

Paranjothy S, Griffiths JD, Broughton HK, et al. Interventions at cesarean sections for reducing risk of aspiration pneumonitis. *Cochrane Database Syst Rev* 2010:CD004943. PMID: 20091567.

ASTHMA DURING PREGNANCY

ESSENTIALS OF DIAGNOSIS

- Most patients are diagnosed with asthma before pregnancy and already are receiving treatment.
- Symptoms suggestive of asthma include cough, dyspnea, chest tightness, and wheezing, particularly when episodes occur episodically.
- Pulmonary function studies are useful to confirm the diagnosis and should be part of the initial investigations.

Pathogenesis

The general prevalence of asthma appears to be increasing. Recent studies report that asthma occurs in up to 9% of the general US population and in 3.7–8.4% of pregnant women. Therefore, asthma has become one of the most common medical illnesses complicating pregnancy. The increased prevalence is reported worldwide, particularly in urban areas, and is generally attributed to industrial pollution. However, marked geographic variations occur, and the extent to which genetic predisposition plays a role is still under active investigation.

Common triggers of asthma include upper respiratory infections (more commonly viral); administration of beta-blockers, aspirin, or nonsteroidal anti-inflammatory drugs; sulfites and other food preservatives; allergens such as pollen, animal dander, mites, or molds; smoking; gastric reflux; and exercise or other causes of hyperventilation. Both cigarette smoking and other major environmental pollutants are specifically associated with fetal damage.

Childhood-onset asthma affects males more often than females. In contrast, adult-onset asthma reportedly occurs more frequently in women. Overall, the prevalence and severity of asthma are consistently reported to be greater in women than in men. Women also are reported to require more frequent emergency room visits and more hospitalizations. Therefore, sex hormones are believed to play a role in the differences observed in the occurrence of asthma, although the exact mechanisms are not completely understood. Asthma shows variations during the menstrual cycle, with premenstrual exacerbation more often reported. Reports on asthma during the menopause are more conflicting, with some studies noting improvement but others reporting more episodes of bronchospasm after 6 months of hormone replacement therapy.

No consistent effect (either worsening or improvement) during pregnancy has been observed, although one-third of women with more severe disease reportedly became worse late in the second trimester or early in the third trimester. Possible factors contributing to improvement include the higher levels of cortisol (anti-inflammatory) and progesterone (smooth muscle relaxant) and for worsening the higher (5–6 times) rate of sinusitis and gastroesophageal reflux during pregnancy. Others speculate that pregnancy does not have an effect on asthma and that the variations observed are simply part of the natural history of the disease or due to variable medication compliance when women find out that they are pregnant. Some become more compliant and their asthma improves, and others stop their medication, fearing for the fetus, and their disease worsens. The responses in subsequent pregnancies are somewhat more consistent and in 60% of women tend to be similar to those that occurred during the first pregnancy.

Clinical Findings

A diagnosis of asthma is usually made on clinical grounds and without much difficulty if an adequate history and physical examination are obtained. Most patients are diagnosed with asthma before pregnancy and already are receiving treatment. Symptoms suggestive of asthma include cough, dyspnea, chest tightness, and wheezing, particularly when episodes occur episodically. Pulmonary function studies are useful to confirm the diagnosis and should be part of the initial investigation and surveillance of disease. The forced expiratory volume in 1 second (FEV_1)/forced vital capacity (FVC) ratio will be <70%, and the airway obstruction can be reversed by administration of a short-acting $beta_2$-agonist preparations.

Asthma currently is classified according to severity as (1) mild intermittent, (2) mild persistent, (3) moderate persistent, and (4) severe persistent. In mild intermittent asthma, symptoms do not occur more often than twice per week, and nocturnal symptoms do not occur more often than twice per month. The peak expiratory flow (PEF) or the FEV_1 is >80% of normal, with <20% variability. In mild persistent asthma, symptoms occur more often than twice per week but not daily, and nocturnal symptoms occur more often than twice per month. The PEF or FEV_1 still is at least 80% of normal, but with greater (20–30%) variability. In moderate persistent asthma, symptoms occur daily, and nocturnal symptoms occur more than once per week. The PEF or FEV_1 is <80% but >60% of normal, with >30% variability. In severe persistent asthma, daytime symptoms occur continually, and nocturnal attacks occur frequently. The PEF or FEV_1 is <60% of normal, with >30% variability.

Differential Diagnosis

Rarely, bronchospasm is caused by a condition other than asthma. These conditions include acute left ventricular heart failure (also called *cardiac asthma*), pulmonary embolism, exacerbation of chronic bronchitis, carcinoid tumors, upper airway obstruction (laryngeal edema, foreign body), gastroesophageal reflux, and cough caused by some medications.

Complications

Potential maternal complications include hyperemesis gravidarum, pneumonia (women with asthma account for >60% of pneumonia cases in pregnancy), preeclampsia, vaginal bleeding, more complicated labors, and more caesarean deliveries. Fetal complications can include intrauterine growth restriction, preterm birth, low birth weight, neonatal hypoxia, and increased overall perinatal mortality. Women with severe asthma are at the highest risk. However, patients are at little or no increased risk when the disease is effectively treated and controlled.

Treatment

A. General Measures

The main goal of therapy is to maintain normal or near normal maternal pulmonary function to allow adequate fetal oxygenation, prevent exacerbations, and allow the patient to maintain her usual activities. In general, pregnant women are receptive to educational interventions that will improve their asthma management, and the benefits are likely to continue after delivery. A good example is learning the proper use of portable peak flow meters to objectively evaluate asthma severity, because clinical symptoms and the patient's own perception of the severity of asthma often are inaccurate. The PEF rate correlates well with FEV_1 and allows the detection of worsening at an early stage before serious symptoms appear as well as the evaluation of response to treatment while the patient is still at home. Avoidance of potential asthma triggers also is extremely important. The general principles of management for pregnant asthmatic women are similar to those for nonpregnant patients and include removing pets if necessary, encasing mattresses and pillows in airtight covers, carefully washing the bedding, keeping ambient humidity <50%, avoid vacuuming (or at least wear a mask), using air conditioning and air filters, avoiding outdoor activities when allergens and air pollution levels are high, and avoiding nonallergen irritants, such as strong odors, food additives, aspirin, beta-blockers, and particularly tobacco smoke. Several recent studies have shown that these measures not only are beneficial, but are cost-effective as well. Every effort should be made to achieve smoking cessation during pregnancy, which is a very serious but modifiable factor associated with adverse outcome.

Patients undergoing immunotherapy may continue doing so during pregnancy but without any further dose increase. Starting immunotherapy de novo during pregnancy is not recommended because uterine contractions are likely to develop if anaphylaxis occurs.

Influenza vaccination is currently recommended for all pregnant women during the flu season. This recommendation is of the utmost importance for pregnant women with asthma. Asthma sufferers also should receive the pneumococcal vaccine but preferably before pregnancy.

Treating rhinitis and sinusitis, which often are associated with asthma and may trigger exacerbations, is important. Treatment of rhinitis includes reducing exposure to antigens (environmental control); intranasal cromolyn sodium, antihistamines (tripelennamine or chlorpheniramine), and intranasal steroids are very beneficial. For treatment of sinusitis, amoxicillin (erythromycin if allergic to penicillin), oxymetazoline (nasal spray or drops), and pseudoephedrine are more often used.

B. Pharmacologic Therapy

Many women have the impression that most, if not all, medications might be harmful to the fetus. However, they should be informed that the risk of uncontrolled asthma is far worse than any of the potential side effects of the most common medications used to treat asthma. Most women with asthma can be managed effectively during pregnancy, and complications are generally confined to patients with uncontrolled asthma.

1. Mild intermittent asthma—These patients do not need daily medications. When symptoms occur, 2 puffs of a short-acting $beta_2$ agonist can be used as needed. More data are available for use of albuterol than for any other $beta_2$ agonist during pregnancy, and no harm to the fetus has been observed to date. These women may still experience severe exacerbations, which may be separated by long asymptomatic periods, and a short course of systemic corticosteroids may be needed.

2. Mild persistent asthma—The preferred therapy for this group of patients is a low-dose inhaled corticosteroid. More experience is available for budesonide use in pregnancy, and the published data regarding its safety and lack of risk for congenital anomalies are reassuring. Less experience is reported with beclomethasone, but the published data also are reassuring. Inhaled corticosteroids suppress and may even prevent airway inflammation, which plays a critical role in the pathogenesis of asthma and may decrease airway responsiveness as well. Because they may decrease and sometimes even obviate the need for systemic steroids, their use is now recommended at earlier stages of asthma. However, the full benefits may not be seen for 2–4 weeks, so they are not recommended as part of the treatment of acute attacks. Use of a mouth spacer to minimize systemic absorption is strongly recommended. Inhaled corticosteroids are likewise beneficial for rhinitis (2 sprays in each nostril twice daily).

Alternative, but not preferred, therapies for this group include inhaled cromolyn sodium, leukotriene receptor antagonists, or sustained-release theophylline. Cromolyn sodium is also anti-inflammatory drug, but its efficacy is less predictable than that of the inhaled corticosteroids, and the benefits may not be seen for 4–6 weeks. Nevertheless, cromolyn sodium seems to be free of side effects for mother or fetus. Few data on the use of leukotriene receptor modifiers during pregnancy are available; they are reported to be safe in animals, but human data are limited. The extensive experience with theophylline during pregnancy indicates that it is safe for the fetus except when maternal levels exceed 12 μg/mL. In these cases, the fetus or newborn may develop jitteriness, tachycardia, and vomiting.

3. Moderate persistent asthma—The preferred treatment is a combination of a low-dose or medium-dose inhaled corticosteroid and a long-acting $beta_2$ agonist. Alternative therapies (but again not preferred) include a low-dose or medium-dose inhaled corticosteroid and either theophylline or a leukotriene receptor antagonist. However, given the limited data on human pregnancy, the use of leukotriene receptor modifiers is reserved for patients who showed a very good response before pregnancy but are not responding well to other medications while pregnant.

4. Severe persistent asthma—The preferred treatment is a high-dose inhaled corticosteroid and a long-acting inhaled $beta_2$ agonist as well as (if needed) a systemic corticosteroid, such as 2 mg/kg/d of prednisone or equivalent steroid not to exceed 60 mg/d, with an attempt to taper to the minimal effective dose. An alternative, but not preferred, treatment includes a high-dose inhaled corticosteroid and sustained-release theophylline (keeping maternal systemic levels at 5–12 μg/mL for the reasons explained previously).

The US Food and Drug Administration has recently issued warnings about the use of long-acting beta-agonists (LABAs). A paradoxical increase in exacerbations in some patients, particularly in children, has been reported mainly with LABA monotherapy. The specific recommendations include (1) not to use LABAs without other asthma-controller medications, (2) stop LABA use once asthma control is achieved and maintain it with other medications, (3) do not use LABAs if the asthma is controlled with inhaled steroids, and (4) use fixed-dose combinations with an inhaled steroid to minimize the likelihood of LABA use alone.

Systemic corticosteroids are used when any of the other drug combinations cannot control the asthma. They usually are given first as a short, rapidly tapering course (eg, 40–60 mg/d of prednisone or equivalent steroid for 1 week, tapering off during the second week). If these courses fail to effectively control symptoms for <2–3 weeks, long-term systemic corticosteroid treatment may be needed. In these cases, the lowest effective dose or alternate-day therapy, if possible, should be used. Potential maternal side effects include impaired glucose tolerance or frank diabetes mellitus, preeclampsia, intrauterine growth restriction, and premature delivery. With prolonged use (>1–2 months) of pharmacologic doses, maternal adrenal insufficiency may occur, and adequate coverage during periods of stress (including labor and delivery) is mandatory. Use during the first trimester is associated with a higher risk for facial clefts (lip and palate). Pregnant women with asthma who are steroid dependent should be managed by an internist/pulmonologist who is experienced in the treatment of asthma during pregnancy.

C. Other Asthma Medications

Nonselective beta agonists such as epinephrine and isoproterenol are sometimes given subcutaneously during acute asthma attacks. Epinephrine use during pregnancy should be avoided because epinephrine causes vasoconstriction and reduces fetal oxygenation. It is teratogenic in animals as well as in humans. Isoproterenol also is teratogenic in animals. Because many other alternative therapies are available, isoproterenol use in humans is best avoided. Iodine-containing medications should be avoided during pregnancy because the fetus may be at risk for developing a goiter, which may become very large and cause airway obstruction and even asphyxia. Nedocromil sodium is similar to cromolyn sodium. No reports on humans are available, but nedocromil sodium has not been observed to be teratogenic in animal experiments. Anticholinergic medications such as atropine (which block bronchoconstriction by inhaled irritants) may accelerate the fetal heart rate and inhibit breathing. Ipratropium has not been reported to be teratogenic in animals, but data on humans are lacking. Glycopyrrolate has been used safely in humans near term, and no defects have been reported in animal experiments.

1. Acute asthmatic attack—During acute exacerbations, dyspnea, cough, wheezing, and chest tightness increase and expiratory flow decreases. A few, well-educated patients with relatively mild attacks might be managed at home, taking advantage of the judicious use of peak flow measurements. However, any serious exacerbation most likely will require hospitalization. Great care should be exercised to maintain a maternal PO_2 >70 mm Hg and O_2 saturation >95%. A maternal PO_2 <60 mm Hg will result in marked fetal hypoxia.

General measures include reassuring the patient and avoiding sedatives, which may depress respiration. Oxygen can be administered by mask or nasal catheter with the goal of maintaining PO_2 >70 mm Hg and O_2 saturation >90% to ensure adequate fetal oxygenation at all times. A few patients may require endotracheal intubation and mechanical ventilation to maintain an adequate oxygen supply. Blood gas determinations are necessary for this purpose. A chest x-ray film should be part of the initial evaluation. Antibiotics are given only if evidence of bacterial infection is present. Some pregnant women receiving large amounts of intravenous fluids, $beta_2$ agonists, and corticosteroids reportedly develop pulmonary edema, so this risk should be considered under these circumstances.

Initial pharmacologic treatment includes an inhaled $beta_2$ agonist administered by a metered-dose inhaler, 2–4 puffs every 20 minutes to a maximum of 3 doses or less if side effects appear. A subcutaneous $beta_2$ agonist (eg, terbutaline 0.25 mg) is also given and can be repeated once 20 minutes later. Systemic corticosteroids are recommended early in the course of treatment of acute exacerbations. The most frequently used corticosteroid is methylprednisolone administered intravenously at an initial dose of 1–2 mg/kg/d. At present, intravenous theophylline is used much less frequently for acute exacerbations because of the early use of corticosteroids. When necessary, the recommended initial loading dose is 5–6 mg/kg given intravenously over 20–30 minutes. The loading dose is not given if the patient was receiving adequate oral doses before the acute attack, or only half the loading dose is given if the patient was receiving theophylline but only intermittently. Maintenance doses are 0.7 mg/kg/h. Serum levels should be monitored to avoid maternal levels in excess of 12 μg/mL.

After admission to the hospital, administration of $beta_2$-agonists is continued by nebulized aerosol every 4–6 hours; administration of intravenous corticosteroids also is continued (eg, methylprednisolone 0.5–1 mg/kg twice daily). If theophylline was started, it is continued per the maintenance dose protocol, with careful monitoring of maternal serum levels to avoid fetal toxicity. As the patient improves, the $beta_2$-agonist aerosols are continued (2 puffs every 4–6 hours), and at this point the inhaled steroids (high dose, per the protocol for the severe persistent asthma) are resumed or the therapy initiated if the patient was not receiving them before the acute attack. If the clinical improvement continues, the systemic steroids can be switched to the oral route (eg, prednisone 0.5 mg/kg/d, with gradual tapering attempted while maximizing inhaled steroid treatment). If theophylline was being given, it also should be changed to the oral route (6 mg/kg), with close monitoring of maternal serum levels.

D. Management During Labor and Delivery

The medications that were being administered before the onset of labor should be continued. Adequate control should be maintained, because labor has been reported to trigger an acute attack in approximately 10% of women with asthma. Peak expiratory flow measurements should be obtained at regular intervals to monitor pulmonary status closely. Adequate hydration should be maintained and pain relief provided as necessary. Fentanyl is considered a good analgesic choice for these patients. Analgesics and/or narcotics, which can cause histamine release, should be avoided because of the possibility of respiratory depression and bronchospasm. Continuous O_2 monitoring is mandatory to ensure that O_2 saturation is >95% at all times.

Medications to avoid include prostaglandin F_2 because it may cause bronchospasm. Prostaglandin E_2, either gel or suppository, is safe for women with asthma and can be used if necessary from the obstetric standpoint. Oxytocin is safe and considered the medication of choice for induction.

Epidural anesthesia is preferred because it reduces O_2 consumption and minute ventilation. General anesthesia may trigger an attack, but the risk may be reduced by pretreatment with atropine (see earlier for potential fetal effects) and glycopyrrolate, which have a bronchodilatory effect. A low concentration of halogenated anesthetic may provide bronchodilation as well. For induction, ketamine is preferred. It is very important that an anesthesiologist experienced in the care of pregnant women be consulted ahead of time when anticipating anesthesia needs.

Ergot derivatives should be avoided because they may precipitate bronchospasm. If postpartum hemorrhage occurs, oxytocin is the best choice. If a prostaglandin is needed, then prostaglandin E_2 is preferred. Aspirin and nonsteroidal anti-inflammatory drugs (eg, indomethacin) may trigger severe bronchospasm as well as ocular, nasal, dermal, and gastrointestinal inflammation in 3–8% of asthmatic patients and are best avoided. Magnesium is safe for asthma but with careful monitoring to avoid respiratory depression.

E. Fetal Monitoring

An ultrasound examination in early pregnancy is useful to confirm dating and to provide a baseline to evaluate future growth assessment. Serial ultrasounds are recommended for women with moderate and severe asthma because they are the most at risk for fetal growth restriction. No specific guidelines have been issued for antepartum fetal surveillance other than very general recommendations such as "when needed in the third trimester to assure fetal well being" and "daily recording of fetal movements is encouraged." Many institutions offer fetal surveillance starting at 32–34 weeks to patients with moderate and severe asthma and at any time during the third trimester when an exacerbation occurs. There is unanimous agreement that all patients with asthma should undergo continuous fetal monitoring during labor and delivery.

F. Breastfeeding

Inhaled $beta_2$ agonists, cromolyn sodium, steroids (inhaled), and ipratropium are safe while breastfeeding. Systemic (oral or parenterally administered) steroids may enter into breast milk but only in small amounts if the total daily dosage contains <40 mg of prednisone (or equivalent steroid).

Asthma and pregnancy—Update 2004. NAEPP working group report on managing asthma during pregnancy: Recommendations for pharmacologic treatment—Update 2004. NIH Publication No. 05-3279. Bethesda, MD: National Institutes of Health; 2004.

Bakhireva LN, Schatz M, Jones KL, Chambers CD. Asthma control during pregnancy and the risk of preterm delivery or impaired fetal growth. *Ann Allergy Asthma Immunol* 2008;101:137–143. PMID: 18727468.

Blais L, Forget A. Asthma exacerbations during the first trimester of pregnancy and the risk of congenital malformations among asthmatic women. *J Allergy Clin Immunol* 2008;121:1379–1384. PMID: 18410961.

Blaiss MS. Management of rhinitis and asthma in pregnancy. *Ann Allergy Asthma Immunol* 2003;90 (Suppl 3):16–22. PMID: 12839108.

Bittoun R, Femia G. Smoking cessation in pregnancy. *Obstet Med* 2010;3:90–93.

Breton MC, Beauchesne MF, Lemiere C, et al. Risk of perinatal mortality associated with asthma during pregnancy. *Thorax* 2009;64:101–106. PMID: 19008298.

Chowdhury BA, Pan GD. The FDA and safe use of long-acting beta-agonists in the treatment of asthma. *N Engl J Med* 2010;362:1169–1171. PMID: 20181964.

Dombrowski MP, Schatz M; ACOG Committee on Practice Bulletins-Obstetrics. ACOG practice bulletin: Clinical management guidelines for obstetrician-gynecologists No. 90, February 2008: Asthma in pregnancy. *Obstet Gynecol* 2008;111:457–464. PMID: 18238988.

Enriquez R, Griffin MR, Carroll KN, et al. Effect of maternal asthma and asthma control on pregnancy and perinatal outcomes. *J Allergy Clin Immunol* 2007;120:625–630. PMID: 17658591.

Hartert TV, Neuzil KM, Shintani AK, et al. Maternal morbidity and perinatal outcomes among pregnant women with respiratory hospitalization during influenza season. *Am J Obstet Gynecol* 2003;189:1705–1712. PMID: 14710102.

Incaudo GA, Takach P. The diagnosis and treatment of allergic rhinitis during pregnancy and lactation. *Immunol Allergy Clin North Am* 2006;26:137–154. PMID: 16443148.

Kallen B, Otterblad Olausson P. Use of anti-asthmatic drugs during pregnancy. Congenital malformations in the infants. *Eur J Clin Pharmacol* 2007;63:383–388. PMID: 17279357.

Kattan M, Stearns SC, Crain EF, et al. Cost-effectiveness of a home-based environmental intervention for inner-city children with asthma. *J Allergy Clin Immunol* 2005;116:1058–1063. PMID: 16275376.

Kwon HL, Triche EW, Belanger K, Bracken MB. The epidemiology of asthma during pregnancy: Prevalence, diagnosis and symptoms. *Immunol Allergy Clin North Am* 2006;26:29–62. PMID: 16443142.

Li YF, Langholz B, Salam MT, Gilliland FD. Maternal and grandmaternal smoking patterns are associated with early childhood asthma. *Chest* 2005;127:1232–1241. PMID: 15821200.

National Asthma Education and Prevention Program. Expert panel report 3: guidelines for the diagnosis and management of asthma. NIH Publication No. 07-4051. Bethesda, MD: National Heart, Lung and Blood Institute; August 2007.

Schatz M, Dombrowski MP, Wise R, et al. Asthma morbidity during pregnancy can be predicted by severity classification. *J Allergy Clin Immunol* 2003;112:283–288. PMID: 12897733.

Tamasi L, Somoskovi A, Muller V, et al. A population-based case-control study on the effect of bronchial asthma during pregnancy for congenital abnormalities in the offspring. *J Asthma* 2006;43:81–86. PMID: 16448971.

PNEUMONIA

ESSENTIALS OF DIAGNOSIS

- Although the incidence of pneumonia in pregnancy is not increased over nonpregnant women, pneumonia is associated with an increased risk of maternal and fetal complications.
- Pneumonia typically presents with fever, chills, and productive cough.

Pathogenesis

Pneumonia is a rare complication of pregnancy, affecting fewer than 1% of all pregnancies. However, it is associated with significant fetal and maternal morbidity. In fact, before the advent of antibiotics, pneumonia in pregnancy was associated with maternal mortality rate of >20%.

A number of different organisms are implicated in causing pneumonia during pregnancy. The most common identifiable organisms are pneumococcus and *Haemophilus influenza*. Viral agents are also implicated in causing pneumonia, including influenza A, infectious mononucleosis, and, less frequently, varicella. Influenza A has been of particular concern in recent years due to well-publicized outbreaks with exceedingly virulent strains. Influenza A has a higher mortality rate in pregnancy than in nonpregnant patients. Pregnant women with viral pneumonia can develop superimposed bacterial infection.

Prevention

One important preventative measure is the injectable influenza vaccine. The intramuscular influenza vaccine consists of inactivated virus. This vaccine is safe when administered during any trimester of pregnancy. It is recommended that pregnant women receive this vaccine during the flu season.

Clinical Findings

Pneumonia usually presents with fever, chills, and productive cough. Patients may also experience pleuritic chest pain and shortness of breath. On physical examination, most women are febrile. Many women will be tachycardic or tachypneic. Chest auscultation reveals rales or decreased breath sounds over the affected fields. With bacterial pneumonia, chest radiograph demonstrates lobar consolidation or infiltrate. With viral pneumonia, chest radiograph may appear normal. Complete blood count reveals leukocytosis with a left shift in most cases.

Differential Diagnosis

Depending on the patient's presenting signs and symptoms, the differential diagnosis includes pulmonary embolism, bronchitis, and uncomplicated influenza.

Complications

Pneumonia during pregnancy increases the risk of a number of fetal and maternal complications, including pulmonary edema and preterm labor.

Treatment

In general, inpatient management is advised for pregnant women with pneumonia. Treatment with antibiotics is the cornerstone of therapy. Community-acquired pneumonia should be treated with azithromycin or azithromycin plus ceftriaxone in severe cases. For patients with varicella pneumonia, acyclovir is recommended. Treatment of influenza and influenza pneumonia during pregnancy is recommended with oseltamivir. For cases of oseltamivir-resistant strains of influenza, zanamivir is recommended. Maternal oxygen saturation should be maintained ≥96% with oxygen nasal canula or face mask if needed.

TUBERCULOSIS

ESSENTIALS OF DIAGNOSIS

- Pregnancy is not associated with an increased risk of contracting tuberculosis or progression from latent tuberculosis to active tuberculosis.
- Pregnancy and prenatal care do provide a unique screening opportunity for women at risk of tuberculosis.
- Effective treatment of tuberculosis during pregnancy and/or in the postpartum period is important to prevent transmission to the neonate.

Pathogenesis

Tuberculosis (TB) was the leading causes of death in the United States for many years until the introduction of effective therapy in the early 1950s. Since then, the number of reported cases declined steadily, until recently, when higher numbers are being identified. This situation is attributed to increased immigration from countries with a high tuberculosis prevalence and particularly to the HIV/acquired immunodeficiency syndrome (AIDS) epidemic. Worldwide, TB is very prevalent, with 8 million new cases and 2 million deaths annually. Eighty percent of TB deaths in women occur during their childbearing years, and pregnant women are not spared from TB effects. Many of these at-risk women will seek health care only when pregnant, thus providing an opportunity for diagnosis and treatment.

Tuberculosis in adults is mainly (>95%) a disease of the pulmonary parenchyma caused by *Mycobacterium tuberculosis,* a nonmotile, acid-fast aerobic rod. Transmission usually occurs by inhalation of droplets produced by infected individuals when coughing. The droplets can remain suspended in the air for prolonged periods (several hours). The persons most at risk for becoming infected are family members and other close contacts, such as coworkers and roommates (elderly residents and employees in long-term care facilities, correctional institutions), homeless individuals, and intravenous drug users. After the initial inhalation, the bacilli multiply in the alveoli and subsequently spread to the regional lymph nodes and to other organs such as the upper lung regions, kidneys, bones, central nervous system, and, rarely, during pregnancy, to the placenta. In most people, the infection is contained by cell-mediated immunity, which develops 2–10 weeks after exposure, when the infected sites are walled off by granulomatous inflammation and the tuberculin tests then becomes reactive. At this stage, these persons are not infectious and are asymptomatic except for the positive tuberculin skin test. After the initial exposure, the risk of developing active disease during the following 2–5 years is generally given as 5–15%, but the risk later falls to very low levels <1–2%. However, active disease may ensue if a person is unable to contain the infection when first exposed or if the person subsequently becomes immunocompromised and the infection is reactivated at a time remote from the initial exposure.

Clinical Findings

Most cases of tuberculosis can be diagnosed on the basis of a history of cough, weight loss, positive tuberculin skin test, and chest x-ray film.

A. Symptoms and Signs

Primary TB infection is usually asymptomatic, except in the rare instances when dissemination occurs. Typical symptoms include cough, sometimes with hemoptysis, low-grade fever, weight loss, fatigue, night sweats, and anorexia, although some patients may have few symptoms. In extrapulmonary TB, the symptoms are related to the organ system involved.

B. Laboratory Findings

The definitive diagnosis is made after positive identification of the bacilli by Ziehl-Neelsen staining and a positive culture, usually from a sputum sample. At times, the sample for culture will be obtained from the urine, other body fluid, or a body tissue. Although acid-fast bacilli can be identified on stained slides, culture confirmation is required, which may take several weeks. Faster detection methods are currently under development.

C. Tuberculin Skin Test

The tuberculin skin test is the most important screening test for tuberculosis. It should be performed early in pregnancy, especially in high-risk populations. An induration of 5 mm or greater is considered positive in individuals with HIV infection; those in close contact of persons with active, infectious tuberculosis; in persons with typical x-ray findings who were never previously treated; and in intravenous drug users. An induration of 10 mm or more is considered positive in persons who have risk factors other than HIV, such as diabetes mellitus, silicosis, chronic use of corticosteroids or other immunosuppressive drugs, cancer (solid tumors as well as leukemias and lymphomas), chronic renal insufficiency, gastrectomy or intestinal bypass, or malabsorption and chronic malnutrition with body weight 10% or less below the ideal. Data are being accumulated on the effectiveness of other methods that could be used as an alternative to the skin test.

D. Chest X-Ray Film

With the abdomen shielded and preferably after the first trimester, a chest x-ray film should be taken in patients in whom skin testing is positive after an earlier negative test and in patients with a suggestive history or physical examination even though skin testing is negative. Findings suggestive of TB include upper lobes or superior lower lobe segments' nodular infiltrates that at times may become cavitary. A calcified hilar node and an also calcified peripheral nodule (Ghon's complex) constitute a healed primary lesion. A small number of patients may initially have a normal x-ray.

Complications

Congenital tuberculosis is rare, although cases of fetal infection have been reported. The infection may occur when the fetus swallows infected amniotic fluid or be bloodborne through the umbilical circulation. The criteria for diagnosis include positive bacteriologic studies occurring within the first few days of life with an exclusion of an extrauterine infection source, as more commonly contamination occurs after birth from an infected mother or a close relative. The most common signs are nonspecific and include fever, failure to thrive, lymphadenopathy, hepatomegaly, and splenomegaly. The disease usually is miliary or disseminated. An early diagnosis is necessary for effective treatment.

Treatment

A. Medical Therapy

Untreated tuberculosis is far riskier to the mother and fetus than any of the potential medications necessary to treat active disease. Treated TB does not seem to lead to adverse maternal or fetal outcomes, whereas untreated cases are associated with intrauterine growth restriction, low birth weight, and lower Apgar scores. A preventive course of isoniazid (isonicotinic acid hydrazide [INH]) is generally recommended for those with a positive skin test and no evidence of active disease. Unless there is high risk of developing TB (eg, close contact with a person with active disease), such preventive therapy is withheld in those older than 35 years and during pregnancy and early postpartum because of an increased risk for INH-related hepatitis, particularly in Latina and African American women. Some authors recommended antepartum INH prophylaxis if there is well-documented evidence of recent (<2 years) TB skin conversion to positive even if there are no other risk factors. The argument is that waiting until after delivery might not be as effective in preventing recurrences, perhaps because the high frequency of noncompliance with medication taking postpartum. When the duration of PPD positivity is unknown, but greater than 2 years, and no active disease, INH prophylaxis is postponed until after delivery. In those at high risk (particularly in cases of HIV/AIDS or close contacts with a person with active TB), preventive INH treatment is initiated as soon as evidence of tuberculosis infection (but no active disease) is documented. The recommended dose of INH is 300 mg/d for 6–9 months as well as pyridoxine (vitamin B_6) to prevent INH-related neuropathy. Periodic evaluation of liver function is recommended to detect hepatotoxicity early if it occurs. Most studies have shown no teratogenic effects of INH.

Active tuberculosis should be treated as soon as the diagnosis is made. Most treatment programs consist of a 3-drug regimen, usually INH 5 mg/kg/d (total 300 mg/d), ethambutol 15 mg/kg/d, and rifampin 10 mg/kg/d (maximum 600 mg/d) for 8 weeks, and the INH and rifampin to complete 9 months. Local public health departments should be consulted to obtain data about drug resistance. These 3 medications cross the placenta, but no adverse fetal side effects have been reported to date. Pyrazinamide has been used in addition to the 3 medications mentioned in areas of highly drug-resistant tuberculosis but is not routinely recommended during pregnancy because of limited safety data. Because of the risk for fetal (and maternal) ototoxicity, streptomycin, kanamycin, and capreomycin should not be used. Isoniazid has many therapeutic advantages (eg, high efficacy, patient acceptability, and low cost) and appears to be the safest drug for use during pregnancy. The major side effects of INH are hepatitis, hypersensitivity reactions, peripheral neuropathy, and gastrointestinal distress. A baseline liver function test should be obtained and then repeated periodically because of higher risk of hepatotoxicity during pregnancy and the first 6 months postpartum. Pyridoxine 50 mg/d should be administered to prevent INH-induced neuritis due to vitamin B_6 deficiency. Optic neuritis is a rare complication reported with ethambutol use. Rifampin may cause hepatitis, hypersensitivity reactions, occasional hematologic toxicity, flulike syndrome, abdominal pain, acute renal failure, and thrombocytopenia. Rifampin may increase the metabolic rate of oral contraceptives through activation of the hepatic P450 enzyme system, so an alternative form of contraception may be necessary after delivery in these patients while they are taking rifampin.

B. Obstetric Management

Routine antepartum obstetric management includes adequate rest and nutrition, family support, correction of anemia if present, and regular follow-up visits. Immediate neonatal contact is allowed if the mother has received treatment for inactive disease and no evidence of reactivation is present. In patients with inactive disease in whom prophylactic INH was not given or those with active disease in whom adequate treatment was given, early neonatal contact may be allowed, provided the mother is reliable in continuing therapy. A mother with active disease should receive at least 3 weeks of treatment before coming into contact with her baby, and the baby must also receive prophylactic INH.

There are no absolute contraindications to breastfeeding once the mother is noninfectious. Although antituberculosis drugs are found in breast milk, the concentrations are low, and the risk of toxicity in the infant is considered to be minimal. However, each case should be judged individually. In general, breastfeeding is not contraindicated while the mother is taking antituberculosis medications.

Immunization of the newborn with bacille Calmette-Guérin (BCG) vaccine remains controversial. If prompt use of INH as prophylaxis is unlikely or if the mother has INH-resistant disease, BCG vaccination of the infant should be considered.

Prognosis

If the pregnant patient is adequately treated with antituberculosis chemotherapy for active disease, tuberculosis generally has no deleterious effect, either during the course of pregnancy or the puerperium or on the fetus. Pregnant women have the same prognosis as nonpregnant women. Tuberculosis is not a reason for recommending a therapeutic abortion, as it was sometimes the case before the advent of effective treatment.

Boggess KA, Myers ER, Hamilton CD. Antepartum or postpartum isoniazid treatment of latent tuberculosis infection. *Obstet Gynecol* 2000;96:(5 Pt 1):757–762. PMID: 11042314.

McCarthy FP, Rowlands S, Giles M. Tuberculosis in pregnancy: Case studies and a review of Australia's screening process. *Aust NZ J Obstet Gynecol* 2006;46:451–455. PMID: 16953862.

Renal & Urinary Tract Disorders in Pregnancy

28

Nathan S. Fox, MD
Andrei Rebarber, MD

For a discussion of normal renal and urinary tract function in pregnancy, see Chapter 6, Normal Pregnancy.

URINARY TRACT INFECTION

Asymptomatic Bacteriuria

ESSENTIALS OF DIAGNOSIS

- Urine culture demonstrating the presence of bacteria in the urine in the absence of maternal symptoms of urinary tract infection

Pathogenesis

Asymptomatic bacteriuria is defined as the presence of actively multiplying bacteria in the urinary tract, excluding the distal urethra, in a patient without any obvious symptoms. The incidence is the same in nonpregnant and pregnant females and averages 2–10%; however, a number of physiologic changes that occur during pregnancy predispose a woman to bacteriuria, including increased glucose concentration in the urine and increased stasis due to the relaxant progesterone effect. Risk factors for developing asymptomatic bacteriuria include low socioeconomic status, parity, age, sexual practice, and medical conditions such as diabetes and sickle cell trait. *Escherichia coli* is the most common offending organism for asymptomatic bacteriuria (approximately 80% of cases). The *Klebsiella-Enterobacter-Serratia* group, *Staphylococcus aureus, Enterococcus,* group B *Streptococcus,* and *Proteus* are responsible for the remainder of cases.

The primary concern with asymptomatic bacteriuria in pregnancy is that it is associated with an increased risk of both maternal and fetal complications during pregnancy (see later).

Prevention

Certain underlying medical disorders may predispose a woman to asymptomatic bacteriuria during pregnancy. Asymptomatic bacteriuria is twice as common in pregnant women with sickle cell trait and 3 times as common in pregnant women with diabetes or with renal transplant as in normal pregnant women. Therefore, we advise that monthly routine urine cultures should be performed in these women when pregnant.

Clinical Findings

The diagnosis of asymptomatic bacteriuria is based on isolation of microorganisms with a colony count $>10^5$ organisms per milliliter of urine in a clean-catch specimen in a woman who is experiencing no symptoms of urinary tract infection. When obtaining a clean-catch specimen, the patient should be instructed to clean the vulvar area from front to back to avoid contamination of the urine sample.

Complications

The main risk of asymptomatic bacteriuria is the development of pyelonephritis. Due to anatomic dilation in the renal system during pregnancy, there is increased stasis of urine in the pregnant urinary tract and a much higher risk of developing an overt infection from the bacteruria. Due to this risk, many authorities advocate screening all pregnant women for bacteruria, and unlike nonpregnant women, a pregnant woman found to have bacteruria should be treated promptly. If asymptomatic bacteriuria is left untreated in pregnancy, up to 40% of patients will develop symptoms of urinary tract infection (UTI), a significant increase from the almost negligible risk in nonpregnant women. Approximately 25–30% of women will develop acute pyelonephritis. With treatment, the rate is less than 10%. Asymptomatic bacteriuria has been associated with preterm delivery, fetal loss, and preeclampsia. Treatment of asymptomatic bacteruria has been associated in large reviews with a reduction in the risk of preterm birth and low birth weight babies. On the other hand, approximately 2% percent of pregnant women with a negative urine culture will develop symptomatic cystitis and pyelonephritis.

Treatment

A midstream urine specimen should be collected for culture at the initial prenatal visit and repeated later in pregnancy. At each prenatal visit, dipstick testing should be performed. If proteinuria is present, urinalysis, culture, or both should be done. A pregnant woman with sickle cell trait should have urine culture and sensitivity testing every 4 weeks. The US Preventive Health Task Force states that single urine culture at 12–16 weeks' gestation has 80% sensitivity. Alternatively, regular dipstick testing for leukocyte esterase and nitrites has a negative predictive value >95% and sensitivity of 50–92%.

Pregnant women should be encouraged to maintain adequate fluid intake and to void frequently.

The initial antibiotic selection should be empiric. Based on the fact that the most common offending pathogen is *E coli,* a sulfonamide, nitrofurantoin, or a cephalosporin is a reasonable choice. These antibiotics should be safe for the mother and fetus, with minimal side effects. A 5- to 14-day course of one of these agents will effectively eradicate asymptomatic bacteriuria in approximately 65% of pregnant patients. A urine culture should be repeated 1–2 weeks after therapy is started. Recurrent infections occur in approximately 30% of patients treated once and in approximately 15% of patients who have been treated twice and/or have not responded to initial therapy.

Nitrofurantoin (US Food and Drug Administration [FDA] category B) should be avoided in mothers with glucose-6-phosphatase deficiency. Additionally, sulfa drugs (FDA category B) are often avoided late in pregnancy because of the theoretical increased likelihood of neonatal hyperbilirubinemia. Tetracyclines (FDA category D) are contraindicated during pregnancy because of dental staining in the exposed child. Trimethoprim (FDA category C) is a folic acid antagonist; therefore, trimethoprim-sulfamethoxazole is generally avoided during organogenesis; it may be used when alternatives are limited.

Suppressive therapy may be appropriate for women with bacteriuria that persists after 2 or more courses of therapy. Nitrofurantoin (50–100 mg orally at bedtime) for the duration of the pregnancy is a commonly used.

Smaill F, Vazquez JC. Antibiotics for asymptomatic bacteriuria in pregnancy. *Cochrane Database Syst Rev* 2007:CD000490. PMID: 17443502.

Acute Cystitis

ESSENTIALS OF DIAGNOSIS

- Urine culture demonstrating the presence of bacteria in the urine in a patient symptomatic for urinary tract infection

Pathogenesis

Acute cystitis is uncommon in pregnancy (approximately 1%). The bacteria causing acute cystitis are similar to those in asymptomatic bacteriuria.

Clinical Findings

Clinically, the patient presents with symptoms of urinary frequency, urgency, dysuria, and suprapubic discomfort. The urine often is cloudy and malodorous and should be cultured to confirm the diagnosis and to identify antibiotic sensitivities. A colony count of $\geq 10^3$ confirms cystitis in a symptomatic patient.

Treatment

The treatment of cystitis is the same as for asymptomatic bacteriuria. A urine culture should be repeated 1–2 weeks after therapy is started. As with asymptomatic bacteriuria, suppressive therapy may be appropriate for women with UTI that persists after 2 or more courses of therapy. Nitrofurantoin (50–100 mg orally at bedtime) for the duration of the pregnancy is commonly used.

Acute Pyelonephritis

ESSENTIALS OF DIAGNOSIS

- The presence of bacteria in urine culture
- Maternal symptoms of flank pain and/or systemic signs of fever, chills, nausea/vomiting

Pathogenesis

Acute pyelonephritis occurs in 1–2% of all pregnant women (usually, although not invariably, in those with previous asymptomatic bacteriuria) and is associated with risk to the mother and fetus. It is one of the most common causes of hospitalization during pregnancy.

Certain anatomic changes that occur during pregnancy predispose pregnant women to pyelonephritis, including increased stasis of the urine in the urinary tract due to smooth muscle relaxation in the ureters.

Prevention

Acute pyelonephritis is best prevented by screening for and treating asymptomatic bacteruria.

Clinical Findings

Clinical manifestations of acute pyelonephritis include fever, shaking chills, costovertebral angle tenderness, flank pain, nausea and vomiting, headache, increased urinary frequency, and dysuria. Patients almost always have pyuria on urinalysis. Urine examination will reveal significant bacteriuria with pyuria and white blood cell casts in the urinary sediment. A count of 1–2 bacteria per high-power field in unspun urine or >20 bacteria in the sediment of a centrifuged specimen of urine collected by bladder catheterization helps in the bedside diagnosis. The absence of pyuria should raise suspicion for another disorder. Due to this, a urine specimen should be obtained and sent for culture before any antibiotics are given in order to properly identify the causative organism and antibiotic susceptibility. Blood cultures may also be sent, as they will be positive 10–20% of the time, although it is unclear whether management should be any different for women with positive blood cultures as outcomes tend to be the same.

Differential Diagnosis

For the patient presenting with back or flank pain, the differential diagnosis includes appendicitis, musculoskeletal pain, costochondritis, and chorioamnionitis. Urinalysis and urine culture can help to differentiate among these disorders.

Complications

Maternal complications include fever, bacterial endotoxemia, endotoxic shock, renal insufficiency, anemia, leukocytosis, thrombocytopenia, and elevated fibrin split product levels. Risk factors for recurrent or severe disease are a history of pyelonephritis, urinary tract malformation, or urinary calculi. The maternal anemia may be due to marrow suppression, increased erythrocyte destruction, or diminished red cell production. Pulmonary dysfunction has been described in association with acute pyelonephritis. Symptoms and signs may range from minimal (mild cough and slight pulmonary infiltrate) to severe (adult respiratory distress syndrome requiring intensive therapy).

Obstetrical complications include preterm labor and prematurity, fetal death, and intrauterine growth restriction.

Treatment

A pregnant woman with pyelonephritis initially should be evaluated in the hospital. Antibiotics should be given parenterally once a urine culture is sent, and hypovolemia should be corrected. Acetaminophen can be used as an antipyretic, if indicated. Vital signs, including respiratory rate, and input and output should be closely monitored. Pulse oximetry may be useful. A first-generation cephalosporin (FDA category B) such as cefazolin 1 g parenterally every 8 hours usually is effective. However, due to increasing antibiotic resistance, the local susceptibilities should be considered when selecting the initial antibiotic. Ceftriaxone 1 g parenterally every 24 hours often is effective for most *Enterobacteriaceae* in this setting. The urine culture and sensitivities guide therapy thereafter. When the patient is afebrile for 48 hours, parenteral therapy may be changed to an effective oral antibiotic. A total course of 14 days of antibiotic is commonly administered. Note that drugs with very high protein binding, such as ceftriaxone, may be inappropriate the day before parturition because of the possibility of bilirubin displacement and subsequent kernicterus.

If no clinical response is seen in 48–72 hours, a resistant organism can be treated by adding an aminoglycoside such as gentamicin 3–5 mg/kg per 24 hours in 3 divided doses given every 8 hours. Failure to respond may be caused by urolithiasis or a structural urinary tract abnormality. Ultrasound imaging of the kidneys and urinary tract usually is the next diagnostic test if the patient does not defervesce after 48 hours of antibiotic therapy. Perinephric abscess causing persistent pain and fever can be identified by ultrasound. Perinephric abscess usually is due to obstruction complicated by infection. The perinephric abscess should have percutaneous drainage (preferably computed tomography or ultrasound-guided) for both diagnostic and therapeutic purposes, in addition to administration of antibiotic therapy. An intravenous pyelogram or computed tomography urogram is often useful if a lack of response continues. A preliminary "scout" film and a film taken 15 minutes after administration of intravenous contrast often are helpful. In selected cases of persistent infection or obstruction, cystoscopy and retrograde pyelography are needed.

Although many women who present with pyelonephritis will have uterine contractions, they are almost always due to the fever and resultant hypovolemia. Tocolytics should be used with extreme caution, as they can greatly increase the risk of respiratory distress. Typically the contractions resolve with the administration of intravenous (IV) fluids and antibiotics.

Respiratory distress is a severe systemic complication of pyelonephritis. It is caused by bacterial endotoxins increasing alveolar permeability and a resultant pulmonary edema. It is more common in women with the following: tachycardia, tachypnea, blood transfusion, fever of 103° degrees, tocolytics, and excessive IV fluids. Patients presenting with respiratory symptoms should be managed aggressively and often require an intensive care setting, as shock can ensue.

Prognosis

Cunningham reported that after an episode of pyelonephritis, recurrent bacteriuria occurred in 28% of women, and pyelonephritis recurred in 10% during the same pregnancy. A more recent study by Wing et al identified that 5% of pregnant

Table 28–1. Antibiotic regimen for pyelonephritis.

Antibiotic	Dosage	Route	Frequency
Ampicillin plus gentamicin	1–2 g	IV	q4–6h
	2 mg/kg, then 1.7 mg/kg	IV	q8h
Ampicillin/sulbactam	3 g	IV	q6h
Cefazolin	1–2 g	IV	q6–8h
Ceftriaxone	1–2 g	IV or IM	q24h
Mezlocillin	3 g	IV	q6h
Piperacillin	4 g	IV	q8h

IM, intramuscular; IV, intravenously; q, every.

patients had urine culture positive for organisms only 2 weeks after completion of initial therapy for pyelonephritis. In the same study, 6.3% had culture positive for organisms later in their antepartum course, and 6.3% developed recurrent pyelonephritis. For this reason, antibiotic suppressive therapy with nitrofurantoin 100 mg orally at bedtime, or a similar regimen, is continued during the pregnancy and during the puerperium, often for 6 weeks (Table 28–1). Monthly urine cultures to identify a recurrent UTI may be similar in effectiveness to antibiotic suppression for patients who are allergic or who prefer not to take antibiotics.

Periodic culture of the urine assists in detection of recurrence. **Relapse** is defined as recurrent infection from the same species and type-specific strain of organism present before treatment; this represents a treatment failure. Most relapses occur <2 weeks after completion of therapy. **Reinfection** is recurrent infection due to a different strain of bacteria after successful treatment of the initial infection, occurring >3 weeks after the completion of therapy.

Hill JB, Sheffield JS, McIntire DD, Wendel GD Jr. Acute pyelonephritis in pregnancy. *Obstet Gynecol* 2005;105:18–23. PMID: 15625136.

URINARY CALCULI

ESSENTIALS OF DIAGNOSIS

- Maternal symptoms of urinary tract obstruction that may include back or flank pain, hematuria, and/or dysuria
- Evidence of urinary tract calculi on imaging studies

Pathogenesis

The incidence of urinary calculi is not altered by pregnancy. The incidence is 0.03–0.35% of pregnancies, and the incidence increases as gestational age advances (only 20% present in the first trimester). Stones cause obstruction, infection, pain, and hematuria (present in 75–95% of patients, one-third of whom have gross hematuria). Recurrent hospitalization, preterm labor and delivery, and need for operative intervention are increased. The causes of urinary calculi are the same in pregnant and nonpregnant women: chronic UTI, hyperparathyroidism or other causes of hypercalciuria, gout (uric acid), and obstructive uropathy. Congenital or familial cystinuria and oxaluria are less common causes. Most stones are composed of calcium, usually calcium phosphate.

The physiologic hydroureter of pregnancy is more prominent on the right side; however, stones occur with equal frequency on either side. The physiologic hydroureter of pregnancy increase the likelihood that a pregnant patient will spontaneously pass her stone(s).

Clinical Findings

Patients may present with a variety of symptoms, including typical renal or ureteric colic, vague abdominal or back pain that may radiate into the groin, fever, nausea, and vomiting. The patient may have a history of recurrent UTI or hematuria. Fever, bacteriuria, and flank pain may suggest coexisting pyelonephritis from obstruction. The differential diagnosis includes other acute abdominal conditions unrelated to pregnancy (eg, appendicitis, biliary colic or tract disease, adnexal torsion) and conditions related to pregnancy (eg, abruption placentae, preterm labor, chorioamnionitis). When fever attributed to pyelonephritis persists beyond 48 hours of parenteral antibiotic treatment, then obstruction due to urolithiasis must be evaluated. Hematuria, ranging from microscopic to gross, is usually present, although it is not pathognomonic for urolithiasis. The index of suspicion should be high in the clinical situations described, in patients in whom urine culture is negative in the setting of suspected pyelonephritis, or in cases of persistent hematuria or recurrent UTI.

Clinical diagnosis is confirmed by ultrasound examination of the urinary tract. In a study by Butler et al in 57 pregnant women had 73 admissions for symptomatic nephrolithiasis over a 13-year period, they noted that calculi were visualized in 21 of 35 (60%) renal ultrasonographic examinations and 4 of 7 (57%) abdominal x-ray studies when these were performed as the initial test. In contrast, urolithiasis was discovered in 93% of cases (n = 8) in which single-shot intravenous pyelography was performed as the initial diagnostic test. In selected cases, excretory urography includes a precontrast scout film and another image obtained 20 minutes after contrast injection. This examination exposes the fetus to 0.2 rad. The common indications for intravenous pyelography include microscopic hematuria and recurrent UTI. Sterile urine culture should be performed when pyelonephritis is suspected. Alternate means of assessing for urinary tract stones during pregnancy if ultrasound is inconclusive include magnetic resonance urography (which involves no radiation exposure to the fetus) and computed tomography urogram.

Differential Diagnosis

The differential diagnosis of urinary tract calculi includes pyelonephritis, appendicitis, chorioamnionitis, cholecystitis, and cholelithiasis. The combination of urinalysis, urine culture, and imaging studies of the abdomen and pelvis can distinguish among these diagnoses.

Complications

A recent retrospective cohort study by Swartz et al found that women admitted for nephrolithiasis during pregnancy had an increased risk of preterm delivery versus those without stones (adjusted odds ratio = 1.8; 95% confidence interval, 1.5–2.1). This finding has potential implications for counseling of pregnant women with kidney stones requiring hospital admission and possible use of biomarkers (eg, cervical length or fetal fibronectin testing) to better identify at-risk pregnancies. Additionally, it may prompt definitive treatment of small, asymptomatic stones in women during reproductive years.

Treatment

Treatment includes hospital admission, adequate hydration, urine culture and Gram stain, appropriate antibiotic therapy, correction of electrolyte imbalances, and systemic analgesia (eg, opioids). Epidural analgesia may be considered for patients with severe pain. Most (75–85%) stones pass spontaneously, due in part to the normally dilated urinary tract of pregnancy. The patient should strain her urine so that a stone can be analyzed. Surgical intervention, such as ureteral stenting, transurethral cystoscopic stone extraction, nephrostomy drainage, or open surgery, can be performed by a urologist if indicated for unremitting pain, sepsis, infection unresponsive to antibiotic therapy, or obstructive uropathy. Shock wave lithotripsy is contraindicated during pregnancy, although it has been performed in 6 pregnancies inadvertently. More recently, ureteroscopy and holmium:YAG laser lithotripsy has been performed successfully in 8 pregnant women with 10 symptomatic stones and 2 encrusted ureteral stents. This device delivers energy to a localized area, can be used with flexible ureteroscopes, and is effective with stones of all compositions. Procedural success was achieved in all but 1 case (91%), with no obstetric or urologic complications.

Ross AE, Handa S, Lingeman JE, Matlaga BR. Kidney stones during pregnancy: An investigation into stone composition. *Urol Res* 2008;36:99–102. PMID: 18470509

Swartz MA, Lydon-Rochelle MT, Simon D, Wright JL, Porter MP. Admission for nephrolithiasis in pregnancy and risk of adverse birth outcomes. *Obstet Gynecol* 2007;109:1099–1104. PMID: 17470589.

Teichman JM. Acute renal colic from ureteral calculus. *N Engl J Med* 2004;350:684–693. PMID: 14960744.

ACUTE RENAL FAILURE

ESSENTIALS OF DIAGNOSIS

- Acute renal failure is defined as sudden reduction in renal function and glomerular filtration rate.
- The most common causes of acute renal failure in pregnancy are severe preeclampsia and placental abruption.

Pathogenesis

Acute renal failure is defined as sudden impairment in kidney function that leads to retention of waste products (eg, urea) and abnormal fluid and electrolyte balance. It occurs infrequently in pregnancy but carries a high mortality rate; therefore, it must be prevented when possible and treated aggressively. Most cases in pregnancy result from acute hypovolemia associated with obstetric hemorrhage (placenta previa, placental abruption, or postpartum hemorrhage), preeclampsia, or sepsis.

Clinically, acute renal failure is a condition in which the kidneys are temporarily unable to perform their excretory and regulatory functions. Blood urea nitrogen and serum creatinine concentrations are increased. Without prompt intervention, the condition may result in abortion, low birthweight, premature labor, and stillbirth. Dialysis may be required. Although hypotension-induced preterm contractions may occur during dialysis, numerous successful pregnancy outcomes have been reported after dialysis during pregnancy. In these cases renal failure most often is the result of intrinsic renal disease.

Similar to nonpregnant patients, acute renal failure can be classified as prerenal, renal, or postrenal. A classic formula in determining the cause of renal failure is the fractional excretion of sodium (FENa). It is defined as the (urine sodium/plasma sodium) divided by (urine creatinine/plasma creatinine). It can also be stated as (urine sodium × plasma creatinine) divided by (urine creatinine × the plasma sodium). Either way, it reflects the amount of sodium excreted as compared with the creatinine. If the renal tubules are working (eg, as in prerenal failure) the sodium excretion should be less than the creatinine, as the kidneys work extra hard to maintain sodium. If the tubules are not working (eg, renal cause, acute tubular necrosis), the kidneys will not be able to resorb sodium and the fractional sodium excreted will be elevated. This can also be measured with urinary sodium levels.

In the prerenal type, acute renal failure occurs due to renal hypoperfusion secondary to maternal hypovolemia (eg, hemorrhage, hyperemesis gravidarum, dehydration, abruptio placentae, septicemia), circulating nephrotoxins (eg, aminoglycosides), aortic or renal artery stenosis or a narrowed off renal arteriole (due to sepsis, nonsteroidal anti-inflammatory drugs [NSAIDs], and certain dyes), mismatched blood transfusion, preeclampsia–eclampsia, disseminated intravascular coagulation, and hypoxemia (eg, chronic lung disease and heart failure). In prerenal failure, the patient typically is clinically hypovolemic with an increased pulse and decreased blood pressure. Laboratory tests show a serum blood urea nitrogen (BUN) to creatinine ratio >20, an FENa <1, urinary sodium <20 mEq/L (often <10) and urinalysis with concentrated urine, few elements in sediment, and positive hyaline casts.

Renal causes can be divided into 4 groups: glomerular, tubular, interstitial and vascular. For all groups, the FENa is >1. Glomerular causes can be from systemic lupus erythematosus (SLE), postinfectious glomerulonephritis, or membranoproliferative glomerulonephritis. In the preceding causes, low complement levels are found. With normal complement levels, the glomerular causes can be immunoglobulin A nephropathy, Goodpasture's syndrome, or rapidly progressive glomerulonephritis. In all glomerular causes, urinalysis shows red blood cell (RBC) casts, dysmorphic RBC's and protein.

When the renal failure is from the tubules, it is called acute tubular necrosis. It can be caused by an ischemic insult, shock, and surgery. It can also be caused by toxins, either endogenous (magnesium, creatinine phosphokinase) or exogenous (drugs, dyes, aminoglycosides). These patients typically have a normal physical exam. Urinalysis may be normal or may have brown pigmented casts. Urinary sodium is >25 mEq/L (often >60). Again, FENa is >1.

Renal failure from the interstitium can be caused by NSAIDs and allergies (often to penicillins and cephalosporins). Eosinophils are found in the blood and urine. The patients typically have a fever and rash. If renal failure is caused by a vasculitis, "telescoped" urinary sediment may be seen, in which red cells, white cells, oval fat bodies, and all types of casts are noted in relatively equal amounts.

The postrenal type is caused by urinary obstruction from ureteric stone, retroperitoneal tumor, and other diseases. Bilateral ureteral obstruction due to polyhydramnios is rare. The BUN to creatinine ratio is usually approximately 10.

Prevention

In obstetric practice, prevention of acute renal failure should be the aim, with appropriate volume replacement to maintain adequate urine output. Proper management of high-risk obstetric conditions (eg, preeclampsia–eclampsia, abruptio placentae, chorioamnionitis), ready blood availability, and avoidance of nephrotoxic antibiotics are important.

Clinical Findings

Acute renal failure is defined as urine output <400 mL in 24 hours (or <0.5 mL/kg/h) or an increase in serum creatinine (at least 1.5 fold). BUN concentrations are also typically increased.

The clinical course has been divided into an oliguric phase, a diuretic phase, and a recovery phase. In the oliguric phase, urine output drops to <30 mL/h, with accumulation of BUN and potassium. The patient becomes acidotic with the increase in hydrogen ion and loss of bicarbonate. In the diuretic phase, large volumes of dilute urine are passed, with loss of electrolytes due to absence of function of the renal tubules. As tubular function returns to normal in the recovery phase, the volume and composition of urine normalize. Clinical manifestations and complications include anorexia, nausea and vomiting, lethargy, cardiac arrhythmia (secondary to electrolyte disturbance), anemia, renal or extrarenal infection, thrombocytopenia, metabolic acidosis, and electrolyte imbalance (hyperkalemia, hyponatremia, hypermagnesemia, hyperphosphatemia, hypocalcemia).

Complications

Without prompt intervention, obstetric complications include pregnancy loss, low birth weight, premature labor, and stillbirth.

Treatment

Specific treatments include the following.

A. Emergency Treatment

Underlying causes of acute renal failure (eg, hemorrhagic shock) may require emergency treatment for correction of the underlying disorder.

B. Surgical Measures

Surgical measures include determination and correction of any obstructive uropathy or sepsis due to infected products of conception. Such problems should be treated as surgically appropriate. If obstructive uropathy is determined to be the cause, the placement of a ureteral stent or nephrostomy is indicated. Infected products of conception can be removed via dilation and curettage. Hypovolemia due to internal bleeding or uterine bleeding may require laparotomy to ligate any bleeding blood vessels or hysterectomy for definitive treatment of uterine bleeding.

C. Routine Measures

Routine measures include achieving fluid and electrolyte balance. Fluid intake can be calculated from urinary output, loss of fluid from other sources (eg, diarrhea, vomiting), and insensible loss of approximately 500 mL/d (correcting for fever may be necessary). Intake and output must be recorded carefully. The patient should be weighed daily and should maintain a constant weight or lose weight slowly (250 g/d assuming a room temperature of 22–23 °C [71–73 °F]). Hyperkalemia is a significant problem that can be controlled by administering glucose and insulin. The diet should be high in calories and carbohydrates, and low in protein and electrolytes. Parenteral feeding may be given in cases of nausea and vomiting. Prophylactic antibiotics should not be used, but known infections can be treated with antibiotics without renal toxicity. Indwelling bladder catheters are to be avoided when possible.

D. Dialysis

Dialysis is indicated if serum potassium levels rise to 7 mEq/L or more, serum sodium levels are 130 mEq/L or less, the serum bicarbonate is 13 mEq/L or less, BUN levels are more than 120 mg/dL or there are daily increments of 30 mg/dL in patients with sepsis, and dialyzable poisons or toxins are present. Different criteria are applied for renal failure in the antepartum period with a continuing pregnancy. In these cases, dialysis is instituted earlier in the process in consideration of fetal well-being. Although specific criteria have not been firmly established, one commonly used figure is a BUN level of 60 mg/dL.

E. Special Circumstances: Thrombotic Thrombocytopenic Purpura–Hemolytic Uremic Syndrome

Thrombotic thrombocytopenic purpura–hemolytic uremic syndrome (TTP-HUS) is characterized by the otherwise unexplained combination of thrombocytopenia and microangiopathic anemia. Renal failure caused by thrombotic microangiopathy may occur. Patients have been traditionally considered to have TTP when neurologic abnormalities are dominant and acute renal failure is minimal or not present, and considered to have HUS when acute renal failure is dominant and neurologic abnormalities are minimal or absent. Renal insufficiency may occur in either pregnancy-associated TTP or HUS, although it is more prevalent among patients with HUS. The optimal therapy of TTP-HUS developing in association with pregnancy includes delivery because distinction from preeclampsia may not be possible but is otherwise the same as for patients who are not pregnant. Patients who were treated with plasma infusion with or without plasma exchange in a series resulted in improved survival.

Schrier RW, Wang W, Poole B, Mitra A. Acute renal failure: Definitions, diagnosis, pathogenesis, and therapy. *J Clin Invest* 2004;114:5–14. PMID: 15232604.

Selcuk NY, Odabas AR, Cetinkaya R, Tonbul HZ, San A. Outcome of pregnancies with HELLP syndrome complicated by acute renal failure (1989–1999). *Ren Fail* 2000;22:319–327. PMID: 10843242.

CHRONIC RENAL DISEASE

ESSENTIALS IN DIAGNOSIS

- Chronic renal disease is defined as persistent kidney damage with impairment in renal function.
- The prognosis for pregnancy outcome depends on the degree of renal impairment.

Pathogenesis

Chronic renal disease, once an absolute contraindication to pregnancy, is now encountered much more often as the prognosis has become much better in the past 30 years. Currently, the best prognostic indicator is the degree of renal disease (mild moderate or severe) present before pregnancy.

For mild disease (creatinine <1.5 mg/dL), the majority of women do well and their pregnancies progress without difficulty. With moderate renal disease (creatinine 1.5–3 mg/dL), fetal outcome is usually good (>90%), but maternal status often deteriorates (up to 40% of these women). With severe disease (creatinine >3 mg/dL), women are usually infertile, and if pregnancy is achieved, the outcome for both the fetus and the patient are poor.

The normal physiologic changes seen in pregnancy are different in women with chronic renal disease. Glomerular filtration rate does increase, but often only in the patients with mild disease. Proteinuria usually more than doubles in women with underlying renal disease. Interestingly, though, even nephrotic range proteinuria is not considered by itself to be harmful to the patient or the fetus.

Despite all of the preceding generalizations, it is difficult to counsel women based on their serum creatinine alone. This is due to the fact that specific renal diseases tend to behave differently from one another. Therefore, it is important to know the patient's underlying condition before managing her during pregnancy. Also, the presence of hypertension before conception, regardless of the patient's renal function and serum creatinine, increases the risk to both mother and fetus. One generalization that can be made, though, is that women with chronic renal disease

Table 28–2. Stages of chronic renal disease.

Stage	Description	GFR (mL/min/1.73 m^2)
1	Kidney damage with normal or increased GFR	≥90
2	Kidney damage with mildly decreased GFR	60–89
3	Moderately decreased GFR	30–59
4	Severely decreased GFR	15–29
5	Kidney failure	<15 or dialysis

GFR, glomerular filtration rate.
(From the National Kidney Foundation: K/DOQI clinical practice guidelines for chronic kidney disease: Evaluation, classification and stratification. *Am J Kidney Dis* 2002;39(Suppl 1):S1–S266.)

are at increased risk of developing gestational hypertension and preeclampsia. Therefore, all of these women should be watched closely for these diseases.

It should be stated that most of the data regarding chronic renal disease and pregnancy are based on retrospective and observational data only.

Clinical Findings

Chronic renal disease can be staged based on the patient's glomerular filtration rate (Table 28–2). Women with chronic renal disease may also demonstrate some degree of elevation in serum creatinine.

Complications

Chronic renal disease is associated with an increased risk of a number of obstetrical complications, including preeclampsia, prematurity, intrauterine growth restriction, and pregnancy loss. The risk of these complications increases with increasing maternal serum creatinine level.

Treatment

General guidelines for management of patients with chronic renal disease begins with preconceptual counseling, if possible. Pregnancy should be discouraged for patients with a serum creatinine above 1.5 (some would allow up to 2.0, especially if the patient is normotensive), or at least the patient should be made fully aware that the pregnancy may have a very poor outcome for her fetus and herself. In fact, approximately 40% of women with this level of chronic kidney disease may experience an irreversible decline in glomerular filtration rate that is greater than predicted based on the patient's previous course. Patients with more than minimal disease should be comanaged by a maternal–fetal medicine specialist and either a nephrologist or an internist familiar with the management of renal diseases. Blood pressure should be strictly controlled. Baseline laboratory values should include serum creatinine, electrolytes, albumin, and cholesterol/triglycerides (for nephritic patients), and some would add baseline liver function tests, uric acid, and lactate dehydrogenase levels to help aid in the subsequent diagnosis of superimposed preeclampsia. A 24-hour urine collection for protein and creatinine clearance should be obtained as well. Patients should have close follow-up and start noninvasive fetal monitoring at approximately 32 weeks. Baby acetylsalicylic acid and calcium therapy for the prevention of preeclampsia may be considered in these patients to start after 10 weeks' gestation.

A. Glomerulonephritis

Acute glomerulonephritis during pregnancy is rare, with an estimated incidence of 1 in 40,000 pregnancies. The condition is associated with increased perinatal loss. The clinical course is variable during pregnancy and may be easily mistaken for preeclampsia. In some patients, the condition resolves early in pregnancy, with return to normal renal function. Microscopic hematuria with RBC casts is a common finding in acute glomerulonephritis. Treatment is similar to that of the nonpregnant patient and consists of controlling blood pressure, preventing congestive heart failure, administering fluids and electrolytes, and close follow-up.

The outcome of pregnancy with chronic glomerulonephritis depends on the degree of functional impairment of the kidneys, blood pressure levels before conception, and the exact histology of the glomerulonephritis. For patients with active glomerulonephritis, the principal risk for pregnancy is superimposed preeclampsia. Conditions associated with poor fetal outcome include preexisting hypertension, severe proteinuria during the first trimester, primary focal and segmental hyalinosis, and sclerosis. Successful pregnancy should be anticipated, although renal function is expected to decrease. The incidence of fetal intrauterine growth restriction, premature labor, abruptio placentae, and intrauterine fetal demise is increased. Routine prenatal care should include periodic renal function tests, control of blood pressure, ultrasonic evaluation of fetal growth, and antepartum testing for fetal well-being. Hypertension at the time of conception correlates with worsening maternal renal function during pregnancy. Early delivery is indicated after evaluation of pulmonary maturity as appropriate.

B. Lupus Nephritis

It is unclear whether patients with SLE are more likely to have a flare during pregnancy. It is known that an exacerbation is more likely if the patient has active disease at conception. Therefore, many people recommend delaying pregnancy until the SLE has been in remission for 6–12 months. This can decrease the risk of flare from 66% to 33%. What seems to be true is that pregnancy itself does not cause the flare. In small controlled studies, the rate of flare is not different between SLE-similar pregnant and nonpregnant women. If a flare does occur, severe renal manifestations can occur. Prednisone and other immunosuppressive agents have been used with success during pregnancy.

SLE patients, like other renal patients, also have a worse prognosis if pregestational hypertension exists. Specific to SLE, however, is the poor prognosis associated with antiphospholipid antibodies and lupus anticoagulant.

C. Systemic Sclerosis and Periarteritis Nodosum

For patients with these diseases, the outcome for the patients and their pregnancies is quite poor. Most of the (scant) literature describes poor fetal outcome, accelerating maternal hypertension, and occasional maternal death. There are some new data showing a better prognosis with angiotensin-converting enzyme (ACE) inhibitor treatment, but at this time most authorities recommend against conception and for early termination, if possible.

D. Diabetic Nephropathy

Diabetic nephropathy refers to diabetic patients with proteinuria of 300 mg/d. It is most commonly seen in pregestational type 1 diabetic patients, but as the pregnant population ages, more women with type 2 diabetes will have diabetic nephropathy by the time they become pregnant.

Currently, perinatal survival in these patients is approximately 95%, compared with 99% in the general population. Pregnancy does not seem to worsen renal function in mildly affected patients at baseline (serum creatinine <1.5, creatinine clearance >80 mL/min), but for those patients with moderate or severe renal dysfunction at baseline, they typically worsen as pregnancy progresses. It is unclear whether pregnancy worsens these patients' *long-term* renal function. Some studies suggest that for women with severe renal dysfunction, those who become pregnant progress to renal failure sooner than those who do not become pregnant.

Some of the renal deterioration can be avoided by strict blood pressure control during pregnancy. Because ACE inhibitors are generally contraindicated in pregnancy, a calcium channel blocker can be used instead to control hypertension, as they also have renal protective properties.

E. Reflux Nephropathy

Reflex nephropathy is a disease of the urinary tract system that starts in childhood. It is a common and generally mild disease. The majority of women have preserved renal function and are normotensive; consequently, their pregnancies are uneventful. The only significant complication that does develop is bacteruria and urinary tract infections. Therefore, they should be frequently screened for bacteruria and treated accordingly. In addition to this, because the disease may be inherited, their children should be evaluated after birth for this condition.

F. Polycystic Kidney Disease

Although the recessive form is quite rare and extremely severe, autosomal dominant polycystic kidney disease is more common and has been studied in pregnancy. Like other renal diseases, these patients do well in pregnancy if they start without hypertension and severe renal dysfunction. Again, like with the other diseases, they are more likely to develop gestational hypertension and preeclampsia. These patients, however, are also more prone to develop urinary tract infections.

G. Solitary Kidney

A solitary kidney may be the result of developmental aberration or disease requiring removal of 1 kidney. A single kidney may be abnormally developed or it may be located low, perhaps even within the true pelvis. A second small, virtually functionless kidney may not be discovered by the usual diagnostic tests. Anatomic and functional hypertrophy of the kidney usually occurs and is augmented by pregnancy. These patients should be evaluated preconceptually for the presence of infection. If renal function is normal, pregnancy is not contraindicated, and good outcomes are expected.

During pregnancy, infection in a solitary kidney must be treated aggressively. An increased rate of preeclampsia with a solitary kidney has been reported.

H. Renal Transplantation

Approximately 0.5% of women who have undergone transplantation in the reproductive age range become pregnant. A number of large series document successful pregnancy outcomes after renal transplantation. Patients with adequate renal function before pregnancy will experience little if any deterioration in graft function during pregnancy. The likelihood of graft rejection during pregnancy remains the same as in nonpregnant graft recipients. For renal transplant patients considering pregnancy, a stable serum creatinine level <1.4 mg/dL identifies a group more likely to experience an uncomplicated obstetric outcome (97% vs. 75% for patients with a higher serum creatinine level). The spontaneous abortion rate is not increased.

Patients should wait 2 years from transplantation to attempt pregnancy. They may wait only 1 year if the kidney is from a living-related donor. This is done to avoid rejection. Despite this recommendation, women who do not wait this period are still likely to have a successful pregnancy. Patients should have a serum creatinine of <2 (and preferably <1.5) as well as no signs of rejection before conception. Patients should not be hypertensive or should be made normotensive with medication before conception.

Antirejection drugs should be reduced to maintenance levels (prednisone ≤15 mg/d and azathioprine ≤2mg/kg/d; a safe dosage for cyclosporine has not been established but should be maintained <5 mg/kg/d if possible). Immunosuppressive levels should be checked frequently, as levels tend to decrease in pregnancy. Patients on steroids should have early glucose intolerance screening. Electrolyte and liver function values should be checked every 6 weeks.

The risk of infection is considerably higher during pregnancy in renal transplant patients. Primary or reactivated herpesvirus or cytomegalovirus infection may be seen. A higher rate of hepatitis B surface antigenemia is seen in dialysis patients as well.

The route of delivery depends primarily on obstetric indications. In patients with aseptic necrosis of the hip joints or other bony dystrophy secondary to long-standing disease, caesarean delivery may be required. Vaginal delivery should be the aim for patients with renal transplant. A transplanted kidney in the false pelvis usually does not cause obstruction leading to dystocia. If a caesarean section becomes indicated, close attention should be made not to damage the transplanted kidney, as it is typically located in the pelvis.

Preterm delivery, both spontaneous and indicated, is common (45–60%). Intrauterine growth restriction and fetal abnormalities caused by immunosuppressive agents taken by the mother may occur.

I. Chronic Renal Disease Requiring Dialysis

As opposed to the horrendous pregnancy outcome noted in older literature, there are data that women on dialysis have approximately a 50% chance of delivering a live infant, albeit often growth restricted or premature. There are a number of pregnancy-related differences in dialysis management:

- Erythropoietin requirements are higher to maintain an appropriate hemoglobin concentration.
- Fetal heart and uterine contraction monitoring are required, as dialysis may induce hypotension or placental insufficiency.
- The placenta produces vitamin D, so the dose of calciferol may need to be reduced to avoid hypercalcemia.
- Since pregnancy is a hypercoagulable state, more heparin may be required during dialysis.

Prognosis

For mild disease (serum creatinine <1.5 mg/dL), the majority of women do well, and their pregnancies progress without difficulty. With moderate renal disease (creatinine 1.5–3 mg/dL), fetal outcome is usually good (>90%), but maternal status often deteriorates (up to 40% of these women). With severe disease (creatinine >3 mg/dL), women are usually infertile, and if pregnancy is achieved, the outcome for both the fetus and the patient are poor.

Armenti VT, Radomski JS, Moritz MJ, et al. Report from the National Transplantation Pregnancy Registry (NTPR): Outcomes of pregnancy after transplantation. In: Cecka JM, Terasaki PI (eds): *Clinical Transplants*. Los Angeles, CA: UCLA Immunogenetics Center; 2002, p. 97. PMID: 12971441.

Bar J, Ben-Rafael Z, Padoa A, Orvieto R, Boner G, Hod M. Prediction of pregnancy outcome in subgroups of women with renal disease. *Clin Nephrol* 2000;53:437–444. PMID: 10879663.

Cohen RA, Brown RS. Microscopic hematuria. *N Engl J Med* 2003;348:2330–2338. PMID: 12788998.

Lindheimer MD, Davison JM, Katz AL. The kidney and hypertension in pregnancy: Twenty exciting years. *Semin Nephrol* 2001;21:173–189. PMID: 11245779.

Gastrointestinal Disorders in Pregnancy

29

Chad K. Klauser, MD
Daniel H. Saltzman, MD

HYPEREMESIS GRAVIDARUM

ESSENTIALS OF DIAGNOSIS

- Hyperemesis gravidarum is defined as unexplained intractable nausea, retching, or vomiting beginning in the first trimester, resulting in dehydration, ketonuria, and typically a weight loss of more than 5% of prepregnancy weight.
- Symptoms typically start between 3 and 5 weeks of pregnancy and 80% resolve by 20 weeks.
- Treatment frequently includes avoidance of noxious stimuli, medications to relieve nausea and vomiting, hydration, and possibly hospitalization.

Pathogenesis

Hyperemesis gravidarum (HEG) affects 0.3–2% of pregnant women. The pathogenesis is largely unknown, with possible contributing factors being increased levels of human chorionic gonadotropin (hCG), estradiol, and possible progesterone. It is more common among younger mothers and those with a history of motion sickness, migraines, and nausea and vomiting associated with oral contraceptives. It is more commonly seen in women carrying multiple gestations, and patients with siblings or a mother with HEG are more likely to be affected.

Clinical Findings

A. Symptoms & Signs

HEG is associated with severe nausea and vomiting that may result in dehydration, weight loss, and frequently social isolation and negative impacts on relationships with family and friends. Patients with HEG, rather than nausea and vomiting of pregnancy, tend to have an earlier onset and longer duration. Excess salivation (ptyalism) may also be seen in a subset of women with HEG.

B. Laboratory Findings

Suppressed thyroid-stimulating hormone/elevated free thyroxine and elevated liver enzymes, bilirubin, amylase, and lipase may all be noted in patients with severe nausea and vomiting; these are transiently abnormal and resolve with improvement of HEG.

C. Imaging Studies

No imaging studies are needed for the diagnosis of hyperemesis; however, they can be used to exclude other conditions such as pancreatitis, cholecystitis, or intracranial lesions.

Differential Diagnosis

Other medical conditions should be suspected if the onset of severe nausea and vomiting is after 9 weeks of gestational age. The differential diagnosis for late HEG should include gastroenteritis, gastroparesis, biliary tract disease, hepatitis, peptic ulcer disease, pancreatitis, appendicitis, pyelonephritis, ovarian torsion, diabetic ketoacidosis, migraines, drug toxicity or withdrawal, psychological conditions, acute fatty liver of pregnancy, and preeclampsia.

Complications

Maternal complications of HEG can include Wernicke's encephalopathy, acute tubular necrosis, central pontine myelinolysis, Mallory-Weiss tear of the esophagus, pneumomediastinum, and splenic avulsion. Additionally, significant psychological burden of the disease has been reported, with depression, anxiety, and lost work frequently seen among those with persistent or severe HEG. Fortunately, no clear fetal complications have been associated with HEG. One study did show that women with HEG who gain <7 kg during the entire pregnancy have a slightly higher risk of low birth weight and preterm birth. However, there are no congenital anomalies or increased risk of miscarriage or stillbirth noted.

Treatment

Treatment of HEG begins with supportive measures including hydration and vitamin supplementation (in particular thiamine to prevent Wernicke's encephalopathy). Nonpharmacologic measures such as acupuncture, hypnotherapy, avoidance of defined nausea triggers, herbal teas, vitamin B_6, and ginger may help alleviate nausea and vomiting in a subset of patients. Antihistamines as a class have been shown to be efficacious and have a long history of safety during pregnancy. Other antiemetics can be used in an algorithm that balances safety and efficacy (Table 29–1). Patients have also been shown to benefit from frequent contact with the health care provider or from an outpatient nursing services program. If weight loss persists despite therapy, nutritional supplementation by enteral tube feeding or parenteral feeding is necessary. If a patient requires hospitalization, it usually occurs prior to 8 weeks.

Prognosis

More than 50% of women have resolution of symptoms by 16 weeks of gestational age and 80% by 20 weeks. However, approximately 10% will be affected to some degree with severe nausea and vomiting for the duration of the pregnancy. HEG has been shown to recur in up to 80% of subsequent pregnancies, although earlier aggressive medical therapy prior to significant symptoms has been demonstrated to reduce both the severity and recurrence rate overall in future pregnancies.

Table 29–1. Safe and effective use of antiemetics.

Nausea or Vomiting Interfering with Daily Routine
Vitamin B_6 10–30 mg TID–QID PO
Continued symptoms after 48 hours: add doxylamine 12.5 mg TID–QID PO
Continued symptoms after 48 hours: substitute doxylamine with other antihistamine:
Promethazine 12.5–25 mg every 4 hours PO or PR
Dimenhydrinate 50–100 mg every 4–6 hours PO or PR
Consider alternative therapies at any point in this sequence:
Acupuncture or acustimulation, ginger tablets 250 mg QID
Persistent Symptoms, with or without Dehydration
Prochlorperazine 25 mg every 12 hours PR
OR
Metoclopramide 5–10 mg every 8 hours PO or IV
OR
Trimethobenzamide 200 mg every 6–8 hours PR
Dehydration or Weight Loss
Thiamine 100 mg IV daily for 3 days; continue thiamine in MVI daily
Ondansetron 8 mg every 8–12 hours IV or PO
OR
Methylprednisolone up to 16 mg TID for 3 days; taper over 2 weeks to lowest effective dose; total duration of therapy 6 weeks
Unable to Maintain Weight
Institute total enteral or parenteral nutrition

IV, intravenously; MVI, multivitamin; PO, oral; PR, per rectum; QID, 4 times a day; TID, 3 times a day.

Bottomley C, Bourne T. Management strategies for hyperemesis. *Best Pract Res Clin Obstet Gynaecol* 2009;23(4):549–564. PMID: 19261546.

Goodwin TM. Hyperemesis gravidarum. *Obstet Gynecol Clin North Am* 2008;35:401–417. PMID: 18760227.

Niebyl JR. Nausea and vomiting in pregnancy. *N Engl J Med* 2010;363:1544–1550. PMID: 20942670.

PEPTIC ULCER DISEASE

ESSENTIALS OF DIAGNOSIS

- Epigastric pain, anorexia, postprandial nausea and vomiting, or abdominal fullness.
- The incidence and severity of peptic ulcer disease (PUD) decrease during pregnancy, whereas symptoms of dyspepsia may be increased among this group.
- Esophagogastroduodenoscopy is generally considered as safe during pregnancy and is recommended for the evaluation of PUD when symptoms are severe and nonresponsive to medical therapy.

Pathogenesis

Peptic ulcers represent an erosion of the gastrointestinal mucosa, extending through the muscularis mucosae. The majority are caused by *Helicobacter pylori* infection or the use of nonsteroidal anti-inflammatory drugs (NSAIDs). These exposures affect the gastric mucosal function and repair through alterations in gastric acid secretion, gastric metaplasia, and immune responses. The incidence of PUD during pregnancy is approximately 1 in 4500 pregnancies, compared with approximately 1 per 1000 of the general population. This finding may be related to the fact that many of the risk factors/exacerbating factors for PUD are less common during pregnancy, including cigarette use, NSAID use, and alcohol intake. Ulcers are 5 times more common in the duodenum than in the stomach.

Prevention

Although PUD is multifactorial, in the absence of *H pylori*, abstaining from cigarette use and limiting the use of aspirin, NSAIDs, and alcoholic beverages may decrease both the incidence of primary occurrence and recurrence.

Clinical Findings

The classic signs of gastric or duodenal ulcer are related to a burning epigastric pain that is relieved by meals or antacids. PUD must be differentiated from reflex esophagitis or simple heartburn, which commonly occurs during pregnancy. Patients with a gastric or duodenal ulcer most often report discomfort rather than pain and describe the feeling as "acid," burning, or indigestion. Pain from a duodenal ulcer occurs several hours postprandially during the day, occurs nocturnally, and is relieved by eating food. Pregnant patients tend to have milder symptoms than nonpregnant patients.

Most commonly, the diagnosis is confirmed by endoscopic visualization of the ulcer crater in the stomach or duodenum. Upper gastrointestinal x-ray films with barium studies usually are avoided during pregnancy because of radiation exposure and because endoscopy is a more direct diagnostic method. The presence of *H pylori* can be confirmed based on biopsy histology, culture, or urease test.

Differential Diagnosis

PUD should be distinguished from other common gastrointestinal problems during pregnancy such as gastroesophageal reflux disease (GERD), nausea and vomiting of pregnancy, HEG, pancreatitis, acute cholecystitis, viral hepatitis, appendicitis, acute fatty liver of pregnancy, and irritable bowel syndrome. GERD is extremely common in pregnancy and may be partially distinguished from PUD by the findings of pain radiating to the neck, pain exacerbated by drinking acidic drinks, and recumbency. Other symptoms more commonly seen with GERD include nocturnal asthma, hoarseness, laryngitis, or periodontal disease. Pancreatitis is marked with pain exacerbated with eating, pain radiating to the back, and presence of leukocytosis or pyrexia. Additionally, serum amylase and lipase levels are generally increased with pancreatitis. Acute cholecystitis is also associated with exacerbation after ingestion of fatty meals, right upper quadrant pain, fever, and leukocytosis. Acute hepatitis is diagnosed serologically, whereas appendicitis typically has an acute onset of abdominal pain, rebound tenderness, pyrexia, leukocytosis, and anorexia.

Complications

Complications of PUD occur in pregnancy much less frequently than in the general population. Case reports have documented complications such as hematemesis, perforation, and gastrointestinal obstruction during pregnancy. The fetus generally is not adversely affected unless significant maternal compromise occurs. One retrospective study proposed a small increased risk of low birthweight and preterm delivery in women diagnosed with PUD when compared to pregnant patients without PUD.

Treatment

Documented PUD is treated symptomatically during pregnancy by avoiding symptom-provoking foods and using antacids and sucralfate. Supportive advice can be given regarding cessation of smoking, bed rest, and avoidance of stress. For persistent symptoms, an H_2 antagonist such as cimetidine or ranitidine can be given. With continued symptoms, a proton pump inhibitor such as lansoprazole can be added to the drug regimen. Eradication of *H pylori* is 90% successful with an antibiotic such as amoxicillin or clarithromycin, a bismuth compound, and a proton pump inhibitor. Both the H_2 antagonists and proton pump inhibitors have been extensively studied for teratogenic effects, and no significant abnormal findings have been associated with their use during pregnancy.

Chen Y, Lin HC, Lou HY. Increased risk of low birthweight, infants small for gestational age, and preterm delivery for women with peptic ulcer. *Am J Obstet Gynecol* 2010;202:164. PMID: 20113692.

Engemise S, Oshowo A, Kyei-Mensah A. Perforated duodenal ulcer in the puerperium. *Arch Gynecol Obstet* 2009;279:407–410. PMID: 18642012.

Parikh N, Howden CW. The safety of drugs used in acid-related disorders and functional gastrointestinal disorders. *Gastroenterol Clin North Am* 2010;39:529–542. PMID: 20951916.

INFLAMMATORY BOWEL DISEASE

ESSENTIALS OF DIAGNOSIS

- Crohn's disease is one subcategory of inflammatory bowel disease (IBD), characterized by insidious onset, episodes of low-grade fever, diarrhea, right lower quadrant pain, and perianal disease with abscess and fistulas formed. Radiographic evidence includes ulceration, stricturing, or fistulas of the small intestine or colon. It may involve any segment of the gastrointestinal tract from the mouth to the anus.
- Ulcerative colitis is the other subcategory of IBD manifesting with bloody diarrhea, lower abdominal cramps, fecal urgency, anemia, and low serum albumin. It is diagnosed with sigmoidoscopy and only involves the colon.

Pathogenesis

Inflammatory bowel disease (IBD) affects approximately 500,000 individuals in the United States at present. There are 2 major categories of IBD: Crohn's disease and ulcerative colitis. Ulcerative colitis is characterized by recurrent episodes of inflammation affecting the mucosal layer of the colon. Lesions are seen to affect the colon in a continuous fashion. In contrast, Crohn's disease is characterized by inflammation affecting the full thickness of the bowel wall and is associated with "skip lesions" in the bowel, lesions separated by unaffected areas. Crohn's disease can affect any area of the gastrointestinal tract from the mouth to the anus, but the most commonly affected site is the distal ileum.

Although the cause of the inflammatory lesions is poorly understood, risk factors have been identified. Most cases of IBD initially present between the ages of 15 and 40 years. Both types of IBD are more common in individuals of Jewish descent. The disease may also have a hereditary component because a family history of IBD increases one's risk of developing IBD.

Clinical Findings

A. Symptoms & Signs

Both Crohn's disease and ulcerative colitis often affect women during their reproductive years and have similar risks in pregnancy as well as with similar treatments. In these conditions, cramping, lower abdominal pain, and diarrhea are the main complaints. Weight loss and anorexia may occur, as well as electrolyte imbalance with severe diarrhea.

B. Diagnostic Studies

Flexible sigmoidoscopy is considered safe during pregnancy and preferred to colonoscopy unless it is felt to be critical for making treatment decisions. The diagnosis is established by finding characteristic intestinal ulcerations and excluding alternative diagnoses.

Differential Diagnosis

The differential diagnosis for IBD includes enteric infection, bowel ischemia, diverticulitis, amyloidosis, diarrhea of acquired immunodeficiency syndrome, celiac sprue, and NSAID-induced changes.

Complications

Poor maternal weight gain, bowel perforation, toxic megacolon, and obstruction are rare complications of IBD during pregnancy. Fertility rates for both ulcerative colitis and Crohn's disease are similar to baseline. Additionally, women with IBD are as likely to flare during pregnancy (34% chance per year) as when not pregnant (32% chance per year).

Both ulcerative colitis and Crohn's disease are associated with an increased risk of first-trimester miscarriage, preterm birth, and small for gestational age infants, as well as an increased caesarean delivery rate. Women who experienced increased disease activity at conception have experienced the most significant increase in these poor obstetrical outcomes. Contradictory findings have been found in regard to congenital anomalies, with some showing an increased risk with ulcerative colitis but not Crohn's disease. These findings are not consistent and may be associated with medications used during the pregnancy.

Treatment

Treatment of IBD typically consists of both dietary changes and medications. Total parenteral nutrition may be required in extreme cases for a period of time during a pregnancy. Sulfasalazine is a frequently used first-line medication that does cross the placenta but has not been associated with an increased risk of birth defects or pregnancy loss. Supplemental folic acid should be given as an adjunct to sulfasalazine. Steroids are also frequently used for moderate to severe cases of IBD, with possible association with low-birth-weight infants and increased risk of oral clefts (when given <10 weeks and at high dose). Immunosuppressive medications such as azathioprine and 6-mercaptopurine can be used in refractory cases, although there are concerns for potential fetal myelotoxicity, as well as miscarriage and preterm birth. Cyclosporine should only be used in those women not responsive to steroids to avoid emergency colectomy; it may be associated with an increased risk of preterm birth and intrauterine growth restriction. Methotrexate is contraindicated in pregnancy secondary to its mutagenic and teratogenic effects. Select antibiotics may be used, especially with Crohn's disease.

In terms of obstetrical management, serial growth ultrasounds and monitoring for preterm labor should be considered in women affected by IBD. Caesarean delivery is generally reserved for obstetrical indications, with the exception of active perianal disease or the presence of an ileoanal pouch.

Prognosis

Symptoms of active IBD during pregnancy are similar to those in the nonpregnant state: abdominal pain, cramping, and rectal bleeding. Pregnancy is not contraindicated with IBD, but when possible, the disorder should be controlled by surgery or medication prior to conception. Pregnancy does not exert an adverse effect on IBD. In most patients, pregnancy and delivery proceed smoothly.

Correia LM, Bonilha DQ, Ramos JD, et al. Treatment of inflammatory bowel disease and pregnancy: A review of the literature. *Arq Gastroenterol* 2010;47:197–201. PMID: 20721468.

Ferguson C, Mahsud-Dornan S, Patterson RN. Inflammatory bowel disease in pregnancy. *BMJ* 2008;337:427. PMID: 18599468.

Habal F, Ravindran NC. Management of inflammatory bowel disease in the pregnant patient. *World J Gastroenterol* 2008;14:1326–1332. PMID: 18322943.

Mahadevan U. Pregnancy and inflammatory bowel disease. *Gastroenterol Clin North Am* 2009;38:629–649. PMID: 19913206.

Reddy D, Murphy SJ, Kane SV, et al. Relapses of inflammatory bowel disease during pregnancy: In-hospital management and birth outcomes. *Am J Gastroenterol* 2008;103:1203–1209. PMID: 18422816.

ACUTE FATTY LIVER OF PREGNANCY

ESSENTIALS OF DIAGNOSIS

- Acute fatty liver of pregnancy (AFLP) is a rare complication of the third trimester of pregnancy involving acute hepatic failure (average gestational age at onset of 36 weeks).
- Symptoms of AFLP include malaise, anorexia, nausea, vomiting, epigastric pain, headache, or jaundice.
- Laboratory abnormalities include thrombocytopenia, elevated transaminases, hyperuricemia, and elevated creatinine. Additionally, hyperbilirubinemia, hypoglycemia, and hyperammonemia are found.
- Other findings may include hypertension, low-grade fever, bleeding from coagulopathy, agitation, or confusion of the patient.

Pathogenesis

Acute fatty liver of pregnancy (AFLP) occurs in approximately 1:10,000 pregnancies and is associated with microvesicular fatty infiltration of the liver and possibly kidney, leading to fatty liver and renal insufficiency. Although it has been diagnosed as early as 23 weeks' gestational age and as late as 1–2 weeks postpartum, it typically occurs in the third trimester, with an average age at diagnosis of 36 weeks. Approximately 50% of patients with AFLP have associated preeclampsia and/or HELLP (hemolysis, elevated liver enzymes, and low platelet count) syndrome. Additionally, it is more common in first pregnancies, multiple gestations, and a male fetus. AFLP has been associated with an inherited defect in mitochondrial beta-oxidation of fatty acids, long-chain 3-hydroxyacyl coenzyme A dehydrogenase deficiency (LCHAD). Both fetal possession and maternal possession of the defect have been linked to a significantly increased risk of developing AFLP, with many women having recurrences in subsequent pregnancies.

Clinical Findings

A. Symptoms & Signs

The patient typically reports malaise and fatigue for 1–2 weeks prior to presentation, with gradual onset of anorexia, worsening nausea and vomiting, headaches, and epigastric/right upper quadrant pain. On physical exam, jaundice may be noted, as well as a deep yellow-orange–colored urine.

B. Laboratory Findings

Laboratory studies typically reveal some degree of thrombocytopenia, as well as low serum glucose and elevated transaminases, bilirubin, creatinine, and ammonia levels. Additionally, varying degrees of coagulopathy can also be found.

C. Imaging Studies

Imaging studies are most useful to exclude other diagnoses such as intrahepatic hemorrhage or hepatic infarct, although changes consistent with nonspecific fatty infiltrations can be seen on computed tomography scan or hepatic ultrasound.

D. Special Tests

Liver biopsy is usually diagnostic, but frequently, coagulation abnormalities preclude this from being done. Moreover, the clinical presentation and laboratory values often lead to a certain diagnosis. Screening both the patient and the neonate after delivery for the LCHAD mutation can greatly assist in the diagnosis and counseling for future pregnancy.

Differential Diagnosis

AFLP is frequently confused with thrombotic thrombocytopenic purpura (TTP), hemolytic-uremic syndrome (HUS), sepsis, HELLP syndrome, or severe preeclampsia. TTP does not typically have significant elevation of liver transaminases, and there is usually a more severe thrombocytopenia present. HUS has an earlier and more severe renal involvement with less hepatic laboratory abnormalities. Hypertensive diseases (preeclampsia/HELLP) may overlap the diagnosis of AFLP frequently; however, increased ammonia levels and a more significant elevation in aspartate transaminase (AST)/alanine transaminase (ALT) and bilirubin are found in AFLP.

Treatment

Patients suspected to have AFLP should be hospitalized in either a labor and delivery unit or intensive care unit, based on maternal/fetal stability. Hypoglycemia should be corrected, and a patient should receive replacement of blood products or coagulation factors as needed. Once the mother is stabilized, delivery should be achieved; induction of labor can be attempted, based on the gestational age, maternal response to resuscitation, and fetal condition since caesarean section may be associated with an increased risk of complications due to maternal coagulopathy. Caesarean section should be performed under general anesthesia, a midline vertical incision should be considered (less dissection, more avascular planes), and placement of a subfascial and subcutaneous drain upon closing the abdomen may be beneficial to track bleeding and decrease hematoma formation. Supportive therapy should be continued in the postpartum period, with special attention to maintaining adequate perfusion to liver, kidneys, and other organs. Pancreatitis can be a lethal complication of AFLP, requiring close monitoring in the postpartum period. Initial improvement is generally is seen within 3–5 days after delivery, with hospitalization of up to 15–20 days not being unusual. Plasmapheresis has been proposed for patients that have worsening hepatic and renal function despite delivery, although the benefit of this is uncertain.

Prognosis

The maternal mortality rate from AFLP and associated complications (eg, infection, disseminated intravascular coagulation) is approximately 10%, which is significantly improved from a historical rate of 70%. Fetal/neonatal mortality is 23%, largely secondary to indicated preterm birth. Liver transplant is a rare but occasionally life-saving procedure for women progressing to fulminant liver failure. As mentioned earlier, the patient, father, and neonate should be screened for the LCHAD mutation. The risk of recurrence in future pregnancies is significant, especially among families with LCHAD deficiency, ranging from 15–70%.

Cappell MS. Hepatic disorders severely affected by pregnancy: Medical and obstetric management. *Med Clin North Am* 2008;92:739–760. PMID: 18570941.

Rajasri AG, Srestha R, Mitchell J. Acute fatty liver of pregnancy (AFLP): An overview. *J Obstet Gynaecol* 2007;27:237–240. PMID: 17664801.

Sibai BM. Imitators of severe pre-eclampsia. *Semin Perinatol* 2009;33:196–205. PMID: 19464511.

Williams J, Mozurkewich E, Chilimigras J, et al. Critical care in obstetrics: Pregnancy-specific conditions. *Best Pract Res Clin Obstet Gynaecol* 2008;22:825–846. PMID: 18775679.

HELLP SYNDROME

ESSENTIALS OF DIAGNOSIS

- HELLP syndrome is a disorder in the spectrum of preeclampsia/eclampsia characterized by hemolysis with a microangiopathic blood smear, elevated liver enzymes, and a low platelet count.
- Up to 20% of patients with HELLP syndrome will be normotensive and/or lack proteinuria.

Pathogenesis

HELLP syndrome complicates up to 1 in 200 pregnancies and is seen in 10–20% of women with preeclampsia. It generally occurs in the third trimester. HELLP syndrome is a disorder characterized by hemolysis, elevated liver enzymes, and low platelets (hence, the acronym HELLP). It is believed to fall within the spectrum of disorders related to preeclampsia, although the absolute cause is unknown.

Clinical Findings

A. Symptoms & Signs

Patients most commonly present with abdominal/epigastric pain, nausea, vomiting, and malaise. Frequently, this is associated with elevated blood pressure and proteinuria (80%). Jaundice, oliguria, and ascites may be seen less frequently.

B. Laboratory Findings

The diagnosis of HELLP syndrome is dependent on the presence of *all* of the following laboratory findings: evidence of hemolysis (demonstrated by the presence of schistocytes on peripheral smear, bilirubin ≥1.2 mg/dL, or serum lactate dehydrogenase ≥600 IU/L), platelet count <100,000, and serum AST ≥70 IU/L. Women who have some but not all of these laboratory abnormalities are given a diagnosis of partial HELLP syndrome. Additionally, mild elevation of prothrombin time (PT)/partial thromboplastin time (PTT) and decrease in fibrinogen may be seen in some women.

Differential Diagnosis

The differential diagnosis includes severe preeclampsia; a significant overlap in symptoms and findings may be seen, but HELLP is diagnosed when the previously mentioned laboratory findings are met. AFLP has abnormal PT/PTT more commonly and more significant liver failure. TTP and HUS do not affect hepatic function as frequently as HELLP syndrome.

Complications

Complications can include disseminated intravascular coagulation (21%), placental abruption (16%), acute renal failure (8%), pulmonary edema (6%), and subcapsular liver hematoma (1%). Hepatic rupture in patients with HELLP syndrome, especially with significant thrombocytopenia, has been associated with a 50% mortality rate. Risk factors for rupture include advanced maternal age, multiparity, and preeclampsia. Blood products may be required in up to 50% of affected pregnancies, and maternal mortality may approach 1%. Neonatal loss rate may range from 7 to 25%, based on gestational age at delivery and presence of growth restriction.

Treatment

Management of the patient diagnosed with HELLP syndrome includes stabilization of the patient/fetus, with replacement of blood and coagulation factors as needed; monitoring urine output/renal function; and treatment of hypertensive disease as necessary. Delivery is the primary treatment and is standard in all but special circumstances. Vaginal delivery is preferred unless there is evidence of fetal growth restriction, placental abruption, or early gestational age with rapidly worsening disease. Antenatal corticosteroids can be given for pregnancies <34 weeks, with some benefit conferred during the labor induction process. If caesarean section is required, a vertical midline incision is recommended secondary to fewer wound separations or infections. HELLP syndrome frequently resolves quickly after delivery, although the platelets and transaminases may nadir up to 36 hours after delivery before improving. Intravenous steroids have not been shown to affect long-term outcome, although one trial demonstrated more rapid recovery of the platelet count with steroids.

Prognosis

Complications of HELLP syndrome can be significant for both the mother and the fetus; however, with prompt recognition and delivery, the vast majority of patients rapidly improve. Recurrence rate for HELLP syndrome ranges from 3 to 25%, whereas the incidence of preeclampsia in subsequent pregnancies ranges from 25 to 75%. Additionally, these women may be at increased risk for cardiovascular disease later in life in the nonpregnant state. Low-dose aspirin prophylaxis has been demonstrated to reduce the recurrence rate in future pregnancies.

Cappell MS. Hepatic disorders severely affected by pregnancy: Medical and obstetric management. *Med Clin North Am* 2008;92:739–760. PMID: 18570941.

Joshi D, James A, Quaglia A, et al. Liver disease in pregnancy. *Lancet* 2010;375:594–605. PMID: 20159293.

Kirkpatrick CA. The HELLP syndrome. *Acta Clinica Belgica* 2010;65:91–97. PMID: 20491358.

OTHER GASTROINTESTINAL DISORDERS IN PREGNANCY

VIRAL HEPATITIS

Hepatitis A

Hepatitis A may occur sporadically or in epidemics. A generalized viremia occurs with the infection that is predominantly hepatic. Symptoms include nausea, headaches, poor appetite, and weight loss. Additionally, diarrhea, fever, and jaundice can be seen. The primary mode of transmission is the fecal–oral route. Excretion of the virus in stool normally begins approximately 2 weeks prior to the onset of clinical symptoms and is complete within 3 weeks after the onset of clinical symptoms. No known carrier state exists for the virus. Both blood and stool are infectious during the 206-week incubation period. Illness during the third trimester may be associated with an increased risk of preterm labor. Vertical transmission of hepatitis A has not been reported, and breastfeeding is encouraged with attention to appropriate hand washing. The hepatitis A vaccine is safe to receive during pregnancy.

Hepatitis B

This virus is typically transmitted by inoculation of infected blood or blood products or through sexual intercourse. The virus is contained in most body secretions, and infection by parenteral and sexual contact has been documented. Groups at risk for hepatitis B infection are intravenous drug users, men who have sex with men, health care personnel, spouses of hepatitis carriers, those with multiple sexual partners, and Southeast Asian emigrants. Approximately 5–10% of people infected with hepatitis B virus become chronic carriers of the virus. The incubation period is 6 weeks to 6 months. The clinical features of hepatitis A and B are similar, although hepatitis B is more insidious. Fulminant hepatitis is rare with hepatitis A but occurs in approximately 1% of patients infected with hepatitis B.

The hepatitis B surface antigen (HBsAg) is the marker usually measured in blood to document prior exposure. This is the first manifestation of viral infection; it usually appears before clinical evidence of the disease and lasts throughout the infection. Persistence of HBsAg after the acute phase of hepatitis usually is associated with clinical and laboratory evidence of chronic hepatitis. The hepatitis B core antibody (HBcAb) is produced against the core of the viral particle and occurs with acute hepatitis B infection at the onset of clinical illness. Hepatitis B e antigen (HBeAg) is found only when HBsAg is present. Pregnant women who are HBeAg positive in the third trimester frequently transmit this infection to the offspring (80–90%), whereas those who are negative have a much lower transmission rate (10–20%).

Treatment of an acute infection during pregnancy is supportive, and there is no associated increased mortality or teratogenicity. Women with elevated hepatitis B viral loads (>10^6 copies/mL) or who are HBeAg positive during the third trimester are frequently treated with lamivudine, which has been demonstrated to significantly decrease the risk of vertical transmission. In addition, newborns born to HBsAg-positive mothers should receive hepatitis B immunoglobulin within 12 hours after birth concurrently with the first pediatric dose of the vaccine. Breastfeeding is not contraindicated in patients with hepatitis B (chronic or acute).

Hepatitis C

Up to 85% of infected individuals become chronic carriers. The incubation period usually is 7–8 weeks, but ranges from 3 to 21 weeks. The course of infection is similar to that of hepatitis B. Hepatitis C antibody is present in approximately 90% of patients. However, the antibody may not be detectable for weeks after infection. Acute or chronic hepatitis C does not adversely affect a pregnancy, with similar rates of miscarriage, growth restriction, preterm delivery, or hypertensive disorders among infected patients and controls. Vertical transmission occurs in 5–8% of infected pregnancies and is increased with concomitant HIV infection (36%). The risk of vertical transmission is increased with higher hepatitis C viral loads. The mode of delivery does not appear to influence transmission rate; however, fetal scalp blood sampling or placement of a fetal scalp electrode for fetal heart rate monitoring should be avoided if possible. Prolonged rupture of membranes increases transmission risk, but in the premature fetus, risks of the gestational age must be balanced against the risk of transmission. Breastfeeding is not contraindicated in women infected with hepatitis C.

Lopez M, Coll O. Chronic viral infections and invasive procedures: Risk of vertical transmission and current recommendations. *Fetal Diagn Ther* 2010;28:1–8. PMID: 20558971.

Panda B, Panda A, Riley LE. Selected viral infections in pregnancy. *Obstet Gynecol Clin North Am* 2010;37:321–331. PMID: 20685556.

Zhongjie S, Yang Y, Ma L, et al. Lamivudine in late pregnancy to interrupt in utero transmission of hepatitis B virus. *Obstet Gynecol* 2010;116:147–159. PMID: 20567182.

CHOLECYSTITIS

Cholecystitis occurs rarely during pregnancy (0.3%) secondary to the relaxing effects of progesterone on the smooth muscle of the gallbladder and biliary duct. Acute inflammation during pregnancy is treated with intravenous fluids and limitation of oral intake. If acute cholecystitis does not resolve or if pancreatitis develops, cholecystectomy should be considered. If this operation can be performed in the second trimester, the fetal loss rate is likely not increased. The laparoscopic approach in pregnancy is widely accepted. After 20 weeks' gestation, it should be performed with special care to avoid injury to the uterus. In the third trimester, surgical intervention can contribute to preterm delivery, and monitoring of uterine contractions should be done after surgery. Additionally, it is generally recommended to have fetal monitoring during the surgical procedure, especially if the pregnancy is past viability. See Chapter 25 (Surgical Disorders in Pregnancy) for an extended review of this topic.

INTRAHEPATIC CHOLESTASIS OF PREGNANCY

Intrahepatic cholestasis of pregnancy is characterized by accumulation of bile acids in the liver with subsequent accumulation in the plasma, causing pruritus and jaundice. It is similar to cholestasis that occasionally occurs during combined oral contraceptive therapy. Estrogens are considered to play a role in its etiology, probably by slowing the enzymes involved in bile transport. Its incidence varies with geographical location and ethnicity (most common in Chile); there is an increased incidence with multiple pregnancies.

The most significant symptom is total-body itching, specifically involving the palms and soles. The differential diagnosis includes hepatitis and biliary tract disease, in addition to AFLP and the HELLP syndrome. Laboratory values show increased levels of alkaline phosphatase, bilirubin, and serum bile acids (chenodeoxycholic acid, deoxycholic acid, cholic acid). AST and ALT levels may be mildly elevated. Patients may be symptomatic weeks before the diagnostic laboratory abnormalities are noted.

Symptomatic treatment of pruritus with antihistamines such as diphenhydramine is useful as an initial therapy. Ursodeoxycholic acid (10–15 mg/kg/d in 2 divided doses) has been shown to inhibit absorption of bile acids and increase their biliary excretion. In doing so, the medication normalizes bile acids, improves liver function tests, and alleviates pruritus. Oral steroids also have been used to relieve symptoms. There is rapid resolution of both laboratory abnormalities and symptoms after delivery.

Intrahepatic cholestasis of pregnancy has been associated with fetal death, spontaneous preterm birth, meconium staining of the amniotic fluid and/or placenta, and postpartum hemorrhage. No specific method of antepartum testing has been demonstrated to prevent fetal demise, although twice-weekly modified biophysical profile testing is suggested by some. Poor obstetrical outcomes seem to be highest in women with total bile acid levels >40 nmol/L. There is no consensus on management of patients with regard to delivery; varying strategies include amniocentesis for fetal lung maturity between 36 and 37 weeks' gestational age, delivery at 37–38 weeks without fetal lung maturity studies, or allowing spontaneous labor to ensue if bile acids are <40 nmol/L and only intervening earlier if the bile acids are higher than this threshold.

See Chapter 30 (Dermatologic Disorders in Pregnancy) for an extended review of this topic.

Greenes V, Williamson C. Intrahepatic cholestasis of pregnancy. *World J Gastroenterol* 2009;15:2049–2066. PMID: 19418576.

Mays JK. The active management of intrahepatic cholestasis of pregnancy. *Curr Opin Obstet Gynecol* 2010;22:100–103. PMID: 20124899.

Pathak B, Sheibani L, Lee RH. Cholestasis of pregnancy. *Obstet Gynecol Clin North Am* 2010;37:269–282. PMID: 20685553.

Dermatologic Disorders in Pregnancy

30

Abigail Ford Winkel, MD

PHYSIOLOGIC SKIN CHANGES IN PREGNANCY

ESSENTIALS OF DIAGNOSIS

- Physiologic changes, especially endocrine processes, result in a variety of effects on the skin in pregnancy.
- Most common changes include hyperpigmentation, striae, vascular changes, and hair loss (postpartum).
- Many changes related to pregnancy resolve postpartum without treatment.

Pathogenesis

Immunologic, metabolic, vascular, and endocrine changes in pregnancy cause cutaneous changes in almost all pregnancies. Hyperpigmentation is related to increased levels of melanocyte-stimulating hormone, estrogen, and progesterone. Vascular changes are related to the effect of estrogen causing congestion, distention, and proliferation of blood vessels.

Prevention

Few interventions have been successful at preventing these changes, which occur as the result of physiologic processes. Judicious use of sunscreen may reduce the appearance of hyperpigmentation and melasma. Varicosities in the legs may be prevented by leg elevation, support hose, and avoiding prolonged sitting or standing.

Clinical Findings

A. Symptoms & Signs

Hyperpigmentation occurs in up to 90% of women, and it is more pronounced in women with darker skin tones. It is most frequently localized in the nipples, areolae, and axillae. The linea alba darkens to become the linea nigra, a dark linear streak on the midline of the abdomen.

Melasma, also known as chloasma or "the mask of pregnancy," is a symmetric brown hyperpigmentation in malar, mandibular, or central facial areas. It is exacerbated by exposure to the sun and certain cosmetics.

Erythema begins in early gestation and appears either diffuse and mottled or focused in the palmar and thenar areas.

Venous congestion and vascular permeability during pregnancy can lead to **varicosities** in up to 40% of women. They result from increased venous pressures by the gravid uterus on femoral and pelvic vessels.

Dilation of arterioles leads to central erythematous spots with fine vessels radiating outward, called **capillary hemangiomas (spider angiomas)**. They are most commonly seen around the gums, tongue, upper lip, and eyelids.

Striae, pinkish or purplish lines, may form on the abdomen, buttocks, and breasts. Striae form as a result of structural changes in the skin caused by weight gain and hormonal influence. Increased activity of the adrenal gland during pregnancy may increase their occurrence.

Nonpitting **edema** of the face, eyelids, and extremities is observed in many pregnant women, with changes most pronounced in the morning and improving throughout the day.

Changes in the distribution and amount of hair are common during pregnancy. Increased hair growth in facial areas and around the breasts occurs, particularly during the second and third trimesters. Importantly, there are no signs of virilization, and hirsutism regresses slightly or remains unchanged postpartum. Increased recruitment of hair follicles into the growing phase (anagen) may result in thickening of scalp hair in late gestation. Postpartum loss of hair is fairly common. During pregnancy, the number of hair follicles in the resting phase (telogen) is decreased by about half and then nearly doubles in the first few weeks postpartum.

Nails may become brittle with transverse grooving, distal onycholysis, and subungual hyperkeratosis. These changes are benign and do not require treatment.

Differential Diagnosis

It is important to distinguish physiologic changes in pregnancy from more worrisome conditions. Erythema, for instance, might be diagnostic of hyperthyroidism, cirrhosis, or systemic lupus erythematosus. Striae are normal findings in pregnancy but may be observed with adrenocortical hyperactivity. Edema, while common, is also an important symptom of preeclampsia, and this condition should be considered in affected women. When pronounced nail onychodystrophy is seen, psoriasis, lichen planus, and onychomycosis should be excluded.

Complications

In general, cutaneous changes of pregnancy are of cosmetic concern only. Some vascular changes result in discomfort that may respond to supportive therapy.

Treatment

Because most changes occurring in pregnancy improve postpartum, no therapy other than reassurance is required. Many remedies have been proposed for striae in pregnancy (vitamin E oil, lubricants, lotions), but none are effective. Laser technology is under investigation as a potential treatment and has shown some promise. If hyperpigmentation does not resolve postpartum, some patients respond to retinoic acid and corticosteroid preparations. Vascular changes are not likely to completely regress postpartum and may be treated with laser, electrodessication, or sclerotherapy.

Prognosis

Hyperpigmentation decreases or, in most cases, disappears postpartum. Vascular changes may become less pronounced but may not resolve completely. Striae usually become silvery-white and sunken, but they rarely disappear. Hair loss usually stops 2–6 months postpartum as the hair follicles enter the growing phase (anagen).

Bremmer M, Driscoll MS, Colgan R. The skin disorders of pregnancy: A family physician's guide. *J Fam Pract* 2010;59: 89–96. PMID: 20141723.

Elsaie ML, Baumann LS, Elsaaiee LT. Striae distensae (stretch marks) and different modalities of therapy: An update. *Dermatol Surg* 2009;35:563–573. PMID: 19400881.

Kumari R, Jaisankar TJ, Thappa DM. A clinical study of skin changes in pregnancy. *Indian J Dermatol Venereol Leprol* 2007;73:141. PMID: 17458033.

DERMATOSES & CUTANEOUS DISORDERS AFFECTED BY PREGNANCY

ATOPIC DERMATITIS

ESSENTIALS OF DIAGNOSIS

- Atopic dermatitis (eczema) is commonly exacerbated in pregnancy.
- Most patients have a history of atopy, but dermatitis may present for the first time in pregnancy.

Pathogenesis

Estrogen and progesterone modulate immune and inflammatory cell functions, including mast cell secretion. This leads to urticaria and exacerbation of cutaneous inflammatory conditions. For some women, atopic dermatitis may improve with pregnancy, but some women experience worsening of or no change in their disease status during pregnancy.

Prevention

Treatment to decrease pruritus can discourage itching, which may improve symptoms. Additionally, maintaining skin hydration with emollients with a low water content (ie, thick creams or petroleum jelly) can protect against the dry, itchy, scaly skin that is associated with atopic dermatitis.

Clinical Findings

A. Symptoms & Signs

In most cases, patients will have a history of atopic dermatitis prior to pregnancy. The diagnosis of atopic dermatitis is a clinical one. The hallmark finding is pruritus. Other clinical manifestations include grouped, crusted erythematous papules and plaques present with excoriations. The skin creases and flexural surfaces are commonly involved.

B. Laboratory Findings

Although there are no laboratory findings specific to the diagnosis of atopic dermatitis, serology, histopathology, and immunofluorescence may show increased levels of immunoglobulin E (IgE).

Differential Diagnosis

Other sources of dermatitis, including contact or allergic dermatitis, tinea infection, and scabies, may mimic these conditions. Additionally, other disorders unique to pregnancy may also manifest in pruritus, including cholestasis of pregnancy and polymorphic eruption of pregnancy. The distribution of any rash can help distinguish between these conditions.

Complications

Bacterial, viral, or fungal superinfections may arise. Patients can have allergic reactions to topical treatments.

Treatment

Symptomatic treatment involves topical corticosteroids, such as hydrocortisone, or systemic antihistamines. For patients who do not respond to topical interventions, oral prednisone may be required. Methotrexate may be used for treatment of severe atopic dermatitis in nonpregnant patients; however, its use is absolutely contraindicated during pregnancy.

Prognosis

Atopic dermatitis is not associated with any adverse effects on the fetus. The prognosis is not affected by pregnancy.

PSORIASIS

ESSENTIALS OF DIAGNOSIS

- Chronic plaque psoriasis is the most common type of psoriasis to develop or worsen in pregnancy.
- Forty percent to 60% of patients with psoriasis improve during pregnancy; only 14% worsen.

Pathogenesis

The pathophysiology is poorly understood. There is a genetic component as well an inciting injury to the skin. The Koebner phenomenon refers to the increased appearance of psoriatic lesions in area of skin trauma. Immune cells move from the dermis to the epidermis, where they stimulate keratinocytes to proliferate. High levels of interleukin-10 in pregnancy may explain the improved prognosis in some patients.

Prevention

No preventative measures have been identified.

Clinical Findings

A. Symptoms & Signs

In chronic plaque psoriasis, red and white scaly patches appear on the top first layer of the epidermis. Skin accumulates in these sites giving a silvery-white appearance, most commonly on elbows and knees, although any surface may be affected.

B. Laboratory Findings

Skin biopsy or scraping can confirm the diagnosis.

Differential Diagnosis

Drug reactions, pityriasis rosea, contact dermatitis, and tinea infections may mimic psoriasis.

Complications

Psoriatic arthritis develops in 10–15% of patients with psoriasis.

Treatment

Phototherapy and topical corticosteroids may be of use. Methotrexate, cyclosporine, and retinoids used in treatment of nonpregnant women are not recommended in pregnancy.

Prognosis

There is currently no cure for psoriasis, but various treatments can help to control the symptoms. Patients have an increased risk of nonmelanoma skin cancers and should be in the regular care of a dermatologist.

CUTANEOUS LUPUS ERYTHEMATOSUS

ESSENTIALS OF DIAGNOSIS

- Chronic cutaneous lupus is rarely affected by pregnancy. Women with systemic lupus erythematosus (SLE) in remission for 3 months or more and who do not have nephropathy or cardiopathy tolerate pregnancy well.
- Cutaneous flares are the most common manifestation of SLE in pregnancy.

Pathogenesis

Binding of autoantibodies to cell membranes in the cutaneous tissues initiates an immunologic cascade that leads to lesion formation.

Prevention

Ultraviolet light may precipitate exacerbations, and avoidance may be helpful in some cases.

Clinical Findings

A. Symptoms & Signs

Erythematous papules or small plaques with slight scaling form. Lesions may expand and merge into larger plaques.

B. Laboratory Findings

Most patients have positive antinuclear antibody screens. Anti-Ro (SS-A) and anti-La (SS-B) should be checked in pregnant patients, as well as complete blood count to screen for anemia, leukopenia, and thrombocytopenia. Decreased complement and elevated erythrocyte sedimentation rate may be observed but are nonspecific.

C. Special Tests

Biopsy of skin shows deposition of immunoglobulin and complement at the dermoepidermal junction. Biopsies of unaffected skin may be higher yield than those of skin lesions. Immunofluorescence may not be helpful with older lesions.

Differential Diagnosis

Drug eruptions and allergic reactions may mimic cutaneous lupus erythematosus.

Complications

If conception occurs during the active phase of systemic lupus erythematosus (SLE), 50% of patients will worsen during pregnancy. Patients with SLE have an increased risk of pregnancy loss, and premature birth is not uncommon. Patients are at increased risk of preeclampsia. Neonatal lupus and congenital heart block may be seen especially in patients with circulating SS-A (anti-Ro) and SS-B (anti-La) antibodies.

Treatment

Topical and intralesional therapy is with steroid treatment. Scarring from lesions may lead to alopecia. Antimalarial treatments such as hydroxychloroquine and systemic corticosteroids may also be used for cases unresponsive to local treatment.

Prognosis

Cutaneous lupus erythematosus without SLE has a good prognosis. Some patients may experience intermittent exacerbations, often in the warmer months of the year, and some patients may experience remission.

CUTANEOUS TUMORS

ESSENTIALS OF DIAGNOSIS

- Tumors may appear for the first time, enlarge, or increase in number during pregnancy.
- Granuloma gravidarum (pyogenic granuloma) is a vascular tumor that occurs in 2% of patients between the second and fifth months of pregnancy.
- Desmoid tumors, leiomyomas, and keloids may grow rapidly during pregnancy.
- Melanocytic nevi may develop, enlarge, or darken during pregnancy.

Pathogenesis

Proliferation of capillaries causes granuloma gravidarum to develop. Molluscum fibrosum gravidarum is also a result of the hormonal effects on vasculature. An increase in estrogen and progesterone receptors has been observed on melanocytes, which may explain changes in melanocytic nevi.

Prevention

No preventative measures have been identified.

Clinical Findings

A. Symptoms & Signs

Granuloma gravidarum is a red or purple nodule that most commonly occurs on gingival surfaces in the mouth but may also occur at other sites such as fingers. Molluscum fibrosum gravidarum are soft fibromas appearing later in pregnancy on the face, neck, and chest wall. Melanocytic nevi are dark, raised nodules of varying size that can occur anywhere on the body.

B. Laboratory Findings

If appearance is classic for a common benign lesion, biopsy is not necessary. Care should be taken in biopsying vascular lesions.

Differential Diagnosis

A wide variety of epidermal, melanocytic, fibroblastic, vascular, follicular, sebaceous, nervous, smooth muscle, and eccrine tumors may be considered. Metastatic tumors should be considered and biopsy performed if suspicion for malignancy exists.

Complications

Complications are limited to maternal cosmetic and physical effects. No fetal impact should be anticipated.

Treatment

In most cases, observation is all that is required. If symptoms exist, surgical resection may be considered.

Prognosis

Many lesions regress postpartum and do not require surgical resection.

Bremmer M, Driscoll MS, Colgan R. The skin disorders of pregnancy: A family physician's guide. *J Fam Pract* 2010;59:89–96. PMID: 20141723.

Clowse ME. Managing contraception and pregnancy in the rheumatologic diseases. *Best Pract Res Clin Rheumatol* 2010;24:373–385. PMID: 20534371.

Kasperska-Zajac A, Brzoza Z, Rogala B. Sex hormones and urticaria. *J Dermatol Sci* 2008;52:79–86. PMID: 18485675.

SPECIFIC DERMATOSES OF PREGNANCY

PRURITIC URTICARIAL PAPULES AND PLAQUES OF PREGNANCY

ESSENTIALS OF DIAGNOSIS

- The most common pruritic dermatosis unique to pregnancy.
- Pruritic, erythematous papules that coalesce into plaques forming usually after the 34th week of gestation.
- The lesions usually appear during the third trimester and disappear completely within 2 weeks after delivery.

Pathogenesis

Pruritic urticarial papules and plaques of pregnancy (PUPPP) are also known as polymorphic eruption of pregnancy. The pathogenesis of PUPPP is still unclear. However, it is likely that overdistension of abdominal connective tissue exposes antigens in collagen bundles that provoke an allergic-type reaction, leading to lesions within the striae gravidarum. It affects approximately 1 in 160 to 1 in 300 pregnancies.

Prevention

No preventative measures have been identified.

Clinical Findings

A. Symptoms & Signs

The diagnosis of PUPPP is based on clinical signs and symptoms. Generally red, unexcoriated papules and plaques are found principally on the abdomen. A marked halo may surround the plaques. Lesions are found on the striae, legs, and arms. Notably, the characteristic papules spare the periumbilical region, leaving what may appear to be a periumbilical "white halo."

B. Laboratory Findings

No relevant laboratory studies yield specific findings for PUPPP. However, immunofluorescence can distinguish PUPPP from pemphigoid gestationis because no immunoglobulin component will be identified with PUPPP.

Differential Diagnosis

Lesions cluster on the striae and tend to spare the umbilical area, differentiating PUPPP from pemphigoid gestationis. The differential diagnosis also includes erythema multiforme, drug reactions, viral syndromes, and scabies.

Complications

This condition poses no real danger for mother or fetus. It is not associated with adverse fetal or maternal outcomes.

Treatment

Symptomatic treatment with antihistamines, topical steroids, and antipruritic medications usually is helpful. Occasionally, oral corticosteroid therapy is necessary for control of extreme pruritus unresponsive to initial treatment.

Prognosis

PUPPP is self-limited and resolves after pregnancy. It is unclear if women who experience PUPPP with one pregnancy are at increased risk of recurrence in future pregnancies.

INTRAHEPATIC CHOLESTASIS OF PREGNANCY

ESSENTIALS OF DIAGNOSIS

- Seen only in pregnancy; results in pruritus and exclusively secondary skin lesions.
- Usually arises after the 30th week of pregnancy.
- Cholestasis is more prominent in South American and Scandinavian populations.

Pathogenesis

Intrahepatic cholestasis of pregnancy (ICP) affects between 0.3 and 5.6% of pregnancies in the United States. The incidence of ICP appears to vary according to ethnicity, with higher incidence rates among Araucanos Indians in Chile and people of Bolivian descent. The cause of ICP is not well understood. Certain genetic mutations have been associated with an increased predisposition to ICP. Alterations in estrogen and progesterone metabolism have also been associated with ICP. Increased levels of both hormones have been associated with ICP. Intrahepatic dysfunction of biliary secretion leads to elevation of bile acids in serum and deposition of bile salts in the skin, causing pruritus. Hormonal factors are likely to contribute to the condition.

Prevention

No preventative measures have been identified.

Clinical Findings

A. Symptoms & Signs

Patients with ICP typically present with a generalized pruritus (often severe) without an identifiable rash focused on palms and soles and sometimes extending to legs and abdomen. Symptoms tend to be worse at night. On physical examination, patients may show signs of excoriations.

B. Laboratory Findings

Testing of serum bile acids and liver function tests should be performed for every pregnant woman with pruritus. Serum total bile acid concentrations are increased in women with ICP. Serum cholic acid is often increased more than chenodeoxycholic acid. Serum aminotransferases may also be elevated. The prothrombin time is usually normal in women with ICP.

Differential Diagnosis

The diagnosis of ICP is made on the basis of pruritus with elevated bile acids and/or abnormal liver enzymes. However, viral hepatitis, gallbladder disease, pemphigus gestationis, and the papular dermatoses of pregnancy should be considered. The absence of a rash helps to distinguish ICP from other dermatoses. The presence of pruritus distinguishes ICP from other causes of abnormal liver function tests.

Complications

ICP is associated with an increased risk of adverse perinatal outcomes, including preterm birth and stillbirth. The earlier in gestation the onset of pruritus, the greater is the risk of prematurity. Patients with higher levels of bile acids have been found to have higher rates of spontaneous preterm birth. Additionally, the incidence of fetal demise appears to be 1–3%. Stillbirths cluster around weeks 37–39 of pregnancy. Although the absolute cause of stillbirth is poorly understood, there is some evidence suggesting that the increased levels of circulating bile acids interfere with cardiac electrical conduction leading to fetal arrhythmia and sudden stillbirth. Because stillbirth in these women appears to be a sudden and unpredictable event, fetal surveillance with nonstress testing and/or biophysical profiles has not been shown to reduce the risk of adverse outcome. Nonetheless, most practitioners advise the initiation of fetal surveillance twice per week once a diagnosis of ICP has been made.

Treatment

Ursodeoxycholic acid (UDCA) may result in a sustained decrease in serum bile acids that improves maternal symptoms. UDCA has not been shown to reduce the risk of stillbirth, primarily because the studies evaluating the effect of UDCA on ICP were not powered to address the effect on fetal/neonatal outcomes. However, in theory, reducing circulating bile acids with UDCA may also reduce the risk of adverse fetal outcomes. Once a diagnosis of ICP is made, fetal surveillance twice per week with nonstress testing and/or biophysical profiles is recommended. The optimal timing of delivery is unclear, but many experts advise delivery at 37–38 weeks or delivery at 36 weeks after confirmation of fetal lung maturity with amniocentesis.

Prognosis

The pruritus typically resolves within days after delivery. ICP is associated with a substantial recurrence risk, which has been reported to be in the range of 40–70%. Women with a history of ICP may also experience recurrent pruritus and cholestasis with oral contraceptives. If a patient with ICP desires oral contraception, a pill with a low dose of estrogen should be prescribed.

PUSTULAR PSORIASIS OF PREGNANCY

ESSENTIALS OF DIAGNOSIS

- Also called impetigo herpetiformis.
- Characterized by a pustular eruption on an erythematous base with total-body distribution.
- This rare condition may represent an acute form of psoriasis that occurs during pregnancy.
- Most patients have personal or family history of psoriasis.

Pathogenesis

Impetigo herpetiformis, or pustular psoriasis of pregnancy, is a very rare skin disorder with few cases described in the medical literature. The pathogenesis is still unclear, although it may be associated with high levels of progesterone and low levels of calcium in the last trimester of pregnancy. Reduced levels of epidermal skin-derived antileukoproteinase (elafin) have been implicated in the formation of pustules.

Prevention

No preventative measures have been identified.

Clinical Findings

A. Symptoms & Signs

Generalized erythematous patches covered with sterile pustules occur. Lesions start on the intertriginous or flexor surfaces and extend centrifugally, including mucosal membranes. Fever, nausea, diarrhea, and malaise often accompany this presentation. Pruritus is not common. Patients may have associated hypocalcaemia.

B. Laboratory Findings

Biopsy confirms presence of spongiform pustules with neutrophils in the epidermis. Immunofluorescence is negative.

Differential Diagnosis

Biopsy and culture can distinguish between pustular psoriasis of pregnancy and other pustular dermatoses and infections such as candidiasis and impetigo. Lesions may become superinfected, causing difficulty with diagnosis.

Complications

Skin lesions that develop superimposed infections may lead to sepsis. Severe hypocalcemia can cause tetany, seizures, and delirium.

Treatment

Treatment generally starts with oral corticosteroids. The steroids are then slowly tapered. Hypocalcemia should be corrected with calcium supplementation.

Prognosis

Increased maternal and perinatal mortality has been reported, but these cases may be related to secondary infection and sepsis. These patients may be at increased risk of placental insufficiency with adverse pregnancy outcomes such as miscarriage, fetal growth restriction, and stillbirth. Consequently, fetal surveillance with biophysical profiles and ultrasound assessment of fetal growth are advised. The skin lesions typically resolve quickly in the postpartum period. Pustular psoriasis of pregnancy may recur with subsequent pregnancies with an earlier gestational age at onset.

PEMPHIGOID GESTATIONIS (HERPES GESTATIONIS)

ESSENTIALS OF DIAGNOSIS

- Rare condition; appears in second and third trimesters.
- Lesions present as erythematous plaques with vesicles that soon form bullae in the periphery of the lesion (herpetiform appearance).
- Lesions start on the trunk and tend to spare the face, palms, and soles.

Pathogenesis

Despite the name, the herpes virus is not the causative agent. An autoimmune reaction against a placental matrix antigen has been implicated. Autoantibodies form that lead to deposition of immune complexes in the skin and complement activation, resulting in tissue damage and blister formation.

Prevention

No preventative measures have been identified.

Clinical Findings

A. Symptoms & Signs

Urticarial papules and plaques usually begin on the trunk and spread to the entire body including the distal extremities. Bullous lesions develop as the disease progresses. Lesions on mucous membranes are uncommon; however, they may occur. The vesicles are not clustered and are more peripheral than herpes. Systemic signs include malaise, fevers, and chills.

B. Laboratory Findings

Biopsy is necessary for diagnosis. Most patients have circulating immunoglobulin G that will fix C3 complement. Immunofluorescence testing of bullous lesions demonstrates C3 in a homogeneous, linear band at the basement membrane zone.

Differential Diagnosis

Pemphigus vulgaris can be excluded by histologic examination. The pustules, fever, and hypocalcemia of impetigo herpetiformis are not present in herpes gestationis. Dermatitis herpetiformis is pruritic, but the clusters of vesicles do not form bullae, and no plaques are present. In herpes gestationis, a crust forms, and a hyperpigmented area, but little or no scarring, occurs after the lesion heals.

Complications

Pruritus can interfere with daily activities and sleep. Ruptured bullae may be painful and develop superficial ulcerations that interfere dramatically with quality of life. Newborns may be small for gestational age at birth, but usually do not have associated morbidity and mortality.

Treatment

Topical or oral corticosteroids are the treatment of choice, typically prednisone 20–60 mg daily. Oral antihistamines may also relieve symptoms. Cyclosporine and intravenous immunoglobulin have been used in refractory conditions.

Prognosis

Exacerbations and remissions occur during pregnancy. The condition usually abates by 6 weeks postpartum, although exacerbations may occur during the postpartum period. Pemphigoid gestationis is associated with placental insufficiency, which increases the risk of intrauterine growth restriction and prematurity. Fetal surveillance with biophysical profiles and ultrasound assessment of fetal growth is advised in these women. The disease tends to recur in subsequent pregnancies.

Bremmer M, Driscoll MS, Colgan R. The skin disorders of pregnancy: A family physician's guide. *J Fam Pract* 2010;59:89–96. PMID: 20141723.

Kumari R, Jaisankar TJ, Thappa DM. A clinical study of skin changes in pregnancy. *Indian J Dermatol Venereol Leprol* 2007;73:141. PMID: 17458033.

Roth MM. Pregnancy dermatoses: Diagnosis, management, and controversies. *Am J Clin Dermatol* 2011;12:25–41. PMID: 21110524.

Diabetes Mellitus & Pregnancy

31

Aisling Murphy, MD
Carla Janzen, MD
Stacy L. Strehlow, MD
Jeffrey S. Greenspoon, MD
Sue M. Palmer, MD

According to the Centers for Disease Control and Prevention, diabetes mellitus was estimated to affect 24 million people in the United States in 2008, an increase of 3 million over the preceding 2 years. Prevalence of diabetes, primarily type 2 disease, is expected to rise even further by 2030, as a consequence of population aging, lifestyle changes, and increasing obesity rates. Approximately 25% of adults with the condition are currently undiagnosed.

Data suggest that this upward trend in prevalence is also affecting pregnant women. Preexisting diabetes affects 1% of all pregnancies, whereas approximately 7% of pregnant women are diagnosed with gestational diabetes mellitus (GDM), a condition traditionally defined as glucose intolerance with onset or first recognition during pregnancy. Even higher rates may be seen in certain minority groups, in particular African American and Hispanic gravidas.

Before the introduction of insulin in 1922, women with preexisting diabetes did not often conceive. When pregnancy did occur, it commonly resulted in the death of the mother. This fact prompted Joseph de Lee to recommend in his seminal 1913 textbook that all such pregnancies be terminated. He observed that "the attempt to carry the pregnancy up to term or even to viability of the child is too perilous."

The introduction of insulin, as well as improvements in general obstetric care, rapidly decreased maternal mortality. However, the risk of stillbirth and neonatal death remained much higher in diabetics than in the general population until the 1960s. Since that time, there has been a dramatic decrease in perinatal mortality due to improved neonatal intensive care, fetal surveillance, and greatly improved diabetic control, the result of self-blood glucose monitoring and intensified insulin regimens. Today, if good glycemic control is achieved, the risk of perinatal mortality approaches that of the general obstetric population. Nevertheless, both preexisting diabetes and GDM continue to pose significant risks during pregnancy.

Currently, the priorities for diabetes care providers are first to identify and control diabetes prior to conception and second to appropriately screen and treat GDM during pregnancy in an effort to prevent maternal and fetal/neonatal complications. Evidence exists that treatment of even mild GDM results in improved outcomes in both mother and baby.

Metabolism in Normal & Diabetic Pregnancy

To accommodate the growth of a healthy fetus, profound metabolic changes occur in all pregnant women during gestation. In particular, it is well established that insulin sensitivity decreases in normal women as gestation advances. However, despite much research, the mechanism behind this phenomenon is unknown. Alterations in maternal cortisol levels, as well as in the placental hormones including estrogen, progesterone, placental growth factor, and human placental lactogen (hPL) (also known as human chorionic somatomammotropin), have all been implicated.

Although some degree of insulin resistance occurs in all women, only a relatively small number develop GDM. Affected women share the same risk factors as patients with type 2 diabetes, and like type 2 disease, GDM is characterized both by insulin resistance and by inadequate insulin secretion. It therefore appears that GDM may be considered as type 2 diabetes that is unmasked by the diabetogenic milieu of pregnancy.

Insulin is an anabolic hormone with essential roles in carbohydrate, fat, and protein metabolism. It promotes the uptake of glucose, storage of glucose as glycogen, lipogenesis, and uptake and utilization of amino acids. A lack of insulin or decreased peripheral responsiveness to insulin results in hyperglycemia and lipolysis. Elevation of free fatty acids leads to an increase in the formation of ketone bodies, acetoacetate, and β-hydroxybutyrate. When blood glucose levels exceed the renal threshold for absorption of filtered glucose, glycosuria occurs and causes an osmotic diuresis with dehydration and electrolyte losses.

In the first trimester of normal pregnancies, insulin sensitivity is unchanged or increased. This appears to be because both estrogen and progesterone levels rise at this time but their effects on insulin activity are antagonistic. Progesterone causes insulin resistance, whereas estrogen has the opposite effect. Because insulin secretion rises while insulin sensitivity is unchanged, the result is a decrease in fasting glucose levels, which reach a nadir by the 12th week. The decrease averages 15 mg/dL; thus, fasting values of 70–80 mg/dL are common by the 10th week of pregnancy.

However, in the second trimester, higher postprandial glucose levels occur, facilitating transfer of glucose across the placenta from mother to fetus. Glucose transfer occurs via a facilitated diffusion that becomes saturated at 250 mg/dL. Fetal glucose levels are 80% of maternal levels. In contrast, maternal amino acid levels are lowered due to active placental transport to the fetus. Lipid metabolism in the second trimester shows continued maternal storage until midgestation, then enhanced mobilization (lipolysis) as fetal fuel demands increase.

hPL, which increases up to 30-fold during pregnancy, is thought to be the hormone mainly responsible for insulin resistance and lipolysis. hPL also decreases the hunger sensation and diverts maternal carbohydrate metabolism to fat metabolism in the third trimester. hPL is similar in structure to growth hormone and acts by reducing the insulin affinity to insulin receptors. The net effect is to favor placental transfer of glucose to the fetus and to reduce the maternal use of glucose. The hPL levels rise steadily during the first and second trimesters, with a plateau in the late third trimester.

Maternal cortisol levels, which likewise rise during pregnancy, may also contribute to insulin resistance by stimulating endogenous glucose production and glycogen storage and decreasing glucose utilization.

Recently, researchers have challenged the view that the insulin resistance of pregnancy is mediated entirely by hormonal changes. Attention has turned to the role adipokines such as tumor necrosis factor-α (TNF-α), adiponectin, and leptin may play. In particular, the change in TNF-α level has been found to be a significant predictor of insulin resistance during pregnancy. TNF-α is produced by the placenta as well as by adipose tissue and may act in a paracrine fashion to impair insulin signaling mechanisms, resulting in decreased insulin sensitivity.

Fetal Effects of Hyperglycemia

Elevated glucose levels are toxic to the developing fetus, producing an increase in miscarriages and major malformations in direct proportion to the glucose level. The mechanism by which teratogenesis occurs has not been definitively established, but oxidative stress as a consequence of fetal hyperglycemia may play a role. These birth defects (Table 31–1), which may be fatal or seriously deleterious to quality of life, are largely preventable by improvement in preconception glucose control.

Table 31–1. Some congenital anomalies of infants of diabetic mothers.

Cardiac	Atrial septal defects
	Ventricular septal defects
	Transposition of the great vessels
	Coarctation of the aorta
	Tetralogy of Fallot
	Truncus arteriosus
	Dextrocardia
	Cardiomegaly
Central nervous system	Neural tube defects
	Anencephaly
	Holoprosencephaly
Renal	Hydronephrosis
	Renal agenesis
	Ureteral duplication
Gastrointestinal	Duodenal atresia
	Anorectal atresia
	Omphalocele
Spinal	Caudal regression syndrome, sacral agenesis

Reprinted, with permission, from Reece EA, Hobbins JC. Diabetes embryopathy, pathogenesis, prenatal diagnosis and prevention. *Obstet Gynecol Surv* 1986;41:325.

Because most malformations occur within the first 8 weeks of gestation, when most women are just beginning prenatal care, preconception care is essential for women with diabetes. Hemoglobin A1c (HbA1c), which reflects the blood glucose concentration over the previous 2 months, can predict the risk for malformations when measured in the first trimester (Table 31–2).

The fetus continues to experience the effects of hyperglycemia beyond the period of organogenesis. Whereas glucose crosses the placenta, insulin does not. This leads to increased fetal production of insulin to compensate for its hyperglycemic environment.

Insulin and insulin-like growth factors promote excessive fetal growth, which may result in macrosomia. Macrosomia, variously defined as a birth weight of more than 4000 g or more than 4500 g, is a risk factor for both maternal and fetal morbidity. Maternal risks include caesarean delivery, vaginal

Table 31–2. Relationship between initial pregnancy value of glycosylated hemoglobin and rate of major fetal congenital malformations.

Initial Maternal Hemoglobin A1c Level	Major Congenital Malformations (%)
≤7.9	3.2
8.9–9.9	8.1
≥10	23.5

laceration, and postpartum hemorrhage. Shoulder dystocia with resultant birth injury, in particular Erb's palsy, is the most feared fetal complication.

There is a disproportionate increase in subcutaneous fat and visceromegaly in macrosomic infants of diabetic mothers, which results in a relatively large abdominal circumference with normal head and skeletal growth. This abnormal growth dynamic appears to predispose these infants to shoulder dystocia. In the presence of maternal diabetes, birth weights of greater than 4500 g have been associated with rates of shoulder dystocia of up to 50% in some studies.

In addition, fetal hyperinsulinemia leads to enlargement of internal organs such as the heart. Ventricular septal hypertrophy may, in rare cases, lead to cardiac failure as a result of left ventricular outflow obstruction.

International Association of Diabetes and Pregnancy Study Groups Consensus Panel, Metzger BE, Gabbe SG, et al. International Association of Diabetes and Pregnancy Study Groups recommendations on the diagnosis and classification of hyperglycemia in pregnancy. *Diabetes Care* 2010;33:676–682. PMID: 20190296.

Metzger BE, Lowe LP, Dyer AR, et al. Hyperglycemia and adverse pregnancy outcomes (HAPO study). *N Engl J Med* 2008;358:1991–2002. PMID: 18463375.

CLASSIFICATION OF DIABETES

The American Diabetes Association (ADA) classifies diabetes mellitus into 4 clinical types:

1. Type 1 diabetes, formerly referred to as insulin-dependent or juvenile-onset diabetes
2. Type 2 diabetes, formerly referred to as non–insulin-dependent or adult-onset diabetes
3. Other specific types of diabetes related to a variety of genetic-, drug-, or chemical-induced diabetes
4. Gestational diabetes

The first 3 categories typically refer to pregestational diabetes or diabetes that has been diagnosed prior to the onset of pregnancy. The severity of pregestational diabetes can be classified according to the White classification system (Table 31–3). This system categorizes diabetes by duration of disease and the presence of end-organ damage, which has prognostic implications for outcomes of women with diabetes mellitus during pregnancy.

Table 31–3. Modified White classification of diabetes complicating pregnancy.

Class	Onset (age in years)	Duration (years)	Type of vascular disease
A1	Gestational - diet-controlled	-	None
A2	Gestational - treated with medication/ insulin	-	None
B	20	<10	None
C	10–19 *or*	10–19	None
D	<10 *or*	20	Benign retinopathy
F	Any	Any	Nephropathy
R	Any	Any	Proliferative retinopathy
T	Any	Any	Prior renal transplant
H	Any	Any	Coronary artery disease

PREGESTATIONAL DIABETES

ESSENTIALS OF DIAGNOSIS

- Abnormal maternal glucose tolerance precedes pregnancy.
- Associated with increased risk of adverse maternal and fetal outcomes including fetal structural malformations.
- Risk of complications correlates with degree of glycemic control.

Pathogenesis

A. Type 1 Diabetes

Type 1 diabetes mellitus, formerly called insulin-dependent diabetes, results from autoimmune destruction of beta cells in the islets of the pancreas, usually leading to an absolute insulin deficiency. Type 1 diabetes accounts for approximately 5–10% of patients with preexisting disease. Although onset generally occurs in the young, type 1 disease can appear in older persons and may occasionally present for the first time during pregnancy.

Type 1 diabetes has multiple identified genetic predispositions. Susceptibility is increased by a gene or genes located near or within the human leukocyte antigen (HLA) locus on the short arm of chromosome 6 (6p). The risk to offspring of developing type 1 with an affected sibling is 5% if 1 haplotype is shared, 13% for 2 haplotypes, and 2% if no haplotypes are shared. If both parents are affected, the risk of the condition is 33%. It is believed that an environmental agent triggers the disease in genetically susceptible individuals. The exact nature of the trigger is, as yet, unknown.

In rare cases, type 1 diabetes is not associated with evidence of autoimmunity and is termed "idiopathic diabetes." Patients with this form of the disorder suffer from episodic attacks of ketoacidosis. They may have an absolute insulin deficiency only during these attacks.

B. Type 2 Diabetes

Type 2 diabetes mellitus, formerly non–insulin-dependent diabetes, is characterized both by insulin resistance and by beta cell dysfunction. This form of the disorder accounts for 90–95% of all patients with diabetes.

Type 2 diabetes is a multifactorial illness that is influenced by heredity, environment, and lifestyle choices. It is typically gradual in onset and may go undiagnosed for many years. Ketoacidosis is rare in this setting. The majority of affected patients are obese.

Although several genes have been associated with the disorder, progression to frank disease can be modified by factors such as diet and exercise. With type 2 diabetes, the risk of diabetes in a first-degree relative is almost 15%, and approximately 30% more will have impaired glucose tolerance. If both parents are affected, the incidence of diabetes in the offspring is 60–75%, although lifestyle modification can decrease the risk.

Clinical Findings

Profound thirst, increased urination, and weight loss or even overt ketoacidosis are the usual symptoms prompting medical evaluation. According to the ADA, there are 4 ways of diagnosing diabetes in nonpregnant patients:

1. Symptoms of diabetes plus random plasma glucose concentration ≥200 mg/dL. The classic symptoms of diabetes include polyuria, polydipsia, and unexplained weight loss.
2. Fasting plasma glucose ≥126 mg/dL. Fasting is defined as no caloric intake for at least 8 hours.
3. Two-hour plasma glucose level ≥200 mg/dL during an oral glucose tolerance test (OGTT). The test uses a glucose load containing the equivalent of 75 g of anhydrous glucose dissolved in water.
4. HbA1c ≥6.5% using a standardized assay.

In the absence of unequivocal hyperglycemia, these criteria should be confirmed by repeat testing on a different day.

Complications

In the case of preexisting disease, poor periconceptional glucose control is associated with an increased risk of spontaneous abortion and fetal malformations. Later in gestation, poor glycemic control may result in intrauterine fetal demise.

Maternal hyperglycemia causes an overproduction of fetal insulin and insulin-like growth factors, which may lead to macrosomia and its attendant risks including operative delivery, shoulder dystocia, and birth injury. Conversely, in diabetic mothers with vascular disease, intrauterine growth restriction may occur.

Neonatal complications in infants of diabetic mothers may include respiratory distress syndrome (RDS), hypoglycemia, hypocalcemia, and hyperbilirubinemia. Additionally, these children may be more likely to develop diabetes and obesity in the long term. The fetus responds to maternal hyperglycemia with pancreatic hyperplasia and increased basal insulin secretion, which are associated with a lifetime increased risk of diabetes. Mothers with diabetes during pregnancy have offspring with higher rates of diabetes at age 20–24 years than do women who develop diabetes after the pregnancy (45% vs. 8.6%). This observation suggests that the hyperglycemia during pregnancy had an effect beyond the mother's genetic tendency.

Pregnant women with diabetes are also at increased risk of complications including preeclampsia, preterm delivery, and, in the case of type 1 disease, diabetic ketoacidosis.

Treatment

Prevention of hyperglycemia through rigorous control of blood glucose level is the mainstay of treatment in the pregnant woman with pregestational diabetes. This is best accomplished by careful preconceptional counseling and achievement of normal HbA1c levels before pregnancy in pregestational diabetics, frequent (usually 4–5 times per day) home glucose level monitoring, adjustment of diet, and regular exercise.

Non–weight-bearing or low-impact exercise can be initiated or continued. Even short episodes of exercise will sensitize the patient's response to insulin for approximately 24 hours. All care providers should stress the importance of diet. Soluble fiber provides satiety and improves both the number of insulin receptors and their sensitivity. Carbohydrate restriction improves glycemic control and may enable a patient to achieve her glycemic goals using diet and activity. Calories are prescribed at 25–35 kcal/kg of actual body weight, generally 1800–2400 kcal/d. Diet should be approximately 40% carbohydrate, 40% fat, and 20% protein usually divided into 3 meals and 2 or 3 snacks per day. A bedtime snack is particularly important to prevent nocturnal hypoglycemia. When postprandial values exceed the targets, it is important to review all recent food intake and to adjust food choice, preparation, and portion size.

Self-monitoring of fasting, 1- or 2-hour postprandial, and nighttime blood glucose levels using a glucose meter provides instant feedback to assess the patient's diet and behavior. When the glycemic goals are met, the feedback is a powerful motivator. Diet and/or activity errors are identified and corrected as needed. Optimal glucose levels during pregnancy are fasting levels of 70–95 mg/dL and 1-hour postprandial values <130–140 mg/dL or 2-hour postprandial values <120 mg/dL.

A minimum of 2 visits to a dietitian improves education and active participation regarding diet. Food records are useful. The dietitian reviews content and calories and suggests how to include favorite ethnic foods to improve compliance. Other family members should be encouraged to participate in the dietary education because their understanding and support increase the chance for a successful diet. Often, the other family members will benefit from the healthful diet changes. Additional follow-up visits between patient and dietitian are important when glycemic goals are not reached, weight change is too great or too small, or the patient is having difficulty maintaining the diet.

When normoglycemia cannot be achieved with diet and exercise alone, medication is added. Although not endorsed by either the American College of Obstetricians and Gynecologists or the ADA, oral hypoglycemic agents such as glyburide and metformin are commonly employed.

Glyburide, a sulfonylurea, is variously categorized as either pregnancy class B or C. It is believed to cross the placenta in only minimal amounts, and studies to date have demonstrated generally favorable results when compared to insulin. Glyburide is commenced at doses of 2.5–5 mg/d and titrated upward to a maximum of 20 mg/d to achieve optimal blood glucose control.

Metformin, a biguanide that suppresses hepatic glucose production and increases insulin sensitivity, has been used for many years as a first-line agent in nonpregnant patients with type 2 diabetes. It is pregnancy category B but is known to cross the placenta and is therefore usually avoided in the first trimester. Studies to date have shown metformin to be a safe and effective treatment for diabetes in pregnancy, although in a randomized controlled trial comparing treatment with metformin to treatment with glyburide, significantly more patients in the metformin group required the addition of insulin in order to achieve euglycemia.

Due to its extensive safety record, insulin remains the first-line treatment of diabetes in pregnancy for many obstetricians. Daily doses of 0.7 U/kg in the first trimester increasing progressively to 1 U/kg later in gestation are commonly employed, although obese women may require significantly higher amounts. Doses are usually divided into basal coverage with intermediate-acting agents such as NPH (neutral protamine Hagedorn) and prandial coverage with rapid-acting or regular insulin. Subcutaneous insulin pumps may also be considered in selected patients.

Preconception Care

Patients with preexisting diabetes should be encouraged to see a physician for care prior to conception. Preconceptional care has been shown to result in improved pregnancy outcomes. Evaluation at the preconceptional visit includes the following:

1. A complete history and physical examination. To provide a risk assessment, a comprehensive review of the patient's history should be performed. Any teratogenic medications such as angiotensin-converting enzyme inhibitors should be discontinued, and prenatal vitamins containing a minimum of 0.4 mg of folic acid should be prescribed.
2. An assessment of glycemic control. Adjustments in medications, diet, and exercise can be made to optimize glycemic control. The goal is to achieve an HbA1c of <7% to minimize the risks of spontaneous abortion and congenital anomalies.
3. An eye examination for retinopathy. Patients with retinopathy should be followed carefully for evidence of progression. If needed, laser therapy can be performed during gestation.
4. An assessment of renal function. Renal function is assessed with a serum creatinine level and a 24-hour urine collection or urinary albumin/creatinine ratio to measure protein excretion. Patients with overt nephropathy should be advised of the risks of pregnancy complications, which include worsening renal function, preeclampsia, fetal growth restriction, and preterm delivery.
5. An assessment of thyroid function. Thyroid function should be assessed, particularly in type 1 diabetics, because of the association between autoimmune thyroid disease and diabetes. In addition patients with longstanding diabetes or hypertension may be screened for ischemic heart disease with an electrocardiogram.

Antenatal Care

After confirmation of pregnancy, patients should have regular antenatal care to assess glycemic control. Evaluation is by self-monitoring of blood glucose, and treatment is adjusted accordingly.

In the first trimester, an ultrasound may be obtained to document viability, particularly if glycemic control is suboptimal. Routine antenatal laboratory evaluations should be undertaken. A urine culture is particularly important because diabetic patients are at increased risk of asymptomatic bacteriuria.

In the second trimester, a fetal ultrasound for anatomy is recommended given the risk of fetal anomalies. Fetal echocardiography is indicated in patients with preexisting diabetes to screen for congenital heart disease.

In the third trimester, further ultrasounds are indicated to assess fetal growth. This also applies to patients who have received a diagnosis of gestational diabetes. In addition, in light of the increased risks of fetal demise, surveillance of fetal well-being is commenced, usually at 32–34 weeks of gestation. This consists of twice weekly nonstress testing or a modified biophysical profile twice weekly. Maternal fetal movement monitoring ("kick counts") using a count to 10 or similar method is recommended for all pregnant women, including those with diabetes, to reduce the stillbirth rate.

Timing of delivery involves balancing the risks of delivery, in particular prematurity and RDS, with the risks of expectant management, namely stillbirth. When fetal assessment is not reassuring, the mature fetus should be delivered. In such cases near term, amniocentesis to obtain amniotic fluid for pulmonary maturity may be helpful. If the fetus is mature, delivery may proceed. If the fetus is immature, then a decision must be made in which the risk of fetal jeopardy is balanced against the risks of preterm birth. Participation of the patient, her partner, and the neonatology and perinatology departments may facilitate a plan.

In the absence of a clear indication for delivery, such as the development of preeclampsia, assessment of fetal lung maturity is recommended for elective delivery prior to 39 weeks. In patients with GDM or preexisting diabetes who require insulin or oral medications to maintain euglycemia, expectant management beyond the due date is generally not recommended.

Preterm labor is more frequent among patients with diabetes. The main goal of tocolysis is to delay delivery so that glucocorticoid therapy to accelerate fetal lung maturation can be administered over 48 hours. Magnesium sulfate tocolysis is widely used. Nifedipine is a reasonable alternative. Beta-adrenergic mimetics such as terbutaline should be avoided if possible because these drugs may cause severe hyperglycemia and, rarely, ketoacidosis. Because glucocorticoids also cause hyperglycemia, a continuous intravenous infusion of insulin may be necessary to maintain normal glucose levels.

Maternal diabetes is not an indication for caesarean section in and of itself; however, if macrosomia coexists, the risk of shoulder dystocia is greatly increased. Therefore, the American College of Obstetricians and Gynecologists recommends that elective caesarean be considered in this setting, in particular if the estimated fetal weight is >4500 g.

American College of Obstetricians and Gynecologists. *Pregestational Diabetes Mellitus. ACOG Practice Bulletin No. 60*. Washington, DC: American College of Obstetricians and Gynecologists; 2005.

American Diabetes Association. Standards of medical care. *Diabetes Care* 2010;33:S11–S61. PMID: 20042772.

Boulot P, Chabbert-Buffet N, d'Ercole C, et al; Diabetes and Pregnancy Group, France. French multicentric survey of outcome of pregnancy in women with pregestational diabetes. *Diabetes Care* 2003;26:2990–2993. PMID: 14578228.

SEVERE HYPERGLYCEMIA & KETOACIDOSIS

The metabolic changes that result in decreased insulin sensitivity during pregnancy also make severe hyperglycemia and ketoacidosis more common. Presenting symptoms of ketoacidosis are similar to the nonpregnant patient and include nausea, vomiting, dehydration, abdominal pain, and confusion. Abnormal laboratory findings include an anion gap metabolic acidosis (arterial pH <7.3), low serum bicarbonate (<15 mEq/L), hyperglycemia, and elevated serum ketones. Management is essentially the same in pregnant and nonpregnant patients and consists of insulin therapy, careful monitoring of potassium level, and fluid replacement. Attention should also be paid to fetal well-being, but diabetic ketoacidosis is not an indication for delivery, because although fetal heart rate monitoring often demonstrates nonreassuring patterns initially, these usually improve as maternal ketoacidosis is corrected.

Intrapartum Management

The goal of intrapartum management is to avoid maternal hyperglycemia and thus minimize the risk of neonatal hypoglycemia after delivery.

Glucose infusion is provided to all patients in labor as 5% dextrose in lactated Ringer's solution or a similar crystalloid. The rate usually is 125 mL/h (providing 6.25 g of glucose per hour) unless the patient requires more. Intravenous fluid bolus prior to conduction anesthesia should not contain glucose.

A bedside glucose monitor can be used to monitor glucose levels every 2–4 hours in early labor and every 1–2 hours in active labor. Patients requiring insulin may receive a continuous infusion of regular insulin, often prepared as 25 U in 250 mL of saline (0.1 U/mL) according to the institution's protocol for intravenous insulin. Most patients require approximately 0.5–2.0 U/h, although rates are adjusted based on the capillary glucose level.

Cervical ripening for induction of labor, if indicated, is conducted in the same manner as for nondiabetic parturients. Continuous electronic fetal monitoring is used. In diabetic pregnancies, the fetus's ability to tolerate the stress of labor may be limited. Fetal heart rate abnormalities should be evaluated with acoustic or scalp stimulation or fetal oxygen saturation monitoring. If fetal well-being cannot be demonstrated, expeditious delivery, often by caesarean section, is indicated. If fetal macrosomia is suspected, operative vaginal delivery should be considered with great caution, if at all. The infant of the diabetic is at increased risk for shoulder dystocia, and this should be anticipated with adequate personnel, obstetric anesthesia, and neonatal resuscitation available at delivery.

If a repeat caesarean delivery or other elective surgery is planned, it should be scheduled for early morning, if possible. The patient should take her evening insulin or oral hypoglycemic dose on the preceding night, but the morning dose should be held. The morning of surgery, the glucose level is monitored and basal insulin needs usually are treated with continuous intravenous insulin to maintain blood glucose between 70 and 120 mg/dL.

Postpartum Care

Postpartum, the patient should start back on an ADA diet as soon as clinically indicated. Insulin sensitivity increases markedly postpartum. In patients with GDM, blood glucose should normalize after delivery. In pregestational patients, as a rule of thumb, insulin doses can be reduced to approximately half the pregnancy dose. Close monitoring of blood glucose should be continued, particularly in the setting of type 1 disease. If the patient underwent surgery, a sliding scale may be implemented until oral intake can be established. The glucose levels should be kept below 140–150 mg/dL to assist the patient in healing. Breastfeeding is strongly encouraged and may be protective against development of childhood diabetes in the infant. Postfeed hypoglycemia can be avoided by increasing caloric intake in the form of snacks.

Contraception

Contraceptive options for diabetic women without vascular complications are the same as for nondiabetic women. In women with an increased risk for embolism, hormonal contraception containing estrogen is not recommended, but progesterone-only methods, including the levonorgestrel intrauterine system, can be offered. Permanent sterilization should be made available to women with diabetes who have completed childbearing.

Prognosis

The prognosis for women with pregestational diabetes is generally not altered by pregnancy. A small percentage of women with end-organ damage related to diabetes prior to pregnancy may experience worsening of their disease. Women with moderate to severe diabetic nephropathy prior to pregnancy (defined as serum creatinine of ≥1.9 mg/dL) are at increased risk of permanent decline in renal function with pregnancy. Approximately 10% of women meeting these criteria progressed to end-stage renal disease. Similarly, diabetic retinopathy worsens in some women during pregnancy. The strict glycemic control achieved during pregnancy is associated with worsening proliferative retinopathy. Laser therapy, however, is an effective treatment of retinopathy and is safe during pregnancy.

GESTATIONAL DIABETES MELLITUS

ESSENTIALS OF DIAGNOSIS

- GDM has been traditionally defined as any degree of glucose intolerance with onset or first recognition during pregnancy.
- The hallmark of GDM is insulin resistance.
- GDM is associated with an increased risk of maternal and fetal/neonatal complications.

Pathogenesis

Approximately 7% of pregnancies are affected by GDM, ranging from 1–14%, depending on the population studied and the diagnostic criteria employed. However, prevalence of the disease is expected to continue to rise as a result of the increasing prevalence of risk factors such as obesity in the gravid population.

The hallmark of GDM is insulin resistance, and as such, it is etiologically similar to type 2 diabetes. Indeed, many patients with a diagnosis of GDM that is made early in gestation may in fact have glucose intolerance that antecedes the pregnancy. Likewise, it is known that as many as 50% of patients with GDM will ultimately go on to develop type 2 diabetes later in life. In recognition of this, the International Association of Diabetes and Pregnancy Study Groups (IADPSG) recently recommended that high-risk women found to have diabetes by standard criteria early in pregnancy be classified as having "overt" rather than "gestational" diabetes.

GDM and type II diabetes are pathogenetically related. In fact, GDM can be considered to be type 2 disease that is unmasked by the metabolic changes of pregnancy. Therefore, it is not surprising that the risk factors for both conditions are similar and include obesity, family history, minority ethnicity, and older age.

The progressive insulin resistance that occurs in normal pregnancies is associated with an increase in insulin release by the beta cells of the pancreas in order to maintain glucose homeostasis. Women with GDM exhibit more insulin resistance than normal patients, which is a function of their prepregnancy metabolic state. GDM becomes manifest when the beta cells are unable to overcome the decreased insulin sensitivity and hyperglycemia results.

Women with GDM continue to demonstrate postpartum defects in insulin action. These defects include the regulations of glucose clearance, glucose production, and plasma-free fatty acid concentrations, together with defects in pancreatic beta cell function, which precede the development of type 2 diabetes.

Clinical Findings

Despite decades of research, the optimal approach to screening and diagnosis of GDM has remained the subject of much controversy. Risk assessment for GDM is performed at the first prenatal visit in all women who do not already have diagnosed diabetes. Women at high risk should undergo screening with plasma glucose as soon as feasible. High-risk characteristics include the following:

1. Age >35–40 years
2. Obesity (nonpregnant body mass index [BMI] >30)
3. Prior history of GDM
4. Heavy glycosuria (>2+ on dipstick)
5. History of unexplained stillbirth
6. Polycystic ovarian syndrome
7. Strong family history of diabetes

If results of testing do not demonstrate diabetes, these women should be retested between 24 and 28 weeks' gestation.

In the past, universal plasma screening was recommended for all women. However, it is acceptable to forgo this in women deemed to be of low risk. A low-risk individual meets all of the following criteria:

1. Age <25 years
2. Not a member of an ethnic group at increased risk (ie, not Hispanic American, African American, Native American, Asian American, or Pacific Islander)
3. BMI ≤25
4. No previous history of abnormal glucose tolerance
5. No previous history of adverse obstetric outcome
6. No known diabetes in a first-degree relative

However, when these criteria are applied, only 10% of the population will be exempt from screening; therefore, many obstetricians believe it is more practical to administer a plasma glucose screen in all pregnant women.

Currently, both the American College of Obstetricians and Gynecologists and the ADA advocate a 2-step approach to screening. Step 1 consists of a 1-hour 50-g oral glucose challenge test (GCT), which is administered between 24 and 28 weeks of gestation. The GCT can be performed at any time of day and without regard to time of prior meal. If this screening test is positive, it is followed by the diagnostic test, a 3-hour 100-g OGTT.

The correct threshold for an abnormal result for the GCT has not been definitively defined. The original blood glucose value for an abnormal screen (>140 mg/dL) was chosen arbitrarily and later validated by its ability to predict future development of diabetes in the mother and not by any correlation with adverse pregnancy outcome. In fact, the blood glucose threshold above which adverse outcomes begin to increase has never been established. The recent Hyperglycemia and Adverse Pregnancy Outcome (HAPO) study addressed this issue and found that no discrete threshold exists. Instead, there is a continuous relationship between blood glucose levels and adverse outcome. This study confirmed that even in women who did not meet the criteria for a diagnosis of GDM, the risk of complications increased in proportion to an increase in blood glucose.

At the blood glucose threshold of 140 mg/dL, 80% of patients with GDM will be detected, but approximately 15% of all patients screened will require further definitive testing. Lowering the threshold from 140 to 130 mg/dL, as many experts advocate, would result in a detection rate of 90%, but would result in false-positive screens in many more women. In patients whose screening result is >200 mg/dL, a diagnosis of GDM can be made without further testing.

Diagnostic testing is usually accomplished by administration of a 3-hour 100-g OGTT after an overnight fast. Two different classification schemes of results are employed, which were adapted from the original O'Sullivan and Mahar whole blood values. There is no clear advantage to one scheme over the other. A diagnosis of GDM is made when 2 or more thresholds are met or exceeded. However, morbidity is increased with even a single abnormal value, and therefore, many physicians advocate initiation of dietary therapy in this scenario.

Outside of the United States, a 1-step approach to testing using a 2-hour 75-g oral glucose load is widely used. In 2010, following publication of the findings of the HAPO study, the IADPSG proposed that this 1-step approach replace the current screening and diagnostic tests. Based on the recommendations of the IADPSG, the diagnosis of GDM can be made if there is 1 or more abnormal value on the 75-g OGTT. Thresholds for both the 100-g and 75-g OGTT are listed in Table 31–4.

Complications

Similar to pregestational diabetes, GDM is associated with an increased risk of maternal and fetal complications including

Table 31–4. Diagnostic criteria for gestational diabetes mellitus.

	100-g GTT Plasma/Serum Level (mg/dL) (Carpenter/Coustan)	100-g GTT Plasma Level (mg/dL) (National Diabetes Data Group)	75-g GTT Plasma Level (mg/dL) (IADPSG)
Fasting	95	105	92
1-hour	180	190	180
2-hour	155	165	153
3-hour	140	145	-

GTT, glucose tolerance test; IADPSG, International Association of Diabetes and Pregnancy Study Groups.

preeclampsia, stillbirth, and macrosomia. Infants born to mothers with gestational diabetes are at increased risk of hypoglycemia, hyperbilirubinemia, hypocalcemia, and RDS.

GDM may also be associated with long-term health consequences for the fetus. Offspring of mothers with GDM appear to be at increased risk of obesity and impaired glucose tolerance later in life.

Unlike offspring of women with pregestational diabetes, fetuses of women with true GDM are not at increased risk of fetal structural malformation.

Treatment

Treatment of women with GDM focuses on achieving rigorous control of blood glucose level and thus minimizing the risk of maternal and fetal complications. At time of diagnosis, dietary counseling is provided, and patients are prescribed a 1800–2400 kcal/d diabetic diet. Diet should be approximately 40% carbohydrate, 40% fat, and 20% protein usually divided into 3 meals and 2 or 3 snacks per day.

Patients are advised to initiate home glucose monitoring of fasting, 1- or 2-hour postprandial, and nighttime blood glucose levels using a glucose meter. Optimal glucose levels during pregnancy are fasting levels of 70–95 mg/dL and 1-hour postprandial values <130–140 mg/dL or 2-hour postprandial values <120 mg/dL. When postprandial values exceed the targets, it is important to review all recent food intake and to adjust food choice, preparation, and portion size. When normoglycemia cannot be achieved with diet and exercise alone, medication is added.

As with pregestational diabetes, treatment of GDM that has failed treatment with dietary modification alone typically starts with insulin as first-line therapy. However, a number of studies have demonstrated that oral hypoglycemics such as glyburide and metformin are efficacious at achieving glycemic control with a favorable safety profile for the fetus. Glyburide, a sulfonylurea, is variously categorized as either pregnancy class B or C. It is believed to cross the placenta in only minimal amounts, and studies to date have demonstrated generally favorable results when compared to insulin. Glyburide is commenced at doses of 2.5–5 mg/d and titrated upward to a maximum of 20 mg/d to achieve optimal blood glucose control.

Antenatal Care

Women with GDM that is well controlled by diet alone usually do not require antenatal fetal testing. In the setting of excellent glycemic control achieved by diet alone, fetal surveillance with nonstress testing or biophysical profiles may be initiated at 40 weeks. However, for women who require medication for control of their blood sugars, who are noncompliant, or who have GDM that is not well controlled, earlier initiation of fetal surveillance and ultrasound assessment of fetal growth are advised.

Intrapartum Management

As with women with pregestational diabetes, the goal of intrapartum management of women with GDM is to avoid maternal hyperglycemia and thus minimize the risk of neonatal hypoglycemia after delivery.

Glucose infusion is provided to all patients in labor as 5% dextrose in lactated Ringer's solution or a similar crystalloid. The rate usually is 125 mL/h (providing 6.25 g of glucose per hour) unless the patient requires more. Intravenous fluid bolus prior to conduction anesthesia should not contain glucose.

A bedside glucose monitor can be used to monitor glucose levels every 2–4 hours in early labor and every 1–2 hours in active labor. Patients requiring insulin may receive a continuous infusion of regular insulin, often prepared as 25 U in 250 mL saline (0.1 U/mL) according to the institution's protocol for intravenous insulin. Most patients require approximately 0.5–2.0 U/h, although rates are adjusted based on the capillary glucose level.

Cervical ripening for induction of labor, if indicated, is conducted in the same manner as for nondiabetic parturients. Continuous electronic fetal monitoring is used. If fetal well-being cannot be demonstrated, expeditious delivery, often by caesarean section, is indicated. If fetal macrosomia is suspected, operative vaginal delivery should be considered with great caution, if at all. The infant of the diabetic is at increased risk for shoulder dystocia, and this should be anticipated with adequate personnel, obstetric anesthesia, and neonatal resuscitation available at delivery.

If a repeat caesarean delivery or other elective surgery is planned, it should be scheduled for early morning, if possible. The patient should take her evening insulin or oral hypoglycemic dose on the preceding night, but the morning dose should be held. The morning of surgery, glucose level is monitored and basal insulin needs usually are treated with continuous intravenous insulin to maintain blood glucose between 70 and 120 mg/dL.

Postpartum Care

Because GDM resolves with delivery of the fetus and placenta, routine postpartum care in the immediate postpartum period is sufficient. For the patient with true GDM, all medications for blood sugar control are discontinued after delivery, as is blood glucose monitoring.

Prognosis

Women diagnosed with GDM are at increased risk to develop type 2 diabetes in the future. They have about a 50% risk of developing the disease within 10–15 years. Lifestyle modification may delay or entirely prevent the onset of diabetes in adults with impaired glucose tolerance, and therefore, counseling of a patient with GDM should include a discussion of the long-term prevention of progression to nongestational diabetes.

Table 31–5. Categories of increased risk for diabetes.

Impaired Fasting Glucose (mg/dL)	Impaired Glucose Tolerance (mg/dL)	Elevated HbA1c
FPG 100–125	2-hour OGTT 140–199	5.7–6.4%

FPG, fasting plasma glucose; HbA1c, hemoglobin A1c; OGTT, oral glucose tolerance test with 75-g glucose load.

All patients with GDM should have a 2-hour, 75-g OGTT approximately 6 weeks postpartum. Those with normal glucose tolerance should be reassessed every 3 years. Those with impaired glucose tolerance or impaired fasting glucose should be reevaluated annually (Table 31–5).

All women should be encouraged to eliminate or reduce any other risk factors (in addition to glucose intolerance) for cardiovascular disease. In practice, this means referral to programs, as needed, to cease smoking and to avoid environmental smoke; to engage in regular physical activity; to consume an appropriate diet; to achieve and maintain a normal weight; and to be treated for individual cardiovascular disease risk factors.

American College of Obstetricians and Gynecologists. *Fetal Macrosomia. ACOG Practice Bulletin No. 22.* Washington, DC: American College of Obstetricians and Gynecologists; 2000.

American College of Obstetricians and Gynecologists. *Gestational Diabetes. ACOG Practice Bulletin No. 30.* Washington, DC: American College of Obstetricians and Gynecologists; 2001.

Centers for Disease Control and Prevention. National diabetes fact sheet: general information and national estimates on diabetes in the United States, 2007. Atlanta, GA: US Department of Health and Human Services, Centers for Disease Control and Prevention; 2008.

Clausen TD, Mathiesen E, Ekbom P, et al. Poor pregnancy outcome in women with type 2 diabetes. *Diabetes Care* 2005;28:323–328. PMID: 15677787.

Dabelea D, Hanson RL, Lindsay RS, et al. Intrauterine exposure to diabetes conveys risks for type 2 diabetes and obesity: a study of discordant sibships. *Diabetes* 2000;49:2208–2211. PMID: 11118027.

Dang K, Homko C, Reece EA. Factors associated with fetal macrosomia in offspring of gestational diabetic women. *J Matern Fetal Med* 2000;9:114–117. PMID: 10902825.

De Lee J. *Principles and Practice of Obstetrics.* 1st ed. Philadelphia, PA: Saunders; 1913.

Eriksson UJ, Borg LA, Cederberg J, et al. Pathogenesis of diabetes-induced congenital malformations. *Ups J Med Sci* 2000;105:53–84. PMID: 11095105.

Jimenez-Moleon JJ, Bueno-Cavanillas A, Luna-Del-Castillo JD, et al. Prevalence of gestational diabetes mellitus: variations related to screening strategy used. *Eur J Endocrinol* 2002;146:831–837. PMID: 12039704.

Jovanovic L, Nakai Y. Successful pregnancy in women with type 1 diabetes: from preconception through postpartum care. *Endocrinol Metab Clin North Am* 2006;35:79–97. PMID: 16310643.

Kamalakannan D, Baskar V, Barton DM, et al. Diabetic ketoacidosis in pregnancy. *Postgrad Med J* 2003;79:454–457. PMID: 12954957.

Kim C, Ferrara A, McEwen LN, et al; TRIAD Study Group. Preconception care in managed care: the Translating Research into Action for Diabetes study. *Am J Obstet Gynecol* 2005;192:227–232. PMID: 13672029.

Landon MB, Spong CY, Thom E, et al. A multicenter, randomized trial of treatment for mild gestational diabetes. *N Engl J Med* 2009;361:1339–1348. PMID: 19797280.

Langer O, Conway DL, Berkus MD, et al. A comparison of glyburide and insulin in women with gestational diabetes mellitus. *N Engl J Med* 2000;343:1134–1138. PMID: 11036118.

Lusignan S, Sismanidis C, Carey IM, et al. Trends in the prevalence and management of diagnosed type 2 diabetes 1994-2001 in England and Wales. *BMC Fam Pract* 2005;6:13. PMID: 15784113.

Moore LE, Clokey D, Rappaport VJ, Curet LB. Metformin compared with glyburide in gestational diabetes: a randomized controlled trial. *Obstet Gynecol* 2010;115:55–59. PMID: 20027034.

Ray JG, O'Brien TE, Chan WS. Preconception care and the risk of congenital anomalies in the offspring of women with diabetes mellitus: a meta-analysis. *QJM* 2001;94:435–444. PMID: 11493721.

Rendell M. Dietary treatment of diabetes mellitus. *N Engl J Med* 2000;342:1440. PMID: 10885301.

Schaefer-Graf UM, Buchanan TA, Xiang A, et al. Patterns of congenital anomalies and relationship to initial maternal fasting glucose levels in pregnancies complicated by type 2 and gestational diabetes. *Am J Obstet Gynecol* 2000;182:313–320. PMID: 10694330.

Shaw JE, Sicree RA, Zimmet PZ. Global estimates of the prevalence of diabetes for 2010 and 2030. *Diabetes Res Clin Pract* 2010;87:4–14. PMID: 19896746.

Strehlow SL, Mestman JH. Prevention of T2DM in women with a previous history of GDM. *Curr Diab Rep* 2005;5:272–277. PMID: 16033678.

Thyroid & Other Endocrine Disorders During Pregnancy

32

Cynthia Gyamfi Bannerman, MD

THYROID DISORDERS

Thyroid diseases are among the most common endocrine disorders encountered during pregnancy. They are challenging both because of pregnancy-related changes in thyroid physiology that make diagnosis of thyroid disorders difficult and because of the limited number of medications used to treat mother and fetus. Screening for subclinical thyroid disorders remains a highly debated topic.

THYROID FUNCTION DURING NORMAL PREGNANCY

The thyroid, a gland that functions to provide thermal and metabolic regulation, develops from the third week in gestation from the primitive pharynx. The gland then migrates to the neck and starts to produce thyroid hormone by 10–12 weeks' gestation.

Maternal thyroid physiology is altered during normal pregnancy. There is glandular hyperplasia with thyroid enlargement. Thyroid volume is increased on ultrasound examination, but the echostructure is unchanged. The normal increase in the renal glomerular filtration rate causes an increase in urinary iodide clearance, necessitating increased intake of dietary iodine in order to make and maintain thyroid hormone concentrations. Both total thyroxine (T_4) and triiodothyronine (T_3) levels increase because the level of their carrier, thyroxine-binding globulin (TBG), becomes elevated. Estrogen causes increased TBG synthesis with decreased TBG clearance. Because of the similar subunits of chorionic gonadotropin and thyrotropin (thyroid-stimulating hormone [TSH]), crossover between these 2 peptides can lead to an increase in free thyroxine (fT_4) in the first trimester. The TSH level is lowest and fT_4 level highest when human chorionic gonadotropin (hCG) levels peak. Elevated fT_4 causes suppression of TSH, which, in turn, causes barely detectable levels of maternal thyrotropin-releasing hormone (TRH). Overall, the demand for T_4 increases by an estimated 1–3% above daily nonpregnant needs. The increased demand starts very early, reaching a plateau at 16–20 weeks. These normal physiologic changes make diagnosis of thyroid disease during pregnancy difficult.

Studies from animal models have helped to elucidate the role of maternal T_4 in the fetus. T_3 is made by conversion of maternal T_4. It has been demonstrated that if maternal T_4 is low, fetal T_3 levels in the brain will be low even in the presence of normal maternal and fetal serum T_3, suggesting that both T_3 and T_4 in the fetal brain are maternal T_4 dependent. Further evidence of a maternal source of T_3 in the fetal brain is that by midgestation, fetal concentration of T_3 is 34% of adult levels. This is much higher than would be expected considering the low circulating fetal serum levels. It is during midgestation that initial growth velocity of the fetal brain occurs, and animal data suggest that the thyroid hormone necessary for this development is primarily maternally derived. Toward the end of the first trimester, the fetal hypothalamic–pituitary–thyroid axis becomes active. By 14 weeks' gestation, fetal production of T_4 is detectable. Normal thyroid hormones levels in the fetus and newborn are crucial for subsequent brain maturation and intellectual development.

HYPERTHYROIDISM

ESSENTIALS OF DIAGNOSIS

- Elevated free T_4 and T_3 levels; suppressed TSH levels
- Signs and symptoms of hyperthyroidism include heat intolerance, fatigue, anxiety, diaphoresis, tachycardia, and a widened pulse pressure

Pathogenesis

The prevalence of hyperthyroidism (also known as thyrotoxicosis) during pregnancy ranges from 0.05 to 0.2%.

The most common cause of hyperthyroidism during pregnancy is Graves' disease. Graves' disease is caused by thyroid-stimulating antibody (TSAb) belonging to the immunoglobulin (Ig) G class, which binds with high affinity to the TSH receptor. TSAb may cross the placenta, bind to fetal TSH receptors, and cause fetal or neonatal hyperthyroidism. However, the placenta acts as a partial barrier, so usually only those with high titers are likely to be affected. Other causes of hyperthyroidism include thyroiditis, thyroid adenoma, and multinodular goiter.

Clinical Findings

The signs and symptoms of hyperthyroidism—heat intolerance, fatigue, anxiety, diaphoresis, tachycardia, and a widened pulse pressure—can all be found during normal pregnancy. Signs specific to hyperthyroidism would be pulse >100 bpm, goiter, and exophthalmos, but these may not be present. Gastrointestinal symptoms such as severe nausea and vomiting may also be present, but these can be related to β-hCG elevations. Laboratory tests will confirm elevated T_4, fT_4, T_3, and free T_3 (fT_3) levels and a suppressed or undetectable TSH level. TSAb titers will be elevated in a significant number of patients. Other laboratory findings may include a normocytic, normochromic anemia, mild neutropenia, and elevated liver enzymes.

Subclinical hyperthyroidism, a condition resulting from suppressed levels of TSH and normal levels of T_4 and T_3, is also seen in pregnancy. It was determined that 1.7% of screened women had subclinical disease. There is no effect of subclinical hyperthyroidism in pregnancy, so screening and treatment for this entity are not warranted.

Complications

The most common complication of hyperthyroidism in pregnancy is preeclampsia. With large amounts of transplacental transfer of thyroid-stimulating immunoglobulins, thyrotoxicosis could develop in the fetus or newborn. Fetal hypothyroidism may also result from overadministration of thioamides. Poorly controlled hyperthyroidism has also been associated with an increased risk of miscarriage, preterm labor, and low-birth-weight infants.

Thyroid storm is a life-threatening complication of women with hyperthyroidism that may result in heart failure if untreated. This complication developed in 8% of women with thyrotoxicosis. Classic findings of thyroid storm include thermoregulatory dysfunction; central nervous system (CNS) effects including agitation, delirium, and coma; gastrointestinal dysfunction; and cardiovascular manifestations such as tachycardia or heart failure. This can be precipitated by labor and delivery, caesarean delivery, infection, or preeclampsia. T_4-induced cardiomyopathy, however, is reversible.

Treatment

Treatment during pregnancy almost always consists of antithyroid medications. Surgery is performed in exceptional situations, such as allergic reactions to all drugs available or lack of response to very large doses ("drug resistance"), which in most cases has been the result of noncompliance. The goals of treatment are to rapidly achieve and maintain euthyroidism with the minimum but effective amount of medication, provide symptomatic relief, and keep fT_4 levels in the upper third of normal. Thionamides are the most commonly prescribed class of medication used for the treatment of hyperthyroidism. The medications available are propylthiouracil (PTU) and methimazole. Both drugs work by blocking thyroid hormone synthesis; however, PTU also blocks peripheral conversion of T_4 to T_3. Some physicians prefer PTU, but reports of large numbers of patients indicate that the 2 drugs are equally effective and have similar side effects. PTU is shorter acting, meaning more pills are required more often; therefore, methimazole may be preferable when compliance is a problem. The initial methimazole dose is 20–40 mg/d, and the initial PTU dose is 200–400 mg/d. The dose is gradually reduced as improvement occurs. Most women can be effectively treated on an outpatient basis; however, hospitalization may be considered in severe, uncontrolled cases in the third trimester because of increased risk for complications. Women who have remained euthyroid while taking small amounts of PTU (≤100 mg/d) or methimazole (≤10 mg/d) for 4 weeks or longer can stop taking the medication altogether by 32–34 weeks' gestation under close surveillance. The purpose is to minimize the risk of fetal/neonatal hypothyroidism, which is otherwise uncommon with PTU doses ≤200 mg/d or methimazole ≤20 mg/d. The therapy is resumed if symptoms recur. Women with large goiters, long-standing hyperthyroidism, or significant eye involvement should remain on treatment throughout pregnancy. Other potential side effects of antithyroid medications are pruritus, skin rash, urticaria, fever, arthralgias, cholestatic jaundice, lupus-like syndrome, and migratory polyarthritis. Leukopenia may be a medication effect but is also seen in untreated Graves' disease; therefore, a white blood cell (WBC) count should be obtained before treatment is started. Agranulocytosis is the most severe complication, but fortunately, it is uncommon and found in only 0.1% of patients. Treatment prior to pregnancy is preferred to treatment during pregnancy because outcomes tend to be better. Recently, methimazole has become the treatment of choice for hyperthyroidism in pregnancy. This is because PTU has been found to cause irreversible liver damage, leading potentially to liver failure.

β-Blockers (propranolol 20–40 mg every 6–8 hours) can be used for symptomatic relief in severe cases but only for short periods (few weeks) and before 34–36 weeks' gestation. They inhibit conversion from T_4 to T_3 but may be related to intrauterine growth restriction and hypoglycemia if used for prolonged periods of time.

Treatment of thyroid storm is aimed at reducing synthesis of thyroid hormone, minimizing release of thyroid hormone from the thyroid gland, and blocking peripheral effects of thyroid hormone. Aggressive treatment for thyroid storm is critical to the patient's survival. PTU or methimazole is started immediately and may be administered via nasogastric tube if the patient has altered mental status. Iodine solution such as potassium iodide (SSKI) or Lugol's solution may also be given. Iodine solution works by inhibiting thyroid hormone release. If the patient has a history of iodine-induced anaphylaxis, then lithium carbonate is given instead. Fluid hydration and nutritional support are also important. β-Blockers are also given for relief of symptoms such as tachycardia and palpitations, and they may also inhibit peripheral conversion of T_4 to T_3. Glucocorticoids may also be used in severe cases to reduce peripheral conversion of T_4 to T_3. Aspirin should be avoided in these patients because it can increase concentrations of fT_4 and T_3.

Prognosis

The maternal and fetal prognosis with hyperthyroidism in pregnancy that is well controlled is generally excellent.

A. Effect of Hyperthyroidism on Pregnancy

Potential complications of hyperthyroidism in the mother include spontaneous abortion, pregnancy-induced hypertension, preterm delivery, anemia, higher susceptibility to infections, placental abruption, and, in severe, untreated cases, cardiac arrhythmias, congestive heart failure, and thyroid storm. In the fetus, possible complications include fetal and neonatal hyperthyroidism, intrauterine growth restriction, stillbirth, prematurity, and morbidity related to antithyroid medications. Most maternal and neonatal complications are seen in cases of uncontrolled or untreated hyperthyroidism.

Approximately 1–5% of infants born to women with Graves' disease have hyperthyroidism at birth due to transplacental transfer of TSAbs. The fetal/neonatal risk correlates with maternal TSAb titer level. Signs of fetal hyperthyroidism include fetal tachycardia (heart rate >160 bpm), fetal goiter, and poor growth. High levels of fetal thyroid hormone detected by cordocentesis have been confirmed in a few cases. Tests of fetal well-being are recommended for poorly controlled cases and for patients with high TSAb titers, even if they are euthyroid. Serial ultrasounds are useful for dating and fetal growth evaluation.

Breastfeeding is allowed if the total daily dose of PTU is ≤150 mg or daily dose of methimazole is ≤10 mg. The medication should be given immediately after each feeding and the infant monitored periodically.

B. Effect of Pregnancy on Hyperthyroidism

Pregnancy is not thought to alter the course of hyperthyroidism.

TRANSIENT HYPERTHYROIDISM OF HYPEREMESIS GRAVIDARUM

ESSENTIALS OF DIAGNOSIS

- Severe nausea and vomiting accompanied by weight loss
- Low serum TSH with mildly elevated fT_4

Pathogenesis

Biochemical hyperthyroidism is seen in most women (66%) with hyperemesis gravidarum. The most likely etiology is thyrotropin receptor stimulation from high serum concentrations of hCG.

Clinical Findings

Laboratory abnormalities include low serum TSH and mildly elevated fT_4. Serum T_3 levels are not elevated in women with transient hyperthyroidism of hyperemesis gravidarum. The degree of thyroid function abnormalities correlates with the severity of vomiting.

Differential Diagnosis

Women in early pregnancy with weight loss, tachycardia, vomiting, and laboratory evidence of hyperthyroidism may be difficult to differentiate from early, true thyrotoxicosis. Women with transient hyperthyroidism of hyperemesis gravidarum have no previous history of thyroid disease, no palpable goiter, and, except for tachycardia, no other symptoms or signs of hyperthyroidism. Test results for thyroid antibodies are negative. With transient hyperthyroidism of hyperemesis gravidarum, TSH level may be suppressed and fT_4 level elevated, but the T_3 level is lower than in true hyperthyroidism. With true hyperthyroidism, both levels are usually elevated.

Treatment

Treatment is symptomatic, and antithyroid medication is not recommended.

Prognosis

The mild hyperthyroidism associated with transient hyperthyroidism of hyperemesis gravidarum usually resolves by 20 weeks' gestation. The time to resolution is widely variable (1–10 weeks).

HYPOTHYROIDISM

ESSENTIALS OF DIAGNOSIS

- Elevated TSH and low free T_4 levels
- Symptoms: modest weight gain, fatigue, sleepiness, lethargy, decreased exercise capacity, depression, and cold intolerance (very unusual in normal pregnancy)

Pathogenesis

Overt hypothyroidism (elevated TSH, low free T_4) has been reported in 1 in 1000 to 1 in 2000 deliveries. A study by Casey and colleagues found that the incidence of overt hypothyroidism in pregnant women was 1.8 per 1000. Subclinical hypothyroidism (elevated TSH, normal fT_4) is more common, with an incidence of 23 per 1000 in pregnancy. This makes the overall incidence of hypothyroidism 2.5%.

The most common cause of hypothyroidism is Hashimoto's thyroiditis, which is found in 8–10% of women of reproductive age. Less common causes are transient hypothyroidism in silent (painless) and subacute thyroiditis, drug induced, high-dose external neck radiation, congenital hypothyroidism, inherited metabolic disorders, and thyroid hormone resistance syndromes. Secondary hypothyroidism may occur in pituitary or hypothalamic disease. Drugs that may cause hypothyroidism by interfering with thyroid hormone synthesis and/or its release include antithyroid drugs (PTU, methimazole), iodine, and lithium. Increased T_4 clearance is caused by carbamazepine, phenytoin, and rifampin. Amiodarone decreases T_4 to T_3 conversion and inhibition of T_3 action. Interference with intestinal absorption is seen with aluminum hydroxide, cholestyramine, ferrous sulfate, calcium, vitamins, soy, and sucralfate. Many pregnant women take ferrous sulfate, and it is important to ensure that T_4 is taken at least 2 hours before (sometimes even 4 hours is recommended) because insoluble ferric–T_4 complexes may form, resulting in reduced T_4 absorption.

Clinical Findings

The clinical diagnosis is difficult and frequently unsuspected except in advanced cases. Symptoms are insidious and may be masked by the hypermetabolic state of pregnancy. Symptoms include modest weight gain, fatigue, sleepiness, lethargy, decreased exercise capacity, depression, and cold intolerance (very unusual in normal pregnancy). Signs include general slowing of speech and movements, dry and pale or yellowish skin, sparse thin hair, hoarseness, bradycardia (also unusual in pregnancy), myxedema, hyporeflexia, prolonged relaxation of reflexes, carpal tunnel syndrome, and a diffuse or a nodular goiter.

The best laboratory test is the TSH level; current sensitive assays allow very early diagnosis and accurate treatment monitoring. Other useful tests include fT_4 and antibody titers. A low fT_4 with an elevated TSH is diagnostic of hypothyroidism. A macrocytic or normochromic, normocytic anemia may be present as well. It usually results from decreased erythropoiesis, but it may result from vitamin B_{12}, folic acid, or iron deficiency. Levels of lipids and creatine phosphokinase (of muscle origin) may be elevated. Hypothyroidism may be seen more commonly in women with type 1 diabetes.

Complications

A. Effect of Hypothyroidism on Pregnancy

Some studies have reported a 2-fold increased rate of spontaneous abortion in women with elevated levels of thyroid antibodies, even if they are euthyroid, but this finding is not universally confirmed. These antibodies (antiperoxidase [TPO], antimicrosomal antibody [AMA], and antithyroglobulin [ATG]) may cross the placenta and cause neonatal hypothyroidism, which, if untreated, may lead to serious cognitive deficiencies. Lower IQs in infants of even very mildly hypothyroid women have been reported. There is an increased risk of preeclampsia, placental abruption, intrauterine growth restriction, prematurity, and intrauterine fetal demise. The severity of the hypertension and other perinatal complications is greater in the more severely hypothyroid woman. Early treatment and close monitoring to ensure euthyroidism will prevent or decrease perinatal complications.

B. Effect of Pregnancy on Hypothyroidism

Pregnancy is known to cause increasing requirement of thyroid hormone. That is the reason for evaluation of maternal TSH levels every trimester, with more frequent evaluation every 4 weeks if changes to dosing are deemed necessary. Requirements usually return to prepregnancy levels postpartum, and dosing can also be adjusted on a monthly schedule after that time.

Treatment

L-Thyroxine has long been the treatment drug of choice. The hormonal content of the synthetic drugs is more reliably standardized, and they have replaced desiccated thyroid as the mainstay of therapy. Administration of T_4 alone is recommended. In the normal physiologic process, T_4 is deiodinated to T_3 in the extrathyroidal tissues. In addition, during early pregnancy, the fetal brain is unable to use maternal T_3. The best time to take L-thyroxine is early in the morning, on an empty stomach. Women experiencing nausea and vomiting should be allowed to take it later in the day until they improve. Numerous reports indicate that T_4 requirements increase during pregnancy. TSH levels should be checked every 4 weeks, with adjustments made until the TSH is at the lower end of the normal range. The initial dose should be 2 μg/kg of actual body weight. Further adjustments are made according to the TSH level. If the TSH level is elevated but <10 μU/mL, add 25–50 μg/d; if the TSH level is >10 but <20, add 50–75 μg/d; and if the TSH level is >20, add 75–100 μg/d. Changes made at less than 4-week intervals may lead to overtreatment. Up to 85% of women receiving T_4 replacement before pregnancy will require higher doses while they are pregnant. The levels should be checked early in pregnancy and then every trimester to maintain euthyroidism. After delivery, the dosage is reduced to the prepregnancy amount, and the TSH level is measured 4–8 weeks postpartum. In women with pituitary disease, the TSH level cannot be used to guide therapy. In these cases, the fT_4 level should be kept in the upper third of normal.

Casey BM, Leveno KJ. Thyroid disease in pregnancy. *Obstet Gynecol* 2006;108:1283–1292. PMID: 17077257.

SUBCLINICAL HYPOTHYROIDISM

ESSENTIALS OF DIAGNOSIS

- Elevated serum TSH with normal fT_4 levels

Pathogenesis

Subclinical hypothyroidism is a condition characterized by an elevated TSH with a normal fT_4. The incidence of this finding is approximately 2.5% in pregnant women and 5% in women of reproductive age. The causes of subclinical hypothyroidism are thought to be the same as overt hypothyroidism.

Clinical Findings

Subclinical hypothyroidism is diagnosed when woman are found to have elevations in TSH and normal fT_4 levels. Women are asymptomatic for thyroid disease.

Complications

The interest in subclinical hypothyroidism and intellectual development in offspring was reignited after several recent publications addressed a possible relationship between the two. Haddow and colleagues performed a study comparing pregnant women with hypothyroidism to pregnant controls with normal thyroid function. They found that children of women with hypothyroidism scored 4 points lower on a standard IQ test when compared to controls ($P = 0.06$). In addition, 15% of cases had an IQ score of 85 or less compared to 5% of controls ($P = 0.08$). Although neither of these values is statistically significant, when the results were sub-analyzed for those women with untreated hypothyroidism, as opposed to those on medication, they found that the IQ scores were 7 points lower in cases than controls ($P = 0.005$), and 19% had IQ scores <85 compared with 5% of controls ($P = 0.007$), suggesting that the greater effect on pediatric neurodevelopment is in the untreated mothers with hypothyroidism. Pop and colleagues had similar results when they studied pediatric neurodevelopment at 10, 12, and 24 months in children of mothers with abnormal thyroid function at 12 weeks' gestation. Note that neither of these studies evaluated infants of women with subclinical hypothyroidism. Haddow evaluated infants of mothers with overt hypothyroidism, whereas Pop evaluated infants of women with hypothyroxinemia, thought to be the more clinically relevant deficiency.

The discrepancy in findings from these 2 studies has led to conflicting position statements regarding the surveillance for hypothyroidism in pregnant women from the American Association of Clinical Endocrinologists, the American Thyroid Association, the Endocrine Society, and the American College of Obstetricians and Gynecologists (ACOG). Current obstetric practice does not involve screening for thyroid disease unless the patient has risk factors, such as pregestational diabetes, or is symptomatic. The most recent joint position statement of the 3 previously mentioned endocrine societies recommends routine TSH evaluation (with fT_4 if TSH is abnormal) both preconceptionally or as soon as pregnancy has been diagnosed. However, ACOG does not support the performance of thyroid function tests in asymptomatic pregnant women. ACOG advises that the current data are limited because of their observational nature. To date, there has not been a clinical trial that specifically addresses isolated subclinical hypothyroidism and neurodevelopmental outcomes, making recommendations regarding the management of this mild thyroid dysfunction difficult. Furthermore, the available clinical literature has not shown that the identification and treatment of women with subclinical hypothyroidism prevents the purported neurodevelopmental sequelae. The National Institute of Child Health and Human Development Maternal-Fetal Medicine Units network is currently conducting a clinical trial to help answer these questions.

Certain pregnant women are at high risk for hypothyroidism and should undergo screening, including those with previous therapy for hyperthyroidism, high-dose neck irradiation, previous postpartum thyroiditis, presence of a goiter, family history of thyroid disease, treatment with amiodarone, suspected hypopituitarism, and type 1 diabetes mellitus.

Treatment

ACOG does not advocate routine screening and treatment for subclinical hypothyroidism at this time.

Haddow JE, Palomaki GE, Allan WC, et al. Maternal thyroid deficiency during pregnancy and subsequent neuropsychological development of the child. *N Engl J Med* 1999;19:549–555. PMID: 10451459.

Pop VJ, Brouwers EP, Vader HL, Vulsma T, van Baar AL, de Vijlder JJ. Maternal hypothyroxinaemia during early pregnancy and subsequent child development: a 3-year follow-up study. *Clin Endocrinol* 2003;59:282–288. PMID: 12919150.

CONGENITAL HYPOTHYROIDISM

ESSENTIALS OF DIAGNOSIS

- Elevated serum TSH and low T_3 and T_4 in the neonate

Pathogenesis

Congenital hypothyroidism is found in 1 in 4000 to 1 in 7000 infants after diagnosis from national screening programs. Congenital hypothyroidism is defined as hypothyroidism in the neonate. Most cases of congenital hypothyroidism are sporadic, resulting from thyroid dysgenesis. However, approximately 15% appear to be hereditary, mostly due to an inborn error in thyroid hormone synthesis. Early and aggressive treatment is critical to improve neonatal outcomes.

Transient congenital hypothyroidism has been described in a number of settings, including iodine deficiency and in utero exposure to antithyroid drugs.

Clinical Findings

Low serum T_4 and high serum TSH levels in the neonate confirm a diagnosis of congenital hypothyroidism. Most neonates are asymptomatic at birth, mainly because some maternal T_4 crosses the placenta. Signs that may present over time include lethargy, slow movement, hoarse cry, poor feeding, and constipation.

Complications

The first report of a possible correlation between thyroid disease and mental retardation in offspring came from iodine-deficient areas of Switzerland in 1915. Mothers of children with mental retardation were noted to have abnormal thyroid function. Choufoer and colleagues then described the effect of maternal thyroid levels on the newborn in 1965. They described pregnancy outcomes related to endemic goiter in iodine-deficient New Guinea. They found neurologic manifestations of cretinism, or physical stunting and mental retardation, in women who were not clinically hypothyroid, but who had a low concentration of thyroid hormone. In this same decade, Man and Jones evaluated a cohort of 1349 children of mothers with hypothyroxinemia, defined in that time as a low serum butanol-extractable with a normal thyroid-binding globulin. They found an association between low BEI and low infant Bayley scores on mental and motor development. The Bayley Scales of Infant Development were designed to test the cognitive, motor, and behavioral development of infants up to 42 months of age. The test has high validity and reliability. These and other observations of maternal thyroid disease led to the landmark double-blind study by Pharoah and colleagues in 1971. They gave alternate families in New Guinea either 4-mL injections of iodized oil or a saline placebo and then returned a year later to initiate periodic evaluation of any offspring delivered after treatment. They concluded that supplementation of iodine in pregnancy prevented subsequent cretinism.

Treatment

Oral thyroid supplementation, usually T_4, is the treatment for congenital hypothyroidism. Treatment is usually starting when screening tests for congenital hypothyroidism return as positive without waiting for result of confirmatory tests.

Prognosis

With early diagnosis and initiation of treatment, long-term outcomes are excellent, with normal growth and development.

Choufeor JC, Vanrhijn M, Querido A. Endemic goiter in western new guinea. II. Clinical picture, incidence and pathogenesis of endemic cretinism. *J Clin Endocrinol Metab* 1965;25:385–402. PMID: 14264263.

Jones WS and Man EB. Thyroid function in human pregnancy. VI. Premature deliveries and reproductive failures of pregnant women with low serum butanol-extractable iodines. Maternal serum TBG and TBPA capacities. *Am J Obstet Gynecol* 1969;15: 909–914. PMID: 4183109.

Pharoah PO, Buttfield IH, and Hetzel BS. Neurological damage to the fetus resulting from severe iodine deficiency during pregnancy. *Lancet* 1971;1:308–310. PMID: 4100150.

POSTPARTUM THYROIDITIS

ESSENTIALS OF DIAGNOSIS

- Postpartum thyroiditis is diagnosed if the serum TSH is either elevated or depressed in the year after delivery.
- This phenomenon has been noted in 5–10% of women in their first postpartum year.
- Women with high thyroid autoantibodies are generally affected, and women with type 1 diabetes are at high risk to develop this complication.

Clinical Findings

The symptoms involve fatigue, palpitations, heat intolerance, and nervousness. There are 2 distinct clinical phases. The first phase lasts from 1–4 months after delivery and is characterized by destruction-induced thyrotoxicosis. Laboratory findings during this phase demonstrate an elevation in free T_4 and suppressed TSH. There is an abrupt onset, and a goiter may be palpable. Approximately two-thirds of these women will become euthyroid. Between 4 and 8 months, the other third will develop hypothyroidism.

Treatment

T_4 replacement is helpful, but about 30% of women will go on to develop permanent hypothyroidism. The clinical course may vary, with some patients experiencing only the hyperthyroid phase and others only the hypothyroid phase. Treatment in the immediate postpartum period is limited to symptomatic patients only (β-blockers for the hyperthyroid phase and low-dose levothyroxine or T_3 for the hypothyroid phase, which is enough to alleviate symptoms and allows recovery of thyroid function when discontinued). Additionally, there is a positive correlation between postpartum depression and postpartum thyroiditis, so these patients should be screened accordingly.

SOLITARY THYROID NODULE DURING PREGNANCY

ESSENTIALS OF DIAGNOSIS

- Thyroid nodule palpable on physical examination

Clinical Findings

Thyroid nodules are frequently first detected during pregnancy when many women see a doctor for the first time. The risk of malignancy for a solitary nodule varies between 5% and 43%, depending on various factors including previous radiation, rate of growth, and patient age.

Treatment

Women with a thyroid nodule diagnosed during pregnancy should undergo fine-needle aspiration of the nodule. Thyroid radionuclide scanning is contraindicated during pregnancy. Women with benign nodules may be followed; in most cases, surgery in these women is deferred until after delivery. Women with thyroid cancer should undergo surgery. Surgery during pregnancy carries a higher risk if it is performed during the first and the third trimesters (miscarriage, premature delivery, and fetal death); surgery during the second trimester reportedly has a lower complication rate. Radioactive iodine should never be given during pregnancy. There is no evidence that thyroid cancer occurs more frequently during pregnancy. However, because of the indolent course of these carcinomas, many practitioners advocate postponing surgery until the postpartum period.

American College of Obstetricians and Gynecologists. ACOG Committee Opinion. Number 381, October 2007. Subclinical hypothyroidism in pregnancy. *Obstet Gynecol* 2007;110:959–960. PMID: 17906045.

Cunningham FG, Leveno KJ, Bloom SL, Hauth JC, Gilstrap LC, Wenstrom KD. *Williams Obstetrics*. 22nd ed. New York, NY: McGraw-Hill; 2005.

Pop VJ, Brouwers EP, Vader HL, Vulsma T, van Baar AL, de Vijlder JJ. Maternal hypothyroxinaemia during early pregnancy and subsequent child development: a 3-year follow-up study. *Clin Endocrinol* 2003;59:282–288. PMID: 12919150.

OTHER ENDOCRINE DISORDERS

HYPERPARATHYROIDISM

ESSENTIALS OF DIAGNOSIS

- Elevated serum parathyroid hormone (PTH) and calcium levels

Pathogenesis

Hyperparathyroidism is a frequently occurring disease but has been uncommonly reported to occur during pregnancy. Just over 120 cases have been reported since 1931, with the first successful surgery performed in 1947. Hyperparathyroidism peaks in incidence from the third to fifth decades; however, it is rare in pregnancy, with an incidence of 0.8%. The PTH level remains unchanged during the first half of pregnancy and then rises gradually until term, coinciding with the time of greatest fetal skeletal calcification. PTH promotes calcium (Ca) transport from mother to fetus. The most potent factor affecting PTH secretion is the free Ca level (inverse correlation), but calcitonin, vitamin D, and magnesium also play a role. Calcitonin is secreted by C cells inside the thyroid, but these cells actually are of neural crest origin and migrate to the thyroid. Calcitonin is a Ca-lowering hormone whose secretion is also mainly affected by free Ca levels, but in this case, the correlation is direct. Its action is antagonistic to that of PTH, and it plays a role in Ca homeostasis and bone remodeling. Vitamin D increases the efficiency of intestinal Ca absorption, plays a role in the maintenance of Ca and phosphorus levels, and has a role in the mineralization of bone matrix. In order to exert its action, vitamin D must be transformed into active metabolites [1,25-$(OH)_2D_3$] in the kidney, and PTH is needed for the process. Hyperparathyroidism is characterized by hypercalcemia, which is a result of elevated PTH. Most patients are asymptomatic, but those with symptoms generally will have nausea, vomiting, renal colic, muscular weakness, mental symptoms, and polyuria.

Whether Ca metabolism during pregnancy is influenced by other hormones, such as estrogen, progesterone, or hCG, is not known. The placenta plays a major role in transporting Ca against a gradient. PTH facilitates this transport, although neither PTH nor calcitonin crosses the placenta. The fetal Ca concentration (both total and free) increases gradually from 5.5 to 11.0 mg/dL from the second trimester to term. In the fetus, the PTH level is suppressed but detectable, and cord levels are 25% lower than in the mother. Calcitonin in cord is higher than in the mother, a combination favoring skeletal growth, which also causes Ca levels in the newborn to fall to normal. Given these findings, all the observed changes in normal pregnancy favor mineralization of the fetal skeleton.

During pregnancy, the etiology of hyperparathyroidism is an adenoma in 89–90% of cases, hyperplasia (of all the glands) in 9%, and carcinoma in 1–2%. The latter should be suspected in severe hyperparathyroidism, particularly if a palpable neck mass is present (palpable neck masses are reported in <5% of parathyroid adenomas). Rarely, it occurs in a familial pattern with or without other endocrine abnormalities (eg, multiple endocrine adenomatosis). Other causes of hypercalcemia during pregnancy are uncommon and include vitamin D toxicity, sarcoidosis, various malignancies, milk-alkali syndrome, thyrotoxicosis, adrenal insufficiency, and secondary hyperparathyroidism in those undergoing chronic hemodialysis or after renal transplantation.

Clinical Findings

The most common presentation of hyperparathyroidism is asymptomatic elevation in serum Ca level. If patients are symptomatic, it is usually related to the hypercalcemia, which may manifest with neuropsychiatric disturbances such as depression and anxiety, constipation, nausea, renal stones, and/or polyuria. Serum intact PTH levels are elevated in most patients with hyperparathyroidism. A diagnosis of hyperparathyroidism can be confirmed with elevated urinary Ca excretion levels.

Differential Diagnosis

Because hyperparathyroidism can be primary (from elevated PTH) or secondary (generally from a cancer-secreting PTH), the differential diagnosis includes a thorough search for malignancy.

Complications

Reported complications include 27.5% fetal mortality and 19% neonatal tetany. Neonatal hypocalcemia is often the initial clue to the presence of maternal hyperparathyroidism. The condition occurs because the high levels of maternal Ca inhibit the activity or the proper development of the infant's parathyroid glands. It develops between days 2 and 14 after delivery, depending on the severity of the maternal hypercalcemia, and usually resolves with appropriate therapy. One case of hypocalcemia persisting for 3 months and another case of hypocalcemia that became permanent have been reported.

Complications in the mother include 36% nephrolithiasis, 19% bone disease, 13% pancreatitis, 13% urinary tract infections and pyelonephritis, 10% hypertension (100% in all cases of carcinoma thus far reported), and 8% hypercalcemic crisis. Maternal deaths have occurred among those with complications of pancreatitis or hypercalcemic crisis. Women who developed hypercalcemic crisis had a 30% maternal death rate and 40% fetal demises. Pancreatitis is reported in only 1.5% of nonpregnant hyperparathyroid patients and in <1% of normal pregnancies. Most pregnant women with hyperparathyroidism (76%) are symptomatic, whereas 50–80% of nonpregnant hyperparathyroid patients are asymptomatic at the time of diagnosis.

Treatment

Treatment of these women involves diuresis with normal saline to increase urine output. Furosemide can be given to block tubular Ca reabsorption. Potassium and magnesium need to be replaced. Additionally, mithramycin can be given to inhibit bone resorption, calcitonin can be given to decrease skeletal release of Ca, and oral phosphorus will lower Ca levels. However, surgery is the treatment of choice for confirmed hyperparathyroidism. In pregnancy, the optimal time for surgery is the second trimester, when the complication risks (abortion or premature labor) are reduced. An experienced surgeon performing the neck exploration will be able to proceed appropriately in case of parathyroid hyperplasia (removal of all glands with parathyroid tissue transplantation); experience helps to lower the complication. Postoperatively, hypocalcemia may occur in patients with significant osteitis fibrosa or if injury occurs to the normal parathyroid glands during surgery. When surgery is not possible, maintaining adequate hydration and administering oral phosphates may be temporary measures until surgery can be safely performed. Preventing hypercalcemic crisis is of utmost importance; if it develops, aggressive treatment is recommended.

Prognosis

Because of Ca shunting to the fetus, pregnancy may improve hyperparathyroidism. Surgical treatment confers the best prognosis, but medical management is a good temporizing measure.

Cunningham FG, Leveno KJ, Bloom SL, Hauth JC, Gilstrap LC, Wenstrom KD. *Williams Obstetrics*. 22nd ed. New York, NY: McGraw-Hill; 2005.

Potts JT. Disease of the parathyroid gland and other hyper- and hypocalcemic disorders. In Braunwald E, Fauci AS, Kasper DL, et al (eds): *Harrison's Principles of Internal Medicine*. 15th ed. New York, NY: McGraw-Hill; 2001:2205.

HYPOPARATHYROIDISM

ESSENTIALS OF DIAGNOSIS

- Low PTH, hypocalcemia, and hyperphosphatemia in the setting of normal renal function
- Clinical signs: dry, scaly skin; brittle nails; coarse hair; and positive Chvostek's (present in 10% of normals) and Trousseau's signs

Pathogenesis

The most common cause of hypoparathyroidism is surgical removal or damage to the parathyroid glands, or their vascular supply, during thyroid surgery. Idiopathic hypoparathyroidism s relatively rare and is seldom seen in pregnancy. It may be isolated or occur in association with agenesis of the thymus or as part of a familial disorder, which includes deficiencies of thyroid, adrenal, and ovarian function; pernicious anemia; and mucocutaneous candidiasis. Pseudohypoparathyroidism (deficient end-organ response to PTH in bone and kidney) is a rare hereditary disorder infrequently encountered during pregnancy. The severity of symptoms depends on the degree of hypocalcemia, and symptoms range from clumsiness (fingers), mental changes (mainly depression), muscle stiffness, parkinsonism, and acral and perioral paresthesias to laryngeal stridor, tetany, and convulsions.

Clinical Findings

Clinical signs include dry, scaly skin; brittle nails; coarse hair; and positive Chvostek's (present in 10% of normals) and Trousseau's signs. Ectopic soft tissue calcifications and a prolonged QT interval on the electrocardiogram may be observed. Pseudohypoparathyroidism is more likely if the patient has unusual skeletal or developmental defects and if other family members are affected. The diagnosis usually is evident from the history and confirmed by a "normal" or low PTH level in the presence of hypocalcemia, hyperphosphatemia, and normal renal function.

Complications

After delivery, hypoparathyroid women may develop hypercalcemia with the same dose of Ca and vitamin D that was effective during pregnancy. Hypersensitivity to vitamin D in lactating women may result from the effect of prolactin on 1α-hydroxylase vitamin D activity. Serum Ca levels should be monitored closely and the doses readjusted as necessary. Vitamin D travels into breast milk, even when low doses are taken, so many physicians discourage breastfeeding in these women.

Treatment

From 1–4 g/d of elemental Ca and 50,000–100,000 U/d of vitamin D usually are recommended. The synthetic vitamin D analogue $1\alpha,25\text{-}(OH)_2D_3$ at doses of 0.25–2 μg/d is considered safer by some authors.

Prognosis

Before the availability of specific therapy, maternal morbidity and mortality rates were high, and termination of pregnancy was frequently recommended. Currently, the prognosis is much improved provided the mother is kept eucalcemic.

ADRENAL DISORDERS

Pregnancy is rarely associated with diseases of the adrenal glands, particularly in those with excessive cortisol secretion, because of the high prevalence of infertility in these women.

CUSHING'S SYNDROME

ESSENTIALS OF DIAGNOSIS

- Signs of glucocorticoid excess, including striae, obesity, hypertension, and glucose intolerance
- Elevated serum and urinary cortisol levels

Pathogenesis

Cushing's syndrome is an unusual diagnosis made during pregnancy because up to 75–80% of women with excess cortisol experience menstrual irregularities and infertility. Excess cortisol, either endogenous or exogenous, suppresses gonadotropin secretion. Cushing's syndrome is usually due to an adrenocorticotropic hormone (ACTH)–producing pituitary tumor (Cushing's disease), ectopic ACTH secretion by a nonpituitary tumor, or cortisol secretion by an adrenal adenoma or carcinoma, although the most common cause of Cushing's syndrome is exogenous corticosteroid treatment. Cushing's disease, bilateral adrenal hyperplasia, is precipitated by corticotropin-producing pituitary adenomas, most of which are microadenomas. About 25% of Cushing's syndrome will be corticotropin independent and caused by an adrenal adenoma.

Clinical Findings

The clinical diagnosis is difficult because the changes occur insidiously. During pregnancy, the diagnosis is even more difficult because weight gain, skin striae (stretch marks), and fatigue are common during normal pregnancy, but all other symptoms and signs will be the same as outside of pregnancy and include hypertension, hirsutism, and glucose intolerance among many others. The laboratory diagnosis also is more difficult during pregnancy. Urinary free cortisol excretion may overlap with that seen in some cases of Cushing's syndrome, and the suppression to exogenous corticosteroids may be incomplete. However, the diurnal variations of both ACTH and cortisol are preserved; therefore, measurement of morning and evening cortisol levels remains very useful. Therefore, the diagnosis may be confirmed by the loss of diurnal variation; elevated levels of urinary free cortisol, particularly if >250 mg per 24 hours; and lack of cortisol suppression to dexamethasone. Measurements of ACTH may be useful as well ("normal" or high in Cushing's disease and suppressed in adrenal tumors). Magnetic resonance imaging (MRI) may confirm the presence of a pituitary or adrenal tumor. A few cases of "pregnancy-induced" Cushing's syndrome with spontaneous resolution postpartum have been reported and attributed to a placental corticotropin-releasing factor. However, long-term follow-up revealed other causes of Cushing's syndrome in most of the women.

Complications

The most common complication (64%) is preterm labor, resulting in considerable fetal morbidity and mortality. Intrauterine growth restriction occurs in 26–37% and fetal losses (spontaneous abortions and stillbirths) in 16%. Little information about the long-term quality of survival of those born premature but alive is available. Hypertension and diabetes mellitus complicate 70% and 32% of these pregnancies, respectively, and unfavorably influence the outcome of these pregnancies if untreated. Maternal mortality has occurred in 5% of cases.

Treatment

An attempt at some form of treatment is advocated given the poor outcome. Surgery in the second trimester can be attempted when a pituitary or adrenal tumor is found. Few reports of these procedures performed during pregnancy are documented. Medical therapy is limited, and the potential side effects of the medications are not well known. Metyrapone, cyproheptadine, aminoglutethimide, and ketoconazole (teratogenic in animals) have been used in a few patients. All efforts should be made to control the hypertension and hyperglycemia that are so commonly seen with excess cortisol. Early delivery in the third trimester as soon as the fetus is mature is recommended, with postponement of definitive treatment of the mother until after delivery.

ADRENAL INSUFFICIENCY (ADDISON'S DISEASE)

ESSENTIALS OF DIAGNOSIS

- Symptoms include weakness, fatigue, nausea and vomiting, and weight loss
- Low serum cortisol levels

Pathogenesis

Primary adrenocortical insufficiency (Addison's disease) often is the result of autoimmune destruction of the adrenal glands (in the era before antibiotics, tuberculosis was the most common cause). More than 90% of the gland has to be destroyed for symptoms to develop. Occasionally, it is associated with other autoimmune endocrine disorders (polyendocrine autoimmune deficiency) such as diabetes, Graves' disease, or Hashimoto's thyroiditis. Secondary adrenal failure results from reduced or absent ACTH secretion caused by various pituitary disorders or inhibition from chronic exogenous steroid use. Causes of partial or complete anterior pituitary insufficiency in women of reproductive age include tumors, pituitary surgery or radiation, and postpartum infarction (Sheehan's syndrome). Less common causes are acute pituitary hemorrhage, infiltration by granulomatous diseases, thalassemia, necrosis from increased intracranial pressure, and lymphocytic hypophysitis. A few cases of pituitary necrosis in pregnant type 1 diabetic women have been reported.

Clinical Findings

Symptoms include weakness, fatigue, nausea and vomiting, and weight loss. On laboratory testing, the patient is found to have low cortisol levels.

Treatment

Since the advent of steroid treatment, most pregnancies have been successfully managed. Even women with anterior pituitary insufficiency may conceive because of advances in infertility treatment and, with proper hormonal replacement, may carry their pregnancies to term. Infants of well-treated mothers with adrenal insufficiency appear to be normal. The daily steroid replacement dose is 20–25 mg/m^2 by mouth (ie, 30–37.5 mg/d of hydrocortisone or equivalent steroid). Two-thirds of the daily dose (20–25 mg) is given in the morning and one-third (10–12.5 mg) in the late afternoon. Usually the daily dosage does not need to be changed during pregnancy. However, compensation is required for periods of stress and during labor and delivery (up to 300 mg of hydrocortisone or equivalent steroid given intravenously in divided doses the first day and gradual tapering to the maintenance dose over the next several days). In secondary adrenal insufficiency, mineralocorticoid replacement is not necessary, but women with primary adrenal disease also should receive fludrocortisone 0.05–0.1 mg/d by mouth.

CONGENITAL ADRENAL HYPERPLASIA

ESSENTIALS OF DIAGNOSIS

- The most common cause is 21-hydroxylase deficiency.
- Elevated serum 17-hydroxyprogesterone is seen.
- Clinical signs include virilization, hirsutism, and menstrual irregularities. Neonates affected by congenital adrenal hyperplasia may present with ambiguous genitalia.

Pathogenesis

Congenital adrenal hyperplasia can be caused by a number of different genetic defects in enzymes involved in cortisol synthesis. These enzymatic deficiencies are inherited as autosomal recessive traits (25% risk of inheriting the condition and 50% of being a carrier). Of the several inherited enzymatic deficiencies of cortisol synthesis that may cause congenital adrenal hyperplasia, the 21-hydroxylase deficiency accounts for 90–95% of cases. In fact, 21-hydroxylase deficiency is one of the most common inherited genetic disorders.

Clinical Findings

Congenital adrenal hyperplasia is typically a diagnosis made in infancy via neonatal screening. Physical signs include virilization and ambiguous genitalia. Affected individuals may have salt wasting. Later in life, women may experience acne, accelerated bone age, hirsutism, and menstrual irregularity. The diagnosis of classic 21-hydroxylase deficiency is made based on high serum concentrations of 17-hydroxyprogesterone. Patients with nonclassic 21-hydroxylase deficiency may have only mild elevations in 17-hydroxyprogesterone yet will have very high values after ACTH stimulation test.

If both parents are known to carry a gene associated with autosomal recessive inheritance of congenital adrenal hyperplasia, prenatal diagnosis is available via chorionic villus sampling or amniocentesis to determine whether the fetus is affected.

Complications

Complications vary depending on whether the mother or the fetus (or both) carry a diagnosis of congenital adrenal hyperplasia. When the fetus is affected, the low cortisol level stimulates excessive ACTH secretion, which in turn causes adrenal enlargement, or hyperplasia. The excessive secretion of androgens leads to masculinization of the external genitalia (congenital sexual ambiguity) and the low cortisol level to adrenal insufficiency. Untreated, these conditions can be life threatening.

In many cases, the diagnosis is made and treatment initiated after birth when the newborn becomes ill. However, prenatal diagnosis (chorionic villous sampling and DNA testing) now is commonplace when both parents are known to be carriers of a mutation associated with congenital adrenal hyperplasia.

Treatment

If the fetus is found to have 21-hydroxylase deficiency and the fetus is female, treatment of the mother with dexamethasone may prevent the development of adrenal hyperplasia and virilization of the external genitalia. The sex of the fetus can be determined by chorionic villous sampling, so early treatment can be initiated. Those born with virilization of the external genitalia will require surgical reconstruction to allow vaginal intercourse.

In affected females, the earlier the treatment is initiated, the higher the likelihood that they will be ovulatory and fertile. During pregnancy, glucocorticoid therapy should be continued and adjusted to avoid excessive androgen levels. Otherwise the steroid management is the same as described for adrenal insufficiency. Genetic counseling should be mandatory for these women, before they consider pregnancy, given the high risk of transmission and the severity of the disease.

If the mother is known to be affected by congenital adrenal hyperplasia, her regimen of glucocorticoid will likely require an increase in dose during pregnancy to maintain levels within the normal range for pregnancy. Additionally, a glucocorticoid that is metabolized by the placenta such as hydrocortisone is suggested to minimize excessive glucocorticoid exposure to the fetus.

Cunningham FG, Leveno KJ, Bloom SL, Hauth JC, Gilstrap LC, Wenstrom KD. *Williams Obstetrics*. 22nd ed. New York, NY: McGraw-Hill; 2005.

PHEOCHROMOCYTOMA

ESSENTIALS OF DIAGNOSIS

- Hypertension with headache and diaphoresis
- Elevated catecholamines and metanephrines on 24-hour urine tests

Pathogenesis

Pheochromocytomas are rare in the general population, but they are a potentially lethal cause of hypertension during pregnancy. They are catecholamine-secreting tumors of the adrenal medulla. However, given the severity of the complications (48% maternal mortality and 55% fetal mortality) if untreated, the possibility of its existence must always be considered in the differential diagnosis.

Clinical Findings

The symptoms are similar to those outside of pregnancy and are caused by excess catecholamines. They include sustained or labile hypertension, headaches, palpitations, diaphoresis, and anxiety. Blurred vision and convulsions are reported more commonly during pregnancy. Elevated levels of free catecholamines and their metabolites metanephrine and vanillylmandelic acid in a 24-hour urine collection confirm the diagnosis. Urinary metanephrine levels >1.2 mg/d are considered highly suggestive of pheochromocytoma. A plasma level of total catecholamines >2000 pg/mL, drawn after the patient has been in the supine position for >30 minutes, also is highly suggestive. For tumor localization, MRI is the test of choice during pregnancy. Most pheochromocytomas are benign and are located in the adrenal glands, but approximately 10% are located elsewhere and difficult to find, and approximately 12% are malignant. In a few patients, the pheochromocytoma may be part of a familial disorder and more likely to be bilateral.

Differential Diagnosis

Differentiation from preeclampsia may be difficult when proteinuria is also present.

Complications

Complications include spontaneous abortion, intrauterine growth restriction, placental abruption, and fetal and maternal death.

Treatment

Few of the reported cases were diagnosed during pregnancy. However, if the diagnosis is made, surgical removal during the second trimester is recommended. Blood pressure control is attempted first with adequate adrenergic blockade (usually phenoxybenzamine), followed by β-adrenergic blockade if necessary, until surgery can be performed in the second trimester or, if after 26–28 weeks, until the fetus is mature. Phenoxybenzamine is considered safe, but it does cross the placenta and has the potential to cause depression and transient hypotension in the newborn. The dose should be started at 10 mg twice daily and increased by 10–20 mg daily until hypertension is controlled. Vaginal delivery is not recommended because of precipitation of hypertensive crisis by mechanical pressure on the tumor from changes in posture, contractions, and fetal movements.

Ahn JT, Hibbard JU, Chapa JB. Atypical presentation of pheochromocytoma as part of multiple endocrine neoplasia IIa in pregnancy. *Obstet Gynecol* 2003;102:1202–1205. PMID: 14607057.

Cunningham FG, Leveno KJ, Bloom SL, Hauth JC, Gilstrap LC, Wenstrom KD. *Williams Obstetrics*. 22nd ed. New York, NY: McGraw-Hill; 2005.

PITUITARY DISORDERS

PROLACTINOMAS

ESSENTIALS OF DIAGNOSIS

- Elevated serum prolactin concentration
- MRI of the head confirming a microadenoma (<10 mm) or macroadenoma (≥10 mm)

Pathogenesis

Prolactinomas are the most common pituitary tumors encountered during pregnancy, particularly since the availability of effective treatments for restoring fertility. They generally arise as lactotroph adenomas from monoclonal expansion of a single cell that has undergone a mutation. Most cases of prolactinomas are sporadic, but they have also been described as a clinical feature of multiple endocrine neoplasia type 1 (MEN1).

Clinical Findings

The most common symptoms include amenorrhea, galactorrhea, and hyperprolactinemia. Bromocriptine has been used successfully to prevent amenorrhea, and thus, many women have had successful pregnancies. The diagnosis usually is made when the prolactin level is high enough to cause galactorrhea, oligomenorrhea, or amenorrhea. MRI confirms the diagnosis. The tumors are divided into microadenomas (<10 mm) or macroadenomas (≥10 mm). The risk of growth during pregnancy is low (1–2%) for microadenomas, in contrast to the 15–25% risk of growth for untreated macroadenomas. Previously treated macroadenomas (bromocriptine, cabergoline, and/or surgery) have a lower risk (4%) of growth during pregnancy.

Differential Diagnosis

There are other tumors that can arise in the parasellar region. These include germ cells tumors, lymphoma, and sarcomas.

Complications

Complications of uncurbed tumor growth include visual disturbances, headache, and diabetes insipidus. Marked tumor growth can lead to blindness.

Treatment

If the tumor enlarges, medical therapy (bromocriptine or cabergoline) is started, and visual field examinations are performed daily. If no rapid response occurs, high-dose steroid therapy is added. If still no response occurs, surgery should be strongly considered. Few reports of surgery during pregnancy are documented, but medical therapy, continued until after delivery, generally has been safe and effective. Serial visual field examinations or MRI is not recommended for microadenomas unless symptoms appear. If severe headache occurs, MRI is recommended even if no visual field defects are detected. MRI should always be performed if visual field defects are detected. Visual field disturbances are more common with macroadenomas. With macroprolactinomas, monthly visual field examinations and MRI are recommended if tumor growth is suspected. In addition to headaches and visual changes, pituitary infarction and diabetes insipidus are rarely seen. Complications of tumor growth are more likely to appear during the first trimester.

Prognosis

Labor and delivery are generally uncomplicated, but shortening the duration of the second stage in women experiencing tumor growth during pregnancy is recommended in an effort to prevent intracranial pressure elevation during the most active pushing. Most women with prolactinomas are allowed to breastfeed. MRI usually is recommended approximately 3–4 months after delivery to reassess tumor size. These women do very well during pregnancy.

ACROMEGALY

ESSENTIALS OF DIAGNOSIS

- Elevated concentrations of growth hormone
- Failure of an oral glucose tolerance test to suppress growth hormone

Clinical Findings

The clinical diagnosis is infrequently made early in the disease because changes in shoe or glove size and coarsening of facial features develop slowly. In normal pregnancy, pituitary growth hormone concentrations will decrease as placental epitopes are secreted. Determination of growth hormone levels during pregnancy requires specific assays able to differentiate growth hormone from pituitary or placental origin. Diagnosis is confirmed if an oral glucose tolerance test fails to suppress pituitary growth hormone.

Complications

Untreated patients with acromegaly can develop hypertension, diabetes, visual loss, cardiomyopathy, and arthritis.

Treatment

In general, medical therapy is stopped when pregnancy is diagnosed. Octreotide has been used successfully. However, bromocriptine administration throughout gestation without untoward effects to mother or infant has been reported. The data for octreotide are limited, so until its safety is determined, octreotide should be stopped when pregnancy is diagnosed. Elective surgery during pregnancy is safer during the second trimester. Emergency surgery is reserved for women with pregnancy-associated tumor enlargement and visual loss.

Prognosis

Early diagnosis and treatment of acromegaly can lead to a good prognosis.

SHEEHAN'S SYNDROME

ESSENTIALS OF DIAGNOSIS

- Panhypopituitarism as defined by decreased levels of TSH, prolactin, follicle-stimulating hormone, luteinizing hormone, and estradiol

Pathogenesis

H.L. Sheehan described the syndrome bearing his name as partial or complete pituitary insufficiency due to postpartum necrosis of the anterior pituitary gland in women with severe blood loss and hypotension during delivery. Nevertheless, up to 10% of cases have no history of bleeding or hypotension. The clinical manifestations depend on the extent of pituitary destruction and hormonal deficiencies. With destruction of 90% or more, symptoms of acute adrenal insufficiency predominate (see Adrenal Insufficiency). Women may present with persistent hypotension, tachycardia, hypoglycemia, and failure to lactate. If the condition is not treated promptly, serious complications and even death may occur. In most cases, the full-blown picture may take longer, even years, to appear. The most common manifestation of this syndrome is in women who have recently delivered and suffered a postpartum hemorrhage. This leads to an infarct in the pituitary due to low blood flow in that region.

Clinical Findings

Failure to lactate, breast involution, and, if untreated, breast atrophy may occur. Fatigue, weight loss, and postural hypotension are common complaints. Hyponatremia and anemia (usually normocytic and normochromic) are frequent laboratory abnormalities. Hormonal deficiencies point to a secondary cause, with low T_4, TSH, estrogen, gonadotropin, cortisol, and ACTH levels. Provocative hormonal testing may be necessary to confirm the diagnosis. Once the diagnosis of secondary hormonal deficiency is established, MRI of the pituitary and hypothalamus is necessary to exclude a tumor or other pathology.

Differential Diagnosis

Other problems that can manifest as hypopituitarism include lymphocytic hypophysitis involving lymphocytic infiltration into the pituitary; hemochromatosis, where iron is deposited into the pituitary; and exogenous causes such as radiation or surgery in that area.

Complications

Untreated Sheehan's syndrome can lead to persistent hypotension, tachycardia, failure to lactate, and hypoglycemia.

Treatment

All deficient hormones must be replaced. However, it is well known that some patients with clear panhypopituitarism may recover TSH and even gonadotropin function after cortisol replacement alone. The mechanism is unknown, but it is speculated that cortisol has a permissive effect on other hypothalamic and pituitary functions. Rare cases of spontaneous recovery have been reported.

Prognosis

The outcome of pregnancy in women with Sheehan's syndrome shows no increased perinatal morbidity or mortality if the mothers are treated properly. Women with persistent amenorrhea and anovulation will require fertility treatment to become pregnant in the future.

DIABETES INSIPIDUS

ESSENTIALS OF DIAGNOSIS

- Polyuria
- Elevated serum sodium
- Water restriction test (excludes primary polydipsia)

Pathogenesis

Diabetes insipidus (DI) is caused by a deficiency of antidiuretic hormone (ADH), called central DI, or by renal tubule resistance to ADH action, called nephrogenic DI. A transient form of DI during pregnancy has been observed with increasing frequency and has been attributed to excessive placental production of vasopressinase, perhaps decreased hepatic clearance, and, because most of the patients reported had abnormal liver function, preeclampsia, fatty liver, or hepatitis. It is possible that some of these cases represent mild preexisting DI unmasked by pregnancy. It usually resolves several weeks after delivery but may recur in subsequent pregnancies, so follow-up is recommended.

The incidence during pregnancy has been reported as 1 in 50,000 to 1 in 80,000 deliveries. Approximately 60% of women with previously known DI worsen, 20% improve, and 20% do not change during pregnancy. Worsening is attributed to excessive placental vasopressinase production. Some women with DI who also develop placental insufficiency show DI improvement, which is attributed to decreased vasopressinase production by the damaged placenta.

A variety of lesions may cause DI, such as pituitary surgery, radiation, trauma, tumors, granulomas, and infections. However, no etiology is found in as many as 50% of patients, and these cases are labeled as "idiopathic."

Clinical Findings

Clinical symptoms include polyuria of 4–15 L/d and intense thirst, particularly for ice-cold fluids. A high-normal plasma sodium concentration is suggestive of DI in the patient with polyuria. The diagnosis of DI is confirmed by the standard water deprivation test. The goal of the water restriction test is to raise plasma osmolality and to assess for the normal physiologic response to water restriction. However, this test may prove hazardous during pregnancy because 3–5% of body weight may be lost during the test. This degree of dehydration, which is required to produce sufficient stimulation for ADH secretion, may lead to uteroplacental insufficiency and fetal distress. Even before fetal distress occurs, uterine contractions and even frank labor may be precipitated, forcing termination of the test before it can be properly interpreted. Uterine contractions respond rapidly to intravenous fluid administration. If the decision is made to perform a water deprivation test, continuous fetal monitoring is recommended.

Differential Diagnosis

The differential includes primary psychogenic polydipsia or osmotic dieresis.

Complications

The primary complications associated with DI are electrolyte imbalance and dehydration.

Treatment

The treatment of choice is intranasal desmopressin (DDAVP). It also can be given subcutaneously when the intranasal route cannot be used. The usual dose is 10–25 μg once or twice daily (or 2–4 μg subcutaneously). The dosage is adjusted according to fluid intake, urinary output, osmolality, and plasma electrolytes. An increased metabolic clearance rate stimulated by vasopressinase may require higher doses of the drug. Close follow-up is necessary to prevent dehydration or the opposite, water intoxication. Many reports indicate that DDAVP is safe during pregnancy and postpartum, even while the mother is breastfeeding. Oxytocin secretion appears to be normal, and no labor difficulties have been reported. No difficulties with lactation have been reported even in women with central DI.

Prognosis

Treated DI has a good prognosis and is not thought to cause long-term complications or change life expectancy.

Molitch MD. Pituitary, thyroid, adrenal, and parathyroid disorders. In Barron WM, Lindheimer MD (eds): *Medical Disorders during Pregnancy*. 3rd ed. St. Louis, MO: Mosby; 2000:101.

Schlechte JA. Prolactinoma. *N Engl J Med* 2003;349:2035–2041. PMID: 14627789

Vaphiades MS, Simmons D, Archer RL, et al. Sheehan syndrome: a splinter of the mind. *Surv Ophthalmol* 2003;48:230–233. PMID: 12686307.

Nervous System & Autoimmune Disorders in Pregnancy

33

Laura Kalayjian, MD
T. Murphy Goodwin, MD
Richard H. Lee, MD

DISORDERS OF THE NERVOUS SYSTEM

CEREBROVASCULAR DISORDERS

ESSENTIALS OF DIAGNOSIS

- Headaches, visual disturbances, syncope, and hemiparesis are among the most common presenting findings.
- Computed tomography scan and magnetic resonance imaging can be used in pregnancy to increase the delineation of cerebrovascular involvement. Arteriography is considered definitive if surgical intervention is being considered because arteriography can more precisely localize the involved area.

Pathogenesis

The causes of cerebrovascular disease include insufficiency *(arteriosclerosis, cerebral embolism, vasospasm from hypertensive disease)* and disorders associated with bleeding into the cerebral cortex *(arteriovenous malformation, ruptured aneurysm)*. The brain becomes infarcted from lack of blood flow, or intracranial bleeding results in a space-occupying lesion. The severity of such disorders can be affected by blood pressure, oxygen saturation (anemia or polycythemia), hypoglycemia, and adequacy of collateral circulation.

The overall incidence of ischemic cerebrovascular accidents in pregnancy is approximately 1 in 20,000 births, with most occurring in the last trimester or immediately postpartum. Etiologic factors for stroke include cardioembolic disorders, cerebral angiopathies, hematologic disorders, and cerebral vein thrombosis. Causes exclusive to pregnancy are eclampsia, choriocarcinoma, and amniotic fluid embolism. Although cerebral ischemic disease can occur in either the arterial or venous system, approximately 75% of occlusive cerebral disease occurs on the arterial side.

Cerebrovascular accidents involving subarachnoid hemorrhage or intraparenchymal hemorrhage similarly occur at a rate of 1 in 20,000 births. These events usually are the result of aneurysms or arteriovenous malformations. The most common aneurysm is the saccular (berry) variety, which protrudes from the major arteries in the circle of Willis, particularly at its bifurcations. Aneurysms have an increasing tendency to bleed as the pregnancy progresses, likely due to changes in hemodynamic factors. Rupture of arteriovenous malformations has been found to occur evenly throughout gestation. No consensus has been reached regarding the increased frequency of bleeding from either an aneurysm or arteriovenous malformation during pregnancy or the immediate postpartum period. Rupture of the malformation appears to be more frequent during pregnancy. Eclampsia can lead to cerebral hemorrhage when elevated blood pressures lead to vasospasm, loss of autoregulatory function, and rupture of the vessel wall.

Clinical Findings

Headaches, visual disturbances, syncope, and hemiparesis are among the most common presenting findings. The pattern of clinical signs and symptoms generally allows recognition of the area of the brain involved. Computed tomography (CT) scan and magnetic resonance imaging (MRI) can be used in pregnancy to increase the delineation of cerebrovascular involvement. Arteriography is considered definitive if surgical intervention is being considered because arteriography can more precisely localize the involved area. Because coagulopathies can also cause intracranial bleeding or may be secondary to the cerebrovascular lesion itself, a coagulation profile should be performed. Additionally, antinuclear antibody (ANA), lupus anticoagulant, factor V Leiden, homocysteine, anticardiolipin, proteins C and S, antithrombin III, and plasminogen levels should be considered with thrombotic cerebral events.

Treatment

The treatment of ischemic or hemorrhagic cerebrovascular disease is best managed supportively; however, surgery is indicated for treatment of some aneurysms and arteriovenous malformations. Anticoagulation with heparin may be required depending on the etiology of the infarction; tissue plasminogen activator is relatively contraindicated in pregnancy, but it has been used successfully according to several case reports. Normalization of blood pressure, adequate respiratory support, therapy for metabolic complications, and treatment of coagulopathies or cardiac abnormalities are crucial. Dexamethasone 10 mg intravenously initially, followed by 5 mg every 6 hours for 24 hours, may decrease cerebral edema and be of some assistance prior to surgery or in recovery. Additionally, hyperventilation, mannitol infusions, phenobarbital coma, and intracerebral pressure monitoring may be helpful with severe cerebral edema. Once the patient's condition has been stabilized, physical therapy and rehabilitation should begin as soon as possible.

Appropriate surgery for aneurysms and arteriovenous malformations should be performed with the pregnancy undisturbed unless fetal maturity allows for caesarean birth just prior to the neurosurgical procedure. On the other hand, inoperable lesions during pregnancy are managed by pregnancy conservation until fetal maturity is sufficient to allow abdominal birth. Once a lesion has been surgically corrected, vaginal delivery can be attempted depending on the practitioner's comfort level. However, the second stage of labor should be modified by regional anesthesia and forceps delivery to reduce cerebral pressures associated with the Valsalva maneuver.

Prognosis

The percentage of patients with venous occlusion who recover from the initial episode without neurologic sequelae during rehabilitation equals that of patients with arterial occlusion. Thrombosis of the superior sagittal sinus is a rare complication. Its incidence is increased in pregnancy, and it has a high mortality rate of approximately 55%.

If the cerebral hemorrhagic disorder is operable, the prognosis is favorable, with few long-term neurologic deficits. In inoperable lesions or when severe maternal cerebral hemorrhage has occurred, the prognosis—although unfavorable—is better for those with aneurysms than for those with arteriovenous fistulas. If a neurosurgical procedure is performed during pregnancy, the fetus usually is not adversely affected, despite the induced hypotension that is often necessary. The prognosis for the mother and fetus is the same as that in a normal gestation once the condition has been corrected.

CEREBRAL NEOPLASMS

ESSENTIALS OF DIAGNOSIS

- The clinical manifestations are generally characterized by a slow progression of neurologic signs with evidence of increased intracranial pressure and headache.
- CT or MRI of the brain reveals a mass lesion within the skull.

Pathogenesis

Cerebral neoplasms occur primarily at the extremes of life; thus, primary cancer or even metastatic tumors are uncommon during the childbearing years. Although brain tumors are not specifically related to gestation, meningiomas, angiomas, and neurofibromas are thought to grow more rapidly with pregnancy. Of the primary neoplasms (half of all brain tumors), gliomas are the most common (50%), with meningiomas and pituitary adenomas accounting for 35%. Of the metastatic cerebral tumors, lung and breast tumors account for 50%. *Choriocarcinoma* commonly metastasizes to the cerebrum.

Clinical Findings

A. Symptoms & Signs

The clinical manifestations, although dependent on the type and location of the tumor, are generally characterized by a slow progression of neurologic signs with evidence of increased intracranial pressure. One of the most frequent signs is headache, which must be differentiated from that occurring in tension and in vascular or inflammatory conditions. Pain that is not relieved by analgesics or muscle relaxants (as a tension headache would be), the absence of a history of migraine headaches, and the lack of signs of infection or meningeal inflammation all point to increased intracranial pressure as a possible cause of the headache. Tumors in the pituitary gland or occipital region may be associated with visual deficits. Other presenting signs and symptoms include nausea, vomiting, double vision, vertigo, seizures, and altered mental status.

B. Imaging Studies

CT scan and MRI are of greatest assistance in revealing space-occupying lesions. MRI is generally preferred during pregnancy, although fetal radiation exposure from CT of the brain is minimal.

C. Laboratory Findings

If the cerebrospinal fluid glucose and protein levels are normal, inflammation or infection of the central nervous system is unlikely. Similarly, an increase in the cerebrospinal fluid human chorionic gonadotropin (hCG) titer raises the suspicion of metastatic choriocarcinoma. Pleocytosis may be present with cerebral neoplasia, but usually it is lymphocytic or monocytic, without an increase in the number of polymorphonucleocytes. Finally, failure to find blood or xanthochromic fluid in the cerebrospinal fluid helps in differentiating a neoplasm from a hemorrhagic lesion, unless the tumor has undergone hemorrhagic necrosis.

Treatment

The treatment of cerebral neoplasms during pregnancy depends on the type of tumor, its location, and the stage of gestation. Anticonvulsants should be used only if seizures have occurred. Steroids can be used to decrease intracranial pressure causing focal neurologic signs or headaches. Deterioration of the patient's status in early pregnancy should prompt a discussion about the risks of continuing the pregnancy. Nevertheless, most such pregnancies can be carried through successfully. During the second trimester, treatment with surgery, chemotherapy, or directed radiation can be started and the pregnancy allowed to continue. Later in gestation, maternal treatment can be delayed until delivery. Pituitary adenomas can be treated with bromocriptine if visual problems or disabling headaches occur.

Prognosis

Brain tumors usually do not affect pregnancy or the fetus unless the neoplasm leads to early delivery or maternal death. When diagnosed in the second or third trimester, the outcome for the fetus is excellent, even though therapy may be initiated during the course of the pregnancy.

MIGRAINE HEADACHE

ESSENTIALS OF DIAGNOSIS

- Headache attacks that last 4–72 hours in duration.
- Headaches may be associated with nausea or vomiting, photophobia, or phonophobia.
- Headaches may also be accompanied by focal neurologic symptoms ("aura").

Chronic migraine headaches decrease during pregnancy in 50–80% of affected patients. Women with classic migraine (migraine with aura) may experience their initial onset during pregnancy.

Clinical Findings

Most often, the patient has a history of migraine headaches, which usually are described as "pounding" and may settle in the eyes, the temporal region, or occiput. The pain can be unilateral or bilateral. Frequently, migraines are associated with gastrointestinal complaints (eg, nausea, vomiting, and diarrhea) or with systemic symptoms (eg, vertigo or syncope). Light sensitivity (photophobia) and noise sensitivity (sonophobia) often accompany the pain. An aura may or may not precede the headache. Aura is characterized by focal neurologic symptoms, most commonly visual changes, that are fully reversible. Sleep often aborts the attack.

The diagnosis of migraine headaches usually is made clinically by the characteristics of the pain, associated symptoms, event triggers (see below), and absence of neurologic signs. Tension and caffeine withdrawal headaches typically are associated with bandlike pressure pain. If vertigo is associated with migraine headaches, it is important to rule out Ménière's disease (labyrinthitis). In the latter, vertigo is accompanied by tinnitus, a fluctuating sensorineural hearing loss, and nystagmus. If vertigo is associated with ataxia of gait, it is almost always central in origin, in which case head trauma, brain tumors, seizure disorders, and multiple sclerosis must be excluded. Syncope (fainting) may occur with migraine or vascular headaches and is common during pregnancy. However, when syncope occurs with migraine headache, it usually is associated with vertigo. Rarely, ocular nerve palsy develops in association with migraine headaches; the third cranial nerve is the most commonly involved, and the palsy usually disappears with abatement of the migraine. It is important to visualize the optic disk to ensure that cerebrospinal fluid pressure is not increased. In cases where the disk borders are not sharp, *pseudotumor cerebri* or an intracranial mass lesion should be considered first.

Treatment

Treatment of migraine headaches initially includes identification of any trigger that precipitates attacks, followed by avoidance of those triggers. Common triggers for some migraine patients include missing meals, stress, aged cheeses, sausage or other nitrates, chocolate, citrus fruit, wine and other sulfites, monosodium glutamate, strong odors, lights or glare, and inadequate sleep. When this environmental manipulation fails to control migraines, drug therapy is indicated. Migraine therapy is either abortive or prophylactic depending on the frequency and severity of attacks. Preferred abortive medications during pregnancy include acetaminophen, acetaminophen and codeine or other narcotics, and magnesium. The following are more effective migraine abortive medications but are not preferred during pregnancy: butalbital, isometheptene, caffeine, aspirin, naproxen, ibuprofen, and triptan drugs (eg, sumatriptan). The nonsteroidal anti-inflammatory drugs should not be used for prolonged periods and should be avoided in the third trimester because of possible oligohydramnios or premature closure of the ductus arteriosus. Prophylactic medications should be instituted if abortive therapy is only partially effective and if disabling migraines are occurring more than once per week. Options include beta mimetic blockers, low-dose tricyclic antidepressants, calcium channel blockers, magnesium, riboflavin, and topiramate. Valproic acid or divalproate should be avoided in pregnancy.

Prognosis

Migraine headaches usually have no deleterious long-term effect on mother or fetus, and treatment of acute exacerbation usually is successful.

EPILEPSY & SEIZURE DISORDERS

ESSENTIALS OF DIAGNOSIS

- Epilepsy is defined as 2 or more unprovoked seizures.
- Seizures associated with epilepsy can be generalized convulsive (tonic-clonic or grand mal), complex partial (loss of awareness or staring with mild motor movements), focal motor or sensory (jacksonian with no loss of awareness), absence or petit mal (brief eye blinking with no postictal confusion), myoclonic jerks, or auras of déjà vu, fear, or abnormal odors.

The onset of epilepsy is not increased during pregnancy. More than 95% of patients who have seizures during pregnancy have a history of epilepsy or have been receiving anticonvulsant therapy. Patients whose seizures are adequately controlled are not likely to experience a deterioration of their condition during pregnancy. On the other hand, patients who have experienced frequent and uncontrolled seizures before pregnancy likely will experience the same pattern, particularly during early pregnancy.

Clinical Findings

A detailed history from the patient and observers helps to distinguish true seizures from other forms of loss of consciousness, such as syncopal episodes, hysteric attacks, or hyperventilation. These problems do not commonly involve a postictal confusional state, nor do they usually involve loss of bladder or bowel control or tongue biting. Non–central nervous system causes, such as hypoxia, hypoglycemia, hypocalcemia, and hyponatremia, also must be excluded. Finally, seizures may result from drug withdrawal, medications, or exposure to toxic substances; thus, appropriate physical examination and screening for toxic substances are important in patients suffering an apparent first seizure during pregnancy.

Detailed neurologic workup is required in patients whose first seizure occurs during pregnancy. Electroencephalogram (EEG), CT scan with shielding or MRI, and lumbar puncture are useful for detailing the cause of the seizure and are not contraindicated during pregnancy. In established epilepsy, EEG is useful to confirm the type of epilepsy and therefore provide the appropriate drug therapy.

Treatment

Treatment of epilepsy should consist of the medication that has been most beneficial for the patient and at the lowest possible dose to maintain seizure control with some caveats. Some antiepileptic agents are more likely to cause birth defects than are others, and attempts to change medications should be made prior to conception.

During pregnancy, anticonvulsant levels change as a result of decreased protein binding, increased plasma volume, and alterations in the absorption and excretion of drugs. In addition, lamotrigine, phenytoin, phenobarbital, and carbamazepine have an increased plasma clearance that probably is related to high hepatic metabolism. These factors most often lead to low antiseizure plasma levels. Noncompliance, morning sickness, and hyperemesis gravidarum are other reasons for low drug levels. Therefore, blood level measurements of antiseizure medications are used to monitor and maintain a therapeutic range. Levels should be checked at least each trimester and prior to delivery. More frequent monitoring may be needed. Because of decreased protein binding, serum-free drug levels rather than routine serum levels will be more accurate. Breakthrough seizures can result from poor sleep in the third trimester because the patient cannot obtain a comfortable sleeping position. For patients with refractory seizures while taking medication, an attempt should be made to maximize the dosage and the level of 1 medication before switching or adding another agent.

In patients with status epilepticus, control of seizures is mandatory for the safety of the patient and fetus. Lorazepam 2 mg intravenous (IV) push followed by 2 mg IV every minute up to 0.1 mg/kg is first-line treatment. If seizures continue, phenytoin 20 mg/kg slow IV push at a rate of 50 mg/min or fosphenytoin 20 phenytoin equivalents/kg IV at 150 phenytoin equivalents/min can be given intravenously. General anesthesia can be considered if seizures persist. In these cases, cerebral edema almost invariably is present and may be reduced with dexamethasone, mannitol, or hyperventilation. Many cases of status epilepticus in pregnancy are the result of inadequate treatment with antiepileptic drugs, abrupt withdrawal of phenobarbital or benzodiazepines, noncompliance, or failure to monitor serum levels.

Antiepileptic drugs and seizures can negatively affect a fetus. Seizures can cause maternal and fetal injury, spontaneous abortion, premature labor, and fetal bradycardia. All antiepileptic drugs cross the placenta, equilibrate rapidly in cord blood, and may have teratogenic effects. The risk of anomalies among infants exposed to anticonvulsants is approximately 2-fold greater than in the general population. The previous thinking that women with seizure disorders had an increased risk of fetal malformations even without exposure to anticonvulsant medication has been disproved. The most common defects fall into 2 categories: major and minor malformations. Major malformations include orofacial clefts, neural tube defects, and congenital heart disease. Minor malformations consist of craniofacial anomalies (eg, low-set ears, widely spaced eyes), short neck, and hypoplastic fingernails. The *fetal hydantoin syndrome* (associated with phenytoin) was the first described association between antiepileptic drugs and birth defects. It affects 3–5% of exposed offspring. It is characterized by mental retardation, small for gestational age size, craniofacial anomalies, and limb defects. A milder phenytoin-associated syndrome may be present at a greater frequency (8–15%) but is detectable only by careful assessment during the first 3 years of life. Use of trimethadione in pregnancy has been abandoned given the high rate of anomalies (up to 30%) associated with intrauterine trimethadione exposure.

The teratogenic potential of specific antiepileptic agents has been the subject of much debate. Prospective pregnancy registries have been established around the world to clarify the risks. The older anticonvulsants—ethosuximide, carbamazepine, phenobarbital, valproic acid, primidone, and phenytoin—are all pregnancy category D because of known increased risk of birth defects in exposed fetuses. Neural tube defects are most common with carbamazepine (0.5–1%) and valproic acid (1–2%). The North American AED (antiepileptic drug) Pregnancy Registry has determined that the overall major malformation rate with exposure to valproic acid is 10.7%. Other pregnancy registries and studies have found the teratogenic potential of valproic acid increases with doses higher than 1000 mg/d or levels higher than 70 μg/mL. Besides neural tube defects, hypospadia, polydactyly, and kidney and heart malformation have been associated with valproic acid, so its use during pregnancy should be avoided if possible. Phenobarbital, previously believed to be safe during pregnancy, has a malformation rate of 6.5%, which is slightly higher than the approximately 3% rate of other antiepileptic drugs such as carbamazepine, phenytoin, and lamotrigine. Less human data on the newer antiepileptic drugs are available, with the exception of lamotrigine and oxcarbazepine. All newer antiepileptic drugs are category C, but more data are needed before they can be deemed safe.

Treatment with 2 or more antiseizure medications approximately doubles the risk for malformations.

Women with existing seizure disorders who are contemplating pregnancy should be tested to determine whether they still require anticonvulsant therapy—particularly if anticonvulsants were started during childhood or if the patient has been seizure-free for 2–5 years. If a pregnant woman requires seizure medication, she should be informed of the likelihood of fetal anomalies associated with each drug, and a discussion regarding the risks and benefits of attempting to switch to a different or safer drug, if available, should ensue. The patient should be counseled regarding folic acid supplementation (4 mg/d) starting at least 3 months preconceptionally to possibly reduce the chance of neural tube defects.

If the patient is taking an antiseizure medication metabolized by the P450 liver enzyme system, she should take vitamin K 10 mg/d from week 36 until delivery to prevent hemorrhage in her baby. This is in addition to the intramuscular vitamin K the infant will receive after delivery.

Antiepileptic drugs pass into the breast milk to varying degrees, depending on protein-binding characteristics. The benefits of breast milk usually outweigh the small risk from the medication to the infant. If a breastfed infant is too sedated and not feeding well, presumably from the medication in the breast milk, breastfeeding should be suspended and supplanted with formula.

Mothers with frequent seizures must be counseled on seizure and infant safety. Sponge baths instead of tub baths and use of a strap on the changing table will decrease potential injury to an infant in case of a maternal seizure.

MULTIPLE SCLEROSIS

ESSENTIALS OF DIAGNOSIS

- Multiple sclerosis is a clinical diagnosis made on the basis of 2 or more clinically distinct episodes of central nervous system dysfunction.
- The diagnosis may be supported by findings on laboratory or imaging studies such as MRI.

Pathogenesis

Multiple sclerosis is an autoimmune demyelinating process in the white matter of the central nervous system. It affects women twice as often as men and usually has its onset between the ages of 20 and 40 years. People in the Northern Hemisphere are more commonly affected. The cause is not known, but possible etiologies include environmental, viral, and genetic.

Clinical Findings

The 2 patterns of disease are relapsing remitting and primary progressive. Findings include weakness in the extremities, sensory loss, difficulty with coordination, and visual problems. Increased reflexes, spasticity, and bladder control problems develop over time. Myasthenia gravis should be ruled out with an anticholinesterase (neostigmine) challenge and acetylcholine receptor antibody testing. Guillain-Barré syndrome should be ruled out if the patient has a history of recent viral infection.

Laboratory tests and imaging should be performed to rule out other possible etiologies. Serum should be checked for vitamin B_{12}, Lyme and HTLV-1 (human T-cell lymphotropic virus type 1) titers, erythrocyte sedimentation rate (ESR), ANA, and rheumatoid factor. An MRI would reveal lesions (plaques) in the white matter of the brain and spinal cord. Active plaques would enhance with contrast materials. An elevated level of immunoglobulin (Ig) G in the cerebrospinal fluid is virtually diagnostic.

Treatment

Treatment options include interferon beta-1a, interferon beta-1b, and glatiramer. These medications decrease relapse rates, decrease disease activity as measured by serial MRI, and decrease disease progression. The interferon beta-1b and -1a multiple sclerosis trials showed an increased rate of spontaneous abortions of exposed fetuses. Although the increased rate did not reach statistical significance, there is good reason for caution. In patients planning to become pregnant, interferon treatment should be switched to glatiramer until conception and then discontinued once pregnancy is established. Symptomatic treatment of spasticity, pain, fatigue, and bowel and bladder dysfunction will be required as well. IV immunoglobulin (IVIG) has been used in the postpartum period to decrease the risk of exacerbation with some success. Short courses of corticosteroids may be helpful if the patient has optic neuritis or other disabling relapse.

Prognosis

The disease is characterized by exacerbations and remissions, with 70% of patients experiencing slow progression over a number of years. Pregnancy does not appear to exert any deleterious effect on multiple sclerosis and may improve the rate of exacerbation. The risk of exacerbations is increased in the first 3 months postpartum. Family planning should be discussed because of the progressive nature of the disease. If so desired, families should be completed or started as soon as possible.

MYASTHENIA GRAVIS

ESSENTIALS OF DIAGNOSIS

- Myasthenia gravis is an autoimmune disorder characterized by antibodies to acetylcholine receptors at the neuromuscular junction.
- It is characterized by muscle weakness, particularly with repetitive movement.

Myasthenia gravis is a chronic disorder of the neuromuscular junction of striate muscles as result of acetylcholine receptor dysfunction. Antibodies to acetylcholine receptors usually are present. It occurs more commonly in females than in males, and its peak occurrence is in the third decade of life. It is characterized by abnormal voluntary muscle function with muscle weakness after repeated effort. Although some cases of myasthenia gravis appear to be hereditary, most adult cases appear to be acquired.

Clinical Findings

The most common symptom is easily fatigued small muscles, most frequently the ocular muscles, which results in double vision. Weakness usually increases as the muscles are used repeatedly. Patients who may not have noticeable symptoms in the morning may be easily diagnosed in the afternoon. Difficulties with swallowing and speech are not uncommon, and the facial muscles are almost always affected.

The diagnosis can be confirmed by administering edrophonium (Tensilon; a total of 10 mg, consisting of 2 mg followed by 8 mg 45 seconds later) to assess improvement in muscular weakness. A radioimmunoassay for the acetylcholine receptor antibody can be performed. Repetitive nerve stimulation would show a decrement >15% in a person with the condition.

One-third of patients with myasthenia gravis experience exacerbation during pregnancy, one-third do not experience a change in disease, and one-third experience remission during pregnancy. The disease does not affect uterine activity because the uterus consists of smooth muscle. The length of labor is not affected. However, an assisted second stage might be considered because of maternal fatigue. Exacerbations are most common during the postpartum period. Placental transfer of acetylcholine receptor antibodies can occur, so the fetus should be monitored at frequent intervals during pregnancy with fetal kick counts and ultrasound. A rare finding in neonates is arthrogryposis multiplex congenita, congenital contractures secondary to lack of movement in utero. Antibodies may affect the fetal diaphragm and lead to pulmonary hypoplasia and polyhydramnios. From 12–15% of newborns will be affected with transient myasthenia gravis. The mean duration of neonatal symptoms is 3 weeks.

Treatment

Treatment with anticholinesterases (eg, neostigmine) is the same as in the nonpregnant state, although dosages must be administered more frequently during pregnancy. Other treatment options include thymectomy, steroids, plasma exchange, and IVIG. During labor, anticholinesterases should be administered parenterally rather than orally. Parenteral and regional anesthesia is not contraindicated in labor. Curare-like agents (eg, aminoglycoside antibiotics) and magnesium sulfate, as well as the older general anesthetics such as ether and chloroform, should be avoided.

Women taking anticholinesterase drugs are advised not to breastfeed.

OTHER NEUROLOGIC DISORDERS AFFECTING PREGNANCY

SPINAL CORD DISORDERS

Spinal cord lesions that are caused by trauma, tumor, infection, or vascular disorders usually do not prevent conception. Diagnosis and therapy should be performed without regard to pregnancy. In general, pregnancy coexisting with trauma to the spinal cord from any cause, even paraplegia, proceeds unremarkably with the exception of an increased frequency of urinary tract infections and sepsis from pressure necrosis of the skin. Fetal growth usually is unimpeded even though initial maternal weight is frequently <100 lb because of muscular wasting. Generally labor proceeds without evidence of fetopelvic disproportion. Women whose paraplegia is related to anterior horn cell damage or to cord lesions below the tenth thoracic level have appropriate perception of labor contractions and may require analgesia or anesthesia. In most patients, rapid, painless labors are the rule, with the only abnormality being a prolonged second stage because of decreased muscular effort. Paraplegic patients may develop autonomic hyperreflexia during labor due to loss of central regulation of the sympathetic nervous system below the level of the lesion. This is best managed with an epidural, continuous monitoring of the cardiac rhythm and blood pressures, antihypertensives, and an assisted second stage.

DISORDERS OF CRANIAL NERVES

Palsies of the facial nerve due to inflammation are called *Bell's palsy.* Although patients may complain of paresthesia over the area of paralysis, this is strictly a motor disorder involving paralysis of the muscles of facial expression on 1 side that are innervated by the facial nerve. Given that approximately one-fifth of cases of Bell's palsy occur during pregnancy or shortly thereafter, it has been suggested that pregnancy increases the frequency of this disorder, although viral infections also have been causally related. Treatment with corticosteroids (prednisone 40–60 mg/d) and acyclovir is helpful if given within 1 week of onset. However, Bell's palsy usually is self-limited. Because the patient is unable to blink or close her eye on the affected side, corneal damage will occur if frequent eye drops and nighttime closure of the eye with patches and lubrication are not instituted. Rarely is surgical decompression of the nerve indicated.

GUILLAIN-BARRÉ SYNDROME

Guillain-Barré syndrome is an acute inflammatory demyelinating polyneuropathy often related to an upper respiratory or gastrointestinal infection or recent immunization. Rapid onset of weakness occurs, most frequently in an ascending pattern involving the extremities first, then respiratory muscles and face. Hospitalization is required, and supportive treatment aimed at preventing respiratory failure is mandatory. If the vital respiratory capacity falls to 800 mL or below, tracheostomy should be performed. Plasmapheresis or IVIG is the treatment of choice to shorten the course of illness. Most patients progress normally through pregnancy and deliver at term, so abortion is not mandated. On the other hand, if respiratory paralysis occurs near term, caesarean delivery may be indicated to improve ventilation.

PERIPHERAL NEUROPATHIES

Carpal tunnel syndrome is a neuropathic disorder related to median nerve compression by swelling of the tissue in the synovial sheaths at the wrist. Symptoms usually are limited to paresthesia over the thumb, index, and middle fingers and the medial portion of the ring finger. Most commonly, symptoms are noted at night and usually are best treated conservatively with elevation of the affected wrist and splinting. The syndrome usually abates postpartum. Surgery and corticosteroids are rarely indicated.

Compression of the femoral or obturator nerve can occur from retraction at the time of caesarean delivery or hysterectomy, but it is most commonly related to pressure of the fetus just before and during vaginal delivery.

Femoral nerve palsy results in weakness of the iliopsoas and quadriceps muscles and sensory loss over the anterior thigh. Obturator nerve palsy is characterized by adduction weakness of the thigh and minimal sensory loss over the medial aspect of the affected limb. *Peroneal neuropathy* reveals footdrop and weakness on dorsiflexion of the foot, occasionally with paresthesia in the foot and second toes. This disorder usually appears 1–2 days postpartum and may be related to prolonged episiotomy repair and to pressure on the nerve from knee stirrups. Women at risk include small women with relatively large babies, those who have had midforceps rotations, and those who have had prolonged labor, especially with abnormally large infants (owing to compression of the L4–5 lumbosacral nerve trunk). The prognosis is excellent with conservative therapy, but occasionally a short leg brace is necessary.

Brachialgia or the *thoracic outlet syndrome* occurs when the brachial plexus and subclavian artery are compressed by the clavicle and first rib. Occurrence in pregnancy is increased because of the greater weight of the breasts and abdomen. The pain is referred to the lateral aspect of the hand and forearm, although motor symptoms are rare. Blanching of the fingers and exacerbation of symptoms when the hands are elevated are diagnostic. The syndrome usually is self-limited; posture instruction and strengthening of shoulder suspension muscles are helpful. Surgical removal of the rib is very occasionally necessary (as in the nonpregnant patient).

Herniation of intervertebral disks occurs more commonly in the lumbar than the cervical region. There are both motor and sensory findings along the distribution of the sciatic nerve. It is limited to 1 extremity and must be differentiated from more serious disorders such as spinal cord tumors and hemorrhage. Diagnosis usually can be made by physical examination and history. MRI of the spine is the best diagnostic modality if needed. Conservative management with bedrest and physical therapy is helpful. The process should cause no problems during pregnancy or vaginal delivery unless the patient has cervical disk disease. In that event, caesarean delivery is advised to prevent herniation and paralysis. Surgical correction should be avoided during pregnancy if possible.

Cunnington M, Tennis P, International Lamotrigine Pregnancy Registry Scientific Advisory Committee. Lamotrigine and the risk of malformations in pregnancy. *Neurology* 2005;64: 955–960. PMID: 15781807.

Holmes LB, Wyszynski DF. North American Antiepileptic Drug Pregnancy Registry. *Epilepsia* 2004;45:1465. PMID: 15509251.

Holms LB, Harvey EA, Coull BA, et al. The teratogenicity of anticonvulsant drugs. *N Engl J Med* 2001;344:1132–1138. PMID: 11297704.

Loder E. Safety of sumatriptan in pregnancy: a review of the data so far. *CNS Drugs* 2003;17:1–7. PMID: 12467489.

Marcus DA, Scharff L, Turk D. Longitudinal prospective study of headache during pregnancy and postpartum. *Headache* 1999;39:625–632. PMID: 11279958.

Sances G, Granella F, Nappi RE, et al. Course of migraine during pregnancy and postpartum: a prospective study. *Cephalalgia* 2003;23:197–205. PMID: 12662187.

Sandberg-Wollheim M, Frank D, Goodwin TM, et al. Pregnancy outcomes during treatment with interferon beta-1a in patients with multiple sclerosis. *Neurology* 2005;65:802–806. PMID: 16093457.

Wiltin AG, Mattar F, Sibai BM. Postpartum stroke: a twenty-year experience. *Am J Obstet Gynecol* 2000;183:83–88. PMID: 10920313.

Wyszynski DF, Nambisan M, Surve T, et al; Antiepileptic Drug Pregnancy Registry. Increased rate of major malformations in offspring exposed to valproate during pregnancy. *Neurology* 2005;64:961–965. PMID: 15781808.

AUTOIMMUNE DISORDERS

RHEUMATOID ARTHRITIS

ESSENTIALS OF DIAGNOSIS

- Inflammatory arthritis involving 3 or more joints
- The presence of certain biomarkers on serum testing such as rheumatoid factor, elevated C-reactive protein, or elevated ESR
- Most patients with rheumatoid arthritis in pregnancy diagnosed prior to pregnancy

Pathogenesis

Rheumatoid arthritis is a chronic autoimmune disease characterized by symmetric inflammatory synovitis. The prevalence in North America is 0.5–3.8%, and it occurs 3 times more frequently in women.

Clinical Findings

Symptoms of rheumatoid arthritis are insidious, with a prodrome of fatigue, weakness, generalized joint stiffness, and myalgias preceding the appearance of joint swelling. The diagnosis can be made when the patient is found to have inflammatory arthritis involving 3 or more joints; the patient has abnormal biomarkers such as rheumatoid factor, elevated C-reactive protein, or elevated ESR, the duration of symptoms is more than 6 weeks; and other diseases have been excluded. Laboratory findings are mild leukocytosis, elevated ESR (which may not always reflect the activity of the disease), and a positive rheumatoid factor (in the majority of patients).

Treatment

Treatment consists of rest, anti-inflammatory drugs, splints, physical therapy, a well-balanced diet, and adequate movement of all joints. Cyclooxygenase (COX)-1 and COX-2 inhibitors should be avoided in pregnancy. If they are used, therapy should be limited to short courses prior to 32 weeks' gestation to avoid premature closure of the ductus arteriosus, and the amniotic fluid index should be followed for oligohydramnios. Low-dose oral corticosteroid therapy, hydroxychloroquine, or sulfasalazine can be substituted safely for COX inhibitors. Tumor necrosis factor (TNF)-α inhibitors, penicillamine, gold, and methotrexate should be avoided. Methotrexate should be stopped 1–3 months prior to conception, and patients on leflunomide should wait to conceive until serum concentrations are undetectable. Symptoms improve during pregnancy in approximately 75% of women. However, many patients relapse within 6 months postpartum. The activity of the disease during pregnancy is best followed by assessment of duration of morning stiffness and the number of joints involved. Levels of Ro/SS-A and La/SS-B antibodies should be obtained to determine the fetal risk for complete heart block. In cases of severe postpartum exacerbation, early termination of breastfeeding may be necessary in order to allow the full range of pharmacologic therapy, including TNF-α inhibitors.

Prognosis

The course is variable and unpredictable, with spontaneous remissions and exacerbations.

SYSTEMIC LUPUS ERYTHEMATOSUS

ESSENTIALS OF DIAGNOSIS

- Systemic lupus erythematosus (SLE) is a multisystem autoimmune disorder with a wide spectrum of disease manifestations.
- The diagnosis can be made when 4 of the following criteria are present: malar rash, discoid rash, photosensitivity, oral ulcers, serositis, renal disorders, neurologic disorders, hematologic disorders (hemolytic anemia, leukopenia, thrombocytopenia), immunologic disorders (anti-DNA, anti-Sm, false-positive Venereal Disease Research Laboratory [VDRL] test), or an abnormal ANA titer.
- As with other autoimmune diseases in pregnancy, the diagnosis of SLE is usually made prior to pregnancy.

Pathogenesis

Systemic lupus erythematosus (SLE) is a chronic inflammatory disease that can affect many different organ systems. It is of interest to obstetricians because it affects women more commonly than men (10:1), and the women it affects tend to be of reproductive age. The cause of SLE is unknown, and the clinical course is variable. Common serologic markers of SLE are present 5 years before the diagnosis is made in up to 50% of women. Complications of pregnancy characteristic of SLE may precede the clinical diagnosis by many years as well.

Clinical Findings

The diagnosis can be made when 4 of the following criteria are present: malar rash, discoid rash, photosensitivity, oral ulcers, serositis, renal disorders, neurologic disorders, hematologic disorders (hemolytic anemia, leukopenia, thrombocytopenia), immunologic disorders (anti-DNA, anti-Sm, false-positive Venereal Disease Research Laboratory [VDRL] test), or an abnormal ANA titer.

Differential Diagnosis

The differential diagnosis includes rheumatoid arthritis, drug-induced SLE syndromes, polyarteritis, chronic active hepatitis, and, late in pregnancy, preeclampsia. Common symptoms at presentation in pregnancy are malaise, fever, myalgias, and weight loss.

Complications

Considerable controversy exists about the effects of pregnancy on SLE and vice versa. Most patients who become pregnant while their SLE is not active for at least 6 months seem to have few problems except for a 2- to 3-fold increased risk of superimposed preeclampsia and fetal growth restriction; the risk of a lupus flare is 20%. Women with active SLE are at very high risk for superimposed preeclampsia (60–80%), fetal growth restriction, preterm birth, and lupus flare (50–80%). Women with preexisting renal disease frequently have some deterioration in renal function, but it is irreversible in only 10% of cases.

Treatment

Management during pregnancy includes a careful history, physical examination, and laboratory evaluation. A history of prior spontaneous abortions or fetal losses should be elicited. The history should note the manifestations of SLE in the past; determination of the severity of disease activity is important in anticipating pregnancy complications. Although the fertility rate of patients with SLE is normal, patients have a higher percentage of total fetal losses. This may be associated with the presence of antiphospholipid antibodies. Physical examination should focus on signs of active disease. Laboratory evaluation should include a complete blood count, serum chemistries, and liver function tests. ANA (if the diagnosis is not previously confirmed), double-stranded DNA, urine protein, C3, C4, and CH_{50} tests should be obtained. Subsequent changes in these values may herald a flare of lupus nephritis. The results of the SS-A, lupus anticoagulant, anticardiolipin antibody, and anti-β_2 glycoprotein 1 tests should be known. The presence of SS-A is associated with neonatal lupus, manifested by cutaneous lesions or congenital heart block. Anticardiolipin antibody and lupus anticoagulant anti-β_2 glycoprotein 1 tests are associated with antiphospholipid antibody syndrome (APS), which predisposes patients to thromboembolic events, fetal death, fetal growth restriction, and preeclampsia. Prophylactic treatment with daily baby aspirin and heparin is recommended when APS is diagnosed. Diagnostic criteria require a clinical event (as listed earlier) plus a positive lupus anticoagulant result, moderate- to high-titer anticardiolipin antibody (>40 IgG phospholipid units or IgM phospholipid units or >99th percentile for the testing laboratory), or anti-β_2 glycoprotein 1 antibodies (IgG or IgM >99th percentile for the testing laboratory). These tests should be positive on 2 occasions 12 weeks apart. Most fetal loss in SLE appears to be due to concomitant APS, which occurs in approximately 30% of patients.

Distinguishing between superimposed preeclampsia in the third trimester and an SLE flare often is difficult. In fact, it is not possible to say with certainty that preeclampsia is not present, but careful consideration can suggest whether an SLE flare is a contributing factor. In a pregnancy remote from term, aggressive empiric therapy of presumed SLE may allow significant prolongation of pregnancy.

Serial ultrasounds for fetal growth and antenatal testing starting at 32–34 weeks should be instituted to ensure fetal well-being. Delivery is often recommended at 39 weeks' gestation. Uterine artery Doppler at midgestation can be used to predict early-onset preeclampsia and fetal growth restriction.

The mainstay of treatment of SLE in pregnancy consists of corticosteroids, hydroxychloroquine, and azathioprine. Corticosteroids appear to be weak teratogens, resulting in 1 extra facial cleft for every 1000 first-trimester exposures. Thereafter, there is a risk of premature rupture of membranes and preterm birth, but usually after 34 weeks' gestation. Corticosteroids also increase the risk for gestational diabetes and maternal hypertension. Medications used to treat SLE that should be avoided during conception and pregnancy include mycophenolate mofetil, cyclophosphamide, methotrexate, and warfarin. Little information on the use of newer agents (eg, rituximab, abatacept) is available. The chance of successful pregnancy outcome for women with SLE has improved dramatically over the years with better understanding of the natural history of the disease and medical therapy in pregnancy.

SCLERODERMA (SYSTEMIC SCLEROSIS)

ESSENTIALS OF DIAGNOSIS

- Scleroderma, or systemic sclerosis, is a rare condition that is uncommonly seen in pregnancy.
- It is a systemic disorder characterized by the presence of thickened, hardened skin, circulatory abnormalities, and often involvement of multiple organ systems.

Clinical Findings

Pregnancy in patients with scleroderma is rare because the disorder occurs most frequently in patients beyond reproductive age. Symptoms include malaise, fatigue, arthralgias, Raynaud's phenomenon, and myalgias. The course of the disease appears to improve or remain unchanged during pregnancy. One study did show an increase in preterm births. Pregnancy progresses normally in otherwise stable disease. When scleroderma-related renal disease and/or hypertension are present, pregnancy is at increased risk of being complicated by preeclampsia or malignant hypertension.

Treatment

Treatment options for women with systemic sclerosis in pregnancy include anti-inflammatory and immunosuppressive drugs such as prednisone, hydroxychloroquine, and nonsteroidal anti-inflammatory drugs.

Arbuckle MR, McClain MT, Rubertone MV et al. Development of autoantibodies before the clinical onset of systemic lupus erythematosus. *N Engl J Med* 2003;349:1526–33. PMID: 14561795.

Cimaz R, Spence DL, Hornberger L, et al. Incidence and spectrum of neonatal lupus erythematosus: a prospective study of infants born to mothers with anti-Ro autoantibodies. *J Pediatr* 2003;142:678–83. PMID: 12838197.

Clark CA, Spitzer KA, Laskin CA. Decrease in pregnancy loss rates in patients with systemic lupus erythematosus over a 40-year period. *J Rheumatol* 2005;32:1709–1712. PMID: 16142865.

Clowse ME, Magder LS, Witter F, et al. Early risk factors for pregnancy loss in lupus. *Obstet Gynecol* 2006;107:293–299. PMID: 16449114.

Clowse ME, Magder LS, Witter F, et al. The impact of increased lupus activity on obstetric outcomes. *Arthritis Rheum* 2005;52:514–521. PMID: 15692998.

Doria A, Ghirardello A, Iaccarino L, et al. Pregnancy, cytokines, and disease activity in systemic lupus erythematosus. *Arthritis Rheum* 2004;51:989–995. PMID: 15593367.

Erkan D, Derksen WJ, Kaplan V, et al. Real world experience with antiphospholipid antibody tests: how stable are results over time? *Ann Rheum Dis* 2005;64:1321–1325. PMID: 15731290.

Janssen NM, Genta MS. The effects of immunosuppressive and anti-inflammatory medications on fertility, pregnancy and lactation. *Arch Intern Med* 2000;160;610–619. PMID: 10724046.

Lassere M, Empson M. Treatment of antiphospholipid syndrome in pregnancy: a systematic review of randomized therapeutic trials. *Thromb Res* 2004;114:419. PMID: 15507273.

Miyakis S, Lockshin MD, Atsumi T, et al. International consensus statement on an update of the classification criteria for definite antiphospholipid syndrome (APS). *J Thromb Haemost* 2006;4:295–306. PMID: 16420554.

Ollier WE, Harrison B, Symmons D. What is the natural history of rheumatoid arthritis? *Best Pract Res Clin Rheumatol* 2001;15:27–48. PMID: 11358413.

Sampaio-Barros PD, Samara AM, Marques Neto JF. Gynecologic history in systemic sclerosis. *Clin Rheumatol* 2000;19:184–187. PMID: 10870650.

Venkat-Raman N, Backos M, Teoh TG, et al. Uterine artery Doppler in predicting pregnancy outcome in women with antiphospholipid syndrome. *Obstet Gynecol* 2001;98:235. PMID: 11506839.

Witter FR, Petri M. Antenatal detection of intrauterine growth restriction in patients with systemic lupus erythematosus. *Int J Gynecol Obstet* 2000;71:67–68. PMID: 11044546.

Yasmeen S, Wilkins EE, Field NT, et al. Pregnancy outcomes in women with systemic lupus erythematosus. *J Matern Fetal Med* 2001;10:91. PMID: 11392599.

Hematologic Disorders in Pregnancy

34

Christina Arnett, MD
Jeffrey S. Greenspoon, MD
Ashley S. Roman, MD, MPH

ANEMIA

Anemia is a significant maternal problem during pregnancy. The Centers for Disease Control and Prevention defines anemia as a hemoglobin concentration of <11 g/dL (hematocrit of <33%) in the first or third trimester or a hemoglobin concentration of <10.5 g/dL (hematocrit <32%) in the second trimester. A pregnant woman will lose blood during delivery and the puerperium, and an anemic woman is at increased jeopardy of blood transfusion and its related complications.

During pregnancy, the blood volume increases by approximately 50% and the red blood cell mass by approximately 33%. This relatively greater increase in plasma volume results in a lower hematocrit but does not truly represent anemia.

Anemia in pregnancy most commonly results from a nutritional deficiency in either iron or folate. Pernicious anemia due to vitamin B_{12} deficiency almost never occurs during pregnancy. Other anemias occurring during pregnancy include anemia of chronic disease; anemia due to hemoglobinopathy; immune, chronic (eg, hereditary spherocytosis or paroxysmal nocturnal hemoglobinuria), or drug-induced hemolytic anemia; and aplastic anemia.

1. Iron Deficiency Anemia

ESSENTIALS OF DIAGNOSIS

- Hypochromic and microcytic anemia with evidence of depleted iron stores

Pathogenesis

Iron deficiency is responsible for approximately 95% of the anemias during pregnancy, reflecting the increased demands for iron. The total body iron consists mostly of (1) iron in hemoglobin (approximately 70% of total iron; approximately 1700 mg in a 56-kg woman) and (2) iron stored as ferritin and hemosiderin in reticuloendothelial cells in bone marrow, the spleen, and parenchymal cells of the liver (approximately 300 mg). Small amounts of iron exist in myoglobin, plasma, and various enzymes. The absence of hemosiderin in the bone marrow indicates that iron stores are depleted. This finding is both diagnostic of anemia and an early sign of iron deficiency. Subsequent events are a decrease in serum iron, an increase in serum total iron-binding capacity, and anemia.

During the first half of pregnancy, iron requirements may not be increased significantly, and iron absorbed from food (approximately 1 mg/d) is sufficient to cover the basal loss of 1 mg/d. However, in the second half of pregnancy, iron requirements increase due to expansion of red blood cell mass and rapid growth of the fetus. Increased numbers of red blood cells and a greater hemoglobin mass require approximately 500 mg of iron. The iron needs of the fetus average 300 mg. Thus, the additional amount of iron needed due to the pregnancy is approximately 800 mg. Data published by the Food and Nutrition Board of the National Academy of Sciences show that pregnancy increases a woman's iron requirements to approximately 3.5 mg/d. This need outstrips the 1 mg/d of iron available from the normal diet.

Prevention

It is unclear whether the well-nourished, nonanemic woman benefits from routine iron supplementation during pregnancy. However, for women with a history of iron deficiency anemia, at least 60 mg/d of elemental iron should be prescribed to prevent anemia during the course of pregnancy and the puerperium.

Clinical Findings

A. Symptoms & Signs

The symptoms may be vague and nonspecific, including pallor, easy fatigability, headache, palpitations, tachycardia, and dyspnea. Angular stomatitis, glossitis, and koilonychia (spoon nails) may be present in longstanding severe anemia.

B. Laboratory Findings

The hematocrit is <33% in the first or third trimesters or <32% in the second trimester. The hemoglobin may fall as low as 3 g/dL, but the red cell count is rarely below $2.5 \times 10^6/mm^3$. The red cells usually are hypochromic and microcytic, with mean corpuscular volumes of <79 fL. Serum ferritin concentrations fall to <15 μg/dL and transferrin saturation to <16%. Serum iron levels usually are <60 μg/dL. The total iron-binding capacity is elevated in both normal pregnancies and pregnancies affected by iron deficiency anemia and, therefore, is of little diagnostic value by itself. The reticulocyte count is low for the degree of anemia. Platelet counts are frequently increased, but white cell counts are normal. Bone marrow biopsy demonstrates lack of stainable iron in marrow macrophages and erythroid precursors but usually is unnecessary in uncomplicated iron deficiency anemia.

Differential Diagnosis

Anemia due to chronic disease or an inflammatory process (eg, rheumatoid arthritis) may be hypochromic and microcytic. Anemia due to thalassemia trait can be differentiated from iron deficiency anemia by normal serum iron levels and ferritin levels, the presence of stainable iron in the marrow, and elevated levels of hemoglobin A_2. Other less common causes of microcytic, hypochromic anemia include sideroblastic anemia and anemia due to lead poisoning.

Complications

Iron deficiency anemia may be associated with intrauterine growth retardation and preterm birth. There also appears to be an association between iron deficiency anemia and an increased risk of postpartum depression.

Angina pectoris or congestive heart failure may develop as a result of marked iron deficiency anemia. **Sideropenic dysphagia (Paterson-Kelly syndrome, Plummer-Vinson syndrome)** is a rare condition characterized by dysphagia, esophageal web, and atrophic glossitis due to long-standing severe iron deficiency anemia.

Severe anemia with hemoglobin <6–7 g/dL has been associated with reduced fetal oxygenation, abnormal fetal heart tracing, low amniotic fluid volume, and intrauterine fetal demise.

Treatment

In an established case of anemia, prompt adequate treatment is necessary.

A. Oral Iron Therapy

Ferrous sulfate 300 mg (containing 60 mg of elemental iron, of which approximately 10% is absorbed) should be given 3 times per day. If this agent is not tolerated, ferrous fumarate or gluconate should be prescribed. Therapy should be continued for approximately 3 months after hemoglobin values return to normal in order to replenish iron stores. Hemoglobin levels should increase by at least 0.3 g/dL/wk if the patient is responding to therapy.

Iron is best absorbed in the ferrous or reduced form from an empty stomach. Administering ascorbic acid via supplement or citrus juice at the time of iron supplementation creates a mildly acidic environment that aids the absorption of iron.

B. Parenteral Iron Therapy

The indication for parenteral iron is intolerance of, or refractoriness to, oral iron. In most cases of moderate iron deficiency anemia, the total iron requirements equal the amount of iron needed to restore hemoglobin levels to normal or near normal plus 50% of that amount to replenish iron stores.

Iron dextran is the most widely available parenteral iron preparation in the United States. While it may be given intramuscularly, it is preferable to administer it intravenously (IV). Each 2-mL vial provides 100 mg of elemental iron. After a 0.5-mL test dose, iron dextran can be administered intramuscularly or IV at a rate not to exceed 100 mg/d of elemental iron. Intramuscular injection must always be given into the muscle mass of the upper outer quadrant of the buttock with a 2-in, 20-gauge needle, using the Z technique (ie, pulling the skin and superficial musculature to one side before inserting the needle to prevent leakage of the solution and subsequent tattooing of the skin). Intramuscular iron raises hemoglobin concentration only slightly faster than oral iron administration due to slow and occasionally incomplete mobilization of iron from the muscle. Risks of parenteral iron administration include anaphylactic reaction (approximately 1% risk), muscle necrosis, fever, and phlebitis.

Other forms of IV iron such as ferric gluconate complex may also be administered IV. Ferric gluconate complex is associated with a lower incidence of adverse reactions.

C. Erythropoietin

Few studies have evaluated the role of erythropoietin in pregnant women with iron deficiency anemia. Although the data are conflicting, erythropoietin administered in conjunction with IV iron may be associated with a shorter time to targeted hematologic indices than IV iron alone. The addition of erythropoietin to iron therapy may be considered in women for whom rapid correction of anemia is desired, particularly women in the third trimester of pregnancy.

D. Blood Transfusion

Blood transfusion is generally reserved for women with coexisting issues such as operative deliver or postpartum hemorrhage or women with evidence of active bleeding. It may also be considered for women with hemoglobin <6–7 g/dL due to the increased risk of obstetrical and fetal complications in women with anemia of this severity.

2. Megaloblastic Anemia of Pregnancy

ESSENTIALS OF DIAGNOSIS

- Macrocytic anemia with low serum levels of folate or vitamin B_{12}

Pathogenesis

Megaloblastic anemia of pregnancy is most commonly caused by folic acid deficiency and is common where nutrition is inadequate. In the United States, access to fresh vegetables and the fortification of grains makes folate deficiency much less common than in the developing world.

In the nonpregnant woman, the minimum daily intake of folate necessary for adequate hematopoiesis and to maintain stores is 50 mg. However, this requirement increases during pregnancy. In order to meet this need and to decrease the neural tube defects associated with folate deficiency, a dietary supplement of at least 400 mg/d of folic acid is recommended.

Additional folic acid may be required in states of heightened DNA synthesis, such as multifetal gestation. Similarly, patients with a chronic hemolytic anemia such as **sickle cell anemia** require additional folate supplementation in order to meet the demand imposed by increased hematopoiesis. Other hemolytic states are also commonly complicated by folic acid deficiency, including **hereditary spherocytosis** and **malaria.**

Folic acid absorption or metabolism may be impaired by the use of oral contraceptives, pyrimethamine, trimethoprim-sulfamethoxazole, primidone, phenytoin, or barbiturates. Alcohol consumption also interferes with folate metabolism. Jejunal bypass surgery for obesity or the malabsorption syndrome (sprue) may impair folic acid absorption.

Megaloblastic anemia may also be caused by vitamin B_{12} deficiency. Women with a history of partial or total gastrectomy or Crohn's disease are at risk of vitamin B_{12} deficiency.

Clinical Findings

A. Symptoms & Signs

The symptoms are nonspecific (eg, lassitude, anorexia, nausea and vomiting, diarrhea, and depression). Pallor often is not marked. Rarely, a sore mouth or tongue is present. Occasionally, purpura may be a clinical manifestation. Megaloblastic anemia should be suspected if iron deficiency anemia fails to respond to iron therapy.

B. Laboratory Findings

Folic acid deficiency results in a hematologic picture similar to that of true pernicious anemia (autoimmune disease that leads to vitamin B_{12} deficiency), which is extremely rare in women of childbearing age.

The hemoglobin may be as low as 4–6 g/dL, and the red cell count may be <2 million/μL in severe cases. Extreme anemia often is associated with leukocytopenia and thrombocytopenia.

The red cells are macrocytic (mean corpuscular volume usually >100 fL) and appear as macro-ovalocytes on peripheral blood smear. However, in pregnancy, macrocytosis may be concealed by accompanying iron deficiency or thalassemia. Up to 70% of folate-deficient patients also lack iron stores.

Serum folate levels <4 ng/mL are suggestive of folic acid depletion in nonpregnant patients. However, in otherwise normal pregnant patients, folate tends to fall slowly to low levels (3–6 ng/mL) with advancing gestation. The red cell folate level in megaloblastic patients is lower, but in 30% of patients, the values overlap. The peripheral white blood cells are hypersegmented. Seventy-five percent of folate-deficient patients have more than 5% neutrophils with 5 or more lobes, but this also may be true for 25% of normal pregnant patients.

The urinary excretion of formiminoglutamic acid (FIGLU) has been used to diagnose folate deficiency, but levels are abnormal only in severe megaloblastic anemia. Bone marrow aspirate demonstrates megaloblastic erythropoiesis but usually is not necessary for diagnosis. Serum iron and vitamin B_{12} levels should be normal.

In women with vitamin B_{12} deficiency, low serum levels of vitamin B_{12} are seen.

Treatment

If the megaloblastic anemia is due to folate deficiency, folic acid 1–5 mg/d orally is initiated. This therapy produces the maximum hematologic response, replaces body stores, and provides the minimum daily requirements. The hematocrit should rise approximately 1% each day, beginning on day 5–6 of therapy. The reticulocyte count should become elevated after 3–4 days of therapy and is the earliest morphologic sign of response. Iron supplementation should be administered as indicated.

For women with vitamin B_{12} deficiency, 1000 μg of vitamin B_{12} should be administered intramuscularly or subcutaneously monthly.

Prognosis

Megaloblastic anemia due to folate deficiency during pregnancy carries a good prognosis if adequately treated.

The anemia usually is mild unless associated with multifetal pregnancy, systemic infection, or hemolytic disease (eg, sickle cell anemia). Low birthweight as well as fetal neural tube defects are known to be associated with maternal folic acid deficiency. The associations with placental abruption, spontaneous abortion, and preeclampsia–eclampsia are not universally accepted. Even without treatment, anemia due to folate deficiency usually resolves after delivery when folate demands normalize.

3. Aplastic Anemia

ESSENTIALS OF DIAGNOSIS

- Pancytopenia
- Empty bone marrow on biopsy

Pathogenesis

Aplastic anemia with primary bone marrow failure during pregnancy is rare. The anemia may be secondary to exposure to known marrow toxins, such as chloramphenicol, phenylbutazone, mephenytoin, alkylating chemotherapeutic agents, or insecticides. In approximately two-thirds of cases, no obvious cause is detected. Idiopathic aplastic anemia in pregnancy may have a spontaneous remission following delivery or pregnancy termination but may recur in subsequent pregnancies. The condition likely is immunologically mediated.

Clinical Findings

The rapidly developing anemia causes pallor, fatigue, tachycardia, painful ulceration of the throat, and fever. The diagnostic criteria are pancytopenia and empty bone marrow on biopsy examination.

Complications

Aplastic anemia in pregnancy may cause increased fetal wastage, prematurity, or intrauterine fetal demise. Increased maternal morbidity and death usually are due to infection and hemorrhage.

Treatment

The patient must avoid any toxic agents known to cause aplastic anemia. Blood product replacement with packed red blood cells and platelets should be used as needed. In some cases, delivery or termination of pregnancy may be necessary. Bone marrow transplantation is performed if remission does not occur following delivery or termination of pregnancy. Other possible treatments include antithymocyte antibody, corticosteroids, or immunosuppressive agents. Infection must be treated aggressively with appropriate antibiotics, but most authorities do not recommend giving prophylactic antibiotics.

Prognosis

Pregnancy generally does not affect the prognosis of aplastic anemia. Prognosis is dependent on degree of bone marrow cellularity and patient age.

4. Drug-Induced Hemolytic Anemia

ESSENTIALS OF DIAGNOSIS

- Anemia with evidence of hemolysis

Pathogenesis

Drug-induced hemolytic anemia usually occurs as a result of drug-mediated immunologic red cell injury. For example, a drug can act as a hapten with an erythrocyte protein to which an antidrug antibody attaches. Hemolysis occurs as a result of the subsequent immune response. Many drugs used in pregnancy can have such an effect, including cephalosporins, acetaminophen, and erythromycin.

In African-American women, drug-induced hemolytic anemia is more likely caused by drug-induced oxidative damage rather than a drug-mediated immune mechanism. The most common congenital erythrocyte enzymatic defect to cause this condition is **glucose-6-phosphate dehydrogenase (G6PD) deficiency**. This X-linked disorder causes a heterozygous state in 10–15% of African-American females, but enzyme activity is variable due to random X-chromosome inactivation.

Decreased G6PD activity in one-third of patients in the third trimester causes an increased risk of hemolytic episodes. More than 40 substances toxic to susceptible people are recognized, including sulfonamides, nitrofurans, antipyretics, some analgesics, sulfones, vitamin K analogues, uncooked fava beans, some antimalarials, naphthalene, and nalidixic acid. Specific laboratory tests to identify susceptible individuals include a glutathione stability test and cresyl blue dye reduction test.

Clinical Findings

The red blood cell count and morphology are normal until hemolysis occurs. Levels of anemia are variable depending on the degree of hemolysis. Hemolysis can be diagnosed based on examination of peripheral smear, which may demonstrate spherocytes, elliptocytes, schistocytes, or helmet cells (fragmented red blood cells). Elevated lactate dehydrogenase (LDH) is also used to diagnose hemolysis. Patients with hemolytic anemia also demonstrate an increase in reticulocyte count.

Complications

Exposure of the G6PD-deficient fetus to maternally ingested oxidant drugs (eg, sulfonamides) may produce fetal hemolysis, hydrops fetalis, and fetal death.

Treatment

Management includes immediate discontinuation of any suspected medications, treatment of intercurrent illness, and blood transfusion where indicated.

SICKLE CELL DISEASE

ESSENTIALS OF DIAGNOSIS

- Abnormal hemoglobin (hemoglobin S) leads to sickling of erythrocytes in the setting of decreased oxygen tension.
- Hemoglobin electrophoresis demonstrates hemoglobin S.
- Pregnancy in women with sickle cell disease is associated with an increased risk of obstetrical complications.

Pathogenesis

Sickle cell hemoglobin (hemoglobin S) results from a genetic substitution of valine for glutamic acid at codon 6 of the β-globin chains. Decreased oxygen tension causes hemoglobin S to form insoluble polymers in curvilinear strands. These polymers deform the normal biconcave structure of the erythrocyte. The process is reversible but eventually leads to cell membrane damage and permanent sickling.

Patients homozygous for the hemoglobin S gene have **sickle cell anemia (SS disease)**, and those who are heterozygous have **sickle cell trait.** Approximately 8–10% of African-Americans carry the sickle cell trait, whereas approximately 1 in 500 has sickle cell anemia.

Other sickling syndromes exist when the gene for hemoglobin S is inherited along with the gene for another abnormal hemoglobin, such as hemoglobin C or thalassemia. Hemoglobin C, also caused by β-globin chain mutation, is less soluble than normal hemoglobin A and has a propensity to form hexagonal crystals. Women who are heterozygous for both the S and C genes have **hemoglobin SC disease.** Maternal mortality rates are as high as 2–3%. Hemoglobin SC disease is peculiarly associated with embolization of necrotic fat and cellular bone marrow with resultant respiratory insufficiency. Neurologic symptoms from fat embolism have been reported with sickle cell disease.

In **hemoglobin S/beta-thalassemia disease,** the patient is heterozygous for both hemoglobin S and beta-thalassemia. The severity of complications during pregnancy is related to hemoglobin S concentrations in this particular disease.

Sickle cell disease is characterized by chronic hemolytic anemia and intermittent crises of variable frequency and severity. Although persons with sickle cell trait are not anemic and usually are asymptomatic, they are at increased risk of developing urinary tract infections during pregnancy and are at higher risk for preeclampsia. Additionally, their red blood cells tend to sickle when oxygen tension is significantly lowered.

Clinical Findings

A. Symptoms & Signs

1. Chronic anemia—Chronic anemia results from the shortened survival time of the homozygous S red blood cells due to circulation trauma and intravascular hemolysis or phagocytosis by reticuloendothelial cells in the spleen and liver.

2. Sickling of red blood cells—Intravascular sickling leads to vaso-occlusion and infarction. Small blood vessels supplying various organs and tissues can be partially or completely blocked by sickled erythrocytes, resulting in ischemia, pain, necrosis, and organ damage.

3. Crises—Crises of variable frequency and severity occur. **Pain crises** involve the bones and joints. They usually are precipitated by dehydration, acidosis, or infection. An **aplastic crisis** is characterized by rapidly developing anemia. The hemoglobin may be as low as 2–3 g/dL due to cessation of red blood cell production. An **acute splenic sequestration** crisis is associated with severe anemia and hypovolemic shock, resulting from sudden massive trapping of red blood cells within the splenic sinusoids.

4. Other manifestations—Other manifestations include increased susceptibility to bacterial infection; bacterial pneumonia and pulmonary infarction; myocardial damage and cardiomegaly; and functional and anatomic renal abnormalities in the form of sickle cell nephropathy or papillary renal necrosis, resulting in hematuria. Central nervous system manifestations include headache, convulsions, hemorrhage, or thrombosis (from vaso-occlusion). Ophthalmologic abnormalities include anoxic retinal damage, retinal detachments, vitreous hemorrhages, and proliferative retinopathy. Hepatosplenomegaly or cholelithiasis may occur.

B. Laboratory Findings

Screening for abnormal hemoglobin is imperative in the population at risk. Hemoglobin electrophoresis ascertains the diagnosis and can differentiate between homozygous and heterozygous states.

Complications

Sickle cell anemia is associated with serious risks for mother and fetus. Pregnant women with sickle cell disease face increased rates of maternal mortality and morbidity from hemolytic and folic acid deficiency anemias, frequent crises, pulmonary complications, congestive heart failure, infection, and preeclampsia–eclampsia. It is encouraging, however, that maternal mortality has decreased to 1% since 1972. There is an increased incidence of early fetal wastage, stillbirth, preterm delivery, and fetal growth restriction. The course of pregnancy is generally more benign in women with hemoglobin SC disease than women with sickle cell disease.

Treatment

Preconception counseling is essential in women with sickle cell disease to optimize the patient's health prior to conception. Many women with sickle cell disease are treated with hydroxyurea. Hydroxyurea use in pregnancy has been associated with fetal structural malformations in animals and is poorly studied in humans. Therefore, it should be discontinued prior to conception. Assessment of preconception health includes maternal echocardiogram to evaluate ejection fraction and to look for signs of pulmonary hypertension. Type and screen should also be tested for any sign of alloimmunization. Many women with sickle cell disease have a history of multiple blood transfusions, which puts them at risk of development of alloantibodies that could affect the fetus.

Additionally, preconception or prenatal genetic counseling is of great importance. If both partners have the gene for S hemoglobin, their offspring have a 1 in 4 chance of having sickle cell anemia. If it is determined that a fetus is at risk of hemoglobinopathy, chorionic villus sampling or amniocentesis can diagnose these disorders in the fetus. Preimplantation genetic diagnosis using single-blastomere DNA analysis prior to in vitro fertilization has allowed for the successful transfer of unaffected embryos.

Optimal prenatal care, including prevention or rapid treatment of complications, is necessary to increase the chance for a good outcome. Pneumococcal polyvalent vaccine has been shown to reduce the incidence of pneumococcal infection in adults with sickle disease and therefore is highly recommended. This vaccine is not contraindicated in pregnancy. Similarly, influenza vaccine should be administered annually. Folic acid 1 mg/d will prevent megaloblastic anemia, which can result from intense hematopoiesis. Serial ultrasonic evaluations are essential to assess fetal growth. Antepartum testing should begin at 32–34 weeks' gestation. Careful surveillance for asymptomatic bacteriuria and demonstration of cure is important for preventing pyelonephritis. Regional anesthesia can be safely administered to patients with sickle cell disease while they are in labor.

In the management of crises, the most common predisposing factors—infection, dehydration, and hypoxia—should be evaluated and treated. Symptomatic treatment of pain crisis consists of IV fluid, oxygen supplementation, and adequate analgesics (eg, morphine). Bacterial pneumonia or pyelonephritis must be treated vigorously with IV antibiotics. Streptococcal pneumonia is common and is a serious complication. In all cases, adequate oxygenation must be maintained by face mask as necessary.

The concentration of hemoglobin S should be <50% of the total hemoglobin to prevent crisis. Blood transfusion should be considered in cases of a fall in hematocrit to <25%, but this decision must be guided by the individual patient history and her status during pregnancy. Important considerations are repeated crisis; symptoms of tachycardia, palpitation, dyspnea, or fatigue; and evidence of inadequate or retarded intrauterine growth.

Randomized controlled trials have shown that administration of prophylactic hypertransfusion or exchange transfusion is not necessary to prevent maternal and fetal complications, except in well-defined circumstances. Transfusion carries the risks of allergic reaction, delayed hemolytic reaction, isoimmunization, and transmission of infection.

Bone marrow transplant has been limited by the complications of infection and graft-versus-host disease but shows promise as a potential long-term solution to sickle cell anemia. In utero stem cell therapy with normal hemoglobin stem cells is a potential future treatment for affected fetuses.

THALASSEMIA

ESSENTIALS OF DIAGNOSIS

- The thalassemias are genetically determined disorders of reduced synthesis of 1 or more of the structurally normal globin chains in hemoglobin.
- Thalassemia is associated with varying degrees of anemia, depending on the type and number of globin chains that are reduced or absent.

Pathogenesis

Thalassemia is found throughout the world but is concentrated in the Mediterranean coastal areas, central Africa, and parts of Asia. The high incidence in these regions may represent a balanced polymorphism due to heterozygous advantage.

All thalassemias are inherited as an autosomal recessive trait. The 2 major groups are the alpha- and beta-thalassemias, both of which affect the synthesis of hemoglobin A, which contains 2 α and 2 β chains. The severity of the anemia varies with the type of hemoglobin abnormality.

Alpha-thalassemia is due to defective production of α-globin chains, resulting in a relative excess of β-globin chains. In beta-thalassemia, hemoglobin β-chain synthesis is defective, but the α chains are produced normally. In both cases, the unbalanced synthesis results in a relative excess of the normally produced chain. The normal globin chains then form tetramers that precipitate within red blood cell precursors in the bone marrow, resulting in ineffective erythropoiesis, red cell sequestration and destruction, and hypochromic anemia. The most severe forms of this disorder may cause intrauterine or childhood death. A person who is heterozygous, or a carrier, for a thalassemia trait may be asymptomatic.

Clinical findings

A. Alpha-Thalassemia

Normally, a patient has 4 functional α-globin genes. Disease severity with alpha-thalassemia varies depending on how many genes are absent or mutated.

1. Alpha-thalassemia-2 trait is seen when 1 of the 4 genes is absent. These patients are not anemic, do not have microcytic red cells, and have a normal hemoglobin electrophoresis.
2. Alpha-thalassemia-1 trait, or alpha-thalassemia minor, is seen when 2 of the 4 genes are absent. These patients may have mild anemia with microcytic red cells, but their hemoglobin electrophoresis is normal.
3. Hemoglobin H (β_4) disease results from deletion of 3 of the 4 α-globin genes. In patients with this disease, some normal hemoglobin A ($\alpha_2\beta_2$) is produced because one of the α-globin genes is present, but the excess of β-globin changes causes the formation of hemoglobin H (β_4) as well. Anemia of variable degree results that usually is worsened in pregnancy. Hemoglobin electrophoresis demonstrates 5–30% hemoglobin H.
4. Hemoglobin Barts is seen with loss of all 4 α-globin genes. This condition is not compatible with extrauterine life. It is associated with fetal hydrops and intrauterine fetal demise.

Maternal hemoglobin H is generally diagnosed prior to pregnancy. Alpha-thalassemia-2 trait and alpha-thalassemia minor may not be diagnosed prior to pregnancy and are relevant in that if the father is a carrier of thalassemia or another hemoglobinopathy, the fetus at risk for significant disease. If the fetus is at risk for thalassemia, prenatal diagnosis is available via DNA testing of fetal cells obtained from amniocentesis or chorionic villus sampling. Preimplantation genetic diagnosis is also available for couples at risk of having a fetus with severe alpha-thalassemia who are undergoing in vitro fertilization.

B. Beta-Thalassemia

Beta-thalassemia results from impaired β-globin chain production. **Beta-thalassemia major** is the homozygous state, in which there is little or no production of β-chains. At birth, the neonate usually is asymptomatic because fetal hemoglobin F ($\alpha_2\gamma_2$) contains no β-globin chain. However, this protection disappears at birth, when fetal hemoglobin production terminates. At approximately 1 year of age, a baby with defective β-globin production usually begins to show signs of thalassemia (anemia, hepatosplenomegaly) and requires frequent blood transfusions. Affected individuals often die in their late teens or early 20s because of congestive heart failure, often related to myocardial hemosiderosis and liver failure. However, improved treatment with transfusion and iron chelation has led to overall improved survival and even to successful pregnancies in women with beta-thalassemia major.

Beta-thalassemia minor, the heterozygous state, is frequently diagnosed only after the patient fails to respond to iron therapy or delivers a baby with homozygous disease. Such patients usually suffer from mild to moderate hypochromic microcytic anemia, with increased red blood cell count, elevated hemoglobin A_2 ($\alpha_2\delta_2$) concentrations, increased serum iron levels, and iron saturation >20%, although hemoglobin electrophoresis may miss a small percentage of patients with beta-thalassemia minor.

Suspected adult cases of thalassemia are diagnosed by hemoglobin electrophoresis. As with alpha-thalassemia, antenatal diagnosis of beta-thalassemia is possible. Molecular hybridization measures the number of intact α-globin structural genes in fetal cells obtained by amniocentesis. Preimplantation genetic diagnosis allows for the transfer of unaffected embryos after in vitro fertilization.

LYMPHOMA & LEUKEMIA

1. Hodgkin's Lymphoma

Hodgkin's lymphoma (previously known as Hodgkin's disease) is the most common lymphoma to affect women of childbearing age. Even so, it is uncommon during pregnancy, affecting only approximately 1 in 6000 pregnancies.

Clinical Findings

Patients may be asymptomatic or have fever, weight loss, and pruritus. The most common finding is peripheral lymphadenopathy. Histologic evaluation of the affected nodes establishes the diagnosis.

Careful staging is essential prior to the initiation of treatment with radiotherapy or chemotherapy. Modifications of standard staging modalities, such as the use of magnetic resonance imaging (MRI), can allow for adequate staging during pregnancy. However, some procedures, such as staging laparotomy, after the first trimester impose risks to the pregnancy.

Complications

Complications associated with Hodgkin's lymphoma during pregnancy are related to treatment of the disease, not the disease itself. Chemotherapy during the first trimester is associated with an increased risk of fetal structural malformation. During the second and third trimesters, chemotherapy is associated with intrauterine growth restriction, preterm birth, stillbirth, and adverse fetal neurodevelopmental outcomes such as mental retardation and learning disabilities. Children exposed to chemotherapy in utero appear to be at increased risk of cancer themselves.

Treatment

Treatment is tailored to the individual based on the extent of disease and the gestational age. Radiotherapy is an effective treatment option if radiation scatter to the fetus can be minimized. Chemotherapy is relatively safe later in gestation but best avoided in the first trimester if the clinical situation allows. Pregnancy termination is an alternative if Hodgkin's lymphoma is diagnosed early in gestation. Although pregnancy itself does not appear to adversely affect the lymphoma, pregnancy termination permits the aggressive radiotherapy and chemotherapy often necessary. Conversely, if the diagnosis is made later in gestation and the patient is asymptomatic, delaying therapy until fetal lung maturity is established may be reasonable.

Women with Hodgkin's lymphoma are extremely susceptible to infection and sepsis. Sequelae of treatment include radiation pneumonitis causing restrictive lung disease, pericarditis leading to congestive heart failure, hypothyroidism, and ovarian failure. Given that 85% of relapses in Hodgkin's lymphoma occur within 2 years, it is generally accepted that pregnancy should be deferred for 2 years following remission. The risk of second malignancies, especially leukemia, is dramatically increased.

2. Non-Hodgkin's Lymphoma

Until recently, non-Hodgkin's lymphomas were encountered infrequently in pregnancy. However, because 5–10% of individuals infected with the human immunodeficiency virus (HIV) will develop a lymphoma, the incidence of non-Hodgkin's lymphomas is rising. Similar to Hodgkin's lymphoma, extensive staging is essential. Treatment with radiotherapy is indicated for localized disease, whereas chemotherapy is used for more extensive disease. Care of the pregnant patient with lymphoma requires a multidisciplinary approach by obstetrician-gynecologists, hematologic oncologists, perinatologists, and neonatologists. With careful treatment, the fetuses of affected women appear to tolerate treatment of lymphoma quite well.

3. Leukemia

Leukemias are malignant proliferations of cells of the hematopoietic system. Acute leukemias are derived from primitive progenitor cells of either the myeloid lineage (**acute myelogenous leukemia** [AML]) or the lymphocytic lineage (**acute lymphocytic leukemia** [ALL]). Chronic leukemias are also derived from either myeloid cells (**chronic myelogenous leukemia** [CML]) or lymphocytic cells (**chronic lymphocytic leukemia** [CLL]). All leukemias are rare before age 40 years with the exception of ALL, a childhood disease with a median age at diagnosis of 10 years.

Clinical Findings

Affected individuals often present with the symptoms of anemia (fatigue, weakness), thrombocytopenia (bleeding, bruising), or neutropenia (infection) caused by the replacement of normal hematopoietic cells with leukemia cells in the bone marrow. White blood cell count in the serum can be low, normal, or extremely elevated. Diagnosis is made by cytochemical, genetic, and immunochemical evaluations of the cells of a bone marrow biopsy or aspirate.

Treatment

Treatment of acute leukemia is based on immediate initiation of chemotherapy. For example, the median survival time of untreated patients with AML is 3 months or less. Exposure to chemotherapy during organogenesis frequently results in fetal death. However, most authorities consider chemotherapy safe in the second and third trimesters. A period of pancytopenia following chemotherapy can be complicated by infection and hemorrhage. Patients often require erythrocyte and platelet transfusions, as well as antibiotic medications.

Acute leukemia during pregnancy is associated with premature delivery, fetal growth restriction, and fetal loss, but these findings are more likely due to chemotherapy and its complications rather than the leukemia itself.

HEMORRHAGIC DISORDERS

Although hemorrhagic disorders (eg, immune thrombocytopenic purpura [ITP], disseminated intravascular coagulation, circulating anticoagulants) are not common during pregnancy, these conditions could cause significant risks for both mother and fetus.

1. Gestational Thrombocytopenia

Incidental thrombocytopenia of pregnancy, also termed *gestational thrombocytopenia,* affects 5% of pregnancies. It is characterized by mild, asymptomatic thrombocytopenia with platelet levels usually >70,000/μL. It usually occurs late in gestation and resolves spontaneously after delivery. Gestational thrombocytopenia has no association with fetal thrombocytopenia. Its etiology is unclear, although some authorities suspect that gestational thrombocytopenia represents a very mild form of ITP. Antiplatelet antibodies are isolated from patients in both groups and therefore do not aid in diagnosis. Routine obstetric management is appropriate.

2. Immune Thrombocytopenic Purpura

In ITP, also called **idiopathic thrombocytopenic purpura,** platelet destruction is secondary to a circulating immunoglobulin (Ig) G antiplatelet antibody that crosses the placenta and may affect fetal platelets.

Clinical Findings

The maternal clinical picture varies from asymptomatic to minor bruises or petechiae, bleeding from mucosal sites, or rarely fatal intracranial bleeding. Splenomegaly may be present. In the peripheral circulation, the platelet count often is between 80,000 and 160,000/μL, but it may be lower. The bone marrow aspirate demonstrates hyperplasia of megakaryocytes, although this test is rarely indicated. The diagnosis can be made once laboratory evaluation demonstrates an isolated thrombocytopenia and other causes, such as drug-induced or HIV-related thrombocytopenia, have been excluded. Antiplatelet antibody testing is not diagnostic.

Complications

Because maternal IgG antiplatelet antibodies cross the placenta, the fetus is at risk for severe thrombocytopenia. Fortunately, only approximately 10% of infants born to women with ITP have platelet counts less than 50,000/μL at birth. Antepartum identification of severely affected fetuses has proved difficult. Maternal and fetal platelet counts do not correlate well, nor do levels of maternal antiplatelet antibody and fetal platelet levels. Given the low incidence of severe neonatal thrombocytopenia and morbidity, most authorities do not recommend direct fetal platelet determination by fetal scalp sampling or umbilical cord blood sampling.

Treatment

The standard management is to initiate treatment when the platelet count falls to <30,000–50,000/μL, although significant bleeding does not begin until platelet levels are <10,000/μL. Glucocorticoids suppress the phagocytic activity in the splenic monocyte-macrophage system, increasing platelet levels in approximately two-thirds of patients. Patients refractory to steroid therapy are candidates for immunoglobulin infusion, which has been a great benefit to most patients who fail glucocorticoid therapy. Splenectomy usually is reserved for patients refractory to prednisone and IV immunoglobulin. Immunosuppressive agents should be used with great caution and only in extraordinary cases of ITP in pregnancy. Transfusion of platelets and whole blood may be necessary to restore losses from acute hemorrhage or to normalize low perioperative platelet counts (<50,000/mL).

THROMBOEMBOLISM

Pathogenesis

Venous thromboembolism (VTE) affects approximately 1 in 1000 pregnancies. Pregnancy and the puerperium are periods of increased risk for these events because they are hypercoagulable states. Indeed, all the elements of **Virchow's triad** (circulatory stasis, vascular damage, and hypercoagulability of blood) are present. Increased venous capacity during pregnancy coupled with compression of large veins by the gravid uterus causes venous stasis. Endothelial damage occurs at delivery and is more extensive after caesarean delivery, contributing to the increased risk of VTE after caesarean section. Coagulation is favored during pregnancy due to estrogen stimulation of coagulation factors and decreased activity of the fibrinolytic.

Inherited thrombophilias such as **activated protein C resistance** (most commonly due to the **factor V Leiden** mutation), prothrombin gene mutation, **antithrombin III deficiency,** and **protein C and protein S deficiency,** along with acquired thrombophilias such as the **antiphospholipid syndrome** (**APS**), have emerged as important risk factors for VTE. Other risk factors include prior VTE, older age, smoking, and immobilization.

1. Superficial Thrombophlebitis

Patients with thrombosis of the superficial veins of the saphenous system present with tenderness, pain, or erythema along a vein. A palpable cord is sometimes present. Because of the possibility of concurrent deep vein thrombosis (DVT), compression ultrasound is reasonable to confirm the diagnosis and exclude DVT. Treatment consists of compression stockings, ambulation, leg elevation, local heat, and analgesic medications. Of note, the superficial femoral vein belongs to the deep venous system despite its name. A thrombus in this vein requires treatment for DVT.

2. Deep Vein Thrombosis

Approximately half of DVT in pregnancy occurs antepartum and half occurs postpartum. Previous clinical practices that contributed to thrombosis, such as prolonged postpartum bed rest, likely falsely elevated the risk of DVT in the puerperium. Greater than 80% of DVT in pregnancy occurs in the left lower extremity rather than the right, a finding attributed to compression of the left iliac vein by the right iliac artery as it branches off the aorta.

Clinical Findings

The presentation of DVT is variable but frequently includes lower extremity tenderness, swelling, color changes, and a palpable cord. **Homan's sign,** pain elicited by passive dorsiflexion of the foot, may be present. Occasionally, the extremity is pale and cool with decreased pulses due to reflex arterial spasm.

Diagnosis

The modality of choice for diagnosis of DVT is real-time ultrasound, used with duplex and color Doppler ultrasound. Venography remains the standard but has been largely replaced by the less invasive diagnostic tests. MRI is used when there is a strong clinical suspicion of thrombus not detected by ultrasound or if the ultrasound results are equivocal. With MRI, anatomy above the inguinal ligament can be evaluated, as can pelvic blood flow.

Treatment

Anticoagulation, bed rest, and analgesia are the fundamental treatments of DVT. Ambulation with elastic stockings begins once all symptoms have abated, usually in 7–10 days. Patients are initially anticoagulated with unfractionated heparin or low-molecular-weight heparin. **Low-molecular-weight heparin** has a longer half-life and increased bioavailability, making administration easier and anticoagulant response more predictable. It is associated with fewer bleeding problems than unfractionated heparin and does not require laboratory monitoring. In the postpartum state, the patient can then transition to warfarin. Due to embryopathy and fetal hemorrhage, warfarin is contraindicated during pregnancy. Antepartum DVT is treated with anticoagulation for the rest of pregnancy and then for 6–12 weeks postpartum for at least a total of 3–6 months of therapy. DVT occurring postpartum should be treated with anticoagulation for 3–6 months.

3. Pulmonary Embolism

Pulmonary embolism accounts for approximately 20% of maternal deaths in the United States. Its antepartum and postpartum prevalence are approximately equal, although postpartum pulmonary embolism is associated with higher mortality rates. Clinical evidence of DVT often precedes pulmonary embolization. However, given the prevalence of thrombosis originating in the iliac veins during pregnancy, antecedent DVT is frequently not clinically apparent.

Prevention

Prophylactic anticoagulation should be considered for women at high risk for thromboembolism during pregnancy. Women with inherited thrombophilias that confer a high risk for thrombosis during pregnancy, such as antithrombin III deficiency, homozygosity for factor V Leiden mutation, or prothrombin gene mutation, or compound heterozygosity for factor V Leiden and prothrombin gene mutations, should be anticoagulated during pregnancy regardless of whether they have an antecedent history of thromboembolism. Women with lower risk thrombophilias, such as protein C or S deficiency and heterozygosity for prothrombin gene mutation (G20210A) or factor V Leiden mutation, *and* a history of thromboembolism should also receive anticoagulation during pregnancy. Women with a prior VTE that was related to a temporary risk factor (eg, prolonged immobilization after injury) do not require anticoagulation during pregnancy. However, for women with a prior thromboembolic event related to pregnancy or estrogen-containing birth control pills and no thrombophilia, consideration may be given to anticoagulation during pregnancy. For this subgroup of women, the American College of Obstetricians and Gynecologists indicates that surveillance without anticoagulation is also acceptable.

Clinical Findings

The most common presenting symptom of pulmonary embolus is dyspnea, followed by pleuritic chest pain, apprehension, cough, syncope, and hemoptysis. Associated signs include tachypnea and tachycardia.

Diagnosis

Initial evaluation of the symptoms associated with pulmonary embolism usually consists of arterial blood gas measurement, chest radiograph, and electrocardiogram. Ventilation–perfusion scintigraphy may be used to evaluate for perfusion defects and ventilation mismatches that suggest pulmonary embolus. The test has negligible fetal radiation exposure. High-probability scans are indicative of pulmonary embolism in 88% of cases. Conversely, in patients with normal or near-normal scans, pulmonary embolism was detected by angiography only 4% of the time. However, the usefulness of this modality is limited by that fact that the majority of results are reported as intermediate- or low-probability scans, categories without much diagnostic value. Because of these limitations, spiral computed tomographic (CT) pulmonary angiography has emerged as a useful, noninvasive modality for the detection of pulmonary embolism but is limited in the detection of small emboli. Pulmonary artery catheterization with angiography remains the gold standard but is used less frequently due to its invasive nature.

Treatment

Treatment of pulmonary embolism is anticoagulation. Guidelines such as those published by the American College of Chest Physicians (2004) should be followed. The factors influencing anticoagulant choice (heparin vs. warfarin [Coumadin]) are the same as those for DVT. First-line therapy during pregnancy is adjusted-dose unfractionated heparin or low-molecular-weight heparin. Therapeutic anticoagulation should be continued for at least 4–6 months to prevent recurrence. Vena caval filter use may be necessary should recurrent embolization occur despite anticoagulation.

SEPTIC PELVIC THROMBOPHLEBITIS

ESSENTIALS OF DIAGNOSIS

- Septic pelvic thrombophlebitis is thrombosis in the veins of the pelvis due to infection.
- It is associated with abdominal pain and high fever.
- CT or MRI can confirm the diagnosis.

Pathogenesis

Septic pelvic thrombophlebitis is thrombosis in the veins of the pelvis due to infection. The most important risk factor is caesarean section, especially if complicated by infection. In fact, almost 90% of cases occur after caesarean delivery. The overall incidence is low, affecting only approximately 1 in every 2000 pregnancies.

Pelvic infection leads to infection of the vein wall and intimal damage. Thrombogenesis occurs at the site of intimal damage. The clot is then invaded by microorganisms. Suppuration follows, with liquefaction, fragmentation, and, finally, septic embolization.

Both the uterine and ovarian veins may be involved, as well as the common iliac, hypogastric, and vaginal veins and the inferior vena cava. The ovarian vein is the most common site of septic thrombosis (40% of cases). The onset of symptoms may be as early as 2–3 days postpartum or as late as 6 weeks after delivery.

Clinical Findings

The condition is suspected when fever persists in the puerperium despite adequate antibiotic therapy for aerobic and anaerobic organisms and no other discernible cause of fever. Abdominal pain and back discomfort are common presenting symptoms. A picket-fence fever curve ("hectic" fevers) with wide swings from normal to as high as 41°C (105.8°F) is seen in 90% of cases. Tachycardia and tachypnea may be present. Leukocytosis usually is present. Blood cultures drawn during fever spikes yield positive results more than 35% of the time.

Pelvic examination often is consistent with a normal postpartum examination and therefore not helpful in diagnosing this condition. However, in approximately 30% of cases, hard, tender, wormlike thrombosed veins may be palpable in the vaginal fornices or in 1 or both parametrial areas. A temperature spike may be noted after examination because of disturbance of infected pelvic veins; this may be considered a diagnostic indication of septic pelvic thrombophlebitis. Chest radiograph often reveals evidence of multiple, small septic emboli. CT or MRI may assist in the diagnosis of pelvic vein thrombosis and eliminate other pelvic causes, such as abscess.

Differential Diagnosis

The differential diagnosis includes pyelonephritis, meningitis, systemic lupus erythematosus, tuberculosis, malaria, typhoid, sickle cell crisis, appendicitis, and torsion of the adnexa.

Complications

The serious complications associated with this condition are septic pulmonary emboli, extension of the venous clot in the pelvis, renal vein thrombosis, ureteral obstruction, and death.

Treatment

The mainstays are anticoagulation with heparin and broad-spectrum antibiotics (including coverage for anaerobes and common Enterobacteriaceae). Within 48–72 hours of initiation of heparin therapy, fever should resolve. Treatment usually is empirically continued for 7–10 days, although the optimal duration of therapy is not well defined.

Alfirevic Z, Mousa HA, Martlew V, et al. Postnatal screening for thrombophilia in women with severe pregnancy complications. *Obstet Gynecol* 2001;97:753–759. PMID: 11339929.

American College of Obstetricians and Gynecologists. *Inherited Thrombophilia in Pregnancy. ACOG Practice Bulletin No. 113.* Washington, DC: American College of Obstetricians and Gynecologists; 2010.

American College of Obstetricians and Gynecologists. *Thromboembolism in Pregnancy. ACOG Practice Bulletin No. 19.* Washington, DC: American College of Obstetricians and Gynecologists; 2000.

Aviles A, Neri N. Hematological malignancies and pregnancy: A final report of 84 children who received chemotherapy in utero. *Clin Lymphoma* 2001;2:173–177. PMID: 11779294.

Bates SM, Greer IA, Hirsh J, et al. Use of antithrombotic agents during pregnancy: the Seventh ACCP Conference on Antithrombotic and Thrombolytic Therapy. *Chest* 2004;126 (3 Suppl):627S. PMID: 15383488.

Bazzan M, Donvito V. Low-molecular-weight heparin during pregnancy. *Thromb Res* 2001;101:V175–V186. PMID: 11342097.

Burlingame J, McGaraghan A, Kilpatrick S et al. Maternal and fetal outcomes in pregnancies affected by von Willebrand disease type 2. *Am J Obstet Gynecol* 2001;184:229–230. PMID: 11174508.

Burns MM. Emerging concepts in the diagnosis and management of venous thromboembolism during pregnancy. *J Thromb Thrombolysis* 2000;10:59–68. PMID: 10947915.

Burrows RF. Platelet disorders in pregnancy. *Curr Opin Obstet Gynecol* 2001;13:115–119. PMID: 11315863.

Choi JW, Pai SH. Change in erythropoiesis with gestational age during pregnancy. *Ann Hematol* 2001;80:26–31. PMID: 11233772.

Gerhardt A, Scharf RE, Beckmann MW, et al. Prothrombin and factor V mutations in women with a history of thrombosis during pregnancy and the puerperium. *N Engl J Med* 2000;342:374–380. PMID: 10666427.

Greer IA. The challenge of thrombophilia in maternal-fetal medicine. *N Engl J Med* 2000;342:424–425. PMID: 10666435.

Haram K, Nilsen ST, Ulvik RJ. Iron supplementation in pregnancy—evidence and controversies. *Acta Obstet Gynecol Scand* 2001;80:683–688. PMID: 11531608.

Murphy M, Wallington TB, Kelsey P, et al; for the British Committee for Standards in Haematology, Blood Transfusion Task Force. Guidelines for the clinical use of red cell transfusions. *Br J Haematol* 2001;113:24–31. PMID: 11328275.

Naylor CS, Steele L, Hsi R, et al. Cefotetan-induced hemolysis associated with antibiotic prophylaxis for cesarean delivery. *Am J Obstet Gynecol* 2000;182:1427–1428. PMID: 10871495.

Nizzi FA Jr, Mues G. Hemorrhagic problems in obstetrics, exclusive of disseminated intravascular coagulation. *Hematol Oncol Clin North Am* 2000;14:1171–1182. PMID: 11005040.

Pejovic T, Schwartz PE. Leukemias. *Clin Obstet Gynecol* 2002;45:866–878. PMID: 12370628.

Rai R, Regan L. Thrombophilia and adverse pregnancy outcome. *Semin Reprod Med* 2000;18:369–377. PMID: 11355796.

Rosenfeld S, Follmann D, Nunez O, et al. Antithymocyte globulin and cyclosporine for severe aplastic anemia: Association between hematologic response and long-term outcome. *JAMA* 2003;289:1130–1135. PMID: 12622583.

Serjeant GR, Loy LL, Crowther M, et al. Outcome of pregnancy in homozygous sickle cell disease. *Obstet Gynecol* 2004;103:1278. PMID: 15172865.

Sermon K, Van Steirteghem A, Liebaers I. Preimplantation genetic diagnosis. *Lancet* 2004;363:1633. PMID: 15145631.

Sloan NL, Jordan E, Winikoff B. Effects of iron supplementation on maternal hematologic status in pregnancy. *Am J Public Health* 2002;92:288. PMID: 11818308.

Spina V, Aleandri V, Morini F. The impact of the factor V Leiden mutation on pregnancy. *Hum Reprod Update* 2000;6:301–306. PMID: 10874575.

Sun PM, Wilburn W, Raynor BD, Jamieson D. Sickle cell disease in pregnancy: twenty years of experience at Grady Memorial Hospital, Atlanta, Georgia. *Am J Obstet Gynecol* 2001;184: 1127–1130. PMID: 11349177.

Tichelli A, Socié G, Marsh J, et al. European Group for Blood and Marrow Transplantation Severe Aplastic Anaemia Working Party. Outcome of pregnancy and disease course among women with aplastic anemia treated with immunosuppression. *Ann Intern Med* 2002;137:164–172. PMID: 12160364.

Xiong X, Buekens P, Alexander S, et al. Anemia during pregnancy and birth outcome: A meta-analysis. *Am J Perinatol* 2000;17:137. PMID: 11012138.

Gynecologic History, Examination, & Diagnostic Procedures

35

Charles Kawada, MD
Drorith Hochner-Celnikier, MD

The gynecologist needs to approach each patient not just as a person requiring medical intervention for a specific presenting problem, but also as one who may have a variety of factors possibly affecting her health. The initial approach to the gynecologic patient and the general diagnostic procedures available for the investigation of gynecologic complaints are presented here. Although other aspects of the general medical examination are left to other texts, concern for the patient's total health and well-being is mandatory.

THE PERIODIC HEALTH SCREENING EXAMINATION

It is now a generally accepted part of the physician's responsibility to advise patients to have periodic medical evaluations. The frequency of visits varies according to the patient's age and specific problem.

The periodic health screening examination helps detect the following ailments of women that are especially amenable to early diagnosis and treatment: diabetes mellitus; urinary tract infection or tumor; hypertension; malnutrition or obesity; thyroid dysfunction or tumor; and breast, abdominal, or pelvic tumor. These conditions can be detected by a review of systems, with specific questions regarding recent abnormalities or any variation in function. Determination of weight, blood pressure, and urinalysis may reveal variations from the previous examination. An examination of the thyroid gland, breasts, abdomen, and pelvis, including a Papanicolaou (Pap) smear, should then be performed. A rectal examination also is advisable, and a conveniently packaged test for occult blood (Hemoccult) is recommended for patients older than 40 years. Patients of an advanced age (>50 years) may undergo blood test for lipid profile, bone density scan, pelvic ultrasound examination, and mammogram.

The physician should be concerned about conditions other than purely somatic ones. Unless a patient's problems require the services of a psychiatrist or some other specialist, the doctor should be prepared to act as a counselor and work with the patient during a mutually agreeable time when it is possible to listen to her problems without being hurried and to give support, counsel, and other kinds of help as required.

HISTORY

To adequately evaluate the gynecologic patient, it is important to establish a rapport during the history taking. The patient needs to tell her story to an interested listener who does not allow body language or facial expressions to imply disinterest or boredom. One should avoid cutting off the patient's story, because doing so may obscure important clues or other problems that may have contributed to the reasons for the visit.

The following outline varies from the routine medical history because, in evaluating the gynecologic patient, the problem often can be clarified if the history is obtained in the following order.

Identifying Information

A. Age

Knowledge of the patient's age sets the tone for the complaint and the approach to the patient. Obviously, the problems and the approach to them vary at different stages in a woman's life (pubescence, adolescence, childbearing years, and premenopausal and postmenopausal years).

B. Last Normal Menstrual Period

The date of onset of the last normal menstrual period (LNMP) is important to define. A missed period, irregularity of periods, erratic bleeding, or other abnormalities may all imply certain events that are more easily diagnosed when the date of onset of the LNMP is established.

C. Gravidity & Parity

The process of taking the patient's obstetric history is detailed in Chapter 6, but the reproductive history should be recorded as part of the gynecologic evaluation. A convenient symbol for recording the reproductive history is a 4-digit code denoting the number of term pregnancies, premature deliveries, abortions, and living children (TPAL) (eg, 2-1-1-3 means 2 term pregnancies, 1 premature delivery, 1 abortion, and 3 living children).

Chief Complaint

The chief complaint usually is best elicited by asking "What kind of problem are you having?" or "How can I help you?" It is important to listen carefully to the way the patient responds to this question and to allow her to fully explain her complaint. The patient should be interrupted only to clarify certain points that may be unclear.

Present Illness

Each of the problems the patient describes must be obtained in detail by questioning regarding what exactly the problem is, where exactly the problem is occurring, the date and time of onset, whether the symptoms are abating or getting worse, the duration of the symptoms when they do occur, and how these symptoms are related to or influence other events in her life. For example, the site, duration, and intensity of pain must be accurately described. Getting a sense of how the pain affects her life often is helpful in evaluating the intensity of pain: "Does the pain prevent you from standing or walking?"

It is important to maintain eye contact with the patient and to listen to every word. Do not rely on a patient's sophistication as a measure of her knowledge of anatomy and medical terminology. It is important for the physician to judiciously adjust the level of terminology according to the patient's knowledge and vocabulary. Communicating with the patient in this manner may help the physician obtain an accurate history and establish rapport.

In addition to physiologic events and the life cycle, symptoms described could be related to starting a new job, the beginning of a new relationship or difficulties in the current relationship, an exercise regimen, new medication, and any emotional changes in the patient's life.

Past History

After the physician is satisfied that all possible information concerning the present illness and the important corollaries has been obtained, the past history should be elicited.

A. Contraception

Continuing with the history, it is important to elicit whether the patient is using or needs some form of contraception. If she is using contraception, her level of satisfaction with her chosen method should be determined. In patients taking oral contraceptives, the history should reflect the agent and dose, whether there is a great variation in the time of day she takes her pill, and any impact of the pill on other physiologic functions. Other forms of hormonal contraceptives, including vaginal rings, dermal patches, and injectable contraceptives, have become available and have their own unique issues. It is extremely important to ask questions during the remainder of the history and to key the physical examination to ascertain whether there are any contraindications to the patient's current form of contraception.

B. Medications & Habits

Any medications, prescribed or otherwise, that are being taken or that were being taken when symptoms first occurred should be described. Particular attention must be directed to use of hormones, steroids, and other compounds likely to influence the reproductive tract. Herbal preparations may not be viewed by the patient as medications, so this question should be specifically asked. In addition to medications, the patient should be questioned concerning her use of street drugs. It must be ascertained whether the patient smokes and, if so, how much and for how long. It is important to ascertain the amount of alcohol ingested, if any. This questioning provides an ideal time to indicate the health risks of various habits.

C. Medical

It is important to discover any history of serious medical and psychiatric illnesses and whether hospitalization was required. Particularly important are illnesses in the major organ systems. It is important to know whether there is a major endocrinopathy in the patient's history. Notable weight gain or loss prior to the onset of the patient's current symptoms should be detailed. Other important details include when she had her last physical examination, including pelvic examination and Pap smear.

D. Surgical

The surgical history includes all operations, the dates performed, and associated postoperative or anesthetic complications.

E. Allergies

Questioning should continue relating any possible allergic reactions to drugs or specific foods. The reaction produced (eg, rash, gastrointestinal upset) must be elicited and the approximate time when it occurred ascertained. Any testing to confirm or deny the observation must be noted. Latex allergy has become more common and severe and should be considered prior to most medical procedures, such as drawing blood samples, pelvic examination, and taking blood pressures.

F. Bleeding & Thrombotic Diatheses

Determining whether or not the patient bleeds excessively in relation to prior surgery or minor trauma is important. A history of easy bruising or of bleeding from the gums while brushing teeth may be useful in this judgment. The patient should be asked whether she or one of her close relatives experienced venous thromboembolism (VTE). A history of VTE may guide the physician as to which treatment to offer. Suspicion of a bleeding or clotting problem indicates the need for further laboratory evaluation.

G. Obstetrics

The obstetric history includes each of the patient's pregnancies listed in chronologic order. The date of birth; sex and weight of the offspring; duration of pregnancy; length of labor; type of delivery; type of anesthesia; and any complications should be included.

H. Gynecologic

The first item in the gynecologic past history is the menstrual history: age at menarche, interval between periods, duration of flow, amount and character of flow, degree of discomfort, and age at menopause. The menstrual history often is an important clue in the diagnosis.

A prior history of sexually transmitted disease (STD) needs to be detailed. Although in the past it was more common to note only gonorrhea and syphilis, it is important to also document exposure to human immunodeficiency virus (HIV), hepatitis, herpesvirus, chlamydia, and papillomavirus. Any treatment or admissions to the hospital for treatment of salpingitis, endometritis, or tubo-ovarian abscess must be carefully documented. Attempts to assess the impact of these processes in relation to ectopic pregnancy, infertility, and type of contraception must be elicited.

Although its significance is less than that of the prior stated diseases, the occurrence of episodes of vaginitis should not be dismissed. Their frequency and the medications used to treat them should be discussed. In the case of such infections, it is important to detail whether or not the episode was pathologic or merely a misinterpreted physiologic circumstance.

I. Sexual

The sexual history should be an integral part of any general gynecologic history. In taking a sexual history, the physician must be nonjudgmental and not embarrassed or critical.

Questions that may be covered include the following. Is she currently sexually active? Is the relationship satisfactory to her and, if not, why not? A question regarding whether the patient is heterosexual or lesbian is important but often difficult to ask because the question may be offensive to some patients. It is important, however, not to assume that a relationship is heterosexual because a lesbian woman will lose all rapport with the physician when the physician is insensitive to such issues.

J. Social

A social history can be an extension of earlier questions pertaining to the marital and sexual history. Knowing the type of work the patient does, the type of educational background, and her community activities may assist in ascertaining the patient's relationship to her entire environment.

The patient's involvement with her own health care should be carefully elicited, including her attention and knowledge concerning diet, health screening examinations, recreation, and the degree of regular physical exercise.

Family History

The patient's family history must include the state of health of immediate relatives (parents, siblings, grandparents, and offspring). In addition to listing these relatives, it is useful in cases where genetic illnesses may be apparent to record a 3-generation pedigree.

The incidence of familial heart disease, hypertensive renal or vascular disease, diabetes mellitus (insulin-dependent or non–insulin-dependent), vascular accidents, and hematologic abnormalities should be ascertained. If the patient has a problem with hirsutism or if she perceives excessive hair growth, it is important to elicit whether anyone in her family has the same distribution of hair growth. Familial history of breast, ovarian, and colon cancers is important to elicit because a close familial history may require additional testing and close follow-up. It is important to relate the time of menopause in the mother or grandmother and to ascertain a history of osteoporosis.

American Cancer Society guidelines for breast cancer screening: update 2003. *CA Cancer J Clin* 2003;53:141–169. PMID: 12809498.

American College of Obstetricians and Gynecologists. Cervical cytology screening. ACOG Practice Bulletin No. 45. *Obstet Gynecol* 2003;102:417.

Marrazzo JM, Stine K. Reproductive health history of lesbians: implications for care. *Am J Obstet Gynecol* 2004;190:1298–1304. PMID: 15167833.

Nustaum MR, Hamilton CD. The proactive sexual health history. *Am Fam Physician* 2002;66:1705–1712. PMID: 12449269.

PHYSICAL EXAMINATION

The physical examination is most useful if it is conducted in an environment that is aesthetically pleasing to the patient. Adequate gowning and draping assist in preventing embarrassment. Often a physician's assistant escorts the patient to the dressing area and gives explicit instructions about what to take off and how to put on her gown and then may assist in draping the patient.

A physician may have a female assistant remain in the examining room to assist when necessary, but whether or not she remains solely as a chaperone depends on local custom and the preference of the patient and the physician. A chaperone is not legally required, but the physician, male or female, must use good judgment, especially during the breast and pelvic examinations. If the patient wants her partner, relative, or a friend to be present, the request should be honored unless, in the physician's judgment, such an arrangement would interfere with the examination or with obtaining an accurate history. It is highly recommended that the physician explain the steps and acts that will be taken, especially during the pelvic examination when the patient might lack a direct eye contact with the physician.

General Examination

If the gynecologist is the primary care physician for the patient, a general physical examination should be performed annually or whenever the situation warrants. A complete examination obviously provides more information, demonstrates the physician's thoroughness, and establishes rapport with the patient.

General Evaluation

A. Vital Signs

As part of every examination—whether for a specific problem, routine annual examination, or a return visit for a previously diagnosed problem—the patient should be weighed and her blood pressure taken. Postmenopausal patients should have their height measured to document any loss of height from osteoporosis and vertebral fractures. Before the patient empties her bladder for the examination, determination should be made as to whether the urine will need to be sent for urinalysis, culture, or pregnancy testing.

The examination of the chest should include visual assessment for any skin lesions and symmetry of movement. Auscultation and percussion of the lungs are important for excluding primary pulmonary problems such as asthma and pneumonia. The examination of the heart includes percussion for size and auscultation for arrhythmias and significant murmurs.

Breast Examination

(See also Chapter 5.)

Breast examination should be a routine part of the physical examination. Breast cancer will occur in 1 in 8 women in the United States during her lifetime. Physicians who treat women should educate patients on the technique of self-examination, because the well-prepared patient is one of the most accurate screening methods for breast disease.

The physical examination provides an ideal time to ascertain the frequency and methodology of breast self-examination. It also is an ideal time to teach the patient how to perform breast self-examination. The patient should be advised to examine herself in the mirror, looking for skin changes or dimpling, and then carefully palpate all quadrants of the breast. Most women prefer to do this with soapy hands while showering or bathing. The examination should be repeated at the same time each month, preferably 1 week after the initiation of the menses, when the breasts are least nodular; postmenopausal women should perform self-examination on the same day each month.

The frequency of mammography or the earlier use of mammography depends on both the individual woman and her family history. Patients with a positive family history of breast cancer should have a mammogram at an earlier age, particularly those whose mother, aunt, or sister developed premenopausal breast cancer. In general, a mammogram should be obtained every 1–2 years from ages 40–50 years and annually thereafter. Ultrasonography now can reliably differentiate solid from cystic lesions; this technique complements but does not supplant mammography. Breast self-examination, physician examination, mammography, and ultrasonography are complementary, and all should be used for the early detection of breast cancer. Annual magnetic resonance imaging (MRI) examination of the breast is indicated only in patients carrying BRCA1/2 mutations or with very strong familial history of breast cancer. However, this examination is complementary to the other techniques for early detection of breast cancer and does not replace them.

The correct technique for breast examination is shown in Figure 35–1. If abnormalities are encountered, a decision should be reached concerning the need for mammography (or other imaging methods) or direct referral to a breast surgeon unless the gynecologist is trained in performing breast biopsies. Skin lesions, particularly eczematous lesions in the area of the nipple, should be closely observed; if they are not easily cured by simple measures, they should be biopsied. An eczematous lesion on the nipple or areola may represent Paget's carcinoma.

Abdominal Examination

The patient should be lying completely supine and relaxed; the knees may be slightly flexed and supported as an aid to relaxation of the abdominal muscles. Inspection should detect irregularity of contour or color. Auscultation should follow inspection but precede palpation because the latter may change the character of intestinal activity. Palpation of the entire abdomen—gently at first, then more firmly as indicated—should detect rigidity, voluntary guarding, masses, and tenderness. If the patient complains of abdominal pain or if unexpected tenderness is elicited, the examiner should ask her to indicate the point of maximal pain or tenderness with 1 finger. Suprapubic palpation is designed to detect uterine, ovarian, or urinary bladder enlargements. A painful area should be left until last for deep palpation; otherwise, the entire abdomen can be guarded voluntarily. As a final part of the abdominal examination, the physician should carefully check for any abnormality of the abdominal organs: liver, gallbladder, spleen, kidneys, and intestines. In some instances, the demonstration of an abnormality of the abdominal muscle reflexes may be diagnostically helpful. Percussion of the abdomen should be performed to identify organ enlargement, tumor, or ascites.

Pelvic Examination

The pelvic examination is a procedure feared by many women, so it must be conducted in such a way as to allay

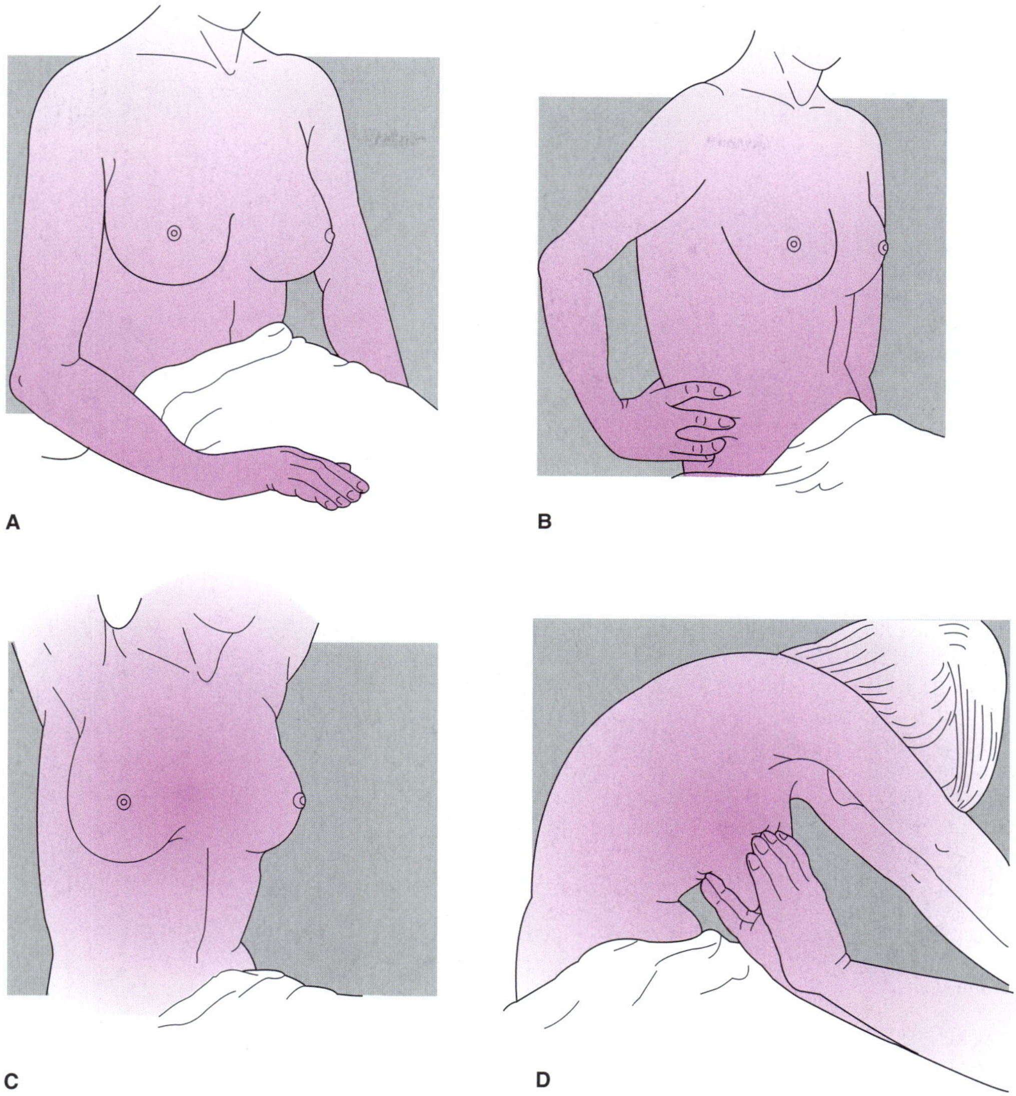

▲ **Figure 35–1.** Breast examination by the physician. **A:** Patient is sitting, arms at sides. Perform visual inspection in good light, looking for lumps or for dimpling or wrinkling of skin. **B:** Patient is sitting, hands pressing on hips so that pectoralis muscles are tensed. Repeat visual inspection. **C:** Patient is sitting, arms above head. Repeat visual inspection of breasts and perform visual inspection of axillae. **D:** Patient is sitting and leaning forward, hands on examiner's shoulders, the stirrups, or her own knees. Perform bimanual palpation, paying particular attention to the base of the glandular portion of the breast.

her anxieties. A patient's first pelvic examination may be especially disturbing, so it is important for the physician to attempt to allay fear and to inspire confidence and cooperation. The empathic physician usually finds that by the time the history has been obtained and a painless and nonembarrassing general examination performed, a satisfactory gynecologic examination is not a problem. Relaxing surroundings; a nurse or attendant chaperone if indicated; warm instruments; and a gentle, unhurried manner with continued explanation and reassurance are helpful in securing patient relaxation and cooperation. This is especially true with the woman who has never before undergone a pelvic examination. In these patients, a 1-finger examination and a narrow speculum often are necessary. In some

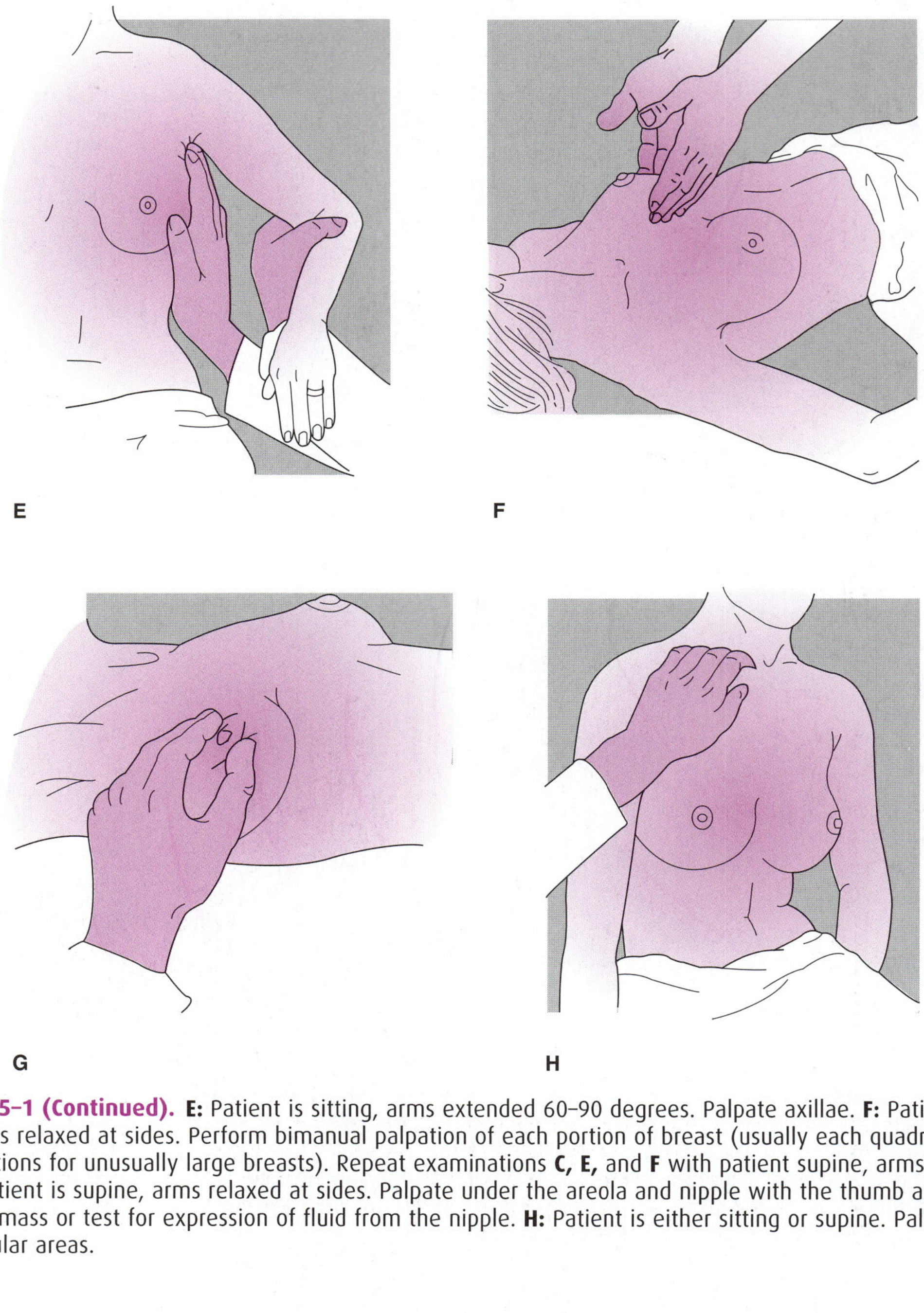

▲ **Figure 35–1 (Continued).** **E:** Patient is sitting, arms extended 60–90 degrees. Palpate axillae. **F:** Patient is supine, arms relaxed at sides. Perform bimanual palpation of each portion of breast (usually each quadrant, but smaller sections for unusually large breasts). Repeat examinations **C, E,** and **F** with patient supine, arms above head. **G:** Patient is supine, arms relaxed at sides. Palpate under the areola and nipple with the thumb and forefinger to detect a mass or test for expression of fluid from the nipple. **H:** Patient is either sitting or supine. Palpate supraclavicular areas.

cases, vaginal examination is not possible; palpation of the pelvic structures by rectal examination is then the only recourse. Occasionally an ultrasound examination may be helpful in ascertaining whether the pelvic organs are normal in size and configuration in patients who cannot adequately relax the abdominal muscles. If a more definitive pelvic examination is essential, it can be performed with the patient anesthetized.

A. External Genitalia (Fig. 35–2)

The pubic hair should be inspected for its pattern (masculine or feminine), for the nits of pubic lice, for infected hair

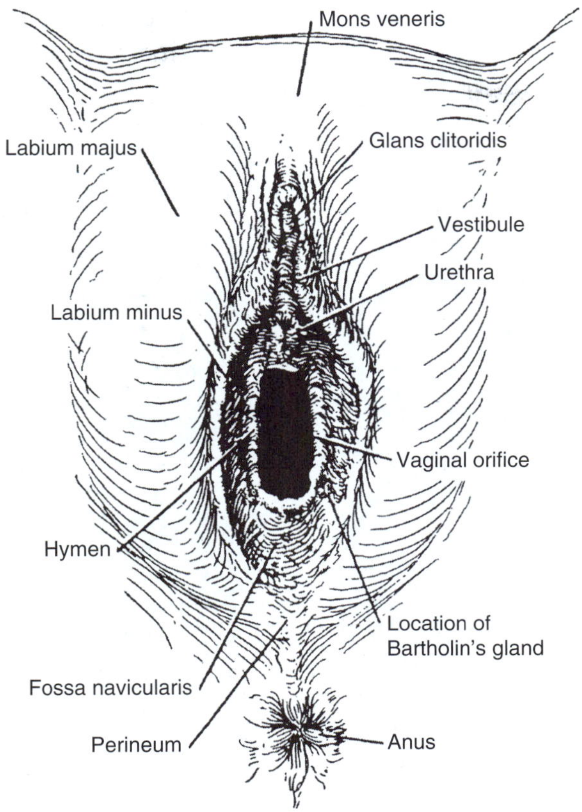

▲ **Figure 35–2.** Normal external genitalia in a mature woman. (Reproduced, with permission, from Pernoll ML. *Benson & Pernoll's Handbook of Obstetrics and Gynecology*. 10th ed. New York, NY: McGraw-Hill; 2001.)

follicles, and for any other abnormalities. The skin of the vulva, mons pubis, and perineal area should be examined for evidence of dermatitis or discoloration. The glans clitoridis can be exposed by gently retracting the surrounding skin folds. The clitoris is at the ventral confluence of the 2 labia; it should be no more than 2.5 cm in length, most of which is subcutaneous. The major and minor labia usually are the same size on both sides, but a moderate difference in size is not abnormal. Small protuberances or subcutaneous nodules may be either sebaceous cysts or tumors. External condylomata are often found in this area. The urethra, just below the clitoris, should be the same color as the surrounding tissue and without protuberances. Normally, vestibular (Bartholin's) glands can be neither seen nor felt, so enlargement may indicate an abnormality of this gland system. The area of vestibular glands should be palpated by placing the index finger in the vagina and the thumb outside and gently feeling for enlargement or tenderness (Fig. 35–3). The perineal skin may be reddened as a result of vulvar or vaginal infection. Scars may indicate obstetric lacerations or surgery. The anus should be inspected at this time for the presence of hemorrhoids, fissures, irritation, or perianal infections (eg, condylomata or herpesvirus lesions).

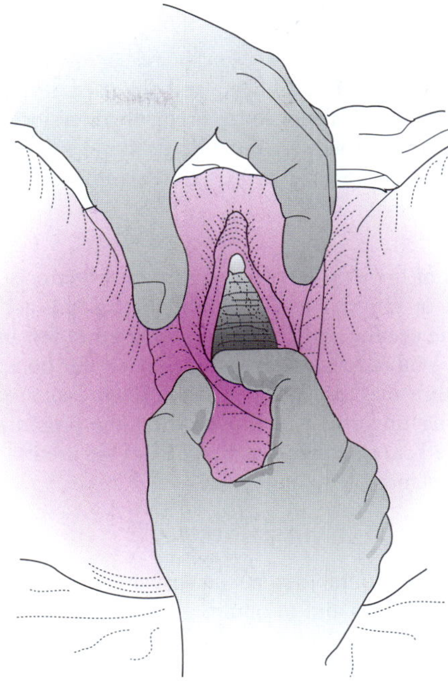

▲ **Figure 35–3.** Palpation of vestibular glands.

B. Hymen

An unruptured hymen may present in many forms, but only a completely imperforate, cribriform, or septate hymen is pathologic. After rupture, the hymen may be seen in various forms (Fig. 35–4). After the birth of several children, the hymen may disappear almost completely.

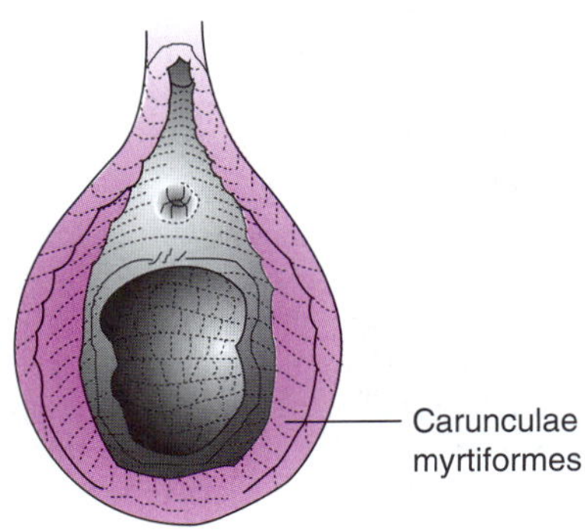

▲ **Figure 35–4.** Ruptured hymen (parous introitus).

C. Perineal Support

To determine the presence of pelvic relaxation, the physician spreads the labia with 2 fingers and tells the patient to "bear down." This will demonstrate urethrocele, cystocele, rectocele, or uterine prolapse, although sometimes an upright position may be necessary to demonstrate significant prolapse.

D. Urethra

Redness of the urethra may indicate infection or a urethral caruncle or carcinoma. The paraurethral glands are situated below the urethra and empty into the urethra just inside the meatus. With the labia spread adequately for better vision, the urethra may be "stripped" (ie, pressure exerted by the examining finger as it is moved from the proximal to the distal urethra) to express discharge from the urethra or paraurethral glands.

Vaginal Examination

The vagina should first be inspected with the speculum for abnormalities and to obtain a Pap smear before further examination. A speculum dampened with warm water but not lubricated is gently inserted into the vagina so that the cervix and fornices can be thoroughly visualized (Fig. 35–5). The cervix should be inspected for discharge, color, erosion, and other lesions. At that time, any discharge can be obtained for test of microbiology, virology, or microscopy and a Pap smear performed. After the Pap smear is prepared, the vaginal wall is again carefully inspected as the speculum is withdrawn (Fig. 35–6). The type of speculum used depends on the preference of the physician, but the most satisfactory instrument for the sexually active patient is the Pederson speculum, although the wider Graves speculum may be necessary to afford adequate visualization (Fig. 35–7). For the patient with a small introitus, the narrow-bladed Pederson speculum is preferable. When more than the usual exposure is necessary, an extra large Graves speculum is available. To visualize a child's vagina, a Huffman or nasal speculum, a large otoscope, or a Kelly air cystoscope is invaluable.

Next, the vagina is palpated; unless the patient's introitus is too small, the index and middle fingers of either hand are inserted gently and the tissues palpated. The vaginal walls should be smooth, elastic, and nontender.

Bimanual Examination

The uterus and adnexal structures should be outlined between the 2 fingers of the hand in the vagina and the flat of the opposite hand, which is placed on the lower abdominal wall (Fig. 35–8). Gentle palpation and manipulation of the structures will delineate position, size, shape, mobility, consistency, and tenderness of the pelvic structures—except in the obese or uncooperative patient or in a patient whose abdominal muscles are taut as a result of fear or tenderness. Tenderness can be elicited either on direct palpation or on movement or stretching of the pelvic structures.

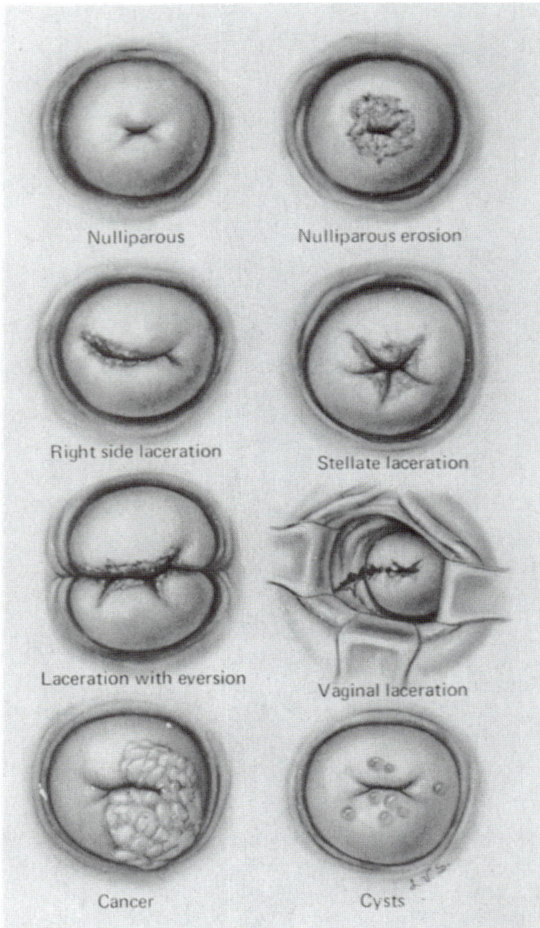

▲ **Figure 35–5.** Uterine cervix: normal and pathologic appearance.

A. Cervix

The cervix is a firm structure traditionally described as having the consistency of the tip of the nose. Normally it is round and approximately 3–4 cm in diameter. Various appearances of the cervix are shown in Figure 35–5. The external os is round and virtually closed. Multiparous women may have an os that has been lacerated. An irregularity in shape or nodularity may be due to 1 or more nabothian cysts. If the cervix is extremely firm, it may contain a tumor, even cancer. The cervix (along with the body of the uterus) normally is moderately mobile, so it can be moved 2–4 cm in any direction without causing undue discomfort. (When examining a patient, it is helpful to warn her that she will feel the movement of her uterus but that ordinarily this maneuver is not painful.) Restricted mobility of the cervix or corpus often follows inflammation, neoplasia, or surgery.

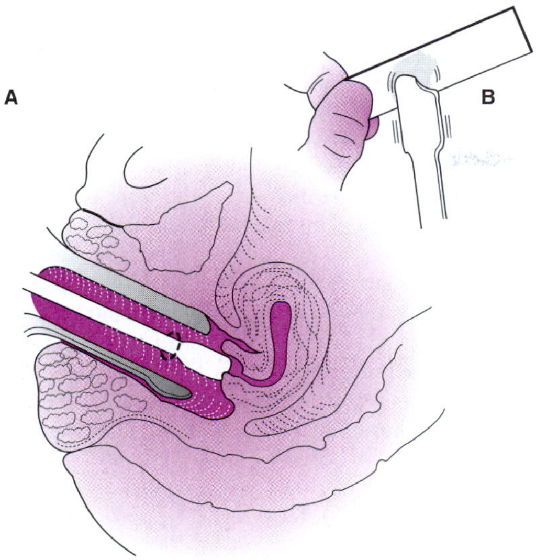

▲ **Figure 35–6.** Preparation of a Papanicolaou (Pap) smear. **A:** Obtain cervical scraping from complete squamocolumnar junction by rotating 360 degrees around the external os. **B:** Place the material 1 in from the end of the slide and smear along the slide to obtain a thin preparation. Place a saline-soaked cotton swab or small endocervical brush into the endocervical canal and rotate 360 degrees. Place this specimen onto the same slide and quickly fix with fixative. (Reproduced, with permission, from Pernoll ML. *Benson & Pernoll's Handbook of Obstetrics and Gynecology*. 10th ed. New York, NY: McGraw-Hill; 2001.)

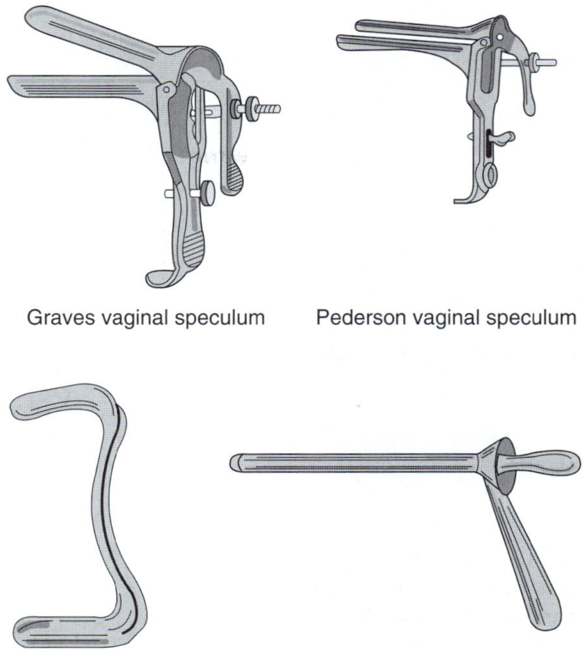

▲ **Figure 35–7.** Specula. (Reproduced, with permission, from Pernoll ML. *Benson & Pernoll's Handbook of Obstetrics and Gynecology*. 10th ed. New York, NY: McGraw-Hill; 2001.)

B. Corpus of the Uterus

The corpus of the uterus is approximately half the size of the patient's fist and weighs approximately 70–90 g. It is regular in outline and not tender to pressure or moderate motion. In most women, the uterus is anteverted; in approximately one-third of women, it is retroverted (see Chapter 42). A retroverted uterus usually is not a pathologic finding. In certain cases of endometriosis or previous salpingitis, the "tipped" uterus may be the result of adhesions caused by the disease process. The uterus usually is described in terms of its size, shape, position, consistency, and mobility.

C. Adnexa

Adnexal structures (fallopian tubes and ovaries) cannot be palpated in many overweight women because the normal tube is only approximately 7 mm in diameter and the ovary is no more than 3 cm in its greatest dimension. In very slender women, however, the ovaries nearly always are palpable and, in some instances, the oviducts are as well. Usually no adnexal structures can be palpated in the postmenopausal woman. Unusual tenderness or enlargement of any adnexal structure indicates the need for further diagnostic procedures; an adnexal mass in any woman is an indication for investigation.

Rectovaginal Examination

At the completion of the bimanual pelvic examination, a rectovaginal examination should always be performed especially after age 40 years. The well-lubricated middle finger of the examining hand should be inserted gently into the rectum to feel for tenderness, masses, or irregularities. When the examining finger has been inserted a short distance, the index finger can then be inserted into the vagina until the depth of the vagina is reached (Fig. 35–9). It is much easier to examine some aspects of the posterior portion of the pelvis by rectovaginal

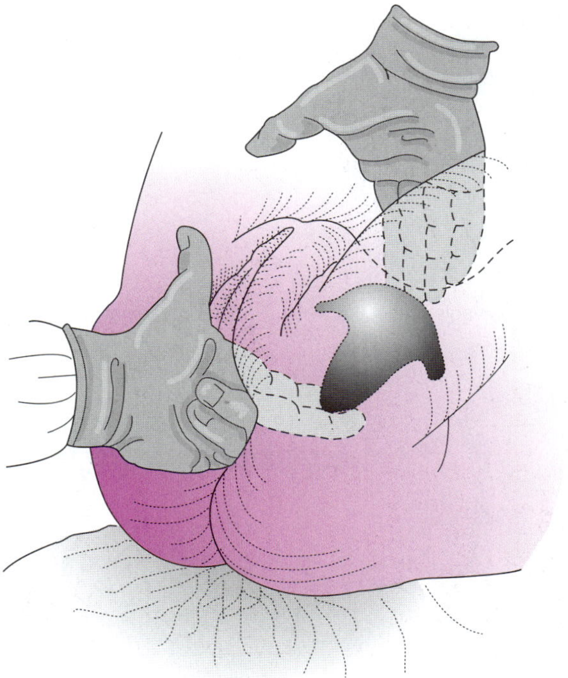

▲ **Figure 35–8.** Bimanual pelvic examination.

examination than by vaginal examination alone. The index finger can now raise the cervix toward the anterior abdominal wall, which stretches the uterosacral ligaments. Usually this process is not painful; if it causes pain—and especially if the finger in the rectum can palpate tender nodules along the uterosacral ligaments—endometriosis may be present.

Occult Bleeding Due to Colorectal Cancer

In the United States, colorectal cancer (CRC) is the third most common cancer diagnosed among men and women and the second leading cause of death from cancer. CRC largely can be prevented by the detection and removal of adenomatous polyps, and survival is significantly better when CRC is diagnosed while still localized. Recent evidence has revealed an unacceptably wide range of sensitivity among strategies aimed at checking the feces for occult blood, with some practices and tests performing so poorly that the large majority of prevalent cancers are missed at the time of screening. Therefore, a single stool sample for fecal occult blood testing obtained by digital rectal examination is not adequate for the detection of CRC and should not be used for CRC screening. Furthermore, it is the physician's role to encourage patients above 50 years of age or those with familial CRC to undergo procedures aimed at prevention of CRC (such as colonoscopy, sigmoidoscopy, or computed tomography [CT] scan) and to not diagnose CRC using methods detecting occult blood in the stool.

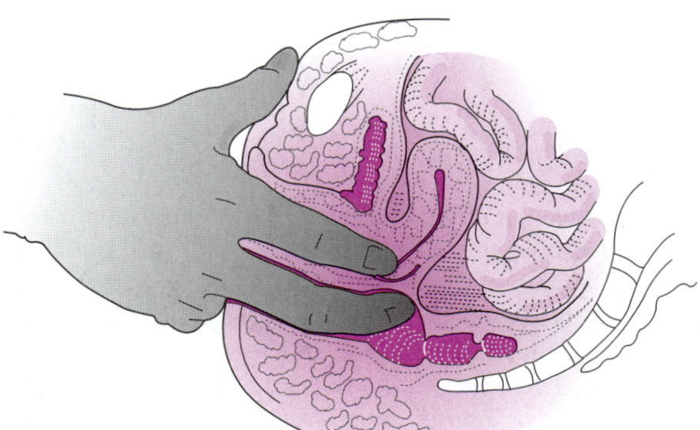

▲ **Figure 35–9.** Rectovaginal examination.

American College of Obstetricians and Gynecologists. *Routine Pelvic Examination and Cervical Cytology Screening. ACOG Committee Opinion No 431*. Washington, DC: American College of Obstetricians and Gynecologists; 2009.

Levin B, Lieberman DA, McFarland B, et al. Screening and surveillance for the early detection of colorectal cancer and adenomatous polyps, 2008. *CA Cancer J Clin* 2008;58:130–160. PMID: 18322143.

DIAGNOSTIC OFFICE PROCEDURES

Certain diagnostic procedures can be performed in the office because complicated equipment and general anesthesia are not required. Other office diagnostic procedures useful in specific situations (eg, tests used in infertility evaluation) can be found in appropriate chapters elsewhere in this book.

Tests for Vaginal Infection

If abnormal vaginal discharge is present, a sample of vaginal discharge should be scrutinized. A culture is obtained by applying a sterile cotton-tipped applicator to the suspect area and then transferring the suspect material to an appropriate culture medium. Because this procedure is inconvenient to perform in the physician's office, most laboratories supply a prepackaged kit that allows the physician to put the cotton-tipped applicator into a sterile container, which is then sent to the laboratory. The vaginal discharge can also be tested for the vaginal pH. An acidic pH of 4–5 is consistent with fungal infection, whereas an alkaline pH of 5.5–7 suggests infections such as bacterial vaginosis and *Trichomonas*. Often an endocervical infection may be perceived as a vaginal infection. Obtaining a swab for gonorrhea and chlamydia testing from the endocervix is warranted.

A. Saline (Plain Slide)

To demonstrate *Trichomonas vaginalis* organisms, the physician mixes on a slide 1 drop of vaginal discharge with 1 drop of normal saline warmed to approximately body temperature. The slide should have a coverslip. If the smear is examined while it is still warm, actively motile trichomonads usually can be seen.

The saline slide can also be used to look for the mycelia of the fungus *Candida albicans*, which appear as segmented and branching filaments. The slide can be useful in looking for bacterial vaginosis by looking for "clue cells," epithelial cells covered from edge to edge by short coccobacilli-type bacteria.

B. Potassium Hydroxide

One drop of an aqueous 10% potassium hydroxide solution is mixed with 1 drop of vaginal discharge on a clean slide and a coverslip applied. The potassium hydroxide dissolves epithelial cells and debris and facilitates visualization of the mycelia of a fungus causing vaginal infection. The slide can be brought near the nose to determine if the discharge has a "fishy" odor. This odor is strongly suggestive of bacterial vaginosis, a common vaginal infection associated with a mixed anaerobic bacterial flora. In addition, this same slide with a coverslip can be magnified with a microscope to visualize mycelia that may have been hidden by debris with just the saline smear.

C. Bacterial Infection

Bacterial infection may be present, especially if there is an ischemic lesion such as occurs after radiation therapy for cervical carcinoma, or if a patient is suspected of having bacterial vaginosis, gonorrhea, or a *Chlamydia trachomatis* infection. Material from the cervix, urethra, or vaginal lesion can be smeared, stained, and examined microscopically, or the material can be cultured.

Fern Test for Ovulation

The fern test can determine the presence or absence of ovulation or the time of ovulation. When cervical mucus is spread on a clean, dry slide and allowed to dry in air, it may or may not assume a frondlike pattern when viewed under the microscope (sometimes it can be seen grossly). The fern frond pattern indicates an estrogenic effect on the mucus without the influence of progesterone; thus, a non-frondlike pattern can be interpreted as showing that ovulation has occurred (Fig. 35–10).

Schiller Test for Neoplasia

Although colposcopy is more accurate, the Schiller test can be performed when cancer or precancerous changes of the cervix or vaginal mucosa are suspected. The suspect area is painted with Lugol's (strong iodine) solution, which interacts and marks the glycogen-rich epithelial cells of the cervix. Any portion of the epithelium that does not accept the dye is abnormal because of the presence of scar tissue,

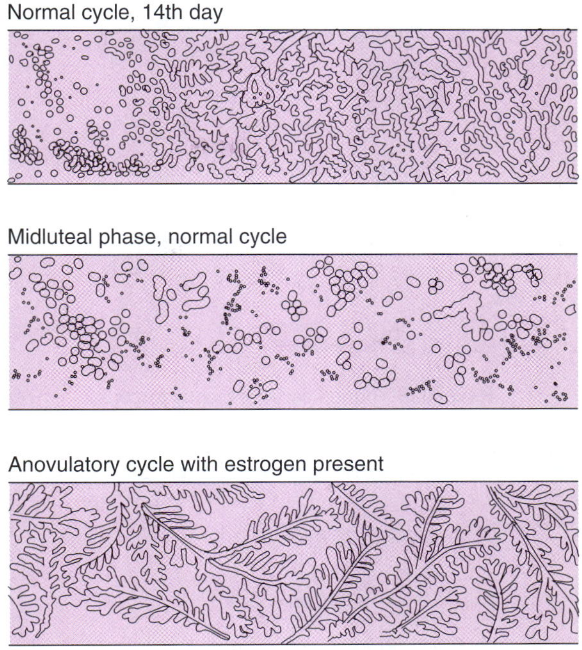

▲ **Figure 35–10.** Patterns formed when cervical mucus is smeared on a slide, permitted to dry, and examined under a microscope. Progesterone makes the mucus thick and cellular. In the smear from a patient who failed to ovulate (**bottom**), there is no progesterone to inhibit the estrogen-induced fern pattern. (Reproduced, with permission, from Ganong WF. *Review of Medical Physiology*. 20th ed. New York, NY: McGraw-Hill; 2003.)

neoplasia and precursors, and columnar epithelium. Biopsy of samples taken from this area should be performed if there is any suspicion of cancer.

Biopsy

A. Vulva & Vagina

For biopsy of the vulva or vagina, a 1–2% aqueous solution of a standard local anesthetic solution can be injected around a small suspicious area and a sample obtained with a skin punch or sharp scalpel. Bleeding usually can be controlled by pressure or by Monsel's solution, but occasionally suturing is necessary.

B. Cervix

Colposcopically directed biopsy is the method of choice for the diagnosis of cervical lesions, either suspected on visualization or indicated after an abnormal Pap smear. Colposcopy should reveal the full columnar–squamous "transformation zone" (TZ) at the juncture of the exocervix and endocervix. In addition, it may be advisable to sample the endocervix by curettage. Specific instruments have been devised for cervical biopsy and endocervical curettage (Fig. 35–11). The cervix is

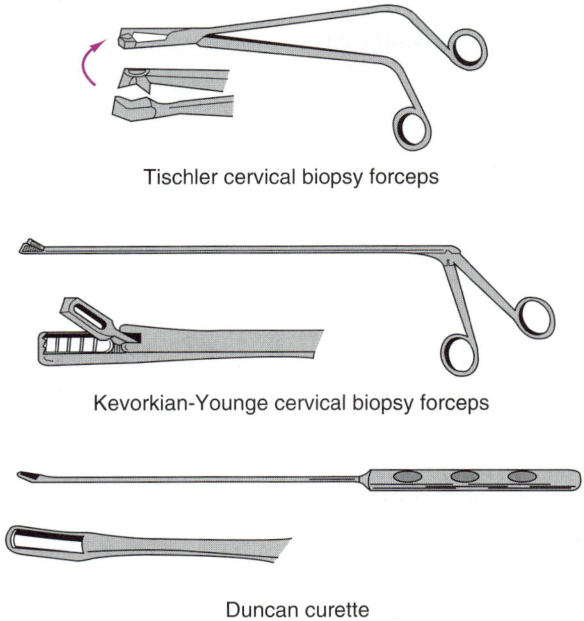

▲ **Figure 35–11.** Biopsy instruments.

less sensitive to cutting procedures than is the vagina, so 1 or more small biopsy samples of the cervix can be taken with no or little discomfort to the patient. Bleeding usually is minimal and controlled with light pressure for a few minutes or by use of Monsel's solution. A "4-quadrant" biopsy sample of the squamocolumnar junction can be taken at 12, 3, 6, and 9 o'clock positions if colposcopy is not available. A Schiller test often may more quickly direct the physician to the area that should be biopsied.

C. Endometrium

Endometrial biopsy can be helpful in the diagnosis of ovarian dysfunction (eg, infertility) or irregular uterine bleeding and as a test for carcinoma of the uterine corpus. Endometrial biopsy can be performed with flexible disposable cannulas, such as the Pipelle, which have replaced most metal curettes previously used (Fig. 35–12). In fact, endometrial biopsies have dramatically reduced the need for formal dilatation and curettage (D&C) because the accuracy of biopsy is nearly the same. Because the procedure causes cramping, the patient should be warned and advised to take a pain medication such as ibuprofen 1 hour prior to the procedure.

DIAGNOSTIC LABORATORY PROCEDURES

Routine procedures that are not discussed here but should be considered with periodic primary care visits include a complete blood count (including differential white cell count), glucose screening, lipid profile, and thyroid function tests. The frequency with which these tests are performed should

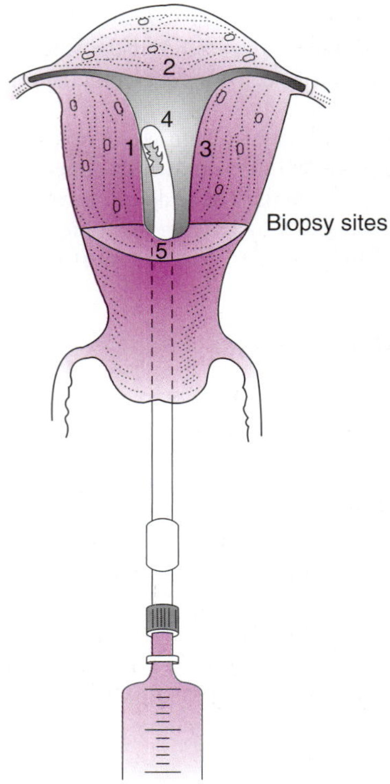

▲ **Figure 35–12.** Sites of endometrial biopsy. (Reproduced, with permission, from Pernoll ML. *Benson & Pernoll's Handbook of Obstetrics and Gynecology*. 10th ed. New York, NY: McGraw-Hill; 2001.)

be at the discretion of the physician, based on risk factors and presenting complaints.

Urinalysis

Urinalysis should be obtained in symptomatic patients and should include both gross and microscopic examinations. A microscopic examination may reveal crystals or bacteria, but unless the specimen is collected in a manner that will exclude vaginal discharge, the presence of bacteria is meaningless (see below).

Urine Culture

Studies have demonstrated that a significant number of women (approximately 3% of nonpregnant women and 7% of pregnant women) have asymptomatic urinary tract infections. Culture and antibiotic sensitivity testing are required for the diagnosis and as a guide to treatment of urinary tract infections.

Reliable specimens of urine for culture often can be obtained by the "clean-catch" method: The patient is instructed to cleanse the urethral meatus carefully with soap and water, to urinate for a few seconds to dispose of urethral contaminants, and then to catch a "midstream" portion of the urine. It is essential that the urine not dribble over the labia, but this may be difficult for some patients to accomplish.

A more reliable method of collecting urine for culture is by sterile catheterization performed by the physician or nurse. However, care must be exercised in catheterization to minimize the risk of introducing an infection.

Other Cultures

A. Urethral

Urethral cultures are indicated if an STD is suspected.

B. Vaginal

A culture usually is unnecessary for the diagnosis of vaginal infections, because visual inspection or microscopic examination usually will enable the physician to make a diagnosis, eg, curdlike vaginal material that reveals mycelia (candidiasis). However, a culture should be obtained in questionable cases. In cases of vaginal candidiasis refractory to the common treatment, it is advisable to characterize the yeast and examine its specific sensitivity to various antimycotic drugs available, enabling elimination of the troublesome infection.

C. Cervical

As in the case of the urethra, the usual indication for a culture of cervical discharge is the suspected presence of an STD.

Specific Tests

A. Herpesvirus Hominis

Herpesvirus hominis (HSV) (herpes genitalis, both types 1 and 2) is a frequently seen vulvar lesion (see Chapter 43). It can be diagnosed by the cytopathologist, who finds typical cellular changes. Other methods that are more accurate and more often used for the detection of HSV infection include culturing and identifying the virus using polymerase chain reaction (PCR) technique.

B. Human Papillomavirus

Human papillomavirus (HPV) infection is associated with the development of genital warts and the occurrence of vaginal and cervical intraepithelial lesions. Some of these lesions are precancerous or cancerous in origin. Different HPV subtypes are linked to either benign or more aggressive epithelial changes. The different subtypes can be identified by the specific fingerprints obtained from the PCR products.

C. Chlamydia & Gonorrheal Infections

These sexually transmitted infections are the 2 most prevalent infections, with chlamydia being the most common. They are found more often in women who have multiple sexual partners and those who do not use barrier methods of contraception. Nucleic acid amplification testing is the most commonly used method of diagnosis, with a sensitivity >90%.

D. Human Immunodeficiency Virus

Acquired immunodeficiency syndrome (AIDS) has become one of the most difficult issues confronting all kinds of clinicians. The need to screen for HIV in the general population has become more pressing given that the largest increase in incidence is seen in young heterosexually active females with no other risk factors. An accurate blood test is available for diagnosis. Prior to drawing the blood, the physician must discuss with the patient the accuracy of the blood test for diagnosing the presence of HIV. The patient must be made aware that there are infrequent false-positive tests and a "window" during which the test may be falsely negative prior to the development of antibodies. At present, a written consent must be signed by the patient prior to drawing the blood.

Other Specific Tests

Specific diagnostic laboratory procedures may be indicated for some of the less common venereal diseases (eg, lymphogranuloma venereum and hepatitis B and C). A screening test for *Streptococcus* B carrier is advocated at 35–37 weeks' gestation. A 1-step culture swab from the lower vagina, followed by the anus, is recommended. These tests are discussed with the specific diseases in other chapters of this book.

Pregnancy Testing

Pregnancy testing is discussed in Chapter 6.

Papanicolaou Smear of Cervix

The Pap smear is an important part of the gynecologic examination. The frequency of the need for this test has been recently revised. Epidemiologic statistics have led the US Preventive Services Task Force to recommend that for the average woman who has had 3 normal Pap smears, a Pap test every 2 or 3 years is adequate. This recommendation is based on the observation that most cervical cancers are slow growing. The American College of Obstetricians and Gynecologists recommends annual Pap smear screenings from 3 years after the start of sexual intercourse but no later than age 21 years. For women aged 30–64 years, the frequency of screening may be reduced to every 2–3 years after 3 consecutive negative Pap smears. Patients at risk, including women with multiple sexual partners, a history of STD, genital condylomata, or prior abnormal Pap smears; women who are receiving immune suppression therapy; women who are infected with HIV; or women who were exposed to diethylstilbestrol (DES) in utero, should continue to be screened annually. Women who are HIV positive should have cervical cytology testing every 6 months after diagnosis, and then annually after 2 consecutive normal test results. HPV vaccination status does not change theses cervical cytology screening recommendations. The physician can consider discontinuing cervical cytology at 65–70 years of age if patient has had 3 or more normal results in a row, no abnormal test results in 10 years, no history of cervical cancer, and no history of DES exposure in utero, is HIV negative, is not immunodepressed, and does not have other risk factors for new acquisition of STDs; if cervical cytology has been discontinued, the physician should review risk factors annually to evaluate the need for re-initiation of screening.

Aside from premalignant and malignant changes, other local conditions often can be suspected by the cytologist. Viral infections, such as HSV, HPV, and condylomata acuminata, can be seen as mucosal changes. Actinomycosis and *Trichomonas* infections can be detected by a Pap smear.

The Pap smear is a screening test only. Positive tests are an indication for further diagnostic procedures, such as colposcopy, endocervical curettage, cervical biopsy or conization, endometrial biopsy, or D&C. The properly collected Pap smear can accurately lead to the diagnosis of carcinoma of the cervix in approximately 95% of cases. The Pap smear also is helpful in the detection of endometrial abnormalities such as endometrial polyps, hyperplasia, and cancers, but it detects fewer than 50% of cases.

The techniques of collection of a Pap smear may vary, but the following is a common procedure.

The patient should not have douched for at least 24 hours before the examination and should not be menstruating. The speculum is placed in the vagina after it has been lubricated with water only. With the cervix exposed, a specially designed plastic or wooden spatula is applied to the cervix and rotated 360 degrees to abrade the surface slightly and to pick up cells from the squamocolumnar area of the cervical os. Next, a cotton-tipped applicator or a small brush is inserted into the endocervix and rotated 360 degrees. These 2 specimens can be mixed or placed on the slide separately according to the preference of the examiner. A preservative is applied immediately to prevent air drying, which would compromise the interpretation. The slide is sent to the laboratory with an identification sheet containing pertinent history and findings (see Fig. 35–6). Another method called ThinPrep automates the preparation of the Pap smear slide so that the variability introduced by the clinician preparing the slide itself is no longer a factor. With this method, the specimen is placed in a liquid-based medium and sent to the laboratory. In addition, the ThinPrep technique decreases the rate of smears showing atypical squamous cells–undetermined significance (ASCUS), thereby decreasing the need for colposcopic evaluations. For these reasons, in many parts of the country, the ThinPrep technique has replaced the conventional Pap smear. However, any advantages of the liquid-based technique over the conventional method in terms of sensitivity and specificity are unclear

The liquid-based medium allows for testing for high-risk HPV, the most common being subtypes 16, 18, 31, 33, and 35. Testing for high-risk HPV has been proposed by the American Society for Colposcopy and Cervical Pathology as a method of evaluating and sorting out patients with ASCUS Pap smear results. If no high-risk HPV is present in the ASCUS Pap smear, then these individuals can be followed-up with a repeat Pap smear in 1 year, similar to those who have a negative Pap smear. Patients known to have a high-risk HPV subtype would undergo colposcopic evaluation.

The laboratory reports the Pap smear using the Bethesda System, which has advocated a standardized reporting system for cytologic reports. Chapter 48 discusses the recently updated nomenclature.

Alternatives to the traditional Pap smear are being evaluated in an attempt to decrease the false-negative and false-positive Pap smear results. Evidence indicates that computerized screening of Pap smears can decrease the likelihood of missing significant pathologies. Various methods of computerized screening have been developed to aid the human eye in picking up abnormalities, although no system has yet achieved widespread acceptance.

Colposcopy

The colposcope is a binocular microscope used for direct visualization of the cervix (Fig. 35–13). Magnification as high as 60× is available, but the most popular instrument in clinical use has 13.5× magnification, which effectively bridges the gap between what can be seen by the naked eye and by the microscope. Some colposcopes are equipped with a camera for single or serial photographic recording of pathologic conditions.

Colposcopy does not replace other methods of diagnosing abnormalities of the cervix; rather, it is an additional and important tool. The 2 most important groups of patients who can benefit by its use are (1) patients with an abnormal Pap smear and (2) DES-exposed daughters, who may have dysplasia of the vagina or cervix (see Chapter 40).

The colposcopist is able to see areas of cellular dysplasia and vascular or tissue abnormalities not visible otherwise, which makes possible the selection of areas most propitious for biopsy. Stains and other chemical agents are also used to improve visualization. The colposcope has reduced the need to perform blind cervical biopsies for which the rate of finding abnormalities is low. In addition, the necessity for a cone biopsy, a procedure with a high morbidity rate, has been greatly reduced. Thus the experienced colposcopist is able to find focal cervical lesions, obtain directed biopsy at the most appropriate sites, and make decisions about the most appropriate therapy largely based on what is seen through the colposcope.

Hysteroscopy

Hysteroscopy enables the gynecologist to examine the uterine cavity through a fiberoptic instrument, called the hysteroscope.

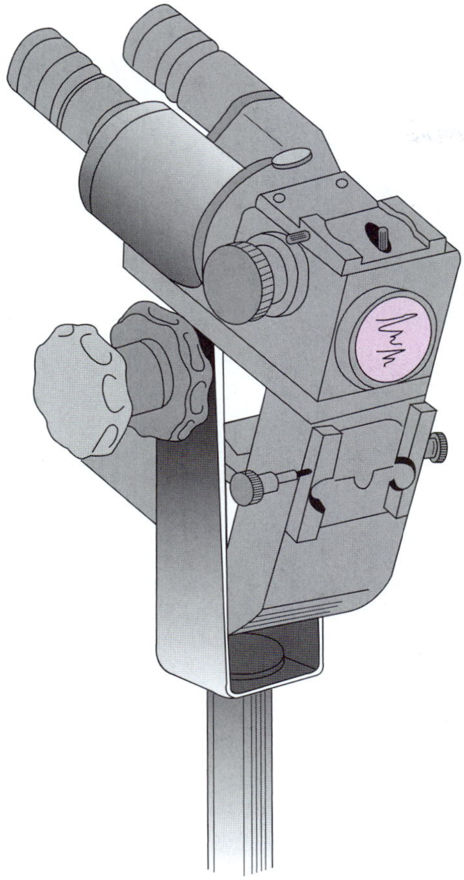

▲ **Figure 35–13.** Zeiss colposcope.

Moreover, surgical interventions such as polypectomy, myomectomy, septectomy, and resection of intrauterine adhesions can be performed via the hysteroscope. In order to inspect the interior of the uterus with the hysteroscope, the uterine cavity is inflated with a solution (usually saline, but other solutions such as glycine or dextran can be used) or by carbon dioxide insufflation. Diagnostic hysteroscopy is usually performed with no sedation; however, intravenous sedation, paracervical block, or general anesthesia is often adequate for operative hysteroscopies.

Hysteroscopic applications include evaluation for abnormal uterine bleeding, resection of uterine synechiae and septa, removal of polyps and intrauterine devices (IUDs), resection of submucous myomas, and endometrial ablation. Most of these therapeutic maneuvers require extensive manipulation, so regional or general anesthesia is required.

Hysteroscopy should be performed only by physicians with proper training. The tip of the instrument should be inserted just beyond the internal cervical os and then advanced slowly, with adequate distention under direct vision. Hysteroscopy is often used in conjunction with other operative procedures, such as curettage and laparoscopy.

Failure of hysteroscopy may be the result of cervical stenosis, inadequate distention of the uterine cavity, bleeding, or excessive mucus secretion. The most common complications include perforation, bleeding, and infection. Perforation of the uterus usually occurs at the fundus. Unless a viscus is damaged or internal bleeding develops, surgical repair may not be required. Bleeding generally subsides, but fulguration following attempts to remove polyps or myomas may be required to stop bleeding in some cases. Parametritis or salpingitis, rarely noted, usually necessitates antibiotic therapy. Intravascular extravasation of fluid or gas from hysteroscopy often does not become clinically significant but has been associated with severe consequences such as hyponatremia, air embolism, cerebral edema, and even death.

Culdocentesis

The passage of a needle into the cul-de-sac—culdocentesis—in order to obtain fluid from the pouch of Douglas is a diagnostic procedure that can be performed in the office or in a hospital treatment room (Fig. 35–14). The type of fluid obtained indicates the type of intraperitoneal lesion (eg, bloody with a ruptured ectopic pregnancy, pus with acute salpingitis, or ascitic fluid with malignant cells in cancer). With refinements in ultrasound technology enabling more definitive evaluation of pelvic pathology, culdocentesis is performed rarely today.

Radiographic Diagnostic Procedures

Many common radiologic procedures may be helpful in the diagnosis of pelvic conditions. The "flat film" shows calcified lesions, teeth, or a ring of a dermoid cyst and indicates other pelvic masses by shadows or displaced intestinal loops. Use of contrast media frequently is indicated to help delineate pelvic masses or to rule out metastatic lesions. Barium enema, upper gastrointestinal series, intravenous urogram, and cystogram may be helpful. With the improvement of technologies such as ultrasound, CT scans, and MRI, the use of "flat films" for the diagnosis of gynecologic abnormalities has become less frequent.

Hysterography & Sonohysterography

The uterine cavity and the lumens of the oviducts can be outlined by instillation of contrast medium through the cervix, followed by fluoroscopic observations or film. The technique was first widely used for the diagnosis of tubal disease as part of the investigation of infertile women. Its use now is being extended to the investigation of uterine disease.

To diagnose tubal patency or occlusion, the medium is instilled through a cervical cannula. Filling of the uterine cavity and spreading of the medium through the tubes are watched via a fluoroscope, with the radiologist taking spot films at intervals for subsequent, more definitive, scrutiny.

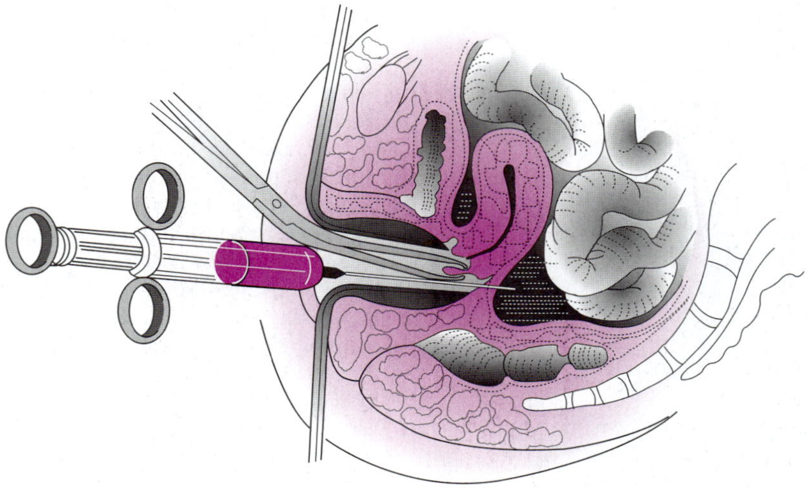

▲ **Figure 35–14.** Culdocentesis.

If no occlusion is present, the medium will reach the fimbriated end of the tube and spill into the pelvis—evidence of tubal patency. This procedure can reveal an abnormality of the uterus (eg, congenital malformation, submucous myomas, or endometrial polyps).

Another technique that is gaining acceptance is sonohysterography, in which the uterine cavity is filled with fluid while ultrasound is used to delineate the architecture of the endometrial cavity and detect a spillage through the fallopian tubes. Thus, it becomes easier to diagnose intrauterine abnormalities, such as polyps or fibroids, and tubal patency.

Angiography

Angiography is the use of radiographic contrast medium to visualize the blood vascular system. By demonstrating the vascular pattern of an area, tumors or other abnormalities can be delineated. Angiography also is used to delineate continued bleeding from pelvic vessels postoperatively, to visualize bleeding from infiltration by cancer in cancer patients, to embolize the uterine arteries in order to treat postpartum hemorrhage following vaginal or caesarean deliveries, to decrease acute bleeding in cases of cervical or cornual pregnancies, and/or to reduce the size of uterine myomas. These vessels then can be embolized with synthetic fabrics to stop the bleeding or indicate therapy that can prevent the need for a major abdominal operation in a highly compromised patient.

Computed Tomography

CT scan is a diagnostic imaging technique that provides high-resolution 2-dimensional images. The CT scan takes cross-sectional images through the body at very close intervals so that multiple "slices" of the body are obtained. The beam transmission is measured and calculated through an array of sensors that are approximately 100 times more sensitive than conventional x-rays. The computer is able to translate the densities of different types of tissues into gray-scale pictures that can be read on an x-ray film or a television monitor.

Contrast media can be given orally, intravenously, or rectally. They are used to outline the gastrointestinal and urinary systems, thus helping to differentiate these organ systems from the pelvic reproductive organs. In gynecology, the CT scan is most useful in accurately diagnosing retroperitoneal lymphadenopathy associated with malignancies. It also has been used to determine the depth of myometrial invasion in endometrial carcinoma as well as extrauterine spread. It is an accurate tool for locating pelvic abscesses that cannot be located by ultrasonography. Often a needle can be placed into an abscess pocket to both drain the abscess and determine what organism may be involved. Pelvic thrombophlebitis often can be diagnosed by CT scan as an adjunct to clinical suspicion. Common abnormalities such as ovarian cysts and myomas are easily diagnosed (Fig. 35–15).

Magnetic Resonance Imaging

MRI is a diagnostic imaging technique that creates a high-resolution, cross-sectional image of the body like a CT scan. The technique is based on the body absorbing radio waves from the machine. A small amount of this energy is absorbed by the nuclei in the various tissues. These nuclei act like small bar magnets and are influenced by the magnetic field created by the machine. These nuclei then emit some of the radio waves back out of the body. The waves are picked up by sensitive and sophisticated receivers, and these signals are translated into images by computer technology.

The advantages of MRI include the fact that it uses nonionized radiation that has no adverse or harmful effects on the body. MRI is superior to CT in its ability to

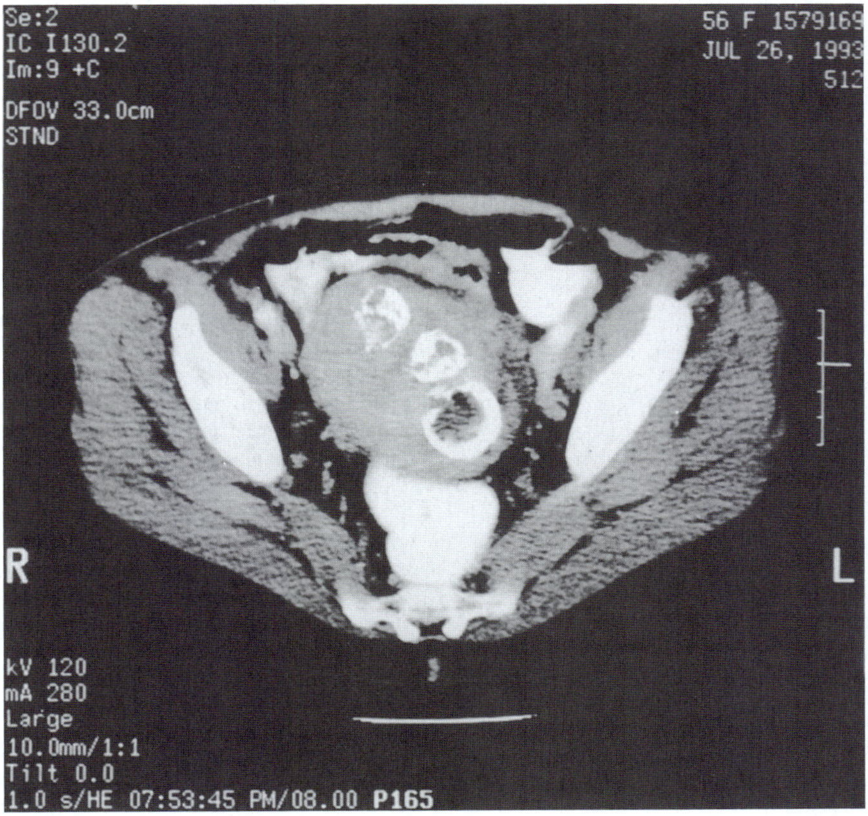

▲ **Figure 35–15.** Computed tomography scan of the pelvis showing a large fibroid uterus with 3 calcified fibroids in the body of the uterus. (Reproduced, with permission, from Dr. Barbara Carter, New England Medical Center, Boston, MA.)

differentiate among various types of tissue, including inflammatory masses, cancers, and abnormal tissue metabolism. Its disadvantages are mainly its high cost and its poor demonstration of calcifications. Its main use in gynecology appears to be staging and follow-up of pelvic cancers. MRI in obstetrics is used mainly as an adjunct to ultrasonic prenatal diagnosis of fetal anomalies. It allows for multiple image cuts that can help decipher complex anomalies. Other potential uses of MRI include evaluation of placental blood flow and accurate performance of pelvimetry.

Ultrasonography

Ultrasonography records high-frequency sound waves as they are reflected from anatomic structures. As the sounds waves pass through tissues, they encounter variable acoustic densities. Each of the tissues returns a different echo, depending on the amount of energy reflected. This echo signal can be measured and converted into a 2-dimensional image of the area under examination, with the relative densities shown as differing shades of gray.

Ultrasonography is a simple and painless procedure that has the added advantage of freedom from any radiation hazard. It is especially helpful in patients in whom an adequate pelvic examination may be difficult, such as in children, virginal women, and obese and uncooperative patients.

The pelvis and lower abdomen are scanned and recorded at regular intervals of distance, using a sector scanner that provides a better 2-dimensional picture than does the linear array scanner (Fig. 35–16). Generally, the abdominal scan is performed with the bladder full; this condition elevates the uterus out of the pelvis, displaces air-filled loops of bowel, and provides the operator with an index of density—a sonographic "window" differentiating the pelvic organs.

Ultrasonography can be helpful in the diagnosis of almost any pelvic abnormality, as all structures, normal and abnormal, usually can be demonstrated. In most instances, a clinical picture has been developed—by history, physical examination, or both—before ultrasonograms are obtained. Thus, the scan often corroborates the clinical impression, but it also may uncover an unexpected condition of which the clinician should be aware.

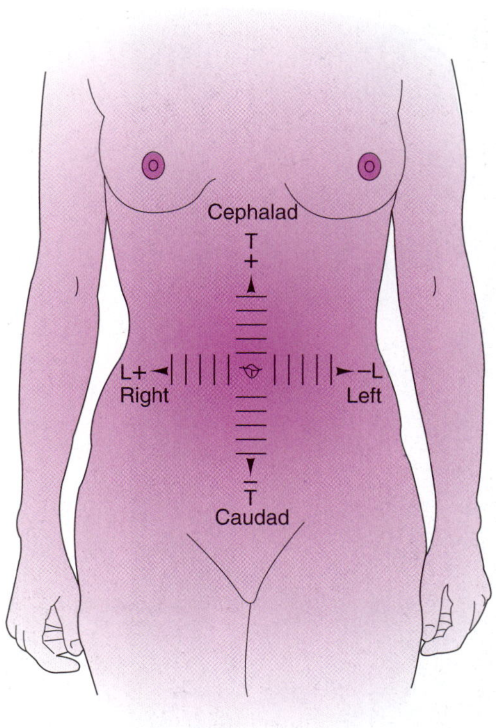

▲ **Figure 35–16.** Planes of ultrasonograms.

There are many indications for ultrasonography. Normal early pregnancy can be diagnosed, as can pathologic pregnancies such as incomplete and missed abortions and hydatidiform moles. Ultrasonography can be extremely helpful in avoiding the placenta and fetus during midtrimester amniocentesis. The uses for ultrasound examination in obstetrics are discussed elsewhere in this book.

Ultrasonography may be used to locate a lost IUD or a foreign body in the vagina of a child. Congenital malformations such as a bicornuate uterus or vaginal agenesis are sometimes, but not always, detected. The development of 3-dimensional CT scan has introduced this technology to the more accurate diagnosis of congenital uterine abnormalities.

Ultrasound examination is useful in the placement of uterine tandems for radiation therapy for endometrial cancer and for guidance during second-trimester abortion procedures.

One of the more common uses for ultrasonography is the diagnosis of pelvic masses. Often because of their location, attachment, and density, myomas can be diagnosed without too much difficulty (Fig. 35–17A).

Adnexal masses can be found with relative ease by ultrasonography, although an accurate diagnosis is more difficult because of the various types of adnexal masses that can be found (Fig. 35–17B and C).

Ovarian cysts can be described as unilocular or multilocular, totally fluid-filled, or partially solid. A common adnexal mass, the dermoid cyst, can have characteristic ultrasound findings because of fat tissue and bone densities seen in these cysts (Fig. 35–17D). Pelvic abscesses can be diagnosed by ultrasonography, especially if a well-encapsulated large abscess pocket is present.

In addition to the traditional abdominal scan, the vaginal probe scan has become a useful modality. The vaginal probe is used for determining early gestations and can diagnose a pregnancy as early as 5 weeks from the LNMP. The vaginal ultrasonographic probe is capable of visualizing ectopic pregnancies quite accurately.

Ultrasonography is commonly used to diagnose ovarian cysts, especially in obese patients in whom abdominal scans are of limited use. The vaginal scan is used often to determine follicular size with in vitro fertilization and to predict the best time for ovum retrieval.

Innovations in ultrasound probes and computerizing processes of the obtained images enable the development of 3-dimensional ultrasound machines. The 3-dimensional images help to accurately evaluate normal and abnormal findings, such as uterine shape and cavity, pelvic masses, and fetal malformations.

Carbon Dioxide Laser

Controlled tissue vaporization by laser is a modality for treatment of cervical, vaginal, or perineal condylomata and dysplasia. It also can be used for conization of the cervix for diagnosis of dysplasia or carcinoma within the cervical canal.

The vaporization procedure is not difficult, but training is essential, especially in the physics of laser light and the potential risks of laser therapy not only to the patient but to the operator and others in the immediate vicinity. Antiseptic preparation of the vagina should be gentle to avoid trauma to the tissue that is to be examined histologically. Local anesthesia, with or without preliminary intravenous sedation, usually is adequate.

Advantages of the laser method of cervical conization include little or no pain; a low incidence of infection because the beam sterilizes the tissues; decreased blood loss, because the laser instrument—at a decreased energy level—is a hemostatic agent; less tissue necrosis than occurs with electrocautery (but probably the same as with excision by a sharp knife); and a decreased incidence of postoperative cervical stenosis.

Loop Electrosurgical Excision Procedure

Loop electrosurgical excision procedure (LEEP) is another modality of therapy for vulvar and cervical lesions. LEEP uses a low-voltage, high-frequency alternating current that limits thermal damage but at the same time has good hemostatic properties. It is most commonly used for excision of vulvar condylomata and cervical dysplasias and for cone biopsies of the cervix. It has displaced sharp knife and laser cone biopsies for treatment of most cervical dysplasias.

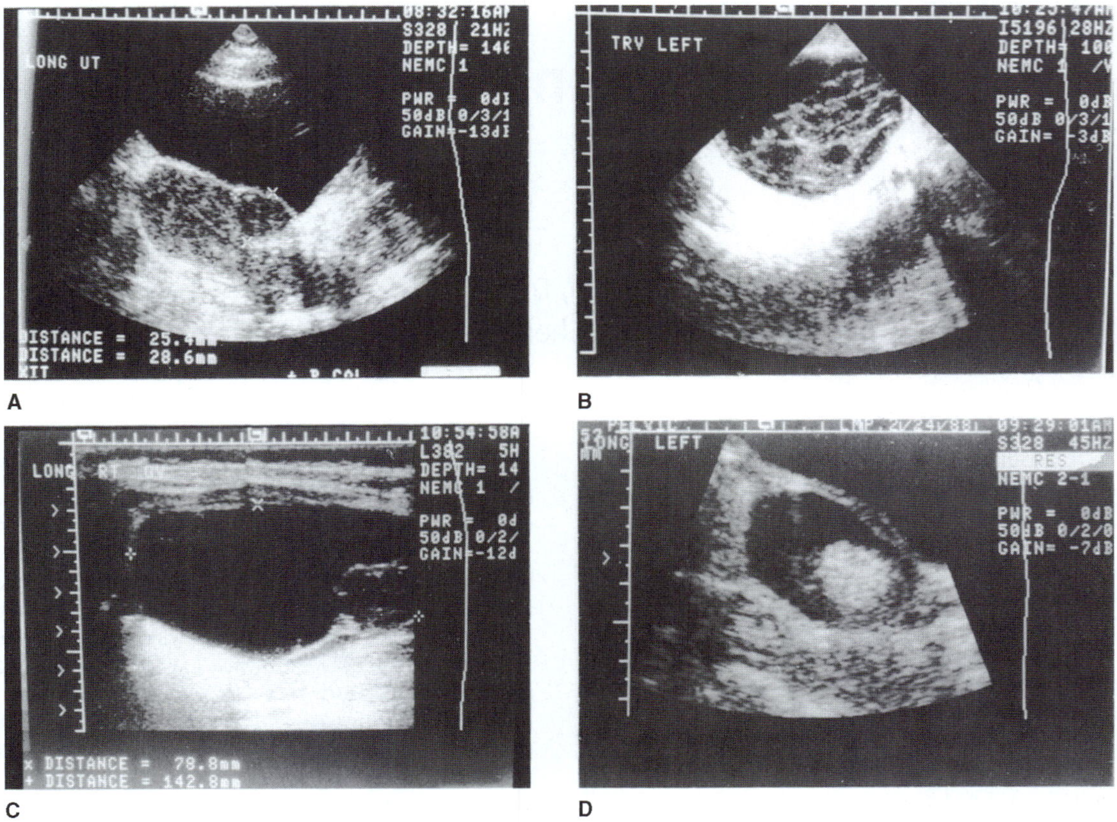

▲ **Figure 35–17.** **A:** Longitudinal view of the uterus with anterior fibroid outlined by the x's; bladder anterior. **B:** Transverse section through an endometrioma with multiple loculations and debris. **C:** Longitudinal view of large ovarian cyst outlined by the +'s and x's with a focal multicystic area. **D:** Longitudinal view of a dermoid cyst showing areas of fat within the cyst.

The technique requires the use of local anesthesia followed by the use of a wire loop cautery unit that cauterizes and cuts the desired tissue. Loops of various sizes are used for specimens of different size. The major advantages of LEEP are its usefulness in an office setting with lower equipment cost, minimal damage to the surrounding tissue, and low morbidity.

Vassilakos P, Schwartz D, de Marval F, et al. Biopsy-based comparison of liquid-based, thin-layer preparations to conventional Pap smear. *J Reprod Med* 2000;45:11–16. PMID: 10664916.

Wright T, Massad LS, Dunton CJ, et al. Interim guidelines for the use of human papillomavirus DNA testing as an adjunct to cervical cytology screening. *Obstet Gynecol* 2004;103:304–309. PMID: 17917566.

36 Imaging in Gynecology

Micah J. Hill, DO
Alan H. DeCherney, MD

CASE REPORT

C.O. is a 29-year-old white woman who presented with a history of infertility for several years, followed by a history of recurrent pregnancy losses.

Her past medical and surgical histories were negative. On gynecologic history, she was remarkable in that she reported severe dysmenorrhea for several years that was relieved by nonsteroidal anti-inflammatory drugs. Her gynecologist found a low luteal phase progesterone level and treated her with 50 mg of clomiphene citrate on days 5–9 of the cycle.

She responded well to the medication, with a subsequent conception. The pregnancy resulted in a spontaneous abortion 5 weeks later. No dilatation and curettage (D&C) was required, and the patient recovered well. She was still unable to conceive on her own and was again given clomiphene citrate therapy. Again, she conceived and had a spontaneous abortion—this time at 7 weeks' gestation. No D&C was performed.

The patient was evaluated for recurrent pregnancy losses. Karyotype was normal for both partners. Hormonal evaluation was normal with the exception of a low midluteal phase progesterone level. Immunologic and infectious screening failed to reveal a cause for the recurrent losses. The hysterosalpingogram (HSG) demonstrated a midline filling defect.

The patient was informed of the results and the potential for future miscarriages. The need for further evaluation and possible repair performed via a hysteroscopic or abdominal approach, together with its risks and benefits, was carefully explained to the patient. She elected to try clomiphene citrate therapy one more time and hoped to avoid surgery.

At 8 weeks' gestation, vaginal ultrasonography (US) revealed positive fetal cardiac activity in an ovulation induced by clomiphene citrate. While still taking micronized progesterone 100 mg 3 times daily, she was referred to her gynecologist for routine obstetric care. At 12 weeks' gestation, the patient had an incomplete abortion that required a D&C. She recovered uneventfully and later returned to the office for further evaluation and treatment.

Several months were allowed to lapse before a hysteroscopy/laparoscopy was performed, which revealed a broad-based intrauterine septum and stage I endometriosis. To evaluate the depth and width of the septum, a LaparoScan (EndoMedix, Irvine, CA) laparoscopic 7.5-Hz probe was used during the procedure. The septum was removed with a hysteroscopic resectoscope loop on a 40-W setting. After the resection, the ultrasonic probe was again used to measure the thickness of the myometrium and to verify the resection of the septum. A 30-mL 18-F Foley catheter with the distal tip resected was placed in the fundus and inflated. The patient was discharged and placed on therapy consisting of a broad-spectrum antibiotic and conjugated estrogen 2.5 mg daily.

DISCUSSION

The new millennium saw a proliferation of imaging techniques used in medical practice. Research into the development, refinement, and application of imaging in gynecology is apparent in the literature.

The HSG has been considered the gold standard for imaging the uterine corpus for benign disorders (submucous myomas, submucous polyps, localization of tubal occlusion, and evaluation of müllerian fusion defects) and malignant disease (endometrial carcinoma). In the case reported, the standard scout film was obtained, and the cervix was prepared after the following were assured: position of the uterus, absence of pelvic tenderness, and negative pregnancy test. The water-soluble contrast medium was injected into the uterine cavity, and oblique and anteroposterior films were obtained. These films showed a midline uterine filling defect of the type usually seen with septate or bicornuate uteri.

US performed on this patient during her pregnancies failed to show the filling defect. If suspected, the septum might have been encountered with more careful scanning.

Table 36–1. Indications for saline infusion sonohysterosalpingogram.

Abnormal x-ray hysterosalpingogram
Abnormal uterine bleeding
Allergies to iodine dyes
Amenorrhea
Infertility

The scans of the last pregnancy revealed only an eccentrically placed pregnancy that might be seen on US even in normally structured uteri. Although not helpful at this point, US examination of the uterus between conceptions might have been helpful if used with a distending medium. This is especially useful in patients allergic to iodine contrast medium (Table 36–1). This technique of ultrasonic HSG is performed by occluding the cervix with a uterine injector and distending the uterus. The method can demonstrate the separate cavities as well as the possible difference between the septate and the bicornuate uterus while demonstrating tubal patency. The technique was adopted for this patient during her uterine septum resection, with the addition of ultrasonic contrast between the endometrial cavity and septum and the myometrium. Readers are referred to the many fine texts on diagnostic pelvic US for instruction and further discussion of these techniques. The development of "sonicated" contrast solutions may add greatly to the usefulness of US.

Using 2 video cameras (1 for the resectoscope and the other for the laparoscope and the LaparoScan laparoscopic US probe), all aspects of the surgery were evaluated. This setup allowed the operating surgeon adequate visualization of the uterine cavity during the resection and enabled other personnel in the operating room to follow the progress of the surgery. The laparoscopic video allowed for careful monitoring of the uterine surface and assured the surgeon that there would be less likelihood of a uterine perforation, a complication that could result in bowel injury. The laparoscopic US probe with a picture within a picture was useful because it allowed visualization of the 2 separate cavities and measurement of the length and width of the septum. It also enabled the operator to demonstrate the complete removal of the septum.

IMAGING OF THE UTERUS & CERVIX

Although plain film radiographs are one of the most common forms of imaging in radiology, they are rarely the test of choice for identifying gynecologic pathology. However, they can be used to detect calcified leiomyomas as well as an intrauterine device (IUD). Such films can help determine if an IUD has been expelled from the uterine cavity or has penetrated the uterine wall and migrated to an ectopic location.

Pelvic US, magnetic resonance imaging (MRI), and computed tomography (CT) imaging are more common modalities in assessment of the uterus and the cervix. Pelvic US is the most common initial imaging approach in diagnosis of uterine disease. Modalities for pelvic US include a transvaginal approach, transabdominal approach, and saline infusion sonohysterosalpingogram. Pelvic US plays a significant role in the diagnosis of uterine leiomyomas (submucosal, intramural, and subserosal) and polyps and in the monitoring of follicular development in assisted reproduction. In more recent years, 3-dimensional (3D) US has been investigated in comparison to 2-dimensional (2D) US and hysteroscopy. Salim and colleagues showed 3D US to be superior over 2D US in the measurement of intramural versus submucosal involvement of leiomyoma. Additionally, US is often the initial test to suggest other pathology such as müllerian anomalies and adenomyosis. Occasionally, the detection and localization of myomas, assessment of their size, and their differential diagnosis are difficult. In the circumstances of adenomyosis, müllerian anomalies, or additional information needed on myomas, it can be useful to perform MRI of the pelvis. MRI produces images with excellent soft tissue resolution and is useful for evaluation of congenital abnormalities of the uterus, leiomyomas, adenomyosis, gestational trophoblastic disease, and endometrial carcinoma diagnosis and staging. MRI can accurately measure the volume of the myoma, which aids in determining whether medical management of myomas has resulted in shrinkage or whether conservatively treated myomas are growing. Malignant degeneration of myomas visualized by MRI, as described by some authors, allows for early and appropriate intervention.

MRI can effectively discern between the septate and the bicornuate uterus, thus avoiding the more costly laparoscopy. MRI may provide a clear anatomic picture of complicated müllerian fusion defects (didelphys with transverse vaginal septum or noncommunicating uterine segment) and allow for proper planning of surgical repair. If pelvic MRI had been performed on the patient in the opening case report, the image probably would have appeared the same as the MRI shown in Figure 36–1. (See review of MRI findings of müllerian fusion defects in Table 36–2.)

Currently, histopathologic evaluation of colposcopic biopsies is required to diagnose cervical cancer and its precursor lesions. However, the technique is expensive and often requires a waiting period before histopathologic results are available and necessary treatment can be scheduled. Several new imaging techniques that evaluate the cervical epithelium are under investigation. Optical techniques, such as elastic backscattering and fluorescence and Raman spectroscopies, have been used to noninvasively examine tissue morphology and the biochemical composition of the cervix. Optical coherence tomography (OCT) is a noninvasive imaging technique that uses coherent light to form images of subsurface tissue structures with 10- to 20-μm resolution and up to 1-mm depth. A study by Zuluaga and colleagues

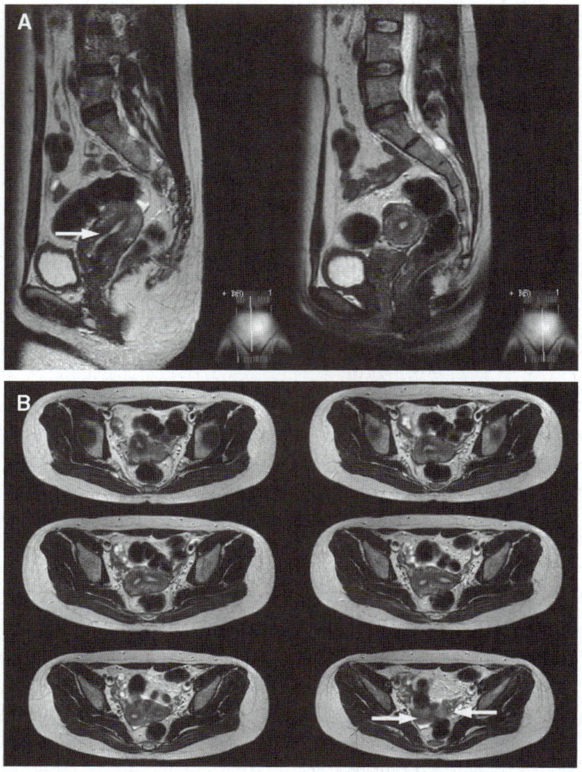

▲ **Figure 36–1.** Magnetic resonance imaging of a bicornuate uterus. (Reproduced, with permission, from (Simons M. Hysteroscopic morcellator system can be used for removal of a uterine septum. *Fertil Steril* 2011;96(2):e118–121.)

showed that simple quantitative analysis of images obtained with an OCT system can be used for noninvasive evaluation of normal and abnormal cervical tissue in vivo. OCT imaging could have broad applications for screening and detection of cervical malignancies and their precursors. It may also aid in surgical planning by allowing surgeons to identify margins in vivo without obtaining frozen sections.

IMAGING OF THE ENDOMETRIUM

Pelvic US has been used to evaluate the uterine cavity, and endometrial thickness has been used as a marker for endometrial pathology. The following guidelines should be used to obtain interobserver consistency in the evaluation of the endometrium. Obtain measurements from the midfundal region in the sagittal plane. Obtain the maximal double-thickness dimension, remembering to exclude the hypoechoic area between the myometrium and the endometrium. Any fluid between the anterior and posterior walls should be subtracted from the total measurement. Endometrial thickness ranges from 4–8 mm during the follicular phase and 7–14 mm during the luteal phase with a uniform echogenic appearance.

Premenopausal women should be evaluated during the early follicular phase, immediately following the menses when the endometrium has a uniform linear appearance. Menopausal women usually have an endometrial stripe <4 mm. Menopausal women on hormone replacement therapy (HRT) may have an endometrial thickness exceeding 8 mm and a small amount of fluid (<1 mm) (Table 36–2).

Approximately one-fifth of patients with abnormal uterine bleeding have submucous myomas or polyps. A study by Tur-Kaspa and colleagues found that 20% of infertile patients had some abnormality on SIS: arcuate uterus (15%), polyps (13%), submucosal fibroids (3%), and adhesions (<1%). These lesions may be detected by irregularities in the endometrial stripe or by saline infusion sonohysterography (SIS), a technique that involves saline infusion to distend the uterine cavity. Using SIS, a polyp appears as a smoothly marginated focal lesion that protrudes into the endometrial cavity. Kelekci and colleagues showed the sensitivities and specificities for detecting cavitary lesions with transvaginal US, SIS, and hysteroscopy to be 56.3% and 72%, 81.3% and 100%, and 87.5% and 100%, respectively. The sensitivity and specificity rates of US in detecting endometrial pathology reportedly increase when color flow and power Doppler imaging are used. However, tissue sampling is required to make a definitive diagnosis and to rule out malignancy in any patient not on HRT with a hyperechogenic endometrial stripe >4 mm.

3D US has been studied for evaluation of the endometrium. The ability of 3D US to produce coronal images of the cornua may increase slightly the sensitivity of SIS for detecting lesions in this location that otherwise might be difficult to evaluate. Endometrial abnormalities that can be seen in women with congenital malformations of the uterus may be imaged to greater advantage with 3D US techniques. 3D US has also been demonstrated to be a valid measurement technique for assessing volume. However, hysteroscopy likely will become the new gold standard for evaluating the endometrium because of the ability of hysteroscopy to directly visualize the endometrium and perform biopsies as indicated. The technique may become more cost effective as use of office hysteroscopy becomes more widespread. Evaluation of the endometrium using transvaginal sonography as the initial screening tool, followed by endometrial biopsy or possibly hysteroscopy, is likely to become the standard of care (Fig. 36–2).

Newer imaging modalities are under investigation to decrease the number of imaging tests often ordered in the evaluation of infertility. These tests seek to evaluate tubal patency, tubal architecture, the uterine cavity, and the myometrium in 1 study. Unterweger and colleagues showed that 3D dynamic magnetic resonance hysterosalpingography (3D dMR-HSG) can evaluate tubal patency in addition to MRI evaluation of the uterus and pelvic structures.

Table 36–2. Types of müllerian anomalies and associated MRI findings.

Class and Type	No.	Finding
I: Segmental agenesis/hypoplasia	7 (24%)	Agenesis: no identifiable organ or small amorphous tissue remnant. Hypoplasia: uterus small for patient's age, maintains adult body/cervix ratio of 2:1, reduced intercornual distance (<2 cm), low signal intensity on T2-weighted images with poor zonal differentiation, endometrial/myometrial width reduced
A. Vaginal	0	
B. Cervical	0	
C. Fundal	0	
D. Tubal	0	
E. Combined	7	
II: Unicornuate uterus	5 (17%)	Banana-shaped uterus, normal width of endometrium and myometrium, endometrial/myometrial ratio preserved
A1. Rudimentary horn with endometrium		
(A) Communicating with main uterine cavity	0	
(B) Not communicating with main uterine cavity	1	
A2. Rudimentary horn without endometrium	1	
B. No rudimentary horn	3	
III: Didelphys	5 (17%)	Double, separate uterus, cervix, and upper vagina; each uterine cavity of normal volume; endometrium and myometrium of normal width; endometrial/myometrial ratio normal
IV: Bicornuate uterus	10 (34%)	Uterine fundus concave or flattened outward, 2 horns visible with increased intercornual distance (>4 cm), high-signal-intensity septum myometrium on T2-weighted images at level of fundus; high-signal-intensity myometrium (7 patients) or low-signal-intensity fibrous tissue at level of lower uterine segment (3 patients)
A. Complete	3	
B. Partial	3	
C. Arcuate	4	
V: Septate	2 (7%)	Uterine fundus convex outward, normal intercornual distance (2–4 cm), each uterine cavity reduced in volume, endometrial/myometrial width and ratio normal, low-signal-intensity septum on T1- and T2-weighted images
A. Complete	1	
B. Incomplete	1	

Because of rounding, the percentages do not add up to 100.
Reproduced, with permission, from Doyle MB. Magnetic resonance imaging in müllerian fusion defects. *J Reprod Med* 1992;37:33.

Virtual hysterosalpingogram (VHSG) and multislice CT hysterosalpingography (MSCT-HSG) are similar tests but use CT technology in place of MRI for evaluation. Although these tests are more expensive than traditional procedures, they can provide the information previously gained from pelvic US, HSG, and MRI/CT in a single radiologic modality.

IMAGING OF THE OVARIES

The flat plate of the abdomen may still be useful in the diagnosis of dermoid cysts of the ovary, which are identified by the presence of calcified teeth. However, cystic and solid structures of the ovary now are better evaluated by transabdominal US, transvaginal US (TVUS), CT, and MRI.

Transvaginal assessment of the ovary is frequently used in assisted reproduction cycles, both in management and prediction of success. Antral follicles measure 2–10 mm in size and appear as small hypoechoic structures within the ovary and are typically measured in a basal state. Hendriks and colleagues have shown that the number of basal antral follicles is superior to follicle-stimulating hormone in predicting poor ovarian response. The ovarian follicles also change size in response to ovarian stimulation, whether exogenous or endogenous. These changes are monitored during assisted reproductive technology (ART) cycles to help in the timing of human chorionic gonadotropin (hCG) injections, oocyte retrieval, management of gonadotropin stimulation, and determining the need for cycle cancellation.

US is frequently used in the evaluation of ovarian pathology. TVUS combined with color flow and Doppler can be used for evaluation of blood flow to the adnexal structures and for diagnosis of ovarian torsion. Venous and lymphatic flow is occluded in early torsion, but arterial flow may be present. Arterial flow ceases completely later in the torsion. Torsion is diagnosed by Doppler study showing no venous or arterial flow, but a study showing arterial blood flow does not necessarily rule out the diagnosis.

Approximately 12,000 women in the United States die annually of ovarian cancer. Unfortunately, the ability of the pelvic examination to detect early ovarian malignancy is

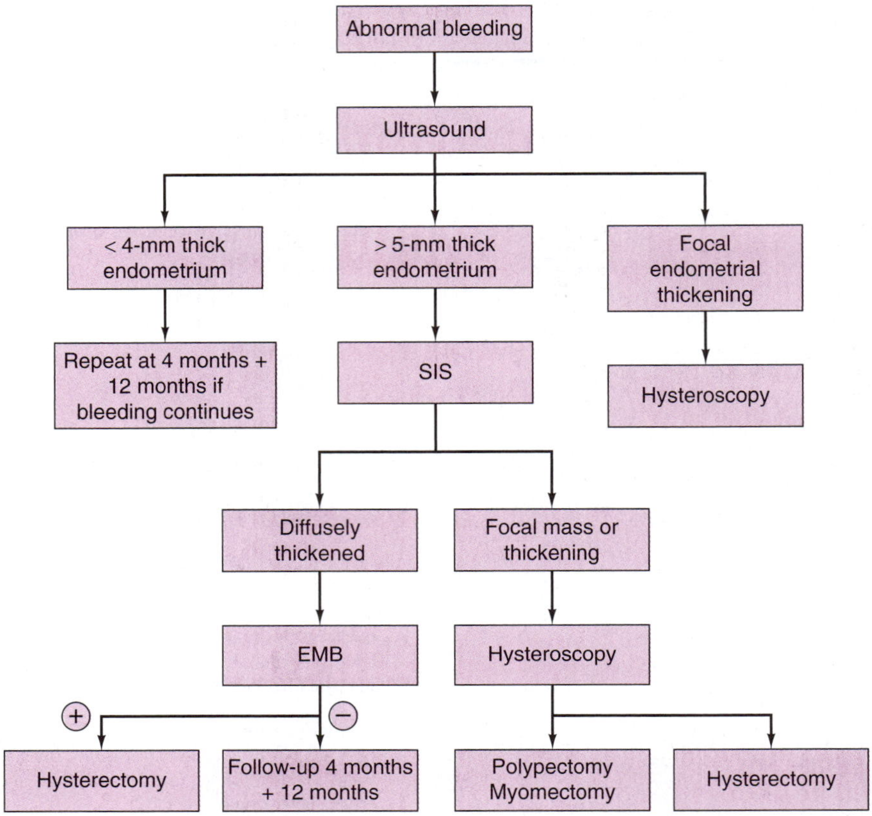

▲ **Figure 36–2.** Proposed algorithm for evaluating women with abnormal vaginal bleeding. EMB, endometrial biopsy; SIS, saline infusion sonohysterography. (Reproduced, with permission, from Davidson KG, Dubinsky TJ. Ultrasonographic evaluation of the endometrium in postmenopausal vaginal bleeding. *Radiol Clin North Am* 2003;41:769–780.)

poor. CA-125 monoclonal marker for ovarian cancer also is a poor predictor of early cases. In an attempt to discriminate between malignant and benign adnexal masses, morphologic criteria have been assigned to increase suspicion concerning US findings when ovarian cancer is suspected. Cysts larger than 4 cm, solid and cystic components, septa, and papillary nodules have all been described (Fig. 36–3). In addition, Doppler flow studies have been used to distinguish between benign and malignant masses (Table 36–3).

CT may be useful for preoperative staging of ovarian cancer or for planning second-look procedures. CT may also be useful for biopsy and drainage in patients with benign-appearing adnexal masses (ovarian cysts or tubo-ovarian abscesses). Contraindications to needle biopsy and drainage include lack of a safe unobstructed path for the needle, bleeding disorders, and lack of a motivated patient. 3D US can be useful in the evaluation of gynecologic diseases. It can reconstruct any plane of interest and is particularly valuable in visualizing abnormalities in the coronal plane. In addition, 3D US is better able to measure volumes than is 2D US and, therefore, is helpful when evaluating patients with conditions ranging from fibroids to infertility. CT can be used in conjunction with pelvic US to diagnose and manage several conditions, such as pelvic inflammatory disease, adnexal torsion, ovarian vein thrombosis, and hemorrhagic ovarian cysts. In addition, MRI has been shown to be particularly useful in the evaluation of ovarian vein thrombosis.

IMAGING OF THE FALLOPIAN TUBES

Endoscopic techniques provide the best direct evaluation of the patency and architecture of the fallopian tubes. HSG provides the best indirect evaluation of tubal function. HSG allows demonstration of tubal patency and visualization of tubal rugations while avoiding the more costly laparoscopic surgery. Some disadvantages of HSG are pelvic infection, dye allergies, failure to detect adnexal adhesions, and false-positive results for tubal occlusion. Salpingitis isthmica nodosa (SIN) is suggested when a honeycombing

Ovarian Tumor Ultrasound-Doppler Classification

Circle all characteristics seen and add numbers in parentheses for a score.

Patient name ________________ Date ________ Institution ___________

	Fluid		Internal Borders		Size
Unilocular	Clear	(0)	Smooth	(0)	
	Internal echoes	(1)	Irregular	(2)	
Multilocular	Clear	(1)	Smooth	(1)	
	Internal echoes	(1)	Irregular	(2)	
Cystic-solid	Clear	(1)	Smooth	(1)	
	Internal echoes	(2)	Irregular	(2)	

Papillary projections	Suspicious	(1)	Definite	(2)
Solid	Homogenous	(1)	Echogenic	(2)
Peritoneal fluid	Absent	(0)	Present	(1)
Laterality	Unilateral	(0)	Bilateral	(1)

Ultrasound Score

≤ 2	Benign
3–4	Questionable
> 4	Suspicious

Color Doppler		RI (resistance index)	
No vessels seen	(0)		(0)
Regular separate vessels	(1)	> 0.40	(1)
Randomly dispersed vessels	(2)	< 0.41	(2)

If suspected corpus luteum, repeat in next menstrual cycle in proliferative phase.

Color Doppler Score

≤ 2	Benign
3–4	Questionable

▲ **Figure 36–3.** Scoring system used to evaluate the morphology of adnexal tumor. RI, resistance index. (Reproduced, with permission, from Kurjak A, Schulman H, Sosic A, et al. Transvaginal ultrasound, color flow, and Doppler waveform of the postmenopausal adnexal mass. *Obstet Gynecol* 1992;80:917–921.)

of the contrast material appears in the tubes during HSG. Hydrosalpinges are suggested when a hypoechoic "sausaging" of the tube is seen on US. Hysterosalpingo-contrast sonography, 3D dMR-HSG, VHSG, and MSCT-HSG are alternatives to laparoscopy, as women with normal findings probably have a normal pelvis.

IMAGING IN ECTOPIC PREGNANCY

Adnexal sonography is a valuable tool in assessing women with suspected ectopic pregnancy (Table 36–4). When hCG levels reach 6500 mIU/mL, most normal intrauterine pregnancies can be detected as a gestational sac by transabdominal US. However, the sonographic appearance of a pseudogestational sac should not be confused with the gestational sac. In the latter, a double ring sign resulting from the decidua parietalis is seen abutting the decidua capsularis.

TVUS, on the other hand, has the advantage of earlier and better localization of the pregnancy, with less pelvic discomfort because the bladder is not painfully distended. An hCG level of 1000–2000 mIU/mL is the discriminatory zone in which an intrauterine pregnancy can be detected by TVUS. The double-ring sign and the yolk sac must be identified to ensure that the pregnancy is intrauterine. When an intrauterine pregnancy is not visualized on TVUS and the hCG level exceeds 1000–2000 mIU/mL, suspicion for an ectopic pregnancy should be high. However, multiple gestations and heterotopic pregnancies may take several more days to be identified. Both of these conditions are more common in patients undergoing ART. Because it is not well established at what hCG levels multiple gestation or

Table 36–3. Histology and blood flow characteristics.

Histology	No.	Flow Detected	RI
Malignant			
Papillary adenocarcinoma	13	12	0.39 ± 0.04
Serous cystadenocarcinoma	3	3	0.30 ± 0.04
Endometrioid adenocarcinoma	4	4	0.38 ± 0.02
Metastatic carcinoma	7	7	0.37 ± 0.07
Theca-granulosa cell	2	1	0.37
Total	29	27	0.37 ± 0.08
Benign			
Simple cyst	25	5	0.75 ± 0.17
Papillary serous cyst	4	1	0.6
Mucinous cyst	5	3	0.62 ± 0.09
Inflammatory mass	2	1	0.62
Parasitic cyst	1	0	0
Fibroma	4	3	0.56 ± 0.03
Thecoma	2	2	0.60
Cystadenofibroma	1	1	0.56
Endometrioma	4	1	0.56
Cystic teratoma	1	1	0.36
Pseudo- and parovarian cyst	4	0	0
Brenner tumor	1	1	0.50
Total	54	19	0.62 ± 0.11[1]

Data are presented as number or mean ± standard deviation.
[1]*P* <.001. RI, resistance index.
Reproduced, with permission, from Kurjak A, Schulman H, Sosic A, et al. Transvaginal ultrasound, color flow, and Doppler waveform of the postmenopausal adnexal mass. *Obstet Gynecol* 1992;80:917–921.

heterotopic pregnancies should be visualized on US, particular caution is needed in evaluating for ectopic pregnancies in ART patients.

IMAGING OF THE PERITONEUM

In recent years, newer imaging modalities have been evaluated for their ability to detect peritoneal pathology, primarily malignant processes and endometriosis. US has limited ability to detect peritoneal pathology, especially smaller processes. Shaw and colleagues concluded that, although MRI may have a role, CT imaging remains the test of choice for the diagnosis of pelvic malignancy. For deep and surface pelvic endometriosis, Bazot and colleagues showed that MRI has a high sensitivity and specificity for diagnosis. Despite these recent advances in peritoneal imaging, laparoscopy remains the gold standard for the diagnosis of peritoneal pathology.

Table 36–4. Criteria for diagnosis of ectopic pregnancy.

Criteria	Sensitivity (%)	Specificity (%)
Extrauterine gestational sac with yolk sac or embryo	8–34	100
Adnexal ring	40–68	100
Complex adnexal mass separate from ovary	89–100	92–99
Any fluid	46–75	69–83
Moderate to large amount of free fluid	29–63	21–96
Echogenic fluid	56	96
Decidual cyst	21	92

Reproduced, with permission, from Harrison BP, Crystal CS. Imaging modalities in obstetrics and gynecology. *Emerg Med Clin North Am* 2003;21:711–735.

IMAGING OF THE PITUITARY GLAND

Although the pituitary gland is located outside the pelvis, imaging of the gland is indicated in gynecologic patients with hyperprolactinemia. Patients with hyperprolactinemia may present with infertility, galactorrhea, decreased libido, and oligomenorrhea. Imaging of the pituitary has been recommended with prolactin levels over 100 ng/mL or in any patient with persistently elevated prolactin levels. A recent study by Bayrak and colleagues showed that while the size of the pituitary prolactinoma does correlate with serum prolactin levels, patients with macroadenomas may present with only moderate prolactin elevations, and therefore, any patient with persistently elevated prolactin levels should undergo pituitary imaging.

Historically, pituitary imaging was performed with a coned-down x-ray film of the sella turcica. MRI has replaced this approach with a greater sensitivity for detecting microadenomas as compared to both x-ray and CT scans. On MRI examination, microadenomas are commonly identified as areas of low-intensity T1 signaling.

CONCLUSION

The imaging techniques prevalent today have proved to be valuable tools in the diagnosis and treatment of benign and malignant gynecologic disorders. To provide the patient with the highest level of medical care, the contemporary practicing gynecologist must constantly keep abreast of the new developments and applications of diagnostic imaging. No matter what technology is used today and in the future, the goal will always be the same: to provide quick, low-risk, accurate diagnosis of gynecologic conditions while keeping in mind the cost effectiveness of the care delivered.

Bayrak A, Saadat P, Mor E, Chong L, Paulson JP, Sokol RZ. Pituitary imaging is indicated for the evaluation of hyperprolactinemia. *Fertil Steril* 2005;84:181–185. PMID: 16009175.

Bazot M, Darai E, Hourani R, Thomassin I, Cortez A, Uzan S, Buy JN. Deep pelvic endometriosis: MR imaging for diagnosis and prediction of extension of disease. *Radiology* 2004;232:379–389. PMID: 15205479.

Davidson KG, Dubinsky TJ. Ultrasonographic evaluation of the endometrium in postmenopausal vaginal bleeding. *Radiol Clin North Am* 2003;41:769–780. PMID: 12899491.

Doyle MB. Magnetic resonance imaging in müllerian fusion defects. *J Reprod Med* 1992;37:33–38. PMID: 1532208.

Harrison BP, Crystal CS. Imaging modalities in obstetrics and gynecology. *Emerg Med Clin North Am* 2003;21:711–735. PMID: 12962355.

Hendriks DJ, Mol BJ, Bancsi LF, Velde DE, Broekmans FJ. Antral follicle count in the prediction of poor ovarian response and pregnancy after in vitro fertilization: a meta-analysis and comparison with basal follicle stimulating hormone level. *Fertil Steril* 2005;83:291–301. PMID: 15705365.

Kelekci S, Kaya E, Alan E, Alan Y, Bilge U, Mollamahmutoglu L. Comparison of transvaginal sonography, saline infusion sonography, and office hysteroscopy in reproductive-aged women with or without abnormal uterine bleeding. *Fertil Steril* 2005;84:682–686. PMID: 16169483.

Kurjak A, Schulman H, Sosic A, et al. Transvaginal ultrasound, color flow, and Doppler waveform of the postmenopausal adnexal mass. *Obstet Gynecol* 1992;80:917–921. PMID: 1148259.

Salim R, Lee C, Davies A, Jolaoso B, Ofuasia E, Jurkovic D. A comparative study of three-dimensional saline infusion sonohysterography and diagnostic hysteroscopy for the classification of submucous fibroids. *Hum Reprod* 2005;20:253–257. PMID: 15498792.

Shaw MS, Healy JC, Reznek RH. Imaging the peritoneum for malignant processes. *Imaging* 2000;12:21–33.

Tur-Kaspa I, Gal M, Hartman M, Hartman J, Hartman A. A prospective evaluation of uterine abnormalities by saline infusion sonohysterography in 1,009 women with infertility or abnormal uterine bleeding. *Fertil Steril* 2006;86:1731–1735. PMID: 17007850.

Unterweger M, Geyter CD, Frohlich FM, Bongartz G, Wiesner W. Three-dimensional dynamic MR-hysterosalpingography; a new, low invasive, radiation-free and less painful radiological approach to female infertility. *Hum Reprod* 2002;12:3138-41. PMID: 12456613.

Zuluaga AF, Follen M, Boiko I, et al. Optical coherence tomography: a pilot study of a new imaging technique for noninvasive examination of cervical tissue. *Am J Obstet Gynecol* 2005;193:83–88. PMID: 16021063.

37 Pediatric & Adolescent Gynecology

Dvora Bauman, MD

Pediatric and adolescent gynecology is a unique subspecialty of gynecology that encompasses reproductive health care of girls and young women under the age of 20 years, although some experts extend the age limit to 22 years.

This field has expanded greatly over the last decades, as increased attention has been directed to disorders of developmental physiology. The spectrum of gynecologic problems that a physician might encounter in young girls is age specific and involves different skills than those applied for adults. Currently, pediatric and adolescent gynecology includes a vast array of diagnoses and treatment modalities for these particular patients.

Pediatric and adolescent gynecology starts with an observation of abnormal external genitalia in a newborn. Later on in childhood, it involves early detection of infections, labial adhesions, congenital anomalies, and even genital tumors. With adolescents, normal pubertal development, evaluation of menstrual disorders, and treatment of genetic and hormonal ailments need to be addressed. Educational approach should be implemented for issues of budding sexuality in teenagers. Concomitantly counseling of proper use of contraceptives is imperative to lower the rates of teen pregnancies and sexually transmitted infections.

The American College of Obstetricians and Gynecologists recommends that adolescents should have their first visit to a gynecologist for health guidance, general physical screening, and the provision of preventive health care services at age 13–15 years. A pelvic examination of adolescents who are sexually active may be deferred until the age of 18 years, unless medically indicated. This first visit should provide an opportunity for the gynecologist to start the physician–patient relationship, recommend proper health behaviors, and dispel myths and fears.

The first gynecologic visit is of paramount importance in establishing a trustful relationship between the young woman and her health care provider for many years to come.

ANATOMIC & PHYSIOLOGIC CONSIDERATIONS

Newborn Infants

During the first few weeks after birth, follicle-stimulating hormone (FSH) rises in the newborn due to the abrupt withdrawal of placental and maternal sex steroid hormones, resulting in hyperestrogenic physiologic effect. Breast budding occurs in nearly all female infants born at term. In some cases, breast enlargement is marked, and there may be fluid discharge from the nipples. No treatment is indicated. The labia majora are bulbous, and the labia minora are thick and protruding (Fig. 37–1). The clitoris is relatively large, with a normal index of 0.6 cm^2 or less.* The hymen initially is turgid, covering the external urethral orifice. Vaginal discharge is common in some cases and can even be bloody for the first 2 weeks, and is composed mainly of cervical mucus and exfoliated vaginal cells. Endometrial cell shedding might occur.

The vagina is approximately 4 cm long at birth. The uterus is enlarged (4 cm in length) and without axial flexion; the ratio between the cervix and the corpus is 3:1. Columnar epithelium protrudes through the external cervical os, creating a reddened zone of physiologic eversion. The ovaries remain abdominal organs in early childhood before descending into the pelvis.

Young Children

In early childhood, the female genital organs receive little estrogen stimulation. The labia majora flatten. The labia minora are thin structures running beside the upper part of vestibule and ending at the 3 and 9 o'clock positions. The hymen become thin (Fig. 37–2) and atrophic. The clitoris remains relatively small, although the clitoral index is unchanged. The vagina, lined with atrophic mucosa with relatively few rugae, offers very little resistance to trauma and infection. The vaginal barrel contains neutral or slightly alkaline secretions and mixed

*Clitoral index (cm^2) = Length (cm) × width (cm). For example, a clitoris 1 cm long and 0.5 cm wide = 0.5 cm^2.

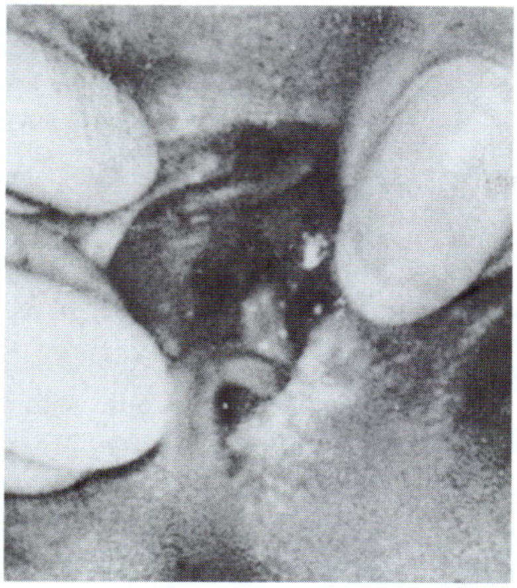

▲ **Figure 37–1.** External genitalia of a newborn female. Note the hypertrophy and turgor of the vulvar tissues. A small catheter is inserted into the vagina to demonstrate patency. (Reproduced, with permission, from Huffman JW. *The Gynecology of Childhood and Adolescence*. New York, NY: WB Saunders; 1968.)

bacterial flora. Because vaginal fornices do not develop until puberty, the cervix in childhood is flush with the vaginal vault, and its opening appears as a small slit. The uterus regresses in size and does not regain the size present at birth until approximately age 6 years. At laparotomy, the uterus may appear as merely a strip of dense tissue in the anteromedial area of the broad ligaments. The ovaries at this age have the volume of 1–2.7 mL with small resting follicles (Table 37–1).

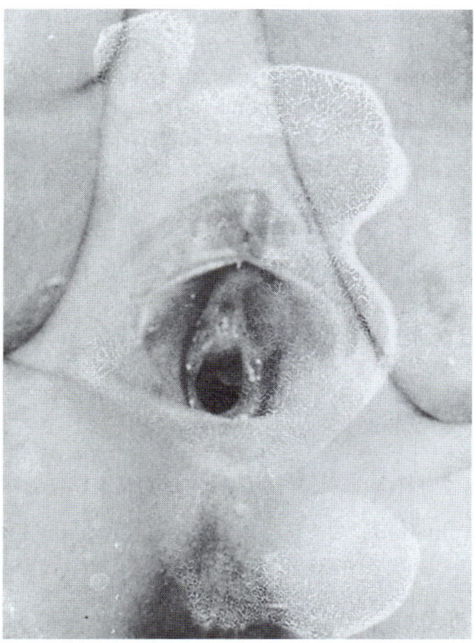

▲ **Figure 37–2.** External genitalia of a child 3 years of age.

Table 37–1. Normal volume of the ovaries and the uterus.

Age	Ovarian Volume (mL)	Uterine Volume (mL)	Uterine Shape	Endometrial Stripe
Neonate	1–3.6	2.6–4	Spade shape	Echogenic
3 months–1 year	1–2.7	0.8–1.3	Tubular shape	Hypoechoic
1–2 years	1–<1.6	0.8–1.3	Tubular shape	Hypoechoic
2–8 years	1–4.3	0.8–1.6	Tubular shape	Hypoechoic
8–16 years	2–18.3	0.8–25	Pear shape after puberty	Cyclical changes after puberty

Adapted and reproduced, with permission, from Stranzinger E, Strouse PJ. Ultrasound of the pediatric female pelvis. *Semin Ultrasound CT MR* 2008;29:98–113.

Older Children

During late childhood (age 7–10 years), the external genitalia again show signs of estrogen stimulation: the mons pubis thickens, the labia majora fill out, and the labia minora become rounded. The hymen thickens, losing its thin, transparent character. The vagina elongates to 8 cm, the mucosa becomes thicker, the corpus uteri enlarge, and the ratio of cervix to corpus becomes 1:1. The cervix remains flush with the vault (Fig. 37–3).

By the time a girl reaches age 9–10 years, uterine growth begins, with alteration in uterine shape resulting primarily from myometrial proliferation. Rapid endometrial proliferation occurs as menarche is imminent. Prior to this time, the endometrium gradually thickens, with modest increases in the depth and complexity of the endometrial glands. As the ovaries enlarge and descend into the pelvis, the number of ovarian follicles increases. Although these follicles are in various stages of development, ovulation generally does not occur.

Young Adolescents

During early puberty (age 10–13 years), the external genitalia take on adult appearance. The major vestibular glands (Bartholin's glands) begin to produce mucus just prior to menarche. The vagina reaches adult length (10–12 cm) and becomes more distensible, the mucosa thickens, vaginal secretions grow more acidic, and lactobacilli reappear. With the development of vaginal fornices, the cervix becomes separated from the vaginal vault, and the differential growth of the corpus and cervix becomes more pronounced. The corpus grows twice as large as the cervix. The ovaries descend into the true pelvis.

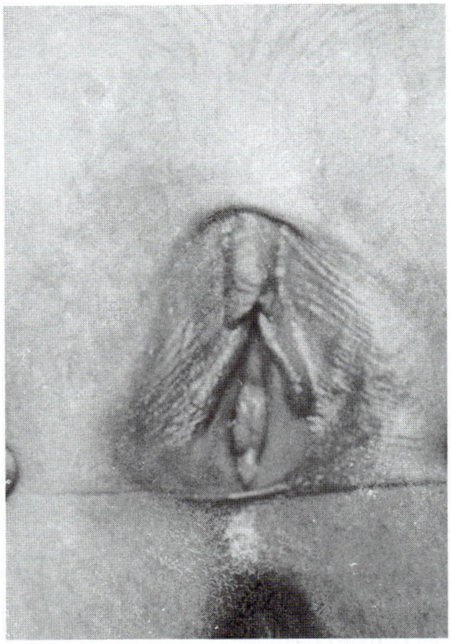

▲ **Figure 37–3.** External genitalia of a child 11 years of age. Early estrogen response is evidenced by the fuller labia, wrinkling of the vulvar mucosa, and thickening of the hymen.

Secondary sexual characteristics develop, often rapidly, during the late premenarchal period. Body habitus becomes more rounded, especially the shoulders and hips. Accelerated somatic growth velocity (the adolescent growth spurt) occurs. At the same time, estrogen increases adipose tissue deposition and initiates stromal and ductal growth in the breasts. Physiologic leukorrhea often is noted.

Pubic hair growth, or pubarche (adrenarche), appears to be under the control of adrenal androgens and is a process that is independent of although associated with gonadarche. Sparse, long, slightly curly, pigmented hair over the pubic area gives way to coarse, pigmented curly hair. The pubic hair pattern assumes the characteristic triangle with the base above the mons pubis. Hair growth in the axilla appears later, also as a result of adrenocorticosteroid stimulation. The development of secondary sexual features described by Marshall and Tanner is summarized in Table 37–2 (see Fig. 4–3).

Table 37–2. Tanner classification of female adolescent development.

Stage	Breast Development	Pubic Hair Development
I	Papillae elevated (preadolescent), no breast buds	None
II	Breast buds and papillae slightly elevated	Sparse, long, slightly pigmented
III	Breasts and areolae confluent, elevated	Darker, coarser, curly
IV	Areolae and papillae project above breast	Adult-type pubis only
V	Papillae projected, mature	Lateral distribution

GYNECOLOGIC EXAMINATION OF INFANTS, CHILDREN, & YOUNG ADOLESCENTS

Examination of the Newborn Infant

Newborns should be examined immediately upon delivery or in the nursery. When an infant is born with ambiguous genitalia, immediate actions should be to counsel the parents and to prevent dehydration, as congenital adrenal hyperplasia accounts for >90% of cases of ambiguous genitalia, and salt-wasting forms may lead to rapid dehydration and fluid imbalances. In most cases, an internal examination is unnecessary, as most gynecologic abnormalities that should be recognized at this stage are limited to the external genitalia.

A. General Examination

As in adults, the first step in a genital evaluation of the newborn is a careful general examination, which may reveal abnormalities suggesting genital anomaly (eg, webbed neck, abdominal mass, edema of the hands and legs, coarctation of the aorta).

B. Clitoris

Clitoral enlargement in the newborn almost always is associated with congenital adrenal hyperplasia. Other causes, such as hermaphroditism and neoplasms, also must be considered.

C. Vulva & Vagina

The vaginal orifice should be evident when the labia are separated or retracted. If the vaginal orifice cannot be located, the infant most likely has an imperforate hymen or vaginal agenesis. Inguinal hernias are uncommon in females, and the presence of bilateral inguinal masses suggests the possibility that the child is a genetic male and may require karyotype testing.

D. Rectoabdominal Examination

Usually, the uterus and adnexa in the newborn cannot be palpated on rectal examination; therefore, is occasionally needed. An ovary that is palpable on abdominal examination denotes enlargement, and the possibility of an ovarian tumor should be investigated, even though pelvic masses in newborns likely represent a Wilms' tumor.

Examination of the Premenarchal Child

The examination of the premenarchal and peripubertal child should focus on the main symptoms identified in this population: pruritus, dysuria, skin color changes, and discharge.

Parents can be helpful during the examination of a young child because they provide a sense of security and they can distract the patient. Placing a child up to age 5 years on her parent's lap affords a better opportunity to perform an adequate examination. Older children can be placed on the examination table so the examiner may have adequate exposure of the genitalia when the patient is asked to flex her knees and abduct her legs. Asking the young patient to assist in the examination may distract the child as well as provide her with a sense of control. In rare cases, the knee–chest position may be useful in visualizing the upper vagina and cervix.

In older girls, explaining procedures and providing health information during the examination may decrease apprehension and help establish a good patient–physician relationship.

A. Physical Examination

1. General inspection—The examination begins with an evaluation of the patient's general appearance, nutritional status, body habitus, and any gross congenital anomalies.

2. Breasts—Breast budding does not normally begin before the age of 7.5–8 years. Prominence of the nipple and breast development at an earlier age may be early signs of sexual precocity. Appropriate monitoring may include assessment of bone age, as well following height and breast development at 3-month intervals.

3. Abdomen—Inspection and palpation of the abdomen should precede examination of the genitalia. If the child is ticklish, having her place one hand on or under the examiner's hand usually will overcome the problem.

The ovary of a premenarchal child is situated high in the pelvis. This location and the small size of the pelvic cavity tend to force ovarian tumors above the true pelvic brim. Thus, large neoplasms of the ovary are likely to be mistaken for other abdominal masses (eg, polycystic kidney). Although inguinal hernias are less common in females than in males (approximately 1:10), they may occur, usually without discomfort. An excellent method of demonstrating an inguinal hernia is to have the child stand up and increase the intra-abdominal pressure by blowing up a balloon.

4. Genitalia—The vulva and vestibule can be exposed by light lateral and downward pressure on each side of the perineum, a technique referred to as *labial separation*. When exposure of the vaginal walls is necessary, the labia can be grasped between the examiner's thumb and forefinger and pulled forward, downward, and sideways, a technique called *labial traction* (Fig. 37–4). Particular attention should be paid to the adequacy of perineal hygiene, because poor hygiene may predispose a child to local inflammation. The examiner should look for skin lesions, perineal excoriations, ulcers, and tumors. Signs of hormonal stimulation in early childhood and absence of such signs later in adolescence are important signs of endocrine disorders associated with precocious or delayed puberty. Enlargement of the clitoris is of diagnostic significance, especially during early pubertal development, because it alerts the clinician to the presence of an endocrinopathy.

The normal hymen has multiple configurations including annular, crescentic, and fimbriated/redundant. Special attention to hymen appearance is given during forensic examination of sexual abuse victims, and the examiner should be familiar with vast variations of normal anatomy.

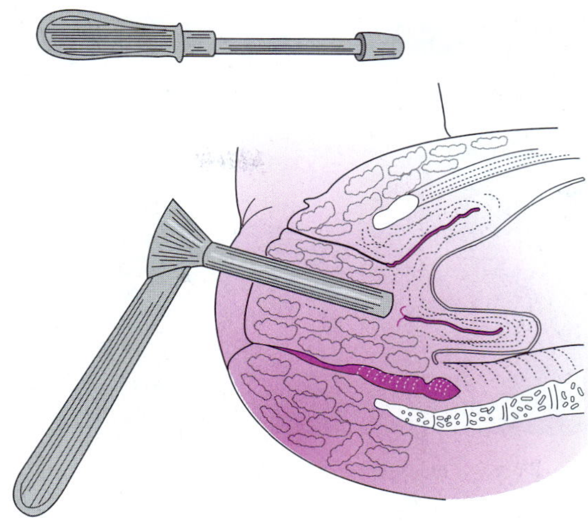

▲ **Figure 37–4.** Huffman vaginoscope used for examination of a premenarchal child.

In some patients, the vestibule or the vaginal orifice may not be visible because of labial adhesions or congenital anomalies. The former condition is frequently mistaken for vaginal agenesis or imperforate hymen.

It is unnecessary to perform a digital vaginal examination in a child whose vagina is very narrow and in whom the hymeneal orifice is small and extremely sensitive. Gentle rectal digital examination can be accomplished, but accurate intrapelvic evaluation is better achieved by other diagnostic procedures such as sonography, computed tomography, vaginoscopy, or laparoscopy.

B. Vaginoscopy

Instrumentation is required when it is necessary to carefully visualize the upper third of the vagina for a source of abnormal vaginal bleeding, to detect and remove foreign bodies, or to exclude penetrating injuries. The water endoscope (hysteroscope, cystoscope) distends the vagina and permits visualization of the vaginal mucosa, while washing away secretions, blood, and debris (Fig. 37–5).

In infancy and childhood, the hymenal orifice normally is smaller than 1 cm. An instrument 0.3–0.4 cm in diameter can be used to examine those girls. Topical lidocaine gel can be used to anesthetize the vulva and provide lubrication in older premenarchal girls. In younger girls and in cases where the aperture is too small to allow instrument passage without patient discomfort, vaginoscopy should not be further attempted without general anesthesia.

Vaginoscopy is a safe and short procedure with few, if any, adverse effects; therefore, it should be used frequently as a diagnostic tool. A "see and treat" approach may be applied to both diagnose and take care of the problem with the same equipment.

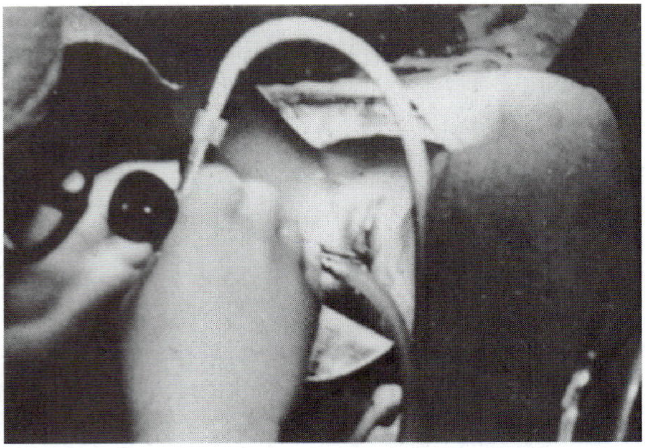

▲ **Figure 37–5.** Performing vaginoscopy under anesthesia using a water cystoscope.

Examination of the Adolescent

The adolescent's first trip to the gynecologist is often laden with fear and apprehension. Time spent putting the patient at ease and winning her confidence will save time and frustration in the examining room. The communicative skills that permit establishment of a good physician–patient relationship with teenagers can be acquired by training. The physician should make it clear that the adolescent is the patient, rather than the accompanying adult, if present. Questions about high-risk behaviors, including sexual behavior and sexually transmitted diseases (STDs), should be asked privately without the presence of the accompanying adult.

The American College of Obstetricians and Gynecologists recommends that adolescents should have their first visit to a gynecologist for health guidance, general physical screening, and the provision of preventive health care services at age 13–15 years. It is reasonable to observe even those who are not sexually active in each stage of adolescence: early adolescence, ages 13–15; middle adolescence, ages 15–17; and late adolescence, ages 17–19.

Unfortunately, many adolescents do not seek health care until after first intercourse. In the United States, the median age of first sexual intercourse is 16.5 years, but as many as 7% of adolescents report their first vaginal intercourse before 13 years of age.

After the history is taken, the patient should be given a brief description of what the examination entails. Girls under the age of 18 years should be informed that pelvic examination is not necessary unless medically indicated, yet an external genital examination can provide an opportunity to familiarize adolescents with normal anatomy and allow the practitioner an opportunity to visualize the perineum for any anomalies. The girl should be assured that any examination will not be painful. While performing the physical examination, the health care provider should reassure the adolescent about her normal anatomy and proper development. Following the examination, the patient is given an opportunity to speak alone with the examiner. Confidentiality is essential to the physician–patient relationship, and problems can be discussed with the patient's guardians only with the patient's consent.

The examination should start with general inspection. A breast examination is an integral part of the physical examination of every female patient, followed by abdominal palpation.

The examination is also used to provide the patient with health maintenance instructions and explanations about her body and its various functions. Many adolescents are not familiar with the appearance of their own genitalia. Some physicians use mirrors during the examination to show normal anatomic details, to demonstrate abnormalities, and to provide explanations regarding health maintenance. Others use a colposcope attached to a video monitor; this provides an enlarged image seen simultaneously by the examiner and the patient and permits direct communication.

The introitus of most virginal adolescents is approximately 1 cm in diameter and will admit a narrow speculum when clinically indicated. The Huffman-Graves and Pedersen specula both are designed to allow for easy inspection of the cervix in adolescents, in whom the vagina is 10–12 cm long (Fig. 37–6). In a patient with a large hymenal opening, bimanual examination is performed by inserting a finger into the vagina. If the hymenal orifice is too small for digital examination, rectal examination can be performed.

All sexually active girls should be screened annually for chlamydia and gonorrhea. Urine-based sexually transmitted infection (STI) testing is an efficient means for accomplishing such screening without speculum examination.

The gynecologic visit serves as an excellent opportunity to review basic health care maintenance. For example, current recommendations advise universal vaccination for hepatitis B for all adolescents at ages 11–12 years, with immunization for older adolescents based on risk status and discussion regarding human papillomavirus vaccine.

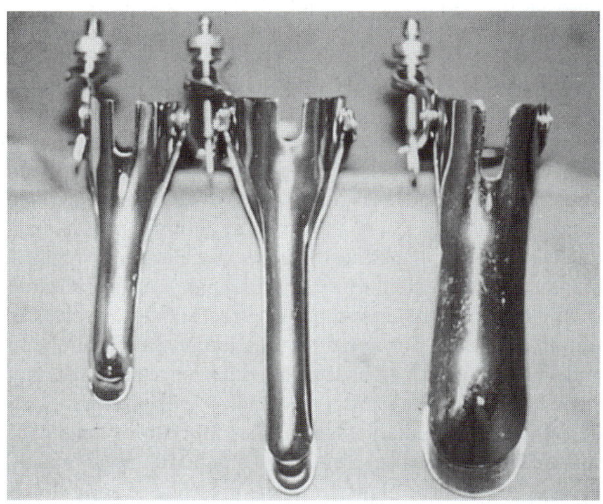

▲ **Figure 37–6.** The Huffman-Graves speculum **(middle)** is as long as the adult Graves speculum **(right)** and as narrow as the short pediatric Graves speculum **(left)**.

In addition, screening for eating disorders, depression, and behavioral risks including sexual activity and tobacco, alcohol, and substance abuse should be done routinely. To assist providers of adolescent health care, the American Medical Association has issued recommendations based on annual health guidance, screening, and immunization schedules. For more information regarding specific legal rights for adolescents, the Guttmacher Institute has established a Web site for practitioner assistance (www.guttmacher.org).

ACOG Committee on Gynecological Practice. ACOG committee opinion No. 431: Routine pelvic examination and cervical cytology screening. *Obstet Gynecol* 2009;113:1190–1193. PMID: 19384150.

Examination of the Young Victim of Sexual Abuse

Studies show that approximately 38% of girls are sexually victimized before age 18 years. Among adolescent girls in grades 9–12, 26% report experiencing physical or sexual abuse. Therefore, all adolescents should be asked about history of abuse. Many children who are possible victims of sexual abuse are brought to a hospital emergency room or to their physician's office for a comprehensive medical evaluation. Statutes vary from state to state as to the need for legal consent from a parent or guardian to perform a genital examination and collect evidence in cases of suspected abuse.

A. History

In some facilities, a designated individual conducts an investigative interview to minimize repetitive questioning of the child. When asking young children about abuse, line drawings, dolls, or other aids are generally used only by professionals trained in interviewing young children. However, this does not preclude the physician from asking relevant questions to obtain a detailed history, a review of systems, and basic information about the assault. An account of the incident is extremely valuable, as it can later be used in court as evidence, or it may reveal an unusual area of injury and thus uncommon sites for collection of evidence. It is important to know how and from whom the patient sustained the injury and whether the child is in a safe environment.

It is imperative that the clinician use questions that are not leading, avoid showing strong emotions such as shock or disbelief, and maintain a "tell me more" or "and then what happened" approach. The courts have allowed physicians to testify regarding specific details of the child's statements obtained in the course of taking a medical history to provide a diagnosis and treatment. The American Academy of Child and Adolescent Psychiatry and the American Professional Society on the Abuse of Children have published guidelines for interviewing sexually abused children.

The examiner should note the patient's composure, behavior, and mental state, as well as how she interacts with her parents and other persons. Victims of physical or sexual abuse must be removed immediately from an unsafe environment.

The information should be recorded carefully, using the patient's own words. Written notes in the medical record or audiotape or videotape should be used to document the questions asked and the child's responses. Although a detailed history is desirable, the victim should not be made to repeatedly recount the incident. When obtaining a history from a very young child is not possible, the physician should obtain accounts of the incident from other sources.

B. Physical Examination

The physical examination has 2 purposes: to detect and treat injuries and to collect samples that later can be used as evidence.

1. Detection of injuries—Nonspecific findings are relatively common in young children. Vulvar irritation is often seen in small children as a result of poor local hygiene, maceration of the skin because of wetness from diapers, or excoriations caused by local infection. Such nonspecific findings should not be regarded as diagnostic of sexual abuse. It is important to remember that the examination is often normal in most children who were sexually abused. In one study of 2384 children who were seen in a tertiary referral center, <5% had genital findings suggesting abuse. The examination was deemed normal in 96.3% of children referred for the evaluation. Even so, interviews of the children indicated that 68% of the girls reported penetration of vagina or anus.

The physician should be familiar with normal genital anatomy, particularly that of the hymen, and should be able to distinguish hymenal trauma. A "clock system" approach is applied to describe hymen lacerations, which usually appear in the form of notches and clefts in the posterior rim between 3 and 9 o' clock. Studies showing that partial tears of the hymen, as well as abrasions and contusions, may heal to leave very little or no sign of previous injury emphasize the importance of urgent evaluations. Additional methods to demonstrate hymenal continuity involve saline irrigation on the posterior rim of the hymen or gentle pulling of Foley catheter balloon against the hymenal margins. In postpubertal girls, penetration and stretch trauma can result in hymeneal remnants.

2. Collection of evidence—During the general inspection, all foreign material (eg, sand and grass) should be removed and placed in clearly labeled envelopes. Scrapings from underneath the fingernails and loose hairs on the skin are collected. Semen can be detected on the skin many hours after the assault. A Wood's lamp can be used to detect the presence of seminal fluid on the patient's body, because the ultraviolet light causes semen to fluoresce. The stain can be lifted off the skin with moistened cotton swabs for further analysis.

If vaginal penetration is suspected, vaginal fluid is collected and sent for sexual disease evaluation, wet-mount preparation, cytology, acid phosphatase determination, and enzyme p30. To avoid additional psychological trauma in a prepubescent child, these specimens can be collected without the insertion of a pediatric speculum, via vaginal aspiration using a feeding tube or Angiocath. An immediate wet-mount preparation done by the examining physician may detect motile sperm.

Culture swabs are obtained from the rectum, vagina, urethra, and pharynx. Current data indicate that a prepubertal child with gonorrhea or trichomonas most likely had genital–genital contact. The mode of transmission of other STIs is controversial. Testing for STIs, including human immunodeficiency virus (HIV), should be offered. In pubertal girls, postcoital contraception should be recommended.

All specimens must be clearly labeled and the containers and envelopes sealed and signed by the examiner. All persons handling the materials must sign for them. Such a system is necessary to maintain the chain of evidence; otherwise, these specimens may not be admissible in court. Some hospitals provide preassembled "rape kits" that guide the examiner in documenting and collecting specimens in a manner suitable for legal uses.

If an STI or other signs of abuse are found, all states require that the findings be reported to child protective service agencies for investigation of sexual abuse. Furthermore, it is important to keep in mind that a normal physical examination does not exclude the possibility of sexual abuse.

CONGENITAL ANOMALIES OF THE FEMALE GENITAL TRACT

The reproductive organs in the female consist of external genitalia, internal duct system (the müllerian ducts), and the gonads. These 3 components originate embryologically from different primordia. External genitalia, including the lower part of vagina, are formed predominantly from the urogenital sinus. The müllerian (paramesonephric) duct system, after complex developmental changes, ends with a final configuration of fallopian tubes, the uterine corpus and cervix, and the upper portion of the vagina. The gonads are derived from the endoderm beneath the coelomic epithelium (detailed embryologic development is described in Chapter 2).

The etiology of these defects is not fully understood. Most forms are of isolated occurrence. Müllerian duct and urogenital sinus malformations are inherited in a polygenic/multifactorial fashion. Considering the influence of embryologic development on adjacent structures (gastrointestinal and urinary systems), one may encounter associated malformations in those systems as well.

ANOMALIES OF EXTERNAL GENITALIA

ANOMALIES OF THE VULVA & LABIA

Minor differences in the contour or size of vulvar structures are not unusual. Often there is considerable variation in the distance between the posterior fourchette and the anus or between the urethra and the clitoris. Rare anomalies of the vulva include bifid clitoris, a caudal appendage resembling a tail; congenital prolapse of the vagina; and variations in the insertion of the bulbocavernosus muscle, which may alter the appearance of the labia majora and at times obliterate the fossa navicularis. Duplication of the vulva is an extremely rare anomaly, which may be associated with duplication of the urinary or intestinal tracts.

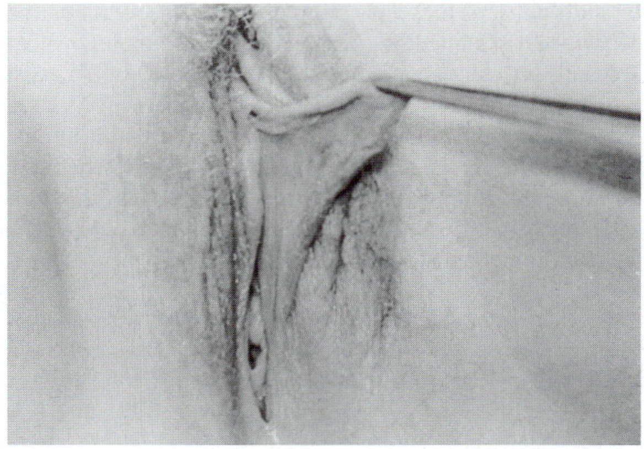

▲ **Figure 37–7.** Labial asymmetry resulting from enlargement of the left labium minor.

There is considerable variation in the size and shape of the labia minora. One of the labia may be considerably larger than the other, or both labia may be unusually large. These variations usually require no treatment (Fig. 37–7). If asymmetry is significant or if large labia are pulled into the vagina during intercourse, the hypertrophied labia can be trimmed surgically to provide a more symmetric appearance or to relieve dyspareunia.

ANOMALIES OF THE CLITORIS

Clitoral enlargement almost invariably suggests exposure to elevated levels of androgens. Such enlargement is often associated with fusion of the labioscrotal folds and could be part of the sexual ambiguity and disorders of sex development. Recklinghausen's neurofibromatosis, lymphangiomas, and fibromas may also involve the clitoris and cause enlargement. When an isolated neoplasm causes enlargement of the clitoris, therapy consists of excision of the neoplasm with reduction of the clitoris to normal size.

In children with disorders of sex development, clitoral reduction is often performed as part of therapy once the diagnosis is made and a female gender is assigned. Many techniques have been described. Although the surgery is often performed in early childhood, the long-term effects on sexual function are unknown. A recent study of 39 adults who had intersex conditions with ambiguous genitalia and who were living as females showed that those who had undergone clitoral surgery had higher rates of nonsensuality and of inability to achieve orgasm. The authors concluded that sexual function of adult females could be compromised by clitoral surgery.

ANOMALIES OF THE HYMEN

Hymenal anomalies result from incomplete degeneration of the central portion of the membrane. Variations include imperforate, microperforate, septate, and cribriform hymens. Hymenal anomalies require surgical correction if they block vaginal secretions or menstrual fluid, interfere with intercourse, or preclude the use of tampons.

Providers should be aware that there have been reports of familial occurrence of hymenal abnormalities and thus alert young women that their daughters may have a similar abnormality.

Imperforate Hymen

Imperforate hymen has an incidence of 1 in 1000 and represents a persistent portion of the urogenital membrane. It occurs when the mesoderm of the primitive streak abnormally invades the urogenital portion of the cloacal membrane. The normal perforation occurs late in fetal life. When mucocolpos develops from accumulation of vaginal secretions behind the hymen, the membrane is seen as a shiny, thin bulge (Fig. 37–8). The distended vagina forms a large mass that may interfere with urination and at times may be mistaken for an abdominal tumor. The diagnosis is quite easy, and resection of the hymen is recommended in the symptomatic infant only. Topical anesthetic is used to prevent discomfort to the newborn, and the central portion of the obstructing membrane is excised. Aspiration should be avoided due to the risks of recurrence and ascending infection. Asymptomatic girls can be monitored throughout childhood, with the optimal time for surgery being just after the onset of puberty.

Imperforate hymen often is not diagnosed until an adolescent presents with complaints of primary amenorrhea and cyclic pelvic pain. It may present as back pain or

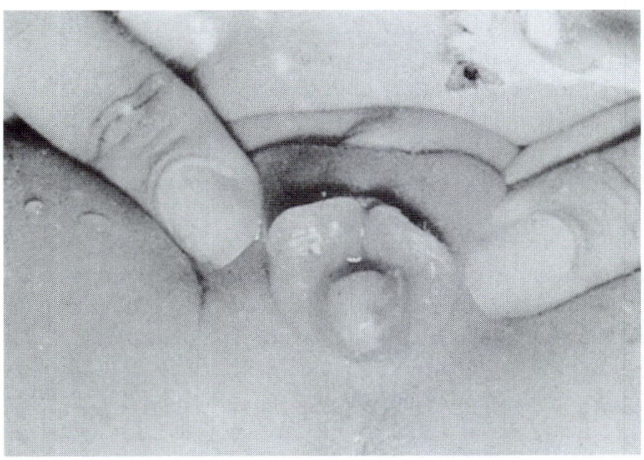

▲ **Figure 37–8.** Mucocolpos in a newborn infant.

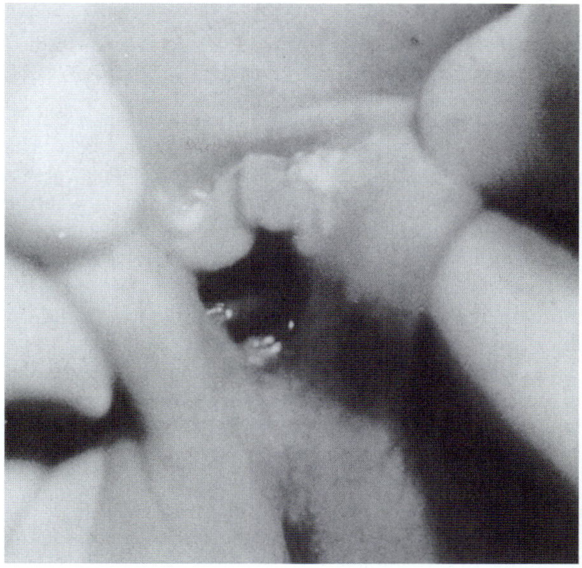

▲ **Figure 37–9.** Newborn infant following excision of an imperforate hymen. Forward traction on the labia majora provides an unimpaired view of the hymenal ring. Note the large opening created. No bleeding was noted, and no sutures were required.

difficulty with defecation or urination secondary to mass effect from vaginal distention. Inspection of the vulva may reveal a purplish-red hymenal membrane bulging outward as a result of accumulation of blood above it (hematocolpos) (Fig. 37–9). Blood may fill the uterus (hematometra) and spill through the fallopian tubes into the peritoneal cavity. Endometriosis and vaginal adenosis are known but not inevitable complications.

The procedure is usually done under general anesthesia with the patient in lithotomy position. A Foley catheter is used to drain the bladder and properly delineate the urethra. A primary small crescentic incision is done in the central part of hymenal bulging membrane; after evacuation of the old blood, the hymenal orifice should be enlarged to allow the egress of menstrual flow, tampon use, and eventually comfortable sexual intercourse. A small incision may coalesce, allowing the obstructing membrane to reform.

ANOMALIES OF INTERNAL DUCT SYSTEM

The actual incidence of müllerian anomalies is not definitively known. An incidence of 3.2% was identified in several studies on fertile women. Urinary tract abnormalities are the most common anomalies associated with müllerian defects, including ipsilateral renal agenesis, duplex collecting systems, renal duplication, and horseshoe kidneys. In female patients with renal anomalies, the incidence of genital defects is estimated to be between 25% and 89%.

ANOMALIES OF THE VAGINA

1. Transverse Vaginal Septum

Transverse vaginal septa result from faulty fusion or canalization of the urogenital sinus and müllerian ducts. The incidence is approximately 1 in 30,000 to 1 in 80,000 women. Approximately 46% occur in the upper vagina, 40% in the midportion, and 14% in the lower vagina. When the septum is located in the upper vagina, it is likely to be patent, whereas those located in the lower part of the vagina are more often complete. The septum is usually less than 1 cm thick and is rarely associated with uterine anomalies.

A complete septum results in signs and symptoms similar to those of an imperforate hymen. Diagnosis is often delayed until after menarche, when menstrual blood is trapped behind an obstructing membrane. An incomplete septum usually is asymptomatic at menarche, as the central aperture allows for vaginal secretions and menstrual flow to egress from the vagina. The first symptoms may appear at the beginning of sexual intercourse, resulting in dyspareunia.

Treatment

If the diagnosis of a complete septum is established prior to menarche, ultrasound or magnetic resonance imaging (MRI) may help define the septum and its thickness preoperatively. It is extremely important to identify a cervix, most reliably seen on MRI, to differentiate between a high septum and congenital absence of the cervix. The corrective surgery consists of septum incision, creating an aperture to allow drainage. Incision of a complete septum is most easily accomplished when the upper vagina is distended and the membrane is bulging, reducing the risk of injury to adjacent structures. Because of the technical difficulties in performing intravaginal surgery on immature structures, it is best to limit the procedure only to allow the establishment of vaginal drainage.

Surgical correction of vaginal narrowing should be performed only when the patient is contemplating initiation of sexual activity. Thin septum can be excised with its surrounding ring of subepithelial connective tissue at the level of partition followed by primary end-to-end anastomosis of the upper and lower vaginal mucosa; thicker septum may require undermining and mobilization of the upper and lower vaginal mucosa before anastomosis. To avoid scar contracture and vaginal stenosis, a circumferential Z-plasty can be helpful. Postoperatively, use of vaginal mold or dilators may further decrease the risk of vaginal stenosis.

2. Longitudinal Vaginal Septum

Longitudinal vaginal septum forms when the distal ends of the müllerian ducts fail to fuse properly. The uterus may be septate or bicornuate, with 1 or 2 cervices (Fig. 37–10). As many as 20% of patients with *longitudinal vaginal septum* may present with associated renal abnormalities and occasionally with anorectal malformations, including imperforated anus with rectovestibular fistula and cloaca.

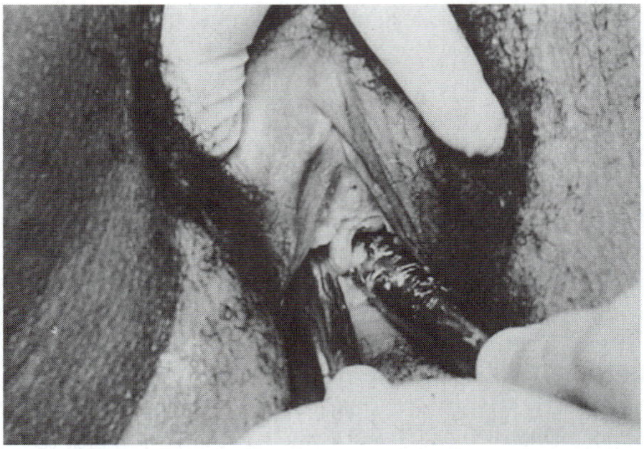

▲ **Figure 37–10.** Longitudinal septum dividing the vagina.

Asymptomatic longitudinal septum requires no treatment. Division of the septum is indicated when dyspareunia is present, vaginal delivery dystocia is anticipated, or worsening of dysmenorrhea occurs. The menstrual pain derives from accumulation of blood in obstructed hemivagina, while normal blood exits from the nonobstructed portion. Care should be taken to avoid damage to the cervix while resecting the upper part of the septum.

3. Vaginal Agenesis (Müllerian Aplasia)

Vaginal agenesis includes the congenital absence of the vagina accompanied by variable müllerian duct development (**Mayer-Rokitansky-Kuster-Hauser [MRKH] syndrome**). The incidence of vaginal agenesis is approximately 1 in 5000. The external genitalia of patients with vaginal agenesis are normal or may reveal only a small dimple at the vaginal introitus (Fig. 37–11). Vaginal agenesis is usually accompanied by cervical and uterine agenesis; however, 7–10% of affected individuals may have a normal uterus or rudimentary uterus with functional endometrium.

Other developmental defects are often present, affecting the urinary tract (45–50%), the spine (10%), and, less frequently, the middle ear and other mesodermal structures. Evaluation of those systems should be performed soon after diagnosis.

Persons with vaginal agenesis typically have normal female karyotypes with normal ovaries and ovarian function; thus, they develop normal secondary sexual attributes. Patients often present with primary amenorrhea or, in women with functioning uteri, with cyclic pelvic pain. Serum testosterone level and karyotyping may identify the rare instances in which müllerian agenesis represents the effects of testicular activity, indicating male pseudohermaphroditism.

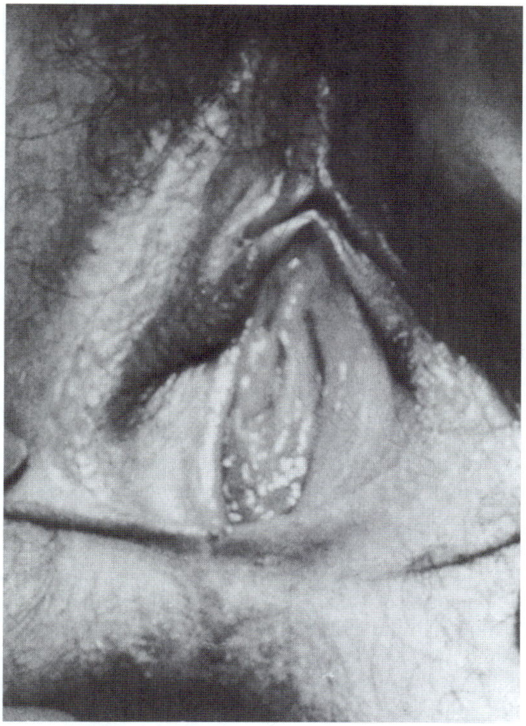

▲ **Figure 37–11.** Vaginal agenesis in a girl 16 years of age.

Treatment

The consultation of the adolescent with vaginal agenesis and her family involves a multidisciplinary approach. It should consist of confirmation of the ability to create a functional vagina and emphasize that she has normal ovarian function and thus preserved fertility with assisted reproductive technology and surrogacy.

Creation of a satisfactory vagina is the objective of treatment of vaginal agenesis. Treatment should be deferred until the patient is contemplating sexual activity. Nonoperative creation of a vagina using serial vaginal dilators, in a method described by Frank and later modified by Ingram, is relatively risk-free but requires patient motivation and cooperation. The procedure takes a few months to complete. Repetitive coitus can also be used to create a functioning vagina. Recent studies have shown that use of dilators resulted in 85–90% success for creation of functional vagina.

Surgical creation of neovagina is another option, and discussion should fully describe that many surgical techniques will require postoperative dilatation to maintain vaginal adequacy. Currently, there are multiple operative methods but no consensus on the best approach.

The modified Abbé–McIndoe vaginoplasty is most commonly performed. The procedure involves the creation of a cavity by surgical dissection between the urethra and bladder anteriorly and the perineal body and rectum posteriorly. The cavity is lined by a split-thickness skin graft overlying a plastic or soft silicone mold. The labia minora are secured around the mold for 7 days prior to removal. Postoperatively, the patient must continue to use dilators for several months to maintain vaginal patency. Patient satisfaction rates greater than 80% have been reported. Complications include graft failure, hematoma, fistula formation, and rectal perforation.

The laparoscopic Davydov technique uses the patient's own pelvic peritoneum to line the neovagina. It involves dissection of the perineum to create a neovaginal space while laparoscopically mobilizing the peritoneum. The peritoneum is then sutured to the introitus, and a purse-string suture closes the cranial end of the neovagina. A vaginal mold is left in situ for 6 weeks, and the patient then begins daily dilation until regularly sexually active. Complications related to laparoscopic injury and fistula formation have occurred; however, patients report similar sexual function to women with a native vagina.

The modified laparoscopic Vecchietti procedure creates a dilation-like neovagina in 7–9 days. It involves placement of an acrylic 2-cm olive-shaped bead onto the vaginal dimple that is gradually pulled superiorly by threads laparoscopically placed that are then connected to the traction device placed on the patient's abdomen. The threads are then gradually tightened approximately 1.0–1.5 cm per day for a week. Postoperatively, the patients must comply with daily vaginal dilation until regularly sexually active.

Bowel vaginoplasty is the preferred method of most pediatric general surgeons, given the immediate and long-term correction of the anomaly. Each bowel segment has advantages and disadvantages. Bowel vaginoplasty is performed by selecting an approximately 10-cm segment of bowel that can be mobilized but retain an adequate vascular pedicle to reach the perineum. Sigmoid vaginoplasty has been the most commonly used bowel segment, given its proximity to the perineum and therefore little difficulty performing a tension-free anastomosis to the introitus.

Postoperative sexual satisfaction has been assessed in a validated fashion in only a relatively small number of patients who underwent bowel vaginoplasty. Seventy-five percent of patients reported satisfaction.

4. Partial Vaginal Agenesis (Atresia)

Vaginal atresia occurs when the urogenital sinus fails to contribute to the lower portion of the vagina. The affected segment of the vagina is replaced by a soft mass of tissue. The cause of this uncommon anomaly is unknown. Absence of the distal vagina may be identified by sonographic visualization of the accumulated blood in the upper vagina, cervix, and uterus.

The symptoms are similar to those associated with imperforate hymen after the menarche. Vulvar inspection reveals findings identical with those of vaginal agenesis, but rectoabdominal palpation reveals a large, boggy pelvic mass. Diagnostic imaging using sonography, computed tomography (CT), or MRI will confirm the diagnosis.

Treatment

Surgery is indicated because obstruction to menstrual flow may occur. In some patients, drainage of the uterus can be achieved through a reconstructed vagina. In others, particularly when the uterus is rudimentary, consideration may be given to performing a hysterectomy.

ANOMALIES OF THE UTERUS

Uterine anomalies result from agenesis of the müllerian duct or a defect in fusion or canalization. The classification by the American Society for Reproductive Medicine (ASRM) is most accepted. These anomalies include bicornuate uterus (37%), arcuate uterus (15%), incomplete septum (13%), uterine didelphys (11%), complete septum (9%), and unicornuate uterus (4%).

Most uterine anomalies are asymptomatic and therefore are not detected during childhood or early adolescence. Symptoms during adolescence are primarily caused by retention of menstrual flow. MRI can be helpful in determining the anatomy in cases complicated by obstructive anomalies and is often considered as the "gold standard" for imaging of anomalies in reproductive tract (Fig. 37–12).

Asymptomatic abnormalities often escape detection until they interfere with reproduction; thus, they are described in more detail in other chapters of this text.

1. Unicornuate Uterus & Rudimentary Uterine Horn

A unicornuate uterus is a single-horned uterus with its corresponding fallopian tube and round ligament. It results from agenesis of 1 müllerian duct, with absence of structures on that side. When the other hemiuterus is present, it often creates a small rudimentary uterine horn. If this rudimentary horn does not communicate with the other uterine cavity or the vagina, menstrual blood cannot escape, resulting in severe dysmenorrhea, hematometra, or pyometra. A pregnancy that occurs in a rudimentary horn may result in rupture, a complication that is potentially fatal for both mother and fetus (Fig. 37–13).

Ideally, a rudimentary horn should be resected before conception. The tube and ovary on the affected side can be preserved, provided that the blood supply is not impaired. If the endometrial cavity of the remaining horn is entered during the operation, caesarean section is a reasonable mode of delivery for any subsequent pregnancies.

As suspected with unilateral impairment in müllerian development, associated renal anomalies are common. Patients with müllerian anomalies with a unicornuate uterus are at increased risk of premature labor and breech presentation. As in other obstructive anomalies, endometriosis and subsequent fertility issues may be significant in patients with an associated obstructed uterine horn or hemiuterus (Fig. 37–14).

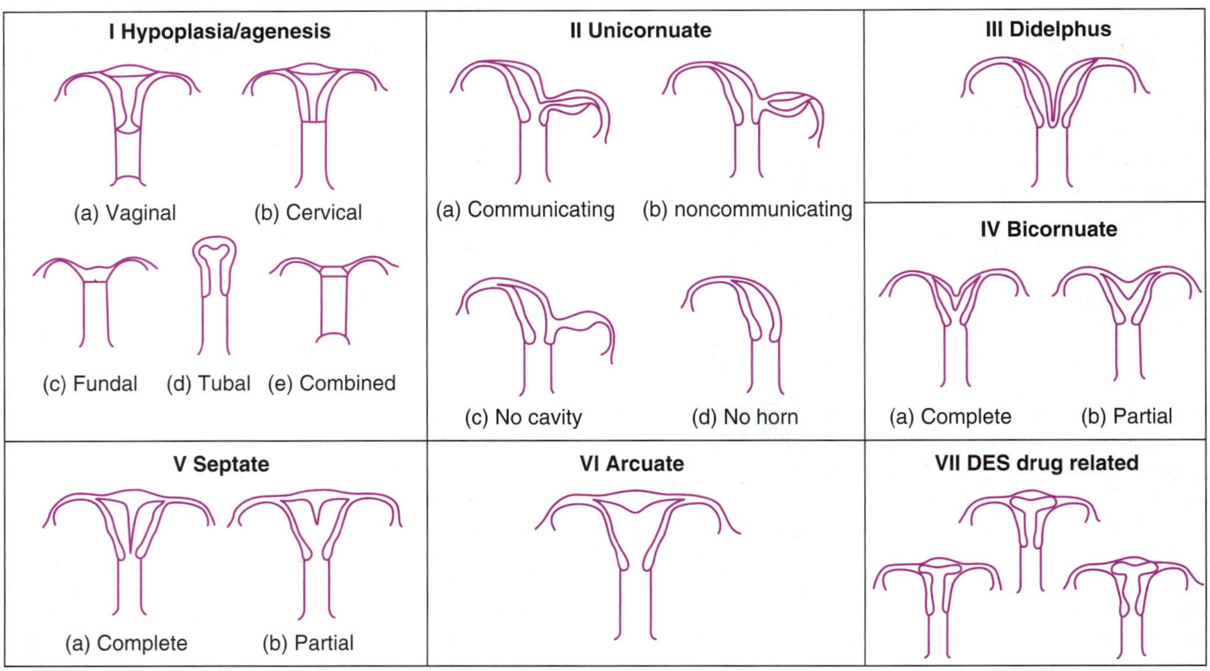

▲ **Figure 37–12.** Classification system of müllerian duct anomalies developed by the American Fertility Society (1998). DES, diethylstilbestrol. (Reproduced, with permission, from the American Society for Reproductive Medicine, copyright 2012.)

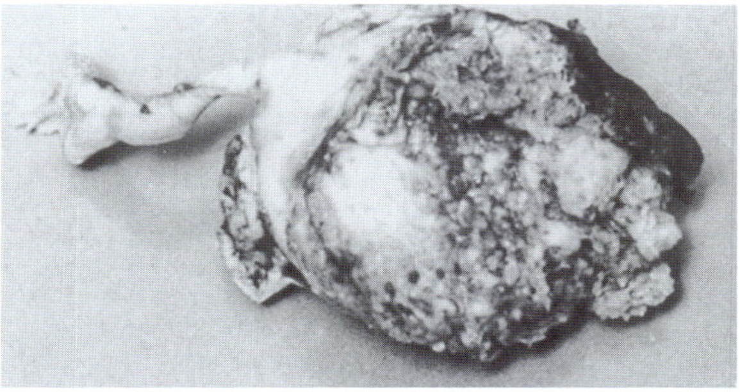

▲ **Figure 37–13.** Pregnancy in a noncommunicating rudimentary uterine horn that has resulted in rupture.

2. Bicornuate Uterus & Septate Uterus

The bicornuate uterus results from partial fusion of the müllerian ducts, leading to varying degrees of separation of the uterine horns. The fundus is deeply indented, often heart-shaped. Presently, no surgical intervention is recommended, and patients are followed closely for obstetric concerns, although reproductive function is good overall. In most cases, the vagina is normal.

The septate uterus has a smooth, normal external surface at the fundus, but the endometrial cavity is split into 2 by a midline septum. There are higher risks for miscarriage and other obstetrical complications. Hysteroscopic resection of septum is currently the technique of choice and almost totally replaces abdominal metroplasty. The surgical correction may improve reproductive performance. However, in young women, the decision to surgically intervene before attempts at pregnancy still remains unclear. The presence of a concomitant vaginal septum may influence the timing of intervention.

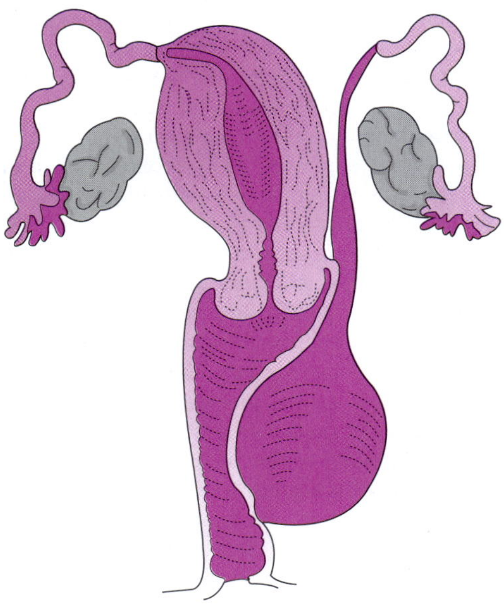

▲ **Figure 37–14.** Unicornuate uterus with obstructed hemivagina. The endometrium lining the obstructed part bleeds at menarche, and the blood filling the lower part of the cyst forms a mass that protrudes into the vagina.

ANOMALIES OF THE OVARIES

During development, the ovaries, which are abdominally located in the neonate, descend to the pelvis at puberty. The ovaries may be drawn by the round ligament into the inguinal canal or the labium major. A firm inguinal mass should alert the examiner to the possible presence of an aberrant gonad, possibly containing testicular elements, even in the presence of female external genitalia. A karyotype should be obtained. At the time of hernia repair, the gonad should be biopsied. If it proves to be an ovary, it should be returned to the peritoneal cavity and the hernia repaired. If a testis is identified, the gonad should be removed. During childhood, the ovary is never at rest, and follicles grow and degenerate continuously.

Gonadal Dysgenesis (Turner's Syndrome)

Turner's syndrome is a disorder in females characterized by the absence of all or part of a normal second sex chromosome. Approximately half of patients have monosomy X (45,X). Most of the rest have mosaicism for 45,X, with 1 or more additional cell lineages, and others (5–10%) have a duplication (isochromosome) of the long arm of 1 X chromosome [46,X,i(Xq)]. Turner's syndrome occurs in 1 in 2500 to 1 in 3000 live-born girls.

The genetic disorder leads to a constellation of physical findings that often includes congenital lymphedema, short stature, and gonadal dysgenesis. In addition, broad chest and small nipples, webbed neck, coarctation of the aorta, renal abnormalities, prominent epicanthal folds, nevi, and other somatic anomalies (eg, short fourth metacarpal) frequently occur. In most adults with gonadal dysgenesis, the normal gonad is replaced by a white fibrous streak, 2–3 cm long and approximately 0.5 cm wide, located in the gonadal ridge. Histologically, the streak gonad is characterized by interlacing waves of dense fibrous stroma, indistinguishable from normal ovarian stroma.

Increased atresia and failure of germ cell formation deplete oocyte supply, but when atresia is incomplete, pubertal changes, spontaneous menstruation, and even pregnancies have been reported.

One-fifth to one-third of affected girls receive a diagnosis as newborns because of puffy hands and feet or redundant nuchal skin. However, in many, the condition is not diagnosed until adolescence when they fail to enter puberty. Turner's syndrome is the most common cause of short stature in otherwise healthy girls; therefore, karyotype testing should be considered in children and adolescents with height stature below the third percentile.

Girls with Turner's syndrome need gonadal hormone therapy for sexual development, enhancement of growth, maintenance of reproductive tissue, and psychosocial health. In addition, prevention of chronic disease, specifically bone loss and possible early heart diseases, needs to be addressed in these girls.

The administration of very-low-dose estradiol (ethinyl estradiol 100 ng/kg/d) in combination with growth hormone at an early age has been shown to assist in enhancing and promoting optimal pubertal height and age-appropriate feminization.

ANOMALIES OF THE URETHRA & ANUS

Failure of a newborn infant to pass meconium or urine demands investigation. Passage of feces or urine through the vagina suggests a fistulous communication, and usually either the urethra or the anus is imperforate.

In general, anomalies are divided into 2 major groups: those that form complete obstruction of the intestinal tract and those that are associated with some type of abnormal opening or fistula.

Because findings are so diverse, only broad generalizations on the management of urogenital anomalies of this type can be offered. Most intestinal and urinary tract obstructions must be corrected soon after birth; however, some associated genital tract anomalies (eg, müllerian anomalies), although diagnosed at the same time, might benefit from postponing final correction until after the onset of puberty.

GYNECOLOGIC DISORDERS IN PREMENARCHAL CHILDREN

VULVOVAGINITIS

Pruritus vulvae and vulvovaginitis are common gynecologic disorders in children. Pruritus vulvae refers to itching of the external female genitalia. Vulvovaginitis, although inconsistently delineated in the literature, generally involves irritation of the skin or mucosal tissue and vaginal discharge. The child is susceptible to both these conditions for several reasons: The prepubertal vulva is thin without labial fat pads and pubic hair, as well as anatomically in close proximity to the anus and its contaminants; the unestrogenized vagina is atrophic with pH ranges excellent for bacterial growth; and perineal hygiene often is suboptimal as supervision declines with age. Table 37–3 lists classification of vulvovaginitis according to cause.

Table 37–3. Classification of vulvovaginitis according to cause.

Nonspecific vulvovaginitis
Polymicrobial infection associated with disturbed homeostasis: secondary to poor perineal hygiene or a foreign body
Vulvovaginitis due to secondary inoculation
Infection resulting from inoculation of the vagina with pathogens affecting other areas of the body by contact or blood-borne transmission: secondary to upper respiratory tract infection or urinary tract infection
Specific vulvovaginitis
Specific primary infection, most commonly sexually transmitted: *Neisseria gonorrhoeae, Gardnerella vaginalis, herpesvirus, Treponema pallidum*, others

Clinical Findings

Acute vulvovaginitis may denude the thin vulvar or vaginal mucosa; however, bleeding usually is minimal. Vaginal discharge may vary from minimal to copious mucopurulent, and at times, it is blood-stained. Symptoms vary from minor discomfort to relatively intense perineal pruritus. The child often complains of a burning sensation, particularly when urine flows, accompanied by a foul-smelling discharge. Vulvovaginitis should be excluded in children prior to treatment for urinary tract infection. The irritating discharge inflames the vulva and often causes the child to scratch the area to the point of bleeding. Inspection of the vagina reveals an area of redness and soreness that may be minimal or may extend laterally to the thighs and backward to the anus.

Diagnosis is suspected by the typical appearance of the inflamed tissue. A wet-mount preparation reveals numerous leukocytes and occasional red blood cells. Culture of vaginal secretions sometimes identifies the offending organism.

Evaluation of the vaginal secretions may include smears for Gram stain, bacterial cultures, cultures for mycotic organisms, wet prep, *Trichomonas*, and parasitic ova.

Improvement of perineal hygiene is important to relieve the symptoms and to prevent recurrences. Most cases of nonspecific pruritus vulvae resolve with improvements in hygiene and avoidance of irritants, including soaps.

Any evidence of pathogens that are usually involved in STIs must be followed by evaluation of sexual abuse.

Amoxicillin (20–40 mg/kg/d in 3 divided doses) is effective against a variety of potentially pathogenic organisms in nonspecific vulvovaginitis. A concomitant tonsillitis should raise the suspicion of genital inoculation by *Streptococcus* group A pathogens and should be treated the same way as the throat infection. In cases with intense perianal pruritus that is especially bothersome during the night, antiparasitic treatment could alleviate the symptoms. Infection with *Candida* species is quite rare in healthy children after diaper weaning until the onset of puberty. When the infection is severe and extensive mucosal damage is seen, a short course of topical estrogen cream is given to promote healing of vulvar and vaginal tissues. When irritation is intense, hydrocortisone cream may be necessary to alleviate the itch. In recurrent infections refractory to treatment or associated with a foul-smelling, bloody discharge, vaginoscopy is necessary to exclude a foreign body or tumor.

FOREIGN BODIES

Vaginal foreign bodies induce an intense inflammatory reaction and result in blood-stained, foul-smelling discharge. Usually, the child does not recall inserting the foreign object or will not admit to it. Radiographs are not reliable for revealing a foreign body because many objects are not radiopaque, the most common being a small piece of reincarnated toilet paper. Foreign bodies in the lower third of the vagina can be flushed out with warm saline irrigation. If the vagina cannot be adequately inspected in the office even after removal of the foreign body, vaginoscopy is indicated to confirm that no other foreign bodies are present in the upper vagina. General anesthesia is applied in some cases, based on the age and psychosocial development of the patient.

URETHRAL PROLAPSE

Occasionally, vulvar bleeding is the result of urethral prolapse. The urethral mucosa protrudes through the meatus and forms a hemorrhagic, sensitive vulvar mass that is separated from the vagina. Treatment consists of warm soaks and a short course of therapy using estrogen cream, when the lesion is small and urination is unimpaired. Resection of the prolapsed tissue should be reserved for a symptomatic child with indwelling catheter inserted for 24 hours after surgery.

LICHEN SCLEROSUS

Lichen sclerosus of the vulva is a hypotrophic dystrophy with prevalence of 1 in 900 girls. It has bimodal age distribution in postmenopausal period and in prepubertal age. Histologically, the findings in both age groups are similar, with flattening of the rete pegs, hyalinization of the subdermal tissues, and keratinization.

The clinical presentation includes a whitish ivory colored lesion that does not extend beyond the middle of the labia majora laterally or into the vagina medially (Fig. 37–15). The clitoris, posterior fourchette, and anorectal areas are frequently involved, forming a figure of 8. Although most lesions are predominantly white, some have pronounced vascular markings. They tend to bruise easily, forming bloody blisters, and they are susceptible to secondary infections. Symptoms consist of intense pruritus, vulvar irritation, and dysuria. Scratching is common and occasionally provokes bleeding or leads to secondary infection and introital distortion.

Histologic confirmation is not necessary in children as opposed to postmenopausal women because of no known malignant potential in this age group. Treatment usually consists of improved local hygiene and reduction of trauma. Currently, the use of ultrapotent topical corticosteroids (clobetasol propionate 0.05%) once or twice daily for 4–8 weeks is accepted as first-line therapy. Occasionally, symptom relief does not occur before 12 weeks of treatment. New treatments with topical calcineurin inhibitors seem to be effective; however, their long-term safety has not been determined. Over half of children improve significantly or recover during puberty.

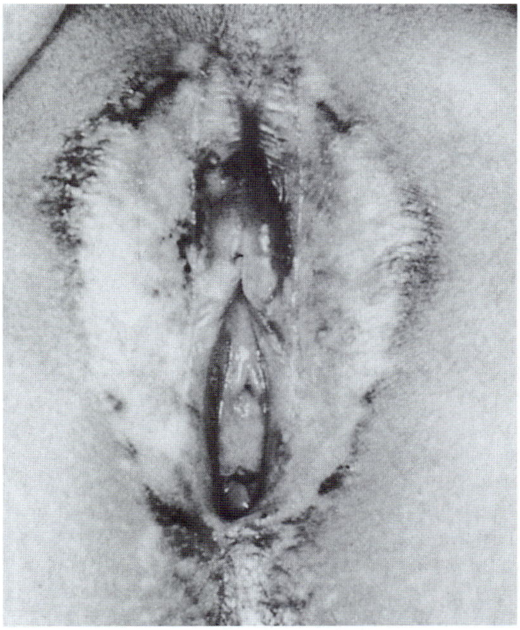

▲ **Figure 37–15.** Lichen sclerosus of the vulva in a 6-year-old child.

LABIAL ADHESION

Labial adhesion is common in prepubertal children with an estimated occurrence of 0.6–3.0% and a peak incidence at 13–23 months. The cause is not known but probably is related to low estrogen levels. The skin covering the labia is extremely thin, and local irritation may induce scratching, which may denude the labia. The labia then adhere in the midline, and re-epithelialization occurs on both sides (Fig. 37–16). It is important to differentiate this condition from congenital absence of the vagina.

Most children with small areas of labial adhesions are asymptomatic. Dysuria and recurrent urinary infections are cardinal symptoms in those with complete or anterior adhesion, although infrequent.

Asymptomatic minimal to moderate labial fusion does not require treatment. Symptomatic fusion may be treated with a course of estrogen cream applied twice daily for 3–12 weeks resulting in successful separation in 50–88% of the cases. When approaching puberty in girls with medical treatment failure or if severe urinary symptoms exist, surgical separation of the labia is indicated. This can be performed in the operating room under anesthesia or as an in-office procedure using 1–2% topical lidocaine (Xylocaine) gel. Because of low estrogen levels, recurrences of labial adhesion are common until puberty. After puberty, the condition resolves spontaneously.

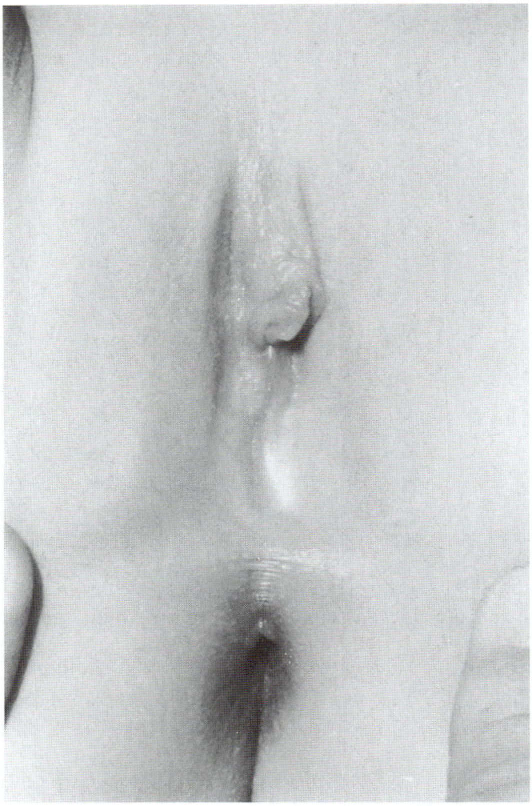

▲ **Figure 37–16.** Labial adhesion in a young girl. Note the translucent vertical line in the center where the labia are fused together.

Improved perineal hygiene and removal of vulvar irritants may help prevent recurrences.

GENITAL INJURIES

Most injuries to the genitalia during childhood are accidental. Many are of minor significance, but a few are life-threatening and require surgical intervention. The physician must determine how the child sustained the injury, bearing in mind that the child requires protection if she is the victim of physical or sexual abuse.

1. Vulvar Injuries

Contusion of the vulva mainly from straddle injury usually does not require treatment. A hematoma manifests as a round, tense, ecchymotic, tender mass (Fig. 37–17). A small vulvar hematoma usually can be controlled by pressure with an ice pack. The vulva should be kept clean and dry. A hematoma that is large or continues to increase in size may require incision, with removal of clotted blood and ligation of bleeding points. If the source of bleeding cannot be found, the cavity should be packed with gauze

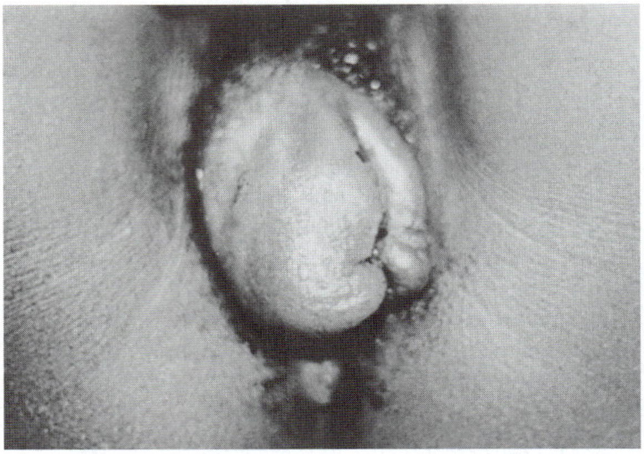

▲ **Figure 37–17.** Large vulvar hematoma secondary to bicycle injury.

and a firm pressure dressing applied. The pack is removed in 24 hours. Prophylactic broad-spectrum antibiotics may be advisable.

When a large hematoma obstructs the urethra, insertion of a catheter is necessary, usually by a suprapubic approach. Radiography of the pelvis may be necessary to rule out pelvic fracture.

2. Vaginal Injuries

Vaginal injuries occur when a girl falls on a sharp object and impales herself; additionally, there is an increasing rate of accidents involving insufflation injuries caused by a fall off jet skis or direct contact with pool or spa jets, allowing pressurized water to enter the vagina. Such injuries might produce no sign of external genital trauma, but careful examination (often under anesthesia) will reveal the extent of injury.

When the hymen is lacerated or other evidence indicates an object has entered the vagina or penetrated the perineum, a detailed examination of the whole vaginal canal is necessary to exclude injuries to the upper vagina or intrapelvic viscera (Fig. 37–18).

Most vaginal injuries involve the lateral walls. Generally, there is relatively little blood loss, and the child does not have much pain if only the mucosa is damaged. If the laceration extends beyond the vaginal vault, exploration of the pelvic cavity is necessary to rule out extension into the broad ligament or peritoneal cavity. Bladder and bowel integrity must be confirmed by catheterization and rectal palpation. Because of the small caliber of the organs involved, special instruments, as well as proper exposure and assistance, may be required for repair of vaginal injuries in young girls. Alternatively, the bleeding may be controlled by angiographic embolization of the bleeding vessel. Many vaginal lacerations are limited to the mucosal and submucosal tissues and are repaired with fine suture material after complete hemostasis is secured.

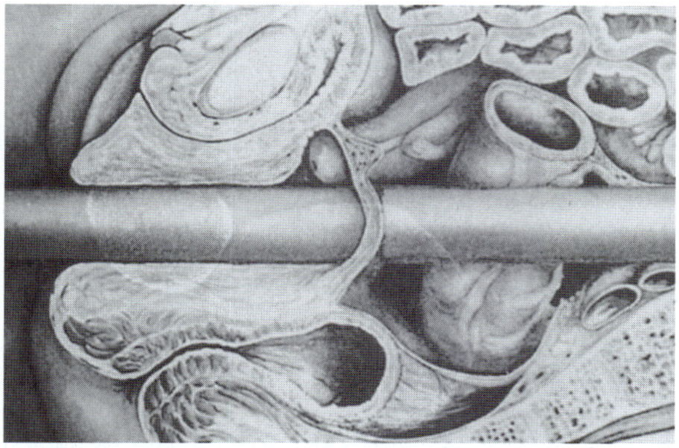

▲ **Figure 37–18.** Transvaginal perforation of cul-de-sac and penetration of peritoneal cavity by a fall on a mop handle. Scanty bleeding from a hymenal tear was the only symptom on admission.

3. Anogenital Injuries Caused by Abuse

Sexual abuse is defined as coerced or forced vaginal, anal, intercrural, and oral–genital fondling or penetration. Many children who are victims of sexual abuse do not sustain physical injuries. The hymen is examined in a "clock"-defined method, being at the 12 o'clock position under the clitoris and 6 o'clock position above the anus, independent of child position during the evaluation. The diagnosis of sex abuse, which was once focused on genital measurements, mainly hymenal configuration, is currently based on descriptive statements made by a child.

The hymen is an elastic structure, and therefore, it does not always demonstrate signs of abuse on examination. In a published study of 2310 children referred for possible sexual abuse, 96.3% of all children had a normal examination. In another study, pregnant adolescents were found to have an intact hymen as well. Unfortunately, even when injured, many of these children may not be seen for weeks, months, or even years after the incident. The delay allows for semen and debris to wash away and for most, if not all, injuries to heal.

Injuries to the vulva may be caused by manipulation of the vulva or introitus, without vaginal penetration, or by friction of the penis against the child's vulva ("dry intercourse"). Erythema, swelling, skin bruising, and excoriations are found on the labia and vestibule. These injuries are superficial and often limited to the vulvar skin; they should resolve within a few days and require no special treatment.

Meticulous perineal hygiene is important in the prevention of secondary infections. Sitz baths should be used to remove secretions and contaminants. In some patients with extensive skin abrasions, broad-spectrum antibiotics should be given as prophylaxis. Large vulvar tears require suturing, which is best performed under general anesthesia. For infected wounds or bites, antitetanus immunization should be given if the child is not already immunized. Broad-spectrum antibiotics should be used for therapy rather than prophylaxis. Most vaginal injuries occur when an object penetrates the vagina through the hymenal opening. A detailed examination including vaginoscopy is necessary to exclude injuries to the upper vagina.

Examination of the anus and rectum is easier than is examination of the vagina, and most children tolerate it well. Because the anal sphincter and anal canal allow for some dilatation, a tear of the anal mucosa or sphincter rarely occurs following a digital assault. However, penetration by a larger object almost always results in some degree of injury, which varies from swelling of the anal verge to gross tearing of the sphincter. In the period immediately following penetration, the main findings are sphincter laxity resulting in anal dilatation, swelling, and small tears of the anal verge. If the sphincter is not severed, it may be in spasm and will not permit a digital examination. Within days, the swelling subsides and the mucosal tears heal, occasionally forming skin tags. If not severed, the anal sphincter regains function. Repeated anal penetration over a prolonged period may cause the anal sphincter to become loose, forming an enlarged opening. The anal mucosa thickens and loses its normal folds. Although some investigators suggest that many children who experience anal assault exhibit perianal scars and tags, longitudinal studies show that anal injuries heal completely in most children.

Occasionally, child victims of abuse contract an STI. The risk of a prepubertal child contracting an STI after sexual assault is relatively low, estimated to range from 2–5%. Treatment of gonorrhea, chlamydia, and syphilis may be deferred until the results of tests become available. A repeat VDRL (Venereal Disease Research Laboratory) test to detect seroconversion is required 6 weeks later. Prophylaxis for hepatitis B with hepatitis B vaccination is recommended following sexual assault. For nonimmune victims with a high-risk exposure, practitioners may also consider adding hepatitis B immune globulin to the regimen. The Sexually Transmitted Diseases Treatment Guidelines do not recommend the routine screening for HIV for all child victims of sexual abuse. Clinicians should try to identify children who are at high risk for HIV exposure and consider offering them counseling and prophylactic therapy. In pubertal girls, the need for postcoital contraception must be addressed. Guidelines for the care of the child and adolescent who has experienced sexual abuse are best found in the literature dedicated to the topic.

Female genital mutilation (female circumcision), which can be viewed as a form of child abuse, is still practiced in some parts of the world. It is estimated that 100–140 million girls and women have undergone some form of female genital mutilation. Victims may suffer from infections, bleeding injury to adjacent tissue, and scarring of the damaged tissue, resulting in urinary and menstrual retention, dyspareunia, and difficulties with childbirth. The World Health Organization and other health organization have openly condemned this practice.

Protective Services & Counseling

It is imperative to ensure that the child will be discharged to a safe environment. When the child is suspected of being a victim of sexual abuse, it is advisable to admit her to the hospital, followed by referral to child protective services for further evaluation.

In the period immediately following sexual assault or disclosure of sexual abuse, the child and her family often require intensive day-to-day emotional support, counseling, and guidance. Child victims often show signs of depression and have feelings of guilt, fear, and low self-esteem. Appropriate referral for counseling is imperative. The major emphasis of emotional support involves strengthening the child's ego, improving her self-image, and helping her to learn to trust others and feel secure again. To begin the strengthening process, the child needs to realize that she was a victim. Often, the child has both positive and negative feelings toward the perpetrator and may need help in sorting out these feelings. The child's relationships with her parents and other family members are critical and may need restructuring. Following this crisis intervention phase, a treatment program using individual and peer-group therapy is initiated.

Adams JA. Guidelines for medical care of children evaluated for suspected sexual abuse: an update for 2008. *Curr Opin Obstet Gynecol* 2008;209:435–441. PMID: 18797265.

Kelly P, Koh J, Thompson JM. Diagnostic findings in alleged sexual abuse: symptoms have no predictive value. *J Paediatr Child Health* 2006;42:112–117. PMID: 16509910.

GENITAL NEOPLASMS

Genital tumors are uncommon but must be considered when a girl is found to have a chronic genital ulcer, nontraumatic swelling of the external genitalia, tissue protruding from the vagina, a fetid or bloody discharge, abdominal pain or enlargement, or premature sexual maturation. Virtually every type of genital neoplasm reported in adults has also been found in girls younger than 14 years. Approximately 50% of the genital tumors in children are premalignant or malignant and account for 1% of all childhood malignancies.

1. Benign Tumors of the Vulva & Vagina

Teratomas, hemangiomas, simple cysts of the hymen, retention cysts of the paraurethral ducts, benign granulomas of the perineum, and condylomata acuminata are some of the benign vulvar neoplasms observed in children and adolescents.

Obstruction of a paraurethral duct may form a relatively large cyst that distorts the urethral orifice. The recommended treatment is surgical intervention.

Teratomas usually present as cystic masses arising from the midline of the perineum. Although a teratoma in this area may be benign, local recurrence is likely. To prevent recurrences, a generous margin of healthy tissue is excised about the periphery of the mass.

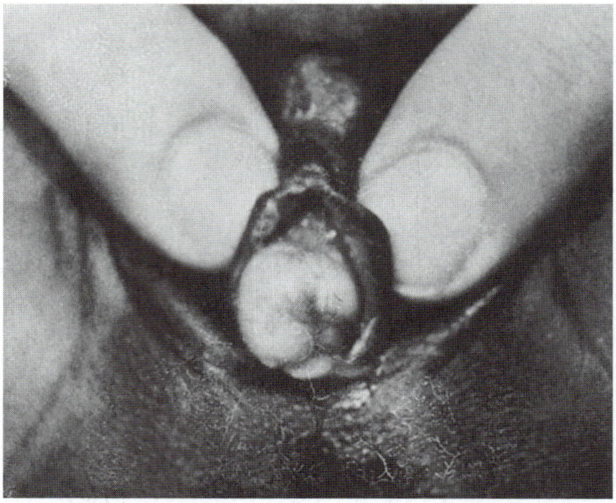

▲ **Figure 37–19.** Simple vulvar or hymeneal cyst arising posterior to the urethra of a newborn infant.

Capillary hemangiomas usually require no therapy except reassurance. However, because of their tendency to bleed, cavernous hemangiomas are best treated surgically.

Most benign tumors of the vagina in children are unilocular cystic remnants of the mesonephric duct (Fig. 37–19) and do not require surgery. Symptomatic cysts (eg, those that block the vagina) can be treated surgically. Removal of a large portion of the cyst wall and marsupialization of the edges, which prevents reaccumulation of fluid, usually are sufficient.

2. Malignant Tumors of the Vagina & Cervix

Botryoid Sarcoma (Embryonal Rhabdomyosarcoma)

Embryonal rhabdomyosarcomas are most commonly seen in very young girls (<3 years old). The tumor usually involves the vagina, but the cervix may be affected as well, particularly in the teenager group, and these tumors have a better prognosis. The clinical presentation is characterized by vaginal bleeding in a child and irregular bleeding in the pubertal girl. Tumors arise in the submucosal tissues and spread rapidly beneath an intact vaginal epithelium. In the early stages, the tumor can be seen by vaginoscopy as 1 or more polypoid projections into the vaginal cavity; later on, it bulges into a series of grapelike growths out of the vestibule (thus the term botryoid sarcoma; Fig. 37–20). The diagnosis is made on the basis of histologic evaluation. Occasionally, electron microscopy may be required to confirm the final diagnosis.

Over the years, there has been a shift in the treatment of this condition from radical surgery to a multimodal approach

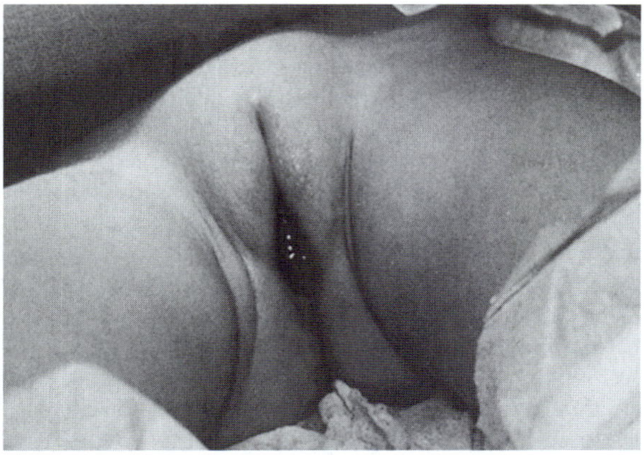

▲ **Figure 37–20.** Botryoid sarcoma presenting as a hemorrhagic growth extruding from the vagina.

involving conservative surgery with chemotherapy and radiotherapy. This approach has been associated with improved survival and preservation of normal anatomy and function.

The operative intervention frequently consists just of cervical conization or simple hysterectomy with preservation of the ovaries. It is then followed by combination chemotherapy (vincristine, dactinomycin, and cyclophosphamide).

Early detection and the combination of surgery, chemotherapy, and occasionally radiation for residual tumor have improved the prognosis of patients, with 2- and 5-year survival rates for early disease reaching >96% and 83%, respectively.

Other Malignant Tumors of the Vagina

Three types of vaginal carcinoma may appear during childhood and the early teens. Endodermal carcinoma occurs most often in young children. Carcinoma arising in a remnant of a mesonephric duct (mesonephric carcinoma) occurs more often in girls 3 years of age or older. Clear cell adenocarcinoma of müllerian origin, often associated with a history of antenatal exposure to diethylstilbestrol (DES), is encountered most frequently in postmenarchal teenage girls. The clinical features and treatment of malignant lesions of the vagina and cervix are similar to those in adult women.

3. Ovarian Tumors

With the increasing use of imaging modalities, greater numbers of ovarian cysts are being diagnosed. The majority of these cysts are asymptomatic and regress spontaneously with time; therefore, many clinicians prefer to observe only. The decision to intervene is based on cyst size, ultrasound characteristics, and clinical symptoms.

Ovarian Torsion

Based on the abdominal location of the ovary and the long utero-ovarian ligament, the adnexa of prepubertal girls are at increased risk of torsion, with a reported prevalence of 3%. The diagnosis is complicated by its vague clinical presentation. The only consistent symptoms are abdominal pain and ovarian enlargement on the same side as demonstrated by sonography. Doppler flow studies may further contribute to the diagnosis; however, even presence of flow in the ovarian vessels should not preclude the clinical impression. When ovarian torsion is suspected, a prompt surgical procedure should be carried out for diagnosis and appropriate management, usually accomplished by operative laparoscopy. During surgery, a conservative approach is advocated because of the enormous revitalization ability of ovarian tissue in these patients and the low rate of true neoplasms; 25% of patients have normal ovaries, and another almost 50% of patients have functional cysts involved. Oophoropexy should be considered in cases of recurrent torsion or single ovary involvement.

Although ovarian tumors are the most common genital neoplasm encountered in children and adolescents, they represent only 1% of all neoplasms in premenarchal children. Ovarian tumors of all varieties (except Brenner's tumors) have been reported in premenarchal children, but in this population, they are rarely malignant.

Benign Tumors

Benign cystic teratomas (dermoid cysts) account for at least 30% of all neoplasms in this age group, with an 18% incidence and bilaterality in 10% of cases. They are usually asymptomatic and diagnosed by abdominal sonography performed for other indications. Expectant management for cysts smaller than 6 cm might be reasonable, considering the low risk for torsion and malignant transformation (<0.17%) and the increased risk of jeopardizing reproductive function with surgical treatment.

Other tumors, such as functional teratoma and gonadoblastoma, are rare and managed by surgical removal.

Malignant Tumors

Seventy percent of ovarian cancers in youth are of germ cell origin, with dysgerminoma accounting for half of them. Although the most common symptoms of ovarian tumors are abdominal pain and an abdominal mass, acute severe pain, peritoneal irritation, or intra-abdominal hemorrhage can be the presenting sign. Despite the advancement in imaging technology applied for exploration of ovarian masses, at least 25% of all childhood ovarian tumors elude diagnosis until exploratory laparotomy is performed. The use of serum markers, such as inhibin or α-fetoprotein, may be helpful in children with ovarian enlargement.

The management of ovarian neoplasms in premenarchal children varies from that in older patients, because continued ovarian function is necessary to complete sexual and somatic maturation in children. In postpubertal patients, surgical intervention should aim, whenever possible, to preserve reproductive potential. Unilateral salpingo-oophorectomy is usually undertaken in young women with stage IA tumors (<10 cm, removed unruptured without evidence of metastatic spread). Approximately 8–15% of dysgerminomas are bilateral, and thus, the contralateral ovary is inspected and any suspicious areas are biopsied. If there is bilateral involvement, then the uterus can be left in situ for future reproduction options with ovum donation. The survival rate for patients treated for dysgerminoma in earlier stage was found to be 96.9%. If a tumor has extended beyond the ovary, more radical surgery (bilateral salpingo-oophorectomy with hysterectomy) is indicated, regardless of age. Germ cell tumors are highly responsive to chemotherapy, with the exception of dysgerminomas, which respond well to radiation; however, multiagent chemotherapy is used in those tumors as well in order to preserve reproductive potential.

Anders JF, Powell EC. Urgency of evaluation and outcome of acute ovarian torsion in pediatric patients. *Arch Pediatr Adolesc Med* 2005;159:532–535. PMID: 15939851.

Libby L, Shadinger MD, Rochelle F, et al. Preoperative sonographic and clinical characteristics as predictors of ovarian torsion. *J Ultrasound Med* 2008;27:7–13. PMID: 18096725.

Panteli C, Curry J, Kiely E, et al. Ovarian germ cell tumours: A 17-year study in a single unit. *Eur J Pediatr Surg* 2009;19: 96–100. PMID: 19360543.

PUBERTY

Puberty is the process by which sexually immature persons become capable of reproduction. These changes occur largely as the result of maturation of the hypothalamic–pituitary–gonadal axis. Puberty is characterized by progressive incline in gonadotropin-releasing hormone (GnRH) production, leading to increasing levels of FSH and luteinizing hormone (LH). These changes are obtained by 2 mechanisms occurring in the hypothalamus: increasing resistance to circulating estrogen levels and a decrease in inhibitory activity of neurotransmitters upon GnRH-secreting neurons. Changes are determined by genetic and environmental factors, such as geographic location and body fat composition, and mediated by the leptin and kisspeptin proteins. As a rule, breast development, which initially may be unilateral, growth of genital hair, and a marked increase in growth rate (*adolescent growth spurt*) precede uterine bleeding by approximately 2 years. The normal sequence of events in sexual development is outlined in Figure 37–21. Pubic and axillary hair may appear before, at about the same time, or well after the appearance of breast tissue. The vaginal mucosa, which in prepubertal girls is a deep red color, takes on a moist pastel pink appearance as estrogen exposure increases. Menarche—the first menstrual shedding of thickened endometrial lining—indicates the process of development of secondary sexual features. Regular ovulatory

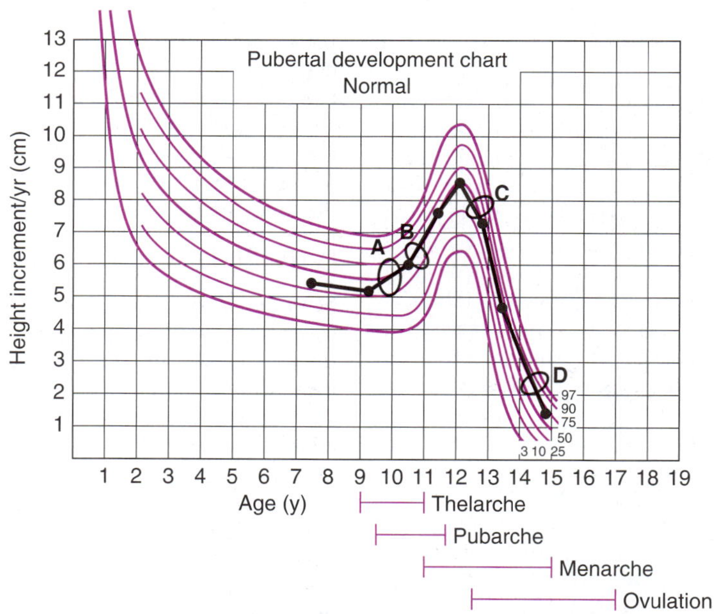

▲ Figure 37–21. Pubertal development chart for a normally developing female adolescent. Growth data are converted to growth velocity and plotted. The growth velocity curve shows initial acceleration in growth, followed by the growth spurt and subsequent deceleration. Superimposed on this curve are the following pubertal events: **A,** thelarche; **B,** pubarche; **C,** menarche; **D,** onset of ovulation. (Reproduced, with permission, from Reindollar RH, McDonough PG. Delayed sexual development: Common causes and basic clinical approach. *Pediatr Ann* 1981;10:178.)

cycles, which usually occur 20 months later, mark the end of pubertal maturation.

The first menstrual period occurs at an average age of 12.43 years in girls in the United States. Although the age of menarche in African-American girls is quite similar, secondary sexual features often occur earlier.

Normal range of menarche is from age 10 to 14 years. In the presence of secondary sexual characteristics, medical intervention can be deferred until 16 years of age.

Roy JR, Chakraborty S, Chakraborty TR. Estrogen-like endocrine disrupting chemicals affecting puberty in humans—a review. *Med Sci Monit* 2009;15:RA137–145. PMID: 19478717.

Shafii T. The adolescent sexual health visit. *Obstet Gynecol Clin North Am* 2009;36:99–117. PMID: 19344850.

Sisk CL, Foster DL. The neural basis of puberty and adolescense. *Nat Neurosci* 2004;7:1040–1047. PMID: 15452575.

DISORDERS OF SEXUAL MATURATION

Precocious Puberty

Sexual precocity is the onset of sexual maturation at any age that is 2.5 standard deviations earlier than the normal age for that population, being usually before the age of 8 years. It may be classified as central, or GnRH-dependent, precocious puberty (true precocious puberty), or peripheral, or GnRH-independent, precocious puberty (pseudoprecocious puberty).

Central Precocious Puberty

Central precocious puberty (CPP), or GnRH-dependent precocious puberty, is normal pubertal development that occurs at an early age. Premature activation of the hypothalamic–pituitary axis is followed by gonadotropin secretion, which in turn stimulates the gonads to produce steroid hormones and, subsequently, pubertal changes. GnRH-dependent precocious puberty is seen more frequently in girls than in boys. The cause of such early development often remains unclear. Most girls suspected of having CPP are otherwise healthy children whose pubertal maturation begins at the early end of the normal distribution curve. In general, the older the child is, the less the chance of finding an organic etiology for CPP. Central nervous system (CNS) imaging studies of these otherwise healthy 6- to 8-year-old girls usually reveal no structural abnormalities.

Occasionally, precocious puberty is associated with CNS abnormalities, including hypothalamic hamartomas, optic gliomas, and neurofibromas, as well as other CNS neoplasms. Cranial irradiation and CNS injuries may also be associated with precocious puberty. Prolonged excessive therapy with exogenous sex steroids or endocrine disorders such as hypothyroidism may accelerate hypothalamic–pituitary axis maturation, resulting in precocious puberty.

The diagnosis is made with the help of a careful history and physical examination in conjunction with radiologic and laboratory evaluations.

Peripheral GnRH-Independent Precocious Puberty

Peripheral precocious puberty, or GnRH-independent precocious puberty, is the appearance of pubertal development, but the presence of sex steroids is independent of pituitary gonadotropin release. Causes of precocious puberty include congenital adrenal hyperplasia, tumors that secrete human chorionic gonadotropin, tumors of the adrenal gland or gonads, McCune-Albright syndrome (MAS), and exposure to exogenous sex steroid hormones.

A. Endogenous Estrogens

The ovary in the newborn female contains 1–2 million primordial follicles, most of which undergo atresia during childhood without producing significant quantities of estrogen. However, large follicular cysts capable of estrogen production occur occasionally and may cause early feminization. Benign tumors of the ovary (eg, teratoma, cystadenoma) may produce estrogen or may induce surrounding ovarian tissue to produce steroids. Circulating sex steroids (estrogen or testosterone) come from either the adrenal gland or the gonad, independent of the hypothalamic–pituitary portion of the pubertal axis. Granulosa cell tumors capable of estrogen production are a rare cause of prepubertal feminization. Other rare tumors of extragonadal origin, including adrenal adenomas and hepatomas, may produce estrogens as well.

B. Exogenous Estrogens

Ingestion of estrogens or prolonged use of creams containing estrogens is a possible, but uncommon, cause of early feminization. A phytoestrogen-enriched diet (mostly soybean extracts) could exert a similar effect. Prompt discontinuation is indicated. Xenoestrogens (endocrine disruptors) found in rivers and soil of industrial regions might stimulate the estrogen receptors as well.

C. McCune-Albright Syndrome

MAS in its classic form consists of at least 2 features of the triad of polyostotic fibrous dysplasia, café-au-lait skin pigmentation (Fig. 37–22), and autonomous endocrine hyperfunction, the most common form of which is GnRH secretion and subsequent precocious puberty. Other endocrine and nonendocrine tissues also may be affected, including the adrenal, thyroid, pituitary, liver, and heart.

MAS is caused by a postzygotic somatic mutation in the gene coding for the subunit of the stimulatory G protein, which is involved in transmitting hormone signals. In patients with MAS, the signaling cascades are activated in the absence of hormone stimulation.

Affected children usually present at a younger age than those with idiopathic precocious puberty. Vaginal bleeding occurs early and, in most, is the first sign of puberty. The diagnosis is made on the basis of skin pigmentation and demonstration of bone lesions or pathologic fractures.

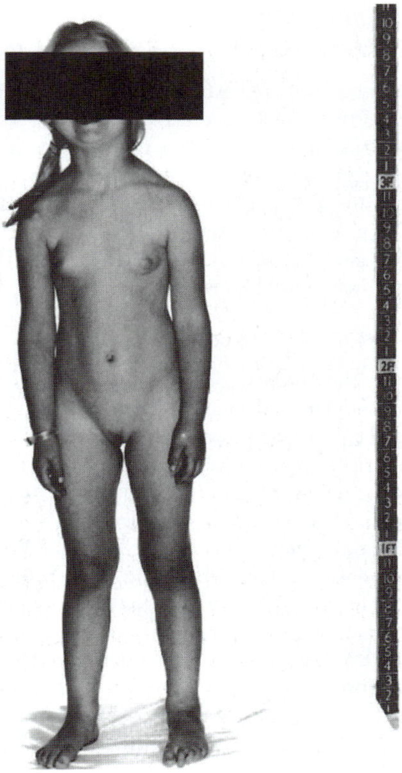

▲ **Figure 37–22.** Four-year-old child with idiopathic precocious puberty.

The prognosis for children with MAS is unfavorable. Adult height is significantly reduced. Multiple endocrinopathies often exist as well. As in adults, most patients have menstrual abnormalities, and many are infertile.

D. Incomplete Forms of Pubertal Development

Occasionally, for reasons that remain unclear, only 1 sign of pubertal development is present. Premature thelarche and premature pubarche, which are more common conditions than true precocious puberty, are 2 benign normal variant conditions that can look like precocious puberty but are nonprogressive or very slowly progressive. It possibly results from transient elevations of the levels of circulating steroid hormones or from extreme sensitivity of the end organ (eg, breast tissue) to the low, prepubertal levels of sex hormones. Such isolated development, however, may represent the initial sign of precocious puberty, and these patients should be re-evaluated at regular intervals.

E. Premature Thelarche

Premature thelarche is the isolated development of breast tissue prior to age 8 years, most commonly occurring between 1 and 3 years of age. It may affect 1 or both breasts (Fig. 37–23). A thorough history, physical examination, and growth curve review can help distinguish this normal variant from true sexual precocity. On examination, the somatic growth pattern is not accelerated and bone age is not advanced. The diagnosis is made by exclusion of other disorders. Occasionally, premature thelarche occurs when the child is exposed to exogenous estrogens.

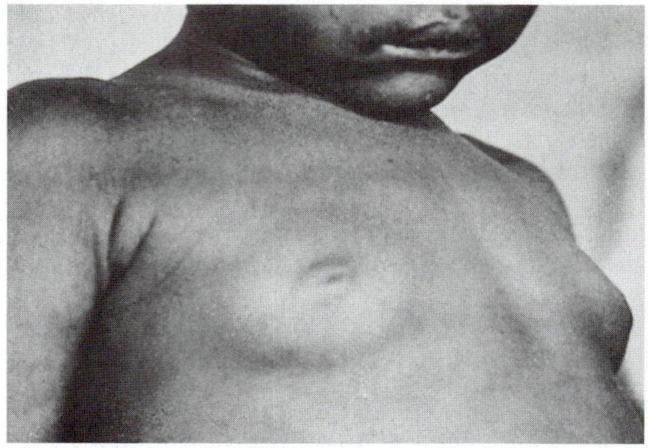

▲ **Figure 37–23.** Premature thelarche in a child 5 years of age.

F. Premature Pubarche

Premature pubarche previously was defined as the appearance of pubic or axillary hair prior to age 8 years, without other signs of precocious puberty (Fig. 37–24). However, new guidelines suggest that this presentation should not be considered precocious unless noted before age 7 years in white girls and before age 6 years in black girls. Such hair growth may be idiopathic and of no clinical significance.

Premature pubarche probably results from an earlier-than-usual increase in the secretion of androgens by the adrenal glands. Regulation of adrenal androgen secretion is distinct from that of gonadal steroids. Early appearance of pubic hair may be a very early sign of developing polycystic ovary disorder and, therefore, should be followed up closely. The diagnosis of idiopathic premature pubarche is made only after thorough evaluation of adrenal and gonadal function that fails to detect an abnormality.

Signs of severe androgen excess (eg, clitoral enlargement, growth acceleration, acne) should prompt further investigation for a rare virilizing tumor (Leydig cell tumor) or a variant form of congenital adrenal hyperplasia.

G. Premature Menarche

Premature menarche denotes the appearance of cyclic vaginal bleeding in children in the absence of other signs of secondary sexual development. The cause is unknown but may be related to increased end-organ sensitivity of

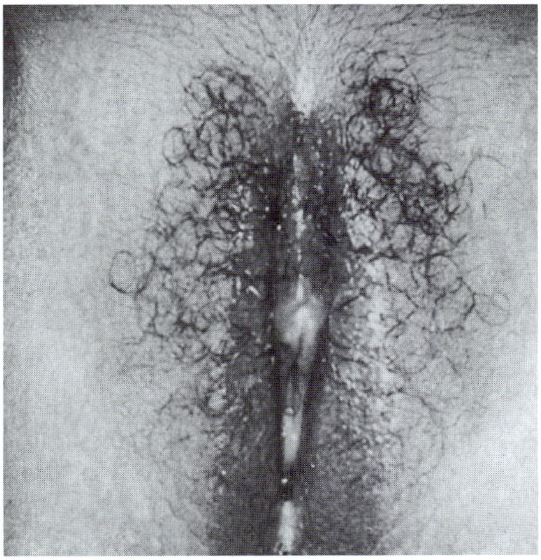

▲ **Figure 37–24.** Premature pubarche in a child 4 years of age.

the endometrium to low prepubertal levels of estrogens. Alternatively, bleeding may be related to transient elevation of estrogens due to premature follicular development. These patients have estradiol levels in the prepubertal range, and when given GnRH, the response of the pituitary gland is similar to that seen in prepubertal children.

Thorough evaluation of the genital tract should be done to exclude other pathologies like tumors, which are seen in up to 20% of patients.

The diagnosis of premature menarche is formulated by exclusion and is confirmed when the cyclic nature of the bleeding becomes apparent. The prognosis is excellent. Adult height is uncompromised, the menstrual pattern is normal, and fertility potential remains unimpaired.

Evaluation of the Patient with Precocious Puberty

When evaluating the patient with sexual precocity, the age at onset, duration, and progression of signs and symptoms constitute important historical information. Family history and review of systems may add important facts.

A. General Changes

Enhancement of general growth and advanced skeletal maturation are coincident with the onset of estrogen-stimulated change acting directly on the growth plate of the bone.

B. Skin

Additional androgen-dependent findings include acne and adult-type body odor.

C. Breast Development

Breast development is at least at Tanner stage II, with the areolae having a broadened, darkened appearance.

D. Genitalia

Genital changes reflect estrogen-induced thickening of the genital tissues. Increased vaginal secretions may result in leukorrhea. Dark, coarse pubic hair may be present.

Diagnosis

The diagnosis of GnRH-dependent precocity requires demonstration of pubertal gonadotropin secretion. The diagnostic evaluation required to document early pubertal development and differentiate central from peripheral causes includes the determination of serum LH, FSH, and estradiol levels, and a GnRH stimulation test. In patients with GnRH-dependent precocious puberty, the results of these tests will be in the normal pubertal range.

With improvements in imaging technology, clinicians often order such studies to help establish the diagnosis. Sonography may aid in the evaluation of the ovaries and adrenal glands. Uterine size and endometrial thickness are estrogen dependent and serve as a good bioassay to determine the length of time and magnitude of estrogen exposure. Ovarian cysts and tumors are also visible. Sonography of the adrenal glands is less sensitive than abdominal CT and MRI. Skeletal imaging to document skeletal age and a bone scan may identify areas of fibrous dysplasia in patients with MAS. Brain MRI is indicated in patients with sexual precocity or with neurologic signs.

Treatment of GnRH-Dependent Precocious Puberty

The treatment of choice for GnRH-dependent precocious puberty is GnRH analogues. Analogues of GnRH are modifications of the native hormone, which have greater resistance to degradation and increased affinity for the pituitary GnRH receptors.

Treatment with GnRH analogues decreases gonadotropins and sex steroids to prepubertal levels, which is followed by regression of secondary sexual features. Treatment also causes a deceleration in the skeletal maturation rate, preserving or even improving predicted height, unless bone age is so advanced that further growth is precluded. The efficacy of GnRH analogs in increasing adult height is undisputed only in girls with early-onset (<6 years old) central precocious puberty. The decision of whether to treat with GnRH analogues is made based on the girl's predicted final height and her emotional maturity. Treatment is continued until puberty is appropriate based on age. Resumption of puberty occurs promptly after discontinuation of GnRH analogue therapy.

DELAYED SEXUAL MATURATION

Delayed sexual development has been defined as the absence of normal pubertal events at an age 2.5 standard deviations later than the mean. The absence of thelarche by age 14 years or the absence of menarche by age 16 years is an indication for investigation. Classification can be based on the gonadotropic level: eugonadotropic, hypogonadotropic, or hypergonadotropic primary amenorrhea.

1. Delayed Menarche with Eugonadotropic Function Including Hyperprolactinemia

Patients with functioning gonads and delayed sexual maturation usually consult a physician while they are in their mid-teens because of amenorrhea. Most have well-formed female configuration with adequately developed breasts. Many of these patients suffer from an inappropriate hypothalamic–pituitary–ovarian feedback mechanism, leading to anovulation and in some cases androgen excess as well. Primary amenorrhea may persist until a progestin challenge is given. Patients should be monitored for continued menstrual shedding. Persistent amenorrhea is treated with progestins administered every other month to prevent endometrial hyperplasia. A sexually active girl should be given oral contraceptives rather than cyclic progestins. Further evaluation is required for diagnosis of adult-onset congenital adrenal hyperplasia and those with polycystic ovarian disease.

The possibility of pregnancy in an adolescent who has not begun to menstruate is highly unlikely but must be borne in mind when considering causes of delayed menarche in patients with normal pubertal development.

Congenital Anomalies

Patients with congenital anomalies of the paramesonephric (müllerian) structures may complain of primary amenorrhea. The most common defect is congenital absence of the uterus and vagina. Other causes are obstructive abnormalities, such as imperforate hymen, transverse vaginal septa, and agenesis of the cervix. Gynecologic examination supplemented by pelvic sonogram or MRI establishes the diagnosis of these congenital anomalies.

Androgen Insensitivity

The complete forms of androgen insensitivity are also associated with amenorrhea and normal breast development. Affected persons have normal testicular function but are not responsive to testosterone, and the development of breasts is secondary to the small amounts of unopposed estrogens produced by the testis. Pubic and axillary hair is scant or often absent. A short blind vaginal pouch is present. Once pubertal development has been completed, surgical extirpation of the gonads and reconstruction of the vagina are necessary. Recent data suggest that regardless of the technique used, sexual function may be impaired in some of these young women. A study of 66 women with complete forms of androgen insensitivity showed that 90% had sexual difficulties, most commonly sexual infrequency and vaginal penetration difficulty.

2. Delayed Puberty with Hypogonadotropic (Hypothalamic) Dysfunction

Hypothalamic–pituitary dysfunction is characterized by low to normal levels of gonadotropins (FSH, LH), similar to prepubertal state.

Constitutional Growth Delay

The onset of puberty depends on an ill-defined stage of maturity that is reflected in skeletal age. Maturation is partly genetically determined but also depends on multiple environmental factors; thus the chronologic age of puberty varies considerably. Statistical limits of normal variation in a defined population group indicate that, by definition, 2.5% of all normal adolescents will develop later than the age defined as "normal." This group has been labeled "late bloomers" or as having a constitutional growth delay (CGD). These girls often have retarded linear growth within the first 3 years of life, and then their growth resumes at a normal rate. As a result, these girls grow either along the lower growth percentiles or beneath the curve but parallel to it for the remainder of the prepubertal years. At the expected time of puberty, the height of children with CGD begins to drift further from the growth curve because of delayed onset of the pubertal growth spurt. Catch-up growth, onset of puberty, and pubertal growth spurt occur later than average, resulting in normal adult stature and sexual development. Although CGD is a variant of normal growth rather than a disorder, absence of signs of puberty (including the growth spurt) often concerns the patient when her adolescent friends have developed secondary sexual features and gained the characteristic increase in height.

The diagnosis of hypothalamic–pituitary dysfunction is made by exclusion of other causes of delayed sexual maturation. Growth charts, bone age, and the GnRH challenge test differentiate constitutional delay from similar conditions associated with GnRH deficiency. Reassurance is the only treatment necessary, but the patient must be kept under observation until regular menstrual cycles are established. Occasionally, an adolescent requires hormonal replacement therapy because of emotional distress over her condition.

Kallmann's Syndrome

Kallmann's syndrome is a genetic condition characterized by hypogonadotropic hypogonadism and anosmia. It affects approximately 1 in 40,000 females, with most presentations of the "sporadic" type. Various forms of Kallmann's syndrome are inherited, and the gene responsible for the X-linked form has been identified.

The clinical features include deficiency of GnRH associated with anosmia. Because GnRH neurons originate extracranially within the olfactory system, both can be simultaneously affected, and the defects are believed to be secondary to abnormalities of neuronal migration during development. Patients with Kallmann's syndrome fail to develop secondary sexual features, and blood levels of gonadotropins are very low.

Patients with Kallmann's syndrome have a diminished gonadotropin response to the GnRH stimulation test. Pulsatile administration of GnRH for 1 week usually restores subsequent pituitary responsiveness to GnRH. All postpubertal-age patients with Kallmann's syndrome are candidates for gonadal steroid replacement therapy in the absence of specific contraindications. Estrogen replacement therapy is used to initiate and sustain sexual development. Induction of ovulation with human menopausal gonadotropins or GnRH is necessary when pregnancy is desired.

Brain Tumors

A pituitary or parasellar tumor, particularly craniopharyngioma or pituitary adenoma, must be considered in the evaluation of a patient with delayed sexual maturation. Craniopharyngiomas are rapidly growing tumors that often develop in late childhood. Pituitary adenomas are slow growing, may become symptomatic during puberty, and may interfere with sexual maturation.

Hyperprolactinemia

An occult pituitary prolactinoma in adolescents with unexplained delayed sexual maturation must be ruled out. Serum prolactin levels should be measured yearly in patients with unexplained delayed sexual maturation.

Eating Disorders

Weight loss due to extreme dieting causes marked decrease of fat tissue concentration, resulting in suppression of GnRH activity, even in cases of almost normal weight without notable loss of muscle (often seen in athletes). It should be emphasized that the very first sign of anorexia nervosa could be primary or secondary amenorrhea.

Heroin addiction may cause amenorrhea, but its effects on sexual maturation have not been documented.

3. Delayed Puberty with Hypergonadotropic Dysfunction

Gonadal Failure

Gonadal failure is characterized by high levels of gonadotropins (FSH, LH), similar to the menopausal state. The common pathway of all ovarian failure disorders is the prominent deficiency of estrogen and the essential need for estrogen-containing replacement therapy in order to achieve normal development and prevent late consequences of estrogen deprivation.

Most patients with gonadal dysgenesis present during adolescence with delayed puberty and primary amenorrhea. For young women with gonadal failure, the most common cause is Turner's syndrome, which occurs with an incidence of 1 in 2500 to 1 in 10,000 live births. The syndrome is sex chromosomal aberration of 45,X monosomy. If untreated, estrogen and androgen levels are decreased, and FSH and LH levels are increased. Estrogen-dependent organs show the predictable effects of hormonal deficiency. Breasts contain little parenchymal tissue, and the areolar tissue is only slightly darker than the surrounding skin. The well-differentiated external genitalia, vagina, and müllerian derivatives remain small. Pubic and axillary hairs fail to develop in normal quantity. These patients should be closely monitored for development of illness caused by affected systems, such as the cardiovascular, urinary, and endocrine systems.

However, normal pubertal development, menstruation, and even pregnancies have been reported in adults with gonadal dysgenesis. It is possible that a few of these persons maintain some germ cells into adulthood. Spontaneous development is more commonly observed in patients with mosaicism with a 46,XX line. The rare offspring of these women probably do not have an increased risk for chromosomal abnormalities. In order to achieve pregnancy in a majority of women with gonadal dysgenesis, ovum donation treatment by using assisted reproductive technology may be offered.

Some patients may have ovarian failure even though they have a normal chromosome complement and 2 intact sex chromosomes (46,XX). An autosomal recessive form of ovarian failure has been demonstrated in some families. A small percentage of ovarian failures may be reversible and may be predicted by detection of anti-müllerian hormone levels, although the assay has not yet demonstrated clinical yield. Other causes of follicular depletion include chemotherapy, irradiation, infections (eg, mumps), infiltrative disease processes of the ovary (eg, tuberculosis), autoimmune diseases, and unknown environmental agents.

A karyotype is necessary to rule out the presence of Y chromosome material. DNA probes and assays for the minor histocompatibility antigen H-Y have also been used to identify Y chromosome material. A high incidence of neoplastic changes in the gonadal ridge has been reported in the presence of a Y chromosome (Fig. 37–25), so prophylactic gonadectomy is recommended. Replacement hormonal therapy is then given in a cyclic manner.

Some patients have similar features, yet follicles are present but unresponsive, a condition called the *resistant ovary syndrome*. It is characterized by delayed menarche or primary amenorrhea, a 46,XX chromosome complement, high

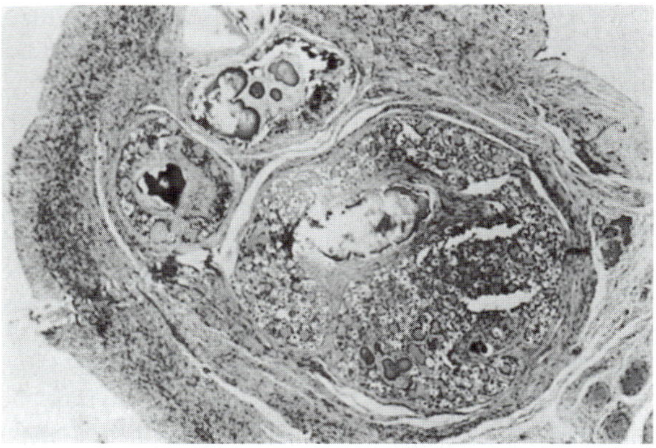

▲ **Figure 37–25.** Gonadoblastoma developing in a gonadal ridge in a patient with gonadal dysgenesis and 45,XO/46,XY karyotype.

FSH levels, and ovaries with apparently normal follicular apparatus that do not respond to endogenous gonadotropins. Absence of follicular receptors for gonadotropins is assumed to be responsible for ovarian dysfunction in these patients. These individuals may have normally developed secondary sexual characteristics. Estrogen replacement therapy is required to prevent long-term complications of estrogen deficiency (eg, vaginal dryness, osteoporosis). Pregnancies have been reported in some patients treated with menotropins or following discontinuation of estrogen therapy.

Evaluation of the Patient with Delayed Sexual Development

Determination of gonadal function can be accomplished by obtaining a medical history and performing a detailed physical examination, supplemented by selected laboratory studies. Historical information should center around previous growth and pubertal development. Linear and velocity growth charts as well as a pubertal development chart clarify previous growth patterns and are useful in subsequent follow-up. Knowledge of previous medical disorders may immediately identify the cause of aberrant puberty.

Physical examination must include height and weight assessments and a careful search for somatic anomalies. Staging of pubertal development by Tanner criteria is most important in the determination of gonadal function. Presence of breast development signifies prior gonadal function. Imaging studies such as pelvic sonogram and CT and MRI are required for confirmation of congenital absence of the vagina and uterus.

Absence of pubic hair is suggestive of the androgen insensitivity syndrome. Karyotype will identify the 46,XY cell line in patients with testicular feminization syndrome. Patients with complete pubertal development and well-formed female configuration ("pear shape") display evidence of continued estrogen production, and normal müllerian systems probably have inappropriate positive feedback and thus chronic anovulation. Progesterone challenge in such patients is helpful. A withdrawal bleed signifies a normal müllerian system and acceptable estrogen production.

Serum gonadotropin assays are performed for further elucidation. Elevated FSH levels suggest gonadal failure. Karyotype determination is crucial in diagnosing the various etiologies of gonadal failure. The presence of a Y chromosome in either group dictates gonadal removal.

Low FSH levels suggest interference with hypothalamic–pituitary maturation and gonadotropin release. Skull films and prolactin assays must be obtained for all patients to rule out the presence of pituitary or hypothalamic tumors. Appropriate endocrine evaluation identifies the occasional patient with hypothyroidism or congenital adrenal hyperplasia and the rare patient with Cushing's syndrome. Diagnosis of Kallmann's syndrome is suspected in hypogonadotropic patients who have an associated anosmia, and the diagnosis is confirmed by GnRH challenge tests. The presumed diagnosis of constitutional delay is made by exclusion of all other causes and by the typical GnRH release patterns after GnRH challenge.

BLEEDING DISORDERS

Vaginal Bleeding in the Premenarchal Child

When vaginal bleeding occurs in children, 2 sources generally should be suspected: (1) the endometrium (bleeding usually is a manifestation of precocious puberty) and (2) a local vulvar or vaginal lesion (eg, vulvovaginitis, foreign bodies, urethral prolapse, trauma, botryoid sarcoma, adenocarcinoma of the cervix or vagina, and vulvar skin disorders).

Vaginal bleeding during childhood should always alert the physician to the possibility of a genital tumor, which could be present in up to 20% of girls with no signs of pubertal maturation. Vaginoscopy and examination under anesthesia are the mainstays of evaluation to exclude the presence of tumors, foreign bodies, and other local lesions. Suspicious lesions require biopsy for diagnosis. Sexual abuse should be always be kept in mind by the physician attending a prepubertal girl with vaginal bleeding.

Disorders of Menstrual Cycle in Adolescents

One of the most common gynecologic complaints of adolescents is a problem with the menstrual period. In most cases, there is no true medical disorder, especially in the first 2 years after menarche, when 50–80% of periods are anovulatory. Dysfunctional uterine bleeding accounts for 95% of abnormal vaginal bleeding in teenagers. Screening for inherited coagulation disorders, such as von Willebrand's disease, may be indicated, as 18% of adolescents hospitalized for menorrhagia have an underlying bleeding disorder.

Pubertal Menorrhagia

In the adolescent, the normal cycle length is 21–45 days, the length of the period is 7 days or less, and product use is no more than 3–6 pads or tampons per day. Menorrhagia is defined as heavy menstrual bleeding that lasts for more than 7 days or results in the loss of more than 80 mL of blood per menstrual cycle.

Heavy bleeding starting from the first menstrual period after menarche might be the first sign of a bleeding disorder, such as von Willebrand's disease (5–20%) or platelet dysfunction.

Pubertal menorrhagia is a result of dysfunctional uterine bleeding more often secondary to anovulation. This is reflection of the immaturity of the hypothalamic–pituitary–ovarian axis; in fact, in 55–82% of adolescents, it takes 24 months for onset of regular ovulatory cycles after menarche. This abnormality is even more common in girls with polycystic ovary syndrome (PCOS), and bleeding disorders such as abnormal platelet function or von Willebrand's disease are the most common inherited bleeding disorders. A positive bleeding history alone had a sensitivity for detecting any bleeding disorder of 82%. It should be followed by initial laboratory evaluation including a complete cell count, prothrombin time, activated partial thromboplastin time (aPTT), and fibrinogen or thrombin clot time, although all of these tests might be normal in patients with VWD. Further evaluation is better done in collaboration with hematologists with expertise in bleeding disorders.

Management of anovulatory bleeding is directed toward controlling symptoms and preventing blood loss based on degree of anemia. Hormonal contraception is the first-line treatment for menorrhagia, and the dosage is adjusted based on severity of the bleeding. Daily administration could reach several pills a day until control of bleeding is achieved, followed by tapering during the following days. Other preparations include medroxyprogesterone acetate and levonorgestrel-secreting intrauterine devices, which have been used by several experts. Consideration of the negative effect on final height caused by the estrogen component must be done based on clinical condition of the patient.

In severe cases, hospitalization and intravenous conjugated equine estrogen in doses of 25 mg every 4–6 hours until bleeding stops for 24 hours have been used successfully. If oral contraceptives are given for secondary amenorrhea, they should be continued for at least 9–12 months before attempting to stop. If menses do not resume within 8 weeks, oral contraceptive pills should be resumed for another 9–12 months.

Adolescents who fail hormonal management should be referred for consideration of hemostatic therapies including desmopressin (DDAVP), antifibrinolytic medications (aminocaproic acid, tranexamic acid), and clotting factor concentrates. In the management of acute severe menorrhagia, every effort is made to preserve future fertility. Invasive intervention should be reserved as a last resort treatment.

POLYCYSTIC OVARIAN SYNDROME IN ADOLESCENTS

The prevalence of PCOS in the general population has been estimated to be 5–10%. The classic presentation is characterized by features of anovulation, amenorrhea, oligomenorrhea, or irregular cycles in combination with signs of androgen excess, acne, hirsutism, or alopecia. It is associated frequently with insulin resistance.

PCOS usually presents at the late pubertal age but may also present before menarche in the form of androgen excess as premature pubarche/adrenarche.

Recent literature has identified a specific biochemical marker (adiponectin) that is significantly lower in concentration in the daughters of women who have PCOS before the onset of hyperandrogenism and may be an early marker of metabolic derangement in adolescent girls.

Primary amenorrhea as the initial feature occurs in 1.4–14% of adolescents with PCOS. As with adults, Rotterdam Criteria should be used to make the diagnosis of PCOS in adolescents; however, some researchers have challenged the consensus of Rotterdam Criteria in adolescents because they may lead to overestimation of the syndrome, because the physiologic process of early puberty is characterized by relative androgenemia, insulin resistance, cystic ovaries, and anovulatory cycles. They have proposed alternative diagnostic criteria in adolescents, which include 4 of the following 5 criteria: (1) oligo- or amenorrhea 2 years after menarche; (2) clinical hyperandrogenism; (3) hyperandrogenemia; (4) insulin resistance or hyperinsulinemia; and (5) polycystic ovaries. The finding of polycystic ovaries in adolescents as the only sign should be considered with caution because 25% of healthy adolescents may present with similar finding.

Adolescents who are obese and have a diagnosis of PCOS should undergo a 2-hour 75-g oral glucose tolerance test (OGTT). This is a more sensitive test than the fasting glucose test to detect diabetes and impaired glucose tolerance, which is a significant risk factor for diagnosis. A fasting glucose/insulin ratio has been proposed as a rapid and easy screening alternative; in adolescents, a ratio of <7 is suggestive as compared with a ratio of <4.5 in adults.

An early diagnosis should be made in order to avoid late health consequences such as diabetes, cardiovascular disease, endometrial hyperplasia, and infertility. Any adolescent with androgen excess should be monitored for evidence of hypertension and hypertriglyceridemia regardless of body weight because of the higher risk for metabolic syndrome.

Treatment

Treatment options for adolescents with PCOS include weight loss for obese girls and lifestyle modifications, including calorie restriction and an increase in formal exercise; symptom-directed therapy to address the main symptoms noted by the adolescent; and metabolic correction of the underlying insulin resistance using insulin-sensitizing medications.

Although weight loss of as little as 5–10% has been shown to result in reduction in testosterone increase in sex hormone-binding globulin and resumption of menses and ovulation, unfortunately, diet and behavioral therapies have been shown to fail in adolescents, with follow-up showing weight regain of 75–121% at 5 years. Obesity can exacerbate the PCOS phenotype in previously asymptomatic individuals. Weight reduction has been shown to improve free androgen levels, insulin sensitivity, and ovulatory function. When menstrual irregularity is accompanied by symptoms such as acne, hirsutism, and obesity, PCOS should be suspected, and treatment may need to address some of these symptoms as well.

Pregnancy should always be considered in a young woman with abnormal bleeding or amenorrhea until proven otherwise. Nonmenstrual causes of bleeding, such as hypothyroidism, cervicitis, condylomas, polyps, cervical cancer, estrogen-producing ovarian tumors, and vaginitis, also should be considered.

ADOLESCENT PREGNANCY AND CONTRACEPTION

Juvenile pregnancy is rare. The youngest known patient was a Peruvian girl aged 5 years 8 months, who in 1939 delivered at term by caesarean section a healthy male infant weighing 2950 g (6 lb 8 oz). Both mother and infant survived. In every reported instance, the underage mothers were sexually precocious, and most had menstruated for several years before becoming pregnant. Juvenile pregnancy per se does not increase the chance of congenital anomalies in the offspring. However, in many cases, the mother is a victim of sexual abuse, and if the pregnancy is the result of incest, there is a greater likelihood of genetic malformations carried by recessive genes.

Most precocious mothers and their babies have not done well, with increased incidences of spontaneous abortion, pregnancy-induced hypertension, and premature labor and delivery. In patients younger than 9 years, <50% have normal labor, with a 35% likelihood of neonatal loss.

The underage mother and her family may need psychiatric counseling, both during pregnancy and after delivery. Lessening the emotional, social, and medical trauma associated with such a gestation is an important task for all who assist in the care of the pregnant child.

For years it has been accepted that adolescent pregnancy is a high-risk pregnancy. Many pregnant adolescents come from low socioeconomic backgrounds and have poor education and perhaps poor general health due to inadequate nutrition, iron deficiency anemia, cigarette smoking, drug abuse, or STDs. Proper education and dietary counseling may improve nutritional status and prevent anemia.

Complications of labor and delivery are highly dependent on the quality of prenatal care. Preeclampsia–eclampsia, which is more common in a first pregnancy, occurs more frequently among adolescents than among adult women. Prematurity and small for gestational age infants are a major problem in adolescent pregnancies. Predisposing factors are high-risk factors such as low prepregnancy weight, poor weight gain, adverse socioeconomic conditions, cigarette smoking, anemia, first pregnancy, and deficient prenatal care, all of which occur more commonly in adolescents. To minimize prenatal complications and to improve maternal and fetal outcome, the young patient should be enrolled in an aggressive prenatal care program. That care should not only improve the pregnancy outcome of adolescents, but also enhance their social, educational, and emotional adjustment.

American Academy of Pediatrics Committee on Adolescence. Contraception and adolescence. *Pediatrics* 2007;120:1135–1148. PMID: 17974753.

Das S, Dhulkota JS, Brook J, et al. The impact of a dedicated antenatal clinic on the obstetric and neonatal outcomes in adolescent pregnant women. *J Obstet Gynecol* 2007;27:464–466. PMID: 17701790.

Lara-Torre E, Schroeder B. Adolescent compliance and side effects with quick start initiation of oral contraceptive pills. *Contraception* 2002;66:81–85. PMID: 12204779.

PREGNANCY TERMINATION

The rate of teenage abortion remains higher in the United States than in other Western countries for which data are available. In many countries, the legal authorities ruled in favor of a minor's right to have an abortion. In others systems, the evacuation of uterine contents can be performed by medical (RU-486) or surgical (dilatation and currettage) technique, both of which are accepted in adolescents; the preferable method is still undetermined. For minors who do not want parental involvement social support is required to perform it on them.

CONTRACEPTION IN ADOLESCENTS

More than 95% of adolescent pregnancies are unintended. By age 18 years, 1 in 4 adolescents experiences a pregnancy. Half of adolescent pregnancies occur in the first 6 months after initiation of sexual activity. Despite a decline in teenage pregnancy rates during the 1990s, teenage pregnancy rates remain higher in the United States than in other Western countries. In addition, teenagers in the United States use contraceptives less frequently and use less effective methods of contraception than do their European counterparts. Although great inroads in adolescent access to health care have been made over the last decade, problems of cost and fears of lack of confidentiality still appear to inhibit young women from obtaining contraceptives, ultimately resulting in high teenage pregnancy rates.

These findings reinforce the importance of addressing contraception during an adolescent's initial health care evaluation.

Postponing sexual activity is an appropriate option to suggest. If this is not realistic, counseling regarding various methods of contraception requires consideration not only of the side effects and efficacy of the various methods but also of the personal requirements of each teenager. Extended regimens such as available 84/7 day and no "placebo" regimens have shown similar efficacy; these may be new options for patient who desire lower frequency of menses such as athletes and military personnel, although studies in adolescents are lacking. Using "Quik Start" (same day of the visit) seems to improve compliance from 56 to 72%.

The common hormonal contraceptive methods are applicable in adolescents with the same success as in adult women; however, teenagers are more likely to forget taking a daily pill, thus resulting in a high failure rate of 9–18% and low long-term compliance of 44%. Long-lasting methods such as the patch, vaginal ring, and hormonal Depo system may be more efficient in preventing pregnancy in young girls. Inserting an IUD in girls before first pregnancy is reasonable under some conditions but still remains controversial. Screening patients for STIs before insertion should be encouraged.

Health benefits of adolescents taking hormonal contraceptive methods include decreased menstrual pain; increased menstrual regularity; decreased risk of pelvic inflammatory disease, anemia, and fibrocystic breast disease; improved long-term fertility; and treatment of acne and hirsutism. The importance of both contraception and STI prevention should be reviewed, and the use of barrier methods together with hormonal method should be encouraged.

Emergency contraception with progestin-only regimens is a highly effective means of preventing pregnancy if taken up to 72 hours after intercourse; despite decreasing efficacy, it should be provided up to 120 hours after unprotected coitus. Improving access through education or prescribing pills in advance or over the telephone may give a young woman a second chance at preventing unintended pregnancy.

SEXUALLY TRANSMITTED INFECTIONS

STIs are the most common infectious diseases in adolescents today. Approximately 25% of all sexually active adolescents aged 13–19 years become infected each year. By age 15 years, 1 in 4 girls in the United States has had sexual relations. The younger the age of first intercourse, the higher is the risk for STIs. Chlamydia is the most prevalent of the bacterial STIs, with almost 30% of inner-city female adolescents aged 12–19 showing positive cultures in a longitudinal 2-year study of family planning, school-based, and STI clinics. Sequelae of chlamydial infections include pelvic inflammatory disease (PID), ectopic pregnancy, and infertility. This age group accounts for 8% of cases of HIV in females, with the majority of these women asymptomatic at the time of positive testing. In the United States, 15- to 24-year-olds accounted for approximately 60% of gonorrhea cases, 25% of syphilis cases, and 17% of hepatitis B cases in 1996. By the time they reach college age, 43% of women are infected with human papillomavirus.

Nearly 70% of patients with PID are younger than 25 years. The estimated incidence of PID in sexually active females is approximately 1 in 8 for 15-year-olds and 1 in 10 for 16-year-olds. PID in adolescents should be treated with hospitalization and intravenous antibiotics. Tubo-ovarian abscess has been found in 2–4% of adolescents with adnexal masses. Treatment includes broad-spectrum antibiotics and possible surgical drainage. Patients who have had PID or tubo-ovarian abscess are at high risk for pelvic pain, pelvic adhesive disease, infertility, and ectopic pregnancy.

CERVICAL CANCER SCREENING & HUMAN PAPILLOMAVIRUS VACCINE IN ADOLESCENTS

Human papillomavirus (HPV) is the most common sexually acquired infection in the world, with a prevalence of 50% among young sexually active adolescents. Most of these infections are self-limiting and harmless, but persistent infection with oncogenic HPV types can cause cervical cancer in women. HPV also causes other anogenital cancers (eg, of the vagina, vulva, and penis), head and neck cancers, and genital warts in both men and women.

The availability of the new vaccine (2006) against carcinogenic types of HPV (mainly types 16 and 18) has led to major changes in the prevention and management of cervical disease. Two vaccines are currently approved for use in humans, and both have shown more than 95% efficacy in preventing cervical dysplasia associated with vaccine type and a high safety profile.

Several organizations, including the American College of Obstetricians and Gynecologists (ACOG), have recommended vaccination for young women aged 9–26 years. Because current HPV vaccines are prophylactic, the greatest impact will be seen by vaccinating girls before they are exposed to HPV and thus before sexual debut.

Some countries introduced the vaccine as a part of scholar vaccination program, which severed the administration of the vaccine from the sexual permissiveness context. The duration of protection seems to be longer than 6 years, but the exact duration of protection and other details on the future of the vaccine are still not clear and need more clinical trials.

Health care providers should encourage vaccinated adolescents to continue with the use of protective methods against other STDs and emphasize the importance of cervical cancer screening with a Papanicolaou (Pap) test. Screening in low-risk adolescent should be initiated 3 years after the onset of sexual activity and not later than age 21 years.

Considering the rarity of cervical cancer among adolescents, the management of abnormal cervical cytology differs from that of the adult population. The American Society for Colposcopy and Cervical Pathology (ASCCP) advises against HPV testing and against treatment of low-grade squamous intraepithelial lesions or cervical intraepithelial neoplasia I. In adherent adolescents, treatment of cervical intraepithelial neoplasia II should also be deferred.

In patients with high-grade lesions or incompliant adolescents with lower grade lesions, ablative or excisional procedures are indicated. Cryotherapy offers a 92–95% cure rate for cervical intraepithelial neoplasia 2–3 in young women. Loop electrosurgical excisional procedure offers similar cure rates and does not appear to impact cervical competence in future pregnancies with depths of excision of 1.5 cm or less.

Adams Hillard PJ. Menstruation in adolescents: what's normal, what's not. *Ann N Y Acad Sci* 2008;1135:29–35. PMID: 18574205.

American College of Obstetricians and Gynecologists. *Guidelines for Women's Health Care: A Resource Manual.* 3rd ed. Washington, DC: American College of Obstetricians and Gynecologists; 2007.

American College of Obstetricians and Gynecologists. *Menstruation in Girls and Adolescents: Using a Menstrual Cycle as a Vital Sign.* Washington, DC: American College of Obstetricians and Gynecologists; 2006.

American Society for Reproductive Medicine Practice Committee. Current evaluation of amenorrhea. *Fertil Steril* 2006;86:148–155. PMID: 17055812.

Bayas J, Costas L, Munoz A. Cervical cancer vaccination, indications, efficacy and side effects. *Gynecol Oncol* 2008;110 (3 Suppl 2):S11–S14. PMID: 18586311.

Beyith Y, Hardoff D, Rom E, et al. A simulated patient-based program for training gynecologists in communication with adolescents girls presenting with gynecological problems. *J Pediatr Adolesc Gynecol* 2009;22:79–84. PMID: 19345912.

Bidet M, Bachelot A, Touraine P. Premature ovarian failure: predictability of intermittent ovarian function and response to ovulation induction agents. *Curr Opin Obstet Gynecol* 2008;20:416–420. PMID: 18660695.

Blank SK, Helm KD, McCartney CR, et al. Polycystic ovary syndrome in adolescence. *Ann N Y Acad Sci* 2008;1135:76–84. PMID: 18574211.

Breech LL, Laufer MR. Mullerian anomalies. *Obstet Gynecol Clin North Am* 2009;36:47–68. PMID: 19344847.

Carel JC, Eugster EA, Rogol A, et al. Consensus statement on the use of gonadotropin-releasing hormone analogs in children. *Pediatrics* 2009;123:e752–e762. PMID: 19332483.

Carmina E, Oberfield SE, Lobo RA. The diagnosis of polycystic ovary syndrome in adolescents. *Am J Obstet Gynecol* 2010;203:201. e1–e5. PMID: 20435290.

Committee on Adolescent Health Care. ACOG Committee Opinion No. 436: evaluation and management of abnormal cervical cytology and histology in adolescents. *Obstet Gynecol* 2009;113:1522–1525. PMID: 19461460.

Dumitrescu CE, Collins MT. McCune-Albright syndrome. *Orphanet J Rare Dis* 2008;19:3–12. PMID: 18489744.

Genazzani AD, Ricchieri F, Lanzoni C, et al. Diagnostic and therapeutic approach to hypothalamic amenorrhea. *Ann N Y Acad Sci* 2006;1092:103–113. PMID: 17308137.

Giannesi A, Marchiole P, Benchaib M, et al. Sexuality after laparoscopic Davydov in patients affected by congenital complete vaginal agenesis associated with uterine agenesis or hypoplasia. *Hum Reprod* 2005;20:2954–2957. PMID: 15979993.

Hertwick SP. Pediatric and adolescent gynecology. *Obstet Gynecol Clin North Am* 2009;36:xv–xvi. PMID: 19344844.

Ibñez L, Díaz R, López-Bermejo A, et al. Clinical spectrum of premature pubarche: links to metabolic syndrome and ovarian hyperandrogenism. *Rev Endocr Metab Disord* 2009;10:63–76. PMID: 18726694.

Ismail IS, Cutner AS, Creighton SM. Laparoscopic vaginoplasty: alternative techniques in vaginal reconstruction. *BJOG* 2006;113:340–343. PMID: 16487208.

James AH. Bleeding disorders in adolescents. *Obstet Gynecol Clin North Am* 2009;36:153–162. PMID: 19344853.

Karateke A, Gurbuz A, Haliloglu B, et al. Intestinal vaginoplasty: is it optimal treatment of vaginal agenesis? A pilot study. Surgical method of sigmoid colon vaginoplasty in vaginal agenesis. *Int Urogynecol J Pelvic Floor Dysfunct* 2006;17:40–45. PMID: 15997363.

Legro RS. Detection of insulin resistance and its treatment in adolescents with polycystic ovary syndrome. *J Pediatr Endocrinol Metab* 2002;15(Suppl 5):1367–1378. PMID: 12510993.

Leung AKC, Robson WLM, Kao CP, et al. Treatment of labial fusion with topical estrogen therapy. *Clin Pediatr* 2005;44: 245–247. PMID: 15821849.

McCann J, Miyamoto S, Boyle C, et al. Healing of hymenal injuries in prepubertal and adolescent girls: a descriptive study. *Pediatrics* 2007;119:E1094–E1106. PMID: 17420260.

Pena A, Levitt MA, Bischhoff A, et al. Rectovestibular fistula: rarely recognized associated gynecologic anomalies. *J Pediatr Surg* 2009;44:1261–1267. PMID: 19524751.

Petermann T, Maliqueo M, Codner E, et al. Early metabolic derangements in daughters of women with PCOS. *J Clin Endocrinol Metab* 2007;92:4637–4642. PMID: 17848407.

Phillipp CS, Faiz A, Dowling N, et al. Age and the prevalence of bleeding disorders in women with menorrhagia. *Obstet Gynecol* 2005;105:61–66. PMID: 15625143.

Poindexter G, Morrell D. Anogenital pruritus: lichen sclerosus in children. *Pediatr Ann* 2007;36:785–791. PMID: 18229519.

Rosenfield RL, Devine N, Hunold JJ. Salutary effects of combining early very low-dose systemic estradiol with growth hormone therapy in girls with Turner syndrome. *J Clin Endocrinol Metab* 2005;90:6424–6430. PMID: 16189255.

Rotterdam ESHRE/tASRM-Sponsored PCOS consensus on diagnostic criteria and long term health risks related to polycystic ovary syndrome. *Hum Reprod* 2004;19:41–47. PMID: 14685514.

Sanfilippo JS, Larra-Torre E. Adolescent gynecology. *Obstet Gynecol* 2009;113:935–947. PMID: 19305342.

Satyaprakash A, Creed R, Ravanfar P, et al. Human papilloma virus vaccines. *Dermatol Ther* 2009;22:150–157. PMID: 19335726.

Solomon LA, Zurawin RK. Vaginoscopic resection for rhabdomyosarcoma of the vagina: a case report and review of the literature. *J Pediatr Adolesc Gynecol* 2003;16:139–142. PMID: 12804937.

Stranzinger E, Strouse PJ. Ultrasound of the pediatric female pelvis. *Semin Ultrasound CT MR* 2008;29:98–113. PMID: 18450135.

Stuart A. Rhabdomyosarcoma. *Indian J Pediatr* 2004;71:331–337. PMID: 15107514.

Sybert VP, McCauley E. Turner's syndrome. *N Engl J Med* 2004;16;351:1227–1238. PMID: 15371580.

Tena-Sempere M. GPR54 and kisspeptin in reproduction. *Hum Reprod Update* 2006;12:631–639. PMID: 16731583.

Troiano RN, McCarthy SM. Müllerian duct anomalies: imaging and clinical issues. *Radiology* 2004;233:19–34. PMID: 15317956.

Complications of Menstruation & Abnormal Uterine Bleeding

38

Asher Shushan, MD

PREMENSTRUAL SYNDROME

ESSENTIALS OF DIAGNOSIS

- Symptoms include mood symptoms (irritability, mood swings, depression, anxiety), physical symptoms (bloating, breast tenderness, insomnia, fatigue, hot flushes, appetite changes), and cognitive changes (confusion and poor concentration).
- Symptoms must occur in the second half of the menstrual cycle (luteal phase).
- There must be a symptom-free period of at least 7 days in the first half of the cycle.
- Symptoms must occur in at least 2 consecutive cycles.
- Symptoms must be severe enough to require medical advice or treatment.

General Considerations

Premenstrual syndrome (PMS) has been defined as "the cyclic occurrence of symptoms that are of sufficient severity to interfere with some aspects of life and that appear with consistent and predictable relationship to the menses." Although the symptoms themselves are not unique, the restriction of the symptoms to the luteal phase of the menstrual cycle is pathognomonic of PMS. It is a psychoneuroendocrine disorder with biologic, psychological, and social parameters that is both difficult to define adequately and quite controversial. One major difficulty in detailing whether PMS is a disease or a description of physiologic changes is its extraordinary prevalence. Up to 75% of women experience some recurrent PMS symptoms; 20–40% are mentally or physically incapacitated to some degree, and 5% experience severe distress. The highest incidence occurs in women in their late 20s to early 30s. PMS is rarely encountered in adolescents and resolves after menopause. Evidence suggests that women who have suffered with PMS and premenstrual dysphoric disorder are more likely to suffer from perimenopausal symptoms.

The symptoms of PMS may include headache, breast tenderness, pelvic pain, bloating, and premenstrual tension. More severe symptoms include irritability, dysphoria, and mood lability. When these symptoms disrupt daily functioning, they are clustered under the name *premenstrual dysphoric disorder* (PMDD).

Other symptoms commonly included in PMS are abdominal discomfort, clumsiness, lack of energy, sleep changes, and mood swings. Behavioral changes include social withdrawal, altered daily activities, marked change in appetite, increased crying, and changes in sexual desire. In all, more than 150 symptoms have been related to PMS. Thus the symptom complex of PMS has not been clearly defined.

Pathogenesis

The etiology of the symptom complex of PMS is not known, although several theories have been proposed, including estrogen–progesterone imbalance, excess aldosterone, hypoglycemia, hyperprolactinemia, and psychogenic factors. A hormonal imbalance previously was thought to be related to the clinical manifestations of PMS/PMDD, but in the most recent consensus, physiologic ovarian function is believed to be the trigger. This is supported by the efficacy of ovarian cyclicity suppression, either medically or surgically, in eliminating premenstrual complaints.

Further research has shown that serotonin (5-hydroxytryptamine [5-HT]), a neurotransmitter, is important in the pathogenesis of PMS/PMDD. Both estrogen and progesterone have been shown to influence the activity of serotonin and gamma-aminobutyric acid (GABA) centrally. Many of the symptoms of other mood disorders resembling the features of PMS/PMDD have been associated with serotonergic dysfunction. Disturbances in cortical GABA neuronal function and modulation by neuroactive steroids have been implicated as potentially important contributors to the pathogenesis of PMS/PMDD. GABA levels are decreased in women with PMS/PMDD during the late luteal phase compared with normal women.

Diagnosis

No objective screening or diagnostic tests for PMS and PMDD are available; thus special attention must be paid to the patient's medical history. Certain medical conditions (eg, thyroid disease and anemia) with symptoms that can mimic those of PMS/PMDD must be ruled out.

The patient is instructed to chart her symptoms during the month. According to the American College of Obstetricians and Gynecologists criteria, PMS can be diagnosed if the patient reports at least 1 affective symptom (depression, angry outbursts, irritability, anxiety, confusion, or social withdrawal) and somatic symptom (breast tenderness, abdominal bloating, headache, or swelling of extremities) during the 5 days before menses in each of the 3 prior menstrual cycles. These symptoms should be relieved within 4 days of the onset of menses, without recurrence until at least cycle day 13, and should be reproducible during 2 cycles of prospective recording.

Clinical Findings

A careful history and physical examination are most important to exclude organic causes of PMS localized to the reproductive, urinary, or gastrointestinal tracts. Most patients readily describe their symptoms, but careful questioning may be needed with some patients who may be reluctant to do so. Although it is important not to lead a patient to exaggerate her concerns, it is equally important not to minimize them.

Symptoms of PMS may be specific, well localized, and recurrent. They may be exacerbated by emotional stress. Migraine-like headaches may occur, often preceded by visual scotomas and vomiting. Symptomatology varies among patients but often is consistent in the same patient.

One of the most common symptoms of PMS is *mastodynia*, or mastalgia (pain, and usually swelling, of the breasts caused by edema and engorgement of the vascular and ductal systems). A positive correlation between degree of ductal dilatation and degree of breast pain has been documented. Mastodynia specifically refers to a cyclical occurrence of severe breast pain, usually in the luteal phase of the menstrual cycle, and it may be the primary symptom of this syndrome in some. It has been shown to be related to high gonadotropin levels. Estrogen stimulates the ductal elements, whereas progesterone stimulates the stroma. An augmented response to prolactin has also been suggested. Examination is always necessary to rule out neoplasm, although most malignant tumors are painless. The presence of solitary or multiple cystic areas suggests fibrocystic change. The diagnosis usually can be confirmed by aspiration, but excisional biopsy occasionally is necessary. Serial mammograms or ultrasound examinations can be used to help monitor these patients (see Chapter 5).

A psychiatric history should be obtained, with special attention paid to a personal history of psychiatric problems or a family history of affective disorders. A mental status evaluation of affect, thinking, and behavior should be performed and recorded. A prospective diary correlating symptoms, daily activities, and menstrual flow can be useful to document changes and to encourage patient participation in her care.

If underlying psychiatric illness is suspected, a psychiatric evaluation is indicated. The most common associated psychiatric illness is depression, which generally responds to antidepressant drugs and psychotherapy. Recall that psychiatric illnesses have premenstrual exacerbations, so medications should be altered accordingly.

Treatment

Treatment of PMS/PMDD depends on the severity of the symptoms. For some women, changes in eating habits—limiting caffeine, alcohol, tobacco, and chocolate intake, and eating small, frequent meals high in complex carbohydrates—may be sufficient. Decreasing sodium intake may alleviate edema. Stress management, cognitive behavioral therapy, and aerobic exercise have all been shown to improve symptoms.

Low-risk pharmacologic interventions that may be effective include calcium carbonate (1000–1200 mg/d) for bloating, food cravings, and pain; magnesium (200–360 mg/d) for water retention; vitamin B_6 (note that prolonged use of 200 mg/d may cause peripheral neurotoxicity) and vitamin E; nonsteroidal anti-inflammatory drugs (NSAIDs); spironolactone for cyclic edema; and bromocriptine for mastalgia. Traditional Chinese herbal medicines are frequently used to treat PMS in China. A recent well-designed study has reported on the effectiveness of Jingqianping in the treatment of PMS. However, currently there is insufficient evidence to support the use of Chinese herbal medicine for PMS.

For symptoms of severe PMS and PMDD, further pharmacologic intervention may be necessary. Large, well-designed, randomized, placebo-controlled trials of fluoxetine and sertraline and smaller trials of several other serotonin reuptake inhibitors have shown clear benefit compared with placebo for women diagnosed with PMDD, with at least moderately beneficial response rates in 50–60% of women taking active drug. This is not a generic antidepressant effect, because agents with different mechanisms are not effective. Treatment should be given 14 days prior to the onset of menstruation and continued through the end of the cycle. Anxiolytics such as alprazolam and buspirone also have been shown to be efficacious, but their side effects and potential for dependence must be seriously considered.

Hormonal interventions have been shown to be effective. Use of selected oral contraceptives and transdermal estradiol patch has been suggested because they suppress ovulation. Recently, the US Food and Drug Administration approved the use of a pill containing drospirenone, which is a progestin derived from spironolactone rather than 19-nortestosterone, for treating PMDD. This approval permits the manufacturer to make claims about the drug's effectiveness in treating PMDD. However, the product label notes that effectiveness after 3 cycles is unknown.

Use of gonadotropin-releasing hormone (GnRH) agonists leads to a temporary "medical menopause" and an improvement in symptoms. Their limitations lie in a hypoestrogenic state and a risk for osteoporosis, although "add-back" therapy with estrogen and progesterone may obviate these problems. There is no conclusive evidence that progesterone can help women with PMS. Danazol may improve mastalgia. Finally, bilateral oophorectomy is a definitive surgical treatment option; again, estrogen replacement would be recommended.

DYSMENORRHEA

Dysmenorrhea, or painful menstruation, is one of the most common complaints of gynecologic patients. Many women experience mild discomfort during menstruation, but the term *dysmenorrhea* is reserved for women whose pain prevents normal activity and requires medication, whether an over-the-counter or a prescription drug.

There are 3 types of dysmenorrhea: (1) primary (no organic cause), (2) secondary (pathologic cause), and (3) membranous (cast of endometrial cavity shed as a single entity). This discussion focuses mainly on primary dysmenorrhea. Secondary dysmenorrhea is discussed elsewhere in this book in association with specific diseases and disorders (eg, endometriosis, adenomyosis, pelvic inflammatory disease, cervical stenosis, fibroids, and endometrial polyps). Membranous dysmenorrhea is rare; it causes intense cramping pain due to passage of a cast of the endometrium through an undilated cervix. Another cause of dysmenorrhea that should be considered is cramping due to the presence of an intrauterine device (IUD).

Pathogenesis

Pain during menstruation has long been known to be associated with ovulatory cycles. The mechanism of pain has been attributed to prostaglandin activity. Advances in the last 3 decades and current understanding suggest that in primary dysmenorrheal there is abnormal and increased prostanoid and possibly eicosanoid secretion, which in turn induces abnormal uterine contractions. The contractions reduce uterine blood flow, leading to uterine hypoxia.

Other studies have confirmed increased leukotriene levels as a contributing factor. Vasopressin was thought to be an aggravating agent, but atosiban, a vasopressin antagonist, has shown no effect on menstrual pain.

Psychological factors may be involved, including attitudes passed from mother to daughter. Girls should receive accurate information about menstruation before menarche; this can be provided by parents, teachers, physicians, or counselors. Emotional anxiety due to academic or social demands may be a cofactor.

Clinical Findings

Reactions to pain are subjective, and questioning by the physician should not lead the patient to exaggerate or minimize her discomfort. History taking is most important and should include the following questions: When does the pain occur? What does the patient do about the pain? Are there other symptoms? Do oral contraceptives relieve or intensify the pain? Does the pain become more severe over time?

Because dysmenorrhea almost always is associated with ovulatory cycles, it does not usually occur at menarche but rather later in adolescence. As many as 14–26% of adolescents miss school or work as a result of pain. Typically, pain occurs on the first day of the menses, usually about the time the flow begins, but it may not be present until the second day. Nausea and vomiting, diarrhea, and headache may occur. The specific symptoms associated with endometriosis are not present.

The physical examination does not reveal any significant pelvic disease. When the patient is symptomatic, she has generalized pelvic tenderness, perhaps more so in the area of the uterus than in the adnexa. Occasionally, ultrasonography or laparoscopy is necessary to rule out pelvic abnormalities such as endometriosis, pelvic inflammatory disease, or an accident in an ovarian cyst.

Differential Diagnosis

The most common misdiagnosis of primary dysmenorrhea is secondary dysmenorrhea due to endometriosis. With endometriosis, the pain usually begins 1–2 weeks before the menses, reaches a peak 1–2 days before, and is relieved at the onset of flow or shortly thereafter. Severe pain during sexual intercourse or findings of adnexal tenderness or mass or cul-de-sac nodularity, particularly in the premenstrual interval, help to confirm the diagnosis (see Chapter 56). A similar pain pattern occurs with adenomyosis, although in an older age group and in the absence of extrauterine clinical findings.

Treatment

NSAIDs or acetaminophen may relieve mild discomfort. Addition of continuous heat to the abdomen in addition to NSAIDs decreases pain significantly. For severe pain, codeine or other stronger analgesics may be needed, and bed rest may be desirable. Occasionally, emergency treatment with parenteral medication is necessary. Analgesics may cause drowsiness at the dosages required.

A. Antiprostaglandins

Antiprostaglandins are now used for treatment of dysmenorrhea. The newer, stronger, faster-acting drugs appear to be more useful than aspirin. Ibuprofen and naproxen, NSAIDs that are available over the counter, have been extremely effective in reducing menstrual prostaglandin and relieving dysmenorrhea. More specific cyclooxygenase-2 (COX-2) inhibitors are now available, but concerns about their adverse effects have recently attracted attention. Rofecoxib, valdecoxib, and lumiracoxib are effective for treating primary dysmenorrhea. Thus far, COX-2 inhibitors are equally effective but not better than naproxen. Given the above considerations, concerns about safety of COX-2 inhibitors, the short duration of therapy for relieving primary dysmenorrhea, and the low costs of NSAIDs, it is prudent to recommend established NSAIDs with track records of long-term safety as the preferred pharmacologic agent. The drug must be used at the earliest onset of symptoms, usually at the onset of, and sometimes 1–2 days prior to, bleeding or cramping.

Antiprostaglandins work by blocking prostaglandin synthesis and metabolism. Once the pain has been established, antiprostaglandins are not nearly as effective as with early use.

B. Oral Contraceptives

Cyclic administration of oral contraceptives, usually in the lowest dosage but occasionally with increased estrogen, prevents pain in most patients who do not obtain relief from antiprostaglandins or cannot tolerate them. The mechanism of pain relief may be related to absence of ovulation or to altered endometrium resulting in decreased prostaglandin production. In women who do not require contraception, oral contraceptives are given for 6–12 months. Many women continue to be free of pain after treatment has been discontinued. NSAIDs act synergistically with oral contraceptive pills to improve dysmenorrhea.

C. Surgical Treatment

In a few women, no medication controls dysmenorrhea. Cervical dilatation is of little use. Laparoscopic uterosacral ligament division and presacral neurectomy are infrequently performed, although some physicians consider these procedures to be important adjuncts to conservative operation for endometriosis.

Adenomyosis, endometriosis, or residual pelvic infection unresponsive to medical therapy or conservative surgical therapy eventually may require hysterectomy with or without ovarian removal in extreme cases. Rarely, a patient with no organic source of pain eventually requires hysterectomy to relieve symptoms.

D. Adjuvant Treatments

Continuous low-level topical heat therapy has been shown to be as effective as ibuprofen in treating dysmenorrhea, although its practicality in daily life may be questionable. Many studies have indicated that exercise decreases the prevalence and/or improves the symptomatology of dysmenorrhea, although solid evidence is lacking.

A recent Cochrane review analyzed 7 randomized controlled trials of transcutaneous electrical nerve stimulation (TENS) compared with placebo or no treatment. Overall, high-frequency TENS is more effective for pain relief in primary dysmenorrhea than placebo TENS.

Currently, there is insufficient evidence to recommend the use of herbal and dietary therapies for dysmenorrhea.

American College of Obstetricians and Gynecologists. *Premenstrual Syndrome. ACOG Practice Bulletin Number 15.* Washington, DC: American College of Obstetricians and Gynecologists; 2000.

Halbreich U. Algorithm for treatment of premenstrual syndromes (PMS): experts' recommendations and limitations. *Gynecol Endocrinol* 2005;20:48–56. PMID: 15969247.

Jing Z, Yang X, Ismail KM, Chen X, Wu T. Chinese herbal medicine for premenstrual syndrome. *Cochrane Database Syst Rev* 2009;1:CD006414. PMID: 19160284.

Johnson S. Premenstrual syndrome, premenstrual dysphoric disorder, and beyond: a clinical primer for practitioners. *Obstet Gynecol* 2004;104:845–859. PMID: 15458909.

Lopez LM, Kaptein A, Helmerhorst FM. Oral contraceptives containing drospirenone for premenstrual syndrome. *Cochrane Database Syst Rev* 2008;1:CD006586. PMID: 18254106.

ABNORMAL UTERINE BLEEDING

ESSENTIALS OF DIAGNOSIS

- Abnormal uterine bleeding includes abnormal menstrual bleeding and bleeding due to other causes such as pregnancy, systemic disease, or cancer.
- In childbearing women, a complication of pregnancy must always be considered.
- Exclusion of all possible pathologic causes of abnormal bleeding establishes the diagnosis of dysfunctional uterine bleeding (nearly 60% of cases).

General Considerations

Abnormal uterine bleeding includes abnormal menstrual bleeding and bleeding due to other causes such as pregnancy, systemic disease, or cancer. The diagnosis and management of abnormal uterine bleeding present some of the most difficult problems in gynecology. Patients may not be able to localize the source of the bleeding from the vagina, urethra, or rectum. In childbearing women, a complication of pregnancy must always be considered, and one must always remember that more than 1 entity may be present, such as uterine myomas and cervical cancer.

Patterns of Abnormal Uterine Bleeding

The standard classification for patterns of abnormal bleeding recognizes 7 different patterns.

1. **Menorrhagia** (**hypermenorrhea**) is heavy or prolonged menstrual flow. The presence of clots may not be abnormal but may signify excessive bleeding. "Gushing" or "open-faucet" bleeding is always abnormal. Submucous myomas, complications of pregnancy, adenomyosis, IUDs, endometrial hyperplasias, malignant tumors, and dysfunctional bleeding are causes of menorrhagia.
2. **Hypomenorrhea** (**cryptomenorrhea**) is unusually light menstrual flow, sometimes only spotting. An obstruction such as hymenal or cervical stenosis may be the cause. Uterine synechiae (Asherman's syndrome) can be causative and are diagnosed by a hysterogram or hysteroscopy. Patients receiving oral contraceptives occasionally complain of light flow and can be reassured that this is not significant.
3. **Metrorrhagia** (**intermenstrual bleeding**) is bleeding that occurs at any time between menstrual periods. Ovulatory bleeding occurs midcycle as spotting and can be documented with basal body temperatures. Endometrial polyps and endometrial and cervical carcinomas are pathologic causes. In recent years, exogenous estrogen administration has become a common cause of this type of bleeding.
4. **Polymenorrhea** describes periods that occur too frequently. This usually is associated with anovulation and rarely with a shortened luteal phase in the menstrual cycle.
5. **Menometrorrhagia** is bleeding that occurs at irregular intervals. The amount and duration of bleeding also vary. Any condition that causes intermenstrual bleeding can eventually lead to menometrorrhagia. Sudden onset of irregular bleeding episodes may be an indication of malignant tumors or complications of pregnancy.
6. **Oligomenorrhea** describes menstrual periods that occur more than 35 days apart. Amenorrhea is diagnosed if no menstrual period occurs for more than 6 months. Bleeding usually is decreased in amount and associated with anovulation, either from endocrine causes (eg, pregnancy, pituitary-hypothalamic causes, menopause) or systemic causes (eg, excessive weight loss). Estrogen-secreting tumors produce oligomenorrhea prior to other patterns of abnormal bleeding.
7. **Contact bleeding** (**postcoital bleeding**) is self-explanatory but must be considered a sign of cervical cancer until proved otherwise. Other causes of contact bleeding are much more common, including cervical eversion, cervical polyps, cervical or vaginal infection (eg, *Trichomonas*), or atrophic vaginitis. A negative cytologic smear does not rule out invasive cervical cancer, and colposcopy, biopsy, or both may be necessary.

Evaluation of Abnormal Uterine Bleeding

Detailed history, physical examination, cytologic examination, pelvic ultrasound, and blood tests are the first steps in the evaluation of abnormal uterine bleeding. The main aim of the blood tests is to exclude a systemic disease, pregnancy, or a trophoblastic disease. The blood tests usually include complete blood count, assay of the β subunit of human chorionic gonadotropin (hCG), and thyroid-stimulating hormone (TSH).

A. History

Many causes of bleeding are strongly suggested by the history alone. Note the amount of menstrual flow, the length of the menstrual cycle and menstrual period, the length and amount of episodes of intermenstrual bleeding, and any episodes of contact bleeding. Note also the last menstrual period, the last normal menstrual period, age at menarche and menopause, and any changes in general health. The patient must keep a record of bleeding patterns to determine whether bleeding is abnormal or only a variation of normal. However, most women have an occasional menstrual cycle that is not in their usual pattern. Depending on the patient's age and the pattern of the bleeding, observation may be all that is necessary.

B. Physical Examination

Abdominal masses and an enlarged, irregular uterus suggest myoma. A symmetrically enlarged uterus is more typical of adenomyosis or endometrial carcinoma. Atrophic and inflammatory vulvar and vaginal lesions can be visualized, and cervical polyps and invasive lesions of cervical carcinoma can be seen. Rectovaginal examination is especially important to identify lateral and posterior spread or the presence of a barrel-shaped cervix. In pregnancy, a decidual reaction of the cervix may be the source of bleeding. The appearance is a velvety, friable erythematous lesion on the ectocervix.

C. Cytologic Examination

Although most useful in diagnosing asymptomatic intraepithelial lesions of the cervix, cytologic smears can help screen for invasive cervical (particularly endocervical) lesions. Although cytology is not reliable for the diagnosis of endometrial abnormalities, the presence of endometrial cells in a postmenopausal woman is abnormal unless she is receiving exogenous estrogens. Likewise, women in the secretory phase of the menstrual cycle should not shed endometrial cells. Of course, a cytologic examination that is positive or suspicious for endometrial cancer demands further evaluation.

Tubal or ovarian cancer can be suspected based on a cervical smear. The technique of obtaining a smear is important, because a tumor may be present only in the endocervical canal and may not shed cells to the ectocervix or vagina. Laboratories should report the presence or absence of endocervical cells. The current use of a spatula and endocervical brush has significantly increased the adequacy of cytologic smears from the cervix. Any abnormal smear requires further evaluation (see Chapter 48).

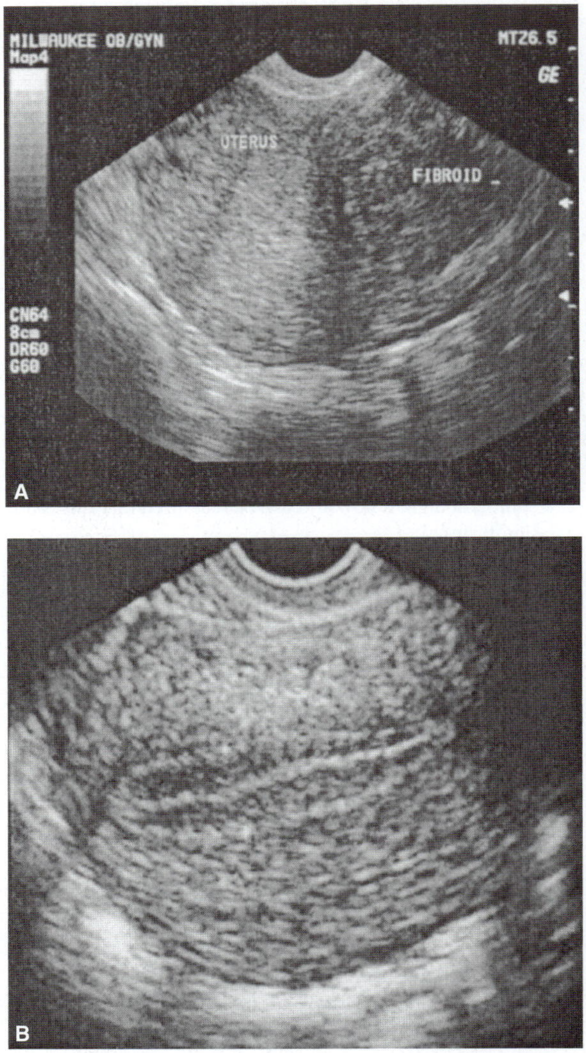

▲ **Figure 38–1.** Typical ultrasound scan of a uterine fibroid (**A**) and normal endometrial lining (**B**).

D. Pelvic Ultrasound Scan

Pelvic ultrasonography has become an integral part of the gynecologic pelvic examination. The scan can be performed either transvaginally or transabdominally. The transvaginal examination is performed with an empty bladder and enables a closer look with greater details at the pelvic organs. The transabdominal examination is performed with a full bladder and enables a wider, but less discriminative, examination of the pelvis. The ultrasound scan can add many details to the physical examination, such as a description of the uterine lining and its width and regularity (Fig. 38–1) and the presence of intramural or submucous fibroids (Fig.38–1), intrauterine polyps, and adnexal masses. Persistent thick and irregular endometrium is one of the preoperative predictors of endometrial pathology and demands further evaluation and tissue biopsy.

Sonohysterography is a modification of the pelvic ultrasound scan. The ultrasound is performed following injection of saline by a thin catheter into the uterus. This technique increases significantly the sensitivity of transvaginal ultrasonography and has been used to evaluate the endometrial cavity for polyps, fibroids, and other abnormalities.

F. Endometrial Biopsy

Methods of endometrial biopsy include use of the Novak suction curette, the Duncan curette, the Kevorkian curette, or the Pipelle. Cervical dilatation is not necessary with these instruments. Small areas of the endometrial lining are sampled.

If bleeding persists and no cause of bleeding can be found or if the tissue obtained is inadequate for diagnosis, hysteroscopy and, in some cases, formal dilatation and curettage (D&C) must be performed.

E. Hysteroscopy

Placing an endoscopic camera through the cervix into the endometrial cavity allows direct visualization of the cavity (Fig. 38–2). Because of its higher diagnostic accuracy and suitability for outpatient investigation, hysteroscopy is increasingly replacing D&C for the evaluation of abnormal uterine bleeding. Hysteroscopy currently is regarded as the gold standard evaluation of pathology in the uterine cavity. Resection attachments allow immediate capability to remove or biopsy lesions.

G. Dilatation & Curettage

For many years, D&C has been regarded as the gold standard for the diagnosis of abnormal uterine bleeding. It can be performed with the patient under local or general anesthesia, almost always in an outpatient or ambulatory setting. With general anesthesia, relaxation of the abdominal musculature is greater, allowing for a more thorough pelvic examination, more precise evaluation of pelvic masses, and more complete curettage. Nevertheless, D&C is a blind procedure, and its accuracy, particularly when the cause of the abnormal uterine bleeding is a focal lesion such as a polyp, is debatable.

General Principles of Management (Fig. 38–3)

In making the diagnosis, it is important not to assume the obvious. A careful history and pelvic examination are vital.

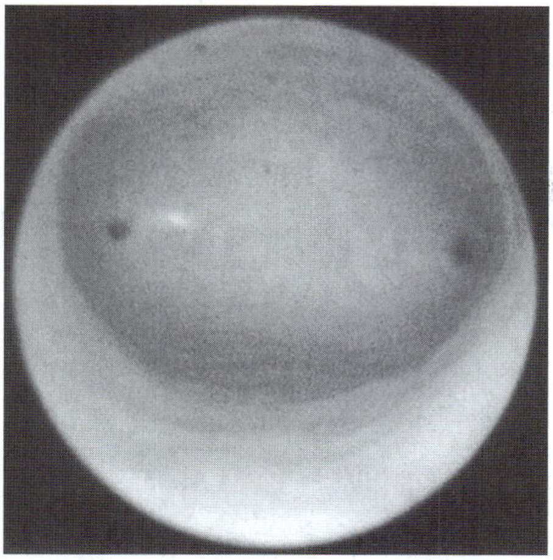

▲ **Figure 38–2.** Hysteroscopic view of the uterine cavity.

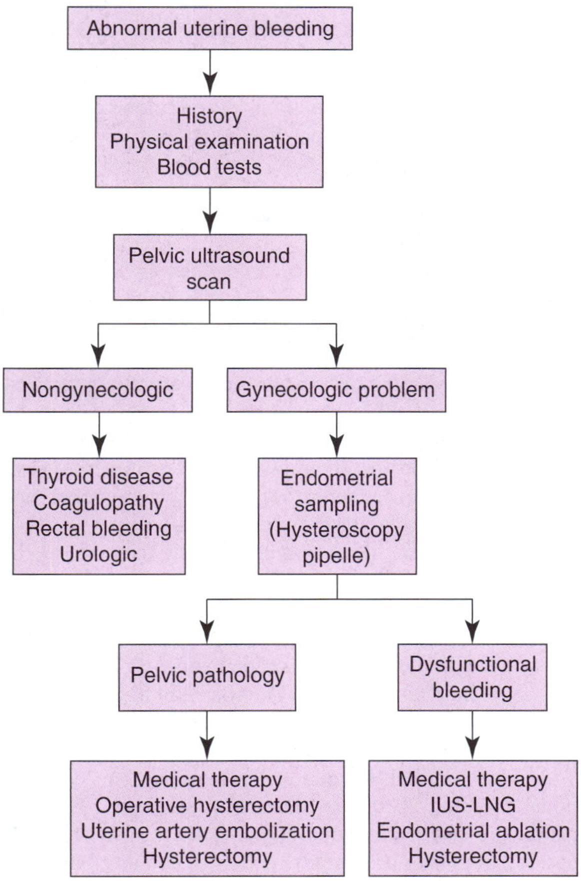

▲ **Figure 38–3.** General principles of management of abnormal uterine bleeding. IUS-LNG, intrauterine system-levonorgestrel releasing.

The possibility of pregnancy must be considered, as well as use of oral contraceptives, IUDs, and hormones.

Another important evaluation during the workup of abnormal uterine bleeding is to decide whether the bleeding is associated with ovulatory or anovulatory cycles. In ovulatory cycles, the bleeding might be due to a persistent corpus luteum cyst or short luteal phase. In anovulatory cycles, the endometrium outgrows its blood supply, partially breaks down, and is sloughed in an irregular manner. In these cases, an organic cause of anovulation must be excluded (eg, thyroid or adrenal abnormalities). Conversion from proliferative to secretory endometrium (by combined oral contraceptive pills or progesterone in the luteal phase) corrects most acute and chronic bleeding problems.

Improved diagnostic techniques and treatment have resulted in decreased use of hysterectomy to treat abnormal bleeding patterns. If pathologic causes (eg, submucous myomas, adenomyosis) can be excluded, if there is no significant risk for cancer development (as from atypical endometrial hyperplasia), and if there is no acute life-threatening hemorrhage, most patients can be treated with hormone preparations or minimally invasive procedures, which are considered as alternatives to hysterectomy. Myomectomy (hysteroscopic, laparoscopic, or conservative) can be suggested for treatment of myoma if the patient wishes to retain her childbearing potential. Endometrial ablation and endometrial resection may offer successful outpatient and in-office alternatives.

For menorrhagia, antifibrinolytic therapy has been shown to significantly decrease blood loss during menses, as have prostaglandin synthetase inhibitors. Long-acting intramuscular progestin administration (Depo-Provera) can be given but may result in erratic bleeding or even amenorrhea. Finally, levonorgestrel-releasing IUDs are as effective as endometrial resection in decreasing blood loss.

1. ABNORMAL UTERINE BLEEDING DURING PREGNANCY

See Chapter 18.

2. ABNORMAL BLEEDING DUE TO NONGYNECOLOGIC DISEASES & DISORDERS

In the differential diagnosis of abnormal bleeding, nongynecologic causes of bleeding (eg, rectal or urologic disorders) must be ruled out, because patients may have difficulty differentiating the source of bleeding. Gynecologic and nongynecologic causes of bleeding may coexist. Systemic disease may cause abnormal uterine bleeding. For example, myxedema usually causes amenorrhea, but less severe hypothyroidism is associated with increased uterine bleeding. Liver disease interferes with estrogen metabolism and may cause variable degrees of bleeding. Both of these conditions are usually clinically apparent before gynecologic symptoms appear. Blood dyscrasias and coagulation abnormalities can also produce gynecologic bleeding. Patients receiving anticoagulants or adrenal steroids may expect abnormalities. Extreme weight loss due to eating disorders, exercise, or dieting may be associated with anovulation and amenorrhea.

3. DYSFUNCTIONAL UTERINE BLEEDING

Exclusion of all possible pathologic causes of abnormal bleeding establishes the diagnosis of dysfunctional uterine bleeding (nearly 60% of cases). Dysfunctional bleeding occurs most commonly at the extremes of reproductive age (20% of cases occur in adolescents and 40% in patients over age 40 years). Management depends on the age of the patient (adolescent, young woman, or premenopausal woman).

Treatment

A. Adolescents

Because the first menstrual cycles frequently are anovulatory, the menses not unusually are irregular, and explanation of the reason is all the treatment that is necessary. Heavy bleeding—even hemorrhage—may occur. Invasive diagnostic procedures usually are not necessary in young patients, but physical (pelvic or rectal if possible) examination, pelvic ultrasonography, and basic blood tests must be performed to exclude pregnancy or pathologic conditions. Estrogens given orally should be adequate for all patients except extremely rare cases requiring curettage to control hemorrhage. Numerous regimens are available, including estrogens followed by progesterone, progesterone alone, or combination oral contraceptives. For acute hemorrhage, high-dose estrogen given intravenously (25 mg conjugated estrogen every 4 hours) gives rapid response. In hemodynamically stable patients, the oral dose of conjugated estrogens is 2.5 mg every 4–6 hours for 14–21 days. Once bleeding has stopped, medroxyprogesterone acetate 5 mg once or twice per day should be given for 7–10 days.

Oral contraceptives, 3–4 times the usual dose, are just as effective and may be simpler to use than sequential hormones. Again, the dose is lowered after a few days, and the lower dose is continued for the next few cycles, particularly to raise the hemoglobin levels in an anemic patient. Medroxyprogesterone acetate 10 mg/d for 10 days can be given to patients who have proliferative endometrium on biopsy. In patients receiving cyclic therapy, 3–6 monthly courses are usually administered, after which treatment is discontinued and further evaluation performed if necessary. In adolescents in whom the bleeding is not severe, oral contraceptives can be used as normally prescribed.

B. Young Women

In patients 20–30 years old, pathologic causes are similarly not very common, and the appropriate diagnostic procedures should be considered after the initial evaluation by history, physical and cytologic examination, and pelvic ultrasound. Hormonal management is the same as for adolescents.

C. Premenopausal Women

In the later reproductive years, even more care must be given to excluding pathologic causes because of the possibility of endometrial cancer. The initial evaluation should be complemented by hysteroscopy and endometrial biopsy and should clearly establish anovulatory or dyssynchronous cycles as the cause before hormonal therapy is started. Recurrences of abnormal bleeding demand further evaluation.

D. Surgical Measures

For patients whose bleeding cannot be controlled with hormones, who are symptomatically anemic, and whose lifestyle is compromised by persistence of irregular bleeding, D&C may temporarily stop bleeding. If bleeding persists, levonorgestrel-releasing IUDs or a minimally invasive procedure such as endometrial ablation may be offered. Studies have shown that approximately 80% of patients scheduled for hysterectomy changed their minds following endometrial ablation. However, if these minimally invasive procedures fail or if the patient prefers a definitive solution, hysterectomy may be necessary. Definitive surgery may also be needed for coexistent endometriosis, myoma, and disorders of pelvic relaxation.

4. POSTMENOPAUSAL BLEEDING

Postmenopausal bleeding may be defined as bleeding that occurs after 12 months of amenorrhea in a middle-aged woman. When amenorrhea occurs in a younger person for 1 year and premature ovarian failure or menopause has been diagnosed, episodes of bleeding may be classified as postmenopausal, although resumption of ovulatory cycles can occur. Follicle-stimulating hormone (FSH) levels are particularly helpful in the differential diagnosis of menopausal versus hypothalamic amenorrhea. An FSH level greater than 30 mIU/mL is highly suggestive of menopause.

Postmenopausal bleeding is more likely to be caused by pathologic disease than is bleeding in younger women and must always be investigated. Nongynecologic causes must be excluded; these causes are more likely to result from pathologic disease in older women, and patients may be unable to determine the site of bleeding. The source of bleeding should not be assumed to be nongynecologic unless there is good evidence or proper evaluation has excluded gynecologic causes.

Neither normal ("functional") bleeding nor dysfunctional bleeding should occur after menopause. Although pathologic disorders are more likely, other causes may also occur. Atrophic or proliferative endometrium is not unusual. Secretory patterns should not occur unless the patient has resumed ovulation or has received progesterone therapy. After nongynecologic causes of bleeding are excluded, gynecologic causes must be considered.

Exogenous Hormones

The most common cause of postmenopausal uterine bleeding is the use of exogenous hormones. In the past, face creams and cosmetics contained homeopathic amounts of estrogens, but today, this cause is highly unlikely. Careful history taking becomes vital, because patients may not follow specific instructions on the use of estrogen and progesterone therapy.

In light of the new caution placed on postmenopausal hormone replacement therapy (HRT) because of cardiovascular risks, long-term estrogen/progesterone administration for prevention of osteoporosis is no longer recommended. Women continue HRT for menopausal symptoms to improve their quality of life. Regular menstrual bleeding may resume if they take HRT agents cyclically. Not uncommonly, these patients present with vaginal bleeding as many as 6–12 months after initiation of HRT. If bleeding is still occurring by that time, further investigation is warranted to determine its etiology. If endometrial hyperplasia is found, specific attention must be paid to the presence of atypia and treatment started by increasing the progesterone component or by hysterectomy.

Vaginal Atrophy & Vaginal & Vulvar Lesions

Bleeding from the lower reproductive tract almost always is related to vaginal atrophy, with or without trauma. Examination reveals thin tissue with ecchymosis. Rarely, a tear at the introitus or deep in the vagina requires suturing. With vulvar dystrophies, a white area and cracking of the skin of the vulva may be present. Cytologic study of material obtained from the cervix and vagina will reveal immature epithelial cells with or without inflammation. After coexisting upper tract lesions are excluded, treatment can include local or systemic estrogen therapy for vaginal lesions. Vulvar lesions require further diagnostic evaluation to determine the proper treatment.

Tumors of the Reproductive Tract

The differential diagnosis of organic causes of postmenopausal uterine bleeding includes endometrial hyperplasias (simple, complex, and atypical), endometrial polyps, endometrial carcinoma or other more rare tumors such as cervical or endocervical carcinoma, uterine sarcomas (including mixed mesodermal and carcinosarcomas), and, even more rarely, uterine tube and ovarian cancer. Estrogen-secreting ovarian tumors also should be considered.

Uterine sampling must be done and tissue obtained. Endocervical curettage should be performed, along with any endometrial sampling technique. If a diagnosis cannot be established or is questionable with office procedures, D&C is necessary. Hysteroscopy performed in the office or operating room may prove helpful in locating endometrial polyps or fibroids that could be missed even by fractional curettage. Pelvic ultrasonography may be extremely helpful in the diagnosis of ovarian tumors and in evaluation of the thickness of the endometrium, as well as in discerning between uterine myomas and adnexal tumors. Recurring episodes of postmenopausal bleeding may rarely require hysterectomy, even when a diagnosis cannot be established by endometrial sampling.

Dawood MY. Primary dysmenorrhea: advances in pathogenesis and management. *Obstet Gynecol* 2006;108:428–441. PMID: 16880317.

Istre O, Qvigstad E. Current treatment options for abnormal uterine bleeding: an evidence-based approach. *Best Pract Res Clin Obstet Gynaecol* 2007;21:905–913. PMID: 17499553.

Jensen JT, Speroff L. Health benefits of oral contraceptives. *Obstet Gynecol Clin North Am* 2000;27:705–721. PMID: 11091985.

Rauramo I, Elo I, Istre O. Long-term treatment of menorrhagia with levonorgestrel intrauterine system versus endometrial resection. *Obstet Gynecol* 2004;104:1314–1321. PMID: 15572496.

Revel A, Shushan A. Investigation of the infertile couple. Hysteroscopy with endometrial biopsy is the gold standard investigation for abnormal uterine bleeding. *Hum Reprod* 2002;17:1947–1949. PMID: 12151418.

Schwayder JM. Pathophysiology of abnormal uterine bleeding. *Obstet Gynecol Clin North Am* 2000;27:219–234. PMID: 10857116.

Telner DE, Jakubovicz D. Approach to diagnosis and management of abnormal uterine bleeding. *Can Fam Physician* 2007;53:58–64. PMID: 17872610.

39 Benign Disorders of the Vulva & Vagina

Jacob Bornstein MD, MPA

Disorders of the vulva and vagina are very common and cause considerable discomfort. Until recently, however, our understanding of vulvar conditions has been scant due to the lack of communication between gynecologists, dermatologists, pathologists, and sex therapists, each with his or her own ideas of the natural history, mode of diagnosis, and preferred therapy. An obvious consequence is the propagation of terms for the same disorders. The establishment in 1970 of the International Society for the Study of Vulvovaginal Disease (ISSVD) fostered exchange of ideas, collective discussion, and understanding of the natural history and modern treatment of vulvar diseases. Common terminology was established. The terminology of benign vulvar and vaginal disorders used in this chapter is based on the guidelines of the ISSVD. The morphologic and functional approach is accessible to the novice in vulvar and vaginal disease. At the same time it emphasizes breakthroughs in the understanding of the different vulvar pain syndromes, the influence of the vaccine against human papillomavirus (HPV) on vulvar diseases, and the modern treatment of the vulvar dermatoses. The premalignant and malignant vulvar and vaginal disorders are discussed in Chapter 47.

ANATOMY & PHYSIOLOGY

The anatomy of the vagina and vulva is described in Chapter 1. In recent years the vulvar vestibule, the site of origin of vestibulodynia, the "provoked" vulvar pain of dyspareunia, has been a focus of attention. Although the vulvar skin is devoid of estrogen receptors, the development of vaginal disorders is influenced by the presence or absence of endogenous or exogenous estrogen. Estrogen thickens the vaginal epithelium, which leads to the accumulation of glycogen in the epithelial cells. The intraepithelial glycogen metabolizes to lactic acid. The resultant vaginal pH of 3.5–4.0 promotes the growth of normal vaginal flora, chiefly lactobacilli and acidogenic corynebacteria. Asymptomatic *Candida* organisms may be present in small quantities.

ESSENTIALS OF DIAGNOSIS

Evaluation of a patient with vulvar and/or vaginal symptoms requires the following:

- A meticulous review of physiologic systems to reveal underlying medical conditions that may lead to vulvar symptoms.
  - Diabetes mellitus may be associated with vulvar pruritus or pain as a consequence of vulvovaginal candidiasis or, in advanced cases, as a result of neuropathic pain.
  - Elevated serum levels of biliary salts, such as in biliary stasis or primary biliary cirrhosis, may cause vulvar pruritus.
  - Hematologic disorders such as polycythemia or lymphoma may be associated with systemic symptoms, including vulvar pruritus.
  - A complete history of potential causes of vulvar irritation, including creams, powders, soaps, type of underwear, and cleansing techniques, should be reviewed.
  - Assessment of compliance to previous prescriptions may help determine whether failure of past treatments is attributable to incorrect diagnosis or to inadequate treatment.
  - Patients sometimes refrain from the use of common medications for vulvar disease due to their high potency or potential for side effects. Typical examples are systemic or potent topical steroids such as clobetasol propionate (Dermovate) and tricyclic antidepressants such as amitriptyline.
  - Information regarding previous infections should be elicited.
  - Sexual activity, although sensitive to both patient and healthcare provider, needs evaluation.
  - The use of feminine hygiene products (eg, douching, soaps, perfumes) and medications (eg, pessaries,

diaphragms, oral contraceptive pills, antibiotics) can alter the normal vaginal flora.
  - Overlying garments made of synthetic fabrics that retain heat and moisture can exacerbate vulvovaginal symptoms.

- Active inquiry about vulvar pain, discharge, and pruritus, as patients may fail to disclose these intimate matters.
- A physical examination including inspection of all mucosal and skin surfaces, because many skin conditions, such as psoriasis, seborrheic dermatitis, pemphigus, and lichen planus, can affect the vulva.
- A vaginal examination including evaluation of the physical, chemical, and microbiologic properties of vaginal discharge. The perianal region should be inspected, as many vulvar disorders affect it. Specimens and cultures may include vaginal wet prep and culture for yeast and bacteria. HPV DNA determination may be required.
- Vulvar examination: although examination of the vulva and vagina may be completed using a magnifying glass, a colposcopic examination (ie, "vulvoscopy," "vaginoscopy" is preferred, especially if a biopsy is to be taken. Two processes are important in the diagnosis of vulvar and vaginal lesions:
  1. Try to assess to which of the 6 morphologic types (Table 39–1) the lesion belongs. Then mentally browse the list of possible causes for that lesion.
  2. Biopsy liberally any suspicious lesion, because in most cases the final diagnosis is based on histopathologic findings. Thus the vulvar biopsy is almost a universal requirement.

PRINCIPLES OF OBTAINING A VULVAR BIOPSY

A satisfactory full-thickness sample of the skin and tumor can be obtained with a dermatologic punch biopsy under local anesthesia. Many vulva experts endeavor not to compress the sample tissue so as to preserve the original morphology of the lesion. Inclusion of the lesion margins helps identify abnormal features. This is also important in case of an ulcer, as its center may be necrotic and noninformative.

Table 39–1. Morphologic classification of vulvovaginal disease.

White lesion
Red lesion
Dark lesion
Ulcer
Small tumor
Large tumor

Table 39–2. Classification of nonneoplastic epithelial disorders of vulvar skin and mucosa.

Lichen sclerosus
Lichen simplex chronicus
Other dermatoses

Hospitalization is not required in most cases. Bleeding can be controlled by local pressure, argentum nitrate application, or, in rare cases, by applying a stitch.

VULVAR DISORDERS

The color of vulvar epithelium or lesions depends principally on the width of keratin layer, vascularity of the dermis, thickness of the overlying epidermis, and the amount of intervening pigment, either melanin or blood pigment.

WHITE LESION

Pathogenesis

The white appearance of a lichenoid lesion of the vulva is primarily due to the maceration of a thickened keratin layer resulting from increased moisture in the vulvar area. The epidermal thickening of neoplasia obscures the underlying vasculature and, in conjunction with the macerating effects of the moist environment, usually produces a hyperplastic white lesion. A diffuse white lesion of the vulva may also occur with the loss or absence of melanin pigmentation as with vitiligo, a hereditary disorder. Leukoderma is a localized white lesion resulting from transient loss of pigment in a residual scar formed after healing of an ulcer.

Formerly, a white lichenoid lesion was termed **leukoplakia**, **kraurosis vulva**, and **senile vulvitis**. In 1976 Jeffcoate introduced the term **dystrophy**, but in 1987 the ISSVD changed the term to **nonneoplastic epithelial disorders of vulvar skin and mucosa** (Table 39–2). This term was coined to emphasize that excision procedures such as vulvectomy are not required, as this condition is not neoplastic. Implied by the term is the need of a biopsy for definitive diagnosis. The use of the term **dystrophy with atypia** has been abandoned, and lesions that contain atypia are now called **vulvar intraepithelial neoplasia** (VIN). They are described in Chapter 47.

LICHEN SCLEROSUS

ESSENTIALS OF DIAGNOSIS

- Lichen sclerosus is the most common nonneoplastic epithelial vulvar disorder.

- Intense pruritus occurs, usually in women older than 60 years.
- The vulvar skin is thin, wrinkled, and white, with areas of lichenification and hyperkeratosis (see Table 39–3 for definitions).
- The anterior parts of the labia minora of both sides agglutinate.
- Erosions, fissures, subepithelial hemorrhages, and ulcerations result from scratching.
- Biopsy is required.

Pathogenesis

Lichen sclerosus, a benign, chronic, inflammatory process, is the most common vulvar dermatologic disorder. Possible etiologic factors of this multifactorial condition include vitamin A deficiency, an autoimmune process, excess of the enzyme elastase, and decreased activity of 5-alpha reductase enzyme, which prevents the conversion of testosterone to dihydrotestosterone (the trophic hormone of the skin) and results in thinning of the skin. The effectiveness of treatment with topical testosterone cream supports the latter hypothesis.

Table 39–3. Dictionary of vulvar terms.

Acanthosis	Abnormal but benign thickening of the prickle-cell layer of the skin
Erosion	Superficial damage to the skin, generally not deeper than the epidermis. Although more superficial than an excoriation, it can bleed mildly.
Excoriation	Erosion caused by mechanical means, appearing in the form of a scratch of the skin. It is commonly seen in skin disorders causing itching/pruritus.
Eczema	A form of dermatitis, or inflammation of the upper layers of the skin. Includes dryness and recurring skin rashes characterized by one or more of the following symptoms: redness, skin edema, itching and dryness, crusting, flaking, blistering, cracking, oozing, or bleeding.
Hyperkeratosis	Excess of keratins in the stratum corneum, thick superficial layer of the skin
Lichenification	Thickening of the skin (or epidermis) with accentuation of the normal lines of the skin, creating an appearance resembling a tree bark. It is commonly seen in chronic eczema (or atopic dermatitis), where there is constant scratching and rubbing of the skin, and in lichen simplex chronicus. Thus lichenification is often associated with pruritic (itching) disorders.
Ulcer	Loss of both epithelium and part of the dermis

Clinical Findings

A. Symptoms & Signs

This disease usually appears in women older than 60 years. Of the rare appearances in childhood, spontaneous resolution at adolescence occurs in approximately half. Most patients present with pruritus. Some complain of vulvar pain or dyspareunia and /or present with asymptomatic white lesions.

The progression and typical clinical characteristics of acute lichen sclerosus include the following:

1. Erythema and edema of vulvar skin
2. Development of white plaques representing lichenification and hyperkeratosis
3. Uniting of white plaques
4. Intense pruritus leading to scratch–itch cycle
5. Telangiectasias and subepithelial hemorrhages resulting from scratching
6. Erosions, fissures, and ulcerations

The progression and typical clinical characteristics of chronic lichen sclerosus include the following:

1. Thin, wrinkled, and white skin with a cigarette-paper appearance
2. Agglutination of the anterior parts of the labia minora of both sides to cover the clitoris and create phimosis (Fig. 39–1)
3. Contraction of the vulvar structures with resultant introital stenosis, previously termed **kraurosis**
4. Involvement of the perianal region in the form of 8: around the vulva and around the anus.
5. Development in some women of islands of hyperplastic epithelia within the atrophic lichen sclerosus epithelium

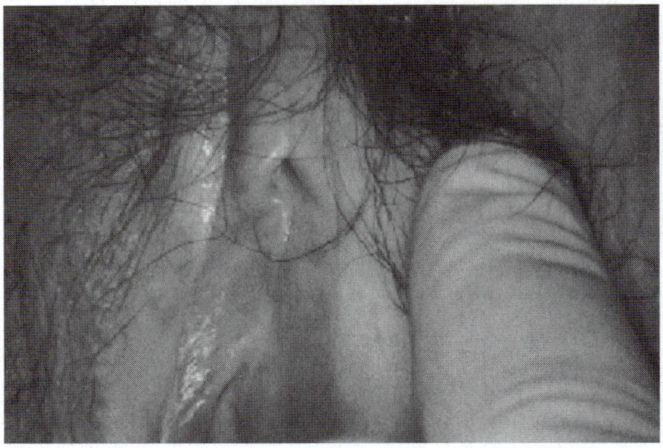

▲ **Figure 39–1.** Advanced lesion of lichen sclerosus. The labia minora and prepuce of the clitoris have blended into the labial skin.

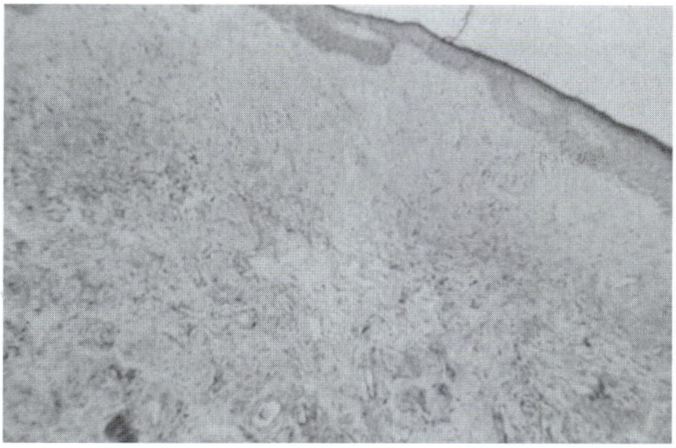

▲ **Figure 39–2.** Microscopic appearance of lichen sclerosus, characterized by hyperkeratosis, flattened epidermis, and hyalinization of the dermis.

Histologic Findings

Definitive diagnosis depends on identification of the following 5 histologic features in the biopsy (Fig. 39–2):

1. Thin hyperkeratotic layer
2. Thinning of the epithelial layer
3. Flattening of the papillae (Rete pegs)
4. Homogenization of the stroma
5. Deep lymphocytic infiltration

Differential Diagnosis

Other causes of a white lesion in the vulva are vitiligo, lichen simplex chronicus, and other dermatoses, such as psoriasis.

Complications

The high rate of squamous cell cancer in women with lichen sclerosus (3–5%) prompts biopsy of all new lesions. Cancer develops mainly in women who continue to suffer from vulvar itch or neglect treatment. It is expected that the introduction of clobetasole, an effective topical treatment for lichen sclerosus, may decrease the incidence of vulvar carcinoma developing from lichen sclerosus lesions.

Treatment

The first step is to stop the itch–scratch cycle and minimize the dermal inflammation. General measures of vulvar hygiene should be applied: avoiding tight undergarments, cleansing daily with mild soap, and drying the vulvar skin with a hair dryer.

A. Medications

An oral antihistamine agent can be taken at bedtime. Although clobetasole dipropionate 0.05% (Dermovate) is a superpotent topical steroid (Table 39–4), it is recommended at the start to obtain immediate relief, stop the itch–scratch cycle, and reinstitute the patient's belief in the health care provider. To prevent or minimize the side effects of this steroid, topical application should be in a small amount, similar to that of toothpaste on a toothbrush, twice daily for 2 weeks, then once daily for 2 weeks, then twice weekly for 2 weeks, and then as needed for the rest of the woman's life. Some recommend tapering to a lower-potency topical steroid for treatment maintenance. Atrophic degeneration of the skin secondary to the steroid is rare.

Table 39–4. Potency of steroids.

Low potency
Hydrocortisone 0.1–1%
Dexamethasone 0.1%
Desonide 0.05%
Medium-level potency
Betamethasone dipropionate 0.05%
Betamethasone valerate 0.1%
Fluocinolone 0.025%
Triamcinolone acetonide 0.1%
High-level potency
Fluocinonide 0.05%
Dexamethasone 0.25%
Maximal potency
Clobetasol dipropionate 0.05%
Betamethasone dipropionate 0.05%

Note: Only representative products are listed.

Some recommend tacrolimus cream, retinoid, antimalarial agents, or photodynamic therapy for these who do not respond to clobetasole. Surgical therapy should be limited to treatment of introital narrowing leading to dyspareunia or associated intraepithelial or invasive squamous cell neoplasia.

When nothing else relieves the itch, either of the following may be tried: intralesional injection of steroids or surgical undermining of the affected skin without excision, with the intention of undercutting the nerve fibers (Mering procedure).

The following 3 treatments, popular in the past, have been discontinued:

1. Topical application of 2% testosterone propionate ointment; less effective than clobetasole, it leads to virilization.
2. Intralesional injection of alcohol, a painful procedure that leads to sloughing of the vulvar tissues.
3. Vulvectomy; after this unnecessary mutilation, the disease tends to recur at the adjacent tissues.

Prognosis

The disease is chronic and usually recurs with cessation of treatment. The introduction of clobetasole dipropionate leads to resolution of symptoms in most patients and reversal of skin changes in approximately half of patients.

VULVAR LICHEN SIMPLEX CHRONICUS

Vulvar lichen simplex chronicus is the current term for the condition that includes the previously designated hyperplastic dystrophy, squamous cell hyperplasia, atopic dermatitis, atopic eczema, and neurodermatitis.

Clinical Findings

A. Symptoms & Signs

Vulvar lichen simplex chronicus is characterized by benign epithelial thickening and hyperkeratosis resulting from chronic irritation, such as from the use of perfumed pads or chronic vulvovaginal infections. The accompanying pruritus leads to rubbing and scratching, which becomes involuntary over time. As epithelial thickening develops, the humid environment of the vulva causes maceration, and a raised white lesion may become diffuse and even involve the adjacent thighs, perineum, or perianal skin.

Histopathologic Findings

Biopsy is necessary to exclude intraepithelial neoplasia and invasive tumor. Histologic examination demonstrates hyperkeratosis and acanthosis (see Table 39–3 for definitions), resulting in thickening of the epithelium and elongation of the rete pegs. In contrast to lichen sclerosus, there is no dermal inflammatory infiltrate.

Differential Diagnosis

Differential diagnosis includes the other nonneoplastic epithelial disorders such as lichen sclerosus, flat condyloma acuminatum, psoriasis, and vulvar intraepithelial neoplasia.

Treatment

Treatment of squamous cell hyperplasia starts with general measures of vulvar hygiene. Sitz baths and lubricants can help restore moisture to cells and reconstruct the epithelial barrier. Oral antihistamines may help relieve pruritus. In addition, topical application of medium-potency steroids twice daily can decrease the inflammation and pruritus. Vulvar epithelium takes at least 6 weeks to heal. For intractable cases, antidepressants or subcutaneous intralesional injection of steroids can be considered.

LICHEN PLANUS

Clinical Findings

Lichen planus rarely affects the vulva. It is a mucocutaneous dermatosis characterized by the presence of sharply marginated flat-topped papules on the skin and less sharply marginated white plaques on oral and genital mucous membranes. The pathogenesis is unknown. In the vulva 2 clinical aspects can be observed: classic leukoplastic lesions and erosive lesions. Vulvar erosive lichen planus seems to be more frequent but is often ignored. The clinical appearance of vaginal erosive lichen planus is similar to that of desquamative inflammatory vaginitis.

Treatment

Treatment of lichen planus is mainly topical, starting with hydrocortisone foam for the vagina (Colifoam). If unsuccessful, fluorinated corticosteroids, ultrapotent corticosteroids, or topical treatment with tacrolimus 0.1% can be tried. Careful and frequent examination of the vagina for formation of adhesions is important. In cases of severe pruritus and intensive mucocutaneous involvement, systemic steroids should be used. Introital stenosis and vaginal adhesions can be treated by use of vaginal dilators in graduated sizes or from surgical release of scars.

RED LESION

The red color of these lesions results from thinning epidermis, revealing capillary vasculature. Other causes are vasodilatation associated with inflammation and neovascularization of a neoplasia. Although they may manifest any acute dermatitis, red lesions are mainly associated with acute candidal vulvovaginitis. Vulvovaginitis is discussed later in this chapter, under Vaginal Disorders. Paget's disease, a nonsquamous intraepithelial neoplasia characterized by an eczematous-like red lesion spreading over the vulvar skin, is discussed in Chapter 47. Other red lesions include seborrheic dermatitis, lupus erythematosus, and some cases of VIN. VIN also presents as a white or dark lesion and as an ulcer or tumor.

PSORIASIS

Psoriasis is a chronic relapsing dermatosis that affects the scalp, the extensor surfaces of the extremities, the trunk, and the vulva. Sometimes the vulvar skin is the only body surface affected. Primary lesions are raised and appear typically erythematous, resembling a candidal infection. Most lesions are sharply demarcated. The silver scaly crusts that characterize psoriasis on other parts of the body are usually absent; hence the lesion is red. Treatment includes topical corticosteroids.

DARK LESION

Dark lesions result from an increased quantity or concentration of melanin or hemosiderin pigments, sometimes subsequent to trauma. A persistent dark lesion on the vulva skin likely represents a nevus or a melanoma.

MELANOSIS OR LENTIGO

Melanosis or lentigo is a benign darkly pigmented flat lesion that may be mistaken for a melanoma. A nevus on the vulvar skin may be flat, slightly elevated, papillomatous, dome-shaped, or pedunculated. Melanomas of the vulva are uncommon neoplasms constituting only 1–3% of vulvar cancers. They are extremely aggressive malignant lesions and may arise from pigmented nevi of the vulva.

CAPILLARY HEMANGIOMA

Senile (cherry) hemangiomas are usually multiple, small, dark blue, asymptomatic papules that are discovered incidentally during examination of the older patient. Excision biopsy is needed only if the hemangiomas bleed repeatedly. A cryosurgical probe or carbon dioxide laser can also be used.

Childhood hemangiomas are usually diagnosed in the first few months of life. They may vary in size from small strawberry hemangiomas to large cavernous ones. They tend to be elevated and bright red or dark, depending on their size and the thickness of the overlying skin. Although tending to increase in size during the first few months of life, they often become static or regress without therapy after age 18 months. Although most of these hemangiomas only require observation, and not therapy, larger ones may require treatment with cryosurgery, argon laser therapy, or sclerosing solutions.

OTHER DARK LESIONS

In some VIN, melanin pigment that is not contained in atypical squamous cells concentrates in local macrophages, causing dark coloration of the tumor. Vulvar epithelium may darken after use of estrogen cream or oral contraceptive pills. Kaposi's sarcoma, dermatofibroma, and seborrheic keratoses are examples of dark lesions. Biopsy of a dark lesion should include the whole lesion, as incomplete removal of melanoma has been suggested as a cause of accelerated spread.

ULCER

The most common cause of ulcerative lesion is a sexually transmitted disease (STD). The most common STD causing vulvar ulcer or erosion is herpes genitalis.

HERPES GENITALIS

ESSENTIALS OF DIAGNOSIS

- Frequently preceded by a prodrome: burning, itching and flu-like symptoms.
- Vesicles develop but erode rapidly, resulting in painful erosions or ulcer.
- Each erosion is surrounded by a red halo (Fig. 39–3).
- Lesions are spread in a serpentine- like fashion.
- Recurrences are common.
- Only 20% of affected patients are diagnosed correctly.
- The gold-standard of diagnosis is viral culture. Other reliable tests are glycoprotein-G–based specific serology and polymerase chain reaction.

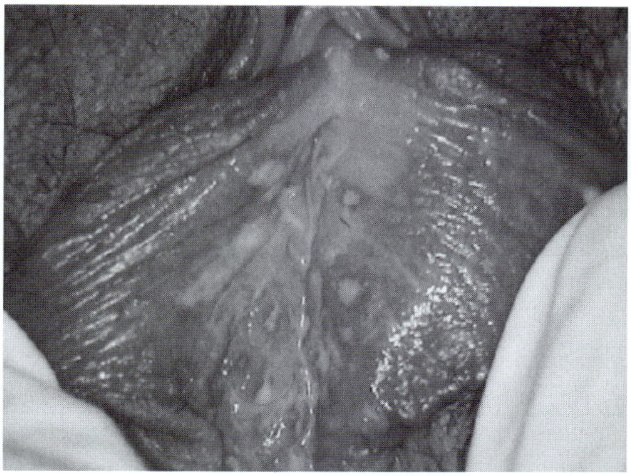

▲ **Figure 39–3.** Ulcers of herpes genitalis. Each is surrounded by a red halo. The lesions are spread in a serpentine-like fashion.

Herpesvirus hominis (herpes simplex virus [HSV], herpes genitalis) is responsible for recurrent and disabling symptomatic disease, venereal transmission, and infection to the neonate (ie, herpes encephalitis). HSV type 1 and type 2 are the variants that affect the vulva and vagina. Serologic prior exposure to HSV type 2 is evident in 20–25% of women. Approximately 83% of patients develop antibodies to HSV type 2 within 21 days of a primary infection. Approximately 60% of primary genital infections are by herpesvirus simplex type 2, and the remainder by type 1.

Pathogenesis

Infection occurs through intimate contact, mainly sexual intercourse. The virus contaminates secretions and mucosal surfaces, entering the skin and mucosa through cracks and other lesions. In turn, the erosions and ulcers of herpes simplex provide a port of entry to other sexually transmitted infections, such as HIV. The virus initially replicates in the dermis and epidermis and then stays latent in a nearby nerve ganglion. Incubation time is 2–7 days. Periods of viral shedding without any symptoms may occur (Table 39–5). This asymptomatic shedding is of particular concern. When unrecognized, the patient continues to have unprotected sexual intercourse, unknowingly transmitting the virus to her partner. This phenomenon is extremely common. For approximately half of the afflicted, asymptomatic viral shedding is identifiable within

Table 39–5. Definition of episode of genital herpes infection.

Definition of Episode	HSV Type Isolated From Lesion	HSV Antigens in the Serum
Primary	HSV-2	None
First, nonprimary	HSV-2	Weakly positive for HSV-1 or HSV-2
Recurrent	HSV-2	Positive for HSV-2
Asymptomatic shedding	HSV-2	Positive for HSV-2

Table 39–6. Oral treatment of herpes genitalis.

First episode of genital herpes Acyclovir 400 mg orally 3 times a day for 7–10 days Acyclovir 200 mg orally 5 times a day for 7–10 days Famciclovir 250 mg orally 3 times a day for 7–10 days
Recurrent genital herpes Acyclovir 400 mg orally 3 times a day for 5 days Acyclovir 800 mg orally twice a day for 5 days Acyclovir 800 mg orally 3 times a day for 2 days
Genital herpes prophylaxis Acyclovir 400 mg orally twice a day Famciclovir 250 mg orally twice a day Valacyclovir 500 mg orally once a day

1 year of the primary outbreak. Later, decreased viral shedding frequency, down to 2% at 10 years, makes detection difficult.

Prevention

Avoidance of direct contact with active lesions prevents spread of the disease. Recommendations for prevention of dissemination are as follows:

- Precautions even in the absence of active lesions, due to asymptomatic shedding of the virus. The most frequent shedding occurs during the year after the first episode.
- Constant use of condoms. However, the condom does not prevent all infections, as lesions may develop in the area outside the tissue covered by the condom.
- The carrier in a serologically discordant couple should consider taking suppressive antiherpetic medication for prolonged periods.
- Administration of a prolonged suppressive therapy for individuals with 6 or more recurrences per year, patients who suffer from distressing prodromes or outbreaks, and men with lesions outside the area that can be protected by a condom (Table 39–6).

Clinical Findings

A. Symptoms & Signs

Prodromal symptoms of tingling, burning, or itching, as well as flu-like feeling with fever, malaise, headaches, and myalgia, may present shortly before the appearance of vesicular eruptions. The vesicles erode rapidly, resulting in painful erosions or ulcers (see Table 39–3 for definitions) distributed in small patches or involving most of the vulvar surfaces. Each lesion is surrounded by a red halo. The lesions appear in a serpentine-like fashion on the vulva, hence the name of the disease: herpes (from Latin, "serpentine, snake-like"). In contrast to the common myth, the typical herpes simplex skin lesion is not a vesicle but rather an erosion or ulcer. Bilateral inguinal adenopathy may be present. Urinary symptoms such as dysuria and urinary retention may develop, necessitating hospitalization and placement of a urinary catheter. In 20% of the cases, the primary infection is asymptomatic (Table 39–5). In 60% of the affected, herpesvirus infection is incorrectly diagnosed as a recurrent yeast infection. Lesions may persist for 2–6 weeks with no subsequent scarring.

Diagnosis

Due to the far-reaching implications on a woman and her relationship with her partner, genital herpes should be carefully diagnosed using the appropriate tests and after all other conditions in the differential diagnosis of vulvar ulcers are excluded.

The gold standard of diagnosis is viral culture on fibroblasts. The virus can be cultured from vesicle fluid or a scraping from an erosion or an ulcer during the acute phase. However, organisms cannot usually be cultured after the primary lesions heal, which occurs within 2 weeks. Although polymerase chain reaction is a sensitive test to detect HSV DNA, its detection in a lesion may indicate a previous outbreak rather than a current event.

A smear scraped from the lesion and stained by Papanicolaou stain or Giemsa (Tzanck test) yields fast results, but is less sensitive and less specific than a culture. Cytologic characteristics of genital herpes include the following:

1. Giant cells
2. Multiple nuclei
3. Molding of the nuclei (compression of one into another)
4. Ground-glass appearance

A. Serologic Tests

Approximately 85% of individuals develop immunoglobulin (Ig) M antibodies to HSV 2 virus within 21 days of exposure. In the past, serologic tests were unreliable because they could not differentiate between herpes virus types 1 and 2, which share approximately 80% of their antigens. New type-specific serologic tests for herpes simplex virus are now available. To distinguish between herpes simplex types 1 and 2, the IgG and IgM antibodies of the type-specific glycoprotein G–based assays should be specifically requested.

Differential Diagnosis

Sometimes the first referral is for a vulvar ulcer of unknown etiology. Although genital herpes is the most frequent cause of vulvar ulcer, other causes, mainly sexually transmitted infections such as syphilis, chancroid, and lymphogranuloma venereum, exist as well (Table 39–7). Noninfectious causes include Behçet's syndrome and desquamative inflammatory vaginitis (DIV), which are discussed later in this chapter. Of particular significance in the differential diagnosis is vulvovaginal candidiasis, recognized as the "great imitator" of genital herpes. Itching and considerable erythema usually present in vulvar and vaginal candidiasis. Persistent scratching can lead to small ulcers or excoriations (see Table 39–3 for definition) that resemble herpetic lesions. Many physicians diagnose any burning, itching, and erythematous lesion in the vulva as vulvar candidiasis and treat with antifungal medications. As a result, many cases of genital herpes are misdiagnosed. Suspicion for genital herpes should increase when a lesion is particularly painful; when there is a complaint about ulcer or erosions, burning vulvar pain, nonspecific influenza-like symptoms, or referred pain to the legs; or when presumed candidiasis does not heal after 1 course of therapy.

Table 39–7. The differential diagnosis of vulvar ulcers.

Infectious Causes		Noninfectious Causes	
STD	Other Infections	Nonneoplastic Diseases	Neoplastic Diseases
Herpes simplex	Tuberculosis	Behçet syndrome	Vulvar intraepithelial neoplasia
Syphilis	Candidiasis	Desquamative inflammatory vaginitis (DIV)	Vulvar cancer
Chancroid		Crohn disease	
Lymphogranuloma venereum		Systemic lupus erythematosus	
Granuloma inguinale		Lichen planus	
		Vesicobullous lesions: Pemphigus, Pemphigoid	

Complications

In addition to pain and discomfort, herpes genitalis entails social and psychologic implications, such as stigmatization and apprehension of recurrent outbreaks during which sexual activity should be abstained. Furthermore, there is a moral obligation to forewarn every partner, before sexual intercourse, of the possibility of infection. The embarassment of self-disclosure may lead to reluctance to start a new relationship. To ease the stress, the health care provider should inform the patient that administration of acyclovir or its valine analog valcyclovir in a continuous prophylactic manner, as suppressive treatment, prevents outbreaks and reduces viral transmission.

A. Neonatal Herpes

The incidence of neonatal herpes simplex virus infection ranges from 1 in 1800 live births in California to 1 in 60,000 in England. Infection of the newborn is associated with a 60% mortality rate, and at least half of the survivors have significant neurologic and/or ocular sequelae. The risk of infection to an infant born vaginally to a woman with active primary genital infection is 40–50% and to one with recurrent infection, 5%. However, most infants who develop herpetic infection are born to women who have no history or clinical evidence of infection during pregnancy. Therefore, identification of women whose infants may be in jeopardy is difficult. All pregnant women should be asked whether they or their partners have had genital herpetic lesions. Women with a history of herpes can deliver vaginally if no clinical signs or symptoms of infection are present. Obtaining routine weekly vaginal cultures to detect herpes is no longer standard procedure. However, some physicians initiate suppressive antiviral therapy at 36 weeks to decrease the need for caesarean section in women with frequent outbreaks.

Treatment

The lesions of herpesvirus infection are self-limiting and heal spontaneously unless they become infected secondarily. Symptomatic treatment includes good genital hygiene, loose-fitting undergarments, cool compresses or sitz baths, and oral analgesics. Indications for hospitalization for a severe primary infection include urinary retention, severe headache or other systemic symptoms, and body temperature exceeding 38.3 °C (101 °F). Immunosuppressed patients are more prone to systemic dissemination and should be carefully managed. Treatment includes intravenous acyclovir for hospitalized patients and oral and/or topical antivirals for ambulatory patients. Recurrent herpes should be treated at the onset of prodromal symptoms or vesicle formation. If initiated early, 1-day treatment may suffice. Once-daily continuous prophylactic (suppressive) dosing for many years may be considered for frequent recurrent outbreaks, with 40–70% of patients free of recurrence at 1 year (Table 39–6).

Prognosis

Despite measurable humoral and cell-mediated immunity, reactivation of the virus occurs. After replication in the skin, the viral particles are transported along the peripheral sensory nerve fibers to the dorsal root ganglion, where latent infection is established. Exogenous factors known to contribute to activation of herpesvirus include fever, emotional stress, and menstruation. Immunocompromised patients are prone to develop extensive local disease and systemic dissemination. Whether frequent coitus promotes recurrent disease is unknown. Type 2 virus is more likely than type 1 to recur. Approximately 50% of patients have a recurrence within 6 months of the primary infection. The recurrent ulcers tend to be smaller, fewer in number, and confined to a constant area in the vulva, cervix, or vagina. Healing is generally complete in 1–3 weeks. The virus is not recoverable within 7 days of healing of recurrent lesions. Inguinal adenopathy and systemic symptoms generally do not occur with recurrent outbreaks. Primary infections can generally be distinguished from secondary infections based on clinical findings. Extragenital sites, such as the fingers (herpetic whitlow), buttocks, and trunk (eczema herpeticum, see Table 39–3), have been described.

BEHÇET'S SYNDROME

Behçet's syndrome is a rare inflammatory disorder characterized by a classic symptom triad: (1) recurrent oral aphthae or ulcers, (2) recurrent genital aphtae or ulcerations, and (3) uveitis. The painful genital ulcers are preceded by small vesicles or papules and last for variable periods. Their borders are irregular. After healing, deep ulcerations may result in scarring or fenestration of the labia. Ocular lesions begin as superficial inflammation and may proceed to iridocyclitis and even blindness. In addition to the classic symptoms, the disease may cause thrombophlebitis or involve the joints in a form of monoarticular arthritis. Central nervous system symptoms manifest in severe disease. Susceptibility to Behçet's disease is strongly associated with the HLA-B51 allele. Prevalence is highest in Eastern Europe and the Mediterranean. Although the exact etiology is unknown, the disease likely represents an underlying autoimmune process.

Behçet's syndrome, together with disseminated lupus erythematosus and pemphigus, should be included in the differential diagnosis of recurrent aphthous ulcers of the oral and vaginal mucosa. Ophthalmic examination and human leukocyte antigen typing can aid in diagnosis. Treatment starts with colchicine tablets. Topical and systemic corticosteroids provide immediate relief.

INVESTIGATION OF A VULVAR ULCER

Patient History

A thorough patient history should be taken, including the general health condition, because debilitating or chronic diseases such as AIDS can lead to chronic infections that generate ulcers. The patient should be asked about outbreaks of vulvar ulcers, as well as previous evaluations and their results. Recurrent lesions are typical of both genital herpes and Behçet's syndrome. Finally, the patient should be asked about any medications she takes. Severe allergic reactions, such as manifested by Stevens-Johnson syndrome, may also cause large ulcers in the vulva and vagina.

Physical Examination

A general physical checkup should include assessment of dermatologic diseases, such as lichen planus, which, in addition to the characteristic dark plaques in the back and limb areas, may appear as extensively desquamated skin and ulcers in the vulva. Pemphigus vulgaris, an autoimmune dermatologic disease with antibodies directed against intercellular sites of stratified squamous epithelium, may present as vesicobullous lesions in the vulva. The oral mucosae should be checked for aphthae or ulcers. Behçet's syndrome, Crohn's disease, lichen planus, and pemphigus vulgaris present as ulcerative lesions in both oral and genital skin and mucosa.

Specific Tests

Using dark-field microscopy, a sample from the base of the ulcer should be investigated for the presence of *Treponema pallidum*, the causative agent of syphilis. Cultures for HSV and serologic tests to exclude chlamydia, systemic lupus erythematosus, HIV, and syphilis should be taken. The absence of a clear diagnosis prompts a biopsy to enable visualization of granulomas and vasculitis apparent in Crohn's disease and Behçet's syndrome and to exclude malignant and premalignant tumors.

SMALL TUMORS

CONDYLOMA ACUMINATUM

ESSENTIALS OF DIAGNOSIS

- Asymptomatic white papillary growths, small at first, tend to coalesce (Fig. 39–4).
- Affects the vulva, vagina, and cervix in women; the penis and scrotum in men; and the pubis, perineum, perianal, and oropharyngeal areas in both sexes.
- A colposcope is necessary to identify small and flat lesions.

- Biopsy may be needed to rule out neoplasia.
- Recurrent respiratory papillomatosis, characterized by laryngeal papillomas on the vocal cords, may develop in infants delivered through an infected vaginal canal.

Pathogenesis

The incubation period ranges from a few weeks to months, and sometimes years. Hence it is impossible to determine the day the viral infection was contracted. Condylomata acuminata (genital warts) are caused by the human papilloma virus (HPV), mainly types 6 and 11. Other types of HPV, particularly 16, 18, 45, 31, and 52, are responsible for intraepithelial and invasive neoplasia in the vagina, cervix, vulva, oropharynx, perineum, and perianal areas. The rate of HPV infection is high and rising. Worldwide, 30 million cases of genital warts (condylomata acuminata) are diagnosed annually. It is estimated that 30–60% of the population has been infected with HPV at some point in their lives. Clinical symptoms, however, present in fewer than 1%. The virus is small and contains all its genetic material on a single double-stranded molecule of DNA. Viral DNA probes have identified more than 35 types of HPV that infect the genital tract. Most HPV types cause asymptomatic infections. The viruses are sexually transmitted and infect both partners.

Prevention

Two vaccines against HPV are available: a bivalent vaccine against high-risk HPV types 16 and 18 and a quadrivalent vaccine against types 6, 11, 16, and 18. Administration is recommended before sexual debut. Both vaccines are intended to protect against cervical cancer and high-grade cervical intraepithelial neoplasia (CIN) caused by HPV 16 and HPV 18. Only the quadrivalent vaccine is designed to prevent condylomata acuminata and low-grade CIN caused by HPV 6 and HPV 11. The quadrivalent vaccine has been approved by the US Food and Drug Administration for women aged 9–45 years and men aged 9–26 years. Both prophylactic vaccines are aimed to prevent primary persistent infection and are targeted against the L1 gene product, which is the major protein of the HPV capsid. The vaccines are produced by inserting the HPV L1 gene into the DNA of the yeast *Saccharomyces cerevisiae* and creating a recombinant DNA. The yeast expresses the L1 capsid protein that spontaneously assembles into a virus-like particle (VLP). The VLP resembles the native HPV virus, but lacks the DNA core. Therefore, it does not carry any infectious or carcinogenic risk. The human immune system recognizes the VLP as if it were HPV itself, thus producing a neutralizing antibody response. The commercial vaccine contains the 97% purified VLP adsorbed onto an aluminum adjuvant, which varies between pharmaceutical companies. The adjuvant system 04 (AS04) of the bivalent vaccine more significantly accelerates an immune reaction.

Both vaccines demonstrate cross-protection, although against different HPV types. Both vaccines are safe and effective.

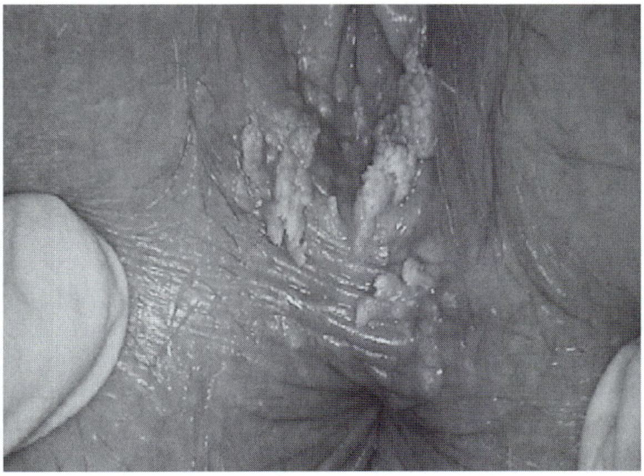

▲ **Figure 39–4.** Vulvar and perineal condylomata acuminata.

Clinical Findings

A. Symptoms & Signs

The typical condyloma is a white, exophytic, or papillomatous growth (Fig. 39–4). Papillary growths, small at first, tend to coalesce and form large cauliflower-like masses that may proliferate profusely. Condyloma acuminata may affect the vagina, cervix, vulva, oropharynx, perineum, and perianal areas.

The florid, papillomatous condyloma is a raised white lesion with fingerlike projections often containing capillaries. Although large lesions can be seen with the naked eye, the colposcope is necessary to identify smaller lesions. Colposcopic examination also permits identification of flat, spiked, and inverted condyloma. Flat condyloma appear as white lesions with somewhat granular surfaces. A mosaic pattern and punctation may also be present, suggesting VIN, which must be excluded by biopsy. Hyperkeratotic lesions present as spiked lesions, with surface projections and prominent capillary tips.

Differential Diagnosis

Other small tumors and cysts of the vulva, to be discussed later in this chapter, should be ruled out before diagnosing condylomata acuminata. In particular, molluscum contagiosum and epidermal and keratin cysts are look-alikes. Condyloma lata, a variation of secondary syphilis, should also be considered in differential diagnosis. Syphilis infection is discussed in Chapter 43.

Definitive diagnosis has medicolegal significance, because condylomata acuminata are sexually transmitted. In children they have been implicated as signs of sexual abuse.

Complications

Condylomatous warts may grow rapidly during pregnancy. Warts at the vaginal introitus may bleed during delivery and predispose the newborn to genital warts or recurrent respiratory papillomatosis (RRP). RRPs are laryngeal papilloma on the vocal cords that may, in rare cases, descend to the pulmonary parenchyma, present as recurrent pneumonia, and become fatal. However, unlike herpetic lesions, vulvar, vaginal, and cervical HPV lesions are not contraindications to a vaginal delivery, but rather require treatment during pregnancy. Condylomata that are recognized early in pregnancy should be treated at 30–32 gestational weeks to allow healing before delivery. When treatment is not successful, or the condylomata cover considerable vulvar area or tend to bleed, delivery by caesarean section should be considered.

Treatment

Before treatment is initiated, the entire lower genital tract should be examined with the colposcope and a cytologic smear taken from the cervix. Lesions may extend to the anal canal or urethral meatus. Treating condylomata only in the vulva, while disregarding others in the vagina or cervix, may result in frequent recurrences. Some recommend testing for syphilis, hepatitis B and C, chlamydia, and HIV due to comorbidity of sexually transmitted diseases. A biopsy may be indicated to rule out intraepithelial or invasive neoplasia. Natural infection after an outbreak produces a low-level, ineffective immune response. Recurrences after treatment may represent reinfection or clinical manifestation of latent disease. The virus presents in normal cells as well as in those with condylomatous changes; therefore, recurrence is common. Biopsy should be considered, especially if the cervix is involved, the condyloma does not respond to standard treatment, or the lesion is pigmented, indurated, fixed, and/or ulcerated. Normal micropapillae of the inner labia minora (vestibular micropapillomatosis) are often confused with papillary HPV and lead to unnecessary therapy. True HPV disease is patchy, with koilocytes, and with more intense acetowhite changes.

During treatment, the patient should keep the area as clean as possible and abstain from sexual intercourse or have her partner use a condom. If clinical disease recurs, then the sexual partner should be examined and treated as necessary. Penile, urethral, and perianal warts in the male may be overlooked.

Whether treatment actually affects the natural progression or eradicates HPV infection is unclear. Concomitant vulvovaginitis should be treated initially. Treatment should be based on patient preference and convenience. Table 39–8 details treatments of condylomata acuminata. If treatment fails with an initial regimen, a different agent can be used. Patients should be informed that, though rare, complications of treatment can result in adhesions, scarring, and loss of pigmentation.

Table 39–8. Treatment of condyloma acuminata.

Applied by health care provider
Bichloracetic acid or trichloroacetic acid, 50–80% solution
Podophyllin 10–25% in tincture of benzoin
Cryosurgery, electrosurgery, simple surgical excision, laser vaporization
Applied by patient
Podofilox 0.5% solution or gel
Imiquimod 5% cream (topically active immune enhancer that stimulates production of interferon and other cytokines)

Treatment may be self-administered by the patient or applied by the health care provider (Table 39–8). Clinical disease may appear on only a small area of the infected surface. Hence some specialists recommend CO_2 laser ablation of all visible lesions, plus a low-dose treatment (brushing), under colposcopic guidance, of a 1-cm margin of normal adjacent skin in all areas where subclinical HPV infection may coexist. Intralesional or systemic interferon has demonstrated effectiveness in refractory cases. Chemotherapeutic agents such as fluorouracil ointment or bleomycin in the form of intralesional injections can also be used as second-line therapies.

During pregnancy, electrocoagulation, cryotherapy, or CO_2 laser therapy should be administered at approximately 32 weeks to avoid, on one hand, post-treatment necrosis, which may last as long as 4–6 weeks, and to prevent, on the other hand, recurrence if treated too early. Podophyllin, podofilox, and imiquimod should not be used during pregnancy.

Prognosis

Recurrences are frequent with all treatment modalities. Prevention of recurrence is particularly difficult in patients who are immunosuppressed or currently receiving long-term corticosteroid therapy. Examination of sexual partners is not necessary because most partners are likely to have subclinical infection. The use of condoms for a few months after treatment may help in reducing "ping-pong" transmission to and from partners who may be infected.

MOLLUSCUM CONTAGIOSUM

These benign epithelial poxvirus-induced tumors are dome-shaped, with a typical umbilicus. Size varies, up to 1 cm. Lesions are often multiple and are mildly contagious. As mentioned above, they are look-alikes of condylomata acuminata. Under the microscope they appear as numerous inclusion bodies (molluscum bodies) in the cytoplasm of cells. Each lesion can be treated by desiccation, freezing, or curettage and chemical cauterization of the base. Topical imiquimod is an alternative therapy. Scarring is frequent.

EPIDERMAL CYSTS

Previously named keratin cysts, these cysts are of epidermal origin. They are lined with squamous epithelium and filled with oily material and desquamated epithelial cells. Epidermal inclusion cysts may result from suturing of skin fragments during closure of the vulvar mucosa and skin after trauma or episiotomy. However, most epidermal cysts arise from occlusion of pilosebaceous ducts. These cysts are usually small, solitary, and asymptomatic, but rarely become irritated or infected.

SEBACEOUS CYSTS

Sebaceous cysts develop when sebaceous gland ducts become occluded and sebaceous material accumulates. These cysts are frequently multiple and almost always involve the labia majora. Although generally asymptomatic, acutely infected cysts may require incision and drainage.

APOCRINE SWEAT GLAND CYSTS

Apocrine sweat glands, abundant in the skin of the labia majora and the mons pubis, become active after puberty. Occlusion of the ducts with keratin results in the extremely pruritic, microcystic Fox-Fordyce disease. This disease should be suspected in patients with consistent vulvar pruritus.

ACROCHORDON

An acrochordon is a flesh-colored, soft polypoid tumor of the vulvar skin, also called a *fibroepithelial polyp* or simply a *skin tag*. The tumor does not become malignant and is of no clinical importance, unless it becomes traumatized, causing bleeding. Simple excisional biopsy in the office is ordinarily adequate therapy.

LARGE TUMORS

BARTHOLIN'S DUCT CYST AND ABSCESS

Clinical Findings

Obstruction of the main duct of Bartholin's gland results in retention of secretions and cystic dilatation. Infection is an important cause of obstruction; however, other causes include inspissated mucus and congenital narrowing of the duct. Secondary infection may result in recurrent abscess formation.

The gland and duct are located deep in the posterior third of each labium major, with the duct opening into the vestibule. Enlargement in the postmenopausal patient may reflect a malignant process (although the incidence is <1%), and biopsy should be considered.

Acute symptoms generally result from infection, which leads to pain, tenderness, dyspareunia, and even difficulty in walking with adducted thighs. The surrounding tissues become edematous and inflamed. A fluctuant, tender mass is usually palpable. Unless an extensive inflammatory process is present, systemic symptoms or signs of infection are unlikely.

Treatment

Primary treatment consists of drainage of the infected cyst or abscess, preferably by marsupialization or by insertion of a Word catheter (an inflatable bulb-tipped catheter). The incision should be made in the vestibule, close to the original orifice of the Bartholin's gland duct. Simple needle aspiration, or incision and drainage, may provide only temporary relief, as recurrent cystic dilatation may recur. Appropriate antibiotics should be administered if considerable inflammation develops. Excision of the cyst may be required in recurrent cases or in the postmenopausal patient.

LEIOMYOMA, FIBROMA, & LIPOMA

Tumors of mesodermal origin present infrequently on the vulva. However, they can become extremely large. Leiomyomas, arising from muscle in the round ligament, appear as firm, symmetric, freely mobile tumors deep in the substance of the labium majus. Fibromas, arising from proliferation of fibroblasts, vary in size from small subcutaneous nodules revealed incidentally to large polypoid tumors. Large tumors often undergo myxomatous degeneration and are very soft and cystic to palpation. Lipomas consist of a combination of mature fat cells and connective tissue. They can be differentiated from degenerated fibromas only by histopathologic examination. Small tumors can be removed under local anesthesia in the office. Large tumors require general anesthesia and operating room facilities. The diagnosis of sarcoma is based on histologic assessment.

NEUROFIBROMA

Neurofibromas are fleshy polypoid lesions that may manifest as solitary, solid tumors of the vulva or be associated with generalized neurofibromatosis (Recklinghausen's disease). Arising from the neural sheath, they are usually small lesions of no consequence. Multiple disfiguring tumors of the vulva may interfere with sexual function and require excision or vulvectomy.

GRANULAR CELL MYOBLASTOMA (SCHWANNOMA)

Granular cell myoblastoma is usually a solitary, painless, slow-growing, infiltrating but benign tumor of neural sheath origin, most commonly found in the tongue or integument. Approximately 7% involve the vulva. The infected area consists of small subcutaneous nodules 1–4 cm in diameter. With increasing size, they erode through the surface and result in ulcerations that may be confused with cancer.

The margins of the tumor are indistinct, and wide local excision is necessary to completely excise the cells extending into contiguous tissues. The area of resection must be periodically re-examined and secondary excision performed promptly if recurrence is suspected.

VARICOSITIES

Clinical Findings

Varicosities of the vulva involve 1 or more veins. Severe varicosities of the legs and vulva may be aggravated during pregnancy. Symptomatic vulvar varices in a woman who is not pregnant are uncommon and may signify an underlying vascular disease, either primary or secondary to a tumor in the pelvis. Rupture of a vulvar varicosity during pregnancy may cause profuse hemorrhage. Pain and tenderness may be caused by acute phlebitis or thrombosis.

Treatment

Treatment of vulvar and vaginal varicosities is seldom necessary. Surgical intervention is generally required only in rare cases of rupture and hemorrhage. Persistent postpartum cases may be alleviated by injection of a sclerosing agent.

HEMATOMA

The vulva has a rich blood supply arising predominately from the pudendal vessels. A ruptured vessel, especially in a pregnant woman, can cause significant bleeding and hematoma formation due to the distensible nature of the vulvar tissue. In rare cases, intercourse leads to laceration with external bleeding or to hematoma that may dissect the tissues in the labia majora or the rectovaginal septum. After trauma, an ice pack should be applied. If the hematoma continues to expand, embolization of the vessel, which is usually a branch of the pudendal artery, is a new, noninvasive approach to control the bleeding. Alternatively, the area should be incised and any bleeders (which may be multiple) ligated. The wound can be packed and left open or closed with a drain in place, if appropriate. Antibiotics should be administered on an individual basis, depending on the initiating event and contamination in the area.

EDEMA

Clinical Findings

The loose integument of the vulva predisposes to the development of edema. Causes of vulvar edema include vascular or lymphatic obstruction resulting from an underlying neoplasm or infection such as lymphogranuloma venereum (LGV), vaginal delivery accompanied by frequent vaginal examinations, trauma from a bicycle accident (saddle injury) in a young girl, and a kick to the pudendum. Severe generalized vulvar edema may represent an underlying systemic illness such as congestive heart failure, nephrotic syndrome, preeclampsia, or eclampsia. Acute edema may result from a systemic or local allergic reaction, immobilization, or ovarian hyperstimulation syndrome.

Treatment

An ice pack applied to the perineum after an acute trauma tends to retard the development of severe edema. Ice application should be restricted to 15 minutes every hour to prevent cold burns. Warm packs or warm sitz baths may then be applied after 1–2 days to help resolve the associated inflammation and/or hematoma.

LYMPHANGIOMA

Lymphangiomas are tumors of the lymphatic vessels. They may be difficult to differentiate from hemangiomas microscopically unless blood cells are present within the blood vessels. Lymphangioma cavernosum may cause a diffuse enlargement of 1 side of the vulva and extend over the remainder of the vulva and perineum. A tumor that is sufficiently enlarged should be surgically excised. Lymphangioma simplex tumors (circumscription tumors) are usually small, soft, white, or purple nodules or small wartlike lesions most commonly seen on the labia majora. Usually asymptomatic, they do not require excision unless intense pruritus and excoriation present. Lymphangioma simplex tumors are not alleviated with topical measures.

OTHER VULVAR TUMORS

A number of other uncommon cystic vulvar tumors must be considered in the differential diagnosis of vulvar tumors. Anteriorly Skene's duct cyst should be differentiated from urethral diverticulum, as careless incision of the latter may damage the urethra and result in urinary incontinence. An inguinal hernia may extend into the labium majus, causing a large cystic dilatation. Suspicion of an inguinal hernia is indication for ultrasound examination of the contents of the labial tumor. The appearance of peristaltic waves is evident that a hernia is in fact present. Occlusion of a persistent processus vaginalis (canal of Nuck) may cause a cystic tumor or hydrocele. Gartner's duct cyst is a dilatation of the mesonephric duct vestiges, always at the lateral vaginal wall. Supernumerary mammary tissue that persists in the labia majora may form a cystic or solid tumor, or even an adenocarcinoma. Engorgement of such tissue in the pregnant patient can be symptomatic.

VULVAR MANIFESTATION OF SYSTEMIC DISEASES

LEUKEMIA

Rarely, nodular infiltration and ulceration of the vulva and rectovaginal septum occur with acute leukemia.

DERMATOLOGIC DISORDERS

Recurrent ulcerations of the mucous membranes of the mouth and vagina may be manifestations of disseminated lupus erythematosus. Bullous eruptions of apparently normal skin and mucous membrane surfaces of the vulva may be early signs of pemphigus vulgaris (a rare, chronic vesicobullous disease, associated with the autoimmune disease, keratinolysis). Contact dermatitis is an inflammatory response of the vulvar tissue to agents that may be either locally irritating or inductive of sensitivity on contact. The local reaction to a systemically administered drug is called dermatitis medicamentosa.

OBESITY

Acanthosis nigricans is a hyperpigmented lesion associated with obesity and is characterized by papillomatous hypertrophy. Although generally benign, it may be associated with an underlying adenocarcinoma. Pseudoacanthosis nigricans is a benign process that may appear on the skin of the vulva and inner thighs in obese and darkly pigmented women. Glucose intolerance, insulin resistance, chronic anovulation, and androgen disorders may be associated.

Intertrigo is an inflammatory reaction involving the genitocrural folds or the skin under the abdominal panniculus. Common in obese individuals, it results from persistent moistness of the skin surfaces. A superficial fungal or bacterial infection may be concomitant. The area may be either erythematous or white from maceration. Maintaining dryness by wearing absorbent cotton undergarments and dusting with cornstarch powder may be helpful.

DIABETES MELLITUS

Diabetes mellitus is the systemic disease most commonly associated with chronic pruritus vulvae. Diabetic vulvitis is caused by chronic vulvovaginal candidiasis. The diagnosis of diabetes should be considered in any patient who responds poorly to antifungal treatment or who has recurrent fungal infections. Such patients should undergo glucose tolerance testing. In rare cases of long-term diabetes mellitus, the associated neuropathy may present as vulvar pruritus or burning. In uncontrolled diabetes, the vulvar epithelium often undergoes lichenification and secondary bacterial infection. Occasionally, vulvar abscesses, chronic subcutaneous abscesses, and draining sinuses develop from a bacterial infection. Treatment should include controlling the underlying diabetes and specific therapy for the bacterial or fungal infection. Suppressive antifungal therapy using fluconazole should be initiated in diabetic patients with recurrent vulvovaginal candidiasis.

Necrotizing fasciitis presents most commonly in diabetics. It is an uncommon, acute, rapidly spreading, sometimes fatal polymicrobial infection of the superficial fascia and subcutaneous fascia. It may appear after a surgical procedure or after minor trauma. It presents as an extremely painful, tender, edematous, and indurated region with central necrosis and peripheral purplish erythema. Treatment requires incision and debridement of involved tissue and broad-spectrum antibiotics.

INFESTATIONS OF THE VULVA

PEDICULOSIS PUBIS

Pathogenesis

The crab louse (*Phthirus pubis*) is transmitted through sexual contact or from shared infected bedding or clothing. The louse eggs are laid at the base of a hair shaft near the skin. The eggs hatch in 7–9 days, and the louse must attach to the skin of the host to survive. The result is intense pubic and anogenital itching.

Clinical Findings

Minute pale-brown insects and their ova may be seen attached to terminal hair shafts.

Treatment

Treatment consists of permethrin 1% cream, lindane 1% shampoo, or pyrethrins with piperonyl butoxide. Lindane is not recommended for pregnant or lactating women or for children younger than 2 years. It is important to treat all contacts and sterilize clothing that was in contact with the infested area.

SCABIES

Pathogenesis

Sarcoptes scabiei causes intractable itching and excoriation (see Table 39–3 for definition) of skin surfaces in the vicinity of minute skin burrows where parasites deposited ova. The scabies mite is transmitted, often directly, from infected persons.

Treatment

The patient should take a hot soapy bath, scrubbing the burrows and encrusted areas thoroughly. Treatment consists of application of permethrin cream (5%) to the entire body from the neck down, with particular attention to the hands, wrists, axillae, breasts, and anogenital region. It should be washed off after 8–14 hours. Alternatively, lindane (1%) in lotion or cream form can be applied in a thin layer to all areas of the body and washed off after 8 hours. All potentially infected clothing or bedding should be washed or dry-cleaned. All people who were in contact must be treated as described to prevent reinfection. Therapy should be repeated in 10–14 days if new lesions develop.

ENTEROBIASIS (PINWORM, SEATWORM)

Clinical Findings

Enterobius vermicularis infection is common in children. Symptoms are nocturnal perineal itching and perianal excoriation. To diagnose, apply adhesive cellulose tape to the anal region, stick the tape to a glass slide, and examine under the microscope for ova.

Treatment

Patients should wash their hands and scrub their nails after defecation. Underclothes must be boiled. Application of ammoniated mercury ointment to the perianal region twice daily relieves itching. Pinworms succumb to systemic treatment with pyrantel pamoate, mebendazole, or pyrvinium pamoate.

MYCOTIC INFECTIONS OF THE VULVA

FUNGAL DERMATITIS (DERMATOPHYTOSES)

Clinical Findings

Tinea cruris is a superficial fungal infection of the genitocrural area that is more common in men than in women. The most common carriers are *Trichophyton mentagrophytes* and *Trichophyton rubrum*. The initial lesions are usually located on the upper inner thighs and are well circumscribed, erythematous, dry, scaly areas that coalesce. Scratching causes lichenification and a gross appearance similar to neurodermatitis. Diagnosis depends on microscopic examination (as for *Candida*) (Fig. 39–5). Culture on Sabouraud's medium confirms diagnosis.

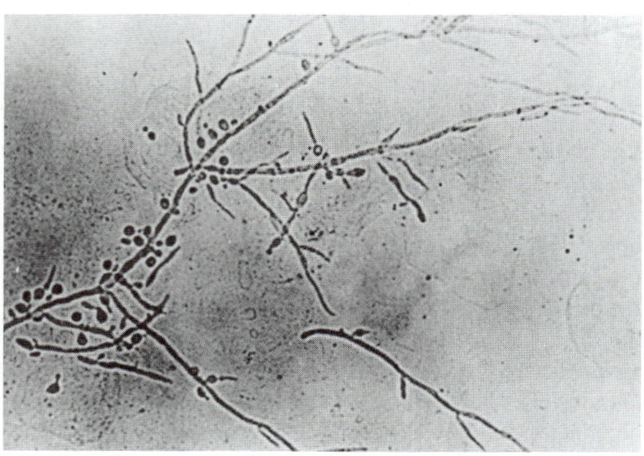

▲ **Figure 39–5.** Potassium hydroxide preparation showing branched and budding *Candida albicans*.

Treatment

Treatment with 1% haloprogin, tolnaftate, or a similar agent is effective. Twice-daily application of topical imidazole preparation for 2–3 weeks is also highly effective.

Tinea versicolor generally involves the skin of the trunk, although vulvar skin is occasionally involved. The lesions are usually multiple and may have a red, brown, or yellowish appearance. Diagnosis is the same as for other fungal infections. Treatment with selenium sulfide suspension daily for 5–7 days is usually effective, as are topical imidazole preparations applied for 4 weeks. Ketoconazole has been used in recalcitrant cases.

DEEP CELLULITIS CAUSED BY FUNGI

Blastomycosis and actinomycosis are examples of deep mycoses that usually affect internal organs but may also involve the skin. Involvement of the vulvar epithelium in these diseases is rare in the United States. Diagnosis is usually by laboratory exclusion of the granulomatous sexually transmitted diseases, tuberculosis, and other causes of chronic infection. Treatment of blastomycosis with amphotericin B or hydroxystilbamidine is not very effective. Penicillin successfully treats actinomycosis in most cases.

OTHER INFECTIONS OF THE VULVA

IMPETIGO

Impetigo is caused by the hemolytic *Staphylococcus aureus* or by streptococci. This autoinoculable disease spreads quickly throughout the body, also to the vulva. The thin-walled vesicles and bullae that develop display reddened edges and crusted surfaces after rupture. The disease is common in children, particularly on the face, hands, and vulva.

The patient must be isolated and the blebs incised or crusts removed aseptically. Neomycin or bacitracin should be applied topically twice daily for 1 week. Bathing with an antibacterial soap is recommended.

FURUNCULOSIS

Vulvar folliculitis is caused by a staphylococcal infection of hair follicles. Furunculosis occurs if the infection spreads into the perifollicular tissues, producing localized cellulitis. Some follicular lesions are palpable as tender subcutaneous nodules that resolve without suppuration. A furuncle begins as a hard, tender subcutaneous nodule that ruptures through the skin, discharging blood and purulent material. After expulsion of a core of necrotic tissue, the lesion heals. New furuncles may appear sporadically over time.

Applications of topical antibiotic lotions effectively treat minor infections. Deeper infections can be treated with hot soaks, followed by incision and drainage of the pustules. Appropriate systemic antibiotics are warranted when extensive furunculosis is present.

ERYSIPELAS

Erysipelas is a rapidly spreading erythematous lesion of the skin caused by invasion of the superficial lymphatics by β-hemolytic streptococci. Erysipelas of the vulva is exceedingly rare and is most commonly seen after trauma to the vulva or a surgical procedure. Systemic symptoms of chills, fever, and malaise associated with an erythematous vulvitis should raise suspicion of this infection. Vesicles and bullae may appear, and erythematous streaks leading to the regional lymph nodes are typical.

Treatment consists of systemic (preferably parenteral) penicillin or large doses of orally administered tetracycline.

HIDRADENITIS SUPPURATIVA

Hidradenitis suppurativa is a refractory process of the apocrine sweat glands, usually associated with staphylococci or streptococci. Inspissation of secretory material and secondary infection occlude ducts of these glands. Multiple pruritic subcutaneous nodules appear and eventually develop into abscesses and then rupture. The process generally involves the skin of the entire vulva, resulting in multiple abscesses and subsequent chronic draining of sinuses and scars. Treatment at an early stage consists of drainage and administration of antibiotics based on organism-sensitivity testing. Long-term therapy with isotretinoin may be considered. Antiandrogen therapy with cyproterone acetate or ethinyl estradiol is an effective alternative treatment. When severe chronic infections do not respond to medical therapy, the involved skin and subcutaneous tissues, down to the deep fascia, must be removed. The area will generally not heal after a primary closure. The wound may therefore be left open and allowed to heal by secondary intention or a split-thickness graft may be placed. Squamous cell carcinoma is rarely associated with hidradenitis suppurativa.

VESTIBULAR DISEASE

VULVAR PAIN SYNDROME

Vulvar pain in the absence of relevant visible physical findings is termed **vulvodynia** (Table 39–9). Women suffering from vulvodynia describe their symptoms as burning, rawness, irritation, dryness, and hyperpathia (pain provoked by very light touch). Approximately 16% of the female population has experienced vulvodynia at some time. The ISSVD has classified vulvodynia by localized vulvodynia (provoked or unprovoked) and generalized vulvodynia (provoked or unprovoked) (Table 39–9).

Table 39–9. Terminology of vulvar pain (ISSVD 2003).

A. Vulvar pain related to a specific disorder
1. Infectious (eg, candidiasis, herpes)
2. Inflammatory (eg, lichen planus, immunobullous disorders)
3. Neoplastic (eg, Paget's disease, squamous cell carcinoma)
4. Neurologic (eg, herpes neuralgia, spinal nerve compression)
B. Vulvodynia
1. Generalized
a. Provoked (sexual, nonsexual, or both)
b. Unprovoked
c. Mixed (provoked and unprovoked)
2. Localized (vestibulodynia, clitorodynia, hemivulvodynia)
a. Provoked (sexual, nonsexual, or both)
b. Unprovoked
c. Mixed (provoked and unprovoked)

LOCALIZED PROVOKED VULVODYNIA, OR VESTIBULODYNIA

ESSENTIALS OF DIAGNOSIS

- Affects mostly young women: 20–30 years old.
- Introital pain on vestibular or vaginal entry (entry dyspareunia).
- Vestibular tenderness—pressure from a cotton-tipped applicator at the vestibule reproduces the pain.
- Erythema is seldom seen. No other lesions are present.

Pathogenesis

Localized provoked vulvodynia, or provoked vestibulodynia (PVD), was formerly known as vulvar vestibulitis and clitorodynia. The vestibule is the nonkeratinized squamous epithelium of the vulva between the labia minora. The "Hart" line is the external perimeter including the hymen (Fig. 39–6). In the vulvar vestibule of PVD, mast cell proliferation and degranulation, hyperinnervation (Fig. 39–7), decreased natural killer cell activity, and enhanced heparanase activity have been detected. Inflammation of the vestibule is related to both mast cell proliferation and hyperinnervation, which act reciprocally, and ultimately increase local inflammation. Mast cells secrete mediators, such as nerve growth factor (NGF), histamine, and serotonin, which have been found to sensitize and induce the proliferation of C-afferent nerve fibers. These nerve

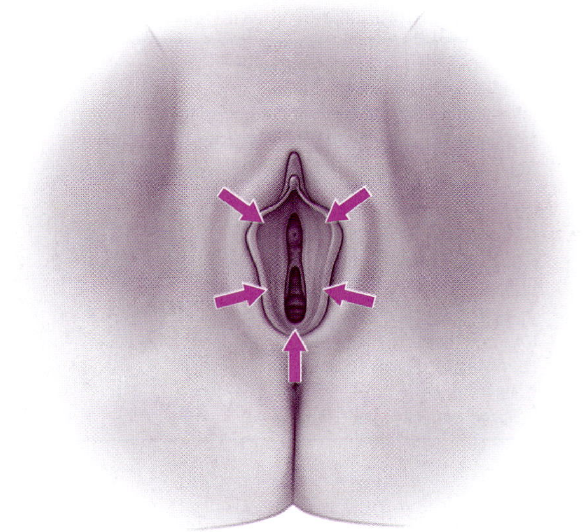

▲ **Figure 39–6.** Hart line is the outer perimeter of the vestibule.

fibers release neuropeptides, including NGF, which increase the proliferation and degranulation of mast cells, cause hyperesthesia, and enhance the inflammatory response. Although mast cells are activated by inflammation, they themselves increase inflammation. This, in turn, increases the density of nerve fibers, leading to further activation of mast cells, and contributing to inflammation. In this way, both inflammatory hyperinnervation and neurogenic

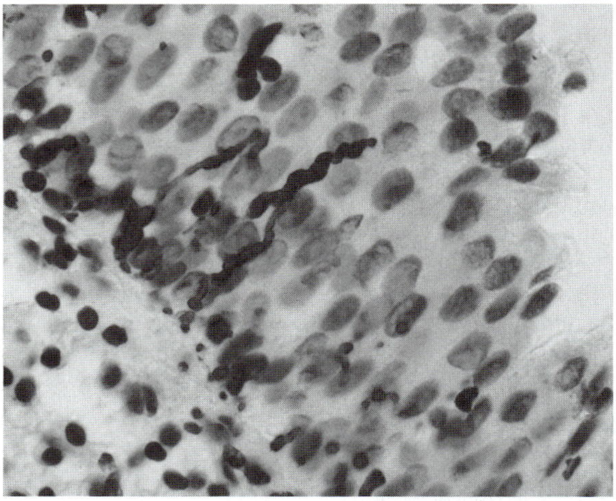

▲ **Figure 39–7.** Hyperinnervation of the vestibular epithelium. Stain by PGP 9,13.

inflammation play significant roles in the cycle, resulting in chronic vulvar pain.

Prevention

There are currently no prophylactic measures.

Clinical Findings

A. Signs & Symptoms

Two clinical criteria only are needed for diagnosis: (1) introital pain on vestibular or vaginal entry (entry dyspareunia), (2) vestibular tenderness—pressure from a cotton-tipped applicator at the vestibule, which reproduces the pain. Originally, a third criterion, vestibular erythema, was used by Friedrich. However, erythema is rarely seen in LPV. Biopsy is not required for diagnosing LPV.

This condition may affect women of all ages, but mainly those between 20 and 30 years of age, who complain of introital dyspareunia (severe pain or burning on vaginal penetration by their partner). However, some women, due to shyness or despair, complain of persistent vaginal discharge. The clue to diagnosis in these cases may be extreme sensitivity at bimanual pelvic examination and expression of fear from speculum insertion. The woman should be questioned in regard to several factors that may be associated with vestibulodynia: prior surgery to the vestibule (ie, episiotomy, vaginal surgery, CO_2 laser treatment), prior infections (eg, HPV, herpes, *Candida*), and associated urologic disorders, mainly interstitial cystitis. Interstitial cystitis and vestibulodynia have similar pathogeneses, including increased mast cell count in the subepithelial tissue.

B. Different Clinical Presentations of Vestibulodynia

- Primary (pain since first attempt at sexual intercourse) or secondary (pain is experienced after an initial period of pain-free intercourse)
- Pure (without concomitant vulvovaginitis) or complicated (with recurrent vulvovaginitis)
- With or without continuous vulvar pain

Differential Diagnosis

Vaginismus is an involuntary contraction of the muscles at the introitus. It is usually secondary to vestibulodynia, but in many cases is erroneously the only diagnosis received by a patient with dyspareunia. Vulvovaginitis should be excluded. Vaginal pH and microscopic examination of vaginal secretions with KOH and normal saline are effective for evaluating vaginitis. Acetowhite changes with application of 5% acetic acid, as well as any distinct lesions, should be biopsied to evaluate for an underlying dermatosis, infection, or neoplastic process. Other causes of vestibular sensitivity should be assessed (Table 39–9).

Complications

Intractable dyspareunia may have a detrimental affect on intimate relationships. Secondary depression is common.

Treatment

Some women, often after consultation with a number of physicians, administer antifungal or antibacterial medications for long periods, to no avail. Frustrated, they become apprehensive of additional treatment failure. Implementation of the following 3-level treatment plan is therefore suggested. Starting with simple measures, this plan should be reevaluated every 3 months.

1. The initial 3 months should focus on pelvic floor physical therapy with biofeedback. The patient should maintain vulvar hygiene, including the use of cotton underwear, drying of the skin, and avoidance of constrictive garments and irritating agents. Topical application of 5% lidocaine cream once daily, and of soothing oils, such as nut oil and tea-tree oil, twice daily, are recommended. In women with a poorly estrogenized vagina due to menopause or to consumption of birth control pills, a daily application of topical estrogenic preparation may be effective. A low-oxalate diet with supplementation of daily calcium citrate may relieve symptoms by decreasing the urinary oxalate crystal concentration that irritates the vulvar vestibule.
2. If, after 3 months, the condition does not improve, oral treatment with the tricyclic antidepressant amitriptyline (Elatrolet) 10–75 mg daily, pregabalin, or gabapentin may be initiated for 3 months.
3. For women who continue to complain of severe dyspareunia after these 2 periods, surgical therapy by vulvar vestibulectomy (Fig. 39–8) with vaginal advancement is the most effective treatment. Vaginal advancement covers the tissue defect and places the mucous-skin junction, which may be sensitive, outside the introitus. The combined sum of complete and partial responses to surgery from 38 studies of surgical treatment is 89%. A high proportion, 93%, of women who underwent vestibulectomy expressed satisfaction with the surgery, stating they would recommend it to another woman experiencing similar symptoms.

Treatments that were proposed in the past but abandoned due to lack of efficacy include intralesional or systemic interferon injection to treat possible HPV, trigger point injections with long-acting injectable anesthetics or steroids, and CO_2 laser vaporization.

New therapies that are currently being evaluated include injections of botulism toxin, topical application of nitroglycerine or nifedipine to treat vaginal muscle spasm as the source of vulvodynia, and topical application of tricyclic antidepressant amitriptyline.

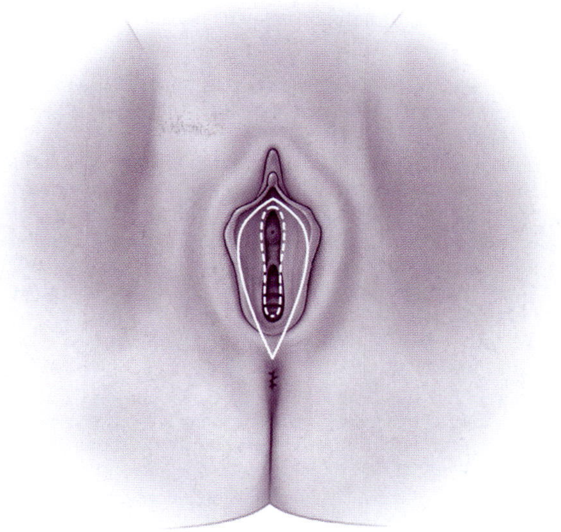

▲ **Figure 39–8.** The outline of vestibulectomy for localized provoked vulvodynia.

Prognosis

Available treatments cure as many as two-thirds of those affected. In recalcitrant cases, women continue to suffer from dyspareunia, even subsequent to surgery. For them, referral to a pain treatment center may be an option.

GENERALIZED UNPROVOKED VULVODYNIA

The etiology of this condition is unknown. The pain involves a larger surface area than does that of localized provoked vulvodynia. The average patient is in her 60s and suffers from hypertension, sometimes receiving various treatments. The pain or burning is usually constant, sometimes with periods of relief and flares. For definitive diagnosis, the following conditions must be excluded: localized provoked vulvodynia, infections and dermatoses, pudendal nerve entrapment, pudendal nerve injury due to childbirth, referred pain from ruptured disk, neuropathic viruses such as herpes simplex or varicella-zoster, and neurologic disease such as multiple sclerosis. A test for allodynia and hyperalgesia using a cotton-tipped swab is usually negative. Therefore, diagnosis of this neuropathic pain is by exclusion.

The most effective treatment for generalized unprovoked vulvodynia is tricyclic antidepressants, mainly amitriptyline (Elatrolet) 10–75 mg daily. Initial relief is expected after a few weeks. In the meantime, topical local anesthetics may be applied. The patient should be counseled on elimination of irritants. If symptoms are not relieved after 3 months, initiation of anticonvulsants such as gabapentin should be considered. If the patient is refractory to such treatment, the next step is referral to a pain clinic, where epidural, other regional blocks, or narcotics may be used.

ACOG Practice Bulletin Number 93, 2008. Diagnosis and management of vulvar skin disorders. *Obstet Gynecol* 2008;111: 1243–1253. PMID: 18448767.

Bornstein J, Cohen V, Zarfati D, Sela S, Ophir E. Involvement of heparanase in the pathogenesis of localized vulvodynia. *J Gynecol Pathol* 2008;27:136–141. PMID: 18156988.

Bornstein J, Goldshmid N, Sabo E. Hyperinnervation and mast cell activation may be used as histopathologic diagnostic criteria for vulvar vestibulitis. *Obstet Gynecol Invest* 2004; 58:171–178. PMID: 15249746.

Edwards L. New concepts in vulvodynia. *Am J Obstet Gynecol* 2003;189:S24–S30. PMID: 14532900.

Goldstein AT, Klingman D, Christopher K, Johnson C, Marinoff SC. Surgical treatment of vulvar vestibulitis syndrome: outcome assessment derived from a postoperative questionnaire. *J Sex Med* 2006;3:923–931. PMID: 16942537.

Gunter J. Vulvodynia: New thoughts on a devastating condition. *Obstet Gynecol Surv* 2007;62:812–819. PMID: 18005458.

Moyal-Barracco M, Lynch PJ. 2003 ISSVD terminology and classification of vulvodynia: A historical perspective. *J Reprod Med* 2004;49:772–777. PMID: 15568398.

Nyirjesy P. Vulvovaginal candidiasis and bacterial vaginosis. *Infect Dis Clin North Am* 2008;22:637–652. PMID: 18954756.

VAGINAL DISORDERS

VAGINITIS

CANDIDIASIS

ESSENTIALS OF DIAGNOSIS

- Intense vulvar pruritus
- A white vaginal discharge
- Vulvar erythema
- Filaments and spores in vaginal discharge can be seen in saline ("wet prep") and KOH preparations
- The gold standard for diagnosis is a vaginal culture

Pathogenesis

Approximately 75% of women experience an episode of vulvovaginal candidiasis during their lifetime. *Candida albicans*, the most common *Candida* species, causes symptomatic vulvovaginitis in approximately 90% of the cases. *C albicans* frequently inhabits the mouth, throat, large intestine, and vagina. Clinical infection is dependent on considerable growth and colonization and may be associated with a systemic disorder (diabetes mellitus, HIV, obesity), pregnancy, medication (antibiotics, corticosteroids, oral contraceptives), and chronic debilitation.

Prevention

Nonabsorbent undergarments should be avoided. The vulva and vaginal area should be kept dry. Controlling any underlying metabolic illnesses, especially diabetes, can prevent candidal growth. Even when diabetes is not present, a low-sugar diet is recommended, as the glucose in a vaginal discharge may promote the growth of the yeast. Complicating medications, especially antibiotics, estrogen, or oral contraceptive, should be discontinued if possible. Some experts recommend administering a prophylactic dose of an antifungal medication simultaneous to every antibiotic administration.

Clinical Findings

A. Symptoms & Signs

Vulvovaginal candidiasis presents with intense vulvar pruritus; a white, cheesy vaginal discharge; and vulvar erythema. A burning sensation may follow urination, particularly if there is excoriation of the skin from scratching. Widespread involvement of the skin adjacent to the labia may suggest an underlying systemic illness. The labia minora may be erythematous and edematous.

B. Wet Prep Evaluation

Diagnosis is based on a normal vaginal pH ≤4.5 and microscopic evaluation of vaginal secretions both in a saline preparation (wet prep) and mixed with 10% KOH solution. Identification of *C albicans* requires detections of filamentous forms (pseudohyphae) of the organism (Fig. 39–5). Spores may be present as well, but the presence of spores alone may indicate a *Candida glabrata* infection. The gold standard for diagnosis is a vaginal culture.

Differential Diagnosis

Genital herpes and localized provoked vulvodynia should be included in the differential diagnosis. Other causes of vaginal discharge are discussed later in this chapter.

Complications

Complications include an entity called complicated vulvovaginal candidiasis, described in Table 39–10.

Treatment

The current medical treatment of candidal infection is by imidazoles, fungistatic agents that interfere with the production

Table 39–10. Classification of vulvovaginal candidiasis (VVC).

Uncomplicated VVC	Complicated VVC
Sporadic or infrequent VVC	Recurrent VVC
Mild-to-moderate VVC	Severe VVC
Likely to be *Candida albicans*	Non-albicans candidiasis
Nonimmunocompromised women	Immunosuppression, or those who are pregnant

of the sterol of the cell wall (Table 39–11). These are available as topical creams, vaginal suppositories, and oral agents. Application of a topical steroid may be beneficial to the patient with severe vulvar itch or edema. In evaluating the patient with complicated candidal vulvovaginitis, underlying predisposing disease processes should be addressed. Additionally, cultures of the vagina should be taken to identify resistant strains. *C glabrata* and *Candida tropicalis*, which are detected with increasing frequency, require prolonged periods of treatment.

Treatment regimens for complicated candidal vulvovaginitis include prolonging antifungal therapy for at least 2 weeks, consistent with the life cycle of yeast; self-medication for 3–5 days upon first evidence of symptoms; and prophylactic treatment for several days before menstruation or during antibiotic therapy. Oral administration of fluconazole 150 mg weekly for 6 months or itraconazole 100 mg daily for 6 months may reduce the frequency of recurrence to 10% during maintenance therapy. Liver function should be monitored during prolonged oral therapy. Treatment of the partner may be considered in cases of symptomatic balanitis. Gentian violet 1%, an aniline dye, has demonstrated effectiveness against *C albicans* and *C glabrata* when painted over vaginal surfaces once weekly. Boric acid compounded in a 600-mg suppository form, administered daily for 6 weeks, is also effective treatment for candidiasis and yeast infestation. Polyenes, such as nystatin, which is not absorbed in the gastrointestinal tract, may be taken orally to reduce intestinal colonization. Flucytosine may be administered in resistant cases.

Table 39–11. Imidazole medications used in the treatment of noncomplicated vulvovaginal candidiasis.

Recommended Regimens
Intravaginal agents
Butoconazole 2% cream 5 g intravaginally for 3 days*
Butoconazole 2% cream 5 g (Butaconazole1-sustained release), single intravaginal application
Clotrimazole 1% cream 5 g intravaginally for 7–14 days*
Clotrimazole 100-mg vaginal tablet for 7 days
Clotrimazole 100-mg vaginal tablet, 2 tablets for 3 days
Miconazole 2% cream 5 g intravaginally for 7 days*
Miconazole 100-mg vaginal suppository, 1 suppository for 7 days*
Miconazole 200-mg vaginal suppository, 1 suppository for 3 days*
Miconazole 1200-mg vaginal suppository, 1 suppository for 1 day*
Nystatin 100,000-unit vaginal tablet, 1 tablet for 14 days
Tioconazole 6.5% ointment 5 g intravaginally in a single application*
Terconazole 0.4% cream 5 g intravaginally for 7 days
Terconazole 0.8% cream 5 g intravaginally for 3 days
Terconazole 80-mg vaginal suppository, 1 suppository for 3 days
Oral agent
Fluconazole 150-mg oral tablet, 1 tablet in single dose

*Over-the-counter preparations.

Prognosis

Recurrent disease may result from insufficient duration of therapy, recontamination, or resistant strains. Unfortunately, in 57% of patients, recurrences present within 6 months of discontinuation of prophylactic treatment.

BACTERIAL VAGINOSIS

ESSENTIALS OF DIAGNOSIS

- Homogeneous vaginal discharge
- Amine (fishy) odor when potassium hydroxide solution is added to vaginal secretions (commonly called the "whiff test")
- Presence of clue cells (more than 20% of epithelial cells) on microscopy (Fig. 39–9)
- Vaginal pH >4.5
- Decrease in lactobacillus, small gram-variable rods, or curved gram-variable rods in gram-stained smear

Pathogenesis

Bacterial vaginosis (BV), previously referred to as *Gardnerella* vaginitis, *Haemophilus* vaginitis, or nonspecific vaginitis, is the most common cause of symptomatic bacterial infection in reproductive-aged women in many countries. This condition is characterized by an alteration in the normal vaginal flora. The concentration of the hydrogen peroxide–producing lactobacillus decreases, and there is overgrowth of *Gardnerella vaginalis, Mobiluncus* spp., anaerobic gram-negative rods (*Prevotella* spp., *Porphyromonas* spp., *Bacteroides* spp.), and *Peptostreptococcus* spp. Whether bacterial vaginosis is a true sexually transmitted disease is controversial, although women who are not sexually active are rarely affected.

Prevention

Maintaining vaginal pH at a normal range may prevent recurrences. The potential benefit of lactobacillus intravaginal suppositories in restoring normal flora, and of acidifying vaginal douching, is being studied.

Clinical Findings

A. Symptoms & signs

Bacterial vaginosis presents as a "fishy" vaginal discharge, which is more noticeable after unprotected intercourse, due to the increased pH caused by the ejaculate. The patient complains of a milky, homogenous, malodorous, usually nonirritating discharge. The term **vaginosis**, rather than **vaginitis**, is used due to the absence of vaginal mucosal inflammation, such as presents in candidal infections.

B. Diagnostic Scales

Two diagnostic scales are often used to diagnose bacterial vaginosis: Amsel's criteria and Nugent's score. According to Amsel's criteria, which establishes accurate diagnosis of bacterial vaginosis in 90% of affected women, 3 of the following 4 criteria must be met:

1. Homogeneous vaginal discharge (color and amount may vary).
2. Amine (fishy) odor when potassium hydroxide solution is added to vaginal secretions (whiff test).
3. Presence of clue cells (>20% of epithelial cells) on microscopy. Clue cells are identified as numerous stippled or granulated epithelial cells (Fig. 39–9). This appearance is caused by the adherence of *G vaginalis* organisms to the edges of the vaginal epithelial cells.
4. Vaginal pH >4.5.

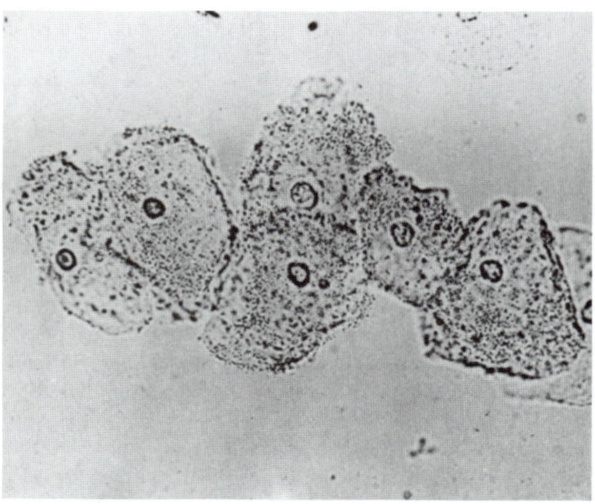

▲ **Figure 39–9.** Bacterial vaginosis. Saline wet mount of clue cells. Note the absence of inflammatory cells.

Nugent's score is a Gram stain scoring system that provides a more sensitive (93%) and specific (70%) diagnosis than does the wet mount. The score is calculated by assessing for the presence of the following:

1. Large gram-positive rods (lactobacillus morphotypes; decrease in lactobacillus, scored 0–4)
2. Small gram-variable rods (*G vaginalis* morphotypes, scored 0–4)
3. Curved gram-variable rods (*Mobiluncus* spp. morphotypes, scored 0–2)

The total score ranges from 0 to 10. A score of 7–10 is consistent with bacterial vaginosis.

C. Other Diagnostic Tests

A culture of *G vaginalis* is not recommended as a diagnostic tool due to low specificity. Cervical Papanicolaou tests have low sensitivity. However, a DNA probe-based test may be clinically useful. Other commercially available tests for the diagnosis of BV include a card test for the detection of elevated pH and trimethylamine and proline aminopeptidase. The home-use of the VI-Sense panty liner has recently demonstrated effectiveness in the early detection of BV and of its recurrences after medical treatment.

Differential Diagnosis

Cervicitis and cervical neoplasia should be considered in the differential diagnosis of bacterial vaginosis.

Complications

BV is reported to increase the risk of preterm delivery. It is unclear whether metronidazole treatment of asymptomatic pregnant women reduces the rates of preterm delivery and adverse pregnancy outcomes. In nonpregnant women, BV is associated with posthysterectomy vaginal cuff cellulitis, postabortion infection, and pelvic inflammatory disease.

Treatment

Treatment should be administered to symptomatic patients and considered in asymptomatic patients. Several treatment regimens exist (Table 39–12). Of importance, intravaginal administration of oil-based clindamycin reduces the effectiveness of condoms and diaphragms. For pregnant women, metronidazole 250 mg orally 3 times daily is recommended for 7 days or, alternatively, clindamycin 300 mg orally twice daily for 7 days. There is no evidence supporting the use of topical agents during pregnancy. Management strategies for recurrent vaginosis include use of condoms, longer treatment periods, prophylactic maintenance therapy, oral

Table 39–12. Treatment of bacterial vaginosis.

Metronidazole 500 mg orally twice a day for 7 days
Metronidazole gel 0.75%, 1 full applicator (5 g) intravaginally, once a day for 5 days
Clindamycin cream 2%, 1 full applicator (5 g) intravaginally at bedtime for 7 days
Alternative regimens Clindamycin 300 mg orally twice a day for 7 days Clindamycin ovules 100 mg intravaginally once at bedtime for 3 days

or vaginal application of yogurt containing lactobacillus acidophilus, intravaginal planting of other exogenous lactobacilli, and acidification of the vagina. Treatment of the male rarely helps in preventing recurrence in the female.

Prognosis

Recurrence is frequent. Overgrowth of candida albicans after antibiotic treatment of bacterial vaginosis may be misinterpreted as recurrent bacterial vaginosis. A "universal" treatment of vulvovaginitis using a combination of clotrimazole and metronidazole in a single vaginal suppository has demonstrated effectiveness. Its use may prevent candida overgrowth.

TRICHOMONAS VAGINITIS

ESSENTIALS OF DIAGNOSIS

- Profuse, frothy, greenish, and foul-smelling discharge
- pH of the vagina usually exceeding 5.0
- Vaginal erythema with multiple small petechiae (strawberry spots)
- Wet mount reveals an increase in polymorphonuclear cells and motile flagellates in 50–70% of zculture-confirmed cases

Pathogenesis

Trichomonas vaginalis is a unicellular flagellate protozoan (Fig. 39–10) that is larger than polymorphonuclear leukocytes but smaller than mature epithelial cells. *T vaginalis* infects the lower urinary tract in both women and men. It is the most prevalent nonviral sexually transmitted disease in the United States. Nonsexual transmission is infrequent because large numbers of organisms are required to produce symptoms.

Clinical Findings

A. Symptoms & Signs

A persistent vaginal discharge is the principal symptom with or without secondary vulvar pruritus. The discharge is profuse, extremely frothy, greenish, and at times foul-smelling. The pH of the vagina usually exceeds 5.0. Involvement of the vulva may be limited to the vestibule and labia minora. The labia minora may become edematous and tender. Urinary symptoms may occur; however, burning with urination is most often associated with severe vulvitis. Examination of the vaginal epithelium and cervix shows generalized vaginal erythema with multiple small petechiae, the so-called strawberry spots, which may be confused with epithelial punctation. Wet mount with normal saline reveals an increase in polymorphonuclear cells and characteristic motile flagellates in 50–70% of culture-confirmed cases.

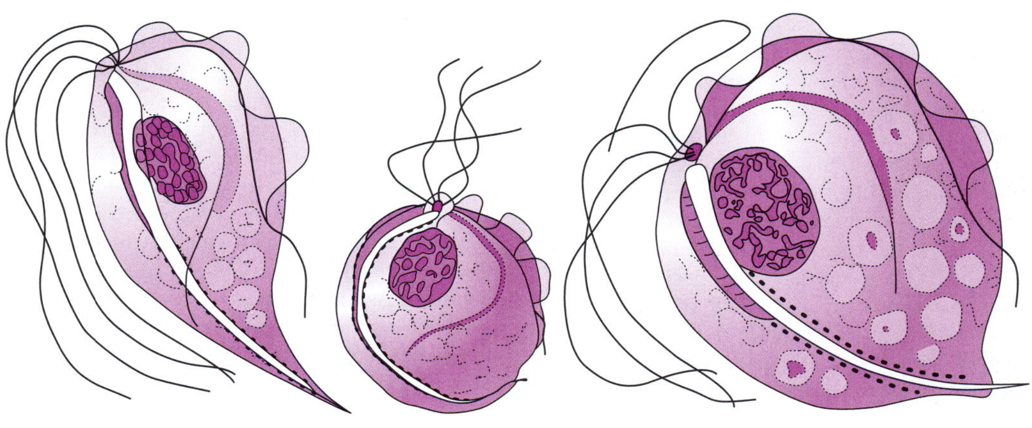

▲ **Figure 39–10.** Trichomonas vaginalis as found in vaginal and prostatic secretions. **A:** Normal trophozoite. **B:** Round form after division. **C:** Common form seen in stained preparation. Cysts not found.(Reproduced, with permission, from Brooks GF, Butel JS, Ornston LN. *Jawetz, Melinick, & Adelberg's Medical Microbiology*. 19th ed. Appleton & Lange; 1991.)

Table 39–13. Treatment of *Trichomonas vaginitis*.

Metronidazole 2 g orally in a single dose
Tinidazole 2 g orally in a single dose
Alternative Regimen Metronidazole 500 mg orally twice a day for 7 days

B. Wet Mount Diagnosis

Vaginal trichomoniasis is usually diagnosed by microscopy of a wet mount preparation of vaginal secretions. Sensitivity is only 60–70%. Immediate evaluation is required, as the heat generated by the microscope light source causes the *T vaginalis* to discontinue its typical movements.

C. Other Diagnostic Tests

Other tests for trichomoniasis include immunochromatographic capillary flow dipstick technology and nucleic acid probing. Sensitivity exceeds 83%, and specificity is 97%. Results of the immunochromatographic Trichomonas Rapid Test are available in 10 minutes, and those of the nucleic acid probe test within 45. False-positive results do occur. Papanicolaou smears have a sensitivity of approximately 60% and also yield false-positive results. Culture is the most sensitive and specific method of diagnosis. In women in whom trichomoniasis is suspected but not confirmed by microscopy, vaginal secretions should be cultured for *T vaginalis*.

Treatment

Systemic therapy with metronidazole is the treatment of choice, because trichomonads sometimes present in the urinary tract system. Partners should be treated simultaneously, with intercourse avoided or a condom used until treatment is completed. US Centers for Disease Control and Prevention recommendations are presented in Table 39–13. If such treatments are not effective, sensitivity of a culture of *T vaginalis* to metronidazole and tinidazole should be determined. Side effects of metronidazole include nausea or emesis with alcohol consumption. Contraindications include certain blood dyscrasias (neutropenia) and central nervous system diseases. An oncogenic effect has been demonstrated in animals but not in humans. Resistance to metronidazole therapy is rare but is rising and can be confirmed in vitro.

Trichomoniasis is associated with a number of perinatal complications and increased incidence in the transmission of HIV. Women with trichomoniasis should be evaluated for other sexually transmitted diseases, including *Neisseria gonorrhoeae, Chlamydia trachomatis*, syphilis, and HIV.

NEISSERIA GONORRHOEAE

Of women infected by *N gonorrhoeae*, 85% are asymptomatic. The glandular structures of the cervix, urethra, vulva, perineum, and anus are most commonly infected. In acute disease, patients present with a copious mucopurulent discharge and gram-negative diplococci within leukocytes. However, diagnosis should be confirmed with nucleic acid amplification or a culture from the endocervix, urethra, rectum, or mouth. An estimated 15–20% of women with lower tract disease develop upper genital tract disease with salpingitis, tubo-ovarian abscess, and peritonitis. Ectopic pregnancy and infertility are classic long-term consequences. If active infection is present during vaginal delivery, the newborn may develop conjunctivitis by contamination. Uncomplicated gonococcal infections of the cervix are treated with ceftriaxone 125 mg administered intramuscularly (IM) in a single dose. Single oral doses of cefixime 400 mg, ciprofloxacin 500 mg, ofloxacin 400 mg, or levofloxacin 250 mg are other recommended regimens. Quinolones are no longer recommended because some strains of *N gonorrhoeae* are quinolone-resistant. Spectinomycin 2 g IM in a single dose is an option for patients sensitive to cephalosporins. Empirical Treatment of *C trachomatis* should be considered, as this infection often coexists.

CHLAMYDIA TRACHOMATIS

The screening of sexually active young women for *C trachomatis* is important because some infections are asymptomatic, and some present with a mucopurulent cervicitis, dysuria, and/or postcoital bleeding. *C trachomatis* can be identified by culture (50–90% sensitivity), a direct fluorescent antibody (50–80% sensitivity), enzyme immunoassay (40–60% sensitivity), or, most recently, by using nucleic acid amplification tests (polymerase chain reaction or ligase chain reaction, 60–100% sensitivity). All tests have a specificity >99%. *C trachomatis* causes atypical cytologic findings on Papanicolaou smear and an ascending infection, salpingitis, in 20–40% of untreated patients. More than 50% of upper tract infections may be caused by *C trachomatis*, leading to tubal occlusion, ectopic pregnancy, or infertility. Untreated *C trachomatis* can also cause neonatal conjunctivitis. *C trachomatis* may present as LGV, which most commonly affects the vulvar tissues. Retroperitoneal lymphadenopathy may present. The initial lesion in LGV presents as a transient, painless vesicular lesion or shallow ulcer at the inoculation site. More advanced disease is characterized by anal or genital fistulas, stricture, or rectal stenosis. The disease is uncommon in the United States, but endemic in Southeast Asia and Africa.

If *C trachomatis* is suspected or diagnosed, both the patient and partner should be treated. They should also be evaluated for concurrent gonococcal infections. Recommended therapy includes azithromycin 1 g orally in a single dose or doxycycline 100 mg orally twice daily for 7 days. Erythromycin base 500 mg orally 4 times daily for 7 days, ofloxacin 300 mg orally twice daily, and levofloxacin 50 mg once daily for 7 days are alternative regimens. Doxycycline, levofloxacin, and ofloxacin should be avoided in pregnancy and during lactation. Patients should abstain from intercourse for 7 days. Test of cure is required in cases of possible reinfection or persistent symptoms and during pregnancy. Repeat testing should be considered 3 weeks after treatment with erythromycin. Rescreening is recommended 3–4 months after treatment. For LGV, the recommended regimen is doxycycline 100 mg twice daily for 21 days.

OTHER INFECTIONS

Mycoplasma hominis and *Ureaplasma urealyticum* also cause genital disease. Polymerase chain reaction is more sensitive than culture. Mycoplasma infections can cause infertility, spontaneous abortion, postpartum fever, salpingitis, and pelvic abscess, as well as nongonococcal urethritis in men. The most effective treatment is doxycycline 100 mg orally twice daily for 10 days.

CONDITIONS MIMICKING VAGINITIS

Cervicitis due to chlamydial infection, cervical polyps, or cervical or vaginal cancer can cause a mucopurulent discharge and bleeding. Adenocarcinoma of the cervix may be missed by cytologic cervical screening and by colposcopy, becasue it generally develops in the endocervical canal rather than at the squamocolumnar junction. Excessive cervical ectropion may cause excessive discharge of cervical mucus from normal endocervical cells. Vaginal adenosis may cause the same type of clear, mucoid-type discharge without associated symptoms. Excessive desquamation of the vaginal epithelium may produce a diffuse gray-white pasty vaginal discharge, which may be confused with candidiasis. Vaginal pH is normal. Microscopic evaluation shows normal bacterial flora, mature vaginal squamae, and no increase in the number of leukocytes. Excessive but normal vaginal discharge should be treated with reassurance and, if required, with cryosurgery, carbon dioxide treatment, or loop conization of the cervix. Continuous use of a tampon should be avoided.

DESQUAMATIVE INFLAMMATORY VAGINITIS

This rare condition of vaginitis should be considered in a patient with hard-to-treat vaginitis. The cause is unknown. Patients complain of a profuse purulent vaginal discharge, burning and pain upon urinating (dysuria) or intercourse (dyspareunia), and occasional spotting. Adherence of both vaginal walls, with gradual stenosis, is a common complication. The disease is a variant of the dermatologic disease lichen planus. In many cases, typical lichen planus layers are found on the skin, oral mucosa, and gums. Upon inspection, the vagina is found to be erythematous, inflamed, and desquamated. A thick discharge and a white membrane cover the vagina. The purulent discharge contains many immature epithelial and pus cells without any identifiable cause. Vaginal erythema is present, and synechiae may develop in the upper vagina, causing partial occlusion. Vaginal pH may be elevated. Wet mount and Gram's stain demonstrate an increased number of parabasal cells, an absence of gram-positive bacilli, and the presence of gram-positive cocci.

The recommended therapy is intravaginal administration of 2% clindamycin cream 5 g daily for 7 days or clindamycin pessaries followed by a foam containing hydrocortisone and pramoxine into the vaginal mucosa to create a protective layer. A second line of therapy is vaginal insertion of corticosteroids in the form of suppository or cream. Recently, application of tacrolimus cream, as an immunosuppressor agent, has also been suggested.

CHEMICAL VAGINITIS

Chemical vaginitis secondary to multiple irritating offenders, including topical irritants (sanitary supplies, spermicides, feminine hygiene supplies, soaps, perfumes); allergens (latex, antimycotic creams), and possibly excessive sexual activity, can cause pruritus, irritation, burning, and vaginal discharge. The etiology may be confused with vulvovaginal candidiasis. Treatment consists of removal of the offending agent. A short course of corticosteroid treatment may be used along with sodium bicarbonate sitz baths and topical vegetable oils.

ATROPHIC VAGINITIS

Clinical Findings

Prepubertal, lactating, and postmenopausal women lack the vaginal effects of estrogen production. The pH of the vagina is abnormally high, and the normally acidogenic flora of the vagina may be replaced by mixed flora. The vaginal epithelium is thinned and more susceptible to infection and trauma. Although most patients are asymptomatic, many postmenopausal women report vaginal dryness, spotting, presence of a serosanguineous or watery discharge, and/or dyspareunia. Some of the symptoms of irritation are caused by a secondary infection. On examination, the vaginal mucosa is thin, with few or absent vaginal folds. The pH is 5.0–7.0. The wet mount shows small, rounded parabasal epithelial cells and an increased number of polymorphonuclear cells.

Treatment

Treatment includes intravaginal application of estrogen cream. Because approximately one-third of the vaginal estrogen is systemically absorbed, this treatment may be contraindicated in women with a history of breast or endometrial cancer. The estradiol vaginal ring, which is changed every 90 days, may provide a preferable route of administration for some women. Estradiol hemihydrate (Vagifem) 1 tablet intravaginally daily for 2 weeks and then twice a week for at least 3–6 months may be more convenient. Systemic estrogen therapy should be considered if there are no contraindications.

FOREIGN BODIES

Pathogenesis

Foreign bodies commonly cause vaginal discharge and infection in preadolescent girls. Paper, cotton, or other materials may be placed in the vagina and cause secondary infection. Children may require vaginoscopy using a small-caliber hysteroscope or vaginal examination under anesthesia to identify or rule out a foreign body or tumor high in the vaginal vault. The vaginal canal can be flushed in the office using a small catheter in an attempt to remove a foreign body. In adults, a forgotten menstrual tampon, a contraceptive device, or a pessary may cause a malodorous discharge. The diagnosis can usually be made by pelvic examination.

Clinical Findings

Clinical symptoms associated with foreign bodies include abnormal malodorous vaginal discharge and intermenstrual spotting. Symptoms are generally secondary to drying of the vaginal epithelium and micro-ulcerations, which can be detected by colposcopy. Ulcerative lesions, particularly associated with tampon use, are typically located in the vaginal fornices and have rolled, irregular edges with a red granulation tissue base (Fig. 39–3). Regenerating epithelium at the ulcer edge may shed cells that may be interpreted as atypical, suggesting dysplasia. The lesions heal spontaneously once tampon use is discontinued. A foreign body retained in the vagina for a prolonged period may erode into the bladder or rectum.

Treatment

Treatment involves removal of the foreign body. Rarely, antibiotics are required for ulcerations or cellulitis of the vulva or vagina. Dryness or ulceration of the vagina secondary to use of menstrual tampons is transient and heals spontaneously.

Toxic shock syndrome is the most serious complication associated with the use of vaginal tampons. It may develop also without tampon use. The syndrome has been linked to staphylococcal vaginal infection in healthy young women who use high-absorbency tampons continuously throughout the menstrual period. Some of the clinical manifestations are secondary to the release of staphylococcal exotoxins. Symptoms consist of a high fever (≥38.9 °C [102 °F]), possibly accompanied by severe headache, sore throat, myalgia, vomiting, and diarrhea. The disease may resemble meningitis or viremia. Palmar erythema and a diffuse sunburn-like rash have been described. The skin rash usually disappears within 24–48 hours, but occasionally a patient has a recurrent maculopapular, morbilliform eruption between days 6 and 10. Superficial desquamation of the palms and soles often follows within 2–3 weeks. Progressive hypotension may occur and proceed to shock levels within 48 hours. Multisystem organ failure may occur, including renal and cardiac dysfunction. The incidence of toxic shock syndrome was 1 in 100,000 among females 15–44 years of age in 1986. Any menstruating woman who presents with sudden onset of a febrile illness should be evaluated and treated for toxic shock syndrome. The tampon should be removed, cultures sent, and the vagina cleansed to decrease the organism inoculum. Appropriate supportive measures should be provided and β-lactamase–resistant penicillin or vancomycin (if the patient is allergic to penicillin) administered. Women who have been treated for toxic shock syndrome are at considerable risk for recurrence. Therefore, these women should avoid tampon use.

VIRAL INFECTIONS

The viruses that affect the vagina are the herpesvirus (herpes simplex, varicella-zoster, and cytomegalovirus), poxvirus (molluscum contagiosum), and papillomavirus types. The main features of these infections have been discussed under Vulvar Diseases.

HERPESVIRUS

The herpesvirus (HSV) may cause erosions, ulcerations, or an exophytic necrotic mass involving the vagina or cervix and causing a profuse vaginal discharge. The cervix may be tender to manipulation and bleed easily. The primary lesion lasts approximately 2 weeks and heals without scarring. Recurrent infections may cause cervical lesions. The virus may be cultured from ulcers or ruptured vesicles. Cervical cytologic examination may reveal multinucleated giant cells with intranuclear inclusions.

HUMAN PAPILLOMAVIRUS INFECTION

As discussed in the section on Vulvar Diseases, condylomata may affect the vagina and cervix as well. Condylomatous vaginitis causes a rough vaginal surface, manifesting white projections from the pink vaginal mucosa. Vaginal discharge resulting from a secondary yeast or bacterial infection is the most common symptom of florid condylomas. Postcoital bleeding may occur. No specific symptoms are related to the other types of condylomas. States of immunosuppression (pregnancy, HIV infection, diabetes, renal transplant) are associated with massive proliferation of condyloma and are often difficult to treat.

PARASITIC INFECTION

Less common causes of vaginitis are parasitic infections with pinworms (*Enterobius vermicularis*) and *Entamoeba histolytica*. Pinworm infection is generally seen in children. Fecal contamination at the introitus is the source of infection. The perineal area is extremely pruritic. The parasite is generally detected by pressing a strip of adhesive cellulose tape to the perineum. The tape is then adhered to a slide, allowing the double-walled ova to be identified under the microscope. *E histolytica* infection of the vagina and cervix is rare in the United States but is quite common in developing countries. Severe infection may resemble cervical cancer, but symptoms are generally due to vulvar involvement. Trophozoites of *E histolytica* may be demonstrated on wet-mount preparations or occasionally on a Papanicolaou smear.

Ahmed AM, Madkan V, Tyring SK. Human papillomaviruses and genital disease. *Dermatol Clin* 2006;24:157–165. PMID: 16677964.

Bornstein J. the HPV vaccines—which to prefer? *Obstet Gynecol Surv* 2009;64:345–350. PMID: 19386141.

Bornstein J. Human papillomavirus vaccine: The beginning of the end for cervical cancer. *Isr Med Assoc J* 2007; 9:156–158. PMID: 17402325.

Geva A, Bornstein J, Dan M, Shoham HK, Sobel JD. The VI-Sense-vaginal discharge self-test to facilitate management of vaginal symptoms. *Am J Obstet Gynecol* 2006;195:1351–1356. PMID: 16769019.

Greer L, Wendel GD. Rapid diagnostic methods in sexually transmitted infections. *Infect Dis Clin North Am* 2008;22: 601–617. PMID: 18954754.

ACOG Practice Bulletin Number 61, 2005. Human papillomavirus. *Obstet Gynecol* 2005;105:905–918. PMID: 15802436.

Moyal-Barracco M, Edwards L. Diagnosis and therapy of anogenital lichen planus. *Dermatol Ther* 2004;17:38–46. PMID: 14756889.

O'Mahony C. Genital warts: Current and future management options. *Am J Clin Dermatol* 2005;6:239–243. PMID: 16060711.

ACOG Practice Bulletin Number 72, 2006. Vaginitis. *Obstet Gynecol* 2006;107:1195–1206. PMID: 16648432.

Val I, Almeida G. An overview of lichen sclerosus. *Clin Obstet Gynecol* 2005;48:808–817. PMID: 16286827.

Centers for Disease Control and Prevention, Workowski KA, Berman SM. Sexually transmitted diseases treatment guidelines, 2006. *MMWR Recomm Rep* 2006;55(rr-11):1–94. PMID: 16888612.

The author thanks Dr. Doron Zarfati for assistance in obtaining some of the figures and Ms Cindy Cohen for assistance in preparing the manuscript.

40 Benign Disorders of the Uterine Cervix

Izabella Khachikyan, MD
Pamela Stratton, MD

CONGENITAL ANOMALIES OF THE CERVIX

The cervix develops from the paramesonephric (müllerian) ducts in the sixth week of embryologic development. The midline fusion and subsequent canalization of the 2 müllerian ducts give rise to the uterine corpus, cervix, and upper vagina (Fig. 40–1). Müllerian duct anomalies result from nondevelopment, defective lateral or vertical fusion, or resorption failure. The most common type of müllerian fusion defect is a lateral fusion defect in which the resulting defective organs can be either symmetrical or asymmetrical and can be obstructed or unobstructed. These fusion defects result from failure of fusion of the müllerian ducts, failure of formation of 1 müllerian duct, or absorption of the intervening septum. Defective resorption of the tissue between the fused müllerian ducts results in a uterine septum that can be partial or extend to the full length to the cervix. The most common lateral fusion defect is a septum. **Vertical fusion** refers to the fusion of the müllerian ducts with the urogenital sinus. The absence of müllerian development results in agenesis of the cervix and uterus. A double cervix is frequently associated with a longitudinal vaginal septum and is an example of lack of fusion. A single hemicervix or septate cervix composed of single muscular septum that can be an extension of a lower uterine segment or vaginal septum is seen with resorption failure. Approximately 20–30% of women with müllerian duct anomalies also have urinary tract abnormalities, a finding that warrants urinary tract imaging. Women with müllerian duct anomalies have normal ovaries and develop normal secondary sex characteristics.

Cervical Agenesis

Isolated cervical agenesis is rare, but cases of an absent uterine cervix with a normal uterine corpus and normal vagina have been reported. These cases presumably result from either failure of müllerian duct canalization or abnormal epithelial proliferation after canalization. More common is absence of the cervix combined with absence of the uterine corpus and upper vagina, known as müllerian agenesis or Mayer-Rokitansky-Kuster-Hauser syndrome, which occurs in approximately 1 in 4000 female births. Because most of the vagina is derived from müllerian ducts, the vagina may be shortened in müllerian agenesis. Female offspring of women with müllerian agenesis have been studied to identify a possible genetic contribution to this disorder. Because no offspring with müllerian agenesis have been reported, this disorder is assumed to result from a polygenic multifactorial inheritance pattern.

Cervical agenesis with a normal functioning uterine corpus must be differentiated from müllerian agenesis (Figs. 40–2 and 40–3). In the former, menstrual blood may accumulate within the uterus or result in retrograde flow and development of endometriosis. Thus cervical agenesis is usually diagnosed at menarche when patients present with primary amenorrhea and cyclic abdominopelvic pain. Suppression of menstruation with continuous combined estrogen/progesterone pills may improve the pain-related complaints. Ultrasonography, magnetic resonance imaging (MRI), and laparoscopy can help with the diagnosis by defining the anatomy.

Women without a cervix or without a cervix and uterus cannot carry a pregnancy. Because women have normally functioning ovaries, they can undergo in vitro fertilization with their partner's sperm. Pregnancy is achieved with use of a surrogate woman who carries the pregnancy.

Women with müllerian or cervical agenesis may have a shortened or absent vagina. Nonsurgical treatment to lengthen or create a vagina involves the use of vaginal dilators that are under constant perineal pressure. One example is using a bicycle stool designed by Ingram that facilitates dilator use under constant perineal pressure. The most common surgical approach to correct vagina agenesis is the McIndoe technique to create a neovagina. The Vecchietti operation combines a surgical and nonsurgical approach to creating a neovagina and is performed by laparoscopy. Other surgical options include colonovaginoplasty using a segment of colon and vaginoplasty using skin flaps.

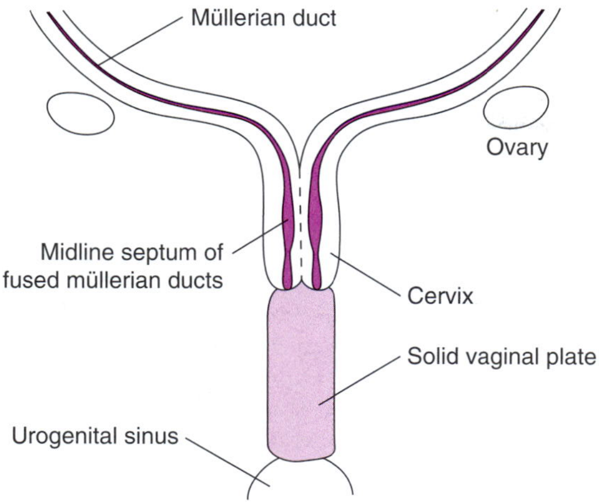

▲ **Figure 40–1.** Fusion of müllerian ducts to form cervix and corpus uteri.

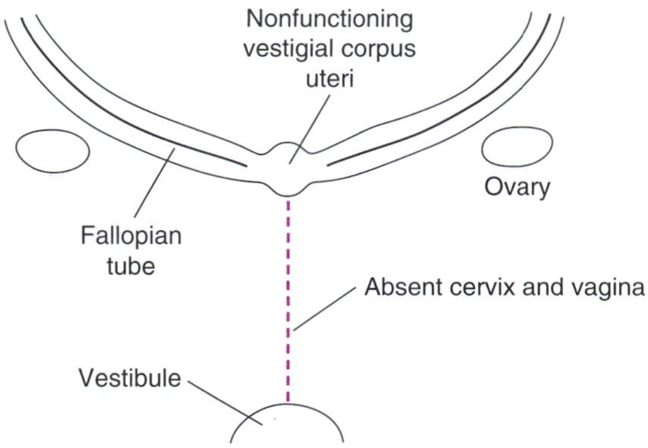

▲ **Figure 40–2.** Congenital absence of vagina.

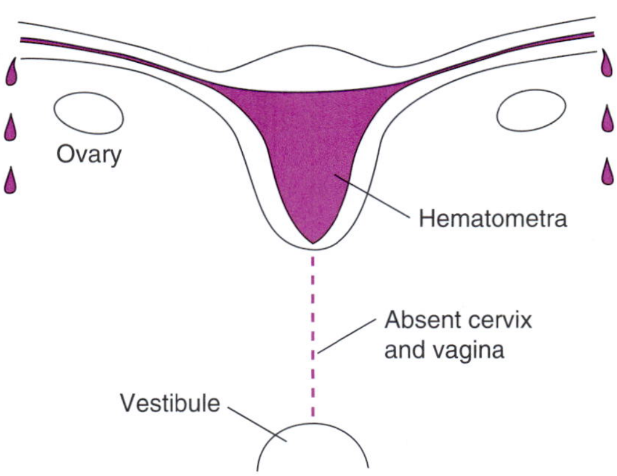

▲ **Figure 40–3.** Cervical agenesis with hematometra and retrograde menstruation.

Incomplete Müllerian Fusion

Congenital uterine anomalies are asymptomatic and thus often are undiagnosed. As with müllerian anomalies in general, these defects arise from agenesis, lateral or vertical fusion defects, or lack of canalization. Complete failure of fusion of the müllerian ducts results in duplication of reproductive structures. One example is uterus didelphys (2 uteri). Uterus bicornuate bicollis (2 cervices) has 2 separate uterine horns, each with a distinct cervix and vagina. The 2 vaginas are separated by a midline, longitudinal septum. If incomplete fusion results in a uterine horn ending blindly, a hematocolpos can develop (Fig. 40–4). Bicornuate uterus and arcuate uterus occur when there is partial or incomplete fusion of the müllerian ducts. In a bicornuate uterus, 2 discrete uterine cavities lead to the same cervix. The arcuate uterus may demonstrate minimal depression of the uterine fundus and is often clinically insignificant.

Women with müllerian fusion defects resulting in uterine anomalies have a higher rate of adverse pregnancy outcome. Premature birth may occur in 15–25%, miscarriage is observed in 25–50%, and malpresentation is similarly common (Fig. 40–5).

Failure of Resorption

Defective resorption of the tissue between the fused müllerian ducts will result in uterine septum formation. The septum consists of fibromuscular tissue and can be either partial or full, extending the length of the uterus (Fig. 40–6). Failure or incomplete resorption of this septum is associated with reproductive and obstetric complications. First- and second-trimester spontaneous miscarriages are common and usually occur between 8 and 16 weeks' gestation. Obstetric complications include premature labor, preterm delivery,

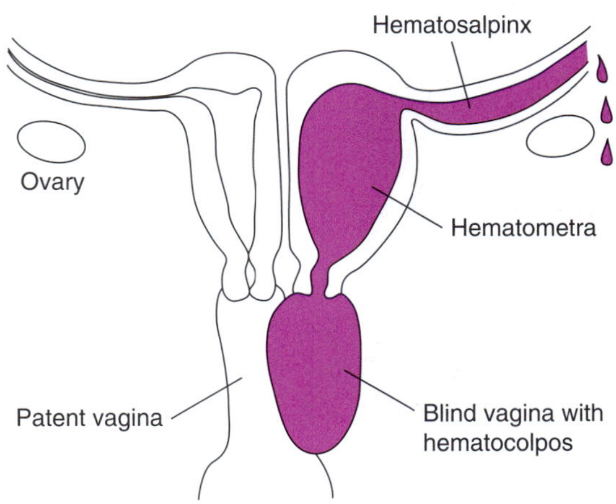

▲ **Figure 40–4.** Uterus didelphys with blind vagina hematocolpos, hematometra, hematosalpinx, and retrograde menstruation.

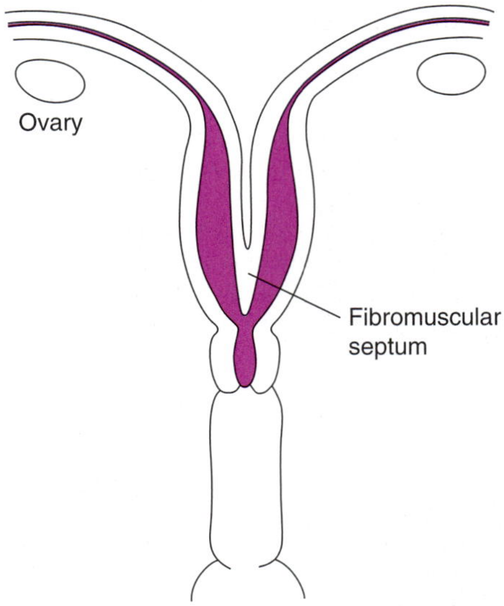

▲ **Figure 40–5.** Complete bicornuate uterus with fibromuscular septum at the level of internal cervical os.

malpresentation, intrauterine growth restriction, and lower term birth rate. Approximately 15–25% of spontaneous miscarriages are due to müllerian abnormalities.

If a septate uterus is identified in association with reproductive or obstetric complications, surgical therapy is recommended because it is hypothesized that the septum interferes with placentation. Hysteroscopic resection of the uterine septum improves reproductive outcome in women with recurrent spontaneous miscarriages. Ultrasound, MRI, sonohysterography, and hysterosalpingogram provide information to differentiate a septate uterus from other uterine abnormalities. Combined laparoscopy and hysteroscopy is the most reliable method to accurately differentiate a septate uterus from a bicornuate uterus.

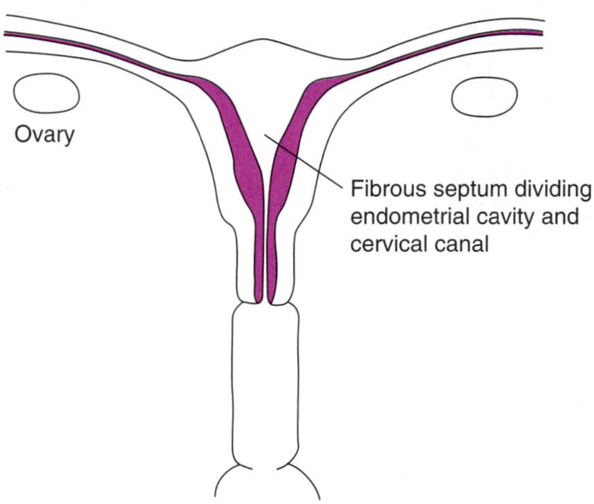

▲ **Figure 40–6.** Complete septate uterus.

CERVICAL ABNORMALITIES DUE TO DIETHYLSTILBESTROL EXPOSURE IN UTERO

Diethylstilbestrol (DES), a synthetic nonsteroidal estrogen, was used between the 1940s and 1971 to prevent premature birth, miscarriages, and other obstetric complications. Although the number of pregnant women treated with DES is unknown, estimates range from 2–10 million. DES crosses placenta and affects reproductive tract cell differentiation. In utero exposure to DES is also associated with vaginal clear cell carcinoma in female offspring, necessitating cytologic and colposcopic screening. Common structural changes of the cervix include collars, hoods, cockscombs, and pseudopolyps, cervical hypoplasia, and transverse septa (Fig. 40–7). Anomalies of the uterus include a T-shaped uterine cavity, hypoplastic uterus, adhesions, and constrictions of uterine cavity.

Women who are exposed to DES in utero and have cervical abnormalities are at increased risk for infertility. These women are also at increased risk for adverse outcomes in pregnancy, including miscarriage, ectopic pregnancy, and premature delivery. The use of prophylactic cervical cerclage for cervical incompetence related to DES exposure in utero is considered based on standard recommendations for cerclage placement.

ACOG Practice Bulletin. Cervical insufficiency. *Obstet Gynecol* 2010;102:1091–1099. PMID: 14672493.

Creighton SM, Davies MC, Cutner A. Laparoscopic management of cervical agenesis. *Fertil Steril* 2006;85:1510.e13–e15. PMID: 16616925.

Deffarges JV, Haddad B, Musset R, Paniel BJ. Utero-vaginal anastomosis in women with uterine cervix atresia: long-term follow-up and reproductive performance. A study of 18 cases. *Hum Reprod* 2001;16:1722–1725. PMID: 11473972.

Folch M, Pigem I, Konje JC. Müllerian agenesis: etiology, diagnosis and management. *Obstet Gynecol Surv* 2000;55:644–649. PMID: 11023205.

Gell JS. Mullerian anomalies. *Semin Reprod Med* 2003;21:375–388. PMID: 14724770.

Homer HA, Li TC, Cooke ID. The septate uterus: a review of management and reproductive outcome. *Fertil Steril* 2000;73:1–14. PMID: 10632403.

Kaufman RH, Adam E, Hatch EE, et al. Continued follow-up of pregnancy outcomes in diethylstilbestrol-exposed offspring. *Obstet Gynecol* 2000; 96:483–489. PMID: 11004345.

Keser A, Bozkurt N, Taner OF, Sensöz O. Treatment of vaginal agenesis with modified Abbe-McIndoe technique: long-term follow-up in 22 patients. *Eur J Obstet Gynecol Reprod Biol* 2005;121:110–116. PMID: 15935544.

Newbold RR. Prenatal exposure to diethylstilbestrol. *Fertil Steril* 2008;89:e55–e56. PMID: 18308064.

Preutthipan S, Herabutya Y. Vaginal misoprostol for cervical priming before operative hysteroscopy: a randomized controlled trial. *Obstet Gynecol* 2000;96:890–894. PMID: 11084173.

Propst AM, Hill JA 3rd. Anatomic factors associated with recurrent pregnancy loss. *Semin Reprod Med* 2000;18:341–350. PMID: 11355792.

Troiano RN, McCarthy SM. Mullerian duct anomalies: imaging and clinical issues. *Radiology* 2004;233:19–34. PMID: 15317956.

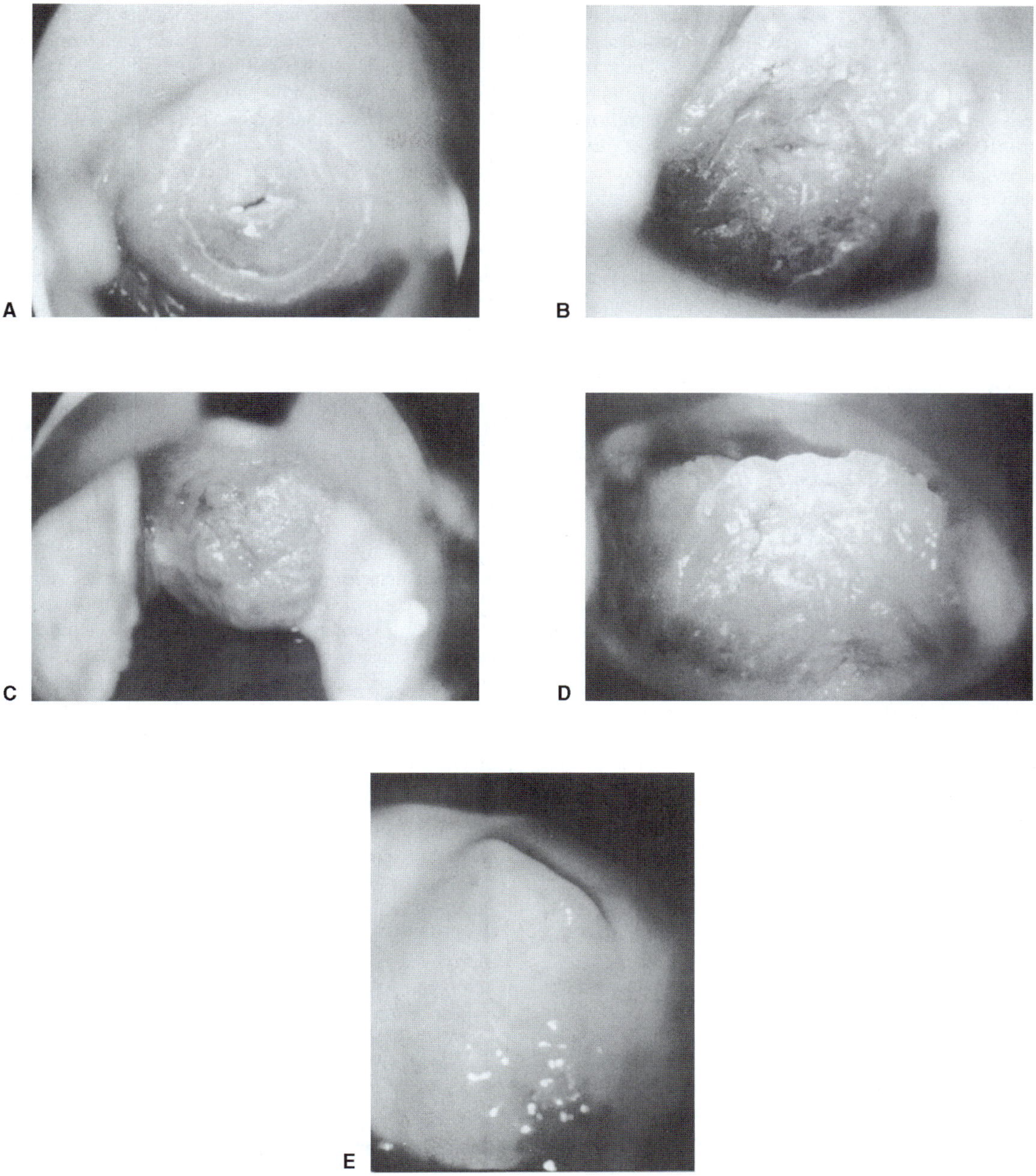

▲ **Figure 40–7.** Cervical changes in women exposed to diethylstilbestrol in utero. **A:** Circular sulcus. **B:** Central depression and ectopy. **C:** Portio vaginalis covered by columnar epithelium (ectopy). **D:** Anterior cervical protuberance (rough). **E:** Anterior cervical protuberance (smooth).

CERVICAL INJURIES

Lacerations

Cervical lacerations are frequent complications of a vaginal delivery. With vaginal deliveries, the most common site of cervical lacerations is the lateral aspect of the cervix. Clinically significant lacerations that are associated with vaginal bleeding or that require suturing complicate less than 5% of vaginal deliveries. Cervical cerclage, precipitous labor, vacuum extraction, nulliparity, and episiotomy are associated with increased risk for clinically significant lacerations. Cervical lacerations that cause abnormal vaginal bleeding or that extend to the lower uterine segment or vaginal wall warrant repair. Careful inspection of the entire cervix after delivery enables identification and repair of these clinically significant lacerations. Asymptomatic lacerations that are small may not need repair. Cervical lacerations do not appear to affect the outcome of subsequent pregnancies.

Performance of dilatation and curettage (D&C), particularly on the postmenopausal patient, can result in cervical laceration, most commonly during dilatation. When a tenaculum tears through the cervix with dilatation, it can easily be repaired by suturing, if needed. Use of cervical laminaria preoperatively may decrease the risk of laceration. Preoperative use of misoprostol to soften the cervix and reduce the force required to dilate it has been reported as an additional strategy.

Cervical lacerations are also reported with operative hysteroscopy, with use of the resecting loop, the roller-ball, and other instruments used to ablate the endometrium.

Perforations

Perforation of the cervix may occur inadvertently during sounding of the uterus, cervical dilatation, insertion of radioactive sources, or conization of the cervix or during self-induced abortion with sharp objects (eg, wires or darning or knitting needles). The urinary bladder and the rectum are at risk for injury because of their close proximity to the cervix. Perforations may involve the entire thickness and result in hemorrhage or hematoma if the uterine vessels are involved.

Ulcerations

Ulceration of the cervix may result from pressure necrosis related to vaginal pessary use. Cervical ulceration may also develop in women with complete uterine prolapse whose cervix protrudes through the vaginal introitus.

Cervical Stenosis

Cervical stenosis may lead to significant symptoms. In premenopausal women, cervical stenosis may obstruct menstrual flow, leading to amenorrhea, pelvic pain, and endometriosis. Additionally, cervical stenosis may impede the movement of semen into the uterus and thus be associated with an increased risk of infertility. Pyometra, although uncommon in women with cervical stenosis, is more common in postmenopausal women. Evacuation of pyometra and biopsy of intrauterine contents to rule out endometrial carcinoma is advised.

Although cervical stenosis may be present from birth, it may be caused by other factors. Cervical surgery such as cone biopsy, loop excision, or cryotherapy for treatment of dysplasia may lead to cervical stenosis. Excision by loop diathermy is less likely to cause cervical stenosis than a cold knife cone biopsy, perhaps because less stroma is removed or because suturing performed with cold knife cone may heal occluding the cervical os. Other causes of stenosis are trauma to the cervix, radiation therapy, and cervical cancer. Cervical atrophy with menopause may result in cervical stenosis.

The diagnosis of cervical stenosis is made clinically, by the inability to pass a small cervical dilator. The obstruction of the cervical canal may be suggested by visualizing intrauterine contents on ultrasonography of the uterus. Treatment of cervical stenosis involves opening or widening the cervical canal. The gentle passage of graduated sounds through the cervical canal at weekly intervals during the intermenstrual phase for 2–3 months after treatment will prevent or correct stenosis. In some circumstances, passing dilators under ultrasound guidance may be helpful. If the stenosis is associated with scar tissue, techniques to vaporize the scar tissue with laser treatment or enlarge the canal with loop diathermy and the resecting loop of the hysteroscope may be performed.

Annular Detachment

Annular detachment of the cervix is an extremely rare obstetric complication in which the cervix is devitalized and torn during labor. Proposed mechanisms include previous cervical damage, failure of the external os to dilate, and compromised blood supply by pressure of the fetal head. The diagnosis may be unrecognized or may be made when the detached ring or portion of cervix is expelled during delivery.

Complications of Cervical Injuries

Cervical injuries can result in immediate and delayed complications. Hemorrhage, although uncommon, is the most immediate and serious complication of cervical laceration. When the cervical tear extends into the lower uterine segment, vaginal bleeding may be present, but occult hemorrhage may occur and result in hypovolemic shock out of proportion to visible blood loss.

Cervical stenosis, cervical incompetence, and failure of the cervical dilation during labor are all sequelae of cone biopsy, and less commonly, unrecognized or improperly repaired lacerations. Repeated or habitual abortion, often occurring during the second trimester of pregnancy, may be due to cervical incompetence.

NORMAL CERVIX

General Considerations

The squamocolumnar junction of the cervix undergoes change over reproductive life. In younger women, the squamocolumnar junction is on the ectocervix. When it extends to replace a large part of the ectocervix, the term **cervical ectopy** is used, and the cervix appears red, granular and inflamed-appearing. Over time, the squamocolumnar

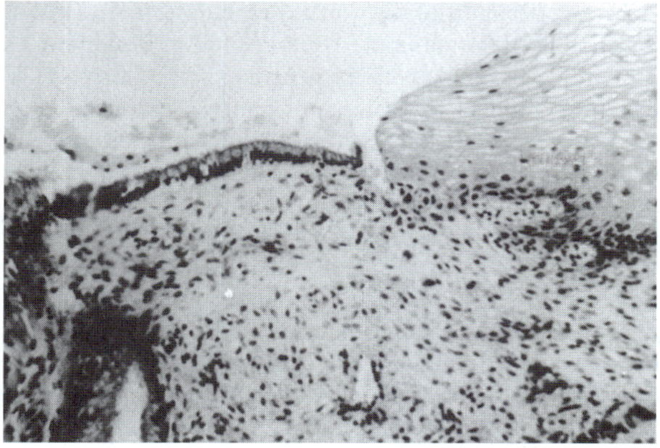

▲ **Figure 40–8.** Abrupt transition, squamocolumnar junction.

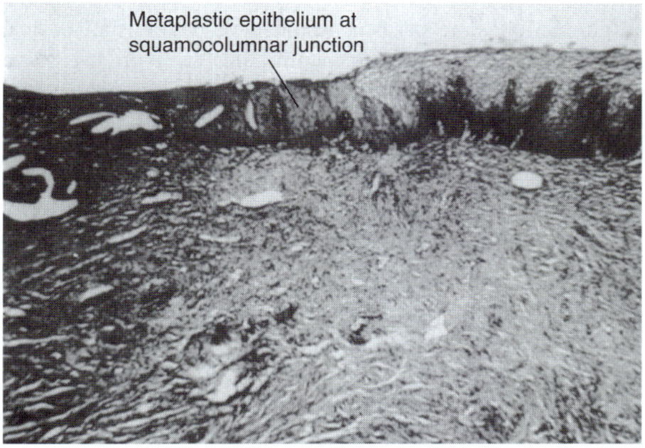

▲ **Figure 40–9.** Metaplastic epithelium at the squamocolumnar junction.

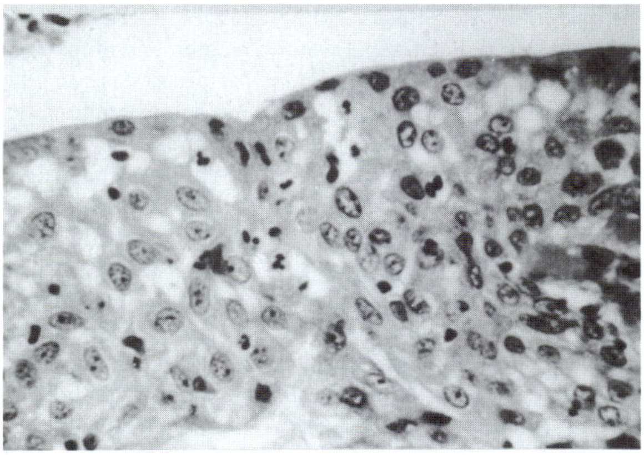

▲ **Figure 40–10.** Squamous epithelium showing histologic changes of human papillomavirus infection.

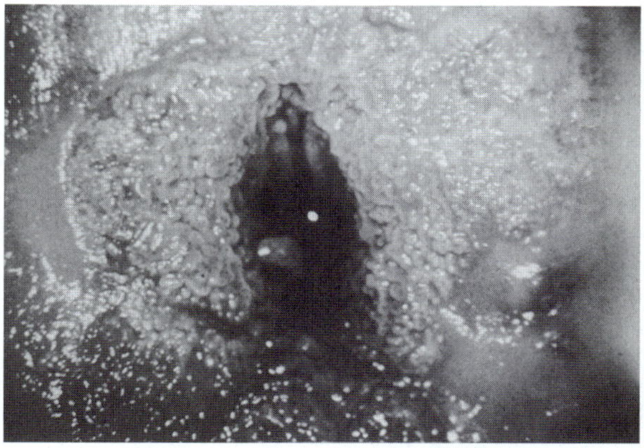

▲ **Figure 40–11.** Colposcopic view of villiform pattern of cervical ectopy.

junction moves toward the external os through the process of squamous metaplasia, in which the columnar epithelium on the ectocervix is gradually converted to stratified squamous epithelium. Initially, the metaplastic epithelium is thin and immature, but it becomes thicker and more mature, eventually becoming stratified squamous epithelium. Microscopically, the squamocolumnar junction rarely demonstrates an abrupt transition from squamous to columnar epithelium, but instead has a zone of immature squamous metaplasia (Figs. 40–8 and 40–9). On colposcopy, cervical ectopy has a fine villiform pattern (Figs. 40–10 and 40–11). This change from a mucous membrane of a single layer of columnar epithelium to one of the stratified squamous epithelium may be accelerated during 3 periods of a woman's life: fetal existence, adolescence, and during the first pregnancy.

By the time a woman reaches her fifth decade, the squamocolumnar junction has receded into the endocervical canal, and the ectocervix is completely covered by squamous epithelium. In the process, the crypts and clefts of columnar epithelium are bridged over and may be occluded, obstructing the egress of mucus, producing the common, typical nabothian cysts of the cervix.

CERVICAL INFECTIONS

General Considerations

Annually 3 million women are diagnosed with cervicitis. Most common causes of infectious cervicitis are *Neisseria gonorrhoeae, Chlamydia trachomatis*, herpes simplex virus (HSV), human papillomavirus (HPV), and trichomoniasis, *Mycoplasma genitalium*, cytomegalovirus, and bacterial vaginosis (covered in Chapter 43). Cervicitis often is asymptomatic and may be undiagnosed for some time. If untreated, cervicitis can result in pelvic inflammatory disease and ultimately lead to a higher risk of infertility, ectopic pregnancy, and chronic pelvic pain. Advances in colposcopy and sensitive testing for infectious diseases have allowed better assessment of the causes of acute and chronic cervicitis. Methods for testing gonorrhea include urethral Gram stain, culture on Thayer-Martin media, DNA probes, and DNA amplification techniques. Testing for chlamydia can be performed using nucleic acid amplification techniques on cervical or urine specimens. For HPV infection, cervical cytology (Pap test) and HPV testing are used with colposcopy and biopsy for detection of HPV disease. The signs of cervicitis are caused by edema and increased vascularity, making the cervix appear swollen and reddened. The presence of hypervascularity, erythema, and ectopy may be found with either squamous metaplasia or inflammatory changes requiring therapy. Cervicitis can be diagnosed histologically when polymorphonuclear leukocytes, lymphocytes, or histiocytes are noted. The cervix is in direct contact with the vagina and is exposed to viral, bacterial, fungal, and parasitic agents. Cervical infections occur in the absence of vaginal disease. Through sexual contact, the cervix may be infected with *N gonorrhoeae, C trachomatis*, HSV, HPV, and *Mycoplasma* spp. Because many women are asymptomatic, screening women in high-risk populations such as those with multiple partners and those with inconsistent use of condoms is important. Patients diagnosed with gonorrhea or chlamydia are at risk for infection with other sexually transmitted diseases (STDs). Counseling and testing should be offered for syphilis, hepatitis B, and HIV, as well as testing for HPV.

Pathogenesis

C trachomatis and *N gonorrhoeae* are sexually transmitted infections (STIs) commonly causing endocervicitis as well as upper reproductive tract infections. More than 1.1 million cases of *C trachomatis* and 350,000 cases of *N gonorrhoeae* were reported in United States in 2007. As *C trachomatis* is often "silent," an undiagnosed, ongoing infection may ascend into the endometrial cavity to the fallopian tubes, causing salpingitis as well as pelvic peritonitis. With the cervix as a reservoir, the organism may infect the fetus during its passage through the birth canal. *C trachomatis* transmitted to the eyes causes trachoma and inclusion conjunctivitis or pneumonia of the newborn.

As with *Chlamydia* infections, *N gonorrhoeae* first causes a cervical infection, which may ascend infecting the endometrium and fallopian tubes. The ascending infection for either agent may occur at the end of menses when there is no protective mucus plug. As with *C trachomatis, N gonorrhea* can be transmitted to newborns during vaginal delivery, causing neonatal ophthalmia.

Fitz-Hugh-Curtis syndrome or perihepatitis is a rare complication usually caused by *C trachomatis* and *N gonorrhoeae* and is characterized by adhesions between the liver and the parietal peritoneum.

There are 2 types of HSV, herpes simplex virus type 1 (HSV-1) and herpes simplex virus type 2 (HSV-2). Although HSV-2 causes most of the genital herpes infections, HSV-1, the etiology of the common cold sore or fever blister, causes some through oral–genital or genital–genital contact. HSV infection produces cervical lesions similar to those found on the vulva. First the lesion is vesicular and then becomes an ulcer. Primary infections may be extensive and severe, producing constitutional symptoms of low-grade fever, myalgia, and malaise lasting approximately 2 weeks. The ulcers heal without scarring. Once infection has occurred, even after healing, the virus continues to reside in the nerve cells of the affected area for life. HSV recurrences are less severe in both symptoms and duration. HSV is found in the lesions caused by HSV infection, but viral shedding can also occur in asymptomatic patients without obvious lesions. Women with either active infection or asymptomatic HSV shedding from normal-appearing skin can infect their infants during vaginal delivery. Those with a positive HSV test near term are advised to undergo caesarean section.

HPV is spread by skin-to-skin contact. Women with vulvar HPV lesions should be assessed for cervical HPV lesions and infection. The cervical lesions are flatter than typical genital warts (condylomata acuminata) seen on the vulva and perianal skin. In fact, they often are invisible to the naked eye, becoming visible only after application of a dilute solution of acetic acid (acetowhite epithelium) or by colposcopic examination (white epithelium, mosaicism, and coarse punctation). There are more than 120 HPV types. Low-risk types 6, 11, 42, 43, 44, 54, and 55 are associated with benign lesions of the cervix, whereas types 16, 18, 31, 33, 35, 39, 45, and 56 are considered high risk and found in association with cervical intraepithelial neoplasia and invasive cancers. Seventy percent of infections resolve in 1 year and 90% by 2 years. Persistent HPV infection may progress to precancerous lesions and, over time, progress to cervical cancer.

Prevention

Abstinence and the use of condoms and barrier methods for protection during coitus are the most important strategies for prevention of cervicitis. Although avoiding sexual contact with infected persons is a sound recommendation, most women do not know whether their partner(s) have an STI, and many of these partners, if infected, are asymptomatic. Because chlamydia and gonorrhea are most prevalent in young adults aged 19 to 25 and have significant long-term complications, annual screening for these 2 infections is advised in high-risk populations, regardless of whether they have symptoms. Other "at risk" populations include those having multiple sexual partners, inconsistently using condoms, with a previous history of STIs, and individuals who engage in other high-risk behaviors (eg, current or prior drug abusers); however, these different risk factors may be difficult to assess.

Because asymptomatic patients are at similar risk of developing complications as symptomatic women, detecting infection in asymptomatic patients is also important.

Treating affected partners at the same time the woman is treated is important to prevent reinfection. Counseling patients and her sexual partner(s) may also be useful.

Detection and treatment of cervicitis in pregnancy has important health benefits for the fetus and newborn. For example, pregnant women should be screened for syphilis and HIV at the first prenatal visit (see Chapter 43). Women with a history of HSV should be screened near term (see Chapter 43). Women at high risk of premature delivery should be screened for bacterial vaginosis (see Chapter 43).

The prompt recognition and proper repair of cervical lacerations lessen the risk of cervical stenosis and cervical incompetence in future pregnancies.

When hysterectomy is performed, if possible, the cervix should be removed to minimize the risk of cervical diseases. Although some recommend retaining the cervix at the time of hysterectomy to maintain sexual function or vaginal support, clinical studies do not provide evidence to support this recommendation.

Clinical Findings

A. Symptoms & Signs

1. Acute Cervicitis—Purulent vaginal discharge is the primary sign and symptom of acute cervicitis. Some women have vaginal bleeding, most frequently after sexual intercourse, although intermenstrual bleeding and bleeding during examination can also occur. The appearance of the discharge varies depending on the pathogen—often thick and creamy discharge is noted in gonorrheal infection, foamy and greenish-white in trichomonal infection, white and curd-like in candidiasis, and thin and gray in bacterial vaginosis. In bacterial vaginosis, an amine or fishy odor is released when the discharge is combined with potassium hydroxide. Vulvar burning and itching may be prominent symptoms of cervicitis.

Chlamydia infections may produce a purulent discharge from a reddened, congested cervix or may be relatively asymptomatic, without visible signs. The muculopurulent discharge of chlamydia infection is often indistinguishable from that of gonorrheal infection. On inspection, the cervix infected by *N gonorrhoeae* reveals an acutely inflamed and edematous cervix with a purulent discharge from the external os. In trichomonal infection, a strawberry-like appearance covers the ectocervix and may extend to the adjacent vaginal mucosa. In candidiasis, a white cheesy exudate may be difficult to wipe away and once wiped off usually leaves punctate hemorrhagic areas.

Gonorrheal or chlamydial cervicitis may be accompanied by urethritis with frequency, urgency, and dysuria. If any infection is associated with acute salpingitis, the symptoms and signs will include pelvic peritonitis. Postcoital bleeding or intermenstrual spotting may occur because of hyperemia of the infected cervix associated with freely bleeding areas. Cervical friability with bleeding occurs when endocervical smears are obtained.

Colposcopic findings of acute cervicitis reveal an altered microangioarchitecture with marked increase in the surface capillaries, which when viewed end-on may show a pattern of diffuse "punctation." Trichomoniasis is typified by characteristic double-hairpin capillaries. In an inflammatory process, the colposcopic picture is diffuse with ill-defined margins in contrast with the localized and sharply demarcated vascular changes associated with intraepithelial neoplasia (Chapter 48). Invasive cancers may be secondarily infected, so in addition to the colposcopic changes associated with malignancy, those related to inflammation are also present.

2. Chronic Cervicitis—In chronic cervicitis, leukorrhea may be the chief symptom. Although not as profuse as in acute cervicitis, the discharge may cause vulvar irritation. The discharge may be frankly purulent and variable in color, or may simply be thick, tenacious, turbid mucus. Intermenstrual or postcoital bleeding may occur. Associated symptoms may be lower abdominal pain, lumbosacral backache, dysmenorrhea, dyspareunia, urinary frequency, urgency, and dysuria.

Inspection of the chronically infected cervix often reveals only abnormal discharge, with the upper vagina appearing normal.

B. Laboratory Findings

1. Stains and Smears—Mucopurulent cervicitis is defined as evidence of purulent material on inspection of an inflamed cervix along with 10 or more polymorphonuclear leukocytes per high-powered microscopic field seen on Gram's stain of the discharge. In acute cervicitis with *N gonorrhoeae,* the sensitivity of Gram's stain for detection of diplococci is only 50%. Thus use of Gram's stain for diagnosis is not recommended in women because of its low sensitivity in detecting infection. Identification of motile flagellated organisms on saline wet smear preparations suggests *Trichomonas vaginalis*. In symptomatic patients, with signs suggesting *Trichomonas*, further testing of nucleic acid amplification, culture testing may be necessary. Bacterial vaginosis can be seen on saline wet mount by the coating of epithelial cells with bacteria called "clue cells." Bacterial vaginosis is diagnosed by using Amsel criteria: thin homogeneous white, yellow discharge, presence of the "clue cells" on microscopy, vaginal pH >4.5, and fishy odor on adding alkaline 10% potassium hydroxide solution. Presence of 3 of these criteria will confirm the diagnosis of bacterial vaginosis. Candidal infections can be seen on potassium hydroxide preparations, with the distinctive presence of hyphae.

2. Detection of Specific Agents Causing Cervical Infections—Previously, culture was the preferred method to detect infection. *N gonorrhoeae* culture is performed on Thayer-Martin or blood agar medium. Although culture has excellent specificity, the sensitivity is no higher than 70% in females. Culture can be influenced by how the specimen was collected, transport conditions, culture procedures, and identification of a positive culture.

More recently, infection is detected more reliably with nucleic acid amplification methods such as polymerase chain reaction (PCR), transcription-mediated amplification, and strand displacement amplification. The benefit of using nucleic acid amplification is its high sensitivity and specificity (82–100%). The specimen can be obtained noninvasively from either a vulvar swab or urine, with non–clean catch urine specimens having greater sensitivity than cervical testing. These tests also allow for simultaneous detection of both *N gonorrhoeae* and *C trachomatis* from the same specimen. Sensitivity with urine and cervical samples is similar for *C trachomatis,* but sensitivity for *N gonorrhoeae* is higher with cervical swab. Enzyme immunoassay and direct fluorescent antibody rely on antigen detection and have a sensitivity ranging from 70–80%, but the specimen still requires invasive testing using a swab from the cervix or urethra.

HSV infection can be detected by viral culture, PCR, and direct fluorescence antibody. Most laboratories are moving toward nonculture assays such as PCR, which offer high sensitivity and specificity.

Syphilis is detected by using nontreponemal rapid plasma reagin (RPR) or Venereal Disease Research Laboratory (VDRL) tests and subsequent confirmation with microhemagglutination assay for *Treponema pallidum* (MHA-TP), fluorescent treponemal antibody-absorption (FTA-ABS) tests.

Combining HPV testing with cervical cytology appears to be the most effective strategy for detecting abnormal cervical pathology. Cervical cytology with HPV testing is first performed in women at 21 years of age regardless of the age of onset of sexual activity because of the low risk of cancer in women under age 21. If cytology is normal and HPV testing is negative, follow-up screening is done in 3 years. If cytology is abnormal, colposcopy with directed biopsy is advised.

3. Blood Studies—In uncomplicated cervicitis not accompanied by salpingitis, the white count may be normal. With salpingitis, a leukocytosis is common with an elevated white count. The erythrocyte sedimentation rate may be slightly elevated.

Cytopathology

Until recently, the Papanicolaou (Pap) smear has been the primary tool to examine the pathologic changes related to cervical neoplasia. Cellular changes of mild dysplasia (low-grade squamous intraepithelial lesion [SIL]), moderate or severe dysplasia (carcinoma in situ [CIS], high-grade SIL), and invasive cancer may be delineated on cytology testing.

Epithelial cell changes associated with cervical inflammation may be difficult to distinguish from those related to neoplastic disease. Nuclear enlargement, clumping of chromatin, hyperchromatism, and nucleoli, as well as cytoplasmic eosinophilia and poorly defined cell membranes, are nonspecific findings of "cytologic atypia." A few inflammatory cells can be seen on the cytology slide, particularly immediately before, during, and immediately after menses. However, large numbers of polymorphonuclear leukocytes or histiocytes indicate an acute cervicitis. When the inflammatory cells are so dense that the epithelial cells are obscured, the smear should be repeated after the inflammatory process has been treated.

Cervical cytology evaluation can also aid in the diagnosis of specific cervical infections. At times, a specific diagnosis can be made either by identifying the infectious organism(s) or by noting changes in the epithelial cells characteristic of a specific type of infection. For example, trichomonads and yeast forms can be identified directly on cytology slides. HPV infection is characterized by squamous epithelial cell enlargement, multinucleation, and the perinuclear "halo" effect of koilocytosis. Enlarged, multinucleated cells with ground-glass cytoplasm and nuclei containing inclusion bodies are indicative of HSV infection.

Histopathology of Cervical Infections

Both *N gonorrhoeae* and *C trachomatis* infections produce a nonspecific acute inflammatory reaction of edema and increased vascularity, and the cervix becomes swollen and reddened. Gross appearance of acute cervicitis must be distinguished clinically and histologically from cervical ectopy. Infection causes the glandular epithelium to hyperfunction, producing a copious purulent or mucopurulent exudate and mucus mixed with inflammatory cells. Microscopically, stromal edema and infiltration by polymorphonuclear leukocytes are seen, and some mucous membrane may be denuded. As the acute infection subsides, swelling and redness disappear, and polymorphonuclear leukocytes are replaced by lymphocytes, plasma cells, and macrophages—the histologic picture of chronic cervicitis. Almost all parous women may have findings characteristic of chronic cervicitis on biopsy that are not significant unless they also have clinical signs and symptoms of cervicitis.

Differential Diagnosis

Noninfectious cervicitis may result from the effects of endogenous or exogenous hormones on the cervicovaginal mucosa. When cervical discharge is noted, bimanual examination may aid in diagnosis of pelvic infection with the clinical signs of cervical motion tenderness and induration.

Infectious cervicitis must be distinguished from cervical intraepithelial neoplasia. This may be hampered because inflammatory conditions may also result in epithelial atypia on cytologic examination. Colposcopy is a useful adjunct (see Chapter 48). Cervical cytology and histologic examination by endocervical curettage and biopsy may help distinguish chronic cervicitis from cervical neoplasia.

Complications

N gonorrhoeae or *C trachomatis* cervicitis is often complicated by salpingitis and pelvic inflammatory disease, which are associated with an increased risk of infertility, ectopic pregnancy, and chronic pelvic pain. The occurrence of gonorrheal or chlamydial cervicitis in HIV-infected women has been reported to be associated with increased shedding of HIV-1 that, in turn, increases the infectiveness of these women. Although a history of genital infections is more common among women with carcinoma of the cervix, these agents do not increase the risk of developing cancer.

Treatment

Selecting the treatment for cervicitis depends on the nature of the infection, whether the patient is pregnant or breastfeeding, her plans for future pregnancy, the severity of the cervical infection as indicated by the presence or absence of complicating factors such as salpingitis, and previous treatment. Instrumentation should be avoided during the acute cervicitis to minimize the risk of ascending infection.

A. Acute Cervicitis

Treatment of acute cervicitis is directed at diagnosing a specific organism; treatment is then directed accordingly.

1. Trichomoniasis—Metronidazole is used to treat *T vaginalis* infection. Metronidazole can be administered as 2 g orally in a single dose or tinidazole 2 g orally in a single dose, or alternatively as metronidazole 500 mg twice daily for 7 days. Any of these regimens have cure rates of approximately 90–95%. Patients should be advised not to use alcohol during treatment. Abstinence from alcohol should continue for 24 hours after treatment with metronidazole and for 72 hours after using tinidazole. Pregnant women should be given 2 g orally as a single dose; those who are breastfeeding should stop breastfeeding for 12–24 hours. Sex partners should be treated and intercourse should be avoided until women and their sex partners are cured. Topical forms of metronidazole are less efficacious (<50%) than the oral preparations.

2. Candidiasis—Candidiasis is most effectively treated with topically applied azole drugs. This will result in relief of symptoms. Treatment course may be 1, 3, or 7 days, depending on the severity of infection. Effective treatments include butoconazole 2% cream 5 g intravaginally for 3 days, clotrimazole 1% cream 5 g intravaginally for 7–14 days, clotrimazole 100 mg vaginal tab for 7 days, miconazole 25 cream 5 g intravaginally for 7 days, miconazole 200-mg vaginal suppository for 3 days or 100 mg for 7 days. A single dose of 150 mg fluconazole by mouth is an effective treatment.

3. Bacterial Vaginosis—See Chapter 43, Sexually Transmitted Diseases and Pelvic Infections.

4. C trachomatis—*C trachomatis* can be treated with azithromycin 1 g orally in a single dose or alternatively with doxycycline 100 mg twice daily for 7 days. Alternative treatments with erythromycin base 500 mg orally 4 times a day for 7 days, erythromycin ethylsuccinate 800 mg orally 4 times a day for 7 days or ofloxacin 300 mg orally twice a day for 7 days, or levofloxacin 500 mg orally once a day for 7 days are suggested. In pregnancy, azithromycin 1 g orally in a single dose or amoxicillin 500 mg orally 3 times a day for 7 days can be given; alternatively erythromycin could be used as well. Doxycycline, ofloxacin, and levofloxacin are contraindicated in pregnancy. Because of the high rate of coinfection with *N gonorrhoeae* and *C trachomatis* (up to 42%), when *N gonorrhoeae* infection is found, it is recommended that patients also receive treatment for *C trachomatis.*

5. N gonorrhoeae—Cervicitis due to *N gonorrhoeae* can be treated with ceftriaxone 125 mg administered intramuscularly in a single dose, cefixime 400 mg orally in a single dose, ciprofloxacin 500 mg orally in a single dose, or ofloxacin 400 mg or levofloxacin 250 mg orally in a single dose. In pregnancy, fluoroquinolones should be avoided. Fluoroquinolones also should not be used in patients residing in or who may have acquired infections in Europe, Middle East, Asia, the Pacific (including Hawaii), or California because of increasing quinolone-resistant *N gonorrhoeae* (QRNG) in these areas (see Chapters 43 and 44 and the 2006 Centers for Disease Control and Prevention guidelines for treatment of STDs for full recommendations).

B. Chronic Cervicitis

Several studies have demonstrated that microscopic findings of 10 or more polymorphonuclear leukocytes per high-power field do not correlate with specific infection using more sensitive testing for *N gonorrhoeae* and *C trachomatis.* Therefore, an asymptomatic patient with chronic cervicitis who does not test positive for an STD does not need to be treated.

Surgical procedures may be useful for treatment of symptomatic chronic cervicitis, especially in the absence of an infectious pathogen or evidence of dysplasia. Cryosurgery, electrocauterization, and laser therapy have been used, although there is a high risk for recurrence and risk for cervical injury.

Treatment of Complications

A. Cervical Hemorrhage

Cervical hemorrhage after surgical procedures such as cone biopsy, electrocauterization, loop excision, cryosurgery, or laser vaporization requires suture ligation of bleeding vessels. For less severe bleeding, directed topical coagulation of bleeding areas with Monsel's solution or silver nitrate is successful. Electrocauterization may also be beneficial.

B. Salpingitis

Inflammation of the fallopian tubes usually necessitates the administration of a broad-spectrum antibiotic. Intravenous administration may be advised to obtain adequate antibiotic levels.

C. Leukorrhea

Persistent cervical discharge after treatment may indicate either persistent infection or reinfection. Testing should be performed and selective antibiotic treatment administered.

D. Cervical Stenosis

Cervical surgery is a common cause of cervical stenosis and secondary amenorrhea after the surgical procedure suggests cervical stenosis. Inability to insert a 2.5-mm diameter dilator is consistent with cervical stenosis. Cervical stenosis is treated by dilating the cervical canal.

E. Infertility

Normally, midcycle cervical mucus enhances transportation of sperm through the cervical canal. Factors that influence production of normal cervical mucus could have an impact on fertility. They include surgical factors (cauterization, freezing, or vaporization) or removal (conization or loop excision) of the endocervical glandular cells and cervical infections. Treatment includes low-dose estrogen for 1 week before ovulation or intrauterine insemination with washed and incubated sperm.

GRANULOMATOUS INFECTIONS OF THE CERVIX

Tuberculosis, tertiary syphilis, and granuloma inguinale rarely present as chronic cervical lesions. When present, cervical nodules, ulcerations, or granulation tissue may produce a chronic inflammatory exudate characterized histologically by lymphocytes, giant cells, and histiocytes. The gross appearance of the cervix may be difficult to distinguish from carcinoma of the cervix.

Tuberculosis

Since 1986, the incidence of tuberculosis in the United States has increased, particularly among African Americans, Hispanics, and Asians. Some of the increase has been attributed to the HIV epidemic. In the past, genital tuberculosis has accounted for only 1% of patients with pelvic inflammatory disease; however, in European and Asian countries, the occurrence ranges from 5–13%. With increasing numbers of immigrants to the United States and with the rise in incidence of AIDS in American women, an increase in the incidence of pelvic tuberculosis may occur. Genitourinary tuberculosis is commonly secondary to infection elsewhere in the body, usually pulmonary, but active pulmonary disease can be documented in only one-third of patients. Vascular dissemination is responsible for infection of the fallopian tubes in almost all patients with genital tuberculosis, and involvement of the endometrium follows in 90%. Cervical disease can occur by direct extension or lymphatic spread but is rare, occurring in only 1% of cases. The chief clinical manifestations of pelvic and cervical involvement are abdominal pain, irregular bleeding, and constitutional symptoms. The cervix may be hypertrophied and nodular, without any visible lesion. Speculum examination may demonstrate either an ulcerative or a papillary lesion, thus resembling neoplastic disease.

The diagnosis of tuberculosis of the cervix must be made by biopsy. Histologically, the disease is characterized by tubercles undergoing central caseation. Because such lesions may be caused by other entities such as amoebiasis, schistosomiasis, brucellosis, tularemia, sarcoidosis, and foreign body reaction, the tubercle bacillus must be demonstrated by acid-fast stains or culture.

The reader is referred to other texts for the details of medical therapy of genital tuberculosis. Most patients are cured by medical management alone. Patients who respond poorly or who have other problems (eg, tumors, fistulas) may require total hysterectomy and bilateral salpingo-oophorectomy after a trial of chemotherapy.

RARE INFECTIOUS DISEASES OF THE CERVIX

Lymphogranuloma venereum, a chlamydial infection, and chancroid, caused by *Haemophilus ducreyi*, may attack the cervix along with other areas of the reproductive tract.

Cervical actinomycosis may occur as a result of contamination by instruments and by intrauterine devices. The cervical lesion may be a nodular tumor, ulcer, or fistula. Prolonged penicillin or sulfonamide therapy is recommended.

Schistosomiasis of the cervix is secondary to involvement of the pelvic and uterine veins by the blood fluke *Schistosoma haematobium*. Cervical schistosomiasis may produce a large papillary growth that ulcerates and bleeds on contact, resembling cervical cancer. In other instances, Schistosomiasis may be found in endocervical polyps and be associated with intermenstrual and postcoital bleeding. An ovum occasionally can be identified in a biopsy specimen taken from the granulomatous cervical lesion. However, the diagnosis usually is made by recovering the parasite from the urine or feces. Chemical, serologic, and intradermal tests for schistosomiasis are available.

Echinococcal cysts may involve the cervix. Treatment consists of surgical excision.

CYSTIC ABNORMALITIES OF THE CERVIX

Nabothian Cysts

Nabothian cysts develop when a cleft or tunnel of columnar endocervical epithelium becomes covered by squamous metaplasia. They appear grossly as translucent or yellow and may vary in diameter from a few millimeters to 3 cm.

Mesonephric Cysts

Microscopic remnants of the mesonephric (wolffian) duct are often seen deep in the lateral vaginal fornices externally in the normal cervix. Occasionally they become cystic, forming structures up to 2.5 mm in diameter, lined by cuboid epithelium. They may be confused with deeply situated nabothian cysts, but their location and the wolffian-type cells lining the cysts serve as useful distinguishing features.

American College of Obstetricians and Gynecologists. Cervical cancer in adolescents: screening, evaluation, and management. *Obstet Gynecol* 2010;116:469–472. PMID: 20664421.

Anttila T, Saikku P, Koskela P, et al. Serotypes of *Chlamydia trachomatis* and risk for development of cervical squamous cell carcinoma. *JAMA* 2001; 285:47–51. PMID: 11150108.

Batalden K, Bria C, Biro FM. Genital herpes and the teen female. *J Pediatr Adolesc Gynecol* 2007;20:319–321. PMID: 18082851.

Black CM, Marrazzo J, Johnson RE, et al. Head-to-head multicenter comparison of DNA probe and nucleic acid amplification tests for *Chlamydia trachomatis* infection in women performed with an improved reference standard. *J Clin Microbiol* 2002;40:3757–3763. PMID: 12354877.

Centers for Disease Control and Prevention. Sexually transmitted disease treatment guidelines. *MMWR Recomm Rep* 2002;51(RR-6):1–78. PMID: 12184549.

Chow TW, Lim BK, Vallipuram S. The masquerades of female pelvic tuberculosis: case reports and review of literature on clinical presentations and diagnosis. *J Obstet Gynaecol Res* 2002;28:203–210. PMID: 12452262.

Cook RL, Hutchison SL, Østergaard L, Braithwaite RS, Ness RB. Systematic review: noninvasive testing for *Chlamydia trachomatis* and *Neisseria gonorrhoeae*. *Ann Intern Med* 2005;142:914–925. PMID: 15941699.

Cuzick J, Clavel C, Petry KU, et al, Overview of the European and North American studies of HPV testing primary cervical cancer screening. *Int J Cancer* 2006;119:1095–1101. PMID: 16586444.

Dalgic H, Kuscu NK. Laser therapy in chronic cervicitis. *Arch Gynecol Obstet* 2001;265:64–66. PMID: 11409476.

Holder NA. Gonococcal infections. *Pediatr Rev* 2008;29;228–234. PMID: 18593752.

Bernal KL, Fahmy L, Remmenga S, Bridge J, Baker J. Embryonal rhabdomyosarcoma (sarcoma botryoides) of the cervix presenting as a cervical polyp treated with fertility-sparing surgery and adjuvant chemotherapy. *Gynecol Oncol* 2004;95:243–246. PMID: 15385139.

Lamba H, Byrne M, Goldin R, Jenkins C. Tuberculosis of the cervix: case presentation and a review of the literature. *Sex Transm Infect* 2002;78:62–63. PMID: 11872864.

Lanham S, Herbert A, Basarab A, Watt P. Detection of cervical infections in colposcopy clinic patients. *J Clin Microbiol* 2001;39:2946–2950. PMID: 11474018.

Marrazzo JM. Mucopurulent cervicitis: No longer ignored, but still misunderstood. *Infect Dis Clin North Am* 2005;19:333–349. PMID: 15963875.

Marrazzo JM, Handsfield HH, Whittington WL. Predicting chlamydial and gonococcal cervical infection: implications for management of cervicitis. *Obstet Gynecol* 2002;100:579–584. PMID: 12220782.

McClelland RS, Wang CC, Mandaliya K, et al. Treatment of cervicitis is associated with decreased cervical shedding of HIV-1. *AIDS* 2001;15:105–110. PMID: 11192850.

Mehta SD, Rothman RE, Kelen GD, Quinn TC, Zenilman JM. Unsuspected gonorrhea and chlamydia in patients of an urban adult emergency department: a critical population for STD control intervention. *Sex Transm Dis* 2001;28:33–39. PMID: 11196043.

Moore SG, Miller WC, Hoffman IF, et al. Clinical utility of measuring white blood cells on vaginal wet mount and endocervical gram stain for the prediction of chlamydial and gonococcal infections. *Sex Transm Dis* 2000;27:530–538. PMID: 11034527.

Myziuk L, Romanowski B, Brown M. Endocervical Gram stain smears and their usefulness in the diagnosis of *Chlamydia trachomatis*. *Sex Transm Infect* 2001;77:103–106. PMID: 11287687.

Nucci MR. Symposium part III: tumor-like glandular lesions of the uterine cervix. *Int J Gynecol Pathol* 2002;21:347–359. PMID: 12352183.

Singh S, Gupta V, Modi S, Rana P, Duhan A, Sen R. Tuberculosis of uterine cervix: a report of two cases with variable clinical presentation. *Trop Doct* 2010;40:125–126. PMID: 20305116.

US Preventive Services Task Force. Screening for Chlamydial infection: Recommendations and rationale. *Am J Prev Med* 2001; 20(3 Suppl):90–94. PMID: 11306237.

Woodman CB, Collins S, Winter H, et al. Natural history of cervical human papillomavirus infection in young women: a longitudinal cohort study. *Lancet* 2001;357:1831–1836. PMID: 11410191.

Wright TC Jr, Subbarao S, Ellerbrock TV, et al. Human immunodeficiency virus 1 expression in the female genital tract in association with cervical inflammation and ulceration. *Am J Obstet Gynecol* 2001;184:279–285. PMID: 11228474.

BENIGN NEOPLASMS OF THE CERVIX

1. CERVICAL POLYPS

ESSENTIALS OF DIAGNOSIS

- Intermenstrual or postcoital bleeding
- A soft, red pedunculated protrusion from the cervical canal at the external os
- Microscopic examination confirms the diagnosis of benign polyp

General Considerations

Cervical polyps are small, pedunculated, often sessile neoplasms of the cervix. Most originate from the endocervix; a few arise from the portio (Fig. 40–12). They are composed of

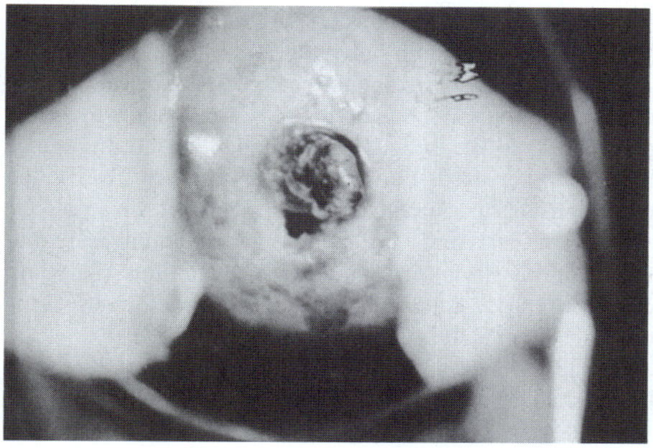

Figure 40–12. Cervical polyp.

a vascular connective tissue stroma and are covered by columnar, squamocolumnar, or squamous epithelium. Polyps are relatively common, especially in multigravidas over 20 years of age. They are rare before menarche, but an occasional polyp may develop after menopause. Asymptomatic polyps often are discovered on routine pelvic examination. Most are benign, but all should be removed and submitted for pathologic examination because malignant change may occur. Moreover, some cervical cancers present as a polypoid mass.

Polyps arise as a result of focal hyperplasia of the endocervix. Whether this is due to chronic inflammation, an abnormal local responsiveness to hormonal stimulation, or a localized vascular congestion of cervical blood vessels is not known. They are often found in association with endometrial hyperplasia, suggesting that hyperestrogenism plays a significant etiologic role. Most polypoid structures are vascular, often are infected, and are subject to displacement or torsion. Increased discharge and postcoital bleeding are common symptoms.

Endocervical polyps usually are red, flame-shaped, fragile growths. The polyps vary from a few millimeters in length and diameter to larger tumors 2–3 cm in diameter and several centimeters long. These polyps usually are attached to the endocervical mucosa near the external os by a narrow pedicle, but occasionally the base is broad. On microscopic examination, the stroma of a polyp is composed of fibrous connective tissue containing numerous small vessels in the center. There is often extravasation of blood and marked infiltration of the stroma by inflammatory cells (polymorphonuclear neutrophils, lymphocytes, and plasma cells). The surface epithelium resembles that of the endocervix, varying from typical picket-fence columnar cells to areas that show squamous metaplasia and mature stratified squamous epithelium. The surface often has many folds, as is much of the normal endocervical mucosa.

Ectocervical polyps are pale, flesh-colored, smooth, and rounded or elongated, often with a broad pedicle. They arise from the outer cells of the cervix and are less likely to bleed than endocervical polyps. Microscopically, ectocervical polyps are more fibrous than endocervical polyps, with few or no mucus glands, and are covered by stratified squamous epithelium.

Metaplastic alteration of both types of polyp is common. Inflammation, often with necrosis at the tip (or more extensively), is typical of both polyp types.

The incidence of malignant change in a cervical polyp is estimated to be <1%. Squamous cell carcinoma is the most common type of malignancy, although adenocarcinomas have been reported. Endometrial cancer may involve the polyp secondarily. Sarcoma rarely develops within a polyp.

Botryoid sarcoma, an embryonal rhabdomyosarcoma tumor of the cervix (or vaginal wall) resembling small pink or yellow grapes, contains striated muscle and other mesenchymal elements. It is extremely malignant.

Because polyps are a potential focus of cancer, they must be examined routinely for malignant characteristics upon removal.

Clinical Findings

A. Symptoms & Signs

Intermenstrual or postcoital bleeding is the most common symptom of cervical polyps. Leukorrhea (white or yellow mucous secretion) and menorrhagia have also been associated with cervical polyps.

Abnormal vaginal bleeding is often reported. Postmenopausal bleeding is frequently described by older women. In the setting of infertility, it is reasonable to remove them as a potential contributing factor.

Cervical polyps appear as smooth, red, fingerlike projections from the cervical canal. They usually are approximately 1–2 cm in length and 0.5–1 cm in diameter. Generally they are too soft to be felt by the examiner's finger.

B. X-Ray Findings

Polyps high in the endocervical canal may be demonstrated by hysterosalpingogram or saline infusion sonohysterography.

C. Laboratory Findings

Vaginal cytology will reveal signs of infection and often mildly atypical cells. Blood and urine studies are not helpful.

D. Special Examination

A polyp high in the endocervical canal may be seen with the aid of a special endocervical speculum or by hysteroscopy. Some polyps are found only at the time of diagnostic D&C in the investigation of abnormal bleeding.

Differential Diagnosis

Masses projecting from the cervix may be polypoid but are not necessarily polyps. Adenocarcinoma of the endometrium or endometrial sarcoma may present as a mass at the external os or extending beyond. Discharge and bleeding usually occur.

Typical polyps are easy to diagnose by gross inspection, but ulcerated and atypical-appearing growths must be distinguished from other small submucous pedunculated myomas or endometrial polyps arising low in the uterus. Any of these growths may result in dilatation of the cervix, presenting just within the os and resembling cervical polyps. Products of conception, usually decidua, may push through the cervix and resemble a polypoid tissue mass, without other signs and symptoms of pregnancy. Condylomata, submucous myomas, and polypoid carcinomas are diagnosed by microscopic examination.

Complications

Cervical polyps may be infected, some by virulent staphylococci, streptococci, or other pathogens. Serious infections occasionally follow instrumentation for the identification or removal of polyps. A broad-spectrum antibiotic should be administered at the first sign or symptom of spreading infection.

Acute salpingitis may be initiated or exacerbated by polypectomy.

It is unwise to remove a large polyp and then perform a hysterectomy several days later. Pelvic peritonitis may complicate the latter procedure. A delay of several weeks or 1 month between polypectomy and hysterectomy is recommended.

Treatment

A. Medical Measures

Appropriate testing for cervical discharge should be performed as indicated and treatment administered if infection is identified.

B. Specific Measures

Most polyps can be removed in the physician's office. The base of the polyp is grasped with forceps and twisted until the growth is avulsed, usually causing little bleeding. When performing polypectomy it is important to cauterize its base to reduce the chances of the bleeding and to decrease the recurrence rate. Large polyps and those with sessile attachments may require excision in an operating room to allow for administration of anesthesia, use of a hysteroscope, and control of any bleeding.

If the cervix is soft, patulous, or definitely dilated and the polyp is large, hysteroscopy should be performed, especially if the pedicle is not readily visible. Exploration of the cervical and uterine cavities with the hysteroscope allows for further identification of other polyps. All tissue must be sent to a pathologist to be examined for possible underlying malignant or premalignant conditions.

Prognosis

Removal of simple, solitary cervical polyps is usually curative.

2. PAPILLOMAS OF THE CERVIX

ESSENTIALS OF DIAGNOSIS

- Asymptomatic
- Papillary projection from the exocervix
- The presence of koilocytes with or without cytologic atypia
- Colposcopic identification

General Considerations

Cervical papillomas are benign neoplasms found on the ectocervix. The neoplasms consist of 2 types: (1) The typical solitary papillary projection from the exocervix composed of a central core of fibrous connective tissue covered by stratified squamous epithelium. This is a true benign neoplasm, and the cause is unknown. (2) Condylomata of the cervix, which may be present in various forms ranging from a slightly raised area on the exocervix that appears white after acetic acid application (on colposcopy) to the typical condyloma acuminatum. These usually are multiple and are caused by HPV infection, an STD. Similar lesions of the vagina and vulva are often, but not always, present. Evidence of HPV infection can be found in 1–2% of cytologically screened women. The incidence is much higher in women attending STD clinics.

Prevention

Contraception with condoms and other barrier methods may prevent primary infection and reinfection.

Clinical Findings

A. Symptoms & Signs

There are no characteristic symptoms of cervical papillomas; they are often discovered on routine pelvic examination or colposcopic examination for dysplasia revealed by Pap smear.

B. Laboratory Findings

Cytologic findings of koilocytes—squamous cells with perinuclear clear halos—are strongly suggestive of HPV infection. Dysplastic squamous cells are frequently found in association with koilocytes. HPV type testing of cervical or vaginal secretions may be used to determine whether there are oncogenic risk types. Biopsy of involved epithelium reveals papillomatosis and acanthosis. Mitoses may be frequent, but in the absence of neoplastic change, the cells are orderly with regular nuclear features. Koilocytes predominate in the superficial cells.

Complications

Intraepithelial neoplasia is associated with certain types of HPV infection (see Cervical Intraepithelial Neoplasia, Chapter 48). Infection with HPV anywhere in the genital tract, vulva, vagina, or cervix increases the risk of developing squamous cell carcinoma of the cervix.

Treatment

Solitary papillomas should be surgically excised and submitted for pathologic examination. Likewise, colposcopically directed biopsies of flat condylomata should be submitted for histopathologic examination. Flat condylomata may be completely removed with a biopsy instrument if they are small. More extensive lesions may require cryotherapy, loop excision, or laser vaporization. Dysplasia associated with HPV infection should be managed according to the severity and extent of the dysplastic process (see Cervical Intraepithelial Neoplasia, Chapter 48).

Prognosis

Because the entire lower genital tract is a target area for HPV infection, long-term follow-up with attention to the cervix, vagina, and vulva is necessary.

3. LEIOMYOMAS OF THE CERVIX

The paucity of smooth muscle elements in the cervical stroma makes leiomyomas that arise in the cervix uncommon. The corpus leiomyoma/cervical leiomyoma ratio is in the range of 12:1.

Although myomas usually are multiple in the corpus, cervical myomas are most often solitary and may be large enough to fill the entire pelvic cavity, compressing the bladder, rectum, and ureters (Fig. 40–13). Grossly and microscopically they are identical to leiomyomas that arise elsewhere in the uterus.

Clinical Findings

A. Symptoms & Signs

Cervical leiomyomas are often silent, producing no symptoms unless they become very large. Symptoms result from pressure on surrounding organs such as the bladder, rectum, or soft tissues of the parametrium, or obstruction of the cervical canal. Frequency and urgency of urination are the result of bladder compression. Urinary retention occasionally occurs as a result of pressure against the urethra. Heavy vaginal bleeding may occur. Hematometra may develop with obstruction of the cervix.

If the direction of growth is lateral, there may be ureteral obstruction with hydronephrosis. Rectal encroachment causes constipation. Dyspareunia may occur if the tumor occupies the vagina. Large cervical leiomyomas in pregnancy, because of their location, unlike those involving the corpus, may cause soft-tissue dystocia, preventing descent of the presenting part in the pelvis. Cervical leiomyomas of significant size can be readily palpated on bimanual examination.

B. Imaging

A plain film may demonstrate the typical mottled calcific pattern associated with cervical leiomyomas. Hysterography may define distortion of the endocervical canal. Intravenous urography may demonstrate ureteral displacement or obstruction. Transvaginal ultrasound or MRI can be helpful in determining the size and location.

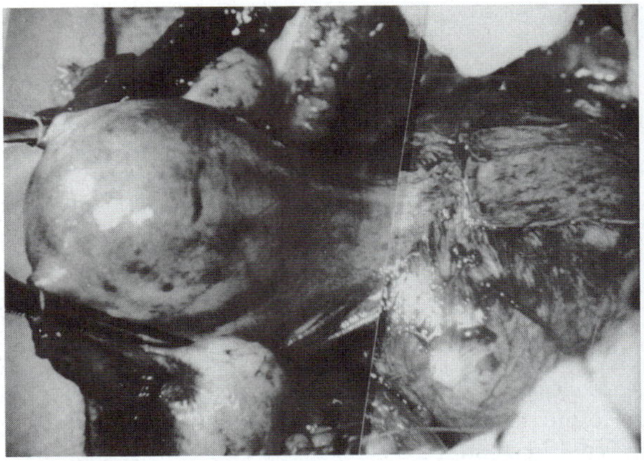

▲ **Figure 40–13.** Large cervical leiomyoma filling true pelvis.

Treatment

Small, asymptomatic cervical leiomyomas do not require treatment. If the leiomyomas become symptomatic, removal may be possible via hysteroscopic resection. If additional multiple leiomyomas are present that cannot be resected with the hysteroscope, uterine artery embolization, abdominal myomectomy, or hysterectomy may be indicated, depending on the patient's desire for preservation of fertility.

Because of the proximity of the pelvic ureter to the cervix, the ureter is at risk of damage in operation involving a cervical leiomyoma. Dissecting the ureters or placement of stent may prevent its injury.

Prognosis

Recurrence of cervical myomas after surgical removal is rare.

Varras M, Hadjilira P, Polyzos D, Tsikini A, Akrivis CH, Tsouroulas M. Clinical considerations and sonographic findings of a large nonpedunculated primary cervical leiomyoma complicated by heavy vaginal haemorrhage: a case report and review of the literature. *Clin Exp Obstet Gynecol* 2003;30:144–146. PMID: 12854862.

Benign Disorders of the Ovaries & Oviducts

41

Ofer Lavie, MD

ESSENTIALS OF DIAGNOSIS

- Benign adnexal mass refers not only to ovarian abnormalities but also to masses originating in the fallopian tube (ectopic pregnancy, pyosalpinx), ovaries (ovarian cyst, tuboovarian abscesses, adnexal torsion), uterine ligaments, lateral uterine masses (myomas), and gastrointestinal tract (diverticulitis, appendicitis) and even the urinary system (pelvic kidney).
- Benign adnexal masses originating from the genital system are common in women in the reproductive age group and are caused by physiologic cysts or benign neoplasms.
- Most adnexal masses are discovered incidentally, and the management of these benign masses is dictated by their presentation.
- The evaluation of these masses should be assessed according to the algorithm shown in Figure 41–1, including a thorough patient history, physical examination, laboratory tests, and imaging modalities.

Clinical Findings

Patient history should include review of patient age and family history in particular for the occurrence of ovarian familial cancers. A full physical examination should be performed, including a node survey and breast, abdominal, and pelvic examination. In many cases the radiologic studies, including ultrasonography of the pelvis and sometimes computed tomography (CT), would be of most importance in the assessment of the patient with an adnexal mass (Fig. 41–1). One way to approach the adnexal mass is to think of it in regard to the patient's age. For the young woman, the majority of ovarian cysts are benign: hemorrhagic corpus luteum follicular cysts and dermoid cysts are common in this age group; however, tubal abnormalities, including ectopic pregnancies, and sequela from tubal infection should be strongly considered (Table 41–1). On the other hand, the majority of ovarian or tubal cancers occur postmenopausally.

Differential Diagnosis

The clinical challenge in assessing an adnexal mass is to distinguish between a benign and malignant mass (Table 41–1) or findings that indicate a need for intervention or treatment versus masses that can be followed up conservatively (Fig. 41–2). Generally, when malignancy is *not* suspected, and if clinically the patient is stable, then expectant management is indicated, as many of these cysts are physiologic in nature and thus are expected to regress over time.

Patients should be re-evaluated 6 weeks after initial presentation, and persistent masses should be considered potentially benign or malignant neoplasms that warrant operative evaluation.

Treatment

Operative intervention is indicated when a patient is symptomatic because of hemorrhage of a ruptured cyst, ovarian torsion, or failure of previous treatments, for example, failure to treat an adnexal abscess. The risk of malignancy must always be assessed and excluded (see Chapter 50 to be checked for proper evaluation). The exclusion of a neoplastic process should be performed mainly through use of imaging modalities. For instance, sonographic indices as suggested in Table 41–2 should indicate whether the adnexal mass is at high risk for involving a neoplastic process.

Pathologic diagnosis by frozen section during surgery can aid in determining what type of treatment is indicated; however, in a young patient, final diagnosis and treatment of an adnexal malignancy should be based on analysis of permanent, rather than frozen sections because pathologic examination of frozen specimens can sometimes lead to incorrect surgical decisions. For most benign ovarian cysts, laparoscopy is the preferred method because of its shorter recovery time, as well as less pain, blood loss, and overall cost compared with

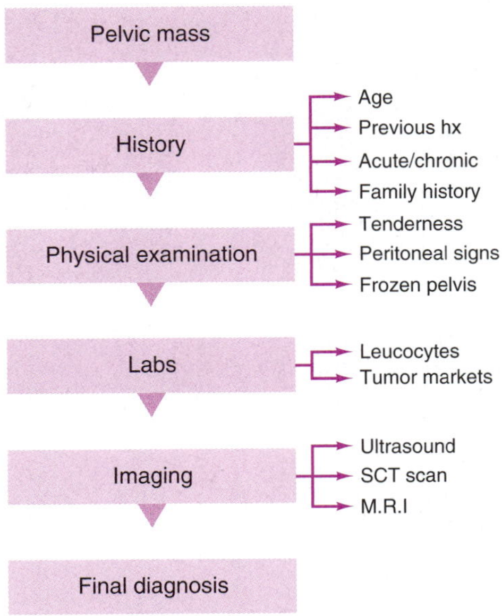

▲ **Figure 41–1.** Triage for evaluation of an adnexal mass.

laparotomy. Even extremely large ovarian cysts (reaching the umbilicus and higher) currently are being managed laparoscopically. A laparoscopic approach is recommended if the cyst appears benign by preoperative evaluation (Table 41–2). For most young patients, ovarian cystectomy is favored over oophorectomy in order to retain fertility.

Ginsburg KA, McGinnis KT. Ovarian cystectomy: Perioperative considerations and operative technique. *Oper Tech Gynecol Surg* 2000;5:224.

Jermy K, Luise C, Bourned T. The characterization of common ovarian cysts in premenopausal women. *Ultrasound Obstet Gynecol* 2001;17:140–144. PMID: 11251923.

Manjunath AP, Pratapkumar, Sujatha K, Vani R. Comparison of three risk of malignancy indices in evaluation of pelvic masses. *Gynecol Oncol* 2001;81:225–229. PMID: 11330953.

Table 41–1. Differential diagnosis of adnexal masses.

Associated with pregnancy
Intrauterine
Tubal
Abdominal
Ovarian or adnexal masses
Functional cysts
Inflammatory masses
Tubo-ovarian complex
Neoplastic Benign Malignant
Paraovarian or paratubal cysts
Intraligmentous myomas
Nongynecologic masses
Diverticular abscess
Appendiceal abscess
Peritoneal cyst
Stool in sigmoid
Less common conditions that must be excluded
Pelvic kidney
Carcinoma of the colon, rectum, appendix
Carcinoma of the fallopian tube
Retroperitoneal tumors (anterior sacral meningocele)
Uterine sarcoma or other malignant tumors

PHYSIOLOGIC ENLARGEMENT: FUNCTIONAL CYSTS

FOLLICULAR CYSTS

ESSENTIALS OF DIAGNOSIS

- The most common functional cyst is the follicular cyst.
- Follicular cysts (Fig. 41–3) vary in diameter from 3 to 8 cm.
- Histologically, they are seen to be lined by an inner layer of granulosa cells and an outer layer of theca interna cells that may or may not be luteinized.

Pathogenesis

These cysts result from a failure in ovulation, most likely secondary to disturbances in the release of the pituitary gonadotropins. The fluid of the incompletely developed follicle is not reabsorbed, producing an enlarged follicular cyst.

Clinical Findings

Typically follicular cysts are asymptomatic, although bleeding and torsion can occur. Large cysts may cause aching pelvic pain, dyspareunia, and occasionally abnormal uterine bleeding associated with a disturbance of the ovulatory pattern.

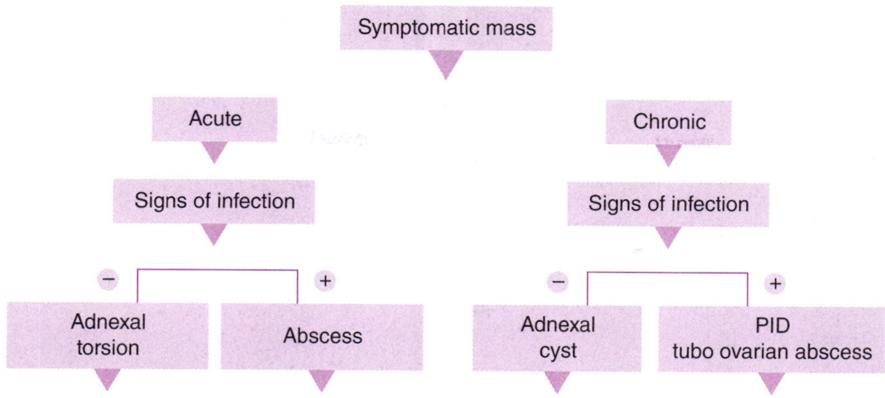

▲ **Figure 41–2.** Triage for making the diagnosis of an adnexal mass

Treatment

Most follicular cysts disappear spontaneously within 60 days without treatment. Use of oral contraceptive pills (OCPs) has often been recommended to help establish a normal rhythm; however, recent data show that this practice may not produce more rapid resolution than expectant management.

Aspiration of follicular cysts was performed in the past; however, recent data suggest that the diagnostic value of this procedure is relatively low and cysts greater than 8 cm in maximal diameter have a 95% tendency to recur after an aspiration procedure.

Allias F, Chanoz J, Blache G, Thivolet-Bejui F, Vancina S. Value of ultrasound-guided fine needle aspiration in the management of ovarian and paraovarian cysts. *Diag Cytopathol* 2000;22:70–80. PMID: 10649515.

Christensen JT, Boldsen JL, Westergaard JG. Functional ovarian cysts in premenopausal and gynecologically healthy women *Contraception* 2002;66:153–157. PMID: 12384202.

MacKenna A, Fabres C, Alam V, Morales V. Clinical management of functional ovarian cysts: a prospective and randomized study. *Hum Reprod* 2000;15:2567–2569. PMID: 11098028.

Table 41–2. Ultrasonographic characteristic for discrimination between benign and malignant adnexal mass.

	Benign	Malignant
Solid components	−	+
Irregularities of outline	−	+
Unilocular	+	−
Septated	−	+
Papillary projections separations	−	+
Doppler Index (Resistance)	High	Low

CORPUS LUTEUM (GRANULOSA LUTEIN) CYSTS

Clinical Findings

These are thin-walled unilocular cysts ranging from 3–11 cm in size. After normal ovulation, the granulosa cells lining the follicle become luteinized. In the stage of vascularization, blood accumulates in the central cavity, producing the corpus hemorrhagicum. Resorption of the blood then results in a corpus luteum, which is defined as a cyst when it grows larger than 3 cm. A persistent corpus luteum cyst may cause local pain or tenderness. It can also be associated with either amenorrhea or delayed menstruation, thus simulating the clinical picture of an ectopic pregnancy. A corpus luteum

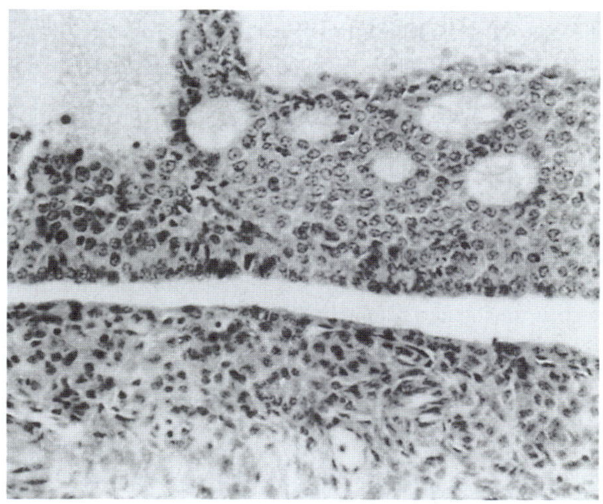

▲ **Figure 41–3.** Wall of a follicular cyst showing the proliferating granulosa cells with tiny cystic Call-Exner bodies in the upper portion of the figure. They have artifactually pulled away from the underlying theca cells.

cyst may be associated with torsion of the ovary, causing severe pain, or it may rupture and bleed, in which case the patient presents with peritoneal signs and acute abdomen.

Treatment

Laparoscopy or laparotomy is usually required to control hemorrhage into the peritoneal cavity and /or to perform detorsion of the adnexa. Unless acute complications develop, symptomatic therapy is indicated. As with follicular cysts, corpus luteum cysts usually regress after 1 or 2 months in menstruating patients, and OCPs have been recommended but may be of questionable benefit.

Iyer V, Farquhar C, Jepson R. Oral contraceptive pills for heavy menstrual bleeding. *Cochrane Database Syst Rev* 2000;CD000154. PMID: 10796696.

Jermy K, Luise C, Bourne T. The characterization of common ovarian cysts in premenopausal women. *Ultrasound Obstet Gynecol* 2001;17:140–144. PMID: 11251923.

THECA LUTEIN CYSTS

Clinical Findings

Elevated levels of chorionic gonadotropin can produce theca lutein cysts and thus are seen in patients with hydatidiform mole or choriocarcinoma and in patients undergoing chorionic gonadotropin or clomiphene therapy. Rarely, they are seen in normal pregnancy. The cysts are lined by theca cells that may or may not be luteinized, and they may or may not have granulosa cells. They are usually bilateral and are filled with clear, straw-colored fluid. Abdominal symptoms are minimal, although a sense of pelvic heaviness or aching may be described. Rupture of the cyst may result in intraperitoneal bleeding. Continued signs and symptoms of pregnancy, especially hyperemesis and breast paresthesias, are reported.

Treatment

The cysts disappear spontaneously after termination of the molar pregnancy, treatment of the choriocarcinoma, or discontinuation of fertility therapy; however, such resolution may take months to occur. Surgery is reserved for complications such as torsion and hemorrhage.

ENDOMETRIOMAS

Clinical Findings

In women with endometriosis, endometriotic foci on the ovarian surface may develop a fibrous enclosure and manifest cyst formation as a result of accumulation of fluid and blood. These endometrial cysts vary from several millimeters to even 10 cm in size. Endometriomas are also referred to as "chocolate cysts" because they contain thick, brown blood debris inside. Filmy or fibroid adhesions from these cysts to the pelvic sidewall, cul-de-sac and fallopian tubes are common and may obscure visualization of the cyst.

Endometriomas are usually associated with chronic pelvic pains, dyspareunia, dysmenorrhea, and infertility.

Differential Diagnosis

The tumor marker CA-125 is commonly elevated in these forms of cysts, which creates a serious clinical problem in distinguishing these cysts from malignant epithelial tumors.

De Ziegler D, Borghese B, Chapron C. Endometriosis and infertility: Pathophysiology and management. *Lancet* 2010:376:730–738. PMID: 20801404.

HYPERTHECOSIS

Clinical Findings

Hyperthecosis, or thecomatosis, commonly produces no gross enlargement of the ovary (Fig. 41–4). Thus the lesions are demonstrable only by histologic examination of the excised gonad. They are characterized by nests of stromal cells demonstrating increased cytoplasm, simulating the changes seen in the normal theca after stimulation by pituitary gonadotropin. In the premenopausal woman, hyperthecosis is associated with virilization and clinical findings similar to those seen in polycystic ovarian disease (see following text). These alterations may also be associated with postmenopausal bleeding and endometrial hyperplasia.

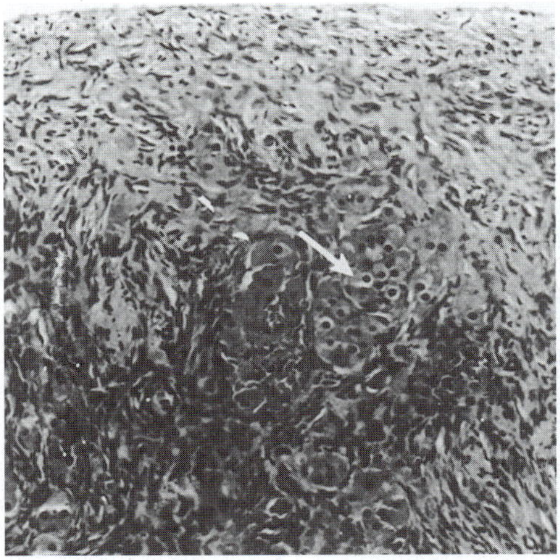

▲ **Figure 41–4.** In hyperthecosis, nests of rounded eosinophilic luteinized stroma cells are found in the ovarian cortex.

POLYCYSTIC OVARIAN SYNDROME (STEIN-LEVENTHAL SYNDROME)

Clinical Findings

Polycystic ovarian syndrome (PCOS) is characterized by persistent anovulation that can lead to clinical manifestations, including enlarged polycystic ovaries, secondary amenorrhea or oligomenorrhea, obesity, hirsutism, and infertility. The syndrome has a prevalence of 5–10%, with variance among races and ethnicities. Approximately 50% of patients are hirsute, and 30–75% are obese. A presumptive diagnosis of PCOS often can be made based on the history and initial examination. According to an international consensus group, the syndrome can be diagnosed if at least 2 of the following conditions are present: oligomenorrhea or amenorrhea, hyperandrogenism, and polycystic ovaries on ultrasound. Polycystic ovaries have been called "oyster ovaries" because they are enlarged and "sclerocystic" with smooth, pearl-white surfaces without indentations. Many small, fluid-filled follicle cysts lie beneath the thickened fibrous surface cortex (Fig. 41–5). Luteinization of the theca interna is usually observed, and occasionally focal stromal luteinization is seen. Laboratory testing often reveals mildly elevated serum androgen levels, an increased ratio of luteinizing hormone to follicle-stimulating hormone (LH/FSH), lipid abnormalities, and insulin resistance. Anovulation is identified in women with persistently high concentrations of LH and low concentrations of FSH, a low day-21 progesterone level, or on sonographic follicular monitoring. PCOS is presumably related to hypothalamic pituitary dysfunction and insulin resistance. A primary ovarian contribution to the problem has not been clearly defined.

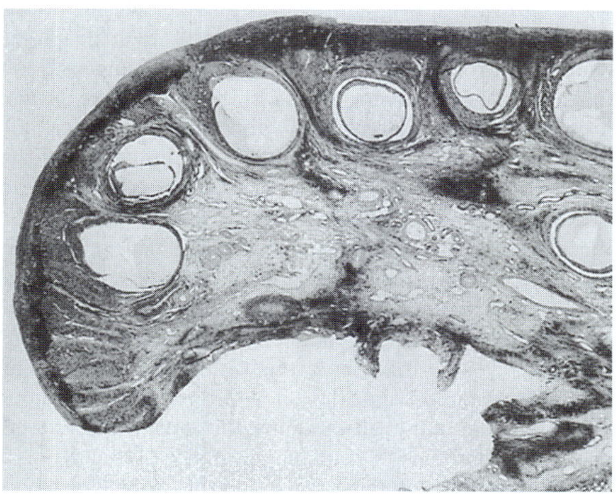

▲ **Figure 41–5.** Polycystic ovary with a thickened capsule and prominent subcapsular cysts. Note lack of corpora lutea or corpora albicantia due to anovulation.

Treatment

Most patients with PCOS seek treatment for either hirsutism or infertility. The hirsutism can be treated with any agent that lowers androgen levels, and OCPs are typically the first choice in patients not desiring pregnancy. Infertility in PCOS patients is often responsive to clomiphene citrate. In the recalcitrant case, the experienced clinician can add human menopausal gonadotropin to produce the desired ovulation. Recent studies indicate that therapy with metformin improves fertility rates both when given alone and, even more so, when given in conjunction with clomiphene. Studies show that a small reduction in body weight, as little as 2–7%, is associated with improved ovulatory function in women with PCOS. As patients with PCOS are chronically anovulatory, the endometrium is stimulated by estrogen alone. Thus endometrial hyperplasia, both typical and atypical, and endometrial carcinoma are more frequent in patients with PCOS and long-term anovulation. Many of these markedly atypical endometrial features can be reversed by large doses of progestational agents, such as megestrol acetate 40–60 mg/d for 3–4 months. Follow-up endometrial biopsy is mandatory to determine endometrial response and subsequent recurrence.

Ehrmann D. Medical progress: Polycystic ovary syndrome. *N Engl J Med* 2005;352:1223–1236. PMID: 15788499.

Lewis V. Polycystic ovary syndrome. A diagnostic challenge. *Obstet Gynecol Clin North Am* 2001;28:1–20. PMID: 11292997.

LUTEOMA OF PREGNANCY

Clinical Findings

Tumorlike nodules of lutein cells may form in the ovaries during pregnancy and are often both multifocal and bilateral. The nodules range up to 20 cm in diameter, but most often they range from 5–10 cm. On section they reveal well-delineated, soft, brown masses with focal hemorrhage. Microscopically, they are formed of sheets of large luteinized cells with abundant cytoplasm and relatively uniform nuclei with occasional mitoses. Clinically, they appear ominous to the obstetrician, who becomes aware of them only when the abdomen is open at the time of caesarean delivery. Unilateral salpingo-oophorectomy can be performed for frozen section in the belief that the large masses are malignant. A confirmatory biopsy is adequate, and follow-up will reveal total regression a few months later.

OVARIAN NEOPLASMS

Evaluation

Ovarian neoplasms may arise from any histologic element of the ovary and are most often benign, especially in premenopausal women. The characteristics of the mass and the age of the patient are important factors guiding diagnosis and treatment. The overall risk of malignancy of an ovarian cyst is 13% in a premenopausal woman versus 45% in a postmenopausal woman. Therefore, vigilant workup of these masses with the aid of ultrasound and close follow-up is essential. Use of cancer antigen-125 (CA-125) for diagnostic purposes is controversial. New tumor markers are being pursued fervently such that soon we may be able to more accurately distinguish malignant from benign adnexal masses. With the increased use of imaging studies has come discovery of incidental, asymptomatic, small ovarian cysts. These cysts should be evaluated by ultrasound. If they do not contain septa or solid components, they can be closely followed. However, any mass that enlarges or changes in character, especially in postmenopausal women, should be explored surgically.

Treatment

The preferred treatment of all ovarian tumors is surgical excision with careful exploration of the abdominal contents. If the risk of malignant neoplasia is confidently low, laparoscopy is preferred. In patients requesting future fertility, cystectomy is performed if possible; otherwise a unilateral oophorectomy is performed. Frozen section is helpful in identifying the type and neoplastic potential of the tumor. However, because adequate sampling of a large ovarian neoplasm often is impossible, final opinion and prognosis *must* be based on analysis of permanent, rather than frozen, sections. Therefore, in a patient desirous of retaining fertility, the surgeon must act on the side of retention of the uterus and contralateral ovary if the pathologist has the slightest doubt as to tumor malignancy.

Canis M, Botchorishvili R, Manhes H, et al. Management of adnexal masses: Role and risk of laparoscopy. *Semin Surg Oncol* 2000;19:28–35. PMID: 10883021.

Canis M, Rabischong B, Houlle C, et al. Laparoscopic management of adnexal masses: A gold standard? *Curr Opin Obstet Gynecol* 2002;14:423–428. PMID: 12151833.

Sagiv R, Golan A, Glezerman M. Laparoscopic management of extremely large ovarian cysts. *Obstet Gynecol* 2005;105: 1319–1322. PMID: 15932823.

EPITHELIAL TUMORS

Clinical Findings

Epithelial tumors account for approximately 60–80% of all true ovarian neoplasms and include the common serous, mucinous, endometrioid, clear cell, and transitional cell (Brenner) tumors, as well as the stromal tumors with an epithelial element. The epithelium of these tumors arises from a common anlage (ie, the mesothelium lining the coelomic cavity and ovarian surfaces). This basic thesis explains the similarity of the epithelia of the upper genital canal—endocervix, endometrium, and endosalpinx—to those found in the ovarian tumors. Most tumors presumably arise from invaginated surface epithelium and proliferation or malignant degeneration in the epithelial lining of the resulting surface inclusion cyst (Fig. 41–6). The epithelial tumors are classified on the basis of their histologic appearance.

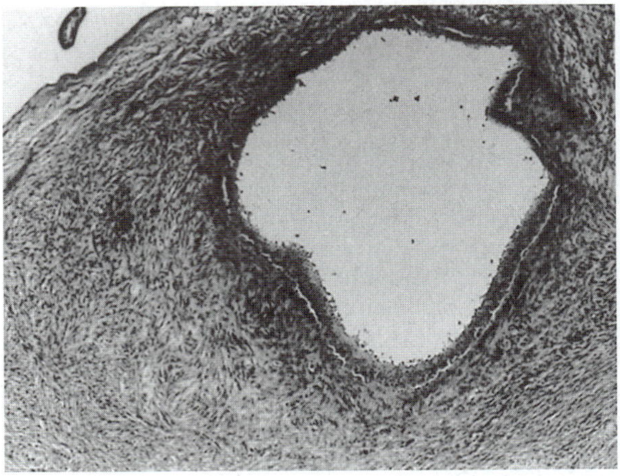

▲ **Figure 41–6.** Most surface (germinal) inclusion cysts, such as the one shown here, undergo a serous (tubal) metaplasia. By definition, cysts larger than 1 cm in diameter are termed cystadenomas.

SEROUS TUMORS

Clinical Findings

Serous tumors have been reported in all age groups and are responsible for approximately 50% of all epithelial ovarian neoplasms. Low-grade neoplasms generally are found in patients in their 20s and 30s, whereas their anaplastic counterparts occur more commonly in perimenopausal and postmenopausal women. Serous cystadenomas are benign lesions, commonly unilocular, with a smooth surface, and containing thin, clear yellow fluid. The cells lining the cyst are a mixed population of ciliated and secretory cells similar to those of the endosalpinx. They may grow large enough to fill the abdominal cavity, but usually they are smaller than their mucinous counterparts. Benign serous tumors are bilateral in approximately 15–20% of cases. Focal proliferation of the underlying stroma may produce firm papillary projections into the cyst, forming a serous cystadenofibroma (Fig. 41–7). These tumors appear to be simple on ultrasonographic evaluation, and although there may be some small internal aches, these are purely cystic in appearance (Table 41–1). It is important to study these papillary projections thoroughly to rule out atypical proliferation. Some serous tumors consist of benign stromal proliferation interspersed with tiny serous cysts; these are known as *serous adenofibromas.*

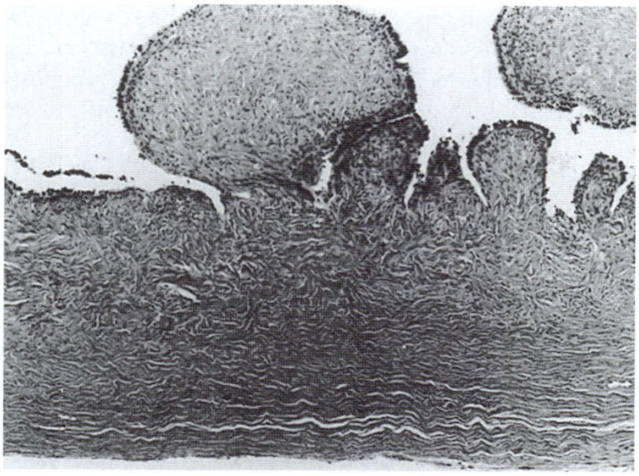

▲ **Figure 41–7.** Serous cystadenofibromas usually form unilocular cysts with firm white papillations protruding into the cyst, seen here microscopically.

MUCINOUS TUMORS

Clinical Findings

Mucinous tumors account for approximately 10–20% of all epithelial ovarian neoplasms, of which approximately 75%–85% are benign. The benign tumors are typically found in women in their 30s through 50s. Bilateral tumor development occurs in 8–10% of all cases, whether the tumors are benign or malignant. They are the largest tumors found in the human body; 15 reported tumors have weighed more than 70 kg (154 lb). Consequently, the more massive the tumor, the greater the possibility that it is mucinous. They generally are asymptomatic, and patients present with either an abdominal mass or nonspecific abdominal discomfort. In postmenopausal patients, luteinization of the stroma rarely may result in hormone production (usually estrogen) leading to associated endometrial hyperplasia with vaginal bleeding. During pregnancy, hormonal stimulation may result in virilization.

Histologically, they are usually smooth-walled; true papillae are rare (compared with the serous variety). The tumors generally are multilocular, and the mucus-containing locules appear blue through the tense capsule (Fig. 41–8). The internal surface is lined by tall columnar cells with dark, basally situated nuclei and mucinous cytoplasm (Fig. 41–9).

The epithelium of mucinous cysts resembles that of the endocervix in approximately 50% of cases; in the other 50%, mucin-containing goblet cells resembling intestinal epithelial cells are present. Careful study of mucinous neoplasms has shown that the histologic appearance may vary greatly from area to area; some areas appear benign, whereas others are of low malignant potential or are frankly malignant. Hence sampling must be more extensive than in the typical serous tumor. Metastases from appendiceal and other primary tumors may simulate closely a mucinous cystadenoma.

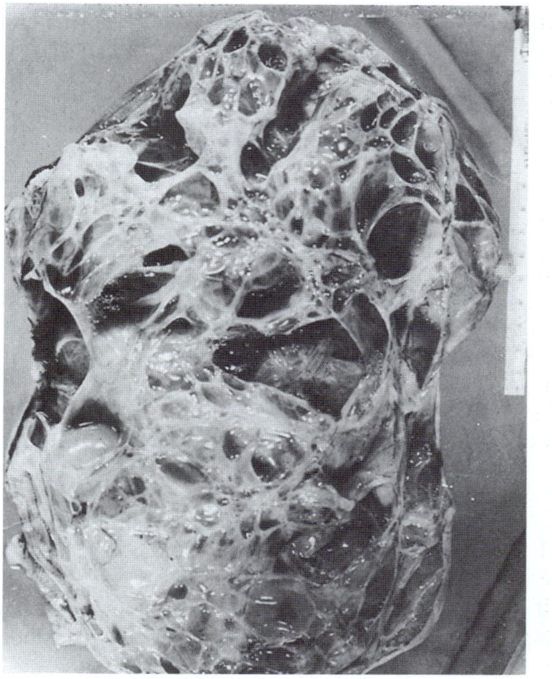

▲ **Figure 41–8.** Multilocular mucinous cystadenoma of the ovary.

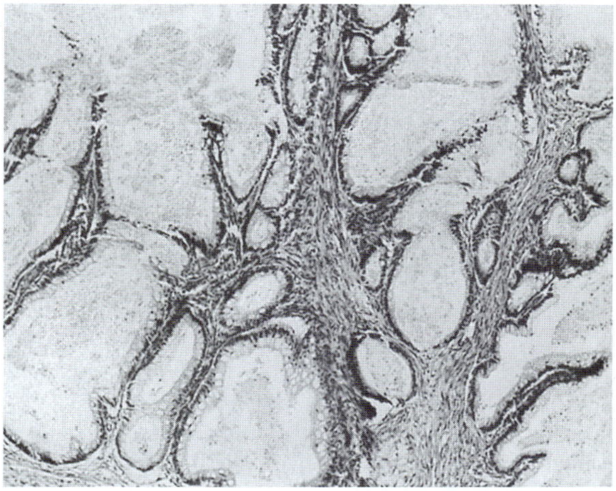

▲ **Figure 41–9.** Mucinous cystadenoma. The lining cells are tall and columnar with basally situated nuclei. Generous sampling of these tumors is necessary to rule out a higher-grade lesion.

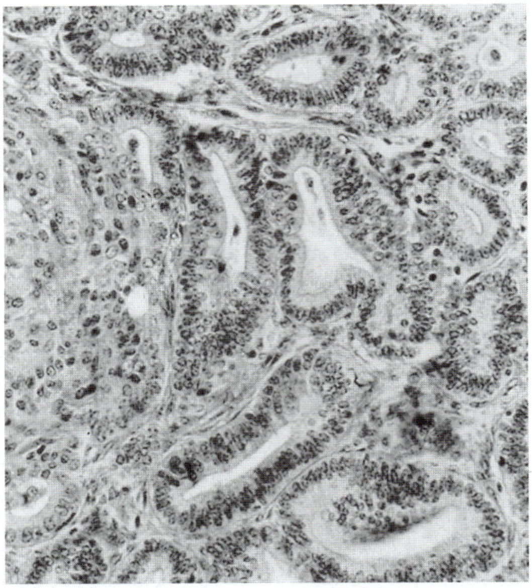

▲ **Figure 41–10.** Endometrioid cystadenomas contain a proliferation of bland endometrial-like glands without the stroma of endometriosis.

ENDOMETRIOID LESIONS

Clinical Findings

Endometrioid tumors are characterized by proliferation of benign nonspecific stroma in which bland endometrial-type glands may be found. The only clearly recognizable benign endometrioid tumors are the uncommon endometrioid adenofibroma and the proliferative endometrioid adenofibroma. If the epithelial growth is exuberant but cytologically benign, it is termed a *proliferative* rather than a low malignant potential tumor, as the prognosis appears to be invariably excellent (Fig. 41–10).

Endometriosis of the ovary (see Chapter 56) represents a benign "tumorlike" condition rather than a true neoplasm. Because pelvic endometriosis may be found in association with endometrioid lesions, one hypothesis is that these lesions arise from preexisting endometriosis.

CLEAR CELL (MESONEPHROID) TUMORS

Clinical Findings

Like the endometrioid tumors, clear cell tumors in their benign form are rare and are virtually limited to clear cell adenofibromas in which a solid proliferation of nonspecific stroma contains small cytologically bland glands formed by columnar cells with clear cytoplasm. The clear cell component usually coexists with another epithelial type. The clear cell histology also is associated with endogenous endometriosis in the pelvic in up to 25% of cases. Clinically, they appear like any other benign ovarian mass and are diagnosed only on histologic examination. The prognosis is excellent.

TRANSITIONAL CELL (BRENNER) TUMORS

Clinical Findings

Transitional cell tumors are adenofibromas in which the proliferating epithelial element has a transitional cell appearance, which represents metaplasia. Brenner tumors account for 1–2% of primary ovarian tumors; more than 98% are benign, and nearly 95% of cases are unilateral. They frequently are so small that they are incidental operative findings. However, the tumor may reach 5–8 cm in diameter and present as an adnexal mass on pelvic examination. On section they are firm and pale yellow or white (Fig. 41–11). The epithelium is composed of nests of cells with ovoid nuclei having a prominent longitudinal groove ("coffee-bean nuclei"; Fig. 41–12). Occasionally there is a mucinous metaplasia of the cells in the center of one or more of these nests, which may account for the 10% incidence of mucinous cystadenomas found associated with Brenner tumors.

Brenner tumors are considered benign, although a malignant variant has been identified.

Christensen JT, Boldsen JL, Westergaard JG. Functional ovarian cysts in premenopausal and gynecologically healthy women. *Contraception* 2002;66:153–157. PMID: 12384202.

Cannistra SA. Cancer of the ovary. *N Engl J Med* 2004;351: 2519–2529. PMID: 15590954.

Jermy K, Luise C, Bourned T. The characterization of common ovarian cysts in premenopausal women. *Ultrasound Obstet Gynecol* 2001;17:140–144. PMID: 11251923.

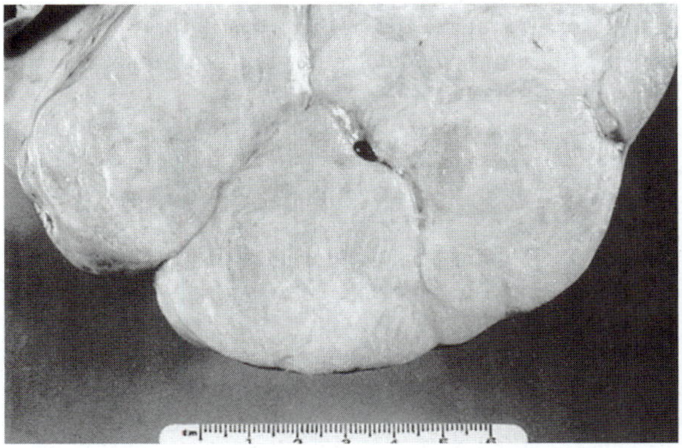

▲ **Figure 41–11.** Cut surface of a Brenner tumor is firm, solid, and yellowish-white and resembles a fibrothecoma.

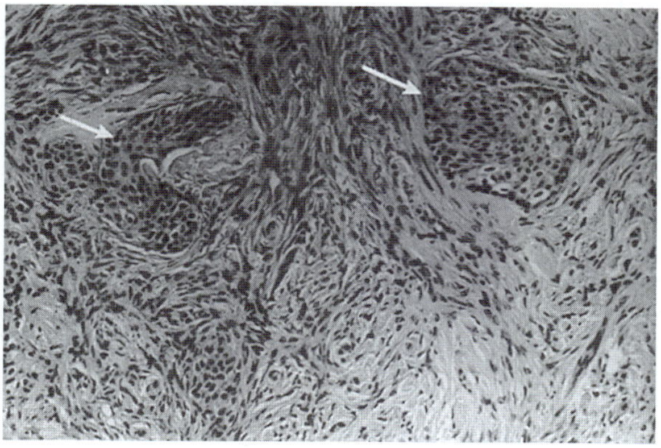

▲ **Figure 41–12.** In a transitional cell (Brenner) tumor, islands of bland transitional cells (arrows) proliferate, accompanied by prominent proliferation of benign spindly fibroblast-like cells.

SEX CORD-STROMAL TUMORS

THECOMA

Clinical Findings

This type of tumor can occur at any age, although they are most commonly found in postmenopausal women. They account for only 2% of all ovarian tumors and may not be a true neoplasm but instead a condition of hyperplasia of the cortical stroma. Histologically, the mass is filled with lipid-containing cells that are similar to theca cells, and the tumor is known to produce estrogen. As such, these tumors often present with dysfunctional uterine bleeding or postmenopausal bleeding. Occasionally they have presented with adenocarcinoma of the endometrium given the unopposed estrogen production by the tumor. The tumors range from nonpalpable to more than 20 cm in size. They are rarely bilateral and rarely malignant.

Treatment

Treatment of thecoma is tailored to patient age and ranges from a total hysterectomy and bilateral salpingo-oophorectomy for menopausal or postmenopausal women to a salpingo-oophorectomy or ovarian cystectomy if possible in patients who desire to retain fertility.

FIBROMA

Clinical Findings

Unlike thecomas, fibromas produce no hormones. They can occur at any age but most often occur in the years before menopause. They range in size from incidental findings to greater than 20 cm. They are multinodular and whorled, and they are formed from bundles of collagen-producing spindle cells. They can be found as part of Meigs' syndrome, in which a patient is found to have a pelvic mass (fibroma or thecoma or granulose cell tumor) in concert with ascites and hydrothorax. Fibromas are also part of a hereditary basal cell nevus syndrome in which basal cell carcinoma is found with mesenteric cysts, calcification of the dura, and keratocysts of the jaw.

HILUS CELL TUMOR

Clinical Findings

These tumors are a subset of Leydig cell tumors, which originate from the ovarian hilum or less frequently from the ovarian stroma. The typical presentation includes hirsutism, virilization, and menstrual irregularities. Hilus cell tumors rarely attain a palpable size. Histologically, groups of steroid cells containing eosinophilic cytoplasm and lipochrome pigment are found. For the tumor to be defined as a Leydig cell neoplasm, elongated eosinophilic crystalloids of Reinke must be found.

GERM CELL TUMORS

MATURE TERATOMAS

Clinical Findings

Mature cystic teratomas, commonly referred to as *dermoid cysts*, compose some 40–50% of all benign ovarian neoplasms. They contain well-differentiated tissue derived from any of the 3 germ cell layers, including hair and teeth as ectodermal derivatives. They account for the majority of benign ovarian neoplasms in reproductive-age women and usually are asymptomatic unless complications such as torsion or rupture occur. Transvaginal ultrasound is known to be very accurate in the diagnosis of dermoid cysts, with the hair and sebum, rather than calcium, creating highly reflective irregular solid components within fluid-containing masses. Up to 15% of cases are bilateral, and these tumors can grow to a large size, weighing several kilograms.

Differential Diagnosis

Although most mature teratomas contain cells from all germ cell layers, a subset of monodermal teratomas exists. Those tumors composed mostly or entirely of thyroid tissue are called *struma ovarii.* These tumors account for only 3% of all teratomas, and only 5% of these will produce symptoms of thyrotoxicosis.

Cases in which immature neuroepithelial tissue is present should always be suspected as immature cystic teratoma, which have some malignant potential.

Treatment

Studies have detailed several advantages to the laparoscopic approach to removal of dermoids, including less postoperative pain and blood loss, shorter hospital stay, and lower overall cost. Recent studies have shown that dermoid cysts can usually be removed laparoscopically without intraperitoneal spillage. If intraoperative spillage does occur, the potential for chemical peritonitis or excess adhesion formation has led to the recommendation of copious saline irrigation until the lavage is clear. The risk of peritonitis, however, is quite low (<0.2%) with laparoscopic removal of dermoid cysts.

Mecke H, Savras V. Laparoscopic surgery of dermoid cyst-intraoperative spillage and complications. *Eur J Obstet Gynecol Reprod Biol* 2001;96:80–84. PMID: 11311766.

Templeman CL, Fallat ME, Lam AM, Perlman SE, Hertweck SP, O'Connor DM. Managing mature cystic teratomas of the ovary. *Obstet Gynecol Surv* 2000;55:738–745. PMID: 11128910.

BENIGN TUMORS OF THE OVIDUCT

Benign lesions of the uterine tube are routinely asymptomatic and rarely large enough to be palpable—with the exception of the paratubal or parovarian cyst—so the diagnosis is made incidentally during a routine ultrasonographic examination or at the operating table or in the pathology laboratory.

CYSTIC TUMORS

Clinical Findings

Hydatid cysts of Morgagni are cystic tumors of the uterine tube located at or near the fimbriated end. They are lined by tubal-type epithelium, filled with clear fluid, and are usually approximately 1 cm in diameter. They are most often found inadvertently during a pelvic operative procedure. On rare occasions, torsion produces an acute surgical emergency.

Occasionally, larger paratubal or parovarian cysts develop, especially in the broad ligament (Fig. 41–13). These cysts are almost always serous tumors of low malignant potential with a benign clinical outcome.

A third type of cyst associated with the fallopian tubes is the *Walthard cell rest*. This type is found as a 1-mm cyst beneath the serosa of the fallopian tube. It appears to represent an inclusion cyst in which the mesothelium has undergone metaplasia similar to transitional cell (Brenner) tumors.

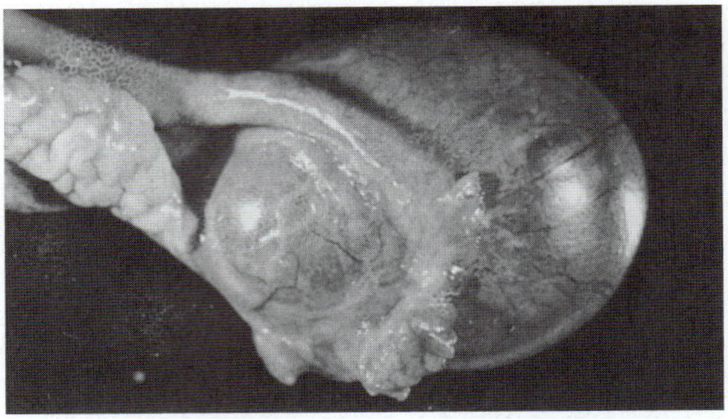

▲ **Figure 41–13.** Parovarian cyst. Note the orientation of the cyst to the fimbriated end of the oviduct.

EPITHELIAL TUMORS

Benign epithelial tumors of the uterine tube are extremely rare. The polyps that occur in the cornual portion appear to be of endometrial rather than tubal origin.

ADENOMATOID TUMORS

The adenomatoid tumor probably is the most common benign tumor found in the uterine tube. It actually represents a benign mesothelioma, but the compact nature of the adenomatous pattern may be mistaken for malignancy. Adenomatoid lesions rarely measure more than 1–1.5 cm. They are always incidental findings when the adnexa are removed for other purposes. Similar lesions, usually cystic, may involve the myometrium or ovary.

OTHER BENIGN TUBAL AND PARATUBAL TUMORS

Other benign tubal tumors, such as leiomyomas and teratomas, are rare, as are benign adnexal tumors of probable wolffian origin. Adrenal cortical nests, however, are common incidental embryologic rests found in the broad ligament, seen as yellowish ovoid nodules 3–4 mm in diameter.

Urinary Incontinence & Pelvic Floor Disorders

42

Christopher M. Tarnay, MD

PELVIC FLOOR DISORDERS

Pelvic floor disorders (PFDs) include urinary incontinence, pelvic organ prolapse, fecal incontinence, and other sensory and emptying abnormalities of the lower urinary and gastrointestinal tracts. Nearly one-quarter of all women and more than one-third of older women reported symptoms of at least 1 pelvic floor disorder. The prevalence of PFDs increase as women age. Advances in modern medicine during the last 80 years have increased the life expectancy of women well into the eighth and ninth decades. We are caring for patients longer and better than ever, effectively managing chronic medical problems such as hypertension, cardiovascular disease, and diabetes, enabling women to enjoy longer and more productive lives. Using US Census data projections, by 2030, more than one-fifth of women will be 65 years of age or older. This will result in a large population of women living up to one-third of their life after menopause, thereby introducing a whole host of medical issues and health concerns.

A prime example of this is the problem of urinary incontinence, which has become more prevalent as the population of aging women grows. Urinary incontinence affects millions adult women in the United States. It is estimated to affect 50% of American women during their lifetime and results in substantial medical, social, and economic burdens. Despite its prevalence and estimated costs in excess of $19.5 billion annually, up to two-thirds of women do not seek help for incontinence, primarily because of social embarrassment or because they are unaware that help is available. Because of increasing awareness by both patients and physicians, the societal concept that incontinence is part of the "normal" aging process is no longer acceptable.

ESSENTIALS OF DIAGNOSIS

- The symptoms of urinary incontinence involve involuntary leakage of urine.
- History and clinical examination can often effectively diagnose the correct condition.
- Two most common types are **stress incontinence** (loss of urine with physical exertion) and **urinary urge incontinence** (sudden urge to urinate and losing urine before toileting).
- The term **overactive bladder** (OAB) is often used to describe the most common symptoms of urinary urgency, usually accompanied by frequency and nocturia, with or without urgency urinary incontinence.
- The use of pads to protect soiling undergarments is the most common coping mechanism for women.
- Behavioral methods such as fluid restriction, avoidance of dietary triggers, and pelvic floor muscle strengthening can be helpful to reduce symptoms.
- Surgery, such as a midurethral sling, can be effective to cure stress urinary incontinence.
- Medications or neuromodulation can be helpful for women with urinary urge incontinence who do not respond to behavioral methods.

ANATOMY

The urinary and reproductive tracts are intimately associated during embryologic development. The lower urinary tract can be divided into 3 parts: the bladder, the vesical neck, and the urethra (Fig. 42–1). The bladder is a hollow muscular organ lined with transitional epithelium designed for urine storage. The bladder musculature consists of layers of smooth muscle, which are densely intertwined and constitute the detrusor muscle. The bladder stays relaxed to facilitate urine storage and contracts periodically to completely evacuate its contents when appropriate and acceptable. At the bladder base is the trigone, which is embryologically distinct from the bladder.

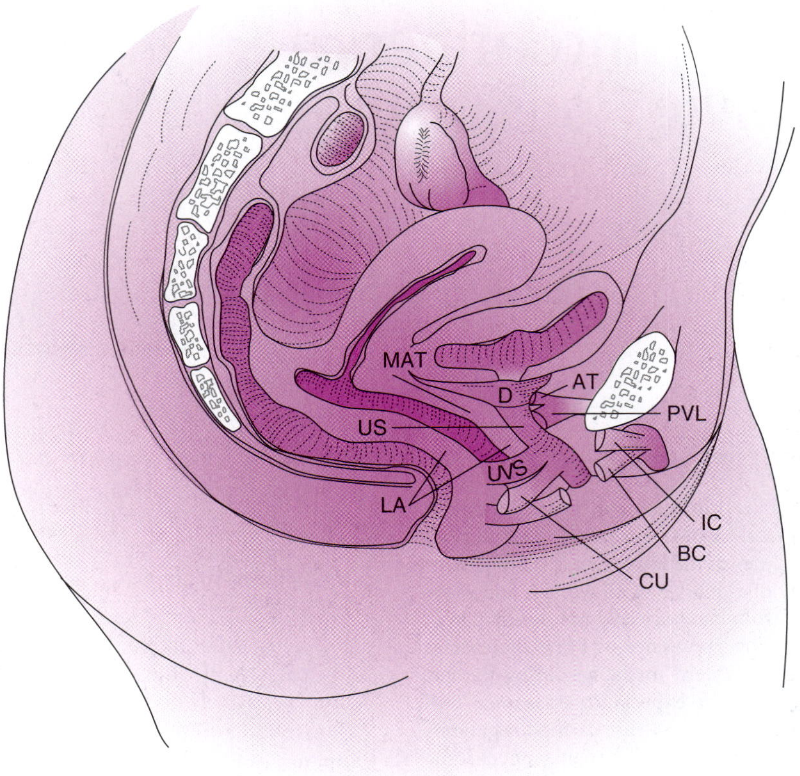

▲ **Figure 42–1.** Interrelationships and approximate location of paraurethral structures. Levator ani muscles are shown as light lines running deep to the pelvic viscera. AT, arcus tendineus fasciae pelvis; BC, bulbocavernosus muscle; CU, compressor urethrae; D, detrusor loop; IC, ischiocavernosus muscle; LA, levator ani muscles; MAT, muscular attachment of the urethral supports; PVL, pubovesical ligament (muscle); US, urethral sphincter; UVS, urethrovaginal sphincter.

The 2 ureteral orifices and the internal urethral meatus form the boundaries of the trigone. The trigone has 2 distinct muscular layers: superficial and deep. The deep layer shares a similar cholinergic autonomic innervation as the detrusor muscle, whereas the superficial layer is densely innervated by noradrenergic nerves. This distinct difference in receptor distribution is important, as it provides opportunities to target more specific sites for pharmacotherapeutic intervention. The superficial detrusor layer extends muscular fibers that contribute to the distal urethra and posterior to the proximal urethra. The urethral "sphincter" itself is not a well-delineated structure; rather, it is a complex and intricate meshwork of intertwining smooth and striated muscle fibers that functionally responds neurophysiologically to variable degrees of vesicle pressures and facilitates urine storage and voiding.

The female urethra is approximately 3–4 cm long. The composition and support of the urethra and bladder neck play key roles in the function and maintenance of urinary continence. Together the striated urethral and periurethral muscles compose the extrinsic urethral sphincter mechanism. The urethral sphincter, along with the levator ani, function in the reflex contraction. The urethra is surrounded by dense vasculature that contributes to the urethral mucosal seal and urethral closure pressure. An abundance of submucosal glands are found along the dorsal surface. Most of the urethral diverticula arise from this area. The uroepithelium is stratified squamous (Fig. 42–2).

Support of the urethra and distal vaginal wall are closely linked. For much of its length, the urethra is fused with the vaginal wall, and the structures that determine urethral position and distal anterior vaginal wall position are the same. The anterior vaginal wall and urethral support system provide a supportive layer on which the proximal urethra and mid urethra rest. The major components of this supportive structure are the vaginal wall, the endopelvic fascia, the arcus tendineus fasciae pelvis, and the levator

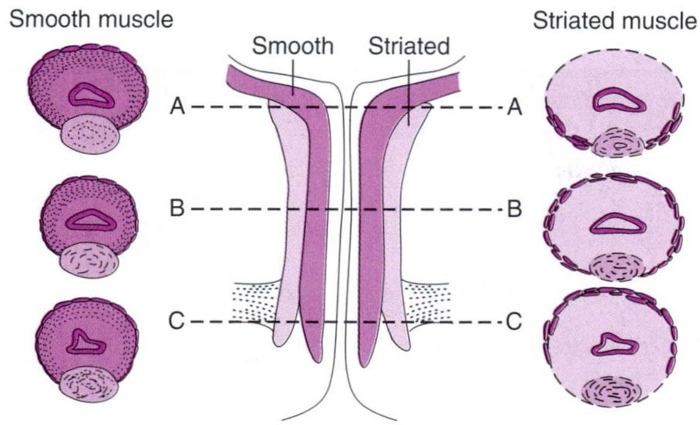

▲ **Figure 42–2.** Urethral anatomy. The submucosal vascular plexus matures after puberty but undergoes great changes after menopause. The amount of smooth and especially striated muscles decreases with age, and the striated components become almost rudimentary. (Reproduced, with permission, from Rud T, Asmussen M. Neurophysiology of the lower urinary tract as measured by simultaneous urethral cystometry. In Ostergard DR, Bent AE (eds): *Urogynecology and Urodynamics: Theory and Practice*. 4th ed. Baltimore, MD: Williams & Wilkins; 1996, p. 55.)

ani muscles (Fig. 42–3). The endopelvic fascia is a dense, fibrous connective tissue layer that surrounds the vagina and attaches it to each arcus tendineus fascia pelvis laterally. Each arcus tendineus fascia pelvis in turn is attached to the pubic bone ventrally and to the ischial spine dorsally.

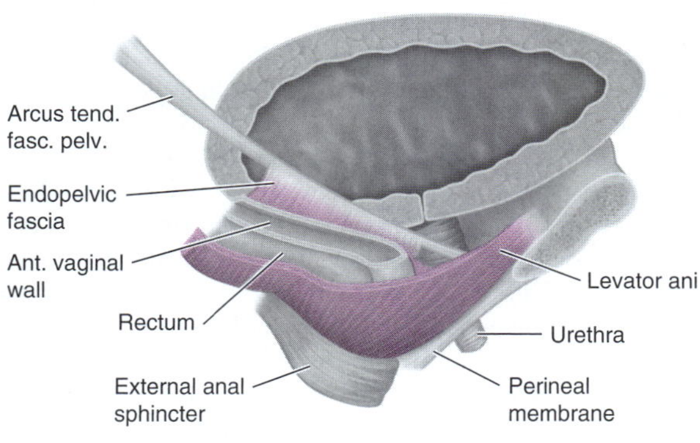

▲ **Figure 42–3.** Lateral view of the components of the urethral support system. Note how the levator ani muscles support the rectum, vagina, and urethrovesical neck. Also note how the endopelvic fascia beside the urethra attaches to the levator ani muscle; contraction of the levator muscle leads to elevation of the urethrovesical neck. Puborectalis muscle is removed for clarity. (Reproduced, with permission, from Ashton-Miller J, DeLancey JOL. Functional anatomy of the female pelvic floor. *Ann NY Acad Sci* 2007;1101:266–296.)

They act like the cable of a suspension bridge that is supported at each end to the pelvis and provides attachment points along the vaginal length, providing the support of the anterior vaginal wall. Although it is well defined as a fibrous band near its origin at the pubic bone, the arcus tendineus fascia pelvis appears as a sheet of fascia as it fuses with the endopelvic fascia, where it merges with the levator ani muscles.

The principal components of the basin-like pelvic floor are the pelvic bones (including the coccyx), the endopelvic fascia, and the levator and perineal muscles. These structures normally support and maintain the position of the pelvic viscera despite great increments in intra-abdominal pressure that occur with straining, coughing, and heavy lifting when the patient is in the erect position. The urogenital hiatus ("anterior levator muscle gap"), which permits the urethra, vagina, and anus to emerge from the pelvis, is a site of potential weakness. Attenuation of the pubococcygeal and puborectal portions of the levator muscles, whether as the result of a traumatic delivery or of involutional changes, widens the levator gap and converts this potential weakness to an actual defect. If there has been a concomitant injury or attenuation of the endopelvic fascia (uterosacral and cardinal ligaments, rectovaginal and pubocervical fascia), heightened intra-abdominal pressure gradually leads to uterine prolapse, along with anterior vaginal prolapse, rectocele, and enterocele. If the integrity of the endopelvic fascia and its condensations has been maintained, the incompetency of the genital hiatus and levator muscles may be associated only with elongation of the cervix.

Neuroanatomy

Neuronal innervation of the lower urinary tract is considered part of the autonomic and somatic nervous systems. The autonomic system (ie, the para-sympathetic and sympathetic components) receives visceral sensation and regulates smooth muscle actively during conscious and involuntary lower urinary tract functions. The autonomic nervous system constitutes the bulk of neural control of the lower urinary tract. Sympathetic contributions from T1–L2 and parasympathetic contributions from S2–4 compose the neuronal control system (Fig. 42–4). Voluntary control of micturition is controlled by the central nervous system. Cortical control of the detrusor muscle rests in the supramedial portion of the frontal lobes and in the genu of the corpus callosum. Receiving both sensory afferent and modulating motor efferent nerves, the net effect is that the brain provides tonic inhibition of detrusor contraction. Lesions in the frontal lobe chiefly cause loss of voluntary control of micturition and thus loss of suppression of the detrusor reflex, resulting in uncontrolled voiding or urge urinary incontinence. The pons and mesencephalic reticular formation in the brainstem constitute the micturition center. A reflex activation in the central brainstem

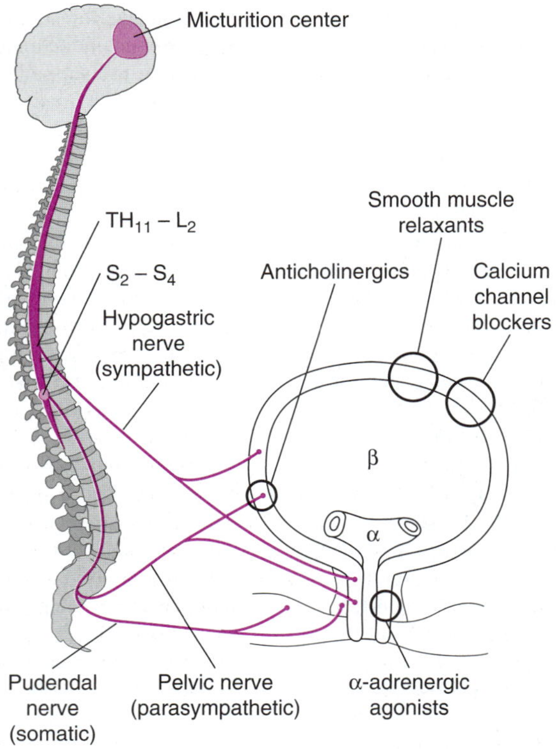

▲ **Figure 42–4.** Schematic neuroanatomy of the lower urinary tract, with major sites of drug action. (Reproduced, with permission, from Sourander LB. Treatment of urinary incontinence. *Gerontology* 1990;36(Suppl 2):19. Copyright Karger S.)

and peripheral spinal cord mediate a coordinated series of events, consisting of relaxation of the striated urethral musculature and detrusor contraction that result in opening of the bladder neck and urethra. Lesions that interrupt these pathways have various effects depending on the level of interruption, essentially resulting abnormal detrusor function.

URINARY INCONTINENCE

Definition

Urinary incontinence as defined by the Consensus Committee on Pelvic Floor Disorders is the complaint of any involuntary leakage of urine. Incontinence can be a sign, a symptom (patient complaint), or a condition diagnosed by an examiner. There are many types and causes of urinary incontinence (Table 42–1). The reported incidence of urinary incontinence varies widely, ranging from 10–70% of women living in a community setting to more than 50% of women living in a nursing home. Incontinence becomes more common as women age, particularly after menopause.

Table 42–1. Differential diagnosis.

Stress incontinence Intrinsic sphincter dysfunction
Urge incontinence Idiopathic Neurologic detrusor hyperreflexia
Mixed incontinence (stress and urge combined)
Overflow incontinence with urinary retention Obstruction Bladder hyporeflexia
Bypass incontinence Genitourinary fistulas
Urethral diverticulum
Congenital urethral abnormalities (eg, epispadias, bladder exstrophy, ectopic ureter)
Functional and transient incontinence Infection Pharmacologic Restricted mobility Dementia/delirium Excessive urine production (diabetes mellitus, diabetes insipidus, resorption of extravascular fluid as with lower extremity edema)

Pathogenesis

PFDs are most assuredly caused by multiple factors. The multifactorial model is the clearest one to explain the incidence of PFD and variety of anatomic findings despite shared risk factors.

For urinary incontinence, numerous factors play a role in maintaining urinary continence; therefore, the development of incontinence is frequently not attributable to any single cause. Sex, age, hormonal status, birthing trauma, and genetic differences in connective tissue all contribute to the development of incontinence. Urinary incontinence is 2–3 times more common in women than in men because of women's shorter urethral length and the risk of connective tissue, muscle, and nerve injury associated with childbirth. Observational studies have consistently noted a high incidence of incontinence in the elderly population, with 1 study finding a 30% higher prevalence for each 5-year increase in age. The association of childbirth with urinary incontinence has long been suspected and has generated new interest in identifying the causes. In 1 study of more than 15,000 women, the risk of developing urinary incontinence was 2.3 times higher in women who had a vaginal delivery compared with nulliparous women. Damage to the pelvic floor neuromusculature during vaginal delivery may lead to loss of pelvic muscle strength and nerve function, resulting in both stress urinary incontinence (SUI) and pelvic floor support defects. Although muscle strength may be regained over time or with the help of pelvic floor muscle exercises, dysfunction may be permanent.

Aging and incontinence are closely associated. The prevalence of incontinence increases as women age, but the specific cause is unclear. Global decrease in the storage capacity, reduced receptor response, general loss in muscle tone, or latent manifestation from denervation during parturition may all be important factors. The state of hypoestrogenism as a woman transitions to menopause may also contribute to urinary incontinence. Although estrogen reduces urinary urgency, results from studies specifically examining menopausal status have been equivocal, with some studies showing a positive association and others showing no association. Abnormalities in the muscular components and innervation of the pelvic floor and the connective tissue to this region likely contribute to the multifactorial etiology of incontinence. Initial observations that the prevalence of abdominal hernias, lower leg varices, and uterine prolapse was higher in women with SUI suggested that connective tissue weakness might identify women at risk for developing incontinence. Subsequent studies have supported a connection between relative collagen deficiencies in the connective tissues of incontinent patients versus continent controls.

Incontinence affects a woman's quality of life, and it is an uncomfortable and embarrassing problem. The psychosocial impact on the patient as well as her family is enormous. Women with urinary incontinence are reported to be more depressed, to have lower self-esteem, and to be ashamed about their appearance and the odor. Urinary incontinence affects sexual desire and reduces sexual activity. This can curb social interactions to the point where individuals become isolated and even entirely homebound.

Prevention

One of the first attempts at the prevention of urinary incontinence was described by Dr. Arnold Kegel in the 1950s. To reduce the risk of postpartum urinary loss, women were taught to contract and thereby strengthen the levator ani muscles in what is now commonly known as a "Kegel" exercise. Other attempts at mitigating the potential detrimental impact of pregnancy and vaginal delivery on the subsequent development of urinary incontinence have led to the increasing prevalence of maternal choice caesarean delivery as a method of perineal preservation. To date there are no high-quality data supporting either empiric pelvic floor strengthening or the avoidance of vaginal delivery as a protective measure against future urinary incontinence.

For urge-related urinary loss, the avoidance of caffeinated beverages, alcoholic drinks, or other potentially irritative foods or beverages can be suggested as a measure to reduce urgency and frequency.

Clinical Findings

The first step in evaluating an incontinent patient is a thorough history. The nature and extent of the patient's lower urinary tract symptoms (LUTS) should be elucidated. Knowledge of the duration, frequency, and severity of the urinary incontinence is essential to understanding the social implications and its impact on the patient's life and aids the clinician in determining the direction and extent of diagnostic and therapeutic measures (Table 42–2). A multitude of diagnostic and imaging studies are available, but taking a thorough but focused urogynecologic history can isolate many of the easily reversible causes of incontinence (Table 42–3). Knowledge of the use of protective items, such as sanitary napkins, panty liners, absorbent pads, or adult diapers, is useful in quantitating urinary loss. Including questions about menopausal status and use of hormone treatment, history of urinary tract infections, previous surgery to remedy incontinence, and the patient's mental and functional status are essential.

Table 42–2. Lower urinary tract symptoms.

Urinary incontinence: the complaint of any involuntary leakage

Stress urinary incontinence: the complaint of involuntary leakage on effort or physical exertion, or on sneezing or coughing

Urge urinary incontinence: the complaint of involuntary leakage accompanied by urgency

Mixed urinary incontinence: the complaint of involuntary leakage associated with urgency and also with exertion, effort, sneezing, or coughing

Postural (urinary) incontinence: the complaint of involuntary loss of urine associated with change of body position, for example, rising from a seated or lying position

Nocturnal enuresis: Complaint of involuntary urinary loss of urine that occurs during sleep

Continuous (urinary) incontinence: Complaint of continuous involuntary loss of urine

Insensible (urinary) incontinence: Complaint of urinary incontinence where the woman has been unaware of how it occurred

Coital incontinence: Complaint of involuntary loss of urine with coitus

Overactive bladder (Urgency) syndrome: Urinary urgency, usually accompanied by frequency and nocturia, with or without urgency urinary incontinence, in the absence of urinary tract infection or other obvious pathology

Increased daytime frequency: the complaint by the patient who considers she voids too often by day

Nocturia: the complaint that the individual has to wake 1 or more times to micturate

Urgency: the complaint of a sudden compelling desire to pass urine that is difficult to defer

Table 42–3. Helpful questions when taking history of incontinence.

Do you leak urine when you cough, sneeze, or laugh?
Do you ever have such an uncomfortably strong need to urinate that if you don't reach the toilet you leak?
How many times during the day do you urinate?
How many times do you get up to urinate during the night after going to bed?
Have you ever wet the bed?
Do you leak during sexual intercourse?
Do you wear a pad to protect your clothing?
If yes, how often do you change the pad: when it has only a few drops, when it is damp, or when it is totally wet?
After you urinate, do you have dribbling or still feel the presence of urine in your bladder?
Does it hurt when you urinate?
Do you lose urine without the urge to go?

A. Patient Questionnaires

Survey instruments can be valuable in helping to identify and determine the severity of patient symptoms. Although initially designed for clinical research, short forms of longer questionnaires exist and can be used for clinical care. Surveys such as the Urinary Distress Inventory (UDI-6) and Incontinence Impact Questionnaire (IIQ-7) can be easily filled out by a patient to facilitate diagnosis and to follow treatment interventions.

B. Voiding Diary

A voiding diary, or urolog, that quantitates frequency and volume is a helpful tool. For a 24- to 48-hour period, the patient records all fluid intake and measures and records all urine output, including frequency and episodes of leakage (Fig. 42–5). Numerous studies have validated the voiding diary as a reliable tool in the diagnosis and management of urinary urgency or urge incontinence. These data are beneficial to the physician because they clarify home voiding patterns, particularly in the elderly. They are often useful to patients as well because they provide a focus on the problem and can serve as a baseline for treatment interventions such as behavioral training, bladder drills, and pharmacologic management.

C. Urinalysis

Examination of the urine is an essential part of the workup of urinary incontinence for any patient with LUTS. Infection is a common cause of urinary complaints, including frequency, urgency, and incontinence. A clean-catch voided specimen is suitable for routine urinalysis; however, a sterile "in and out" catheterized specimen is appropriate for patients unable to correctly perform collection or if urine culture has been previously equivocal because of skin flora contamination.

Urinary protein, glucose, ketones, hemoglobin, casts, and nitrates can indicate primary renal disease or injury. Microscopic evaluation of the urinary sediment may indicate renal tubular damage with the presence of casts or indicate infection by the presence of leukocytes and red blood cells. More than 6–8 white blood cells per high-power field along with the presence of bacteria are very suggestive of urinary tract infection.

D. Physical Examination

A general gynecologic and neurologic examination should be performed on all patients, with a focus on the vaginal walls and pelvic floor. The patient should come to the clinic with a comfortably full bladder for spontaneous uroflowmetry and postvoid residual assessment. An examination should be performed with the patient in the lithotomy position. The examination should begin with an assessment of the vulvar area. In postmenopausal patients, atrophy and change in labial architecture may be due to estrogen deficiency. Vulvar dermatoses may be coexistent with vulvar complaints ascribed to incontinence. The presence of inflammation or irritation from chronic moisture or pad usage should be noted. The presence of discharge should be noted because this may mimic urinary incontinence. Examination of the urethra with palpation of the anterior vaginal wall under the urethra for fluctuance, masses, or discharge may reveal signs of urethral diverticulum, infection of the urethra, or rarely carcinoma. Tenderness may point to urethral pain syndrome, a condition marked by episodic urethral pain usually with voiding, and by daytime frequency and nocturia.

Vaginal wall integrity must be assessed. Vaginal rugae, or the folds in the epithelium, are normal and tend to be absent if the underlying supportive endopelvic fascia is detached. The presence of anterior wall defects (cystoceles), posterior vaginal wall defects (rectoceles), and apical defects (uterine prolapse or enteroceles) can be quantified. The uterocervical position, or, if the woman has had a hysterectomy, the cuff position and its descent should be recorded. The position of the vaginal walls should be noted in the lithotomy position at rest and with Valsalva's/straining maneuver. A Sims' speculum or the lower blade of a Graves' speculum allows easy visualization of either the anterior or posterior vaginal wall. The severity of vaginal laxity, which may be masked in the supine position, can often best be elicited by repeating the examination in the standing position while the patient places 1 foot on the step of the examination table or on a small portable step.

Mobility at the level of the bladder neck is often seen in women with urinary incontinence. Urethral hypermobility must be interpreted with caution because it may be present

Urolog

Date	Time	Fluids (type and how much) ounces	Urine (how much) ounces or mL	Accidents/ Leaks
example 9/1/00	8:00	Water 8 oz		
9/1/00	8:30		150 mL	

▲ **Figure 42–5.** Urinary diary (urolog).

in women without incontinence. In the absence of mobility, the physician must question the diagnosis of stress incontinence and entertain the possibility of a fixed and damaged urethral sphincter (**intrinsic sphincteric deficiency**) to explain stress-related urinary loss.

E. Urinary Cough Stress Test

Having the patient perform Valsalva's maneuver or to cough forcefully multiple times to reproduce urine loss at the beginning of the examination may reveal the presence of incontinence. Observation of urine lost immediately with the cough or Valsalva's maneuver may obviate the need for more complex urodynamic testing if the complaint is minor. If no urine loss is exhibited, the patient is asked to stand with legs shoulder width apart and asked to cough. Immediate loss of urine suggests a diagnosis of SUI.

Bimanual examination to evaluate the uterine size, position, and descent within the vaginal canal and palpation of the ovaries should be performed. A rectovaginal examination permits adequate assessment of the posterior vaginal wall. Anal sphincter tone can be assessed at rest and with anal tightening. The presence of fecal impaction must be ruled out because this condition has been shown to be a contributing factor to urinary incontinence, particularly in the elderly population.

F. Neurologic Examination

The control of micturition is complex and multitiered, with both autonomic and voluntary control. In addition to a complete history and screening for neurologic symptoms, a thorough physical examination is important because many neurologic diseases may present with voiding dysfunction in the absence of overt neurologic findings.

Mental status, motor strength, sensory function, deep tendon reflexes, and sacral spinal cord integrity should all be assessed. Testing the patient's orientation to place and time and assessing speech and comprehension skills will help to ascertain her mental status. Motor control may be diminished in focal brain or cord lesions, most commonly Parkinson's disease, multiple sclerosis, and cerebrovascular accident. Motor strength is tested in the lower extremities by assessing hip, knee, and ankle flexion, as well as ankle eversion and inversion. Deep tendon reflexes are tested at the patella, ankle, and foot planus. Sensation can be tested at the dermatomes using light touch and pin-prick over the perineum and thigh area. Deficits should be noted, but it should be kept in mind that there is considerable overlap in sensory innervation in the sensory nerve roots. The sacral spinal cord nerve roots 2–4 contain vital neurons controlling micturition. The anal wink reflex and the bulbocavernosus reflex can confirm integrity of neurovisceral and urethral reflex functions. These reflexes can be evoked by stroking the perianal area and looking for an external anal sphincter contraction, and by tapping or gently squeezing the clitoris and watching for contraction of the bulbocavernosus muscle, respectively. These reflexes are often easier to elicit at the beginning of the examination, but their absence is not always indicative of neurologic deficit. Clinically observed neurologic deficits should lead to a neurologic consultation.

G. Urodynamics

A urodynamic study is any test that provides objective dynamic information about lower urinary tract function. Many methods and tests are available (Table 42–4). Some methods are simple, such as diaries that track frequency and volume of urination, and some methods are more complex, requiring special equipment and training. A cystometrogram can aid in the discovery of an unstable bladder, overflow incontinence, reduced bladder capacity, or abnormalities of bladder sensation. A cystometrogram can be performed using water manometry or more advanced methods. Complex urodynamic testing increases the diagnostic accuracy and may often identify the reason for failure of previous therapy. Uroflowmetry can be performed to measure detrusor pressure and flow rate to evaluate for voiding dysfunction. If a poorly functioning urethra, such as in intrinsic sphincter deficiency (ISD), is suspected, urethral pressure profile (UPP) or abdominal leak point pressure (ALPP) can be measured to evaluate urethral closure pressures. Such testing is particularly helpful in difficult or complex cases.

The indications for more complex testing in the form of multichannel urodynamics are not standardized, and each patient must be assessed individually (Table 42–5). However, some basic criteria, if met, indicate a need for urodynamic evaluation, which can aid in more accurate diagnosis and thus appropriate medical or surgical management.

H. Cystourethroscopy

Endoscopic evaluation is an invaluable adjunct for the diagnosis and management of the urogynecologic patient. It is a simple office procedure that can yield important data when performed by experienced operators. Cystourethroscopy is indicated for hematuria and irritative voiding symptoms, particularly in the presence of previous continence surgery, obstructive voiding, suspicion of diverticula or fistula, or persistent incontinence and as a preoperative evaluation before reconstructive pelvic surgery.

Table 42–4. Urodynamic testing methods.

Test	Purpose	Indications
Simple cystometry	Measures bladder pressure and volume	Useful in patients with clear-cut symptoms
Complex cystometry	Multiple parameters: bladder volume, filling rate, bladder pressure, abdominal pressure, and subtracted detrusor pressure	More accurate information on bladder function; most common type of urodynamics test
Uroflowmetry	Measures flow rate with special electronic flowmeters	Useful for general impression of voiding function
Pressure-flow	Combines complex cystometry and uroflowmetry; measures bladder pressure, abdominal pressure, subtracted detrusor pressure, and uroflow	Provides accurate means of differentiating detrusor contraction, straining, and pelvic relaxation as mechanisms of urination
Leak point pressure	Using abdominal or bladder pressures, urethral resistance to abdominal strain is measured	Used in assessing urethral sphincter function
Urethral pressure profilometry	Using a dual transducer catheter, simultaneous bladder and urethral pressure can be recorded	Used in assessing urethral sphincter function
Electromyography	Surface or needle electrodes to determine striated muscle activity of the pelvic floor or the anal or urethral sphincters	Useful in patients with abnormal voiding patterns

Table 42–5. Indications for multichannel urodynamic testing.

Complicated symptoms and history
Use when considering surgery for correction of incontinence or pelvic organ prolapse
Underlying neurologic disease
Urge incontinence refractive to initial conservative therapies
Continuous leakage
Previous continence surgery
Clinical findings do not correlate with symptoms
Elderly patients >65 years old

I. Imaging Tests

Radiologic studies can be an integral component of the evaluation of lower urinary tract dysfunction and abnormalities. However, these modalities are of limited use in the evaluation of all but the most complex of incontinent patients. Ultrasound has become an increasingly frequent adjunct investigation for pelvic floor disorders both in the office and in the urodynamic laboratory. Magnetic resonance imaging (MRI) has become more extensively used in patients with PFDs and prolapse. As the technique becomes less costly, applications for the uses of MRI to aid in the urogynecologic workup will expand.

Differential Diagnosis

See Table 42–1.

STRESS URINARY INCONTINENCE

Stress urinary incontinence (SUI) is defined as the complaint of involuntary leakage on effort or physical exertion or on coughing or sneezing. Normally, at rest the intraurethral pressure is greater than the intravesical pressure. The pressure difference between the bladder and the urethra is known as the **urethral closure pressure**. If intra-abdominal pressure increases, as it does with a cough, sneeze, or strain, and if this pressure is not equally transmitted to the urethra, then continence is not maintained and leakage of urine occurs. What is thought to cause this inequity of pressure transmission is not universally accepted; however, surgical therapy directed at stabilization of the suburethral support appears to be the mechanism for long-term correction.

Treatment

A. Nonsurgical Measures

For most patients with SUI, consideration of the simplest, least invasive, and least costly interventions is appropriate (Table 42–6). Dietary measures can be instituted, with identification of items that can be modified. Reduction in consumption of caffeinated beverages and alcoholic drinks should be encouraged. Fluid restriction in patients without chronic medical problems, such as cardiovascular, renal, or endocrinologic disease, can be attempted. Timed voiding to prevent filling the bladder to a capacity that causes urine loss should be undertaken with the use of a urine diary. The diary can also facilitate discussion between patient and clinician as therapy progresses.

Table 42–6. Nonsurgical management of urinary incontinence.

Behavioral therapy
Fluid management
Bladder training
Pelvic floor muscle training • Biofeedback • Vaginal cones
Functional electrical stimulation
Anti-incontinence pessary
Pharmacotherapy
Sacral neuromodulation

Pelvic floor muscle exercises or Kegel exercises have been found to be extremely helpful in patients with mild to moderate forms of incontinence. Focused repetitive voluntary contractions of the levator ani muscles (pubococcygeus, coccygeus, and iliococcygeus) created by having the patient contract or "squeeze" the muscle as if to prevent the passage of rectal gas is an effective therapy. The contractions exert a closing force on the urethra and increase muscle support to the pelvic organs. The patient should be provided written and verbal instructions on performing the exercises. Repetitions, with each contraction held for 3–5 seconds alternated with periods of relaxation, should be begun at 45–100 repetitions daily. In settings in which the patient is motivated and has individual instruction and thorough follow-up and support, results for cure or improvement of bladder control (reduction in urine loss) can be up to 75%.

1. Biofeedback—Biofeedback is an adjunct to pelvic floor exercises that is used to facilitate the patient's comprehension of the proper muscles to contract. By using a pressure catheter and myographic monitoring, a visual or auditory signal of the physiologic response can be provided to the patient to help refine exercise skills. Using surface electromyography on the perineum to measure levator contraction and a pressure monitor in the vagina or rectum to indicate abdominal pressure, the patient can be instructed to preferentially contract the pelvic floor without concomitant abdominal contraction. Studies using a variety of techniques demonstrate a 54–95% cure rate or improvement in SUI. The efficacy of this modality is highly dependent on patient motivation and compliance. Pelvic floor muscle exercises with or without biofeedback require continued implementation and practice or effectiveness will wane.

2. Electrical stimulation—As an alternative to active patient contraction of the levator muscles, electrical stimulation of the muscles via small electrical currents can be used to help both SUI and mixed incontinence. Using intravaginal or transrectal electrodes with stimulators, the pelvic muscles automatically contract and are thereby artificially "trained." When used long term, weakened muscles are strengthened and innervation re-established during activation. Experiences with the devices are variable, but they generally show a positive impact on incontinence and acceptable patient tolerance.

3. Pessaries—Intravaginal devices or pessaries to correct the anatomic deficits associated with stress incontinence have long been used to address this vexing problem. Many devices have been proffered, but long-term solutions to incontinence have yet to be proven in the general population. Pessaries, traditionally used for treatment of genital prolapse, have also been shown to have a potential role in supporting the bladder neck and urethra and preventing stress incontinence. Many pessary devices designed to fit within the vagina and elevate the bladder neck are available. Continence can often be achieved because many devices adequately obstruct the bladder neck and urethra. As with all intravaginal devices, maintenance is essential to avoid urinary obstruction and vaginal erosion if the pessary is too compressive.

B. Surgical Management

Surgical treatment may be offered for moderate to severe incontinence. Urinary incontinence is not a life-threatening condition, and the decision to operate must be based on the patient's symptoms and the impact on daily life. Many patients are able to tolerate slight urine loss, and what often provokes a desire for treatment is an increase in loss above a tolerable threshold. If medical management to improve bladder control is possible and symptoms are reduced to below this threshold, then medical management is most desirable. If not, surgery should be considered.

At least 130 operative procedures have been described for treatment of female urinary stress incontinence. It is therefore not surprising that many of these procedures have not resulted in long-term success. For patients who desire surgical correction, the options can be categorized by method of surgical approach (Table 42–7). Common to most surgical procedures is restoration of bladder neck support by elevation of the urethrovesical junction. Some procedures reconstruct bladder neck supports and provide a stable suburethral layer.

Table 42–7. Surgical treatment of stress urinary incontinence.

Retropubic urethropexy
  Burch (open or laparoscopic)
  Marshall-Marchetti-Krantz

Suburethral sling

Midurethral sling
  Retropubic
  Transobturator
  Single incision

Urethral bulking agents

Assessment of the cure rate of any surgical treatment for genuine stress incontinence must take into account the selection of patients, accuracy of the preoperative diagnosis, length of postoperative follow-up, and criteria for cure. Reported cure rates for procedures range from 60–100%, with 75–90% being the generally accepted rate. Most failures appear to result from incorrect preoperative diagnosis, poor surgical technique, and healing failures.

1. Abdominal Retropubic Colpopexy—The Marshall-Marchetti-Krantz (MMK) and Burch's colposuspension are the 2 classic retropubic surgeries for incontinence. They share the same mechanism of correction. First, both suspend the periurethral and paravaginal tissue at the level of the urethrovesical junction, and second, both use a firm point of attachment for fixation of these suspension sutures. In the MMK procedure, the sutures are fixed to the periosteum of the pubic bone, and in Burch's procedure, the iliopectineal ligament (Cooper's ligament) (Fig. 42–6). Burch's colposuspension has been a longstanding treatment of patients with hypermobility of the bladder neck and genuine SUI. In both longitudinal studies and randomized comparative trials against other procedures, Burch's procedure maintains high objective and subjective cure rates of 80% after 5 years and 68% after 10 years of follow-up.

A laparoscopic approach to Burch's colposuspension offers the benefit of minimally invasive surgery with the same level of efficacy.

2. Suburethral Slings—The suburethral sling was one of the original surgical procedures developed for correction of SUI. The concept of restoring continence by encircling the urethra with supportive tissue, either from the patient or foreign material, was introduced at the beginning of the 20th century. Contemporary techniques have used a patient's own fascia harvested from the leg or rectus fascia, or donor fascia in the form of cadaveric fascia lata. Cure rates of suburethral sling procedures for genuine stress incontinence vary from 70–95%. Reported rates vary because of the heterogeneity of

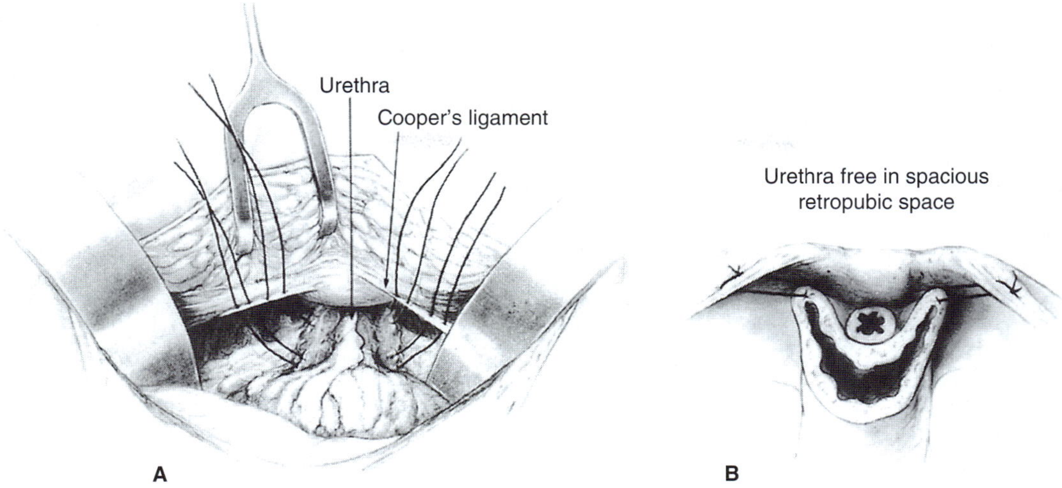

▲ **Figure 42–6.** Abdominal surgical procedure to correct stress incontinence. **A:** Anterior vaginal wall has been mobilized. Two sutures have been placed on either side and far lateral from the midline. Distal sutures are opposite the midurethra. Proximal sutures are at the end of the vesicourethral junction. Sutures are attached to Cooper's ligament. **B:** Cross-section shows urethra free in the retropubic space, with anterior vaginal wall lifting and supporting it. (Reproduced, with permission, from Tanagho EA. Colpocystourethropexy. *J Urol* 1876;116:751. Copyright 1976 by Williams & Wilkins.)

patients, and many are previous surgical failures. Variations in sling material and technique have made cure rates among sling techniques difficult to interpret. Furthermore, most studies vary in the definition of cure and may not distinguish between cure and improvement.

In a large prospective trial comparing suburethral fascial slings versus Burch's procedure, at 24 months, success rates were higher for women who underwent the sling procedure than for those who underwent Burch's procedure (66% vs. 49%, respectively). These efficacy results are notable; in a review study summarizing cure rates of surgical treatments for SUI, 16 studies comparing sling procedures with colposuspension were reviewed. Of the 4 that were randomized controlled trials comprising 150 patients, none reported a difference in cure.

3. Midurethral Slings—This recent modification of the sling is the use of tension-free vaginal mesh made of polypropylene placed at the level of the midurethra. This technique, developed in Sweden, was introduced to the United States in the late 1990s. Use of tension-free vaginal tape (TVT) (Fig. 42–7) was developed as a minimally invasive technique for surgical correction of genuine SUI. The initial study had an 84% cure rate in 75 women with 2-year follow-up. The success rates of this procedure that have been reported in trials range from 86% to 99%, with up to 10-year follow-up. Because these results have been reproduced, most clinicians consider the midurethral sling as the gold standard for continence surgery.

Because of the success of TVT midurethral sling, numerous other devices using the same principles and technique are available. All use a polypropylene mesh but have different designs of delivery needle/trocar, mesh construction, and sheath type. Comparative data between devices are scanty.

An alternate to retropubic passage is the transobturator route, in which the sling is passed through the obturator foramen laterally. This creates a more lateral point of fixation. The purported advantage is reduction in bladder, bowel, or major vascular injury because this method avoids the space of Retzius and does not traverse the peritoneal space. Studies suggest 2-year cure rates comparable to those of retropubic passage (94%). There are reservations regarding the transobturator approach as it relates to correcting SUI due to a poorly functioning urethra and in complications related to groin pain, particularly in thin patients (Fig. 42–7).

A more recent introduction is the **single-incision slings**, in which instead of passing externally through the obturator foramen, the mesh sling is anchored internally into the fascia/muscle of the obturator.

C. Periurethral and Transurethral Injection

Periurethral or transurethral injection of a bulking agent into the submucosal space of the bladder neck causes narrowing or coaptation of the proximal urethra and bladder neck opening. This increases urethral resistance to involuntary urine loss without changing resting urethral closure

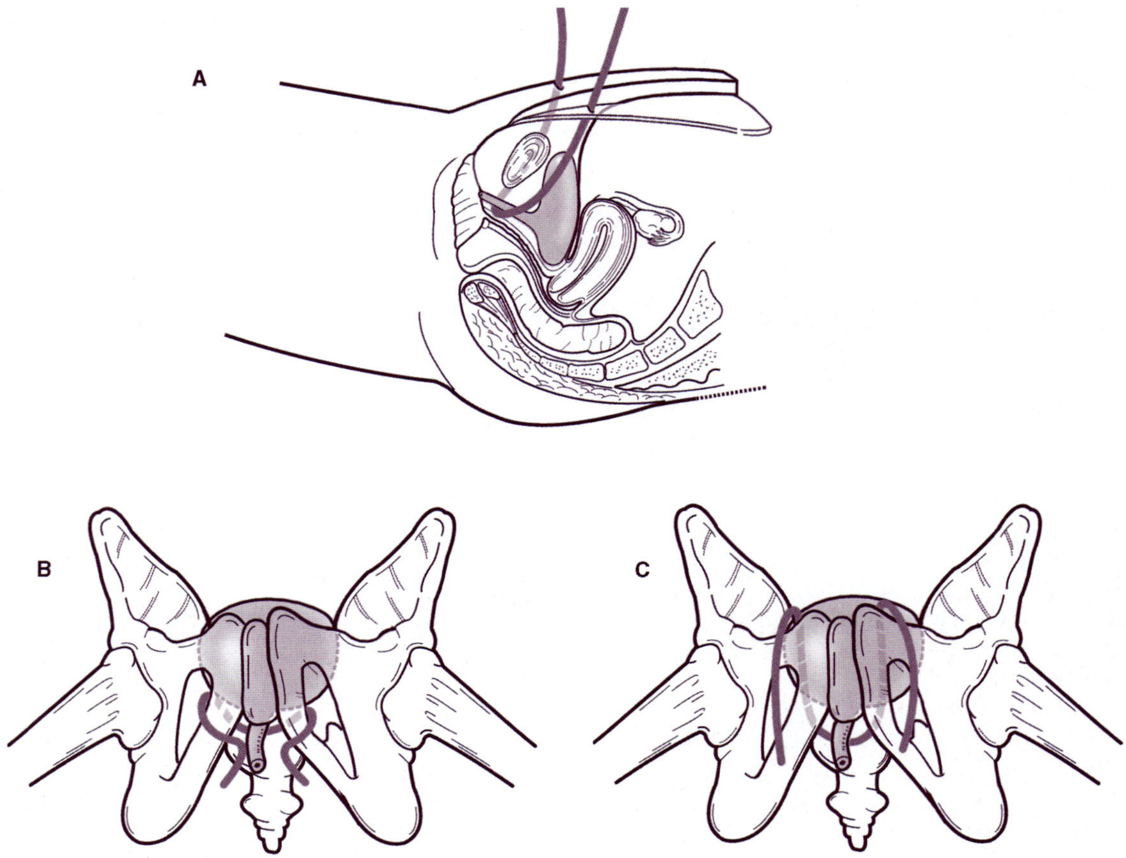

▲ **Figure 42–7.** **A:** Placement of midurethral sling in the sagittal view. **B:** Retropubic passage of midurethral sling. **C:** Transobturator passage of midurethral sling.

pressure. Currently glutaraldehyde cross-linked bovine collagen and calcium hydroxyl apatite are the most commonly used materials. This procedure is generally reserved for genuine SUI caused by intrinsic sphincteric deficiency. The injections can be performed with the patient under sedation with local anesthetic in an outpatient or office setting. These materials are biologic and resorb over time. Improvement and cure rates are 53–66% in the short term, and complications are minimal.

D. Artificial Sphincters

The artificial urethral sphincter is an effective option for patients with incontinence not amenable to standard surgical treatment because of urethral scarring or atony. The artificial urinary sphincter is best used in patients with incontinence due to poor urethral sphincter function. The sphincter obstructs the urethra by compressing the bladder neck via a pressure-regulated balloon and releases the compression when the patient desires to void. Reported success rates are up to 91%, but complication rates are high, with 21% of patients requiring surgical replacement of parts or the entire sphincter.

URGE URINARY INCONTINENCE

Urge urinary incontinence is the complaint of involuntary leakage accompanied by urgency. Urge urinary incontinence may be associated with involuntary contractions of the bladder or detrusor contractions; however, most often it is attributable to increased sensation with strong urge. The term **overactive bladder** (OAB) is often used to describe the most common symptoms of urinary urgency, usually accompanied by frequency and nocturia, with or without urgency urinary incontinence, in the absence of urinary tract infection or other obvious pathology. Not all patients with OAB have detrusor overactivity, and neither will all patients with detrusor overactivity have OAB. OAB is a term that lends itself to encompassing all conditions related to bladder urgency and frequency with and without incontinence. OAB has become a preferred clinical term because it comprises the spectrum of related symptoms.

Pathogenesis

The incidence of OAB varies depending on the population studied and the definition applied. Consequently, the reported prevalence varies widely from 8–50% in the general population, and in women older than 65 years, it is estimated to be at least 38%. An important concept is that involuntary detrusor contractions for bladder emptying are normally overridden by cortical inhibition of reflex bladder activity. In the majority of cases the cause of OAB symptoms is unknown. Patients with underlying neurologic disease may manifest with urinary incontinence. Although neurologic disease is not a common cause of OAB, multiple sclerosis, cerebrovascular disease, Parkinson's disease, and Alzheimer's disease are most often associated with involuntary bladder contractions.

Clinical Findings

OAB is suggested by urinary frequency often associated with a strong urge or a sense of impending urine loss. Incontinence often occurs before reaching the toilet. Physical or environmental stimuli, such as running water, cold weather, or hand washing, may elicit an urge. Patients often describe "key in lock" syndrome. This is typically characterized by an uncontrollable urge to void when unlocking the door after returning from a trip out of the house. The first thing done upon return is to immediately rush to the toilet or risk losing urine.

Treatment

Adequate therapy depends greatly on accuracy of diagnosis of OAB. History is most often suggestive, and the diagnosis can be supported by urinary diary or confirmed with office cystometry or more precisely with multichannel urodynamics.

Patients with OAB first should be offered simple treatments. Behavioral modifications and medical treatment are the standard first-line therapy for urge urinary incontinence.

A. Behavioral Therapy

Behavioral therapy includes bladder training, timed voiding, and pelvic floor muscle exercises. Bladder training is an educational program that combines written and verbal instruction to educate patients about the mechanisms of normal bladder control with the teaching of relaxation and distraction skills to resist premature signals to urinate. Creating a voiding schedule for which the patient urinates at preset intervals while attempting to ignore the urge to urinate may progressively lead to re-establishment of cortical voluntary control over the micturition reflex.

Timed voiding is a form of bladder retraining that again mandates regularly scheduled voiding and attempts to match the person's natural voiding schedule. No effort is made to motivate the patient to delay voiding by resisting the urge. This method is geared more toward elderly patients with more challenging problems who have skilled help available.

Pelvic floor exercises may aid in the treatment of OAB. Evidence supports the utility of this modality in all types of incontinence. Particularly when augmented with biofeedback, pelvic floor exercises can greatly reduce symptoms of urinary frequency and urge incontinence, by up to 54–85%.

B. Pharmacologic Therapy

One of the most effective and popular treatments for urge urinary incontinence and OAB is drug therapy. Numerous agents for the treatment of these patients have been tried over the years, but only a few have demonstrated substantial impact on reduction of symptoms in controlled trials. One of the main difficulties in treating OAB is that the cause of OAB is still under investigation. The drugs available can be divided into classes by mechanism of action (Table 42–8).

Antimuscarinics, or anticholinergics, have become the mainstay of drug treatment of OAB. Acetylcholine is the primary neurotransmitter involved with bladder contraction. The detrusor muscle of the bladder is heavily populated with cholinergic receptors. Anticholinergic activity, therefore, is a property of most drugs used to treat OAB. The mainstays of drug therapy for OAB include oxybutynin chloride and tolterodine. Oxybutynin chloride has been shown in randomized placebo-controlled trials to be effective in increasing bladder capacity, decreasing the frequency of detrusor contractions, and improving symptoms of urinary urgency in approximately 70% of patients. It is effective for both idiopathic and neuropathic etiologies of detrusor instability.

Tolterodine is a medication designed specifically for OAB. It also has anticholinergic activity with specificity for the bladder, and it acts through muscarinic receptors as well as smooth muscle relaxation. In a multicenter randomized controlled trial, the medication compared favorably with oxybutynin in terms of reducing the number of micturitions in 24 hours and the number of incontinent episodes. Because of its bladder specificity, tolterodine has a more favorable side effect profile than oxybutynin. It is also dosed less frequently and improves patient compliance. Both are available in immediate-release and long-acting formulations. Oxybutynin is also available for delivery in a transdermal patch.

A large randomized comparative trial evaluating the performance of the long-acting formulations of oxybutynin and tolterodine demonstrated similar efficacy. Adverse events were similar, but the occurrence of dry mouth was higher in the oxybutynin group.

Other antimuscarinics are available. All significantly improve OAB symptoms compared with placebo. Evidence suggests that medications such as darifenacin, solifenacin, trospium chloride, and fesoterodine have side effects similar to or lower than those of traditional antimuscarinics. Comparative trials exist essentially demonstrating comparable efficacy and

Table 42–8. Pharmacologic treatment of urge incontinence.

Drug Name	Trade Name	Drug Type	Dosage	Potential Side Effects
Oxybutynin chloride	Ditropan	Anticholinergic (antimuscarinic)/ smooth muscle relaxant; tertiary amine	15–30 mg daily	Dry mouth, blurry vision, constipation, tachycardia, drowsiness, dizziness
Oxybutynin chloride (OROS)	Ditropan XL	See above	5–30 mg daily	See above, less CNS side effects
Transdermal oxybutynin	Oxytrol	See above	3.9 mg/day patch	See above
Tolterodine	Detrol	Antimuscarinic/smooth muscle relaxant	1–2 mg BID	See above
Tolterodine (long acting)	Detrol LA	See above	2–4 mg Q day	See above
Trospium chloride	Sanctura	Antimuscarinic; quaternary amine	20 mg BID	Dry mouth, constipation, headache
Darifenacin	Enablex	Antimuscarinic selective; tertiary amine	7.5–15 mg QD	Dry mouth, constipation, blurred vision, reduced CNS effects
Solifenacin	Vesicare	Antimuscarinic selective	5–10 mg daily	Dry mouth, constipation, blurred vision
Fesoterodine	Toviaz	Antimuscarinic	4–8 mg daily	Dry mouth, constipation, blurred vision

BID, twice per day; CNS, central nervous system; QD, once per day.

adverse event profiles. Most of the clinical effectiveness of antimuscarinics, however, is limited by side effects. Long-term compliance of these medications appears to be imperfect at best.

C. Sacral Neuromodulation

Electrical stimulation to the nerves that control the bladder have been used in people with OAB. An electrode is placed via the sacral foramen alongside a sacral nerve (usually S3). In a second procedure, the electrode is connected by cables under the skin to an implanted programmable pulse generator that provides stimulation within set stimulation parameters. Implantation of the pulse generator is usually carried out only after a successful trial. The technology has been used for patients with OAB, urgency incontinence, and voiding (retention of urine) difficulties, and for some patients with defecation problems. It has also been used in the management of chronic pelvic pain, and it is approved for fecal incontinence, but this indication is not included in this review.

In patients with urge urinary incontinence caused by detrusor overactivity, sacral neuromodulation seems to act primarily by activation of nonmuscular afferent sacral nerve fibers that inhibit parasympathetic motor neurones in the cord through interneurons. It appears that any change induced by implanted electrodes persists only while the stimulator is turned on, returning to baseline when the stimulation is stopped. A longer lasting benefit has, however, been reported for stimulation via vaginal or anal plug electrodes, persisting after active treatment stops. These devices are expensive, the surgery is invasive, and many people need another operation.

It is not clear how best to use these devices. However, implantable stimulators that provide continuous electrical stimulation to the nerves or nerve roots supplying the bladder and pelvis, or to the peripheral nerves that share the same nerve roots, can benefit selected patients with difficult-to-control urinary problems.

MIXED INCONTINENCE

Mixed incontinence occurs when both stress incontinence and urge incontinence occur simultaneously. Patients may present with symptoms of both types of incontinence. These patients present both a diagnostic and therapeutic dilemma. The prevalence of mixed incontinence is more common than most practitioners realize. A detailed history will reveal symptoms of SUI with urine loss associated with cough, sneeze, or other increase in Valsalva's pressure, as well as urinary urgency, frequency, and concomitant incontinence. The coexistence of these 2 conditions may be brought about by many causes. Patients with SUI often preemptively urinate to avoid a full bladder and subsequent urine loss, thereby conditioning the bladder to habituate to a low functional capacity. This may promote premature signaling of bladder fullness and result in frequent urge symptoms.

Treatment

For mixed incontinence, treatment should be based on the patient's worst symptoms. Often patients can prioritize their symptoms, stating that one component impacts their life more than the other. By having the patient separate the symptoms, a practical management plan with realistic expectations can be devised. A great disservice can be done by operating on a patient to restore bladder neck support and remove stress symptoms when the patient's main concern is daily urge incontinence while she is at work. Conservative measures should be tried first, and if symptoms do not improve, surgical measures can be entertained to target alleviation of the stress component; however, there is a 50–60% chance that urge symptoms may resolve after a midurethral sling is performed.

OVERFLOW INCONTINENCE

Overflow incontinence is the involuntary loss of urine associated with bladder overdistention in the absence of detrusor contraction.

Pathogenesis

This condition classically occurs in men who have outlet obstruction secondary to prostatic enlargement that progresses to urinary retention. In women this is a relatively uncommon cause of urinary incontinence. When it does occur, it can be from increased outlet resistance from advanced vaginal prolapse causing a "kink" in the urethra or after an anti-incontinence procedure that has overcorrected the problem. Additionally, it can result from bladder hyporeflexia from a variety of neurologic causes (Table 42–9).

Overflow incontinence most often occurs due to postoperative obstruction if the bladder neck is overcorrected or with a hyporeflexic bladder due to neurologic disease or spinal cord injury. The normal act of voiding is controlled centrally by sacral and pontine micturition centers.

Table 42–9. Causes of overflow incontinence.

Neurologic	Anatomic	Iatrogenic
Spinal cord trauma	Extrinsic compression (prolapse in women)	Surgery
Cerebral cortical lesions	Urethral mass	Obstetric
Diabetes mellitus		Anesthetic
Multiple sclerosis		
Infectious	**Pharmacologic**	
Cystitis	Anticholinergics	
Urethritis	α-Adrenergics	

Impaired emptying can be the result of disruption of either central or peripheral neurons mediating detrusor function. Failure to identify the cause early may lead to permanent dysfunction and may lead to injury to the detrusor muscle or compromise in the parasympathetic ganglia in the bladder wall.

Clinical Findings

Usually symptoms are loss of urine without awareness or intermittent dribbling and constant wetness. Suprapubic pressure or pain may be associated. Patients will often note a sensation of a full bladder and the need to strain in order to empty or apply suprapubic pressure to void. Patients are at risk for urinary tract infection secondary to persistent residual urine in the bladder, which acts as a medium for bacterial growth. It is commonly seen after a bladder neck suspension. Complaints of poor urinary stream and sense of incomplete emptying combined with having to strain or apply hand pressure to void are likely.

Evaluation should always include a postvoid residual and, if the diagnosis is questionable, voiding pressure flow studies. An imaging study of the upper urinary tract to evaluate the ureters and kidney should follow, because persistent high-volume retention can lead to reflux and hydroureter or hydronephrosis and renal injury if left unchecked.

Treatment

Bladder drainage to relieve retention is the first priority. Self-intermittent or prolonged catheterization may be necessary, depending on resolution of the inciting cause. In cases of postoperative urinary retention, bladder function can be evaluated by serial postvoid residual urine determinations. Although no normal volume for residual urine is universally accepted, less than 100 mL is generally considered to be within normal limits and greater than 150 mL is considered abnormal. More than 1 value is needed because persistently high residual volumes will require prolonged catheterization.

When urinary retention occurs in the setting of neurologic disease, diabetes, or stroke, correction of the underlying cause is often impossible; therefore, the goal is to prevent injury or damage to the upper urinary tract. Intermittent self-catheterization is preferable to an indwelling catheter, which may predispose to infection, bladder spasms, or erosion.

Medical therapy may assist in the care of these patients. Acetylcholine agonists can stimulate detrusor contractions in patients who have vesical areflexia. α-Adrenergic blockers can facilitate bladder emptying by relaxing tone at the bladder neck.

Behavior modification in the form of timed voiding on a preset schedule to empty regardless of urge will prevent accumulation of excess urine. Usually a voiding pattern of every 2–3 hours is preferable. In bladder areflexia, manual pressure or abdominal splinting may facilitate emptying.

BYPASS INCONTINENCE

Urinary loss due to abnormal anatomic variations is uncommon but extremely important to consider in the evaluation of the incontinent woman. Bypass incontinence may often mimic other forms of urinary incontinence but usually presents as constant dribbling or dampness. Patients may complain of positional loss of urine without urge or forewarning. Diagnosing this type of incontinence requires a high level of suspicion and an understanding of the underlying anatomic deviation in the lower urinary tract. Genitourinary fistulas (vesicovaginal or ureterovaginal) can be a debilitating cause of incontinence and are formed because of poor wound healing after a traumatic insult (eg, obstetric laceration, pelvic surgery, perineal trauma, or radiation exposure). Leakage due to fistulas is generally continuous, although it may be elicited by position change or stress-inducing activities. Evaluation should include a careful examination of the vaginal walls for fistulas. This can be facilitated by filling the bladder with milk or dilute indigo carmine dye and looking for pooling in the vaginal canal. Pad testing can be performed by having the patient ingest 200 mg of oral phenazopyridine hydrochloride (Pyridium) several hours before a subsequent examination. By placing a tampon in the vagina and on the perineum, the diagnosis may be confirmed by inspection of the pads after a period of time. Further imaging (intravenous urography) and cystoscopy can identify the exact location of the aberrant communication. If diagnosis is made early, the fistulous tract may heal with prolonged catheterization. However, if this procedure is unsuccessful or if diagnosis is made late, surgical correction is generally the only hope for cure.

Urethral Diverticula

Another important but uncommon cause of involuntary urine loss is urethral diverticula. Diverticula are essentially weaknesses or "hernias" in the supportive fascial layer of the bladder or urethra. Urethral diverticulum is most likely to cause symptoms of urinary loss. It has an incidence of 0.3–3% in women and is thought to be largely an acquired condition resulting from obstruction and expansion of the paraurethral Skene's glands. The symptoms of constant small amounts of leakage or urethral discharge are often described. A suburethral mass is visible and palpable on physical examination. Urine or discharge may often be "milked" by palpation of the suburethral mass. Treatment is usually surgical excision of the diverticulum.

FUNCTIONAL AND TRANSIENT INCONTINENCE

Incontinence may be caused by factors outside the lower urinary tract and is particularly significant in the geriatric population, because often a multitude of special circumstances affect the health of the elderly. Physical impairment, cognitive function, medication, systemic illness, and bowel function are all factors that may contribute to incontinence. Many immobile patients are incontinent because of the inability to toilet. Cognitive disturbances limit a patient's ability to respond normally to the sensation to void. Numerous medications have effects on the bladder that may reduce capacity, inhibit bladder function, increase diuresis and bladder load, or relax the urinary sphincter. Additionally, stool impaction and constipation both have been associated with increased prevalence of urinary incontinence. Treatments should first identify the etiologic factors of the incontinence and then reduce or remove the cause.

PROGNOSIS

Urinary incontinence is fundamentally a condition that affects quality of life. The natural history of incontinence is generally that of stability or progression. Excluding transient causes, spontaneous resolution is not a feature of this condition. Most women learn coping skills (pad use, frequent toileting, timed voiding) and adaptive measures (fluid restriction or toilet mapping) to handle the detriment in quality of life. Although bothersome and even socially debilitating, the extent of treatment is dependent on patient direction. One example of true health risk with incontinence is in the instance of outlet obstruction and urinary retention with resultant overflow incontinence. Chronic urinary retention may lead to upper urinary tract dilation and ultimately lead to reduction in urinary function, therefore intervention in this setting is warranted.

Albo M, Richter HE, Brubaker L, et al. Burch colposuspension versus fascial sling to reduce urinary stress incontinence. *N Engl J Med* 2007;356:2143–2155. PMID: 17517855.

American Urogynecologic Society. www.augs.org. Accessed March 13, 2012.

Ashton-Miller J, DeLancey JOL. Functional anatomy of the female pelvic floor. *Ann NY Acad Sci* 2007;1101:266–296. PMID: 17416924.

Brubaker L, Nygaard I, Richter HE, et al. Two-year outcomes after sacrocolpopexy with and without burch to prevent stress urinary incontinence. *Obstet Gynecol* 2008;112:49–55. PMID: 18591307.

Burgio KL, Goode PS, Richter HE, et al. Combined behavioral and individualized drug therapy versus individualized drug therapy alone for urge urinary incontinence in women. *J Urol* 2010;184:598–603. PMID: 20639023.

Diokno A, Sampselle CM, Herzog AR, et al. Prevention of urinary incontinence by behavioral modification program: A randomized, controlled trial among older women in the community. *J Urol* 2004;171:1165–1171. PMID: 14767293.

Diokno AC, Appell RA, Sand PK, et al. OPERA Study Group. Prospective, randomized, double-blind study of the efficacy and tolerability of the extended-release formulations of oxybutynin and tolterodine for overactive bladder: Results of the OPERA trial. *Mayo Clin Proc* 2003;78:687–695. PMID: 12934777.

Elkelini MS, Abuzgaya A, Hassouna MM. Mechanisms of sacral neuromodulation. *Int Urogynecol J* 2010;21(Suppl 2):S439–S446. PMID: 20972548.

Holmgren C, Nilsson S, Lanner L, Hellberg D. Long-term results with tension-free vaginal tape on mixed and stress urinary incontinence. *Obstet Gynecol* 2005;106:38–43. PMID: 15994615.

Holroyd-Leduc JM, Straus SE. Management of urinary incontinence in women: Scientific review. *JAMA* 2004;291:986–995. PMID: 14982915.

National Association for Continence. www.nafc.org. Accessed March 13, 2012.

Novara G, Galfano A, Secco S, D'Elia C, Cavalleri S, Ficarra V, Artibani W. A systematic review and meta-analysis of randomized controlled trials with antimuscarinic drugs for overactive bladder. *Eur Urol* 2008;54:740–763. PMID: 18632201.

Ogah J, Cody JD, Rogerson L. Minimally invasive synthetic suburethral sling operations for stress urinary incontinence in women. *Cochrane Database Syst Rev* 2009;CD006375. PMID: 19821363.

Richter H, Albo ME, Zyczynski HM, et al. Retropubic versus transobturator midurethral slings for stress incontinence. *N Engl J Med* 2010;362:2066–2076. PMID: 20479459.

Rortveit G, Daltveit AK, Hannestad YS, Hunskaar S. Norwegian EPINCONT Study. Urinary incontinence after vaginal delivery or cesarean section. *N Engl J Med* 2003;348:900–907. PMID: 12621134.

Ulmsten U. An introduction to tension-free vaginal tape (TVT)—A new surgical procedure for treatment of female urinary incontinence. *Int Urogynecol J Pelvic Floor Dysfunct* 2001;12(Suppl 2):S3–S4. PMID: 11450978.

Voices for PFD. www.mypelvichealth.org. Accessed March 13, 2012.

Ward K, Hilton P; United Kingdom and Ireland Tension Free Vaginal Tape Trial Group. Prospective multicentre randomised trial of tension-free vaginal tape and colposuspension as primary treatment for stress incontinence. *BMJ* 2002;325:67. PMID: 12114234.

PELVIC ORGAN PROLAPSE

Pelvic organ prolapse (POP), including anterior vaginal and posterior vaginal prolapse, uterine prolapse, and enteroceles, is a common group of clinical conditions affecting women. The prevalence rates increase with age, and POP currently affects millions of women. In the United States, POP is responsible for more than 200,000 surgeries per year. The lifetime risk that a woman will undergo surgery for prolapse or urinary incontinence is 11%, with a third of surgeries representing repeat procedures. The risk of requiring a repeat procedure for POP may be as high as 29%. As our population ages, quality-of-life–altering conditions such as POP will demand more attention from our health care services. Prolapse can be asymptomatic or manifest with severe debility and associated bladder, bowel, or sexual dysfunction. The ability to screen, diagnose, and treat these entities will become increasingly important for clinicians.

Defects in the pelvic supporting structures result in a variety of clinically evident pelvic relaxation abnormalities.

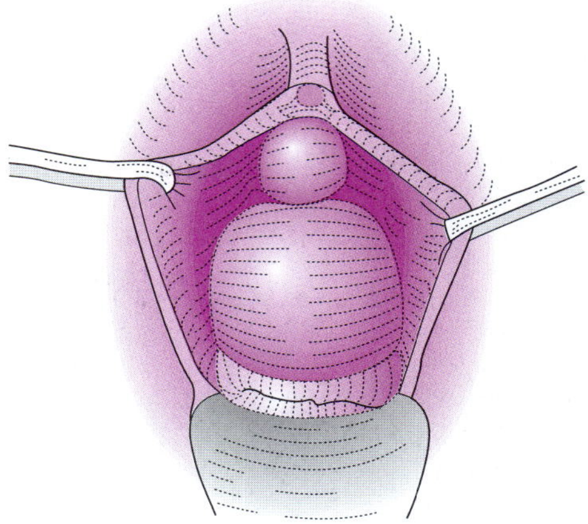

▲ **Figure 42–8.** Anterior vaginal prolapse, known as a cystocele.

Pelvic support defects can be classified by their anatomic location.

Anterior Vaginal Wall Defects

ESSENTIALS OF DIAGNOSIS

- **Anterior vaginal prolapse** describes an anterior vaginal wall defect in which the bladder is associated with the prolapse. It is also known as a cystocele (Fig. 42–8).
- **Paravaginal/midline/transverse prolapse** are terms used to indicate the location of anterior vaginal wall defects (Fig. 42–9).

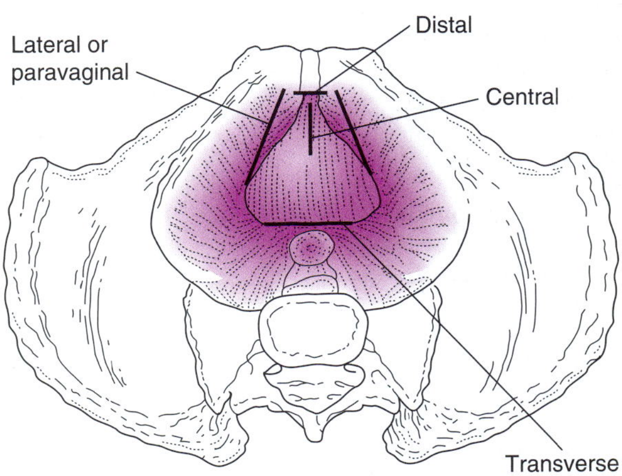

▲ **Figure 42–9.** Four areas in which pubocervical fascia can break or separate—4 defects.

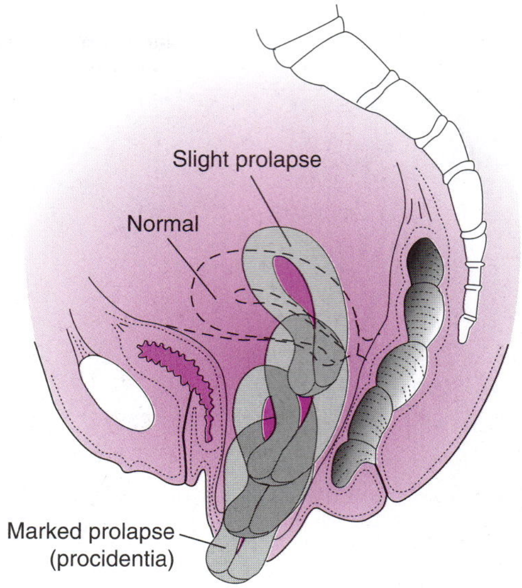

▲ **Figure 42–10.** Prolapse of the uterus.

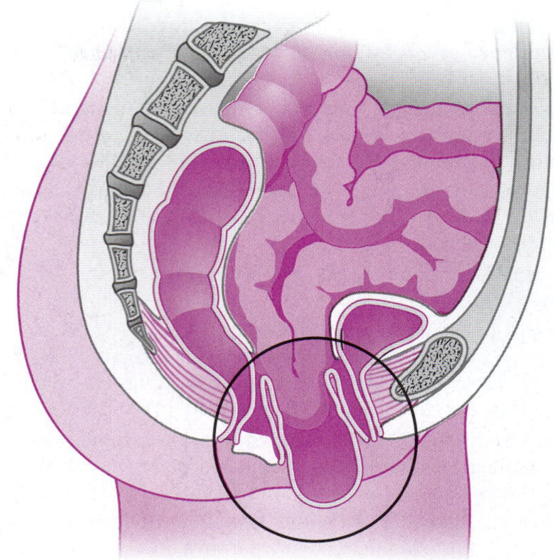

▲ **Figure 42–11.** Enterocele and prolapsed uterus.

Apical Prolapse

ESSENTIALS OF DIAGNOSIS

- **Uterine prolapse** is shown in Figure 42–10.
- **Vaginal vault prolapse** (posthysterectomy)
- **Enterocele** describes an apical vaginal wall defect in which bowel is contained within the prolapsed segment (Fig. 42–11). Generally occurs in posthysterectomy women, but can occur with the uterus in situ.

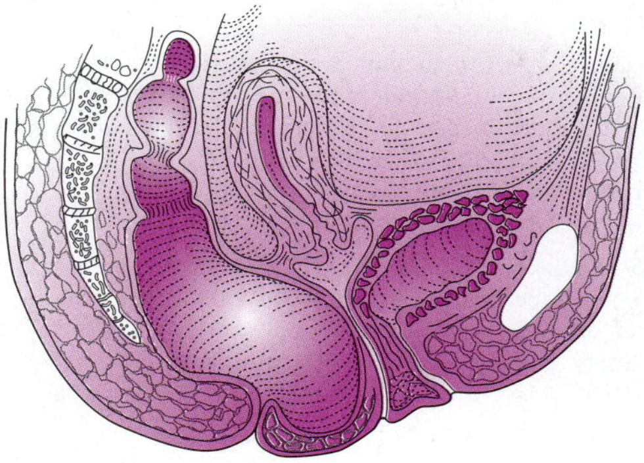

▲ **Figure 42–12.** Posterior vaginal prolapse.

Posterior Vaginal Wall Prolapse

ESSENTIALS OF DIAGNOSIS

- **Posterior vaginal wall prolapse** describes a posterior vaginal wall defect. It is also known as a rectocele (Figs. 42–12 and 42–13).

Description and Staging of Pelvic Organ Prolapse

Two general classifications are used to describe and document the severity of pelvic organ prolapse. The most current system employs objective measurements from fixed anatomic points. The Pelvic Organ Prolapse Quantification

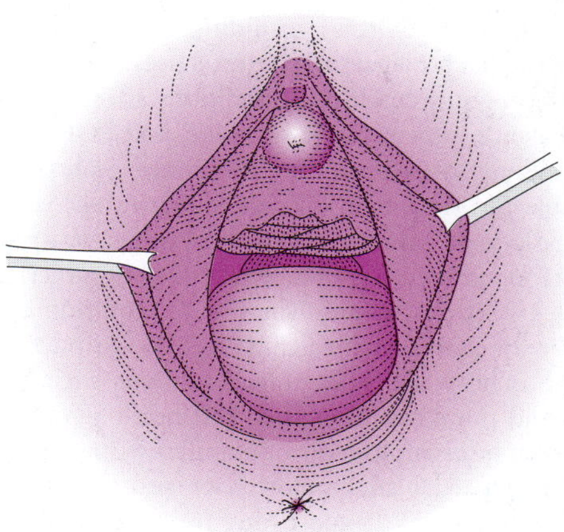

▲ **Figure 42–13.** Posterior vaginal prolapse, known as rectocele.

(POP-Q) system standardizes terminology of female pelvic organ prolapse. This is accepted as the most objective method for quantifying prolapse as it provides a more precise description of the anatomy. This descriptive system contains a series of site-specific measurements of vaginal and perineal anatomy. Prolapse in each segment is evaluated and measured relative to the hymen, which is a fixed anatomic landmark that can be consistently identified. The anatomic position of the 6 defined points for measurement should be in centimeters above the hymen (negative number) or centimeters beyond the hymen (positive number). The plane at the level of the hymen is defined as 0 (Fig. 42–14 and Table 42–10). Stages are assigned according to the most severe portion of the prolapse when the full extent of the protrusion has been demonstrated. An ordinal system is used for measurements of different points along the vaginal canal that facilitates communication among clinicians and enables objective tracking of surgical results. The POP-Q system has generally replaced the "1/2 way" system designed by Baden and Walker.

A better understanding of the pathophysiology of the pelvic supportive defects, their causes, and clinical presentations allows the individualization of the therapy most likely to successfully affect long-term outcome for each patient. Because POP is a disease impacting the quality of life, obtaining a detailed symptom history is an essential starting point.

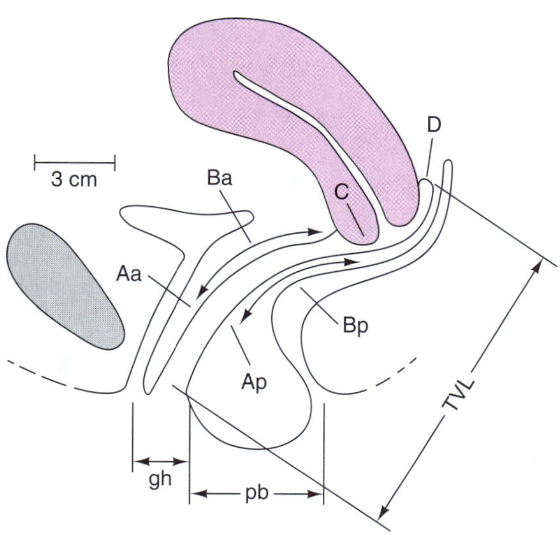

▲ **Figure 42–14.** Six sites (points *Aa, Ba, C, D, Bp,* and *Ap*), genital hiatus (*gh*), perineal body (*pb*), and total vaginal length (*TVL*) used for pelvic organ quantitation. (Reproduced with permission from Bump RC, Mattiasson A, Bø K, et al. The standardization of terminology of female pelvic organ prolapse and pelvic floor dysfunction. *Am J Obstet Gynecol* 1996;175:10–17.)

Table 42–10. Staging of pelvic organ prolapse.

Stage 0	No prolapse is demonstrated. Points Aa, Ap, Ba, and Bp are all at -3 cm and either point C or D is between -TVL (total vaginal length) cm and -(TVL-2) cm (ie, the quantitation value for point C or D is ≤-[TVL-2] cm).
Stage I	The criteria for stage 0 are not met, but the most distal portion of the prolapse is >1 cm above the level of the hymen (ie, its quantitation value is <-1 cm).
Stage II	The most distal portion of the prolapse is ≤1 cm proximal to or distal to the plane of the hymen (ie, its quantitation value is ≥1 cm but ≤+1 cm).
Stage III	The most distal portion of the prolapse is >1 cm below the plane of the hymen but protrudes no further than 2 cm less than the TVL in centimeters (ie, its quantitation value is >+1 cm but <+[TVL-2] cm).
Stage IV	Essentially, complete eversion of the total length of the lower genital tract is demonstrated. The distal portion of the prolapse protrudes to at least (TVL-2) cm (ie, its quantitation value is ≥+[TVL-2] cm). In most instances, the leading edge of stage IV prolapse is the cervix or vaginal cuff scar.

Reproduced, with permission, from Bump RC, Mattiasson A, Bø K, et al. The standardization of terminology of female pelvic organ prolapse and pelvic floor dysfunction. *Am J Obstet Gynecol* 1996;175:10–17.

General Considerations

Anterior and posterior vaginal relaxation, as well as incompetence of the perineum, often accompanies prolapse of the uterus. Large anterior vaginal prolapse is more common than posterior vaginal prolapse because the bladder is more easily carried downward than is the rectum. Before menopause, the prolapsed uterus hypertrophies and is engorged and flaccid. After the menopause, the uterus atrophies. In procidentia, the vaginal mucosa thickens and cornifies, coming to resemble skin.

ESSENTIALS OF DIAGNOSIS

The symptoms of POP are in general not unique to any particular vaginal defect. Often the symptoms are a reflection of only the most prominent point of prolapse. Most women become symptomatic only when the prolapse nears the vaginal opening. A critical concept is that the functional complaints may not always relate to the anatomic findings.

Symptoms of POP include:

- Sensation of vaginal fullness, pressure, heaviness, "something falling out"
- Sensation of "sitting on a ball"

- Discomfort in the vaginal area
- Presence of a soft, reducible mass bulging into the vagina and distending through vaginal introitus
- With straining or coughing, there is increased bulging and descent of the vaginal wall.
- Back pain and pelvic pain are often also associated with POP. It is important in women with these complaints to investigate other causes, as a direct link in mild to moderate prolapse is unproven.
- Urinary symptoms are also common:
  - Feeling of incomplete emptying of the bladder
  - Stress incontinence
  - Urinary frequency
  - Urinary hesitancy
  - Perhaps a need to push the bladder up in order to void (splinting)
  - Patients with advanced prolapse may have "potential" stress urinary incontinence. A condition in which underlying urinary incontinence is masked by kinking of the urethra and causing functional continence.

Defecatory symptoms may also occur, more commonly in posterior vaginal prolapse. The sense is one of incomplete emptying, need to strain, or manually splint in the vagina or on the perineal body (space between vagina and anus) in order to defecate. The history may include prolonged, excessive use of laxatives or frequent enemas. Other nonspecific symptoms such as low back pain, dyspareunia, or even fecal and gas incontinence may be reported.

Symptoms of sexual function may also be elicited. Coital laxity or a sense of feeling "loose" may be reported. Avoiding intercourse as a consequence of embarrassment may occur. Attention to this aspect of a woman's symptoms is especially critical if any surgical intervention is considered.

Pathogenesis

For pelvic organ prolapse, proven risk factors include age, increasing parity, obesity, and history of pelvic surgery, specifically hysterectomy. Additionally, certain lifestyle or disease conditions can promote the development of POP. Chronic coughing from lung disease and straining from chronic constipation, for example, may increase the pressures on the pelvic floor. Acting as a constant piston, driving forces exerted onto the pelvic support tissues can cause herniation of the vaginal walls. In a similar manner, occupational activity requiring repetitive heavy lifting (eg, environmental service workers or care providers of the elderly) may promote the development of POP with this daily insult of frequent pelvic pressure.

Furthermore, menopausal status, physical debilitation, and even neurologic decline can contribute to the development of POP. Yet even with a multitude of risk factors, certain women are predisposed to developing POP. As prolapse has been demonstrated in women with no identifiable risk factors, the inherent quality of a woman's connective tissue plays a large role in the susceptibility to the development of prolapse and related conditions. Investigating the genotype, consistency, and composition of the endopelvic "fascial" tissues and the interplay of enzymatic remodeling is an area of intense interest and current research.

Parity has long been recognized as a prime risk factor for the development of POP. Not surprisingly, it is also strongly associated with anal and urinary incontinence as well. Parity is clearly associated with POP, as case-controlled studies show vaginal parity as an independent risk factor with a 3-fold increased risk for POP among parous women compared with nullipara controls. This risk increases up to 4.5-fold with more than 2 vaginal deliveries. The question of whether it is the pregnancy, the size of the baby, or the mode of delivery that plays the largest role in the development of POP is still not clear. During labor, as the vertex descends through the vagina, the physical forces on the pelvic tissues can be severe. The muscles, viscera, connective tissue, and nerves are all potentially susceptible to injury. Forces of compression and stretching combine to injure pelvic-floor nerves, leading to ischemia and neurapraxia. Myofascial fibers can be disrupted or torn because of distention of the fetal head and body. When tissues are injured, the body will repair them. Factors impairing adequate tissue repair and wound healing may also play an as yet undetermined role in the development of POP.

Clinical Findings

A. Physical Examination

Examination for pelvic organ prolapse should begin in the dorsal lithotomy position. Inspection of the vulva and perineum should focus on evaluation of vulvar architecture and the presence of pressure ulceration or erosions or other skin lesions. Epithelial skin lesions, particularly in the elderly, should be biopsied.

At first, with the patient at rest, the labia should be separated and any prolapse noted (Figs. 42–8 and 42–13). Examination of the patient with vaginal prolapse reveals a relaxed and open genital hiatus with a thin-walled, rather smooth, bulging mass. Vaginal rugae are normally present. A loss of rugation denotes disruption of the connective tissue attachment below the epithelium.

During evaluation for urinary incontinence, a stress test is performed at this initial portion of the examination. The patient should be asked to cough forcefully, and any loss of urine is noted.

For prolapse assessment, when using the POP-Q system, the genital hiatus, perineal body, and vaginal length can be recorded. (Use of a wooden PAP spatula and tape measure can be helpful.) Vaginal support can then be assessed with strain (cough or Valsalva's maneuver), and the point of maximal protrusion should be noted in centimeters relative to the hymen and recorded. A speculum can also be used to "usher" the prolapse out during straining. This is also the most effective way to evaluate uterocervical support. In posthysterectomy patients, the cuff can often be visualized by the presence of "dimples" in the vaginal epithelium at the apex. Discriminate examination of the vaginal walls using the posterior blade of a Graves' speculum or Sims' retractor should then be used to evaluate the anterior and posterior walls separately, again noting the point of maximal prolapse during strain. For evaluation of the anterior wall, compress the posterior wall and have the patient strain. For evaluation of the posterior wall, elevate the anterior wall and have the patient strain. Complete examination should also include a rectovaginal palpation. In this way, one can evaluate for the presence of concurrent enterocele in addition to a rectocele. The septal defect may involve only the lower third of the posterior vaginal wall, but it often happens that the entire length of the rectovaginal septum is thinned out. The finger in the rectum confirms sacculation into the vagina. A deep pocket into the perineal body may be noted, so that on apposition of the finger in the rectum and the thumb on the outside, the perineal body seems to consist of nothing but skin and rectal wall.

Assessment of anal sphincter tone should also be performed both at rest and with squeeze contraction. The presence of perianal lesions or hemorrhoids should be noted.

If during examination the prolapse is not able to be reproduced based on symptoms, examination with the woman in the standing position should be performed. With the patient facing the seated examiner, knees slightly bent, and with strain, prolapse not demonstrable in the supine position because of poor Valsalva's maneuver can often be confirmed in the upright position.

Assessment of the pelvic floor strength is accomplished by vaginal or rectovaginal palpation of the levator ani musculature. Within 2 to 3 cm from the hymen, the bulk of the pubococcygeus component of the levator ani muscle can be palpated. The patient should be asked to contract the muscle, and the tone, symmetry, and duration of contraction should be recorded. This portion of the examination is often a valuable time to provide feedback to the patient about the volitional ability to contract the pelvic floor muscles. If the patient's ability to identify and contract the muscles is inadequate, the examiner may facilitate isolation of the proper muscles using verbal cues and manual feedback.

Evaluation of urinary function is also important in patients with POP. This is most germane in patients with large anterior vaginal defects. With prolapse of the anterior vagina, the bladder and urethra may herniate into the vagina. The urethra can bend and kink as it is fixed distally at the level of the pubourethral ligament. This "kinking" can alter normal voiding function in 2 fundamental ways. First, it will increase outflow resistance and impair normal emptying. After voiding, simple catheterization or ultrasonographic measure should be performed and the residual volume measured. Although not standardized, postvoid residual volumes greater than 100 mL are considered elevated and may indicate abnormal voiding and require referral for more sophisticated testing.

The second way urethral kinking can impact voiding is by masking underlying stress urinary incontinence. With increased outflow resistance, functional continence is created. Reduction of the prolapse during examination can be performed (elevation of anterior segment with a pessary, ring forceps, or speculum). The patient strains/coughs and the presence of urinary loss confirms the condition of SUI. This is termed **stress incontinence on prolapse reduction** and may be addressed with an anti-incontinence procedure at the same time if surgery is offered for POP.

B. Imaging Studies

In general, a complete discriminative gynecologic examination is all that is necessary to accurately assess pelvic organ prolapse. In certain cases, further diagnostic studies can be used.

Recent advances in radiologic medicine have allowed assessment of the pelvic floor with sonography and MRI. Despite newer techniques, intravenous pyelogram or computed tomography urogram still hold great value, as they are simple and safe methods to visualize the urinary tract. They can be used to evaluate the bladder and ureters. The course of the ureters can be identified preoperatively if obstruction caused by pelvic mass or scarring is suspected. These imaging tests can be used to evaluate for fistulae, congenital anomalies, or suspected damage as a result of operative injury. However, they lack sensitivity in imaging the pelvic floor and its associated defects, do not yield much information regarding vaginal support and pelvic floor musculature, and lack dynamic capabilities.

Ultrasound techniques can be an important tool to the urogynecologist. Compared with other radiologic techniques, ultrasound is noninvasive and inexpensive and does not require contrast media. Its main disadvantage is that the quality of the study depends heavily on the skill of the operator. When performed transabdominally, transvaginally, or transperineally and combined with Doppler or endoluminal transducers, the bladder, urethra, and surrounding structures can be visualized with detail.

1. Videocystourethrography (VCUG)—VCUG combines a fluoroscopic voiding cystourethrogram with simultaneous recording of intravesical, intraurethral, and intra-abdominal pressure and urine flow rate. The contrast in the bladder allows dynamic evaluation of the bladder and bladder support.

2. Magnetic Resonance Imaging—MRI has evolved into an important tool for the evaluation of the pelvic floor. It is an ideal modality because its resolution of soft tissues is superior to that of other radiologic techniques. The capability to image in multiple planes is also an advantage, particularly when visualizing the complex 3-dimensional relationships of the pelvic floor. Dynamic straining can be used to demonstrate prolapse under pressure and is often useful in surgical planning. As this modality becomes less costly and techniques evolve to allow evaluation of patients in the upright position, the information provided by MRI will be invaluable in increasing our knowledge and understanding of functional pelvic support.

Differential Diagnosis

Prolapse of the vagina is generally a straightforward diagnosis. However, less common disease entities may present as bulges in the vagina. Tumors of the urethra and bladder are often more indurated and fixed than is anterior vaginal prolapse.

A large urethral diverticulum may look and feel like an anterior vaginal prolapse but usually is more focal and may be painful. With urethral diverticulum, compression may express some purulent material from the urethral meatus. Anterolateral defects can represent embryologic remnants such as a Gartner's duct cyst.

Skene's and Bartholin's glands can become obstructed and enlarge to form cysts or abscesses. Rarely, hemangiomas will present as vaginal bulging, although they will often have characteristic purple discoloration on the overlying epithelium.

Soft tumors (lipoma, leiomyoma, sarcoma, myofibroblastoma) of the vagina are more fixed and are nonreducible.

Cervical tumors—as well as endometrial tumors (pedunculated myoma or endometrial polyps)—if prolapsed through a dilated cervix and presenting in the lower third of the vagina, may be confused with mild or moderate uterine prolapse. Myomas or polyps may coexist with prolapse of the uterus and cause unusual symptoms.

Despite the variety of possibilities, the history and physical findings in vaginal or uterine prolapse are so characteristic that diagnosis is usually not a challenge.

Prevention

Prevention of genital prolapse is the focus of much debate. Antepartum, intrapartum, and postpartum exercises, especially those designed to strengthen the levator and perineal muscle groups (Kegel), often help improve or maintain pelvic support. Obesity, chronic cough, straining, and traumatic deliveries must be corrected or avoided. Estrogen therapy after menopause may help to maintain the tone and vitality of pelvic musculofascial tissues; however, evidence is lacking to support its benefit to prevent or postpone the appearance of anterior vaginal prolapse and other forms of relaxation.

Treatment

Pelvic organ prolapse, except in rare situations, is a condition that impacts only the quality of life. Consequently, the extent and type of treatment should reflect and be commensurate with the degree of impact on the quality of life the patient experiences. Patient perception is also a critical component, and self-image and conceptual discomfort are relevant to any discussion of therapy. Common reasons to intervene are when function is impaired because of the prolapse. Anterior prolapse can contribute to urinary incontinence or, when severe, urinary obstruction. Bulging vaginal epithelium can come into contact with undergarments and clothing and over time develop pressure sores and erosions. A posterior vaginal defect can become so large that fecal evacuation is difficult, or the patient finds it necessary to manually reduce the posterior vaginal wall into the vagina to expedite expulsion of feces. Mobility can be impaired by a large prolapse. All of the preceding complaints are reasons to discuss surgical repair.

Chronic decubitus ulceration of the vaginal epithelium may develop in procidentia. Urinary tract infection may occur with prolapse because of anterior vaginal prolapse, and partial ureteral obstruction with hydronephrosis may occur in procidentia. Hemorrhoids result from straining to overcome constipation. Small-bowel obstruction from a deep enterocele is rare.

A. Conservative Measures

The patient with a small or moderate-sized POP requires reassurance that the pressure symptoms are not the result of a serious condition and that, in the absence of urinary retention or severe skin pressure ulceration, no serious illness will result. The natural history of POP is such that it either will stay the same or progress. There is some evidence that a small subset of patients may experience regression of the prolapse after menopause or postpartum if the prolapse is noted shortly after delivery. Reassurance and observation of prolapse should be encouraged in the absence of symptoms.

If prolapse presents in the reproductive years, surgical correction of POP is rarely indicated in women who are not family complete. If the young woman does present with significant symptoms related to POP or with a disturbing degree of urinary incontinence, then temporary medical measures may provide adequate relief until she has completed childbearing, whereupon a definitive operative procedure can be accomplished.

1. Pessary—Pessary use in selected patients may provide adequate relief of symptoms. There are a variety of available pessary types and sizes that allow for individualization of therapy (Fig. 42–15). For the most common type of POP of the anterior or apical segment, a ring pessary is usually a sensible starting point for treatment. For the patient with

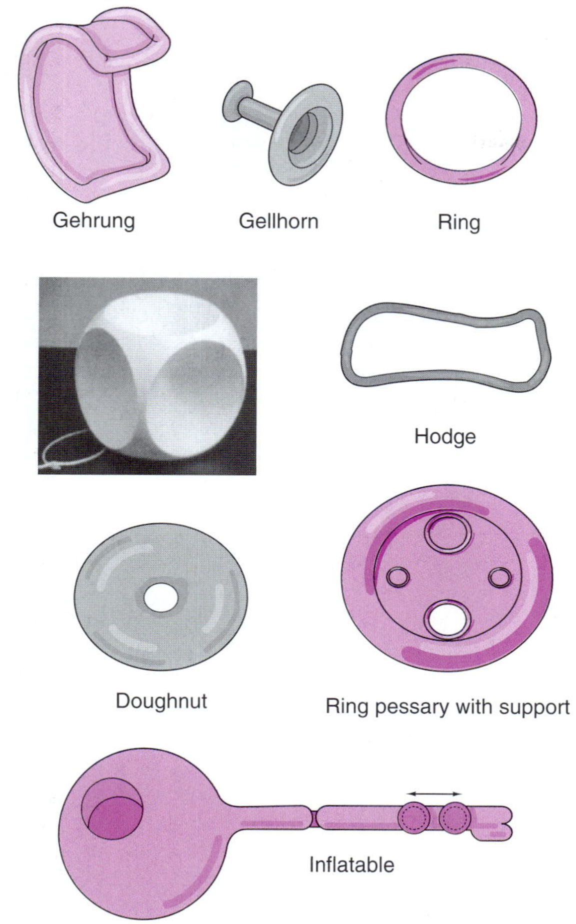

▲ **Figure 42–15.** Types of pessaries.

complicating medical factors who is a poor operative risk, the temporary use of a vaginal pessary may provide relief of symptoms until her general condition has improved.

Prolonged use of pessaries, if improperly managed, may lead to pressure necrosis and vaginal ulceration. The vaginal pessary is a prosthesis of ancient lineage, now made of rubber, plastics, and silicone-based material, often with a metal band or spring frame. Many types have been devised, but fewer than a dozen are basically unique and specifically helpful.

Pessaries are principally used to support the uterus and vaginal walls. They are effective because they reduce vaginal prolapse and increase the tautness of the pelvic floor structures. Little or no leverage is involved. Either by placement behind the pubic bone and perineal body or by filling the vaginal vault, pessaries remain in place to hold up the prolapsing vaginal walls or uterus. In most cases, adequate support anteriorly and a reasonably good perineal body are required; otherwise, the pessary may slip from behind the symphysis and extrude from the vagina.

Pessaries are contraindicated in acute genital tract infections and in adherent retroposition of the uterus.

Several pessary types are available:

- A **ring pessary** with or without support provides relief of uterine prolapse or anterior vaginal prolapse.
- **Gellhorn pessaries** are uniquely shaped like a collar button and provide a ringlike platform for the cervix or apex. The pessary is stabilized by a stem that rests on the perineum. These pessaries are used to correct marked prolapse when the perineal body is reasonably adequate.
- The **doughnut** is made of soft rubber or silicone, and this type of pessary provides support for severe uterine prolapse or vault prolapse.
- The **Gehrung pessary** resembles 2 firm letter *U*s attached by crossbars. It rests in the vagina with the cervix cradled between the long arms; this arches the anterior or posterior vaginal wall and helps reduce the vaginal prolapse.
- The **Hodge pessary (Smith-Hodge, or Smith and other variations)** is an elongated, curved ovoid. One end is placed behind the symphysis and the other in the posterior vaginal fornix. The anterior bow is curved to avoid the urethra; the cervix rests within the larger, posterior bow. This type of pessary is used to hold the uterus in place after it has been repositioned.
- The **inflatable pessary** functions much like a doughnut pessary. The ball valve is moved up and down; when the ball is in the down position, air inflates the pessary; when in the up position, the air is sealed in and inflation is maintained.
- The **cube** is a flexible rubber cube with suction cups on each of its 6 sides that adhere to the vaginal walls. This is useful in women with severe prolapse. However, vaginal erosions are common and can be severe. Frequent monitoring initially to identify pressure ulcers is critical.

A. Fitting of pessaries—Medicine is known as both an art and a science. Pessary fitting (Fig. 42–16) falls into the art category. Pessaries that are too large cause irritation and ulceration; those that are too small may not stay in place and may protrude.

In general, fitting a pessary is very much a trial-and-error endeavor. Once a type is selected based on the defects in the vaginal anatomy and on symptoms, sizing is best done with an office sizing set. This task is somewhat complicated as each pessary has its own measurement system, but familiarity with each pessary over time simplifies this task. The pessary should be lubricated and inserted with its widest dimension in the oblique diameter of the vagina to avoid painful distention at the introitus. With a finger of the opposite hand, depress the perineum to widen the introitus. Each pessary type has an optimal method for insertion.

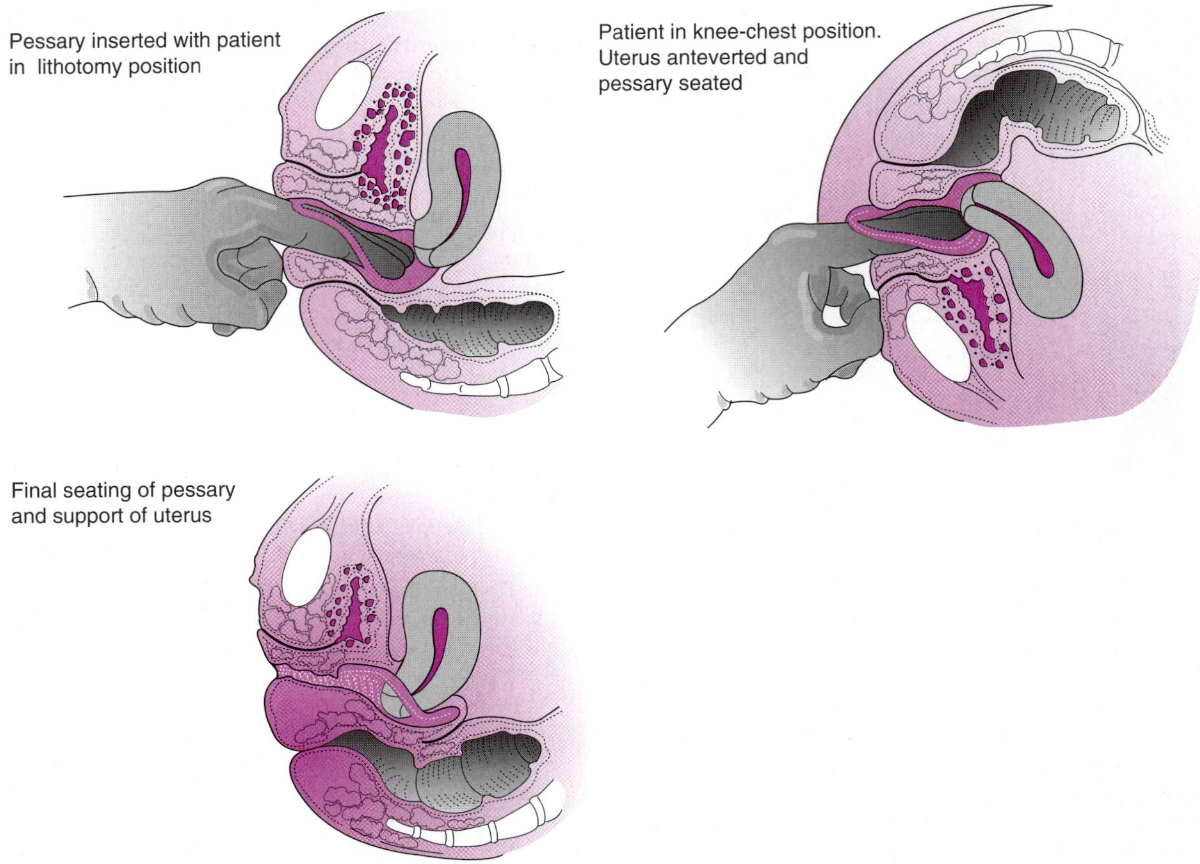

▲ **Figure 42–16.** Insertion of Hodge-type pessary.

Once a pessary is in place, the forefinger should pass easily between the sides of the frame and the vaginal wall at any point; if it cannot, the pessary is too large. After the pessary has been fitted, the patient should be asked to stand, walk, and squat to determine whether pain occurs or whether the pessary becomes displaced. The patient should be shown how to withdraw the pessary if it becomes displaced or is uncomfortable and cautioned that a contraceptive vaginal diaphragm cannot be used while a vaginal pessary is in place.

During the initial period of pessary wear, any discomfort, bleeding, or disturbance in defecation or urinary function should be reported immediately. The patient should be examined 1–2 weeks after insertion to inspect for the presence of pressure and inflammatory or allergic reactions. A repeat exam in 4 weeks can be done; then visits should be done at 3- to 6-month intervals to assess for continued proper fit and to evaluate for vaginal erosion and inflammation as a result of pessary use. For women who are unable to remove and clean the pessary themselves, the pessary should be changed approximately every 2–3 months.

The pessary should be maintained with an acidic pH gel such as Trimo-San (Milex Products, Chicago, IL). In postmenopausal patients, topical estrogen can vitalize the vaginal mucosa and reduce ulceration. An estrogen-containing ring can also be used in conjunction by "piggybacking" the ring with the pessary and then changing it every 3 months.

Vaginal pessaries are not curative of prolapse, but they may be used for months or years for palliation with proper supervision.

A neglected pessary may cause fistulas or promote genital infections, but there is no clear evidence that cancer occurs as a result of wearing a modern pessary.

2. Pelvic Floor Muscle Exercises—In some patients, improvement of pressure symptoms and of urinary control may be obtained by using pelvic floor muscle exercises, also referred to as Kegel exercises. These exercises are aimed to tighten and strengthen the pubococcygeus muscles. Evidence strongly supports use of Kegel exercises as first-line management in the treatment of urinary and fecal incontinence; however, they may also have some benefit in the relief of POP symptoms. Kegel exercises work best after specific instruction on how to perform them as most women do not perform them either correctly or in optimal fashion without supervised instruction and feedback.

3. Estrogens—In postmenopausal women, local estrogen therapy for a number of months may improve the tone, quality, and vascularity of the musculofascial supports. It is available in cream, parvule, and ring insert forms. With counseling, local estrogen can be offered to all postmenopausal women to reduce urogenital atrophy. For postmenopausal patients with exposed prolapse, who are awaiting surgery, or using a pessary, local therapy should be recommended to promote healthy epithelium particularly in preparation for surgery.

B. Surgical Measures

1. Anterior Vaginal Prolapse

A. ANTERIOR VAGINAL COLPORRHAPHY—Anterior vaginal colporrhaphy is the most common surgical treatment for anterior vaginal prolapse (Fig. 42–17). Traditional anterior colporrhaphy (anterior repair) is a vaginal approach that involves dissecting the vaginal epithelium from the underlying fibromuscular connective tissue and bladder, and then plicating the vaginal muscularis across the midline. Excess vaginal epithelium may be excised and the wound closed. Recurrence of anterior prolapse as high as 52% has been reported and has always been a limitation of all reparative procedures. Modifications involving permanent suture material and graft materials have been introduced in the hope of increasing durability.

B. PARAVAGINAL REPAIR—The etiology of the anterior vaginal prolapse has been much debated, beginning with White in 1912. The repair of defects in the anterior vaginal segment has traditionally been done by midline plication. An alternative method based on the anatomic observations by Richardson and colleagues advocates identification of the specific defect in the pubocervical fascia underlying the anterior vaginal epithelium and repairing the discrete breaks (Fig. 42–9). This relationship and a lack of correction of apical defects may help explain why no single operative repair should be universally applied to patients with anterior vaginal wall defects and why traditional repair has resulted in high recurrence rates.

Paravaginal repair is performed for anterior vaginal prolapse that is confirmed to be a result of detachment of the pubocervical fascia from its lateral attachment at the arcus tendineus fascia pelvis (white line). This defect can be unilateral or bilateral. It can be confirmed preoperatively by noting loss of the lateral sulci and lack of rugation over the epithelium along the base of the bladder and elongation to the anterior vaginal wall. Clinically, vaginal examination using a speculum reveals a preponderance of the prolapse lateralized to 1 side as the speculum is withdrawn. In addition, a ring forceps can be used by gently exerting anterior traction along the vaginal sulci. If the defect is reduced, then the defect is consistent with a paravaginal defect and can be approached with a paravaginal repair technique.

The surgery can be performed either abdominally or vaginally. Both require identification of the white line and placement of serial sutures from the medial portion of the pubocervical fascia to the lateral side-wall at the level of the white line as it runs from the ischial spine over the obturator

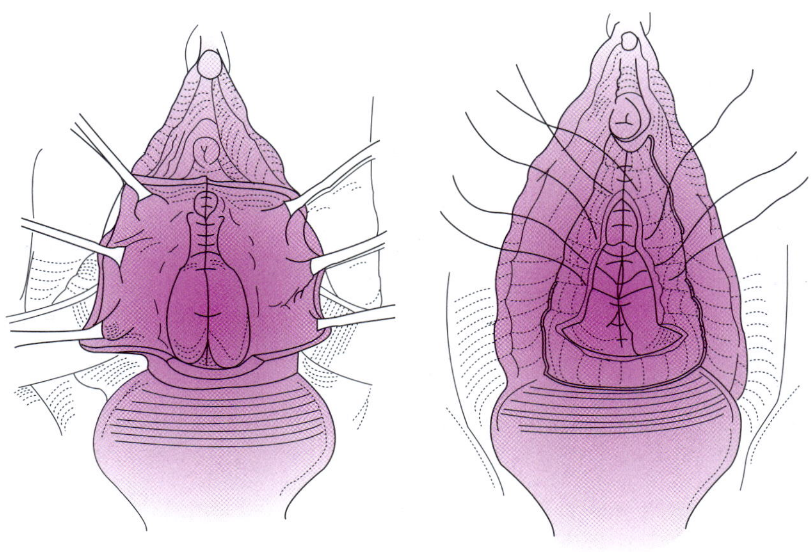

▲ **Figure 42–17.** Repair of anterior vaginal prolapse.

internus muscle to the posterior and inferior aspect of the pubic bone on the ipsilateral side. Reapproximation of the detached pubocervical fascia should reduce the anterior vaginal prolapse. This procedure can be done with other reconstructive procedures in the vagina as well as surgery to alleviate incontinence. Short-term surgical studies have shown good results, but no long-term or comparative data exist for this repair.

A transabdominal approach to the paravaginal repair may be elected to correct the anterior vaginal prolapse when an abdominal approach is necessary for other pelvic conditions such as abdominal hysterectomy, adnexal surgery, or, most commonly, with sacral colpopexy for apical prolapse repair.

2. Posterior Vaginal Prolapse—The traditional repair (Fig. 42–18) involves posterior midline incision, often high, to the level of the posterior fornix. The vaginal epithelium is separated off the underlying fibromuscular layer and endopelvic fascia. This fibromuscular layer is then serially plicated across the midline. Some describe adding levator muscle plication as well. No attempt at identifying specific fascial defects is made.

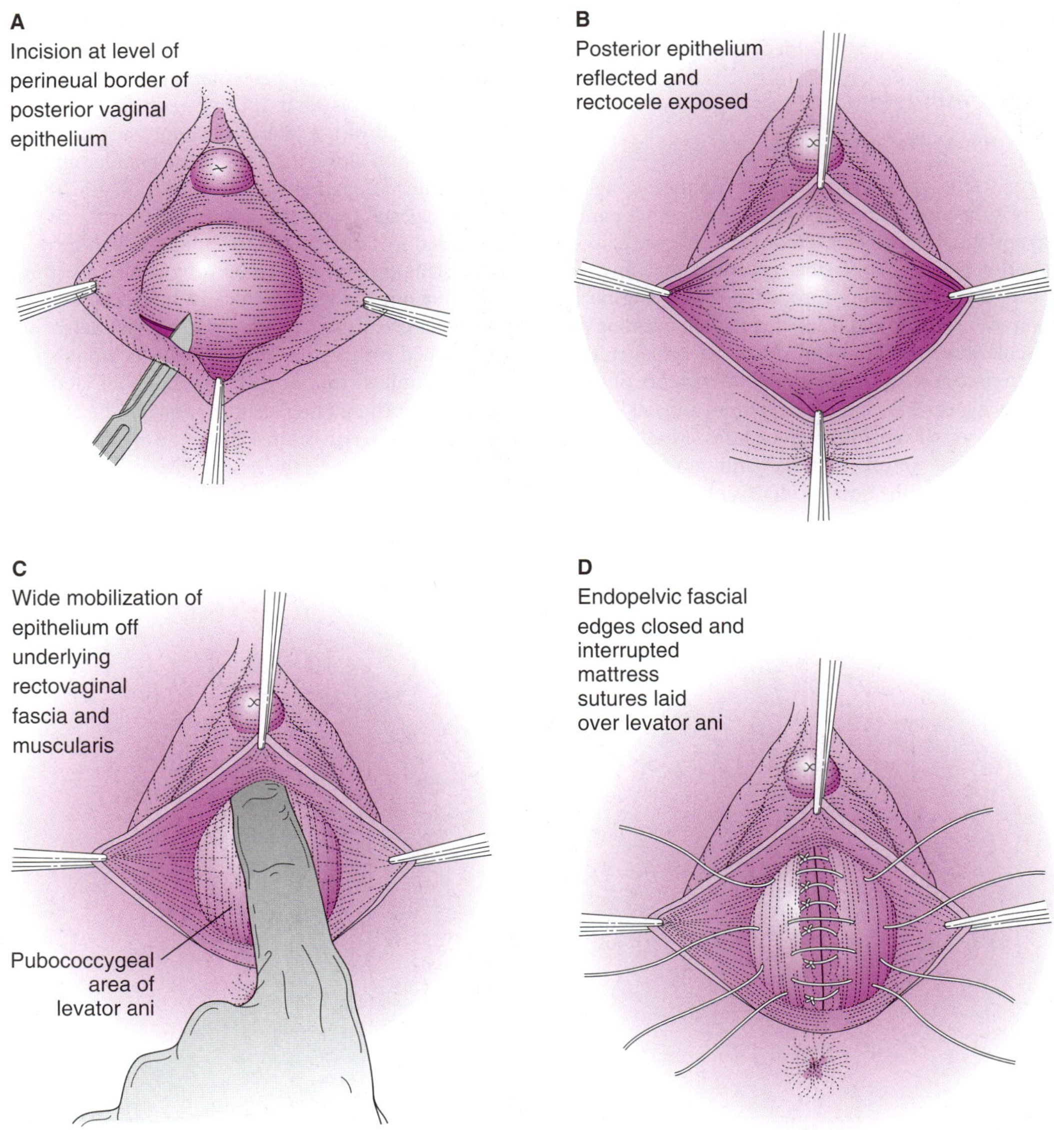

▲ **Figure 42–18.** Repair of rectocele.

An alternate method of posterior vaginal defect (rectocele) repair relies on the identification of discrete defects in the rectovaginal fascia (Fig. 42–19). The surgeon inserts a finger of the nondominant hand into the rectum to inspect the rectovaginal fascia for defects. The rectal wall is brought forward to distinguish the uncovered muscularis (fascial defect) from the muscularis that was covered by the smooth semitransparent rectal vaginal septum. The defects are then repaired with interrupted sutures to plicate over the rectal wall. In this manner, the isolated defects are repaired, and the functional anatomy is optimally restored. Notably absent is any effort to plicate the levator ani musculature, as this often results in a bandlike stricture over the posterior wall—a likely cause of dyspareunia. Randomized trials do not support improved outcomes using this technique.

Perineorrhaphy is generally combined with posterior vaginal repairs. This procedure is principally aimed at restoring the perineal body and reducing the vaginal outlet (genital hiatus) to more normal caliber. Reapproximation of the superficial transverse perinei muscle and the bulbocavernosus muscle rebuilds the perineum and lengthens the distance between vaginal opening and anal verge.

A. Postoperative factors—The prognosis after vaginal repair is excellent in the absence of a subsequent pregnancy or comparable factors (eg, constipation, obesity, large pelvic tumors, bronchitis, bronchiectasis, heavy manual labor) that increase intra-abdominal pressure. The recurrence of the POP is probable when a specific defect of pelvic supports has been overlooked or ignored; in such cases, subsequent progression of the overlooked site may itself lead to new symptoms or even to disruption of the previously repaired segment.

Postoperative avoidance of straining, coughing, and strenuous activity is advisable. Careful instruction about

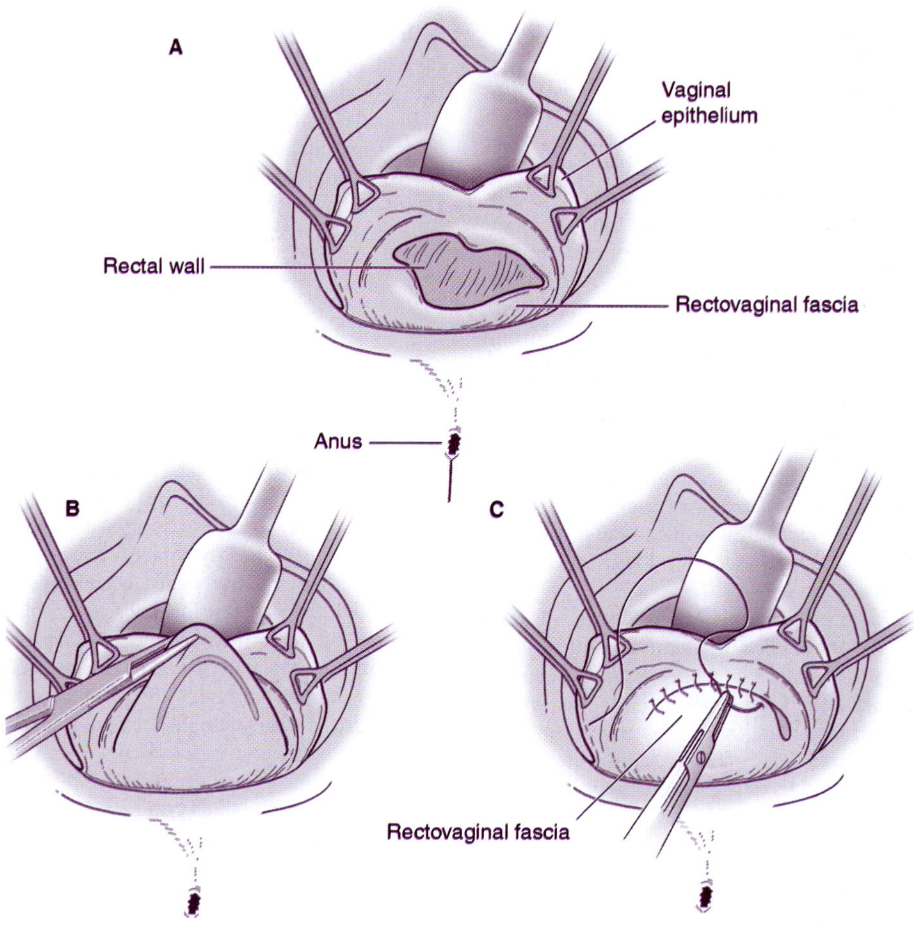

▲ **Figure 42–19.** Site-specific repair of posterior vaginal prolapse. **A:** Dissection below vaginal epithelium exposes defect in rectovaginal (RV) fascia. **B:** Reflection of detached RV fascia. **C:** Restoration of the continuity of RV fascia by reapproximation with delayed absorbable suture.

diet to avoid constipation, about intake of fluids, and about the use of stool-softening laxatives and lubricating suppositories is necessary to ensure durable integrity of the rectocele repair.

B. Mesh augmentation in vaginal surgery—Efforts to reduce prolapse recurrence rates have ushered in a dramatic increase in the use of mesh for vaginal repairs. Current evidence would only support the use of synthetic mesh to augment anterior vaginal repairs but at the expense of increased rates of complications. Clinically significant rates of vaginal erosions, painful intercourse, and pelvic pain have all been reported with the use of permanent mesh materials.

3. Apical vaginal repair—Prolapse of the vaginal apex includes:

- Uterine prolapse
- Posthysterectomy vaginal cuff prolapse
- Enterocele

All of the preceding clinical conditions indicate a failure of apical support. The procedures used to address surgical repair require knowledge of the specific support structures available to reestablish normal anatomy.

Uterine prolapse is almost always accompanied by some degree of enterocele, and, as the degree of uterine descent progresses, the size of the hernial sac increases. Similarly, posthysterectomy prolapse of the vaginal vault may be the result of poor repair and identification of cuff support structure at the time of hysterectomy or may develop as a result of an enterocele that was overlooked (not repaired). Consequently, it is critical to always address apical cuff support at the time of surgery if a hysterectomy is being performed. Less common, after hysterectomy, the enterocele is located anterior to the vaginal vault, where it may be easily confused with typical anterior vaginal prolapse.

Apical vaginal repair may be accomplished transabdominally or transvaginally. A review of vaginal operations includes, among others, sacrospinous ligament suspension, iliococcygeal fixation, and high uterosacral ligament suspension (high McCall culdoplasty).

Because the normal vaginal axis is directed some distance posteriorly (almost horizontally when the patient is in an erect position) over the levator plate, operative correction by any means, whether by the vaginal or the abdominal route, should restore a normal vaginal axis. This is accomplished by suspension of the vaginal apex far back on the uterosacral ligaments, the presacral fascia, or the sacrospinous ligaments.

A. Sacrospinous ligament fixation—A popular method of vaginal vault suspension is that of unilateral or bilateral fixation to the sacrospinous ligament. In this technique, the vaginal epithelium is separated from the rectovaginal tissues. Perforation through the rectal pillar is accomplished by directing blunt dissection toward the ischial spine through the loose areolar tissue. After an appropriate location on the sacrospinous ligament is identified (usually 2–3 cm medial to the ischial spine), one of several techniques may be used to safely pass 2 or more permanent (or delayed absorbable) ligatures through the ligament to the submucosal apex of the vagina. Tying the sutures brings the vaginal apex to that sacrospinous ligament, and a posterior colporrhaphy is then performed (as noted previously). Closing the dead space by intermittently suturing the vaginal mucosa to the underlying reconstituted rectovaginal septum may be useful.

Vaginal vault suspension to 1 or both sacrospinous ligaments has the potential of injury to the pudendal nerve or pudendal vessels and is often technically difficult. Because gluteal and posterior leg pain is a potential complication of this procedure, particularly if the branches of the sacral plexus are disturbed by suturing deep to the ligament, the procedure requires a skilled vaginal surgeon and should be undertaken only by those familiar with the technique.

B. Iliococcygeal vaginal suspension—First described in 1962, this procedure uses the fascia overlying the iliococcygeal muscle. Although not nearly as commonly used as other procedures, this point of attachment allows reliable apical fixation without the need to gain peritoneal access. It is generally a safe procedure requiring a posterior vaginal incision in the midline with wide dissection of the overlying epithelium. Bilateral placement of permanent or delayed absorbable suture can be used.

C. Bilateral uterosacral ligament suspension—The use of the uterosacral ligaments to attach the vaginal cuff has become a re-appreciated technique in apical repairs. Several modifications of the procedure have been described since its introduction in 1938. This technique, as with the other vaginal procedures, can be done at the time of vaginal hysterectomy or to correct posthysterectomy apical cuff prolapse. After entrance into the peritoneum is complete, traction on the ipsilateral posterior vaginal wall with rectal digital examination will facilitate transperitoneal identification of the uterosacral ligament. Placement of a pair of permanent sutures in a lateral-to-medial fashion, 1 at the level of the ischial spine and another placed more cephalad, can be performed bilaterally. These sutures are then brought to the ipsilateral vaginal apices. Fixation of the cuff at this level reproduces cuff placement to the normal position of the cervicovaginal junction. Anterior vaginal repair should be performed before tying down the vaginal cuff.

A risk of this procedure is medial displacement and kinking of the ureters, which has been reported to occur in up to 11% of patients undergoing this procedure. Cystoscopic assessment of ureteral function without and with tension on the fixation sutures, before tying down the vaginal apices, is critical to identify any potential compromise intraoperatively. If ureteral flow reduction is identified, then removal of the sutures on the affected side will often restore normal function.

D. Abdominal sacrocolpopexy—Vaginal vault suspension can also be performed abdominally by attaching the vaginal cuff to the sacral promontory. Abdominal sacrocolpopexy is an excellent primary procedure for apical vaginal prolapse and enterocele and is the procedure of choice for those who are already having an abdominal approach for hysterectomy or for another indication. In this procedure, a laparotomy is performed, and the cul-de-sac and peritoneum overlying the sacrum are visualized. A window in the peritoneum over the sacral promontory is created, and 2 permanent sutures are placed through the anterior longitudinal ligament, approximately at the level of S1. The vaginal cuff is then exposed by dissecting off the overlying peritoneum. Fixation of a graft over the anterior and posterior vagina is then performed fashioning a Y-shape or 2 individual strips of graft. This Y graft is then brought posteriorly along the hollow of the sacrum and affixed to the anterior longitudinal ligament sutures overriding the sacral promontory. Avoidance of undue tension is critical to prevent postoperative dyspareunia.

Dissection and suture placement over the sacrum may introduce risk of operative hemorrhage. During placement of the sacral sutures, the nearby fragile sacral veins may be lacerated. Bleeding from these veins is difficult to control if the veins retract into the bone. Use of sterile thumbtacks to occlude these veins has been an operative technique used to stem potentially life-threatening hemorrhage.

Many different graft types have been described, as well as different methods of attaching these grafts to the vagina. Biologic grafts, however, have high failure rates when placed at the apex. Synthetic grafts are effective; however, they have erosion complication rates between 5% and 10%. As graft technologies continue to evolve, identification of the optimal graft material that maximizes durability and compatibility may materialize.

Numerous studies demonstrate this colpopexy to be highly curative of apical/uterine prolapse. Most surgeons consider the sacrocolpopexy to be the gold standard for apical repair. In the largest prospective evaluation of sacrocolpopexy outcome, the success rates are more than 95%. The procedure can also be performed laparoscopically. A prospective study evaluating outcomes of this approach in more than 100 women describe no apical recurrences and no mesh complication. Another retrospective study of 188 cases resulted in a 10% erosion rate; however, 13 of the 19 erosions occurred with concomitant hysterectomy.

The addition of robotic assistance has been introduced to facilitate the technical aspects of laparoscopic repair. To date no prospective trial exists on efficacy.

E. Obliterative vaginal operations (colpocleisis and Le Fort's operation)—These are used primarily for severe uterovaginal prolapse in elderly patients and chronically ill patients who no longer desire coital function. It has the advantage of being done with either regional or local anesthesia. These procedures are highly effective and generally well tolerated. Traction produced by the obliterating scar tissue under the bladder neck and the urethra that may actually cause or aggravate stress incontinence is associated with these operations. Closing the genital hiatus may reduce the chance of recurrence and can be achieved by performing an "extended" perineorrhaphy concomitantly (Table 42–11).

Table 42–11. Follow-up and cure rate after abdominal sacral colpopexy.

Author (Year)	Duration of Follow-Up (months)	No. of Patients	No. Cured (%)
Cowan and Morgan (1980)	≤60	39	38 (97)
Addision et al (1985)	6–126	56	54 (96)
Baker et al (1990)	1–45	51	51 (100)
Snyder and Krantz (1991)	≥6	116	108 (93)
Timmons et al (1992)	9–216	162	161 (99)
Iosif (1993)	12–120	40	39 (96)
Grunberger et al (1994)	3–91	48	45 (94)
Valatis and Stanton (1994)	3–91	41	38 (96)

Adapted and reproduced, with permission, from Walters MD, Karram MM. *Urogynecology and Reconstructive Pelvic Surgery*. 2nd ed. St. Louis, MO: Mosby; 1999.

Burrows LJ, Meyn LA, Walters MD, Weber AM. Pelvic symptoms in women with pelvic organ prolapse. *Obstet Gynecol* 2004;104(5 Pt 1):982–988. PMID: 15516388.

Fitzgerald MP, Richter HE, Siddique S, Thompson P, Zyczynski H; Ann Weber for the Pelvic Floor Disorders Network. Colpocleisis: A review. *Int Urogynecol J Pelvic Floor Dysfunct* 2006;17:261–271. PMID: 15983731.

Handa VL, Garrett E, Hendrix S, Gold E, Robbins J. Progression and remission of pelvic organ prolapse: A longitudinal study of menopausal women. *Am J Obstet Gynecol* 2004;190:27–32. PMID: 14749630.

Haylen BT, de Ridder D, Freeman RM, et al. An International Urogynecological Association (IUGA)/International Continence Society (ICS) joint report on the terminology for female pelvic floor dysfunction. *NeuroUrodyn* 2010;29:4–20. PMID: 19941278.

Luber KM, Boero S, Choe JY. The demographics of pelvic floor disorders: Current observations and future projections. *Am J Obstet Gynecol* 2001;184:1496–1501. PMID: 11408873.

Lukacz ES, Lawrence JM, Contreras R, Nager CW, Luber KM. Parity, mode of delivery, and pelvic floor disorders. *Obstet Gynecol* 2006;107:1253–1260. PMID: 16738149.

Maher C, Feiner B, Baessler K, Adams EJ, Hagen S, Glazener CM. Surgical management of pelvic organ prolapse in women. *Cochrane Database Syst Rev* 2010;CD004014. PMID: 20393938.

Morgan DM, Larson K. Uterosacral and sacrospinous ligament suspension for restoration of apical vaginal support. *Clin Obstet Gynecol* 2010;53:72–85. PMID: 20142645.

NIH State-of-the-Science Conference Statement on cesarean delivery on maternal request. *NIH Consens Sci Statements* 2006; 23:1–29. PMID: 17308552.

Nygaard IE, McCreery R, Brubaker L, et al. Abdominal sacrocolpopexy: A comprehensive review. *Obstet Gynecol* 2004;104:805–823. PMID: 15458906.

Nygaard I, Barber MD, Burgio KL, et al. Prevalence of symptomatic pelvic floor disorder in U.S. women. *JAMA* 2008;300: 1311–1316. PMID: 18799443.

The Simon Foundation. www.simonfoundation.org. Accessed March 13, 2012.

Sung VW, Hampton BS. Epidemiology of pelvic floor dysfunction. *Obstet Gynecol Clin North Am* 2009;36:421–443. PMID: 19932408.

Sexually Transmitted Diseases & Pelvic Infections

43

Gillian Mackay, MD

SEXUALLY TRANSMITTED DISEASES

The term **sexually transmitted diseases** (STDs) is used to describe disorders spread by intimate contact. Although this usually means sexual intercourse, it also includes close body contact, kissing, cunnilingus, anilingus, fellatio, mouth–breast contact, and anal intercourse. Many STDs can also be transmitted to the fetus in utero by transplacental spread or passage through the birth canal and via lactation during the neonatal period. The organisms involved are adapted to growth in the genital tract and are present in body secretions or blood. Having one STD increases the risk of coinfection with other STDs; therefore, full screening should be offered to all patients with a new STD diagnosis.

Physicians have a critical role in the prevention and treatment of STDs. The clinician's role is to understand the microbiology of STDs in order to appropriately diagnose and treat patients. Treatment is aimed at alleviating symptoms and preventing future sequelae, as well as the prevention of transmission to others and providing appropriate patient education and counseling, as the mainstay of prevention is through lifestyle and behavioral modification. Multiple cohort studies have demonstrated the protective effects of both male and female condoms in the prevention of most STDs.

Most treatment regimens detailed below are based on guidelines issued by the US Center for Disease Control and Prevention (CDC).

VULVAR LESIONS & GENITAL ULCERS

Genital herpes, syphilis, and, less commonly, chancroid are the most prevalent genital ulcerative lesions in the United States. The diagnosis is difficult to make by physical examination alone. Thus the workup for all genital ulcers should include serologic screening for syphilis, culture/antigen testing for herpes simplex virus (HSV)-1 and HSV-2, and culture for *Haemophilus ducreyi* in areas where chancroid is prevalent. More than 1 infectious etiology may be present in a single lesion.

HERPES SIMPLEX

ESSENTIALS OF DIAGNOSIS

- Most commonly caused by HSV-2 but increasingly also caused by HSV-1
- Painful genital ulcers
- Chronic, lifelong, relapsing condition
- Transmissible even in the absence of lesions
- Antivirals improve symptoms, speed healing of lesions, and may decrease asymptomatic viral shedding

Pathogenesis

Genital herpes simplex virus (HSV) is a chronic viral infection cause by 2 types of virus: HSV-1 and HSV-2. Most cases of recurrent genital herpes are caused by HSV-2, and at least 50 million persons in the United States are infected with this type of genital herpes. However, an increasing proportion of genital herpes infections in some populations (eg, young women and men who have sex with men) have been attributed to infection by HSV-1.

Most patients infected with HSV-2 have not been diagnosed with genital herpes. Many of these patients have mild or unrecognized infections but shed virus intermittently in the genital tract. As a result, the majority of genital herpes infections are transmitted by persons unaware that they have the infection or who are asymptomatic when transmission occurs.

Prevention

Counseling at the time of diagnosis is essential in order to educate the patient regarding the high probability of recurrence and the prevention of transmission to sexual partners.

Sex partners of patients with genital herpes should be evaluated and counseled. Patients should be counseled that viral shedding can occur during asymptomatic periods and that this can lead to transmission. Consistent condom use is associated with a decline in transmission of genital HSV infection. For patients with symptomatic genital HSV-2 infection and an uninfected partner, chronic suppressive therapy to reduce clinical recurrences and viral transmission should be considered. Valacyclovir (500 mg daily) is the best-studied regimen for this specific indication and offers the convenience of once-daily dosing; however, acyclovir may be a reasonable alternative.

For prevention of neonatal herpes, see Genital Herpes in Pregnancy.

Clinical Findings

A. Symptoms & Signs

The clinical diagnosis of genital herpes is often difficult or inaccurate. Classically, patients present with multiple painful vesicular or ulcerative lesions on the genitals. However, these are absent in many cases, particularly in infections caused by HSV-1. After initial infection, the virus remains dormant, but can be reactivated at a future time, which manifests as a recurrent, symptomatic episode with painful ulceration. Recurrences and subclinical shedding are much less frequent for genital HSV-1 infection than for genital HSV-2 infection.

Patients with a primary HSV infection may, in addition to painful ulceration, have multiple constitutional symptoms such as fever, headaches, and malaise.

B. Laboratory Findings

Cell culture and polymerase chain reaction (PCR) are the preferred tests for HSV in symptomatic patients. The sensitivity of viral culture is low, especially for recurrent lesions, and declines rapidly as lesions begin to heal. PCR assays for HSV DNA are more sensitive and are increasingly used. PCR is the test of choice for detecting HSV in spinal fluid for diagnosis of HSV infection of the central nervous system (CNS). Viral culture isolates should be typed to determine which type of HSV is causing the infection. Failure to detect HSV by culture or PCR does not indicate an absence of HSV infection, because viral shedding is intermittent.

Both type-specific and non–type-specific antibodies to HSV develop during the first several weeks after infection, persist indefinitely, and can be tested for serologically. Immunoglobulin (Ig)M testing for HSV is not useful, because the IgM tests are not type-specific and might also be positive during recurrent episodes of herpes.

Because nearly all HSV-2 infections are sexually acquired, the presence of type-specific HSV-2 antibody implies anogenital infection and should prompt appropriate counseling. The presence of HSV-1 antibody alone is more difficult to interpret. In most cases, the presence of HSV-1 antibody indicates oral HSV infection acquired during childhood, which might be asymptomatic. However, acquisition of genital HSV-1 is increasing and can be asymptomatic. Lack of symptoms in an HSV-1 seropositive person does not distinguish anogenital from orolabial or cutaneous infection, and regardless of site of infection, these persons remain at risk for acquiring HSV-2.

Type-specific HSV serologic assays may be useful in the evaluation of the following situations: patients with recurrent genital symptoms or atypical symptoms with negative HSV cultures, patients with a clinical diagnosis of genital herpes without laboratory confirmation, and patients who have a partner with genital herpes.

Differential Diagnosis

Differential diagnosis includes other causes of genital ulceration such as syphilis and chancroid among infectious causes and drug eruptions and Behçet's disease among noninfectious causes.

Complications

Urinary retention can occur due to severe dysuria associated with extensive genital lesions. Rarely patients can develop severe herpes infection manifesting as disseminated infection, pneumonitis, hepatitis, or CNS complications such as meningoencephalitis. These patients should be hospitalized for close monitoring and intravenous antiviral administration.

Treatment

Systemic antiviral drugs can help to control the symptoms of herpes episodes and may also be used as daily suppressive therapy. However, these drugs neither eradicate latent virus nor affect the risk, frequency, or severity of recurrences after the drug is discontinued.

A. First Clinical Episode of Genital Herpes

1. Recommended regimens—Choose one of the following:

1. Acyclovir 400 mg orally 3 times a day for 7–10 days
2. Acyclovir 200 mg orally 5 times a day for 7–10 days
3. Famciclovir 250 mg orally 3 times a day for 7–10 days
4. Valacyclovir 1 g orally twice a day for 7–10 days

Treatment can be continued for longer than 10 days if lesions are not resolved.

B. Suppressive Therapy for Recurrent Genital Herpes

Suppressive therapy reduces the frequency of genital herpes recurrences by 70–80% in patients who have frequent recurrences. Treatment also is effective in patients with less frequent recurrences. Treatment with valacyclovir 500 mg daily decreases the rate of HSV-2 transmission in discordant, heterosexual couples in which the source partner has a history of genital HSV-2 infection. Suppressive antiviral therapy also is likely to reduce transmission when used by persons who have multiple partners and by those who are HSV-2 seropositive without a history of genital herpes.

1. Recommended Regimens—Choose one of the following:

1. Acyclovir 200 mg orally twice a day
2. Famciclovir 250 mg orally twice a day
3. Valacyclovir 500 mg orally once a day (may be less effective than the other regimens in patients with >10 episodes per year)
4. Valacyclovir 1g orally once a day

C. Episodic Therapy for Recurrent Genital Herpes

Effective treatment of recurrences requires initiation of therapy within 1 day of lesion onset or during the prodrome that precedes some outbreaks; therefore, patients should be provided with a supply of drug or a prescription in order to be able to start therapy in a timely fashion should a recurrence occur.

1. Recommended regimens—Choose one of the following:

1. Acyclovir 400 mg orally 3 times a day for 5 days
2. Acyclovir 800 mg orally twice a day for 5 days
3. Acyclovir 800 mg orally 3 times a day for 2 days
4. Famciclovir 125 mg orally twice a day for 5 days
5. Famciclovir 1 g orally twice a day for 1 day
6. Famciclovir 500 mg once, followed by 250 mg twice daily for 2 days
7. Valacyclovir 500 mg orally twice a day for 3 days
8. Valacyclovir 1 g orally once a day for 5 days

D. Genital Herpes in Pregnancy

Most mothers of infants who acquire neonatal herpes do not have a history of clinically evident genital herpes. The risk for transmission to the neonate from an infected mother is dependent on when in pregnancy they acquire the infection. In women who acquire genital herpes near the time of delivery, transmission is high (30–50%); conversely, in women with a history of recurrent herpes at term or who acquire genital HSV during the first half of pregnancy, the risk of transmission is low (<1%). However, because recurrent genital herpes is much more common than initial HSV infection during pregnancy, the proportion of neonatal HSV infections acquired from mothers with recurrent herpes is significant.

Prevention of neonatal herpes depends both on preventing acquisition of genital HSV infection during late pregnancy and avoiding exposure of the infant to herpetic lesions during delivery. Women without known genital herpes should be counseled to abstain from intercourse during the third trimester with partners known or suspected of having genital herpes. In addition, pregnant women without known orolabial herpes should be advised to abstain from receptive oral sex during the third trimester with partners known or suspected to have orolabial herpes. Type-specific serologic tests may be offered to uninfected women whose sex partner has HSV infection.

All pregnant women should be asked whether they have a history of genital herpes. At the onset of labor, all women should be questioned carefully about symptoms of genital herpes, including prodromal symptoms, and all women should be examined carefully for herpetic lesions. Women without symptoms or signs of genital herpes or its prodrome can deliver vaginally. Although caesarean section does not completely eliminate the risk for HSV transmission to the infant, women with recurrent genital herpetic lesions at the onset of labor should deliver by caesarean section to prevent neonatal HSV infection.

Acyclovir can be administered orally to pregnant women with first-episode genital herpes or severe recurrent herpes. Acyclovir treatment late in pregnancy reduces the frequency of caesarean sections among women who have recurrent genital herpes by diminishing the frequency of recurrences at term and should be offered to patients for suppression from approximately 36 weeks of gestation.

E. Genital Herpes and HIV

HIV-positive patients can have prolonged or severe episodes of genital, perianal, or oral herpes. HSV shedding is also increased in HIV-infected persons. Suppressive or episodic therapy with oral antiviral agents is effective in decreasing the clinical manifestations of HSV in this population.

1. Recommended regimens—Choose one of the following:

A. SUPPRESSION

1. Acyclovir 400–800 mg orally 2–3 times a day
2. Famciclovir 500 mg orally twice a day
3. Valacyclovir 500 mg orally twice a day

B. EPISODIC INFECTION

1. Acyclovir 400 mg orally 3 times a day for 5–10 days
2. Famciclovir 500 mg orally twice a day for 5–10 days
3. Valacyclovir 1 g orally twice a day for 5–10 days

Prognosis

HSV is a chronic, relapsing condition. Suppressive therapies are effective at reducing the number of outbreaks in patients with recurrent episodes.

CONDYLOMATA ACUMINATA

See Chapter 39.

CHANCROID

ESSENTIALS OF DIAGNOSIS

- Caused by gram-negative rod *Haemophilus ducreyi*
- Painful, tender genital ulcer
- Suppurative inguinal adenopathy

Pathogenesis

Chancroid prevalence has declined in the United States in recent years. Worldwide prevalence has also declined, but it may still be found in areas of Africa and the Caribbean. The causative organism is the highly infectious gram-negative rod *Haemophilus ducreyi*. Exposure is usually through coitus, but accidentally acquired lesions of the hands have been reported. The incubation period is typically 4–10 days. Chancroid is a reportable disease.

Prevention

Sexual partners should be treated, regardless of symptoms, if they have had sexual contact in the 10 days preceding the patient's onset of symptoms.

Clinical Findings

A. Symptoms & Signs

The chancroid lesion begins as an erythematous papule that evolves into a pustule and ultimately degenerates into a saucer-shaped ragged ulcer circumscribed by an inflammatory wheal. Typically, the lesion is very tender and produces a heavy, foul discharge that is contagious. Patients typically have more than 1 ulcer, and these are almost exclusively confined to the genital region.

Painful inguinal adenitis is noted in approximately 50% of cases, although this may occur less often in women. The nodes may undergo liquefaction, producing fluctuant buboes that may become necrotic and drain spontaneously.

B. Laboratory Findings

Definitive diagnosis is by identification of *H ducreyi* on specialized culture media that is not widely available from commercial sources and has sensitivity of less than 80%. There is no PCR test available in the United States that has been approved by the US Food and Drug Administration (FDA), although many labs have developed their own PCR test. However, this test may not be available at many centers due to cost. Therefore, in many cases the diagnosis is presumptive, based on symptoms of multiple painful ulcers with inguinal adenopathy and negative testing for other ulcerative diseases such as HSV and syphilis.

Differential Diagnosis

Syphilis, herpes simplex, granuloma inguinale, lymphogranuloma venereum, and Behçet's disease.

Complications

Inguinal scarring or fistula formation may occur from draining buboes.

Treatment

A. Local Treatment

Good personal hygiene is important. The early lesions should be cleansed with mild soap solution. Sitz baths are beneficial. Fluctuant lymph nodes should be needle aspirated or incised and drained through normal adjacent skin to prevent fistula formation or secondary ulcers from spontaneous rupture.

B. Antibiotic Treatment

The susceptibility of *H ducreyi* to antimicrobial agents varies regionally.

1. Recommended regimens—Choose one of the following. The course may have to be repeated.

1. Azithromycin 1 g orally in a single dose
2. Ceftriaxone 250 mg intramuscularly (IM) in a single dose
3. Ciprofloxacin 500 mg orally twice daily for 3 days (in nonpregnant patients over age 17 years who are not lactating)
4. Erythromycin base 500 mg orally 3 times daily for 7 days

Prognosis

Chancroid usually responds quickly to antibiotic therapy, with symptom improvement in 3 days and clinical improvement in 7 days. If there has been no improvement after 7 days, the patient should be re-evaluated. Given the difficulty in isolating *H ducreyi*, consideration should be given to the following possibilities: whether the original diagnosis was correct, existence of STD coinfection, poor compliance to treatment if a multidose regimen was selected, or antibiotic resistance. HIV-positive patients with chancroid may experience a higher rate of treatment failure, slower healing, and the need for prolonged antibiotic therapy. If the ulcers are not adequately treated, deep scarring may occur.

GRANULOMA INGUINALE (DONOVANOSIS)

ESSENTIALS OF DIAGNOSIS

- Painless, ulcerative vulvitis, chronic or recurrent
- Donovan bodies revealed by Wright's or Giemsa's stain

Pathogenesis

Granuloma inguinale is a chronic ulcerative granulomatous disease that usually develops in the vulva, perineum, and inguinal regions (Fig. 43–1). The disease is rare in the United States, being most common in India, Papua New Guinea, the Caribbean, central Australia, and southern Africa. The causative organism is *Klebsiella granulomatis* (formerly known as *Calymmatobacterium granulomatis*). The incubation period is 8–12 weeks. Granuloma inguinale is a reportable disease.

Prevention

Personal hygiene is the best method of prevention. Therapy immediately after exposure may abort the infection. Sex partners must be considered for treatment. Partners who had sexual contact during the 60 days preceding the onset of symptoms or are clinically symptomatic should be examined and offered treatment.

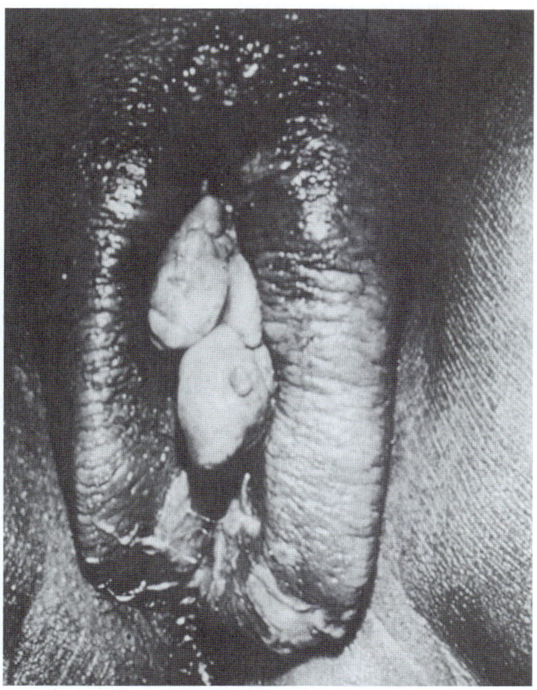

▲ **Figure 43–1.** Granuloma inguinale.

Clinical Findings

A. Symptoms & Signs

Clinically, the disease is characterized as painless, slowly progressive ulcerative lesions on the genitals or perineum without regional lymphadenopathy. Although granuloma inguinale most often involves the skin and subcutaneous tissues of the vulva and inguinal regions, cervical, uterine, orolabial, and ovarian sites have been reported. A malodorous discharge is characteristic. The disorder often begins as a papule, which then ulcerates, with the development of a beefy-red granular zone with clean, sharp edges. The lesions are highly vascular and bleed easily, with poor healing, and are susceptible to secondary bacterial infection. Rarely, granuloma inguinale present as chronic cervical lesions. These lesions usually take the form of redness or ulceration, or they form granulation tissue. They produce a chronic inflammatory exudate characterized histologically by lymphocytes, giant cells, and histiocytes. They may mimic carcinoma of the cervix and must be distinguished from this as well as other neoplastic diseases.

B. Laboratory Findings

The causative organism is difficult to culture, and diagnosis requires visualization of dark-staining Donovan bodies on tissue crush preparation or biopsy. Donovan bodies are bacteria encapsulated in mononuclear leukocytes and are best seen in Wright-stained smears as small round or rod-shaped particles that stain purple in traditional hematoxylin and eosin preparations. Initial testing may be done with direct smear from beneath the surface of an ulcer, but if these are negative, a biopsy specimen should be taken. Biopsy of the lesion generally shows granulation tissue infiltrated by plasma cells and scattered large macrophages with rod-shaped cytoplasmic inclusion bodies. Pseudoepitheliomatous hyperplasia often is seen at the margin of the ulcer. No FDA-cleared molecular tests for the detection of *K granulomatis* DNA exist at this time.

Differential Diagnosis

Syphilis, herpes simplex, chancroid, lymphogranuloma venereum, and Behçet's disease.

Complications

Scarring may cause introital contraction, which may make coitus difficult or impossible; walking or sitting may also become painful.

Treatment

Several antimicrobial regimens have been effective. Treatment has been shown to slow progression of lesions, and healing typically proceeds inward from the ulcer margins. Prolonged therapy is sometimes necessary to permit adequate granulation and re-epithelialization.

1. Recommended regimen—Doxycycline 100 mg twice daily for at least 3 weeks and until all ulcers are completely healed.

2. Alternative regimens—Choose one of the following. All regimens are for 3 weeks or until all lesions are healed.

1. Azithromycin 1 g orally once per week
2. Ciprofloxacin 750 mg orally twice daily
3. Erythromycin base 500 mg orally 4 times a day
4. Trimethoprim-sulfamethoxazole 1 double strength (160 mg/800 mg) tablet orally twice daily

Sulfonamides, doxycycline, and ciprofloxacin are contraindicated in pregnant women. The addition of an aminoglycoside (eg, gentamicin 1 mg/kg intravenously [IV] every 8 hours) to these regimens can be considered if improvement is not evident within the first few days of therapy or for known HIV-positive patients.

Prognosis

Prognosis is good. Prolonged therapy is often required, but in most cases it is ultimately effective.

LYMPHOGRANULOMA VENEREUM

ESSENTIALS OF DIAGNOSIS

- Tender inguinal lymphadenopathy
- Genital ulcer is often not evident
- Diagnosis suggested by positive complement fixation test

Pathogenesis

The causative agent of lymphogranuloma venereum (LGV) is one of the aggressive L serotypes (L1, L2, or L3) of *Chlamydia trachomatis*. It is encountered more frequently in the tropical and subtropical nations of Africa and Asia but is also seen in the southeastern United States. Transmission is via sexual contact; men are affected more frequently than women (6:1). The incubation period is 7–21 days. Presence of this infection is strongly associated with HIV-positive status in men who have sex with men, with positive HIV found in up to 75% of this population with a diagnosis of LGV. LGV is a reportable disease.

Prevention

Avoiding infectious contact with a carrier is achieved by use of a condom or by refraining from coitus. Sexual contacts of a patient who has LGV within the 60 days before onset of the patient's symptoms should be examined, tested for urethral or cervical chlamydial infection, and treated with a chlamydia regimen.

Clinical Findings

A. Symptoms & Signs

In heterosexuals the most common presentation is tender, usually unilateral inguinal and/or femoral lymphadenopathy. A genital ulcer sometimes occurs at the site of inoculation (Fig. 43–2), although this has often disappeared by the time patient seeks care. Rectal exposure can result in proctocolitis, including mucoid and/or hemorrhagic rectal discharge, pain, constipation, fever, or tenesmus. In the late phase, systemic symptoms such as fever, headache, arthralgia, chills, and abdominal cramps may develop.

B. Laboratory Findings

Diagnosis is based on clinical suspicion, epidemiologic information, and the exclusion of other etiologies for proctocolitis, inguinal lymphadenopathy, or genital or rectal ulcers.

The diagnosis can be proved only by isolating *C trachomatis* from genital or lymph node specimens and confirming the immunotype. These procedures are seldom available, so less specific tests are used.

A complement fixation test using a heat-stable antigen that is group-specific for all *Chlamydia* species is available. A titer of >1:64 is considered positive, whereas a titer of <1:32 is considered negative. If acute or convalescent sera are available, a rise in titer is particularly helpful in making the diagnosis. Application of a microimmunofluorescent test may also be useful.

Differential Diagnosis

As with any disseminated disease, the systemic symptoms of LGV may resemble meningitis, arthritis, pleurisy, or peritonitis. The cutaneous lesions must be differentiated from those of granuloma inguinale, tuberculosis, early syphilis, and chancroid. In the case of colonic lesions, proctoscopic

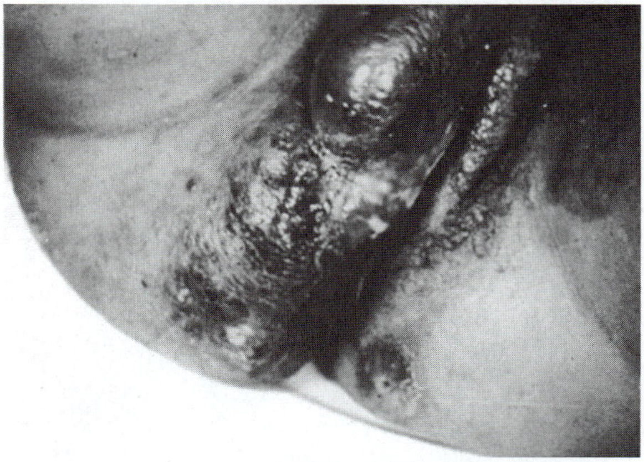

▲ **Figure 43–2.** Lymphogranuloma venereum. Note involvement of perineum and spread over buttocks.

examination and mucosal biopsy are needed to rule out carcinoma, schistosomiasis, and granuloma inguinale.

Complications

LGV is an invasive, systemic infection, and if it is not treated early, LGV proctocolitis can lead to chronic, colorectal fistulas and strictures, which can involve the entire sigmoid. Vulvar elephantiasis can cause marked distortion of the external genitalia. Vaginal narrowing and distortion may result in severe dyspareunia.

Treatment

A. Chemotherapy

1. Recommended regimen—Doxycycline 100 mg twice daily orally for 21 days. If disease persists, the course should be repeated.

2. Alternative regimen—Erythromycin 500 mg orally 4 times daily for 21 days.

B. Local & Surgical Treatment

Anal strictures should be dilated manually at weekly intervals. Severe stricture may require diversionary colostomy. If the disease is arrested, complete vulvectomy may be done for cosmetic reasons. Abscesses should be aspirated.

Prognosis

Treatment cures infection and prevents ongoing tissue damage, although tissue reaction to the infection can result in scarring.

SYPHILIS

ESSENTIALS OF DIAGNOSIS

Primary Syphilis

- Painless genital sore (chancre) on labia, vulva, vagina, cervix, anus, lips, or nipples
- Painless, rubbery, regional lymphadenopathy followed by generalized lymphadenopathy in the third to sixth weeks
- Dark-field microscopic findings
- Positive serologic test in 70% of cases

Secondary Syphilis

- Bilaterally symmetric extragenital papulosquamous eruption
- Condyloma latum, mucous patches
- Dark-field findings positive in moist lesions
- Positive serologic test for syphilis
- Lymphadenopathy

Tertiary Syphilis

- Cardiac, neurologic, ophthalmic, and auditory lesions
- Gummas

Latent Syphilis

- History or serologic evidence of previous infection
- Absence of lesions
- Serologic test usually reactive; titer may be low

Pathogenesis

Syphilis is a chronic, systemic disease caused by the spirochete *Treponema pallidum*, which is transmitted by direct contact with an infectious moist lesion. In the majority of cases it is sexually acquired, although it can also be vertically transmitted from mother to fetus. The disease has been divided into several stages based on clinical presentation in order to guide best treatment. It is transmissible in the primary or secondary stages. Treponemes pass through intact mucous membranes or abraded skin, and 10–90 days later, a primary lesion, or chancre, develops (median incubation period is 21 days). Two weeks to 6 months (average of 6 weeks) after the primary lesion appears, the generalized cutaneous eruption of secondary syphilis may appear. Latent syphilis may follow the secondary stage and may last a lifetime, or tertiary syphilis may develop. The latter usually becomes manifest 4–20 or more years after disappearance of the primary lesion. Syphilis is a reportable disease.

Prevention

If a patient is known to have been exposed to syphilis, preventative treatment should not be delayed by waiting for symptoms to develop, although every effort should be made to reach a diagnosis, including a complete physical examination. Any patient who has been exposed and becomes symptomatic within 90 days of sexual contact should be treated regardless of negative serologies, and similarly, if it has been >90 days since exposure with positive titers, treatment should be initiated. If the duration since exposure is unknown and the treponemal antibody titer is greater than 1:32, treatment is indicated.

All pregnant women should undergo routine serologic testing for syphilis at the first prenatal visit, and this should be repeated at 28–32 weeks' gestation in high-risk regions. If the test result is positive, attention must be given to the patient's prior serologic test and therapy (if any) for syphilis. If doubt exists regarding whether the patient has active syphilis, repeat therapy is far better than the risk of congenital syphilis.

Syphilis is still a serious public health problem, and education is still the best method of control. Use of a condom, together with soap and water decontamination after coitus, would prevent most cases. Screening people at high risk for acquiring syphilis (men who have sex with men, who engage in high-risk behaviors, commercial sex workers, persons who exchange sex for drugs, and those in adult correctional facilities) is a recommended strategy.

Clinical Findings

A. Symptoms & Signs

1. Primary syphilis—The chancre (Fig. 43–3) is an indurated, firm, painless papule or ulcer with raised borders. Groin lymph nodes may be enlarged, firm, and painless. Genital lesions are not usually seen in women unless they occur on the external genitalia; however, careful examination may reveal a cervical or vaginal lesion. Primary lesions may occur on any mucous membrane or skin area of the body (nose, breast, perineum), and dark-field examination is required for all suspect lesions. Serologic tests should be done every week for 6 weeks or until positive.

2. Secondary syphilis—Signs of diffuse systemic infection become evident as the spirochetes spread hematogenously. A "viral syndrome" presentation, often with diffuse lymphadenopathy, is not uncommon. The characteristic dermatitis appears as diffuse, bilateral, symmetric, papulosquamous lesions that often involve the palms and soles. Lesions may also cover the trunk and be macular, maculopapular, papular, or pustular. Other systemic manifestations include patchy alopecia, hepatitis, and nephritis. Moist papules can be seen in the perineal area (condyloma lata). Mucous patches may also be seen; like condyloma lata, they are dark-field–positive, infectious lesions. Serologic tests for syphilis are invariably reactive in this stage.

3. Latent syphilis—With resolution of the lesions of primary and secondary infection or the finding of a reactive serologic test without a history of therapy, a patient passes into latency. Persons are infectious in the first 1–2 years of latency, with clinical relapses resembling the secondary stage occurring in approximately 25% of cases in the first year. Latent syphilis acquired within the preceding year is referred to as early latent syphilis. All other cases of latent syphilis are referred to as either late latent syphilis or latent syphilis of unknown duration.

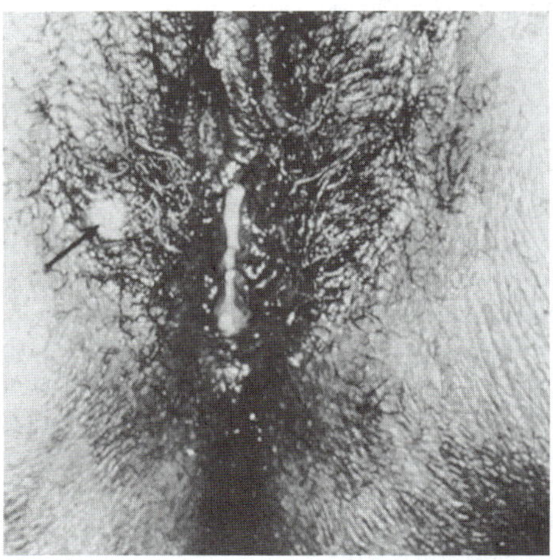

▲ **Figure 43–3.** Chancre of primary syphilis (arrow).

4. Neurosyphilis—Although the CNS is always vulnerable to *T pallidum*, it is most commonly infected during latent syphilis. Neurologic involvement of ophthalmic and auditory systems can be detected. Cranial nerve palsy and meningeal signs should be evaluated on physical examination.

5. Syphilis during pregnancy—The course of syphilis is unaltered by pregnancy, but misdiagnoses are common. The chancre is often unnoticed or internal and not brought to medical attention. Chancres, mucous patches, and condyloma lata are often thought to be herpes genitalis.

The effect of syphilis on pregnancy outcome can be profound. The risk of fetal infection depends on the degree of maternal spirochetemia (greater in the secondary stage than in the primary or latent stages) and the gestational age of the fetus. Treponemes may cross the placenta at all stages of pregnancy, but fetal involvement is rare before 18 weeks. After 18 weeks, the fetus is able to mount an immunologic response, and tissue damage may result. The earlier in pregnancy the fetus is exposed, the more severe the fetal infection and the greater the risk of premature delivery or stillbirth. Antepartum infection in late pregnancy does not necessarily result in congenital infection; only 40–50% of such infants will have congenital infection. Placental infection can occur, with resultant endarteritis, stromal hyperplasia, and immature villi. Grossly, the placenta looks hydropic (pale yellow, waxy, and enlarged). Because polyhydramnios is frequently associated with symptomatic congenital infection, fetuses are ultrasonographically followed throughout pregnancy.

6. Congenital syphilis—Most infants with congenital syphilis are born to women of low socioeconomic status with inadequate or no prenatal care. Either these neonates may be affected at birth from intrauterine infection (hepatosplenomegaly, osteochondritis, jaundice, anemia, skin lesions, rhinitis, lymphadenopathy, nervous system involvement), or symptoms may develop weeks or months later. The clinical spectrum of congenital infection is analogous to adult secondary disease, as the disease is systemic from onset due to transplacental hematogenous inoculation. The specifics of congenital syphilis are beyond the scope of this text.

B. Laboratory findings

1. Identification of the organism—Definitive diagnosis of *T pallidum* is by identification of spirochetes by dark-field examination of specimens from cutaneous lesions. When this specimen is not available, diagnosis depends on the history and serologic tests. An immunofluorescent technique is now available for dried smears. Silver staining for *T pallidum* of biopsy specimens, placental sections, or autopsy material may confirm the diagnosis in difficult cases. Motile spirochetes can be identified in amniotic fluid obtained transabdominally in women with syphilis and fetal death. PCR is extremely specific for detection of *T pallidum* in amniotic fluid and neonatal serum and spinal fluid. Newer techniques involving molecular methods are now being used to diagnosis early syphilis.

2. Serologic tests—Diagnostic tests after the primary or secondary moist lesion has disappeared are confined largely to serologic testing. Serologic tests become positive several weeks after the primary lesion appears.

A. NONTREPONEMAL TESTS—These tests measure reaginic antibody detected by highly purified cardiolipin-lecithin antigen. They can be performed rapidly, easily, and inexpensively. Nontreponemal tests are used principally for syphilis screening, but due to their nonspecific nature, false positives can occur. Nontreponemal tests currently in use are the Venereal Disease Research Laboratory (VDRL), the Rapid Plasma Reagin test (RPR) and the Toluidine Red Unheated Serum Test (TRUST).

These antibody titers may correlate with disease activity, and results should be reported quantitatively. A 4-fold change in titer (equivalent to a change of 2 dilutions: eg, from 1:16 to 1:4 or from 1:8 to 1:32) is considered necessary to demonstrate a clinically significant difference between 2 nontreponemal test results that were obtained using the same serologic test. Sequential serologic tests in individual patients should be performed using the same testing method (eg, VDRL or RPR), preferably by the same laboratory. Nontreponemal test titers usually decline after treatment and might become nonreactive with time; however, in some persons, nontreponemal antibodies can persist for a long period of time.

The VDRL test generally becomes positive 3–6 weeks after infection, or 2–3 weeks after the appearance of the primary lesion, and is invariably positive in the secondary stage. False-positive serologic reactions are frequently encountered in a wide variety of situations, including collagen diseases, infectious mononucleosis, malaria, many febrile diseases, leprosy, drug addiction, old age, and possibly pregnancy. False-positive reactions are usually of low titer and transient and may be distinguished from true-positive results by specific treponemal antibody tests.

B. TREPONEMAL ANTIBODY TESTS—The fluorescent treponemal antibody absorbed test (FTA-ABS) and microhemagglutination assay for *Treponema pallidum* (MHA-TP) detect antibody against *Treponema spirochetes.* Both tests are generally more sensitive and specific than nontreponemal tests. These tests remain positive despite therapy, so they are not given in titers or used to follow serologic response to treatment (Table 43–1).

Differential Diagnosis

Syphilis has often been called "the great imitator" because so many of the signs and symptoms are indistinguishable from those of other diseases. Amongst others, primary syphilis must be differentiated from chancroid, granuloma inguinale, lymphogranuloma venereum, herpes genitalis, carcinoma, scabies, trauma, lichen planus, psoriasis, drug eruption, aphthosis, mycotic infections, Reiter's syndrome, and Bowen's disease. Secondary syphilis must be differentiated from pityriasis rosea, psoriasis, lichen planus, tinea versicolor, drug eruption, perlèche, parasitic infections, iritis, neuroretinitis, condyloma acuminatum, acute exanthems, infectious mononucleosis, alopecia, and sarcoidosis.

Complications

In one-third of untreated cases, the destructive lesions of tertiary syphilis develop. These may involve skin or bone (gummas), the cardiovascular system (aortic aneurysm or insufficiency), and the nervous system (meningitis, tabes dorsalis, paresis). The complications of tertiary syphilis are fatal in almost one-fourth of cases. However, another one-fourth never show any ill effects.

Treatment

Penicillin G, administered parenterally, is the preferred drug for treating all stages of syphilis. The preparation, dosage, and length of treatment depend on the stage and clinical manifestations of the disease. Selection of the appropriate penicillin preparation is important, because *T pallidum* can reside in sequestered sites that are poorly accessed by some forms of penicillin.

Table 43–1. Percent sensitivity of serologic tests in untreated syphilis.

	Stage of Disease			
Type of Test	**Primary**	**Secondary**	**Latent**	**Late**
VDRL	59–87	100	73–91	37–94
FTA-ABS	86–100	99–100	96–99	96–100
MHA-TP	64–87	96–100	96–100	94–100

Reproduced, with permission, from Holmes KK, et al (eds). *Sexually Transmitted Diseases*. New York, NY: McGraw-Hill; 1984.

A. Early Syphilis & Contacts

Includes primary, secondary, and early latent syphilis (<1 year's duration):

1. Recommended regimen—Benzathine penicillin G 2.4 million units IM in a single dose.

B. Late Syphilis

Includes latent syphilis of indeterminate duration or more than 1 year's duration, gumma, and cardiovascular syphilis, but not neurosyphilis.

1. Recommended regimen—Benzathine penicillin G 2.4 million units IM weekly for 3 successive weeks (7.2 million units total).

C. Neurosyphilis

1. Recommended regimen—Aqueous crystalline penicillin G 18–24 million units per day, administered as 3–4 million units IV every 4 hours or continuous infusion, for 10–14 days.

2. Alternative regimen—Procaine penicillin 2.4 million units IM once daily plus probenecid 500 mg orally 4 times a day, both for 10–14 days.

D. Penicillin Allergy

Data to support the use of alternatives to penicillin in the treatment of early syphilis are limited. However, several therapies might be effective in nonpregnant, penicillin-allergic patients who have primary or secondary syphilis:

1. Recommended regimens—Choose one of the following:

1. Doxycycline 100 mg orally twice daily for 14 days
2. Tetracycline 500 mg orally 4 times daily for 14 days

Some limited studies suggest that ceftriaxone 1 g daily either IM or IV for 10–14 days is effective for treating early syphilis. However, the optimal dose and duration of ceftriaxone therapy have not been defined.

Azithromycin as a single 2-g oral dose is effective for treating early syphilis; however, azithromycin resistance and treatment failures have been documented in several geographical areas in the United States. Therefore, the use of azithromycin should be used with caution only when treatment with penicillin or doxycycline is not feasible. Close follow-up of persons receiving any alternative therapies is essential. Patients with a penicillin allergy whose compliance with therapy or follow-up cannot be ensured should be desensitized and treated with benzathine penicillin.

E. Syphilis in Pregnancy

Parenteral penicillin G is the only therapy with documented efficacy for syphilis during pregnancy. Pregnant women with syphilis in any stage who report penicillin allergy should be desensitized and treated with penicillin. If serologic tests are equivocal (eg, possible biologic false-positive result), it is better to err on the side of early treatment. Because of an increased risk for treatment failure, a second dose of 2.4 million units of penicillin IM is often recommended in pregnancy.

F. Congenital Syphilis

Adequate maternal treatment before 16–18 weeks' gestation prevents congenital syphilis. Treatment thereafter may arrest fetal syphilitic infection, but some stigmata may remain. Penicillin treatment with varying regimens and preparations is recommended for most cases depending on clinical presentation of the infant and results of serologic, laboratory, and radiologic testing. The details of the management of congenital syphilis are beyond the scope of this text.

G. Jarisch-Herxheimer Reaction

The Jarisch-Herxheimer reaction occurs in 50–75% of patients with early syphilis treated with penicillin. It is a febrile reaction accompanied by myalgias and headaches that occurs 4–12 hours after injection and is completed by 24 hours. The cause is uncertain but likely involves a release of treponemal toxic products upon organism lysis. The reaction is generally benign but may trigger labor or fetal distress in pregnancy. Prophylaxis with antipyretics or corticosteroids is of unknown value.

H. Coexisting Infection With HIV

Syphilis and HIV coinfection is alarmingly common; therefore, all patients with syphilis should be tested for HIV and vice versa. No specific changes in management for HIV-positive patients is recommended, but closer follow-up is necessary to ensure adequate treatment.

▶ Prognosis

Untreated syphilis may progress to tertiary or neurosyphilis with resultant sequelae. Treatment with penicillin is highly effective at curing this infection.

VAGINITIS

BACTERIAL VAGINOSIS

ESSENTIALS OF DIAGNOSIS

- White homogenous vaginal discharge with fishy odor
- Presence of clue cells on wet preparation microscopy
- Vaginal pH >4.5

Pathogenesis

Bacterial vaginosis is the most prevalent vaginal infection, although almost 50% of affected women are asymptomatic. The term **bacterial vaginosis** refers to the changes of vaginal bacterial flora with a loss of lactobacilli, an increase in vaginal pH, and an increase in multiple anaerobic and aerobic bacteria. It is a polymicrobial infection, and commonly involved organisms include *Gardnerella vaginalis, Ureaplasma, Mycoplasma, Prevotella* spp., and *Mobiluncus* spp. *G vaginalis*, the predominant organism involved, is a small, nonmotile, nonencapsulated, pleomorphic rod. The characteristic fishy odor of bacterial vaginosis is due to anaerobic bacteria.

Bacterial vaginosis is associated with multiple sex partners, new sex partner, douching, lack of condom use, and lack of vaginal lactobacilli.

Prevention

Condom use and avoidance of douching will help to prevent bacterial vaginosis. It is not necessary to treat male sexual partners of affected women. Women with bacterial vaginosis who have sex with women should have their partners screened and, if positive, treated.

Clinical Findings

Patients usually complain of a vaginal discharge with an odor. Clinical criteria for diagnoses include (1) homogeneous white, noninflammatory discharge, (2) microscopic presence of clue cells, (3) vaginal discharge with pH >4.5, and (4) fishy odor with or without addition of 10% potassium hydroxide. Three of these 4 criteria are required to make a clinical diagnosis of bacterial vaginosis. Clue cells are the unstained vaginal cells in a wet preparation that appear to be dusted with many small dark particles, which are the *G vaginalis* organisms.

Gram stain is the gold standard for diagnosis, which shows a relative lack of lactobacilli and presence of gram-negative and gram variable rods and cocci.

Differential Diagnosis

Trichomoniasis, atrophic vaginitis, and desquamative inflammatory vaginitis should be considered in the differential diagnosis of bacterial vaginosis.

Complications

Observational studies have consistently shown an association between bacterial vaginosis and adverse pregnancy outcomes, including preterm delivery, preterm premature rupture of membranes, spontaneous abortion, and preterm labor. However, 2 large randomized, placebo-controlled trials demonstrated that treatment of bacterial vaginosis in asymptomatic pregnant women with metronidazole does not prevent preterm deliveries. Nevertheless, the CDC recommends that pregnant women with a history of preterm delivery and asymptomatic bacterial vaginosis be evaluated for treatment.

Treatment

Therapy should be initiated for symptomatic relief. Pregnant women who are at high risk for preterm labor may benefit from treatment. Treatment is recommended for low-risk groups during pregnancy if patients are infected and symptomatic. Lastly, patients who may also benefit from therapy are asymptomatic carriers before scheduled pelvic/abdominal surgery.

1. Recommended regimens—Choose 1 of the following:

1. Metronidazole 500 mg orally twice daily for 7 days
2. Metronidazole gel 0.75%, 1 full applicator (5 g) intravaginally once daily for 5 days
3. Clindamycin cream 2%, 1 full applicator (5 g) intravaginally at night for 7 days

2. Alternative regimens—Choose 1 of the following:

1. Tinidazole 2 g orally once a day for 2 days
2. Tinidazole 1 g orally once a day for 5 days
3. Clindamycin 300 mg orally twice daily for 7 days
4. Clindamycin ovules 100 mg intravaginally once at night for 3 days

During pregnancy, oral treatment is preferred to local agents due to the possibility of subclinical upper genital tract infection.

3. Recommended regimens in pregnancy—Choose 1 of the following:

1. Metronidazole 500 mg orally twice daily for 7 days
2. Metronidazole 250 mg orally 3 times a day for 7 days
3. Clindamycin 300 mg orally twice daily for 7 days

Prognosis

Thirty percent of patients with an initial response to therapy will have recurrent symptoms within 3 months, and greater than 50% will have recurrence within 12 months. If a patient has had multiple recurrences, suppressive therapy may be beneficial.

TRICHOMONIASIS

ESSENTIALS OF DIAGNOSIS

- Common infection caused by the flagellated protozoan *Trichomonas vaginalis*
- Purulent, malodorous, thin vaginal discharge
- Diagnosis by wet-prep, point-of-care tests or culture
- High rate of reinfection

Pathogenesis

Trichomoniasis is caused by the flagellated protozoan *Trichomonas vaginalis*. It is common, accounting for up to 35% of vaginitis in symptomatic patients, and should be considered in all women presenting with vaginal discharge. It is virtually always sexually transmitted, although it is usually transient and self-limited in male partners. The incubation period is thought to be 4–28 days.

Prevention

Use of condoms, limiting the number of sexual partners, and possibly good vulvar hygiene reduce the risk of acquiring trichomoniasis. Sex partners of patients with *T vaginalis* should be treated, and patients should abstain from sexual intercourse until both partners are treated and asymptomatic.

Clinical Findings

A. Symptoms & Signs

Symptoms include a purulent, malodorous, thin discharge (70%) with associated burning, pruritus, dysuria, frequency, and dyspareunia. Postcoital bleeding can occur. The urethra is also infected in the majority of women. The classically described green, frothy, foul-smelling discharge is found in fewer than 10% of symptomatic women. Many women, however, will be asymptomatic.

Physical examination often reveals erythema of the vulva and vaginal mucosa with observation of yellow-green discharge. Punctate hemorrhages may be visible on the cervix ("strawberry cervix") in 2% of cases.

B. Laboratory Findings

Diagnosis of vaginal trichomoniasis is usually performed by immediate wet preparation microscopy of vaginal secretions. However, this has a sensitivity of only 60–70%.

FDA-cleared point-of-care tests for trichomoniasis exist and include OSOM Trichomonas Rapid Test, an immunochromatographic capillary flow dipstick technology, and the Affirm VP III, a nucleic acid probe test that evaluates for *T vaginalis*, *G vaginalis*, and *Candida albicans*.

Culture on Diamond's medium is another sensitive and highly specific method of diagnosis. Among women in whom trichomoniasis is suspected but not confirmed by microscopy, vaginal secretions can be cultured for *T vaginalis*.

Differential Diagnosis

Bacterial vaginosis, atrophic vaginitis, and desquamative inflammatory vaginitis should be considered in the differential diagnosis of trichomoniasis.

Complications

Trichomoniasis is a risk factor for development of posthysterectomy cellulitis, tubal infertility, and cervical neoplasia. In pregnancy it is associated with preterm premature rupture of membranes and preterm delivery.

Treatment

1. Recommended regimens—Choose 1 of the following:

1. Metronidazole 2 g orally in a single dose
2. Tinidazole 2 g orally in a single dose

2. Alternative regimen—Metronidazole 500 mg orally twice a day for 7 days.

Prognosis

The recommended metronidazole regimens result in cure in 90–95% of cases. However, there is a high reinfection rate (approximately 17% in the first 3 months); therefore, rescreening of patients 3 months after treatment may be considered.

URETHRITIS & CERVICITIS

GONORRHEA

ESSENTIALS OF DIAGNOSIS

- May be asymptomatic
- Purulent vaginal discharge
- Urinary frequency and dysuria
- Diagnosis by Gram's stain, culture on selective media, or nucleic acid amplification tests
- May progress to pelvic infection or disseminated infection

Pathogenesis

Neisseria gonorrhoeae is a gram-negative diplococcus that may be recovered from the urethra, cervix, anal canal, or pharynx. The columnar and transitional epithelium of the genitourinary tract is the principal site of invasion. The organism may enter the upper reproductive tract (Fig. 43–4), causing salpingitis with its associated complications. Approximately 700,000 new infections occur each year. After exposure to an infected partner, 20–50% of men and 60–90% of women become infected. Without therapy, 10–17% of women with gonorrhea develop pelvic infection. The incubation period is 3–5 days. Gonorrhea is a reportable disease.

Prevention

Gonorrhea is a reportable disease that can be controlled only by the detection and treatment of asymptomatic carriers and their sexual partners. All high-risk populations should be screened by routine cultures, including all sexually

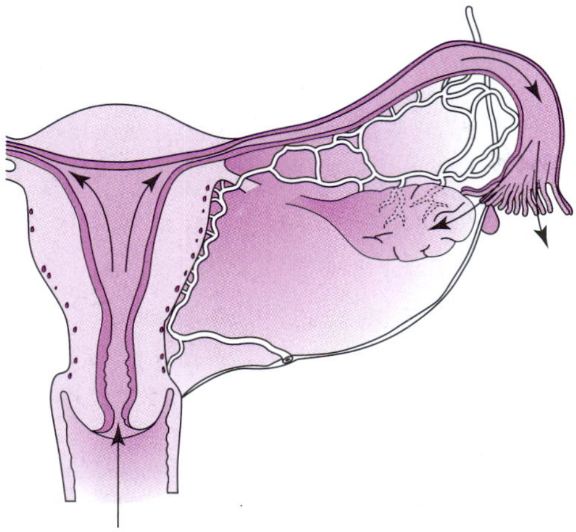

▲ **Figure 43–4.** Intra-abdominal spread of gonorrhea and other pathogenic bacteria.

active women age 25 years or less. Use of condoms will protect against gonorrhea. Sex partners of patients with *N gonorrhoeae* infection whose last sexual contact with the patient was within 60 days of the onset of symptoms or of diagnosis of the infection should be evaluated and treated for *N gonorrhoeae* and *C trachomatis* infections. If a patient's last sexual intercourse was >60 days before onset of symptoms or diagnosis, the patient's most recent sexual partner should be treated. Patients should be instructed to abstain from sexual intercourse until therapy is completed and until they and their sex partners no longer have symptoms.

For prevention of ophthalmia neonatorum, all newborns should receive erythromycin ophthalmic ointment 0.5% to each eye in a single application shortly after delivery.

Clinical Findings

A. Symptoms & Signs

Many women with gonorrhea are asymptomatic. When symptoms occur, they are generally localized to the lower genitourinary tract and include vaginal discharge, urinary frequency or dysuria, and rectal discomfort. The vulva, vagina, cervix, and urethra may be inflamed and may itch or burn. Unilateral swelling in the inferior lateral portion of the introitus suggests involvement of Bartholin's duct and gland. Anal itching, pain, discharge, or bleeding occurs rarely. Acute pharyngitis and tonsillitis rarely occur. Conjunctivitis can occur; in adults this is usually due to autoinoculation. Ophthalmia neonatorum may result from delivery through an infected birth canal.

Some asymptomatic carriers can develop systemic infection. A triad of polyarthralgia, tenosynovitis, and dermatitis may be present, or purulent arthritis without dermatitis. Septicemia can occur in the former clinical setting and *N gonorrhoeae* cultured from joint aspirates in the latter. Endocarditis and meningitis have been described.

Gonococcal invasion of nonkeratinized membranes in prepubertal girls produces severe vulvovaginitis. The typical sign is a purulent vaginal discharge with dysuria. The genital mucous membranes are red and swollen. Infection is commonly introduced by adults, and in such cases the physician must consider the possibility of sexual abuse.

B. Laboratory Findings

A presumptive diagnosis of gonorrhea can be made based on examination of the stained smear; however, confirmation requires positive identification on selective media. Secretions are examined under oil immersion for presumptive identification. Gram-negative diplococci that are oxidase-positive and obtained from selective media (Thayer-Martin) usually signify *N gonorrhoeae*. However, this test is not completely sensitive so cannot completely rule out infection if negative. Specific diagnosis of infection with *N gonorrhoeae* can be performed by testing endocervical, vaginal, or urine specimens. Culture, nucleic acid hybridization tests, and nucleic acid amplification testing (NAATs) are also available for the detection of genitourinary infection with *N gonorrhoeae*.

Because nonculture tests cannot provide antimicrobial susceptibility results, in cases of suspected or documented treatment failure, clinicians should perform both culture and antimicrobial susceptibility testing.

Differential Diagnosis

Chlamydia, urinary tract infection, and pelvic inflammatory disease should be considered in the differential diagnosis.

Complications

The major complication is salpingitis, which may result in tubal scarring, infertility, and increased risk for ectopic gestations. *N gonorrhoeae* can be recovered from the cervix in approximately 50% of women with salpingitis. Asymptomatic carriers can also develop these complications. Resistant strains of *N gonorrhoeae* have emerged in some geographic areas; therefore, follow-up cultures are essential in these settings.

Treatment

Patients diagnosed with uncomplicated gonorrhea who are treated with any of the recommended or alternative regimens do not need a test-of-cure. It is crucial to instruct patients to abstain from sexual relations for the 7 days after therapy is initiated.

Dual therapy to cover for chlamydia infection has contributed greatly to the declining prevalence of chlamydial infections. Therefore, if chlamydial infection is not ruled out, the following regimens should be given with doxycycline (for nonpregnant patients) or azithromycin.

Quinolone-resistant gonorrhea is now widespread in the United States as well as many other regions. For this reason, quinolones are no longer recommended for treatment of gonorrhea.

A. Uncomplicated Infections

1. Recommended Regimens

- Ceftriaxone 250 mg IM in a single dose, **or**
- Cefixime 400 mg orally in a single dose, **plus**
- Azithromycin 1 g orally in a single dose, **or**
- Doxycycline 100 mg orally twice daily for 7 days (for *C trachomatis* coverage)

B. Pelvic Inflammatory Disease

See Pelvic Inflammatory Disease.

C. Disseminated Infections

Patients with disseminated gonococcal infection should be hospitalized. Evidence of endocarditis or meningitis should be sought, and the patient should be closely monitored.

1. Recommended regimen—Ceftriaxone 1 g IM or IV every 24 hours.

2. Alternative regimens—Choose 1 of the following:

1. Cefotaxime 1 g IV every 8 hours
2. Ceftizoxime 1 g IV every 8 hours

All of these regimens should be continued for 24–48 hours after improvement begins, at which time therapy can be switched to cefixime 400 mg orally twice daily to complete at least 1 week of antimicrobial therapy. No treatment failures have been reported with these recommended regimens.

D. β-Lactamase Allergy

Reactions to first-generation cephalosporins occur in only 5–10% of patients with a history of penicillin allergy and occur less frequently with third-generation cephalosporins. In patients with a history of penicillin allergy, the use of cephalosporins is contraindicated only in those with a history of a severe reaction to penicillin (eg, anaphylaxis, Stevens-Johnson syndrome, or toxic epidermal necrolysis).

Because data are limited regarding alternative regimens for treating gonorrhea among persons who have severe cephalosporin allergy, treatment of these individuals should be undertaken in consultation with an infectious disease specialists. Azithromycin 2 g orally is effective against uncomplicated gonococcal infection, but due to emerging antimicrobial resistance to macrolides, its use should be limited. Cephalosporin desensitization is possible but impractical in most clinical settings.

Prognosis

The prognosis is excellent for patients with gonorrhea who receive prompt treatment, although infertility may result from even a single episode.

CHLAMYDIA

ESSENTIALS OF DIAGNOSIS

- Mucopurulent cervicitis
- Salpingitis
- Urethral syndrome
- May progress to pelvic inflammatory disease
- May cause infection in neonates born to infected mothers

Pathogenesis

Chlamydia trachomatis is the most commonly reported infectious disease in the United States, with highest prevalence found in people age ≤25 years. Higher number of sexual partners and lower socioeconomic status are also associated with increased rates of chlamydial infection rates.

Chlamydiae are obligate intracellular organisms that have a cell wall similar to that of gram-negative bacteria. They are classified as bacteria and contain both DNA and RNA. They divide by binary fission, but like viruses they grow intracellularly. With the exception of the L serotypes, chlamydiae attach only to columnar epithelial cells without deep tissue invasion. *C trachomatis* infections are associated with many adverse sequelae due to chronic inflammatory changes as well as fibrosis. Chlamydia is a reportable disease.

Prevention

Many patients who have *C trachomatis* infection are asymptomatic. Therefore, screening with subsequent treatment of infection is the mainstay of prevention, as well as condom use. The CDC recommends annual screening of sexually active women age ≤25 years and older women with risk factors (eg, new or multiple sex partners).

Patients who test positive for chlamydia should be instructed to refer their sex partners for evaluation, testing, and treatment if they had sexual contact with the patient during the 60 days preceding onset of the patient's symptoms or chlamydia diagnosis. In addition, the most recent sex partner should be evaluated and treated, even if the time of the last sexual contact was >60 days before symptom onset or diagnosis.

Clinical Findings

A. Symptoms & Signs

Women with chlamydial infection are often asymptomatic. Women with cervical infection may have a mucopurulent discharge with hypertrophic cervical inflammation. Salpingitis may cause pelvic pain or be asymptomatic.

B. Laboratory Findings

C trachomatis infection can be diagnosed either by testing urine or by collecting specimens from the endocervix or vagina. Rectal and oral *C trachomatis* infections in persons that engage in receptive anal or oral intercourse can be diagnosed by swabbing those areas. NAATs, cell culture, direct immunofluorescence, enzyme immunoassay, and nucleic acid hybridization tests are available for the detection of *C trachomatis*. NAATs are the most sensitive test for endocervical specimens and are also FDA approved for use on urine. Some NAATs are FDA approved for vaginal swabs. Most tests are not FDA approved for use on oropharyngeal or rectal specimens, although NAATs have been shown to have improved sensitivity and specificity compared with culture.

Differential Diagnosis

Mucopurulent cervicitis is frequently caused by *N gonorrhoea*, and selective cultures for this organism should be performed.

Complications

Adverse sequelae of chlamydia result from upper genital tract involvement. Salpingitis and pelvic inflammatory disease may lead to infertility due to tubal obstruction and ectopic pregnancy. Occasionally, patients with chlamydia infection develop perihepatitis (also known as Fitz-Hugh Curtis syndrome), an inflammation of the liver capsule and adjacent peritoneal surfaces. Adhesions may be seen in this area, which resemble "violin strings." Perihepatitis is more commonly seen in pelvic inflammatory disease. The pathogenesis of this entity is not fully understood but may involve either direct extension of infected material from the cul-de-sac through the peritoneum and/or lymphatics or an immunologically mediated mechanism.

Perihepatitis should be suspected in persons with right-upper quadrant pain or pleuritic pain, in the clinical context of a lower genital tract infection. There are typically no associated liver enzyme abnormalities. Treatment is supportive, usually with nonsteroidal anti-inflammatory agents.

Pregnant women with cervical chlamydial infection can transmit infections to their newborns, and up to 50% of infants born to such mothers will have conjunctivitis. In 10% of infants, an indolent chlamydial pneumonitis develops at 2–3 months of age. This pathogen may also cause otitis media in the neonate.

Chlamydial infection in pregnancy is a risk factor for premature delivery and postpartum infections, particularly when it is acute. It is hypothesized that asymptomatic cervicitis predisposes to mild amnionitis. This event activates phospholipase A_2 to release prostaglandins, which cause uterine contractions that may lead to premature labor. Chlamydial infection is associated with higher rates of early postpartum endometritis as well as delayed infection from *Chlamydia* that may present several weeks postpartum.

Treatment

Dual therapy to cover for *N gonorrhea* is appropriate due to high rates of coinfection.

A. Recommended Regimens

- Azithromycin 1 g orally in a single dose, **or**
- Doxycycline 100 mg orally twice daily for 7 days, **plus**
- Ceftriaxone 250 mg IM in a single dose, **or**
- Cefixime 400 mg orally in a single dose (for *N gonorrhea* coverage)

B. Alternative regimens

Choose 1 of the following:

1. Erythromycin base 500 mg orally 4 times a day for 7 days
2. Erythromycin ethylsuccinate 800 mg orally 4 times a day for 7 days
3. Levofloxacin 500 mg orally once daily for 7 days
4. Ofloxacin 300 mg orally twice daily for 7 days

In pregnancy, amoxicillin 500 mg orally 3 times a day for 7 days is the recommended alternative regimen to azithromycin. Levofloxacin and ofloxacin should not be used in pregnant patients.

Except in pregnancy, test-of-cure (repeat testing 3–4 weeks after completing therapy) is not advised for persons treated with the recommended or alterative regimens, unless therapeutic compliance is in question, symptoms persist, or reinfection is suspected. However, patients should be rescreened approximately 3 months after treatment or, if this is not possible, whenever persons next present for medical care in the 12 months after initial treatment.

Prognosis

Treatment of chlamydial infection is usually effective, although reinfection can occur, particularly if sexual partners are inadequately treated. Long-term sequelae are discussed under Complications and are related to postinflammatory scar tissue formation.

BLOODBORNE INFECTIONS

HEPATITIS B

ESSENTIALS OF DIAGNOSIS

- Caused by hepatitis B virus (HBV)
- Acute illness is often asymptomatic
- Can lead to chronic carrier state—more likely if acquired earlier in life
- Treatment of acute illness is supportive
- Vaccination available
- Hepatitis B immunoglobulin indicated for postexposure prophylaxis along with vaccination

Pathogenesis

Hepatitis B is caused by infection with hepatitis B virus (HBV), an hepadnavirus. The incubation period is 6 weeks to 6 months. Concentration of HBV is highest in blood, with lower concentrations found in other body fluids such as wound exudates, semen, vaginal secretions, and saliva. HBV is more infectious and relatively more stable in the environment than other bloodborne pathogens such as hepatitis C virus (HCV) and HIV.

HBV is transmitted by percutaneous or mucous membrane exposure to blood or body fluids that contain blood. The primary risk factors associated with infection among adolescents and adults are unprotected sex with an infected partner, history of other STDs, and illegal injected-drug use. HBV is a reportable disease.

Prevention

Two products are available for hepatitis B prevention: hepatitis B immune globulin (HBIG) and hepatitis B vaccine. HBIG provides temporary (3–6 months) protection from HBV infection and is typically used as postexposure prophylaxis, either as an adjunct to hepatitis B vaccination in previously unvaccinated persons or alone in persons who have not responded to vaccination. HBIG is prepared from plasma known to contain high concentrations of anti-HBs. The recommended dose of HBIG is 0.06 mL/kg.

Hepatitis B vaccine contains hepatitis B surface antigen (HBsAg) produced by recombinant DNA technology and provides protection from HBV infection when used for both pre- and postexposure vaccination. There are multiple vaccines available, which have different schedules depending on the specific product. All products require a series of multiple doses over varying time frames, and which regimen is selected depends on local availability and the age of the patient. The vaccine should be administered IM in the deltoid muscle and can be administered simultaneously with other vaccines.

Prevention of perinatal infection can be achieved through routine screening of all pregnant women for HBsAg and immunoprophylaxis (both HBIG and hepatitis B vaccine) of infants born to HBsAg-positive mothers or mothers whose HBsAg status is unknown. Prevention in infancy and childhood can be achieved by routine infant vaccination, and vaccination of previously unvaccinated children and adolescents through age 18 years. Adults who are previously unvaccinated but at increased risk for HBV, such as health care workers, sex workers, men who have sex with men, persons in correctional facilities, intravenous drug users, or household contacts of persons known to carry HBV, should also be vaccinated. Hepatitis B vaccination is recommended for all unvaccinated adolescents, all unvaccinated adults at risk for HBV infection, and all adults seeking protection from HBV infection. Hepatitis B vaccine should be offered to all unvaccinated persons attending STD clinics or seeking treatment for STDs in other settings. This vaccine may be administered in pregnancy if necessary.

Unvaccinated persons or those known not to have responded to a complete hepatitis B vaccine series should receive both HBIG and hepatitis vaccine as soon as possible (preferably ≤24 hours) after a discrete, identifiable exposure to blood or body fluids that contain blood from an HBsAg-positive source. Hepatitis B vaccine should be administered simultaneously with HBIG at a separate injection site, and the vaccine series should be completed by using the age-appropriate vaccine dose and schedule. Exposed persons who are in the process of being vaccinated but who have not completed the vaccine series should receive HBIG and complete the vaccine series. Exposed persons who are known to have responded to vaccination are considered protected.

Patients known to be chronic carriers of HBV should be counseled to have their household contacts and sex partners immunized, use condoms for sexual intercourse, and cover cuts and skin lesions to prevent transmission to others.

Clinical Findings

A. Symptoms & Signs

Approximately 70% of patients with acute hepatitis B are asymptomatic, with the remainder having jaundice. Rarely patients will present with fulminant hepatic failure.

A serum sickness-like syndrome may develop during the prodromal period, followed by constitutional symptoms, anorexia, nausea, jaundice, and right upper quadrant discomfort. The symptoms and jaundice generally disappear after 1 to 3 months, but some patients have prolonged fatigue even after normalization of serum aminotransferase concentrations.

Patients with chronic hepatitis B are generally asymptomatic, unless they develop significant cirrhosis or have extra hepatic manifestations. Patients may report nonspecific symptoms such as fatigue. Physical examination may be normal, or there may be stigmata of chronic liver disease, or decompensated cirrhosis.

B. Laboratory Findings

Diagnosis of acute or chronic HBV infection is by serology. Because HBsAg is present in both acute and chronic infection, the presence of IgM antibody to hepatitis B core antigen (IgM anti-HBc) is diagnostic of acute or recently acquired HBV infection. Antibody to HBsAg (anti-HBs) is produced after a resolved infection and is the only HBV antibody marker present after vaccination. The presence of HBsAg and total anti-HBc, with a negative test for IgM anti-HBc, indicates chronic HBV infection. The presence of anti-HBc alone might indicate a false-positive result or acute, resolved, or chronic infection.

Differential Diagnosis

The differential diagnosis of hepatitis B is broad and includes any other cause for hepatitis such as other infectious causes, genetic causes of liver disease, alcoholic hepatitis, autoimmune hepatitis, and medications.

Complications

The most serious, yet rare complication is acute liver failure and death, which occurs in 1% of reported cases. Becoming a chronic carrier of HBV is also a potential complication of acute infection. Risk for chronic infection is inversely related to age at acquisition; approximately 90% of infected infants and 30% of infected children aged <5 years become chronically infected, compared with 2–6% of persons who become infected as adults. Among persons with chronic HBV infection, the risk for premature death from cirrhosis or hepatocellular carcinoma is 15–25%.

Treatment

The treatment of acute HBV is supportive care. There are no specific effective antiviral drugs available at this time.

Patients who have chronic HBV infection should be managed by physicians with specific expertise of chronic liver disease. The agents interferon, lamivudine, adefovir, dipivoxil, telbivudine, and entecavir may be used to treat chronic HBV infection.

Prognosis

Acute hepatitis B is usually a self-limited condition, and if the affected patient does not become a chronic carrier, complete recovery is expected in the majority of cases. Chronic carrier status is associated with the potential complications previously described.

HEPATITIS C

ESSENTIALS OF DIAGNOSIS

- Caused by hepatitis C virus (HCV), an RNA virus
- Primarily transmitted by parenteral route; rarely sexually transmitted
- Up to 85% of affected patients become chronic carriers; of these, up to 70% will develop chronic liver disease
- No effective vaccine
- No effective treatment for acute disease
- Chronic HCV can be treated with combination therapy of pegylated interferon and ribavirin

Pathogenesis

Hepatitis C is caused by hepatitis C virus (HCV), a small single-stranded RNA virus. HCV RNA can be detected in blood 1–3 weeks after exposure, and antibodies to HCV (anti-HCV) may be detected in the blood as early as 8–9 weeks postexposure. As with hepatitis B, hepatitis C may manifest as an acute or chronic illness and is the most common chronic bloodborne infection in the United States, with approximately 3.2 million people affected.

HCV is transmitted through parenteral exposures to contaminated blood, usually through use of injected drugs and, to a lesser extent, through exposures in health care settings as a consequence of inadequate infection-control practices. Transmission rarely follows receipt of blood, tissues, and organs from HCV-infected donors who were not identified during routine screening activities, which have been mandated in the United States since 1992. Occupational and perinatal exposures can also result in transmission of HCV.

Sexual transmission of HCV had been considered to occur rarely, although it is observed, especially among HIV-infected persons. Ten percent of patients with acute HCV infection report contact with a known HCV-infected sex partner as their only risk for infection. HCV is a reportable disease.

Prevention

No vaccine for hepatitis C is available, and prophylaxis with immune globulin is not effective in preventing HCV infection after exposure. Therefore, prevention is focused on reducing transmission and reducing chronic liver disease in HCV-infected persons by identifying them and providing medical management and antiviral therapy, as indicated.

Although sexual transmission occurs rarely, condom use is still advisable. Screening of patients who are at risk of HCV is the key to reducing transmission. Patients presenting to STD clinics or in correctional facilities should be offered screening for HCV. All patients with HIV infection should also be screened. Other risk factors for which HCV testing is recommended include prior blood transfusion or solid organ transplant before July 1992, prior transfusion of clotting factor concentrates produced before 1987, long-term dialysis, and signs and symptoms of liver disease.

To reduce the risk for transmission to others, HCV-positive persons should be advised not to donate blood, body organs, or semen; not share any personal items that might have blood on them (eg, toothbrushes and razors); and cover cuts and sores.

HCV-positive women do not need to avoid pregnancy or breastfeeding. However, they should be advised that approximately 6 of every 100 infants born to HCV-infected woman become infected. This infection occurs predominantly during or near delivery, and no treatment or delivery method has been demonstrated to decrease this risk. The risk is increased by the presence of maternal HCV viremia at delivery and also is greater if the woman is coinfected with HIV. HCV has not been shown to be transmitted through breast milk, although HCV-positive mothers should consider abstaining from breastfeeding if their nipples are cracked or bleeding. Infants born to HCV-positive mothers should be tested for HCV infection and, if positive, evaluated for the presence of chronic liver disease.

Clinical Findings

A. Symptoms & Signs

Patients newly infected with HCV typically are either asymptomatic or have a mild clinical illness. As a result, most infected persons remain unaware of their infection because they feel well and therefore serve as a source of transmission to others as well as being at risk for chronic liver disease and other HCV-related chronic diseases for decades to come.

B. Laboratory Findings

Testing for antibodies to HCV (anti-HCV) is recommended for screening of asymptomatic persons based on risk factors or a recognized exposure. Multiple FDA-approved tests are commercially available. Nucleic acid PCR testing to detect HCV RNA is necessary to confirm the diagnosis of current HCV infection in a patient with a positive anti-HCV. Elevated ALT levels are suggestive of chronic liver disease.

Differential Diagnosis

The differential diagnosis of hepatitis C is broad and includes any other cause for hepatitis such as other infectious causes, genetic causes of liver disease, alcoholic hepatitis, autoimmune hepatitis, and medications.

Complications

Chronic HCV infection develops in up to 85% of HCV-infected persons, and of these, up to 70% will develop evidence of active liver disease.

Treatment

Patients who have been determined to be anti-HCV positive should be evaluated for the presence of active infection, presence or development of chronic liver disease, and possible treatment.

Combination therapy with pegylated interferon and ribavirin is the treatment of choice for patients with chronic hepatitis C. Providers should consult with gastroenterology or infectious disease specialists who are familiar with the most current management options for HCV.

Prognosis

Cirrhosis occurs in up to 50% of chronically infected patients. In patients with cirrhosis, there is a risk of subsequent hepatic decompensation and also of hepatocellular carcinoma, the latter risk being up to 3% per year. Death may occur as a consequence of these complications.

HIV INFECTION AND ACQUIRED IMMUNE DEFICIENCY SYNDROME

ESSENTIALS OF DIAGNOSIS

Asymptomatic Infection

- HIV antibody, antigen, or ribonucleic acid or culture
- Mononucleosis-like syndrome with weight loss, fever, night sweats
- Lymphadenopathy
- Pharyngitis
- Erythematous maculopapular rash
- Extragenital lymphadenopathy.

Acquired Immunodeficiency Syndrome (AIDS)

- Opportunistic infections
- Cognitive difficulties or depression
- Kaposi's sarcoma
- CD4 counts below 200
- Cervical neoplasia

Pathogenesis

HIV infection represents a spectrum of disease that begins with a brief acute viral syndrome that typically transitions to a chronic and clinically latent illness. Without treatment, this illness eventually progresses to a symptomatic, life-threatening immunodeficiency disease known as AIDS. In untreated patients, the time between initial HIV infection and the development of AIDS varies significantly from a few months to many years, with an estimated median time of approximately 11 years.

HIV is a single-stranded RNA retrovirus that attaches to the CD4 receptor of the target cell and integrates into the host genome. Its replication is present during all stages of the infection. This progressively depletes CD4 lymphocytes, which are essential for maintenance of effective immune function. When the CD4 cell count falls below 200 cells/μL, patients are at high risk for life-threatening AIDS-defining opportunistic infections. In the absence of treatment, virtually all HIV-infected persons will die of AIDS.

HIV infection can be acquired by sexual contact, parenteral exposure to blood or body fluids, or transmission from an infected woman to her fetus or infant. Sexual transmission risk is greatest for the female sexual partners of men with AIDS. Other factors that increase the risk for heterosexual acquisition of HIV infection are the number of exposures to high-risk sexual partners, anal-receptive intercourse, and infection with other STDs such as syphilis, genital herpes, chancroid, and condylomata acuminata. The reason for these findings is due to the high concentration of HIV in semen and the fact that coitus causes more breaks in the introital mucosa than in the penile skin. These breaks in the mucosa, similar to those that occur with anal-receptive intercourse, increase the chances for acquiring HIV through sexual contact. The presence of a genital ulcerative disease also increases the risk of infection in a similar fashion.

More than 80% of the female AIDS cases occur in women of reproductive age, making heterosexual and perinatal transmission important concerns. Minorities are disproportionately represented in the reported AIDS cases. In the United States most cases are due to HIV-1, with HIV-2 prevalence being very low. HIV-2 is endemic in parts of West Africa and has been reported increasingly in Angola, Mozambique, Portugal, and France. AIDS is a reportable disease.

Prevention

Primary prevention is based on condom use for sexual intercourse, avoiding the sharing of needles in persons who use IV drugs, universal precautions in occupations where blood of body fluid exposure is possible (ie, health care workers), and good prenatal care of HIV-infected pregnant women. In the latter group, antiretroviral therapy in pregnancy, in addition to peripartum intravenous antiretroviral therapy, caesarean section in selected cases, and avoidance of breastfeeding, can significantly decrease the risk of vertical transmission. In the third world, breastfeeding is still recommended for these women due to the risks associated with contaminated water for formula.

Secondary prevention guidelines for seropositive patients include refraining from donating blood, plasma, organs, or tissue and maintaining a mutually monogamous sexual relationship with condom use for all sexual activity. Circumcision decreases the transmission of HIV and is recommended in areas with high prevalence of HIV infection such as Africa.

Screening high-risk populations is essential in order to properly practice these prevention strategies. HIV serologic testing should include pre- and post-test counseling about interpretation of test results. HIV testing should be offered to persons that use or have used IV drugs, engaged in prostitution, have sex partners who are HIV-infected or are at risk for HIV infection, have other STDs, have lived in communities or were born in countries where the prevalence of HIV infection is high, have received blood transfusions between 1978 and 1985, have been inmates in correctional systems, or who are pregnant.

Clinical Findings

A. Symptoms & Signs

As many as 45–90% of patients develop an acute HIV-induced retroviral infection in the first few months after infection. This is similar to mononucleosis, with symptoms of weight loss, fever, night sweats, pharyngitis, lymphadenopathy, erythematous maculopapular rash, and extragenital lymphadenopathy. Critical awareness of this acute syndrome is important because of improved prognoses associated with early antiretroviral treatment. This syndrome usually resolves within several weeks, and the patient becomes asymptomatic. HIV-infected individuals ultimately show evidence of progressive immune dysfunction and the condition progresses to AIDS as immunosuppression continues and systemic involvement becomes more severe and diffuse. Characteristic opportunistic infections may occur, such as *Pneumocystis carinii* pneumonia, esophageal candidiasis, Kaposi's sarcoma, disseminated *Mycobacterium avium* infection, tuberculosis, cytomegalovirus, recurrent bacterial pneumonia, toxoplasmosis, chronic cryptosporidiosis, disseminated histoplasmosis, invasive cervical cancer, and chronic HSV.

The CDC definition of AIDS is an HIV-infected person with a specific opportunistic infection (eg, *P carinii* pneumonia, CNS toxoplasmosis), neoplasia (eg, Kaposi's sarcoma), dementia, encephalopathy, wasting syndrome, rapid progression of cervical dysplasia to cancer, or CD4 lymphocyte count less than 200/μL.

B. Laboratory Findings

The diagnosis of HIV infection is usually by HIV-1 antibody tests. Routine testing for HIV-2, other than at blood banks, is currently not recommended unless a patient is at risk for HIV-2 infection or has clinical findings of HIV disease and has had a negative HIV-1 antibody test. In general, the enzyme-linked immunosorbent assay (ELISA) functions as a screening test for exposure to HIV. Most patients exposed to HIV develop detectable levels of antibody against the virus by 12 weeks after exposure. The presence of antibody indicates current infection, although the patient may be asymptomatic for years. The sensitivity and specificity of the ELISA test is 99% when it is repeatedly reactive.

The probability of a false-negative test in an uninfected woman is remote unless she is in the "window" before antibody is produced. Individuals in high-risk groups should be retested in 3 months.

Rapid HIV testing can be used to identify HIV infection in women who arrive at labor and delivery with undocumented HIV status and to provide an opportunity to begin prophylaxis of previously undiagnosed infection before delivery. Test results are available within a few hours. Most rapid assays have a sensitivity and specificity comparable to that of ELISA.

Viral load (evaluated by PCR) is useful in determining the activity level of the disease. In the acute infective period the viral load is usually extremely high. The CD4 count will also determine disease activity, as it decreases as the disease progresses.

Differential Diagnosis

The differential diagnosis of acute HIV infection includes mononucleosis due to Epstein-Barr virus or cytomegalovirus, toxoplasmosis, rubella, syphilis, viral hepatitis, disseminated gonococcal infection, and other viral infections. Opportunistic infections seen in HIV-infected patients may also present in patients with immunodeficiency of other etiologies.

Complications

Complications relate to the opportunistic infections that can occur in patients with HIV infection as well as development of cancers such as Kaposi's sarcoma, lymphoma, and cervical carcinoma.

Treatment

A. General Considerations

The specifics of treatment of HIV-infected patients is beyond the scope of this text, and these patients should be managed by specialists in infectious disease medicine. However, the general approach is to use combination highly active antiretroviral therapy (HAART) in order to increase disease-free survival through suppression of HIV replication and improvement in immunologic function. The CD4 count is the main indicator of immune function in HIV-infected patients, and this value is used to determine when to initiate HAART and chemoprophylaxis for opportunistic infections, as well as being a valuable prognostic indicator. Patients with a CD4 count of less than 200/μL should be initiated on HAART. Patients with CD4 counts of 200–500/μL may also benefit from HAART, although the benefit is less pronounced than with more immunosuppressed patients. Patients with a history of an AIDS-defining illness or patients who are pregnant should also be treated with HAART.

For selected patients with a CD4 cell count greater than 500/μL, HAART may be considered. Appropriate patients include those who are motivated to start lifelong therapy, and these patients should be advised that there is less evidence for the potential benefits of treatment at earlier stages of HIV infection. The decision to treat should be balanced against potential toxicities of long-term therapy.

The specifics of the HARRT regimens are outside the scope of this text, but in general, 2 nucleoside reverse transcriptase inhibitors and 1 non-nucleoside reverse transcriptase inhibitor or a protease inhibitor are used in combination.

Antibiotic prophylaxis against various opportunistic infections should be initiated in patients who have CD4 counts of less than 200/μL. The specific coverage depends on how low the CD4 count is, and these decisions should be made by specialists in infectious disease medicine.

B. HIV and Pregnancy

Maternal transmission of HIV can occur transplacentally before birth, peripartum by exposure to blood and bodily fluids at delivery, or postpartum through breastfeeding. Therefore, all pregnant women should be offered HIV testing. In the absence of any intervention, an estimated 15–30% of mothers with HIV infection will transmit the infection during pregnancy and delivery, and 10–20% will transmit the infection through breast milk. Vertical transmission of HIV-1 occurs mostly during the intrapartum period (50–70%) but also can occur in the antepartum period (15–30%), especially in untreated women who seroconvert during pregnancy. The mode of delivery may play a role in increasing or decreasing the risks of developing pediatric AIDS. It is recommended that membranes not be ruptured longer than 4 hours. Fetal scalp electrodes and scalp sampling are contraindicated.

Prenatal care must be individualized, with referral to support systems ideally occurring during the pregnancy rather than postpartum. Screening for other STDs is important. HIV-infected patients should undergo shielded chest radiography, a tuberculin skin test with controls, and cytomegalovirus and toxoplasmosis baseline serologic tests. Susceptible patients should receive hepatitis B virus, pneumococcal, and influenza vaccines. CD4 cell counts should be monitored each trimester, as should plasma viral load (HIV-1 RNA).

Zidovudine (ZDV) administered during the second and third trimesters, during labor, and for 6 weeks to the newborn has been shown to decrease vertical transmission from 25–30% to 5–8%. Combination HAART has been shown to reduce the overall transmission to approximately 1.2%.

Caesarean section before onset of labor and rupture of membranes further decreases the risk of vertical transmission; however, the risk of vertical transmission is related to the viral load. When the viral load is less than 1000 copies per milliliter, the perinatal transmission rate approaches zero. Therefore, it is reasonable to offer scheduled caesarean section before onset of labor and rupture of membranes to HIV-infected women with viral loads greater than 1000 copies per milliliter. The American College of Obstetricians and Gynecologists (ACOG) recommends that a scheduled caesarean section be performed at 38 weeks' gestation in order to prevent HIV transmission. ZDV infusion should be started 3 hours preoperatively. The increased maternal morbidity associated with caesarean section must be taken into account, however, when making decisions regarding mode of delivery. Whether caesarean section is beneficial when the mother has received HAART and/or has low to undetectable viral loads is unclear. Also unclear is whether caesarean section after rupture of membranes or onset of labor confers a decrease in HIV transmission.

In resource-rich settings, patients should be counseled against breastfeeding in order to further decrease the risk of transmission.

Prognosis

Although early mortality was nearly certain for most HIV-infected patients in the beginning of the epidemic in the

1980s, the introduction of potent combination therapy has resulted in profound reductions in morbidity and mortality.

American College of Obstetricians and Gynecologists. Scheduled cesarean delivery and the prevention of vertical transmission of HIV infection. ACOG Committee Opinion No. 234. Washington, DC: ACOG; 2000.

Anderson JR (ed). *A Guide to the Clinical Care of Women with HIV*. Washington, DC: US Department of Health and Human Services, HIV/AIDS Bureau; 2001, pp. 1, 77.

Blattner W, et al. Effectiveness of potent antiretroviral therapies on reducing perinatal transmission of HIV-1. XIII International AIDS Conference, Durban, South Africa, July 9–14, 2000. [Abstract LbOr4]

PELVIC INFECTIONS

Because of their common occurrence and often serious consequences, infections are amongst the most important problems encountered in the practice of gynecology. A wide variety of pelvic infections, ranging from uncomplicated gonococcal salpingo-oophoritis to septic shock after rupture of a pelvic abscess, confront the general physician as well as the gynecologist. Pelvic infection can be due to processes in the following categories and will be discussed in the following section.

- Pelvic inflammatory disease, including tubo-ovarian abscess (TOA)
- Puerperal infections
- Postoperative pelvic infection after gynecologic surgery
- Abortion-associated infections
- Secondary to other infections

PELVIC INFLAMMATORY DISEASE

ESSENTIALS OF DIAGNOSIS

- Inflammation of upper female genital tract
- Usually polymicrobial
- Often diagnosed clinically based on the presence of cervical motion tenderness or uterine or adnexal tenderness
- Criteria exist to determine whether to manage patient as an inpatient or outpatient
- May result in pelvic scarring and infertility

Pathogenesis

Pelvic inflammatory disease (PID) comprises a spectrum of inflammatory disorders of the upper female genital tract, including any combination of endometritis, salpingitis, tubo-ovarian abscess, and pelvic peritonitis. Sexually transmitted organisms, particularly *N gonorrhoeae* and *C trachomatis*, are implicated in many cases. However, microorganisms that comprise the vaginal flora (eg, anaerobes, *G vaginalis*, *Haemophilus influenzae*, enteric gram-negative rods, and *Streptococcus agalactiae*) are also associated with PID, which is often polymicrobial. More uncommonly, cytomegalovirus, *Mycoplasma hominis*, *Ureaplasma urealyticum*, and *Mycoplasma genitalium* can cause PID. All women who have acute PID should be tested for *N gonorrhoeae* and *C trachomatis* and should be screened for other STDs.

Prevention

Screening and treating sexually active women and their sex partners for chlamydia and gonorrhea reduces their risk for PID. Early diagnosis and eradication of minimally symptomatic disease can also prevent salpingitis. Sex partners of women with PID should be examined and treated if they had sexual contact with the patient during the 60 days preceding the patient's onset of symptoms. If a patient's last sexual intercourse was >60 days before onset of symptoms or diagnosis, the patient's most recent sex partner should be treated. Patients should be instructed to abstain from sexual intercourse until therapy is completed and until they and their sex partners no longer have symptoms.

Clinical Findings

A. Symptoms & Signs

Acute PID is difficult to diagnose due to a wide variation in symptoms and signs. Many women with PID have subtle or mild symptoms. Delay in diagnosis and treatment contributes to inflammatory sequelae in the upper reproductive tract. Consequently, a diagnosis of PID usually is based on clinical findings, although clinical diagnosis is imprecise, and many cases of PID go unrecognized.

Patients may complain of insidious or acute onset of lower abdominal and pelvic pain, which is usually bilateral. There may be a sensation of pelvic pressure or back pain. There is often an associated purulent vaginal discharge.

Nausea may occur, with or without vomiting. Headache and general lassitude are common complaints. Fever is not necessary for the diagnosis of acute salpingitis, although its absence may indicate other disorders. In one study, only 30% of women with laparoscopically confirmed acute salpingitis had fever.

Abdominal tenderness is often encountered, usually in both lower quadrants. The abdomen may be somewhat distended, and bowel sounds may be hypoactive or absent. Pelvic examination may demonstrate inflammation of the periurethral (Skene) or Bartholin's glands as well as a purulent cervical discharge. Bimanual examination typically elicits extreme tenderness on movement of the cervix and uterus and palpation of the parametria.

Based on the CDC guidelines, the diagnosis of PID should be made and empiric treatment initiated in sexually active young women and other women at risk for STDs if they are experiencing pelvic or lower abdominal pain, if no cause for the illness other than PID can be identified, and if 1 or more of the following minimum criteria are present on pelvic examination: cervical motion tenderness, uterine tenderness, or adnexal tenderness.

B. Laboratory Findings

Saline microscopy of vaginal fluid may reveal abundant white blood cells. Complete blood count may reveal a leukocytosis with a shift to the left. Erythrocyte sedimentation rate and C-reactive protein may be elevated. Endocervical swabs may be positive for infection with *N gonorrhoeae* or *C trachomatis*. However, all these tests may be normal in a patient with PID; therefore, should be used as supportive evidence only, not as definitive diagnostic tools. Endometrial biopsy is more specific and usually shows histopathologic evidence of endometritis. In practice, however, this is often not done, although it may be particularly useful in women who have undergone laparoscopy with no visual evidence of salpingitis, as endometritis may be the only sign of PID in some cases.

C. Imaging

Transvaginal sonography or magnetic resonance imaging techniques showing thickened, fluid-filled tubes with or without free pelvic fluid or tubo-ovarian complex or Doppler studies suggesting pelvic infection (eg, tubal hyperemia) are quite specific for PID, although in less complicated cases, imaging may be normal.

D. Laparoscopy

Diagnostic laparoscopy can be used to obtain a more accurate diagnosis of salpingitis and a more complete bacteriologic diagnosis. However, this tool may not be available at some sites, and it may not be appropriate when symptoms are mild or vague. Laparoscopy will not detect endometritis and may not detect subtle inflammation of the fallopian tubes. It remains, however, a useful adjunct when the diagnosis is in question.

Differential Diagnosis

PID must be differentiated from other acute abdominal processes such as acute appendicitis, ectopic pregnancy, ruptured corpus luteum cyst with hemorrhage, diverticulitis, infected septic abortion, torsion of an adnexal mass, degeneration of a leiomyoma, endometriosis, acute urinary tract infection, regional enteritis, and ulcerative colitis.

Complications

Complications of acute salpingitis include pelvic peritonitis or generalized peritonitis, prolonged ileus, septic pelvic thrombophlebitis, abscess formation with adnexal destruction and subsequent infertility, and intestinal adhesions and obstruction. Rarely, dermatitis, gonococcal arthritis, or bacteremia with septic shock occurs.

Treatment

PID treatment regimens provide empiric, broad spectrum coverage of likely pathogens and should be given as soon as a presumptive diagnosis is made. Several antimicrobial regimens have been effective in achieving clinical and microbiologic cure in randomized clinical trials with short-term follow-up. However, the data on long-term outcomes and frequency of complications such as tubal infertility and ectopic pregnancy are limited.

All regimens used to treat PID should also be effective against *N gonorrhoeae* and *C trachomatis* because negative endocervical screening for these organisms does not rule out upper reproductive tract infection.

The majority of women with a clinical diagnosis of PID have symptoms of mild to moderate severity that usually respond well to outpatient antibiotic therapy. Hospitalization usually is warranted for women who are more severely ill, as well as the following cases:

- Patient in whom surgical emergencies (eg, appendicitis) cannot be excluded
- Patient who are pregnant
- Patients who have not responded well to outpatient oral therapy
- Patients who are unable to tolerate or comply with outpatient therapy
- Patients who have severe illness, nausea and vomiting, or high fever
- Patients with tubo-ovarian abscess

A. Outpatient Therapy

1. Recommended regimens

- Ceftriaxone 250 mg IM in a single dose (or other parenteral third-generation cephalosporin), **plus**
- Doxycycline 100 mg orally twice a day for 14 days, **with** or **without**
- Metronidazole 500 mg orally twice a day for 14 days

or

- Cefoxitin 2 g IM in a single dose and probenecid 1 g orally in a single dose administered concurrently, **plus**
- Doxycycline 100 mg orally twice a day for 14 days, **with** or **without**
- Metronidazole 500 mg orally twice a day for 14 days

Data on alternative regimens are limited. Amoxicillin/clavulanic acid and doxycycline may be used, as well as ceftriaxone 250 mg IM single dose and azithromycin 1 g orally once a week for 2 weeks. When considering alternative regimens, the addition of metronidazole should be considered. As a result of the emergence of quinolone-resistant *N gonorrhoeae*, regimens that include a quinolone agent are no longer recommended for the treatment of PID. If parenteral cephalosporin therapy is not feasible, use of fluoroquinolones (levofloxacin 500 mg orally once daily or ofloxacin 400 mg twice daily for 14 days) with or without metronidazole (500 mg orally twice daily for 14 days) can be considered if the community prevalence and individual risk for gonorrhea are low.

If a response to therapy is not observed after 72 hours, the patient should be re-evaluated to confirm the diagnosis and consideration made to admitting the patient for inpatient therapy.

B. Inpatient Therapy

1. Recommended regimen A

- Cefotetan 2 g IV every 12 hours, **or** cefoxitin 2 g IV every 6 hours, **plus**
- Doxycycline 100 mg orally or IV every 12 hours

2. Recommended regimen B

- Clindamycin 900 mg IV every 8 hours, **plus**
- Gentamicin loading dose IV or IM (2 mg/kg body weight) followed by a maintenance dose (1.5 mg/kg) every 8 hours. Single daily dosing (3–5 mg/kg) can be substituted.

3. Alternative regimens

- Ampicillin/sulbactam 3 g IV every 6 hours, **plus**
- Doxycycline 100 mg orally or IV every 12 hours

Oral doxycycline is preferable due to pain associated with IV infusion and similar bioavailability of oral and parenteral preparations.

Parenteral agents can be discontinued 24 hours after clinical improvement is observed, but oral therapy with doxycycline should be continued to complete a course of 14 days of treatment. When tubo-ovarian abscess is present, metronidazole or clindamycin should be added to the inpatient or outpatient regimen to provide adequate anaerobic coverage.

C. Special Circumstances

All pregnant women with suspected PID should be hospitalized and treated with parenteral antibiotics. Doxycycline should not be used in pregnancy.

Patients with intrauterine devices (IUDs) with suspected PID do not necessarily need to have the IUD removed, particularly if the patient is at high risk of unintended pregnancy. However, caution should be exercised if the IUD remains in place, and close clinical follow-up is required. Re-evaluation for IUD removal should be considered if the patient is not clinically improving. Of note, the risk of PID is not increased in IUD users other than in the first 21 days after insertion, after which it is uncommon. The levonorgestrel-releasing IUD may have a protective effect against PID due to thickening of cervical mucus. If an IUD is removed due to PID, a new one may be reinserted 3 months after resolution of the infection if the patient is not at ongoing risk of PID.

Actinomyces israelii is a normal anaerobic commensal of the gastrointestinal tract but can be associated with pelvic infection and abscess. It is present on the Papanicolaou test of approximately 7% of IUD users. Most patients are asymptomatically colonized. If actinomyces is present, the patient should be examined, and if asymptomatic, there is no indication to administer antibiotics or remove the IUD. If the patient demonstrates symptoms of PID or tubo-ovarian abscess, antibiotics should be commenced and the IUD removed, as actinomyces preferentially grow on foreign bodies.

Actinomyces is sensitive to penicillin; a 14-day course of penicillin G (500 mg 4 times per day), or doxycycline (100 mg twice per day) in patients with penicillin allergy, may be adequate treatment for a very early, local infection, but prolonged IV therapy (weeks to months) is indicated for tubo-ovarian abscess or disseminated infection. Surgical drainage is usually required for actinomycotic abscesses, which are often the result of intestinal infections such as appendicitis but may be associated with IUD use.

Prognosis

A favorable outcome is directly related to the promptness with which adequate therapy is begun. A single episode of salpingitis has been shown to cause infertility in 12–18% of women. Follow-up care and education are necessary to prevent reinfection and complications. In some cases patients may experience recurrent or chronic pelvic infection resulting in chronic pelvic pain.

TUBO-OVARIAN ABSCESS

ESSENTIALS OF DIAGNOSIS

- Usually preceded by PID
- Lower abdominal and pelvic pain of varying degrees
- Nausea and vomiting
- Complex multiloculated adnexal mass on imaging
- Requires inpatient IV antibiotic therapy
- Ruptured tubo-ovarian abscess is a surgical emergency

Pathogenesis

Tubo-ovarian abscess (TOA) is part of the spectrum of PID and can be acute or more chronic in nature. TOA formation may occur after an initial episode of acute salpingitis, but it is usually seen with recurrent infection superimposed on chronically damaged adnexal tissue. Fallopian tube necrosis and epithelial damage by bacterial pathogens create an environment conducive to anaerobic invasion and growth. The adjacent ovary may become involved with an ovulation site serving as the portal of entry for infection and subsequent abscess formation. Pressure of the purulent exudate may cause rupture of the abscess with resultant fulminating peritonitis, necessitating emergency laparotomy.

Slow leakage of the abscess may cause formation of a cul-de-sac abscess. TOAs may occur in association with diverticulitis or in the presence of granulomatous infection. Disease can be bilateral, although unilateral disease is more common. Abscesses are usually polymicrobial.

Clinical Findings

A. Symptoms & Signs

The clinical spectrum varies greatly and may range from total absence of symptoms in a woman who, on routine pelvic examination, is found to have an adnexal mass to a moribund patient presenting with acute abdomen and septicemic shock.

Patients with TOA are often young, of low parity, with a history of previous pelvic infection, although it can occur in women of any age. Patients typically report pelvic and abdominal pain, fever, and nausea and vomiting developing over a week or so. Physical examination may reveal abdominal tenderness and guarding. Adequate pelvic examination is often difficult due to tenderness, but an adnexal mass may be palpated. If the patient has a ruptured TOA, she will likely present with symptoms and signs of an acute surgical abdomen and may develop signs of septic shock.

B. Laboratory Findings

Laboratory findings are generally of little value. The white count may vary from leukopenia to marked leukocytosis. Urinalysis may demonstrate pyuria without bacteriuria. An elevated erythrocyte sedimentation rate or C-reactive protein is suggestive of a diagnosis of TOA in the presence of an adnexal mass.

C. Imaging

Ultrasonography is the radiologic modality of choice and will typically demonstrate complex multiloculated adnexal masses that obscure normal adnexal structures. These masses may contain internal echoes consistent with inflammatory debris.

Computed tomography (CT) may be preferable in a patient in whom other abdominal pathology cannot be excluded, such as diverticulitis or appendicitis. CT findings consistent with TOAs include multilocular, thick walled, rim-enhancing adnexal masses containing increased fluid density.

Differential Diagnosis

An unruptured TOA must be differentiated from an ovarian cyst or tumor with or without torsion, unruptured ectopic pregnancy, periappendiceal abscess, uterine leiomyoma, hydrosalpinx, perforation of a diverticulum or diverticular abscess, perforation of peptic ulcer, urinary tract infection or calculi, and any systemic disease that causes acute abdominal distress.

Complications

Unruptured TOA may be complicated by rupture in 15% of cases. Other complications include sepsis (10–20%), reinfection at a later date, and subsequent bowel obstruction, infertility, and ectopic pregnancy due to pelvic adhesions.

Ruptured TOA is a surgical emergency and may be complicated by septic shock, intra-abdominal abscess, and septic emboli with renal, lung, or brain abscess.

Treatment

A. Unruptured TOA

Treatment is similar to that of inpatient management of PID (see prior section), although total duration of therapy may be longer, depending on the size of the abscess and clinical response (up to 4–6 weeks, although an optimal duration of therapy has not been established). Patients should be monitored on an inpatient basis for 48–72 hours. Minimally invasive radiologic-guided drainage of abscesses is appropriate for large abscesses or for patients who are not worsening, but not improving on medical treatment alone. The drained fluid should be sent for culture so that ongoing antimicrobial therapy can be pathogen directed. If a patient is not improving despite these measures, or is worsening, surgical management should be considered, which generally involves exploratory laparotomy by an experienced gynecologic surgeon, as these cases are usually technically extremely challenging due to the inflammatory process, which destroys normal tissue planes. The extent of resection depends on the extent of disease, the patient's age, and the patient's desire for future fertility. A total abdominal hysterectomy and bilateral salpingo-oophorectomy is the optimal surgery in order to remove all areas of infected tissue. Surgical drains are often left in place.

Close follow-up is essential after initial hospitalization, with repeat imaging as indicated.

B. Ruptured TOA

This is an acute life-threatening emergency requiring immediate surgery in conjunction with antibiotic therapy. Total abdominal hysterectomy and bilateral salpingo-oophorectomy via a vertical midline incision is the procedure of choice, in association with aggressive fluid resuscitation. Careful surgical technique is necessary to avoid perforation of the bowel or transection of the ureters. Surgical drains should be left in place. Postoperatively, consideration should be made to placing the patient in the intensive care unit, where vital signs and urine output can be closely monitored and antibiotic treatment should be continued.

C. Special Considerations

Patients with a TOA and an IUD should have the IUD removed.

The majority of TOAs are found in premenopausal women, but when a postmenopausal women is found to have a TOA, there is a high risk of concurrent malignancy. Therefore, these patients should be counseled regarding this potential and consented for full staging.

TOA in pregnancy is rare, but is managed no differently from outside of pregnancy, with the exception of the avoidance of antibiotics with teratogenic potential.

Prognosis

Generally the patient with an unruptured abscess has an excellent prognosis. Medical therapy, followed by judicious surgical treatment, yields good results in most cases. Fertility may be greatly reduced, with an increased risk for ectopic pregnancy. The risk of reinfection must be considered if definitive surgical treatment has not been performed.

Before effective means of treating overwhelming septicemia became available and the need for immediate surgical intervention was recognized, the mortality rate from ruptured TOA was 80–90%. However, with modern therapeutic resources, both medical and surgical, the mortality rate is less than 2%.

POSTPARTUM ENDOMYOMETRITIS

ESSENTIALS OF DIAGNOSIS

- Common cause of fever in the postpartum patient
- Diagnosis is clinical
- Fever and uterine tenderness
- Laboratory tests are of limited use
- IV broad-spectrum antibiotics are mainstay of therapy and are continued until the patient has been afebrile for 24–48 hours

Pathogenesis

Puerperal infections refer primarily to postpartum infections of the uterus, which may involve the deciduas (endometritis), myometrium (endomyometritis), or parametria (parametritis). It is a common cause of postpartum fever and is usually a polymicrobial process involving a mixture of organisms from the genital tract. It can occur after either vaginal delivery or caesarean section.

Prevention

There are a number of strategies that can be used to decrease the rate of postpartum endomyometritis, including the use of prophylactic antibiotics at the time of caesarean section (both elective and nonelective) and avoidance of manual delivery of the placenta at caesarean section. Intrapartum chorioamnionitis increases the risk of postpartum endomyometritis; therefore, factors that decrease the risk of chorioamnionitis (eg, decreased number of internal vaginal examinations, shorter labor length) should also decrease the risk of postpartum endometritis.

Clinical Findings

A. Symptoms & Signs

Diagnosis is clinical and is suspected when a postpartum patient presents with fever and uterine tenderness.

B. Laboratory Findings

Laboratory tests are of limited value. Leucocytosis may be present, although this can be a normal finding in a postpartum patient. Endometrial cultures are not usually performed, as it is nearly impossible to obtain an uncontaminated specimen. Bacteremia can occur in 10–20% of cases, so consideration of blood cultures should be made.

Differential Diagnosis

The differential diagnosis of fever in a postpartum patient includes mastitis, surgical site infection, urinary tract infection, pneumonia, and deep vein thrombosis.

Complications

Peritoneal infection and pelvic abscess can occur as a result of endomyometritis, which may lead to pelvic adhesions and tubal occlusion.

Treatment

Administration of broad-spectrum antibiotics is the mainstay of therapy. Common practice is to use clindamycin 900 mg IV every 8 hours with gentamicin 1.5 mg/kg IV every 8 hours. This regimen is generally continued until the patient has been afebrile for 24–48 hours. For patients known to be colonized with group B streptococcus from universal screening, the addition of ampicillin 2 g IV every 6 hours is recommended. Subsequent oral antibiotic therapy is not required. Alternative regimens include cefotetan, cefoxitin, ceftriaxone, cefotaxime, and piperacillin, although data are limited.

Prognosis

The majority of patients will respond to therapy within 48–72 hours. A minority will have persistent fevers and require further evaluation.

POSTOPERATIVE PELVIC INFECTIONS

ESSENTIALS OF DIAGNOSIS

- Recent pelvic surgery
- Pelvic or low abdominal pain or pressure
- Fever and tachycardia
- Purulent, foul discharge
- Constitutional symptoms often present
- Vaginal cuff tenderness with cellulitis or abscess

Pathogenesis

Patients who have undergone gynecologic surgery, particularly hysterectomy, may develop postoperative infections of the remaining pelvic structures. These infections include vaginal cuff cellulitis, infected vaginal cuff hematoma, salpingitis, pelvic cellulitis, septic pelvic thrombophlebitis, and TOA with or without rupture. The incidence of such infections has been significantly reduced by the use of single-dose, perioperative antibiotic prophylaxis for hysterectomy.

The pathogenesis of posthysterectomy infection is simple. The apex of the vaginal vault consists of crushed, devitalized tissue, and the loose areolar tissue in the parametrial areas usually oozes postoperatively. These conditions provide an ideal medium for the myriad of pathogens that normally inhabit the vagina and are inoculated into the operative site during surgery. The term **pelvic cellulitis** implies that the soft tissue of the vaginal apex and adjacent parametrial tissues have been invaded by bacteria. Serum and blood at the cuff apex may become infected, resulting in an infected hematoma or cuff abscess. Infection may extend via lymphatic channels to the adnexa, resulting in salpingitis. Pelvic veins may become involved in the infectious process, particularly if *Bacteroides* or anaerobic streptococci are predominant pathogens.

Prevention

Many attempts have been made to decrease infectious morbidity after gynecologic surgical procedures. None have been uniformly successful, but the following measures may be helpful:

- Preoperative treatment of cervicitis, bacterial vaginosis, or vulvovaginitis if present
- Preparation of the vagina with hexachlorophene or povidone-iodine solution immediately before surgery
- Meticulous attention to hemostasis and gentle handling of tissues intraoperatively
- If hemostasis is less than desirable but is maximal under given circumstances, suction drains to that area should be placed
- Antimicrobial prophylaxis beginning preoperatively. For hysterectomy the antibiotic of choice is cefazolin 1–2 g IV administered not more than 60 minutes before surgical start time.
- Severe, more advanced infections may be prevented by early diagnosis, drainage, and prompt treatment of mild infections.

Clinical Findings

A. Symptoms & Signs

Fever due to postoperative pelvic infection usually does not occur before the third or fourth postoperative day. The vaginal cuff may appear hyperemic and edematous, and there is often a purulent exudate. When palpated, this site is usually indurated and tender. If infection involves the tubes and ovaries or intra-abdominal abscess forms, the patient may complain of lower abdominal, pelvic, or back pain. Abdominal distention due to ileus may develop, as may urinary symptoms due to perivesical irritation.

The diagnosis of septic pelvic thrombophlebitis is rare and usually is not apparent until after the sixth postoperative day, at which time the patient usually has high spiking fevers with a diurnal variation. The pelvic findings are usually unrevealing except for mild pelvic tenderness.

An infected pelvic hematoma may only be evident by recurrent fevers. Rarely do these patients have symptoms, and their examination is may be unremarkable.

B. Laboratory Findings

Due to the polymicrobial nature of these infections, it is usually not possible to isolate a specific organism in a reasonable time. For this reason, broad-spectrum empirical antimicrobial administration is necessary. However, blood cultures or culture of any drained purulent material should be sent in order to assist with directing therapy in the case of poor clinical improvement.

Serial complete blood counts usually demonstrate leukocytosis but occasionally enable the physician to detect concealed hemorrhage, which may harbor a large pelvic abscess. Urinalysis is rarely helpful.

C. Imaging

Pelvic ultrasound is helpful in detecting hematomas or abscesses that develop as a complication of cuff infection. CT scan is the imaging modality of choice for septic pelvic thrombophlebitis, although a negative study does not necessarily exclude the diagnosis.

Differential Diagnosis

The differential diagnosis of postoperative fever includes pulmonary atelectasis, aspiration pneumonitis, deep vein thrombophlebitis, superficial phlebitis due to an indwelling venous catheter, urinary tract infection, wound infection, and drug fever.

Complications

Complications of postoperative pelvic infection include pelvic or intra-abdominal abscesses, TOA with or without rupture, intestinal adhesions and obstruction, septic pelvic thrombophlebitis, and septicemia.

Treatment

If an infected cuff hematoma or abscess is found, adequate drainage can be established by separating the opposed vaginal edges with ring forceps or some other suitable instrument. The usual supportive measures are instituted, and broad-spectrum antibiotic therapy commenced. Pelvic abscesses in other locations may be drained with CT or ultrasound guidance and a drain left in place.

Septic pelvic thrombophlebitis is generally a diagnosis of exclusion when a patient has persistent fevers after 7–10 days of broad-spectrum antibiotics. The recommended treatment is systemic anticoagulation with either IV unfractionated heparin or subcutaneous low-molecular-weight heparin. In the absence of documented thromboses or underlying hypercoagulable state, anticoagulation is generally discontinued after resolution of fever for at least 48 hours. If pelvic branch vein thromboses are documented radiographically, anticoagulation with low-molecular-weight heparin is usually continued for at least 2 weeks. If septic emboli or extensive pelvic thromboses (eg, thrombosis involving the ovarian vein, iliac veins or vena cava) are documented radiographically, anticoagulation with low-molecular-weight heparin or warfarin for at least 6 weeks is recommended. Follow-up imaging to evaluate for persistence or resolution of thromboses should be obtained to guide subsequent management.

Prognosis

With prompt diagnosis and treatment, postoperative infections usually resolve completely without long-term sequelae.

ABORTION-ASSOCIATED INFECTIONS

ESSENTIALS OF DIAGNOSIS

- Incidence of postabortion infection is decreased with preprocedure antibiotic prophylaxis.
- Septic abortion is rare.
- There is a rare association with *Clostridium sordellii*.

Pathogenesis

Postabortal endometritis occurs in 5–20% of patients undergoing elective termination of pregnancy who do not receive prophylactic antibiotics; this rate is halved if antibiotics are used. It may occur in the presence or absence of retained products of conception. It is usually polymicrobial.

Septic abortion usually refers to intrauterine infection that leads to spontaneous abortion and is uncommon. Patients are usually extremely unwell compared with patients with postabortal endometritis. Infection is usually due to *Staphylococcus aureus*, gram-negative bacilli, or some gram-positive cocci. The infection may spread, leading to salpingitis, generalized peritonitis, and septicemia. Rarely septic abortion be associated with a foreign body, such as an IUD; invasive procedures, such as amniocentesis; or maternal bacteremia.

A small number of septic deaths related to *Clostridium sordellii* have been reported with medical abortion. Overall, infection rates after medical abortion are much lower than with surgical abortion. However, in 2005, 4 septic deaths were reported. They all occurred in California within 1 week of medical abortion. *C sordellii* infection was diagnosed in all 4 cases. Subsequently, 5 more deaths from clostridial sepsis after medical abortion in the United States and Canada have been reported, 2 from *Clostridium perfringens* and 3 from *C sordellii*. Interestingly, no abortion-related deaths from *Clostridial* infection have been reported in Europe, where mifepristone is widely used.

Reports are rare of fulminant lethal clostridial sepsis in women of childbearing age, but there is generally an association with childbirth, abortion, or cervical or uterine procedures. Sepsis related to *C sordellii* is unusual because of its subtle clinical manifestations and rapid progression to death. A causal relationship between mifepristone/misoprostol and *Clostridium* sepsis has not been established.

Prevention

Prophylactic antibiotics are the cornerstone of prevention. The agent recommended by ACOG for prophylaxis for induced abortion is doxycycline 100 mg orally 1 hour before the procedure and 200 mg orally after the procedure. An alternative regimen is metronidazole 500 mg orally twice a day for 5 days.

Clinical Findings

A. Symptoms & Signs

Signs and symptoms of postabortal endometritis include fever, enlarged and tender uterus, lower abdominal tenderness, and vaginal bleeding greater than expected. Common clinical features of septic abortion include fever, chills, malaise, abdominal pain, vaginal bleeding, and discharge, which is often sanguinopurulent. Physical examination may reveal tachycardia, tachypnea, lower abdominal tenderness, and a boggy, tender uterus with dilated cervix.

Patients with *C sordellii* sepsis after medical abortion generally present without fever, bacteremia, rash, or significant findings on pelvic examination, but have dramatic leukocytosis with a marked left shift, hemoconcentration, tachycardia, hypotension crampy abdominal pain, pleural/peritoneal effusion, and general malaise (weakness, nausea, vomiting, diarrhea).

B. Imaging

Pelvic ultrasound may reveal retained products of conception or may be unremarkable.

Differential Diagnosis

Other causes of infection such as PID, vaginitis, cervicitis, appendicitis, and urinary tract infection, should be excluded.

Complications

Postabortion infection can lead to intrauterine or intra-abdominal scarring and in severe cases can lead to sepsis and rarely death.

Treatment

If retained products are demonstrated, suction dilatation and curettage should be performed to evaluate this infected material. In the absence of retained products, or after uterine evacuation, broad-spectrum antibiotics should be commenced, such as cefotetan 2 g IV every 12 hours plus doxycycline 100 mg orally twice a day. This course can be completed as an outpatient with doxycycline 100 mg orally twice a day with or without metronidazole 500 mg orally twice a day for a total of 14 days.

Patients who are demonstrating signs and symptoms of sepsis should be aggressively managed with fluid resuscitation, broad-spectrum antibiotics, uterine evacuation, assessment for uterine perforation, and supportive care in an intensive care unit.

Optimal therapy for *C sordellii* is unknown, but probably includes surgical debridement, removal of infected organs (eg, hysterectomy), and antibiotics with good anaerobic activity.

Prognosis

With prompt diagnosis and treatment, most abortion-associated infections are effectively cured. *C sordellii* is extremely rare, but its onset is insidious with subsequent rapid progression to severe illness and death; therefore, the index of suspicion should remain high, particularly in cases of recent medical abortion.

American College of Obstetricians and Gynecologists. ACOG Practice Bulletin Number 104. Antibiotic Prophylaxis for Gynecologic Procedures. Washington, DC: ACOG; 2009.

Cohen AL, Bhatnagar J, Reagan S, et al. Toxic shock associated with *Clostridium sordellii* and *Clostridium perfringens* after medical and spontaneous abortion. *Obstet Gynecol* 2007;110:1027–1033. PMID: 17978116.

Fischer M, Bhatnagar J, Guarner J, et al. Fatal toxic shock syndrome associated with *Clostridium sordellii* after medical abortion. *N Engl J Med* 2005;353:2352–2360. PMID: 16319384.

Meites E, Zane S, Gould C. C. sordellii Investigators. Fatal *Clostridium sordellii* infections after medical abortions. *N Engl J Med* 2010;363:1382–1383. PMID: 20879895.

Sinave C, Le Templier G, Blouin D, Léveillé F, Deland E. Toxic shock syndrome due to *Clostridium sordellii*: A dramatic postpartum and postabortion disease. *Clin Infect Dis* 2002;35:1441–1443. PMID: 12439811.

Wiebe E, Guilbert E, Jacot F, Shannon C, Winikoff B. A fatal case of *Clostridium sordellii* septic shock syndrome associated with medical abortion. *Obstet Gynecol* 2004;104(5 Pt 2):1142–1144. PMID: 15516429.

PELVIC TUBERCULOSIS

ESSENTIALS OF DIAGNOSIS

- Often results in infertility
- Associated with active or healed pulmonary tuberculosis
- Diagnosis by hysterosalpingogram or laparoscopy
- Recovery of *Mycobacterium tuberculosis* from either menstrual fluid or biopsy specimen

Pathogenesis

In the United States, pelvic tuberculosis is a rare entity. When it does occur, it usually represents secondary invasion from a primary lung infection via lymphatic or hematogenous spread. The overall incidence of pelvic tuberculosis in patients with pulmonary tuberculosis is approximately 5%. Prepubertal tuberculosis rarely results in genital tract infection.

After the pelvic organs become affected (Fig. 43–5), direct extension to adjacent organs may occur. The endometrium is involved in more than 90% of cases, with fallopian tube involvement in only 5%.

Prevention

Prevention is largely based on screening populations at risk of tuberculosis for active or latent disease in order to treat pulmonary tuberculosis early to prevent systemic spread and transmission to others. Populations at risk include foreign-born persons from areas with high tuberculosis prevalence, homeless populations, residents of correctional or long-term care facilities, health care workers who work with high-risk populations, low-income and medically underserved populations, and patients with immunocompromise.

Clinical Findings

A. Symptoms & Signs

The only complaint may be infertility, although dysmenorrhea, pelvic pain, and evidence of tuberculous peritonitis may also be present. Endometrial involvement may result in amenorrhea or other disturbance of the menstrual cycle.

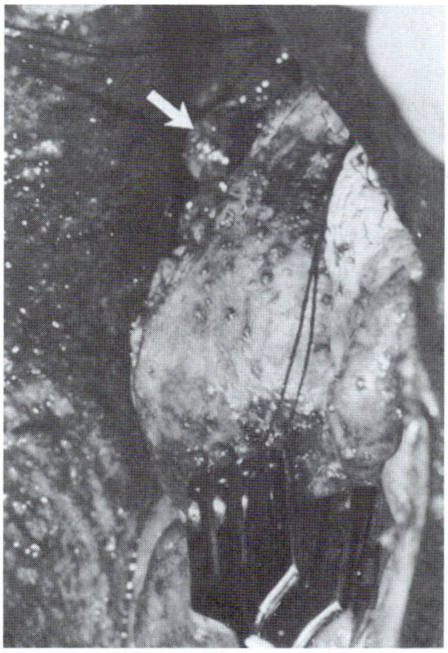

▲ **Figure 43–5.** Miliary tuberculosis involving the uterus and peritoneum.

Abdominal or pelvic pain may be associated with low-grade fever, fatigue, and weight loss. Gross ascites may be present in tuberculous peritonitis.

Pelvic tuberculosis may be encountered in the course of a gynecologic surgery performed for other reasons. Although pelvic tuberculosis may be mistaken for chronic pelvic inflammation, some distinguishing features usually can be found: extremely dense adhesions without planes of cleavage, segmental dilatation of the tubes, and lack of occlusion of the tubes at the ostia.

B. Laboratory Findings

Diagnosis can be established on the basis of a complete history and physical examination, chest x-ray, and appropriate tests such as a tuberculin (Mantoux) test, sputum smears, and cultures. The best direct method of diagnosis in suspected genital tuberculosis is detection of acid-fast bacteria by Ziehl-Neelsen stain followed by culture on Lowenstein-Jensen medium. The specimen may be from menstrual discharge, from curettage or biopsy, or from peritoneum.

C. X-Ray Findings

A chest x-ray film should be obtained in any patient with proven or suspected tuberculosis of other organs or tissues. Upper lobe infiltrates and hilar adenopathy may be seen. A hysterosalpingogram may demonstrate irregular tubal lining and areas of dilatation. Saccular diverticula extending from the ampulla and giving the impression of a cluster of currants are characteristic of granulomatous salpingitis.

Differential Diagnosis

Pelvic tuberculosis should be differentiated from schistosomiasis, enterobiasis, lipoid salpingitis, carcinoma, chronic pelvic inflammation, and mycotic infections.

Complications

Sterility and tuberculous peritonitis are possible sequelae of pelvic tuberculosis.

Treatment

A. Medical Measures

To prevent the emergence of drug-resistant strains, the initial therapy of tuberculous infection should include 4 drugs. The drug regimen for the first 2 months of treatment should include isoniazid, rifampin, pyrazinamide, and streptomycin or ethambutol. Once drug susceptibility results are available, the drug regimen can be adjusted. The specifics and duration of treatment should be determined in conjunction with an infectious disease specialist.

B. Surgical Measures

The primary mode of treatment for pelvic tuberculosis is medical therapy; however, surgical intervention may be necessary. Medical therapy should be attempted for 12–18 months before evaluation for surgery. The ultimate indications for surgery include (1) masses not resolving with medical therapy, (2) resistant or reactivated disease, (3) persistent menstrual irregularities, and (4) fistula formation.

Prognosis

The prognosis for life and health is excellent if chemotherapy is instituted promptly, although the prognosis for fertility is poor.

TOXIC SHOCK SYNDROME

ESSENTIALS OF DIAGNOSIS

- High fever
- Diffuse macular rash
- Desquamation 1–2 weeks after onset of illness; particularly affects palms and soles
- Hypotension or orthostatic syncope
- Involvement of 3 or more of the following organ systems: gastrointestinal, muscular, mucous membrane, renal, hepatic, hematologic, CNS

Pathogenesis

Toxic shock syndrome (TSS) is a rare entity caused by exotoxins produced by the ubiquitous aerobic gram-positive coccus, *Staphylococcus aureus*. It was first described in 1978 in children, but was quickly identified as an illness occurring primarily in menstruating women. Cases can be menstrual or nonmenstrual. For the purposes of this chapter, menstrual cases will be discussed.

TSS is associated with the use of highly absorbent tampons, and since these types of tampons have been withdrawn from the market, the incidence has decreased. Since 1986 the incidence of menstrual TSS is 1 in 100,000 women (declined from 9 in 100,000 in 1980). However, tampon use is still a risk factor. Women who develop TSS are more likely to have used tampons with higher absorbencies, used tampons continuously for more days of their menstrual cycle, and kept a single tampon in place for a longer period of time. Nonmenstrual TSS has been reported with diaphragm use and after delivery.

The cause of toxic shock syndrome is preformed toxins produced by *S aureus* after colonization or infection by this microorganism. A pyrogenic toxin induces high fever and may enhance susceptibility to endotoxins that cause shock as well as liver, kidney, and myocardial damage. Other unrecognized toxins may play a role. How toxins gain access to the circulatory system is unknown. Tampon use has been associated with this syndrome, but evidence for the mechanism of toxin entry remains obscure. Insertion could cause mucosal damage. Vaginal ulcerations due to pressure changes usually are not observed, although vaginal erythema commonly is present. Superabsorbent tampons may obstruct the vagina, resulting in retrograde menstruation and peritoneal absorption of bacteria or toxin. Tampons may be associated with increased numbers of aerobic bacteria due to oxygen trapped in interfibrous spaces. The longer a tampon is left in place, the greater the risk for development of this syndrome.

Clinical Findings

A. Symptoms & Signs

The clinical manifestations of TSS are diverse based on the action of the *S aureus* toxin. The symptoms and signs typically develop rapidly, often in otherwise healthy individuals. Commonly affected patients have fever, hypotension, and skin manifestations. Additional symptoms and signs include chills, malaise, headache, sore throat, myalgias, fatigue, vomiting, diarrhea, abdominal pain, and orthostatic dizziness or syncope.

During the initial 48 hours of hospitalization, patients may develop diffuse erythroderma, severe watery diarrhea, decreased urine output, cyanosis, and edema of the extremities. Neurologic symptoms such as somnolence, confusion, irritability, agitation, and hallucinations may occur secondary to cerebral ischemia and edema.

A vaginal examination should be performed; if a tampon is present, it must be removed. Mucosal lesions should be sought, and a culture for *S aureus* performed. During convalescence, desquamation can be striking.

B. Laboratory Findings

Clinical laboratory test abnormalities usually reflect shock and organ failure. Leukocytosis may not be present, but the total number of mature and immature neutrophils usually exceeds 90%. Thrombocytopenia and anemia are present during the first few days, and abnormal coagulation studies may be observed. Disseminated intravascular coagulation can develop.

Other laboratory abnormalities may reflect multiorgan failure with elevated blood urea nitrogen and creatinine, elevated liver function tests, and an elevated creatine phosphokinase. Most laboratory tests will return to normal within 7–10 days of disease onset.

Although the majority of patient with TSS will have *S aureus* isolated from mucosal or wound sites, this finding is not required to make the diagnosis, which is largely clinical. *S aureus* is rarely isolated from blood cultures. Cultures from mucosal and wound sites should be obtained in order to try to isolate toxins production from *S aureus*. These tests are usually only available in specialized laboratories.

Differential Diagnosis

Other systemic diseases characterized by rash, fever, and systemic complications should be considered. Most patients will not have an obvious source of infection, such as a recent incision, soft-tissue abscess, or osteomyelitis, but these should be sought. Kawasaki's disease of young children is similar but not as severe. Scarlet fever must be excluded. Rocky Mountain spotted fever, leptospirosis, and measles can be excluded by appropriate serologic tests.

Complications

Recurrences of TSS can occur. Often these cases are in patients who have not been treated with appropriate courses of antistaphylococcal antimicrobials or who fail to develop an appropriate antibody response to staphylococcal toxins. Recurrent episodes are generally milder than the initial disease. Recurrence may occur days to months after the initial episode.

Treatment

Aggressive supportive therapy is the mainstay of successful treatment, and patients should be managed in an intensive care setting. Aggressive fluid resuscitation is required and may be up to 10–20 L per day. Vasopressors, packed red blood cells, and coagulation factors may be necessary. Any foreign body in the vagina such as tampon or contraceptive device should be removed. Mechanical ventilation or hemodialysis may be necessary if acute respiratory syndrome or renal failure develop.

Although it is unclear whether antimicrobials alter the course of TSS, antistaphylococcal antibiotics are important in eradicating the infection and preventing recurrences. Antibiotics such as clindamycin that suppress protein synthesis and, therefore, toxin synthesis are more efficacious than cell wall active agents such as β-lactams. Current recommendations based on animal studies and clinical case series are as follows. Treatment is usually for 10–14 days.

1. Empiric therapy for all patients with suspected TSS—Clindamycin 600 mg IV every 8 hours **plus** vancomycin 30 mg/kg per day IV in 2 divided doses.

2. Patient With TSS and Culture/Sensitivity Results Available

A. METHICILLIN-SUSCEPTIBLE *S AUREUS*—Clindamycin 600 mg IV every 8 hours **plus** oxacillin **or** nafcillin 2 g IV every 4 hours.

B. METHICILLIN-RESISTANT *S AUREUS*—Clindamycin 600 mg IV every 8 hours **plus either** vancomycin 30 mg/kg per day IV in 2 divided doses **or** linezolid 600 mg oral or IV every 12 hours.

Prognosis

Death associated with TSS usually occurs within the first few days of hospitalization but may occur as late as 15 days after admission. Fatalities have been attributed to refractory cardiac arrhythmias, cardiomyopathy, irreversible respiratory failure, and rarely bleeding caused by coagulation defects, demonstrating the importance of good supportive care. The TSS-related mortality rate in menstrual cases has decreased since the syndrome was first recognized in 1980, from 5.5% in 1987 to 1.8% in 1996.

Workowski KA, Berman S. Centers for Disease Control and Prevention (CDC). Sexually transmitted diseases, treatment guidelines, 2010. *MMWR Recomm Rep* 2010;59:1–110. PMID: 21160459.

44 Antimicrobial Chemotherapy

Shmuel Benenson, MD
Lisa Green, MD, MPH
Alan H. DeCherney, MD

Microbial infection has always been a grave threat to obstetric and gynecologic patients. Developments in antimicrobial therapy, however, have led to decreases in puerperal and postoperative morbidity and perinatal mortality. Indeed antibiotic development is one of the most important advances in medicine in the 20th century. Empiric antibiotics for bacterial infections improve clinical symptoms and outcome. As a consequence, clinicians prescribe antibiotics very frequently and sometimes even when it is not necessary. This approach has led to huge overuse of antibiotics, which in turn has led to the appearance of multidrug-resistant bacteria. Clinicians need to adopt an approach where effective antibiotic treatment is given to those who have bacterial infections, while at the same time antibiotic use is limited when not indicated.

SELECTION OF ANTIMICROBIAL DRUGS

Several considerations are pertinent to most infections encountered in obstetric and gynecologic practice. First, the majority of patients are generally healthy and free of debilitating illness, with the exception of some elderly and oncology patients. Second, the lower genital tract (vagina and cervix) contains a complex flora (eg, anaerobes, gram-positive and gram-negative aerobes, and *Candida*), whereas the upper genital tract (uterus, fallopian tubes, and ovaries) is sterile. Infections in the upper genital tract usually result from spread of the lower genital tract flora when the upper tract is anatomically disrupted (eg, by sexually transmitted disease, by surgery, or during delivery). For this reason, most infections, such as postpartum or postoperative infection and pelvic inflammatory disease, are polymicrobial. Third, cultures must be obtained when infection is suspected (eg, pelvic abscess, chorioamnionitis), and empiric antibiotic therapy targeted at the potential organisms is usually indicated before culture results are available. However, in some gynecologic infections, because of laboratory limitations, culture results may not be available in a timely fashion, or tests may not even be performed at all. In some cases, surgical intervention ("source control") rather than antibiotic treatment ("antibiotic control") is the main component of treatment. Fourth, when selecting antibiotic agents in a pregnant woman, the potential risk for the fetus should be taken into account.

To serve as a guide to antibiotic selection, 5 tables are provided. Tables 44–1 and 44–2 provide the classification and dosages of selected β-lactam antibiotics and antibiotics from other classes. Table 44–3 presents the main or serious adverse events of antibiotics commonly used in obstetric-gynecologic practice and risk categories of antimicrobials in pregnancy. Table 44–4 shows recommended drugs and alternatives against selected bacteria encountered in obstetric-gynecologic practice. Finally, Table 44–5 shows suggested regimens for main clinical diagnoses.

The following steps merit consideration in each patient.

A. Infectious Diagnosis?

The physician must attempt to decide on clinical grounds whether the patient has an infection or whether the symptoms and signs are caused by a noninfectious cause.

B. Diagnostic Microbiology

Before beginning antimicrobial drug treatment for a suspected infection, always attempt to obtain appropriate clinical specimens for culture in order to identify the causative infectious organism and its susceptibility to antimicrobial drugs. Gram stains of sterile body fluids or abscess fluid are one of the most useful tools available to direct an empiric antibiotic treatment. Cultures should be obtained from the suspected site of infection, and if infection is severe, blood cultures should be taken.

C. The Pathogen

The most likely pathogen (or pathogens) causing infection should be defined. This assessment is based on clinical

Table 44–1. Antibiotic dosage of selected β-lactam agents.

Class, Agent	Usual Adult Dosage in Normal Renal Function	Class, Agent	Usual Adult Dosage in Normal Renal Function
Natural penicillins		**Carbapenems**	
Benzathine penicillin G	600,000–1.2 million units IM	Ertapenem	1 g IV q24h
Penicillin G	2–4 million units IV q4h	Imipenem	0.5 g IV q6h; for *Pseudomonas aeruginosa* 1 g IV every 6–8 hours
Penicillin V	0.25–0.5 g PO bid-qid	Meropenem	0.5–1 g IV q8h
Antistaphylococcal penicillins		**Cephalosporins, first generation**	
Cloxacillin	0.25–0.5 g PO q6h; 1–2 g IV q4h	Cefadroxil	0.5–1 g PO q12h
Dicloxacillin	0.125–0.5 g PO q6h	Cephalexin	0.25–0.5 g PO q6h
Nafcillin	1–2 g IV q4h	Cefazolin	1–2 g IV q8h
Oxacillin	1–2 g IV q4h	**Cephalosporins, second generation**	
Aminopenicillins		Cefaclor	0.25–0.5 g PO q8h
Amoxicillin	250 mg–1 g PO tid	Cefuroxime	0.25–0.5 g PO q12h; 0.75–1.5 g IV q8h
Ampicillin	0.25–0.5 g PO qid; 1–2 g IV q4h	Cefotetan	1–3 g IV q12h
Antipseudomonal penicillins		Cefoxitin	IV 1 g q8h–2 g q4h
Piperacillin	3–4 g IV every 4–6 hours	**Cephalosporins, third generation**	
Ticarcillin	3 g IV every 4–6 hours	Cefixime	400 mg PO every 12–24 hours
β-lactam + β-lactamase inhibitor		Cefotaxime	1–2 g IV q8h
Amoxicillin/clavulanic acid	500 mg/125 mg 1 tab PO tid; 875 mg/125 mg 1 tab PO bid; 1 g/200 mg IV every 6–8 hours	Ceftriaxone	1 g IV once daily; bacterial meningitis 2 g q12h
Ampicillin/sulbactam	1.5–3 g IV q6h	Ceftazidime	1–2 g IV q8h
Piperacillin/tazobactam	3.375 g or 4.5 g IV every 6–8 hours	**Cephalosporins, fourth generation**	
Ticarcillin/clavulanic acid	3.1 g IV every 4–6 hours	Cefepime	1–2 g IV q12h
Monobactams			
Aztreonam	1–2 g IV every 6–8 hours		

bid, twice a day; IM, intramuscular; IV, intravenous; PO, per os (by mouth); qid, 4 times a day; tid, 3 times a day.

information and epidemiology (eg, age, organ involved, community-acquired vs. hospital-acquired infection; Table 44–5).

D. Pathogen-Oriented Empiric Antibiotic Treatment

Selecting appropriate initial antimicrobial therapy is of high priority. Based on the probable pathogen causing the infection and the local susceptibility patterns, the physician should choose a drug (or drug combination) that is likely to be effective against the suspected microorganism.

E. Other Factors Influencing the Antibiotic Choice

1. Are there antibiotic allergies?
2. Pregnancy: Choose antibiotics in a pregnant woman in accordance with the US Food and Drug Administration's (FDA) use-in-pregnancy drug rating system (Table 44–3).
3. Renal failure may affect not only the choice of antibiotic but also its dosages.
   a. Dosages of antibiotics primarily excreted by the kidneys (eg, β-lactams, aminoglycosides, and

Table 44–2. Antibiotic dosage of selected antimicrobial agents other than β-lactams.

Class, Agent	Usual Adult Dosage in Normal Renal Function
Aminoglycosides[1]	
Gentamicin, tobramycin	5 mg/kg once daily; 1.7 mg/kg every 8 hours
Amikacin	15 mg/kg once daily; 7.5 mg/kg every 12 hours
Fluoroquinolones	
Ciprofloxacin	250–500 mg PO bid; 400 mg IV bid[2]
Ofloxacin	200–400 mg PO/IV bid
Gatifloxacin	200–400 mg PO/IV every 24 hours
Levofloxacin	250–750 mg PO/IV every 24 hours
Moxifloxacin	400 mg PO/IV every 24 hours
Macrolides	
Erythromycin	0.25–0.5 g PO every 6 hours; 0.25–1.0 g IV every 6 hours
Roxithromycin	150 mg PO every 12 hours
Clarithromycin	0.25–0.5 g PO every 12 hours
Azithromycin	PO or IV. Tabs of 250 mg. Dose varies with indication. See text.
Tetracyclines	
Doxycycline	100 mg PO (or IV) once or twice daily
Tetracycline	250–500 mg PO every 6 hours
Tigecycline	100 mg IV, then 50 mg IV every 12 hours
Clindamycin	300–450 mg PO every 6–8 hours; 600–900 mg IV every 8 hours
Metronidazole	500 mg PO (or IV) every 8 hours
Glycopeptides	
Vancomycin[1]	15–20 mg/kg IV every 12 hours
Linezolid	600 mg PO/IV every 12 hours
Trimethoprim-sulfamethoxazole	For UTI, 960 mg PO every 12 hours
Urinary antiseptics	
Nitrofurantoin	100 mg PO qid[3]
Fosfomycin	Single dose of 3 g PO

bid, twice a day; IV, intravenous; PO, per os (by mouth); qid, 4 times a day; tid, 3 times a day; UTI, urinary tract infection.
[1]Serum drug level monitoring is required.
[2]For *Pseudomonas aeruginosa*, 400 mg every 8 hours
[3]Nitrofurantoin as a combination of macrocrystals/monohydrate salt, 100 mg (nitrofurantoin capsules, Macrobid) is given every 12 hours.

fluoroquinolones) should be modified based on the creatinine clearance.

b. Renal function should be monitored in patients treated with antibiotics that are potentially nephrotoxic (eg, aminoglycosides).

c. Serum antibiotic levels should be monitored every 2 to 4 days when an aminoglycoside or vancomycin is used.

4. Severity of illness: In those who are seriously ill, the spectrum of the empiric antibiotic regimen needs to include coverage of potentially resistant pathogens.

F. Route of Administration

Intravenous (IV) antibiotics are preferred in serious infections. Oral therapy is effective for mild to moderately severe infections and for completion of therapy initially treated with IV antibiotics. For some antibiotics, absorption after oral administration depends on the proximity to other food intake (eg, amoxicillin-clavulanate and doxycycline should be taken immediately after eating food, whereas trimethoprim-sulfamethoxazole should be taken between meals).

G. Laboratory Results and Clinical Response

Based on the laboratory results (eg, culture and susceptibility) and on the patient clinical response, the desirability of changing the antimicrobial drug regimen should be considered. Conversion from a broad-spectrum to a narrow-spectrum drug should be carried out if possible. It is important to assess the clinical response of the patient before making changes based on culture results. Laboratory results should not automatically overrule clinical judgment.

H. Duration of Antimicrobial Therapy

In general, effective antimicrobial treatment results in marked clinical improvement within a few days. However, continued treatment for varying periods may be necessary to effect cure. The duration of therapy depends on clinical judgment. For most infections, the duration ranges from 5–7 to 10–14 days. For most postoperative and postpartum infections, IV antibiotics can be discontinued after the patient has been afebrile for 24–48 hours. Transfer from IV to oral can be made if the patient can eat and the absorption is not interrupted.

I. Adverse Reactions

The administration of antimicrobial drugs is occasionally associated with untoward reactions (Table 44–3). These reactions can be divided into 3 main groups.

1. Hypersensitivity—The most common reactions are fever and skin rashes. Hematologic or hepatic disorders and anaphylaxis are rare.

Table 44–3. Main or serious adverse events of antibiotics commonly used in obstetric-gynecologic practice and pregnancy risk categories.

Antibiotic	Main or Serious Adverse Events	FDA Pregnancy Categories[1]
β-Lactams (penicillins, cephalosporins, carbapenems)	Late-type hypersensitivity (rash, fever); immediate-type (anaphylaxis); seizures in high concentrations	B (imipenem, C)
Aminoglycosides	Nephrotoxicity, ototoxicity	D
Fluoroquinolones	GI; QT prolongation	C
Macrolides	GI; drug-drug interactions (major concern - prolonged QT)	Erythromycin/azithromycin, B Clarithromycin, C
Tetracyclines	GI; esophagitis (take drug while sitting and with adequate amount of fluids); phototoxicity (avoid intense sun exposure)	D
Clindamycin	GI; *Clostridium difficile*-associated disease[2]	B
Metronidazole	Alcohol intolerance; metallic unpleasant taste; rarely, peripheral neuropathy with prolonged use	B
Vancomycin	"Red man syndrome" (if infused rapidly, not allergic); allergic rash in 5%; nephrotoxicity (if high doses are used or coadministration with aminoglycosides)	C
Linezolid	Reversible myelosuppression (ie, thrombocytopenia, anemia, and neutropenia); most often after more than 2 weeks of therapy	C
TMP-SMX	Skin rash (more rarely Stevens-Johnson syndrome); GI; hemolysis in G6PD deficiency	C
Nitrofurantoin	Skin rashes (1–5%); pneumonitis and polyneuropathies (more common in the elderly)	B
Fluconazole	Rash; nausea and vomiting	C
Acyclovir, famciclovir, valacyclovir	Intravenous acyclovir may cause phlebitis; nephrotoxicity (5%). Adequate prehydration may prevent it.	B

FDA, Food and Drug Administration; G6PD, glucose-6-phosphate dehydrogenase; GI, gastrointestinal; TMP-SMX, trimethoprim-sulfamethoxazole.
[1]FDA categories: **A**, studies in pregnant woman, no risk; **B**, animal studies no risk, no adequate studies in pregnant women; **C**, animal studies show toxicity, no adequate studies in humans, but potential benefits may warrant use of the drug in pregnant women despite potential risks; **D**, evidence of human risk, but benefits may outweigh; **X**, risks clearly outweigh potential benefits.
[2]*Clostridium difficile*-associated disease (pseudomembranous colitis) may result from use of any antibiotic.

2. Direct toxicity—Most common are nausea, vomiting, and diarrhea. More serious toxic reactions are impairment of renal, hepatic, or hematopoietic function.

3. Suppression—Suppression of normal microbial flora and "superinfection" by drug-resistant microorganisms (such as *Clostridium difficile*).

J. Failure to Improve

When the patient is not improving despite adequate antibiotic treatment as determined by culture results, the following possibilities should be considered:

1. Presence of an undrained abscess, hematoma, or foreign body
2. Inappropriate antibiotic dose or route of administration
3. Low antibiotic concentration at the site of infection (eg, central nervous system [CNS])
4. Emergence of drug-resistant or -tolerant organism
5. Involvement of 2 or more microorganisms in the infectious process, of which only 1 was originally detected and used for drug selection

ANTIMICROBIAL DRUGS

1. Penicillins

The penicillins are among the most widely used antimicrobial drugs. The term penicillin is the generic term for a large group

Table 44–4. Recommended and alternative antimicrobial drugs against selected bacteria encountered in obstetric-gynecologic practice.

Suspected or Proved Etiologic Agent	Recommended Drug(s)	Alternative Drug(s)
Gram-negative cocci		
Neisseria gonorrhoeae	Cefixime, ceftriaxone	Spectinomycin, azithromycin. High prevalence of quinolone resistance in Asia and United States. Treat also *Chlamydia trachomatis*
Gram-positive cocci		
Streptococcus pneumoniae	Penicillin[1]	First/second-generation cephalosporins, macrolide, clindamycin, vancomycin
β-Hemolytic *Streptococcus* (eg, groups A, B, C, G)	Penicillin (some add clindamycin in severe groups A or B infections)	All β-lactams, macrolide
Enterococcus faecalis	Ampicillin + gentamicin (or streptomycin)	Vancomycin + gentamicin (or streptomycin)
Staphylococcus aureus, methicillin susceptible	Oxacillin, nafcillin	First-generation cephalosporin, vancomycin, clindamycin
Staphylococcus aureus, methicillin resistant	Vancomycin	TMP-SMX, linezolid, daptomycin, tigecycline
Gram-negative rods		
Acinetobacter baumannii	Imipenem (resistance increasing)	Ampicillin/sulbactam; colistin
Enterobacteriaceae (eg, *Escherichia coli*, *Klebsiella pneumoniae*, *Enterobacter* species etc.)	Agents vary with clinical setting. See text.	
Pseudomonas aeruginosa	Antipseudomonal β-lactam (eg, piperacillin, ceftazidime); ciprofloxacin; imipenem; meropenem	For serious infection, use a combination of antipseudomonal β-lactam + aminoglycoside (eg, gentamicin, amikacin)
Gram-positive rods		
Listeria monocytogenes	Ampicillin ± gentamicin	TMP-SMX
Anaerobes		
Actinomyces israelii	Ampicillin or penicillin	Doxycycline, ceftriaxone
Oropharyngeal anaerobes	Penicillin	Metronidazole, clindamycin cephalosporin
Bacteroides fragilis	Metronidazole	Cefoxitin, cefotetan, β-lactam + β-lactamase inhibitors, carbapenem (Resistance to clindamycin ~20%)
Clostridium difficile	Metronidazole	PO vancomycin (in severe cases)
Clostridium perfringens	Penicillin G ± clindamycin	Doxycycline
Miscellaneous		
Chlamydia trachomatis	Doxycycline/azithromycin	IV clindamycin
Chlamydia pneumoniae	Doxycycline	Macrolide, quinolone
Haemophilus ducreyi	Ceftriaxone, azithromycin	Ciprofloxacin
Mycoplasma species	Macrolide, quinolone	Doxycycline

[1]For penicillin intermediate-susceptible strains, use high-dose penicillin (except for meningitis). For penicillin-resistant strains, use vancomycin.
IV, intravenous; PO, per os (by mouth); TMP-SMX, trimethoprim-sulfamethoxazole.

Table 44–5. Treatment regimens for selected infections in obstetric-gynecologic practice.

Clinical Diagnosis	Etiologies	Recommended Regimen	Alternative Regimen/Comments
Chancroid	*Haemophilus ducreyi*	Ceftriaxone 250 mg IM single dose or azithromycin 1 g PO single dose	Ciprofloxacin 500 PO bid × 3 days
Non gonococcal urethritis	Common: chlamydia, *Mycoplasma hominis*. Other: *Trichomonas*, herpes simplex virus (HSV), *Mycoplasma genitalium*	Doxycycline 100 mg PO bid × 7 days or azithromycin 1 g PO single dose Evaluate and treat sex partner	Ofloxacin 300 mg PO bid × 7 days or levofloxacin 500 mg PO once daily × 7 days
Gonorrhea urethritis/cervicitis	*Neisseria gonorrhoeae* (50% have concomitant *Chlamydia trachomatis*; treat for both)	(Ceftriaxone 125 mg IM single dose or cefixime 400 mg PO single dose) PLUS (Azithromycin 2 g PO single dose or doxycycline 100 mg PO every 24 hours × 7 days)	Spectinomycin 2 g IM × 1 for *Neisseria gonorrhoeae*
Genital herpes			
Initial episode	Herpes simplex virus	Acyclovir 400 mg PO tid × 7–10 days or valacyclovir 1 g PO bid × 7–10 days or famciclovir 250 mg PO tid × 7–10 days	IV acyclovir (5 mg/kg q8h × 5–7 days) can be used in hospitalized patients with severe primary HSV infection
Periodic recurrences	Episodic therapy. Initiate therapy within 1 day of lesion onset or during the prodrome.	Acyclovir 800 mg PO tid × 2 days or valacyclovir 500 mg PO bid × 3 days or famciclovir 1 g PO bid × 1 day	Activity and side effects of valacyclovir and famcyclovir are similar to acyclovir
Frequent recurrences	Chronic suppressive therapy	Acyclovir 400 mg PO bid or famciclovir 250 mg PO bid or valacyclovir 1 g PO q24h	
Lymphogranuloma venereum	*Chlamydia trachomatis* (serovars L1–3)	Doxycycline 100 mg PO bid × 21 days	Erythromycin 500 mg PO qid × 21 days
Syphilis			
Early: less than 1 year	*Treponema pallidum*	Benzathine penicillin G, 2.4 million units IM × 1. In pregnancy, it is the only option. Desensitize if there is penicillin allergy.	Doxycycline 100 mg PO bid × 14 days or ceftriaxone 1 g IM/IV q24h × 10 days
Late: more than 1 year		Benzathine penicillin G 2.4 million units IM every week × 3	Doxycycline 100 mg PO bid × 28 days. Consider neurosyphilis.
Amnionitis, septic abortion, early postpartum endometritis	Bacteroides, streptococci (groups A, B), *Chlamydia Trachomatis*, Enterobacteriaceae	Lots of options: [Cefoxitin or (cefuroxime + metronidazole) or β-lactam + β-lactamase inhibitor] + doxycycline	Clindamycin + gentamicin
Actinomycosis (tubo-ovarian abscess)	*Actinomyces israelii*	Penicillin G 10–20 million units/d IV × 4–6 weeks, then penicillin V 2–4 g/d PO × 3–6 months	Doxycycline or ceftriaxone or clindamycin Remove intrauterine device

(*Continued*)

Table 44–5. Treatment regimens for selected infections in obstetric-gynecologic practice. (Continued)

Clinical Diagnosis	Etiologies	Recommended Regimen	Alternative Regimen/Comments
Pelvic inflammatory disease			
Outpatient	*Neisseria gonorrhoeae*, chlamydia, *Bacteroides*, streptococci, Enterobacteriaceae	(Ceftriaxone 250 mg IM/IV × 1 dose) then (doxycycline 100 mg PO bid ± metronidazole 500 mg PO bid × 14 days)	(Amoxicillin-clavulanate 875 mg PO bid + doxycycline 100 mg PO bid) × 14 days
Inpatient		(Cefoxitin 2 g IV every 6 hours + doxycycline 100 mg PO bid) × 14 days	(Clindamycin 900 mg IV q8h + gentamicin 5 mg/kg once daily + doxycycline 100 mg PO bid) × 14 days
Vaginitis			
Candidiasis	*Candida albicans* most common (other, *Candida glabrata*, *Candida tropicalis*)	Fluconazole 150 mg PO single dose (For recurrent episodes, fluconazole 150 mg PO every week)	Intravaginal azoles (variety of preparations) For azole-resistant, boric acid
Trichomoniasis	*Trichomonas vaginalis*	Metronidazole 2 g PO as single dose or 500 mg PO bid × 7 days	Treat male sexual partner
Bacterial vaginosis	*Gardnerella vaginalis*, other anaerobes	Metronidazole 0.5 g PO bid × 7 days or vaginal gel × 5 days	Clindamycin 0.3 g PO bid × 7 days or clindamycin vaginal cream or ovules
Urinary tract infection			
Acute uncomplicated	Enterobacteriaceae, *Staphylococcus saprophyticus*, enterococci (uncommon)	TMP-SMX 960 mg PO bid × 3 days (if local resistance to TMP-SMX >20%, ciprofloxacin 250 mg PO bid × 3 days)	Nitrofurantoin 100 mg PO bid × 5 days or single 3 g fosfomycin
Recurrent (in young women)	Same	Eradicate infection, then TMP-SMX 480 mg PO q24h long term	Single dose of TMP-SMX 2 tabs of 960 mg at symptom onset or 1 tab of 960 mg postcoitus; nitrofurantoin 50–100 mg PO daily at bedtime or postcoital

bid, twice a day; IM, intramuscular; IV, intravenous; PO, per os (by mouth); qid, 4 times a day; tid, 3 times a day; TMP-SMX, trimethoprim-sulfamethoxazole.

of antimicrobial substances, all of which share a common chemical nucleus consisting of a thiadolizine ring, the β-lactam ring, and a side chain; hence the synonym "β-lactams" for the whole group (ie, penicillins, cephalosporins, and carbapenems). The ring is essential for antibacterial activity, whereas the side chain determines the antibacterial spectrum and pharmacologic properties of a particular penicillin (Table 44–1). As a result of the common ring, the potential for allergic cross-sensitivity among penicillins is high. All β-lactam antibiotics inhibit formation of microbial cell wall. By binding to proteins in the cell wall (penicillin-binding proteins), they block the final transpeptidation reaction in the synthesis of cell wall peptidoglycan. This reaction results in bacterial cell death; thus, penicillin is bactericidal.

The most common mechanism of bacterial resistance against penicillin is the production of a β-lactamase enzyme, which destructs the β-lactam ring. This is the principal mechanism of penicillin resistance in *Staphylococcus aureus*, *Bacteroides fragilis*, and Enterobacteriaceae. When penicillin is combined with a β-lactamase inhibitor, the penicillin may escape breakdown.

Pharmacokinetics (Absorption, Distribution, & Excretion)

Acid-labile compounds are poorly absorbed and hence administered only parenterally (penicillin G, antipseudomonal penicillins). Acid-stable compounds vary in the proportion of absorption after oral administration (50% for cloxacillin, 60% for penicillin V, and 75% for amoxicillin). To minimize binding to foods, most oral penicillins should not be preceded or followed by food for at least 1 hour.

After absorption, penicillins are widely distributed in body fluids and tissues (lung, liver, kidney, muscle, bone, and placenta). The levels of penicillins in abscesses and peritoneal fluids are sufficient in the presence of inflammation. In many tissues, penicillin concentrations are equal to those in serum. Lower levels are found in the CNS; however, with active inflammation of the meninges, as in bacterial meningitis, penicillin levels in the cerebrospinal fluid exceed 1–10% of serum concentrations.

Most penicillins are rapidly excreted by the kidneys into the urine—90% by tubular secretion, which results in very high levels in the urine. Significant reduction in renal function must be taken into account in the administration of most penicillins.

Indications, Dosages, & Routes of Administration

A. Penicillin G, Penicillin V

In obstetric-gynecologic practice, penicillin is the drug of choice for treatment of infections caused by groups A and B streptococci, *Treponema pallidum* (causing syphilis), clostridia, and actinomycosis. Severe infections caused by enterococci should be treated by a synergistic combination of ampicillin (or penicillin G) and gentamicin. Penicillin is *not* recommended to treat *Neisseria gonorrhoeae* because of widespread resistance.

1. **Aqueous penicillin G** is given intravenously and produces high blood levels but is excreted rapidly. Therefore, for serious infections, it should be given every 4 hours (6 times daily). In adults with normal renal function, a dose of 18–24 million units a day is used in severe infections and 9–12 million units in other infections.
2. **Benzathine penicillin G** is an insoluble salt that is injected intramuscularly to establish a depot that yields very low drug levels for prolonged periods of time (ie, 3–4 weeks). An injection of 2.4 million units intramuscularly once per week for 1 or 3 weeks is the recommended treatment for early and late syphilis, respectively.
3. **Penicillin V** is made by a mild modification of the side chain of penicillin G, which allows it to resist gastric acid breakdown and thus can be given orally. Penicillin V is indicated in minor infections (eg, group A *Streptococcus* pharyngitis) in daily doses of 1–2 g (500 mg of penicillin V equals 800,000 units).

B. Amoxicillin, Ampicillin, Ticarcillin, Piperacillin

Several side-chain modifications of penicillin have been made to provide enhanced activity of these "broad-spectrum" penicillins.

1. **Amoxicillin** and **ampicillin**, in addition to being active against penicillin-susceptible organisms, are more active than penicillin against enterococci and *Listeria monocytogenes*. Due to widespread bacterial resistance among Enterobacteriaceae, these drugs can be given against Enterobacteriaceae (eg, to treat urinary tract infections) only after susceptibility studies are available. They are ineffective against *Pseudomonas aeruginosa*.

   Amoxicillin is available only for oral use in daily doses of 1.0 g every 8 hours. Amoxicillin has replaced oral ampicillin. IV ampicillin is given in a dose of 1–2 g every 4 hours (ie, 6–12 g daily) depending on the organism involved and the severity and site of infection.
2. **Ticarcillin and piperacillin** were introduced for gram-negative bacteria. They are active against many Enterobacteriaceae and also *P aeruginosa*. Because resistance emerges rapidly, susceptibility testing is required. Their anti–gram-positive spectrum mimics that of ampicillin. For severe *P aeruginosa* infection, piperacillin is preferred (it is 4 times more active against *P aeruginosa*), and addition of an aminoglycoside is required in order to decrease the likelihood of emergence of resistance.

   These drugs are administered IV only: piperacillin 4 g every 6 hours and ticarcillin 3 g every 4 hours.

C. β-Lactamase–Resistant Penicillins

These agents, which are resistant to destruction by β-lactamase, are used primarily to treat infections caused by β-lactamase–producing *S aureus*. They are also active against other gram-positive aerobes (eg, group A *Streptococcus*, *Streptococcus pneumoniae*) but are inferior to penicillin for them. They are not active against the Enterobacteriaceae or enterococci.

1. Oral—Cloxacillin or dicloxacillin can be given in doses of 0.25–1.0 g every 6 hours in mild or localized staphylococcal infections. Food markedly interferes with absorption, and hence, they should not be preceded or followed by food for at least 1 hour.

2. IV—Nafcillin, **oxacillin**, and **cloxacillin** are the drugs of choice for the treatment of serious systemic methicillin-sensitive *S aureus* (MSSA) infections. The usual dose is 6–12 g/d (1–2 g every 4 hours), depending on the severity of the infection. Because these drugs are excreted primarily by hepatic mechanisms, dose reduction is not needed in renal failure (mild reduction of cloxacillin is needed in severe renal failure), but in hepatic failure, dose reduction is required.

D. Combinations of Penicillins plus β-Lactamase Inhibitors

Because the primary bacterial resistance mechanism against penicillin is through β-lactamase production, a β-lactamase inhibitor was combined with several penicillins. This inhibitor binds irreversibly to the β-lactamase, and thus allows the free penicillin to exert its antibacterial activity.

In addition to being active against the penicillin component–susceptible organisms (eg, streptococci, enterococci), these combinations are effective also against MSSA, *B fragilis* and many Enterobacteriaceae (some species of Enterobacteriaceae produce β-lactamases that are resistant to these inhibitors). They are not active against methicillin-resistant *S aureus* (MRSA) or vancomycin-resistant enterococci (VRE) because their mechanism of resistance is different.

Because of their wide spectrum of activity against bacteria involved in pelvic infections (eg, anaerobes, Enterobacteriaceae, enterococci), these combinations have been successful in many circumstances.

1. Oral—Amoxicillin-clavulanate is the only oral combination agent available. It should be administered at the start of the meal to decrease gastrointestinal side effects. The dose is 500 mg amoxicillin and 125 mg clavulanate given 3 times a day or 875 mg amoxicillin and 125 mg clavulanate given every 12 hours.

2. IV—Four parenteral combinations are available that are different in their anti–gram-negative spectrum of activity. **Amoxicillin-clavulanate** (amoxicillin 1.0 g, clavulanate 200 mg) and **ampicillin-sulbactam** (ampicillin 2.0 g, sulbactam 1.0 g) are administered 3 times daily and are active against many gram-negative organisms but not *P aeruginosa*. Ampicillin-sulbactam is sometimes active against resistant *Acinetobacter baumannii*. **Ticarcillin-clavulanate** (ticarcillin 3.0 g, clavulanate 0.1 g) given 4 to 6 times daily and **piperacillin-tazobactam** (piperacillin 4.0 g, tazobactam 0.5 g) given 3 to 4 times daily are active also against *P aeruginosa*. Piperacillin-tazobactam is the widest spectrum anti–gram-negative agent among these 4 agents.

Adverse Effects of Penicillins

Most of the serious side effects of the penicillins are due to hypersensitivity.

A. Allergy

Allergic reactions to penicillin occur in 1–10% of patients.

1. The most frequent (80–90%) are late reactions, which occur days after initiation of therapy. The common clinical signs are morbilliform rash and fever but also eosinophilia and interstitial nephritis (gastrointestinal symptoms are not a sign of allergy).
2. Immediate reactions (within 1 hour) occur as a result of histamine release from immunoglobulin (Ig) E–sensitized mast cells. These are the most dangerous reactions but fortunately are rare (0.05%). Immediate reactions may be associated with urticaria, angioedema, laryngeal edema, bronchospasm, and anaphylaxis.
3. Accelerated reactions occur in the first 1–72 hours and, except for laryngeal edema, are not life threatening.

The penicillin-allergic patient (any agent of the penicillin group; consider both trade and generic names) should be presumed to be allergic to other penicillins (unless skin tests prove otherwise). The risk of cross-allergy to a cephalosporin is estimated to be 10% and to a carbapenem 1%. In a patient with a history of delayed mild reaction to penicillin, cephalosporins can be used. When there is a history of immediate penicillin allergy, cephalosporins should not be administered (unless a cephalosporin skin test has been performed).

In circumstances where penicillin is the clear drug of choice and where alternatives are likely to be less effective, an oral desensitization protocol may be used safely. One such indication is the treatment of a pregnant woman with syphilis.

B. Toxicity

High penicillin blood levels may lead to high spinal fluid levels. This may occur when high doses are given in the presence of renal failure and may lead to seizures. Large doses of penicillins given orally may lead to gastrointestinal upset, particularly nausea and diarrhea. These symptoms are most marked with oral amoxicillin or amoxicillin-clavulanate. Penicillins can cause pseudomembranous colitis.

2. Cephalosporins

The cephalosporins are bactericidal agents that inhibit bacterial cell wall synthesis, similar to the penicillins, and are part of the β-lactam family. They consist of a β-lactam ring attached to a dihydrothiazoline ring. Substitutions of chemical groups at various positions on the basic structure have resulted in a proliferation of drugs with varying pharmacologic properties and antimicrobial activities. In patients with impaired renal function, dosage adjustment is required for most cephalosporins (not including ceftriaxone).

Cephalosporins have been divided into 3 (or 4) major groups or "generations" based mainly on their antibacterial activity (Table 44–1):

1. First-generation cephalosporins have good activity against aerobic gram-positive organisms (streptococci, MSSA; excluding enterococci) and many community-acquired gram-negative organisms.
2. Second-generation drugs have a slightly extended spectrum against gram-negative bacteria (eg, cefuroxime) and some also against anaerobes (eg, cefoxitin).
3. Third- and fourth-generation cephalosporins can be divided into 2 subsets: one type (ie, ceftriaxone, cefotaxime) has significant anti–gram-positive activity and also anti–community-acquired gram-negative activity (not *P aeruginosa*); the other type (ie, ceftazidime) is

less active against gram-positive organisms but has broad-spectrum anti–gram-negative bacteria activity, including *P aeruginosa*. The fourth-generation agent cefepime is active against both gram-positive and gram-negative organisms, including *P aeruginosa*.

Not all cephalosporins fit neatly into this grouping, and there are exceptions to the general characterization of the drugs in the individual generations. However, the generational classification of cephalosporins is useful for discussion purposes. In this part, only a limited number of agents that are particularly useful will be discussed.

The most common mechanisms for resistance are production of β-lactamases, alteration of the penicillin-binding proteins (PBPs), and changes in the outer membrane. Some of the β-lactamases are plasmid mediated, and others are inducible and chromosomal mediated (*Enterobacter* species, *Citrobacter* species, *P aeruginosa*), which lead to treatment failure and emergence of resistance in isolates initially susceptible. The resistance of *S aureus* to methicillin and cephalosporins is mediated by change of the PBP. Extended-spectrum β-lactamases (ESBLs) have been recognized in the early 1980s. They confer resistance to almost all cephalosporins and penicillins (even to those that seemed sensitive in vitro) but not to carbapenems. The clue for the presence of ESBL is resistance of an Enterobacteriaceae to 1 or all third-generation cephalosporins. Today, most laboratories are performing a specific test (double disc diffusion) in order to identify an ESBL producer.

Indications, Dosages, & Routes of Administration

A. First-Generation Cephalosporins

These drugs are active against gram-positive cocci, including *S pneumoniae*, viridans streptococci, groups A and B streptococci, and MSSA. They are also active against many community-acquired gram-negative bacteria. They are inactive against enterococci and MRSA (like all other cephalosporins) and *P aeruginosa*. Oral anaerobic bacteria are usually sensitive, but most bowel anaerobes (ie, *B fragilis*) are not.

1. Oral—In general, these agents are rapidly and thoroughly absorbed. They are useful for mild to moderate MSSA and group A streptococcal infections of the skin and soft tissue (eg, cellulitis).

1. **Cephalexin** and **cephradine** are given orally in doses of 0.25–0.5 g 4 times daily. When treating a significant *S aureus* infection, a dose of 1.0 g 4 times daily should be used initially.
2. **Cefadroxil** can be given in doses of 0.5–1 g twice daily.

2. IV—**Cefazolin** is the most commonly used agent.

1. It is among the drugs of choice for surgical prophylaxis in gynecologic operations and caesarean section.
2. It serves as an alternative to β-lactamase–resistant penicillins (eg, nafcillin, oxacillin) for known or suspected MSSA infections (eg, cellulitis).
3. Cefazolin is an alternative to penicillin for group B streptococcal prophylaxis in patients with a delayed mild allergic reaction to penicillin.

Cefazolin can be given in doses of 0.5–2 g every 8 hours (depends on the severity of the infection).

B. Second-Generation Cephalosporins

These drugs are active against organisms also covered by first-generation drugs, but they have an extended anti–gram-negative activity (community acquired). In addition, cefoxitin and cefotetan are active against bowel anaerobes, especially *B fragilis*. They have no activity against enterococci, MRSA, and *P aeruginosa*.

1. Oral—They are useful for respiratory tract infections and for simple cystitis. **Cefuroxime axetil** or **cefprozil** is given orally in doses of 0.25–0.5 g twice daily.

2. IV—Due to the spectrum of activity, these drugs can be used to treat obstetric and gynecologic infections. They have no advantage over first-generation cephalosporins for perioperative prophylaxis.

1. **Cefuroxime** is given in doses of 750 mg to 1.5 g 3 times daily. For intra-abdominal polymicrobial infections, an antianaerobic drug (ie, metronidazole) should be added to cefuroxime.
2. **Cefoxitin** and **cefotetan** have enhanced anaerobic activity and hence can generally be used alone for intra-abdominal infections. These drugs should not be relied on as monotherapy in patients with bacteremia due to *B fragilis* because they may not be active against 5–30% of these isolates. Cefoxitin is given in doses of 2 g every 6–8 hours, and cefotetan is given in a dose of 1–2 g twice daily.

C. Third-/Fourth-Generation Cephalosporins

Third-/fourth-generation cephalosporins have the broadest anti–gram-negative spectrum of all cephalosporins. In addition to anti–gram-negative activity, ceftriaxone, cefotaxime, and cefixime have significant anti–gram-positive activity (less than that of first and second generations), whereas ceftazidime (which is less active against gram-positives) is active also against *P aeruginosa*. The fourth-generation agent cefepime is active against both gram-positive and gram-negative organisms, including *P aeruginosa*. None of these agents has good activity against the bowel anaerobe *B fragilis*. Most of these drugs are active against *N gonorrhoeae*.

Ceftriaxone is eliminated primarily by biliary excretion, and no dosage adjustment is required in renal insufficiency. The other drugs in this generation are eliminated by the kidneys and thus require dosage adjustments in renal insufficiency.

1. Oral—Cefixime is used in a very limited fashion. In obstetric-gynecologic practice, this agent can be used to treat uncomplicated gonococcal infection by 400 mg given once (combined with doxycycline or azithromycin for cotreatment of chlamydia).

2. IV

1. **Ceftriaxone** is a widely used agent due to its broad spectrum of activity against community-acquired infections and its long half-life, allowing a once-daily regimen (except for CNS infections). One dose of ceftriaxone 250 mg intramuscularly is used for treating uncomplicated gonorrhea (combined with doxycycline or azithromycin for cotreatment of chlamydia). For non-CNS infections (eg, community-acquired pneumonia, abdominal/gynecologic infections, and urinary tract infections), a once-daily dose of 1 g is given.
2. **Ceftazidime** is, for practical purposes, exclusively an antiaerobic gram-negative agent. It has an excellent anti–*P aeruginosa* activity and is used to treat hospital-acquired infections where *P aeruginosa* is an option. Ceftazidime is given in doses of 1–2 g every 8 hours.
3. **Cefepime** is an extended-spectrum cephalosporin that has activity against gram-positive organisms comparable with ceftriaxone and anti–gram-negative activity comparable to ceftazidime, including an excellent activity against *P aeruginosa*. It is used to treat hospital-acquired infections where gram-positive and gram-negative organisms are a possibility. In many centers, it has replaced ceftazidime due to its wider spectrum. As with all cephalosporins, it is not active against MRSA, *B fragilis*, and enterococci. Cefepime is given in doses of 1–2 g every 12 hours.

Adverse Effects of Cephalosporins

A. Allergy

Cephalosporins, both oral and IV formulations, are very well tolerated. There is approximately a 1–3% rate of primary allergic reactions to cephalosporins (rashes, fever, and eosinophilia). Anaphylaxis is rare, occurring in less than 0.02% of recipients. The incidence of cross-allergy between cephalosporins and penicillins is estimated to be approximately 10%. In a patient with a history of delayed mild reaction to penicillin, cephalosporins are commonly used. With a history of an immediate reaction to penicillin (eg, bronchospasm, hypotension), cephalosporins should be avoided. The risk with third-generation cephalosporins in this setting is as low as 1%, similar to those without that history.

B. Toxicity

Positive Coombs reaction occurs in 3%. Other uncommon adverse effects include nephrotoxicity and hematologic effects (granulocytopenia and thrombocytopenia).

C. Superinfection

Pseudomembranous colitis caused by *C difficile* may occur more frequently in recipients of second- and third-generation cephalosporins.

3. Unique β-Lactam Antibiotics

Monobactams (Aztreonam)

Aztreonam is active against most gram-negative aerobes (including *P aeruginosa*) but not against gram-positive organisms or anaerobes. Aztreonam resembles aminoglycosides in activity without their nephrotoxicity. Because it is active against gram-negative aerobes only, combination therapy is necessary for suspected mixed infections with gram-positive organisms and/or anaerobes. The usual dose is 1–2 g IV every 6–8 hours. Although aztreonam has potentially less toxicity than gentamicin, gentamicin is much less expensive, and the majority of obstetric-gynecologic patients are at low risk for gentamicin toxicity. It is an alternative anti–gram-negative agent in patients with allergy to penicillins or cephalosporins because there is little risk of cross-sensitivity.

Carbapenems

Carbapenems have the broadest antibacterial spectrum of the β-lactam class, largely because they are so β-lactamase stable. Four carbapenems—**ertapenem**, **doripenem**, **imipenem**, and **meropenem**—are in clinical use. All have excellent activity against gram-positive cocci, excluding MRSA. Imipenem is active against *Enterococcus faecalis* but not the other carbapenems. The carbapenems have the broadest anti–gram-negative spectrum, including *P aeruginosa* (except for ertapenem), and are the drugs of choice for ESBL gram-negative producers. Carbapenems are highly active against most anaerobic species including the bowel anaerobes (eg, *B fragilis*). Generally speaking, doripenem, imipenem, and meropenem are therapeutically equivalent and interchangeable in most clinical situations; ertapenem is different in its lack of activity against *P aeruginosa* and *A baumannii*. During the past decade, carbapenem resistance in Enterobacteriaceae and *A baumannii* has emerged, mostly mediated by a β-lactamase that hydrolyses carbapenems.

All the carbapenems must be administered parenterally. They are well distributed to various body compartments and penetrate well into most tissues. The usual doses are ertapenem 1 g once daily; doripenem 500 mg every 8 hours; imipenem 500 mg every 6 hours; and meropenem 0.5–1 g every 8 hours. Dosage adjustment is required in renal insufficiency.

Because carbapenems have an unusual spectrum, they should be reserved for serious nosocomial infections for the treatment of highly resistant organisms. They should not be used as a first-line treatment for pelvic infections.

Carbapenems generally are well tolerated. The most common adverse effects of imipenem are nausea, vomiting, diarrhea, and skin rashes. All carbapenems, particularly imipenem, have been associated with seizures. The cross-allergy between carbapenems and penicillins is probably low (ie, ~1%).

4. Aminoglycosides

These agents are in most instances bactericidal. They penetrate the cell wall and membrane and inhibit protein synthesis by binding irreversibly to the 30S subunit of the bacterial ribosome. The most commonly used aminoglycosides are **gentamicin**, **tobramycin**, and **amikacin**.

Aminoglycosides are active against almost all gram-negative rods including *P aeruginosa*. Among resistant gram-negative bacilli, amikacin is the most frequently active, tobramycin is the next frequently active, and gentamicin is the least frequently active. Aminoglycosides have some activity against some gram-positive aerobes (eg, staphylococci, enterococci) but are never given alone for these bacteria but are administered together with a β-lactam agent. Gentamicin, together with penicillin or ampicillin, usually is bactericidal against enterococci, but the incidence of high-level resistance of enterococci to gentamicin is increasing. Anaerobes are not susceptible to aminoglycosides.

General Properties of Aminoglycosides

A. Pharmacokinetics

Aminoglycosides are not absorbed from the gut. The IV route is preferred, although the intramuscular route can be used if thrombocytopenia is absent. They are distributed widely in tissues and achieve reasonable concentrations in bone, synovial fluid, and peritoneal fluid. Urinary concentrations are high and exceed serum concentrations by 100 times. They have limited penetration into the CNS and probably intra-abdominal abscesses. There is a variation in the volume of distribution and rate of excretion of aminoglycosides in individual patients with normal renal function. Thus, it is important to monitor serum levels in all patients every 3–4 days. Aminoglycoside excretion is entirely renal, mandating dose adjustment for renal failure. The serum half-life is 2–3 hours.

B. Dosing & Serum Level Monitoring

Aminoglycosides demonstrate a postantibiotic effect (ie, persistent suppression of bacterial growth after short antibiotic exposure) against aerobic gram-negative bacilli. Hence aminoglycosides can be administered as a single daily dose (SDD) or with the conventional multiple daily dosing regimen. The SDD approach appears to be comparable in efficacy to the traditional multiple daily dosing, is simpler to administer, and is less toxic. Some clinicians prefer to continue to use multiple daily dosing in the pregnant patient.

Creatinine clearance should be calculated before aminoglycoside administration, and doses should be corrected accordingly. In normal renal function, once-daily dose of gentamicin or tobramycin is 5 mg/kg and amikacin 15 mg/kg, given over 60 minutes. In conventional dosing, 1.7 mg/kg of gentamicin or tobramycin is given every 8 hours, and 7.5 mg/kg of amikacin is given every 12 hours.

In patients treated by SDD, trough level should be obtained before the next dose every 3–4 days. In patients treated by multiple daily dosing, peak levels (30 minutes after completion of the infusion, to ensure that enough quantity of drug was administered) and trough levels (before the next dose) should be monitored. If trough levels are elevated, the next dose needs to be reduced or the interval prolonged.

C. Clinical Use in Obstetrics & Gynecology

1. Aminoglycosides are used to treat complicated **urinary tract infections** (ie, pyelonephritis). Gentamicin is a primary agent unless the patient has recently received gentamicin and is possibly infected with a relatively resistant gram-negative bacterium; in this situation, amikacin should be used while awaiting culture results.
2. Aminoglycosides are used to treat **intra-abdominal infections** (combined with antianaerobic agent).
3. Gentamicin can be used to treat ***P aeruginosa* infections** in combination with piperacillin.
4. Amikacin is used empirically to treat gram-negative bacteria in **hospital-acquired infections** especially in specialized areas (eg, intensive care units).
5. Aminoglycoside effectiveness is not optimal for sterilization of abscesses and in lower respiratory tract infections because of poor activity in the presence of low pH.

D. Adverse Effects

1. Hypersensitivity reactions are uncommon.
2. All aminoglycosides can cause varying degrees of **nephrotoxicity**, expressed by a rising blood urea nitrogen and creatinine. Changes are usually reversible with discontinuation, and rational use can prevent it. Risk factors for nephrotoxicity (and ototoxicity) include concomitant liver disease, concomitant use of other potentially nephrotoxic drugs (eg, vancomycin, nonsteroidal anti-inflammatory drugs), and prior renal disease. Prevention includes the following: use aminoglycosides for the shortest appropriate course, correct hypovolemia, avoid in the presence of risk factors, use SDD regimen, and monitor levels and serum creatinine. Serum creatinine levels should be obtained every 2–4 days.
3. **Ototoxicity** (eg, hearing loss, vertigo and loss of balance, or nystagmus) is frequently irreversible. Older patients are at greater risk.

5. Fluoroquinolones

All fluoroquinolones (FQs) inhibit bacterial DNA gyrase, a bacterial enzyme essential for DNA replication. They promote gyrase-mediated DNA breakage at specific sites, which leads to cell death. Quinolones are categorized based on spectrum of antimicrobial activity:

1. First-generation FQs (eg, nalidixic acid) are no longer used.
2. The second-generation agents, **ciprofloxacin** and **ofloxacin**, are very active against gram-negative organisms. Ciprofloxacin is the most potent FQ against *P aeruginosa*. They lack consistent activity against gram-positive cocci and anaerobes. There is increasing resistance of *N gonorrhoeae* against ciprofloxacin, once considered the drug of choice, and thus, FQs are no longer recommended in the United States for this indication.
3. Third- and fourth-generation FQs (**gatifloxacin**, **levofloxacin**, and **moxifloxacin**) have, in addition to anti–gram-negative activity (modest activity against *P aeruginosa*), enhanced anti–gram-positive activity, but limited activity against anaerobes. All FQs lack activity against MRSA and multidrug nosocomial gram-negative organisms.

All FQs are active against atypical respiratory pathogens (ie, *Chlamydia pneumoniae*, *Mycoplasma pneumoniae*, and *Legionella pneumophila*).

Their wide spectrums of activity, along with their excellent bioavailability, good tissue penetration, and safety, have made the FQs very attractive. The challenge is to limit their use to the appropriate setting where their enhanced spectrum is required, in order to reduce the risk of resistance selection and to lengthen their useful life.

Pharmacokinetics

Most FQs can be administered both orally and IV. Due to their excellent bioavailability, oral regimens provide similar serum levels as IV formulations, and thus, the oral route should be used preferentially whenever possible (ie, the patient is allowed to eat and does not have active nausea or vomiting). FQs have good tissue penetration. They are excreted mainly by the kidneys and require dose reduction in renal dysfunction (except moxifloxacin).

Clinical Use

1. **Urinary tract infections (UTIs):** Use of quinolones for uncomplicated community-acquired UTI should be reserved for infection due to organisms resistant to first-line treatment with trimethoprim-sulfamethoxazole (TMP-SMX). Ciprofloxacin is preferred when *P aeruginosa* is suspected. FQs are very useful in complicated UTI (eg, pyelonephritis).
2. **Pelvic inflammatory disease** as part of the antibiotic regimen. When *N gonorrhoeae* is a possibility, ceftriaxone is preferred over FQs due to increased resistance. In this setting, azithromycin or doxycycline should be added to treat the possibility of chlamydia.
3. **Intra-abdominal infections:** Ciprofloxacin plus metronidazole is a reasonable option (although usually, anti–*P aeruginosa* treatment is unnecessary) because this combination provides good anti–gram-negative and anaerobic activity.
4. **Community-acquired pneumonia (CAP):** The advanced-generation FQs (eg, gatifloxacin, levofloxacin, and moxifloxacin) are active against the common pathogens causing CAP (ie, *S pneumoniae*, *Haemophilus influenzae*, *Moraxella catarrhalis*, *Mycoplasma* and *Chlamydia* species, and *L pneumophila*). Consequently, they are included as a therapeutic option ("respiratory quinolones") in the guidelines of CAP. However, in order to avoid the development of bacterial resistance, macrolides are preferred.

Dosing in Normal Renal Function

See Table 44–2.

Adverse Effects

FQs are well tolerated. The most common adverse effects are gastrointestinal symptoms, primarily nausea (5%), and CNS symptoms (1–4%) mainly in the elderly (eg, headache, dizziness, sleep disturbance, alteration of mood). The third- and fourth-generation FQs can cause QT prolongation and arrhythmia. Quinolone use may be associated with tendon rupture (eg, Achilles, shoulder, or hand) and hence should be discontinued with the first sign of tendon pain.

Quinolones should be avoided in pregnancy and nursing mothers because of the potential effect on developing cartilage.

Resistance

With widespread use of the FQs (partially due to their oral administration), the emergence of quinolone-resistant bacteria resulted (eg, *P aeruginosa*, nosocomial Enterobacteriaceae, *N gonorrhoeae*, *Salmonella* species).

6. Macrolides

The macrolides inhibit protein synthesis by reversibly binding to the 50S ribosomal subunit. Although generally bacteriostatic, they may be bactericidal under certain conditions or against certain microorganisms. Because their structure is different from that of β-lactams, macrolides are useful for β-lactam–allergic patients. Dose reduction is not necessary in mild to moderate renal failure (for azithromycin, no dose adjustment is needed even in severe renal failure). Resistance to one macrolide implies cross-resistance to other macrolides.

1. **Erythromycin**, the first macrolide, is active against many gram-positive bacteria (streptococci, MSSA, but *not* enterococci). *Campylobacter jejuni*, *Bordetella pertussis*, *Haemophilus ducreyi*, *Mycoplasma*, *Chlamydia*, and *Legionella* are also susceptible. It is not active against Enterobacteriaceae. It can be administered orally (250–500 mg every 6 hours) or IV (250 mg–1 g every 6 hours). Because of its common gastrointestinal side effects, the newer macrolides are often preferred.
2. **Roxithromycin** has a similar spectrum of activity as erythromycin. It is given solely by the oral route (150 mg twice daily) with fewer gastrointestinal side effects. It is not available in the United States.
3. The spectrum of activity of **clarithromycin** is similar to that of erythromycin except for enhanced activity against respiratory gram-negative bacteria (eg, *H influenzae*) and atypical mycobacteria. Only oral preparations are available (250–500 mg twice daily). Clarithromycin is relatively nontoxic.
4. **Azithromycin** is a macrolide compound with unique properties—high and sustained tissue antibiotic levels (which are much greater than the serum antibiotic levels) and prolonged tissue half-life (between 2 and 4 days), which decrease the duration of therapy needed. Its spectrum of activity is similar to that of clarithromycin. Both oral (250-mg tablet commonly distributed in a pack containing 6 tablets) and IV formulations are available. The dose and duration of treatment vary with the indication (eg, CAP: 500 mg on first day, then 250 mg once daily; chlamydia cervicitis: 1 g orally as a single dose).

Clinical Use

1. Community acquired pneumonia (CAP)
2. Sexually transmitted diseases:
   a. Azithromycin (1 g orally once) is as effective as doxycycline (100 mg twice daily for 7 days) in treating chlamydia urethritis and cervicitis; cotreatment with single-dose ceftriaxone (250 mg intramuscularly) is necessary.
   b. *H ducreyi* (chancroid) genital ulcer disease has been treated with a single dose of azithromycin 1 g orally.
   c. Azithromycin may be used to treat *Chlamydia trachomatis* in pelvic inflammatory disease.
3. Macrolides are an alternative, in β-lactam–allergic patients, for the treatment of infections caused by groups A and B streptococci and MSSA.
4. Clarithromycin is active against *Helicobacter pylori* in duodenal/gastric ulcer as part of a combination therapy.

Adverse Effects

Gastrointestinal side effects (eg, nausea, vomiting, diarrhea) may occur; mostly with erythromycin. Allergic reactions are uncommon and are generally mild. Drug interactions are important (eg, elevation of warfarin blood levels) and have been reviewed elsewhere. Azithromycin has the least drug interactions of all the macrolides.

7. Tetracycline Group

The tetracyclines are bacteriostatic and act by interfering with protein synthesis at the ribosomal level (ie, 30S subunit). All have common basic chemical structures and antimicrobial activity. **Doxycycline** is the tetracycline of choice due to its superior pharmacokinetic properties, enhanced compliance, and lesser toxicity. Recently, a new generation (ie, glycylcyclines) that is also active against resistant bacteria has been developed. The clinical candidate of this class is **tigecycline**.

Antimicrobial Activity

Tetracyclines are active against a wide variety of organisms including the following:

1. Community-acquired respiratory tract pathogens (ie, *S pneumoniae*, *H influenzae*, *M catarrhalis*, and *Mycoplasma*, *Legionella*, and *Chlamydia* species)
2. *C trachomatis*
3. *Treponema pallidum* (syphilis)
4. The drug of choice for the treatment of *Rickettsia* and *Brucella* (with gentamicin)
5. They are *not* reliably active against *N gonorrhoeae.*
6. Tigecycline is also active against a variety of gram-positive and gram-negative organisms (including VRE, MRSA, and *N gonorrhoeae*, but not *P aeruginosa*).

Pharmacokinetics

The oral route is most commonly used, except for treatment of severe pelvic inflammatory disease (PID). Absorption is improved if the antibiotic is taken 1 hour before or 2 hours after meals. Doxycycline's long half-life permits dosing every 12 to 24 hours, thus improving compliance. Tetracyclines are excreted via the urine, except for doxycycline, which is excreted in the feces (therefore, there is no need for doxycycline dose adjustment in renal failure). Oral contraceptive efficacy may be decreased with simultaneous use of tetracyclines.

Clinical Use in Obstetrics & Gynecology

Doxycycline is the drug of choice for genital infections caused by *C trachomatis* (eg, PID, cervicitis, lymphogranuloma venereum) in nonpregnant women.

1. In mucopurulent cervicitis, doxycycline 100 mg twice daily orally is given for 7 days (or single-dose

azithromycin 1 g) in addition to a single dose of intramuscular ceftriaxone 250 mg (to treat *N gonorrhoeae*).

2. For PID, doxycycline 100 mg twice daily orally is given for 14 days (in combination with ceftriaxone and metronidazole). It can be administered IV with the same dosing regimen, but the oral route is preferred whenever possible.
3. Doxycycline is an alternative to penicillin for the treatment of syphilis (*not* in pregnant woman or in neurosyphilis).

The equivalent dose of **tetracycline** is 250–500 mg (orally only) every 6 hours.

Adverse Effects & Contraindications

1. Hypersensitivity reactions with fever or skin rashes are uncommon.
2. Toxic photosensitivity reactions consisting of a red rash on areas exposed to sunlight can occur. Patients should avoid intense sun exposure during doxycycline treatment.
3. Esophageal ulceration can occur with doxycycline. Patients should be told to take the drug while sitting and with adequate amount of fluids.
4. Thrombophlebitis can occur with IV doxycycline use.
5. Superinfection with Candida of the anogenital region can occur.
6. Tetracyclines should be avoided by pregnant women due to a possible hepatotoxicity to the mother and dental deformities in the child (also during lactation).

8. Clindamycin

Clindamycin inhibits protein synthesis at the ribosomal level (ie, 50S subunit) and is generally bacteriostatic. Its spectrum of activity includes gram-positive cocci (groups A and B streptococci, MSSA) and anaerobes, although there is increasing resistance of *Bacteroides* species to clindamycin. It is *not* active against gram-negative aerobes (eg, Enterobacteriaceae) or enterococci.

Pharmacokinetics

Clindamycin is well absorbed from the gastrointestinal tract, and food does not decrease its absorption. Therapeutic blood levels can be achieved by the oral or parenteral routes of administration. It penetrates most body tissues well, but not the cerebrospinal fluid. It is metabolized primarily by the liver; therefore, doses of clindamycin should be reduced in severe hepatic insufficiency. Dose adjustment is *not* required in renal failure. The oral dose is 300–450 mg every 6–8 hours. The IV dose is 600–900 mg every 8 hours.

Clinical Use in Obstetrics & Gynecology

1. In intra-abdominal/pelvic infections (eg, tubo-ovarian abscess), clindamycin (which is active against gram-positive cocci and anaerobes) must be combined with an agent active against gram-negative organisms (eg, gentamicin, ciprofloxacin). Because *B fragilis* plays an important role in these infections and there is increasing resistance of *B fragilis* to clindamycin, many experts turned to metronidazole.
2. Clindamycin is an option for mixed aerobic and anaerobic perineal infection (ie, soft tissue infection) in combination with an agent active against gram-negative organisms.
3. Clindamycin is an alternative drug for the treatment of groups A and B streptococci and MSSA in patients allergic to both penicillin and cephalosporins.
4. Clindamycin is the drug of choice (in combination with high-dose penicillin) for the treatment of necrotizing fasciitis caused by group A Streptococcus.
5. Clindamycin 300 mg orally twice a day or 2% vaginal cream 5 g intravaginally at bedtime (both for 7 days) or clindamycin ovules 100 mg intravaginally at bed time for 3 days is an alternative to metronidazole for treatment of bacterial vaginosis.

Adverse Effects

1. Diarrhea is the most significant side effect of clindamycin: Antibiotic-associated diarrhea occurs in up to 20% of patients; *C difficile*–associated diarrhea (CDAD) occurs less frequently. When CDAD occurs, clindamycin should be discontinued if possible and oral (or IV) metronidazole or (in severe cases) oral vancomycin started.
2. Allergic reactions (eg, rash and fever) can occur.
3. Minor reversible elevations of hepatocellular enzymes are frequent.

9. Metronidazole

Metronidazole is mainly an agent for the treatment of anaerobic infections including *B fragilis* and *Gardnerella vaginalis*. It also has antiparasitic activity, including *Entamoeba histolytica*, *Giardia lamblia*, and *Trichomonas vaginalis*. Metronidazole inhibits DNA synthesis and is rapidly bactericidal.

Pharmacokinetics

The drug is absorbed very well and can be taken with food. Serum levels are similar after equivalent oral and IV doses. It has excellent penetration into almost all tissues. The drug is metabolized in the liver and excreted in the kidney. The usual daily dose is 500 mg orally or IV every 8 hours.

Dose reduction is required in severe renal failure and significant hepatic impairment.

Clinical Use in Obstetrics & Gynecology

1. Metronidazole is the drug of choice for *Bacteroides* species, *C difficile*-associated disease, *G vaginalis*, *E histolytica*, and *G lamblia*.
2. It is indicated (in combination) for mixed aerobic/anaerobic infections (eg, intra-abdominal and pelvic infections).
3. For Trichomonas vaginitis, the recommended dose is 2 g orally as a single dose or 500 mg twice daily for 7 days. Both sexual partners should be treated.
4. For bacterial vaginosis, the recommended regimens are 500 mg orally twice daily for 7 days or vaginal gel (1 applicator intravaginally) for 5 days. Treatment of sexual partners is not recommended unless balanitis is present. Topical treatment of bacterial vaginosis is not recommended in pregnancy.

Adverse Effects

In general, metronidazole is well tolerated.

1. Alcoholic beverages should not be consumed while taking metronidazole because of a disulfiram-like effect (ie, nausea, vomiting, and headaches).
2. Patients complain of a metallic unpleasant taste while on oral therapy.
3. With prolonged use, peripheral neuropathy may develop.

10. Vancomycin

Vancomycin is the first glycopeptides antibiotic. The primary effect of glycopeptides is inhibition of cell wall synthesis. Vancomycin is active *only* against gram-positive organisms. Except for enterococci, vancomycin is bactericidal; however, the addition of gentamicin increases the bactericidal activity against enterococci. The excessive use of vancomycin has contributed to the emergence of VRE and also *S aureus* with intermediate resistance or complete resistance to vancomycin. Prudent use of vancomycin is essential to preserve the effectiveness of this important antibiotic.

Pharmacokinetics & Dosage

Vancomycin is poorly absorbed. Very high stool concentrations after oral administration make it active against *C difficile*-associated disease (CDAD). The route of administration is mostly IV with diverse tissue penetration. Initial doses are based on actual weight, 15–20 mg/kg IV every 12 hours (over 1–2 hours to avoid the "red man syndrome"). Subsequent doses are based on measured trough serum levels. Target trough level in serious infections should be 15–20 μg/mL. Because vancomycin is excreted primarily by the kidneys, in renal failure, the dose must be reduced or the interval between doses increased.

Clinical Use in Obstetrics & Gynecology

Vancomycin is less active than β-lactam antibiotics (eg, nafcillin, oxacillin) for MSSA, and thus, β-lactam antibiotics should be preferred in this setting.

1. Vancomycin is the treatment of choice for MRSA infections.
2. It is an alternative for the treatment of MSSA and groups A and B Streptococcus in patients with a history of anaphylaxis to β-lactam antibiotics.
3. For severe cases of *C difficile* diarrhea, vancomycin 125 mg every 6 hours for 10–14 days is indicated instead of metronidazole. Discontinue other antibiotic agents if possible.

Adverse Effects

1. If vancomycin is infused too rapidly, it may cause flushing of the face, neck, or torso ("red man syndrome"), pruritus, and hypotension. To avoid this, vancomycin should be infused no more rapidly than 500 mg/h. Because this reaction is not immunologically mediated, it does not preclude further use.
2. Allergy (rashes other than red man syndrome) occurs in 5% of patients.
3. Nephrotoxicity and ototoxicity are very uncommon (occur mostly when vancomycin is used in combination with another nephrotoxic or ototoxic drug such as an aminoglycoside).

11. Linezolid

Linezolid belongs to the oxazolidinones; it interferes with bacterial protein synthesis by binding at the 50S ribosomal subunit. It is bacteriostatic and active only against gram-positive bacteria including MRSA and VRE, which are the main indications for use (although MRSA and VRE resistance to linezolid was described). Oral drug is 100% bioavailable. The oral and IV doses are 600 mg every 12 hours; no dose modification is required for renal or hepatic failure. Reversible myelosuppression (ie, thrombocytopenia, anemia, and neutropenia) has been reported, most often after more than 2 weeks of therapy. Its use in obstetric and gynecologic practice currently is limited.

12. Spectinomycin

Spectinomycin structure is similar (but not identical) to the aminoglycosides. It inhibits ribosomal protein synthesis and is bactericidal. Spectinomycin is used *only* as an alternative agent for the treatment of *N gonorrhoeae* when the drugs of choice (eg, cephalosporin or azithromycin) cannot be used or in resistant strains. One injection of 2 g intramuscularly is given. No dose adjustment is required in renal failure. There are no known serious adverse reactions.

13. Trimethoprim-Sulfamethoxazole

The combination of trimethoprim and sulfamethoxazole (TMP-SMX) inhibits 2 sequential steps in the synthesis of folic acid by bacteria. Alone, each agent is bacteriostatic, but together, they are synergistic and bactericidal. The combination is available in oral and IV forms of 80 mg trimethoprim and 400 mg sulfamethoxazole. There are also double-strength (DS) tablets (160 mg trimethoprim and 800 mg sulfamethoxazole).

Antimicrobial Activity

1. TMP-SMX has a wide spectrum of activity against gram-positive cocci (including some strains of MRSA) and gram-negative bacteria.
2. It is *not* active against enterococci, *P aeruginosa*, or anaerobes.
3. It is active against *L monocytogenes*, *Nocardia* species, and *Pneumocystis* (*carinii*) *jiroveci*.

Pharmacokinetics

Because oral TMP-SMX is well absorbed, the oral route is usually preferred. Each component is distributed widely to most tissues. It is excreted mainly by the kidneys; therefore, dose reduction is required in renal failure. The long half-life allows twice-daily dosing.

Clinical Use in Obstetrics and Gynecology

1. TMP-SMX is used to treat acute uncomplicated UTI (cystitis) in females (in the presence of <20% resistance of local *Escherichia coli*). The dose is 960 mg twice a day for 3 days.
2. It is useful for susceptible pathogens in the treatment of pyelonephritis.
3. In a young woman with recurrent episodes of uncomplicated UTI (3 or more episodes per year), TMP-SMX 1 single-strength tablet orally every 24 hours long term, after eradication of infection, is a possibility. An alternative is self-administered single-dose treatment (TMP-SMX DS, 2 tablets, 320/1600 mg) at symptom onset or 1 DS tablet after coitus.
4. TMP-SMX is an alternative in *L monocytogenes* infection (eg, meningitis or amnionitis) in a penicillin-allergic patient.
5. It is considered the drug of choice for the treatment and prevention of *P jiroveci* (*carinii*) pneumonia.

Toxicity & Side Effects

Although skin rashes are common, this combination usually is well tolerated.

1. Mild gastrointestinal symptoms occur in 3%.
2. Skin rashes occur in 3–5%; most are benign; however, severe skin rashes (eg, exfoliative dermatitis, Stevens-Johnson syndrome) may occur. Rashes are more common in HIV patients.
3. Thrombocytopenia and neutropenia can occur. Complete blood count should be performed weekly.
4. It should be avoided in patients with glucose-6-phosphate dehydrogenase deficiency because hemolysis can be precipitated.
5. If TMP-SMX is used in patients receiving warfarin, it enhances the response to warfarin; thus, the risk of bleeding is increased.

14. Urinary Antiseptics (Nitrofurantoin, Fosfomycin)

Urinary antiseptics are agents that concentrate in the urine but do not produce therapeutic levels in the serum. Therefore, they are useful only for the treatment of lower UTIs. This feature has advantages, including reduced suppression of normal flora.

Nitrofurantoin

Nitrofurantoin is active for both gram-negative (eg, Enterobacteriaceae) and gram-positive (eg, enterococci, coagulase-negative staphylococci) bacteria causing UTI. *Pseudomonas* species are resistant. It is well absorbed (preferably taken with food) but reaches therapeutic concentrations only in urine. The drug is contraindicated in creatinine clearance of <40 mL/min (because the excretion to urine is reduced and the drug accumulates in the serum) and in hepatic insufficiency. The urine should *not* be alkalinized because the drug effect is reduced in alkaline urine.

For uncomplicated UTI, nitrofurantoin is taken for 3–7 days at 100 mg twice daily. For the prophylaxis of recurrent uncomplicated UTI, it can be given daily at bedtime or postcoital as a single 50- or 100-mg dose, but pulmonary toxicity is a risk with long-term use. Nitrofurantoin may be administered as a combination of macrocrystals/monohydrate salt (nitrofurantoin capsules, Macrobid). The usual dose of this combination is 100 mg every 12 hours.

Skin rashes occur in 1–5% of patients and are reversible. Major adverse effects include pneumonitis and polyneuropathies. Because these are more common in the elderly, Macrodantin should be administered with caution to people 60 years of age or older.

Fosfomycin

Fosfomycin is used as a single oral dose of 3 g for treatment of uncomplicated UTI in women. The drug acts on the bacterial cell wall. It is active against the common pathogens of community-acquired UTI (eg, Enterobacteriaceae, *Staphylococcus saprophyticus*, and enterococci). *P aeruginosa* are usually resistant.

It is absorbed rapidly and excreted unchanged in the urine. Bactericidal concentrations persist for 24–48 hours in the urine. It is generally well tolerated, with diarrhea occurring in 9%. It may play a useful role in settings were compliance is a problem. Its high cost compared to the 3-day effective course of TMP-SMX is a limitation.

15. Antifungal Drugs

There are 3 main groups of antifungal agents: polyenes (eg, amphotericin B), azoles (eg, fluconazole), and echinocandins (eg, caspofungin). The major agents will be discussed briefly.

Amphotericin B

Amphotericin B is active and bactericidal against most invasive fungal pathogens (eg, *Candida* species and molds). It is poorly absorbed; hence, systemic infections must be treated IV. The dose for seriously ill patients is 0.7–1.0 mg/kg/d, typically infused over 4 hours. Thrice-weekly regimens may be used to minimize side effects. Elimination occurs via the biliary tract. Although amphotericin B is nephrotoxic, it does not accumulate in renal failure, and dose adjustments are made to minimize toxicity.

Fever and chills during infusion are common and usually diminish after the first week of treatment. Pretreatment by acetaminophen or ibuprofen is often used to reduce these symptoms. Nephrotoxicity is the main serious drug effect that limits its use. The incidence of renal failure may be reduced by saline infusion before each dose. Renal failure is usually reversible. The FDA pregnancy risk category is B.

To overcome the adverse effect–related dosage limitation, a liposomal delivery system was developed (eg, liposomal amphotericin [AmBisome]), allowing treatment with higher doses without increased systemic toxicity.

Triazoles (Fluconazole, Voriconazole)

These fungistatic agents are effective and less toxic alternatives to amphotericin B for the treatment of many systemic fungal infections. There are also some topical preparations and vaginal suppositories (eg, clotrimazole). They act by inhibition of the biosynthesis of ergosterol in the fungal cell membrane and, as a result, inhibition of cell growth.

Fluconazole

Fluconazole is available in both IV and oral preparations. Because absorption is excellent, the daily doses for oral and IV therapy are the same. It is excreted mainly in the kidneys; hence, dose adjustment is required in renal failure. It is active against yeasts (eg, *Candida species*, *Cryptococcus species*) but *not* against molds. The usual daily dose is 200–400 mg orally or IV once daily. In gynecology, it is often used to treat *Candida* vaginitis with a single oral dose of 150 mg. Alternatively, for this indication, there are many preparations of intravaginal azoles (eg, clotrimazole, miconazole) that are administered from one dose to 7–14 days. Fluconazole is well tolerated; side effects include rash (in <5%) and nausea and vomiting.

Voriconazole

Voriconazole is active against yeasts but also against molds. It is the drug of choice for the treatment of invasive aspergillosis. Voriconazole is available in both IV and oral preparations with excellent bioavailability. A loading dose of 6 mg/kg IV every 12 hours is followed by a maintenance dose of 4 mg/kg every 12 hours. With creatinine clearance of less than 50 mL/min, switch to oral therapy (due to accumulation of IV vehicle). The oral dose is 200 mg twice daily for patients who weigh more than 40 kg. Dose adjustment is necessary in hepatic insufficiency. The most frequent side effects include reversible visual disturbances and rash, both in 20%.

Echinocandins

Caspofungin is the first echinocandin. Its mechanism of action is inhibition of glucan (ie, an integral component of the fungal cell wall) synthesis. It is used to treat invasive candidiasis and invasive aspergillosis (an alternative to voriconazole). It is only available as IV formulation. Dose adjustment is necessary for patients with liver failure but *not* in renal failure. Caspofungin 70 mg IV on day 1 is followed by 50 mg IV once daily for maintenance. It is remarkably *not* toxic. There are also new agents in this class like **anidulafungin**. The FDA pregnancy risk category of the echinocandins is C.

16. Antiviral Drugs (Acyclovir, Valacyclovir, Famciclovir)

Only antiherpesvirus drugs will be discussed and *not* antiretrovirals or anticytomegalovirus agents.

Acyclovir acts by inhibition of viral DNA polymerase and thus blocks viral DNA synthesis. It is activated by the viral thymidine kinase. The antiviral spectrum of acyclovir is limited to herpesviruses (eg, herpes simplex virus [HSV] and varicella-zoster virus [VZV]). **Valacyclovir** is a prodrug of acyclovir. **Famciclovir** is a prodrug of penciclovir with similar spectrum of activity as acyclovir. The bioavailability of oral acyclovir is low (15–20%). Valacyclovir and famciclovir are readily absorbed after oral administration (bioavailability of 54–70% and 77%, respectively) and rapidly converted to their active form (acyclovir and penciclovir, respectively). Dose adjustment is required for these drugs in renal failure.

Clinical Use in Obstetrics & Gynecology

Acyclovir is the agent of choice for HSV and VZV and can be administered both orally and IV. Valacyclovir and famciclovir are comparably effective as oral alternatives and offer more convenient dosing regimen.

1. Acyclovir is effective in primary genital HSV infections. In outpatients, oral acyclovir (400 mg every 8 hours for 7–10 days) is used. Alternatively, oral valacyclovir or famciclovir (1,000 mg twice a day and 250 mg 3 times a day, respectively, both for 7–10 days) may be used. Topical acyclovir is less effective, and its use is discouraged. IV acyclovir (5 mg/kg every 8 hours for 5–7 days) can be used in hospitalized patients with severe primary HSV infections.
2. In recurrent genital HSV infections, patient-initiated treatment during the prodrome or at the first lesion appearance is associated with 2-day reduction in duration of symptoms. The options are acyclovir 800 mg 3 times a day for 2 days; valacyclovir 500 mg twice a day for 3 days; and famciclovir 1000 mg twice a day for 1 day.
3. Suppressive therapy reduces the frequency of genital HSV recurrences by 70–80% among patients who suffer frequent recurrences (ie, >6 per year). Effective regimens include acyclovir 400 mg twice a day, famciclovir 250 mg twice a day, and valacyclovir 1 g once daily.
4. Acyclovir treatment late in pregnancy reduces the frequency of caesarean sections among women who have recurrent genital herpes by diminishing the frequency of recurrences at term; the effect of antiviral therapy late in pregnancy on the incidence of neonatal herpes is not known. No data support the use of antiviral therapy among HSV-seropositive women without a history of genital herpes.
5. High-dose acyclovir is effective treatment for chickenpox and VZV in older adults.
6. For cytomegalovirus (CMV) infections, these agents are ineffective.

Toxicity & Side Effects

Oral agents (ie, acyclovir, valacyclovir, and famciclovir) are generally well tolerated. IV acyclovir may cause phlebitis and, in 5%, nephrotoxicity. Adequate prehydration may prevent it.

Available data do not indicate an increased risk for major birth defects in women treated with acyclovir during the first trimester, compared with the general population. However, data regarding prenatal exposure to valacyclovir and famciclovir are too limited to provide useful information on pregnancy outcomes.

Babinchak T, Ellis-Grosse E, Dartois N, Rose GM, Loh E; Tigecycline 301 Study Group; Tigecycline 306 Study Group. The efficacy and safety of tigecycline for the treatment of complicated intra-abdominal infections: analysis of pooled clinical trial data. *Clin Infect Dis* 2005;41(Suppl 5):S354–S367. PMID: 16080073.

Betts RF, Chapman SW, Penn RL, eds. *A Practical Approach to Infectious Diseases*. 5th ed. Philadelphia, PA: Lippincott Williams & Wilkins; 2003.

Centers for Disease Control and Prevention. Sexually transmitted diseases treatment guidelines. *MMWR Recomm Rep* 2010;59(RR-12): 1–110. PMID: 21160495.

Centers for Disease Control and Prevention. Update to CDC's sexually transmitted diseases treatment guidelines, 2006: fluoroquinolones no longer recommended for treatment of gonococcal infections. *MMWR Morb Mortal Wkly Rep* 2007;56:332–336. PMID: 17431378.

Gilbert DN, Mollering RC, Eliopolus GM, Chambers HF, Saag MS. *The Sanford Guide to Antimicrobial Therapy*. 40th ed. Sperryville, VA: Antimicrobial Therapy, Inc.; 2010.

Mandell GL, Bennett JE, Dolin R, eds. *Principle and Practice of Infectious Diseases*. 7th ed. New York, NY: Churchill Livingstone; 2010.

Romano A, Viola M, Guéant-Rodriguez RM, Gaeta F, Pettinato R, Guéant JL. Imipenem in patients with immediate hypersensitivity to penicillins. *N Engl J Med* 2006;354:2835–2837. PMID: 16807429.

Society of Obstetricians and Gynaecologists of Canada. Screening and management of bacterial vaginosis in pregnancy. Available at: http://www.sogc.org/guidelines/documents/gui211CPG0808.pdf. Accessed August 2008.

ANTIMICROBIAL PROPHYLAXIS IN SURGERY

Indications

Antimicrobial prophylaxis reduces the incidence of wound infection after certain operations. It should be used only for procedures with high infection rates such as clean contaminated procedures (ie, involving mucosal surfaces such as the vagina), operations involving implantation of prosthetic material (eg, general surgeries where meshes are used, artificial joints), and procedures where the consequences of infection are serious.

Organisms Involved

For most gynecologic surgical site infections, the source of pathogens is the endogenous flora of the patient's skin or vagina. Gynecologic surgical procedures, such as laparotomies or laparoscopies, do not breach surfaces colonized with bacteria from the vagina, and infections after these procedures more commonly result from skin bacteria only. The major pathogen in these clean surgeries is *S aureus*. Procedures breaching the endocervix, such as hysterosalpingogram, intrauterine device (IUD) insertion, endometrial biopsy, chromotubation, and dilation and curettage, may seed the endometrium and the fallopian tubes with microorganisms found in the upper vagina and endocervix (eg, Enterobacteriaceae, group B *Streptococcus*).

Timing

To be optimally effective, antibiotics must be given so that good tissue levels are present at the time of incision and for the duration of the operation. To achieve that goal, antibiotics should be started preferably less than 1 hour before incision for most agents (except for vancomycin and quinolones because they are infused over an hour). A convenient time to administer antibiotic prophylaxis is just before induction of anesthesia.

However, timing of antibiotic prophylaxis has historically been different with regard to caesarean delivery; the prophylactic antibiotic was given only after clamping of the umbilical cord. The rationale for this was to avoid exposure of the neonate to the antibiotics and to prevent any masking of newborn culture results in cases of a suspected newborn infection. In 2007, Sullivan and colleagues reported results from a randomized, prospective, double-blind trial comparing the administration of cefazolin an hour prior to skin incision with administration after cord clamping. The group receiving the earlier antibiotics had less overall infectious morbidity and less endometritis, with no associated increase in neonatal adverse effects. Other similar studies have found comparable results. In September 2010, this evidence prompted the American College of Obstetricians and Gynecologists (ACOG) to issue a Committee Opinion advocating that all patients undergoing caesarean delivery be given appropriate prophylactic antibiotics *prior* to skin incision.

Duration

In most instances, a single dose is sufficient. For procedures lasting more than 2 half-lives of prophylactic agent, intraoperative supplementary dose(s) may be required. In most cases, prophylaxis is not extended beyond 24 hours.

Antibiotic Prophylaxis Choices in Selected Procedures

1. Hysterectomy, either vaginal or abdominal: IV cefazolin 1–2 g 30 minutes before incision.
2. Cesarean section: IV cefazolin 1–2 g 30 minutes *before* incision.
3. Surgical abortion: first trimester, doxycycline 100 mg before procedure and 200 mg after; second trimester, IV cefazolin 1–2 g before procedure.
4. *No* antibiotic prophylaxis is indicated during IUD insertion, hysteroscopy, and endometrial biopsy.

An alternative in patients with immediate hypersensitivity to penicillins is clindamycin plus gentamicin. MRSA should be considered when it is prevalent in the community or in institutions where the rate of postoperative MRSA infection is high; in these circumstances, vancomycin should be considered.

ACOG Committee Opinion No. 465: antimicrobial prophylaxis for cesarean delivery: timing of administration. *Obstet Gynecol* 2010;116:791–792. PMID: 20733474.

ACOG Practice Bulletin No. 104: antibiotic prophylaxis for gynecologic procedures. *Obstet Gynecol* 2009;113:1180–1189. PMID: 19384919.

Camann W, Tuomala R. Antibiotic prophylaxis for cesarean delivery: always before skin incision! *Int J Obstet Anesth* 2011;20:1–2. PMID: 21126866.

45 Perioperative, Intraoperative, & Postoperative Complications in Gynecologic Surgery

Cecilia K. Wieslander, MD
Danielle D. Marshall, MD

PREOPERATIVE COMPLICATIONS

One of the main purposes of the preoperative history and physical exam is to identify any preoperative medical comorbidity that may lead to an increased perioperative morbidity or mortality. If comorbidities are identified, the surgeon should obtain medical consultation to ensure that the patient's medical conditions are optimized and stable enough to proceed with surgery at an acceptable risk.

CARDIOVASCULAR DISEASE

Clinical Findings

Most gynecologic surgeries fall in the low (<1%) or intermediate (1–5%) risk of cardiac death or nonfatal myocardial infarction (Table 45–1). It is crucial to obtain a careful preoperative history to discover cardiac and/or comorbid diseases that would place the patient in a high surgical risk category. If the patient is found to have active cardiac conditions, such as unstable coronary syndrome, decompensated heart failure, significant arrhythmias, or severe valvular disease, the surgery should be delayed or cancelled (unless emergent), and the patient should be evaluated and treated (Table 45–2). One should also determine if the patient has a prior history of a pacemaker, implantable cardioverter-defibrillator, orthostatic intolerance, or other clinical risk factors that are associated with increased perioperative cardiovascular risk (Table 45–2). If the patient has a history of cardiac disease, any recent change in symptoms must be elicited. In addition, one should record current medications including doses and any use of alcohol, tobacco, and over-the-counter and illicit drugs. The history should also include the patient's functional capacity (Table 45–3). Assessing a person's capacity to perform common daily tasks correlates well with maximum oxygen uptake by treadmill testing.

The American College of Cardiology/American Heart Association 2007 Guidelines on Perioperative Cardiovascular Evaluation and Care for Noncardiac Surgery recommend a stepwise approach to perioperative cardiac assessment.

Step 1: Does the patient need emergency noncardiac surgery? If yes, one should proceed with surgery and perioperative surveillance and postoperative stratification and risk factor management. If no, one should proceed with step 2.

Step 2: Does the patient have active cardiac conditions (see Table 45–2)? If yes, the surgery should be postponed and the conditions evaluated and treated. If no, proceed with step 3.

Step 3: Is the planned procedure a low-risk surgery (see Table 45–1)? If yes, proceed with the planned surgery. If no, proceed with step 4.

Step 4: Does the patient have good functional capacity (≥4 metabolic equivalents [MET]; see Table 45–3) without symptoms? If yes, proceed with planned surgery. If no, proceed with step 5.

Step 5: If the patient has poor functional capacity, is symptomatic, or has unknown functional capacity, then the presence of active clinical risk factors determines the need for further evaluation. Clinical risk factors include a history of heart disease, compensated or prior heart failure, cerebrovascular disease, diabetes mellitus, and renal insufficiency.

- ≥3 clinical risk factors + high-risk surgery: testing should be considered if it will change management.
- ≥3 clinical risk factors + intermediate surgery: proceed with planned surgery with heart rate control with beta-blocker or consider noninvasive testing if it will change management.
- 1 or 2 clinical risk factors + high-risk surgery: proceed with planned surgery with heart rate control with beta-blocker or consider noninvasive testing if it will change management.

Table 45–1. Cardiac risk (cardiac death and nonfatal myocardial infarction) for noncardiac procedures.

Risk Stratification	Examples of Procedures
High (vascular surgery) (reported risk >5%)	Aortic and other major vascular surgery Peripheral vascular surgery
Intermediate (reported risk 1–5%)	Intraperitoneal surgery Intrathoracic surgery Carotid endarterectomy Head and neck surgery Orthopedic surgery Prostate surgery
Low risk (reported risk <1%)	Endoscopic procedures Superficial procedures Cataract surgery Breast surgery Ambulatory surgery

Modified and reproduced, with permission, from Fleisher LA, Beckman JA, Brown KA, et al. ACC/AHA 2007 guidelines on perioperative cardiovascular evaluation and care for noncardiac surgery: executive summary. *J Am Coll Cardiol* 2007;50:1707–1732.

- 1 or 2 clinical risk factors + intermediate surgery: proceed with planned surgery with heart rate control with beta-blocker or consider noninvasive testing if it will change management.
- No clinical risk factors: proceed with planned surgery.

Treatment

A. Coronary Artery Disease

In patients with known or previous occult coronary artery disease, one has to determine the amount of myocardium in jeopardy, the ischemic threshold, the ventricular function, and whether the patient's condition is optimized. Selective noninvasive testing can be used to determine the patient risk of ischemia during surgery.

B. Hypertension

Induction of anesthesia causes an increase in blood pressure and heart rate due to sympathetic activation. These changes are more pronounced in patients with untreated hypertension than in patients with well-controlled hypertension. Elective surgery should be delayed for stage 3 hypertension (systolic blood pressure ≥180 mm Hg and diastolic blood pressure ≥100 mm Hg). If emergent surgery is needed, rapid-acting intravenous agents should be used to control the blood pressure perioperatively.

Patients should continue taking their antihypertensive medications with a sip of water the morning of surgery, and medications should be resumed postoperatively. Some physicians recommend withholding angiotensin-converting enzyme inhibitors and angiotensin receptor antagonists the morning of surgery. These medications can be restarted postoperatively after the patient is euvolemic to decrease the risk of perioperative renal dysfunction.

Postoperatively, reversible causes of hypertension, such as pain, anxiety, hypervolemia, hypercarbia, hypoxia, and

Table 45–2. Clinical risk factors for increased perioperative cardiovascular complications (myocardial infarction, heart failure, death).

Active cardiac conditions that require intensive management and may result in delay or cancellation of surgery unless the surgery is emergent
Unstable coronary syndromes
Including unstable or severe angina or recent myocardial infarction (within 30 days)
Decompensated heart failure
Including NYHA functional class IV or worsening or new-onset heart failure
Significant arrhythmias
Including high-grade AV block, Mobitz II AV block, third-degree AV block, symptomatic ventricular arrhythmias, supraventricular arrhythmias (including atrial fibrillation) with uncontrolled ventricular rate (>100 bpm at rest), symptomatic bradycardia, newly recognized ventricular tachycardia
Severe valvular disease
Including severe aortic stenosis (mean pressure gradient >40 mm Hg, aortic valve area <1.0 cm^2, or symptomatic), symptomatic mitral stenosis (progressive dyspnea on exertion, exertional presyncope, or heart failure)
Other clinical risk factors that require careful assessment of current cardiovascular status
History of heart disease
History of compensated or prior heart failure
History of cerebrovascular disease
Diabetes mellitus
Renal insufficiency

AV, atrioventricular; NYHA, New York Heart Association.
Modified and reproduced, with permission, from Fleisher LA, Beckman JA, Brown KA, et al. ACC/AHA 2007 guidelines on perioperative cardiovascular evaluation and care for noncardiac surgery: executive summary. *J Am Coll Cardiol* 2007;50:1707–1732.

Table 45–3. Estimated energy requirements for various activities.

Metabolic Equivalent (MET)	Questions to Determine Functional Capacity
1 MET	Can you take care of yourself? Can you eat, dress, or use the toilet?
>1 MET, <4 METS	Can you walk indoors around the house? Can you walk a block or two on level ground at 2–3 mph?
4 METS	Can you do light work around the house like dusting or washing dishes? Can you walk a flight of stairs or walk up a hill? Can you walk on level ground at 4 mph?
>4 METS, <10 METS	Can you run a short distance? Can you do heavy work around the house like scrubbing floors or lifting or moving heavy furniture? Can you participate in moderate recreational activities like golf, bowling, dancing, doubles tennis, or throwing a baseball of football?
>10 METS	Can you participate in strenuous sports like swimming, singles tennis, football, basketball, or skiing?

Modified and reproduced, with permission, from Fleisher LA, Beckman JA, Brown KA, et al. ACC/AHA 2007 guidelines on perioperative cardiovascular evaluation and care for noncardiac surgery: executive summary. *J Am Coll Cardiol* 2007;50:1707–1732.

bladder distension should be treated. Patients on chronic antihypertensive medications should restart their usual medications as needed. Patients with sustained systolic blood pressure greater than 180 mm Hg or diastolic blood pressure greater than 110 mm Hg should be treated once reversible causes have been addressed.

C. Valvular Heart Disease

In patients with symptomatic aortic stenosis, elective noncardiac surgery should be postponed or cancelled because the mortality risk is approximately 10%. Such patients require aortic valve replacement before elective but necessary noncardiac surgery. If the aortic stenosis is severe but asymptomatic, the surgery should be postponed or cancelled if the valve has not been evaluated within the year.

Significant mitral stenosis increases the risk of heart failure. When the stenosis is severe, the patient may benefit from balloon mitral valvuloplasty or open surgical repair before high-risk surgery. However, in general, preoperative surgical correction is not indicated, unless the valvular condition should be corrected to prolong survival.

Patients with atrial fibrillation who are at risk for thromboembolism should be given preoperative and postoperative intravenous heparin or low-molecular-weight heparin to cover periods of subtherapeutic anticoagulation.

Patients with mechanical prosthetic valves need careful anticoagulation management when they undergo surgery. Perioperative heparin is recommended for patients in whom the risk of bleeding with oral anticoagulation is high and the risk of thromboembolism without anticoagulation is also high. These patients include patients with mechanical heart valve in the mitral position, Bjork-Shiley valve, recent (<1 year) thrombosis or embolus, or 3 or more of the following risk factors: atrial fibrillation, previous embolus at any time, hypercoagulable condition, mechanical prosthesis, and left ventricular ejection fraction less than 30%.

Recommendations regarding endocarditis prophylaxis in patients with mechanical heart valves have recently been changed. The American Heart Association no longer recommends endocarditis prophylaxis in patients undergoing genitourinary or gastrointestinal surgery, including gynecologic surgery, or vaginal delivery or caesarean section. The only exception is in a patient with an infection that could cause bacteremia, such as chorioamnionitis or pyelonephritis. In these cases, the underlying infection should be treated in the usual fashion, and the treatment should include a regimen effective for infective endocarditis prophylaxis (Table 45–4). In addition to prosthetic heart valves, the American Heart Association only recommends endocarditis prophylaxis for previous infective endocarditis and congenital heart disease (Table 45–5).

Fleischer LA, Beckman JA, Brown KA, et al. The ACC/AHA 2007 guidelines on perioperative cardiovascular evaluation and care for noncardiac surgery: executive summary. *J Am Coll Cardiol* 2007;50:1707–1732. PMID: 17950159.

Wilson W, Taubert KA, Gewitz M, et al. Prevention of infective endocarditis: guidelines from the American Heart Association: a guideline from the American Heart Association Rheumatic Fever, Endocarditis and Kawasaki Disease Committee, Council on Cardiovascular Disease in the Young, and the Council on Clinical Cardiology, Council on Cardiovascular Surgery and Anesthesia, and the Quality of Care and Outcomes Research Interdisciplinary Working Group. *Circulation* 2007;116:1736–1754. PMID: 17446442.

VENOUS THROMBOEMBOLISM

In patients with a prior history of venous thromboembolism (VTE; pulmonary embolism or deep vein thrombosis

Table 45–4. Antibiotic prophylaxis for infective endocarditis.

Treatment	Antibiotic	Regimen (single dose 30–60 minutes before procedure)
Oral	Amoxicillin	2 g
Intravenous	Ampicillin or Cefazolin/Caftriaxone	2g intravenous 1g intravenous
Allergic to penicillin or ampicillin	Cefazolin or ceftriaxone or clindamycin	1 g intravenous 600 mg intravenous

Modified and reproduced, with permission, from Wilson W, Taubert KA, Gewitz M, et al. Prevention of infective endocarditis: guidelines from the American Heart Association: a guideline from the American Heart Association Rheumatic Fever, Endocarditis and Kawasaki Disease Committee, Council on Cardiovascular Disease in the Young, and the Council on Clinical Cardiology, Council on Cardiovascular Surgery and Anesthesia, and the Quality of Care and Outcomes Research Interdisciplinary Working Group. *Circulation* 2007;116:1736–1754.

[DVT]), it is important to weigh the risk of a thromboembolic event during interruption of anticoagulation against the risk of bleeding when antithrombotic therapy is administered in close proximity to surgery. Patients can be divided into risk strata according to their suggested risk for perioperative thromboembolism:

High risk:

- Recent (within 3 months) VTE
- Severe thrombophilia (eg, deficiency of protein C, protein S or antithrombin, antiphospholipid antibodies, or multiple abnormalities)

Moderate risk:

- VTE within the past 3–12 months
- Nonsevere thrombophilic conditions (eg, heterozygous factor V Leiden mutation, heterozygous factor II mutation)
- Recurrent VTE
- Active cancer (treated within 6 months or palliative)

Low risk:

- Single VTE occurred >12 months ago and no other risk factors

For patients undergoing a major surgical procedure, vitamin K antagonists (warfarin) should be stopped 5 days and antiplatelet drugs (aspirin, clopidogrel) 7–10 days before the procedure. Nonsteroidal anti-inflammatory drugs (NSAIDs) cause reversible inhibition of platelet-mediated cyclooxygenase activity. NSAIDs with a short half-life (eg, ibuprofen, indomethacin) should be stopped on the day before surgery, whereas NSAIDs with an intermediate half-life (eg, naproxen, celecoxib) should be stopped 2–3 days before surgery. NSAIDs with a long half-life (>20 hours) should be stopped 10 days before surgery. If the international normalized ratio (INR) is still elevated (ie, ≥1.5) 1–2 days before surgery, low-dose (ie, 1–2 mg) oral vitamin K can be administered to normalize the INR. Vitamin K antagonists should be restarted approximately 12–24 hours after surgery and when there is adequate hemostasis. Similarly, antiplatelet drugs should be resumed approximately 24 hours (or the next morning) after surgery when there is adequate hemostasis.

Patients at high or moderate risk (see risk strata) for perioperative thromboembolism need bridging anticoagulation with therapeutic-dose subcutaneous low-molecular-weight heparin (LMWH) or intravenous unfractionated heparin

Table 45–5. Cardiac conditions for which prophylaxis for obstetric-gynecologic procedures associated with infection or dental procedures is reasonable.

Cardiac Condition
Prosthetic cardiac valve or prosthetic material used for cardiac repair
Previous infective endocarditis
Congenital heart disease (CHD)
Unrepaired cyanotic CHD, including palliative shunts and conduits
Completely repaired congenital heart defects with prosthetic material or device, whether placed by surgery or by catheter invention, during the first 6 months after the procedure
Repaired CHD with residual defects at the site or adjacent to the site of a prosthetic patch or prosthetic device (which inhibit endothelialization)
Cardiac transplant recipient who develop cardiac valvulopathy

Modified and reproduced, with permission, from Wilson W, Taubert KA, Gewitz M, et al. Prevention of infective endocarditis: guidelines from the American Heart Association: a guideline from the American Heart Association Rheumatic Fever, Endocarditis and Kawasaki Disease Committee, Council on Cardiovascular Disease in the Young, and the Council on Clinical Cardiology, Council on Cardiovascular Surgery and Anesthesia, and the Quality of Care and Outcomes Research Interdisciplinary Working Group. *Circulation* 2007;116:1736–1754.

(UFH). Patients at low risk for perioperative thromboembolism can use low-dose subcutaneous LMWH or no bridging. Bridging with LMWH can be easily administrated outside the hospital and does not require laboratory monitoring. A common regimen is enoxaparin 1 mg/kg twice a day. The last dose of therapeutic LMWH should be given the morning prior to the day of surgery, thus holding the evening dose. Therapeutic LMWH can be restarted in 24 hours for patients undergoing minor surgical or other invasive procedures but should be held for 48–72 hours in patients undergoing major surgery. Bridging using therapeutic-dose intravenous UFH is performed by achieving a target activated partial thromboplastin time (aPTT) of 1.5–2.0 times the control aPTT value. The infusion is stopped approximately 4 hours before the surgery and is restarted during the initial 24 hours postoperatively. Bridging with LMWH is preferred to intravenous UFH in an outpatient setting.

In patients who are receiving vitamin K antagonists and require an urgent surgical procedure, the anticoagulant effect can be reversed with low-dose (2.5–5 mg) intravenous or oral vitamin K. If an immediate reversal effect is needed, the patient can be given fresh-frozen plasma or other prothrombin concentrate in addition to vitamin K. Because there is no pharmacologic agent that can reverse the antithrombotic effect of aspirin, clopidogrel, or ticlopidine, transfusion of platelets or the administration of other prohemostatic agents can be given to patients who are undergoing surgery and have excessive or life-threatening bleeding.

Douketis JD, Berger PB, Dunn AS, et al. The perioperative management of antithrombotic therapy: American College of Chest Physicians Evidence-Based Clinical Practice Guidelines (8th Edition). *Chest* 2008;133(6 Suppl):299S–339S. PMID: 18574269.

PULMONARY DISEASE

Complications

Postoperative pulmonary complications, such as atelectasis, pneumonia, respiratory failure, and exacerbation of underlying chronic lung disease, occur at similar rates to cardiac complications. In a study of 2964 patients undergoing elective noncardiac surgery, postoperative pulmonary and cardiac complications occurred in 2.0% and 2.2%, respectively.

All patients undergoing noncardiothoracic surgery should be evaluated for the presence of significant risk factors for postoperative pulmonary complications in order to receive pre- and postoperative interventions to reduce pulmonary risk. These risk factors include (1) chronic obstructive pulmonary disease, (2) age older than 60 years, (3) American Society of Anesthesiologists (ASA) class II or greater, (4) functionally dependent, (5) and congestive heart failure. Chronic obstructive pulmonary disease is the most commonly identified risk factor for postoperative pulmonary complications, with an odds ratio of 1.79. Advancing age is an important predictor of postoperative pulmonary complications, even after adjusting for comorbid conditions. The risk for pulmonary complications increases 2-fold for patients age 60–69 and 3-fold for patients age 70–79. The ASA classification (Table 45–6) has been proven to predict both postoperative pulmonary and cardiac complications. An ASA class of II or higher has a 4.9 times higher risk of pulmonary complications compared to ASA class I. Similarly, an ASA class of II or greater has a 2.3 times higher risk of pulmonary complications than ASA class of I or II combined. Functional dependence also increases the risk of postoperative pulmonary complications. Total dependence (inability to perform any activities of daily living) increases the risk by 2.5 times, whereas partial dependence (need for equipment or devices and assistance from another person for some activities of daily living) increases the risk by 1.7 times. Finally, congestive heart failure increases the risk of postoperative pulmonary complications by almost 3 times. Cigarette smoking has only a modest increased risk of pulmonary complications, with an odds ratio of 1.26. Contrary to previous beliefs, obesity and mild to moderate asthma are not significant risk factors for postoperative pulmonary complications.

Table 45–6. American Association of Anesthesiologists (ASA) classification.

ASA Class	Class Definition
I	A normal healthy patient
II	A patient with mild systemic disease
III	A patient with systemic disease that is not incapacitating
IV	A patient with an incapacitating systemic disease that is a constant threat to life
V	A moribund patient who is not expected to survive for 24 hours without or with operation

Modified and reproduced, with permission, from Smetana GW, Lawrence VA, Cornell JE. Preoperative pulmonary risk stratification for noncardiothoracic surgery: systematic review for the American College of Physicians. *Ann Intern Med* 2006;144:581–595.

Procedure-related risk factors are another important consideration when trying to reduce postoperative pulmonary complications. Certain procedures carry a higher risk of complications. These procedures include aortic aneurysm repair, thoracic surgery, abdominal surgery (especially upper abdominal surgery), neurosurgery, prolonged surgery, head and neck surgery, emergency surgery, and vascular surgery. The duration of surgery also affects postoperative pulmonary complications. A prolonged surgery lasting over 3–4 hours doubles the rate of postoperative pulmonary complications. Finally, general anesthesia and emergency surgery increase the risk of postoperative pulmonary complications by an odds ratio of 1.83 and 2.21, respectively.

Laboratory testing to estimate surgical risk has not been shown to be better than a careful history and physical exam.

Therefore, the American College of Physicians does not recommend preoperative spirometry or chest radiography to predict risk for postoperative pulmonary complications. Spirometry is recommended for thoracic surgery only, and studies of preoperative chest radiographs have shown that 10–23% of chest radiographs are abnormal but only 1.3–3% were clinically significant. Interestingly, a low serum albumin of <3.5 mg/dL is a powerful marker of increased risk for postoperative pulmonary complications and should be measured in all patients who are suspected of having hypoalbuminemia. Measurements should be considered in patients with 1 or more risk factors for pulmonary complications.

Treatment

All patients who are found to be at higher risk for postoperative pulmonary complications after perioperative evaluation should receive treatment to reduce postoperative complications. These treatments include (1) deep breathing exercises or incentive spirometry and (2) selective use of a nasogastric tube in patients for postoperative nausea and vomiting, inability to tolerate oral intake, or symptomatic abdominal distension.

Smetana GW, Lawrence VA, Cornell JE. Preoperative pulmonary risk stratification for noncardiothoracic surgery: systematic review for the American College of Physicians. *Ann Intern Med* 2006;144:581–595. PMID: 16618956.

ENDOCRINE DISEASE

Endocrine disorders are common in patients presenting for elective surgery. This section will discuss the perioperative management of diabetes, hyper- and hypothyroidism, and corticosteroid-induced adrenal insufficiency.

1. Diabetes Mellitus

Clinical Findings

Diabetes is the most common endocrine disorder affecting almost 20 million Americans. Fifty percent of these patients are estimated to require surgery during their lifetime. All patients with diabetes should have a careful preoperative assessment. The physician should ask about existing diabetic complications, such as neuropathies (peripheral sensory, bladder dysfunction, gastroparesis, and hypoglycemic unawareness), retinopathy, nephropathy, hyperlipidemia, and hypertension. Preoperative glucose control should be evaluated, since elevated blood sugar >150 mg/dL leads to macrophage dysfunction. This increases the risk of infection and delayed wound healing. Glycosylated hemoglobin (HbA1c) value is an indicator of glycemic level over 120 days but is strongly related to the level over the last 2–3 months. A normal value is up to 6%, and the goal of the American Diabetes Association is an HbA1c level less than 7% (considered adequate control). HbA1c values over 8% correspond to average blood glucose levels greater than 180 mg/dL and are an indication of poor glycemic control. Because diabetes is the leading cause of renal failure, it is important to measure the renal function preoperatively. Impaired renal function increases the risk of perioperative hypoglycemia because it prolongs the half-life of insulin and sulfonylureas. The major goal of perioperative management in patients with diabetes is to minimize hyperglycemia and avoid hypoglycemia, hypovolemia, and hypo- or hyperkalemia. Surgery and anesthesia invoke a stress response that leads to a hypersecretion of counterregulatory hormones culminating in hyperglycemia. This may lead to diabetic ketoacidosis (DKA) in patients with type 1 diabetes and hyperosmolar hyperglycemia nonketosis (HHNK) in patients with type 2 diabetes. There are no current guidelines on perioperative glycemic control, but a reasonable approach is to maintain blood glucose levels at less than 200 mg/dL intraoperatively and less than 150 mg/dL postoperatively, but avoid levels less than 80 mg/dL.

Treatment

Perioperative management of antihyperglycemic medications can be challenging, especially if the patient is required to be NPO (nothing by mouth) perioperatively. Thiazolidinedione (rosiglitazone, pioglitazone, and troglitazone) can be held the morning of surgery and sulfonylureas (glipizide and glyburide) must be held preoperatively. The biguanide metformin, which has been associated with the development of lactic acidosis, should be withheld 24 hours preoperatively and restarted 48–72 hours postoperatively once normal renal function has been documented. Thiazolidinedione and sulfonylureas can be restarted once enteral intake is permitted.

Patients who routinely use insulin should preferably be scheduled as the first case of the day to minimize hyper- or hypoglycemia. Patients with type 1 diabetes need basal insulin at all times to avoid DKA. The night before the procedure, the patient should take usual oral intake and continue the usual dose of evening glargine/NPH or a mixture. Patients using insulin pumps should continue the usual overnight basal rate. During the morning of the procedure, short-acting hypoglycemics should not be given unless the blood sugar is greater than 200 mg/dL and greater than 3 hours preoperatively. If the patient takes glargine insulin (long-acting), the usual dose of glargine can be given or the patient can be placed on an insulin drip. Patients using an insulin pump should continue the usual basal rate and infuse D5 throughout the operation. If the patient takes NPH (intermediate-acting) or other insulin mixture, the following steps should be taken. No short-acting insulin should be given within 3–4 hours of the procedure (ie, no mixture preoperatively). Half the usual dose of intermediate-acting insulin, with D5 at a controlled rate, should be given throughout the procedure. If performing an operation without continuous D5, insulin should not be given preoperatively. During emergency surgery, bolus of short-acting insulin should not be given preoperatively. Instead, frequent (every 30–60 minutes) monitoring of blood sugars should be performed throughout the operation. An insulin drip should be started for blood sugars greater than 200 mg/dL.

2. Hyperthyroidism

Clinical Findings

Untreated hyperthyroidism causes an increase in blood pressure, heart rate, and circulating blood volume, which leads to an increased cardiac output of 50–300%. These changes may limit the patient's ability to respond to the stress of surgery and can lead to thyroid storm and cardiovascular collapse. Therefore, thyroid function tests should be evaluated in all patients with hyperthyroidism preoperatively.

Treatment

Patients with uncontrolled hyperthyroidisms who present for elective surgery should have their surgery postponed until they have been stabilized medically. If a patient needs urgent or emergent surgery, the anesthesiologist should have drugs available that block the systemic effects of excess thyroid hormones, such as beta-blockers, antithyroid medications (propylthiouracil and methimazole), and iodine. The patient should take their antithyroid medications on the morning of surgery and resume the medications postoperatively when they tolerate enteral intake.

Complications

The most serious perioperative complication is thyroid storm, which usually arises from undiagnosed or undertreated hyperthyroidism. It can occur at any time in the perioperative period but usually occur intraoperatively or in the first 48 hours. Symptoms of thyroid storm are nonspecific and include fever (up to 41.1°C), tachycardia, and delirium. The mortality rate is 10–75%, and the patient must be treated in a critical care environment. Treatment includes thionamides, beta-blockers, antipyretics, and external cooling measures.

3. Hypothyroidism

Clinical Findings

Hypothyroidism is a common endocrine disorder that affects 1% of all patients. Patients with well-controlled hypothyroidism and patients with mild to moderately controlled hypothyroidism can usually undergo elective surgery without an increase in their perioperative risk. The physician should monitor closely for symptoms of worsening hypothyroidisms including delirium, prolonged ileus, infections without fever, and myxedema coma. Due to the long half-life of levothyroxine (1 week), it is not necessary for the patient to take their dose the morning of surgery. Levothyroxine can be restarted postoperatively once the patient tolerates enteral intake.

Treatment

Patients with severe hypothyroidism (myxedema coma) should be stabilized medically before any elective surgery. Myxedema coma is rare and usually presents postoperatively. It has a reported mortality rate of 80% and is precipitated by insults such as infection, cold exposure, and medications (sedatives and analgesics). Myxedema coma is characterized by severely depressed mental status (sometimes coma or seizures), hypothermia, bradycardia, hyponatremia, heart failure, and hypopnea. Myxedema coma is a medical emergency requiring intensive care admission and urgent administration of intravenous levothyroxine. Dehydration is often present, and aggressive fluid resuscitation with dextrose and normal saline should be performed. Intravenous glucocorticoids should be given because concomitant adrenal insufficiency is often present. Resolution of symptoms should be seen within 24 hours.

4. Adrenal Insufficiency

Adrenal insufficiency (AI) limits a patient's ability to respond to stress during surgery.

Pathogenesis

Primary AI is caused by autoimmune adrenalitis, infection, adrenalectomy, and sepsis, whereas secondary AI is due to pituitary depression, damage, and tumors. Tertiary AI is caused by exogenous glucocorticoid administration, which suppresses hypothalamic corticotropin-releasing hormone and pituitary adrenocorticotropic hormone (ACTH). These patients may need perioperative steroid supplementation (stress dose steroids).

Treatment

There is a wide variability in individual response to a particular dose and length of treatment. However, in general, patients who have received the equivalent of 20 mg/d of prednisone for greater than 5 days may be at risk for AI. If the patient has been on therapy for 1 month or longer, they may have AI for up to 6–12 months after stopping therapy. Patients who have been on an equivalent dose of prednisone 5 mg (or less) for any period of time will usually not have AI and will not need to receive stress dose steroids. The treatment of patients taking more than 5 mg/d of prednisone or equivalent is controversial. Some experts recommend performing a short ACTH stimulation test preoperatively in patients receiving steroid equivalents of 20 mg/d. Only patients who do not respond appropriately would receive stress dose steroids perioperatively. Others perform the ACTH stimulation test for patients receiving 6–19 mg/d of prednisone while giving patients taking 20 mg/d or higher stress dose steroids. Finally, some authors recommend giving all patients taking more than 5 mg/d of prednisone equivalent-dose stress dose steroids. In our practice, we treat all patients taking more than 5 mg/d of prednisone with stress dose steroids perioperatively. Patients taking 5 mg/d or less of prednisone should continue their usual maintenance dose orally or intravenously as the clinical situation mandates.

Coursin DB, Wood KE. Corticosteroid supplementation for adrenal insufficiency. *JAMA* 2002;287:236–240. PMID: 11779267.

Kohl BA, Schwartz S. Surgery in the patient with endocrine dysfunction. *Med Clin N Am* 2009;93:1031–1047. PMID: 19665618.

RENAL DISEASE

Clinical Findings

Preoperative laboratory studies should include a measure of the glomerular filtration rate (GFR) to ensure that the correct dosage of medications excreted by the kidney is given. A complete blood count and a type and screen should be performed because many patients with chronic renal disease have anemia and some patients may require a preoperative blood transfusion. Electrolytes should be checked because electrolyte disturbances are common. Up to 50% of patients have hyperkalemia, and some studies suggest that acute intervention should be reserved for potassium levels greater than 6.5 mmol/L.

Complications

Patients with chronic renal disease have a 2- to 5-fold higher risk of postoperative death and cardiovascular events than those with normal kidney function. Patients receiving dialysis are at the highest risk of such events.

During the preoperative assessment, the physician should establish the type and severity of kidney disease, any comorbid conditions, any complications related to the level of kidney function, risk for loss of kidney function, and risk for cardiovascular disease. Modifiable risk factors should be optimized prior to surgery. A mean arterial blood pressure of 110 mm Hg is associated with increased rates of cardiovascular and renal complications. Therefore, the preoperative blood pressure goal should be 130/80 mm Hg. To minimize the risk of volume overload, electrolyte imbalances, and uremic bleeding, patients requiring dialysis should receive it within 24 hour of surgery. Angiotensin-converting enzyme inhibitors (ACEIs) and angiotensin II antagonists (ARAs) are associated with intraoperative hypotension, especially with induction of general anesthesia. It is recommended to discontinue ACEIs and ARAs for at least 10 hours before general anesthesia.

Treatment

If a patient needs contrast media intraoperatively or during a radiologic study, a nonionic contrast agent is recommended to reduce the risk of contrast-induced nephropathy. In addition, the patients should be well hydrated, other nephrotoxic drugs and hypotension should be avoided, and medications such as *N*-acetylcysteine (Mucomyst 600 mg orally twice daily on the day before and/or on the day of the procedure) can be given. Laparoscopy reduces renal blood flow and can cause hypotension (which can further aggravate reduced renal blood flow). To mitigate these changes, abdominal insufflation pressures should not exceed 15 mm Hg, and adequate fluid replacement is recommended.

Jones DR, Lee HT. Surgery in the patient with renal dysfunction. *Med Clin North Am* 2009;93:1083–1093. PMID: 18299098.

Mathew A, Devereaux PJ, O'Hare A, et al. Chronic kidney disease and postoperative mortality: a systematic review and meta-analysis. *Kidney Int* 2008;73:1069–1081. PMID: 19665621.

HEPATIC DISEASE

Clinical Findings

Management of the surgical patient with liver disease should begin with a careful history and physical exam. This also serves as a screening test for patients with asymptomatic disease. One should ask about a history of prior surgeries, jaundice or blood transfusions, use of alcohol and other recreational drugs, sexual history, and a review of systems. The review of systems should include pruritus, easy fatigability, excessive bleeding after minor trauma, abdominal distension, and weight gain. The physical exam should include signs of liver disease, such as icterus, pallor, ascites, hepatomegaly, splenomegaly, palmar erythema, and spider nevi. If there is any suspicion of liver disease, blood testing for hepatic function should be performed including coagulation studies, electrolytes, and liver enzymes. However, routine preoperative testing of liver function is not recommended due to its low yield of abnormal results (<1%).

Complications

Older studies have reported high mortality rates in patients with acute hepatitis. It is therefore recommended to postpone elective surgery in these patients until the liver function tests have normalized. Surgery is generally considered safe in patients with chronic hepatitis. In general, patients with fatty liver tolerate surgery well, while patients with alcoholic hepatitis and cirrhosis have increased postoperative morbidity and mortality. Patients with a history of alcohol abuse have an increased risk of postoperative complications, such as poor wound healing, infections, bleeding, and delirium. Patients should refrain from using alcohol to improve liver function and should be monitored closely for signs of alcohol withdrawal.

Patients with cirrhosis have a high postoperative mortality of 10–80%. These patients may have nutritional disorders, ascites, abnormal coagulation profile, renal dysfunction, and encephalopathy. Five factors that significantly affect mortality in patients with cirrhosis include ascites, albumin, bilirubin, encephalopathy, and nutritional status. Cirrhotic patients benefit from aggressive preoperative treatment of coagulopathy, ascites, and encephalopathy. Coagulopathy can be managed preoperatively with vitamin K (10 mg subcutaneous); however, vitamin K does not correct the prothrombin time if there is decreased hepatic synthesis. In these cases, fresh-frozen plasma (FFP) infusion usually brings the prothrombin time to normal limits. If vitamin K and FFP fail to reduce the prothrombin time to within 3 seconds of normal, cryoprecipitate should be given. Cirrhotic patients are at high risk of developing encephalopathy postoperatively. Constipation, infection, upper gastrointestinal bleeding, uremia, alkalosis, and overuse of sedatives are known precipitating factors of encephalopathy. Ascites can cause respiratory compromise and wound dehiscence. It should be treated aggressively preoperatively with diuretics and paracentesis. Increasing evidence suggests that laparoscopic procedures have decreased operative morbidity and mortality compared with open procedures in patients with cirrhosis.

Rizvon MK, Chou CL. Surgery in the patient with liver disease. *Med Clin North Am* 2003;87:211–227. PMID: 12575891.

RHEUMATOLOGIC DISEASE

Complications

Two common challenges in the perioperative management of patients with rheumatologic disease are surgical positioning and perioperative management of antirheumatic medications. Patients with rheumatologic disease often have restricted joint mobility and pain. To decrease the risk of postoperative pain exacerbation and intraoperative injury to joints, it is important to preoperatively access the mobility of the joint. In addition, it is helpful to position these patients awake (ie, in lithotomy position) to ensure that the joints are not hyperflexed or hyperextended.

Treatment

When deciding on whether or not to stop an antirheumatic medication, one must weigh the risk of impaired wound healing and postoperative complications with maintaining disease control. Methotrexate has been extensively studied and should be continued in otherwise healthy patients. Compared with patients who discontinued the drug, patients who continued methotrexate had fewer infections and less flares. There are only a limited number of studies on leflunomide, and the results are conflicting. However, due to the very long half-life of leflunomide, its discontinuation would be necessary for a long time and is probably not necessary. Data on hydroxychloroquine do not show an increased risk of infection, and the drug has a long half-life. Clinical data are lacking on the perioperative use of sulfasalazine. The drug has a short half-life and is eliminated primarily via the kidneys. Some authors suggest withholding sulfasalazine at least the day of surgery. Three studies on azathioprine did not show the drug to be associated with any postoperative complications, and it is considered safe. Although preliminary data on tumor necrosis factor (TNF)–blocking agents show that the risk of infections may be lower than initially expected, it is still recommended to discontinue the drugs before surgery for several weeks. TNF-blocking agent should not be restarted until wound healing is complete. There are no data available on the drugs anakinra, rituximab, or abatacept. NSAIDs and aspirin should be discontinued as previously described in this chapter, whereas glucocorticoids should not be discontinued preoperatively. Patient with a suspected suppression of the hypothalamic–pituitary–adrenal axis should receive stress dose steroid supplementation, as previously described.

Pieringer H, Stuby U, Biesenback G. Patients with rheumatoid arthritis undergoing surgery: how should we deal with antirheumatic treatment? *Semin Arthritis Rheum* 2007;36:278–286. PMID: 17204310.

INTRAOPERATIVE COMPLICATIONS

Intraoperative complications can occur even in the most experienced surgeon's hands. Several factors, such as a surgeon's experience, technique, and knowledge of the pelvic anatomy, may prevent some of these complications. However, a surgeon must always be prepared to recognize and treat injuries when they occur in an organized and timely fashion. The complications listed in the following sections comprise some of the most common and serious complications encountered in gynecologic surgery.

URINARY TRACT INJURIES

1. Bladder Injury

Bladder injuries most commonly occur while dissecting down the bladder during abdominal or laparoscopic hysterectomy. The bladder may also be injured when attempting to enter the anterior cul-de-sac during vaginal hysterectomy. Bladder laceration can be confirmed by filling the bladder with either sterile milk or methylene blue retrograde through a urethral catheter. The bladder defect is repaired with 2 layers of absorbable suture. The Foley catheter is left in place for several days (5–7 days if injury is at the dome and 7–10 days if injury is at the bladder base) to prevent bladder distention and to allow the repair to heal. Another procedure that may result in bladder injury is retropubic suburethral slings used to treat stress urinary incontinence. The risk is approximately 5%. Therefore, this procedure includes routine cystoscopy to detect these injuries. If a cystotomy is present, the surgeon must replace the trocar and then continue Foley catheter drainage for 2–3 days. Very small injuries to the bladder such as a veress needle injury generally does not require repair and may be treated conservatively with Foley catheter drainage.

2. Ureteral Injury

Clinical Findings

Ureteral injuries are rare but recognized complications in gynecologic surgery. The incidence associated with hysterectomies ranges from 0.03–1.5%. Many of these intraoperative injuries go unrecognized and cause significant morbidity, including pyelonephritis, urine peritonitis, ureterovaginal fistula, and loss of a functioning kidney. Rates of injury are increased with operations for pelvic organ prolapse and in women with adhesions from endometriosis or prior surgery, distorted pelvic anatomy from malignancy, and enlarged uteri.

Common sites of ureteral injuries are at the level of the infundibulopelvic ligament, as the ureter courses under the uterine artery, at the distal uterosacral ligaments, and at the lateral apex of the vagina before its insertion into the bladder. Mechanisms for ureteral damage include transecting, ligating, kinking, burning, devascularizing, or crushing the ureters. Some of these injuries can be detected during surgery; however, the majority of injuries are unsuspected and diagnosed postoperatively. Early recognition of an injury is crucial to preserve the function of that kidney, and repair is most likely to be successful if done during the initial surgery.

Intraoperative cystoscopy with intravenous indigo carmine offers confirmation of bilateral ureteral patency. If efflux of blue dye is sluggish or absent from a ureteral orifice, then a ureteral injury should be suspected. If injury is confirmed, a urology consultation is recommended. If an abdominal procedure is being performed and a cystoscope is unavailable, another method of evaluating the ureteral function is through a purposeful cystotomy using an endoscope. In that case, a purse-string suture is placed at the dome of the bladder, and a small purposeful cystotomy is made within it. The 0- or 30-degree endoscope is then placed through the cystotomy to evaluate the bladder and ureteral orifices. Once the endoscope is removed, the purse-string suture is tied and a second imbricating layer is placed. The bladder should be drained postoperatively for 5–7 days using a Foley catheter. If cystoscopy is not diagnostic or there is strong suspicion of an injury, then transurethral stenting may be required and the appropriate consultation service should be called intraoperatively.

Studies on universal cystoscopy during routine hysterectomies have not been shown to be cost effective given the low rates of ureteral injury. However, if the patient is at higher risk or there is suspicion, cystoscopy should be performed.

If a patient develops flank pain in the postoperative period, a ureteral injury should be suspected. Urinary tract injury can be detected by an intravenous pyelogram (IVP). A renal ultrasound may reveal hydronephrosis or hydroureter. If a fluid collection is noted in the abdomen, it may be a urinoma from a transected ureter. Clear fluid draining from the surgical wound or from the vagina may be from a fistula. If this fluid is sent for creatinine levels, fluid from a urine leak would demonstrate a much higher creatinine concentration than the patient's serum creatinine levels.

Ibeanu OA, Chesson RR, Echols KT, et al. Urinary tract injury during hysterectomy based on universal cystoscopy. *Obstet Gynecol* 2009;113:6–10. PMID: 19104353.

Visco AG, Taber KH, Weidner AC, et al. Cost-effectiveness of universal cystoscopy to identify ureteral injury at hysterectomy. *Obstet Gynecol* 2001;97(5 Pt 1):685–692. PMID: 11339916.

GASTROINTESTINAL TRACT INJURY

Bowel is susceptible to injury during all types of gynecologic, abdominal, laparoscopic, and vaginal surgeries. Patients at highest risk include those with adhesions from previous surgery, endometriosis, tubo-ovarian abscess, or advanced malignancy.

Small Bowel

Patients with adhesions from previous surgery are particularly at risk, especially upon entry into the peritoneal cavity. Small bowel can be injured from electrocautery or via enterotomy. Small defects of the serosal or muscularis may be repaired using interrupted 3-0 silk or synthetic absorbable sutures in 1 or 2 layers. Suture repair lines should be perpendicular to the long axis of the bowel to prevent narrowing of the bowel lumen. Larger injuries and thermal injuries may require segmental resection with reanastomosis or with use of stapling devices.

Large Bowel

Large bowel injury is repaired in a similar fashion as the small bowel. Suture repair and resection with reanastomosis are techniques used in repair. However, if bowel reanastomosis is not possible due to extensive damage or pathology, a diverting colostomy may be needed. Injury to bowel results in spillage of bowel contents into the peritoneal cavity, which causes peritonitis. If unrecognized, the patient usually develops fever, abdominal distention, and pain from peritonitis in the immediate postoperative period. An unrecognized thermal bowel injury from electrocautery may have a delayed onset of symptoms. Any unrecognized bowel injury could potentially be lethal.

Stany MP, Farley JH. Complications of gynecologic surgery. *Surg Clin North Am* 2008;88:343–359. PMID: 18381117.

VASCULAR INJURY

Major Vessel Injury

Injury to a major blood vessel, such as the iliac vessels, aorta, or vena cava, is a rare but catastrophic complication of pelvic surgery. Compared to the muscular walls of the major arteries, the thin-walled veins, such as the external iliac vein, may be more prone to injury during a lymph node dissection. If injury occurs, direct pressure should be applied. This allows time to allow adequate exposure for repair, to call for blood products, and to call a consulting surgeon if needed. If a major catastrophic vascular injury occurs to the aorta or iliac vessels during laparoscopy with a trocar or veress needle, a vertical exploratory laparotomy should be performed. Pressure should be placed over the area with a laparotomy sponge to tamponade the hemorrhage until vascular surgeons are available.

Hemorrhage

Intraoperative hemorrhage is defined as blood loss exceeding 1000 mL or blood loss of more than 25% of the patient's blood volume. At the onset of heavy or uncontrolled bleeding, the first step is to apply pressure to the site either with a finger or a moist laparotomy sponge. Good communication with the surgical team, including the anesthesiologist and scrub and circulating nurses, is essential in responding to a hemorrhage and calling for blood products if needed.

Once pressure has been applied, the sponges should be removed slowly in attempt to visualize the bleeding vessels. Knowledge of the pelvic anatomy is crucial to avoid damage to the surrounding major vessels, nerves, and ureter. After identification of vital structures in the surrounding area, the bleeding vessels should be isolated and ligated. Specific areas prone to hemorrhage include the retroperitoneum during lymph node dissections, dissection close to the uterine artery during hysterectomy, and dissection in the presacral space, which can cause bleeding from presacral venous plexus during abdominal sacral colpopexy.

A technique that may control hemorrhage is hypogastric artery ligation or internal iliac artery ligation. This will decrease the pulse pressure at the distal bleeding site. Another technique that may be useful in controlling hemorrhage after caesarean section is bilateral uterine artery ligation by placing a large stitch through the uterine wall at the level of the cervical isthmus to ligate the uterine artery. During this technique, one must be careful of the ureter running inferior to the uterine artery. Topical hemostatic agents, cautery, clips, and sutures may also control the bleeding.

Goustout BS, Cliby WA, Podratz KC. Prevention and management of acute intraoperative bleeding. *Clin Obstet Gynecol* 2002;45:481–491. PMID: 12048406.

Stany MP, Farley JH. Complications of gynecologic surgery. *Surg Clin North Am* 2008;88:343–359. PMID: 18381117.

NEUROLOGIC INJURY

Incorrect positioning of a patient while under anesthesia can cause significant neurologic injury resulting in sensory and motor deficits. These complications are rare, usually transient, and usually resolve spontaneously with minimal intervention. However, long-term disability occasionally occurs. During pelvic surgery, injury can involve components of the lumbosacral nerve plexus, specifically the femoral nerve, the obturator nerve, the sciatic nerve, the iliohypogastric nerve, the ilioinguinal nerve, the genitofemoral nerve, the lateral femoral cutaneous nerve, and the pudendal nerve.

Gynecologic surgery is the most common cause of iatrogenic femoral nerve injury. Injury can occur with prolonged compression by retractor blades, when the hip is hyperflexed and hyperabducted in lithotomy position or due to direct injury associated with surgical dissection. Injury most commonly occurs when self-retaining retractors rest on the psoas muscle compressing the femoral or genitofemoral nerves. Symptoms from impaired motor function of the femoral nerve include weakness or inability to flex at the hip or extend at the knee. Sensory impairment includes paresthesia over the anterior and medial thigh and medial aspect of the calf. The obturator nerve may be injured during retroperitoneal dissection, such as lymph node dissection for gynecologic malignancies. This nerve injury will present with sensory loss in the upper medial thigh and motor weakness in hip adductors.

Other nerves compromised during incorrect positioning in lithotomy include the sciatic and peroneal nerves. Sciatic nerve compression and stretch occur with prolonged hyperflexion of the thigh. The common peroneal nerve courses across the lateral head of the fibula and therefore is susceptible to compression injury if the lateral aspect below the knee rests firmly against lithotomy stirrups. As for positioning of the upper extremities during gynecologic surgery, care should be taken to avoid hyperabduction to minimize risk for brachial plexus injury.

Two nerves at risk during a low transverse abdominal incision are the ilioinguinal and iliohypogastric nerves. They are susceptible to injury when a Pfannenstiel incision is extended beyond the border of the oblique muscle, and they also can be incorporated into the fascial repair resulting in nerve entrapment syndrome. This can cause a sharp burning pain or paresthesia over the nerve distribution. Therefore, careful positioning and placement of retractor blades are the best defenses against neurologic injuries.

Irvin W, Andersen W, Taylor P, et al. Minimizing the risk of neurologic injury in gynecologic surgery. *Obstet Gynecol* 2004;103:374–382. PMID: 14754710.

POSTOPERATIVE COMPLICATIONS

ACUTE HEMORRHAGE

Acute hemorrhage in the postoperative period can occur after many different procedures. This may occur as a result of an unrecognized trocar injury to the inferior epigastric vessels, a high cervical laceration from a dilatation and curettage, or a loose suture on a uterine artery pedicle after vaginal hysterectomy. In the recovery room, if a patient is persistently hypotensive despite fluid resuscitation, an internal hemorrhage should be suspected. One should respond by resuscitating the patient, checking blood count and coagulation studies, and ordering blood products for transfusion. If the patient does not respond, the patient may need to return to the operating room. Emergent uterine artery embolization has also shown to be a successful technique for postoperative bleeding.

THROMBOEMBOLIC COMPLICATIONS

1. Deep Vein Thrombosis

DVT is a serious and potentially preventable complication of major gynecologic surgery. Patients at increased risk include those with malignancy, obesity, immobility, previous VTE, thrombophilia, smoking, estrogen-containing hormone therapy use, and increasing age. Untreated DVT can lead to a fatal pulmonary embolus.

ESSENTIALS OF DIAGNOSIS

- Diagnosis can usually be made with compression ultrasonography.
- If ultrasonography is negative but there is still a high suspicion for DVT, contrast venography is the gold standard and should be performed.

Clinical Findings

A careful history and physical is important in the diagnosis of DVT. Patients usually present complaining of unilateral leg swelling and calf or leg pain. Physical exam may reveal ipsilateral leg edema, calf tenderness, warmth, or erythema. During the exam, a cord can be palpated indicating a thrombosed vein. Homan's sign is pain with dorsiflexion of the foot. However, this sign is unreliable. A discrepancy in the calf diameter can be of some value in raising the suspicion for DVT.

Treatment

Patients with DVT should be treated with anticoagulants immediately. This is done as soon as DVT is confirmed by objective testing. If there is a delay in diagnostic testing and the clinical suspicious is high, therapy should be started before such testing. Several options are available for the initial treatment of DVT according to the American College of Chest Physicians Guidelines: (1) LMWH, administered subcutaneous, without monitoring; (2) intravenous (IV) UFH, with monitoring; (3) subcutaneous UFH, with monitoring; (4) weight-based subcutaneous UFH, without monitoring; and (5) subcutaneous fondaparinux, without monitoring. For those treatments requiring monitoring, coagulation studies such as INR and partial thromboplastin time (PTT) should be measured at baseline. With UFH, the PTT should be kept 1.5–2.5 times the control value.

Anticoagulation therapy is continued for 3–6 months. Therefore, oral anticoagulants, particularly warfarin, are often started at the same time as initial treatment with the LMWH or UFH therapies above. Oral anticoagulants do not exert their full effect for 48–72 hours. Warfarin is generally started a dose of 5 mg daily, and subsequent doses are adjusted to maintain the INR value at 2.5 (range 2.0–3.0). Therefore, the LMWH or UFH therapy is continued for at least 5 days until the warfarin takes effect and the INR is ≥2.0 for 24 hours. For patients in whom bleeding is a particular risk or laboratory monitoring is problematic, LMWH can be used for long-term treatment instead of warfarin. Due to more predictable pharmacokinetics, LMWH, such as enoxaparin, can be administered subcutaneous once or twice daily without laboratory monitoring in the majority of patients. This treatment, as well as oral anticoagulation, allows initial treatment of DVT as an outpatient. Recommended long-term therapy for distal or calf vein thrombosis includes 3 months of anticoagulation. Long-term treatment for a proximal DVT is 3–6 months of anticoagulation.

Surgical treatment, such as thrombectomy, occasionally can be considered for persistent severe swelling in the extremity. An inferior vena cava filter can be placed for patients who develop DVT or pulmonary embolism that occurs despite adequate anticoagulation or in patients who have contraindications to anticoagulation therapy.

2. Pulmonary Embolism

Laboratory and radiologic imaging is helpful in evaluating a patient for a pulmonary embolus (PE). With arterial blood gas, a low arterial Po_2 should raise suspicion for a PE. D-dimer assays are usually elevated and have a high negative predictive value in ruling out a PE. However, recent surgery can elevate D-dimer levels and, therefore, may have little value in the workup.

Chest radiograph findings frequently show no abnormalities. However, a peripheral lung density, enlargement of the main pulmonary artery, or a small pleural effusion can be seen. Chest radiograph can rule out other diagnoses on the differential, such as pneumonia. Electrocardiogram is helpful in ruling out myocardial infarction. It can also show characteristic changes of PE, such as S1Q3T3 patterns, right bundle branch block, and T-wave inversions in leads V1 through V4.

Spiral chest computed tomography (CT) is now the diagnostic procedure of choice for PE. It can frequently visualize the emboli and has high sensitivity and specificity. Pulmonary angiography is the "gold standard" test but is used less frequently given it is an invasive procedure. It is reserved in patients with a high clinical suspicion for PE despite a negative or nondiagnostic spiral CT. Another imaging modality is the ventilation-perfusion (V/Q) scan.

It is not the tests of choice because the results are frequently equivocal. It is useful in diagnosis in patients who cannot receive IV contrast.

Clinical Findings

PE is a potentially fatal complication of gynecologic surgery and usually occurs suddenly as a complication of a pelvic or lower extremity DVT. Risk factors are the same as noted earlier for DVT. Symptoms usually occur abruptly and include pleuritic chest pain, dyspnea, tachypnea, and tachycardia. A large embolus may result in hypotension, shock, and even sudden death from cor pulmonale. The symptoms are not specific for PE, and the differential diagnosis includes atelectasis, pneumonia, myocardial infarction, and pneumothorax.

Prevention

There is ample evidence that primary thromboprophylaxis reduces DVT and PE and that fatal PE can be prevented. Recommendations based on guidelines from the American College of Chest Physicians include prophylaxis with low-dose UFH, LMWH, or intermittent pneumatic compression (IPC) devices for the extremities. For a low-risk patient undergoing a brief procedure <30 minutes, prophylaxis is not necessary. For brief procedures and laparoscopy, in patients who have risk factors for VTE, prophylaxis may be indicated. During any major gynecologic procedure, prophylaxis is recommended with low-dose heparin twice daily; LMWH, such as enoxaparin, once daily; or IPC. This prophylaxis is started just prior to surgery and is used continuously until discharge. For patients with malignancy, who are particularly at high risk, the recommendation is to continue prophylaxis with LMWH once daily or low-dose heparin 3 times daily for 2 to 4 weeks after discharge.

Treatment

Cardiopulmonary resuscitation should be instituted if necessary, and the patient should be closely monitored. Due to the risk of mortality, patients with strong clinical suspicion of PE should get immediate treatment with anticoagulation. Treatment regimens for DVT and PE are similar given they are manifestations of the same disease process and are described earlier.

According to the American College of Chest Physicians and their guidelines, in patients with acute nonmassive PE, recommendations include initial treatment with LMWH over IV UFH. In patients with massive PE, where there is concern for subcutaneous absorption, the guidelines suggest IV UFH over LMWH. For patients with a massive PE with evidence of hemodynamic compromise, thrombolytic therapy with urokinase, streptokinase, or recombinant tissue plasminogen activator is also recommended in addition to anticoagulation. Patients who are highly compromised and cannot receive thrombolytic therapy due to bleeding risks may be candidates for surgical pulmonary embolectomy.

ACOG Practice Bulletin No. 84: prevention of deep vein thrombosis and pulmonary embolism. Committee on Practice Bulletins–Gynecology, American College of Obstetricians and Gynecologist. *Obstet Gynecol* 2007;110(2 Pt 1):429–440. PMID: 17666620.

Geerts WH, Bergqvist D, Pineo GF, et al. Prevention of venous thromboembolism: American College of Chest Physicians Evidence-Based Clinical Practice Guidelines (8th edition). *Chest* 2008;133:381S–453S. PMID: 18574271.

Kearon C, Kahn SR, Agnelli G, et al. Antithrombotic therapy for venous thromboembolic disease: College of Chest Physicians Evidence-Based Clinical Practice Guidelines (8th edition). *Chest* 2008;133:454S–545S. PMID: 18574272.

GASTROINTESTINAL TRACT COMPLICATIONS

1. Ileus

Ileus is defined as a pattern of bowel dysmotility that results in accumulation of gas and fluid in the gastrointestinal tract. During abdominal or pelvic surgery, there usually is some degree of ileus for 3–6 days postoperatively. This is due to an increase in sympathetic tone, which causes inhibition in bowel motility. Bowel manipulation during surgery causes an inflammatory reaction resulting in an ileus. Opiate pain medications also have an inhibitory effect and can prolong an ileus.

Clinical Findings

The patient usually complains of abdominal pain and may have nausea or vomiting. Clinical findings include abdominal distention with decreased or absent bowel sounds. On plain abdominal radiographs, there is generalized dilatation and gaseous distention of both the small and large bowel.

Treatment

If nausea, vomiting, and abdominal distention are severe, the patient should be restricted of oral intake. A nasogastric (NG) tube should also be inserted into the stomach. IV fluids should be administered, and electrolytes should be monitored. Although an NG tube is sometimes used for treatment, routine use in all patients does not prevent ileus. Early feeding in the postoperative period does not cause ileus and shortens hospital stays. Thoracic epidural analgesia use postoperatively has shown to promote quicker return to bowel function. The use of NSAIDs and opioid receptor antagonists has not been proven to decrease ileus.

2. Small Bowel Obstruction

Small bowel obstruction can result as a complication of an intraperitoneal operation. This is usually due to the formation of adhesions, which can trap or kink a segment of small intestine. Other causes include herniation through a laparoscopic trocar site, internal herniation, or an inflammatory process such as an abscess. Obstruction can occur in the immediate postoperative period or several years later due to dense adhesions. This results in partial or complete bowel obstruction and can cause bowel strangulation and perforation.

Plain abdominal radiographs are very sensitive in the diagnosis of small bowel obstruction. They usually reveal air-fluid levels of differential height within the same loop of bowel. In patients with inconclusive radiograph films, a CT scan (with IV and oral contrast) is sensitive and specific and can give incremental information on the grade of obstruction. Signs of bowel obstruction or strangulation on CT include continuous dilation of proximal small bowel with a discrete transition zone, serrated beak sign, mesenteric fluid and ascites, and intraluminal fluid. The colon usually contains little or no gas. Enteroclysis or small bowel follow-through study with oral contrast, as well as CT enterography and magnetic resonance imaging (MRI) contrast studies, are also available as diagnostic tests.

Clinical Findings

Obstruction is characterized by abdominal pain, vomiting, abdominal distention, and obstipation. On examination, the abdomen is distended and tender with high-pitched bowel sounds. It can be difficult to differentiate from a postoperative ileus and may require diagnostic studies.

Treatment

Small bowel obstruction requires immediate intervention to prevent bowel ischemia and infarction. If the patient has no signs of bowel strangulation or peritonitis, conservative treatment can be used. This includes bowel rest, IV fluid hydration, electrolyte replacement, and bowel decompression with an NG tube. Patients with leukocytosis, fever, peritonitis, metabolic acidosis, and continuous pain suggest bowel strangulation and require operative intervention. In patients who received conservation management, if there is no improvement in symptoms within 48 hours, operative intervention is recommended with either exploratory laparotomy or laparoscopy.

3. Constipation

Constipation and a reduction in the number of bowel movements are expected in the early postoperative period given low food intake, ileus, and narcotic use. If a bowel obstruction is not suspected, stool softeners and mild laxatives can be prescribed. An enema can also be used. Fecal impaction can also be present and cause diarrhea in the postoperative patient. It is diagnosed by digital rectal examination, and treatment involves disimpaction of the firm fecal masses.

4. Diarrhea

Pathogenesis

Most postoperative diarrhea is caused by antibiotic administration or oral contrast for radiographic studies. This is usually mild and self-limiting. Antibiotics can alter the bacterial flora in the gastrointestinal tract. If overgrowth with *Clostridium difficile* occurs, a more serious infection can occur. *C difficile* may be a complication after treatment with antibiotics such as clindamycin, penicillins, cephalosporins, or fluoroquinolones. If untreated, *C difficile* infection can progress to fulminant colitis, ileus, obstruction, perforation, and toxic megacolon; therefore, prompt diagnosis and treatment are essential.

Clinical Findings

Clinical findings include diarrhea, fever, and leukocytosis. If *C difficile* infection is suspected, the stool should be sent for cytotoxin assay. If the infection is strongly suspected despite negative toxin stool toxin assays, colonoscopy can be performed to detect pseudomembranous changes in the colon. Toxic megacolon is a clinical diagnosis based on dilatation of the colon >7 cm on plain films, accompanied by severe systemic toxicity.

Treatment

C difficile is becoming increasingly pathogenic and contagious. Once diagnosed, the patient should be placed in isolation with infection precautions. Management includes first withdrawal of the implicated antibiotic, and then treatment with preferably oral metronidazole or vancomycin. However, oral metronidazole is preferred in order to reduce vancomycin resistance and to reduce cost. If the infection is unresponsive to antibiotics and progresses to toxic megacolon, surgical intervention with colectomy may be necessary.

Diaz JJ Jr, Bokhari F, Mowery NT, et al. Guidelines for management of small bowel obstruction. *J Trauma* 2008;64:1651–1664. PMID: 18545135.

Hookman P, Barkin JS. *Clostridium difficile* associated infection, diarrhea and colitis. *World J Gastroenterol* 2009;15:1554–1580. PMID: 19340897.

Stewart D, Waxman K. Management of postoperative ileus. *Am J Ther* 2007;14:561–566. PMID: 18090881.

URINARY TRACT COMPLICATIONS

1. Urinary Retention

Postoperative urinary retention is the inability to void in the presence of a full bladder. Risk factors for development of postoperative urinary retention include prolonged duration of surgery and the use of regional anesthesia or epidural analgesia. The patient may complain of suprapubic discomfort with the inability to void. The bladder may be palpable on abdominal exam if severely distended. Retention is likely if the patient is unable to void within 8 hours after surgery or 8 hours after bladder catheter removal. The diagnosis is confirmed if a bladder ultrasound displays 500 mL of urine or if a postvoid residual is 500 mL or greater. If retention is present, complications and bladder dysfunction may result. An overdistended bladder can cause pain and an autonomic response, resulting in vomiting, hypotension, bradycardia, and cardiac dysrhythmias. Infection can also be a direct complication or an indirect complication due to an indwelling bladder catheter. Severe overdistention for prolonged periods may cause ischemia and long-term bladder dysfunction.

Treatment

Standard treatment for retention is immediate bladder drainage with sterile catheterization. Although intermittent in-out catheters are an alternative, most patients have an indwelling bladder catheter placed while in the hospital. The catheter is placed for approximately 24 hours, and then a void trial is performed. With incontinence procedures, such as suburethral slings, there may be retention due to overcorrection of the bladder neck requiring outpatient treatment with a catheter for several days.

2. Urinary Tract Infection

In the immediate postoperative period, patients are at risk for urinary tract infection (UTI). They are at risk of UTI due to urinary retention that follows surgery and anesthesia, as well as due to instrumentation or catheterization during surgery. Catheter-associated UTI is one of the most common nosocomial infections.

Cystitis and UTI can cause increased frequency of urination, urgency, and dysuria. White blood cells, leukocyte esterase, and nitrites can be seen on urine analysis. When fever is present, pyelonephritis should be considered. If untreated, pyelonephritis can progress to urosepsis.

In patients suspected of having a UTI, a urine specimen should be sent for culture. Appropriate antibiotic therapy should be instituted and adjusted based on culture and sensitivity results. In patients with urinary retention, a bladder catheter is recommended. However, in patients without urinary retention, removal of the bladder catheter at the earliest possible time is important in treating and preventing UTIs.

3. Lower Urinary Tract Fistula

A lower urinary tract fistula is a rare complication of gynecologic surgery and obstetric trauma. These fistulas include vesicovaginal and ureterovaginal fistulas. Risk factors for fistula include malignancy, radiation therapy, intraoperative injury to bladder or the ureter, and obstructed labor. Most lower urinary tract fistulas in the Unites States occur after hysterectomies.

A lower urinary tract fistula can present perioperatively as gross hematuria or urinoma noted after surgery. In the postoperative period, patients with fistulas usually present 1 to 3 weeks after surgery complaining of urinary incontinence or persistent vaginal discharge. A speculum exam may reveal a fluid collection in the vagina and scarring at the apex. If a vesicovaginal fistula cannot be seen, a "tampon test" can be performed in the clinic. This test is performed by instilling methylene blue transurethrally into the bladder after placing vaginal sponges or a tampon in the vagina. The patient is then asked to walk around and perform the Valsalva maneuver. Intravenous indigo carmine or oral phenazopyridine can be given to exclude an ureterovaginal fistula. A voiding cystourethrogram can also be performed to diagnose and evaluate the size and location of a vesicovaginal fistula.

Cystoscopy is indicated in all cases to evaluate the size, location, and number of fistulas and the condition of the tissue. Radiologic imaging such an IVP or cystoscopic retrograde urogram is recommended to exclude a ureterovaginal fistula or hydronephrosis.

If a vesicovaginal fistula is diagnosed early, conservative management can be attempted. Although the timing, fistula size, and success rate remain unclear, limited data suggest that fistulas less than 1 cm in size diagnosed within 3 weeks of surgery can close spontaneously after bladder drainage. In 1 study, 39% of fistulas closed with bladder drainage if diagnosed within 3 weeks of surgery, while only 3% closed if diagnosed greater than 6 weeks after surgery. The duration of bladder drainage remains unclear, but some authors recommend 4 weeks of continuous drainage.

Ureteral fistulas are usually treated with ureteral stents for 6 to 8 weeks. An IVP is performed after 4 to 6 weeks to evaluate if the fistula has healed. If the fistula has healed, the stent is removed and IVP is performed at 3, 6, 12, and 24 months to rule out stricture formation. If the fistula has not healed, the stent is left in place for 8 weeks and the IVP repeated. If the fistula is not healed in 8 weeks, surgical repair is recommended.

The timing of vesicovaginal fistulas is controversial. Ideally, the fistula should be repaired within 72 hours of injury, before inflammation and induration take place. Some surgeons recommend waiting 3 to 6 months until the fistula has matured. Other surgeons have successfully closed fistulas earlier, after the initial inflammation has subsided. Timing of surgical repair should be individualized and based on cystoscopic evidence of healing, including the fistula site and adjacent tissue being pliable, noninflamed, epithelialized, and free of granulation tissue and necrosis. Vesicovaginal fistulas can be repaired vaginally or abdominally, but the surgical technique is beyond the scope of this chapter.

Baldini G, Bagry H, Aprikian A, et al. Postoperative urinary retention: anesthetic and perioperative considerations. *Anesthesiology* 2009;110:1139–1157. PMID: 19352147.

Bazi T. Spontaneous closure of vesicovaginal fistulas after bladder drainage alone: a review of the evidence. *Int Urogynecol J Pelvic Floor Dysfunct* 2007;18:329–333. PMID: 17036168.

Karram MM. Lower urinary tract fistulas. In Walters MD, Karram MM, eds. *Urogynecology and Reconstructive Surgery*. 3rd ed. Philadelphia, PA: Mosby Elsevier; 2007.

INFECTIOUS COMPLICATIONS

Bacterial contamination of the operative site is a common occurrence in major gynecologic surgery. Hysterectomies are classified as "clean contaminated" cases due to the entrance into the genital tract and contamination with endogenous vaginal flora. Although antibiotic prophylaxis decreases the risk of postoperative infection, it still remains one of the most common postoperative complications. The diagnosis of a postoperative infection is generally made when there is pain and tenderness in the area contiguous with the infection and an oral temperature of ≥38°C on 2 separate occasions at least 6 hours apart or of >38.5°C at any time.

Prevention

Antibiotic prophylaxis is usually only indicated for hysterectomy and urogynecology procedures. Cefazolin (1 g) is the most commonly used agent and is given within 30 minutes of the start of the procedure. A second dose of intraoperative antibiotic may be given if the duration of the surgery approaches 3 hours or in cases with increased blood loss (>1500 mL). Doxycycline is also used before and after surgical abortion. For procedures such as laparoscopy or exploratory laparotomy that do not directly enter the genital tract, antibiotic prophylaxis is not indicated.

1. Hematoma & Pelvic Abcess

Clinical Findings

An abscess should be considered in the postoperative patient with fever and no other source or in a patient who has failed initial antibiotic treatment. The patient usually presents with fever and abdominal pain. Clinical findings may include a mass palpated on pelvic examination. Pelvic hematomas that become infected can also present in a similar manner.

Treatment

If an abscess is suspected, imaging should be performed with ultrasound or a CT scan with contrast. If confirmed, treatment involves parenteral antibiotics. Some regimens include gentamicin and clindamycin; ampicillin, gentamicin, and metronidazole; imipenem/cilastatin; and levofloxacin and metronidazole. Parenteral antibiotics are continued until the patient has been afebrile for 24 to 48 hours, and then patients are switched to oral antibiotics. Many abscesses, especially large ones, require drainage for adequate treatment. Percutaneous drainage of the fluid collection is often possible with insertion of a large-caliber "pigtail" catheter under ultrasound or CT guidance. An infected cuff hematoma or abscess can sometimes be managed by reopening the cuff. If the abscess does not respond to the above treatment, the patient may need a laparotomy with opening of the abscess, irrigation, and drain placement.

2. Wound Infection

A wound infection is usually localized to the skin and fatty tissue above the fascia. The diagnosis of a postoperative wound infection is usually made several days after surgery, on postoperative day 4 or 5.

Clinical Findings

With wound infections or cellulitis, skin erythema (redness and warmth), subcutaneous induration, and fever are usually present. If there is incisional drainage present, there may be an abscess or fluid collection beneath the incision.

Treatment

Cellulitis alone is usually treated with a single agent that is effective against streptococci, staphylococci, and most gram-negative organisms, such as a cephalosporin. If there is a fluid collection presenting with purulent drainage from the wound, it should be opened to allow drainage and debridement if necrotic tissue is present. The wound should be gently probed to check for fascial integrity. If the fascia is intact, the wound should be packed with moist gauze dressings 2 or 3 times daily.

3. Wound Dehiscence & Evisceration

Wound dehiscence is a postoperative wound separation that involves all layers of the abdominal wall. Risk factors include age, malnutrition, diabetes, smoking, malignancy, chronic steroid use, and obesity. Wound infection also predisposes the wound to disruption. Evisceration includes disruption of these layers with protrusion of intestines through the incision. The hallmark of this complication is profuse serosanguinous discharge from the abdominal incision. This is a surgical emergency that requires immediate closure in the operating room.

4. Necrotizing Fasciitis

ESSENTIALS OF DIAGNOSIS

- Diagnosis is based on physical findings of a rapidly progressing infection.
- Radiologic tests, such as CT, MRI, or plain films, will display gas in the subcutaneous tissue.
- Surgical exploration will confirm the diagnosis, which reveals necrotic subcutaneous tissue and fasciae.

Pathogenesis

Necrotizing fasciitis is a rare and often fatal infection that is characterized by extensive necrosis of the fascia and adjacent subcutaneous tissue. Predisposing factors include advanced age, obesity, hypertension, arteriosclerosis, diabetes, malnutrition, renal failure, immunosuppression, and trauma. The bacteria that cause these infections include group A *Streptococcus* and other anaerobes such as *Clostridium perfringens*.

Clinical Findings

The clinical triad includes sepsis, inordinate pain, and unilateral edema. On physical examination, patients may appear septic with a fever and leukocytosis. The skin around the incision site is usually cool, gray, and boggy, and may reveal crepitus. Usually, the wound will display a marked degree of subcutaneous edema and varying degrees of cutaneous discoloration. There also may be a sensory deficit over the area of infection.

Treatment

The most important treatment includes early and aggressive surgical debridement of the infection. This includes removal of all the necrotic tissue that is not bleeding and discolored. Healing is usually by secondary intention, with skin grafts often being necessary. Therefore, a gynecologic oncologist or plastic surgeon is usually involved. Treatment also includes broad-spectrum antibiotics, including a penicillin. Hyperbaric oxygen treatment can also lead to a decrease in the morbidity of these infections.

ACOG Practice Bulletin No. 104: antibiotic prophylaxis for gynecologic procedures. ACOG Committee on Practice Bulletins–Gynecology. *Obstet Gynecol* 2009;113:1180–1189. PMID: 19384149.

Gallup DG, Freedman MA, Mequiar RV, et al. Necrotizing fasciitis in gynecologic and obstetric patients: a surgical emergency. *Am J Obstet Gynecol* 2002;187:305–310. PMID: 12193917.

Larsen JW, Hager WD, Livengood CH, et al. Guidelines for the diagnosis, treatment and prevention of postoperative infections. *Infect Dis Obstet Gynecol* 2003;11:65–70. PMID: 12839635.

Therapeutic Gynecologic Procedures

46

Cecilia K. Wieslander, MD
Keri S. Wong, MD

The 4 most commonly performed gynecologic procedures in the United States are abdominal and vaginal hysterectomy, tubal sterilization, and dilation and curettage. This chapter will review these procedures, as well as other therapeutic operations. Indications, contraindications, technique, and complications will be discussed for each procedure.

Agency for Healthcare Research and Quality. HCUP Nationwide Inpatient Sample (NIS), Procedures. Healthcare Cost and Utilization Project (HCUP). 2006. Rockville, MD: Agency for Healthcare Research and Quality. http://www.hcupnet.ahrq.gov/HCUPnet.jsp.

DILATION & CURETTAGE

Indications

The procedure of cervical dilation and uterine curettage (D&C) is usually performed for 1 of the following indications: diagnosis and treatment of abnormal uterine bleeding, management of abortion (incomplete, missed, or induced), or diagnosis of cancer of the uterus. The diagnosis of abnormal bleeding is discussed in Chapter 38; D&C as a method of induced abortion is discussed in Chapter 58. This section will discuss the remaining therapeutic uses of D&C.

Technique

A. Cervical Dilation

Dilation of the cervix may be conducted under paracervical, epidural, spinal, or general anesthesia, depending largely on the indication for the procedure. Perioperative antibiotic prophylaxis is not recommended, but venous thromboembolism prophylaxis should be used in patients 40 years and older or with additional risk factors. Cervical dilation usually precedes uterine curettage but may be performed in a patient with cervical stenosis prior to insertion of an intrauterine contraceptive device (IUD) or radium device for treatment of cancer. Dilation may also precede hysterosalpingogram or hysteroscopy.

The patient is placed in the dorsal lithotomy position, with the back and shoulders supported and the extremities padded. The inner thighs, perineum, and vagina are prepared as for any vaginal operation; the surgeon and assistant should adhere to surgical principles of asepsis. A thorough pelvic examination under anesthesia is mandatory prior to performing cervical dilation, in order to determine the size and position of the cervix, uterus, and adnexa and the presence of any abnormalities. The patient voids normally before the operation if possible; urinary catheterization is used only if significant residual urine is suspected.

A right-angle retractor is placed anteriorly to gently retract the bladder. A weighted speculum is placed posteriorly to reveal the cervix. Under direct vision, the anterior lip of the cervix is grasped with a tenaculum, avoiding the vascular supply at 3 and 9 o'clock. The cervix is grasped firmly but with care taken not to compromise, or especially perforate, the endocervical canal. With gentle traction, the cervix can be brought down toward the introitus. Before proceeding further, a complete visual examination should be made of the cervix and the 4 vaginal fornices, because the latter areas (especially posteriorly) are otherwise difficult to examine. Areas that appear abnormal (even benign inclusion cysts) should be noted and followed as appropriate. Areas that are clearly abnormal should be biopsied. After the cervix and vagina are evaluated, the uterine cavity is examined. A uterine sound is gently inserted into the endocervix and then advanced into the uterine cavity in the plane of least resistance and most compatible with the position of the uterus as revealed by pelvic examination. The depth of the uterine cavity is recorded as well as any abnormalities such as leiomyomas or septa.

Perforation of the uterus during D&C is most likely to occur at the time of uterine sounding or cervical dilation. Recognized uterine perforations during D&C occur at a rate of 0.63–1.0% according to 2 large classical studies.

The majority of perforations are thought to be due to misdirected or excessive force. Perforation is more likely to occur if the woman is postmenopausal (1 in 38), has cancer (1 in 48), or is post pregnancy (1 in 122). Other risk factors include having a retroverted or anteverted uterus or having cervical stenosis. Unless there is evidence of hemorrhage, injury to the bowel, or evulsion of the omentum, conservative treatment of uterine perforation is best.

If severe cervical stenosis is suspected from the preoperative office examination, cervical softening agents such as misoprostol or *Laminaria* tents may be used. Both oral and vaginal misoprostol and *Laminaria* tents have demonstrated a benefit over placebo in the ease of cervical dilation in pregnant and premenopausal women. In a systematic review of 10 randomized controlled trials involving premenopausal women undergoing hysteroscopy compared preprocedure misoprostol versus placebo to aid in cervical dilation, preprocedure misoprostol resulted in a reduced need for cervical dilation (relative risk [RR], 0.6; 95% confidence interval [CI], 0.5–0.7), a lower rate of cervical laceration (RR, 0.22; 95% CI, 0.1–0.6), and an increase in cervical dilatation (RR, 2.66; 95% CI, 1.7–3.5), but a higher rate of side effects (vaginal bleeding, cramping, and elevated temperature). For every 4 premenopausal women who received misoprostol prior to hysteroscopy, 1 avoided the need for further cervical dilation. For every 12 premenopausal women receiving misoprostol, 1 cervical laceration was avoided. The vaginal route of misoprostol may be more effective than oral misoprostol as shown by 1 study. In postmenopausal women and women who have been pretreated with gonadotropin-releasing hormone, randomized controlled trials have produced inconclusive results.

The most common dilators used are the Hegar, Pratt, and Hank dilators. Hegar dilators are relatively blunt, gently curved, and numbered sequentially according to width (ie, a No. 7 dilator is 7 mm wide). Pratt and Hank dilators differ from Hegar dilators in being more gradually tapered ("sharper"); they may have a solid core (Pratt) or a hollow center (Hank), allowing egress of trapped blood and air. Pratt or Hank dilators are measured in French sizes (a No. 20F Hank dilator is approximately the same diameter as a No. 9 Hegar dilator). The choice of dilator is largely based on surgical training; many prefer not to use the more pointed Hank dilators in a small postmenopausal uterus.

B. Endocervical Curettage

Fractional curettage should be used for abnormal uterine bleeding or if genital tract neoplasia is suspected. The cervical canal should be curetted prior to dilation of the cervix and curettage of the endometrial cavity, in order to preserve the histologic characteristics of the endocervix and prevent contamination of the endometrial sample with endocervical cells. If cervical conization is planned for diagnosis or treatment of cervical intraepithelial neoplasia, uterine sounding precedes conization, but cervical dilation and fractional curettage follow in order to minimize denuding of the endocervical epithelium. The Gusberg curette is a small, slightly curved instrument particularly well suited for endocervical curettage. The curette is placed in the endocervical canal to the level of the internal os; with a firm touch, each of the 4 walls is curetted with a single stroke, with the specimen delivered onto a coated cellulose sponge with a twirling motion of the curette. (The coated cellulose sponge is preferred over ordinary surgical sponges because tissue is less likely to adhere to it.) The cervix is then dilated as described earlier and curettage of the endometrium performed. The endocervical and endometrial specimens are immersed in fixative in separate containers and submitted to the pathologist.

Complications from endocervical curettage are rare in nongravid patients. Because of obvious risks to the fetus and membranes, endocervical curettage is contraindicated in pregnant women. Healing of the curetted endocervix may take 3 weeks or more; the cervical epithelium commonly takes 2 weeks to heal following a routine Papanicolaou (Pap) smear. Tissue should be allowed to heal before follow-up Pap smears are taken because regenerating cells are often mistaken for dysplastic cells.

C. Endometrial Polypectomy

The uterine cavity is explored with polyp forceps prior to diagnostic or therapeutic endometrial curettage. It is easier to remove polyps prior to curettage, preserving the histologic integrity necessary to differentiate benign uterine polyps from neoplasia. In a large series advocating routine exploration of the endometrial cavity preceding curettage, 64% of 130 diagnosed endometrial polyps were removed by ureteral stone forceps. Thirty-nine percent of the polyps were removed with exploring forceps after the curettage had been carried out. Pedunculated or submucous leiomyomas, intrauterine and intracervical synechias, and uterine anomalies may be first suspected at passage of the polyp forceps.

The technique of polypectomy includes gentle insertion of the forceps in the plane most compatible with the position of the uterus (as for uterine sounding). The forceps are opened slightly, rotated 90 degrees, and removed. Many clinicians repeat this procedure through 360 degrees, completely exploring the uterine cavity.

Skillful use of hysteroscopy for diagnosis and treatment of synechias, septa, leiomyomas, and polyps is preferred to blind polypectomy and curettage. With the new, narrow hysteroscope, the procedure is easily done as an office procedure similar to colposcopy for biopsy or laser conization.

D. Endometrial Curettage

Endometrial curettage is often both diagnostic and therapeutic. It is indicated for treatment of complications of pregnancy, including incomplete or missed abortion, postpartum retention of products of conception, and placental polyps. The procedure is also useful in women with menorrhagia who are hypovolemic and refractory to medical management to stop the acute bleeding. D&C should not be used to treat dysfunctional uterine bleeding in women without hypovolemia, because it has no effect on mean blood loss in subsequent periods (with the exception of the first period following the D&C) and is inferior to medical management. D&C is inferior to hysteroscopy in diagnosing and treating abnormal uterine bleeding due to uterine fibroids or endometrial polyps. It is contraindicated in infection, such as acute endometritis, salpingitis, and pyometra. If infected placental tissue must be removed, the D&C should follow a period of parenteral antibiotics. The technique of endometrial curettage is tailored to the individual patient. In determining the hormone responsiveness of the endometrium, a small but representative sample may be obtained from the anterior and posterior walls. When curettage is being performed therapeutically, a systematic, thorough approach is indicated. The largest sharp curette that can comfortably fit through the dilated cervix is chosen. A serrated curette may cause injury to the underlying basalis layer of the endometrium and myometrium. The anterior, lateral, and posterior walls are scraped with firm pressure in a clockwise or counterclockwise fashion from the top of the uterine fundus down to the internal os. The top of the cavity is curetted with a side-to-side motion. The curettings are retrieved onto the waiting gauze and immersed in fixative as soon as possible. If endometrial curettage is being used for diagnosis of infection (eg, tuberculous endometritis), a portion of the curettings should be placed in containers appropriate for culture (without fixative).

A single curettage will not remove the entire endometrium. Thorough curettage by an experienced gynecologist often removes 50–60% of the endometrium, as determined by immediate postcurettage hysterectomy. If risk factors for endometrial cancer are present and clinical suspicion for neoplasia persists despite a histologic diagnosis of benign endometrium, further evaluation with hysteroscopically guided biopsy or hysterectomy is indicated.

Perforation of the uterus occurred in 0.63% of a large series of D&Cs. Perforation is suspected when the sound or curette meets no resistance at the point expected by uterine size, consistency, and position determined by preoperative bimanual examination. Curettage may be continued if the area of suspected perforation is avoided. Should suction curettage be associated with perforation, laparoscopy must be used to continue the procedure to avoid aspiration of bowel into the uterine cavity. In the case of suspected perforation, the patient should be observed for at least 24 hours in the hospital for possible infection or hemorrhage. In a series of 70 uterine perforations, 55 were treated expectantly, and only 1 patient developed complications (pelvic abscess drained via colpotomy). In 7 patients, hysterectomy was elected but not indicated by operative findings. Today, laparoscopy is the method of choice for evaluating perforations in the hemodynamically stable patient.

E. Endometrial Biopsy

Outpatient curettage, or endometrial biopsy, should always be a diagnostic and not a therapeutic technique. The many techniques available, all compared to D&C under adequate anesthesia, are discussed in Chapter 35.

American College of Obstetricians and Gynecologists. Antibiotic prophylaxis for gynecologic procedures. ACOG Practice Bulletin No. 104. *Obstet Gynecol* 2009;113:1180–1189. PMID: 19384149.

American College of Obstetricians and Gynecologists. Prevention of deep venous thrombosis and pulmonary embolism. ACOG Practice Bulletin No. 84, 2007. *Obstet Gynecol* 2007;110(2 Pt 1): 429–440. PMID: 17666620.

Aronsson A, Helstrom L, Gemzell-Danielsson K. Sublingual compared with oral misoprostol for cervical dilation prior to vacuum aspiration: a randomized comparison. *Contraception* 2004;69:165–169. PMID: 14759623.

Batukan C, Ozgun MT, Ozcelik B, et al. Cervical ripening before operative hysteroscopy in premenopausal women: a randomized, double-blind, placebo-controlled comparison of vaginal and oral misoprostol. *Fertil Steril* 2008;89:966–973. PMID: 17681307.

Bunnasathiansri S, Herabutya Y, O-Prasertsawat P. Vaginal misoprostol for cervical priming before dilation and curettage in postmenopausal women: a randomized controlled trial. *J Obstet Gynaecol Res* 2004;30:221–225. PMID: 15210047.

Crane JM, Healey S. Use of misoprostol before hysteroscopy: a systematic review. *J Obstet Gynaecol Can* 2006;28:373–379. PMID: 16768880.

Josey WE. Routine intrauterine forceps exploration at curettage. *Obstet Gynecol* 1958;11:108–111. PMID: 13504642.

McElin TW, Bird CC, Reeves BD, et al. Diagnostic dilation and curettage. A 20-year study. *Obstet Gynecol* 1969;33:807–812. PMID: 5770554.

Ngai SW, Chan YM, Ho PC. The use of misoprostol prior to hysteroscopy in postmenopausal women. *Hum Reprod* 2001;16:1486–1488. PMID: 11425834.

Stock RJ, Kanbour A. Prehysterectomy curettage. *Obstet Gynecol* 1975;45:537–541. PMID: 1124168.

Thomas JA, Leyland N, Durand N, et al. The use of oral misoprostol as a cervical ripening agent in operative hysteroscopy: a double-blind, placebo-controlled trial. *Am J Obstet Gynecol* 2002;186:876–879. PMID: 12015500.

Word B, Gravlee LC, Wideman GL. The fallacy of simple uterine curettage. *Obstet Gynecol* 1958;12:642–648. PMID: 13613649.

HYSTEROSCOPY

This section will discuss the therapeutic uses of hysteroscopy.

Indications & Contraindications

See Table 46–1.

Table 46–1. Indications and contraindications for hysteroscopy.

Indications	
	Abnormal premenopausal or postmenopausal uterine bleeding
	Desire for endometrial ablation
	Endometrial thickening or polyps
	Submucosal myomas
	Endocervical lesions
	Suspected müllerian anomalies
	Intrauterine adhesions
	Retained intrauterine device or other foreign body
	Desire for sterilization via tubal occlusion (Essure)
	Retained products of conception
Absolute contraindications	
	Viable intrauterine pregnancy
	Active pelvic infection (including genital herpes infection)
	Known uterine or cervical cancer
Relative contraindications	
	Heavy bleeding limiting visual field

Technique

Hysteroscopes exist as both flexible and rigid models. Operative hysteroscopes are rigid and typically 8–10 mm in external diameter. The outer sleeve encloses a fiberoptic light source, a channel used to introduce a medium to distend the uterus, and a channel through which probes, forceps, and electrocautery or laser instruments may be visually directed in the uterine cavity. Viewing angles vary from 0 to 70 degrees.

The uterine cavity, which is normally collapsed, must be distended by a medium. Carbon dioxide is used in the outpatient setting for diagnostic purposes. Low-viscosity, electrolyte-poor fluids include glycine 1.5%, sorbitol 3%, and mannitol 5%. These fluids can be used with monopolar devices during electrosurgery because they do not conduct electricity. Glycine 1.5% and sorbitol 3% are hypo-osmolar solutions. The use of these fluids can cause hyponatremia and decreased serum osmolality, which can lead to cerebral edema and death. Mannitol 5% is iso-osmolar and acts as its own diuretic. It may cause hyponatremia but not decreased serum osmolality. Low-viscosity electrolyte fluids include normal saline and lactated Ringer's solution. These fluids are isotonic, which decreases the risk of hyponatremia and decreased serum osmolality. Pulmonary edema can still occur, and therefore, careful attention should be paid to the fluid deficit. Two disadvantages to the use of electrolyte solutions are mixing of blood, which limits visualization, and the inability to use monopolar electrosurgery because these solutions are electroconductors. However, it is possible to conduct electrosurgery in electrolyte fluids using bipolar electrosurgical systems.

High-viscosity fluids include dextran-70, which is a colorless, viscous, polysaccharide solution. The advantage of using dextran is that it is immiscible with blood, which allows for clear visualization in the presence of bleeding. The disadvantage is that it is sticky, and when dry, can harden and crystallize into the equipment. Dextran can cause rare but serious complications including anaphylactic reactions, fluid overload, pulmonary edema, and coagulopathy. The manufacturer recommends that patients be followed closely for pulmonary edema in the following situations: the procedure lasts >45 minutes, absorption of more than 250 mL of dextran-70, resection of large areas of endometrium, or administration of intravenous fluids at more than maintenance rate. If pulmonary edema develops, the patient may need plasmapheresis, because dextran-70 contains mainly high-molecular-weight molecules that are excreted slowly or not at all from the kidneys. Beet sugar allergy is an absolute contraindication to using dextran-70. The volume of dextran-70 is usually limited to 300 mL but must not exceed 500 mL.

An abundance of instruments are available for use in hysteroscopic procedures, including blunt probes, microscissors, alligator clamps, rollerball electrode, wire loop for excision and coagulation (resectoscope), and devices for nonresectoscopic system endometrial ablation. Local or general anesthetics are chosen on the basis of expected hysteroscopic findings or procedures, concomitant operations planned, and the desires and cooperation of the patient. Most hysteroscopic examinations and virtually all therapeutic procedures are performed under general anesthesia. Following administration of anesthesia, the urinary bladder is drained, and the anterior lip of the cervix is grasped with a tenaculum. The cervix should then be gradually dilated to the same diameter as the external sleeve of the hysteroscope in order to provide a snug fit. An assistant must be constantly present during hysteroscopy to monitor uterine insufflation so that the pressure never exceeds 100 mm Hg and the flow rate of the distending medium never exceeds 100 mL/min. The chance of fluid overload is markedly increased when the mean infusion pressure exceeds the mean arterial pressure. The lowest infusion pressure needed to obtain good visualization should be used. The assistant and surgeon must monitor the fluid deficit closely to prevent volume overload. The surgeon should be sitting comfortably, with all instruments available to perform the hysteroscopic procedure safely and expeditiously. Following the procedure, intrauterine instruments should be inspected for their integrity. The microscissors in particular are delicate and could break within the uterus. If dextran is used, it must be immediately flushed from the hysteroscope before it is allowed to dry.

Complications

Hysteroscopic surgery is generally safe in experienced hands. The most common complications include cervical laceration

(1–11%), hemorrhage (2.4%), and fluid overload (1.5%). Other complications include uterine perforation, visceral injury, carbon dioxide and air embolism, and rarely death. With laparoscopic observation, the serious complication of uterine perforation can almost always be prevented. If overt bleeding occurs during resection of a septum, polyp, or leiomyoma, the laparoscopic probe can be held against the uterine vessels to slow the blood flow. Alternatively, the bleeding area can be electrocoagulated, or a Foley catheter may be inserted into the uterine cavity and inflated to provide a tamponade. Infection is an unusual complication following hysteroscopy, and prophylactic antibiotics are not recommended. Air and carbon dioxide emboli are rare but serious complications that can result in circulatory collapse. Signs and symptoms of embolization include chest pain and dyspnea in the awake patient, sudden hypotension, decrease in oxygenation and/or in end-tidal carbon dioxide, or cardiac dysrhythmias in the anesthetized patient. Other findings include the presence of a "mill wheel" cardiac murmur, hypotension, tachycardia, or bradycardia. If gas embolization occurs, the patient should be placed in the left lateral decubitus position with the head tilted downward 5 degrees. This position favors movement of gas in the right ventricle toward the apex of the right ventricle. The gas may then be aspirated via cardiocentesis or by passing a catheter down the jugular vein into the right ventricle.

Complications of distending media include hyponatremia and pulmonary edema if an excessive amount results in vascular intervasation. The American College of Obstetricians and Gynecologists (ACOG) has adopted the following guidelines for fluid monitoring. (1) Hydration of patients should be monitored closely pre- and postoperatively. (2) If low-viscosity, electrolyte-poor fluids are used, the fluid deficit should be monitored at an extremely close interval when a deficit of 750 mL is reached. The procedure should be terminated in elderly patients, in patients with comorbid conditions, and in patients with cardiovascular compromise. (3) If fluid deficit reaches 1000–1500 mL of a nonelectrolyte solution or 2500 mL of an electrolyte solution, the procedure should be terminated. Electrolytes should be obtained, administration of diuretics should be considered, and further diagnostic and therapeutic interventions should begin as indicated. (4) In an outpatient setting with limited acute care and laboratory services, consideration should be given to terminate the procedure at a lower fluid deficit threshold. (5) An automated fluid monitoring system facilitates early recognition of excessive deficit in real-life totals. (6) In the absence of automated fluid monitoring, an individual should be designated to frequently measure intake and outflow and report the deficit to the operative team. Patients who need treatment for fluid overload from hypotonic agents may require transfer to an acute care facility and consultation. Seizure, permanent brain damage, and death have been reported with serum sodium levels of 112–118 mmol/L. If hyponatremia has existed for <24 hours, rapid correction can be made. However, if hyponatremia has existed for over 48 hours, rapid correction should not be undertaken due to the risk of neurologic compromise, seizures, and death. Consultation is strongly encouraged in these circumstances.

Prognosis

With proper selection of patients, hysteroscopic surgery has high success rates. Small pedunculated leiomyomas and polyps are usually retrieved by an experienced, patient surgeon. Submucous leiomyomas may be destroyed if they are not too vascular. In the treatment of intrauterine adhesions, the chance for success and restoration of a normal endometrial cavity depends on the density and extent of the adhesions and the area of normal endometrium remaining after dissection. Following hysteroscopic surgery for infertility in which the endometrium is denuded, postoperative estrogen therapy is prescribed by many physicians to promote rapid endometrial growth.

Both resectoscopic and nonresectoscopic endometrial ablation techniques exist and appear to be equivalent with respect to successful reduction in menstrual flow and patient satisfaction at 1 year (Table 46–2). Despite the high satisfaction rate, both resectoscopic and nonresectoscopic endometrial ablations are associated with hysterectomy rates of at least 24% within 4 years of the procedure.

American College of Obstetricians and Gynecologists. Endometrial ablation. ACOG Practice Bulletin No. 81. *Obstet Gynecol* 2007;109:1233–1248. PMID: 17470612.

American College of Obstetricians and Gynecologists. Hysteroscopy. ACOG Technology Assessment in Obstetrics and Gynecology No. 4. *Obstet Gynecol* 2005;106:439–442. PMID: 16055609.

Cooper JM, Brady RM. Intraoperative and early postoperative complications of operative hysteroscopy. *Obstet Gynecol Clin* 2000;27:347–366. PMID: 10857125.

Hatfield JL, Brumsted JR, Cooper BC. Conservative treatment of placenta accreta. *J Minim Invasive Gynecol* 2006;13:510–513. PMID: 17097571.

Loffer FD, Bradley LD, Brill AI, et al. Hysteroscopic fluid monitoring guidelines. The Ad Hoc Committee on Hysteroscopic Training Guidelines of the American Association of Gynecologic Laparoscopists. *J Am Assoc Gynecol Laparosc* 2000;7:167–168. PMID: 10648762.

Price TM, Harris JB. Fulminant hepatic failure due to herpes simplex after hysteroscopy. *Obstet Gynecol* 2001;98:954–956. PMID: 11704219.

Propst AM, Liberman RF, Harlow BL, et al. Complications of hysteroscopic surgery: predicting patients at risk. *Obstet Gynecol* 2000;96:517–520. PMID: 11004351.

Sharp HT. Assessment of new technology in the treatment of idiopathic menorrhagia and uterine leiomyomata. *Obstet Gynecol* 2006;108:990–1003. PMID: 17012464.

Stoloff DR, Isenberg RA, Burns WN, et al. Venous air and gas emboli in operative hysteroscopy. *J Am Assoc Gynecol Laparoscop* 2001;8:181–192. PMID: 11342722.

Table 46–2. Patient satisfaction and amenorrhea rates associated with nonresectoscopic endometrial ablation compared with resectoscopic ablation at 12 months.[1]

Device	Satisfaction Rate (%) NR/R Ablation[2]	Amenorrhea Rate (%)[3] NR/R Ablation[2]
ThermaChoice (thermal balloon)	96/99[4]	13.9/24.4
Hydro ThermAblator (heated free fluid)	–/–[5]	35.3/47.1
Her Option (cryotherapy)	86/88[6]	22.2/46.5
NoveSure (radiofrequency electricity)	92/93[4]	36/32.2
Microwave Endometrial Ablation System (microwave energy)	99/99[4]	55.3/45.8

[1]Based on US Food and Drug Administration pivotal trials.
[2]NRA/RA, nonresectoscopic/resectoscopic ablation.
[3]Based on intent to treat.
[4]Patients reported being satisfied or very satisfied.
[5]Quality-of-life scores compared with baseline only.
[6]Patients reported being very or extremely satisfied.
Modified with permission from Sharp HT. Assessment of new technology in the treatment of idiopathic menorrhagia and uterine leiomyomata. *Obstet Gynecol* 2006;108:990–1003.

LAPAROSCOPY

Laparoscopy is a transperitoneal endoscopic technique that provides excellent visualization of the pelvic structures and often permits the diagnosis of gynecologic disorders and pelvic surgery without laparotomy.

Laparoscopes range in diameter from 3–12 mm and have lenses with a viewing angle ranging from 0–135 degrees. The instrument has an effective length of over 25 cm and can be used with a fiberoptic light box. To facilitate visualization, carbon dioxide (CO_2) must be instilled into the peritoneal cavity to distend the abdominal wall.

Use of a pneumatic insufflator permits continuous monitoring of the rate, pressure, and volume of the gas used for inflation. In addition to the equipment used for observation, a variety of other instruments for resection, biopsy, coagulation, aspiration, and manipulation can be passed through separate ports or inserted through the same port as the laparoscope. Laparoscopic ports range in diameter from 3–20 mm in diameter. A laser (CO_2 or Nd:YAG) may be used with the laparoscope.

The laparoscope has become an invaluable tool in both diagnostic and operative gynecologic procedures. However, its use requires considerable expertise, and it should always be used by a surgeon familiar with the management of complications. Laparoscopic procedures are *major* intra-abdominal operations performed through small incisions. This technique is rapidly performed and has a low morbidity rate and a short convalescence period. In many cases, laparoscopy may replace conventional laparotomy for diagnosis and treatment of gynecologic problems. It is a cost-effective outpatient procedure.

Indications

The indications will increase with the clinician's experience and as technical innovations permit even more complicated procedures.

A. Diagnosis

1. Differentiation between ovarian, tubal, and uterine masses (eg, ectopic pregnancy, ovarian cyst, salpingitis, myomas, endometriosis, and tuberculosis)
2. Pelvic pain (eg, possible adhesions, endometriosis, ectopic pregnancy, ovarian torsion or hemorrhagic ovarian cyst, salpingitis, appendicitis, and nongynecologic pelvic pain)
3. Genital anomalies (eg, ovarian dysgenesis, müllerian anomalies)
4. Ascites (eg, ovarian diseases vs. cirrhosis)
5. Pelvic injuries after penetrating or nonpenetrating abdominal trauma
6. Diagnosis of occult cancer

B. Evaluation

1. Infertility (eg, tubal patency, ovarian biopsy)
2. "Second look" after tubal surgery or treatment of endometriosis
3. Peritoneal washings for cytology study
4. Peritoneal culture (eg, *Actinomyces* or tuberculosis)
5. Evaluation of uterine perforation
6. Evaluation of pelvic viscera to determine the feasibility of vaginal hysterectomy

C. Therapy

1. Tubal sterilization:
   a. Electrical: Unipolar or bipolar technique
   b. Mechanical: Silastic bands or rings, metal clips
2. Lysis of adhesions, with or without laser
3. Fulguration of endometriosis by laser or thermal cautery
4. Removal of extruded IUD
5. Uterosacral ligament division (denervation)

6. Treatment of ectopic pregnancy
7. Myomectomy
8. Salpingostomy for phimotic fimbria
9. Removal of tuboplastic hoods or splints
10. Ova collection for in vitro fertilization
11. GIFT (gamete intrafallopian transfer for fertilization)
12. Mini-wedge resection of ovary
13. Biopsy of tumor, liver, ovary, spleen, omentum, etc
14. Placement of intraperitoneal clips as markers for radiotherapy
15. Oophorectomy
16. Ovarian cystectomy
17. Laparoscopic-assisted vaginal hysterectomy, laparoscopic subtotal hysterectomy, and laparoscopic hysterectomy
18. Reconstructive surgery for pelvic organ prolapse and urinary incontinence

Contraindications

A. Absolute

Intestinal obstruction, generalized peritonitis, massive hemorrhage.

B. Relative

Severe cardiac or pulmonary disease, previous periumbilical surgery, shock, cancer involving anterior abdominal wall.

Additional factors weighing against performing laparoscopic surgery include extremes of weight, intrauterine pregnancy after the first or early second trimester, presence of a large mass, inflammatory bowel disease, and known severe intraperitoneal adhesions.

Preparation for Laparoscopy

Careful explanation of the risks and benefits of the planned procedure must be given to each patient prior to surgery. The risk of visceral and vascular injuries and the need to convert to laparotomy should be discussed with all patients. Patients with prior abdominal surgery, prior pelvic inflammation (appendicitis and pelvic inflammatory disease), or radiation therapy should be told that they are at increased risk of visceral or vascular injury or conversion to laparotomy. Preparation includes no solid food for at least 8 hours prior to surgery, no liquids for more than 6 hours preoperatively, a history and physical examination, and routine blood studies. Preoperative bowel cleansing can aid in visualization during surgery by decompressing the small bowel and sigmoid colon. Abdominal or perineal shaving is usually unnecessary, but skin preparation with an antiseptic is routine. Antibiotic prophylaxis is not recommended because the frequency of wound infection is low.

Anesthesia

Local anesthesia, local anesthesia with systemic analgesia, spinal or epidural block techniques, or general anesthesia with or without endotracheal intubation may be used. Special hazards of anesthesia exist (eg, reduced diaphragmatic excursion because of the pneumoperitoneum and because the patient may be operated on in the Trendelenburg position). Because of these factors, most procedures in the United States are performed with the patient under general anesthesia with endotracheal intubation. With adequate understanding of the physiology involved, effective anesthesia and laparoscopy can be accomplished safely.

An alternative to general anesthesia is local anesthesia with intravenous sedation. The patient may experience transient discomfort during manipulation of the uterine tubes, but in selected patients, this discomfort is easily tolerated.

Surgical Technique

The patient should be placed with her arms at her sides in the dorsal lithotomy position and draped after induction of anesthesia and preparation of the abdomen and pelvic area. The video monitor should be placed in a position that allows for easy viewing by the surgeon, usually at the patient's feet or side. The bladder must be emptied by catheterization to decrease the risk of injury during subsequent introduction and use of other instruments. After careful bimanual examination, a tenaculum is attached to the cervix, and a uterine manipulator (Hasson, HUMI, Hulka, etc.) is placed into the cervical canal to elevate the uterus, which places tissue on tension. A 1-cm incision is made within or immediately below the umbilicus. The peritoneal cavity is entered blindly with a veress needle advanced at a 45-degree angle toward the hollow of the sacrum. Alternatively, the pelvis can be entered by using a trocar-cannula system or under direct visualization via a mini-laparotomy called "open laparoscopy." Direct insertion of a cannula-trocar system can be accomplished safely if there have been no previous peritonitis or abdominopelvic surgeries. Open laparoscopy minimizes the risk of vascular injuries but does not eliminate intestinal injuries. Carbon dioxide should then be introduced and monitored by the pneumatic insufflator. The amount of gas insufflated will vary with the patient's size, the laxity of the abdominal wall, and the planned procedure. In most patients, 2–3 L of gas will be needed to obtain adequate visualization. The maximum insufflation pressure should not exceed 15 mm Hg. If a veress needle is used, it is withdrawn and the laparoscopic trocar and cannula inserted. After proper abdominal entry, the trocar may be withdrawn and replaced with the fiberoptic laparoscope. The examiner manipulates the intrauterine cannula so that the pelvic organs can be observed. To test for tubal patency, methylene blue or indigo carmine solution can be injected through the intrauterine cannula. Direct observation of a lack of dye leakage attests to tubal patency. A second trocar with a cannula may be inserted under direct laparoscopic vision through a 5-mm transverse midline incision at the pubic hairline. Additional punctures are used as necessary for the placement of other instruments. A number of instruments are available including irrigators, the harmonic scalpel, forceps, scissors, staple applicators, and several vessel sealing and transection systems. Surgical knots may be tied and sutures placed using specially made equipment.

The operation is terminated by evacuating the insufflated gas through the cannula, followed by removal of all instruments and closure of the incisions. The skin can be closed with 3-0 subcuticular suture, skin glue, or steri-strips. Incisions >10 mm require fascial closure to avoid incisional hernias. A small dressing is applied to the wound.

A. Sterilization

Electrical cautery, Silastic rings or bands, and metal spring clips achieve sterilization by occluding the fallopian tubes. The advantages or disadvantages of the different techniques are of less significance than the skill with which a physician can perform any one technique; therefore, choice of method should depend on which technique is most comfortable for the physician. The failure rate of most sterilization methods is greater in women <28 years old.

1. Cautery—Laparoscopic sterilization with electrical cautery is one of the most common laparoscopic sterilization methods. Unipolar coagulation has a significantly lower pregnancy rate than bipolar coagulation (7.5/1000 vs. 24.8 over 10 years); however, bipolar coagulation is less likely to cause injury to adjacent structures (eg, bowel). At least 3 cm of the isthmic portion of the tube must be completely coagulated by using sufficient energy (25 W) delivered in a cutting waveform when using bipolar coagulation. The use of a current meter more accurately indicates complete coagulation than visual inspection. Generally, the tube is burned at 2 to 3 different locations, and division of the tube by cutting is not necessary.

2. Silastic Bands—Tubal occlusion with Silastic bands or rings results in a slightly higher pregnancy rate (17.7/1000 over 10 years) but fewer ectopic pregnancies. Mechanical problems in placement of the bands and bleeding from the tubes during the procedure are more common.

3. Clips—Tubal occlusion with clips (Hulka or Filshie clips) has a wide range of failure. Failure rates are higher for the Hulka clip (36.5/1000 over 10 years) than for the Filshie clip (0–4/1000 over 6–10 years). The advantages of using clips are that only a small portion of the tube is damaged (thus increasing the chance of successful sterilization reversal if the patient has regret) and that inadvertent burn injury to the bowel is avoided.

4. Interval Partial Salpingectomy—Compared to postpartum tubal ligation, interval partial salpingectomy has a higher failure rate of 20.1/1000 over 10 years.

B. Infertility

In procedures of sterilization reversal, laparoscopic visualization may be needed prior to reanastomosis, particularly if the ligation procedure involved electrocautery. Peritubal adhesions may be lysed with electric scissors, and salpingostomy may be accomplished. The minimal trauma of these procedures using laparoscopy and the saving of a major operative procedure are obvious benefits. Laparoscopy should be considered for women with complaints of abnormal bleeding and unexplained pelvic pain. More liberal use of the laparoscope has led to the diagnosis of many unsuspected cases of endometriosis.

Electrical fulguration of areas of endometriosis or laser destruction of these diseased areas by laparoscopy is a safe, effective, and rapid treatment. The use of laser obviously allows implants on structures such as bowel, bladder, and the fallopian tubes to be treated with a fairly wide margin of safety. Relief may be immediate and striking, whether the woman has complained of dysmenorrhea, dyspareunia, or generalized pelvic pain.

In infertility, the laparoscope has been important for ova collection for in vitro fertilization, GIFT, and other procedures. However, it is used less frequently now because most egg retrievals for in vitro fertilization are performed under ultrasound guidance.

C. Ectopic Pregnancy

In hemodynamically stable patients, laparoscopic linear salpingostomy is the preferred method for conservative management of tubal pregnancies. According to a recent Cochrane Database systematic review, the laparoscopic approach is less successful than the open approach in the elimination of tubal pregnancy due to the higher rate of persistent trophoblast tissue. However, it is feasible in virtually all patients, safe, and less costly compared to the open approach. Long-term follow-up shows a comparable intrauterine pregnancy rate and a lower repeat ectopic pregnancy rate. Persistent trophoblast tissue after laparoscopic salpingostomy can be significantly reduced after a prophylactic single dose of systemic methotrexate. An alternative conservative approach for those who meet the criteria is methotrexate administration.

D. Laparoscopic Hysterectomy

Laparoscopy can be used for total laparoscopic hysterectomy, laparoscopic-assisted vaginal hysterectomy, and laparoscopic subtotal hysterectomy (see section on hysterectomy). Other procedures that can be done via the laparoscope include vault suspension and pelvic reconstruction such as retropubic Burch colposuspension and abdominal sacral colpopexy.

E. Abdominal & Pelvic Pain

Laparoscopy has proved invaluable in differentiating various causes of acute and chronic pain. The technique may save the patient the necessity of a major exploratory operation. Fluid aspiration and tissue biopsy are possible through laparoscopy. Also, pelvic and intestinal disease can be differentiated. The appendix may be visualized and acute appendicitis may be diagnosed. Numerous cases of pain caused by intra-abdominal adhesions also have been diagnosed by laparoscopy, and relief has been obtained following laparoscopic adhesion resection.

F. Trauma

In cases of intra-abdominal trauma, laparoscopy can be used to exclude the need for a major abdominal operation.

G. Miscellaneous

"Missing" IUDs have been removed from the intra-abdominal cavity. Mulligan plastic hoods from tuboplasty procedures, "lost" drains, and other foreign material have been removed from the abdomen by operative laparoscopy.

Postsurgical Care

Patients may be sent home following full recovery from anesthesia, usually in 1–2 hours. Recovery from more extensive procedures such as laparoscopic hysterectomy may require a longer hospital stay of 1–2 days. Postoperative pain is usually minimal, and patients are discharged with a prescription for a simple oral analgesic. The most common complaint is shoulder pain secondary to subdiaphragmatic accumulation of gas. Patients are encouraged to resume full activity, except for sexual relations, the day following surgery. Sexual relations may be resumed several days postoperatively after a simple procedure (eg, tubal ligation). Following extensive operative laparoscopy or other gynecologic procedures, coitus should be delayed for an appropriate interval (ie, until it is unlikely to cause discomfort or damage to the operative site). Patients should routinely be seen in the office 1–2 weeks postoperatively.

Complications

A review of the world experience of laparoscopic gynecologic operations, including 1,549,360 patients, showed an overall complication rate ranging from 0.2–10%. Higher complications rates were noted with prospective studies. The frequency of complications was less for nonoperative or minor procedures (0.06–7.0%) than for major operations (0.6–18%). Complications requiring conversion to laparotomy have been estimated to be 2.1% and are most commonly due to major vascular and intestinal injuries. The readmission rate to the hospital has been quoted to be 0.4–0.5%. The mortality rate for laparoscopy including 1,374,827 patients is 4.4 per 100,000 laparoscopies. The major causes of death are due to intestinal and vascular complications and anesthesia.

A. Vascular injuries

Major vascular injuries are infrequent (0.01–0.5%) and are almost 5 times more frequent during blind entry than during the laparoscopic operation itself. Catastrophic bleeding can occur if the aorta; inferior vena cava; or common, internal, or external iliac arteries and veins are injured. The mortality rate due to major vascular injuries is between 9 and 17%, and immediate conversion to laparotomy is almost always needed. Massive bleeding is often concealed in large retroperitoneal hematomas, and often only a small amount of intraperitoneal bleeding is seen. Open laparoscopic technique minimizes the risk of major vascular injury, but aortic injury has been reported in thin patients caused by the scalpel during the skin incision. The incidence of abdominal wall bleeding is 0.5%, and most injuries involve the inferior epigastric vessels (deep and superficial) and muscular vessels. Major bleeding requiring transfusion has been observed. The inferior epigastric vessels run in the lateral umbilical ligaments, and contrary to common belief, the inferior epigastric vessels cannot be seen via transillumination by the laparoscope. These are best avoided by placing the trocars lateral to the insertion of the round ligament into the anterior abdominal wall or 1–2 cm lateral to McBurney's point (one-third the way between the anterior superior iliac spine and the umbilicus).

B. Intestinal Injury

Bowel injuries are uncommon (0.03–0.5%) but have a mortality rate of 2.5–5%. The colon and small bowel are injured at about the same rate, and they can be injured sharply or via thermal burns. About one-third are related to entry, and the rest are due to operative procedures. Unfortunately, most bowel injuries are not recognized intraoperatively (mean 4.4 postoperative days), likely due to the fact that most patients with laparoscopic intestinal injury do not present with the typical clinical signs of bowel perforation. Most patients present with low-grade fever, leukopenia, or normal leukocyte count. Pain at the trocar site near the injury, abdominal distention, and diarrhea with normal bowel sounds were commonly seen. Peritoneal signs, severe pain, nausea, vomiting, and ileus were uncommon, in a review of 266 cases of intestinal injury. Open laparoscopy has a similar rate of bowel injuries, but they are recognized more commonly intraoperatively.

C. Urinary Injuries

Urinary injuries during laparoscopy have a similar rate to open procedures (0.02–1.7%). Bladder injuries are more common than ureteral injuries and are recognized more frequently intraoperatively. About two-thirds of urinary injuries occur during laparoscopic-assisted vaginal hysterectomy.

D. Hernia at Site of Abdominal Wall Trocar

Ventral hernia formation is about 10 times lower with laparoscopy compared with laparotomy (0.06–1% vs. 11–13%). Five-millimeter trocar wounds do not require closure, whereas larger trocar wounds do. Most surgeons close incisions greater than 10 mm, due to the high rate of hernias. Richter's hernias, where only a portion of the intestinal wall is entrapped in a defect of the peritoneum or posterior fascia, can be difficult to diagnose, since an externally visible bulge is often absent. The condition needs a high index of suspicion and can be diagnosed with an ultrasound or computed tomography scan.

E. Subcutaneous Emphysema & Gas Embolisms

Localized or generalized subcutaneous emphysema occurs in 0.3–2% of cases and generally has no clinical consequences. However, subcutaneous emphysema of the neck, face, and chest may be a manifestation of a pneumothorax or pneumomediastinum.

F. Postoperative Shoulder Pain

Pain from diaphragmatic irritation can be referred to the shoulder causing discomfort. Irritation of the diaphragm by the formation of carbonic acid (due to use of CO_2), stretching of the phrenic nerve by pneumoperitoneum, or pressure from the abdominal organs during Trendelenburg position are possible etiologies. It can be treated with mild analgesics and reassurance.

Chi DS, Abu-Rustum NR, Sonoda Y, et al. Ten-year experience with laparoscopy on a gynecologic oncology service: analysis of risk factors for complications and conversion to laparotomy. *Am J Obstet Gynecol* 2004;191:1138–1145. PMID: 15507933.

Hajenius PJ, Mol BW, Bossuyt PM, et al. Interventions for tubal ectopic pregnancy. *Cochrane Database Syst Rev* 2007;1:CD0000324. PMID: 17253448.

Jansen FW, Kolkman W, Bakkum EA, et al. Complications of laparoscopy: an inquiry about closed- versus open-entry technique. *Am J Obstet Gynecol* 2004;190:634–638. PMID: 15041992.

Magrina JF. Complications of laparoscopic surgery. *Clin Obstet Gynecol* 2002;45:469–480. PMID: 12048405.

Meeks GR. Advanced laparoscopic gynecologic surgery. *Surg Clin North Am* 2000;80:1443–1464. PMID: 11059713.

Munro MG. Laparoscopic access: complications, technologies, and techniques. *Curr Opin Obstet Gynecol* 2002;14:365–374. PMID: 12151825.

Penfield AJ. The Filshie clip for female sterilization: a review of world experience. *Am J Obstet Gynecol* 2000;182:485–489. PMID: 10739495.

Peterson HB. Sterilization. *Obstet Gynecol* 2008;11:189–203. PMID: 18165410.

Tittel A, Treutner KH, Titkova S, et al. New adhesion formation after laparoscopic and conventional adhesiolysis: a comparative study in the rabbit. *Surg Endosc* 2001;15:44–46. PMID: 11178761.

OPERATIONS FOR STERILIZATION OF WOMEN & MEN

Sterilization is a permanent method of contraception and is the most commonly used contraceptive method used in the United States. Approximately 700,000 tubal sterilizations and 500,000 vasectomies are performed in the United States annually.

TUBAL STERILIZATION

Thirty-three percent of US women use sterilization as their contraceptive method, and of those, 27% had tubal sterilization and 9% had partners who had a vasectomy. Table 46–3 lists the most common methods of tubal sterilization and their failure rates.

Preoperative Counseling

Clear, comprehensive counseling is essential for women who are considering tubal sterilization. Possible medical and psychological complications must be carefully outlined (see Complications, later); women are more likely to regret having had the operation if they do not know what to expect. The physician should be alert to signs that the patient is undecided about having the operation or is being pressured by her partner or others. Regret or dissatisfaction is more common if the procedure is done postpartum than at another time, and these women are more than twice as

Table 46–3. Overall failure rates with tubal sterilization over 10 years.

Procedure	Failure Rate (%) (per 1000 procedures)
Postpartum partial salpingectomy	7.5
Unipolar coagulation	7.5
Bipolar coagulation	24.8
Spring clip	36.5
Silicone rubber band	17.7
Interval partial salpingectomy	20.1
All methods	18.5

Modified with permission from Peterson HB, Xia Z, Hughes JM, et al. The risk of pregnancy after tubal sterilization: Findings from the U.S. Collaborative Review of Sterilization. *Am J Obstet Gynecol* 1996;174:1161–1168.

likely to feel that preoperative counseling was inadequate. Temporary stress associated with the pregnancy may have influenced a premature decision for sterilization in these women.

Patients should be told that tubal sterilization is usually not reversible. Some methods are sometimes reversible (see Chapter 58). Most studies estimate that about 1–2% of women who undergo tubal sterilization request reversal. The major risk factor for subsequent regret of sterilization is young maternal age (younger than age 30 years) at the time of sterilization. Collaborative Review of Sterilization (CREST) study data showed that women who were younger than 30 years at the time of sterilization were twice as likely to seek information about reversal as women between age 30 and 34. Another major risk factor for regret is marital disharmony at the time of sterilization. In addition, women who have postpartum sterilization are more prone to regret than are women who have interval sterilization. Parity has not been found to be a significant risk factor for regret when controlling for maternal age. Pregnancy rates after tubal ligation reversals range from 55–90% by laparotomy and 31–78% via laparoscopy. Success of tubal ligation reversal depends on the woman's age at the timer of reversal (<35 years old) and length of remaining fallopian tube segment (>4 cm). Some studies have found improved pregnancy results when the initial sterilization procedure was performed using mechanical techniques rather than electrocautery.

Complications

Pain and menstrual disturbances (postbilateral tubal ligation syndrome) have been reported following tubal sterilization. The theory holds that destruction of the mesosalpinx might alter the blood supply and subsequent gonadotropin delivery to the ovary. Ovarian function and hormone production may then be altered. However, prospective controlled studies show that these problems are no more common than in women who have not undergone sterilization. Menstrual changes seem to be related to use of contraceptives—before sterilization. Oral contraceptives are associated with decreased menstrual flow and relief of dysmenorrhea. Once they are discontinued, heavier flow and pain may recur. Complaints of menstrual changes are much less frequent in the second half of the first postoperative year. Patients should be told that pelvic pain or menstrual disturbances may develop after tubal sterilization but are no more common than in other women of similar age and parity.

Patients who have undergone tubal sterilization require hysterectomy more frequently than patients who have not undergone this procedure. This is probably because most women who have tubal sterilizations have had children and are therefore more likely to have disorders typically treated with hysterectomy (eg, symptomatic pelvic relaxation, adenomyosis). Patients may have been sterilized secondary to medical reasons and gynecologic disorders that might eventually require further surgery. Some studies suggest that women are more likely to accept a surgical treatment if they have been sterilized.

Failure of sterilization is most often secondary to poor technique, for example, improper application of a clip or ring. Fistula formation may occur. A complication of failure is ectopic pregnancy (7.3 per 1000).

An association between decreased risk of ovarian cancer and tubal sterilization has been shown in several studies.

Technique (See Figs. 46–1 through 46–4).

Postpartum tubal ligation uses a small infraumbilical incision to access the tubes. Mini-laparotomy involves a 2- to 3-cm incision made above the symphysis pubis. The incision is closed in 2 layers.

HYSTEROSCOPIC MICROINSERT PLACEMENT

A hysteroscopic tubal sterilization technique (Essure) was approved by the US Food and Drug Administration in 2002 (Fig. 46–5). It consists of a fallopian tube implant and a delivery catheter. The implant is a spring-like device 40 mm in length and 0.8 mm in diameter. It is made of titanium, stainless steel, and nickel that contain Dacron fibers that induce an inflammatory response and final fibrosis of the intramural tubal lumen. The implant is placed into the fallopian tube using a standard hysteroscope (<5 mm) with a 5-French working channel with continuous flow of normal saline. When released, the outer coil expands, which anchors the implant into the fallopian tube. Three to 8 coils should remain in the uterus for optimal placement. The procedure can be performed in the outpatient setting using oral analgesics alone or under local anesthesia with or without intravenous sedation. Hysterosalpingogram should be performed 3 months after the procedure to confirm closure of the fallopian tubes. The patient needs to use an alternative form of contraception until tubal occlusion is documented.

A recent systematic review showed that the bilateral placement success rate was 81–90% with up to 2 attempts. At 3 months postprocedure, 3.5% of patients did not show tubal occlusion, but after 6 months, all women with successful placement showed total occlusion. The Essure system has been shown to be safe, but unintended pregnancies have been reported (64 in 50,000 procedures). The majority of unintended pregnancies occurred in patients with inappropriate follow-up. However, misinterpreted hysterosalpingograms, undetected preprocedure pregnancies, and failure to follow product-labeling guidelines have also led to unintended pregnancies.

OTHER METHODS OF FEMALE STERILIZATION

Because of relatively high morbidity and mortality rates in comparison with tubal occlusion procedures, hysterectomy is justified for sterilization only if there is another unequivocal indication for hysterectomy. Transvaginal

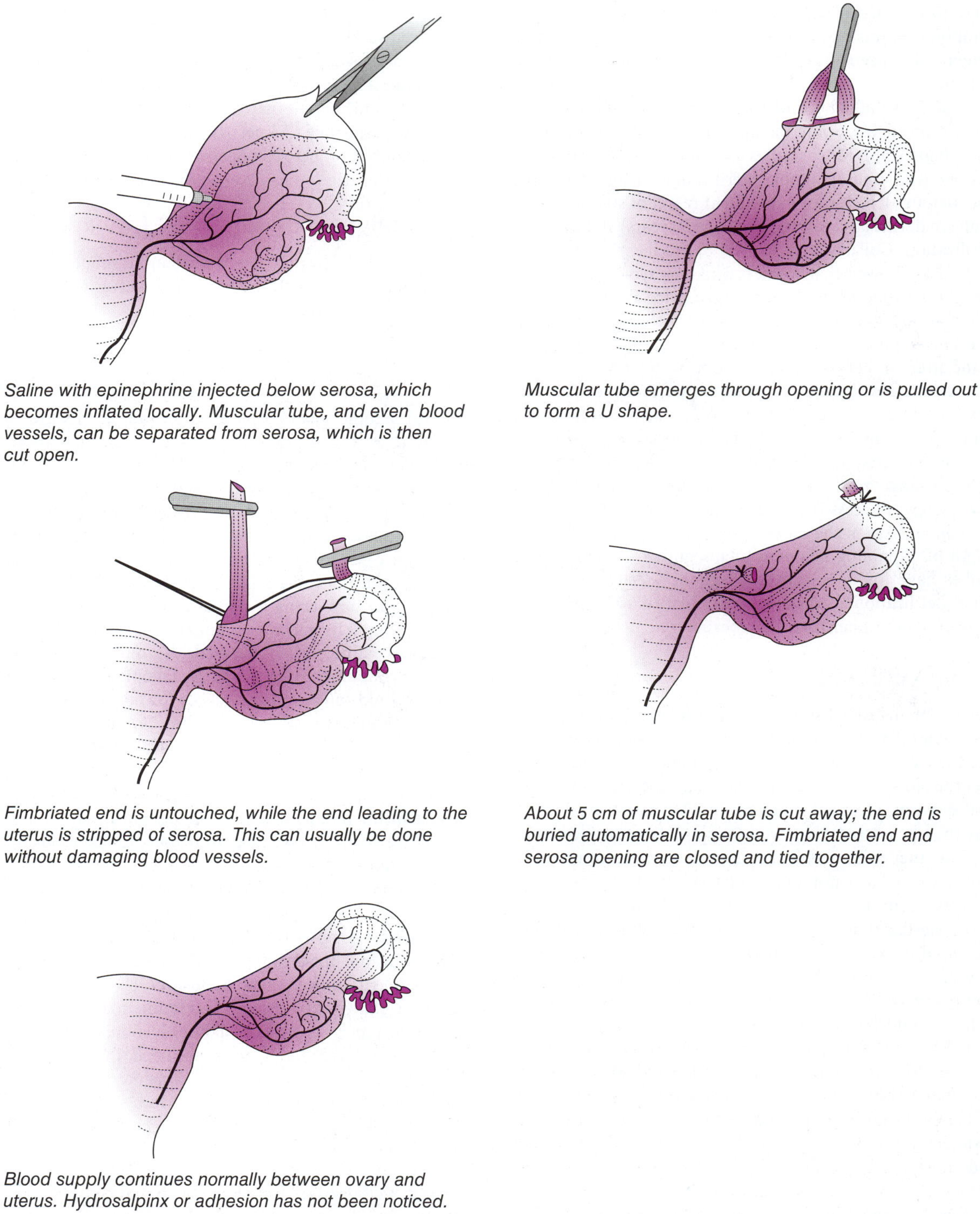

▲ **Figure 46–1.** Uchida method of sterilization. (Reproduced, with permission, from Benson RC. *Handbook of Obstetrics & Gynecology*. 8th ed. New York, NY: Lange; 1983.)

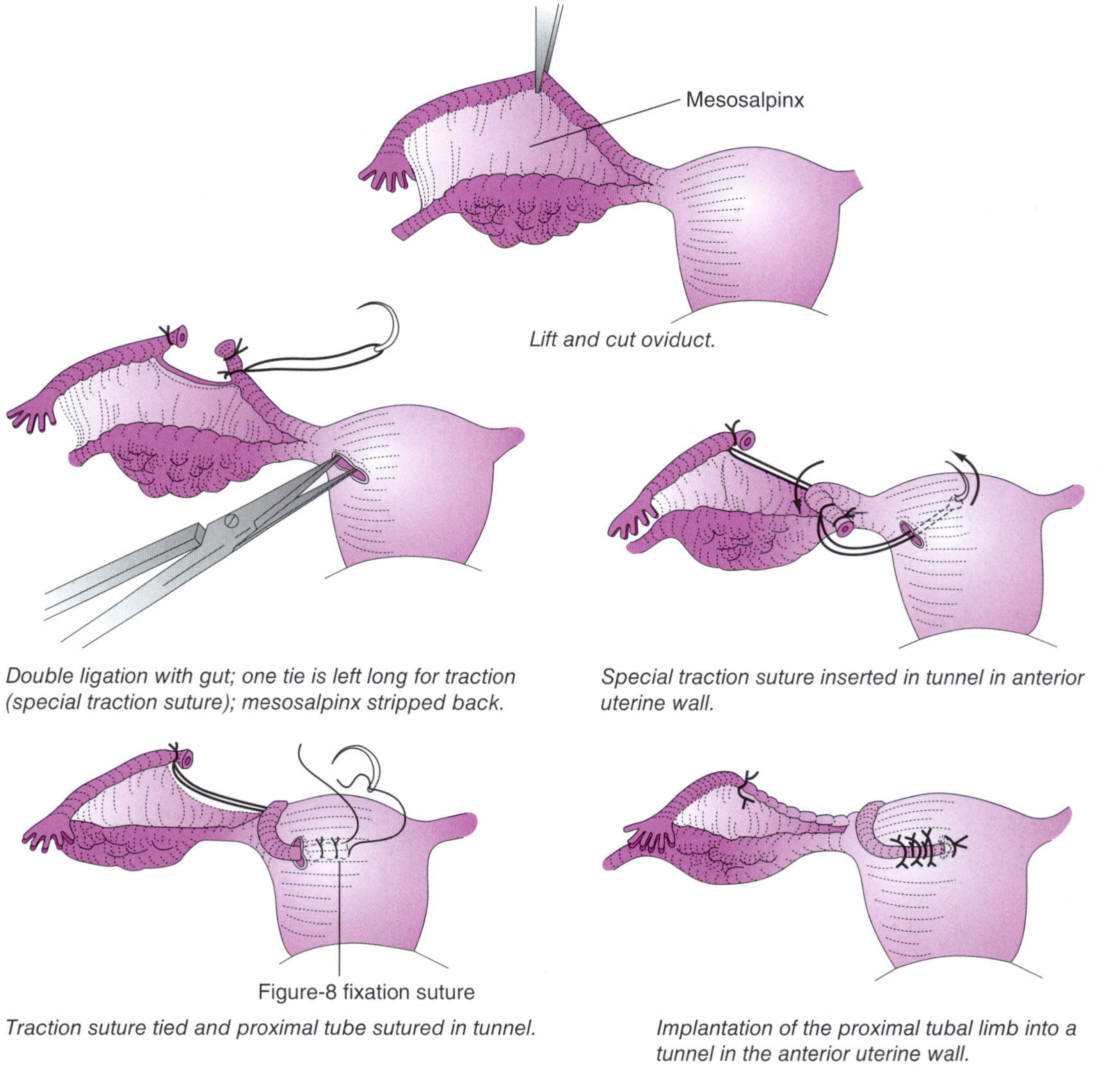

▲ **Figure 46–2.** Irving method of sterilization. (Reproduced, with permission, from Benson RC. *Handbook of Obstetrics & Gynecology*. 8th ed. New York, NY: Lange; 1983.)

tubal ligation via culdotomy or culdoscopy is technically more difficult than transabdominal sterilization and has a higher infection rate. However, there may be less discomfort postoperatively.

VASECTOMY

Vasectomy, or vas occlusion, accounts for 9% of sterilizations in the United States. Partial vasectomy is usually done under local anesthesia via a small incision in the upper outer aspect of the scrotum (Fig. 46–6). Sutures or clips are placed tightly around the vas, demarcating a 1- to 1.5-cm segment, which is then excised. The ligated and fulgurated ends are tucked back into the scrotal sac, and the incision is closed. The same procedure is performed on the opposite side. The no-scalpel technique requires no incision because a sharpened dissection forceps is used to pierce the skin and dissect the vas. Microscopic examination confirms excision of vasal tissue.

Vasectomy is as effective as tubal sterilization with a reported failure rate of <1%. Half of the vasectomy failures in the CREST study occurred within 3 months of the procedure. Thus, sterility is assumed only after ejaculates are completely free of sperm after 3 months and after periodic microscopic analysis.

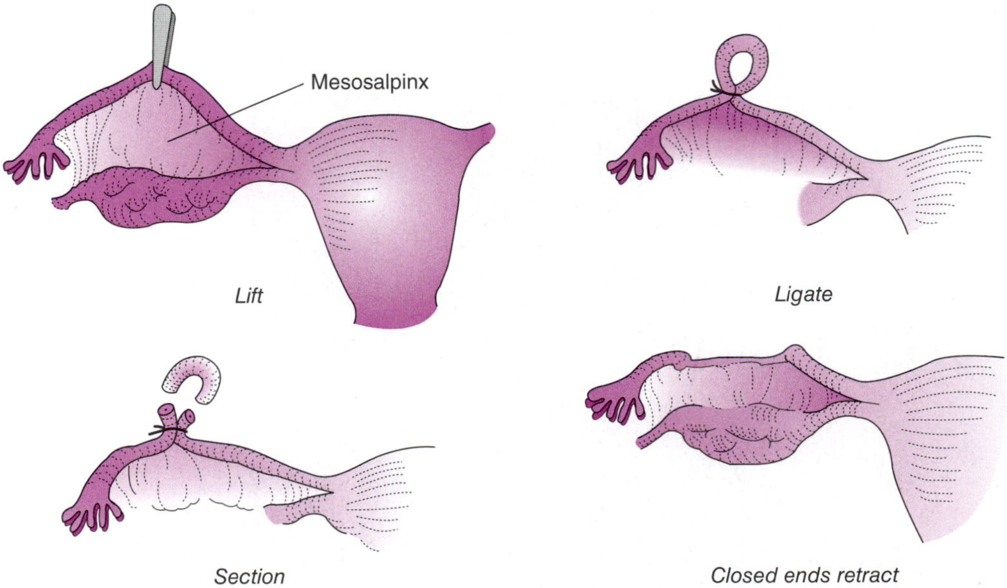

▲ **Figure 46–3.** Pomeroy method of sterilization. (Reproduced, with permission, from Benson RC. *Handbook of Obstetrics & Gynecology*. 8th ed. New York, NY: Lange; 1983.)

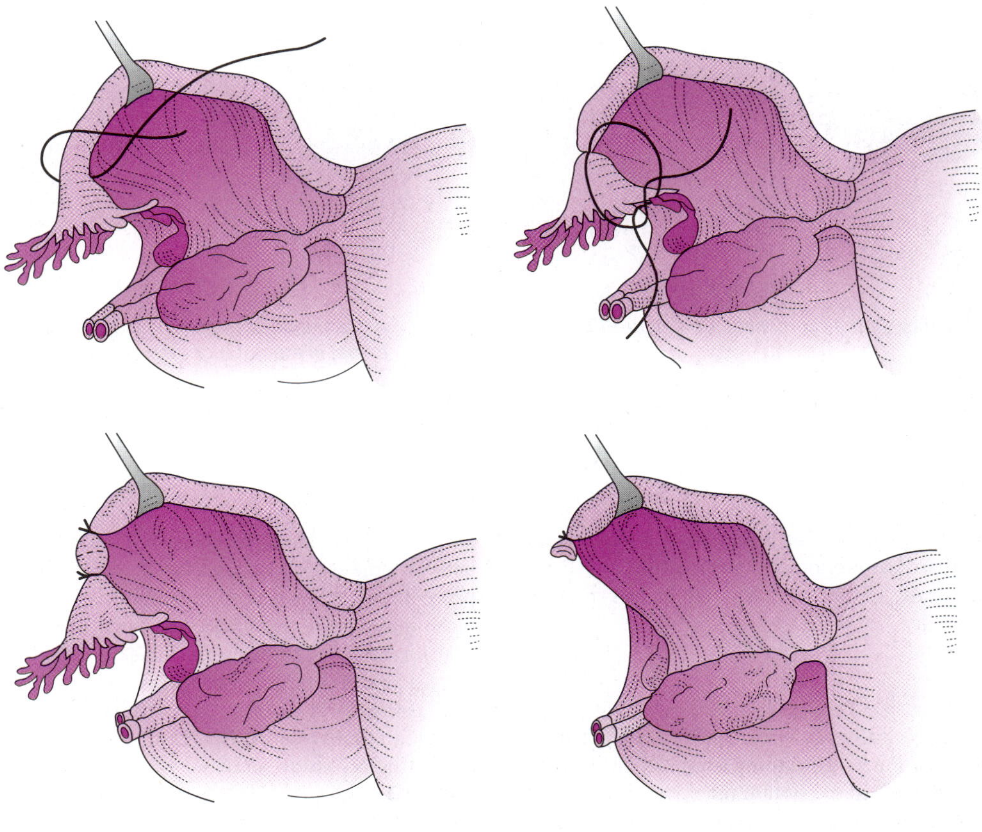

▲ **Figure 46–4.** Sterilization by fimbriectomy.

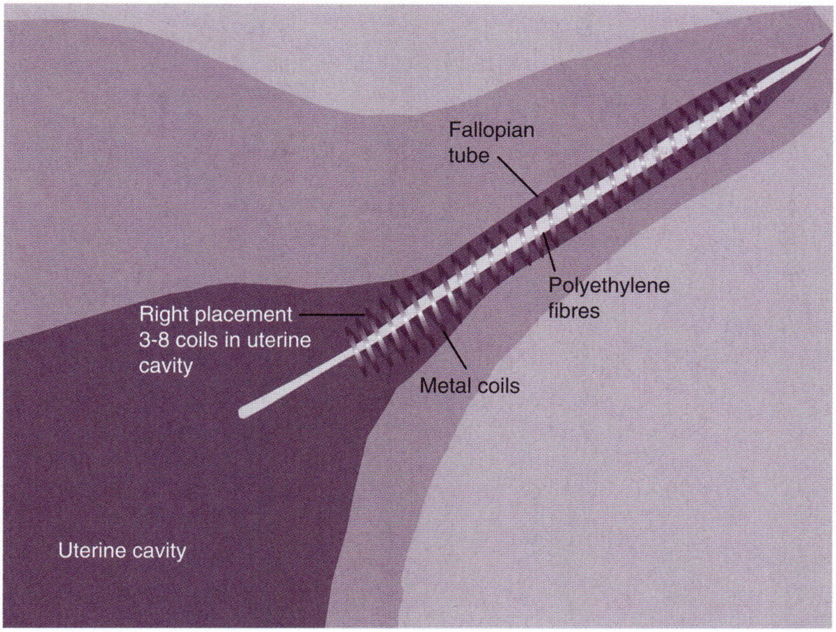

▲ **Figure 46–5.** Hysteroscopic microinsert placement. (Reproduced, with permission, from Hurskainen R, Hovi SL, Gissler M, et al. Hysteroscopic tubal sterilization: Systematic review of the Essure system. *Fertil Steril* 2010;94:16–19.)

Complications are infrequent, usually involving slight bleeding, hematoma formation, skin infection, and reactions to sutures or local anesthetics.

American College of Obstetricians and Gynecologists. Benefits and risks of sterilization. ACOG Practice Bulletin No. 46. *Obstet Gynecol* 2003;102:647–658. PMID: 12962966.

Hurskainen R, Hovi S-L, Gissler M, et al. Hysteroscopic tubal sterilization: a systematic review of the Essure system. *Fertil Steril* 2010;94:16–19. PMID: 19409549.

Jamieson DJ, Costello C, Trussel J, et al. The risk of pregnancy after vasectomy. *Obstet Gynecol* 2004;103:848–850. PMID: 15121555.

Peterson HB, Xia Z, Hughes JM, et al. The risk of pregnancy after tubal sterilization: findings from the U.S. Collaborative Review of Sterilization. *Am J Obstet Gynecol* 1996;174:1161–1168. PMID: 8623843.

Van Voorhis BJ. Comparison of tubal reversal procedures. *Clin Obstet Gynecol* 2000;43:641–649. PMID: 10949765.

HYSTERECTOMY

Hysterectomy is complete surgical removal of the uterus. It is the most common gynecologic surgery and second most common major operation performed in the United States with over 600,000 hysterectomies performed between 2003 and 2004. With advancements in medical and conservative surgical therapy of gynecologic conditions, the need for hysterectomy has declined, with small decreases in rates between 1997 and 2004. More women now wish to avoid major surgery if equally efficacious alternatives exist. Regulatory boards of gynecologists now support the use of hysterectomy as treatment for conditions refractory to more conservative management.

Indications

The indications for hysterectomy can be practically divided into those for the treatment of gynecologic cancer, benign gynecologic conditions, and obstetric complications. Hysterectomy for cancer of the uterus, ovary, and cervix is discussed in Chapters 47–50. Hysterectomy for obstetric complications, including excessive bleeding and molar pregnancy, is becoming less common (see Chapter 21).

The most common benign diseases and disorders (the indication for >90% of surgeries) that warrant hysterectomy are shown in Table 46–4.

Preoperative Evaluation

A. Diagnostic Tests to Detect Occult Cancer

Prior to hysterectomy, all patients should have a baseline evaluation to detect occult cancer. A Pap smear should be performed within 3 months before operation, and abnormalities should be followed with colposcopic examination with biopsy and endocervical curettage before surgery.

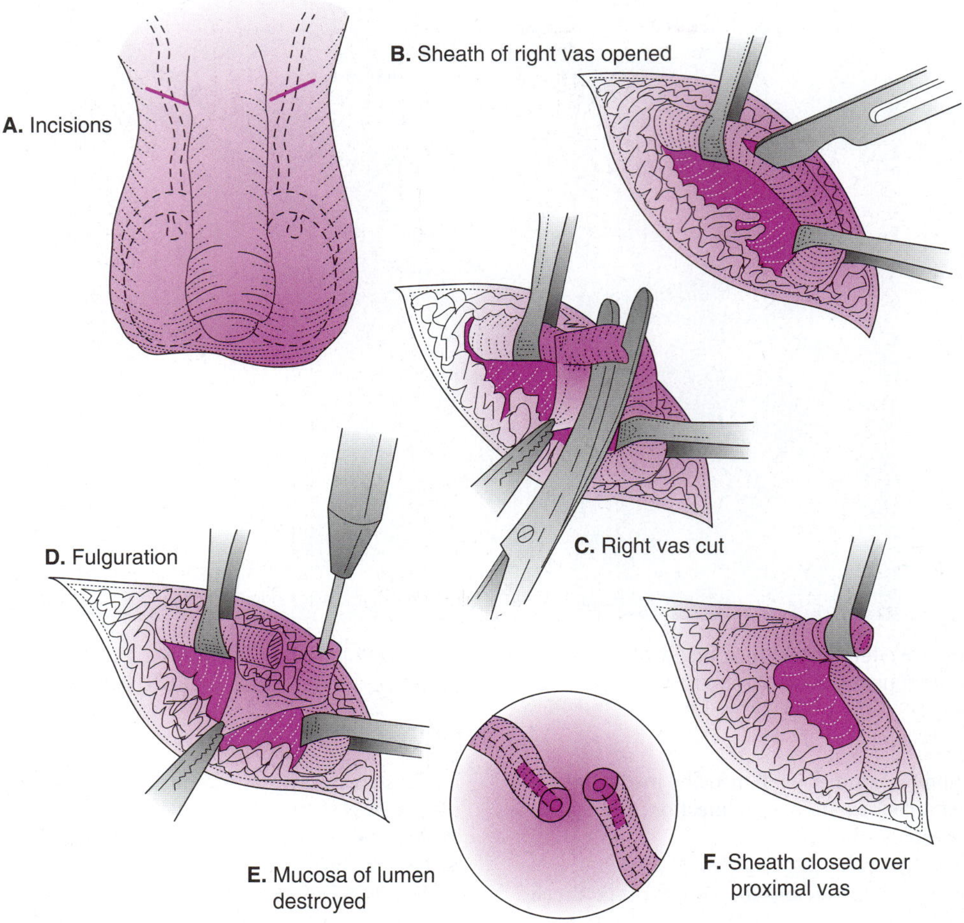

▲ **Figure 46–6.** Steps in vasectomy. (Modified with permission from a drawing by S. Taft. Reproduced, with permission, from Schmidt S. Vasectomy should not fail. *Contemp Surg* 1974;4:13)

Cervical conization is indicated prior to hysterectomy if (1) colposcopy fails to demonstrate the entire squamocolumnar junction, where cervical cancers typically arise; (2) colposcopically guided biopsies reveal cervical intraepithelial neoplasia I or less after a preceding high-grade squamous intraepithelial lesion Pap smear; (3) endocervical curettage demonstrates atypical endocervical cells; and (4) biopsy reveals microinvasive squamous cell carcinoma or squamous adenocarcinoma in situ. Cervical conization for the last scenario is performed to ensure that occult invasive cancer is not present. Frozen-section analysis of cervical conization tissue correlates well enough with "permanent" (hematoxylin and eosin) slide analysis that if intraepithelial neoplasia with clear margins is found, the surgeon may, with reasonable certainty, perform a hysterectomy that will totally include the tumor.

Biopsy for endometrial neoplasia must also be considered in certain clinical scenarios. Generally any woman over age 35 who presents with abnormal uterine bleeding should undergo endometrial evaluation (endometrial biopsy with pipelle, D&C, or hysteroscopy with directed biopsies) before hysterectomy. However, certain clinical situations that produce an unopposed estrogen effect on the endometrium warrant preoperative endometrial evaluation at any age: chronic anovulation and secondary oligomenorrhea, unopposed estrogen therapy for menopause, and known ovarian disorders associated with endometrial neoplasia (eg, polycystic ovarian syndrome, granulosa cell tumors). Unfortunately, frozen-section analysis of endometrial curettings is neither practical nor accurate, so hysterectomy usually must wait for permanent section.

Table 46–4. Benign diseases and disorders for which hysterectomy may be performed.

Uterine leiomyomas Symptomatic (abnormal bleeding or pelvic pressure) Asymptomatic (presenting as a large uterus obscuring palpation of the adnexa and ultrasound unavailable) Rapid growth of uterus (suspected leiomyosarcoma) Failed conservative management of abnormal bleeding or uterine pain
Symptomatic adenomyosis refractory to medical management
Symptomatic endometriosis refractory to conservative surgical or medical management
Symptomatic pelvic organ prolapse
Chronic incapacitating central pelvic pain disorder refractory to conservative treatment in a woman with a normal urologic and gastrointestinal evaluation
Definite treatment of severe pelvic inflammatory disease if conservative therapy is not possible or desired by the patient

Occult cancer may also be present outside the genital tract. All patients should have their stool checked for occult blood preoperatively. In women 40 years of age or older, mammography is standard.

B. Preoperative Evaluation of the Pelvis

In the woman with a small, mobile uterus with mobile adnexa, little diagnostic evaluation beyond bimanual examination is indicated. However, pelvic disease may have caused disturbance of normal tissue planes that endanger the urologic and gastrointestinal tracts. The following conditions may indicate the need for more extensive evaluation of the pelvis prior to hysterectomy: (1) pelvic inflammatory disease, especially if repeated, chronic, or associated with a tubo-ovarian complex; (2) endometriosis; (3) pelvic adhesions due to other causes of pelvic inflammation (eg, appendicitis, cholecystitis, previous pelvic surgery); (4) chronic pelvic pain; (5) questionable origin of a palpable pelvic mass; and (6) clinical suspicion of cancer (eg, palpable adnexa in a postmenopausal woman).

The most commonly used preoperative adjunctive diagnostic evaluation is pelvic ultrasound, which has advantages over computed tomography (CT) scan. Ultrasound is helpful in detecting masses in the difficult-to-examine patient (eg, obese) and in confirming a pelvic mass detected on bimanual examination.

Intravenous pyelography (IVP) or CT urogram is helpful in delineating the course of the ureters through the pelvis especially in the setting of inflammatory conditions that could distort or obstruct the ureters. Also, patients with known genital developmental anomalies should have preoperative imaging to look for concomitant urologic anomalies.

Prehysterectomy evaluation of the colon (beyond screening for occult blood in the stool) is indicated in any patient with symptoms for rectal disease. In most cases, proctoscopy or flexible proctosigmoidoscopy is sufficient. In cases of severe pelvic inflammation, chronic pelvic pain, or suspected cancer, complete colonoscopy or barium enema is indicated. Preoperative diagnosis of bowel disease will aid in the selection of the incision. If necessary, a consultant gastrointestinal surgeon can be present during the operation.

C. Preoperative Bowel Preparation

Preoperative bowel preparation is not required prior to hysterectomy. It has been a common practice in the past to use a mechanical bowel preparation prior to hysterectomy in patients where the likelihood of bowel injury is high. However, recent data in the colorectal literature have refuted these practices. Preoperative mechanical bowel preparation is associated with increased spillage of bowel contents during elective colon resection and leads to a higher rate of anastomotic leaks and wound infections compared to no mechanical bowel preparation.

D. Prophylactic Antibiotics

The incidence of febrile morbidity is approximately 14% in patients undergoing hysterectomy. Certain risk factors are associated with a higher likelihood of operative site infection. These factors include an abdominal surgical approach, blood loss greater than 750 mL, and no preoperative antibiotics. ACOG also recommends giving additional doses of intraoperative antibiotics during lengthy operations, given at intervals of 1 or 2 half-lives of the drug. A second dose of the prophylactic antibiotic may also be given in surgical cases with a blood loss >1500 mL. Patients diagnosed with a vaginal infection during preoperative evaluation should be treated prior to surgery.

A broad-spectrum antibiotic should be chosen that is effective against common (but not necessarily *all*) pathogens causing pelvic infection. The agent should have a low incidence of toxicity and side effects and should be easily administered and cost-effective. The proper dosage should be administered 30 minutes prior to incision to achieve therapeutic levels in tissue at the surgical site. It should *not* be an antibiotic reserved for serious infection. ACOG recommends intravenous (IV) cefazolin (1–2 g IV), clindamycin (600 mg IV), plus either gentamicin 1.5 mg/kg IV) or quinolone (400 mg IV) or aztreonam (1 g IV), or metronidazole (500 mg IV) plus gentamicin (1.5 mg/kg IV) or quinolone (400 mg IV) prior to vaginal or abdominal hysterectomy.

E. Thromboembolism Prophylaxis

Hysterectomy is a major surgical procedure, carrying at least a moderate risk of thromboembolism. The risk of calf vein thrombosis, proximal vein thrombosis, and pulmonary embolism can be minimized with the use of graduated compression stockings perioperatively and early ambulation postoperatively. Sequential compression devices will help prevent stasis as well. Compression stockings and devices should be in use prior to administration of anesthesia for optimal effect. For patients at high risk for thromboembolic disease, a dose of 5000 U subcutaneous heparin is given preoperatively and then every 8–12 hours postoperatively while in the hospital. Risk factors include malignancy, obesity, previous radiation therapy, immobilization, estrogen use, prolonged anesthesia, radical surgery, history of thromboembolism, nephrotic syndrome, HIV, and personal or family history of hypercoagulability (inherited thrombophilia). Low-molecular-weight heparin may also be used postoperatively.

F. Blood Products

It is not necessary to preoperatively cross-match all patients undergoing hysterectomy. Women who are not at particular risk of needing a transfusion during hysterectomy should at least have blood typing and antibody screening prior to surgery. Patients undergoing peripartum hysterectomy or hysterectomy for gynecologic cancer are more likely to need blood transfusion. Patients undergoing elective hysterectomy are more likely to need a transfusion if the starting hematocrit is low (30%), if they have pelvic inflammatory disease or pelvic abscess or adhesions, or if colporrhaphy is performed at the time of vaginal hysterectomy.

G. Informed Consent

Many women desire, and most insurance companies require, a second opinion prior to scheduling an elective hysterectomy. The patient must understand the diagnosis and be aware of alternative therapies (medical or conservative surgical options) and the risks and benefits of the operation. Common risks of surgery such as wound infection, cuff cellulitis, and blood loss are usually explained during preoperative counseling. The current medicolegal climate mandates the discussion of unusual complications, including the possibility of completing a vaginal or laparoscopic operation via an abdominal route and the risks of viral illness following transfusion, severe postoperative infection (including adnexal abscess), and vaginal vault prolapse.

Technique

A. Vaginal Versus Abdominal Hysterectomy

The route of hysterectomy is chosen according to the following guidelines.

1. Pelvic anatomy—The ideal candidate for vaginal hysterectomy has a gynecoid pelvis with a wide pubic arch and a vaginal apex >2 fingerbreadths at the apex. Some descent of the uterus is helpful but not mandatory; procidentia makes for a more complicated vaginal hysterectomy because of the greater vulnerability of the prolapsed ureters.

2. Uterine size—Most gynecologists will perform vaginal hysterectomy on a uterus equivalent in size to a uterus at 12 weeks' gestation or smaller or a uterine weight of <280 g. More experienced surgeons have successfully removed uteri of up to 1200 g vaginally using bivalve and morcellation techniques.

3. Adnexa—In patients with symptoms or pelvic findings suggesting adnexal disease that may indicate adnexectomy, the abdominal route for hysterectomy is preferred. In addition, most surgeons offer patients the option of prophylactic removal of the ovaries after age 45 years old to decrease the risk of ovarian cancer, in spite of the lack of supporting evidence. Such patients may still undergo vaginal removal or laparoscopic-assisted vaginal hysterectomy if otherwise a good candidate for these routes.

4. Gastrointestinal tract—Especially in older patients or those with significant history of gastrointestinal complaints, the abdominal approach offers an opportunity for complete examination of the bowel.

5. Urologic disorders—Symptomatic or potential stress urinary incontinence can be treated vaginally (suburethral sling) or abdominally (retropubic urethropexy; see Chapter 42). The route of the hysterectomy should depend on the size of the uterus and not on the planned surgical procedure for the incontinence.

6. Pelvic organ prolapse—Pelvic organ prolapse can be treated via a vaginal, laparoscopic, robotic, or abdominal approach, and the choice of route is often surgeon dependent (see Chapter 42)

7. Medical disorders—In patients with significant heart or lung disease, the vaginal or laparoscopic approach is preferable when possible because of a lower incidence of postoperative pulmonary complications and earlier ambulation.

8. Previous surgery—Most surgeons are willing to perform a vaginal hysterectomy in patients with previous tubal ligation or caesarean section. The surgery would be more problematic in patients with a history of multiple caesarean births or complications (eg, postpartum endomyometritis) or with probable abdominal adhesions from previous laparotomy. Laparoscopic-assisted vaginal hysterectomy may be used in these situations.

The preceding guidelines may certainly be adjusted to the individual patient based on the surgeon's experience and abilities. An examination performed under anesthesia when the physician first sees the patient may help to decide on the approach. Uterine size can be assessed with transvaginal ultrasound. Laparoscopic evaluation of the adnexa will further aid in the decision. All patients anticipating vaginal hysterectomy, laparoscopic hysterectomy, or laparoscopic-assisted vaginal hysterectomy should be told that the operation may have to be completed abdominally if difficulties arise.

B. Abdominal Hysterectomy

The technique of abdominal hysterectomy varies according to the indication for the operation, the size and placement of vital structures including the ureters (which may be distorted), and the pelvic anatomy. A standard, well-organized approach to abdominal hysterectomy is essential to avoid incidental injury. Modifications are made as necessary, always within an organized plan of operation.

The anesthetic of choice typically includes general endotracheal intubation, an inhalation agent, and an analgesic. Hysterectomies are of such duration and risk that using a mask alone is unwise. In patients with pulmonary compromise, spinal or epidural anesthesia may be used.

A sterile scrub of the abdomen and vagina is done, and a urinary catheter is placed so that the anesthesiologist can monitor urine output intraoperatively. The choice of incision is based on the suspected disease, prior surgeries/incisions, patient preference, and uterine size; in general, a midline incision extending from 2 fingerbreadths above the pubic symphysis to the umbilicus offers the greatest exposure. One modification of the low transverse incision to improve exposure is the Maylard muscle-splitting procedure or the Cherney detachment of the rectus muscles from their insertion on the pubic symphysis. For an uncomplicated hysterectomy with a small uterus, a Pfannenstiel incision is usually sufficient.

The surgeon and assistants should rinse excessive talcum powder from their gloves before making the incision to prevent granulomatous tissue reaction in the wound. Once the incision is complete, peritoneal fluid may be aspirated if the possibility of gynecologic cancer exists. The pelvic organs are then inspected and the upper abdomen palpated in a systematic fashion: right gutter, right hemidiaphragm, liver, gallbladder, pancreas, stomach (assessing the position of the indwelling gastric decompression tube if present), and spleen and right hemidiaphragm (gently, because of the risk of trauma to the spleen), left gutter, para-aortic lymph nodes, and omentum. Excessive bowel manipulation should be avoided to decrease the severity of postoperative adynamic ileus; at the least, the appendix and cecum should be inspected as well as the terminal meter of ileum. Older patients and those with gastrointestinal complaints would benefit from careful palpation and inspection of the bowel from rectum to ligament of Treitz. If desired, the wound may be protected with moist towels, a self-retaining retractor placed, and the bowel packed into the upper abdomen.

The classic extrafascial hysterectomy performed by Richardson remains the mainstay of surgical technique in abdominal hysterectomy. Choice of suture and needle is made according to surgeon experience and preference; 2-0, 0, or 1 absorbable sutures on half-curved taper needles are standard choices. The uterus is grasped either by the fundus with a Massachusetts double-toothed clamp or at the cornua with Ochsner or Kocher clamps. The round ligament is grasped proximal to the uterus; at its midportion, it is ligated by suture, and the suture is tagged with a small hemostat. The round ligament is divided about 0.5 cm proximal to the suture, thus opening the broad ligament at its apex. The anterior uterine peritoneum may be incised at the vesicouterine junction in preparation for advancement of the bladder. The peritoneum only should be incised; the potentially vascular areolar tissue should be avoided. When this procedure is repeated on the contralateral side, the anterior leaves of the broad ligament are opened; the uterine vessels first become apparent. Attention is then directed to the posterior leaf of the broad ligament.

The posterior leaf of the broad ligament is incised beginning at the ligated round ligament. The extent of the incision is determined by the decision to preserve or remove the adnexa. If the adnexa are to be removed, the peritoneum is incised parallel to the infundibulopelvic ligament to the pelvic sidewall; the loose areolar tissue is dissected medial to the internal iliac (hypogastric) artery, which is typically 0.5 cm thick with a visually appreciable (and certainly palpable) pulse. The dissection will reveal a clear area of peritoneum under the infundibulopelvic ligament; below this area at a variable distance lays the ureter on this medial leaf of peritoneum.

The intimate proximity of the ureters to the uterus makes ureteral identification important. Whereas the ureter is usually 4–6 cm deep to the infundibulopelvic ligament at the lateral margin of the uterus, it is only 0.5–2 cm below this vascular bundle at the level of the pelvic brim. Observing the ureter through the peritoneum or palpating the characteristic "snap" of the ureter should serve only to guide dissection and should not be a substitute for identification of the entire ureter through its pelvic course. The ureter tolerates careful dissection well as long as its blood-carrying adventitia is not stripped away. The ureter can always be found and dissection begun at the pelvic brim, where the ureter passes over the bifurcation of the iliac artery. The most serious ureteral injury is the unrecognized insult. The most common ureteral injuries during hysterectomy occur during ligation of the infundibulopelvic ligament, clamping and suture ligation of the uterosacral–cardinal ligament complex, placement of vaginal angle sutures, ligation of the vesicouterine ligament, ligation of the hypogastric artery as an adjunctive measure to lessen operative blood loss, and reperitonealization of the pelvic floor.

Once the course of the ureters is well established, the adnexal component of the operation is completed. If the adnexa are to be removed, the infundibulopelvic ligament is clamped, divided, and double ligated. The ligament may then be ligated again adjacent to the uterus to avoid back bleeding; the infundibulopelvic ligament is divided and the peritoneum incised to the back of the uterine fundus, always cognizant of the proximity of the ureter. If the adnexa are to be preserved, a hole is made in the avascular portion of the posterior leaf of the broad ligament superior to the ureter. The utero-ovarian ligament and fallopian tube are doubly clamped, divided, and ligated, with care taken to avoid incorporation of ovarian tissue into the ligature.

The peritoneal incision can be extended posteriorly around the uterus between the medial portions of the uterosacral ligaments. If the incision of the posterior leaf of the broad ligament is extended over the uterosacral ligaments, there is typically significant bleeding just lateral to the insertion of the ligament at the uterus. The advantages of making an incision between the uterosacral ligaments include clear identification of the rectum and its separation from the uterus, ease of suturing the vaginal cuff, and improved mobility of the peritoneum to allow reperitonealization under less tension.

The bladder is advanced down off of the lower uterine segment prior to clamping the uterine vessels. Surgeons-in-training have more difficulty with advancement of the bladder than with other aspects of abdominal hysterectomy. The principal difficulty in mobilization of the bladder is failure to identify the proper cleavage plane between the bladder and the uterus. At the attachment of the bladder to the lower uterine segment, a median raphe is variably present; it is typically a 1-cm long longitudinal band of thick connective tissue. The raphe is attenuated in pregnant or postmenopausal patients. The raphe is divided at midportion, and loose avascular fibroareolar tissue is seen immediately between the cervix and bladder. The uterus is retracted posteriorly and superiorly, roughly at an angle of 30 degrees to the long axis of the vagina. The midpoint of the peritoneal incision of the bladder flap is gently lifted with forceps; the avascular plane of the vesicovaginal and vesicocervical areolar spaces is continuous once the median raphe is divided. Metzenbaum scissors are pointed to the uterus, and sharp dissection reveals the shiny white pubocervical fascia overlying the cervix. Properly done, the dissection is bloodless, and the plane is recognized by the ease with which the bladder falls away from the cervix. The vesicouterine space is developed 2 cm beyond the anterior vaginal fornix. Care must be exercised in any dissection laterally, because the vesicouterine ligaments ("bladder pillars") may bleed because of the paracervical and paravaginal veins present laterally.

The uterine vessels may be skeletonized by separating the loose avascular areolar connective tissue from the vessels. The intraligamentous course of the ureter is again checked; it is typically 2–3 cm inferolateral to the insertion of the uterine vessels into the uterus. The uterine vessels are clamped with a curved crushing clamp (eg, Heaney, Zeppelin, or curved Ballantine clamp). Double clamping may be used for larger vessels. It is not necessary to place another clamp on the uterine side of the pedicle to prevent back bleeding if the uterine arteries on both sides of the uterus are clamped before either pedicle is incised. The clamp is applied at the level of the internal os, with the tip of the clamp at a right angle to the long axis of the cervix; the temptation to clamp the entire cervix and "slide off" dragging paracervical tissue into the pedicle should be avoided in order to minimize the risk of the pedicle slipping out of the clamp. The uterine vessels are then ligated by suture at the tip of the clamp. Occasionally, a second application of the curved clamp is necessary to complete ligation of the uterine vessels.

Next, the cardinal ligament is assessed. On occasion, a single application of a straight clamp (Ochsner, Kocher, or Ballantine clamp) will include the cardinal ligament to the level of its attachment at the lateral edge of the cervix and upper vagina. However, with an elongated cervix, multiple pedicles need to be taken before the upper vagina is encountered. A deep knife is often useful in dividing the cardinal ligament adjacent to the uterus, leaving a larger pedicle, which is less likely to slip out of the suture than one remaining after cutting with scissors flush to the clamp. The uterosacral ligaments are clamped at their insertion into the lower cervix, divided at their insertion, and ligated. Alternatively, they may be transected with large Mayo scissors while the vagina is entered posterolaterally. If division and suture ligation of either pedicle of the cardinal–uterosacral ligament complex fails to enter the vagina, the safest approach is to enter the vagina with the knife in the midline, either anteriorly or posteriorly, at the confluence of the vagina with cervix. Once entered, the cervix is circumferentially incised, with long Ochsner clamps used to control point bleeders and elevate the vaginal cuff. The vaginal cuff can also be cross-clamped with a curved clamp (Heaney or Zeppelins) from either side just below the cervix and amputated with Jorgenson's scissors. The cervix is inspected to ensure complete excision. If the cervix is amputated without cross-clamping the vagina, sutures are placed at each lateral vaginal angle to ligate small paravaginal vessels coursing upward through the paravaginal tissues and to provide vaginal vault support. The suture is begun inside the vagina 1 cm from the upper border, then incorporates the cardinal and uterosacral ligaments, and finally transverses the vagina again to end up within the vagina. This suture is tagged, and the procedure is repeated on the contralateral side.

Surgical management of the cuff is individualized. In the case of marked pelvic inflammation and persistent oozing, the cuff may be left open to afford retroperitoneal drainage or allow egress of a closed drain system. In most cases, closing the cuff may reduce granulation tissue and possibly minimize ascension of bacteria from the vagina. The cuff may be closed with either interrupted figure-of-eight sutures or a double running suture; the key points with either closure are inversion of the cut edges into the vagina and hemostasis. If the vagina apex is cross-clamped prior to amputating the cervix, the cuff is closed with either a Heaney suture placed at the tip of each clamp, or with a running suture over each clamp. If a defect remains at the middle of the cuff, this can be closed with interrupted or figure-of-eight sutures.

The pelvis is irrigated and hemostasis checked in a systematic fashion from one lateral pedicle to the ipsilateral round ligament pedicle to the cuff and on to the other side. Small bleeding vessels must be ligated to minimize the risk of retroperitoneal hematoma formation, which may expand or become infected. For diffuse oozing, hemostatic agents such as thrombin powder or thrombostatic absorbable sponges may be useful. There is no advantage to closing the parietal peritoneum. Retained ovaries may be suspended to minimize the risk of torsion and adherence to the vaginal cuff. The utero-ovarian ligament can be conveniently attached to the round ligament stump to suspend the ovaries above the pelvis without placing the infundibulopelvic ligament under tension.

The abnormal appendix should be removed. In cases of hysterectomy for endometriosis, appendectomy will reveal microscopic endometriotic foci in some 3% of cases.

C. Supracervical Hysterectomy

Supracervical/subtotal hysterectomy, or removal of the uterine corpus without the cervix, made up 95% of hysterectomies prior to the 1940s. Despite Papanicolaou's introduction of his cervical smear, concern over neoplastic changes occurring in the retained cervix made total abdominal hysterectomy (TAH) the leading approach to surgery from the 1950s and on. Several studies have addressed the debate about which approach leads to decreased morbidity. Proponents of supracervical hysterectomy believe that there is less damage to sympathetic and parasympathetic innervation that might occur with paracervical dissection. Thus, bladder function and orgasm are less likely to be affected with supracervical hysterectomy. However, 2 randomized controlled trials assessing psychosocial outcome and resultant sexual function found no difference between the 2 groups. A meta-analysis failed to detect a significant difference in stress or urge incontinence after supracervical versus total hysterectomy. Another randomized, double-blind, controlled trial showed no statistically significant difference in bladder, bowel, and sexual function between women who had undergone total versus supracervical hysterectomy. It has also been proposed that by leaving the cervix, vault prolapse and vaginal shortening might be avoided. Yet, a recent study performed on cadavers found equal resistance to forces applied to the vaginal apex after supracervical and total hysterectomy.

Those in favor of TAH suggest that it decreases the risk of cervical cancer, especially in women who might not follow up for routine Pap smears. In fact, a malignant or premalignant condition of the cervix or uterine corpus is an absolute contraindication to a supracervical hysterectomy. It also eliminates the small risk of cyclical bleeding (6.8%) that can occur after supracervical hysterectomy if residual endometrium is left behind.

Supracervical hysterectomy does decrease length of surgery, blood loss, and febrile morbidity. Current indications for supracervical hysterectomy include difficulty dissecting the cervix, distorted anatomy secondary to pelvic inflammatory disease or endometriosis, and compromised medical condition.

Following ligation of the uterine vessels, the uterine fundus may be amputated from the cervix; the level of amputation should be below the internal cervical os to avoid postoperative uterine bleeding from endometrial remnants. The endocervical canal can be resected or ablated to further avoid cyclical bleeding. The cervical stump is closed with figure-of-eight sutures.

D. Vaginal Hysterectomy

Vaginal hysterectomies are performed under general or regional anesthesia. Following administration of the anesthetic, a bimanual examination is mandatory before beginning surgery. The perineum is shaved or trimmed as necessary and a sterile wash performed. The patient is placed in a low lithotomy position and draped; the surgeon should participate in proper positioning of the patient, because excessive flexion of the hips can stretch the sciatic nerve and compress the femoral nerve and excessive extension of the knee can jeopardize the peroneal nerves. All bony prominences and soft tissues in contact with the leg stirrups should be carefully padded.

The urinary bladder may be drained by catheter, but this step is optional. The cervix is grasped with a tenaculum. As the surgeon exerts gentle traction downward on the cervix, 2 assistants maintain exposure with lateral vaginal retractors and protect the bladder with an anterior Heaney retractor. If desired, the junction of the vagina and cervix can be injected with a 1% 1:1000 epinephrine solution to minimize blood loss during incision of the cervix. Beginning posteriorly to minimize obscuring the field with blood, the surgeon circumferentially incises the cervix down to the level of the pubovesicocervical fascia. Gentle traction with the bladder retractor and downward traction of the cervix will allow exposure of the fibers of fascia between bladder and cervix, which are incised. When the bladder has been advanced up off of the cervix, attention is given to the posterior attachment of the cervix. While the assistant pulls the uterus upward, the posterior vaginal mucosa is tented away from the cervix. With the patient in the Trendelenburg position to allow as much emptying of the posterior cul-de-sac as possible, the posterior cul-de-sac is incised with a single stroke of the scissors. A retractor is placed within the opening, exposing the uterosacral ligaments. The uterosacral ligaments are grasped with Heaney clamps, making certain that the peritoneum posterior to the ligament is within the clamp. The ligament is cut and ligated with 2-0 or 0 absorbable suture and tagged with a hemostat for later manipulation of the cuff.

The cardinal ligament may next be clamped if the bladder is safely advanced; likewise, the uterine vessels are included in the next application of the Heaney clamps. The anterior cul-de-sac is entered by blunt and sharp dissection to the anterior vesicouterine fold of peritoneum. The anterior retractor is placed within this opening, and the bladder is gently lifted upward. The surgeon now clamps, incises, and ligates in pedicles the remaining portions of the broad ligaments bilaterally, incorporating the tissue between the anterior and posterior leaves of the broad ligament. The round ligament, utero-ovarian ligament, and fallopian tube are excised from the uterus and incorporated into these pedicles, and the uterus is removed from the field. A larger uterus may require special manipulation for delivery through the vaginal introitus (eg, bivalving the uterus in the midline, morcellation of the uterus into multiple extractable segments, or myomectomy). Rarely, in the event of a narrow introitus, an episiotomy may be performed to facilitate in the delivery of the uterus. The final suture on the utero-ovarian ligament is tagged to allow careful inspection of the tubes and ovaries. If ovarian disease is suspected or if prophylactic oophorectomy is planned, a clamp is placed above the ovary and uterine tube on the infundibulopelvic ligament for suture ligature, while traction is placed on the last stay suture. The entire ovary must be removed, because an ovarian remnant may become cystic and produce pain many years after the hysterectomy.

Once all pedicles are inspected and found to be hemostatic, some surgeons advocate closing the peritoneum with a running 2-0 absorbable suture, incorporating the cardinal and uterosacral ligament pedicles for support of the vaginal vault. Lateral vaginal angle sutures are placed from the vaginal mucosa at 2 o'clock, inside the cuff and including the uterosacral pedicle, then out through the cuff to the 4 o'clock position. If anterior or posterior colporrhaphy is planned, that operation is completed prior to complete closure of the cuff. The cuff may be closed in either a horizontal or vertical manner, grasping full vaginal thickness, by an interrupted absorbable 0 suture or a running simple suture. One small randomized controlled trial showed improved preservation of vaginal length with vertical closure. The goals of closure are obliteration of the cuff's dead space back to the peritoneum and approximation of the cut edges of the vagina to afford healing and minimize postoperative granulation tissue. Modifications of the just-described technique are made by virtually every gynecologic surgeon based on operative findings and experience. Some surgeons will close the posterior cul-de-sac to prevent development of an enterocele or will shorten the uterosacral ligaments to suspend the vaginal vault. As in abdominal hysterectomy, the cuff can be left open to promote drainage with a running locked absorbable 0 suture. Another technique to drain the closure is insertion of a T-tube above the cuff, which is associated with a demonstrable reduction in postoperative febrile morbidity.

After the operation is completed, the vagina and perineum are gently cleansed. An indwelling bladder catheter is inserted and a vaginal pack may be placed. The patient is returned slowly to the dorsal supine position.

E. Laparoscopic Hysterectomy

The laparoscope can be used to aid vaginal hysterectomy by freeing abdominal adhesions (laparoscopic-assisted vaginal hysterectomy; LAVH) or to free the uterus in its entirety with removal via the vagina with the assistance of uterine manipulators (ie, V-care). Supracervical hysterectomy can also be done laparoscopically with morcellation and removal by culdotomy or through extended trocar sites. Advantages to laparoscopic hysterectomy (LH) include decreased length of hospital stay, decreased postoperative analgesia, and decreased convalescence period. There may be a lower complication rate compared to TAH, but there is no difference versus vaginal hysterectomy. Advantages of LH include the ability to inspect the peritoneal cavity and ovaries. Studies present conflicting data on whether there is a benefit of LH compared to vaginal hysterectomy in respect to hospital stay and blood loss. However, the laparoscopic approach requires significantly more operating time and a well-trained, experienced surgeon. Because of the costs for the endoscopic equipment, LH has been found to be more expensive despite the shorter hospital stay.

Complications with LH include hemorrhage and bowel or urinary tract damage. Conversion to abdominal hysterectomy may occur, especially in cases with large leiomyomas obstructing access to upper pedicles.

Postoperative Care of the Hysterectomy Patient

The details of postoperative care are dictated by the indications for surgery and the individual patient's overall medical condition. General guidelines include the following:

1. A Foley catheter is left indwelling for 24 hours, but ideally not longer to decrease the risk of urinary tract infections.
2. Prophylactic postoperative antibiotics are not necessary unless there is concern for an underlying infection diagnosed at time of surgery.
3. Hydration, 2–3 L/d of balanced electrolyte solution, is given intravenously, depending on blood loss and intraoperative replacement.
4. Sips of water may be given the first night, followed by clear liquids or regular diet on the next postoperative day depending on the patient's appetite. The absence of bowel sounds and flatus should not delay the advancement of diet.

5. Prophylactic heparin therapy, sequential compression device, or antiembolic stockings are used in patients according to risk for thromboembolic complications.
6. Ambulation is begun on the first postoperative day.
7. Adequate analgesia is given parenterally. Once the patient can tolerate a regular diet, she can be switched to oral analgesics.

Complications

Perioperative deaths may be due to cardiac arrest, coronary occlusion, or respiratory paralysis. Postoperative deaths are usually the result of hemorrhage, infection, pulmonary embolus, or intercurrent disease. A recent study of the morbidity of more than 10,000 hysterectomies found the mortality rate to be <0.1% with equal rates in the abdominal, laparoscopic, and vaginal groups. Mortality rates increase with age and medical complications for both vaginal and abdominal hysterectomies.

The bladder may be injured in 1–2% of all hysterectomies. Consequences are slight if the injury is to the dome of the bladder—which is usually the case away from the trigone. Ureteral injury occurs in 0.7–1.7% of abdominal hysterectomies and 0–0.1% of vaginal hysterectomies. The essential point is to recognize urologic injuries and correct them intraoperatively, avoiding the serious postoperative complications that occur from urinary extravasation.

Damage to the bowel occurs in 0.2–0.5% of all hysterectomies. A preoperative mechanical bowel preparation has not been shown to decreased morbidity after bowel resections; however, bowel preparation is preferred for laparoscopic hysterectomy to assist with bowel decompression. Small bowel injuries, assuming no obstruction, can be closed in a single layer or multiple layers depending on surgeon preference. The injury should be closed perpendicular to the long axis of the bowel. If multiple-layer closure is used, an interrupted or running layer of 3-0 silk or absorbable sutures is used to reapproximate the mucosa followed by interrupted 2-0 absorbable or silk sutures in the serosa. Bowel resection and anastomosis may be required for larger injuries. Large bowel injuries are repaired in the same fashion as small bowel injuries. Lack of a mechanical bowel preparation is not an indication for a colostomy. Large injuries may require bowel resection and reanastomosis. After the repair, the pelvis is copiously irrigated and a drain is used by some surgeons.

The most serious postoperative complication is hemorrhage (0.2–2% of patients). Bleeding usually originates at the lateral vaginal angles and is amenable to vaginal resuturing in most cases. Blood products are replaced as needed.

Infection remains the most common complication following hysterectomy. Even with immaculate technique and careful patient selection, the gynecologic surgeon can still expect a 10% rate of postoperative febrile morbidity. A postoperative temperature of 38°C (100.4°F) or higher on 2 consecutive determinations 6 hours apart must be investigated by (1) careful interview of the patient for localizing symptoms (eg, productive cough, intravenous line pain), (2) thorough physical examination (including pelvic examination for inspection and palpation of the cuff), and (3) appropriate laboratory studies (eg, urinalysis, chest x-ray, gram-stained smear of sputum, or complete blood count). Antibiotics are begun only if a focus of infection is identified or highly suspected. Broad-spectrum antibiotics covering anticipated pathogens are prescribed; single-agent semisynthetic penicillins (eg, piperacillin) and cephalosporins (eg, cefoxitin) offer sufficient coverage. In the presence of sepsis, multiagent comprehensive coverage (eg, penicillin, an aminoglycoside, and an anaerobic agent such as clindamycin or metronidazole) must be prescribed.

Granulation of the vaginal vault is part of the normal healing process and is evident on speculum examination in over half of cases. The granulation is rarely troublesome; light cauterization with silver nitrate sticks or electrocautery eliminates the granulation tissue promptly in most cases. Many suggestions have been made on ways to minimize granulation, including management of the cuff (open vs. closed), choice of suture (plain gut vs. chromic vs. newer synthetics), and drainage techniques. The most important common denominator is close apposition of the cut vaginal edges, which can be accomplished with any of the techniques.

American College of Obstetricians and Gynecologists. ACOG Practice Bulletin No. 99: management of abnormal cervical cytology and histology. *Obstet Gynecol* 2008;112:1419–1444. PMID: 19037054.

Candiani M, Izzu S, Bulfoni A, et al. Laparoscopic vs vaginal hysterectomy for benign pathology. *Am J Obstet Gynecol* 2009;200(4):368.e1–7. PMID: 19136094.

Charoenkwan K, Phillipson G, Vutyanich T. Early versus delayed (traditional) oral fluids and food for reducing complications after major abdominal gynaecological surgery. *Cochrane Database Syst Rev* 2007;4:CD004508. PMID: 17943817.

Cosson M, Lambaudie E, Boukerrou M, et al. Vaginal, laparoscopic, or abdominal hysterectomies for benign disorders: immediate and early postoperative complications. *Eur J Obstet Gynecol Reprod Biol* 2001;98:23–26. PMID: 115574137.

Flory N, Bissonnette F, Amsel RT, et al. The psychosocial outcomes of total and subtotal hysterectomy: a randomized controlled trial. *J Sex Med* 2006;3:483–491. PMID: 16681474.

Kovac SR. Transvaginal hysterectomy: rationale and surgical approach. *Obstet Gynecol* 2004;103:1321–1325. PMID: 15172872.

Kuppermann M, Summitt RL, Varner RE, et al. Sexual functioning after total compared with supracervical hysterectomy: a randomized controlled trial. *Obstet Gynecol* 2005;105:1309–1318. PMID: 15932822.

Lethaby A, Ivanova V, Johnson NP. Total versus subtotal hysterectomy for benign gynaecological conditions. *Cochrane Database Syst Rev* 2006;2:CD004993. PMID: 16625620.

Mahajna A, Krausz M, Rosin D, et al. Bowel preparation is associated with spillage of bowel contents in colorectal surgery. *Dis Colon Rectum* 2005;48:1626–1631. PMID: 15981063.

Makinen J, Johansson J, Tomas C, et al. Morbidity of 10,110 hysterectomies by type of approach. *Hum Reprod* 2001;16:-1473–1478. PMID: 11425832.

Peipert JF, Weitzen S, Cruickshank C, et al. Risk factors for febrile morbidity after hysterectomy. *Obstet Gynecol* 2004;103:86–91. PMID: 14704250.

Rahn DD, Marker AC, Corton MM, et al. Does supracervical hysterectomy provide more support to the vaginal apex than total abdominal hysterectomy? *Am J Obstet Gynecol* 2007;197:650.e1–4. PMID: 18060966.

Robert M, Soraisham A, Sauve R. Postoperative urinary incontinence after total abdominal hysterectomy or supracervical hysterectomy: a metaanalysis. *Am J Obstet Gynecol* 2008;198:264.e1–5. PMID: 18199420.

Vassallo BJ, Culpepper C, Segal JL, et al. A randomized trial comparing methods of vaginal closure at vaginal hysterectomy and the effect on vaginal length. *Am J Obstet Gynecol* 2006;195:1805–1808. PMID: 17132483.

Whiteman MK, Hillis SD, Jamieson DJ, et al. Inpatient hysterectomy surveillance in the United States, 2000-2004. *Am J Obstet Gynecol* 2008;198:34.e1–7. PMID: 17981254.

Wille-Jorgensen P, Guenaga KF, Matos D, et al. Pre-operative mechanical bowel cleansing or not? An updated meta-analysis. *Colorectal Dis* 2005;7:304–310. PMID: 15932549.

Wu JM, Wechter ME, Geller EJ, et al. Hysterectomy rates in the United States, 2003. *Obstet Gynecol* 2007;110:1091–1095. PMID: 17989124.

Premalignant & Malignant Disorders of the Vulva & Vagina

47

Amer Karam, MD

PREINVASIVE DISEASE OF THE VULVA

ESSENTIALS OF DIAGNOSIS

- Possibly 1–2% of young women with cervical dysplasia have multifocal disease that tends to involve the upper third of the vagina and the vulva, perineum, and perianal areas—these surfaces arising from a common cloacogenic origin.
- A spectrum of disease may be found ranging from mild dysplasia to carcinoma in situ. Involvement may not be appreciated without careful inspection with and without the green colposcopy filter. Clinically, the appearance of vulvar intraepithelial neoplasia can be quite variable.
- Lesions are typically white and hyperkeratotic, but may also appear gray, pink, or brown.
- Colposcopy and biopsy of any suspicious lesion should be performed and is considered the gold standard for diagnosis.
- An abnormal vascular pattern is most frequently associated with a severe degree of dysplasia, carcinoma in situ, or early invasive disease.

General Considerations

The vulvar skin is 1 component of the anogenital epithelium, extending from the distal vagina to the perineum and perianal skin. The lower genital tract epithelium is of common cloacogenic origin. Neoplasia of the vulvar skin is often associated with multiple foci of dysplasia in the lower genital tract. A strong association exists between sexually transmitted diseases and vulvar intraepithelial neoplasia (VIN), primarily human papillomavirus (HPV), but also human immunodeficiency virus (HIV). Approximately 90% of VIN lesions are positive for HPV; multicentric VIN is primarily associated with high oncogenic risk HPV subtypes such as types 16, 18, and 31, whereas vulvar condylomata and low-grade VIN are frequently associated with low-risk HPV subtypes 6 and 11. Other risk factors include smoking and other genital precancers or cancers. VIN can also be classified into viral and nonviral etiologies. Younger women are more commonly affected by viral VIN than older women and are also more likely to exhibit multifocal disease. The incidence of VIN has increased over the past decade due to the increased incidence of HPV infections in young women. The incidence of vulvar carcinoma has increased as well but at a relatively slower rate. The long-term risk of malignant transformation of treated VIN III has been estimated at 3.4–7%, and the risk for progression of untreated VIN is thought to be higher.

Premalignant lesions of the vulva occur in both premenopausal and postmenopausal women, with the median age being approximately 40 years. The average age is shifting toward younger women, with 75% of lesions occurring during the premenopausal period. There is no racial predisposition to VIN, and the disease process is often asymptomatic. The most common presenting symptom is pruritus, which is seen in more than 60% of patients with VIN. The diagnosis is made by careful inspection of the vulvar area followed by biopsy of suspicious lesions.

Pathogenesis

Previously, the standard for reporting of vulvar dysplastic lesions was to classify VIN according to the degree of epithelial cellular maturation, with VIN I defined as immature cells occurring in the lower one-third of the epithelium and VIN III as complete loss of cellular maturation in the full thickness of epithelium, which is synonymous with carcinoma in situ of the vulva or Bowen's disease. VIN II was designated as intermediate between VIN I and VIN III. In 2004, the International Congress of the International Society for the Study of Vulvar Disease (ISSVD) recommended that the

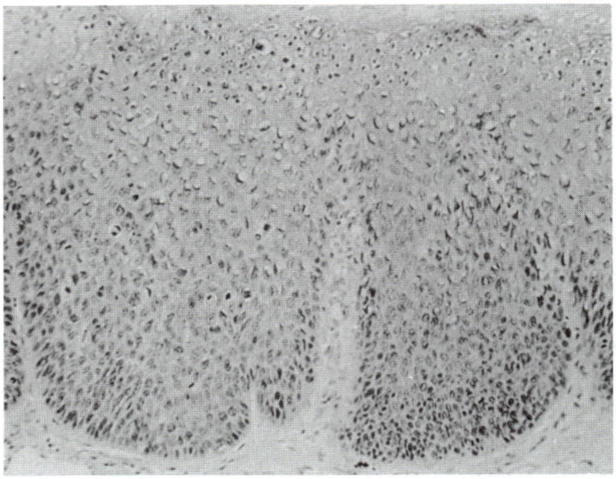

▲ **Figure 47–1.** Carcinoma in situ demonstrating hyperkeratosis, acanthosis, and parakeratosis. The rete ridges are elongated and thickened, and individual cells are atypical.

designation of VIN be reserved for high-grade lesions such as VIN II and III, which are at higher risk of progression to invasive disease.

In contrast to intraepithelial carcinoma of the cervix, which seems to arise from a single point of origin, dysplasia of the vulva is often multicentric. These lesions may be discrete or diffuse, single or multiple, and flat or raised. They even form papules and vary in color from the white appearance of hyperkeratotic tumors to a velvety red or black.

The microscopic appearance of dysplastic vulvar lesions is characterized by cellular disorganization and loss of stratification that involves essentially the full thickness of the epithelium. Cellular density is increased, and individual cells vary greatly in size, with giant and multinucleated cells, numerous mitotic figures, and hyperchromatism (Fig. 47–1). HPV cytopathic changes, such as perinuclear halos with displacement of nuclei, are also common.

Treatment

Treatment options for VIN are individualized based on biopsy results and include wide local excision, laser ablation, topical application of 5-fluorouracil (5-FU) or imiquimod, or superficial vulvectomy with or without split-thickness skin grafting. Untreated VIN has the potential for progression to invasive carcinoma. This risk may be high for women older than age 40 years. In younger patients, spontaneous regression may occur.

Treatment modality depends on the extent of involvement of the vulva, perineum, and perianal skin, which is defined by colposcopy. Wide local excision of small foci of VIN is preferred. For unifocal lesions, a 1-cm margin of uninvolved skin is usually curative. Carbon dioxide laser may be used for multifocal disease. Disadvantages of the laser include painful recovery and lack of pathology specimens. The incidence of foci of microinvasion in VIN III has been reported to range from 10 to 22% in different series. Extensive disease may be best treated by superficial vulvectomy. The surgical goal is to preserve as much of the normal anatomy as possible. In the superficial "skinning" vulvectomy procedure, the excised vulvar skin can be closed with fine suture or may need to be replaced with a split-thickness skin graft (Figs. 47–2 and 47–3) if the defect is too large.

Topical application of imiquimod cream, which stimulates local cytokine release and enhances cell-mediated immunity, can be attempted in order to preserve vulvar anatomy, particularly in younger patients or around sensitive areas such as the clitoris. A recent review of published trials looking at topical imiquimod therapy for high-grade VIN reported a complete response rate of 51% with an additional 25% partial response rate. The use of 5-FU has fallen out of favor due to poor tolerance, with a significant proportion of patients reporting significant burning, pain, and ulcerations. Cryotherapy, photodynamic therapy, and

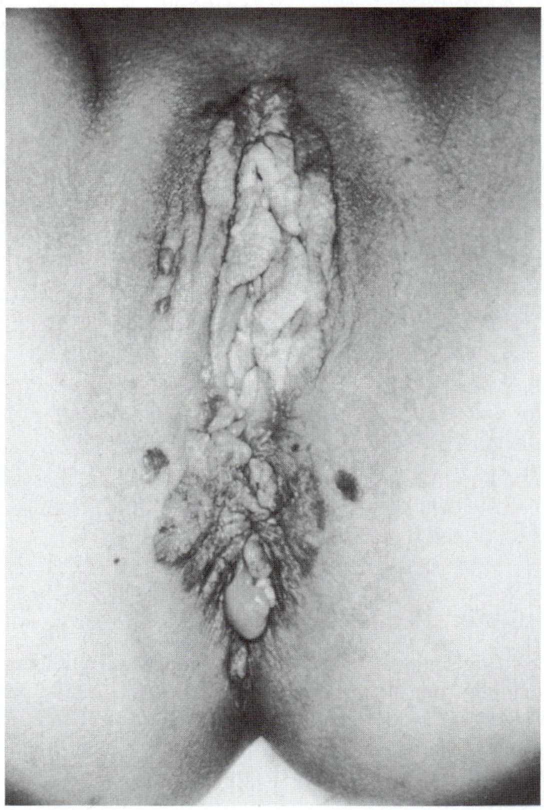

▲ **Figure 47–2.** Diffuse, hypertrophic carcinoma in situ of the vulva and perianal skin. A skinning vulvectomy was performed.

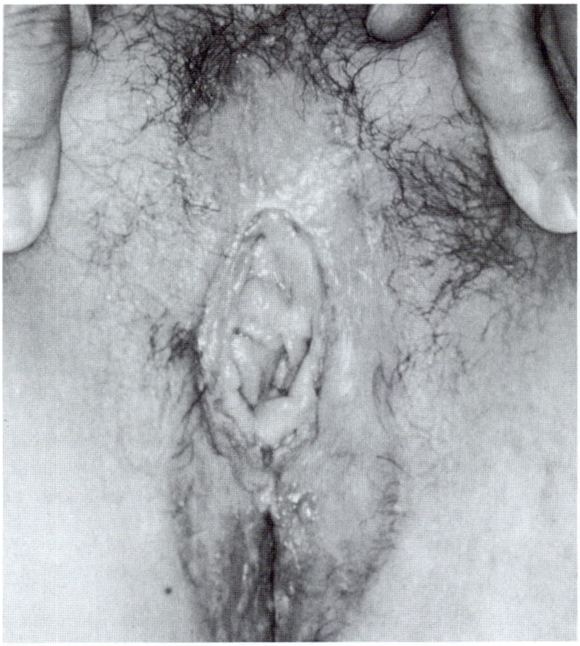

▲ **Figure 47–3.** Appearance after skinning vulvectomy and split-thickness skin grafting of the lesion shown in Figure 47–2.

ultrasonic surgical aspiration have each historically been proven useful in the treatment of some lesions, but remain investigational.

Follow-Up

Intraepithelial carcinoma of the vulva is often one manifestation of multifocal disease. For this reason, affected patients must be examined periodically for a number of years. Recommended follow-up includes thorough pelvic examinations with colposcopy every 3–4 months until the patient is disease free for 2 years. If the patient is disease free for a 2-year period, examinations can be done every 6 months.

EXTRAMAMMARY PAGET DISEASE

ESSENTIALS OF DIAGNOSIS

- Pruritus and vulvar soreness are the most frequent symptoms.
- These symptoms may persist for years before the patient seeks medical attention.
- The lesion may be localized to 1 labium or involve the entire vulvar area.
- The lesion usually has an eczematoid appearance macroscopically and usually begins on the hair-bearing portions of the vulva.
- It is not unusual for the disease process to extend beyond the vulva to involve the perirectal area, buttocks, thighs, inguinal area, and mons.
- Intraepithelial extramammary Paget's disease presents as a lesion with hyperemic areas associated with a superficial white coating to give the impression of "cake icing."
- Although these lesions can be very extensive, most are confined to the epithelial layer.
- The diagnosis is made by vulvar biopsy. It is important to palpate the lesion in its entirety.
- A generous biopsy should be taken of any area that appears to be thickened to rule out an underlying adenocarcinoma.

General Considerations

Paget's disease of the skin is an intraepithelial neoplasia, or adenocarcinoma in situ, and accounts for <1% of all vulvar malignancies occurring mostly in Caucasian patients in their 60s and 70s. Reports of long-term survival suggest that the in situ stage of the disease persists for a long time or that invasive disease is a different clinicopathologic entity. At present, most experts posit that extramammary Paget's disease (EMPD) arises as either an intraepithelial neoplasia that may progress to a dermally invasive carcinoma (primary EMPD) or epidermal infiltration of malignant cells from an underlying or distant carcinoma (secondary EMPD) such as primary adenocarcinoma of an underlying apocrine gland, Bartholin's gland, or anorectum. Unlike mammary Paget's disease, <20% of vulvar Paget's disease is associated with an underlying adenocarcinoma. Paget's disease with an underlying adenocarcinoma metastasizes frequently to regional lymph nodes and distally. Paget's disease without an underlying adenocarcinoma behaves like an intraepithelial neoplasia and can be treated as such. However, patients with Paget's disease should be carefully examined for the presence of synchronous primaries elsewhere; 20–30% of these patients will be found to have carcinomas at other sites, including the breast, rectum, bladder, cervix, ovary, and urethra.

Pathogenesis

The initial lesion may be confused with a number of benign forms of chronic vulvar pruritus. It is a pruritic, slowly spreading, velvety-red discoloration of the skin that eventually becomes eczematoid in appearance with secondary maceration and development of white plaques; it may spread to involve the skin of the perineum, the perianal area,

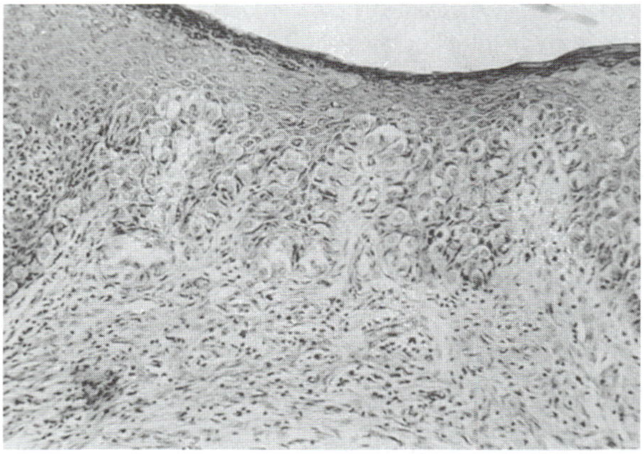

▲ **Figure 47–4.** Paget's disease with typical cells in the basal layer of the epidermis.

and the adjacent skin of the thigh. Grossly, the lesion gives the impression of "cake icing." Because of the serpiginous growth pattern of Paget cells in the basal layer of the epidermis, the true extent of disease is difficult to assess.

Paget's disease of the vulvar skin is an intraepithelial disease. The typical Paget cell, pathognomonic of the disease process, apparently arises from abnormal differentiation of the cells of the basal layer of the epithelium (Fig. 47–4). The appearance of malignant cells varies from that of the clear cell of the apocrine gland epithelium to a totally undifferentiated basal cell. It has been suggested that there may be both an intraepithelial and an invasive variety of the disease. The intraepithelial stage of the disease persists for years without evidence of an underlying adenocarcinoma.

Treatment

Wide local excision is the primary treatment modality for this disease process. The lesion needs to be excised in its entirety; however, wide margins need to be removed around the primary lesion as disease often extends beyond the clinically visible erythematous area. The underlying dermis should be removed for adequate histologic evaluation. Often such a resection involves a complete vulvectomy. Careful histologic examination of the entire operative specimen is necessary to delineate the true extent of disease, ensure free surgical margins, and detect the remote possibility of underlying adenocarcinoma. For this reason, laser therapy is unsatisfactory. Patients who have Paget's disease with underlying adenocarcinoma should be treated with radical local excision of the vulva and bilateral inguinal lymph node dissection as they would for any other invasive tumor involving the vulvar area.

Prognosis

Paget's disease of the vulva has a great propensity for local recurrence even with negative resection margins, which may represent persistence of the disease or development of new disease in the remaining vulvar skin. EMPD characteristically requires repeated local excisions of recurrent disease after treatment of the primary disease by total vulvectomy. Invasive disease without evidence of lymph node metastases has a favorable prognosis; however, with nodal metastases, the disease is almost invariably fatal.

Black D, Tornos C, Soslow RA, Awtrey CS, Barakat RR, Chi DS. The outcomes of patients with positive margins after excision for intraepithelial Paget's disease of the vulva. *Gynecol Oncol* 2007;104:547–550. PMID: 17067662.

Kanitakis J. Mammary and extramammary Paget's disease. *J Eur Acad Dermatol Venereol* 2007;21:581–590. PMID: 17447970.

McCarter MD, Quan SH, Busam K, Paty PP, Wong D, Guillem JG. Long-term outcome of perianal Paget's disease. *Dis Colon Rectum* 2003;46:612–616. PMID: 12792436.

Parker LP, Parker JR, Bodurka-Bevers D, et al. Paget's disease of the vulva: pathology, pattern of involvement, and prognosis. *Gynecol Oncol* 2000;77:183–189. PMID: 10739709.

Pierie JP, Choudry U, Muzikansky A, Finkelstein DM, Ott MJ. Prognosis and management of extramammary Paget's disease and the association with secondary malignancies. *J Am Coll Surg* 2003;196:45–50. PMID: 12517548.

Shepherd V, Davidson EJ, Davies-Humphreys J. Extramammary Paget's disease. *BJOG* 2005;112:273–279. PMID: 15713139.

CANCER OF THE VULVA

ESSENTIALS OF DIAGNOSIS

- Typically occurs in postmenopausal women
- Long history of vulvar irritation with pruritus, local discomfort, and bloody discharge
- Appearance of early lesions like that of chronic vulvar dermatitis
- Appearance of late lesions like that of a large cauliflower or a hard ulcerated area in the vulva
- Biopsy necessary for diagnosis

General Considerations

Cancer of the vulva may arise from the skin, subcutaneous tissues, or glandular elements of the vulva. Approximately 90% of these tumors are squamous cell carcinomas. Less common tumors are EMPD with underlying adenocarcinoma, carcinoma of Bartholin's gland, basal cell carcinoma, melanoma, sarcoma, and metastatic cancers from other sites.

Cancer of the vulva is uncommon, accounting for approximately 4% of gynecologic cancers. Vulvar cancer is more common in the poor and elderly in most parts of the world, and no race or culture is spared. Vulvar cancer is primarily a disease of postmenopausal women, with a peak incidence in women ages 60–70 years. The average age at the time of diagnosis is 65 years, and 75% of patients are older than age 50 years. In general, the mean age of patients with carcinoma in situ is approximately 10 years less than that for patients with invasive cancer. Intraepithelial cancer of the vulva in women ages 20–40 years has increased remarkably in recent years. Two independent pathways for the development of vulvar carcinoma are thought to exist. HPV infection is strongly associated in younger women with vulvar cancer, whereas in older women, vulvar dystrophy and chronic inflammation are thought to be the prevailing carcinogenic pathways. Older women are more likely to have squamous hyperplasia in the tissue adjacent to the tumor.

Considering that cancer of the vulva is a disease of a body surface readily accessible to diagnostic procedures, early diagnosis should be the rule. This is not the case, however, and a 6- to 12-month delay in reporting symptoms of discovery of a tumor is common. Despite the advanced age of many of these patients and the frequent finding of a moderately large tumor, the disease is usually amenable to surgical therapy. In stage I and II disease, the corrected 5-year survival rate is >90%. A 75% corrected 5-year survival rate for all stages of vulvar cancer is reported by most institutions.

Risk factor most frequently associated with carcinoma of the vulva are cigarette smoking, immunodeficiency syndromes, a history of cervical carcinoma or dysplasia, HPV infection, and chronic vulvar irritation secondary to diabetes mellitus, granulomatous venereal disease, or vulvar dystrophy.

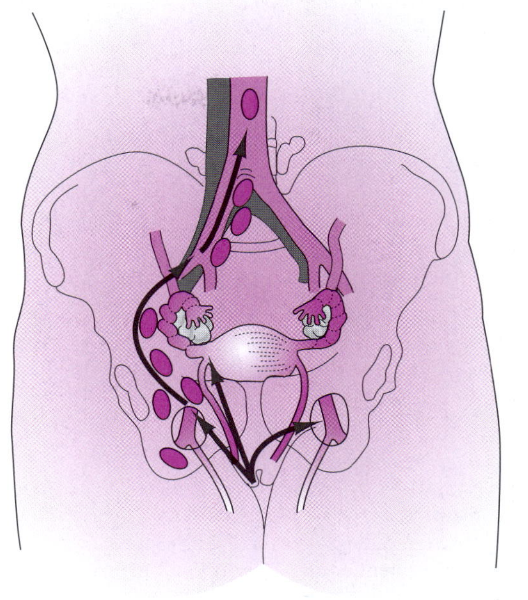

▲ **Figure 47–5.** Lymphatic spread of cancer of the vulva.

Pathogenesis

The gross appearance of vulvar cancer depends on the origin and histologic type. These tumors spread by local extension and, with few exceptions, by lymphatic embolization. The primary route of lymphatic spread is by way of the superficial inguinal, deep femoral, and external iliac lymph nodes (Fig. 47–5). Contralateral spread may occur as a result of the rich intercommunicating lymphatic system of the vulvar skin. Direct extension to the deep pelvic lymph nodes, primarily the obturator nodes, occurs in approximately 3% of patients and seems to be related to midline involvement around the clitoris, urethra, or rectum, or to cancer of a vestibular (Bartholin's) gland. Extension of the tumor to the lower and middle thirds of the vagina may also allow access of tumor cells to lymph channels leading to the deep pelvic lymph nodes.

The following sections describe the gross and histologic appearance of the various types of vulvar cancers.

A. Squamous Cell Carcinoma

Squamous cell carcinoma is by far the most common type of tumor and most frequently involves the anterior half of the vulva. In approximately 65% of patients, the tumor arises in the labia majora and minora, and in 25%, the clitoris or perineum is involved. More than one-third of tumors involve the vulva bilaterally or are midline tumors. These tumors are most frequently associated with nodal spread, particularly bilateral nodal metastases. Midline tumors that involve the perineum do not worsen the outlook unless they extend into the vagina or to the anus and rectum.

Squamous cell carcinoma of the vulva varies in appearance from a large, exophytic, cauliflowerlike lesion to a small ulcer crater superimposed on a dystrophic lesion of the vulvar skin (Figs. 47–6 and 47–7). Ulcerative lesions may begin as a raised, flat, white area of hypertrophic skin that subsequently undergoes ulceration. Exophytic lesions may become extremely large, undergo necrosis, and become secondarily infected and malodorous. A third variety arises as a slightly elevated, red, velvety tumor that gradually spreads over the vulvar skin. There does not appear to be a positive correlation between the gross appearance of the tumor and either histologic grade or frequency of nodal metastases. The primary determinant of nodal metastases is tumor size.

Squamous cell cancers may be graded histologically from I to III. Grade I tumors are well differentiated, often forming keratin pearls; grade II tumors are moderately well differentiated; grade III tumors are composed of poorly differentiated cells. The extent of underlying inflammatory cell infiltration into the stroma surrounding the invasive tumor is variable. The histologic grade of the tumor may be of some significance in tumors <2 cm in diameter.

A variant of squamous cell carcinoma, **verrucous carcinoma**, is a locally invasive tumor that seldom metastasizes to regional lymph nodes. Grossly, the tumor looks like a mature condylomatous growth. It is distinguished from

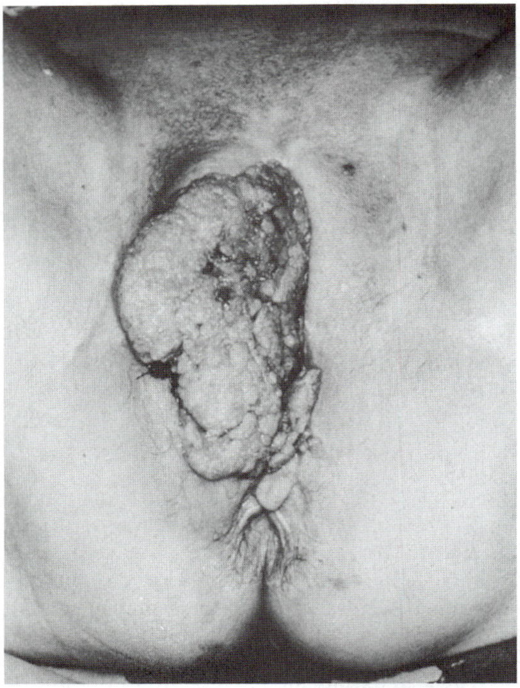

▲ **Figure 47–6.** Large, exophytic, squamous cell carcinoma of the vulva, which was treated by radical vulvectomy and regional lymphadenectomy.

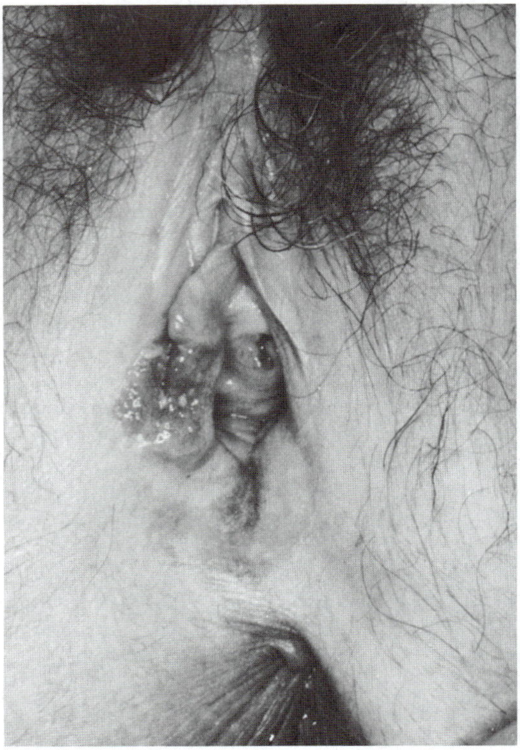

▲ **Figure 47–7.** Ulcerative squamous cell carcinoma of the vulva.

squamous cell cancer by histopathology of the tumor base, which reveals papillary fronds without a central core. Local recurrence is common if a wide vulvectomy is not performed; lymphadenectomy is usually not recommended unless suspicious nodes are encountered. Radiation therapy is usually contraindicated as it can induce an anaplastic transformation increasing the risk of metastases.

Depth of stromal penetration has proved to be the key factor in determining invasive potential of the tumor. The ISSVD, International Federation of Gynecology and Obstetrics (FIGO), and Tumor, Node, Metastasis (TNM) staging defined stage IA carcinoma of the vulva as a single lesion measuring 2 cm or less in diameter and exhibiting 1 focus of invasion to a depth of 1 mm or less. The depth of invasion was measured from the epidermal–stromal junction of the most superficial dermal papilla to the deepest point of tumor invasion.

B. Carcinoma of Bartholin's Gland

Carcinoma of Bartholin's gland accounts for approximately 1% of vulvar cancers and, although rare, is the most common site for vulvar adenocarcinoma. Approximately 50% of Bartholin's gland tumors are squamous cell carcinomas. Other types of tumors arising in the Bartholin's glands are adenocarcinoma, adenoid cystic, adenosquamous, and transitional cell carcinomas.

Because inflammatory disease of the Bartholin's gland is uncommon after age 40, older women with a mass in this location undergo biopsy to rule out cancer. Because of its location deep in the substance of the labium, a tumor may impinge on the rectum and directly spread into the ischiorectal fossa. Consequently, these tumors have access to lymphatic channels draining directly to the deep pelvic lymph nodes as well as to the superficial channels draining to the inguinal lymph nodes.

C. Basal Cell Carcinoma

Basal cell carcinomas account for 1–2% of vulvar cancers. Most tumors are small elevated lesions with an ulcerated center and rolled edges, so-called "rodent" ulcers. Some are described as pigmented tumors, moles, or simply pruritic maculopapular eruptions. These tumors arise almost exclusively in the skin of the labia majora, although occasionally a tumor can be found elsewhere in the vulva. The tumor is derived from primordial basal cells in the epidermis or hair follicles and is characterized by slow growth, local infiltration, and a tendency to recur if not totally excised.

On microscopic examination, the typical tumor consists of nodular masses and lobules of closely packed, uniform-appearing basaloid cells with scant cytoplasm and spherical or oval dark nuclei. Peripheral margination by columnar cells is usually prominent. In larger tumor nodules, there may be areas of central degeneration and necrosis.

If a sufficiently wide local excision is not performed, there is a tendency for local recurrence, estimated to be approximately 20%. A lymphadenectomy is rarely indicated as these tumors, although sometimes locally aggressive, rarely metastasize.

D. Malignant Melanoma

Approximately 5% of vulvar cancers are malignant melanomas, the second most common vulvar cancer. Because only 0.1% of all nevi in women are on vulvar skin, the disproportionate frequency of occurrence of melanoma in this area may be a result of the fact that nearly all vulvar nevi are of the junctional variety. Malignant melanoma most commonly arises in the region of the labia minora and clitoris, and there is a tendency for superficial spread toward the urethra and vagina. A nonpigmented melanoma may closely resemble squamous cell carcinoma on clinical examination. A darkly pigmented, raised lesion at the mucocutaneous junction is a characteristic finding; however, the degree of melanin pigmentation is variable, and amelanotic lesions do occur. The lesion spreads primarily through lymphatic channels and tends to metastasize early in the course of the disease; local or remote cutaneous satellite lesions may be found. In contrast to squamous cell cancers, melanoma is staged according to depth of invasion. All small pigmented lesions of the vulva are suspect and should be removed by excision biopsy with a 0.5- to 1-cm margin of normal skin. In the case of large tumors, the diagnosis should be confirmed by a generous biopsy.

Clinical Findings

The patient with vulvar cancer characteristically has had infrequent medical examinations. Approximately 10% are diabetic, and 30–50% are obese or hypertensive or demonstrate other evidence of cardiovascular disease. The incidence of complicating medical illness exceeds that expected in the age group under consideration.

Invasive squamous cell cancer is a disease mainly of the seventh and eighth decades of life, although approximately 15% of patients are age 40 years or younger. Approximately 20% of patients have a second primary cancer that was diagnosed prior to, at the time of, or subsequent to the diagnosis of vulvar cancer; 75% of these second primary cancers are in the cervix.

A. Symptoms & Signs

Vulvar pruritus and/or a vulvar mass are frequent complaints and are present in more than 50% of patients with vulvar cancer. Other patients complain of bleeding or vulvar pain, whereas approximately 20% of patients have no complaints, and the tumor is found incidentally during routine pelvic examination. Approximately 25% of patients have seen a physician and received various medical treatments without benefit of a biopsy of the tumor. The importance of performing a biopsy of any vulvar lesion cannot be overemphasized. A biopsy should be taken from the area that appears to be the most abnormal, and multiple biopsies may be necessary in the event of multifocal disease.

B. Differential Diagnosis

The differential diagnosis includes epidermal inclusion cysts, acrochordons, seborrheic dermatoses, lichen sclerosus and other vulvar dystrophies, condyloma acuminate, granulomatous venereal diseases (eg, syphilis, herpes, or granuloma inguinale), pyogenic infections, or benign tumor, such as a granular cell myoblastoma.

C. Unusual Vulvar Malignancies

Sarcomas of the vulva constitute a variety of malignant neoplasms that account for 1–2% of vulvar cancers. The most common is leiomyosarcoma, followed in frequency of occurrence by the fibrous histiocytoma group and an array of other sarcomas. Clinically, sarcoma may present as a subcutaneous nodule or may be exophytic and fleshy. Prognosis is usually poor and depends on histologic type, extent of local invasion, and treatment. In general, radical vulvectomy and regional lymphadenectomy are indicated, with the exception of tumors such as dermatofibrosarcoma protuberans, which is a locally aggressive tumor that tends to recur locally but does not metastasize.

Adenocarcinoma of the vulva is exceptionally rare unless it arises from the Bartholin's gland or the urethra. Primary cancer of the breast from ectopic breast tissue has been reported. Rarely, a malignant tumor will arise from a vulvar sweat gland.

Metastatic cancers of the vulva constitute 8% of all vulvar tumors. They usually originate from a genital tract tumor, and 18% arise from the kidney or urethra. Advanced cervical cancer is the most common primary tumor. Other primary tumors have been reported, including malignant melanoma, choriocarcinoma, and adenocarcinoma of the rectum or breast. Cloacogenic carcinoma is primarily an anorectal neoplasm, occurring twice as often in women than in men; it may arise in anal ducts and present as a submucosal mass.

Metastatic epidermoid cancer tends to form nests of cells within the dermis. Adenocarcinoma, regardless of the primary site, invades the surface squamous epithelium. Because these tumors are a manifestation of advanced disease, the prognosis is uniformly grave.

Complications

A. Operative Morbidity & Mortality

The most frequently encountered complication is wound breakdown, which occurs in well over 50% of patients undergoing radical vulvectomy and bilateral inguinal dissection. This complication is related to the amount of skin removed during the procedure, particularly at the groin areas. Separate groin incisions and careful handling of skin flaps have reduced the incidence of wound breakdown. Vigorous wound care with debridement almost always results in adequate healing.

Lymphedema occurs in up to 65% of patients who have had inguinofemoral lymph node dissection. Hemorrhage, lymphocyst formation, thromboembolic disease, urinary tract infections, and sexual dysfunction are other commonly associated morbidities.

Treatment

Staging and treatment for vulvar cancer are surgical (Table 47–1). The primary treatment for invasive vulvar cancer is complete surgical removal of all tumor whenever possible. The recent trend is toward a more conservative surgical approach, departing from traditional en bloc resections.

The number of preoperative studies ordered prior to surgery depends on the extent of disease and the general condition of the patient. A complete history and a thorough physical examination that includes cytologic study of the cervix and vulvoscopy should be performed. A large tumor may interfere with adequate pelvic examination. Bleeding may be caused by a lesion higher in the genital tract rather than the obvious vulvar tumor. In that case, the pelvic examination may be performed under anesthesia, and endometrial biopsy or dilatation and curettage (D&C) may be considered.

Chest radiography and other studies such as proctoscopy, pyelography, barium enema, and computed tomography (CT) scans are ordered on an individual basis, especially in the event of locally advanced disease or suspected metastases. Enlarged lymph nodes do not require biopsy; they will be excised by lymphadenectomy or thoroughly sampled at the time of operation.

Historically, the basic operation was radical vulvectomy and regional lymphadenectomy. The trend, however, is shifting away from standard en bloc radical vulvectomy and bilateral lymph node dissection toward wide radical local excision of the primary tumor with inguinal lymph node dissection. For a unifocal stage I lesion with <1 mm stromal invasion, wide radical local excision with surgical margins of at least 1–2 cm should be performed. Patients with unilateral lesions with a depth of invasion ≥1 mm should undergo ipsilateral groin dissection in addition to the above to determine nodal status. For patients with bilateral lesions, lesions impinging on or crossing the midline, or stage II or greater disease or if lymph node metastases are discovered at the time of unilateral lymphadenectomy, bilateral inguinal femoral lymphadenectomy can be performed. When disease has spread to lymph nodes, adjuvant radiation therapy is generally recommended; pelvic lymph node dissection is not required for staging or therapy. In general, lymphatic spread occurs in a sequential manner from the superficial to the deep inguinal lymph nodes.

Table 47–1. International Federation of Gynecology and Obstetrics (FIGO) staging of vulvar cancer.

TNM Category	FIGO Stage	Definition	
Primary tumor size (T)			
Tis	0	Carcinoma in situ, intraepithelial carcinoma	
T1a	IA	Tumor confined to the vulva and/or perineum, 2 cm or less in greatest dimension with stromal invasion 1.0 mm or less	
T1b	IB	Tumor more than 2 cm or tumor of any size in greatest dimension with more than 1.0 mm of stromal invasion confined to the vulva and/or perineum	
T2	II	Tumor of any size with adjacent spread to the lower 1/3 of the urethra or vagina, or the anus	
T3	IVA	Tumor of any size with extension to any of the following: upper/proximal 2/3 urethra or vagina, bladder or rectal mucosa, or fixed to the pelvic bone	
Regional lymph nodes (N)			
N1a	IIIA	One or two lymph node metastases 5 mm or less each	
N1b	IIIA	One lymph node metastasis 5 mm or more	
N2a	IIIB	Three or more lymph node metastases each <5 mm	
N2b	IIIB	Two or more lymph node metastases 5 mm or more	
N2c	IIIC	Lymph node metastasis with extranodal spread	
N3	IVA	Fixed or ulcerated regional lymph node metastasis	
Distant metastasis (M)			
M1	IVB	Any distant metastasis including pelvic lymph nodes	
FIGO Stage/TNM Classification			
Stage 0	Tis	N0	M0
Stage IA	T1a	N0	M0
Stage IB	T1b	N0	M0
Stage II	T2	N0	M0
Stage IIIA	T1, T2	N1a, N1b	M0
Stage IIIB	T1, T2	N2a, N2b	M0
Stage IIIC	T1, T2	N2c	M0
Stage IVA	T1, T2	N3	
Stage IVA	T3	Any N	M0
Stage IVB	Any T	Any N	M1

Reproduced, with permission, from International Federation of Gynecology and Obstetrics. Annual Report on the results of treatment in gynecologic cancer. *Int J Gynecol Obstet*, 1991;36(Suppl):132. Copyright 1991, with permission from the International Federation of Gynecology & Obstetrics.

Consequently, if the superficial nodes harbor no metastatic disease, there is reasonable assurance that the deeper nodes are not involved. The role of sentinel node mapping is also being evaluated for patients with squamous vulvar carcinoma and melanomas and should be reserved for investigational use.

Postoperative radiation therapy is usually reserved for patients with more than 1 microscopically involved lymph node or if 1 of more lymph nodes are macroscopically involved. Radiation therapy can also be considered for patients with negative lymph nodes who are at high risk of local recurrence (tumors measuring >4 cm, positive or close margins, lymphovascular invasion).

When the disease involves the anus, rectum, rectovaginal septum, proximal urethra, or bladder, an adequate surgical resection is only possible with pelvic exenteration combined with radical vulvectomy. Operative mortality is high for these procedures, and the postoperative psychological impact is significant. In addition, with advanced-stage disease where ulcerated or fixed lymph nodes are palpated, attempts at lymphadenectomy have yielded very poor results. Based on data from the Gynecologic Oncology Group, this group of patients may benefit from preoperative chemoradiation, resulting in higher rates of successful resection and reduced need for more radical surgery. Chemotherapeutic agents such as cisplatin and 5-FU have been combined with radiation therapy. These chemotherapeutic agents are used as radiation sensitizers in large necrotic tumor beds, enhancing the radiation effects.

There is controversy concerning the extent of surgery required for treatment of malignant melanoma of the vulva. For some years, standard treatment consisted of vulvectomy with superficial and deep inguinal and pelvic lymphadenectomy. It is also generally treated with a more conservative surgical approach. If depth of the vulvar lesion is <1 mm, vulvar melanoma may be adequately treated with local incision using a 1-cm margin. However, if the depth of invasion is between 1 and 4 mm, excision requires a 2-cm margin in addition to a bilateral groin node dissection. Advanced or recurrent melanoma may be best treated with chemotherapy, radiation, or immunotherapy.

Radical wide local resection with wide surgical margins is the standard treatment for most vulvar sarcomas. Inguinofemoral lymphadenectomy should be performed for suspected metastases because the risk of lymphatic spread is low. The primary determinant of cure appears to be adequate wide removal of the primary lesion.

Follow-Up

After the immediate postoperative period, patients should be examined every 3 months for 2 years and every 6 months thereafter to detect recurrent disease or a second primary cancer. Nearly 80% of recurrent vulvar cancer occurs in the first 2 years. Treatment modalities depend on the location of recurrence. Malignant melanomas and sarcomas may recur locally or metastasize to the liver or lungs.

Prognosis

The principal prognostic factors in cancer of the vulva are the presence or absence of regional lymph node metastases, size and location of the lesion, and the histologic type. A 5-year survival rate of 75% and a 10-year survival rate of approximately 58% should be expected after complete surgical treatment of primary invasive squamous vulvar cancer. Lymph node status is the most important prognostic variable. Overall, the survival rate for patients with vulvar cancer and negative inguinal femoral nodes is 90%, whereas rates drop to almost 40% with nodal metastasis. Several authors have reported no deaths from cancer among patients who were found to have negative lymph nodes. With tumors <2 cm in diameter, the incidence of nodal metastases is 10–15%. In general, approximately 30% of patients undergoing surgery will have positive lymph nodes. With nodal metastases, the approximate 5-year cure rates are as follows: 1 node, 94%; 2 nodes, 80%; and 3 nodes or more, <15%. Patients who have 3 or more positive lymph nodes in the groin usually demonstrate palpably suspicious nodes preoperatively. These patients have a high incidence of metastases to the pelvic lymph nodes; however, pelvic lymphadenectomy does not improve survival rates. Involvement of contiguous organs such as the bladder or rectum increases the incidence of nodal metastases and worsens the prognosis accordingly.

The cure rate for adequately treated cancer of Bartholin's gland has not been established. There is a propensity for unresectable local recurrences under the pubic ramus despite a thorough primary operation.

Wide local excision of basal cell carcinoma should be curative. Some authors have reported an approximately 20% recurrence rate after local excision that may represent cases of incomplete excision.

Results of treatment of malignant melanoma are related to the level of penetration of the tumor into the dermis of the vulvar skin or the lamina propria of the vaginal mucosa and to the presence or absence of nodal metastases. The 5-year survival rate ranges from 24 to 70%. The prognosis of patients with metastases to groin lymph nodes is generally poor. Amelanotic cutaneous melanomas are particularly virulent tumors. The survival rate for patients with superficial spreading melanomas is much better than for those with the nodular variety, which tend to have a smaller diameter and exhibit aggressive vertical invasion, increased incidence of nodal metastases, treatment failures, and distant recurrences. The most common site of recurrence is at the site of resection or the groin lymph nodes (if not previously resected).

Sarcomas of the vulva tend to recur locally, particularly if the initial resection is not extensive, and metastasize to the liver and lungs.

Al-Ghamdi A, Freedman D, Miller D, et al. Vulvar squamous cell carcinoma in young women: a clinicopathologic study of 21 cases. *Gynecol Oncol* 2002;84:94–101. PMID: 11748983.

American Joint Committee on Cancer. Vulva. In: *AJCC Cancer Staging Manual*. 7th ed. New York, NY: Springer; 2010.

Beller U, Quinn MA, Benedet JL, et al. Carcinoma of the vulva. FIGO 6th Annual Report on the Results of Treatment in Gynecological Cancer. *Int J Gynaecol Obstet* 2006;95 (Suppl 1):S7–27. PMID: 17161169.

Beller U, Sideri M, Maisonneuve P, et al. Carcinoma of the vagina. *J Epidemiol Biostat* 2001;6:141–152. PMID: 11385774.

Gadducci A, Cionini L, Romanini A, Fanucchi A, Genazzani AR. Old and new perspectives in the management of high-risk, locally advanced or recurrent, and metastatic vulvar cancer. *Crit Rev Oncol Hematol* 2006;60:227–241. PMID: 16945551.

Gonzalez Bosquet J, Kinney WK, Russell AH, Gaffey TA, Magrina JF, Podratz KC. Risk of occult inguinofemoral lymph node metastasis from squamous carcinoma of the vulva. *Int J Radiat Oncol Biol Phys* 2003;57:419–424. PMID: 12957253.

Gonzalez Bosquet J, Magrina JF, Gaffey TA, et al. Long-term survival and disease recurrence in patients with primary squamous cell carcinoma of the vulva. *Gynecol Oncol* 2005;97:828–833. PMID: 15896831.

Hillemanns P, Wang X, Staehle S, Michels W, Dannecker C. Evaluation of different treatment modalities for vulvar intraepithelial neoplasia (VIN): CO(2) laser vaporization, photodynamic therapy, excision and vulvectomy. *Gynecol Oncol* 2006;100:271–275. PMID: 16169064.

Joura EA, Losch A, Haider-Angeler MG, Breitenecker G, Leodolter S. Trends in vulvar neoplasia. Increasing incidence of vulvar intraepithelial neoplasia and squamous cell carcinoma of the vulva in young women. *J Reprod Med.* 2000;45:613–615. PMID: 10986677.

Judson PL, Habermann EB, Baxter NN, Durham SB, Virnig BA. Trends in the incidence of invasive and in situ vulvar carcinoma. *Obstet Gynecol* 2006;107:1018–1022. PMID: 16648405.

Kunos C, Simpkins F, Gibbons H, Tian C, Homesley H. Radiation therapy compared with pelvic node resection for node-positive vulvar cancer: a randomized controlled trial. *Obstet Gynecol* 2009;114:537–546. PMID: 19701032.

Leminen A, Forss M, Paavonen J. Wound complications in patients with carcinoma of the vulva. Comparison between radical and modified vulvectomies. *Eur J Obstet Gynecol Reprod Biol* 2000;93:193–197. PMID: 11074142.

Montana GS, Thomas GM, Moore DH, et al. Preoperative chemoradiation for carcinoma of the vulva with N2/N3 nodes: a gynecologic oncology group study. *Int J Radiat Oncol Biol Phys* 2000;48:1007–1013. PMID: 11072157.

Rodolakis A, Diakomanolis E, Vlachos G, et al. Vulvar intraepithelial neoplasia (VIN)—diagnostic and therapeutic challenges. *Eur J Gynaecol Oncol* 2003;24:317–322. PMID: 12807248.

Rouzier R, Haddad B, Atallah D, Dubois P, Paniel BJ. Surgery for vulvar cancer. *Clin Obstet Gynecol* 2005;48:869–878. PMID: 16286833.

Selman TJ, Luesley DM, Acheson N, Khan KS, Mann CH. A systematic review of the accuracy of diagnostic tests for inguinal lymph node status in vulvar cancer. *Gynecol Oncol* 2005;99:206–214. PMID: 16081147.

Sideri M, Jones RW, Wilkinson EJ, et al. Squamous vulvar intraepithelial neoplasia: 2004 modified terminology, ISSVD Vulvar Oncology Subcommittee. *J Reprod Med* 2005;50:807–810. PMID: 16419625.

Stang A, Streller B, Eisinger B, Jockel KH. Population-based incidence rates of malignant melanoma of the vulva in Germany. *Gynecol Oncol* 2005;96:216–221. PMID: 15589604.

Sugiyama VE, Chan JK, Shin JY, Berek JS, Osann K, Kapp DS. Vulvar melanoma: a multivariable analysis of 644 patients. *Obstet Gynecol* 2007;110:296–301. PMID: 17666603.

van de Nieuwenhof HP, van der Avoort IA, de Hullu JA. Review of squamous premalignant vulvar lesions. *Crit Rev Oncol Hematol* 2008;68:131–156. PMID: 18406622.

van Seters M, van Beurden M, de Craen AJ. Is the assumed natural history of vulvar intraepithelial neoplasia III based on enough evidence? A systematic review of 3322 published patients. *Gynecol Oncol* 2005;97:645–651. PMID: 15863172.

PREINVASIVE DISEASE OF THE VAGINA

ESSENTIALS OF DIAGNOSIS

- Almost all lesions of vaginal intraepithelial neoplasia are asymptomatic.
- Lesions often accompany HPV infection, so patients may complain of vulvar warts. An abnormal Papanicolaou (Pap) smear is usually the first sign of disease.
- The diagnosis is made by colposcopic examination of the vagina with a directed biopsy.
- Colposcopic examination of the vagina can be difficult to perform, particularly if a hysterectomy has already been done, because lesions can lay hidden within the recesses of the vaginal cuff.
- Techniques similar to those used for colposcopic examination of the cervix are used for examination of the vagina.
- After application of 3–5% acetic acid to the vagina, a lesion under the colposcope may appear as white epithelium and may have mosaicism or punctuation.
- Lugol's iodine may also help to identify the borders of a lesion.
- Lesions are often located along the vaginal ridges; they may appear to be raised or have spicules.
- Because the disease process tends to be multifocal, a thorough examination of the vagina from the introitus to the apex must be conducted.

General Considerations

Vaginal intraepithelial neoplasia (VAIN) can occur as an isolated lesion, but multifocal disease is more common. Although little is known regarding the natural history of VAIN, it is thought to be similar to that of cervical intraepithelial neoplasia (CIN). Many patients may have similar intraepithelial neoplastic lesions involving the cervix or vulva.

At least one-half to two-thirds of patients with VAIN have been treated for similar disease in either the cervix or the vulva. In addition, VAIN can reappear several years later, necessitating long-term follow-up in these patients. Several investigators have recognized a "field effect" involving the squamous epithelium of the lower genital tract including the cervix, vagina, and vulva to be affected simultaneously by the same carcinogenic agent. The vagina lacks a transformation zone, whereas in the cervix, immature epithelial cells are infected with HPV. The upper third of the vagina is where the majority of these lesions are diagnosed. As in cervical and vulvar intraepithelial neoplasia, several investigators have found that smoking is associated with an increased risk of high-grade VAIN. Controversy still exists regarding the role of prior irradiation in the pathogenesis of vaginal neoplasia.

Condylomatous lesions of the lower genital tract often demonstrate associated dysplasias. For this reason, a biopsy should be made of condylomatous growth of the vagina prior to treatment.

Pathogenesis

As with other intraepithelial neoplasias occurring in the lower genital tract, VAIN is characterized by a loss of epithelial cell maturation. This is associated with nuclear hyperchromatosis and pleomorphism with cellular crowding. The thickness of the epithelial abnormality designates the various lesions as VAIN I, II, or III. VAIN III is synonymous with carcinoma in situ of the vagina.

Treatment

The primary treatment modality for VAIN is surgical excision or carbon dioxide laser ablation. VAIN I lesions usually do not require treatment, as lesions typically regress, and usually close clinical observation is sufficient. VAIN II and III can be treated by laser ablation or excision. VAIN III lesions are more often associated with an early invasive lesion; therefore, adequate sampling should be performed before any ablative procedure is employed. If the lesion is focal, it is best removed in its entirety with local excision. When carcinoma in situ of the cervix extends to the upper vagina, the upper third of the vagina can be removed at the time of hysterectomy. If multifocal disease is present, a total vaginectomy may be performed with a split-thickness skin graft vaginal reconstruction. Topical 5-FU may also be used in treating multifocal VAIN. Approximately 80% of patients can expect to have evidence of regression of disease after 1 to 2 courses of treatment. Several small series have also reported success in using topical application of imiquimod for the treatment of high-grade VAIN, although the treatment remains investigational.

Follow-Up

VAIN tends to be multifocal, with involvement of the cervix and vulva in many cases. These lesions can be difficult to eradicate with only 1 treatment modality or treatment session. This group of patients must be monitored closely every 4–6 months with cytologic smears and HPV testing and close examination of not only the vagina but also the entire lower genital tract.

CANCER OF THE VAGINA

ESSENTIALS OF DIAGNOSIS

- Asymptomatic: abnormal vaginal cytology
- Early: painless bleeding from ulcerated tumor
- Late: bleeding, pain, weight loss, swelling

General Considerations

Primary cancers of the vagina are rare, representing approximately 0.3% of gynecologic cancers. Approximately 85% are squamous cell cancers, and the remainder, in decreasing order of frequency, are adenocarcinomas, sarcomas, and melanomas. A tumor should not be considered a primary vaginal cancer unless the cervix is uninvolved or only minimally involved by a tumor obviously arising in the vagina. By convention, any malignancy involving both cervix and vagina that is histologically compatible with an origin in either organ is classified as cervical cancer. Secondary carcinoma of the vagina is seen more frequently than primary vaginal cancers. Secondary, or metastatic, tumors may arise from cervical, endometrial, or ovarian cancer, breast cancer, gestational trophoblastic disease, colorectal cancer, or urogenital or vulvar cancer. Extension of cervical cancer to the vagina is probably the most common malignancy involving the vagina. In general, invasive vaginal carcinoma shares the same risk factors as cervical neoplasia such as smoking, HPV infection, multiple sexual partners, and a history of lower genital tract neoplasia. In addition, in utero diethylstilbestrol (DES) exposure is associated with an increased risk of primary vaginal adenocarcinoma, namely the clear cell variant.

Pathogenesis

Squamous cell carcinoma may be ulcerative or exophytic. It usually involves the posterior wall of the upper third of the vagina, but may be multicentric. Direct invasion of the bladder or rectum may occur. The incidence of lymph node metastases is directly related to the size of the tumor. The route of nodal metastases depends on the location of the tumor in the vagina. Tumors in the lower third metastasize like cancer of the vulva, primarily to the inguinal lymph nodes (Fig. 47–8). Cancers of the upper vagina, which is the most common site, metastasize in a manner similar to cancer of the cervix. The lymphatic drainage of the vagina consists of a fine capillary meshwork in the mucosa and submucosa with multiple anastomoses. As a consequence,

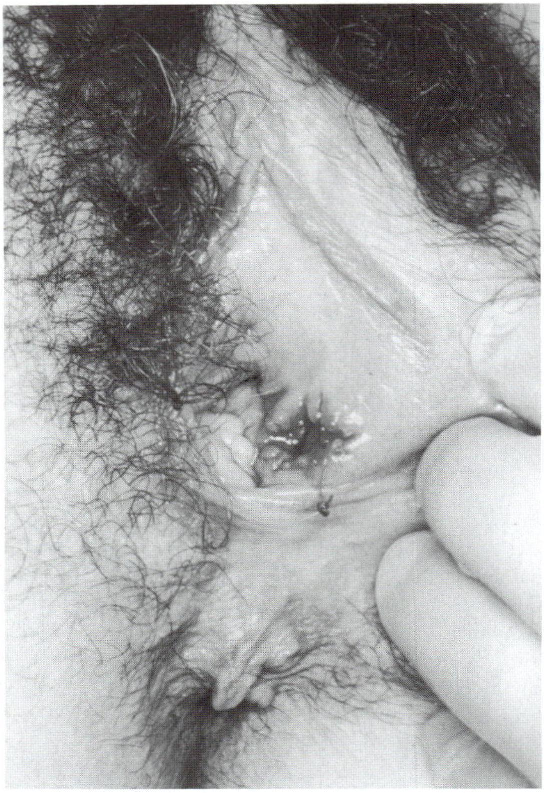

▲ **Figure 47–8.** An ulcerated epidermoid cancer of the lower third of the vagina.

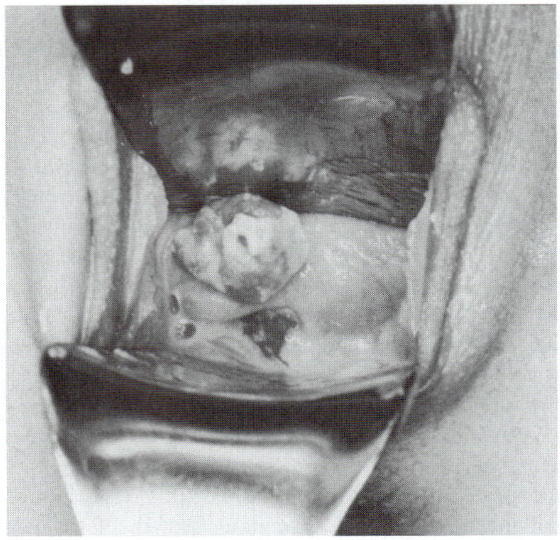

▲ **Figure 47–9.** A clear cell adenocarcinoma of the vagina in a 19-year-old patient. The lesion is on the posterior wall of the upper third of the vagina.

lesions in the middle third of the vagina may metastasize to the inguinal lymph nodes or directly to the deep pelvic lymph nodes.

Adenocarcinomas account for the great majority of primary vaginal malignancies in young patients and may arise in areas of vaginal adenosis, endometriosis, wolffian duct remnants, or periurethral glands. In addition, the clear cell variant has been associated with a history of exposure to DES in utero (Fig. 47–9) with a mean age at diagnosis of 19 years. The risk of developing clear cell adenocarcinoma by age 24 years has been calculated to be 0.14–1.4 per 1000 exposed female fetuses.

Melanomas of the vagina are rare and most frequently arise from the anterior surface and lower half of the vagina and almost always occur in Caucasian patients. Nevi rarely occur in the vagina; therefore, any pigmented lesion of the vagina should be excised or biopsied. Primary vaginal melanomas behave aggressively and tend to recur locally with distant spread and generally poor long-term survival.

The most common primary vaginal sarcoma is embryonal rhabdomyosarcomas or sarcoma botryoides, a highly aggressive tumor that occurs in infancy or early childhood replacing the vaginal mucosa with polypoid, edematous, "grapelike" masses that may protrude from the vaginal introitus. The outcome of these patients has improved with advent of multimodality treatment with chemotherapy, surgery, and radiation therapy. Leiomyosarcomas, endometrial stromal sarcomas, and carcinosarcomas occur in older women. The upper anterior vaginal wall is the most common site of origin. The appearance of these tumors depends on the size and the extent of disease at the time of diagnosis. In general, melanomas and sarcomas spread like squamous cell cancer, although hematogenous spread with liver and pulmonary metastases is more common.

Metastatic adenocarcinoma to the vagina may arise from the urethra, Bartholin's gland, the rectum or bladder, the endometrial cavity, the endocervix, or an ovary, or it may be metastatic from a distant site. Hypernephroma of the kidney characteristically metastasizes to the lower third of the anterior wall of the vagina.

Clinical Findings

Vaginal cancer is often asymptomatic, discovered by routine vaginal cytologic examination, and confirmed by biopsy after delineation of the location and extent of the tumor by colposcopy.

Postmenopausal vaginal and/or postcoital bleeding are the most common presenting symptoms. Other common symptoms include vaginal discharge, a vaginal mass, or urinary symptoms. Approximately 50% of patients with invasive vaginal cancer report for examination within 6 months after symptoms are noted. Less commonly, advanced tumors may impinge upon the rectum or bladder or extend to the pelvic wall, causing pain or leg edema.

A diagnosis of primary cancer of the vagina cannot be established unless metastasis from another source is

Table 47–2. International Federation of Gynecology and Obstetrics (FIGO) staging of carcinoma of the vagina.

Preinvasive carcinoma	
Stage 0	Carcinoma in situ, intraepithelial carcinoma.
Invasive carcinoma	
Stage I	The carcinoma is limited to the vaginal mucosa.
Stage II	The carcinoma has involved the subvaginal tissue but has not extended to the pelvic wall.
Stage III	The carcinoma has extended to the pelvic wall.
Stage IV	The carcinoma has extended beyond the true pelvis or has involved the mucosa of the bladder or rectum. A bullous edema as such does not permit allotment of a case to stage IV.
Stage IVA	Spread of the growth to adjacent organs.
Stage IVB	Spread to distant organs.

Reprinted, with permission, from Benedet JL, Bender H, Jones H 3rd, Ngan HY, Pecorelli S. FIGO staging classifications and clinical practice guidelines in the management of gynecologic cancers. *Int J Gynecol Obstet* 2000;70:209–262.

eliminated. A complete history and physical examination should be performed, including a thorough pelvic examination, cervical cytologic examination, endometrial biopsy when indicated, complete inspection of the vagina, including colposcopy, and biopsy of the vaginal tumor. Careful bimanual examination with palpation of the entire length of the vagina can detect small submucosal nodules not visualized during the examination. Biopsy should be performed to establish a histologic diagnosis.

The staging system for cancer of the vagina is clinical and not surgical (Table 47–2).

Differential Diagnosis

Benign tumors of the vagina are uncommon, are usually cystic, arise from the mesonephric (wolffian) or paramesonephric ducts, and are usually an incidental finding on examination of the anterolateral wall of the vagina (Gartner's duct cyst).

An ulcerative lesion may occur at the site of direct trauma, following an inflammatory reaction caused by prolonged retention of a pessary or other foreign body, or, occasionally, following a chemical burn. Granulomatous venereal diseases seldom affect the vagina but may be diagnosed with appropriate laboratory studies and a biopsy.

Endometriosis that penetrates the cul-de-sac of Douglas into the upper vagina cannot be differentiated from cancer except by biopsy.

Treatment

Following biopsy confirmation of disease, all patients should undergo a thorough physical examination and evaluation of the extent of local and metastatic disease. Pretreatment evaluation may include the following studies: chest radiography, intravenous pyelogram, cystoscopy, proctosigmoidoscopy, and CT scan of the abdomen and pelvis. The optimal treatment of patients with invasive vaginal cancer is still controversial and should take into account the proximity of adjacent structures that preclude a proper surgical margin and the desire to preserve a functional vagina. In general, surgery is reserved for those patients with stage I lesions affecting the upper vagina incorporating a radical hysterectomy with an upper vaginectomy and a bilateral pelvic lymphadenectomy if a hysterectomy had not been previously performed. Otherwise the treatment consists of primary radiotherapy with brachytherapy for small superficial lesions and external beam radiotherapy with or without intracavitary radiotherapy for larger lesions. Interstitial therapy is commonly used unless there exists a small vault lesion, which may be adequately managed by a tandem and ovoid implant.

For locally advanced cancers, because of the poor outcomes associated with radiation therapy alone, concurrent chemotherapy sensitization has been proposed, although the data are still lacking. An exenterative procedure with removal of the vagina, uterus, tubes, ovaries, rectum, pelvis, and/or bladder and urethra with or without vaginal reconstruction may be considered for patients with a central recurrence after radiation therapy or select patients with stage IVA tumors, especially if a rectovaginal or vesicovaginal fistula is present.

The principles of treatment of primary adenocarcinoma of the vagina are the same as those for squamous cell cancer. However, preferred therapy for clear cell carcinoma of the vagina and cervix in young women has not been established. Approximately 60% of tumors occur in the upper half of the vagina, and the remainder occur in the cervix. The incidence of nodal metastases is approximately 18% in stage I and 30% or more in stage II disease. If the disease is found sufficiently early and is confined to the upper vagina and cervix, radical abdominal hysterectomy, upper vaginectomy, and pelvic lymphadenectomy with ovarian preservation can be performed. More advanced lesions are treated with irradiation.

For sarcoma botryoides, primary radiation therapy and local excision have historically yielded poor results. Primary chemotherapy with vincristine, dactinomycin, and cyclophosphamide plus radiation has led to excellent results in treating patients with this disease. Melanoma of the vagina may be treated with radiation, conservative excision, and/or radical surgery.

Prognosis

The size and stage of the disease at the time of diagnosis are the most important prognostic indicators in squamous cell cancers. The 5-year survival rate is approximately 77% in patients with stage I disease, 45% in patients with stage II disease, 31% in patients with stage III disease, and 18% in patients with stage IV disease.

Melanomas—even small ones—are very malignant, and few respond to therapy. The tumor recurs locally and metastasizes to the liver and lungs. Chemotherapy and immunotherapy have been used as adjunctive treatment.

Too few sarcomas of the vagina have been reported to generate survival data. Except for sarcoma botryoides, these tumors have a propensity for local recurrence and distant metastases, and the prognosis is usually poor.

Benedet JL, Bender H, Jones H 3rd, Ngan HY, Pecorelli S. FIGO staging classifications and clinical practice guidelines in the management of gynecologic cancers. FIGO Committee on Gynecologic Oncology. *Int J Gynaecol Obstet* 2000;70:209–262. PMID: 11041682.

Cardosi RJ, Speights A, Fiorica JV, Grendys EC Jr, Hakam A, Hoffman MS. Bartholin's gland carcinoma: a 15-year experience. *Gynecol Oncol* 2001;82:247–251. PMID: 11531274.

Conley LJ, Ellerbrock TV, Bush TJ, Chiasson MA, Sawo D, Wright TC. HIV-1 infection and risk of vulvovaginal and perianal condylomata acuminata and intraepithelial neoplasia: a prospective cohort study. *Lancet* 2002;359:108–113. PMID: 11809252.

Daling JR, Madeleine MM, Schwartz SM, et al. A population-based study of squamous cell vaginal cancer: HPV and cofactors. *Gynecol Oncol* 2002;84:263–270. PMID: 11812085.

de Koning MN, Waddell K, Magyezi J, et al. Genital and cutaneous human papillomavirus (HPV) types in relation to conjunctival squamous cell neoplasia: a case-control study in Uganda. *Infect Agent Cancer* 2008;3:12. PMID: 18783604.

Frank SJ, Jhingran A, Levenback C, Eifel PJ. Definitive radiation therapy for squamous cell carcinoma of the vagina. *Int J Radiat Oncol Biol Phys* 2005;62:138–147. PMID: 15850914.

Frega A, French D, Piazze J, Cerekja A, Vetrano G, Moscarini M. Prediction of persistent vaginal intraepithelial neoplasia in previously hysterectomized women by high-risk HPV DNA detection. *Cancer Lett* 2007;249:235–241. PMID: 17070990.

Hellman K, Lundell M, Silfversward C, Nilsson B, Hellstrom AC, Frankendal B. Clinical and histopathologic factors related to prognosis in primary squamous cell carcinoma of the vagina. *Int J Gynecol Cancer* 2006;16:1201–1211. PMID: 16803507.

Iavazzo C, Pitsouni E, Athanasiou S, Falagas ME. Imiquimod for treatment of vulvar and vaginal intraepithelial neoplasia. *Int J Gynaecol Obstet* 2008;101:3–10. PMID: 18222451.

Jemal A, Siegel R, Xu J, Ward E. Cancer statistics, 2010. *CA Cancer J Clin* 2010;60:277–300. PMID: 20610543.

Samant R, Lau B, E C, Le T, Tam T. Primary vaginal cancer treated with concurrent chemoradiation using cis-platinum. *Int J Radiat Oncol Biol Phys* 2007;69:746–750. PMID: 17512130.

Sherman JF, Mount SL, Evans MF, Skelly J, Simmons-Arnold L, Eltabbakh GH. Smoking increases the risk of high-grade vaginal intraepithelial neoplasia in women with oncogenic human papillomavirus. *Gynecol Oncol* 2008;110:396–401. PMID: 18586314.

Srodon M, Stoler MH, Baber GB, Kurman RJ. The distribution of low and high-risk HPV types in vulvar and vaginal intraepithelial neoplasia (VIN and VaIN). *Am J Surg Pathol* 2006;30:1513–1518. PMID: 17122506.

Tjalma WA, Monaghan JM, de Barros Lopes A, Naik R, Nordin AJ, Weyler JJ. The role of surgery in invasive squamous carcinoma of the vagina. *Gynecol Oncol* 2001;81:360–365. PMID: 11371123.

Troisi R, Hatch EE, Titus-Ernstoff L, et al. Cancer risk in women prenatally exposed to diethylstilbestrol. *Int J Cancer* 2007;121:356–360. PMID: 17390375.

Vinokurova S, Wentzensen N, Einenkel J, et al. Clonal history of papillomavirus-induced dysplasia in the female lower genital tract. *J Natl Cancer Inst* 2005;97:1816–1821. PMID: 16368943.

von Gruenigen VE, Gibbons HE, Gibbins K, Jenison EL, Hopkins MP. Surgical treatments for vulvar and vaginal dysplasia: a randomized controlled trial. *Obstet Gynecol* 2007;109:942–947. PMID: 17400858.

Premalignant & Malignant Disorders of the Uterine Cervix

48

Christine H. Holschneider, MD

CERVICAL INTRAEPITHELIAL NEOPLASIA

ESSENTIALS OF DIAGNOSIS

- The cervix often appears grossly normal.
- Infection with the human papillomavirus is present.
- Dysplastic or carcinoma in situ cells are noted in a cytologic smear preparation (traditional Pap smear or liquid-based cytology).
- Colposcopic examination reveals an atypical transformation zone with thickened epithelium, coarse punctate, or mosaic patterns of surface capillaries.
- Iodine-nonstaining (Schiller-positive) area of squamous epithelium is typical.
- Biopsy diagnosis of cervical intraepithelial neoplasia (dysplasia or carcinoma in situ).

General Considerations

Lower genital tract squamous intraepithelial neoplasia is often multicentric (ie, affecting multiple anatomic sites that embryologically are derived from the same anogenital epithelium): cervical intraepithelial neoplasia (CIN), vaginal intraepithelial neoplasia (VAIN, see Chapter 47), vulvar intraepithelial neoplasia (VIN, see Chapter 47), and perianal intraepithelial neoplasia (PAIN). Approximately 10% of women with CIN have concomitant preinvasive neoplasia of the vulva, vagina, or anus. Conversely, 40–60% of patients with VIN or VAIN have synchronous or metachronous CIN.

CIN, formerly called dysplasia, means disordered growth and development of the epithelial lining of the cervix. There are various degrees of CIN. Mild dysplasia, or CIN I, is defined as disordered growth of the lower third of the epithelial lining. Abnormal maturation of the lower two-thirds of the lining is called moderate dysplasia, or CIN II. Severe dysplasia, CIN III, encompasses more than two-thirds of the epithelial thickness with carcinoma in situ (CIS) representing full-thickness dysmaturity. While histologically evaluated lesions are characterized using the CIN nomenclature, cytologic smears are classified according to the Bethesda system, which was most recently revised in 2001. Briefly, atypical squamous cells are divided into those of undetermined significance (ASC-US) and those in which a high-grade lesion cannot be excluded (ASC-H). Low-grade squamous intraepithelial lesion (LSIL) encompasses cytologic changes consistent with koilocytic atypia or CIN I. High-grade squamous intraepithelial lesion (HSIL) denotes the cytologic findings corresponding to CIN II and CIN III. CIN may be suspected because of an abnormal cytologic smear, but the diagnosis is established by cervical biopsy. Spontaneous regression, especially of CIN I, occurs in a significant number of patients, allowing for expectant management with serial cytologic smears in the reliable patient. A certain percentage of high-grade lesions will progress to an invasive cancer if left untreated. Because it is not presently possible to predict which lesions will progress, it is recommended that all patients with CIN II and CIN III be treated when diagnosed. The only 2 exceptions to this recommendation concern adolescents, in whom CIN II may be followed, as spontaneous regression is substantial and the risk of cancer almost nil, as well as pregnant women, in whom treatment should be deferred to the postpartum period.

Pathogenesis

Prevalence figures for CIN vary according to the socioeconomic characteristics and geographic area of the population studied, from as low as 1.05% in some family planning clinics to as high as 13.7% in women attending sexually transmitted disease (STD) clinics. CIN is most commonly detected in women in their 20s; the peak incidence of CIS is in women ages 25–35 years, whereas the incidence of cervical cancer rises most significantly after the age of 40 years.

The epidemiologic risk factors for CIN are similar to those for cervical cancer and include multiple sexual partners, early onset of sexual activity, a high-risk sexual partner (history of multiple sexual partners, human papillomavirus [HPV] infection, lower genital tract neoplasia, or prior sexual exposure to someone with cervical neoplasia), a history of sexually transmitted infections (STIs), cigarette smoking, human immunodeficiency virus (HIV) infection, acquired immunodeficiency syndrome (AIDS), other forms of immunosuppression, multiparity, and long-term oral contraceptive pill use.

HPVs are a prime etiologic factor in the development of CIN and cervical cancer. In fact, most of the above behavioral and sexual risk factors for cervical neoplasia become statistically insignificant as independent variables after adjusting for HPV infection. Analyses of cervical neoplasia lesions show the presence of HPV in more than 80% of all CIN lesions and in 99.7% of all invasive cervical cancers. The 2 most common high-risk HPV types are HPV-16, found in 50–70% of cervical cancers, and HPV-18, found in 7–20% of cases.

Infection with HPV is extremely common and varies with the patient's age. In the United States, the prevalence of detectable HPV infection rises from 1% in newborns, to 20% in teenagers, to 40% in women 20–29 years of age, with a slow decline thereafter to a plateau of 5% in women age 50 years and older. A women's lifetime risk for infection with HPV is approximately 50–80%. Condoms are not as protective against HPV as they are against other STDs because transmission can occur from labial-scrotal contact. Regular and consistent condom use is necessary to achieve a 60% protection against infection.

There are about 130 HPV types, about 30–40 of which infect the anogenital epithelium. Based on their malignant potential, HPV subtypes are categorized into low-risk and high-risk types. Low-risk HPV types (eg, types 6, 11, 42, 43, and 44) are associated with condylomata and low-grade lesions (CIN I), whereas high-risk HPV types (eg, types 16, 18, 31, 33, 35, 39, 45, 51, 52, 56, 58, 59, and 68) are associated with invasive cancer in addition to high-grade lesions (CIN II and CIN III),

More than 90% of immunocompetent women will have a spontaneous resolution of their HPV infection over a 2-year period, and only approximately 5% will have cytologically detectable CIN. About 10% of women will have a persistent high-risk HPV infection, which places them at increased risk for developing CIN II/III and cervical cancer.

The vast majority of women infected with HPV do not develop CIN or cervical cancer. This suggests that infection with HPV alone is insufficient for the development of CIN or cervical cancer and underscores the importance of other cofactors, such as cigarette smoking or immunosuppression.

Cigarette smoking and HPV infection have synergistic effects on the development of CIN, and cigarette smoking is associated with a 2- to 4-fold increase in the relative risk for developing cervical cancer. Cigarette smoke carcinogens have been found to accumulate locally in the cervical mucus, and the cumulative exposure as measured by pack-years smoked is related to the risk of developing CIN or CIS. However, the mechanisms by which cigarette smoking contributes to cervical carcinogenesis are poorly understood.

The incidence of cervical neoplasia is increased in HIV-infected women, who, in some studies, have a 20–30% incidence of colposcopically confirmed CIN. With increasing immunosuppression, there is an increased risk of de novo HPV infection, persistent HPV infection, and progressive cervical neoplasia. Since 1993, invasive cervical cancer has been included as an AIDS-defining illness.

Prevention

A. HPV Vaccination

Two HPV vaccines are currently approved by the Food and Drug Administration (FDA), a quadrivalent vaccine (Gardasil) against HPV-16, -18, -6, and -11 and a bivalent vaccine (Cervarix) against HPV-16 and -18. In clinical trials, the efficacy of these vaccines for preventing CIN II or worse due to HPV types included in the vaccine was 93–100% in the HPV-naïve study population. In the entire study cohorts (those with or without prior HPV infection), the efficacy of either vaccine for preventing CIN II or worse was only 30–44%. Among HPV-naive populations, these vaccines also provided approximately 20–50% protection against CIN II or worse due to nonvaccine HPV types. The Centers for Disease Control and Prevention (CDC) Advisory Committee on Immunization Practices (ACIP) recommends that all girls 11–12 years of age should be routinely offered HPV vaccination, as well as girls and women age 13–26 who have not yet been vaccinated (catch-up population) and girls as young as 9 years, if indicated. In 2009, the FDA approved the use of the quadrivalent vaccine in males, and ACIP states that the quadrivalent vaccine may be given to males age 9–26 years to reduce their likelihood of acquiring genital warts and prevent the development of anal intraepithelial neoplasia and anal cancer.

These HPV vaccines are prophylactic and not therapeutic. Thus, immunization with HPV vaccine is most effective in female or male individuals who have not been infected with HPV (eg, before sexual debut). These recommendations are not altered if a girl or woman in the qualifying age group is found to have an abnormal Pap or a positive HPV test for the following reason: By their mid-20s, approximately 25% of women test positive for 1 of the 4 HPV types in the quadrivalent vaccine, but only 1% test positive for HPV-16 and -18, and only 0.1% test positive for all 4 HPV types. Thus, the bivalent or quadrivalent HPV vaccine should offer benefit to almost all individuals in the indicated age range. There is no evidence that HPV vaccine is harmful during pregnancy. However, HPV vaccination is not recommended during pregnancy due to limited safety data. Women who have started the vaccination series but became pregnant before completion or women who received the vaccination before knowing they were pregnant should be reassured and advised to resume the vaccination series postpartum. It is safe to offer HPV vaccination during lactation.

B. Screening for CIN & Cervical Cancer

Following the implementation of population-based screening programs and treatment of preinvasive and early invasive disease, there has been a 75% reduction in the incidence and mortality of cervical cancer in developed countries. In the United States, more than half of women who develop cervical cancer either have never had cervical cytology, have been screened only sporadically, or have not been screened within the previous 5 years. It is critical that women, whether vaccinated or not, follow current cervical cancer screening guidelines.

1. Cervical cytology screening—In 2012 new and generally consistent cervical cancer screening recommendations for the general population, HPV vaccinated and unvaccinated, were released by two separate groups: the U.S. Preventive Services Task Force (USPSTF) and the multidisciplinary partnership of the American Cancer Society, American Society for Colposcopy and Cervical Pathology, and American Society for Clinical Pathology (ACS/ASCCP/ASCP).

A. ONSET OF SCREENING—Cervical cytology screening should not begin before age 21 regardless of the age at onset of sexual intercourse. This recommendation is based on the fact that invasive cervical cancer is very rare in women younger than 21 years of age; yet there is significant potential for adverse effects associated with the follow-up of abnormal cervical cytology including anxiety, cost, morbidity and long-term consequences of overuse of follow-up procedures. In young women, there is a high prevalence of HPV infection shortly after the onset of intercourse, commonly associated with abnormal cervical cytology and followed by a very high subsequent spontaneous clearance rate of both HPV infection and dysplasia.

B. FREQUENCY OF SCREENING—Cervical cytology screening is recommended every 3 years for women 21–29 years of age. HPV testing should not be performed in this age group. Women age 30 or older should be screened with cytology and HPV co-testing every 5 years or cytology alone every 3 years.

C. DISCONTINUATION OF SCREENING—Screening should be discontinued in women older than 65 years with negative consecutive screening in the preceding 10 years. Screening should not be resumed for any reason. However, women who have completed their post-treatment surveillance for CIN 2/3 or worse, should continue routine screening for at least 20 years, even if that extends screening past age 65. Cytology testing should be discontinued in women who have had a total hysterectomy and do not have a prior history of CIN 2/3 or worse. Evidence of adequate negative prior screening is not required.

D. SPECIAL POPULATIONS—Based on 2009 ACOG guidelines, women who are HIV positive should be screened twice in the first year after diagnosis and annually thereafter. Women who are immunosuppressed for other reasons or had in utero DES exposure should be screened annually.

As previously discussed, the Pap test results are reported using the 2001 Bethesda nomenclature.

2. HPV testing—Currently, there are 2 US FDA-approved HPV tests in clinical practice. They test for the presence of 1 or more of 13 or 14 high-risk HPV types. High-risk HPV testing is currently being used in the United States for cervical cancer screening in the following scenarios:

- As a triage test for ASC-US cervical cytology in women 21 years of age or older with reflex-HPV testing on the residual preservative of the liquid-based cytology.
- As a triage test for LSIL in postmenopausal women.
- As a follow-up test after CIN I or negative colposcopy in women with ASC-US, ASC-H, LSIL, or atypical glandular cells (AGCs).
- In follow-up after treatment for CIN II/III.
- As an adjunct to cytology for the primary screening in women older than 30 years. HPV testing combined with a cervical cytology smear has been approved as a primary screening approach in the patient age 30 years and older, who still has her uterus and has no immunosuppression. If both results are negative, combined screening should not be repeated for 5 years. If cytology and HPV testing are positive, triaging to colposcopy is as outlined earlier. If cytology is normal, but HPV test is positive, repeat cytology and HPV testing in 6–12 months is recommended, with colposcopy at that point if either test is abnormal. Type-specific testing for HPV-16 and HPV-18 has recently been FDA approved and can be used as an adjunct for women with negative cytology results but positive high-risk HPV test.

3. Visual screening in low-resource settings—Visual inspection of the cervix is being used as a screening tool in low-resource settings with no access to HPV testing or cytology screening. It has limited specificity but is economical and provides immediate results. Visual inspection can be performed by direct visual inspection or by performing cervicoscopy using acetic acid, toluidine blue, or Lugol's iodine as an adjunct.

Clinical Findings

A. Symptoms & Signs

There are usually no symptoms or signs of CIN, and the diagnosis is most often based on biopsy findings following an abnormal routine cervical cytology smear. Because high-grade dysplasia is a transitional phase in the pathogenesis of many cervical cancers, early detection by following the previously described screening guidelines is extremely important. If during pelvic examination, a cervical lesion is visualized, it should be promptly biopsied.

B. Pathology

On cytologic examination, the dysplastic cell is characterized by anaplasia, an increased nuclear-to-cytoplasmic ratio (ie, the nucleus is larger), hyperchromatism with changes in the nuclear chromatin, multinucleation, and abnormalities in differentiation.

Histologically, involvement of varying degrees of thickness of the stratified squamous epithelium is typical of dysplasia. The cells are anaplastic and hyperchromatic and show a loss of polarity in the deeper layers as well as abnormal mitotic figures in increased numbers. Benign epithelial alterations, particularly those of an inflammatory nature, the cytopathic effects of HPV, and technical artifacts may be mistaken for CIN I and CIN II.

The columnar epithelium of the mucus-secreting endocervical glands can also undergo neoplastic transformation. Adenocarcinoma in situ (ACIS) is defined as the presence of endocervical glands lined by atypical columnar epithelium that cytologically resembles the cells of endocervical adenocarcinoma, but that occur in the absence of stromal invasion. The diagnosis of ACIS can be made only by cone biopsy.

C. Special Examinations

All abnormal cervical cytology tests require further evaluation, such as visual inspection of the cervix, repeat cytology, HPV testing, staining with Lugol's solution (Schiller test) or toluidine blue, colposcopy, directed biopsy, endocervical sampling, or diagnostic conization (see Treatment section) (Fig. 48–1). The objective is to exclude the presence of invasive carcinoma and to determine the degree and extent of any CIN.

1. Repeat cervical cytology—There are 3 acceptable initial evaluation steps for patients with minimally abnormal cervical cytology smears (eg, ASC-US, postmenopausal LSIL): accelerated serial cytology smears, triage to colposcopy based on a positive HPV testing result, or immediate referral to colposcopy. All patients with ASC-H, premenopausal LSILs, HSILs, AGCs, or smears suspicious for cancer should be referred for immediate colposcopy.

Prior to performing a repeat smear for a patient with ASC-US, she should be evaluated and treated for potential underlying conditions that might contribute to an atypical smear, such as antimicrobials for infections or hormones for atrophic vaginitis. The cervical cytology smear should be

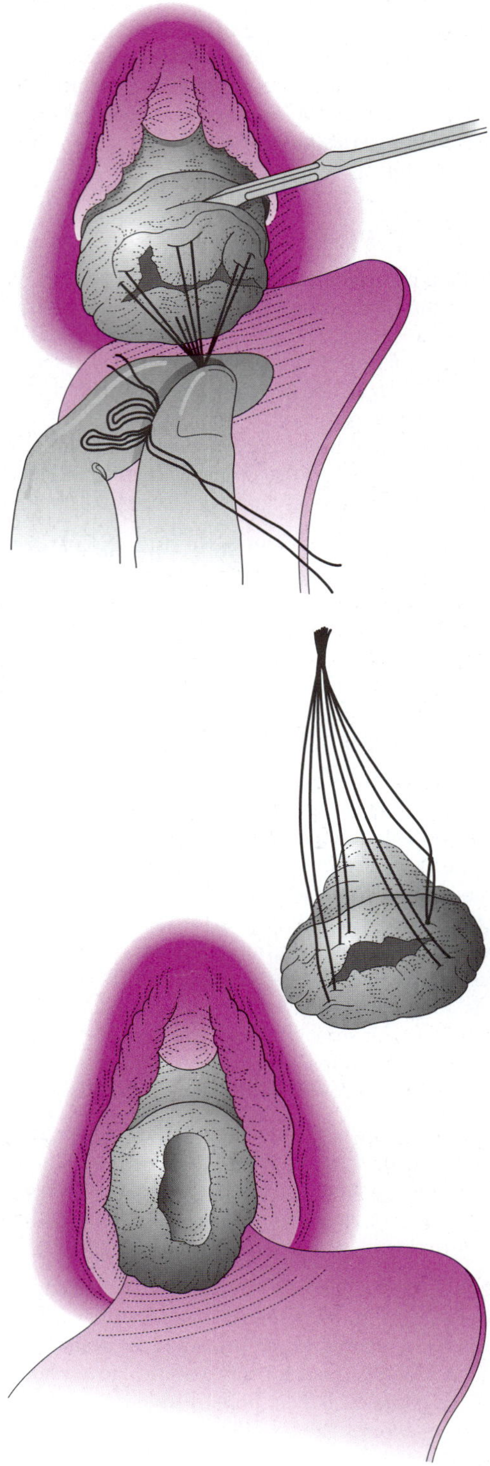

▲ **Figure 48–1.** Conization of the cervix.

repeated every 6 months until there are 2 consecutive normal smears. The use of serial cytologic smears is important, as the false-negative rate of a single repeat smear following an ASC-US diagnosis is as high as 33% for biopsy-proven HSILs (CIN II/III). A second abnormal smear (atypical squamous cell [ASC] or worse) should be evaluated by colposcopy.

2. HPV testing—Testing for low-risk HPV types has no role in cervical cancer prevention. Testing for high-risk HPV types has become an integral part of the management of some abnormal cervical cytology smears (ie, ASC-US, postmenopausal LSIL). For patients with ASC-US, reflex HPV testing is the preferred approach, with triage of women who test positive for high-risk HPV to colposcopy. Reflex HPV testing refers to the concurrent collection of a specimen for cervical cytology and HPV testing, with the HPV testing being performed only in case of an abnormal cytologic screen. For ASC-US, this approach is the most cost-effective and has an equal or higher sensitivity for CIN II/III at the lowest referral rate to colposcopy compared to the 2 alternate approaches (accelerated serial cytology or immediate colposcopy). Women with an ASC-US smear and a negative HPV test are followed with a cervical cytology smear at 1 year. The value of HPV testing for the triage of premenopausal patients with LSIL is limited because nearly 85% of the lesions are HPV positive.

3. Schiller test—The Schiller test is based on the principle that normal mature squamous epithelium of the cervix contains glycogen, which combines with iodine to produce a deep mahogany-brown color. Nonstaining, therefore, indicates abnormal squamous (or columnar) epithelium, scarring, cyst formation, or immature metaplastic epithelium, and constitutes a positive Schiller test. Lugol's solution is an aqueous iodine preparation and is commonly used for the Schiller test.

4. Colposcopic examination—Colposcopy is the primary technique for the evaluation of an abnormal cervical cytology smear. The colposcope is an instrument that uses illuminated low-power magnification (5–15×) to inspect the cervix, vagina, vulva, or anal epithelium. Abnormalities in the appearance of the epithelium and its capillary blood supply often are invisible to the naked eye but can be identified by colposcopy, particularly after the application of 3–5% aqueous acetic acid solution. CIN produces recognizable abnormalities of the cervical epithelium in the majority of patients.

Indications for colposcopy are:

1. Abnormal cervical cytology smear or HPV testing;
2. Clinically abnormal or suspicious-looking cervix;
3. Unexplained intermenstrual or postcoital bleeding;
4. Vulvar or vaginal neoplasia; or
5. History of in utero DES exposure.

Details of the colposcopy technique are described in Chapter 40.

Normal colposcopic findings are those of:

1. The original squamous epithelium, which extends from the mucocutaneous vulvovaginal junction to the original squamocolumnar junction.
2. The transformation zone, which is the metaplastic squamous epithelium between the original squamocolumnar junction and the active squamocolumnar junction. The original squamocolumnar junction is the junction between the stratified squamous epithelium of the vagina and ectocervix and the columnar epithelium of the endocervical canal. In two-thirds of female infants, this original squamocolumnar junction is located on the ectocervix, in close to a third in the endocervical canal, and in a very small subset out in the vaginal fornices. During a woman's life cycle, the squamocolumnar junction "migrates" as a consequence of various hormonal and environmental influences that alter the cervical volume and cause squamous metaplasia of everted endocervical columnar cells. Following menarche, the squamocolumnar junction is generally found on the ectocervix, with further eversion during pregnancy. In the postmenopausal patient, the squamocolumnar junction is frequently within the endocervical canal. This squamous metaplasia is a dynamic process, and cervical neoplasia almost invariably originates within the transformation zone. If the new squamocolumnar junction is visualized in its entirety, the colposcopic examination is called satisfactory; if it cannot be fully visualized, the examination is called unsatisfactory.
3. The columnar epithelium of the endocervical canal.

Abnormal findings indicative of dysplasia and CIS are those of:

1. Leukoplakia or hyperkeratosis, which is an area of white, thickened epithelium that is appreciated prior to the application of acetic acid and may indicate underlying neoplasia.
2. Acetowhite epithelium, which is epithelium that stains white after the application of acetic acid.
3. Mosaicism or punctation reflecting abnormal vascular patterns of the surface capillaries. As a general rule, capillary thickness and intercapillary distances correlate with the severity of the lesion and thus tend to be larger and coarser in higher grade lesions.
4. Atypical vessels with bizarre capillaries with so-called corkscrew, comma-shaped, or spaghetti-like configurations suggest early stromal invasion (Figs. 48–2 through 48–4).

Colposcopically directed punch biopsy of the abnormal areas should be done. The transformation zone extends into

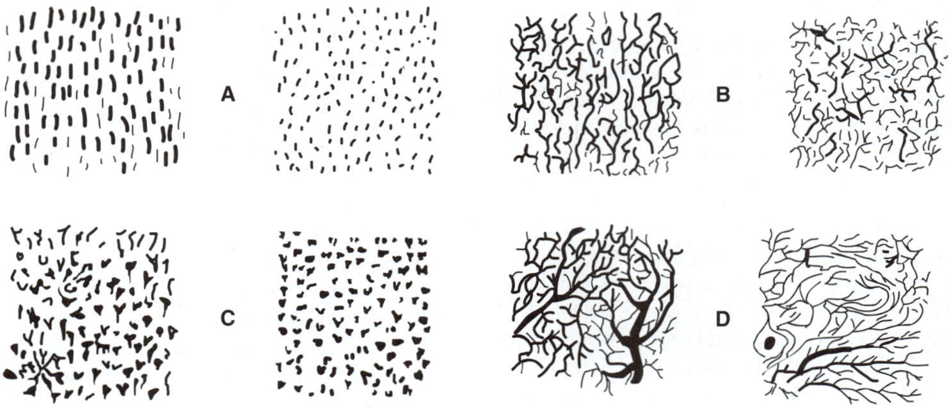

▲ **Figure 48–2.** Schematic of different types of terminal vessels as observed in the normal squamous epithelium: hairpin capillaries (**A**), network capillaries (**B**) both found in normal states, double capillaries (**C**) seen in *Trichomonas* inflammation, and branching vessels (**D**) seen in the transformation zone. (Reproduced, with permission, from Johannisson E, Kolstat P, Soderberg G. Cytologic, vascular, and histologic patterns of dysplasia, carcinoma in situ and early invasive carcinoma of the cervix. *Acta Radiol Suppl* [Stockh] 1966;258:1.)

the endocervical canal beyond the field of vision in 12–15% of premenopausal women and in a significantly higher percentage of postmenopausal women. Evaluation of the nonvisualized portion of the endocervical canal by endocervical sampling should be performed using a brush or curette, at a minimum, in every case in which colposcopy is unsatisfactory, where the lesion is extending into the endocervical canal, where the colposcopic impression does not explain the cervical cytology findings, or where ablative therapy is contemplated. Endocervical sampling is not indicated in pregnancy. In up to 20% of patients with CIN, the endocervical sampling is positive for dysplasia.

5. Diagnostic conization—Following expert colposcopic evaluation, diagnostic conization of the cervix (Fig. 48–1) is indicated if colposcopy is unsatisfactory, if the lesion extends into the cervical canal beyond the view afforded by the colposcope, if there is dysplasia on the endocervical sampling,

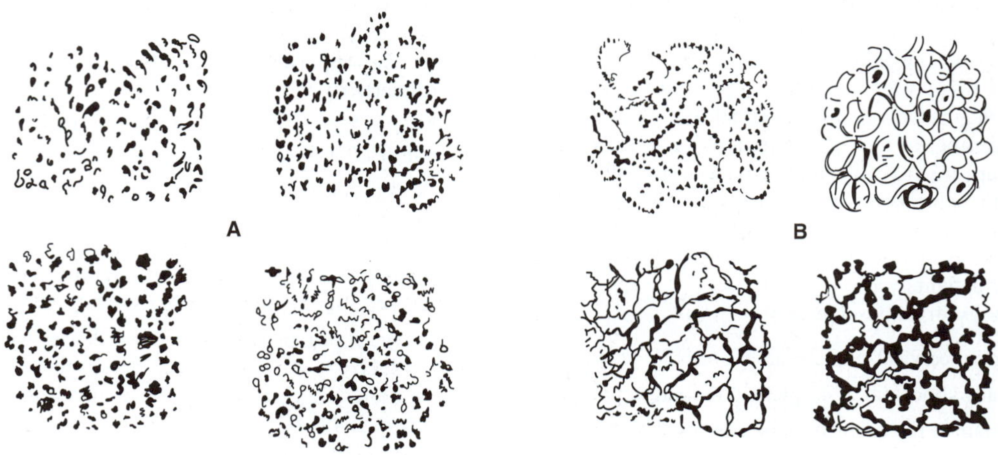

▲ **Figure 48–3.** Schematic of punctation terminal vessels (**A**) and mosaic terminal vessels (**B**). (Reproduced, with permission, from Johannisson E, Kolstat P, Soderberg G. Cytologic, vascular, and histologic patterns of dysplasia, carcinoma in situ and early invasive carcinoma of the cervix. *Acta Radiol Suppl* [Stockh] 1966;258:1.)

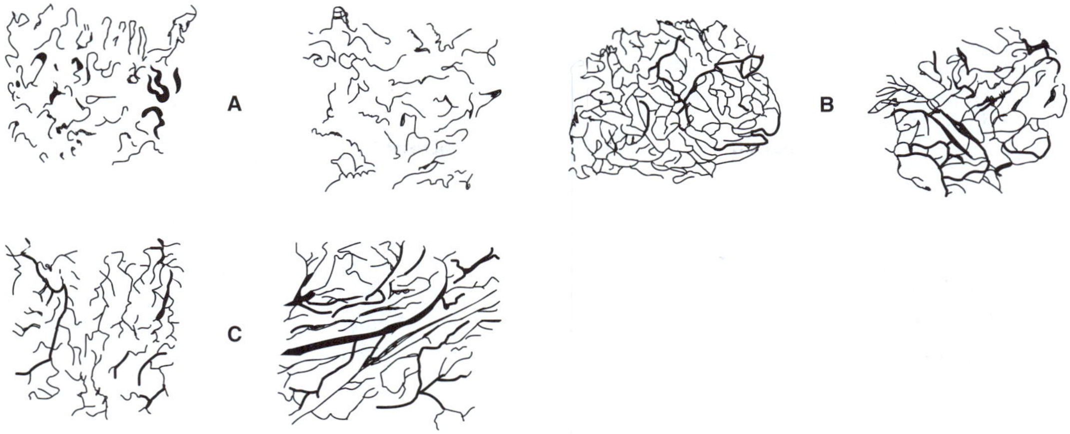

▲ **Figure 48–4.** Schematic of atypical vessels: hairpinlike (**A**); networklike (**B**); and branching type (**C**). (Reproduced, with permission, from Johannisson E, Kolstat P, Soderberg G. Cytologic, vascular, and histologic patterns of dysplasia, carcinoma in situ and early invasive carcinoma of the cervix. *Acta Radiol Suppl* [Stockh] 1966;258:1.)

if there is a significant discrepancy between the histologic diagnosis of the directed biopsy specimen and the cytologic examination, if ACIS is suspected, or if microinvasive carcinoma is suspected.

Differential Diagnosis

As CIN is generally asymptomatic, it is suspected based on an abnormal cervical cytology test, and diagnosis is confirmed by colposcopy-directed cervical biopsy or endocervical sampling. Abnormal cells on a cervical cytology smear may at times arise from locations other than the uterine cervix, including the vulva, vagina, and, especially in case of abnormal glandular cells, the endometrium and adnexae.

Complications

Understanding the natural history of the various degrees of CIN is central to the appropriate clinical management of these patients. In addition to the degree of dysplasia, it is likely that the course of a specific lesion is also influenced by a number of other factors, such as the patient's age, the inciting HPV type, the patient's immune competence, and smoking habits. For individuals who do not clear an HPV infection, longitudinal natural history studies suggest that the time from detection of an infection with high-risk HPV to development of CIN II/III is about 3–5 years and that another 10–20 years pass before the progression to cancer. It is estimated that 30–40% of CIN III actually progresses to cancer.

As summarized in Table 48–1, the majority of CIN I lesions will spontaneously regress without treatment. However, 9–16% of patients with untreated CIN I are diagnosed with CIN II/III over a 2-year follow-up. Spontaneous regression rates of CIN I overall are 60%; in young women, the rates are as high as 91%. Therefore, it is generally reasonable to expectantly follow the compliant patient with CIN I using enhanced surveillance to allow for spontaneous resolution (see following Treatment section). The majority of high-grade lesions will persist or progress (Table 48–1), so immediate treatment is generally warranted.

Treatment

Patient management is based on the results of the cervical cytology smear, findings at colposcopy, biopsy and endocervical sampling results, and individual patient characteristics, such as age, wishes regarding future pregnancies, HIV infection, and the likelihood of compliance with management recommendations. Consensus guidelines for the management of women with CIN have been developed and can be

Table 48–1. Approximate rates of spontaneous regression, persistence, and progression of CIN.

	CIN I	CIN II	CIN III
Regression to normal	60%	40%	30%
Persistence	30%	35%	48%
Progression to CIN III	10%	20%	–
Progression to cancer	<1%	5%	30–40%

CIN, cervical intraepithelial neoplasia.

found online at the American Society for Colposcopy and Cervical Pathology Web site (www.asccp.org). Management options fall into 2 general categories: expectant management or treatment. Expectant management is appropriate for CIN I when preceded by a cervical cytology smear suggestive of a low-grade lesion (ASC-US, LSIL, or ASC-H). These women have a high chance of spontaneous regression. About 12–13% will be diagnosed with CIN II/III or worse in the subsequent 2 years. Thus, expectant management of these patients entails enhanced surveillance with either 2 cervical cytology specimens every 6 months or 1 HPV test at 12 months and a referral to repeat colposcopy if cytology reveals ASC or worse or the HPV test is positive. If the 2 cervical cytology specimens are normal and/or the HPV test is negative, routine screening may be resumed. Follow-up of women with CIN I beyond 24 months has shown that spontaneous regression or progression continues to occur. There are no data to suggest that it is unsafe to continue close clinical follow-up of a compliant patient with persistent CIN I.

Because we currently lack the means to identify individuals at risk for progressive disease, immediate treatment might be appropriate for high-risk patients likely to be lost to follow-up. On the other hand, CIN I preceded by HSIL or AGC–not otherwise specified has a high prevalence of underlying CIN II/III or worse and is thus managed more aggressively. Acceptable options include a diagnostic excisional procedure, review of all findings, or for patients who desire future childbearing, observation with cytology and colposcopy at 6-month intervals for 1 year. If colposcopy is unsatisfactory or endocervical sampling is positive, a diagnostic excisional procedure should be performed. In this setting, immediate excisional procedure is also the preferred approach for any patients who are beyond childbearing. CIN II and III are high-grade lesions, and prompt treatment is generally recommended except in adolescent and pregnant patients (see later Special Situations section).

Treatment options fall into 1 of 2 main categories: procedures that ablate the abnormal tissue and do not produce a tissue specimen for additional histologic evaluation and procedures that excise the area of abnormality, allowing for further histologic study. Prior to any therapeutic intervention, an assessment has to be made as to whether a patient qualifies for ablative therapy (eg, satisfactory diagnostic evaluation has excluded invasive disease) or if she requires an excisional procedure (conization) for further diagnostic workup. In most cases, conization is also the appropriate therapeutic intervention. If the intraepithelial lesion is confined to the ectocervix, treatment with cryotherapy, laser ablation, or a superficial excision by the loop electrosurgical excision procedure (LEEP) is appropriate. If the lesion extends into the endocervical canal, the endocervical curettage contains dysplastic epithelium, or the colposcopic examination is otherwise unsatisfactory, the endocervical canal must be included in the treatment by a deeper LEEP or cone biopsy (Fig. 48–5). A conization procedure is also indicated in cases of a significant discrepancy between cervical cytology and colposcopy/biopsy results, in cases of suspected microinvasive carcinoma or adenocarcinoma in situ.

The 5 most common techniques for the treatment of CIN include 2 ablative techniques—cryotherapy and laser ablation—and 3 excisional procedures—cold knife conization, laser cone excision, and LEEP. Evidence from controlled trials shows that these techniques are of equal efficacy, averaging 80–90% success rates in the treatment of CIN. Cure depends on the size of the lesion, endocervical gland involvement, margin status of any excisional specimen, and endocervical curettage results.

A. Cryotherapy

In cryotherapy, an office procedure not requiring anesthesia, nitrous oxide or carbon dioxide is used as the refrigerant for a supercooled probe. The cryoprobe is positioned on the ectocervix where it must cover the entire lesion, which at times is not easily achieved. It is then activated until blanching of the cervix extends at least 7 mm beyond the probe in all directions in order to assure that freezing extends beyond the depth of the crypts of the glands into which the dysplasia might be extending. Introduction of a 2-cycle freeze–thaw–freeze technique has improved efficacy. The advantages of cryotherapy include ease of use, low cost, widespread availability, and a low complication rate. Side effects include mild uterine cramping and a copious watery vaginal discharge for several weeks. Infection and cervical stenosis are rare. Follow-up colposcopic examinations can be unsatisfactory because of the inability to visualize the squamocolumnar junction.

B. Carbon Dioxide Laser

Carbon dioxide (CO_2) laser can be used either to ablate the transformation zone or as a tool for cone biopsies. The laser destroys tissue with a very narrow zone of injury around the treated tissue and is therefore both precise and flexible. The tissue is vaporized to a depth of at least 7 mm to assure that the bases of the deepest glands are destroyed. Posttreatment vaginal discharge may last 1–2 weeks, and bleeding that requires reexamination can occur in a small percentage of patients. The technique is expensive and requires significant training and attention to safety, as well as local or general anesthesia.

C. Loop Electrosurgical Excision Procedure

LEEP is frequently used for treating CIN II and CIN III because of its ease of use, low cost, and provision of additional tissue for histologic evaluation. LEEP uses a small, fine, wire loop attached to an electrosurgical generator to excise the tissue of interest. Various sizes of wire loop are available. Following LEEP excision of the transformation

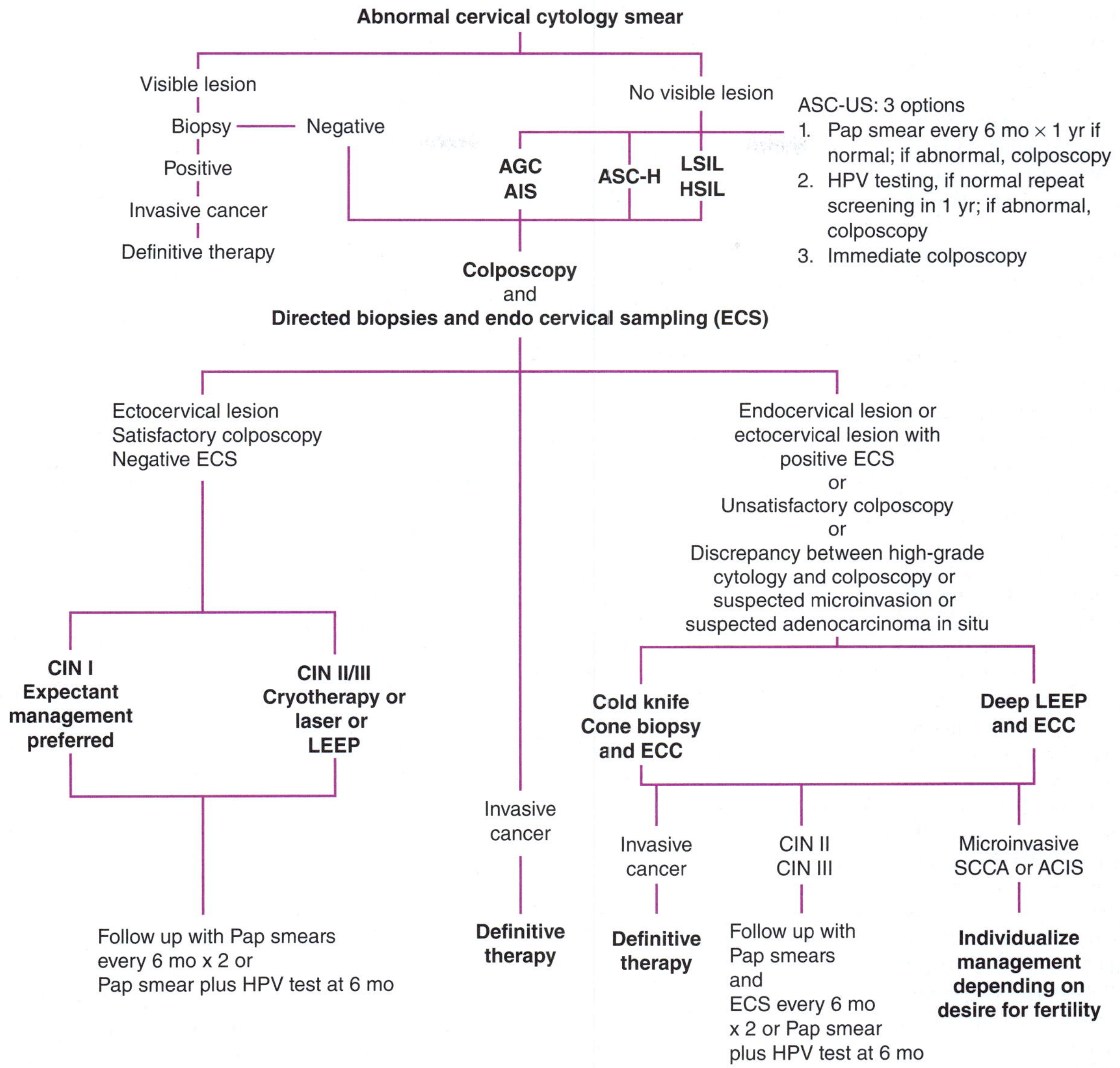

▲ **Figure 48–5.** Plan for management of the abnormal cytologic smear with visible or no visible cervical lesion. SCCA, squamous cell carcinoma.

zone, frequently an additional narrow endocervical specimen ("top hat") is removed to allow for histologic evaluation while avoiding excessive damage to the cervical stroma. Fulguration with a roller ball electrode is then used to achieve complete hemostasis in the excision bed. LEEP can be performed as an office procedure under local anesthesia. An insulated speculum to prevent conduction of electricity, a grounding pad, and a vacuum to remove the smoke are necessary. Complications are less frequent than with cold knife conization and include bleeding, infection, and cervical stenosis.

D. Cold Knife Conization

Cold knife conization of the cervix refers to the excision of a cone-shaped portion of the cervix using a scalpel.

This technique can be individualized to accommodate the cervical anatomy and the size and shape of the lesion. For example, a wide, shallow cone specimen can be obtained from a young patient whose squamocolumnar junction is on the ectocervix. In an older patient, in whom the squamocolumnar junction tends to move more cephalad into the endocervical canal, a narrower, deeper cone is preferable. An endocervical sampling is performed after the conization to assess the remaining endocervical canal. Cervical cone biopsy is generally done in the operating room under local or general anesthesia. Complications include bleeding, infection, cervical stenosis, and cervical insufficiency. The need to perform the procedure in the operating room and a higher complication rate are distinct disadvantages of cold knife conization. However, it results in a specimen devoid of any thermal artifact that may complicate the histologic diagnosis and margin assessment seen with LEEP and laser conization. This becomes particularly important with suspected microinvasive carcinoma and adenocarcinoma in situ.

Prognosis

Controlled trials show 80–90% success rates in the treatment of CIN, regardless of treatment modality used. Patients with larger lesions, endocervical gland involvement, positive margins, or positive endocervical curettage after an excisional procedure are at higher risk for persistent/recurrent disease than are women with negative margins. Most treatment failures are diagnosed within the first 1–2 years after therapy. A number of follow-up protocols have been advocated including HPV testing, serial cytology, endocervical sampling, colposcopy, or various combinations thereof. HPV testing at 6–12 months posttreatment is highly sensitive at detecting persistent/recurrent CIN and is more sensitive than cytology alone. A recent long-term multicohort study of 435 women treated for CIN II/III demonstrated the value of combined cervical cytology and high-risk HPV testing at 6 and 24 months postprocedure at a referral threshold for further evaluation and treatment if either the cytology test showed ASC or worse or the HPV test was positive: If both tests were negative at 6 months, the risk of persistent or recurrent CIN II/III was 4.6%; if both tests were negative at 6 and 24 months, the risk was 1.8%. In contrast, if either test was positive at 6 months, the risk of persistent CIN II/III or worse was 45–60%, indicating the need for immediate evaluation and treatment for these patients.

Outpatient therapy for CIN can reduce the risk of cervical cancer by 95%. However, the risk of invasive cancer among these patients remains increased for at least 20–25 years, necessitating long-term annual surveillance.

Management of recurrent dysplasia follows the same guidelines outlined in Figure 48–5. If a woman has completed childbearing, recurrent dysplasia can be treated by a simple hysterectomy after invasion has been ruled out. Women with a history of cervical dysplasia have a higher incidence of vaginal dysplasia. These women continue to need Pap tests after hysterectomy.

Impact of Treatment of CIN on Subsequent Fertility & Pregnancy

For women with CIN who desire future childbearing, management priorities are to diagnose and treat preinvasive disease and prevent cervical cancer while minimizing the impact on future fertility and pregnancy. Potential treatment-associated effects on future reproductive outcome include cervical stenosis, alteration of the cervical mucus, and removal or destruction of the collagen matrix of the cervical stroma. It appears that the cervix is better preserved following ablation compared with excision.

One of the main concerns for future pregnancy is the potential for treatment-associated preterm delivery with its associated neonatal morbidity and mortality from prematurity. These risks appear to vary by the type of treatment procedure, and many experts believe the risks are largely related to the amount and depth of tissue removed. Cold knife conization increases the risk of second-trimester pregnancy loss, preterm delivery, and perinatal mortality approximately 3-fold. The risk of preterm delivery increases further with the number of procedures performed. The data on LEEP are more conflicting. While in some studies, LEEP did not increase the risk of preterm delivery and perinatal mortality, others found that LEEP nearly doubles the risk of preterm premature rupture of membranes and preterm delivery. Cryotherapy does not appear to have such strong association with preterm delivery. Thus, strong consideration should be given to offer cryotherapy treatment to women who desire future pregnancy and are candidates for ablative therapy (as discussed earlier).

Special Situations

A. Adolescents & Young Women

Adherence to the ACOG/USPSTF/ACS/ASCCP cervical cancer screening guidelines, which recommend initiation of screening at 21 years of age, should largely obviate the need for the special management algorithms for adolescents and young women found at the American Society for Colposcopy and Cervical Pathology Web site (www.asccp.org), which rest on the guiding principle that expectant management is preferred in females age 20 years old or younger.

B. Pregnancy

Pregnant women routinely undergo cervical cytology screening at their first prenatal visit. As a result, it is not uncommon that an abnormal cervical cytology smear is first discovered during pregnancy. Colposcopy is generally performed for the same indications as in the nonpregnant patient. However, biopsies are limited unless there are colposcopic signs suggestive of high-grade dysplasia, CIS, or invasive disease. Endocervical curettage is not performed in pregnancy because of the potential risk of abortion and infection. The physiologic changes of pregnancy render the transformation zone easily accessible for satisfactory colposcopy by 20 weeks' gestation in almost all women. Colposcopy during pregnancy can be challenging because pregnancy may produce changes in the cervical epithelium that mimic those of cervical dysplasia. Although the gravid cervix is more vascular, directed ectocervical biopsies can be performed safely with minimal increase in the risk of significant bleeding. After the diagnosis of CIN II/III has been established, the patient can be carefully followed with colposcopic examinations and cervical cytology smears each trimester. Repeat biopsies are only performed for progressive lesions. Treatment is deferred into the postpartum period. Even high-grade lesions discovered during pregnancy have a high rate of regression in the postpartum period. Conization during pregnancy is indicated only if early invasive disease is suspected and the timing and extent of the procedure during pregnancy are individualized. Complications of a cone biopsy in pregnancy include abortion, hemorrhage, infection, and incompetent cervix.

C. HIV Infection

HIV-infected women are more likely to have persistent HPV infection, and CIN is common in HIV-infected women. Based on ACOG guidelines, women who are infected with HIV should undergo cervical cytology screening twice in the first year after diagnosis of HIV infection and then annually. Women with advanced HIV appear to be more likely to have persistent HPV and CIN than those with early HIV infections. Use of highly active antiretroviral therapy (HAART) has been suggested to reduce the risk of CIN and cervical cancer. However, data are conflicting.

Cytologic abnormalities in HIV-infected women should be evaluated in the same manner as in uninfected women. Management of CIN in the HIV-infected patient presents a great challenge. Primary treatment of CIN in HIV-infected women is generally similar to the approach used in HIV-negative women. Generally, expectant management of CIN I is acceptable in HIV-infected women. LEEP excision of the cervix appears to be most appropriate for patients with CIN II/III, and topical 5-fluorouracil cream is recommended by some experts as adjunctive therapy in this setting. Following treatment, the risk of recurrent CIN is high, especially in the immunocompromised patient with low CD4 counts and high viral loads. Recurrence rates may reach 80% within 3 years in markedly immunocompromised women. Thus, surveillance with cervical cytology and colposcopy is recommended by some experts as frequently as every 3 months.

D. Atypical Glandular Cells on Cervical Cytology Smear

Patients with AGCs on a cervical cytology smear have up to a 50% risk of having significant underlying pathology. Nine to 38% of women with AGC have significant neoplasia (CIN II/III, ACIS), and 3–17% have invasive cancer.

The 2001 Bethesda System divides glandular cell abnormalities into AGCs, AGC–favor neoplasia, endocervical ACIS, and adenocarcinoma. Given the high risk for significant pathology, any patient with glandular cell abnormalities on a cervical cytology smear requires immediate evaluation, which includes, at a minimum, colposcopy with careful endocervical sampling. Assessment of the endometrium is recommended in all patients older than age 35 years, in patients at any age with conditions associated with chronic anovulation, in those at increased risk for endometrial cancer, in any women with abnormal bleeding, in women with AGC–endometrial cells, and in women with AGC–nonspecified cell type. Diagnostic conization is indicated in all cases of AGC–favor neoplasia, ACIS, or suspected adenocarcinoma as well as persistent AGC–not otherwise specified, unless a definitive diagnosis has been made on the colposcopy-directed biopsy or endometrial sampling.

E. Adenocarcinoma In Situ

ACIS of the cervix is a precursor of adenocarcinoma of the cervix, which comprises about 25% of cervical cancers in the United States. The incidence of both in situ and invasive disease is rising, especially in young women, with up to 30% of cases occurring in women younger than 35 years of age. As with squamous intraepithelial neoplasia, HPV infection is almost universally found. ACIS has no pathognomonic clinical, cytologic, or colposcopic features. The lesion is not grossly visible on examination. Management is difficult. The lesion is usually at the transformation zone but may be located high in the endocervical canal, involve the deeper portions of the endocervical clefts, or be multifocal with skip lesions. Ten to 13% of ACIS is multifocal, defined as foci of ACIS separated by at least 2 mm of normal mucosa. Nearly half of women with ACIS have concomitant squamous CIN or cancer. Conization with negative margins is required to make the diagnosis of ACIS.

Follow-up surveillance after conization is difficult, as cervical cytology, endocervical curettage, or endocervical cytobrush sampling each have a sensitivity of only approximately 50%. This is of particular concern because the incidence of residual ACIS or invasive adenocarcinoma following conization for ACIS is as high as 45% with positive conization margins and 27% with negative conization margins. Therefore, conservative management should be undertaken only in the young patient with a negative conization margin and negative endocervical sampling who is fully counseled and desires to maintain her fertility. After completion of childbearing, hysterectomy is generally recommended. In all other patients, hysterectomy should be performed as a definitive therapeutic intervention. Approximately 7% of patients with positive and 2% of patients with negative conization margins will have invasive disease on the hysterectomy specimen. Thus, extrafascial hysterectomy can be recommended for those patients with negative conization margins. If conization margins are positive, prehysterectomy repeat conization is recommended or consideration can be given to the performance of a modified radical hysterectomy, especially if there is significantly altered anatomy following prior conization procedures or extensive disease and positive margins were found on the preceding conization specimen.

Ahdieh L, Muñoz A, Vlahov D, et al. Cervical neoplasia and repeated positivity of human papillomavirus infection in human immunodeficiency virus-seropositive and -seronegative women. *Am J Epidemiol* 2000;151:1148–1157. PMID: 10905527.

American College of Obstetricians and Gynecologists Committee on Practice Bulletins–Gynecology. ACOG Practice Bulletin no. 109: cervical cytology screening. *Obstet Gynecol* 2009;114: 1409–1420. PMID: 20134296.

Arbyn M, Buntinx F, Van Ranst M, et al. Virologic versus cytologic triage of women with equivocal Pap smears: a meta-analysis of the accuracy to detect high-grade intraepithelial neoplasia. *J Natl Cancer Inst* 2004;96:280–293. PMID: 14970277.

Arbyn M, Kyrgiou M, Simoens C, et al. Perinatal mortality and other severe adverse pregnancy outcomes associated with treatment of cervical intraepithelial neoplasia: meta-analysis. *BMJ* 2008;337:a1284. doi: 10.1136/bmj.a1284. PMID: 18808168.

Arends MJ, Buckley CH, Wells M. Etiology, pathogenesis, and pathology of cervical neoplasia. *J Clin Pathol* 1998;51:96–103. PMID: 9602680.

Atypical Squamous Cell of Undetermined Significance/Low-Grade Squamous Intraepithelial Lesions Triage Study (ALTS) Group. Human papillomavirus testing for triage of women with cytologic evidence of low-grade squamous intraepithelial lesions: baseline data from a randomized trial. *J Natl Cancer Inst* 2000;92:397–402. PMID: 10700419.

Atypical Squamous Cell of Undetermined Significance/Low-Grade Squamous Intraepithelial Lesions Triage Study (ALTS) Group. Results of a randomized trial on the management of cytology interpretations of atypical squamous cells of undetermined significance. *Am J Obstet Gynecol* 2003;188:1383–1392. PMID: 12824967.

Centers for Disease Control and Prevention (CDC). FDA licensure of bivalent human papillomavirus vaccine (HPV2, Cervarix) for use in females and updated HPV vaccination recommendations from the Advisory Committee on Immunization Practices (ACIP). *MMWR Morb Mortal Wkly Rep* 2010;59:626–629. PMID: 20508593.

Denehy TR, Gregori CA, Breen JL. Endocervical curettage, cone margins, and residual adenocarcinoma in situ of the cervix. *Obstet Gynecol* 1997;90:1–6. PMID: 9207802.

FUTURE II Study Group. Quadrivalent vaccine against human papillomavirus to prevent high-grade cervical lesions. *N Engl J Med* 2007;356:1915–1927. PMID: 17492945.

Gage JC, Hanson VW, Abbey K, et al. Number of cervical biopsies and sensitivity of colposcopy. *Obstet Gynecol* 2006;108:264–272. PMID: 16880294.

Harper DM, Franco EL, Wheeler C, et al. Efficacy of a bivalent L1 virus-like particle vaccine in prevention of infection with human papillomavirus types 16 and 18 in young women: a randomised controlled trial. *Lancet* 2004;364:1757–1765. PMID: 15541448.

Ho GY, Bierman R, Beardsley L, et al. Natural history of cervicovaginal papillomavirus infection in young women. *N Engl J Med* 1998;338:423–428. PMID: 9459645.

Holowaty P, Miller AB, Rohan T, To T. Natural history of dysplasia of the uterine cervix. *J Natl Cancer Inst* 1999;91:252–258. PMID: 10037103.

Im DD, Duska LR, Rosenshein NB. Adequacy of conization margins in adenocarcinoma in situ of the cervix as a predictor of residual disease. *Gynecol Oncol* 1995;59:179–182. PMID: 7590468.

Kocken M, Helmerhorst TJ, Berkhof J, et al. Risk of recurrent high-grade cervical intraepithelial neoplasia after successful treatment: a long-term multi-cohort study. *Lancet Oncol* 2011;12:441–450. PMID: 21530398.

Koutsky LA, Ault KA, Wheeler CM, et al. A controlled trial of a human papillomavirus type 16 vaccine. *N Engl J Med* 2002; 347:1645–1651. PMID: 12444178.

Kyrgiou M, Koliopoulos G, Martin-Hirsch P, et al. Obstetric outcomes after conservative treatment for intraepithelial or early invasive cervical lesions: systematic review and meta-analysis. *Lancet* 2006;367:489–498. PMID: 16473126.

Lea JS, Shin CH, Sheets EE, et al. Endocervical curettage at conization to predict residual cervical adenocarcinoma in situ. *Gynecol Oncol* 2002;87:129–132. PMID: 12468353.

Martin-Hirsch PL, Paraskevaidis E, Kitchener H. Surgery for cervical intraepithelial neoplasia. *Cochrane Database Syst Rev* 2000;2:CD001318. PMID: 10796771.

McCredie MR, Sharples KJ, Paul C, et al. Natural history of cervical neoplasia and risk of invasive cancer in women with cervical intraepithelial neoplasia 3: a retrospective cohort study. *Lancet Oncol* 2008;9:425–434. PMID: 18407790.

McIndoe WA, McLean MR, Jones RW, et al. The invasive potential of carcinoma in situ of the cervix. *Obstet Gynecol* 1984;64:451–458. PMID: 6483293.

Melnikow J, Nuovo J, Willan AR, et al. Natural history of cervical squamous intraepithelial lesions: a meta-analysis. *Obstet Gynecol* 1998;92:727–735. PMID: 9764690.

Moscicki AB, Shiboski S, Hills NK, et al. Regression of low-grade squamous intraepithelial lesions in young women. *Lancet* 2004;364:1678–1683. PMID: 15530628.

Moyer VA, on behalf of the U.S. Preventive Services Task Force. *Ann Int Med* 2012 Mar 14 [Epub ahead of print].

Munoz N, Bosch FX, de Sanjosé S, et al. Epidemiologic classification of human papillomavirus types associated with cervical cancer. *N Engl J Med* 2003;348:518–527. PMID: 12571259.

Noehr B, Frederiksen K, Tabor A, et al. Loop electrosurgical excision of the cervix and subsequent risk for spontaneous preterm delivery: a population-based study of singleton deliveries during a 9-year period. *Am J Obstet Gynecol* 2009;114:511–515. PMID: 19701028.

Olsen AO, Dillner J, Skrondal A, Magnus P. Combined effect of smoking and human papillomavirus type 16 infection in cervical carcinogenesis. *Epidemiology* 1998;9:346–349. PMID: 9583429.

Paavonen J, Naud P, Salmerón J, et al. Efficacy of human papillomavirus (HPV)-16/18 AS04-adjuvanted vaccine against cervical infection and precancer caused by oncogenic HPV types (PATRICIA): final analysis of a double-blind, randomised study in young women. *Lancet* 2009;374:301–314. PMID: 19586656.

Poynor EA, Barakat RR, Hoskins WJ. Management and follow-up of patients with adenocarcinoma in situ of the uterine cervix. *Gynecol Oncol* 1995;57:158–164. PMID: 7729727.

Prokopczyk B, Cox JE, Hoffmann D, et al. Identification of tobacco-specific carcinogen in the cervical mucus of smokers and nonsmokers. *J Natl Cancer Inst* 1997;89:868–873. PMID: 9196253.

Saslow D, Runowicz CD, Solomon D, et al. American Cancer Society guideline for the early detection of cervical neoplasia and cancer. *CA Cancer J Clin* 2002;52:342–362. PMID: 12469763.

Saslow D, Solomon, Lawson HW et al. American Cancer Society, American Society for Colposcopy and Cervical Pathology, and American Society for Clinical Pathology Screening Guidelines for the Prevention and Early Detection of Cervical Cancer. *CA Cancer J Clin* 2012;62:147–172. PMID: 22422631.

Solomon D, Davey D, Kurman R, et al. The 2001 Bethesda system terminology for reporting results of cervical cytology. *JAMA* 2002;287:2114–2119. PMID: 11966386.

Solomon D, Schiffman M, Tarone R. Comparison of three management strategies for patients with atypical squamous cells of undetermined significance: baseline results from a randomized trial. *J Natl Cancer Inst* 2001;93:293–299. PMID: 11181776.

Soutter WP, de Barros Lopes A, Fletcher A, et al. Invasive cervical cancer after conservative therapy for cervical intraepithelial neoplasia. *Lancet* 1997;349: 978–980. PMID: 9100623.

Stanley M. Pathology and epidemiology of HPV infection in females. *Gynecol Oncol* 2010;117(2 suppl):S5–S10. PMID: 20304221.

Wallin KL, Wiklund F, Angström T, et al. Type-specific persistence of human papillomavirus DNA before the development of invasive cervical cancer. *N Engl J Med* 1999;341:1633–1670. PMID: 10572150.

Wolf JK, Levenback C, Malpica A, et al. Adenocarcinoma in situ of the cervix: significance of cone biopsy margins. *Obstet Gynecol* 1996;88:82–86. PMID: 8684768.

Wright TC Jr, Massad LS, Dunton CJ, et al. 2006 consensus guidelines for the management of women with abnormal cervical cancer screening tests. *Am J Obstet Gynecol* 2007;197:346–355. PMID: 17904957.

Wright TC Jr, Massad LS, Dunton CJ, et al. 2006 consensus guidelines for the management of women with cervical intraepithelial neoplasia or adenocarcinoma in situ. *Am J Obstet Gynecol* 2007;197:340–345. PMID: 17904956.

Ylitalo N, Sørensen P, Josefsson AM, et al. Consistent high viral load of human papillomavirus 16 and risk of cervical carcinoma in situ: a nested case-control study. *Lancet* 2000;355:2194–2198. PMID: 10881892.

Yost NP, Santoso JT, McIntire DD, et al. Postpartum regression rates of antepartum cervical intraepithelial neoplasia II and III lesions. *Obstet Gynecol* 1999;93:359–362. PMID: 10097949.

CANCER OF THE CERVIX

ESSENTIALS OF DIAGNOSIS

- Early disease is frequently asymptomatic, underscoring the importance of cervical cytology screening.
- Abnormal uterine bleeding and vaginal discharge are the most common symptoms.
- A cervical lesion may be visible on inspection as a tumor or ulceration; cancer within the cervical canal may be occult.
- Diagnosis must be confirmed by biopsy.

General Considerations

In the United States, an estimated 12,710 new cases of invasive cervical cancer are diagnosed annually, and there are 4290 deaths from the disease. In contrast, with more than 529,000 new cases diagnosed annually and a >50% mortality rate, cervical cancer is the second most common cause of cancer-related morbidity and mortality among women in developing countries. This dichotomy is largely the result of a 75% decrease in the incidence of cervical cancer in developed countries following the implementation of population-based screening programs and treatment of preinvasive disease. The average age at diagnosis of patients with cervical cancer is 51 years. However, the disease can occur in the second decade of life and during pregnancy, and nearly 20% of cervical cancers are diagnosed in women age 65 or older. More than 95% of patients with early cancer of the cervix can be cured.

Pathogenesis

The major epidemiologic risk factors for cervical cancer are the same as those for CIN and were discussed earlier. HPV is central to the development of cervical neoplasia. HPV DNA is found in 99.7% of all cervical carcinomas. HPV-16 is the most prevalent HPV type in squamous cell carcinoma and adenocarcinoma, followed by HPV-18 and HPV-45. Other associated risk factors are tobacco use, immunosuppression, infection with HIV or a history of other STIs, high parity, and oral contraceptive use.

HPV is epitheliotropic. Once the epithelium is acutely infected with HPV, 1 of 3 clinical scenarios ensues:

1. Asymptomatic latent infection;
2. Active infection in which HPV undergoes vegetative replication but not integration into the genome (eg, leading to condyloma or CIN I); or
3. Neoplastic transformation following integration of oncogenic HPV DNA into the human genome.

The virus infects a subset of primitive basal cells in the epithelium where it will undergo replication. The infected cell then enters the proliferating epithelial component. Active infection, in which HPV undergoes replication but remains episomal, is characterized by minimal viral oncogene expression. However, integration of HPV into the human genome is associated with cell immortalization, allowing for malignant transformation. This involves an upregulation of the viral oncogenes E6 and E7. These oncoproteins interfere with cell-cycle control in the human host cell. E6 and E7 have the ability to complex with the tumor suppressor genes p53 and Rb, respectively. The disabling of these 2 major tumor suppressor genes is thought to be central to host cell immortalization and transformation induced by HPV and the observed increased genetic instability.

Table 48–2. Risk of any lymph node metastasis for patients with microscopic squamous cell carcinoma of the cervix.

Depth of Tumor Invasion	Risk of Lymph Node Metastasis
FIGO stage IA1	
Early stromal invasion (<1 mm)	3/1543 (0.2%)
Microinvasion (1–3 mm)	5/809 (0.6%)
FIGO stage IA2	
Microscopic 3–5 mm invasion	14/214 (6.5%)

FIGO, International Federation of Gynecology and Obstetrics.

Incipient cancer of the cervix is generally a slowly developing process. Most cervical cancers probably begin as a high-grade dysplastic change (see previous section) or CIS with gradual progression over a period of several years. At least 90% of carcinomas of the cervix develop from the intraepithelial layers, almost always within 1 cm of the squamocolumnar junction of the cervix either on the portio vaginalis of the cervix or slightly higher in the endocervical canal.

Early stromal invasion (stage IA1) up to a depth of 3 mm below the basement membrane is a localized process, provided there is no pathologic evidence of lymphovascular space involvement. Penetration of the stroma beyond this point carries an increased risk of lymphatic metastasis (Table 48–2). When the lymphatics are involved, tumor cells are carried to the regional pelvic lymph nodes (parametrial, hypogastric, obturator, external iliac, and sacral) (Fig. 48–6). The more pleomorphic or extensive the local disease, the greater is the likelihood of lymph node involvement. As the tumor grows, it also spreads by direct extension to the parametria.

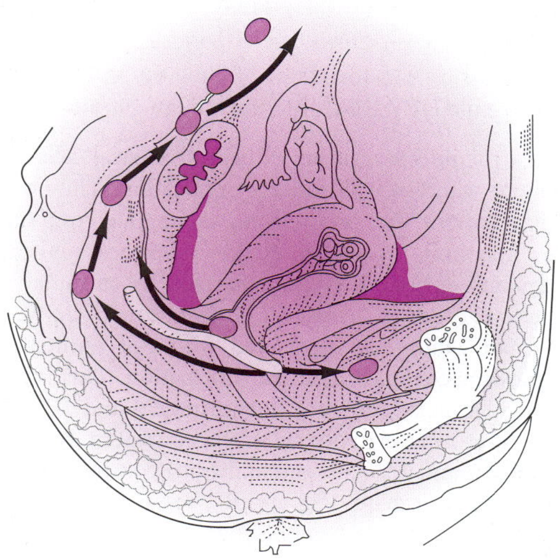

▲ **Figure 48–6.** Lymphatic spread of carcinoma of the cervix.

Squamous cell carcinoma clinically confined to the cervix involves the regional pelvic lymph nodes in 15–20% of cases. When the cancer involves the parametrium (stage IIB), tumor cells can be found in the pelvic lymph nodes in 30–40% of cases and in the para-aortic nodes in approximately 15–30% of cases. The more advanced the local disease, the greater is the likelihood of distant metastases. The para-aortic nodes are involved in approximately 45% of patients with stage IVA disease.

Ovarian involvement is rare, occurring in approximately 0.5% of squamous cell carcinomas and 1.7% of adenocarcinomas. The liver and lungs are the most common sites of blood-borne metastasis, but the tumor may involve the brain, bones, bowels, adrenal glands, spleen, or pancreas.

When cancer of the cervix is untreated or fails to respond to treatment, death occurs in 95% of patients within 2 years after the onset of symptoms. Death can occur from uremia, pulmonary embolism, or hemorrhage from direct extension of tumor into blood vessels. Life-threatening sepsis from complications of pyelonephritis or vesicovaginal and rectovaginal fistulas is possible. Large bowel obstruction from direct extension of tumor into the rectosigmoid can be the terminal event. Pain from perineural extension is a significant management problem of advanced disease.

Pathology

Approximately 70–75% of cervical carcinomas are squamous cell; the remainder are composed of various types of adenocarcinomas (20–25%), adenosquamous carcinomas (3–5%), and undifferentiated carcinomas.

A. Squamous Cell Carcinomas

Cervical squamous cell carcinomas have been classified according to the predominant cell type: large cell nonkeratinizing, large cell keratinizing, and small cell carcinomas. The large cell nonkeratinizing variety accounts for the majority of tumors.

B. Verrucous Squamous Carcinoma

Verrucous squamous carcinoma, which has been associated with HPV-6, is a rare subtype of well-differentiated squamous carcinoma. It is a slow-growing, locally invasive neoplasm. Histologically, this tumor is composed of well-differentiated squamous cells with frondlike papillae and little apparent stromal invasion, but it is potentially lethal. Radical resection is the mainstay of therapy.

C. Papillary Squamous Carcinoma

Papillary squamous carcinoma of the cervix is characterized by highly dysplastic squamous cells forming papillary fronds with thin fibrovascular cores. The gross appearance of this lesion may be warty or fungating.

D. Adenocarcinoma

Adenocarcinoma of the cervix is derived from the glandular elements of the cervix. The incidence of adenocarcinomas, including the mucinous, endometrioid, clear cell, and serous types, has been rising over the last several decades, especially in women younger than 35 years of age. Part of this increase may be a result of an increasing prevalence of HPV infection, and part may be a result of improvements in screening and prevention of squamous preinvasive disease, thus leading to a histologic shift toward adenocarcinoma. When the initial growth of adenocarcinoma of the cervix is within the endocervical canal and the ectocervix appears normal, this lesion might not be diagnosed until it is advanced and ulcerative. Cervical adenocarcinoma is subdivided into endocervical type (usual type; minimal deviation adenocarcinoma [adenoma malignum] and well-differentiated villoglandular adenocarcinoma), endometrioid type, clear cell type, papillary serous type, intestinal type, mesonephric type, and mixed type. The clear cell type may be related to in utero exposure to DES. It has a prognosis comparable to that of other adenocarcinomas of the cervix.

E. Minimal Deviation Adenocarcinoma (Adenoma Malignum)

Adenoma malignum, or minimal deviation adenocarcinoma, is an extremely well-differentiated adenocarcinoma that may be difficult to recognize as a malignant process. It represents approximately 1% of adenocarcinomas of the cervix and has been associated with Peutz-Jeghers syndrome. It occurs mainly in the fifth and sixth decades of life. Diagnosis is often delayed because of frequently normal cervical cytology smears. Punch biopsies are often nondiagnostic, requiring conization for further evaluation.

F. Adenoid Cystic Carcinoma

Another uncommon variant of adenocarcinoma is adenoid cystic carcinoma. This lesion is considered more aggressive than most cervical adenocarcinomas and occurs more commonly in black women of high parity in their sixth and seventh decades of life. It should not be confused with adenoid basal carcinomas, which have an indolent growth pattern.

G. Adenosquamous Carcinoma

Adenosquamous carcinomas contain an admixture of malignant squamous and glandular cells; subtypes include the mature type, signet-ring type (mucoepidermoid carcinoma), and glassy cell type. Glassy cell carcinoma is a poorly differentiated form of adenosquamous carcinoma and is considered to have an extremely aggressive course. It accounts for approximately 1–2% of cervical cancers. Synchronous adenocarcinomas and squamous cell carcinomas that invade each other are called collision tumors.

H. Neuroendocrine Carcinomas

Approximately one-third of small cell carcinomas of the cervix stain positive for neuroendocrine markers (neuron-specific enolase, chromogranin, synaptophysin). These tumors need to be distinguished from small cell type of squamous tumors. They have a high frequency of lymphovascular space invasion, lymph node metastases, recurrence, and poor survival. Neuroendocrine carcinomas are not limited to the small-sized tumor cells. Poorly differentiated large cell carcinomas may express neuroendocrine differentiation by immunohistochemistry. Carcinoid tumors, arising from the argyrophil cells of the endocervical epithelium, are malignant but have rarely been associated with the carcinoid syndrome. Because of their propensity for early systemic spread, systemic chemotherapy is an integral part of the treatment of neuroendocrine tumors of the cervix.

I. Other Malignant Tumors

Direct extension of metastatic tumors to the cervix includes those originating from the endometrium, rectum, and bladder. Lymphatic or vascular metastases occur less often but are associated with endometrial, ovarian, gastric, breast, colon, kidney, and pancreas carcinomas. Sarcomas, lymphomas, choriocarcinomas, and melanomas are encountered rarely in the cervix.

Prevention

Until now, prevention of morbidity and death from cervical cancer largely involved recognition and treatment of preinvasive and early invasive disease. Over 60% of women who develop cervical cancer in developed countries either never have been screened or have not been screened in the preceding 5 years. Risk factors must be recognized, and screening, treatment intervention, and patient education must be modified.

Universal cytologic screening of all women age 21 years or older must be continued on a regular basis until better, more sensitive and specific means of screening are found and outreach into underserved areas is improved. Women with preinvasive cervical neoplasia should be treated and followed up closely (Fig. 48–5). It is important to remember that cervical cytology smears are of limited value in detecting frankly invasive disease, with some studies finding false-negative rates up to 50%. Sexual abstinence is an effective but impractical prophylactic measure. Education of young women and men about risk factors and the necessity for regular screening, as well as information about the association of HIV infection and smoking with the development of cervical cancers, is crucial.

The role of HPV vaccination has been discussed earlier.

Clinical Findings

A. Symptoms & Signs

Abnormal vaginal bleeding is the most common symptom of invasive cancer and may take the form of a blood-stained leukorrheal discharge, scant spotting, or frank bleeding. Leukorrhea, usually sanguineous or purulent, odorous, and nonpruritic, is frequently present. A history of postcoital bleeding may be elicited on specific questioning.

Pelvic pain, often unilateral and radiating to the hip or thigh, is a manifestation of advanced disease, as is the involuntary loss of urine or feces through the vagina, a sign of fistula formation. Weakness, weight loss, and anemia are characteristic of the late stages of the disease, although acute blood loss and anemia may occur in a bulky or ulcerating stage I lesion.

Physical examination findings include a grossly normal-appearing cervix with preclinical disease. As the local disease progresses, physical signs appear. Infiltrative cancer produces enlargement, irregularity, and a firm consistency of the cervix and eventually of the adjacent parametria. The growth pattern can be endophytic, leading to a barrel-shaped enlargement of the cervix, or exophytic, where the lesion generally appears as a friable, bleeding, cauliflowerlike lesion of the portio vaginalis. Ulceration may be the primary manifestation of invasive carcinoma; in the early stages, the change often is superficial, so that it may resemble an ectropion or chronic cervicitis. With further progression of the disease, the ulcer becomes deeper and necrotic, with indurated edges and a friable, bleeding surface. The adjacent vaginal fornices may become involved next. Eventually, extensive parametrial involvement by the infiltrative process may produce a nodular thickening of the uterosacral and cardinal ligaments with resultant loss of mobility and fixation of the cervix.

B. Biopsy

Because of the failure of malignant cells to desquamate and the obscuring effect of inflammatory cells, it is not uncommon for an invasive carcinoma of the cervix to exist despite a negative cytologic smear. Any suspicious lesion of the cervix should be sampled by adequate biopsy, regardless of cytologic examination result. Biopsy of any Schiller-positive areas or of any ulcerative, granular, nodular, or papillary lesion provides the diagnosis in most cases. Colposcopically directed biopsies with endocervical sampling or conization of the cervix may be required when reports of suspicious or probable exfoliated carcinoma cells are made by the pathologist and a visible or palpable lesion of the cervix is not evident. Colposcopic warning signs of early invasive cancer in a field of CIN include capillaries that are markedly irregular, appearing as commas, corkscrews, and spaghetti-shaped vessels with great variation in caliber and abrupt changes in direction, often causing acute angles. Ulcerations or a markedly irregular appearance of the cervix with a waxy, yellowish surface and numerous bizarre, atypical blood vessels are common. Bleeding may occur also after slight irritation.

C. Conization

In the setting of a biopsy revealing CIS, where invasion cannot be ruled out, or in the setting of a negative colposcopy in the face of a significantly abnormal cervical cytology smear, conization of the cervix should be performed to determine the presence or absence of invasion. If a cervical biopsy shows microinvasive cancer (<3 mm of invasion), a cone biopsy is necessary to rule out deeper invasion. The conization specimen should be properly marked for the pathologist (eg, with a pin or small suture), so that the area of involvement can be specifically localized in relation to the circumference and margins of the cervix. Conization for a lesion grossly suggestive of invasive cancer is not indicated, as it only delays the initiation of appropriate therapy and predisposes the patient to serious pelvic infections and bleeding. The diagnosis of such a lesion can almost always be confirmed by simple cervical biopsy.

D. Radiologic Findings

Chest radiographs are indicated in all patients with cervical cancer and an intravenous pyelogram (IVP) or computed tomography (CT) urogram should be performed to determine if there is any ureteral obstruction producing hydroureter and hydronephrosis. Magnetic resonance imaging (MRI), CT scan, lymphangiography, or positron emission tomography (PET) scanning may demonstrate involvement of the pelvic or periaortic lymph nodes or other sites of metastases. The sensitivities of CT, MRI, and PET for lymph node metastases in cervical cancer are approximately 45%, 60%, and 80%, respectively. Integrated PET CT appears to have a slightly higher sensitivity for detecting nodal metastases than PET alone. Although the latter imaging studies are not used to assign disease stage in the International Federation of Gynecology and Obstetrics (FIGO) classification, they may be of value for planning treatment, particularly the extent of the radiation therapy field or scope of surgery.

Clinical Staging

It is important to estimate the extent of the disease not only for prognostic purposes, but also for treatment planning. Clinical staging also affords a means of comparing methods of therapy for various stages of the disease worldwide. The classification adopted by FIGO is the most widely used staging system (Table 48–3). Cervical cancer is staged by clinical examination and evaluation of the bladder, ureters, and rectum. If the lesion is clearly confined to the cervix by office examination, only chest radiography and evaluation of the ureters by IVP or CT scan with intravenous contrast are necessary to assign the stage. If it is not possible to evaluate the extent of local disease in the office, examination under anesthesia with cystoscopy and proctoscopy may be necessary. Although CT scan, MRI, lymphangiography, and PET scan may offer information helpful for treatment planning, these findings do not change the FIGO stage of

Table 48–3. 2009 International Federation of Gynecology and Obstetrics (FIGO) staging of cervical cancer.

FIGO Stage	Definition
Stage 0	Carcinoma in situ
Stage I	Cervical carcinoma confined to the cervix (extension to the corpus should be disregarded)
Stage IA[1]	Invasive cervical cancer diagnosed by microscopy only
Stage IA1	Stromal invasion no deeper than 3 mm, no wider than 7 mm in horizontal spread
Stage IA2	Stromal invasion >3, but no more than 5 mm and no wider than 7 mm in horizontal spread
Stage IB	Clinically visible lesion confined to the cervix or microscopic disease greater than stage IA
Stage IB1	Clinically visible lesion not >4 cm
Stage IB2	Clinically visible lesion >4 cm
Stage II	Tumor extends beyond uterus but not to pelvic sidewall or lower third of vagina
Stage IIA	Vaginal involvement without parametrial involvement
Stage IIA1	Clinically visible lesion not >4 cm
Stage IIA2	Clinically visible lesion >4 cm
Stage IIB	Parametrial involvement
Stage III	Tumor extends to pelvic sidewall and/or causes hydronephrosis and/or extends to lower third of vagina
Stage IIIA	Involvement of lower third of vagina with no extension to sidewall
Stage IIIB	Extension to pelvic sidewall and/or hydronephrosis
Stage IV	Extension beyond the true pelvis or into mucosa of rectum or bladder
Stage IVA[2]	Extension into adjacent organs
Stage IVB	Distant metastases

[1]The depth of invasion should be no more than 5 mm from the epithelial basement membrane of the adjacent most superficial epithelial papilla to the deepest point of invasion where the cancer originates. Vascular space invasion, venous or lymphatic, does not affect staging, but should be noted because it may affect future therapy. All macroscopically visible lesions (even with superficial invasion only) are allotted to stage IB.

[2]The presence of bullous edema is not sufficient to classify a tumor as stage IVA. The finding of malignant cells in cytologic bladder washings requires further histologic confirmation in order to be considered stage IVA.

Reproduced, with permission, from Sergio Pecorelli, Lucia Zigliani, Franco Odicino. Revised FIGO staging for carcinoma of the cervix. *Int J Gynecol Obste.* 2009;105:107-108.

disease. The FIGO stage of disease is also not changed by surgicopathologic findings of metastatic disease at the time of radical hysterectomy or lymphadenectomy.

Differential Diagnosis

A variety of lesions of the cervix can be confused with cancer. Entities that must sometimes be ruled out include cervical ectropion, acute or chronic cervicitis, condyloma acuminata, cervical tuberculosis, ulceration secondary to STD (syphilis, granuloma inguinale, lymphogranuloma venereum, chancroid), abortion of a cervical pregnancy, metastatic choriocarcinoma or other cancers, and rare lesions such as those of actinomycosis or schistosomiasis. Histopathologic examination is usually definitive.

Complications

The complications of cervical cancer, for the most part, are those related to tumor size or invasion, necrosis of the tumor, infection, and metastatic disease. The natural history of the disease was outlined earlier. There are also problems pertaining to treatment of the disease (eg, radical surgery or radiation therapy; see next section, Treatment).

Treatment

Invasive carcinoma of the cervix spreads primarily by direct extension and lymphatic dissemination. The therapy of patients with cervical cancer needs to address not only the primary tumor site, but also the adjacent tissues and lymph nodes. This is generally accomplished by either radical hysterectomy and pelvic lymphadenectomy, radiation with concomitant chemotherapy, or a combination thereof.

A. Treatment of Early-Stage Disease (Stage IA2 to IIA2)

Patients with early-stage cervical cancer may be treated either with radical hysterectomy and pelvic lymphadenectomy or with primary radiation with concomitant chemotherapy. The overall 5-year cure rates for surgery and for radiation therapy in operable patients are approximately equal. The advantages of surgery are that the ovaries may be left intact and be transposed out of the radiation field if adjuvant postoperative therapy appears necessary, that the extent of disease can be determined surgicopathologically, and that grossly metastatic lymph nodes can be resected. Furthermore, surgery may be more appropriate in sexually active women with early-stage disease as radiation causes vaginal stenosis and atrophy. Adjuvant radiation with or without concomitant chemotherapy is administered to selected patients at increased risk for recurrence following radical hysterectomy.

1. Radical hysterectomy & therapeutic lymphadenectomy—Radical hysterectomy (techniques initially described by Wertheim, Meigs, and Okabayashi) with pelvic lymphadenectomy is the surgical procedure for invasive cancer limited

Table 48–4. Types of hysterectomy based on radicality.

Type of Hysterectomy	Principles of Procedure
Type I	Extrafascial hysterectomy with removal of all cervical tissue without dissecting into the cervix itself.
Type II	The uterine artery is ligated where it crosses over the ureter. The uterosacral and cardinal ligaments are divided midway toward their attachment to sacrum and pelvic sidewall. The upper third of the vagina is resected.
Type III	The uterine artery is ligated at its origin from the superior vesical or internal iliac artery. Uterosacral and cardinal ligaments are resected at their attachments to the sacrum and pelvic sidewall. The upper half of the vagina is resected.
Type IV	The ureter is completely dissected from the vesicouterine ligament, the superior vesical artery is sacrificed, and three-fourths of the vagina is resected.
Type V	Involves the additional resection of a portion of the bladder or the distal ureter with ureteral reimplantation into the bladder.

to the cervix and upper vagina (stages I and II). The operation is technically difficult and should be performed only by those experienced in radical pelvic surgery. Surgery involves dissection of the ureters from the paracervical structures so that the ligaments supporting the uterus and upper vagina can be removed. When the operation is done vaginally, a deep Schuchardt (paravaginal) incision is required for exposure. Five different types of hysterectomy have been described based on the extent of parametrial dissection and vaginal tissue removed (Table 48–4). Typically, a type I hysterectomy is indicated for patients with stage IA1 disease. An alternative treatment is cervical conization in the young patient wishing to preserve fertility. Stage IA2 to IIA2 can be treated with a type II (modified radical) or type III (radical) hysterectomy. It is rarely necessary to remove as much vaginal tissue as was initially recommended. As long as complete tumor clearance can be provided, a modified radical hysterectomy appears to provide therapeutic outcomes comparable to a radical hysterectomy for stage IB and IIA disease, but with shorter operating time and lower urologic morbidity. Full pelvic lymphadenectomy is indicated at the time of radical hysterectomy, followed by para-aortic lymphadenectomy for tumors larger than 2 cm or those with suspicious pelvic lymph nodes. Resection of all grossly involved lymph nodes provides a distinct survival advantage. Microscopic evaluation of the lymph nodes allows for tailoring of the postoperative radiation field, if indicated.

2. Adjuvant postoperative radiation with or without concomitant chemotherapy—Postoperative adjuvant radiation therapy with concomitant chemotherapy is indicated in women with localized cervical cancer at high risk for recurrent disease, such as positive lymph nodes, positive or close resection margins, or microscopic parametrial involvement. In this setting, adjuvant radiation with platinum-based chemotherapy is superior to adjuvant radiation alone, with an improvement in the 4-year progression-free interval from 63% to 80%. Women with intermediate-risk factors for recurrent disease, such as large tumor size, deep cervical stromal invasion, and lymphovascular space invasion, also benefit from postoperative adjuvant radiation. These patients have an improved 2-year recurrence-free survival of 88% with adjuvant radiation versus 79% without adjuvant therapy. Whether the addition of chemotherapy to the adjuvant radiation further improves outcomes for women with intermediate-risk factors is currently under investigation.

3. Primary radiation with concomitant chemotherapy—For the treatment of early cervical cancer (stages IA to IIA), primary therapy with definitive radiation or radical surgery followed by tailored radiation if indicated by the surgical findings produces comparable outcomes. The choice of treatment depends on the tumor size, the general condition of the patient, and patient preferences. Surgery is often preferred for young patients in the hope of preserving ovarian function. If it is likely that the patient will need postoperative radiation therapy, transposition of the ovaries to a location outside the radiation field can be performed. The main argument for primary chemoradiation exists in patients with larger tumors, due to the added morbidity of triple-modality therapy (see later section Special Situations; bulky stage IB2 and IIA2 cervical cancer). For primary radiation of cervical cancer, external-beam radiation is used in combination with intracavitary irradiation (see Chapter 52). At least 5 controlled trials have demonstrated the superiority of radiation with concomitant platinum-based chemotherapy over radiation alone. This has led to the adoption of radiation plus concomitant chemotherapy as the standard of care whenever radiation therapy is given for the treatment of cervical cancer over a broad spectrum of disease stages.

B. Treatment of Locally Advanced Disease (Stage IIB to IVA)

Patients with locally advanced cervical cancer are best treated with primary radiation (external beam plus brachytherapy; see Chapter 52) with concomitant chemotherapy. Extended-field radiation should be considered in the presence of para-aortic lymph node metastases documented at surgical staging or by imaging, especially when biopsy confirmed and in the absence of other systemic metastases. The benefit of cisplatin-based combined-modality therapy over radiation alone for advanced disease has been demonstrated in at least 3 randomized controlled trials, which found a 30–50% reduction in the risk of death from cervical cancer for patients treated with chemoradiation compared to those treated with radiation alone. This difference is most significant for patients with stage II disease (and bulky IB disease) in whom, in 1 study, chemoradiation, compared to radiation alone, improved 5-year survival rates from 58% to 77%. For patients with more advanced disease, there is still significant benefit, but it appears to be less pronounced. The optimal drug regimen is not known. Many experts recommend weekly cisplatin concomitantly with radiation. A recent study suggested the superiority of weekly combination cisplatin/gemcitabine during chemoradiation. However, the experimental group also received 2 additional cycles of adjuvant cisplatin/gemcitabine after brachytherapy and toxicity was significant. It is unclear what proportion of the improvement in outcome can be attributed to the multiagent chemoradiotherapy versus the adjuvant chemotherapy. This question is currently being investigated by the Gynecologic Cancer Intergroup.

C. Treatment of Disseminated Primary (Stage IVB) & Persistent or Recurrent Disease

The use of chemotherapeutic agents in the treatment of cervical carcinoma has been discouraging. This is partly because most patients who may be candidates for this type of treatment either present with disseminated disease or have cancer that has already failed to respond to radical surgery or radiation therapy. In this setting, chemotherapy is generally palliative and not curative. Modest activity in recurrent or disseminated cervical cancer has been observed with single-agent cisplatin, ifosfamide, paclitaxel, and vinorelbine. If the patient can tolerate it, multiagent chemotherapy is preferred as it is associated with significantly higher response rates and longer progression-free survival. There is also a small overall survival advantage to multiagent chemotherapy with cisplatin and topotecan. Combination therapy using paclitaxel and platinum offers very similar outcomes, with response rate and median survival time of 36% and 9.7 months, compared to 27% and 9.6 months, respectively, for cisplatin and topotecan. Other acceptable combination regimens include cisplatin/vinorelbine and cisplatin/gemcitabine. Surgical resection of lung metastases is an alternative to palliative chemotherapy for highly selected patients with isolated, potentially resectable pulmonary metastases. Palliative radiation therapy may be indicated, especially for the control of symptoms, such as pain or hemorrhage. If a patient develops a palpable mass in the left supraclavicular region, it can be palliated with radiation therapy with concomitant chemotherapy, with or without resection.

D. Total Pelvic Exenteration for Isolated Central Pelvic Recurrence of Disease

Patients who develop a central recurrence of cervical cancer after primary therapy with radiation or after surgery followed by radiation may be candidates for this extensive, potentially curative surgical procedure if a complete evaluation fails to reveal evidence of metastatic disease. In a small proportion of patients with cancer of the cervix treated initially with radiation, a small recurrence of the cancer may be noted centrally within the cervix. A radical hysterectomy may be an alternative to total pelvic exenteration in this selected subgroup of patients. Surgery is the only potentially curative method of treating cancers that persist or recur centrally following adequate radiation therapy. In such instances, pelvic exenteration is often necessary to make certain that all of the cancer has been removed.

Pelvic exenteration is one of the most formidable of all gynecologic operations and requires removal of the bladder, rectum, and vagina, along with the uterus if hysterectomy has not yet been performed. This is followed by the reconstructive phase of the procedure. Urinary diversion needs to be provided, necessitating the creation of either a continent ileocolonic pouch or a noncontinent ileal conduit. In either case, a stoma is created in the anterior abdominal wall. If extensive rectal resection was required, a sigmoid colostomy serves for the passage of feces. If a low rectal anastomosis could be accomplished, a temporary diverting colostomy is recommended for all patients who have received prior radiation. The vagina can be reconstructed using various myocutaneous flaps, such as vertical rectus abdominis or gracilis myocutaneous flaps. Depending on the location of the lesion, an anterior (preservation of the rectosigmoid) or posterior (preservation of the bladder) exenteration is at times an alternative.

Because of the high surgical morbidity and mortality rates, stringent criteria are necessary to justify these procedures. Pelvic exenteration should be reserved primarily for problems that cannot be effectively managed in any other manner. In essence, this means (1) a biopsy-proven persistence or recurrence of cervical cancer following an adequate course of radiation therapy or radical surgery in which the recurrent or persistent tumor occupies the central portion of the pelvis (without metastases) and is completely removable; and (2) a patient who is able to cope with the urinary and fecal stomas in the abdomen created by the operation. Both psychological and physical preparation of the patient for this operation and its aftermath are of vital importance. Because of the extreme difficulties encountered in making an accurate assessment preoperatively, only about half of the patients explored for a total pelvic exenteration will intraoperatively be confirmed to have resectable, nonmetastatic disease. Favorable prognostic factors in addition to an isolated central pelvic recurrence with no side wall fixation are a long disease-free interval and size of the recurrence < 3 cm in diameter. The 5-year survival rate following pelvic exenteration for recurrent cervical cancer averages 30–40%.

E. Palliative Care

Comprehensive care of a patient with cancer involves, in addition to antitumor therapy, good symptom relief and personal and family support. The palliative care for patients with progressive cervical cancer poses many challenges. The emphasis should be to facilitate comfort, dignity, autonomy, and personal rehabilitation and development, especially in the face of an incurable disease.

Most patients with progressive cervical cancer eventually develop symptoms related principally to the site and extent of the malignant disease. Ulceration of the cervix and adjacent vagina produces a foul-smelling discharge. Tissue necrosis and slough may initiate life-threatening hemorrhage. If the bladder or rectum is involved in the tissue breakdown, fistulas result in incontinence of urine and feces. Pain caused by involvement of the lumbosacral plexus, soft tissues of the pelvis, or bone is frequently encountered in advanced disease. Ureteral compression leading to hydronephrosis and, if bilateral, to renal failure and uremia is a common terminal event. The comfort and well-being of the patient can be considerably enhanced even though cure cannot be effected. A foul, purulent discharge may be ameliorated by astringent douches and antimicrobial vaginal creams or suppositories. Hemorrhage from the vagina often can be controlled by packing the area with gauze impregnated with a hemostatic agent; occasionally, emergent radiation or hypogastric artery embolization is indicated.

Current management of severe pain combines the use of a long-acting narcotic such as morphine or a transdermal fentanyl patch with short-acting narcotics for breakthrough pain and nonsteroidal anti-inflammatory agents. Anxiolytics and antidepressants may be of considerable value. For patients with significant pain who are no longer responding to oral medications, a subcutaneous or intravenous morphine drip can be started. In patients with lower back or extremity pain, a peridural catheter can be placed and connected to a subcutaneous pump with a reservoir for continuous morphine instillation. This method gives pain relief without the sedating effects of oral and parenteral narcotics.

Radiation therapy may be very helpful in the relief of pain caused by bony metastases and in the treatment of lesions that recur following primary surgical treatment of cervical cancer. In general, if initial therapy was accomplished by adequate radiation therapy, retreatment is contraindicated because it does little good and carries the potential of massive radiation necrosis.

Special Situations

A. Stage IA1 Disease

The definitive diagnosis of microinvasive carcinoma of the cervix can only be made by conization. These patients may be treated by simple abdominal or vaginal hysterectomy. For a young woman desiring to maintain fertility, conization only is an acceptable treatment modality for microinvasive carcinoma with a depth of invasion of 3 mm or less, if the conization margins are negative, and if there is no evidence of lymphovascular space invasion. If conization margin and endocervical sampling are positive, the risk of residual disease is as high as 33%. In this case, repeat conization should be performed if uterine preservation is the goal. FIGO staging is not influenced by the presence of lymphovascular space invasion, which occurs in close to 10% of patients with stage IA1 disease. These patients have a small but significant risk for lymph node metastases to parametrial and pelvic lymph nodes. This subgroup of patients should therefore be treated like patients with stage IA2 disease.

B. Radical Trachelectomy

Over the past 2 decades, radical trachelectomy has evolved as an alternative to radical hysterectomy in carefully selected young women with early-stage (IA2 or small IB1) cervical cancer and no evidence of lymph node metastases who wish to preserve fertility. A preoperative MRI is critical for treatment planning as it allows for measurement of the distance between the upper margin of the lesion and the isthmus. The radical trachelectomy can be performed transvaginally or abdominally via open or robotic approach; ideally the cervix is amputated 1 cm above the tumor to optimize oncologic outcome and 1 cm below the isthmus to maintain some cervical function for future pregnancies. An open or minimally invasive therapeutic lymphadenectomy is performed, and following radical resection of the cervix, a cerclage is placed. Experience with this technique is growing, and the oncologic outcome, with recurrence rates <5% and mortality rates of 2–3%, is comparable in carefully selected patients to radical hysterectomy. A review of pregnancy outcomes in women who underwent radical trachelectomy revealed that 40% of women conceived following radical trachelectomy. Of those women who do conceive, 16–20% have a first-trimester abortion, close to 10% have a second-trimester pregnancy loss, 25% have a preterm delivery, and 42% deliver a live born infant at term. The majority of successful pregnancy outcomes have occurred with a cerclage in place.

C. Bulky Cervical Cancer

The management of patients with stage IB2 and bulky IIA2 disease is a matter of considerable debate. Proposed management strategies include the following.

1. Primary radiation therapy with concomitant chemotherapy & the option of a subsequent adjuvant extrafascial hysterectomy—Radiation therapy is usually recommended for patients with bulky cervical cancers with the addition of concomitant chemotherapy. Many of these tumors, however, contain hypoxic central areas that do not respond well to radiation, as is reflected in a 15–35% pelvic failure rate. This provides the rationale for the performance of an adjuvant hysterectomy following radiation, which is associated with a significant reduction in pelvic recurrences to 2–5%. However, the impact of adjuvant hysterectomy on extrapelvic recurrences and survival is less well established.

2. Primary radical hysterectomy & therapeutic lymphadenectomy, followed by tailored radiation with concomitant chemotherapy when indicated by pathologic findings—The potential benefits of this approach include the removal of the large primary tumor, complete surgical staging with the opportunity to resect any grossly involved lymph nodes, and the preservation of ovarian function as ovarian transposition can be performed if adjuvant radiation therapy is likely. If postoperative radiation becomes necessary, the radiation field can be tailored to the surgicopathologic findings. The resection of macroscopically involved lymph nodes has a therapeutic benefit because it improves survival to that of patients with microscopic lymph node metastases only. A primary surgical approach should be taken in patients with acute or chronic pelvic inflammatory disease, an undiagnosed coexistent adnexal mass, or anatomic alterations that make radiation therapy difficult.

3. Neoadjuvant chemotherapy followed by radical hysterectomy and lymphadenectomy & subsequent chemoradiation when indicated by pathologic findings—Neoadjuvant chemotherapy, frequently 3 cycles of platinum-based combination therapy followed by radical hysterectomy and lymphadenectomy, has been proposed as a treatment strategy for these patients. Neoadjuvant chemotherapy is reported to improve the resectability of bulky lesions, pelvic disease control, and possibly long-term survival. Although this is a provocative treatment strategy, in most studies, patients ultimately received multimodality treatment with chemotherapy, radical surgery, and radiation, and it remains unclear whether the use of neoadjuvant chemotherapy followed by surgery gives superior long-term results in the era of modern chemoradiotherapy. This question is currently being studied in phase III trials by the European Organization for the Research and Treatment of Cancer.

D. Carcinoma of the Cervix during Pregnancy

Invasive carcinoma of the cervix in pregnancy is found more frequently in areas where routine prenatal cytologic examination is done. Abnormal cervical cytology in pregnancy calls for immediate colposcopic evaluation and any other diagnostic modalities necessary to exclude invasive cancer (see section on preinvasive disease).

Invasive cervical cancer complicates approximately 0.05% of pregnancies. As is the case with nonpregnant patients, the principal symptom is bleeding, but the diagnosis is frequently missed because the bleeding is assumed to be related to the pregnancy rather than to cancer. The possibility of cancer must be kept in mind. The diagnosis and management of invasive cervical cancer during pregnancy present the patient and the physician with many challenges. Pregnancy does not appear to affect the prognosis for women with cervical cancer, and the fetus is not affected by the maternal disease, but may suffer morbidity from its treatment (eg, preterm delivery).

If the pregnancy is early and the disease is stage I to IIA, radical hysterectomy and therapeutic lymphadenectomy can be performed with the fetus left in situ, unless the patient is unwilling to terminate the pregnancy. Women at a gestational age closer to fetal viability or who are unwilling to lose the baby may decide to continue the pregnancy after careful discussion regarding the maternal risks. With early-stage disease (≤stage IB1/IIA1), the literature supports expectant management with careful serial examinations to exclude disease progression as a reasonable choice. With more advanced disease (≥ stage IB2/IIA2), neoadjuvant chemotherapy may offer an opportunity to delay definitive therapy until fetal maturity while reducing maternal risks potentially associated with treatment delay. Delivery in patients with cervical dysplasia and CIS may be via the vaginal route. Patients with invasive cervical cancer should be delivered by caesarean section to avoid potential cervical hemorrhage and dissemination of tumor cells during vaginal delivery. A caesarean radical hysterectomy with therapeutic lymphadenectomy is the procedure of choice for patients with stages IA2–IIA disease as soon as fetal maturity is established.

As in the nonpregnant patient, radiation with concomitant chemotherapy is used for the treatment of more advanced disease. Irradiation may be carried out with the expectation of spontaneous abortion. In selected cases with locally advanced disease in which the patient declines pregnancy termination, consideration may be given to neoadjuvant chemotherapy in an effort to prevent disease progression during the time needed to achieve fetal maturity. Delivery should be by caesarean section. A lymphadenectomy can be performed at the same time. Postpartum the patient should receive chemoradiation following guidelines established for the nonpregnant patient.

E. Carcinoma of the Cervical Stump

About 2% of all cervical cancers occur in the cervical stump. Early-stage cervical cancer noted on a cervical stump (left in situ following supracervical hysterectomy for an unrelated indication) should be treated with radical trachelectomy and therapeutic lymphadenectomy in the medically fit patient. Surgery is preferred over chemoradiation in this setting as the delivery of an adequate radiation dose may be difficult in a patient with a short cervical stump. However, radiation with concomitant chemotherapy is the preferred treatment modality for patients with more advanced disease.

F. Cervical Cancer Incidentally Diagnosed after Simple Hysterectomy

Women who are found to have microinvasive disease after a simple hysterectomy do not require any additional therapy. Patients with invasive disease who do not have gross parametrial disease are candidates for a radical parametrectomy, upper vaginectomy, and lymphadenectomy. This approach may be particularly desirable for young women in whom ovarian function can be preserved or for any surgically fit women with enlarged lymph nodes that should be resected prior to chemoradiation. Indications for chemoradiation follow the same guidelines as outlined earlier. Chemoradiation may be associated with less morbidity and comparable oncologic outcomes.

Complications of Therapy

A. Radical Surgery

The operative mortality rate in radical hysterectomy with lymphadenectomy has been reduced to <1%. The most common complication is prolonged bladder dysfunction. Approximately 75% of patients have adequate recovery of bladder function within 1–2 weeks after radical hysterectomy, and most patients will have satisfactory voiding function by 3 weeks. Serious complications include fistula formation; ureterovaginal fistula is the most common type (1–2%), followed by vesicovaginal and rectovaginal fistulas. Modified radical hysterectomy, as compared to radical hysterectomy, is associated with a shorter operating time, a more rapid return of bladder function, and fewer fistulas. Other complications are urinary tract infections, lymphocysts and lymphedema, wound sepsis, dehiscence, thromboembolic disease, ileus, postoperative hemorrhage, and intestinal obstruction.

The surgical mortality rate from pelvic exenteration has been reduced from approximately 25% to <5%, but as many as 50% of patients experience major morbidity. Complications include intraoperative and postoperative hemorrhage, infectious morbidity, urinary fistulas or obstruction, urinary pouch dysfunction, pyelonephritis, bowel obstruction or intestinal leaks and fistulas, stomal retraction, electrolyte disturbances, and other less common occurrences.

B. Radiation Therapy with Concomitant Chemotherapy

See Chapter 52.

Posttreatment Follow-Up

Approximately 35% of patients with invasive cervical cancer will have recurrent or persistent disease following therapy. Approximately 50% of deaths from cervical cancer occur in the first year after treatment, another 25% in the second year, and 15% in the third year. This explains the generally accepted schedule of posttreatment surveillance in asymptomatic patients with more frequent visits initially. Symptomatic patients should be evaluated with appropriate examinations immediately when symptoms occur. The most common signs and symptoms of recurrent malignant disease are a palpable tumor in the pelvis or abdomen, ulceration of the cervix or vagina, pain in the pelvis, back, groin, and lower extremity, unilateral lower extremity edema, vaginal

Table 48–5. Cervical cancer surveillance recommendations.

	0–12 Months	12–24 Months	24–36 Months	3–5 Years	>5 Years
Review of symptoms and physical exam					
Low risk (early stage, treated with surgery alone, no adjuvant therapy)	Every 6 mo	Every 6 mo	Every 6 mo*	Every 6 mo*	Every 6 mo*
High risk (advanced stage, treated with primary chemo/RT or surgery plus adjuvant therapy)	Every 3 mo	Every 3 mo	Every 3 mo	Every 3 mo	Every 3 mo*
Pap test/cytology	Yearly†	Yearly†	Yearly†	Yearly†	Yearly†
Routine radiographic imaging (CXR, PET/CT, MRI)	Insufficient data to support routine use	Insufficient data to support routine use	Insufficient data to support routine use	Insufficient data to support routine use	Insufficient data to support routine use
Recurrence suspected	CT and/or PET scan	CT and/or PET scan	CT and/or PET scan	CT and/or PET scan	CT and/or PET scan

chemo, chemotherapy; CT, computed tomography; CXR, chest x-ray; MRI, magnetic resonance imaging; PET, positron emission tomography; RT, radiotherapy.

*May be followed by generalist or gynecologic oncologist.

†Insufficient evidence for cancer recurrence but may have value in detection of other lower genital tract neoplasia.

Reproduced, with permission, from Salani R, Backes FJ, Fung MF, et al. Posttreatment surveillance and diagnosis of recurrence in women with gynecologic malignancies: Society of Gynecologic Oncologists recommendations. *Am J Obstet Gynecol* 2011;204:466–478.

bleeding or discharge, supraclavicular lymphadenopathy, ascites, unexplained weight loss, progressive ureteral obstruction, and cough (especially with hemoptysis or chest pain).

The Society of Gynecologic Oncologists has recently developed risk-stratified recommendations for the posttreatment follow-up of patients with cervical cancer. These are summarized in Table 48–5.

Prognosis

The major prognostic factors affecting survival are stage, lymph node status, tumor volume, depth of cervical stromal invasion, lymphovascular space invasion, and to a lesser extent, histologic type and grade. After stage of disease, lymph node status is the most important prognostic factor. For example, following radical surgery, patients with stage IB or IIA disease have a 5-year survival of 88–96% with negative lymph nodes, compared to 64–73% in the presence of lymph node metastases.

Table 48–6 summarizes survival rates by stage of disease. These are based on the FIGO Annual Report on the Results of Treatment in Gynecological Cancer, in which results of treatment for each stage of cervical cancer are reported by more than 100 participating institutions worldwide. The results are equated in terms of 5-year cure rates, or those patients who are living and show no evidence of cervical cancer 5 years after beginning therapy. Recurrences following radiation therapy are not often centrally located and thus amenable to exenteration procedures. Only approximately 25% of recurrences are localized to the central portion of the pelvis. The most common site of recurrence is the pelvic side wall.

Table 48–6. Survival of patients with cervical cancer based on International Federation of Gynecology and Obstetrics (FIGO) stage.

Stage	Number of Patients (%)	Survival		
		1 Year	2 Years	5 Years
IA1	860	99.8%	99.5%	98.7%
IA2	227	98.2%	97.7%	95.9%
IB	3480	98.1%	94.0%	86.5%
IIA	881	94.1%	85.6%	68.8%
IIB	2375	93.3%	80.7%	64.7%
IIIA	160	82.8%	58.8%	40.4%
IIIB	1949	81.5%	62.2%	43.3%
IVA	245	56.1%	35.6%	19.5%
IVB	189	45.8%	23.9%	15.0%

American Cancer Society. Cancer Facts and Figures 2011. Available at: http://www.cancer.org/Research/CancerFactsFigures/CancerFactsFigures/cancer-facts-figures-2011. Accessed September 10, 2011.

Anderson B, LaPolla J, Turner D, et al. Ovarian transposition in cervical cancer. *Gynecol Oncol* 1993;49:206–214. PMID: 8504989.

Ault KA. Vaccines for the prevention of human papillomavirus and associated gynecologic diseases: a review. *Obstet Gynecol Surv* 2006;61(6 Suppl 1):S26–S31. PMID: 16729901.

Averette HE, Nguyen HN, Donato DM, et al. Radical hysterectomy for invasive cervical cancer: a 25-year prospective experience with the Miami technique. *Cancer* 1993;71:1422–1437. PMID: 8431876.

Benedet JL, Bender H, Jones H 3rd, et al. FIGO staging classifications and clinical practice guidelines in the management of gynecologic cancers. FIGO Committee on Gynecologic Oncology. *Int J Gynaecol Obstet* 2000;70:209–216. PMID: 11041682.

Benedet JL, Odicino F, Maisonneuve P, et al. FIGO annual report: carcinoma of the cervix uteri. *Int J Gynaecol Obstet* 2003; 83(Suppl 1):41–47. PMID: 14763169.

Chemoradiotherapy for Cervical Cancer Meta-analysis Collaboration (CCCMAC). Reducing uncertainties about the effects of chemoradiotherapy for cervical cancer: individual patient data meta-analysis. *Cochrane Database Syst Rev* 2010;1:CD008285. PMID: 20091664.

Cosin JA, Fowler JM, Chen MD, et al. Pretreatment surgical staging of patients with cervical carcinoma: the case for lymph node debulking. *Cancer* 1998;82:2241–2248. PMID: 9610715.

Dargent D, Martin X, Sacchetoni A, et al. Laparoscopic vaginal radical trachelectomy: a treatment to preserve the fertility of cervical carcinoma patients. *Cancer* 2000;88:1877–1882. PMID: 107607665.

Dueñas-González A, Zarbá JJ, Patel F, et al. Phase III, open-label, randomized study comparing concurrent gemcitabine plus cisplatin and radiation followed by adjuvant gemcitabine and cisplatin versus concurrent cisplatin and radiation in patients with stage IIB to IVA carcinoma of the cervix. *J Clin Oncol* 2011;29:1678–1685. PMID: 21444871.

Eifel PJ, Thoms WW Jr, Smith TL, et al. The relationship between brachytherapy dose and outcome in patients with bulky endocervical tumors treated with radiation alone. *Int J Radiat Oncol Biol Phys* 1994;28:113–118. PMID: 8270431.

Feeney DD, Moore DH, Look KY, et al. The fate of the ovaries after radical hysterectomy and ovarian transposition. *Gynecol Oncol* 1995;56:3–7. PMID: 7821844.

FIGO Committee on Gynecologic Oncology. Revised FIGO staging for carcinoma of the vulva, cervix, and endometrium. *Int J Gynecol Obstet* 2009;105:103–104. PMID: 19367689.

Gallion HH, van Nagell JR Jr, Donaldson ES, et al. Combined radiation therapy and extrafascial hysterectomy in the treatment of stage IB barrel-shaped cervical cancer. *Cancer* 1985; 56:262–265. PMID: 4005798.

Hacker NF, Wain GV, Nicklin JL. Resection of bulky positive lymph nodes in patients with cervical carcinoma. *Int J Gynaecol Cancer* 1995;5:250–256. PMID: 11578485.

Hellström AC, Hellman K, Pettersson BF, et al. Carcinoma of the cervical stump: fifty years of experience. *Oncol Rep* 2011; 25:1651–1654. PMID: 21431283.

Hopkins MP, Lavin JP. Cervical cancer in pregnancy. *Gynecol Oncol* 1996;63:293. PMID: 8946860.

Hricak H, Gatsonis C, Chi DS, et al. Role of imaging in pretreatment evaluation of early invasive cervical cancer: results of the intergroup study American College of Radiology Imaging Network 6651-Gynecologic Oncology Group 183. *J Clin Oncol* 2005;23:9329–9337. PMID: 16361632.

Jemal A, Bray F, Center MM, et al. Global cancer statistics. *CA Cancer J Clin* 2011;61:69–90. PMID: 21296855.

Jolley JA, Battista L, Wing DA. Management of pregnancy after radical trachelectomy: case reports and systematic review of the literature. *Am J Perinatol* 2007;24:531–539. PMID: 17899494.

Keys HM, Bundy BN, Stehman FB, et al. Cisplatin, radiation, and adjuvant hysterectomy compared with radiation and adjuvant hysterectomy for bulky stage IB cervical carcinoma. *N Engl J Med* 1999;340:1154–1161. PMID: 10202166.

Landoni F, Maneo A, Cormio G, et al. Class II versus class III radical hysterectomy in stage IB–IIA cervical cancer: a prospective randomized study. *Gynecol Oncol* 2001;80:3–12. PMID: 11136561.

Landoni F, Maneo A, Colombo A, et al. Randomised study of radical surgery versus radio-therapy for stage IB–IIA cervical cancer. *Lancet* 1997;350:535–540. PMID: 9284774.

Lazo PA. The molecular genetics of cervical carcinoma. *Br J Cancer* 1999;80:2008–2018. PMID: 10471054.

Lee YN, Wang KL, Lin MH, et al. Radical hysterectomy with pelvic lymph node dissection for treatment of cervical cancer: a clinical review of 954 cases. *Gynecol Oncol* 1989;32:135–142. PMID: 2910773.

Long HJ 3rd, Bundy BN, Grendys EC Jr, et al. Randomized phase III trial of cisplatin with or without topotecan in carcinoma of the uterine cervix: a Gynecologic Oncology Group study. *J Clin Oncol* 2005;23:4626–4631. PMID: 15911865.

Metcalf KS, Johnson N, Calvert S, Peel KR. Site specific lymph node metastasis in carcinoma of the cervix: is there a sentinel node? *Int J Gynecol Cancer* 2000;10:411–414. PMID: 11240707.

Monk BJ, Sill MW, McMeekin DS, et al. Phase III trial of four cisplatin-containing doublet combinations in stage IVB, recurrent, or persistent cervical carcinoma: a Gynecologic Oncology Group study. *J Clin Oncol* 2009;27:4649–4655. PMID: 17920909.

Moore DH, Blessing JA, McQuellon RP, et al. Phase III study of cisplatin with or without paclitaxel in stage IVB, recurrent, or persistent squamous cell carcinoma of the cervix: a Gynecologic Oncology Group study. *J Clin Oncol* 2004;22:3113–3119. PMID: 15284282.

Morris M, Eifel PJ, Lu J, et al. Pelvic radiation with concurrent chemotherapy compared with pelvic and para-aortic radiation for high-risk cervical cancer. *N Engl J Med* 1999;340:1137–1143. PMID: 10202164.

Omura GA. Chemotherapy for stage IVB or recurrent cancer of the uterine cervix. *J Natl Cancer Inst Monogr* 1996;21:123–126. PMID: 9023841.

Omura GA, Blessing JA, Vaccarello L, et al. Randomized trial of cisplatin versus cisplatin plus mitolactol versus cisplatin plus ifosfamide in advanced squamous carcinoma of the cervix: a Gynecologic Oncology Group study. *J Clin Oncol* 1997;15: 165–171. PMID: 8991638.

Parkin DM, Pisani P, Ferlay J. Global cancer statistics. *CA Cancer J Clin* 1999;49:33–64. PMID: 10200776.

Perez CA, Grigsby PW, Camel HM, et al. Irradiation alone or combined with surgery in stage IB, IIA, and IIB carcinoma of uterine cervix: update of a nonrandomized comparison. *Int J Radiat Oncol Biol Phys* 1995;31:703–716. PMID: 7860381.

Peters WA III, Liu PY, Barrett RJ 2nd, et al. Concurrent chemotherapy and pelvic radiation therapy compared with pelvic radiation therapy alone as adjuvant therapy after radical surgery in high-risk early-stage cancer of the cervix. *J Clin Oncol* 2000;18: 1606–1613. PMID: 10764420.

Piver MS, Rutledge F, Smith JP. Five classes of extended hysterectomy for women with cervical cancer. *Obstet Gynecol* 1974;44:265–272. PMID: 4417035.

Plante M, Renaud MC, François H, et al. Vaginal radical trachelectomy: An oncologically safe fertility-preserving surgery. An updated series of 72 cases and review of the literature. *Gynecol Oncol* 2004;94:614–623. PMID: 15350349.

Plante M, Renaud MC, Hoskins IA, et al. Vaginal radical trachelectomy: a valuable fertility-preserving option in the management of early-stage cervical cancer. A series of 50 pregnancies and review of the literature. *Gynecol Oncol* 2005;98:3–10. PMID: 15936061.

Roman LD, Felix JC, Muderspach LI, et al. Risk of residual invasive disease in women with microinvasive squamous cancer in a conization specimen. *Obstet Gynecol* 1997;90:759–764. PMID: 9351760.

Rose PG, Bundy BN, Watkins EB, et al. Concurrent cisplatin-based radiotherapy and chemotherapy for locally advanced cervical cancer. *N Engl J Med* 1999;340:1144–1153. PMID: 10202165.

Rotman M, Sedlis A, Piedmonte MR, et al. A phase III randomized trial of postoperative pelvic irradiation in stage IB cervical carcinoma with poor prognostic features: follow-up of a gynecologic oncology group study. *Int J Radiat Oncol Biol Phys* 2006;65:169–174. PMID: 16427212.

Salani R, Backes FJ, Fung MF, et al. Posttreatment surveillance and diagnosis of recurrence in women with gynecologic malignancies: Society of Gynecologic Oncologists recommendations. *Am J Obstet Gynecol* 2011;204:466–478. PMID: 21752752.

Sardi JE, Giaroli A, Sananes C, et al. Long-term follow-up of the first randomized trial using neoadjuvant chemotherapy in stage IB squamous carcinoma of the cervix: the final results. *Gynecol Oncol* 1997;67:61–69. PMID: 9345358.

Sasieni PD, Cuzick J, Lynch-Farmery E. Estimating the efficacy of screening by auditing smear histories of women with and without cervical cancer. The National Coordinating Network for Cervical Screening Working Group. *Br J Cancer* 1996;73: 1001–1005. PMID: 8611418.

Sedlis A, Bundy BN, Rotman MZ, et al. A randomized trial of pelvic radiation therapy versus no further therapy in selected patients with stage IB carcinoma of the cervix after radical hysterectomy and pelvic lymphadenectomy: a Gynecologic Oncology Group study. *Gynecol Oncol* 1999;73:177–183. PMID: 10329031.

Sood AK, Sorosky JI, Mayr N, et al. Cervical cancer diagnosed shortly after pregnancy: prognostic variables and delivery routes. *Obstet Gynecol* 2000;95:832–838. PMID: 10831976.

Sutton GP, Bundy BN, Delgado G, et al. Ovarian metastases in stage IB carcinoma of the cervix: a Gynecologic Oncology Group study. *Am J Obstet Gynecol* 1992;166:50–53. PMID: 1733218.

Tewari K, Cappuccini F, Gambino A, et al. Neoadjuvant chemotherapy in the treatment of locally advanced cervical carcinoma in pregnancy: a report of two cases and review of issues specific to the management of cervical carcinoma in pregnancy including planned delay of therapy. *Cancer* 1998;82:1529–1543. PMID: 9554531.

Vizcaino AP, Moreno V, Bosch FX, et al. International trends in the incidence of cervical cancer: I. Adenocarcinoma and adenosquamous cell carcinomas. *Int J Cancer* 1998;75:536–545. PMID: 9466653.

Walboomers JM, Jacobs MV, Manos MM, et al. Human papillomavirus is a necessary cause of invasive cervical cancer worldwide. *J Pathol* 1999;189:12–19. PMID: 10451482.

Whitney CW, Sause W, Bundy BN, et al. Randomized comparison of fluorouracil plus cisplatin versus hydroxyurea as an adjunct to radiation therapy in stage IIB–IVA carcinoma of the cervix with negative para-aortic lymph nodes: a Gynecologic Oncology Group and Southwest Oncology Group study. *J Clin Oncol* 1999;17:1339–1348. PMID: 10334517.

Wright JD, NathavithArana R, Lewin SN, et al. Fertility-conserving surgery for young women with stage IA1 cervical cancer: safety and access. *Obstet Gynecol* 2010;115:585–590. PMID: 20177290.

49 Premalignant & Malignant Disorders of the Uterine Corpus

Nicole D. Fleming, MD
Oliver Dorigo, MD, PhD

ENDOMETRIAL HYPERPLASIA & CARCINOMA

ESSENTIALS OF DIAGNOSIS

- Abnormal uterine bleeding: menorrhagia, metrorrhagia, or postmenopausal bleeding
- Risk factors: hyperestrogenism—long-term exposure to unopposed estrogens (polycystic ovarian syndrome, chronic anovulation, late menopause, and exogenous estrogens); metabolic syndrome including diabetes, hypertension, and obesity; nulliparity; increasing age; history of breast cancer; genetic predisposition (hereditary nonpolyposis colon cancer syndrome)
- Diagnosis: endometrial sampling, ultrasonography

Pathogenesis

Endometrial cancer is the most common gynecologic malignancy. The American Cancer Society estimates that over 43,000 new cases will be diagnosed in 2010, and over 7900 women will die from endometrial cancer. In the United States, white women have a lifetime risk of endometrial carcinoma of 2.4% compared with 1.3% for black women; however, survival for white women is about 8% greater at each stage of diagnosis compared to black women. The peak incidence of onset is in the seventh decade, but 25% of cancers occur in premenopausal women, and the disease has even been reported in women ages 20–30 years.

Most endometrial carcinomas arise on the background of endometrial hyperplasia and are well-differentiated tumors. There are 2 major types of endometrial cancer. Type I tumors are more common (85%) and tend to occur in younger women. These are associated with either endogenous or exogenous unopposed estrogen exposure and usually consist of a low-grade or well-differentiated tumor with a favorable prognosis. Type II tumors grow independent of estrogen, are associated with endometrial atrophy, and occur in an older population. Poorly differentiated endometrioid or nonendometrioid, such as papillary serous and clear cell, histologies are included in type II tumors and confer a high risk of relapse with poor prognosis. Gene expression profiles have also been shown to be different between type I and II tumors, with PTEN mutations more common in type I and p53 overexpression more common in type II tumors.

Estrogens and progesterone are the 2 main hormones that influence the metabolic and proliferative state of the endometrium. In general, estrogens stimulate the endometrium, unlike progesterone, which has an antiproliferative effect. Long-term exposure to estrogens can lead to endometrial hyperplasia and, subsequently, to hormone-driven atypical endometrial hyperplasia and endometrial cancer. Clinical circumstances with chronically high levels of estrogenic stimulation include obesity, metabolic syndrome, polycystic ovary syndrome, exogenous and unopposed estrogen replacement therapy, and chronic anovulation in the premenopausal women. Granulosa cell tumors of the ovary can produce high levels of estrogens and can be associated with endometrial hyperplasia or cancer. The selective estrogen receptor modulator (SERM) tamoxifen used for adjuvant therapy in breast cancer has a weak estrogenic effect on the endometrium and increases the incidence of endometrial cancer by about 2- to 3-fold. However, the benefit of tamoxifen therapy for breast cancer outweighed the potential increase in endometrial cancer reported with a 38% reduction in the 5-year cumulative hazard rate in the tamoxifen-treated group.

More than a dozen case-control studies indicate an association between estrogen administration and endometrial carcinoma. These studies report a 2- to 10-fold increase in the incidence of endometrial carcinoma in women receiving exogenous unopposed estrogens. The risk of cancer is related to both the dose and the duration of exposure and diminishes with cessation of estrogen use. The risk seems to be neutralized by the addition of cyclic progestin for 10 days at least every 1–3 months. In women without a hysterectomy, progestin should be added to the treatment to oppose the effect of estrogens on the endometrium. Endometrial biopsies to rule out endometrial hyperplasia or pelvic ultrasonography to evaluate the thickness of the endometrial stripe should be obtained if abnormal bleeding occurs.

About 5–6% of endometrial cancer cases develop on a genetic background. Women with a personal history of ovarian, colon, or breast cancer as well as those with a family history of endometrial cancer may be at higher risk. In hereditary nonpolyposis colorectal cancer (HNPCC) or Lynch syndrome, there is an autosomal dominant pattern of inheritance for colon and endometrial cancers most commonly, and rectal, ovarian, small bowel, and renal cancers less frequently. Patients with Lynch syndrome have an up to 70% lifetime risk of developing endometrial cancer, and a 10–12% risk of developing ovarian cancer. Most cases of HNPCC are a result of alterations in mismatch repair genes MSH2, MLH1, or MSH6.

Surgical Staging

In 1988, the Cancer Committee of the International Federation of Gynecology and Obstetrics (FIGO) introduced a surgical staging system for endometrial carcinoma based on abdominal exploration, pelvic washings, total hysterectomy with salpingo-oophorectomy, and selective pelvic and periaortic lymph node biopsies. This was revised by the FIGO Committee on Gynecologic Oncology in 2009 (Table 49–1). The grade of the tumors refers to the architecture and nuclear atypia on histology. The architecture of the tumor is judged by the percentage of differentiated (glandular) versus nondifferentiated (solid) elements within the tumor specimen. Grade 1 tumors consist of at least 95% glandular tissue and have <5% of a nonsquamous solid growth pattern. Areas of squamous differentiation are not considered to be solid tumor growth. Grade 2 tumors contain 6–50% of a nonsquamous solid growth pattern. Tumors with more than 50% of a solid pattern are classified as grade 3. The nuclear grade depends on the appearance of the nucleus (size of nucleus, chromatin pattern) and is more subjective. An architectural grade of 1 or 2 is raised by 1 point in the presence of significant nuclear atypia (nuclear grade 3).

Surgical stage I tumors account for 75% of all endometrial carcinomas, which explains the relatively good overall prognosis. Eleven percent of cancers are surgical stage II, and the remaining 11% and 3% are surgical stages III and IV, respectively.

Table 49–1. International Federation of Gynecology and Obstetrics (FIGO) surgical staging of carcinoma of the corpus uteri (2009).

Stage I: Tumor confined to the corpus uteri Stage IA: No or less than half myometrial invasion Stage IB: Invasion equal to or more than half of the myometrium
Stage II: Tumor invades cervical stroma, but does not extend beyond uterus (endocervical glandular involvement considered stage I)
Stage III: Local and/or regional spread of the tumor Stage IIIA: Tumor invades serosa of the corpus uteri and/or adnexa Stage IIIB: Vaginal and/or parametrial involvement Stage IIIC: Metastases to pelvic and/or para-aortic lymph nodes Stage IIIC1: Positive pelvic nodes Stage IIIC2: Positive para-aortic nodes with or without positive pelvic nodes
Stage IV: Tumor invades bladder and/or bowel mucosa, and/or distant metastases Stage IVA: Tumor invades bladder and/or bowel mucosa Stage IVB: Distant metastases including intra-abdominal and/or inguinal lymph nodes

*Positive cytology has to be reported separately without changing the stage.

Reproduced, with permission, from International Federation of Gynecology and Obstetrics. Revised FIGO staging for carcinoma of the vulva, cervix, and endometrium. *Int J Gynecol Obstet* 2009; 105:103–104.

A. Endometrial Hyperplasia

The glandular hyperplasias of the endometrium are benign conditions that can be classified as simple or complex and either with or without atypia. Because of their association with hyperestrogenic states, the atypical hyperplasias are considered premalignant lesions. Because endometrial hyperplasia and endometrial carcinoma present clinically as abnormal bleeding, thorough endometrial sampling or fractional curettage is always necessary when hyperplasia is present to rule out coexisting carcinoma.

1. Hyperplasia without atypia—Microscopically, this type of hyperplasia shows crowding of glands in the stroma without nuclear atypia. This type of hyperplasia is frequently asymptomatic and found incidentally in hysterectomy specimens. When followed without treatment over a 15-year period, approximately 1% progressed to endometrial cancer, whereas 80% spontaneously regressed.

Simple hyperplasia without atypia describes enlarged glands with an irregular outline. Long-term follow-up reveals a 1% risk of progression to carcinoma if untreated. Complex hyperplasia without atypia (previously designated "adenomatous hyperplasia") describes a complex, crowded back-to-back glandular appearance with intraluminal papillae. Complex hyperplasia regresses under progestin therapy in approximately 85% of cases but progresses to cancer in 3–5% if untreated.

2. Hyperplasia with atypia—The histology of hyperplasia with atypia is characterized by endometrial glands that are lined with enlarged cells. An increased nuclear-to-cytoplasmic ratio is a sign of increased nuclear activity (eg, transcription). The nuclei may be irregular with coarse chromatin clumping and prominent nucleoli. These hyperplasias are generally considered premalignant. Progression to carcinoma occurs in 10% of simple atypical and in 30% of complex atypical hyperplasias. The majority of lesions regress with progestin therapy but have a higher rate of relapse when therapy is stopped compared to lesions without atypia. In peri- and postmenopausal patients with atypical hyperplasias who relapse after progestin therapy or who cannot tolerate the associated side effects, vaginal or abdominal hysterectomy is recommended.

A recent prospective cohort study by the Gynecologic Oncology Group (GOG) demonstrated that in patients with untreated atypical endometrial hyperplasia on preoperative biopsy, 42.6% had a concurrent endometrial carcinoma at hysterectomy. In the subset of women who had biopsies interpreted as less than atypical endometrial hyperplasia who underwent hysterectomy, 18.9% had cancer.

The term **atypical endometrial hyperplasia** should be applied to endometrial neoplasia without invasion. Severe atypical endometrial hyperplasia and adenocarcinoma in situ describe preinvasive histologies that are frequently difficult to distinguish from early invasive endometrial cancer. It is still a matter of debate whether the term **adenocarcinoma in situ** should be used for endometrial pathology. In contrast, the precursor lesion for serous carcinomas in endometrial intraepithelial carcinoma shows pleomorphic tumor cells in the epithelium of the endometrial surface and the underlying glands without stromal invasion.

In recent years, the term **endometrial intraepithelial neoplasia (EIN)** has been used to describe premalignant lesion of the uterine lining that predisposes to endometrioid endometrial adenocarcinoma. EIN lesions have been discovered by molecular, histologic, and clinical outcome studies and comprise a subset of endometrial hyperplasia lesions. EIN should not be confused with intraepithelial carcinoma (EIC), which is an early stage of papillary serous adenocarcinomas originating from the glandular endometrium.

B. Endometrial Carcinoma

Endometrial cancer is characterized by obvious hyperplasia and anaplasia of the glandular elements, with invasion of underlying stroma, myometrium, and vascular spaces. Although atypical complex hyperplasia is thought to be a precursor lesion, only approximately 25% of patients with endometrial carcinoma have a history of hyperplasia.

Important prognostic factors include stage, histologic grade and cell type, depth of myometrial invasion, presence of lymphovascular space involvement (LVSI), lymph node status, involvement of the lower uterine segment, and size of tumor.

Endometrial cancers of endometrioid histology of any grade with no myometrial invasion are almost never associated with lymph node metastases. The depth of myometrial invasion and histologic grade are correlated with the incidence of pelvic and aortic lymph node metastases. In the surgical pathology study GOG-33, nodal disease was more frequent with increasing grade (3% grade 1, 9% grade 2, 18% grade 3), depth of invasion (1% endometrium only, 5% inner one-third, 6% middle one-third, 25% outer one-third myometrial invasion), and LVSI (27% with LVSI, 7% without LVSI). Patients with poorly differentiated deeply invasive cancers have about a 35% incidence of involved pelvic nodes and a 10–20% incidence of aortic node metastases. Because patients with lymph node metastases are at very high risk for recurrence, these pathologic features have serious implications for treatment planning.

Endometrial cancer can spread by 4 possible routes: direct extension, lymphatic metastases, peritoneal implants after transtubal spread, and hematogenous spread. Undifferentiated lesions (grade 3) may spread to the pelvic and aortic nodes while still confined to the superficial myometrium. In serous and clear cell subtypes, the spread pattern is similar to that of ovarian cancer, and upper abdominal metastases are common. Hematogenous metastases to the lungs are uncommon with primary tumors limited to the uterus but do occur with recurrent or disseminated disease. Endometrial cancer spreads via a dual pathway to the pelvic and aortic lymph nodes (Fig. 49–1). The aortic nodes are rarely involved when the pelvic nodes are free of metastases.

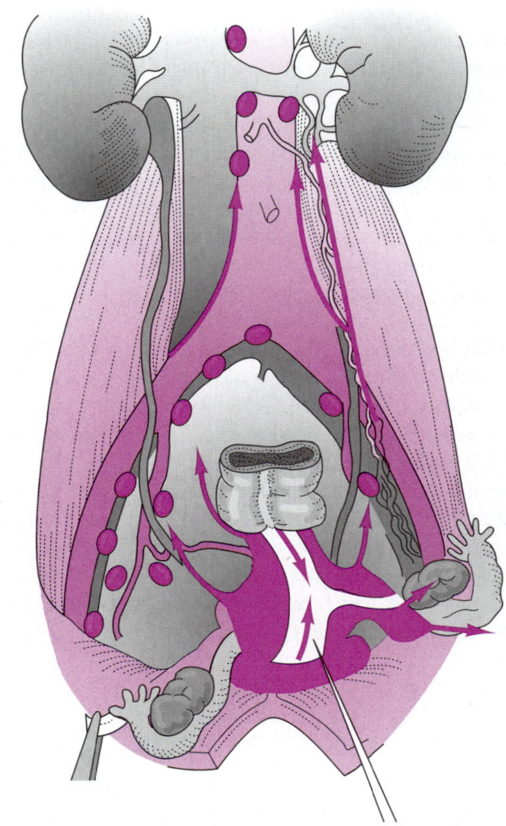

▲ **Figure 49–1.** Dual lymphatic spread pattern of endometrial carcinoma.

The lymph nodes most commonly involved in endometrial cancer are found in the obturator space.

Vaginal metastases occur by submucosal lymphatic or vascular metastases in approximately 3–8% of patients with clinical stage I disease. The concept that these metastases occur by spillage of tumor through the cervix at the time of surgery lacks convincing support. However, vaginal metastases are more common with higher histologic grade and with lower uterine segment or cervical involvement.

Pathologists recognize various histologic types of endometrial carcinoma. Approximately 80% of all endometrial cancers are of the endometrioid type with several variants: villoglandular, secretory, with squamous differentiation, and with ciliated cells. These types have similar presenting symptoms and signs, patterns of spread, and general clinical behavior. For this reason, they can be considered collectively for purposes of clinical workup, differential diagnosis, and treatment. Endometrial adenocarcinomas of the nonendometrioid phenotype show mucinous, serous, clear cell, squamous, small cell, mixed, or transitional cell differentiation.

1. Adenocarcinoma—The most common type of endometrial carcinoma is adenocarcinoma, composed of malignant glands that range from well-differentiated (grade 1) to anaplastic carcinoma (grade 3). To determine stage and prognosis, the tumor is usually graded by the most undifferentiated area visible under the microscope (Fig. 49–2). In the United States, adenocarcinoma comprises 80% of endometrial carcinomas.

2. Adenocarcinoma with squamous differentiation—Approximately 25% of endometrioid carcinomas contain focal to extensive squamous elements, ranging from bland squamous cells to foci that could be viewed as squamous carcinoma. The behavior of the tumors with squamous differentiation is dependent on the grade of the glandular component.

3. Serous carcinoma—Histologically, this cancer is identical to the complex papillary architecture seen in serous carcinomas of the ovary. Serous carcinoma represents approximately 10% of endometrial carcinomas. Women with serous carcinoma are more likely to be older and less likely to have hyperestrogenic states. These tumors account for 50% of all relapses in stage I tumors. Serous tumors spread early and involve peritoneal surfaces of the pelvis and abdomen. The tumors also have a propensity for myometrial and lymphatic invasion. The prognosis is unfavorable, and patients with serous tumors should be treated in a manner similar to that of patients with ovarian tumors.

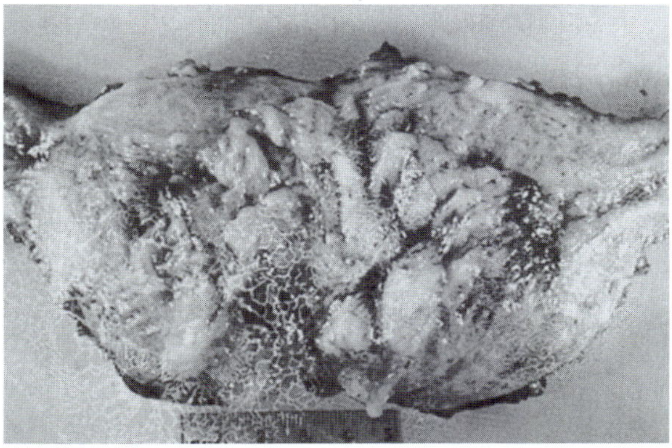

▲ **Figure 49–2.** Adenocarcinoma of the endometrium. Note the sharp demarcation of the tumor at the isthmus.

4. Clear cell carcinoma—This subtype is not associated with clear cell carcinomas of the cervix and vagina that are seen in young women with diethylstilbestrol exposure. Clear cell carcinomas encompass approximately 1–4% of all endometrial carcinomas. Its microscopic appearance is significant for clear cells or hobnail cells. Solid, papillary, tubular, and cystic patterns are possible. Clear cell carcinoma is commonly high grade and aggressive with deep invasion and is seen at an advanced stage. The mean age at diagnosis is approximately 67 years, which is similar to the serous subtype, and it is not associated with a hyperestrogenic state.

5. Miscellaneous subtypes—Mucinous carcinomas make up 1–9% of endometrial adenocarcinomas. The cytoplasm is positive for mucin, carcinoembryonic antigen, and periodic acid-Schiff stain. Secretory carcinoma, present in 1–2% of cases, exhibits subnuclear or supranuclear vacuoles resembling early secretory endometrium. These rare cancers behave in a manner similar to that of typical endometrial carcinomas. Pure squamous cell carcinomas are extremely rare (<1%) and are associated with cervical stenosis, pyometra, and chronic inflammation.

Prevention

A doubling of the incidence of endometrial cancer in the 1970s correlated with unopposed estrogen use in hormone replacement and sequential oral contraceptives over the previous 10 years. The declining incidence in the 1980s paralleled progesterone use in hormone replacement regimens and low-dose estrogen combination birth control pills.

Estrogens are implicated as a causative factor in endometrial carcinoma based mainly on the high incidence of this disease in patients with presumed alterations in estrogen metabolism and in those who take exogenous estrogens. Furthermore, patients with anovulatory cycles are at higher risk of developing endometrial cancer because of prolonged periods of estrogenic stimulation of the endometrium without the opposing effects of progesterone. Progesterone has an antiproliferative effect on the endometrium and can induce apoptosis of endometrial cells.

Classically, endometrial carcinoma affects the obese, nulliparous, infertile, hypertensive, and diabetic white woman, but it can occur in the absence of all these factors. Unlike cervical cancer, it is not related to sexual history.

Prophylactic hysterectomy and bilateral salpingo-oophorectomy have been shown to be effective strategies for preventing endometrial and ovarian cancer in these high-risk patients.

Several modifiable risk factors for endometrial carcinoma have been described, including obesity, diabetes, hypertension, and nulliparity. Prevention of endometrial cancer is primarily based on weight control, physical exercise, adequate control of diabetes and hypertension, and increased surveillance of women at high risk. In addition, a careful family history of each patient will help identify patients with a genetic predisposition for endometrial cancer, for example, as part of the HNPCC syndrome. If appropriate, these patients should undergo genetic counseling and genetic testing. A hysterectomy after the completion of childbearing is appropriate for patients with HNPCC syndrome given the lifetime risk for endometrial cancer of up to 70%. Hormone therapy in postmenopausal patients without hysterectomy should always include a progestational agent to oppose the action of estrogens on the endometrium. Estrogens should be administered either continuously or cyclically using the lowest dose that controls symptoms. Progesterone (10 mg of medroxyprogesterone acetate or 200 mg of micronized progesterone) should be added for the last 10–14 days of the cycle to neutralize the risk of endometrial carcinoma. Alternatively, if estrogen and progesterone are administered continuously, 2.5 mg of medroxyprogesterone acetate is given daily.

Clinical Findings

The onset of endometrial bleeding facilitates detection in the earlier stages of disease. The most common presenting symptom is abnormal vaginal bleeding, particularly postmenopausal bleeding. Less frequently, severe cramps from hematometra or pyometra caused by an obliterated endocervical canal in elderly patients may be the presenting symptom.

A. Symptoms & Signs

Abnormal bleeding occurs in approximately 80% of patients and is the most important and early symptom of endometrial carcinoma. An abnormal vaginal discharge, especially after menopause or intermittent spotting, is reported by some patients. During the premenopausal years, the bleeding is usually described as excessive flow at the time of menstruation. However, bleeding may occur as intermenstrual spotting or premenstrual and postmenstrual bleeding. Approximately 5–10% of patients with postmenopausal bleeding have underlying cancer, but the probability increases with age and depends on underlying risk factors. Approximately 10% of patients complain of lower abdominal cramps and pain secondary to uterine contractions caused by detritus and blood trapped behind a stenotic cervical os (hematometra). If the uterine contents become infected, an abscess develops and sepsis may occur.

Physical examination is usually unremarkable but may reveal medical problems associated with advanced age. Speculum examination may confirm the presence of bleeding, but because it may be minimal and intermittent, blood might not be present. Atrophic vaginitis is frequently identified in these elderly women, but postmenopausal bleeding should never be ascribed to atrophy without a histologic sampling of the endometrium to rule out endometrial carcinoma. Bimanual and rectovaginal examination of the uterus in the early stages of the disease will be normal unless hematometra or pyometra is present. If the cancer is extensive at the time of presentation, the uterus may be enlarged and may be misdiagnosed as a benign condition such as leiomyomata. In advanced cases, the uterus may be fixed and immobile from parametrial extension.

Vaginal, vulvar, or inguinal–femoral lymph node metastases are rarely identified in early disease but are not uncommon in advanced cases or with recurrence following treatment. Ovarian metastases may cause marked enlargement of these organs.

B. Laboratory Findings

Routine laboratory findings are normal in most patients with endometrial carcinoma. If bleeding has been prolonged or profuse, anemia may be present. Cytologic study of specimens taken from the endocervix and posterior vaginal fornix can reveal adenocarcinoma in symptomatic patients. More important, endometrial carcinoma will be missed in 40% of symptomatic patients by routine cytologic examination. Accuracy has been greatly increased by aspiration cytologic study or biopsy (discussed under Special Examinations). Nevertheless, the Papanicolaou (Pap) smear is an integral part of the examination of all patients, because it identifies a small but definite percentage of patients with asymptomatic disease. Furthermore, the presence of benign endometrial cells in the cervical or vaginal smear of a menopausal or postmenopausal woman is associated with occult endometrial carcinoma in 2–6% of cases and in up to 25% with postmenopausal bleeding. Thus, any postmenopausal woman who shows endometrial cells on a routine cervical Pap smear requires evaluation for endometrial cancer, including endometrial sampling.

Routine blood counts, urinalysis, endocervical and vaginal pool cytology, chest radiography, stool guaiac, and sigmoidoscopy are useful ancillary diagnostic tests in patients with endometrial carcinoma. Liver function tests, blood urea nitrogen, serum creatinine, and a blood glucose test (because of the known relationship to diabetes) are considered routine. Serum CA-125 (cancer antigen-125), a well-established tumor marker for epithelial ovarian cancer, might be useful for endometrial cancer. Approximately 20% of patients with clinical stage I disease (preoperatively, the tumor appears to be confined to the uterus) have an elevated CA-125. In cases with extensive intraperitoneal spread or enlarged uterus, the tumor marker CA-125 may be markedly elevated. However, in contrast to patients with ovarian cancer, the value of CA-125 in the management of patients with endometrial cancer is limited.

C. Imaging Studies

Chest radiography might reveal metastases in patients with advanced disease but is rarely positive in the early stages. Colonoscopy is usually unnecessary in a patient with a negative stool guaiac test and normal sigmoidoscopic examination but should always be performed in the patient with gross or occult gastrointestinal bleeding or symptoms. In patients from families with HNPCC, a colonoscopy should be performed preoperatively, particularly if the patient screens positive for the HNPCC-associated DNA mismatch repair gene mutations.

Hysteroscopy can increase the diagnostic accuracy over office endometrial biopsy or dilatation and curettage. Hysteroscopy promotes the transtubal spread of tumor cells into the peritoneal cavity. However, the presence of a positive peritoneal cytology after hysteroscopy does not seem to alter the prognosis. Computed tomography is useful in assessing pelvic anatomy, visualizing enlarged lymph nodes in the pelvis and periaortic areas and diagnosing distant metastasis in the liver and lungs. Magnetic resonance imaging (MRI) is particularly helpful in identifying myometrial invasion and lower uterine segment or cervical involvement.

D. Special Examinations

1. Fractional curettage—Dilatation and fractional curettage (D&C) is the definitive procedure for diagnosis of endometrial carcinoma. It should be performed with the patient under anesthesia to provide an opportunity for a thorough and more accurate pelvic examination. It is carried out by careful and complete curettage of the endocervical canal followed by dilatation of the canal and circumferential curettage of the endometrial cavity. When obvious cancer is present with the first passes of the curette, the procedure should be terminated as long as sufficient tissue for analysis has been obtained from the endocervix and endometrium. Perforation of the uterus followed by intraperitoneal contamination with malignant cells, blood, and bacteria is a common complication in patients with endometrial carcinoma and can usually be avoided by gentle surgical technique and limitation of the procedure to the extent necessary for accurate diagnosis and staging. D&C is never considered curative in these circumstances and should not be performed with the same vigor as therapeutic curettage.

2. Endometrial biopsy—This procedure is attractive because it can be performed in an outpatient setting, resulting in a substantial savings in cost. It can usually be done without anesthesia, although paracervical block is effective when necessary. Results of endometrial biopsies (EMB) correlate well with endometrial curettings with the accuracy to detect cancer between 91% and 95%. The accuracy of identifying cancers with EMB is higher in postmenopausal patients than in premenopausal patients. There is a false-negative rate of approximately 10%, and all symptomatic patients with a negative EMB need to undergo a formal

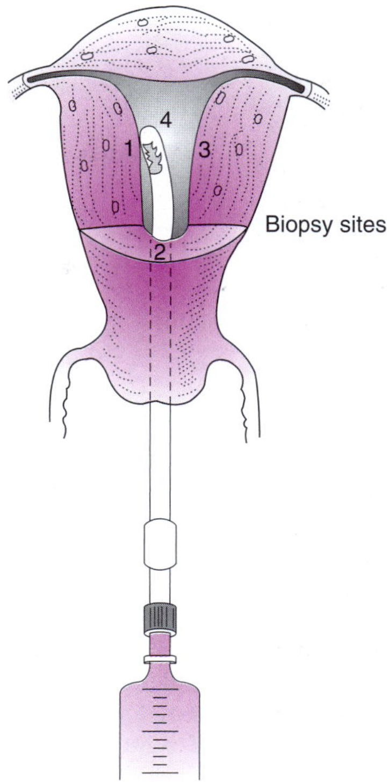

▲ **Figure 49–3.** Technique of endometrial biopsy with Novak curet.

D&C. There are many types of office biopsy techniques including a Pipelle, Novak curet (Fig. 49–3), and Vabra aspirator (Fig. 49–4). All types of EMB are notoriously inaccurate for diagnosing polyps and will miss a significant number of cases of endometrial hyperplasia as well.

3. Pelvic ultrasonography—Ultrasonography can be helpful in the surveillance of asymptomatic, high-risk patients (eg, breast cancer patients on tamoxifen and women with strong family histories of endometrial cancer). Pelvic and transvaginal ultrasonography yield information about the size and shape of the uterus, as well as the thickness and surface contour of the endometrium. Transvaginal ultrasound measuring the lining thickness of the endometrium has an excellent negative predictive value for ruling out endometrial cancer or hyperplasia when the thickness is <5 mm, but provides less information when >5 mm. In postmenopausal women, an endometrial thickness of more than 5 mm is considered to be suspicious for hyperplasia or malignancy and should be further evaluated with an EMB. Transvaginal ultrasound, however, can yield a high false-positive rate in women who have been on tamoxifen for more than 2 years. The subendometrial edema that develops from tamoxifen use is indistinguishable from a thickened endometrial stripe. A sonohysterogram, which involves instilling sterile saline into the endometrial cavity prior to transvaginal ultrasound,

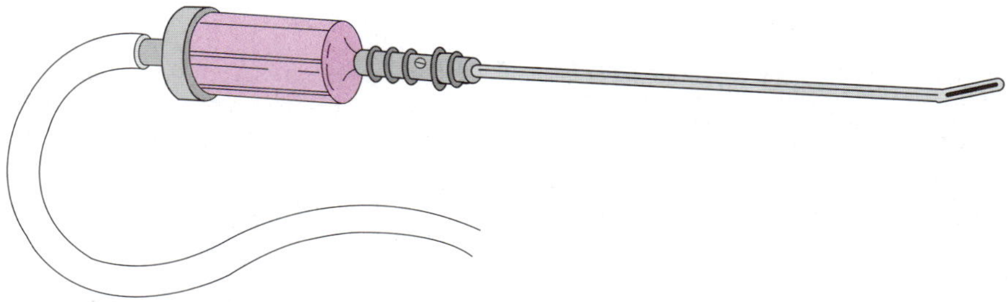

▲ **Figure 49–4.** Vabra aspirator.

can reduce false-positive results and better delineate the endometrial cavity.

4. Estrogen and Progesterone Receptor Assays— Estrogen and progesterone receptor assays should be obtained from the neoplastic tissue. This information helps in planning adjuvant or subsequent hormone therapy. Estrogen and progesterone receptor content are inversely proportional to histologic grade. In general, patients with tumors positive for 1 or 2 receptors have longer survival than patients with receptor-negative tumors. Furthermore, patients with receptor-positive tumors might be candidates for hormone-based therapy of recurrent tumor disease.

Differential Diagnosis

In the asymptomatic patient, a diagnosis may be made incidentally from an abnormal Pap smear, but cytologic discovery of endometrial cancer is not consistent and should not be relied on for early diagnosis. Screening for endometrial cancer in the general population is not recommended but should be performed for patients with a Lynch or HNPCC syndrome.

Clinically, the differential diagnosis of endometrial carcinoma includes all the various causes of abnormal uterine bleeding. In the premenopausal patient, complications of early pregnancy, such as threatened or incomplete abortion, must be considered initially. Other causes of bleeding in premenopausal patients are leiomyomata, endometrial hyperplasia and polyps, cervical polyps, an intrauterine device, and various genital or metastatic cancers. Cervical, endometrial, tubal, and ovarian neoplasms all can cause abnormal uterine bleeding. Although rare, metastatic cancers from the bowel, bladder, and breast have also been reported to cause abnormal uterine bleeding. After exclusion of anatomic causes for vaginal bleeding, a workup for hemophilias should be performed. In the postmenopausal age group, the differential diagnosis includes atrophic vaginitis, exogenous estrogens, endometrial hyperplasia and polyps, and various genital neoplasms. The likelihood of cancer increases with age. In the patient with a normal pelvic examination and recurrent postmenopausal bleeding following a recent negative D&C, tubal and ovarian cancer must be strongly considered. Patients with recurrent unexplained episodes of postmenopausal uterine bleeding should be considered for total hysterectomy and bilateral salpingo-oophorectomy.

Complications

Patients with advanced disease and deep myometrial invasion may present with severe anemia secondary to chronic blood loss or acute hemorrhage. If bleeding is significant and continuous, a short-term boost of radiation therapy is usually effective in slowing the hemorrhage.

The presence of a hematometra can be confirmed by sounding the uterus under anesthesia, followed by dilatation of the cervix to allow adequate drainage. When a pyometra is present, the patient may present with peritonitis or generalized sepsis, with all the consequent complications.

Perforation of the uterus at the time of D&C or EMB is not an uncommon problem. If the perforating instrument is large, loops of small bowel may be inadvertently retrieved through the cervical canal. A large perforation warrants laparoscopy or laparotomy to evaluate and repair the damage. If significant contamination of the peritoneal cavity with blood or necrotic tumor has occurred, the patient should be treated with broad-spectrum antibiotics to prevent peritonitis. Perforation in the patient with endometrial cancer should be viewed as a serious complication, as spillage of tumor into the peritoneal cavity may alter her prognosis.

Treatment

The mainstay of treatment is surgery, including a total hysterectomy with bilateral salpingo-oophorectomy and staging with pelvic and periaortic lymphadenectomy. Further postoperative therapy depends on the particular histologic characteristics and the extent of the tumor.

The majority of endometrial cancer cases are diagnosed at an early stage and can be treated with high cure rates. The most important treatment modality is surgery with total hysterectomy, bilateral salpingo-oophorectomy, and staging, including pelvic and periaortic lymphadenectomy. Primary radiation therapy is used only in patients with medical contraindications for surgery or advanced pelvic disease. It has been repeatedly demonstrated that radiation therapy can cure endometrial carcinoma in some patients. However, radiation therapy averages about a 20% lower cure rate compared to surgery in stage I disease. Primary chemotherapy is used infrequently and mostly in patients with metastatic disease. High-dose progesterone therapy, commonly with medroxyprogesterone acetate or megestrol acetate, may be used for patients who are inoperable or in younger patients who elect for fertility preservation. The overall response to high-dose progesterone therapy is up to 75% in grade 1 endometrial cancer cases limited to the endometrium. To verify that the patient is responding to therapy, regular endometrial sampling needs to be performed.

Adjuvant treatment is dependent on the results of surgical staging and histology. For example, adjuvant radiation therapy is frequently used in high-risk endometrial cancers of endometrioid histology to prevent pelvic recurrences. Advanced pelvic disease may be treated with radiation followed by systemic chemotherapy. Serous cancers of the endometrium behave biologically similar to ovarian cancer and are treated with adjuvant platinum-based chemotherapy possibly in conjunction with radiation.

A. Emergency Measures

Patients with endometrial adenocarcinoma may present with severe anemia after prolonged periods of vaginal bleeding. Acute and massive blood loss may lead to hypovolemic shock. The management of these patients includes stabilization of vital signs with volume substitution and blood transfusion. A tamponade of the uterus using vaginal packing might be useful, particularly in the presence of a bleeding cervical or vaginal tumor. Monsel's solution or silver nitrate can further aid in obtaining hemostasis. An emergency D&C might help to control the bleeding but has to be performed with great caution to avoid perforation. If bleeding does not subside, a high-dose radiation boost to the whole pelvis is usually the treatment of choice to acutely control uterine bleeding in this situation. Rarely, in the face of very advanced lesions, embolization of the hypogastric arteries via percutaneous selective angiography may be required to control hemorrhage before treatment can be initiated. Hysterectomy should always be considered if it can be accomplished safely without jeopardizing curative therapy.

Elderly patients may present with severe lower abdominal pain and cramping secondary to hematometra or pyometra; these complications result from endometrial carcinoma in more than 50% of cases. When adequate blood levels of broad-spectrum antibiotics are established, the cervix should be dilated and the endometrial cavity adequately drained. In this setting, vigorous D&C is contraindicated because of the high risk of uterine perforation. If the cervix is well dilated, an indwelling drain is usually unnecessary, but if sepsis is not controlled within 24–48 hours, the patient should be re-examined to ascertain cervical patency. Once the infection has completely subsided and the patient has been afebrile for 7–10 days, gentle fractional curettage should be performed if the diagnosis was not confirmed at the initial procedure.

B. Radiation Therapy

Radiation therapy is used as primary therapy in patients considered too medically unstable for laparotomy. Adjuvant preoperative radiation is no longer used unless the patient presents with gross cervical involvement. In this situation, after preoperative whole-pelvic radiation and an intracavitary implant, an extrafascial hysterectomy is performed. Relative contraindications to preoperative radiation therapy include the presence of a pelvic mass, a pelvic kidney, pyometra, history of a pelvic abscess, prior pelvic radiation, and previous multiple laparotomies (see Chapter 52).

Adjuvant radiation therapy has been shown to significantly improve locoregional control in early-stage, high-risk endometrial cancer. Two randomized controlled clinical trials, one conducted in the United States by the GOG (GOG-99) and the other one conducted in Europe (PORTEC trial), demonstrated that the addition of postoperative external-beam radiation therapy (EBRT) in early-stage, high-risk endometrial cancers decreased the rate of vaginal and pelvic recurrences versus surgery alone. However, local radiation alone did not result in improvement of overall survival.

Accordingly, in the presence of extrauterine extension, lower uterine segment or cervical involvement, poor histologic differentiation, papillary serous or clear cell histology, or myometrial invasion greater than one-third of the full thickness, adjuvant radiation therapy is recommended. In the absence of these findings, it is difficult to justify the risk and morbidity of any additional treatment beyond simple total abdominal hysterectomy and bilateral salpingo-oophorectomy. In stage III and IV disease, the optimal adjuvant therapy has also been of much debate. Management options in advanced-stage disease can include systemic chemotherapy alone or in addition to radiation therapy to improve locoregional control. Overall, adjuvant therapy in patients with early-stage, high-risk endometrioid endometrial cancers should be individualized based on stage and grade, on whether surgical lymph node staging was performed, and on the risk of nodal versus vaginal recurrence.

C. Surgical Treatment

Because bleeding is usually an early sign of endometrial carcinoma, most patients present with early disease and can be adequately and completely treated by simple hysterectomy. Staging includes a bilateral salpingo-oophorectomy, peritoneal washings for cytology, and removal of pelvic and periaortic lymph nodes. Recently, minimally invasive methods, including laparoscopic-assisted and robotic-assisted endometrial cancer staging procedures, have been successfully performed. Laparoscopic surgery is currently the preferred management for patients with endometrial cancer, because patient outcome is equivalent to open surgery. In addition, length of hospital stay and recovery time are both shorter.

Pelvic and para-aortic lymphadenectomy play an important role in the surgical staging of endometrial cancer. A gross pathologic assessment of the uterus should be performed during surgery to determine the need for surgical staging in patients with grade 1 or 2 endometrioid adenocarcinomas. Patients who require surgical staging are patients with stage I disease with grade 3 lesions, tumors >2 cm in maximum dimension, tumors with >50% myometrial invasion, cervical extension, and evidence of extrauterine spread. Furthermore, staging should be performed in clear cell and papillary serous carcinomas in all cases because of a high incidence of lymphatic spread. However, the criteria for lymphadenectomy are not universally accepted and are under constant investigation. The therapeutic role of lymphadenectomy is still under investigation. Several studies have suggested that EBRT may be omitted or the radiation field reduced to the central pelvis if the lymph nodes are negative. Bulky, positive nodes, which are unlikely to respond to EBRT, should be removed during surgery.

Radical hysterectomy for stage II tumors is an accepted procedure that has the potential to omit adjuvant radiation therapy. A radical hysterectomy can also be an effective treatment for patients with recurrence following treatment with radiation therapy alone or for those who have previously received therapeutic doses of pelvic radiation therapy for other pelvic cancers. The increased risk of bowel or urinary tract injury in this setting must be understood and accepted by both patient and physician.

Patients who present with significant cervical involvement or vaginal and parametrial involvement should receive initial pelvic radiation. Exploratory laparotomy should then be considered in patients whose disease seems resectable. Hormonal therapy or chemotherapy is most appropriate for patients with clinical evidence of extrapelvic metastases. Palliative radiation to bone or brain metastases is beneficial for symptomatic relief. Pelvic radiation can be helpful for local tumor control and alleviation of bleeding.

D. Hormone Therapy

Progesterone has shown some efficacy in the treatment of recurrent endometrial carcinoma not amenable to irradiation or surgery. This type of therapy can be administered orally or parenterally. Oral megestrol, parenteral medroxyprogesterone acetate suspension, and parenteral hydroxyprogesterone caproate appear to have similar effectiveness with response rates of approximately 25%. Overall, approximately 13% of patients with recurrent disease appear to achieve long-term remission with progesterone therapy. The average duration of response is 20 months, and up to 30% of responders survive for 5 years. In general, the clinical response is better in patients with localized recurrence, well-differentiated tumors, long disease-free intervals, and positive estrogen or progesterone receptor status. Because some patients do not achieve remission until after 10–12 weeks of therapy, the minimum duration of treatment should be longer than 3 months. Although progesterones have a somewhat encouraging record in the treatment of recurrent endometrial adenocarcinoma, they are disappointing as prophylactic agents. They have not improved survival or decreased recurrence when used following definitive treatment of early-stage disease.

Tamoxifen, either alone or in combination with progesterone, has been used in advanced or recurrent endometrial cancer. Patients with well-differentiated, estrogen receptor–positive tumors and long disease-free intervals tend to have a better response to tamoxifen. Tamoxifen is administered orally at 10–20 mg twice daily. For single-agent tamoxifen, the overall response rate is approximately 15–20%. Studies using combination tamoxifen–progestin therapy suggest a possibly better clinical response of up to 40%.

E. Chemotherapy

Doxorubicin and cisplatin are the 2 most active agents in the treatment of advanced or recurrent endometrial cancer. Doxorubicin used as a single agent has an overall response rate of 38%, with 26% of the patients achieving a complete response. The combination of cisplatin and doxorubicin shows slightly longer survival than either agent alone. The addition of paclitaxel to cisplatin and doxorubicin shows an overall response rate of 57% with improved long-term survival compared to the same regimen without paclitaxel. More recently, the combination of paclitaxel and carboplatin has shown comparable response rates and less side effects. Other agents with antitumor activity against endometrial cancer include cyclophosphamide, hexamethylmelamine, and 5-fluorouracil.

Prognosis

The overall prognosis is considerably better than for the other major gynecologic cancers with 5-year survival rates of 96%, 67%, and 17% for local, regional, and distant disease at diagnosis, respectively.

The most important prognostic factors for endometrial cancer are stage, histologic type, grade, myometrial invasion, and the presence of lymphovascular space invasion. Identification of these risk factors is crucial for treatment decisions, surveillance, and counseling of the patient. The prognosis is worse with increasing age, higher pathologic grade, advanced-stage disease, increasing depth of myometrial invasion, and presence of lymphovascular space invasion. Because the prognosis for each patient is dependent on a variety of factors, overall 5-year survival stratified by stage is indicated as a range of percentages. The overall 5-year survival rates are 81–95% for surgical stage I, 67–77% for stage II, 31–60% for stage III, and 5–20% for stage IV.

These figures underline the increasing risk for treatment failure and recurrence with increasing bulk and extension of tumor. In the absence of risk factors, a simple total abdominal hysterectomy and bilateral salpingo-oophorectomy should result in survival >95% at 5 years. However, in the presence of risk factors, a more aggressive surgical approach and using adjuvant radiation and chemotherapy may be warranted.

Amant F, Moerman P, Neven P, et al. Endometrial cancer. *Lancet* 2005;366(9484):491–505. PMID: 16084259.

American Cancer Society. American Cancer Society Facts and Figures 2010. Available at: http://www.cancer.org/Research/CancerFactsFigures/CancerFactsFigures/cancer-facts-and-figures-2010.

Cao QJ, Belbin T, Socci N, et al. Distinctive gene expression profiles by cDNA microarrays in endometrioid and serous carcinomas of the endometrium. *Int J Gynecol Pathol* 2004;23:321–329. PMID: 15389101.

Creutzberg C, van Putten WL, Koper PC, et al. Surgery and postoperative radiotherapy versus surgery alone for patients with stage 1 endometrial carcinoma: multicentre randomized trial. *Lancet* 2000;355:1404–1411. PMID: 10791524.

Dijkhuizen FP, Mol BW, Brölmann HA, Heintz AP. The accuracy of endometrial sampling in the diagnosis of patients with endometrial carcinoma and hyperplasia: a meta-analysis. *Cancer* 2000;89:1765–1772. PMID: 11042572.

Duska LR, Berkowitz R, Matulonis U, et al. Pilot trial of TAC (paclitaxel, doxorubicin, and carboplatin) chemotherapy with filgrastim (r-metHuG-CSF) support followed by radiotherapy in patients with "high-risk" endometrial cancer. *Gynecol Oncol* 2005;96:198–203. PMID: 15589601.

FIGO Committee on Gynecologic Oncology. Revised FIGO staging for carcinoma of the vulva, cervix, and endometrium. *Int J Gynecol Obstet* 2009;105:103–104. PMID: 19367689.

Fung MFK, Reid A, Faught W, et al. Prospective longitudinal study of ultrasound screening for endometrial abnormalities in women with breast cancer receiving tamoxifen. *Gynecol Oncol* 2003;91:154–159. PMID: 14529676.

Karamursel BS, Guven S, Tulunay G, et al. Which surgical procedure for patients with atypical endometrial hyperplasia? *Int J Gynecol Cancer* 2005;15:127–131. PMID: 15670307.

Keys HM, Roberts JA, Brunetto VL et al. A phase III trial of surgery with or without adjunctive external pelvic radiation therapy in intermediate risk endometrial adenocarcinoma: a Gynecologic Oncology Group study. *Gynecol Oncol* 2004; 92:744–751. PMID: 14984936.

Koh WJ, Tran AB, Douglas JG, Stelzer KJ. Radiation therapy in endometrial cancer. *Baillieres Best Pract Res Clin Obstet Gynaecol* 2001;15:417–432. PMID: 11476563.

Lalloo F, Evans G. Molecular genetics and endometrial cancer. *Baillieres Best Pract Res Clin Obstet Gynaecol* 2001;15:355–363. PMID: 11476568.

Lu K, Dinh M, Kohlman W, et al. Gynecologic cancer as a "sentinel cancer" for women with hereditary nonpolyposis colorectal cancer syndrome. *Obstet Gynecol* 2005;105:569–574. PMID: 15738026.

Mariani A, Webb MJ, Keeney GL, Podratz KC. Routes of lymphatic spread: a study of 112 consecutive patients with endometrial cancer. *Gynecol Oncol* 2001;81:100–104. PMID: 11277658.

Montz FJ. Significance of "normal" endometrial cells in cervical cytology from asymptomatic postmenopausal women receiving hormone replacement therapy. *Gynecol Oncol* 2001;81:33–39. PMID: 11277646.

Nout RA, Smit VT, Putter H, et al. Vaginal brachytherapy versus pelvic external beam radiotherapy for patients with endometrial cancer of high-intermediate risk (PORTEC-2): an open-label non-inferiority, randomized trial. *Lancet* 2010;375:816–823. PMID: 20206777.

Pothuri B, Ramondetta L, Martino M, et al. Development of endometrial cancer after radiation treatment for cervical carcinoma. *Obstet Gynecol* 2003;101:941–945. PMID: 12738155.

Ramirez P, Frumovitz M, Bodurka DC, et al. Hormonal therapy for the management of grade 1 endometrial adenocarcinoma: a literature review. *Gynecol Oncol* 2004;95:133–138. PMID: 15385122.

Sakuragi N, Hareyama H, Todo Y, et al. Prognostic significance of serous and clear cell adenocarcinoma in surgically staged endometrial carcinoma. *Acta Obstet Gynecol Scand* 2000;79:311–316. PMID: 10746868.

Schmeler K, Lynch H, Chen L, et al. Prophylactic surgery to reduce the risk of gynecologic cancers in the Lynch syndrome. *N Engl J Med* 2006;354:261–269. PMID: 16421367.

Takeshima N, Nishida H, Tabata T, et al. Positive peritoneal cytology in endometrial cancer: enhancement of other prognostic indicators. *Gynecol Oncol* 2001;82:470–473. PMID: 11520142.

Thigpen JT, Brady MF, Homesley HD, et al. Phase III trial of doxorubicin with or without cisplatin in advanced endometrial carcinoma: a Gynecologic Oncology Group study. *J Clin Oncol* 2004;22:3902–3908. PMID: 15459211.

Trimble CL, Kauderer J, Zaino R, et al. Concurrent endometrial carcinoma in women with a biopsy diagnosis of atypical endometrial hyperplasia: a Gynecologic Oncology Group study. *Cancer* 2006;106:812–819. PMID: 16400639.

Walker JL, Piedmonte MR, Spirtos NM, et al. Laparoscopy compared with laparotomy for comprehensive surgical staging of uterine cancer: a Gynecologic Oncology Group Study Lap 2. *J Clin Oncol* 2009;27:5331–5336. PMID: 19805679.

SARCOMA OF THE UTERUS (LEIOMYOSARCOMA, ENDOMETRIAL SARCOMAS)

ESSENTIALS OF DIAGNOSIS

- Bleeding: metrorrhagia, menorrhagia, postmenopausal or preadolescent bleeding
- Mass: rapid enlargement of the uterus or a leiomyoma
- Pain: pelvic discomfort as a result of mass effect from the enlarged uterus
- Malignant tissue: histology confirmed by D&C or in hysterectomy specimen

Pathogenesis

The uterine sarcomas are mesodermally derived highly malignant tumors and account for approximately 3–4% of all uterine malignancies. No common etiology has been identified in uterine sarcomas, but prior pelvic radiation therapy is associated with the mixed forms of uterine sarcoma.

Sarcomas can occur at any age but are most prevalent after age 40. A bimodal age distribution has been seen with uterine sarcomas, with a premenopausal or perimenopausal

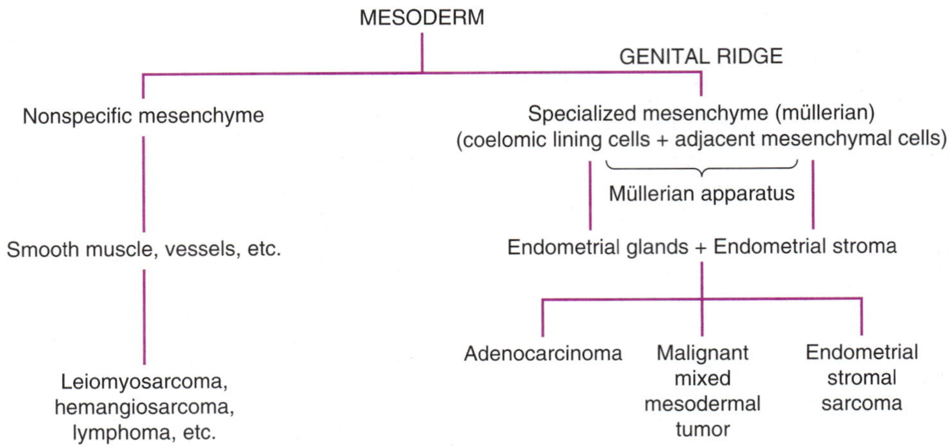

▲ **Figure 49–5.** Histogenesis of uterine sarcomas.

peak for patients with leiomyosarcoma and a postmenopausal peak for patients with carcinosarcoma. Sarcomas are well known as a source of hematogenous metastases, but with the exception of leiomyosarcomas, lymphatic permeation and contiguous spread are probably the most common methods of extension. Endometrial sarcomas can usually be diagnosed by EMB or D&C, but the sarcomas derived from the myometrium (leiomyosarcoma) frequently require hysterectomy to obtain adequate tissue for analysis.

In general, uterine sarcomas follow a very aggressive growth pattern with early metastasis to the abdomen, liver, and lung. There is no universal agreement on the histologic features that determine outcome, but most authorities agree that the number of mitotic figures per high-power field, vascular and lymphatic invasion, serosal extension, and degree of anaplasia are all helpful. Surgery is the most common primary treatment approach, followed by radiation and chemotherapy. Chemotherapeutic agents reported to be active against sarcomas include doxorubicin, cisplatin, ifosfamide, gemcitabine, and the taxanes. Clinical response rates for combination chemotherapy in recurrent and advanced disease are reported to be as high as 54%. However, most responses are partial and only temporary.

Histogenesis, Classification, & Staging

Although several classification systems exist for uterine sarcomas, they can be separated into 4 major categories: leiomyosarcomas (LMSs), endometrial stromal sarcomas (ESSs), malignant mixed mesodermal tumors (MMMTs), and adenosarcomas. LMSs are thought to arise from the myometrial smooth muscle cell or a similar cell lining blood vessels within the myometrium. ESS and MMMT arise from undifferentiated endometrial stromal cells, which retain the potential to differentiate into malignant cell lines that histologically appear native (homologous) or foreign (heterologous) to the human uterus. Because the undifferentiated stromal cells of the endometrium arise from specialized mesenchymal cells of the müllerian apparatus in the genital ridge, and ultimately from the mesoderm during embryogenesis, endometrial sarcomas have been variously termed "mesodermal," "müllerian," or "mesenchymal" sarcomas. The prognoses of patients with homologous and heterologous tumors are similar stage for stage, and this terminology has limited clinical usefulness. ESSs have been categorized in the older literature as "pure" and homologous endometrial sarcomas because they are composed of a single cell line. MMMTs, previously designated as "mixed" because they contain 2 or more cell lines, arise from an undifferentiated malignant stem cell. MMMTs contain both a carcinomatous or epithelium-derived element and a sarcomatous or mesenchymal element and have also been called "carcinosarcomas." The carcinomatous element is usually an undifferentiated adenocarcinoma. The concept of this terminology is better understood by study of Figure 49–5, which graphically represents the histogenesis of uterine sarcomas. Table 49–2 combines the prevailing histogenetic

Table 49–2. Classification of uterine sarcomas.

Leiomyosarcoma (tumors of the uterine smooth muscle)
Endometrial stromal sarcoma (pure homologous endometrial sarcoma) Undifferentiated Low grade (endolymphatic stromal myosis)
Malignant mixed mesodermal tumor (mixed epithelial/stromal tumors) Homologous carcinosarcoma Heterologous carcinosarcoma
Adenosarcoma (mixed epithelial/stromal tumors) Homologous Heterologous

terminology for endometrial sarcomas and depicts the various possibilities in each category.

Pure heterologous sarcomas, such as rhabdomyosarcoma, chondrosarcoma, osteosarcoma, and liposarcoma, are extremely rare. Other uterine sarcomas, like hemangiosarcomas, fibrosarcomas, reticulum cell sarcomas, and lymphosarcomas, are indistinguishable from identical sarcomas elsewhere in the body and are therefore not considered specialized tumors of the uterus.

Recently, a new FIGO classification and staging system has been specifically designed for uterine sarcomas in an attempt to reflect their different biologic behavior (Table 49–3). Carcinosarcomas should continue to be staged as carcinomas of the endometrium.

Major Types of Sarcomas of the Uterus

A. Leiomyosarcomas

LMSs make up 35–40% of all uterine sarcomas and 1–2% of all uterine cancers. LMS usually occurs between ages 25 and 75 years, with a mean incidence at about age 50 years. Younger patients with this disease seem to have a more favorable outcome than postmenopausal women. Like the benign leiomyomas, LMSs are 1.5 times more common in African American patients than in the white population. Leiomyomas are commonly identified in uteri containing LMSs, but the incidence of malignant transformation of a leiomyoma is only 0.1–0.5%. Only approximately 5–10% of LMSs are reported to originate in a leiomyoma.

Abnormal uterine bleeding is the most common symptom of LMS, occurring in approximately 60% of patients; pelvic or abdominal pain and discomfort are reported by approximately 50% of all patients. Only approximately 10% of patients are aware of an abdominal mass. The deeply situated intramural position of most tumors impedes diagnosis by D&C, which is accurate in only 25% of cases. Abnormal cells might be identified on Pap smear. The diagnosis is more commonly made after pathologic analysis of a hysterectomy specimen.

LMSs spread by contiguous growth, invading the myometrium, cervix, and surrounding supporting tissues. Lymphatic dissemination is common in the late stages. Pelvic recurrence and peritoneal dissemination following resection are also common. In the more malignant types, hematogenous metastasis to the lungs, liver, kidney, brain, and bones probably occurs early but is clinically evident only in the lungs until the advanced stages.

The clinical behavior of the tumor is generally aggressive, with some correlation with the number of mitotic figures identified on microscopic examination. Low-grade LMSs are those with <5 mitoses per 10 high-power fields, with pushing rather than infiltrating margins. LMSs with 5–10 mitoses per 10 high-power fields are considered to be of intermediate grade, and tumors with mitotic counts >10 per 10 high-power fields are highly malignant and usually lethal; <20% of these patients are alive at 5 years. Tumor size and mitotic index are useful prognostic indicators, but other factors have to be taken into account. An invasive pattern, particularly into the blood and lymphatic vessels and the surrounding smooth muscle, is important. By contrast, cellular characteristics, such as atypia, anaplasia, and giant cells, are not accurate prognosticators of aggressive behavior. Clinically, the most reliable prognostic feature of LMS is stage. The prognosis of patients with extrauterine disease is much worse compared to patients with disease confined to the uterus. Patients with LMS mostly present at stage I. A pelvic

Table 49–3. International Federation of Gynecology and Obstetrics (FIGO) staging of uterine sarcomas (2009).

(1) Leiomyosarcomas and Endometrial Stromal Sarcomas
Stage I Tumor limited to the uterus IA ≤5 cm IB >5 cm
Stage II Tumor extends beyond uterus, within the pelvis IIA Adnexal involvement IIB Involvement of other pelvic tissues
Stage III Tumor invades abdominal tissues IIIA One site IIIB More than one site IIIC Metastasis to pelvic and/or para-aortic lymph nodes
Stage IV IVA Tumor invades bladder and/or rectum IVB Distant metastasis
(2) Adenosarcomas
Stage I Tumor limited to uterus IA Tumor limited to endometrium/endocervix with no myometrial invasion IB Less than or equal to half myometrial invasion IC More than half myometrial invasion
Stage II Tumor extends beyond the uterus, within the pelvis IIA Adnexal involvement IIB Tumor extends to extrauterine pelvic tissue
Stage III Tumor invades abdominal tissues IIIA One site IIIB More than one site IIIC Metastasis to pelvic and/or para-aortic lymph nodes
Stage IV IVA Tumor invades bladder and/or rectum IVB Distant metastasis
(3) Carcinosarcomas (MMMT)
Carcinosarcomas should be staged as carcinomas of the endometrium

MMMT, malignant mixed mesodermal tumor.
Reproduced, with permission, from FIGO Committee on Gynecologic Oncology. FIGO staging for uterine sarcomas. *Int J Gynecol Obstet* 2009;104:179.

MRI can help delineate the extent of uterine involvement and can help in the preoperative determination of a benign versus a malignant smooth muscle tumor by evidence of scattered foci of hemorrhage and necrosis and absence of calcifications. Benign leiomyomata have sharp boundaries, whereas sarcomas have infiltrating borders on MRI imaging.

Other unusual smooth muscle tumors of the uterus such as benign metastasizing leiomyoma and intravenous leiomyomatosis should be considered low-grade LMS or smooth muscle tumors of uncertain malignant potential (STUMP). Although they are histologically benign, they are notorious for local recurrence and can cause death by compression of contiguous or distant vital structures. Intravenous leiomyomatosis has been known to grow up the vena cava into the right atrium, impeding venous return and precipitating congestive heart failure. Because of their slow growth, they can frequently be controlled by repeated local excision. The metastatic lung lesions of benign metastasizing leiomyoma have disappeared following resection of the primary lesion in some cases, perhaps indicating hormone dependency.

B. Endometrial Sarcomas

1. Endometrial stromal sarcomas—ESSs make up 8% of all sarcomas. They occur predominantly in postmenopausal women. Patients with these tumors most commonly present with bleeding or lower abdominal discomfort and pain. The diagnosis can be made accurately by D&C in approximately 75% of cases. Although no etiologic relationship to hormones has been established, a small number of metastatic lesions have responded to progesterone therapy.

ESSs can be divided into 3 distinct subtypes: low-grade ESS, endometrial stromal nodules, and undifferentiated endometrial sarcomas previously known as high-grade ESS. The indolent low-grade ESSs—also called endolymphatic stromal myosis—have fewer than 10 mitoses per 10 high-power fields, with infiltrating margins and myometrial invasion. A benign form, the stromal nodule, contains pushing rather than infiltrating margins and fewer than 3 mitoses per 10 high-power fields, with no vascular or myometrial invasion.

The mean age at onset for low-grade ESS is 5–10 years earlier than for undifferentiated endometrial sarcomas. This tumor infiltrates surrounding structures and is characterized by indolent growth and a propensity to vascular invasion. Patients frequently present with yellowish wormlike extensions into the periuterine vascular spaces. Under such circumstances, it may be confused grossly with intravenous leiomyomatosis, as previously described. It tends to recur late, sometimes after 5–10 years, and can often be controlled by repeated local excisions. Low-grade ESSs frequently express estrogen and progesterone receptors. Adjuvant targeted hormonal treatment can be considered to reduce recurrence.

The undifferentiated endometrial sarcoma displays infiltrating margins and vascular and myometrial invasion and contains more than 10 mitoses per 10 high-power fields. These tumors are highly malignant and are associated with a poor prognosis, particularly when they extend beyond the uterus at the time of diagnosis. They spread by contiguous growth via the serosal uterine surface and lymphatic metastasis. Distant hematogenous metastases to the lungs and liver are usually a late event.

2. Carcinosarcoma (malignant mixed mesodermal tumors)—MMMTs account for 50% of all uterine sarcomas and 3–6% of all uterine tumors. They characteristically occur in postmenopausal women, with the exception of embryonal rhabdomyosarcoma of the cervix or vagina (sarcoma botryoides), which occurs also in infants and children. The incidence is about 3 times greater in black than in white women. Radiation therapy may be a predisposing cause, but the etiology of MMMTs is unknown. Many published series are available containing a significant number of patients with a history of pelvic radiation for benign or malignant conditions (Fig. 49–6).

As with the other types, the presenting symptom of MMMT is usually bleeding. Abdominal discomfort and pain or a large, bulky polypoid mass filling the uterine cavity and prolapsing through the cervical os also occurs. Because the tumors are endometrial in origin, approximately 75% can be diagnosed accurately by D&C. Histologically, MMMTs are usually highly anaplastic, with many bizarre nuclei and mitotic figures. They contain a carcinomatous or epithelial component and a sarcomatous component, hence the term *malignant mixed mesodermal tumor*, or carcinosarcoma. The carcinomatous component is usually serous (two-thirds) or endometrioid (one-third), and rarely clear cell, mucinous, or squamous cell carcinoma. If the sarcomatous component is derived from the smooth muscle tissue of the uterus, they are called homologous MMMTs. If the sarcomatous component contains bone, striated muscle, cartilage, or fat, the term heterologous MMMT is applied. The most common heterologous elements are malignant skeletal muscle or cartilage resembling either pleomorphic rhabdomyosarcoma or embryonal rhabdomyosarcoma. Presence of the heterologous elements is a poor prognostic factor in stage I patients.

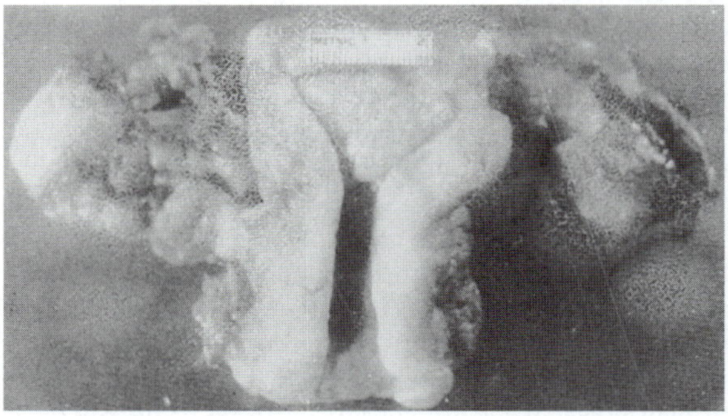

▲ **Figure 49–6.** Mixed sarcoma of the uterine fundus. Prior full-pelvic radiation therapy had little effect on the tumor.

MMMTs spread by contiguous infiltration of the surrounding tissues and by early hematogenous and lymphatic dissemination. The metastatic deposits are usually composed of the epithelial malignant glands, but sarcomatous elements have been identified in some cases. The prognosis depends mainly on the extent of the tumor at the time of primary surgery; there are virtually no long-term survivors among those whose tumor has extended beyond the confines of the uterus at the time of diagnosis. Treatment includes total abdominal hysterectomy with bilateral salpingo-oophorectomy, lymphadenectomy, and tumor debulking if necessary and technically feasible. Active chemotherapeutic agents include cisplatin, ifosfamide, doxorubicin, epirubicin, carboplatin, paclitaxel, and gemcitabine.

C. Adenosarcomas

Adenosarcoma is a distinctive mixed müllerian tumor of low malignant potential that accounts for 1–2% of uterine sarcomas. It arises from the endometrium and is composed of a combination of benign-appearing glands and a stromal sarcoma or fibrosarcoma. Adenosarcomas usually occur in the postmenopausal age group but have been reported in adolescents and women of reproductive age. Bleeding is the most common symptom and has been associated with prior tamoxifen or radiation therapy. Recurrence occurs in 25% of patients and is usually late. The primary treatment is total abdominal hysterectomy and bilateral salpingo-oophorectomy. Postoperative radiation therapy is recommended for those tumors with deep myometrial invasion.

D. Other Uterine Sarcomas

Embryonal rhabdomyosarcoma of the cervix (sarcoma botryoides), which occurs in infants and children, was previously lethal. However, combination therapy using surgery, radiation, and chemotherapy has considerably improved the outlook for these patients.

Fibrosarcoma, hemangiosarcoma, reticulum cell sarcoma, hemangiopericytoma, and other esoteric and bizarre uterine sarcomas are rare. In general, these sarcomas behave like the other intermediate-grade uterine sarcomas, but treatment must be individualized according to age, histologic type, and the patient's state of health.

Prevention

Indiscriminate use of radiation therapy for benign conditions in the pelvis should be avoided, as several clinical studies have suggested an etiologic role of pelvic radiation in the development of MMMT.

Clinical Findings

A. Symptoms & Signs

Abnormal uterine bleeding is the most common manifestation of uterine sarcoma. Other recurring complaints include pelvic discomfort or pain, constipation, urinary frequency and urgency, and the presence of a mass low in the abdomen. Uterine sarcoma should be suspected in any nonpregnant woman with a rapidly enlarging uterus. Severe uterine cramps may exist if the tumor has prolapsed into the endometrial cavity or through the cervix. Pelvic examination may reveal the characteristic grapelike structures of sarcoma botryoides protruding from the cervix or the presence of velvety fronds of ESS in the cervical canal. A necrotic fungating mass at the vaginal apex should suggest an infarcted myoma, LMS, or MMMT. The uterus is usually enlarged and often soft and globular. If the cancer has involved the cervix, cul-de-sac, or cardinal ligaments, fixation or asymmetry of the parametria may be found. In advanced cases, inguinal or supraclavicular node metastases may be evident. Patients with advanced uterine sarcomas may present with a large omental mass or ascites secondary to abdominal carcinomatosis.

B. Laboratory Findings

Standard laboratory evaluation of patients with uterine sarcoma should include a complete blood count and urinalysis, liver function studies (especially serum alkaline phosphatase, prothrombin time, and serum lactic dehydrogenase), blood urea nitrogen, and serum creatinine. CA-125 may be elevated. Estrogen and progesterone receptor analysis may indicate which patients are likely to respond to hormone therapy. Office EMB or punch biopsy of a prolapsed vaginal mass is helpful only if positive.

C. Radiograph Findings

The chest radiography may contain metastatic coin lesions characteristic of uterine sarcomas. Because uterine sarcomas commonly metastasize to the lung, a chest computed tomography (CT) scan should be considered when the routine films are negative, particularly before any radical extirpative surgery in the pelvis is performed. CT scan of the abdomen and pelvis is helpful in assessing the extent of abdominal disease, evaluating the kidneys for hydronephrosis, identifying enlarged retroperitoneal nodes, and identifying liver metastases. MRI scans are not routinely performed but may provide an accurate preoperative assessment of uterine size and degree of involvement.

D. Special Examinations

Pelvic ultrasonography may confirm the presence of a pelvic mass or help to differentiate an adnexal from a uterine mass in the obese patient. Sigmoidoscopy should always be performed in older women, and in young women if gastrointestinal bleeding or masses suspected of being malignant are present. Cystoscopy is indicated in locally advanced disease or in the presence of gross or microscopic hematuria.

Differential Diagnosis

The clinical diagnosis of uterine sarcoma is frequently overlooked. Diagnostic accuracy can be increased if the physician keeps these tumors in mind while investigating any pelvic mass. The tumor frequently does not present the classic picture of abnormal bleeding accompanied by a symmetrically enlarged soft globular uterus. It can masquerade as any condition causing uterine enlargement or a pelvic mass; of these, pregnancy, leiomyoma, adenomyosis, and adherent ovarian neoplasms or pelvic inflammatory disease are most likely to cause misinterpretation. When cytologic studies, EMB, or D&C fail to provide the diagnosis—a situation not uncommon with LMS—laparotomy is necessary. At laparotomy, thorough evaluation is critical to the future management of the patient with uterine sarcoma and must include inspection (where possible) and palpation of all abdominal viscera, peritoneal and mesenteric surfaces, liver, both diaphragms, and retroperitoneal structures, especially the pelvic and aortic lymph nodes. Cytologic examination of peritoneal exudate is indispensable for treatment planning; if no free fluid is present, samples may be obtained by instilling 50–100 mL of normal saline into the abdominal cavity (pelvic washings). If a sarcoma is identified on frozen section of the hysterectomy specimen, suspicious lymph nodes should be removed. This information, gathered at the time of the initial exploration and carefully documented in the operative records, is critical for identification and staging of the neoplasm and for predicting outcome.

The pathologic diagnosis of uterine sarcoma is often extremely difficult and may require consultation with a gynecologic pathologist familiar with these tumors. As each cancer becomes more anaplastic, the parent cell or tissue becomes more difficult to identify histologically. Because proper treatment is predicated on accurate histologic diagnosis, every effort should be expended to identify the cell of origin.

Complications

Severe anemia from chronic blood loss or acute hemorrhage may be present. The severity and extent of other complications caused by uterine sarcomas are directly related to the size and virulence of the primary tumor. A pedunculated mass may protrude into the uterine cavity or prolapse through the cervix, causing bleeding or uterine cramps as the uterus attempts to expel the tumor. Infarction with subsequent infection and sepsis may ensue. Rupture of the uterus as a consequence of rapidly growing uterine sarcomas has been reported. Obstructed labor and postpartum uterine inversion secondary to endometrial sarcomas have also been noted. Extensive pulmonary metastases can produce hemoptysis and respiratory failure. Ascites is common in advanced disease with peritoneal metastases.

A wide variety of complications has been reported secondary to pressure or compression of a neighboring viscus or resulting from extension or metastases to other vital structures. Urethral elongation caused by stretching of the bladder over a rapidly growing mass can simultaneously produce obstruction and loss of sphincter control, with subsequent overflow incontinence. Colon compression may result in ribbon stools and, eventually, complete bowel obstruction. Ureteral obstruction is common, especially with recurrent pelvic sarcomas. Urinary diversion or colostomy may be required prior to treatment if life-threatening viscus obstruction is present in an untreated patient, but urinary diversion should not be performed unless there is some hope for cure or meaningful palliation, because it precludes a painless death from uremia.

Treatment

A. Emergency Measures

Hemorrhage from uterine sarcomas can be severe and requires prompt attention. In acute hemorrhage, blood volume should be replaced rapidly, using packed red blood cells, crystalloid solutions, volume expanders, and fresh-frozen plasma.

Emergency D&C should be used only to obtain tissue for analysis. Vigorous curettage is likely to aggravate or provoke bleeding. High-dose bolus radiation is a more reliable and safe method of controlling bleeding. A dose of 400–500 cGy administered daily to the whole pelvis over 2–3 days usually controls acute hemorrhage; this does not appreciably interfere with future management. If these measures are not successful, emergency embolization or ligation of the hypogastric arteries sometimes controls hemorrhage when hysterectomy is not indicated or technically feasible.

B. Surgical Measures

Extirpative surgery provides the best chance for long-term palliation or cure for patients with uterine sarcomas. Surgery is the cornerstone of the treatment plan and should be the central focus of attack against these cancers.

Because low-grade uterine sarcomas (some LMSs, endolymphatic stromal myosis, intravenous leiomyomatosis) have a propensity for isolated local spread and central pelvic recurrence, such patients should be considered for radical hysterectomy and bilateral salpingo-oophorectomy. The benefits of this type of therapy have not been conclusively shown, but, theoretically, the problem of local recurrence should be improved by more radical excision of the primary tumor. Lymph node metastases in these low-grade tumors are negligible; consequently, pelvic lymphadenectomy can be reserved for patients with enlarged or suspicious nodes. Pelvic recurrences of low-grade uterine sarcomas have been successfully treated by repeated excisions of all resectable tumor. Patients have been known to survive for many years following this type of conservative treatment. Partial or complete pelvic exenteration may occasionally be useful for recurrence of indolent tumors.

The high-grade uterine sarcomas (some LMSs, ESSs, all MMMTs) display early lymphatic, local, and hematogenous metastases, even when apparently confined to the uterus. For this reason, radical surgery has been abandoned in favor of simple total abdominal hysterectomy and bilateral salpingo-oophorectomy preceded or followed by adjunctive radiation therapy. At the time of surgical exploration, a thorough examination and evaluation of the abdominal contents must be performed and documented. Cytologic specimens and omental tissue should be obtained, and suspicious papillations, excrescences, and adhesions should be excised for pathologic analysis. A thorough staging procedure is important for prognosis and a postoperative treatment plan.

When uterine sarcomas recur in the lung and the metastatic survey is negative, unilateral isolated metastases can be excised after a chest CT scan has ruled out other lesions not apparent on the routine chest radiograph. Considering all sources, resection of isolated sarcoma metastases to the lung carries about a 25% 5-year cure rate.

C. Chemotherapy

Adjuvant single-agent doxorubicin has been shown to have a 25% response rate for LMS. Recent data suggest that use of combination gemcitabine and docetaxel in LMS improves progression-free survival and reduces risk of recurrence.

Because of the high hormone receptor content in ESS, adjuvant progestin or aromatase inhibitors are recommended. For receptor-negative tumors, doxorubicin- or ifosfamide-based chemotherapy is used. Tamoxifen and estrogen replacement therapy should be avoided in patients with ESS.

Doxorubicin, cisplatin, carboplatin, paclitaxel, gemcitabine, and ifosfamide display significant activity against MMMTs. Cyclophosphamide and vincristine also show activity. Some data suggest that combination chemotherapy is more effective than single-agent therapy. In advanced or metastatic disease, adjuvant combination chemotherapy is recommended. Trabectedin, a new agent, has been actively evaluated in sarcomas and appears to show some modest promise. Treatment with tyrosine kinase inhibitors like imatinib or sorafenib has shown response in some patients.

D. Radiation Therapy

When used as the only modality of treatment for uterine sarcomas, radiation has produced dismal results—very few survivors are reported in the literature following treatment with radiation therapy alone for any of the uterine sarcomas. Radiation therapy does provide local tumor control and reduces local recurrences when used in combination with surgery for the treatment of some endometrial sarcomas. However, it is unclear whether a combined surgical and radiation approach changes overall survival. Collected data indicate that adjuvant radiation therapy improves the 2-year survival rate in patients with ESS by approximately 20% and may also improve survival for those with MMMTs, although less convincingly. Although an occasional 5-year survivor with LMS has been reported following radiation therapy alone, analysis of large numbers of patients from different institutions does not support its use for these tumors. Nevertheless, in advanced forms of LMS, radiation may prove useful for palliation and control of pelvic symptoms such as massive bleeding or pain.

Prognosis

In determining the prognosis for patients with uterine sarcomas, a constellation of factors must be examined simultaneously. Such considerations as the patient's age, state of health, and ability to withstand major surgery or radiation therapy (or both) must be evaluated. The most important clinical characteristic—and probably the overriding prognostic feature affecting the prognosis of these patients—is the stage of the disease at the time of diagnosis. In the high-grade sarcomas (LMS and mixed endometrial sarcoma), the presence of tumor outside the uterus at the time of diagnosis is a clear prognostic omen: Fewer than 10% of patients survive 2 years. Even when the disease is apparently limited to the uterus, the prognosis is poor: 10–50% survive 5 years. In intermediate-grade LMS and undifferentiated endometrial sarcoma, the outcome is improved, with up to 80–90% of patients surviving 5 years if the disease is clinically limited to the uterus at the time of surgery. Low-grade ESS and low-grade LMS have a generally favorable outcome: 80–100% of patients survive 5 years following complete excision of the uterus. Low-grade stromal tumors have been known to recur locally after 10–20 years; this confuses the survival statistics. Undoubtedly, these patients must be followed closely for life.

Brooks SE, Zhan M, Cote T, Baquet CR. Surveillance, epidemiology, and end results analysis of 2677 cases of uterine sarcoma 1989–1999. *Gynecol Oncol* 2004;93:204–208. PMID: 15047237.

D'Angelo E, Prat J. Uterine sarcomas: a review. *Gynecol Oncol* 2010;116:131–139. PMID: 19853898.

Demetri GD. ET-743: the US experience in sarcomas of the soft tissues. *Anticancer Drugs* 2002;13:S7. PMID: 12173492.

Dinh TA, Oliva EA, Fuller AF Jr, et al. The treatment of uterine leiomyosarcoma. Results from a 10-year experience (1990–1999) at Massachusetts General Hospital. *Gynecol Oncol* 2004;92: 648–652. PMID: 14766261.

Ferguson SE, Tornos C, Hummer A, et al. Prognostic features of surgical stage I uterine carcinosarcoma. *Am J Surg Pathol* 2007;31:1653–1661. PMID: 18059221.

Giuntoli RL, Metzinger DS, DiMarco CS, et al. Retrospective review of 208 patients with leiomyosarcoma of the uterus: prognostic indicators, surgical management, and adjuvant therapy. *Gynecol Oncol* 2003;89:460–467. PMID: 12798172.

Hensley ML, Ishill N, Soslow R, et al. Adjuvant gemcitabine plus docetaxel for completely resected stages I-IV high grade leiomyosarcoma: results of a prospective study. *Gynecol Oncol* 2009:112;563–567. PMID: 19135708.

Kushner D, Webster KD, Belinson JL, et al. Safety and efficacy of adjuvant single-agent ifosfamide in uterine sarcoma. *Gynecol Oncol* 2000;78:221–227. PMID: 10926807.

Look KY, Sandler A, Blessing JA, et al. Phase II trial of gemcitabine as second line chemo-therapy of uterine leiomyosarcoma: an Gynecologic Oncology Group (GOG) study. *Gynecol Oncol* 2004;92:644–647. PMID: 14766260.

Manolitsas TP, Wain GV, Williams KE, et al. Multimodality therapy for patients with clinical stage I and II malignant mixed müllerian tumors of the uterus. *Cancer* 2001;15:1437–1443. PMID: 11301390.

O'Meara AT. Uterine sarcomas: have we made any progress? *Curr Opin Obstet Gynecol* 2004;16:1–4. PMID: 15128000.

50 Premalignant & Malignant Disorders of the Ovaries & Oviducts

Gary Levy, MD
Karen Purcell, MD, PhD

OVARIAN CANCER

ESSENTIALS OF DIAGNOSIS

- ▶ Early-stage ovarian cancer often presents with vague and ill-defined symptoms.
- ▶ Late-stage disease presents with abdominal pain or bloating, early satiety, and/or urinary urgency or frequency.
- ▶ The majority of women present with late-stage disease.
- ▶ Pelvic ultrasound findings show complex adnexal mass(es).
- ▶ The mean age of diagnosis for epithelial ovarian cancer is in the mid-50s, with the majority diagnosed between ages 40 and 65.
- ▶ Hereditary causes of ovarian cancer diagnosed at earlier age by almost a decade.
- ▶ Nonepithelial ovarian tumors are more common in girls and younger women.

▶ Pathogenesis

Although there are many different cell types present in the normal adnexa, the majority of adnexal cancers arise from the surface epithelial cells of the ovary (epithelial ovarian cancer [EOC]). Fewer ovarian cancers develop from the remaining cell types (sex cord-stromal, germ cell, or mixed cell type tumors) (Table 50–1), and even fewer adnexal cancers arise from the fallopian tubes, although recent evidence has shown that they account for a greater percentage than previously thought. The specific events leading to the transition of normal tissue to malignancy have not been established, nor has a definitive precursor lesion been identified. For sporadic tumors, molecular events leading to the inactivation of tumor suppressor genes (PTEN, p16, p53) or the activation of oncogenes (HER-2, c-myc, K-ras, Akt) have been described. For the small proportion of genetically heritable cancers, germline mutations in BRCA1, BRCA2, and other genes have been described, but the molecular pathway leading to tumorigenesis has not been elucidated. It is likely that epigenetic events also contribute to the transformation to cancer.

A. Epithelial Ovarian Cancer

The most prominent theory for the development of EOC associates the repeated trauma and repair to the ovarian epithelium during normal ovulation with subsequent genetic alterations and further progression to malignant transformation. This is supported by evidence that suppression of ovulation leads to a decreased incidence of EOC. A second theory invokes high serum concentrations of gonadotropins, estrogen, androgen, or inflammatory agents, leading to epithelial proliferation and subsequent transformation.

EOCs account for more than 90% of all malignant ovarian tumors and include serous, mucinous, endometrioid, clear cell, transitional cell types, and undifferentiated neoplasms. **Serous cystadenocarcinomas** represent 75–80% of EOCs. They present with extraovarian spread 85% of the time and are bilateral in half the cases. The tumors are typically large at the time of diagnosis, most being larger than 15 cm in diameter, with the unilocular or multilocular cystic structures containing papillae projecting into the lumen. Histologic sections resemble the endosalpinx with nuclear atypia in the stratified squamous epithelium. Psammoma bodies with irregular lamellar calcifications are frequently seen in these tumors. The grade of differentiation is based on the degree of preservation of the papillary architecture, the majority of which is poorly differentiated at the time of diagnosis.

Mucinous cystadenocarcinomas represent 10% of all EOCs, are typically unilateral, and are notable for the ability to attain very large sizes. Histologic sections resemble endocervical epithelium with large hyperchromatic nuclei

Table 50–1. Categories of ovarian cancer.

Epithelial (90%)	Low Malignant Potential	Sex Cord-Stromal (5–8%)	Germ Cell (2–5%)	Metastatic to the Ovary
Serous (75–80%)	Serous	Granulosa cell (70%)	Dysgerminoma (30–40%)	Breast
Mucinous (10%)	Mucinous	Fibroma	Endodermal sinus tumor	Colon
Endometrioid (10%)		Thecoma	Teratoma (immature, mature, specialized)	Stomach
Clear cell (1%)		Sertoli-Leydig cell	Embryonal	Endometrium
Transitional cell (Brenner's) (1%)		Gynandroblastoma	Choriocarcinoma	Lymphoma
Undifferentiated (<10%)			Gonadoblastoma	
			Mixed germ cell	
			Polyembryoma	

and prominent nucleoli. The variability within the tumor requires extensive sampling to determine the most malignant focus. Given the similar cell architecture, they are often difficult to distinguish from metastatic tumors from the colon, appendix, endocervix, and pancreas. Thus after diagnosis of a mucinous tumor, an evaluation of the gastrointestinal (GI) tract is recommended.

Mucinous tumors, whether from ovarian origin or appendix, can be associated with a condition called pseudomyxoma peritonei where progressive accumulation of mucin within the abdominal cavity occurs and often leads to significant protracted morbidity secondary to bowel obstruction.

Endometrioid neoplasms of the ovary occur bilaterally in 30–50% of cases and account for 10% of EOCs. Histologic sections reveal an adenomatoid pattern with the degree of differentiation determined by the extent to which the glandular architecture is preserved. Rarely, this tumor arises within a focus of endometriosis, but not uncommonly, patients with endometrioid tumors of the ovary will have a synchronous endometrial carcinoma.

Clear cell carcinoma of the ovary, or mesonephroid carcinoma, accounts for <1% of EOCs. They typically present at a smaller size than the serous or mucinous cystadenocarcinomas. These tumors are aggressive and may be associated with hypercalcemia or hyperpyrexia. Histologic sections show features of "clear cells," similar to renal cell carcinomas; occasionally, they are difficult to differentiate from mucinous neoplasms, although a weak staining pattern with the periodic acid-Schiff reaction is useful.

Transitional cell carcinoma, or Brenner's tumor, accounts for <1% of EOCs. Histologic sections resemble low-grade transitional cell carcinoma of the urinary bladder. Compared to other types of EOCs, these patients have a poorer prognosis.

Undifferentiated carcinomas account for <10% of EOCs and are characterized by the absence of any microscopic features to define them as another type.

B. Germ Cell Tumors of the Ovary

Although EOCs typically occur in women near or in menopause, germ cell tumors tend to present in the second and third decades of life. Also different from EOCs, these tumors often have a good prognosis. Because they arise from the germ cell elements of the ovary, they often secrete hormones or proteins that can be used to monitor response to therapy (Table 50–2).

Dysgerminomas account for 30–40% of the germ cell tumors. They occur in young females and most often are unilateral at presentation. Although they are solid tumors, they may have areas of softening due to degeneration. At the time of surgery, they appear smooth and thinly encapsulated, with a brown or grayish-brown color. On histologic sections, nests of germ cells, which appear as large, rounded cells with central nuclei, are surrounded by undifferentiated stroma. If lymphocytic infiltration is present, it is considered a favorable prognostic indicator.

Immature teratomas are the malignant counterpart of mature cystic teratomas, or dermoids, and are the second most common germ cell malignancy. Histologic sections show a disordered collection of tissues derived from all 3 germ layers, with some components having an immature, embryonic appearance. The grade of the tumor is determined by the amount of immature neural tissue present, which correlated with prognosis and guidelines for chemotherapy. Typical presentation occurs in females <20 years old. They are usually unilateral, although the contralateral ovary may contain a mature teratoma. These tumors often secrete α fetoprotein (AFP).

Endodermal sinus tumors, or yolk sac tumors, are the third most common germ cell tumor. This is the most rapidly growing neoplasm that occurs at any site, and patients may present with an acute abdomen given they are friable, necrotic, and often hemorrhagic. These tumors are almost always bilateral and, on histologic section, resemble the

Table 50–2. Biologic markers associated with ovarian tumors.

Type	Histology	Tumor Markers						
		AFP	hCG	LDH	CA-125	Estrogen	Androgens	Inhibin
Epithelial ovarian carcinoma					+/−			
Germ cell								
	Dysgerminoma	+/−	+/−	+				
	Endodermal sinus tumor (yolk sac)	+	−	+				
	Immature teratoma	+/−	+/−	+/−				
	Mixed germ cell tumor	+/−	+/−	+/−				
	Choriocarcinoma	−	+	+/−				
	Embryonal cancer	+/−		++/−				
	Polyembryoma	+/−	+	−				
Sex cord-stromal						+/−	+/−	
Granulosa cell tumor								+

AFP, α fetoprotein; hCG, human chorionic gonadotropin; LDH, lactate dehydrogenase.

primitive gut and liver; Schiller-Duval bodies, which show a single papilla lined by tumor cells with a central blood vessel, and the production of AFP are characteristic.

Embryonal carcinoma presents at a mean age of 15 years old and has a highly aggressive growth pattern. Histologic sections show solid sheets of large polygonal cells with pale, eosinophilic cytoplasm that give the appearance of a syncytium. Biologic markers of AFP, human chorionic gonadotropin (hCG), and estrogens are often secreted.

Choriocarcinoma of the ovary is a rare germ cell tumor. Unlike gestational choriocarcinoma, this primary ovarian tumor produces lower levels of hCG and may cause precocious puberty, uterine bleeding, or amenorrhea. Histologic sections show cytotrophoblasts, intermediate trophoblasts, and syncytiotrophoblasts.

Gonadoblastoma is a rare germ cell tumor that presents in the second decade of life and is located more commonly in the right ovary over the left. Patients have abnormal gonadal development with the presence of a Y chromosome. Histologic sections show nests of germ cells and sex cord derivatives surrounded by connective tissue stroma.

Mixed germ cell tumors account for 10% of germ cell neoplasms and contain 2 or more germ cell elements. The most frequent composition includes dysgerminoma and endodermal sinus tumor. Careful sectioning by the pathologist is necessary to determine all different components in order to correctly determine the chemotherapeutic regimens.

Polyembryoma is extremely rare and is seen in premenarchal girls with signs of pseudopuberty. It secretes AFP and hCG and histologically will contain the 3 somatic layers of early embryonic differentiation.

C. Sex Cord-Stromal Tumors of the Ovary

Sex cord-stromal tumors of the ovary account for 5–8% of all ovarian malignancies. **Granulosa cell tumors** account for 70% of this class of tumors. Because they secrete high levels of estrogen, they may cause precocious puberty in young girls or adenomatous hyperplasia and vaginal bleeding in postmenopausal women. Microscopically, the granulosa cells exhibit characteristic grooved or coffee bean nuclei; Call-Exner bodies represent multiple small cavities that contain eosinophilic fluid. Theca cells are present in varying amounts. Granulosa cell tumors are characterized by inhibin secretion, and this tumor marker can be used for monitoring tumor progression and response to therapy.

Like granulosa cell tumors, ovarian **thecomas** are associated with hyperestrogenism. This mostly benign ovarian tumor consists of lipid-laden stromal cells, which confer a yellow appearance on cut section.

Sertoli-stromal cell tumors are rare, consisting of testicular structures at different stages of development and therefore are usually virilizing. The average age at diagnosis is 25, and they are rarely bilateral. Microscopically, both

Sertoli and Leydig cells are present. A variety of architectural patterns have been described.

D. Borderline Tumors of the Ovary

For 10% of women with malignant ovarian neoplasms, the histologic pattern shows atypical epithelial proliferation without stromal invasion. These tumors are termed serous tumors of low malignant potential (LMP) or noninvasive borderline tumors. They tend to have similar genetic alterations and molecular pathways to low-grade carcinomas, which are different from those seen with high-grade serous carcinomas. Although this has led some to hypothesize that the borderline tumors and low-grade carcinomas are a part of a progression to high-grade carcinomas, most believe they are 2 separate entities rather than a continuum of tumor progression often seen with other gynecologic malignancies. There is no evidence that low-grade serous carcinomas arise from serous tumors of LMP.

E. Metastatic Disease to the Ovary

Approximately 5% of ovarian tumors are due to metastases, with the primary tumor being located in the female genital tract, breast, or gastrointestinal tract. Traditionally, Krukenberg tumors signaled metastases from the stomach, although now the term is used more loosely to define ovarian tumors from any location in the gastrointestinal tract.

F. Hereditary Ovarian Cancer Syndromes

Although the majority of ovarian cancers are defined as sporadic, approximately 10–15% of cases are attributed to genetic causes. Breast–ovarian cancer syndrome is one such cause, with the majority of patients having mutations in BRCA1 or BRCA2. Germline mutations in BRCA1 confer a 35–45% lifetime risk of ovarian cancer, whereas BRCA2 mutations confer a 15–24% risk of ovarian cancer. Within the United States, approximately 1 in 800 women are carriers, and this rate is increased for women of Ashkenazi Jewish, French Canadian, or Icelandic descent.

A second syndrome is Lynch II syndrome, or hereditary nonpolyposis colorectal cancer (HNPCC). These women have a 12% risk of developing ovarian cancer and are also at increased risk of developing cancers of the colon, breast, and endometrium. Several gene mutations have been detected in families with Lynch II, including PMS1, PMS2, MSH2, MSH3, MSH6, and MLH1. Each of these is known to be involved in DNA mismatch repair.

G. Cancer of the Fallopian Tubes

Primary carcinoma of the fallopian tube is the least common cancer arising in the female genital tract, accounting for approximately 0.3% of all such cancers. Fallopian tube cancers are similar to EOC with regard to clinical presentation and biologic behavior. At least 95% of all primary carcinomas of the fallopian tube are papillary carcinomas. Bilaterality is found in 40–50% of cases, and this is believed to represent synchronous neoplasms rather than metastatic disease from one tube to the other. Grossly, the affected tube is fusiform or sausage-shaped. On initial inspection, these neoplasms resemble pyosalpinx or tubo-ovarian inflammatory disease. However, there is usually little associated serosal reaction with adhesion formation, as is noted with an inflammatory process.

Classically, the neoplastic fallopian tube contains solid or necrotic cancer tissue and a dark-brown or serosanguinous fluid. The fimbriated end of the fallopian tube is patent in as many as 50% of cases, and often tumor extrudes from the ostium to adhere to adjacent structures. Histologically, papillary carcinomas may exhibit papillary, papillary–alveolar, and alveolar growth patterns. There is no prognostic significance attached to these differences. Of note, women with BRCA1 and BRCA2 mutations are at substantially higher risk of fallopian tube cancer; consequently, women who have prophylactic oophorectomies should also have complete resection of the oviducts.

de Waal YR, Thomas CM, Oei AL, Sweep FC, Massuger LF. Secondary ovarian malignancies: frequency, origin, and characteristics. *Int J Gynecol Cancer* 2009;19:1160. PMID: 19823050.

Lalwani N, Shanbhogue AK, Vikram R, et al. Current update on borderline ovarian neoplasms. *AJR Am J Roentgenol* 2010; 194:330. PMID: 20093592.

Roett MA, Evans P. Ovarian cancer: an overview. *Am Fam Physician* 2009;80:609. PMID: 19817326.

Shih IM, Davidson B. Pathogenesis of ovarian cancer: clues from selected overexpressed genes. *Future Oncol* 2009;5:1641. PMID: 20001801.

Prevention

The lifetime risk of ovarian cancer in the general population is 1.7%, and the majority of known risks factors are not amenable to change, with age, early menarche (prior to age 12), and late menopause (after age 50) being the most prominent. Ethnic differences confer variable risk. Caucasians have the highest age-adjusted annual incidence per 100,000 women in the United States with a rate of 14.3. Hispanics are less, at 11.5, then African-Americans at 10.1 and Asians at 9.7. Infertility is also a risk factor, whereas fertility treatment is unlikely to be a risk factor. Endometriosis is an independent risk factor of EOC; malignant transformation occurs in approximately 2.5% of patients, who are typically younger. The prognosis is typically better because the tumors are more often well-differentiated, low-stage carcinomas. Nulligravidity is a major risk factor for EOC.

Certain protective factors have been identified. The use of oral contraceptive pills (OCPs) decreased the risk of ovarian cancer, with increasing protection conferred by longer duration of use. The risk is reduced to half by 15 years of use, and the protection persists after discontinuing medication, although the effects become attenuated over time. Low-dose OCPs, with ≤ 35 μg of ethinyl estradiol are as effective as the higher dose OCPs. Women who have undergone tubal ligation were found to have a decreased risk by about a third to a half, with the effect being synergistic with a history of OCP use. However, caution must be taken when suggesting this as a preventive measure, especially in patients with hereditary syndromes because occult malignancies within the fallopian tubes are often present in women carrying a genetic mutation. Breastfeeding and progesterone use have also been shown to have a protective effect.

One environmental factor, current or past cigarette smoking, is known to increase the risk of mucinous ovarian cancer but not other types of EOC. The contribution of diet is uncertain, as most published studies have potential biases. The effects of exercise are also without a clear relationship to the risk of ovarian cancer. Obesity may lead to an increased risk of ovarian cancer. Previous studies had implicated talc use as leading to a small increased risk of ovarian cancer, although recent studies have not substantiated this.

Prevention by screening methods is currently not possible. The lack of sensitivity or specificity of available testing negates their use to identify women at risk of developing ovarian cancer, and therefore, screening by any modality is not recommended.

Risk Reduction in Women with Familial Ovarian Cancer Syndromes

One of the strongest known risk factors for ovarian cancer is a family history of the disease. A family pedigree of at least 3 generations should be evaluated by a geneticist to provide counseling and consent for potential genetic testing. Although a woman with a family history of ovarian cancer has an increased personal lifetime risk of 2–6%, women with a familial ovarian cancer syndrome are at significantly greater lifetime risk of 25–50%.

Efforts to find effective screening, through use of ultrasound or multimodal techniques encompassing humoral markers, have been disappointing. Thus prophylactic bilateral salpingo-oophorectomy (BSO) has been advocated to reduce the risk for patients with a familial ovarian cancer syndrome. This procedure leads to a significant reduction in the risk of ovarian cancer (80–90% for BRCA carriers) as well as decreased overall mortality; however, the gains in life expectancy are dependent on the age at the time of the procedure, with little gain for women undergoing the procedure after the age of 60. The decision to proceed with prophylactic BSO requires a careful discussion of consequences of infertility and premature menopause. Most suggest performing the procedure as soon as childbearing is complete or by age 35.

An alternative preventive measure may be the use of OCPs containing a high-potency progestin. Although results have been mixed, the majority show an appropriate reduction in risk of ovarian cancer in these women.

Mourits MJ, de Bock GH. Managing hereditary ovarian cancer. *Maturitas* 2009;64:172. PMID: 19811881.

Clinical Findings

A. Symptoms & Signs

Early-stage EOC is associated with poorly defined or vague symptoms, which often are not severe enough to prompt a woman to seek medical attention. For later stage disease, which accounts for more than 70% of all diagnoses, the most common symptoms include an increased abdominal girth, pelvic or abdominal pain, bloating, urinary symptoms of frequency or urgency, or early satiety. Occasionally patients will have nausea or anorexia secondary to ascites or bowel metastases. Patients may also present with dyspnea due to pleural effusions. Rarely do patients present with paraneoplastic phenomena such as subacute cerebellar degeneration, seborrheic keratoses (sign of Leser-Trelat), Trousseau's syndrome (migratory thrombophlebitis), or hypercalcemia of malignancy.

Approximately 15% of reproductive-age patients will present with menstrual abnormalities. Abnormal vaginal bleeding may occur in the presence of a synchronous endometrial carcinoma or as a consequence of metastatic disease to the lower genital tract. Excess androgens or estrogens may be present due to stimulation of normal theca, granulosa, or hilar cells that surround the neoplasm or due to secretion by a germ cell tumor or sex cord-stromal tumor. Ovarian stromal hyperplasia or hyperthecosis may also be associated with excess androgen production.

A pelvic exam will often reveal a solid, fixed, irregular adnexal mass. Unilateral, cystic masses in reproductive-age women are benign in up to 95% of cases. These masses, particularly when <6–8 cm in size, are observed through a menstrual cycle because many represent functional cysts that spontaneously resolve. An enlarging mass or one that is associated with pain merits prompt intervention. A cystic, somewhat immobile adnexal mass may represent a hydrosalpinx or tubo-ovarian abscess. Fixed, bilateral masses and firm masses with nodularity are suggestive of, but not diagnostic of, an ovarian malignancy (Table 50–3).

Although several benign lesions may also present with similar findings, the presence of ascites or an upper abdominal mass are very suggestive of ovarian cancer. Abdominal distention is one of the more common findings. The presence of flank fullness and shifting dullness implies the presence of

Table 50–3. Characteristics to be noted on physical exam of a pelvic mass.

	Benign	Malignant
Location	Unilateral	Bilateral
Mobility	Mobile	Fixed
Consistency	Cystic	Solid or firm
Cul-de-sac	Smooth	Nodular

ascites or a large pelvic-abdominal mass. Together with these signs, tympanitic percussion noted over the lateral abdomen is consistent with a large mass that displaces the bowel to the periphery. In contrast, a central tympanitic percussion note is suggestive of ascites. Recent eversion of the umbilicus in a patient with abdominal distention may result from an increase in intra-abdominal pressure secondary to ascites.

A rectal exam evaluating the presence of occult blood in the stool should also be performed given the possibility of a primary gastrointestinal malignancy with metastases to the ovary. Similarly, a breast exam should be performed, and the presence of a breast mass warrants a mammogram, given the possibility of a primary breast cancer with ovarian metastases. Particular attention should be paid to the lymph node–bearing areas, particularly the supraclavicular and inguinal areas. Metastatic disease to the skin rarely occurs in the presence of ovarian cancer. Sister Mary Joseph's nodule refers to a metastatic implant in the umbilicus.

For patients with carcinoma of the fallopian tube, presentation typically occurs in the fifth or sixth decade of life, and the signs and symptoms are often similar to those noted in patients with ovarian cancer. In fact, it is difficult to differentiate tubal from ovarian carcinomas preoperatively. Fewer than 15% of patients are noted to have the classic triad of symptoms and signs associated with fallopian tube cancer including **hydrops tubae profluens** (a watery vaginal discharge), pelvic pain, and a palpable adnexal mass. Positive vaginal cytology in the absence of endometrial or cervical neoplasia suggests the possibility of a tubal cancer, but this is rarely diagnostic.

B. Laboratory Findings

The best characterized tumor marker in EOC is cancer antigen-125 (CA-125). CA-125 is a secreted glycoprotein present in fetal amniotic and coelomic epithelium, and its level can be detected in serum using immunoassay. The accepted upper limit of normal is 35 IU/mL, but this is a rather arbitrary cutoff. CA-125 is elevated in many patients with ovarian cancer, especially with serous histology, but is also elevated in other malignancies such as pancreatic, colon, breast, stomach, fallopian, or endometrial cancer. In addition, it is also elevated in certain benign conditions such as endometriosis, leiomyoma, or pelvic inflammatory disease, although rarely above 200 IU/mL. Therefore, it can be a useful adjunct in postmenopausal women, but not very useful in premenopausal women given the low incidence of EOC and greater incidence of benign lesions. Additionally, a normal CA-125 does not exclude the diagnosis of cancer and does not represent a reason to delay surgery.

In young girls and adolescents presenting with an adnexal mass, serum AFP, lactate dehydrogenase (LDH), and hCG should be measured as potential biomarkers given the greater likelihood of a malignant germ cell tumor.

In all patients, a complete blood count (CBC), serum electrolyte test, and hCG level should be drawn. For patients with apparent ascites, a paracentesis is not advocated as a routine procedure once renal, cardiac, and hepatic failure have been excluded. False-negative results may occur in as many as 40% of patients with widespread intra-abdominal disease. In contrast to paracentesis, diagnostic thoracentesis for cytology is recommended for staging purposes; the presence of a malignant pleural effusion confirms stage IV disease.

Table 50–4. Ultrasonographic features to aid diagnosis of benign and malignant adnexal masses.

Benign	Malignant
Simple cyst, <10 cm in size	Solid or both solid and cystic
Septations <3 mm in thickness	Multiple septations <2 mm
Unilateral	Bilateral
Calcification, especially teeth	Ascites
Gravity-dependent layering of cyst contents	

C. Imaging Studies

Pelvic ultrasound helps delineate the presence of a benign or malignant adnexal mass (Table 50–4), and a number of different scoring systems have been used, although there is no standardized system for evaluation of ovarian masses. Typical characteristics of ovarian cancer include a solid component, which is often nodular or papillary, septations, and ascites. Angiogenesis accompanying malignancy results in vascular abnormalities and increased blood flow compared with the vascular architecture and patterns of blood flow in nonmalignant lesions. The addition of color flow Doppler studies that evaluate the vascular patterns of adnexal masses improves the sensitivity and specificity of the radiographic diagnosis of benign and malignant lesions. However, even when combined with laboratory or physical findings, ultrasound is limited in making a definitive diagnosis, and surgery is required to document malignancy histologically.

Characterization of adnexal masses by computed tomography (CT) or magnetic resonance imaging (MRI) may provide clinically useful information in select instances. CT scanning provides information about the retroperitoneal structures in addition to the pelvic organs. MRI scans can add more information regarding the nature of the ovarian neoplasm. Because of the high cost and questionable benefit, this diagnostic procedure is infrequently used for ovarian tumors. However, it may be of particular benefit in the evaluation of pregnant patients because it avoids radiation exposure of the fetus.

A patient with suspected ovarian malignancy should undergo a radiograph of the chest to exclude metastatic parenchymal disease and to detect a pleural effusion. If the patient notes a change in bowel habits or if guaiac-positive stools are detected, a barium enema should be obtained. Patients who appear to have advanced ovarian cancer, evidenced by a nodular pelvic mass with or without ascites, may actually have colon cancer. Because of the genetic links among ovarian cancer, colon cancer, and breast cancer, a patient with a suspected ovarian malignancy should also undergo a screening mammogram study.

Twickler DM, Moschos E. Ultrasound and assessment of ovarian cancer risk. *AJR Am J Roentgenol* 2010;194:322. PMID: 20093591.

Differential Diagnosis

The differential diagnosis of a pelvic mass is influenced by the age of the patient, the characteristics of the mass on pelvic examination, and the radiographic appearance of the mass. In general, the prepubescent child and the postmenopausal woman are at greatest risk for a malignant ovarian neoplasm. The reproductive-age woman is more likely to have a functional ovarian cyst or endometrioma. Although functional cysts are typically mobile, both endometriomas and tubo-ovarian abscesses can present as an adnexal mass that is fixed, solid, and irregular.

Mature teratomas or dermoids are common ovarian neoplasms, occurring primarily in women ages 20–30 years. They represent the most common neoplasm diagnosed during pregnancy. Less than 1% of all teratomas are malignant.

An ovarian fibroma is another benign tumor that is noteworthy because of its association with Meigs' syndrome. Meigs' syndrome refers to the occurrence of an ovarian fibroma, ascites, and pleural effusion, which collectively mimic the presentation of ovarian cancer.

For masses diagnosed by ultrasound, pathologies such as pedunculated fibroids, hydrosalpinx, peritoneal inclusion cyst, and paraovarian cysts also need to be considered. Persistence of ultrasonic findings on a repeat scan after 4–6 weeks may help reduce the false-positive rate associated with ovarian masses.

Givens V, Mitchell GE, Harraway-Smith C, Reddy A, Maness DL. Diagnosis and management of adnexal masses. *Am Fam Physician* 2009;80:815. PMID: 19835343.

Complications

The majority of complications from ovarian cancer arise secondary to metastases. Metastases often arise from exfoliation into the peritoneal cavity and then migrate along the circulatory pattern of peritoneal fluid from the right paracolic gutter toward the upper abdomen. Additionally, hematogenous dissemination may occur. The bulk of the tumor, especially within the omentum, may lead to bowel obstruction or nutritional deficits. Removal of the mass may produce significant fluid shifts in women with advanced ovarian cancer.

Patients are at an increased risk of venous thromboembolism (VTE) if metastatic disease, medical comorbidities, or clear cell histology exist. Additionally, the first 3 months after diagnosis give rise to an increased risk of VTE. For patients undergoing surgical intervention, VTE prophylaxis is given.

Treatment

A. Surgical Intervention for Epithelial Ovarian Cancers

Surgical staging and tumor removal are required for all patients, unless the performance status of the patient limits surgical intervention. Initial surgical staging provides the definitive histologic diagnosis as well as the extent of disease. Obtaining the true stage of disease allows appropriate treatment and subsequent prognosis. Table 50–5 lists the current staging of ovarian cancer approved by the International Federation of Gynecology and Obstetrics (FIGO).

Intraoperatively, several features have been described that assist in the differentiation of malignant from benign adnexal masses (Table 50–6). However, gross examination of a mass is never a substitute for histologic examination. Whenever the pathology of a pelvic or adnexal mass is in question, a frozen-section pathologic study should be requested. In the hands of experienced pathologists, false-positive and false-negative diagnoses occur in <5% of cases. Patients diagnosed with ovarian cancer have to undergo surgical staging to reduce the amount of disease and evaluate the extent of spread. Removal of the primary tumor, as well as the associated metastatic disease, is referred to as tumor debulking or cytoreductive surgery. In early stages and when fertility is desired, removal of the involved adnexa alone may be considered.

Surgical staging for ovarian cancer is performed by laparotomy. Initial recovery of ascites or pelvic free fluid is sent for cytologic evaluation. If no free fluid is present, "peritoneal washings" are obtained by instilling 50–100 cc of saline in the cul-de-sac, paracolic gutters, and underneath each hemidiaphragm. An exploratory laparotomy is then performed in a systematic and thorough manner, evaluating the pelvic organs, omentum, intestines, mesentery, gallbladder, liver, diaphragm, spleen, and entire peritoneum. The kidneys, pancreas, and lymph nodes are also evaluated in the retroperitoneum. Complete surgical staging of ovarian cancer requires the biopsy of pelvic and para-aortic lymph nodes. It is emphasized that the palpation of the retroperitoneal node-bearing areas is inaccurate and is not a substitute for biopsy and histologic examination. Table 50–7 lists the procedures included in surgical staging of ovarian cancer.

Removal of the tumor burden is also therapeutic. The extent of surgical resection is dependent on the stage of

Table 50–5. International Federation of Gynecology and Obstetrics (FIGO) staging.

Stage I		Growth limited to the ovaries
	IA	Limited to 1 ovary; no ascites with malignant cells; capsule intact; no tumor on external surface of ovary
	IB	Limited to both ovaries; no ascites with malignant cells; capsules intact; no tumor on external surfaces of the ovaries
	IC	Either IA or IB but tumor present on external ovarian surface, ruptured capsule, or malignant cells present in ascites or peritoneal washings
Stage II		Growth involving 1 or both ovaries with pelvic extension
	IIA	Extension or metastases to uterus and/or tubes
	IIB	Extension to other pelvic tissues
	IIC	Either IIA or IIB but tumor present on external ovarian surface, ruptured capsule, or malignant cells present in ascites or peritoneal washings
Stage III		Peritoneal implants outside the pelvis and/or positive retroperitoneal or inguinal nodes; superficial liver metastases; tumor limited to true pelvis but histologic extension to small bowel or omentum
	IIIA	Tumor grossly limited to true pelvis, negative nodes but microscopic seeding of abdominal peritoneal surfaces
	IIIB	Histologically confirmed abdominal peritoneal surface implants ≤2 cm; negative nodes
	IIIC	Abdominal implants >2 cm in diameter and/or positive retroperitoneal or inguinal nodes
Stage IV		Distant metastasis; pleural effusion contains cytologic evidence of metastasis; parenchymal liver involvement

Reproduced, with permission, from International Federation of Gynecology and Obstetrics. Reprinted from *Int J Gynecol Obstet* 2000;70:207–312.

the disease as well as the age of the patient. If possible, complete removal of the tumor burden should be attempted as optimal cytoreduction or debulking improves subsequent systemic chemotherapy; large bulky tumors are often poorly vascularized and thus more resistant to chemotherapy and radiation therapy. Large tumor masses also consist of a higher proportion of cells in the resting phase of the cell cycle. However, even if complete resection is not possible, decreasing the tumor burden provides other benefits such as an improvement in symptoms (abdominal pain, bloating, satiety, or dyspnea) as well as a potential improvement in immune competence because ovarian tumors often produce immunosuppressive cytokines.

In general, the contralateral adnexa should be removed even when they are grossly normal. They are often the site

Table 50–6. Intraoperative features of benign and malignant masses.

Benign	Malignant
Simple cyst	Adhesions
Unilateral	Rupture
No adhesions	Ascites
Smooth surfaces	Solid areas
Intact capsule	Areas of hemorrhage or necrosis Papillary excrescences Multiloculated mass Bilateral

Table 50–7. Procedure to stage and remove ovarian cancer.

Evaluation of peritoneal free fluid	Collect and send for cytologic evaluation
Peritoneal washings if no free fluid	Instill 50–100 cc of saline to collect from cul-de-sac, paracolic gutters, and bilateral diaphragm
Exploratory evaluation of pelvis and abdomen	Systematically evaluate pelvic organs, peritoneum, omentum, bowel, mesentery, liver, gallbladder
Biopsy	All suspicious lesions or adhesions to be biopsied Multiple biopsies obtained from cul-de-sac, paracolic gutters, bladder, intestinal mesentery, and diaphragm if no visualized lesions
Resect tumor	Intact removal of tumor
Hysterectomy	
Resect omentum	From transverse colon
Evaluated nodes	Biopsy
Retroperitoneal nodes	Biopsy; resect if suspicious
Para-aortic, mesenteric artery nodes	Biopsy; resect if enlarged
Pelvic nodes	Biopsy; resect if enlarged
Cytoreductive surgery	Remove all visible disease

of occult metastatic disease, and there is a significant risk of subsequent cancer. Exceptions to this generalization are made for young women with an apparent stage I epithelial ovarian neoplasm. If future fertility is desired and the patient is informed about a higher risk of recurrent disease, a more conservative surgical approach may be chosen. The histology and grade of the neoplasm, as well as the findings at the time of surgery, guide these decisions. Well-differentiated stage I lesions are associated with a much better 5-year survival rate than are moderately and poorly differentiated lesions. Mucinous and endometrioid neoplasms are associated with a better prognosis than serous and clear cell carcinomas of the ovary. If the frozen section during surgery does not reveal a reliable diagnosis of malignancy, the surgical procedure should be limited until the pathology results are finalized.

An infracolic omentectomy is recommended, even in the absence of gross tumor involvement, because it is a common site of microscopic metastatic disease. Removal of the omentum facilitates the distribution of intraperitoneal agents, may decrease the rate of accumulation of ascites postoperatively, and provides palliation to patients with omental metastases.

A hysterectomy is generally performed because the uterus is a common site for metastatic disease. There is also a risk of synchronous endometrial cancer in patients with endometrioid carcinoma of the ovary. In addition, removal of the uterus facilitates subsequent follow-up examinations and obviates potential problems secondary to uterine bleeding.

B. Surgical Intervention for Germ Cell Neoplasms

In contrast to epithelial ovarian neoplasms, most germ cell neoplasms are early stage at the time of diagnosis. This observation, in conjunction with the low incidence of bilaterality and the young age of most patients, for whom future fertility is desired, influences the surgical management of this group of neoplasms. For young women with a germ cell neoplasm of the ovary, removal of the involved adnexa with preservation of the normal-appearing contralateral adnexa and uterus is generally advocated. In view of the low incidence of bilaterality, biopsy or bivalving the contralateral ovary is not recommended because of the risk of peritubal and periovarian adhesions. Complete surgical staging of germ cell neoplasms is the same as for epithelial ovarian neoplasms and should be performed in all cases.

Certain characteristics unique to germ cell neoplasms make an impact on their surgical management. Dysgerminoma of the ovary has a propensity to metastasize to the pelvic and para-aortic lymph nodes in the absence of other evidence of metastatic disease. Performing a biopsy of these structures is particularly important. Endodermal sinus tumor of the ovary is the most rapidly growing neoplasm known to occur at any site. This diagnosis must be considered in a young woman with a rapidly enlarging pelvic or abdominal mass. Immature teratoma of the ovary may present with numerous peritoneal implants consistent with metastatic disease. It is important to adequately sample these lesions to determine whether or not they contain malignant elements.

C. Medical Intervention for Epithelial Ovarian Cancer

After the initial surgical intervention and definitive staging, subsequent treatment can be established. Almost all patients with EOC will receive chemotherapy. The 1 exception is for stage IA disease and grade 1 tumors, where a discussion of the risks and benefits of chemotherapy should be undertaken because chemotherapy after the initial surgical treatment may have no influence on survival. For all other stages, chemotherapy is indicated. Agents shown to be active against EOC include cisplatin, carboplatin, cyclophosphamide, and paclitaxel. Combination therapies have been demonstrated to be superior to single-agent treatment. Typically, chemotherapy is started 4–6 weeks after surgical intervention. Earlier administration has not been shown to provide a benefit.

Currently the most effective regimen uses a combination of paclitaxel and carboplatin. This combination has replaced the former treatment with cyclophosphamide and cisplatin because it was shown to be more efficacious in a number of clinical trials. A typical regimen includes systemic administration of carboplatin and paclitaxel for 6 cycles at 3-week intervals. Potential toxicities of this treatment include nausea, vomiting, diarrhea, alopecia, nephrotoxicity, and myelosuppression (see Chapter 52).

Carboplatin is a second-generation platinum analogue that shows clinical efficacies and survival rates similar to cisplatin when used in combination with paclitaxel. However, the frequency of gastrointestinal side effects and neurotoxicity associated with carboplatin was found to be lower compared to cisplatin.

The route of administration may vary depending on the stage. Patients with optimally cytoreduced stage III EOC are offered intraperitoneal (IP) or systemic intravenous (IV) administration of the chemotherapeutic agents. The IP route has been shown to increase survival, although an increase in side effects is also noted. For patients with suboptimally cytoreduced disease or stage IV disease, systemic IV administration is the preferred route.

Occasionally, chemotherapy will be offered in patients with stage IV disease prior to surgical staging. This is termed neoadjuvant chemotherapy and may be useful to lessen the tumor burden, thereby decreasing the morbidities associated with surgical resection of advanced disease. It may also increase the chance of optimal debulking.

Assessment of response to combination chemotherapy is based on physical examination, changes in size of palpable or radiographically measurable lesions, and changes in the CA-125 level. Although the preoperative CA-125 level does not correlate with tumor burden, changes in response to chemotherapy appear to be of some prognostic benefit.

An elevated CA-125 (>35 IU/mL) predicts persistent disease at second look in more than 97% of patients. However, a normal CA-125 level does not completely exclude the possibility of residual, subclinical disease.

Most patients develop resistance to platinum-based regimens during the course of treatment. Salvage therapy for ovarian cancer is rarely curative, although significant prolongation of survival may be achieved in some instances. The response to re-treatment with platinum-based chemotherapy is influenced by the time interval between completion of the initial regimen and subsequent disease recurrence: The greater the interval, the greater is the likelihood of a beneficial response, with platinum resistance defined as recurrence <6 months after completion of combination chemotherapy or progression on treatment.

D. Medical Intervention for Germ Cell Neoplasms

Significant advances have been made in the treatment of germ cell neoplasms of the ovary. Once associated with 5-year survival rates of <20–30%, these neoplasms are now considered curable in a majority of cases following the introduction and refinement of combination chemotherapy.

Dysgerminoma is the most radiation-sensitive neoplasm identified. Historically, it has been treated with whole abdominal radiation therapy with excellent results. More recently, chemotherapy with cisplatin-containing regimens has been administered with excellent results. A significant advantage of chemotherapy is the potential to preserve future reproductive potential compared with radiation therapy.

The other germ cell neoplasms are rare, and the optimal chemotherapy and duration of therapy have not been established. Regimens such as vinblastine/bleomycin/cisplatin, vincristine/dactinomycin/cyclophosphamide, and bleomycin/etoposide/cisplatin have been used with encouraging results. Response to chemotherapy is based on physical examination and the decrease in serum tumor markers, if initially elevated.

E. Radiation Therapy

With respect to germ cell neoplasms, radiation therapy has been used successfully in the treatment of patients with dysgerminoma. For patients with EOC, radiation therapy plays a limited role mainly because of radiation damage to the small bowel, liver, and kidneys. Radioisotopes such as intraperitoneal phosphorus-32 may be of benefit in patients with stage IC disease and those with microscopically positive second-look operations.

F. Intervention for Fallopian Tube Cancers

The surgical therapy of fallopian tube carcinoma is the same as that recommended for EOC. In addition, the same type of surgical staging should be performed if for no other reason than it is often not clear at the time of surgery whether the primary cancer is of ovarian or fallopian tube origin. The staging system for ovarian cancer is often applied to neoplasms of the fallopian tube, although this is by custom rather than FIGO recommendations.

Chemotherapy for fallopian tube cancer has evolved along the same lines as that for EOC. The currently used chemotherapeutic regimen is similar to that of EOC and includes platinum combination chemotherapy. Radiation may also be used in select cases with no residual disease after surgery. Because there are little data on well-staged tubal lesions, it is unclear if patients with early-stage disease benefit from adjuvant therapy.

G. Alternative Therapies

A number of alternative therapies have been applied for the treatment of EOC. Cytokines like interleukin-2 and interferon-γ, either alone or in combination with chemotherapy, have shown some promising effects. Monoclonal antibodies directed against ovarian cancer–associated antigens, including CA-125, HMFG (human milk-fat globulin), and HER-2/*neu*, have been used with variable clinical responses. Recently, antibodies against vascular endothelial growth factor (VEGF) have shown efficacy in patients with ovarian cancer. Anti-VEGF antibodies are currently being tested in combination with carboplatin and paclitaxel in first-line chemotherapy for ovarian cancer patients. Gene therapy trials have used different antitumor approaches, including the delivery of tumor suppressor gene p53 via recombinant adenovirus into the peritoneal cavities. The early trials have not shown significant clinical response, mainly as a result of the inefficiency of intraperitoneal and intratumoral gene transfer.

Gardner GJ. Ovarian cancer cytoreductive surgery in the elderly. *Curr Treat Options Oncol* 2009;10:171. PMID: 19806460.

Marchetti C, Pisano C, Facchini G, et al. First-line treatment of advanced ovarian cancer: current research and perspectives. *Expert Rev Anticancer Ther* 2010;10:47. PMID: 20014885.

Schwartz PE. Contemporary considerations for neoadjuvant chemotherapy in primary ovarian cancer. *Curr Oncol Rep* 2009;11:457. PMID: 19840523.

Prognosis

Ovarian cancer is the second most common gynecologic malignancy, yet the most common cause of death in women with such a malignancy. The prognosis for patients with ovarian cancer is primarily related to the stage of disease (Table 50–8). Within each stage of disease, other factors such as cell type and response to chemotherapy are also important in determining disease-free survival and overall survival. In general, patients with well-differentiated, diploid neoplasms with an S-phase fraction of <8–10% do better than patients

Table 50–8. Overall survival rates for patients with epithelial ovarian cancer.

Stage	1-Year Survival	5-Year Survival
I	96–100%	83–90%
II	93–94%	65–71%
III	85–88%	33–47%
IV	72%	19%

who have poorly differentiated, aneuploid, rapidly proliferating (eg, high S-phase fraction) neoplasms.

In general, germ cell tumors are associated with better 5-year survival rates than epithelial ovarian neoplasms. Patients with dysgerminoma have a 5-year survival rate of 95%. Immature teratomas are associated with 5-year survival rates of 70–80%. An endodermal sinus tumor is associated with a 5-year survival rate of 60–70%. Embryonal carcinoma, choriocarcinoma, and polyembryoma are very rare lesions, and it is difficult to assess 5-year survival estimates. Epithelial ovarian neoplasms of low malignancy potential are characterized by 5-year survival rates of 95%, reflecting their protracted and indolent biologic behavior.

The prognosis for patients with fallopian tube carcinoma is based on the stage of disease. The overall 5-year survival rate is approximately 56%. The prognosis for early-stage disease is much better than for advanced disease, as 5-year survival is 84% with stage I disease, 52% with stage II, and 36% with stage III.

Gestational Trophoblastic Diseases

51

Paola Aghajanian, MD

ESSENTIALS OF DIAGNOSIS

- Uterine bleeding in first trimester
- Absence of fetal heart tones and fetal structures
- Rapid enlargement of the uterus or uterine size greater than anticipated by dates
- Human chorionic gonadotropin titers greater than expected for gestational age
- Vaginal expulsion of vesicles
- Hyperemesis gravidarum
- Theca lutein cysts
- Onset of preeclampsia in the first trimester

Pathogenesis

The spectrum of gestational trophoblastic disease includes hydatidiform moles (complete and partial) and gestational trophoblastic neoplasia comprising invasive moles, choriocarcinomas, and placental-site trophoblastic tumors (PSTT). These tumors are unique in that they develop from an aberrant fertilization event and hence arise from fetal tissue within the maternal host. They are composed of both syncytiotrophoblastic and cytotrophoblastic cells, with the exception of PSTT, which is derived from intermediate trophoblastic cells. In addition to being the first and only disseminated solid tumors that have proved to be highly curable by chemotherapy, they elaborate a unique and characteristic tumor marker, human chorionic gonadotropin (hCG).

A. Hydatidiform Mole

Hydatidiform mole is the most common form of gestational trophoblastic disease and is benign in nature. Its incidence varies worldwide from 1 in 125 deliveries in Mexico and Taiwan to 1 in 1500 deliveries in the United States. The incidence is higher in women younger than 20 and older than 40 years of age, in nulliparous women, in patients of low socioeconomic status, and in women whose diets are deficient in protein, folic acid, and carotene. Blood group A women impregnated by group O men have an almost 10-fold greater risk of subsequently developing gestational trophoblastic neoplasia than group A women impregnated by group A partners. Furthermore, women with blood group AB tend to have a relatively worse prognosis.

Two distinct forms of hydatidiform mole exist: complete and partial moles. Table 51–1 outlines the clinical, pathologic, and genetic characteristics of both. Cytogenetic studies demonstrate that complete moles are usually euploid, paternal in origin, and sex chromatin-positive—46 XX or 46 XY. They arise when an empty ovum (with an absent or inactivated nucleus) is fertilized by a haploid sperm that duplicates its chromosomes or by two haploid sperm. A partial mole, on the other hand, is triploid—69 XXY (70%), 69 XXX (27%), or 69 XYY (3%)—arising when an ovum with an active nucleus is fertilized by a duplicated sperm or two haploid sperm. Both of these processes result in a homozygous conceptus with a propensity for altered growth.

Hydatidiform mole is thought to arise from extraembryonic trophoblasts. Histologic similarities between molar vesicles and chorionic villi support the view that one is derived from the other. Detailed morphologic studies of hysterectomy specimens containing intact molar pregnancies suggest that transformation of the embryonic inner cell mass at a stage just prior to the laying down of endoderm gives rise to hydatidiform moles. At this stage in embryogenesis, the inner cell mass has the potential to develop into trophoblasts, ectoderm, or endoderm. If normal development is interrupted, such that the inner cell mass loses its capacity to differentiate into embryonic ectoderm and endoderm, a divergent development pathway is created. This pathway may then result in production of extraembryonic mesoderm and molar vesicles with loose primitive mesoderm in their villous core.

Table 51–1. Comparison of complete and partial hydatidiform moles.

	Complete	Partial
Karyotype	Diploid (46,XX or 46,XY)	Triploid (69,XXX or 69,XXY)
Fetus	Absent	Often present
Villi	Diffusely hydropic	Focally hydropic
Trophoblasts	Diffuse hyperplasia	Mild focal hyperplasia
Implantation-site trophoblast	Diffuse atypia	Focal atypia
P57, PHLDA2 immunostaining[1]	Negative	Positive
Fetal RBCs	Absent	Present
β-hCG (mIU per milliliter)	High (>50,000)	Slight elevation (<50,000)
Frequency of classic clinical symptoms[2]	Common	Rare
Risk for persistent GTT	20–30%	<5%

GTT, gestational trophoblastic tumor.
[1]PHLDA2 is the product of a paternally imprinted, maternally expressed gene stained by p57 immunohistochemistry. Complete moles stain negative, as their genome is exclusively paternally derived and cannot express PHLDA2.
[2]Hyperemesis, hyperthyroidism, excessive uterine enlargement, anemia, and preeclampsia. The frequency of these symptoms has decreased as a consequence of earlier diagnosis of molar pregnancies through evaluating hCG levels and ultrasonography.

Grossly, a hydatidiform mole is characterized by multiple grapelike vesicles filling and distending the uterus, usually in the absence of an intact fetus (Fig. 51–1). Most hydatidiform moles are recognizable on gross examination, but some are small and may seem to be ordinary abortuses. Microscopically, moles may be identified by three classic findings: edema of the villous stroma, avascular villi, and nests of proliferating trophoblastic elements surrounding villi (Figs. 51–2 and 51–3). The likelihood of malignant sequelae is higher in patients whose trophoblastic cells show increased proliferation and anaplasia. Although histologic studies of the trophoblast provide some basis for predicting a benign or malignant course for the mole, the correlation is not absolute.

Today, with earlier detection, the classic pathologic presentation of molar pregnancies is less common. Therefore, it can be more difficult to differentiate histologically between a complete mole, a partial mole, and a nonmolar hydropic abortion. Use of flow cytometry can determine ploidy (eg, diploid versus triploid). Additionally, p57 immunohistochemistry staining can be used to stain for PHLDA2, a paternally imprinted, maternally expressed gene product that is absent in complete moles but present in partial moles and hydropic abortuses.

B. Invasive Mole

Invasive mole is reported in 10–15% of patients who have had a hydatidiform mole. Although considered a benign neoplasm, invasive mole, as its name implies, is locally invasive and invades the myometrium and adjacent structures. Additionally, it has the potential to completely penetrate the myometrium and cause subsequent uterine rupture and hemoperitoneum. However, it also has the ability to spontaneously regress. The microscopic findings are similar to that of a hydatidiform mole. Because adequate myometrium is rarely obtained at curettage and

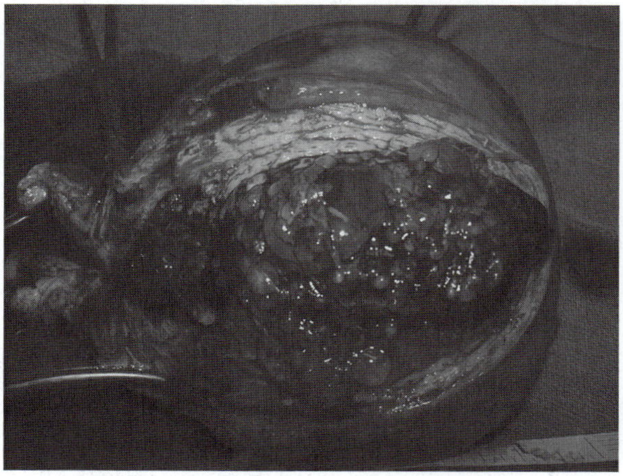

▲ **Figure 51–1.** Hysterectomy specimen of a complete mole with anterior wall incised, displaying typical clear, "grapelike" vesicles filling the uterine cavity. Hysterectomy was performed as primary treatment for molar gestation. (Reproduced, with permission, from *Emiliano Chavira, MD.*)

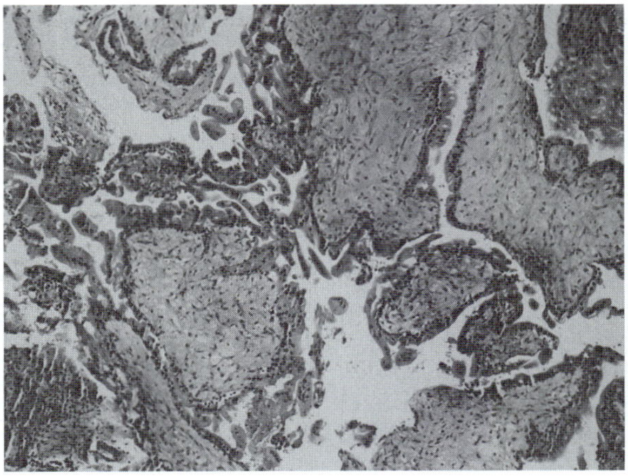

▲ **Figure 51–2.** A complete mole characterized by enlarged, avascular chorionic villi with exuberant cytotrophoblastic and syncytiotrophoblastic proliferation. Magnified 100x. (Reproduced, with permission, from *Wenxue Xing, MD.*)

fewer hysterectomies are being performed in patients with trophoblastic disease, the diagnosis is less often made by histologic analysis.

C. Choriocarcinoma

Choriocarcinoma is reported in 2–5% of all cases of gestational trophoblastic neoplasia. The incidence in the United States is 1 in 40,000 pregnancies, but it is higher in Asia. It

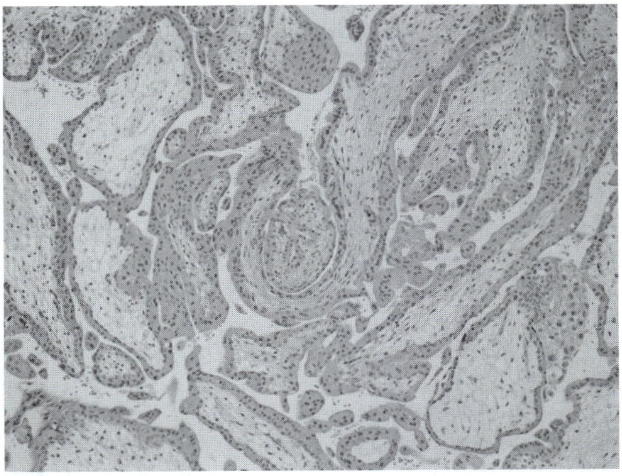

▲ **Figure 51–3.** A partial mole showing a biphasic population of small, normal appearing, and enlarged villi with irregular contours. The large villi exhibit mild to moderate syncytiotrophoblastic proliferation. Fetal red blood cells can be appreciated in the villous capillaries. Magnified 100x. (Reproduced, with permission, from *Wenxue Xing, MD.*)

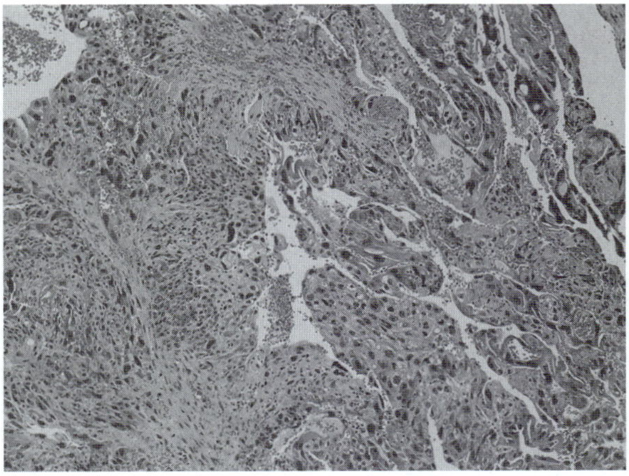

▲ **Figure 51–4.** This choriocarcinoma demonstrates the typical avillous trophoblastic proliferation that characterizes this neoplasm. Masses of markedly atypical cytotrophoblasts are intimately associated with multinucleated syncytiotrophoblasts. Mitotic figures are readily identified. Magnified 100x. (Reproduced, with permission, from *Wenxue Xing, MD.*)

may accompany or follow any type of pregnancy. In about half of choriocarcinoma cases, the antecedent gestational event is a hydatidiform mole. Another 25% follow a term pregnancy, and the remaining 25% occur after an abortion.

Choriocarcinoma is a pure epithelial tumor composed of syncytiotrophoblastic and cytotrophoblastic cells. It usually presents as late vaginal bleeding in the postpartum period. An enlarged uterus, enlarged ovaries, and vaginal lesions may be noted during the physical examination.

Histologic evaluation of the tumor discloses sheets or foci of trophoblasts on a background of hemorrhage and necrosis, but no villi (Fig. 51–4). Assessment of trophoblastic tissue following or accompanying pregnancy may prove difficult because of the histologic similarities of the trophoblastic patterns in very early pregnancy and choriocarcinoma. Consequently, the curettage specimen must be processed in its entirety, as the specimen may contain only small, isolated areas of choriocarcinoma. A histopathologic diagnosis of choriocarcinoma in any site is an indication for prompt treatment after confirmation by gonadotropin excretion measurements.

D. Placental-Site Trophoblastic Tumor

PSTT is a rare variant of gestational trophoblastic tumor. It may arise months to years after a hydatidiform mole or, less commonly, following a normal term pregnancy. The tumor is generally confined to the uterus, but local invasion may occur into the myometrium, lymphatics, or vasculature. It metastasizes late in its course. PSTT is derived from the intermediate trophoblasts of the placental bed, with minimal or absent syncytiotrophoblastic tissue. As syncytiotrophoblastic cells are generally absent from this tumor, minimal amounts of hCG are released in relation to the tumor burden. However, human placental lactogen is secreted, and its levels can be monitored to follow response to therapy.

Prevention

The only way to prevent the occurrence of gestational trophoblastic diseases is abstinence from sexual intercourse.

Clinical Findings

A. Symptoms & Signs

Abnormal uterine bleeding, usually during the first trimester, is the most common presenting symptom, occurring in more than 90% of patients with molar pregnancies. Three-fourths of these patients present before the end of the first trimester. Nausea and vomiting have been reported in 14–32% of patients with hydatidiform mole and may be confused with nausea and vomiting of pregnancy or hyperemesis gravidarum. Ten percent of these patients may have nausea and vomiting severe enough to require hospitalization.

About half of patients will have a uterine size that is greater than expected for their gestational age. However, in one-third of patients, the uterus may be smaller than expected. Multiple theca lutein cysts causing enlargement of one or both ovaries are seen in 15–30% of women with molar pregnancies. In about half of these cases, both ovaries are enlarged and may be a source of pain. Involution of the cysts proceeds over several weeks and usually parallels the decline of hCG values. In studies, patients with theca lutein cysts appear to have a greater likelihood of developing malignant sequelae of gestational trophoblastic neoplasia.

Preeclampsia in the first trimester or early second trimester—an unusual finding in normal pregnancies—has been said to be pathognomonic for a molar pregnancy. Hyperthyroidism from stimulation of thyrotropin receptors by hCG can also occur in 10% of patients, although the disease is usually subclinical, and most patients remain asymptomatic. Treatment involves evacuation of the mole. An occasional patient may require brief antithyroid therapy.

Because of the earlier diagnosis of molar pregnancies, the classic presenting symptoms and signs of gestational trophoblastic disease are now less prevalent. For instance, at the New England Trophoblastic Disease Center, the incidence of excessive uterine enlargement, hyperemesis, and preeclampsia was 28%, 8%, and 1%, respectively. The incidence of hyperthyroidism and respiratory insufficiency was negligible. Although the number of cases presenting with these classic signs and symptoms has decreased, the incidence of persistent postmolar gestational trophoblastic disease has remained static.

This highlights the importance of vigilant postmolar hCG surveillance. Any woman with a recent history of molar pregnancy, abortion, or normal pregnancy who presents with vaginal bleeding or a tumor in any organ should have a thorough physical examination and at least one hCG assay to ensure that gestational trophoblastic neoplasia is not the cause. This is of utmost importance given that the cure rate of properly treated gestational trophoblastic neoplasia approaches 90%.

B. Laboratory Findings

The principal characteristic of gestational trophoblastic neoplasms is their capacity to produce hCG. This hormone may be detected in the serum or urine of virtually all patients with hydatidiform mole or malignant trophoblastic disease, and its levels correlate closely with the presence of viable tumor cells. Consequently, monitoring of hCG levels is a necessary tool for the diagnosis, treatment, and surveillance of the disease process.

The usefulness of a serum gonadotropin assay depends on the hCG titer and the sensitivity of the test. Today, sensitive and specific immunoassays are available to differentiate hCG from luteinizing hormone by measuring the β chain of hCG. Serial β-hCG levels are best monitored in the same laboratory using the same immunoassay technique.

The rate of decline in hCG titers is also important. Normal postmolar pregnancy hCG regression curves highlighting the weekly hCG levels in patients undergoing spontaneous remission have been constructed, hence providing a reference for the comparison of random or serial values. In most instances, the hCG values exhibit a progressive decline to nondetectable levels within 14 weeks after evacuation of a molar pregnancy. If the hCG titer rises or plateaus, it must be concluded that viable tumor continues to persist. If the levels of hCG are very low and not responsive to treatment, a false-positive hCG result or "phantom hCG," caused by cross-reaction of heterophilic antibodies with the hCG test, should be considered.

C. Ultrasonographic Findings

The simplicity, safety, and reliability of ultrasonography define it as the diagnostic method of choice for patients with suspected molar pregnancy. In a complete molar pregnancy, the characteristic ultrasound pattern consists of multiple hypoechoic areas corresponding to hydropic villi, at times described as a "snowstorm" pattern (Fig. 51–5). A normal gestational sac or fetus is not present. Theca lutein cysts may be visualized. In a partial mole, focal areas of trophoblastic changes and fetal tissue may be noted. Focal cystic changes in the placenta are also a hallmark finding. On the other hand, an ultrasonogram of a choriocarcinoma may reveal an enlarged uterus with a necrotic and hemorrhagic pattern, whereas that of PSTT may show an intrauterine mass.

A pelvic ultrasound should be obtained in any patient who presents with bleeding in the first half of pregnancy and/or has a uterus greater than the gestational size. Even when the uterus is appropriate for gestational age, ultrasonography

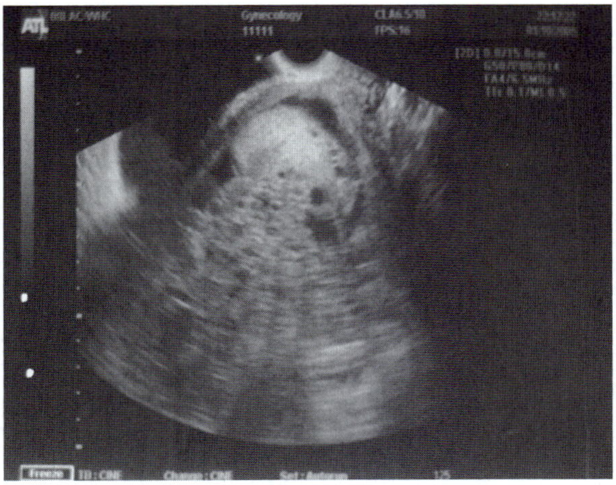

▲ **Figure 51–5.** Vaginal ultrasound of patient in Figure 51–1 demonstrating the characteristic intrauterine hypoechoic areas corresponding to hydropic villi, at times described as a "snowstorm" pattern. (Reproduced, with permission, from *Emiliano Chavira, MD.*)

can be key in differentiating between a normal pregnancy and a hydatidiform mole.

Differential Diagnosis

Gestational trophoblastic disease must be distinguished from a normal pregnancy, an aborting pregnancy, and an ectopic pregnancy. Ultrasonography is a useful tool in this respect. Quantitative hCG levels improve the accuracy of the diagnosis. Analysis of tissue obtained from a dilatation and evacuation for histology and DNA content will prove invaluable.

Complications

The maternal–fetal barrier contains leaks large enough to permit passage of cellular and tissue elements. As a result, deportations of trophoblastic tissue to the lungs are frequent. Spontaneous regression of these ectopic trophoblastic tissues can occur. Less commonly, this results in a syndrome of acute pulmonary insufficiency. Symptoms of dyspnea and cyanosis, due to massive deportation of trophoblasts to the pulmonary vasculature and subsequent formation of pulmonary emboli, can present within 4–6 hours after evacuation of a molar pregnancy. Pulmonary edema leading to high-output congestive heart failure may complicate excessive fluid administration, preeclampsia, anemia, or hyperthyroidism.

Treatment

A. Hydatidiform Mole

1. Evacuation—After the diagnosis has been confirmed, blood type, hematocrit, and thyroid, liver, and renal function tests should be obtained. A chest radiograph can rule out metastasis to the lungs. Subsequently, the molar pregnancy should be terminated. Suction curettage under general anesthesia is the method of choice once the patient is deemed stable. This can be safely accomplished even when the uterus is the size of a 28-week gestation. Local or regional anesthesia may be an option for the stable, cooperative patient with a small uterus. Intravenous oxytocin should be administered after dilation of the cervix but before the start of evacuation and may be continued, if necessary, for 24 hours post-evacuation. Tissue should be submitted for pathologic study. Blood loss usually is moderate, but precautions should be taken for the possibility of hemorrhage requiring a transfusion. When a large hydatidiform mole (>12 weeks in size) is evacuated by suction curettage, a laparotomy setup should be readily available, as hysterotomy, hysterectomy, or bilateral hypogastric artery ligation may be necessary if perforation or hemorrhage occurs. After the completion of the evacuation, all Rh-negative patients should receive Rh immune globulin.

Hysterectomy continues to remain an option for good surgical candidates not desirous of future pregnancy and for older women (who are more likely to develop malignant sequelae). If theca lutein cysts are encountered at laparotomy, the ovaries should remain intact, as regression to normal size will occur with diminishing hCG titers. Surgical treatment of these cysts is indicated only if rupture, torsion, or hemorrhage occurs or if the enlarged ovaries become infected.

It is important to note that hysterectomy does not eliminate the need for careful postsurgical surveillance with hCG testing, although the likelihood of metastatic disease following hysterectomy for gestational trophoblastic disease decreases from 20 to 3.5%. Current recommendations restrict hysterotomy to cases complicated by hemorrhage. Medical induction of labor with prostaglandins, oxytocin, or intra-amniotic instillation of prostaglandin or hypertonic solutions is no longer an acceptable method for evacuation of a molar pregnancy.

2. Prophylactic chemotherapy—Controversy surrounds the use of prophylactic chemotherapy (with methotrexate or dactinomycin) after a complete molar pregnancy. Several studies indicate that the incidence of postmolar gestational trophoblastic neoplasia may be decreased with prophylactic chemotherapy. However, further studies are required to determine whether the potential side effects warrant such treatment in noncompliant patients and in those at high risk for persistent gestational trophoblastic disease (age >35 years, history of prior molar pregnancy, trophoblastic hyperplasia).

3. Surveillance—Despite earlier diagnosis of molar pregnancies, the incidence of persistent gestational trophoblastic disease has not decreased. Three-fourths of patients with malignant nonmetastatic trophoblastic disease and half of patients with malignant metastatic disease develop these tumors following a hydatidiform mole. In the remainder, disease arises subsequent to a term pregnancy, abortion, or ectopic pregnancy. Several clinical features of hydatidiform moles are recognized as having a high association with malignant trophoblastic neoplasia. In general, at diagnosis, the larger the uterus and the higher the hCG titer, the greater the risk for malignant gestational trophoblastic disease. The combination of theca lutein cysts and uterine size excessive for gestational age is associated with an extremely high risk of malignant sequelae. Pathologic specimens with marked nuclear atypia, necrosis, hemorrhage, or trophoblastic proliferation may also increase the risk of persistent disease.

Regardless of the method of termination (suction curettage or hysterectomy) or presence of high-risk features, close monitoring with serial hCG titers is essential for every patient, as the incidence of malignant sequelae approaches 20–30%. After evacuation of the molar pregnancy, the patient should undergo serial hCG determinations, beginning within 48 hours after evacuation and then at weekly intervals until hCG values decline to undetectable levels (<5 mIU per milliliter) on three successive assays. If titer remission occurs spontaneously within 14 weeks and without a titer plateau, the hCG titer should then be repeated monthly for at least 6 months to 1 year before the patient is released from close medical supervision. Thereafter, the patient may enter into a routine gynecologic care program.

A gynecologic examination should be done 1 week after evacuation, at which time blood may be taken for the hCG titer. Estimates of uterine size, presence of adnexal masses (theca lutein cysts) and presence of vulvar, vaginal, or cervical lesions should be noted. Unless symptoms develop, the examination may be repeated at 4-week intervals throughout the observation period. If pre-evacuation chest radiography has revealed pulmonary metastases, chest radiographs should be repeated at 4-week intervals until spontaneous remission is confirmed, then at 3-month intervals during the remainder of the surveillance period.

Effective contraceptive measures should be implemented and maintained throughout the period of surveillance. Studies have not shown an increased risk of persistent gestational trophoblastic neoplasia after a molar pregnancy with the use of oral contraceptives. Therefore, they remain the most widely used method of birth control. A patient who has entered into spontaneous remission with negative titers, examinations, and chest radiographs for 6 months to 1 year and who is desirous of becoming pregnant may terminate contraceptive practices. Successful pregnancy is the norm, and complications are similar to those of the general population.

Therapy for persistent gestational trophoblastic neoplasia after evacuation of a hydatidiform mole is usually instituted because of an abnormal hCG regression curve. The most critical period of observation is the first 4 to 6 weeks post-evacuation. Although the hCG titer usually returns to normal by 1–2 weeks after evacuation of a hydatidiform mole, it should normalize in most women by the eighth week.

Approximately 70% of patients achieve a normal hCG level within 8 weeks of evacuation. Very few patients whose hCG titers normalize during this interval will require future treatment. In the past, therapy for persistent disease was initiated for the 30% of women whose hCG titer remained elevated at or beyond 8 weeks post-termination. However, current data suggest that half of these patients will demonstrate a continuous decline in titers and ultimately achieve normal hCG levels without further treatment. The remaining half will experience a rising or plateauing titer with histologic evidence of an invasive mole or choriocarcinoma.

Delayed postevacuation bleeding is uncommon after a molar pregnancy and signifies the presence of an invasive mole or choriocarcinoma. It is invariably attended by an enlarging uterus and an abnormal hCG regression pattern. In some cases, curettage is effective in stopping the bleeding, although little intracavitary tissue will be present in most of these cases. The mainstay of treatment is chemotherapy.

B. Malignant Gestational Trophoblastic Neoplasia

According to the 2002 criteria established by the International Federation of Gynecology and Obstetrics (FIGO), malignant gestational trophoblastic neoplasia may be diagnosed in the setting of (1) a rise in hCG levels of 10% or greater for ≥3 values over 2 weeks; (2) a plateau in ≥4 hCG values over 3 successive weeks; (3) hCG levels elevated at 6 months postevacuation; or (4) a tissue diagnosis of choriocarcinoma.

Once the diagnosis of malignant trophoblastic disease is suspected or established, an accurate history and physical examination are crucial. Most patients will have an enlarged uterus as well as ovarian enlargement caused by theca lutein cysts. Sites of metastasis must be sought, especially in the lower genital tract. A chest radiograph can diagnose lung metastases, although a chest computerized tomography (CT) will miss fewer pulmonary metastatic lesions. Liver metastases may be diagnosed with ultrasonography or CT scan. Brain metastases are best evaluated with a CT scan or magnetic resonance imaging (MRI). The ratio of serum hCG values to the concentration of hCG in cerebrospinal fluid (normal >60:1) may also prove helpful. Baseline hematologic counts, coagulation studies, and hepatic and renal function tests are critical in later assessing the risk of drug toxicity. After all sites of metastases have been identified and the patient's desires for preservation of reproductive function are determined, specific therapy should be initiated.

1. Nonmetastatic malignant gestational trophoblastic disease—Trophoblastic disease confined to the uterus is the most common malignant lesion seen in gestational trophoblastic neoplasia. The diagnosis is usually made during the postmolar surveillance period. Therapy for patients with nonmetastatic malignant trophoblastic disease includes (1) single-agent chemotherapy or (2) combination chemotherapy and hysterectomy, with surgery performed on the third day of drug therapy for patients who do not wish to preserve reproductive function.

Table 51–2. Chemotherapy regimens for nonmetastatic or low-risk metastatic gestational trophoblastic disease.

Drug/dosage:
Methotrexate 30–60 mg/m² IM once a week.[1]
Methotrexate 0.4 mg/kg/d IV or IM for 5 days, repeat every 14 days
Methotrexate 1 mg/kg IM on days 1, 3, 5, and 7 and folinic acid 0.1 mg/kg IM on days 2, 4, 6, and 8, repeat every 15–18 days
Dactinomycin 1.25 mg/m² IV every 14 days
Dactinomycin 10–12 μg/kg/d IV for 5 days, repeat every 14 days
Follow-up:
Follow β-hCG titer weekly. Switch to alternative drug if β-hCG titer rises 10-fold or more, titer plateaus at an elevated level, or new metastasis appears.
Obtain labs daily during treatment cycle or weekly as indicated. Hold chemotherapy for WBC count <3000 (absolute neutrophil count <1500); platelets <100,000; significantly elevated BUN, Cr, AST, ALT, or bilirubin; or for significant side effects (severe stomatitis, gastrointestinal ulceration, or febrile course).
Oral contraceptive agents or other form of birth control should be taken concurrently and continued for at least 1 year after remission.
Chemotherapy continued for 1 course after negative β-hCG titer.
Follow-up program: β-hCG titer weekly until 3 consecutive normal titers; monthly β-hCG titer for 12 months thereafter; β-hCG titer every 2 months for 1 additional year or at 6-month intervals indefinitely.
Physical examination including pelvic examination and chest radiography monthly until remission is induced; at 3-month intervals for 1 year thereafter; then at 6-month intervals indefinitely.

ALT, alanine transaminase; AST, aspartate transaminase; Cr, creatinine; BUN, blood urea nitrogen; IM, intramuscular; IV, intravenous.
[1]For nonmetastatic disease only.

Table 51–2 summarizes the recommended chemotherapeutic regimens available for nonmetastatic gestational trophoblastic neoplasia. Single-agent chemotherapy using methotrexate or dactinomycin has demonstrated clear-cut superiority over other protocols. A randomized trial conducted by the Gynecologic Oncology Group concluded that biweekly IV dactinomycin 1.25 mg/m² achieved a higher complete response rate as compared to weekly IM methotrexate 30 mg/m². The methotrexate dose used in this trial, however, was lower than the weekly dose of 50 mg/m² given typically to most low-risk patients and may have accounted for the superiority of the dactinomycin. Therefore, the regimen of choice in this group of patients has yet to be determined.

Treatment failure or intolerable side effects should result in administration of the alternative agent or regimen. Each treatment cycle should be repeated as soon as normal tissues (bone marrow and gastrointestinal mucosa) have recovered, with a minimum 7-day window between the last day of one course and the first day of the next course. Overall, the complete response rate to single-agent therapy ranges from 60 to 98%, with salvage rates approaching 100%. Methotrexate is contraindicated in the presence of hepatocellular disease or when renal function is impaired.

During treatment, weekly quantitative hCG titers and complete blood counts should be obtained. Before each course of therapy, liver and renal function assessments should be assessed. At least 1 additional course of drug therapy should be given after attainment of the first normal hCG value. The number of treatment cycles necessary to induce remission is proportionate to the magnitude of the hCG concentration at the start of therapy. An average of 3 or 4 courses of single-agent therapy is usually required. After remission has been induced and treatment is completed, hCG assays should be obtained monthly for 1 year.

2. Metastatic gestational trophoblastic disease— Treatment in metastatic disease uses either single-agent chemotherapy (Table 51–2) or multiagent chemotherapy in cases in which resistance to a single agent is anticipated. Several systems have been developed to determine at onset which patients will require more aggressive therapy. The National Cancer Institute system is used in the United States to determine whether the patient will have a good or poor prognosis in response to single-agent chemotherapy (Table 51–3).

Table 51–4 highlights the World Health Organization (WHO) scoring system in which patients are categorized into low- or high-risk groups based on risk factors such as age, type of antecedent pregnancy, interval from antecedent pregnancy to initiation of chemotherapy, pretreatment hCG level, size of largest tumor, site of metastases, number of metastases, and prior chemotherapy. A total score of 0–6 is considered low risk and a total score ≥7 is categorized as high risk.

The revised 2002 FIGO staging system combines the use of both anatomic and nonanatomic factors (Table 51–5).

Table 51–3. Categorization of gestational trophoblastic neoplasia.

A. Nonmetastatic disease: No evidence of disease outside uterus.
B. Metastatic disease: Any disease outside uterus. **1. Good-prognosis metastatic disease (low risk)** a. Short duration (<4 months) b. Serum β-hCG < 40,000 mIU/mL c. No metastasis to brain or liver d. No significant prior chemotherapy **2. Poor-prognosis metastatic disease (high risk)** a. Long duration (>4 months) b. Serum β-hCG >40,000 mIu/mL c. Metastasis to brain or liver d. Unsuccessful prior chemotherapy e. Gestational trophoblastic neoplasia after term pregnancy

Table 51–4. Modified WHO prognostic scoring system as adapted by FIGO.

	0	1	2	4
Age, years	<40	≥40	—	—
Antecedent pregnancy	Mole	Abortion	Term	—
Interval months from index pregnancy	<4	4–<7	7–<13	≥13
Pretreatment serum hCG (IU/mL)	$<10^3$	10^3–$<10^4$	10^4–$<10^5$	$\geq 10^5$
Largest tumor size (including uterus)	—	3–<5 cm	≥5 cm	—
Site of metastases	Lung	Spleen, kidney	Gastrointestinal	Liver, brain
Number of metastases	—	1–4	5–8	>8
Previous failed chemotherapy	—	—	Single drug	2 or more drugs

FIGO, International Federation on Gynecology and Obstetrics, WHO, World Health Organization.
(Reproduced, with permission, of the FIGO Committee Report. FIGO staging for gestational trophoblastic neoplasia 2000. *Int J Gynecol Obstet* 2002;77:286, Table 4.)

A patient is assigned a stage based on the anatomic location of disease and given a risk factor score based on the WHO prognostic scoring system. The goal of the revised FIGO staging is to improve the assessment and clinical management of patients and to unify staging to allow for international comparisons in treatment success.

A. Good-prognosis patients—Based on the clinical classification of malignant disease, patients can be expected to respond satisfactorily to single-agent chemotherapy if (1) metastases are confined to the lungs or pelvis, (2) serum hCG levels are below 40,000 mIU/mL at the onset of treatment, and (3) therapy is started within 4 months of apparent onset of disease. The most common site of metastasis in gestational trophoblastic disease is the lungs. When a patient develops pulmonary metastasis with elevation of the hCG titer, choriocarcinoma is a more likely cause than metastatic invasive mole, although the latter can also metastasize to the lungs.

Table 51–5. FIGO anatomic staging.

Stage I	Disease confined to the uterus
Stage II	GTN extends outside of the uterus, but is limited to the genital structures (adnexa, vagina, broad ligament)
Stage III	GTN extends to the lungs, with or without known genital tract involvement
Stage IV	All other metastatic sites

FIGO, International Federation on Gynecology and Obstetrics; GTN, gestational trophoblastic neoplasia.
(Reproduced, with permission, of the FIGO Committee Report. FIGO staging for gestational trophoblastic neoplasia 2000. *Int J Gynecol Obstet* 2002;77:286, Table 1.)

The advantage of single-agent chemotherapy over multiagent therapy lies in its more favorable toxicity profile, with fewer total side effects, and a lower likelihood that these effects would be irreversible. It is important to keep in mind that despite the "good-prognosis" designation of low-risk disease, failure of drug therapy does occur in 10% of cases. Therefore, meticulous care by a knowledgeable physician such as a gynecologic oncologist is necessary for optimal outcomes.

In good-prognosis patients, single-agent chemotherapy (Table 51–2) with methotrexate is considered the drug of choice. Ideally, the 5-day treatment course is given every other week, as the possibility of tumor regrowth increases with treatment gaps >2 weeks. Once negative titers have been achieved, an additional course is administered before beginning the period of surveillance. In cases in which resistance to methotrexate occurs, as manifested by rising or plateauing titers or by the development of new metastases, or cases in which negative titers are not achieved by the fifth course of methotrexate, the patient should be given dactinomycin. Dactinomycin should also be the agent of choice for patients who experience severe side effects with methotrexate.

B. Poor-prognosis patients—Poor-prognosis patients, based on the Clinical Classification of Malignant Disease, are those with any of the following risk factors: (1) serum hCG titers >40,000 mIU/mL at the onset of treatment, (2) diagnosis of disease more than 4 months after molar pregnancy,

(3) brain or liver metastases, (4) prior unsuccessful chemotherapy, or (5) onset after term gestation. These patients respond poorly (<40% response rate) to single-agent therapy. A poor response is also seen in patients with advanced revised FIGO stages and WHO scores ≥7. These patients present a serious challenge to the clinician, as many have been previously treated with chemotherapy, have developed resistance to key agents, and/or have accumulated considerable toxicity with depleted bone marrow reserves. In fact, prior unsuccessful chemotherapy is considered to be one of the worst prognostic factors.

Generally, poor-prognosis patients are managed by a gynecologic oncologist and may require prolonged hospitalization and multiple courses of chemotherapy. They often need multispeciality care and other life-support measures, including hyperalimentation, antibiotics, and transfusions to correct the effects of marrow depression.

Central nervous system involvement, particularly brain metastases with focal neurologic signs, commonly occurs with choriocarcinoma. Because patients with brain or liver metastases are at high risk of sudden death from hemorrhagic lesions, it is standard practice to institute whole-brain or whole-liver irradiation concomitantly with combination chemotherapy. Uncertainty remains regarding whether radiation therapy exerts its beneficial effects by destroying tumor in combination with drug therapy or by preventing fatal hemorrhage and thus keeping the patient alive until remission with chemotherapy has been achieved. For acute bleeding episodes, surgical intervention or angiographic embolization should be considered.

Cerebral metastases are treated over a 2-week period with radiation given at a dosage of 3 Gy daily, 5 days a week, to a total organ dose of 30 Gy. Whole-liver irradiation is usually accomplished over 10 days to attain a 20-Gy whole-organ dose given at a rate of 2 Gy daily, 5 days a week. Other treatment options include selective hepatic artery chemotherapy infusion.

Previously, patients with poor prognosis or high-risk gestational trophoblastic neoplasia were treated with methotrexate, dactinomycin, and chlorambucil or cyclophosphamide and the modified Bagshawe protocol (cyclophosphamide, hydroxyurea, methotrexate, vincristine, cyclophosphamide, and dactinomycin). Currently, etoposide, methotrexate, dactinomycin, cyclophosphamide, and vincristine (EMACO) chemotherapy (Table 51–6) repeated every 2 weeks provides the best response rate (approximately 80%) with the lowest side-effect profile. Monitoring for drug toxicity is the same as that in single-agent therapy but with higher vigilance due to the possibility of combined toxicity.

Treatment of malignant trophoblastic disease must be continued with repeated courses of combination chemotherapy until hCG titers return to undetectable levels (<5 mIU/mL). Complete remission is documented only after 3 consecutive weekly normal hCG titers have been achieved. It is recommended that all high-risk patients receive at least 3 courses of multiagent chemotherapy after hCG titers have returned to normal. After remission is achieved, follow-up is the same as for hydatidiform moles and metastatic good-prognosis disease.

Salvage therapy for disease not responsive to EMACO substitutes cisplatin and etoposide for cyclophosphamide and vincristine (EP-EMA) (Table 51–6). Close monitoring of renal function is required because of nephrotoxicity

Table 51–6. Current treatment regimens for high-risk metastatic gestational trophoblastic disease.

EMA/CO[1]		
Day		
1	Etoposide Dactinomycin Methotrexate[2]	100 mg/m² IV (infused over 30 min) 0.5 mg IV bolus 100 mg/m² IV bolus 200 mg/m² IV (infused over 12 h)
2	Etoposide Dactinomycin Folinic acid	100 mg/m² IV (infused over 30 min) 0.5 mg IV bolus 15 mg IM infusion or orally every 12 hours for 4 doses beginning 24 hours after start of methotrexate
8	Cyclophosphamide Vincristine	600 mg/m² IV infusion 1 mg/m² IV bolus
Other options:		
Salvage therapy: Substituting etoposide (100 mg/m² IV) and cisplatin (80 mg/m² IV) (EMA-EP) for cyclophosphamide and vincristine. Adjuvant surgery (hysterectomy and thoracotomy) for chemotherapy-resistant disease.		
With failure of EMA-EP, treatment with: BEP (cisplatin 20 mg/m² IV, etoposide 100 mg/m² IV on days 1–4 every 21 days, with bleomycin 30 units IV on day 1 then every week), G-CSF (granulocyte colony-stimulating factor) 300 μg SC on days 6–14.		
VIP (etoposide 75 mg/m² IV, ifosfamide 1.2 g/m² IV, cisplatin 20 mg/m² IV each day for 4 days every 21 days). Mesna 120 mg/m² IV bolus before first ifosfamide dose, followed by 1.2 mg/m² 12-hour IV infusion daily after each ifosfamide dose, G-CSF 300 μg SC on days 6–14.		
High-dose chemotherapy with autologous bone marrow transplantation.		
Taxanes (paclitaxel and docetaxel) and camptothecins (topotecan and irinotecan).		

G-CSF, granulocyte colony-stimulating factor; IM, intramuscular; IV, intravenous; SC, subcutaneous.

[1]Mild toxicity with 5-year survival 80%. Repeat cycles on days 15, 16, and 22 (every 2 weeks).

[2]Increase to 1 g/m² as 24-h infusion with central nervous system metastases, with folinic acid increased to 15 mg every 8 h for 9 doses beginning 12 h after completion of methotrexate infusion. Also may receive methotrexate 12.5 mg by intrathecal injection on day 8. Another option is whole-brain irradiation 3000 cGy in 200-cGy fractions given over 10–14 days during chemotherapy.

secondary to cisplatin and renally excreted methotrexate. Other treatment options include paclitaxel, topotecan, and high-dose chemotherapy with autologous bone marrow transplantation. As stated previously, chemotherapy should be continued for at least 3 cycles after a negative hCG is achieved. In resistant cases, adjunctive measures along with chemotherapy may include hysterectomy, resection of metastatic tumors, or irradiation of unresectable lesions.

During and after treatment, a thorough discussion about birth control and reproductive options is of utmost importance. Oral contraceptive pills should be used if not contraindicated. Contraceptive efforts should be continued for at least 1 year after remission.

3. Placental-Site Trophoblastic Tumor—As treatment of PSTT is generally resistant to chemotherapy, hysterectomy is the recommended route of treatment. Partial uterine resection involving the tumor is possible if the patient desires future fertility. Chemotherapy is indicated in cases of metastatic disease. EP-EMA is the preferred regimen over EMACO, with paclitaxel and topotecan used when resistance develops. The greatest adverse outcomes are associated with an interval of >2 years from the antecedent pregnancy to diagnosis.

Prognosis

The prognosis for molar pregnancies treated with evacuation is uniformly excellent, although close surveillance is needed, as outlined previously. After spontaneous normalization of hCG values after evacuation, recurrence rates are <0.5%. The prognosis for malignant nonmetastatic disease with appropriate therapy is also quite good, as almost all patients are cured. More than 90% of these patients can preserve reproductive function, but first-line therapy fails in 6.5%.

Additionally, more than 90% of patients with good-prognosis or low-risk metastatic disease respond to single-agent chemotherapy. Virtually all patients with this type of disease can be cured without the need for hysterectomy. In poor-prognosis or high-risk metastatic disease, the best results are achieved with the EMACO chemotherapy regimen and concurrent radiation. Approximately 75–85% of patients achieve remission with a 69% salvage rate. This is a similar response rate to agents used previously but with fewer side effects. Women with nonpulmonary metastases have the worst prognosis, with reports of survival ranging from 0 to 60% for hepatic involvement and 50–80% for central nervous system involvement. Survival decreases to <20% when prior chemotherapeutic agents have been administered or if brain metastasis develops while undergoing treatment. In metastatic disease that is in remission, relapse can occur in 8% of patients, usually in the first several months after termination of therapy but even as late as 3 years.

Over the years, deaths from chemotherapeutic drug toxicity have decreased considerably. However, multiagent chemotherapy, specifically a regimen containing etoposide, is associated with a 50% increased risk for secondary tumors. One retrospective study found that the relative risk for developing myeloid leukemia and colon cancer was 16.6 and 4.6, respectively. When survival exceeded 25 years, the relative risk for developing breast cancer was 5.8.

Subsequent pregnancies are not at increased risk for complications such as preterm labor, congenital anomalies, or stillbirth. These pregnancies should, however, be monitored early with ultrasonography and hCG levels as there is a 1% risk of recurrent gestational trophoblastic disease after 1 molar pregnancy and a 15% risk of recurrence after 2 molar pregnancies. After delivery, the placenta should be sent to pathology and an hCG level checked at the 6-week postpartum visit.

In cases in which pregnancy occurs before completion of standard postmolar surveillance, the pregnancy may be continued with close observation, and the risks discussed with the patient. Most of these pregnancies have a favorable outcome, but a small risk exists for delayed diagnosis of recurrent gestational trophoblastic disease.

ACOG Committee on Practice Bulletins. Practice Bulletin Number 53: Diagnosis and treatment of gestational trophoblastic disease. *Obstet Gynecol* 2004, reaffirmed 2008;104:1422. PMID: 15172880.

Baergen RN, Rutgers JL, Young RH, et al. Placental site trophoblastic tumor: a study of 55 cases and review of the literature emphasizing factors of prognostic significance. *Gynecol Oncol* 2006;100:511. PMID: 16246400.

Berkowitz RS, Goldstein DP. Current management of gestational trophoblastic diseases. *Gynecol Oncol* 2009;112:654. PMID: 18851873.

Berkowitz RS, Goldstein DP. Molar pregnancy. *N Engl J Med* 2009;360:1639. PMID: 19369669.

Chiang JW, Berek JS. Gestational trophoblastic disease: epidemiology, clinical manifestations and diagnosis. www.uptodate.com. Version 17.1, February 2009.

Deng L, Yan X, Zhang J, et al. Combination chemotherapy for high-risk gestational trophoblastic tumour. *Cochrane Database Syst Rev* 2009;2:CD005196. PMID: 19370618.

Dorigo O, Berek JS. Gestational trophoblastic disease: pathology. www.uptodate.com. Version 17.1, July 2008.

Garner EIO. Malignant gestational trophoblastic disease: staging and treatment. www.uptodate.com. Version 17.1, November 2008.

Garner EIO. Gestational trophoblastic disease: management of hydatidiform mole. www.uptodate.com. Version 17.1, February 2009.

Garrett LA, Garner EI, Feltmate CM, et al. Subsequent pregnancy outcomes in patients with molar pregnancy and persistent gestational trophoblastic neoplasia. *J Reprod Med* 2008;53:481. PMID: 18720922.

Hoekstra AV, Lurain JR, Rademaker AW, et al. Gestational trophoblastic neoplasia: treatment outcomes. *Obstet Gynecol* 2008;112:251. PMID: 18669719.

Horowitz NS, Goldstein DP, Berkowitz RS. Management of gestational trophoblastic neoplasia. *Semin Oncol* 2009;36:181. PMID: 19332252.

Kerkmeijer LGW, Wielsma S, Massuger LFAG, et al. Recurrent gestational trophoblastic disease after hCG normalization following hydatidiform mole in The Netherlands. *Gynecol Oncol* 2007;106:142. PMID: 17462723.

Osborne RJ, Filiaci V, Schink JC, et al. Phase III Trial of Weekly Methotrexate or Pulsed Dactinomycin for Low-Risk Gestational Trophoblastic Neoplasia: A Gynecologic Oncology Group Study. *J Clin Oncol* 2011;29:825. PMID: 21263100.

Smith HO, Kohorn E, Cole LA. Choriocarcinoma and gestational trophoblastic disease. *Obstet Gynecol Clin North Am* 2005;32:661. PMID: 16310678.

Soper JT. Gestational trophoblastic disease. *Obstet Gynecol* 2006;108:176. PMID: 16816073.

Wang KL, Yang YC, Wang TY, et al. Treatment of gestational trophoblastic neoplasia according to the FIGO 2000 staging and scoring system: a 20 years' experience. *Acta Obstet Gynecol Scand* 2009;88:204. PMID: 19031297.

52 Radiation and Chemotherapy for Gynecologic Cancers

Wafic M. ElMasri, MD
Oliver Dorigo, MD, PhD

Two European discoveries in the late 1800s led to future radiation treatment of human malignancies. While studying the penetrating power of cathode ray emission in Germany, Wilhelm Roentgen discovered x-rays on November 8, 1895. In France, the Curies isolated radium from uranium ore in 1898. Soon thereafter, Robert Abbe of New York City introduced radium for medical therapy, and Howard Kelly of Baltimore pioneered radium treatment of cervical cancer. Since then, radiation therapy has evolved to become a major modality in the treatment of many cancers, particularly those of the female reproductive tract.

RADIATION PRINCIPLES

Radiation therapy is used for definitive or palliative treatment of cancer and may be defined as therapeutic delivery of radiation to a target tissue, which results in tissue damage. Radiation causes breaks in DNA and generates free radicals from cell water that may damage cell membranes, proteins, and organelles. Such radiation may be electromagnetic or particulate, both of which transfer energy to the electrons or nuclei of the target atoms.

Electromagnetic radiation is energy that is transmitted at the speed of light through oscillating electric and magnetic fields. The energy contained in these fields can be described as discrete units known as photons. The energy of each photon is proportional to the frequency of the wave associated with that photon. Because radiation with a shorter wavelength has greater frequency, it carries greater energy per photon, allowing deeper tissue penetration. The most clinically relevant forms of electromagnetic radiation are x-rays and gamma rays. For therapeutic applications, x-rays are mechanically produced by linear accelerators that accelerate electrons to very high energies. These electrons then strike a target within the accelerator, usually tungsten, to produce a beam of x-rays that is targeted at the patient. Gamma rays are produced by the decay of radioactive substances. Currently, the most commonly used radioisotopes for gynecologic cancer treatments are cesium-137 and iridium-192.

Particulate radiation uses subatomic particles (electrons, neutrons, protons), instead of photons, to deliver the dose of radiation. Compared with electromagnetic radiation, particle-beam therapy enables more precise dose localization and better depth-dose distribution.

Interaction of Photons with Matter

The first step in the absorption of an incident photon with matter is the conversion of the energy of that photon into the kinetic energy of an electron, or electron–positron pair. Depending on the energy of the photon, this conversion takes place either through the photoelectric effect, the Compton effect, or pair production. In the lower range of energy transfer, the photoelectric effect predominates, whereas in the transfer of higher levels of energy, the Compton effect and pair production are more prevalent.

Photoelectric effect: an incident low-energy photon (0.5–100 kV) interacts with a tightly bound inner shell electron of the target tissue. The energy is completely absorbed by this electron, which is ejected from the atomic orbit with kinetic energy equal to the photon energy. The product electron then ionizes the surrounding tissue. The lower the energy of the incoming photon and the higher the atomic number of the tissue, the more likely photoelectric effect will occur. Absorption is directly proportional to the atomic number of the target. Tissues bearing elements of higher atomic numbers (eg, calcium in bone) absorb proportionately higher levels of radiation, which may lead to toxicity.

Compton effect: an incident mid-energy photon (100 kV–20 MV) transfers energy to an outer-shell electron in the target tissue, causing ejection of this electron. The photon's energy is incompletely absorbed; instead, the photon is scattered at an angle to its original path. Both the product electron and the scattered incoming photon (which now has lower energy) continue with ionizing interactions (Fig. 52–1). The Compton effect is inversely proportional to the energy of the incoming photon and is independent of atomic number (ie, all tissue absorbs the same amount of energy). The Compton

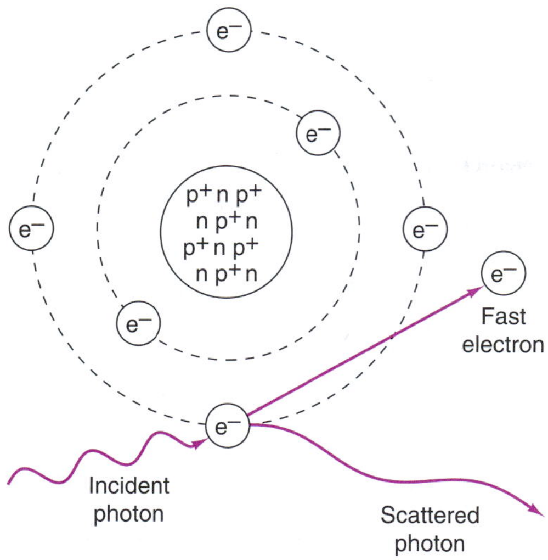

▲ **Figure 52–1.** Absorption of an x-ray photon by the Compton process. The photon interacts with a loosely bound planetary electron of an atom of the absorbing material. Part of the photon energy is given to the electron as kinetic energy. The photon, deflected from its original direction, proceeds with reduced energy. e^-, electron; p^+, proton; n, neutron. (Reproduced, with permission, from Hall EJ. *Radiobiology for the Radiologist.* 4th ed. Philadelphia, PA: JB Lippincott; 1994, p. 7.)

effect accounts for the biologic effects on tissues seen in radiation therapy.

Pair production: refers to a complex interaction between an incident high-energy photon (>1.02 MV) with the nucleus of a target atom resulting in formation of a pair of electron–positron (e+) and negatively charged electron (e–) that scatters in the opposite direction. Because the pair production interaction typically predominates at energy levels above the range that is usually used in therapy, it plays a small role in most clinical settings.

Interaction of Photons with Tissue

As a radiation beam travels through a patient, it deposits energy in the tissue through interactions such as the Compton effect. The depth of tissue penetration is dependent on the energy. At 100% depth dose, 250 KeV will be reached at the skin level, 1.25 MeV at 5 mm, 6 MeV at 1.2 cm, and 20 MeV at 10 cm.

These interactions set secondary electrons in motion, which result in further ionizations. These ionizations lead to the breakage of chemical bonds and subsequent damage to DNA and cellular structures. The result is reproductive cell death and apoptosis in case of excessive damage.

The most critical target for damage within the cell is DNA. Direct damage occurs when a photon becomes absorbed by an atom in the DNA resulting in DNA breaks that are beyond the cell's repair machinery. More commonly, however, DNA breaks are indirect. The water surrounding the DNA is ionized by the radiation, creating oxygen radicals, hydroxyl radicals, peroxide, and hydrated electrons. These highly reactive species then interact with the DNA to cause damage.

Dosage Theory

Normal tissues as well as malignant cells are susceptible to toxicity induced by radiation therapy, the extent of which depends on total dose, fractionization, and tumor volume.

After exposure to radiation, tissue survival follows a predictable curve that essentially constitutes the number of viable clone cells (Fig. 52–2). The shoulder represents the cell's enzymatic ability to reverse radiation-induced damage. As radiation increases, cells become incapable of self-repair, and a logarithmic pattern of cell destruction occurs. Importantly, for every increase in dosage that occurs beyond the shoulder, a constant fraction of cells is eliminated (**log-kill hypothesis**).

The implications of these observations provide some of the rationale for dividing (fractionating) the total dose of radiation therapy administered in the clinical setting. It is helpful to consider the so-called 4 Rs of radiobiology to understand the effects of fractionated doses at the cellular level:

A. Repair

Fractionation into small doses allows for sublethal injury repair (shoulder repetition) and results in the higher total dose necessary to achieve the same biologic effect. When a specified radiation dose is divided into ≥2 doses given at separate times, the number of cells surviving is higher than that seen when the same total dose is given at 1 time. However, fractionation allows the administration of a divided radiation dose that would not be tolerated by surrounding normal tissue if the specified dose were to be given in only 1 treatment.

B. Repopulation

The reactivation of stem cells that occurs when radiation is stopped is necessary for further tissue growth. Repopulation is cellular proliferation during delivery of a radiation therapy course. If the cancer repopulates slower than acutely responding normal tissue, fractionated radiation will be successful in eliminating tumor cells. The shorter the doubling time of tumor cells, the higher total dose of radiation will have to be delivered. Prolonged and unnecessary delays between radiation fractions decrease the effectiveness of the total radiation dose delivered.

C. Reoxygenation

Hypoxic cells are known to be relatively resistant to radiation. Oxygenated cells are 3 times more sensitive than cells irradiated under anoxic conditions (Fig. 52–2). Malignant cells located farther than 100 mm from capillary flow are at risk for

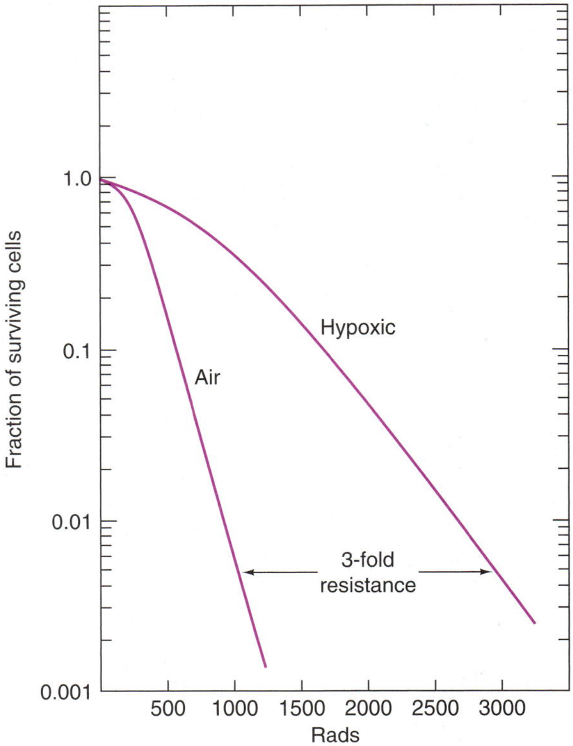

▲ **Figure 52–2.** Typical radiation survival curve for mammalian cells. These cells have been irradiated and then plated out in culture, and the number of survivors has been determined by measuring the colonies (clones) of cells that survive. The curve is characterized by an initial shoulder followed by a log-linear region. Cells irradiated in air are considerably more sensitive than those irradiated in nitrogen (hypoxic), and the difference between the levels of killing is frequently about 3-fold. It is believed that most clinically demonstrable tumors have areas of hypoxia that lead to radioresistance. (Reproduced, with permission, from Morrow CP, Curtin JP, Townsend DE (eds). *Synopsis of Gynecologic Oncology.* 4th ed. New York: Churchill Livingstone; 1993, p. 449.)

hypoxia and may not be killed by radiation therapy. For this reason, it is important to correct anemia in patients undergoing radiation treatment so that tissue oxygen perfusion will be enhanced and tissues will become more radiosensitive. Fractionated radiation results in better oxygenation of initially hypoxic tumor cells. As tumor shrinks with radiation treatments, the percentage of hypoxic cells decrease and the percentage of radiation sensitive cells is increased.

D. Redistribution

Radiation-induced synchrony allows for cellular progression into a more radiosensitive part of the cell cycle during interfraction intervals. Within an asynchronous tumor cell population, fractionated radiation kills radiosensitive cells (late G_2 and M phase), leaving radioresistant cells (early G_1 and mid-late S phase) with little damage. Interfraction intervals allow for cell-cycle synchronization (progression to G_2 and M phase) and leads to higher overall cell death with each subsequent fraction. Cell killing is more effective with shorter cell-cycles.

Dosimetry

Dosimetry is the measurement of the amount of radiation absorbed by target tissue. The unit of absorbed dose is the Gray (Gy), which is defined as the joules of energy absorbed in a kilogram of tissue (J/kg). One Gy is equal to 100 rads. External pelvic irradiation is expressed in those terms, whereas internal irradiation (intracavitary) is also described in milligram-radium-equivalent hours (mgRaEq-hr). This latter unit is calculated by multiplying the mgRaEq of cesium or radium in the system by the number of hours the radioactive sources are left in place during treatment.

The amount of radiation used in radiation therapy varies depending on the type and stage of cancer. The typical dose for the primary treatment of solid epithelial tumors including advanced cervical cancer ranges from 60 to 85 Gy, whereas the lower doses between 20 and 40 Gy are used for lymphomas.

Adjuvant radiation therapy is used in selected cases after surgery for cervical and endometrial cancer. The radiation doses are typically lower compared with primary treatment, ranging between 45 and 60 Gy in 1.8- to 2-Gy fractions. Factors to be considered when planning radiation and selection of a dose include concurrent chemotherapy and patient comorbidities.

Planning of radiation treatment involves specialized treatment planning software that incorporates the radiation delivery method and several angles or sources to optimize the dose to the tumor and minimize the radiation effect on the surrounding healthy tissues. Computer-directed dosimetry permits the calculation of isodose curves, points of equal dose surrounding a radioactive source that permit critical considerations in avoiding overdose to the bladder and rectum. Unfortunately, the radiation tolerance of the bladder and rectum is close to the dosage levels required for curative radiation therapy of common pelvic cancers.

Fractionation

Fractionation is an important principle of radiation biology and treatment. The total radiation dose is given over a period of time at approximately 1.8–2 Gy per day over 5 days a week. Fractionation allows time for normal cells to recover and repair radiation-induced DNA damage. Tumor cells usually have dysfunctional repair mechanisms and are therefore preferentially effected by the radiation. In addition, fractionation allows tumor cells that were relatively radiation resistant during one treatment to enter a radiation sensitive phase of the cell cycle before the next fraction is given. Another tumor cell selective killing mechanism relates to hypoxia-induced radiation resistance. Hypoxic tumor cells might reoxygenate between fractions, therefore improving the effect of radiation during the next treatment.

TREATMENT METHODS

For gynecologic cancers, therapeutic radiation is delivered as external radiation (teletherapy), internal radiation (brachytherapy), or a combination of both.

External Irradiation (Teletherapy)

Early radiation therapists used electric x-ray sources that were basically modifications of Roentgen's experimental apparatus. Electrons were accelerated across a vacuum tube to strike a tungsten target with the subsequent liberation of photons. These orthovoltage (140–400 keV) units were limited in their power to penetrate tissue effectively because of their relatively low energy output. Consequently, pronounced fibrotic skin changes and high absorbed bone radiation levels limited their usefulness in some patients.

As units generating higher levels of energy were developed, the penetrating power of the x-rays produced was enhanced, and less scattering of radiation was seen at the margins of the treatment area. The surface skin dose was also diminished, of particular importance in the treatment of obese patients, and less toxic bone radiation was achieved (Fig. 52–3).

The goal of external radiation treatment is to ensure that radiation is delivered to the target tissue without affecting uninvolved tissues and that the amount of radiation received is as uniform as possible. Traditionally, the planning of radiation treatment has been done in 2 dimensions (height and width). Today, this is achieved by optimized 3-dimensional conformal planning to more precisely target a tumor with radiation beams (height, width, and depth). Patients undergo computed tomography (CT) scanning

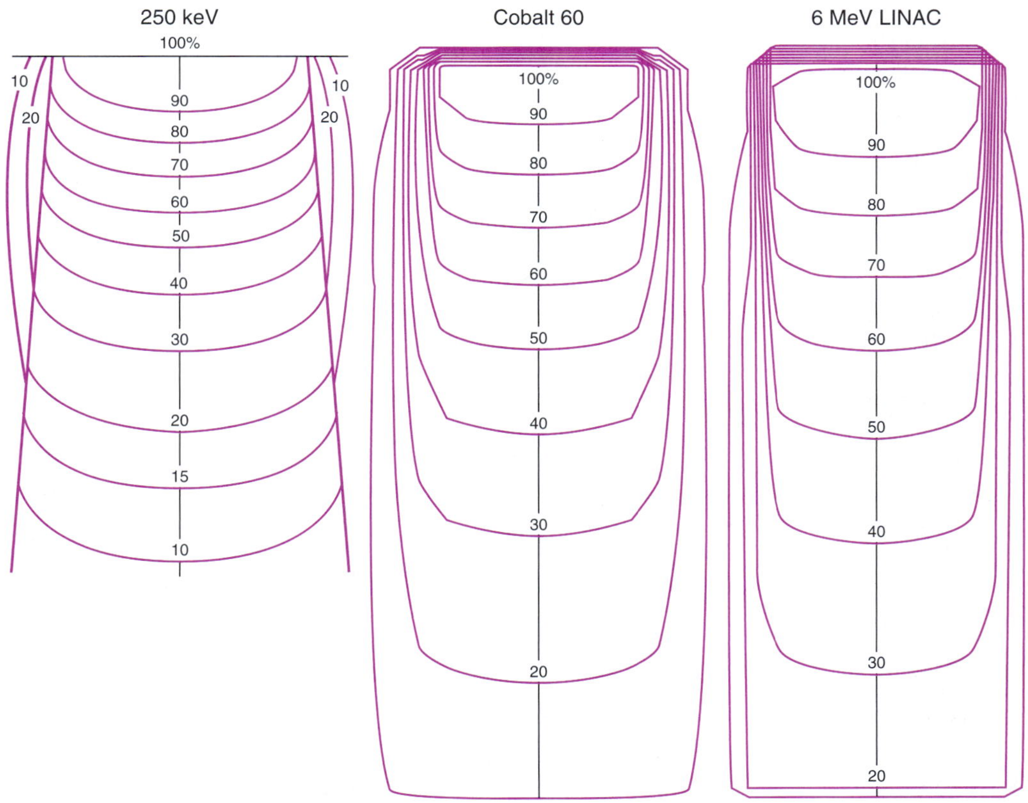

▲ **Figure 52–3.** Typical isodose curves for orthovoltage (250 keV), cobalt 60, and a 6-MeV linear accelerator (LINAC). The most important difference between the megavoltage (cobalt 60 and LINAC) beams in comparison with the 250-keV beam is the movement of the 100% isodose line several millimeters beneath the surface. This results in elimination of the severe skin reactions characteristic of earlier radiation sources. In addition, the higher energy leads to deeper penetration as the energy of the beam increases.

in the treatment position, and the volume of abnormal tissue, that is, the gross tumor volume (GTV), is delineated. Given the possibility of microscopic extension along tissue planes, a margin of tissue is added to the GTV. This larger volume, the clinical tumor volume, is the volume of tissue to be irradiated. Using information from these images, special computer programs design radiation beams that "conform" to the shape of the tumor.

Internal Irradiation (Brachytherapy)

Brachytherapy is radiation therapy in which the source of therapeutic ionizing radiation is placed close to the treatment area. The chief advantage of local irradiation is that a relatively high dose of radiation can be applied to a limited anatomic region. The **inverse square law** has critical implications in clinical applications. The principle of the inverse square law states that the intensity of radiation is inversely proportional to the square of the distance from the source. An important implication is that the rapid falloff of radiant energy supplied by a central source precludes the achievement of cancerocidal doses at the margins of the pelvis. Consequently, external therapy must be used to provide adequate radiation to eliminate tumor at the periphery of large lesions and at the pelvic side walls, where metastatic disease may be present.

Brachytherapy can be delivered using an intracavitary approach with a variety of applicators, or via an interstitial approach using needles or catheters. Most applicators for intracavitary brachytherapy consist of an intrauterine tandem and paired colpostats or ovoids, which are placed in the lateral vaginal fornices. Interstitial applicators consist of multiple needles that are inserted into the tissue at or near the target site. Radioactive isotopes are then loaded into the applicators at the beginning of the treatment.

Several isotopes are available for brachytherapy. The most commonly used in the United States is a low-dose rate (LDR) approach employing cesium-137. However, acceptance of a high-dose rate (HDR) therapy, usually with iridium-192, is quickly gaining acceptance. HDR brachytherapy offers some significant advantages over LDR, as it can be used on an outpatient basis, eliminates radiation exposure to medical personnel, and has shorter treatment times.

TREATMENT OF GYNECOLOGIC CANCER

Cervical Cancer

Treatment of cervical cancer is considered a prime example of the successful application of radiation therapy. The relative accessibility of a central cervical lesion, a predictable metastatic and local spread pattern, and the radiation tolerance of the cervix and surrounding tissues often permit the administration of curative therapy in cases of cervical carcinoma.

Radiation therapy with curative intent uses both external-beam and intracavitary radiation. Palliative radiation for advanced or recurrent cervical cancer may use either modality for control of bleeding, management of disease in the pelvis, and relief of pain.

The size of the radiation field used to treat a patient with carcinoma of the cervix must be carefully designed to encompass those structures at risk for regional spread of the cancer. The goal of external irradiation in is to sterilize metastatic disease to pelvic lymph nodes and the parametria and/or to decrease the size of the cervical lesion to allow optimal placement of intracavitary radioactive sources. A standard radiation field for external-beam radiation therapy extends inferiorly to the midpubis or 3–4 cm below the most distal disease, superiorly to the interface between the fourth and fifth interlumbar vertebrae, and lateral at least 1 cm lateral to the bony pelvic markings. The dose for external-beam radiation therapy is approximately 40–45 Gy.

The rationale for external-beam radiation therapy is the treatment of the lymphatic lymph node chain along the pelvic side walls, but it also induces shrinkage of the primary cervical tumor. However, in order to deliver a curative dose to the tumor, brachytherapy needs to follow external-beam radiation therapy. This is done mainly by HDR radiation therapy applied directly to the tumor via a vaginal applicator. The doses of radiation are commonly calculated based on 2 reference points. Point A defines a point 2 cm lateral and 2 cm superior to the external cervical os in the plane of the implant. Point B is located 3 cm lateral to point A. The total dose for the primary treatment of cervical cancer ranges between 75 and 90 Gy when external and brachytherapy doses are combined.

Definitive radiation therapy is an acceptable alternative to radical surgery for women with early-stage disease (stages IA, IB1, and nonbulky IIA) and is the treatment of choice in more advanced stages. Concurrent cisplatin-based chemotherapy is synergistic and leads to better tumor control and clinical response. Numerous studies show that concomitant radiation therapy and chemotherapy (chemoradiation) improves overall and progression-free survival in patients with cervical cancer.

Concurrent chemotherapy does not generally lead to treatment delays, and it sensitizes cervical cancer cells to the effects of radiation therapy. Its proposed mechanisms of action include interference with and modification of sublethal injury repair, cell phase distribution, tumor vascularity, hypoxic cells, repopulation, cell survival curve, and apoptosis all culminating in maximal cellular lethal damage.

The treatment volume for women undergoing external-beam radiation therapy after radical surgery usually involves the whole pelvis. Patients with known or suspected metastatic disease to periaortic lymph nodes may be considered for extended-field irradiation that includes a para-aortic radiation field.

Endometrial Cancer

The decision to use radiation treatment for endometrial cancer is often made after comprehensive surgical staging has been performed and is dependent on the estimated risk of recurrent disease. Patients have been traditionally divided into different risk groups for adjuvant treatment decisions based on the likelihood of recurrence.

In general, low-risk patients have disease confined to the endometrium. Adjuvant radiation should be considered in patients over 60 years of age and patients with poorly differentiated tumors (grade 3), lower uterine segment involvement, or large tumor size. However, these criteria are controversial, and the decision to administer adjuvant radiation in early-stage disease is made at the physician's discretion.

Intermediate-risk patients have cancers that are confined to the uterus but invade the myometrium or demonstrate occult cervical involvement. Other adverse prognostic factors that increase the risk for recurrence include invasion of the outer one-third of the myometrium, poor histologic differentiation, and the presence of lymphovascular invasion. The presence of these risk factors might prompt the administration of adjuvant pelvic radiation to reduce the rates of local recurrence.

Patients with **high risk of recurrence** have tumors with stromal cervical involvement (stage II), extrauterine disease (stage III and IV), or high-risk histologies (papillary serous or clear cell tumors). High-risk histologies have a propensity for lymphovascular and upper abdominal spread and are associated with a worse outcome than the hormone-dependent, more frequent endometrioid adenocarcinomas. When high-risk disease is present and confined to the pelvis, whole-pelvis radiation with or without vaginal brachytherapy should be considered. In the presence of distant disease, a combination of radiation and chemotherapy will be necessary to achieve tumor control.

Primary radiation therapy may be used in women who are considered to be at high surgical risk, such as the elderly and those with significant comorbidities. Patients with well-differentiated adenocarcinoma may be managed with tandem and ovoids or intrauterine Simon capsules. Patients with moderately or poorly differentiated cancers or those with involvement of the cervix are at risk for parametrial and pelvic lymph node spread and should receive whole-pelvic irradiation before brachytherapy.

Ovarian Cancer

The role of radiation therapy in the management of ovarian cancer is minor. There are no well-structured trials that demonstrate the benefit of external-beam radiation in the treatment of ovarian cancer. Several studies have compared the use of intraperitoneal chromic phosphate (^{32}P) with platinum-based chemotherapy in early-stage ovarian cancer. None of these trials showed a difference in 5-year survival rates, but the gastrointestinal complication rate was significant in the radiation group. Local radiation therapy is occasionally used for the treatment of isolated recurrences in ovarian cancer.

Vaginal Cancer

Radiotherapy remains the primary treatment for vaginal cancer, which is one of the rarest human malignancies and historically one of the gravest. A 1954 review of a published series of 992 patients reported an overall 5-year survival rate of 18%. More recent studies, however, have shown overall 5-year cure rates of 40–50%. Such improvement in survival rates is attributed to megavoltage external-beam therapy along with physical and technical advances in local irradiation. Despite radiation therapy being the primary treatment modality for vaginal cancers, there are no standardized treatment protocols. With squamous cell carcinoma comprising the most common form of vaginal cancer, most of these patients undergo whole-pelvic radiation therapy followed by intracavitary or interstitial brachytherapy. Patients with lesions involving the lower third of the vagina should have the inguinal and femoral lymph nodes included in the external-beam treatment field. Extended-field radiation to include periaortic lymph nodes may be needed if imaging studies reveal bulky pelvic or periaortic disease.

Vulvar Cancer

Slightly more common than vaginal cancer (5% vs. 2% of female malignancies), vulvar cancer is usually squamous cell in origin. The mainstay of treatment of stages I and II vulvar cancer is surgical, often consisting of radical vulvectomy plus inguinofemoral lymphadenectomy. Adjuvant pelvic radiation therapy benefits patients with close or positive surgical margins, as well as patients with positive inguinofemoral lymph nodes. In patients with more advanced vulvar squamous cancer (stage III or IV), chemoradiation may reduce the need for more radical surgery, including primary pelvic exenteration.

Complications of Radiation Therapy

Radiation therapy regimens are formulated to maximize the chances for cure while incurring the smallest amount of damage to normal tissues. The effects of radiation on normal tissue are what limit the doses of therapeutic radiation that can be administered. In gynecologic cancers, the most serious complications are those involving the gastrointestinal or genitourinary systems.

Planning of radiation dosimetry takes in account the sensitivity of the pelvic organs, which varies greatly between the different tissues. The vaginal mucosa tolerates 20,000–25,000 cGy in the area of the vaginal vault, whereas the bladder mucosa only tolerates 7000 cGy of total radiation. The rectum mucosa is even more sensitive, with 5000–6000 cGy as the maximum-tolerated dose. The most sensitive pelvic organs are the ovaries, which will cease all hormone production when a dose of 2000 cGy is reached. However, approximately 50% of all ovaries stop hormone production when about half of this dose is delivered.

Complications of radiation therapy are classified as early or delayed. **Early** radiation reactions result from direct damage of parenchymal cells in organs that are sensitive to radiation. These include enteritis, proctosigmoiditis, cystitis, vulvitis, and, occasionally, depression of bone marrow elements. Bowel side effects usually comprise cramping and diarrhea that require dietary adjustments and the judicious use of antidiarrheal agents. Such problems usually respond to appropriate medication, but occasionally radiation therapy must be interrupted or curtailed because of fulminant acute reactions.

Delayed radiation reactions are believed to be caused by slow vascular damage along with direct damage of parenchymal cells. Such injury may be manifested by chronic proctosigmoiditis, hemorrhagic cystitis, small- and large-bowel strictures, and the formation of rectovaginal and vesicovaginal fistulas. Pelvic fibrosis and loss of ovarian function may affect sexual activity in younger patients.

In order to protect the pelvic organs from radiation injury, isodose curves have to be calculated very carefully to minimize the radiation to the bladder and rectum. In young, fertile patients who require radiation therapy to the pelvis, the ovaries can surgically be moved from their location within the radiation field and area along the paracolic gutters (oophoropexy). In many cases, this will preserve ovarian function after radiation. When brachytherapy is administered using a vaginal applicator, the vagina is packed with gauze around the applicator, therefore creating a greater distance between the radiation source and the bladder and rectum.

NEW DIRECTIONS IN RADIATION THERAPY

Novel, improved radiation treatment strategies are under development. These include more effective radiation sensitizers, neutron beam therapy, and altered fractionation schemes. Intensity-modulated radiotherapy (IMRT) has emerged as a new teletherapy technique. IMRT improves the ability to conform the treatment volume to the 3-dimensional tumor shapes. The radiation beam's intensity varies according to the shape of the tumor. The radiation dose intensity is increased in areas of gross tumor volume, whereas radiation to the surrounding tissue is significantly decreased. This tumor tailored radiation dose is intended to maximize tumor dose while protecting the surrounding normal tissue. As newer computer-imaging technologies continue to improve, further advances in anatomic contouring for planning and treatment are expected to translate into better local control rates, as well as improved survival with a wider margin of safety.

Ahamad A, Jhingran A. New radiation techniques in gynecological cancer [review]. *Int J Gynecol Cancer* 2004;14:569–579. PMID: 15304149.

Brown AK, Madom L, Moore R, Granai CO, DiSilvestro P. The prognostic significance of lower uterine segment involvement in surgically staged endometrial cancer patients with negative nodes. *Gynecol Oncol* 2007; 105:55–58. PMID: 17157904.

Cardenes H, Randall ME. Integrating radiation therapy in the curative management of ovarian cancer: Current issues and future directions. *Semin Radiat Oncol* 2000;10:61–70. PMID: 10671660.

Cmelak AJ, Kapp DS. Long-term survival with whole abdominopelvic irradiation in platinum-refractory persistent or recurrent ovarian cancer. *Gynecol Oncol* 1997;65:453–460. PMID: 9190975.

Creutzberg CL, van Putten WL, Koper PC, et al. Surgery and postoperative radiotherapy versus surgery alone for patients with stage-1 endometrial carcinoma: Multicentre randomised trial. PORTEC Study Group. Post Operative Radiation Therapy in Endometrial Carcinoma. *Lancet* 2000;355:1404–1411. PMID: 10791524.

Eifel PJ, Winter K, Morris M, et al. Pelvic irradiation with concurrent chemotherapy versus pelvic and para-aortic irradiation for high-risk cervical cancer: an update of radiation therapy oncology group trial (RTOG) 90-01. *J Clin Oncol* 2004;22:872–880. PMID: 14990643.

Frank SJ, Jhingran A, Levenback C, Eifel PJ. Definitive radiation therapy for squamous cell carcinoma of the vagina. *Int J Radiat Oncol Biol Phys* 2005;62:138–147. PMID: 15850914.

Frumovitz M, Sun CC, Schover LR, et al. Quality of life and sexual functioning in cervical cancer survivors. *J Clin Oncol* 2005;23:7428–7436. PMID: 16234510.

Green JA, Kirwan JM, Tierney JF, et al. Survival and radiotherapy for cancer of the uterine cervix: A systematic review and meta-analysis. *Lancet* 2001;358:781–786. PMID: 11564482.

Greven KM, Corn BW. Endometrial cancer. *Curr Prob Cancer* 1997;21:65–127. PMID: 9128804.

Grigsby P, Russell A, Bruner D, et al. Late injury of cancer therapy on the female reproductive tract. *Int J Radiat Oncol Biol Phys* 1995;31:1289–1299. PMID: 7713788.

Hareyama M, Sakata K, Oouchi A, et al. High-dose-rate versus low-dose-rate intracavitary therapy for carcinoma of the uterine cervix: A randomized trial. *Cancer* 2002;94:117–124. PMID: 11815967.

Hasselle MD, Rose BS, Kochanski JD, et al. Clinical outcomes of intensity-modulated pelvic radiation therapy for carcinoma of the cervix. *Int J Radiat Oncol Biol Phys* 2010;80:1436–1445. PMID: 20708346.

Keys H, Bundy BN, Stehman FB, et al. Cisplatin, radiation, and adjuvant hysterectomy compared with radiation and adjuvant hysterectomy for bulky stage IB cervical carcinoma. *N Engl J Med* 1999;340:1154–1161. PMID: 10202166.

Kidd EA, Siegel BA, Dehdashti F, et al. Clinical outcomes of definitive intensity-modulated radiation therapy with fluorodeoxyglucose-positron emission tomography simulation in patients with locally advanced cervical cancer. *Int J Radiat Oncol Biol Phys* 2010;77:1085–1091. PMID: 19880262.

Klopp AH, Eifel PJ. Chemoradiotherapy for cervical cancer in 2010. *Curr Oncol Rep* 2010;13:77–85. PMID: 21042887.

Landoni F, Maneo A, Colombo A, et al. Randomised study of radical surgery versus radiotherapy for stage Ib-IIa cervical cancer. *Lancet* 1997;350:535–540. PMID: 9284774.

Lertsanguansinchai P, Lertbutsayanukul C, Shotelersuk K, et al. Phase III randomized trial comparing LDR and HDR brachytherapy in treatment of cervical carcinoma. *Int J Radiat Oncol Biol Phys* 2004;59:1424–1431. PMID: 15275728.

Moore DH, Thomas GM, Montana GS, Saxer A, Gallup DG, Olt G. Preoperative chemoradiation for advanced vulvar cancer: A phase II study of the Gynecologic Oncology Group. *Int J Radiat Oncol Biol Phys* 1998;42:79–85. PMID: 9747823.

Morris M, Eifel PJ, Lu J, et al. Pelvic radiation with concurrent chemotherapy compared with pelvic and para-aortic radiation for high-risk cervical cancer. *N Engl J Med* 1999;340:1137–1143. PMID: 10202164.

Nag S, Chao C, Erickson B, et al. The American Brachytherapy Society recommendations for low-dose-rate brachytherapy for carcinoma of the cervix. *Int J Radiat Oncol Biol Phys* 2002;52:33–48. PMID: 11777620. [Erratum: *Int J Radiat Oncol Biol* Phys 2002;52:1157.]

Nag S, Erickson B, Thomadsen B, Orton C, Demanes JD, Petereit D. The American Brachytherapy Society recommendations for high-dose-rate brachytherapy for carcinoma of the cervix. *Int J Radiat Oncol Biol Phys* 2000;48:201–211. PMID: 10924990.

National Institutes of Health Consensus Development Conference Statement on Cervical Cancer. *Gynecol Oncol* 1997;66:351–361. PMID: 9312522.

Okada M, Kigawa J, Minagawa Y, et al. Indication and efficacy of radiation therapy following radical surgery in patients with stage IB to IIB cervical cancer. *Gynecol Oncol* 1998;70:61–64. PMID: 9698475.

Peters WA 3rd, Liu PY, Barrett RJ 2nd, et al. Concurrent chemotherapy and pelvic radiation therapy compared with pelvic radiation therapy alone as adjuvant therapy after radical surgery in high-risk early-stage cancer of the cervix. *J Clin Oncol* 2000;18:1606–1613. PMID: 10764420.

Pickel H, Lahousen M, Petru E, et al. Consolidation radiotherapy after carboplatin-based chemotherapy in radically operated advanced ovarian cancer. *Gynecol Oncol* 1999;72:215–219. PMID: 10021304.

Pinilla J. Cost minimization analysis of high-dose-rate versus low-dose-rate brachytherapy in endometrial cancer. *Int J Radiat Oncol Biol Phys* 1998;42:87–90. PMID: 9747824.

Rose P, Bundy BN, Watkins EB, et al. Concurrent cisplatin-based radiotherapy and chemotherapy for locally advanced cervical cancer. *N Engl J Med* 1999;340:1144–1153. PMID: 10202165.

Thomas G, Dembo A, Ackerman I, et al. A randomized trial of standard versus partially hyper-fractionated radiation with or without concurrent 5-fluorouracil in locally advanced cervical cancer. *Gynecol Oncol* 1998;69:137–145. PMID: 9600821.

US Department of Health and Human Services. *Concurrent Chemoradiation for Cervical Cancer*. Bethesda, MD: National Cancer Institute Clinical Announcement; February 1999.

Wang X, Liu R, Ma B, et al. High dose rate versus low dose rate intracavity brachytherapy for locally advanced uterine cervix cancer. *Cochrane Database Syst Rev*. 2010:CD007563. PMID: 20614461.

Young RC, Brady MF, Nieberg RK, et al. Adjuvant treatment for early ovarian cancer: A randomized phase III trial of intraperitoneal ^{32}P or intravenous cyclophosphamide and cisplatin—A Gynecologic Oncology Group study. *J Clin Oncol* 2003;21:4350–4355. PMID: 14645424.

Infertility

53

Shahin Ghadir, MD
Gayane Ambartsumyan, MD, PhD
Alan H. DeCherney, MD

ESSENTIALS OF DIAGNOSIS

- Both male and female evaluation are needed to reach diagnosis.
- Male partner:
  - History
  - Semen analysis
  - If semen analysis abnormal, referral to urology, endocrine evaluation, and karyotyping in severe cases
  - State-mandated infectious disease panel if treatment includes intrauterine insemination or in vitro fertilization
- Female partner:
  - History, confirm ovulation
  - Physical exam to assess cervix, uterus, and adnexa for pathology
  - Cycle day 3 blood work and ultrasound to assess ovarian reserve
  - Hysterosalpingogram to evaluate uterine cavity and fallopian tubes
  - Possible saline sonogram to evaluate uterine cavity
  - Laparoscopy to assess endometriosis when indicated
  - State-mandated infectious disease panel if undergoing in vitro fertilization

The number of infertility visits has increased over the past decades. In some cases, couples have voluntarily delayed childbearing in favor of establishing careers and may experience an age-related decline in fertility. There have been significant advances in assisted reproductive technologies (ART), from improved embryo culture media to intracytoplasmic sperm injection (ICSI) and preimplantation genetic diagnosis (PGD), which have resulted in remarkable increases in in vitro fertilization–embryo transfer (IVF-ET) pregnancy rates. These advances coupled with increasing public awareness and acceptance of ART have spurred women or couples with infertility to seek medical care.

Definition

Infertility is defined as the inability of a couple to conceive within 1 year. **Sterility** implies an intrinsic inability to achieve pregnancy, whereas infertility implies a decrease in the ability to conceive and is synonymous with **subfertility. Primary infertility** applies to those who have never conceived, whereas **secondary infertility** designates those who have conceived at some time in the past.

Fecundity is the probability of achieving a live birth in 1 menstrual cycle. **Fecundability** is expressed as the likelihood of conception per month of exposure. Fertility, as well as infertility, of a woman or couple is best perceived as fecundability, as few infertile patients are sterile. It also allows for a direct comparison of treatment options over a more functional time frame.

The prevalence of women diagnosed with infertility is approximately 13%, with a range from 7 to 28%, depending on the age of the woman. It has remained stable over the past 40 years; ethnicity or race appears to have little effect on prevalence. However, the incidence of primary infertility has increased, with a concurrent decrease in secondary infertility, most likely as a result of social changes such as delayed childbearing.

In normal fertile couples having frequent intercourse, the fecundability is estimated to be approximately 20–25%. Approximately 85–90% of couples with unprotected intercourse will conceive within 1 year. Sterility affects 1–2% of couples.

PATHOGENESIS

Infertility can be due to either partner or both. Overall, an etiology for infertility can be found in 80% of cases with an even distribution of male and female factors, including couples with multiple factors. A primary diagnosis of male factor is made in approximately 25% of cases. Ovulatory dysfunction and tubal/peritoneal factors comprise the majority of female factor infertility. In 15–20% of infertile couples, the etiology cannot be found, and a diagnosis of unexplained infertility is made.

PREVENTION

Prevention of infertility is difficult to achieve and thus discuss, as a couple isn't really aware of the diagnosis until they try to achieve pregnancy. Although difficult to do, there are a few steps one can take to possibly decrease risk of infertility.

Although infertility is defined as the failure to achieve pregnancy after 12 months or more, earlier evaluation may be justified depending on one's history and is warranted for women over the age of 35. Because fertility is related to aging in women and perhaps in men after the age of 50, one should be aware of these risks when considering delaying childbearing. Therefore, it is the responsibility of the primary care provider or gynecologist to openly discuss fertility and aging during a well-woman visit. The new techniques of oocyte cryopreservations hold a great promise for women who would like to delay childbearing and should be addressed with women to increase awareness.

Weight extremes have also been associated with infertility in women, mainly due to anovulation. Thus a healthy lifestyle may improve fertility for women with ovulatory dysfunction. However, beyond what has been mentioned previously, there is little evidence that dietary variations enhance fertility. Women should also be advised to take folic acid supplement (at least 400 μg daily) when trying to conceive.

Smoking has a substantial adverse effect on female fertility demonstrated by a recent meta-analysis and also causes abnormalities in male semen parameters. Thus couples who smoke and are trying to conceive should be advised accordingly. Moderate alcohol and caffeine consumption has no adverse effect on fertility; however. higher levels of alcohol and recreational drugs should be discouraged for couples trying to conceive.

Lastly, couples trying to conceive should be advised to avoid using vaginal lubricants as these can be toxic to sperm based on their effect demonstrated in vitro. If needed, it may be better to recommend mineral oil, canola oil, or hydroxyethylcellulose-based lubricants.

Practice Committee of the American Society for Reproductive Medicine. Smoking and infertility. *Fertil Steril* 2006;86:S172–S177. PMID: 17055816.

DIFFERENTIAL DIAGNOSIS & CLINICAL FINDINGS

The armamentarium of diagnostic tests available for the evaluation of an infertile couple is large. Therefore, a clinician should be judicious in his/her use of tests. The history and physical exam shape the endocrinologic and radiologic testing algorithm specific to each patient. Other factors to consider include patient age, risks associated with the test, invasiveness, expense, and probabilities of significant findings (Table 53–1). The patient(s) should be included in the decision-making process.

New Patient Assessment

The initial aspect of the interview includes discussion of the factors (ie, ovulation, sperm concentration, ovarian reserve, etc.) that affect fertility so that the patient(s) is aware of the potential etiologies. In this light, the physician can present an algorithm for the diagnostic evaluation that the patient will understand. This will help the patient grasp the peculiarities of the specific tests, such as timing the hysterosalpingogram to the day of the menstrual cycle, and provide an opportunity for the patient(s) to ask fertility-related questions and to address any information learned from friends, family, or the Internet.

The initial clinical assessment should begin with a thorough history of both partners. Factors to consider while obtaining the medical history are outlined in Table 53–2 for the female and in Table 53–3 for the male. The history should guide the physical examination beyond the general evaluation; for example, a rectovaginal exam to detect uterosacral ligament nodularity associated with endometriosis is indicated if a woman presents with a history of severe dysmenorrhea. However, a thorough physical exam may divulge key information such as acanthosis nigricans and its association with insulin resistance.

The laboratory and radiologic tests assess 4 key aspects for fertility in a couple: the sperm (male factor), the oocyte (ovulatory factor and ovarian reserve), transport (pelvic factor including fallopian tubes), and implantation of ova (uterus). In many cases, the couple will be attempting to absorb significant amounts of information, some of which may be highly technical, at a time of heightened emotion. It is therefore helpful to offer literature or a written summary of the discussion. Frequently, the initial history will indicate a probable diagnosis or a contributing cause of infertility, but it is important to complete a basic evaluation of all of the major factors so a secondary diagnosis is not ignored.

Evaluation of Male Partner

Male factor is diagnosed in 25–40% of infertile couples. The majority of the diagnoses involve testicular pathology such as varicocele. Although validation is incomplete, there is a trend toward increasing use of molecular techniques to quantify the fertility potential of semen as our knowledge of fundamental molecular genetics expands. Experience and investigation have relegated several tests previously used to assess fertilization to historical interest. Beyond the history and physical exam, the initial evaluation of male factor is through semen analysis. If abnormal, the semen analysis should be repeated in 4 weeks or more to confirm findings. Normal semen analysis excludes any important male factor,

Table 53–1. Causes of infertility.

Male Factor	
Endocrine disorders	
	Hypothalamic dysfunction (Kallmann's syndrome)
	Pituitary failure (tumor, radiation, surgery)
	Hyperprolactinemia (drug, tumor)
	Exogenous androgens
	Thyroid disorders
	Adrenal hyperplasia
Anatomic disorders	
	Congenital absence of vas deferens
	Obstruction of vas deferens
	Congenital abnormalities of ejaculatory system
Abnormal spermatogenesis	
	Chromosomal abnormalities
	Mumps orchitis
	Cryptorchidism
	Chemical or radiation exposure
Abnormal motility	
	Absent cilia (Kartagener's syndrome)
	Varicocele
	Antibody formation
Sexual dysfunction	
	Retrograde ejaculation
	Impotence
	Decreased libido
Ovulatory Factor	
Central defects	
	Chronic hyperandrogenemic anovulation
	Hyperprolactinemia (drug, tumor, empty selia)
	Hypothalamic insufficiency
	Pituitary insufficiency (trauma, tumor, congenital)
Ovulatory Factor (cont.)	
Peripheral defects	
	Gonadal dysgenesis
	Premature ovarian failure
	Ovarian tumor
	Ovarian resistance
Metabolic disease	
	Thyroid disease
	Liver disease
	Renal disease
	Obesity
	Androgen excess, adrenal or neoplastic
Pelvic Factor	
Infection	
	Appendicitis
	Pelvic inflammatory disease
	Uterine adhesions (Asherman's syndrome)
Endometriosis	
Structural abnormalities	
	Diethylstilbestrol (DES) exposure
	Failure of normal fusion of the reproductive tract
	Myoma
Cervical Factor	
Congenital	
	DES exposure
	Müllerian duct abnormality
Acquired	
	Surgical treatment
	Infection

Table 53–2. Medical history for female factor infertility.

In utero diethylstilbestrol (DES) exposure
History of pubertal development
Present menstrual cycle characteristics (length, duration, molimina)
Contraceptive history
Prior pregnancies, outcomes
Previous surgeries, especially pelvic
Prior infection
History of abnormal Papanicolaou (Pap) smear, treatment
Drugs and medications
General health (diet, weight stability, exercise patterns, review of systems)

whereas abnormal semen analysis suggests the need for further evaluation (endocrine, urological, or genetic).

A. Semen Analysis

The male partner should abstain from coitus for 2–5 days before collecting the sample, and the specimen should be received in the lab within 1 hour of collection. Table 53–4 lists normal sperm values. If fundamental parameters of count and motility are normal, the assessment of the morphology of the sperm becomes more critical. Specialized expertise in determining sperm morphology and strict application of criteria should be used before declaring the semen normal.

The semen parameters in normal fertile males may vary significantly over time, and the first response to any abnormal result should be to wait an interval of several weeks and repeat the test. A normal semen analysis will usually exclude significant male factor. Although low counts, decreased motility, and increased numbers of abnormal forms are most frequently associated with infertility, unfavorable semen parameters may still be found in 20% of males undergoing vasectomy after having completed their families. If the semen analysis reveals abnormal or borderline parameters, the history should be reviewed for any proximate cause of an abnormality, keeping in mind that the cycle of spermatogenesis takes approximately 74 days. A male with <5 million sperm per milliliter warrants an endocrinologic evaluation including follicle-stimulating hormone (FSH), luteinizing hormone (LH), and testosterone, or a karyotype in selected cases. The patient should be referred to a urologist with a special interest and expertise in infertility as indicated.

Table 53–3. Medical history for male factor infertility.

Congenital abnormalities
Undescended testes
Prior paternity
Frequency of intercourse
Exposure to toxins
Previous surgery
Previous infections, treatment
Drugs and medications
General health (diet, exercise, review of systems)
Decreased frequency of shaving

Table 53–4. Normal semen parameters.

Liquefaction	30 minutes
Count	20 million/mL or more
Motility	>50%
Volume	2 mL or more
Morphology	
WHO criteria	>30% normal
Kruger Strict Criteria	>14% normal
pH	7.2–7.8
White blood cell count	<1 million/mL

B. DNA Assays

Several tests, including sperm chromatin structure assay (SCSA), comet, and terminal deoxyuridine triphosphate (dUTP) nick-end labeling (TUNEL), have been developed to quantify the damage to DNA or chromatin (packaged DNA). There is some evidence associating increased DNA damage as determined by these tests with poor fertility outcome. The SCSA determines the percent of chromatin that is fragmented by exposing sperm DNA to acid denaturation (fragmented DNA is more vulnerable). Clinical experience has not matched initial expectations, although the test may be useful for couples with unexplained infertility with repeated in vitro fertilization (IVF) failures. The comet assay consists of placing the sperm DNA on gel electrophoresis; DNA with increased strand breaks will be smaller and therefore travel further on the slide. The TUNEL assay identifies DNA strand breaks by their incorporation of labeled dUTP. The comet and TUNEL assay are not in wide clinical use.

C. Other Tests

More detailed assessment of sperm function may include postcoital test, antibody studies, a sperm penetration assay (hamster egg penetration assay). Such assessments are designed to investigate more subtle problems or abnormalities of function not revealed by the assessment of sperm number and motility. Although helpful in some cases, the sensitivity of these assays in detecting fertility is still uncertain and varies with the particular laboratory where the test is performed. Because no universal methodology has yet been accepted, the interpretation of these tests requires close communication with the laboratory selected.

Cervical mucus is a heterogeneous secretion containing more than 90% water. It has intrinsic properties including consistency, spinnbarkeit (stretchability), and ferning. When mucus is obtained from the cervical canal in the preovulatory phase, it normally exhibits a response to the high estrogen environment. The mucus is thin, watery, and acellular; it dries in a crystalline pattern (ferning), and acts as a facilitative reservoir for the sperm.

The functional sperm must interact normally with the egg and surrounding cells in the uterine tube. The normal migration of sperm is affected by attrition and filtering, and it is estimated that fewer than 1000 sperm will be found in the environment of the oocyte. The initial interaction of sperm and female genital tract can be determined by postcoital examination of the cervical mucus (Sims-Huhner test).

The purpose of the postcoital test is to determine the number of active spermatozoa in the cervical mucus and the length of sperm survival (in hours) after coitus. The test should be performed as close to ovulation as possible, but not after. The test involves aspirating cervical mucus with a syringe 6–8 hours after coitus and checking under a microscope for the number and the motility of the sperm; fewer than 10 motile sperm per high-power field is considered abnormal. The postcoital test is controversial and has limited use in the infertility workup. Its value in assessing cervical hostility to sperm has never been proven.

Tests developed to predict the fertilizing ability of sperm include the zona-free hamster egg penetration test (the sperm penetration assay) and the hemizona test. These assays compare the ability of sperm to penetrate the zona-free hamster egg (a hamster egg in which the zona pellucida has been enzymatically digested) or to bind to human zona with sperm from a known fertile donor. The value of these tests remains controversial, and they are not in general clinical use.

Sperm possess antigens and semen may contain antibodies including sperm-agglutinating, sperm-immobilizing, or cytotoxic antibodies. The antibodies can be measured in semen or in serum. The immunobead test is the antibody assay used in most labs and is considered positive when only 20% or more of motile spermatozoa have immunobead binding. However, the test is considered to be clinically significant when 50% of sperm are coated with immunobeads.

Evaluation of Female Partner

A. Ovulatory Factor

An ovulatory dysfunction is responsible for approximately 20–25% of infertility cases (~40% of female factor infertility). The problem should be investigated first by review of historical factors, including the onset of menarche, present cycle length (intermenstrual interval), and presence or absence of premenstrual symptoms (molimina), such as breast tenderness, bloating, or dysmenorrhea. Signs and symptoms of systemic disease, particularly of hyperthyroidism or hypothyroidism, and physical signs of endocrine disease (ie, hirsutism, galactorrhea, and obesity) should be noted. The degree and intensity of exercise, a history of weight loss, and complaints of hot flushes all are clinical clues to possible endocrine or ovulatory dysfunction.

1. Follicular pool—Early in gestation, the germ cells undergo mitosis to produce oogonia. The oogonia undergo meiosis in their transformation to oocytes but arrest at prophase of meiosis I until the time of ovulation. A layer of granulosa cells encircles the oocytes, creating the follicle. A female will have the highest number of germ cells, approximately 6 million, in her ovaries at 20 weeks' gestational age. Henceforth, atresia depletes the follicular pool at a brisk pace, with only 1–2 million oocytes remaining at the time of birth. The ovaries contain approximately 500,000 oocytes at the time of first ovulation. Menopause signals the complete depletion of germ cells, with a woman having ovulated approximately 500 oocytes during her reproductive years.

2. Ovarian reserve—An inverse relationship exists between fecundity and the age of the woman. The decline in fecundity is a result of progressive follicular atresia through apoptosis, which accelerates in the early thirties and progresses rapidly in the late thirties and early forties. Concomitantly, there is a decrease in follicular quality as a result of an increase in oocytes with chromosomal anomalies and progressive deletions in mitochondrial DNA. The concept of ovarian reserve represents the remaining follicular pool of the ovaries. As ovarian reserve decreases, the ovaries' responsiveness to gonadotropins decreases, necessitating higher amounts of FSH to achieve follicular growth and maturation.

Ovarian reserve should be evaluated in women older than 35 years of age who are seeking fertility. Evaluation of the level of FSH and estradiol in the early follicular phase (cycle days 2–4) may provide helpful guidance in terms of the likelihood of achieving success, as mild elevations in either FSH or estradiol may precede overt ovulatory dysfunction but still indicate a poor prognosis for successful pregnancy. Use of the clomiphene challenge test has gone out of favor, whereas newer tests such as inhibin-B and anti-müllerian hormone (AMH) remain to be validated in large studies. The specific cause of oligo-ovulation or anovulation is determined by the history, the physical examination, and appropriate laboratory studies.

3. Confirmation of ovulation—If the patient reports a history of mittelschmerz and/or regular menses with molimina (headaches, bloating, cramping, and emotional lability) and mild dysmenorrhea occurring at intervals of 28–32 days, the likelihood of the patient having regular ovulatory cycles is very high. Otherwise, ovulation can be confirmed with a serum progesterone assay performed in the mid-luteal phase or the third week of the cycle. Progesterone levels of 3 ng/mL or greater are consistent with ovulation.

Pelvic **ultrasonography** can provide evidence for ovulation. In the follicular phase, the developing follicle can be monitored to maturation and subsequent rupture. The disappearance of, or change in, the follicle and free fluid in the cul-de-sac can document ovulation.

To detect the LH surge, the patient can use commercially available urinary LH kits or serum LH assay. Ovulation occurs 24–36 hours after the onset of the LH surge and 10–12 hours after the peak of the LH surge. The kits can be used to time intercourse or intrauterine insemination.

The **basal body temperature** (BBT) is the temperature obtained in the resting state and should be taken shortly after awakening in the morning after at least 6 hours of sleep and before ambulating. Progesterone has a central thermogenic effect; it elevates the BBT by an average of 0.8 °F during the luteal phase. The luteal phase is thus characterized by a temperature elevation lasting about 10 days. When a biphasic monthly temperature pattern is recorded, it is confirmatory evidence of luteinization, but the absence of a biphasic pattern may be seen in ovulatory cycles.

The finding of secretory endometrium confirms ovulation. The use of an **endometrial biopsy** (EMB) near the end of the luteal phase can provide reassurance of an adequate maturational effect on the endometrial lining. Within 48 hours of ovulation, the **cervical mucus** changes under the influence of progesterone to become thick, tacky, and cellular, with loss of the crystalline fernlike pattern on drying.

The only absolute documentation of release of an oocyte is pregnancy. In the case of oligomenorrhea, amenorrhea, short or very irregular menstrual cycles, or when ovulation is not confirmed, evaluation of the hypothalamic–pituitary–ovarian axis is warranted. A usual initial assessment includes the serum concentrations of FSH, estradiol, prolactin, and thyroid-stimulating hormone.

4. Luteal phase defect—The subject of the inadequate luteal phase remains an area of controversy. There is disagreement on how to make the diagnosis, when the diagnosis is significant, and how best to treat the problem if diagnosed. Luteal phase defect is a histologic diagnosis made when the endometrium lags 3 days or more behind the expected pattern at the time of EMB. EMB to assess luteal phase defect is rarely performed nowadays due to high levels of variability in histologic diagnosis.

B. The Pelvic Factor

The pelvic factor includes abnormalities of the uterus, fallopian tubes, ovaries, and adjacent pelvic structures. Factors in the **history** that are suggestive of a pelvic factor include any history of pelvic infection, such as pelvic inflammatory disease or appendicitis, use of intrauterine devices, endometritis, and septic abortion. Endometriosis is included as a pelvic factor in infertility and may be suggested by worsening dysmenorrhea, dyspareunia, or previous surgical reports. Any history of ectopic pregnancy, adnexal surgery, leiomyomas, or exposure to diethylstilbestrol (DES) in utero should be noted as possibly contributory to the diagnosis of a pelvic factor. A **pelvic examination** can be informative, yielding information such as a fixed uterus suggestive of adhesions, leiomyomas, or adnexal masses.

A transvaginal **ultrasound** examination can be an efficient means of supplementing information gained from the standard bimanual examination. Hydrosalpinges, leiomyoma, and ovarian cysts, including endometriomas, can often be observed, and the appropriate focused evaluations initiated.

A **hysterosalpingogram** (HSG) is a fluoroscopic study performed by instilling radiopaque dye into the uterine cavity through a catheter to determine the contour of the endometrial cavity and patency of the fallopian tubes. Sensitivity and specificity of an HSG are approximately 65% and 85%, respectively. Abnormal findings include congenital malformations of the uterus, submucous leiomyomas, intrauterine synechiae (Asherman's syndrome), intrauterine polyps, salpingitis isthmica nodosa, and proximal or distal tubal occlusion. The hysterosalpingogram can be obtained in an outpatient setting with minimal analgesia consisting of premedication with a nonsteroidal anti-inflammatory drug. The test is usually scheduled for the interval after menstrual bleeding and before ovulation. Either water- or oil-based dye may be selected; Table 53–5 summarizes the advantages and disadvantages of each. There is evidence for a fertility-enhancing effect of HSG using the oil-based dye.

Peritonitis is a risk of the procedure observed in up to 1–3% of patients; many clinicians use a short-course doxycycline during the immediate period before and after the procedure to minimize risk. An HSG is contraindicated in the presence of an adnexal mass or an allergy to iodine or radiocontrast dye.

A sonohysterogram, a transvaginal ultrasound of the uterus with instillation of saline into the uterine cavity, is a sensitive and specific test for the detection of intrauterine lesions, specifically space-occupying lesions. Hysterosalpingo contrast sonography, transcervical injection of sonopaque material during ultrasonography, is used to determine tubal

Table 53–5. Comparison of oil-based versus water-based dye used in the hysterosalpingogram.

Fertility enhancement	Oil: higher pregnancy rates
Patient discomfort	Water: less cramping
Image quality	Water: rugae seen Oil: better image
Embolization	Minimal risk with either dye
Granuloma	Greater risk for retained oil

patency as well as detect intrauterine defects; more commonly used in Europe, the procedure's sensitivity is comparable to that of HSG.

Laparoscopy with chromotubation (dye instillation) is the gold standard for the evaluation of tubal factor, and when performed in conjunction with hysteroscopy, information on uterine contour can be obtained simultaneously. Tubal abnormalities such as agglutinated fimbria or adhesions (which restrict motion of the tubes) or peritubal cysts may suggest tubal disease that would not necessarily be detected on hysterosalpingogram. The diagnosis of endometriosis is usually based on laparoscopic findings.

The necessity of laparoscopy in an infertility workup is controversial. There is significant evidence that pelvic pathology may exist in almost one-third of patients with normal HSG and ultrasound; consequently, some believe that with laparoscopy one can treat the pathology (such as adhesions) found at the time of procedure or can spare a patient needless cycles of ovulation induction that are unlikely to succeed by providing knowledge of severe pelvic disease. Others believe that although pelvic disease may be present, a stepwise empiric approach is more cost-effective.

C. The Cervical Factor

A cervical factor may be indicated by a history of abnormal Papanicolaou (Pap) smears, postcoital bleeding, cryotherapy, conization, or DES exposure in utero. The major evaluation of the cervical factor is by speculum examination, which may reveal evidence of cervicitis that may require further evaluation and treatment, or cervical stenosis, especially in a patient with prior history of cervical conization. If none of these findings are present, it is unlikely that cervical mucous presents a major obstacle. The postcoital test has been part of the assessment of cervical factor for many years in the past; however, the current consensus is that it is no longer required due to high variability in its methodology and interpretation. Moreover, treatment for otherwise unexplained infertility generally is a combination of ovarian stimulation and intrauterine insemination (IUI), which therefore bypasses the cervical factor. Therefore, postcoital test may only be reserved for patients in whom results will actually influence the treatment strategy.

Combined Factors & Unexplained Infertility

After the completion of the diagnostic workup, the findings should be reviewed with the patients and a treatment plan finalized based on guidance from the physician and input from the patient(s). In approximately 20% of couples, a combination of factors found may be suboptimal, and multiple therapies may need to be instigated, either sequentially or simultaneously.

Diagnosis of unexplained infertility, on the other hand, generally implies normal uterine cavity, bilateral patent tubes, normal semen analysis, and evidence of ovulation. Postcoital tests and endometrial biopsy are no longer necessary in order to diagnose unexplained infertility. For the couple with unexplained infertility, an empiric stepwise approach is an excellent option. However, depending on the history, workup, and individual situation, additional test(s) including surgery to rule out endometriosis should be discussed.

Coutifaris C, Myers ER, Guzick DS, et al. NICHD National Cooperative Reproductive Medicine Network. Histological dating of timed endometrial biopsy tissue is not related to fertility status. *Fertil Steril* 2004;82:1264–1272. PMID: 15533340.

Domingues TS, Rocha AM, Serafini PC. Tests for ovarian reserve: reliability and utility. *Curr Opin Obstet Gynecol* 2010;22:271–276. PMID: 20543692.

Jacobson TZ, Duffy JM, Barlow D, Farquhar C, Koninckx PR, Olive D. Laparoscopic surgery for subfertility associated with endometriosis. *Cochrance Database Syst Rev* 2010;20:1398. PMID: 20091519.

Practice Committee of the American Society for Reproductive Medicine. Definitions of infertility and recurrent pregnancy loss. *Fertil Steril* 2008:89:1603. PMID: 18485348.

The Practice Committee of American Society of Reproductive Medicine. Optimal evaluation of infertile female. Birmingham, AL: American Society of Reproductive Medicine; 2006.

TREATMENT

Male Factor Infertility

Treatment options progress from least to most invasive or use of donor sperm. Mild to moderate disease can be treated with **intrauterine insemination** (IUI). Before the insemination, the semen is prepared to select for highly motile sperm, concentrate sperm, and remove seminal fluid (with prostaglandins). The prepared sperm is transcervically injected into the uterus.

ICSI is used in conjunction with IVF for treatment of severe disease (<2 million motile sperm or <4% normal sperm). In this procedure, a sperm is individually injected into each oocyte. The sperm can be retrieved from the testes by microsurgical epididymal sperm aspiration (MESA) or testicular sperm aspiration (TESA); a minimum number of sperm is necessary.

Indications for ICSI include poor semen analysis parameters (low number of motile sperm, poor morphology), fertilization failure with standard IVF, and spermatozoal defects leading to poor fertilization. A decade of experience with the procedure has proven its overall safety. However, offspring conceived using ICSI may be at increased risk of imprinting disorders (eg, Angelman's syndrome), and male children are at risk for inheriting the genetic disorder (eg, Y chromosome microdeletions) that rendered their father infertile.

The initial evaluation of FSH, LH, testosterone, and prolactin helps to differentiate between obstructive defects, primary hypogonadism (testicular defect), and secondary hypogonadism (hypothalamic or pituitary). **Obstructive defects** may be addressed through surgical reanastomosis or through retrieval of sperm via MESA or TESA for use with ICSI. **Retrograde ejaculation** can be treated with alpha sympathomimetics or urine can be centrifuged to collect sperm for IUI. Patients with **primary hypogonadism** should have a karyotype, as Klinefelter's syndrome (47,XXY) is the most common etiology.

Secondary hypogonadism, or hypogonadotropic hypogonadism, may be a result of a pituitary lesion such as prolactinoma or a hypothalamic etiology such as Kallmann's syndrome. Most prolactinomas respond to medical management. Pulsatile gonadotropin-releasing hormone (GnRH) administration with a pump or FSH replacement restores testosterone and sperm production in disorders leading to hypogonadotropic hypogonadism.

A **varicocele** is a dilatation of scrotal veins in the pampiniform plexus and is postulated to impair fertility through elevation of scrotal temperature. A clinical varicocele is one that is detected by examination and is present in 15% of men. Subclinical varicoceles can be detected by ultrasound or venography. There is contradicting evidence regarding whether ligation of clinical varicoceles leads to improved pregnancy rates; infertility is a questionable indication for the correction of subclinical varicoceles.

When male infertility is not amenable to therapy, **donor sperm** for insemination or IVF offers an opportunity for pregnancy. The use of donor sperm is common in clinical practice, and experience has lessened some of the medical, emotional, ethical, and legal issues. The American Society for Reproductive Medicine (ASRM) advocates use of frozen semen to reduce risk of transmission of infectious disease.

Female Factor Infertility

A. The Ovulatory Factor

The treatment and success of specific ovulatory disorders is determined by the age of the patient and the etiology of the anovulation. A stepwise approach, from least to most invasive (and expensive), usually starts with clomiphene citrate and progresses to ovulation induction with gonadotropins and, ultimately, IVF. The risk to the patient, cost of therapy, and fecundability increase with each step closer to IVF. If premature ovarian failure or early menopause is the etiology, the options include oocyte or embryo donation.

Induction of ovulation can be accomplished in 90–95% of patients with chronic anovulation, normal ovarian reserve, and absence of other endocrine abnormalities (eg, hyperprolactinemia or hypothyroidism). Clomiphene citrate is the agent of choice for women younger than 36 years of age with oligomenorrhea or amenorrhea and normal FSH, including women with polycystic ovary syndrome (PCOS). Clomiphene citrate blocks the feedback inhibition of estradiol on the hypothalamus and pituitary, leading to an increase in endogenous FSH. It is administered orally for 5 days starting on day 3–5 of the cycle; approximately half of the patients will ovulate at 50 mg/d and another 25% at 100 mg/d. Ultrasonographic and hormonal monitoring of follicular development is an option, which provides more information and allows greater control of the cycle. After a regimen has achieved ovulation, 3 cycles with either timed intercourse or IUI should be attempted. Side effects with clomiphene are common, including hot flushes, emotional lability or depression, bloating, and visual changes; most are mild and all disappear with discontinuation of the drug. The incidence of twin gestation is 8% and triplets or higher-order multiple pregnancy is <1%.

Aromatase inhibitor letrozole is an alternative option for patients who do not respond to clomiphene citrate or instead of clomiphene citrate. It was first used to induce ovulation in 2001. Letrozole works by inhibiting estrogen biosynthesis, thus releasing the hypothalamus/pituitary from negative feedback and increasing endogenous FSH secretion by the pituitary. It is also administered orally for 5 days starting on day 3–5. The starting dose is 2.5 mg, but studies have revealed improved response and higher pregnancy rates with 5 mg. The dose can be increased to up to 7.5 mg daily. As in the case of clomiphene citrate, ultrasound and hormonal monitoring is an option and may provide more information on individual response and how to proceed with future cycles. Letrozole has fewer side effects than clomiphene, and studies reveal at least similar if not better success rates than clomiphene. Lastly, letrozole has less thinning effect on the endometrium than clomiphene.

A patient in whom there is no response to clomiphene or letrozole, response but no pregnancy, pituitary insufficiency, or hypothalamic insufficiency should undergo ovulation induction with gonadotropins, often used in conjunction with IUI. Human menopausal gonadotropin (hMG) consists of FSH and LH isolated from the urine of postmenopausal women to various levels of purification (and LH content); recombinant FSH (rFSH) contains purely FSH. Gonadotropins are administered by subcutaneous (rFSH) or intramuscular injection (hMG), and the overall evidence indicates that the 2 preparations have similar efficacy.

Because of an increased risk of side effects such as multiple gestation and ovarian hyperstimulation syndrome (OHSS), the use of gonadotropins requires close monitoring with ultrasonography and estradiol levels. Consequently, it is more time-consuming and expensive than clomiphene or letrozole. The monitoring reveals both the number of developing follicles and their level of maturity. Mimicking the effects of the LH surge, human chorionic gonadotropins (hCG) is used to trigger ovulation. With perseverance, cumulative pregnancy rates of 45–90% can be achieved over 3–4 cycles with gonadotropin treatment; but even with careful monitoring there is a 25% risk of a multiple gestation. OHSS is a rare complication that occurs in <2% of cycles.

If pregnancy is not achieved with ovulation induction, IVF/embryo transfer (ET) is the next modality in the treatment algorithm. Development of the follicular cohort is induced with higher doses of FSH (hMG or rFSH). Follicular growth is monitored by ultrasonography and estradiol levels. When the leading follicles are mature, ovulation is triggered with hCG. The oocytes are retrieved from the follicles before ovulation by ultrasound-guided transvaginal aspiration of the follicular fluid. The oocytes are incubated with sperm for fertilization. Alternatively, ICSI is performed if male factor is also a concern. On average, several (from 1 to >3) embryos are transferred into the uterine cavity on day 3–5 after retrieval of the oocytes. OHSS is minimized by withholding hCG if there is a high number of follicles or elevated estradiol levels. Another option to limit the extent of OHSS is to cryopreserve the embryos for transfer at a later time, as pregnancy can prolong the course of OHSS.

When modification of lifestyle or body habitus does not successfully restore ovulation in the patient diagnosed with hypothalamic insufficiency, pulsatile GnRH is another viable option with high likelihood of restoring normal ovulation. Normal fertility is then restored during cycles of treatment, and most pregnancies occur within 3–6 cycles.

Hypothyroidism and hyperprolactinemia can lead to ovulatory dysfunction. Primary hypothyroidism leads to elevated thyroid-stimulating hormone levels, which is a secretogogue of prolactin. Elevated prolactin levels inhibit GnRH secretion, causing oligomenorrhea or amenorrhea. If elevated prolactin levels are detected in a woman with normal thyroid function, a full workup including thorough history (to rule out drugs such as psychotropics), physical exam (galactorrhea), and imaging (magnetic resonance imaging to rule out a prolactinoma or other central nervous system tumors) is likely to reveal the etiology. The elevated prolactin can be medically managed with dopamine agonist, leading to normalization of the cycle.

B. The Pelvic Factor

Adhesions resulting from **endometriosis** or **tubal occlusion** after salpingitis are 2 of the most common problems confronting infertile couples. With increasing pregnancy rates, IVF represents improved fecundability and lower risk over surgical repair except in unique circumstances. The role of surgical treatment is mostly limited to what can be accomplished at the time of diagnostic laparoscopy. There is some evidence to suggest that resection of mild endometriosis results in improved pregnancy rates. Laparoscopic resection or ablation of moderate or advanced endometriosis enhances fecundity in infertile women for the period immediately after surgery. Reversal of tubal sterilization is indicated in young women with adequate residual tubal length. Tubal interruption or resection increases IVF pregnancy rates in women with hydrosalpinx.

The role of **fibroids** in infertility is unclear, and most surgeons reserve myomectomy for treatment of recurrent abortion, repeated implantation failure, or with distortion of the endometrial cavity by a submucosal leiomyoma. The fibroids that distort the endometrial cavity are considered to be significant. These may be diagnosed by hysterosalpingogram, sonohysterogram, hysteroscopy, or magnetic resonance imaging.

C. The Cervical Factor

The absence of nurturing mucus at midcycle can be treated by bypassing the mucus with IUI. When the cervical mucus appears to be affected by cervicitis and inflammatory changes, some physicians advocate empiric treatment of patient and partner with doxycycline. When the cervix is altered by congenital malformation or past surgical treatment that has rendered endocervical glands absent or nonfunctional, IUI with washed sperm can be anticipated to result in pregnancy in 20–30% of patients per cycle in each of the first 3 cycles of treatment. Cervical factor patients who do not respond to these therapies can be offered IVF, gamete intrafallopian transfer (GIFT), or zygote intrafallopian transfer (ZIFT), although GIFT and ZIFT are now rarely used.

Unexplained Infertility

A diagnosis of unexplained infertility is assigned to couples with normal results of a standard infertility workup. The main treatment options include expectant observation with timed intercourse, ovarian stimulation with or without IUI, and IVF. Studies support the use of clomiphene with IUI for up to 4 cycles. The next step is usually hMG with intrauterine insemination for 3 cycles; if unsuccessful, IVF should be considered. The rationale for treatment with superovulation in women with documented ovulation is that by increasing the number of oocytes available, the likelihood of pregnancy is increased. In instances in which unexplained infertility may be the result of a fundamental defect in fertilization or in embryo transfer to the uterus, IVF may play a role in treatment. Donor oocytes or donor sperm may be considered in couples with continued difficulties in achieving pregnancy. For many, the hardest course to contemplate is no therapy at all.

French DB, Desai NR, Agarwal A. Varicocele repair: does it still have a role in infertility treatment? *Curr Opin Obstet Gynecol* 2008;20:269–274. PMID: 18460942.

Kolankaya A, Arici A. Myomas and assisted reproductive technologies: when and how to act? *Obstet Gynecol Clin North Am* 2006;33:145–152. PMID: 16504812.

Nadalini M, Tarozzi N, Distratis V, Scaravelli G, Borini A. Impact of intracytooplasmic morphologically selected sperm injection on assisted reproduction outcome: a review. *Reprod Biomed Online* 2009;19:45–55. PMID: 20034423.

The Practice Committee of American Society of Reproductive Medicine. The clinical utility of sperm DNA integrity testing. *Fertil Steril* 2008;90:S178–S180. PMID: 19007622.

Practice Committee of the American Society for Reproductive Medicine. Optimizing natural fertility. *Fertil Steril* 2008:90: S1–S6. PMID: 19007604.

Pritts EA. Letrozole for ovulation induction and controlled ovarian hyperstimulation. *Curr Opin Obstet Gynecol* 2010;22:289–294. PMID: 20592587.

Santos MA, Kuijk EW, Macklon NS. The impact of ovarian stimulation for IVF on the developing embryo. *Reproduction* 2010;139:23–24. PMID: 19710204.

World Health Organization. *WHO Laboratory Manual for the Examination and Processing of Human Semen*. 5th ed. Geneva: World Health Organization; 2010.

COMPLICATIONS

The major complication associated with ovarian stimulation is OHSS. It has a broad spectrum of disease, ranging from mild to extremely severe cases. The pathophysiology of the disease is due to increased capillary permeability resulting in fluid shift from the intravascular to extravascular spaces. Risk factors for OHSS include young age, PCOS, higher doses of gonadotropins, and high serum estradiol levels. Severe cases of hyperstimulation warrant very careful monitoring and hospitalization, as it can lead to electrolyte abnormalities, abnormal liver function tests, respiratory distress, and hyponatremia. There are several methods used nowadays in order to prevent OHSS, including gentler stimulation protocols, coasting until lower estradiol levels are achieved, and most recently, GnRH agonist instead of hCG trigger.

There is also a concern about a possible association between ovulation induction agents, specifically >12 cycles of clomiphene citrate, and **ovarian cancer**. The possibility that ovulation induction increases the risk of ovarian cancer remains unproven. Primary infertility and endometriosis are independent risk factors for ovarian cancer. Although additional investigation is necessary, the low incidence of ovarian cancer makes it difficult to design an adequate study to detect an association of infertility drugs with ovarian cancer.

PROGNOSIS

The success rates of treatment for infertility depends on a variety of factors, including cause of infertility, woman's age, duration of infertility, and treatment modality. Health insurance plans vary a great deal in the amount and type of infertility treatments that are covered. For those couples without infertility coverage, treatment choices are dictated by medical and financial considerations. Not uncommonly, infertility treatment does not actually make the difference between conceiving and not conceiving, but allows for conception in the more immediate future rather than at a delayed point of time (increasing fecundability).

Gelbaya TA. Short and long-term risks to women who conceive through in vitro fertilization. *Hum Fertil* 2010;13:19–27. PMID: 19929571.

Humaidan P, Quartarolo J, Papanikolaou EG. Preventing ovarian hyperstimulation syndrome; guidance for the clinician. *Fertil Steril* 2010;94:389–400. PMID: 20416867.

Amenorrhea

54

Alex Simon, MD
Wendy Y. Chang, MD
Alan H. DeCherney, MD

ESSENTIALS OF DIAGNOSIS

- Amenorrhea is literally defined as the absence of menses.
- **Primary amenorrhea** (seen in approximately 2.5% of the population) is clinically defined as the absence of menses by age 13 years in the absence of normal growth or secondary sexual development, or the absence of menses by age 15 years in the setting of normal growth and secondary sexual development.
  - Traditionally, evaluation was usually initiated by age 16 years if normal growth and secondary sexual characteristics were present, and at age 14 years if absent.
  - Because of secular trends toward earlier menarche over the past half century, the evaluation should begin at age 15 years, the age when more than 97% of girls should have experienced menarche.
  - The decision to evaluate should be made with a full understanding of the patient's clinical presentation.
  - Evaluation should not be delayed in the setting of neurologic symptoms (suggestive of hypothalamic-pituitary lesion) or pelvic pain (suggestive of outflow obstruction).
- **Secondary amenorrhea** is clinically defined as the absence of menses for more than 3 cycle intervals, or 6 consecutive months, in a previously menstruating woman.
  - The incidence of secondary amenorrhea can be quite variable, from 3% in the general population to 100% under conditions of extreme physical or emotional stress.
  - Table 54–1 lists the most common causes of secondary amenorrhea.

Pathogenesis

Menstruation has long been an important societal marker of female sexual development, as well as one of the most tangible signs of female endocrine and reproductive tract maturation. Regular and spontaneous menstruation requires (1) functional hypothalamic–pituitary–ovarian endocrine axis, (2) an endometrium competent to respond to steroid hormone stimulation, and (3) an intact outflow tract from internal to external genitalia.

The human menstrual cycle is susceptible to environmental influences and stressors. Thus missing a single or occasional menstruation rarely reflects a significant pathology. However, prolonged or persistent absence of menses may be one of the earliest signs of neuroendocrine or anatomic abnormality.

Diagnosing and treating amenorrhea is important because of the implications for future fertility; risks of unopposed estrogen, including endometrial hyperplasia and neoplasia; risks of hypoestrogenism, including osteoporosis and urogenital atrophy; and impact on psychosocial development. Because of their significant overlap in etiology and treatment, primary and secondary amenorrhea are discussed collectively in this chapter.

Pregnancy is the most common cause of amenorrhea and must be considered in every patient presenting for evaluation of amenorrhea. Amenorrhea caused by aberrations of the normal menstrual cycle is discussed in Chapter 4. Chapters 37 and 55 discuss developmental anomalies of the reproductive organs and masculinization, respectively. This chapter discusses amenorrhea associated with 46, XX and 46, XY karyotypes, anatomic defects, and dysfunction of the hypothalamic–pituitary–ovarian axis, as well as systemic disorders that affect menstruation.

Both primary and secondary amenorrhea can result from abnormalities in the compartments linked with the occurrence of menses. This includes the hypothalamic–pituitary axis, the ovaries, and the outflow tract, namely the uterus, cervix, and vagina.

Table 54–1. Causes of secondary amenorrhea.

Common
Pregnancy
Hypothalamic amenorrhea
Pituitary amenorrhea
Androgen disorders: polycystic ovarian syndrome, adult-onset adrenal hyperplasia
Galactorrhea-amenorrhea syndrome
Less Common
Premature ovarian failure
Asherman's syndrome
Sheehan's syndrome
Drug-induced amenorrhea
Rare
Diabetes
Hyperthyroidism or hypothyroidism
Cushing's syndrome or Addison's disease
Cirrhosis
Infection (tuberculosis, syphilis, encephalitis/meningitis, sarcoidosis)
Chronic renal failure
Malnutrition
Irradiation or chemotherapy
Hemosiderosis
Surgery

Clinical Findings

A. Hypothalamic–Pituitary Dysfunction

Gonadotropin-releasing hormone (GnRH)–secreting neurons of the hypothalamus originate in the olfactory bulb and migrate along the olfactory tract into the mediobasal hypothalamus and the arcuate nucleus. Under normal physiologic circumstances, the arcuate nucleus releases pulses of GnRH into the hypophyseal portal system approximately every hour. Discharge of GnRH releases luteinizing hormone (LH) and follicle-stimulating hormone (FSH) from the pituitary; LH and FSH, in turn, stimulate ovarian follicular growth and ovulation. The ovarian hormones estradiol and progesterone stimulate the development and shedding of the endometrium, culminating in the withdrawal bleeding of menses. Anovulation and amenorrhea occur as a result of interference with GnRH transport, GnRH pulse discharge, or congenital absence of GnRH (Kallmann's syndrome). Any of these situations leads to hypogonadotropic hypogonadism, resulting in amenorrhea.

1. Defects of GnRH transport—Interference with the transport of GnRH from the hypothalamus to the pituitary may occur with pituitary stalk compression or destruction of the arcuate nucleus. Pituitary stalk transsection from trauma, compression, radiation, tumors (craniopharyngioma, germinoma, glioma, teratomas), and infiltrative disorders (sarcoidosis, tuberculosis) may either destroy areas of the hypothalamus or prevent transport of hypothalamic hormones to the pituitary.

2. Defects of GnRH pulse production—The metabolic consequence of any significant reduction in the normal GnRH pulse frequency or amplitude is that little or no LH or FSH can be released, with the result that no ovarian follicles develop, virtually no estradiol is secreted, and the patient is amenorrheic. This is the biochemical status in normal prepubertal girls and those with constitutional delayed puberty, such as in anorexia nervosa, severe stress, extreme weight loss, or prolonged vigorous athletic exertion, and in hyperprolactinemia. Amenorrhea on this basis may also be an idiopathic phenomenon.

Less severe reductions in GnRH pulse amplitude and frequency result in diminished LH and FSH secretion with some follicular stimulation. The stimulation is insufficient to result in full follicular development and ovulation, but estradiol is secreted. This may occur with stress, hyperprolactinemia, as a result of vigorous athletic activity, or in the early stages of eating disorders. It may also be idiopathic.

Functional or hypothalamic amenorrhea results from abnormal hypothalamic GnRH secretion in the absence of pathologic processes. As a result, patients demonstrate decreased gonadotropin pulsations, absent follicular development and ovulation, and low estradiol secretion. Serum FSH levels are usually in the normal range; the setting of high FSH:LH ratio is consistent with prepubertal patterns. A number of environmental stressors are associated, including eating disorders and physical or psychologic stress. Weight loss, especially to a level of at least 10% below ideal body weight, and excessive exercise are also associated with hypothalamic amenorrhea. The female athlete triad syndrome is defined by amenorrhea, eating disorder, and osteopenia or osteoporosis.

Congenital GnRH deficiency is called idiopathic hypogonadotropic hypogonadism when it occurs as an isolated phenomenon and **Kallmann's syndrome** when it is associated with anosmia. These patients lack GnRH secretion and express low, prepubertal levels of serum gonadotropins. Follicular recruitment and ovulation do not occur. Although more than 60% of cases are sporadic, congenital GnRH deficiency can also be inherited in an autosomal dominant trait or X-linked recessive pattern.

Autosomal recessive mutations of the GnRH receptor gene have also been reported. This defect appears to produce a wider spectrum of physical symptoms than with the other gene defects, and the defect lies in the ability of the pituitary gland to recognize GnRH, rather than the ability of the hypothalamus to produce GnRH. It is debatable whether this is in fact Kallmann's syndrome, as the GnRH receptor development is not related to anosmia. More common in boys with delayed puberty, **constitutional delay** of puberty is an uncommon etiology of primary amenorrhea in girls. Patients demonstrate delayed adrenarche and gonadarche, but ultimately go on to have normal, albeit delayed, pubertal development.

B. Pituitary Defects

Pituitary causes of amenorrhea are rare; most are secondary to hypothalamic dysfunction. However, acquired pituitary dysfunction can ensue from previous local radiation or surgery. Excess iron deposition due to hemochromatosis or hemosiderosis may destroy gonadotropes.

1. Congenital pituitary dysfunction—Congenital absence of the pituitary is a rare and lethal condition. Isolated defects of LH or FSH production do occur (rarely), resulting in anovulation and amenorrhea.

2. Acquired pituitary dysfunction—Sheehan's syndrome, characterized by postpartum amenorrhea, results from postpartum pituitary necrosis secondary to severe hemorrhage and hypotension and is a rare cause of amenorrhea. Surgical ablation and irradiation of the pituitary as management of pituitary tumors also can cause amenorrhea.

Iron deposition in the pituitary may result in destruction of the cells that produce LH and FSH. This occurs only in patients with markedly elevated serum iron levels (ie, hemosiderosis), usually resulting from extensive red cell destruction. Thalassemia major is an example of a disease that causes hemosiderosis.

Pituitary microadenomas and macroadenomas also lead to amenorrhea because of elevated prolactin levels, but the mechanism(s) underlying this cause of amenorrhea are unclear. Isolated hyperprolactinemia in the absence of adenoma is an uncommon cause of primary amenorrhea. However, the diagnosis is strongly suggested by a history of galactorrhea. Diagnosis is readily made by evaluating a serum prolactin level. Drugs given to treat medical conditions may induce hyperprolactinemia to result in amenorrhea. Discontinuation of the medication if possible or adequate treatment to reduce prolactin level may solve the problem. Table 54–2 lists the most common drugs associated with hyperprolactinemia.

Hypothyroidism may also lead to elevated prolactin levels and thereby lead to amenorrhea.

Table 54–2. Drug-induced hyperprolactinemia.

Antipsychotic
Haloperidol
Chlorpromazine
Thioridazine
Thiothixene
Risperidone
Antidepressant
Tricyclics: Amitriptyline, desipramine, clomipramine, amoxapine
SSRI: Sertraline, fluoxetine, paroxetine
MAO-I: Pargyline, clorgyline
Prokinetics
Metoclopramide
Domperidone
Antihypertensive
Alpha-methyldopa
Reserpine
Verapamil
Opiates
Morphine
H2 Antagonists
Cimetidine
Ranitidine
Others
Fenfluramine
Physostigmine
Chemotherapeutics

C. Ovarian and Ovulatory Dysfunction

A variety of gonadal disorders can result in amenorrhea. The most common cause of primary amenorrhea is gonadal dysgenesis. This group of disorders is usually associated with sex chromosomal abnormalities, resulting in streak gonad development, premature depletion of ovarian follicles and oocytes, and absence of estradiol secretion. Patients usually present with hypergonadotropic amenorrhea regardless of degree of pubertal development. Primary ovarian failure is characterized by elevated gonadotropins and low estradiol (**hypergonadotropic hypogonadism**). Secondary ovarian failure is almost always caused by hypothalamic dysfunction and is characterized by normal or low gonadotropins and low estradiol (**hypogonadotropic hypogonadism**).

Table 54–3 lists the causes of primary ovarian failure.

1. Ovarian dysgenesis—If the primitive oogonia do not migrate to the genital ridge, the ovaries fail to develop. Streak gonads, which do not secrete hormones, develop instead, and the result is primary amenorrhea. Cytogenetic abnormalities of the X chromosome account for the majority of abnormal ovarian development and function, and studies show that 2 intact X chromosomes are required to maintain normal oocytes. Fetuses with 45,X karyotype demonstrate normal oocyte number at 20–24 weeks' gestation, but there is rapid atresia resulting in absence of oocytes at birth. Similarly, women with deletions in either the long or short arm of one X chromosome also develop either primary or secondary amenorrhea.

A. GONADAL DYSGENESIS WITH NO Y CHROMATIN—-Turner's syndrome (45,XO or 45,XO,XX mosaics) and 46,XX gonadal dysgenesis are the most common karyotypes. Patients with Turner's syndrome usually present with primary amenorrhea. However, some patients with mosaic abnormalities may menstruate briefly, and a few have conceived.

B. GONADAL DYSGENESIS WITH Y CHROMATIN—Normal female sexual differentiation depends on testicular secretion of antimüllerian hormone (AMH) by Sertoli cells and testosterone by Leydig cells. AMH causes regression of

Table 54–3. Causes of primary ovarian failure (hypergonadotrophic hypogonadism).

Idiopathic premature ovarian failure
Steroidogenic enzyme defects (primary amenorrhea) Cholesterol side-chain cleavage 3β-ol-dehydrogenase 17-hydroxylase 17-desmolase 17-ketoreductase
Testicular regression syndrome
True hermaphroditism
Gonadal dysgenesis Pure gonadal dysgenesis (Swyer's syndrome) (46,XY) Turner's syndrome (45,XO) Turner variants
Mixed gonadal dysgenesis
Ovarian resistance syndrome (Savage's syndrome)
Autoimmune oophoritis
Post infection (eg, mumps)
Post oophorectomy (also wedge resections and bivalving)
Post irradiation
Post chemotherapy

müllerian structures, whereas testosterone and its metabolite dihydrotestosterone (DHT) promote differentiation of male internal and external genitalia, respectively. A variety of disorders can result in the presentation of amenorrhea in phenotypic females possessing Y chromatin material.

The vanishing testes syndrome occurs in 46,XY males with failed gonadal development. Although anorchia commonly occurs at approximately 7 weeks' gestational age, the patient's presentation depends on the timing of gonadal regression. Failure occurring later in development might result in male genitalia at birth, but absence of puberty as a consequence of gonadal failure. On the other hand, typical early gonadal failure before testicular development would result in absent secretion of testis-determining factor (TDF) and AMH. These patients would demonstrate feminization of internal and external genitalia and primary amenorrhea.

Swyer's syndrome, which presents as a form of early-onset vanishing testes syndrome, results from a deletion mutation in the TDF region of Y chromosome. These patients possess the 46,XY genotype but do not secrete testosterone or AMH, resulting in feminization of internal and external genitalia. Patients present with primary amenorrhea and gonadal failure. The syndrome is diagnosed by DNA hybridization studies showing abnormality in the short arm of the Y chromosome.

2. Premature Ovarian Failure—Menopause occurs when the ovaries fail secondary to depletion of ova. If this occurs before age 40 years, it is considered premature and affects 1–5% of women. It is marked by amenorrhea, increased gonadotropin levels, and estrogen deficiency. Woman presented with premature ovarian failure (POF) should be tested for karyotype to rule out sex chromosome translocations, short arm deletions, or the presence of an occult Y chromosome fragment, which is associated with an increased risk of gonadal tumors. Approximately 16% of women having fragile X permutation experience POF. Thus this permutation as well as other genetic trait reported to be associated with POF should be tested in some patients. Surgery affecting the ovaries, chemotherapy, and pelvic irradiation are iatrogenic causes of POF and should be discussed with the patient in order to use modalities aimed at preserving fertility.

3. Steroid Enzyme Defects—Figure 54–1 depicts normal steroidogenesis in the ovary. Genetic females with defects in enzymes 1–4 have normal internal female genitalia and 46,XX karyotype. However, they cannot produce estradiol, and thus they fail to menstruate or have breast development.

Congenital lipoid adrenal hyperplasia describes 1 of 15 known defects in the steroidogenic acute regulatory protein, which facilitates cholesterol transport from the outer to the inner mitochondrial membrane. This enzyme catalyzes an early, rate-limiting step in tropic hormone-stimulated steroidogenesis. Patients thus present with hyponatremia, hyperkalemia, and acidosis in infancy. Both XX and XY individuals are phenotypically female. These patients can survive into adulthood given appropriate glucocorticoid and mineralocorticoid supplementation. XX patients may exhibit some secondary sexual characteristics at puberty, but present with amenorrhea and premature ovarian failure due to intraovarian accumulation of cholesterol.

4. Ovarian resistance (Savage's Syndrome)—Patients with this syndrome have elevated LH and FSH levels, and the ovaries contain primordial germ cells. A defect in the cell receptor mechanism is the presumed cause.

5. Polycystic ovary syndrome—One of the most common causes of secondary amenorrhea is **polycystic ovary syndrome (PCOS)**. PCOS is the most common cause of ovulatory dysfunction in reproductive-age women. After exclusion of other etiologies (congenital adrenal hyperplasia, androgen-secreting tumors, Cushing's syndrome), the diagnosis is based on the presence of at least 2 of the following characteristics: (a) oligo- or anovulation, (2) clinical and/or biochemical signs of hyperandrogenism, (3) polycystic ovaries. Although the exact mechanism is unknown, it appears that insulin resistance and hyperinsulinemia play a permissive role. Abnormally elevated baseline insulin leads to increased androgens via decreased sex hormone-binding globulin and stimulation of ovarian insulin and insulinlike growth factor-I receptors. Insulin-sensitizing agents such as metformin and rosiglitazone are used as a sole or adjuvant agent for ovulation induction in PCOS.

D. Anatomic Abnormalities Associated With Amenorrhea (see Chapter 37)

1. Müllerian dysgenesis—Müllerian dysgenesis is characterized by congenital absence of the uterus and the upper two-thirds of the vagina. Affected individuals may ovulate regularly, have normal development of the secondary sex characteristic, and have a 46, XX karyotype.

2. Vaginal agenesis—Vaginal agenesis is characterized by failure of the vagina to develop.

3. Transverse vaginal septum—This anomaly results from failure of fusion of the müllerian and urogenital sinus-derived portions of the vagina.

4. Imperforate hymen—If the hymen is complete, menstrual efflux cannot occur.

5. Asherman's syndrome—In Asherman's syndrome, amenorrhea is caused by intrauterine synechiae. The usual cause is a complicated dilatation and curettage (D&C) (eg, infected products of conception, vigorous elimination of the endometrium), but the syndrome can occur after myomectomy, caesarean section, and tuberculous endometritis.

E. Amenorrhea in Women With 46, XY Karyotype

The details of embryonic sexual differentiation are discussed in Chapter 2. Briefly, the sexually undifferentiated male fetal testis secretes müllerian-inhibiting factor (MIF) and testosterone. MIF promotes regression of all müllerian structures: the uterine tubes, the uterus, and the upper two-thirds of the vagina. Testosterone and its active metabolite DHT are responsible for embryonic differentiation of the male internal and external genitalia.

1. Testicular feminization—In testicular feminization, a condition also addressed as complete androgen insensitivity syndrome, all müllerian-derived structures are absent because MIF is present. The external genital and mesonephric ducts cannot respond to androgens, because androgen receptors are either absent or defective. Affected individuals are therefore phenotypic females lacking a uterus and a complete vagina. They produce some estrogen, develop breasts, and are reared as girls and therefore present with primary amenorrhea. The syndrome is inherited in an X-linked recessive trait. In contrast to other dysgenetic gonads with a Y chromosome, the occurrence of gonadal malignancy is late (rarely before the age of 25) and the incidence is less, approximately 5–10%. Therefore, the removal of the nonfunctioning testes can be postponed until the age of 16–18 years to allow completion of puberty.

2. Pure gonadal dysgenesis (Swyer Syndrome)—If the primitive germ cells do not migrate to the genital ridge or the SRY gene is not functioning harboring a mutation, a testis will not develop, and a streak gonad will be present. Affected individuals have normal female internal and external genitalia, as neither MIF nor androgens are secreted by the streaks. Because these individuals produce no estrogen, they will not develop breasts. They are reared as girls and present clinically with either delayed puberty or primary amenorrhea. Removal of the streak gonads should be done as soon as the diagnosis is made to prevent the possible development of tumor in such gonads.

3. Anorchia—If the fetal testes regress before 7 weeks' gestation, neither MIF nor testosterone is secreted, and affected individuals will present with a clinical picture identical to that of pure gonadal dysgenesis. Individuals whose testes regress between 7 and 13 weeks' gestation present with ambiguous genitalia.

4. Testicular steroid enzyme defects—A testis with defective enzymes 1–4 will produce MIF but not testosterone (Fig. 54–1). Affected individuals have female external genitalia and no müllerian structures. They will be reared as girls and present clinically with either delayed puberty or primary amenorrhea.

A defect in enzyme 6 (17-hydroxysteroid dehydrogenase) results in ambiguous genitalia and virilization at puberty.

Differential Diagnosis

Figures 54–2 and 54–3 summarize the diagnostic workup for primary and secondary amenorrhea, respectively. It is important at the outset to determine which organ is dysfunctional and then to identify the exact cause. Medical history, patient symptoms and complaints, and physical examination will lead to the correct diagnosis. Applying other assisting tests will substantiate the diagnosis. Once this has been done, specific therapy can be planned.

Any patient with amenorrhea who has a uterus should be tested for pregnancy and for serum levels of thyroid-stimulating hormone (TSH) and prolactin. Galactorrhea should be identified or ruled out by physical examination.

A. Diagnosis of Primary Amenorrhea

Figure 54–2 outlines the diagnostic scheme for primary amenorrhea. Pelvic examination should be done to establish the presence of a vagina and uterus and no vaginal septum or imperforate hymen that might account for the failure of appearance of menses. Because pelvic examination of an adolescent girl may be difficult, pelvic ultrasound or examination under anesthesia may be required to establish the presence of a uterus. Other diagnostic tools, namely pelvic computed tomography (CT) scan and magnetic resonance imaging (MRI), may be helpful.

If no uterus is present, serum testosterone levels should be measured and karyotyping done to differentiate between müllerian agenesis and testicular feminization.

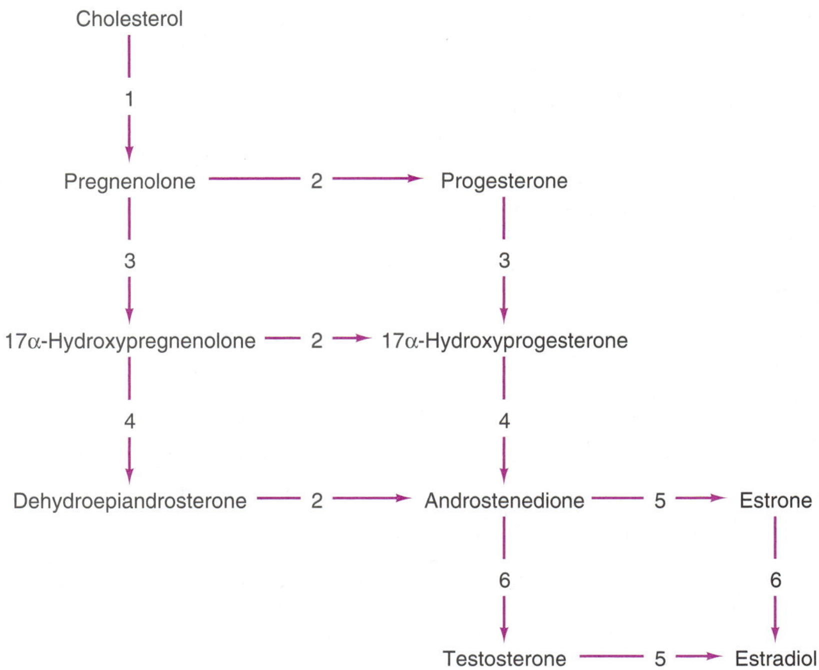

Key to enzymes
1 = Cholesterol 20- and 22-desmolase and 20-hydroxylase
2 = 3β-Hydroxysteroid dehydrogenase
3 = 17α-Hydroxylase
4 = 17- and 20-Desmolase
5 = Aromatase
6 = 17-Hydroxysteroid dehydrogenase

▲ **Figure 54–1.** Steroidogenesis in the ovary.

B. Diagnosis of Amenorrhea Associated With Galactorrhea-Hyperprolactinemia

Figure 54–3 outlines the diagnostic workup of patients with galactorrhea or hyperprolactinemia. Table 54–4 summarizes the differential diagnosis of galactorrhea-amenorrhea.

Patients with primary hypothyroidism have elevated thyroid-releasing hormone (TRH) levels. TRH acts to stimulate the release of prolactin and may thereby lead to galactorrhea-amenorrhea syndrome. TSH is also elevated and easier to measure and thus is the screening test for hypothyroidism.

Once hypothyroidism is adequately treated, serum prolactin must be measured again after thyroid function has become normal. If prolactin remains elevated or is initially higher than 50–200 ng/mL, the patient should be further studied via cone view of the sella or CT or MRI scan of the sella to rule out pituitary micro- or macroadenoma.

A meticulous history must be taken to ascertain whether the hyperprolactinemia is caused by ingestion of drugs. Prolactin secretion is inhibited by dopamine and stimulated by serotonin and TRH. Any drug that blocks the synthesis or binding of dopamine will increase the prolactin level. Prolactin is increased by serotonin agonists and decreased by serotonin antagonists. Pituitary macroadenoma should be ruled out if prolactin levels are higher than 50–100 ng/mL, even if the patient is taking drugs that lead to raised prolactin levels.

C. Diagnosis of Amenorrhea Caused by Primary Ovarian Failure

Table 54–3 lists the causes of primary ovarian failure.

Karyotyping is indicated for all women who present with premature menopause, particularly if their amenorrhea is primary. Patients with primary amenorrhea may have a steroid enzyme defect. Autoimmune oophoritis is a reversible cause of ovarian failure that must be investigated.

D. Diagnosis of Amenorrhea Associated with Hypothalamic–Pituitary Dysfunction

Table 54–5 summarizes the differential diagnosis of hypoestrogenic amenorrhea. The category includes amenorrhea associated with athletic activity, weight loss, or stress. Differentiation of hypothalamic from pituitary dysfunction can be achieved by giving GnRH, but is generally not a worthwhile effort, as pituitary causes are rare and can often be diagnosed on the basis of the history. Moreover,

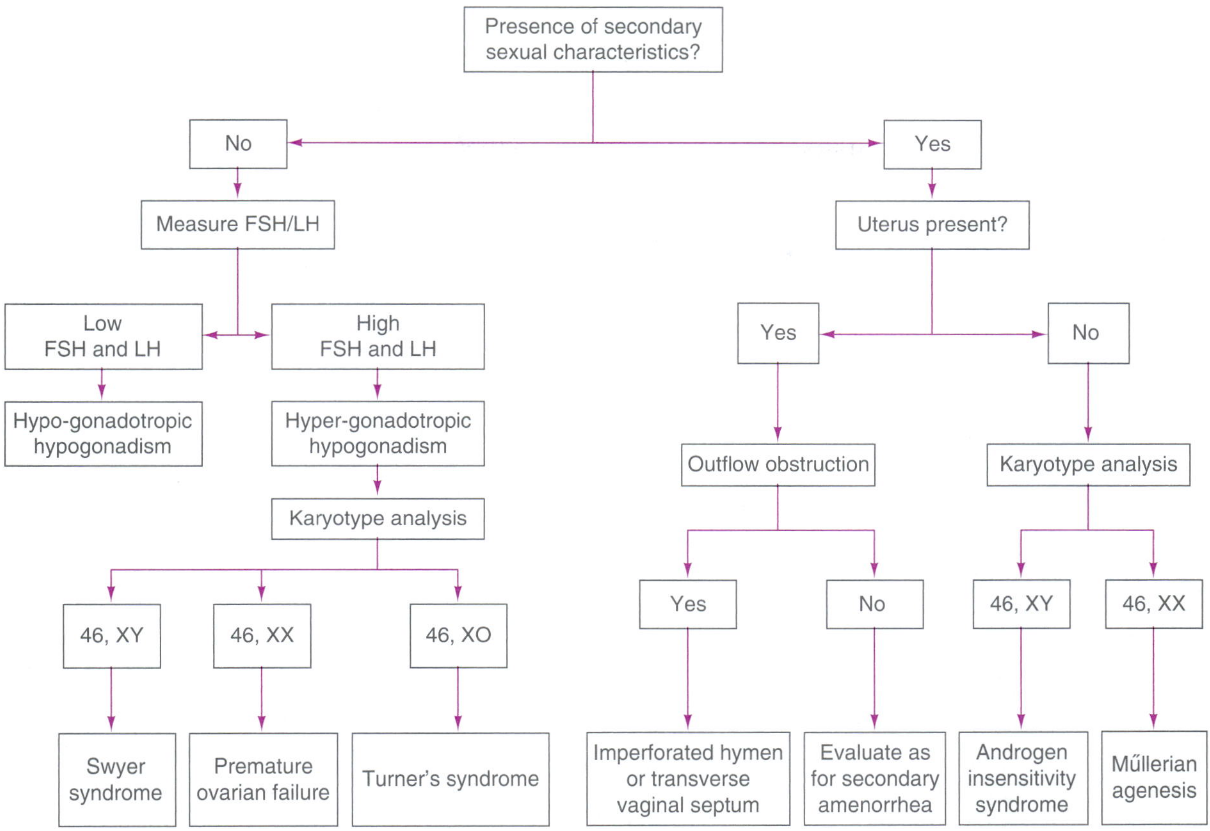

▲ **Figure 54–2.** Workup for patients with primary amenorrhea.

in Kallmann's syndrome, a single bolus dose of GnRH may not elicit a normal response. Up to 40 doses of GnRH have been required to prime the pituitary so that it will respond normally. A GnRH pump also has been used.

If there is a significant history consistent with Sheehan's syndrome, pituitary function testing is indicated in order to determine the functional capacity of the gland—particularly the integrity of the pituitary–adrenal axis.

In girls with primary amenorrhea, observing the pattern of LH and FSH release after administration of GnRH will help to determine whether the patient is undergoing late pubertal changes.

E. Diagnosis of Secondary Amenorrhea

These patients are studied according to the scheme outlined in Figure 54–3. The first step is the progestin challenge, which indirectly determines whether the ovary is producing estrogen. If the endometrium has been primed with estrogen, exogenous progestin will produce menses. Give either medroxyprogesterone acetate 10 mg orally daily for 5–7 days, or progesterone 100 mg intramuscularly as a single dose. Other progestative preparations can be used as well (Table 54–6). If vaginal bleeding follows, the ovaries are secreting estrogen. If it does not, it can be concluded that there is no estrogen or that the patient has Asherman's syndrome.

From a practical standpoint, if a patient has not had a D&C, it is virtually impossible for her to have Asherman's syndrome, so the diagnostic steps summarized in the following paragraphs can be disregarded.

Asherman's syndrome can be ruled out by administration of conjugated estrogen 2.5 mg orally daily or estradiol 4 mg daily for 21 days, followed by a progestational agent for 7–10 days (Table 54–6). Patients with Asherman's syndrome do not bleed after this regimen.

Asherman's syndrome can also be diagnosed by weekly serum progesterone tests. Any value in the ovulatory range (>3 ng/mL) not associated with menses is indicative of Asherman's syndrome. Hysterosalpingography, sonohysterography, and hysteroscopy can also lead to a diagnosis of Asherman's syndrome. Three dimensional ultrasound (3D US) is a non invasive tool and may also help in diagnosis. In a patient who does not have Asherman's syndrome and who does not respond to the progestin challenge, ovarian dysfunction may be of hypothalamic or ovarian origin.

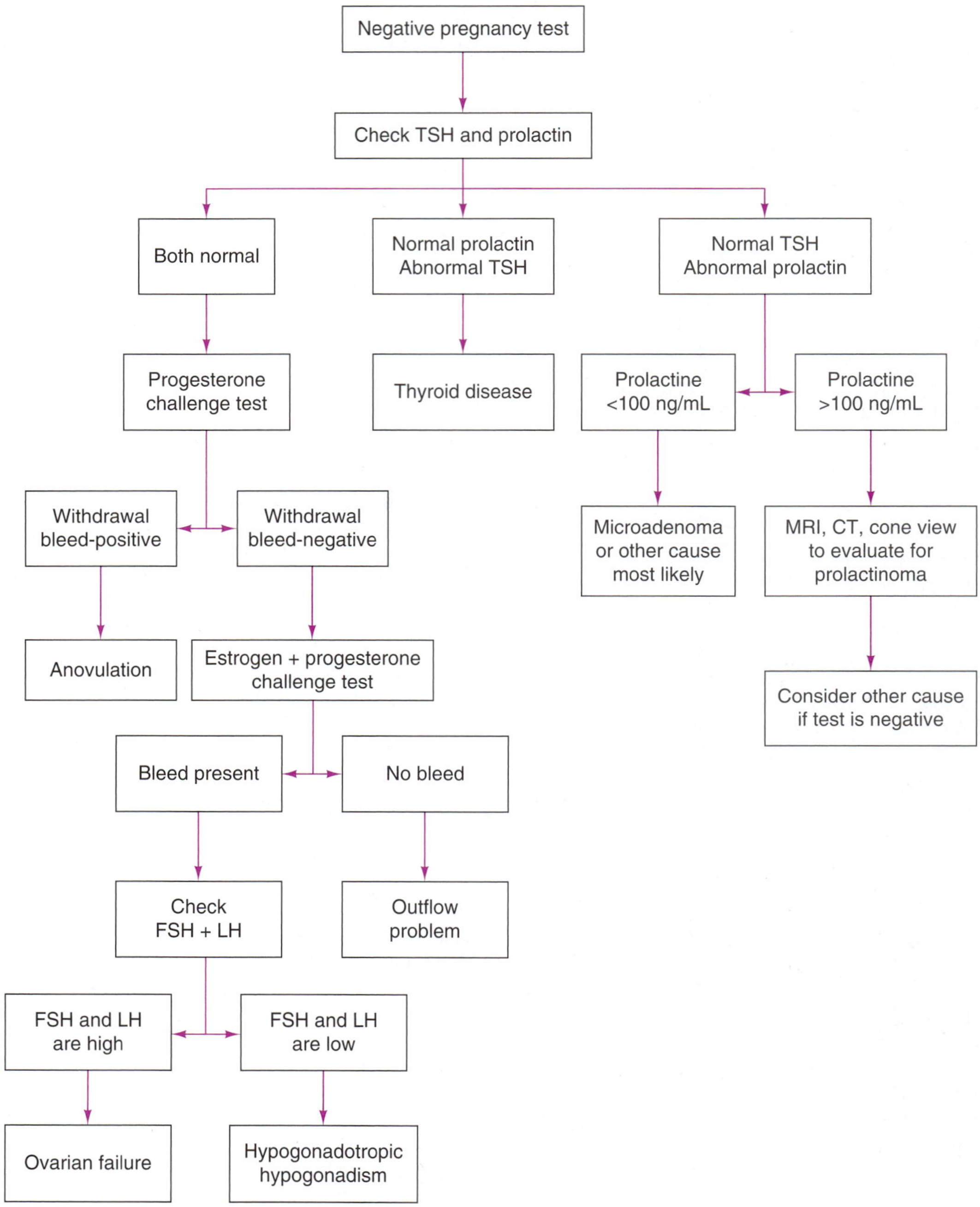

▲ **Figure 54–3.** Workup for patients with secondary amenorrhea.

The distinction is based on the FSH level. Primary ovarian dysfunction resulting in low estradiol secretion is associated with high serum FSH. Values vary in different laboratories, but in general an FSH level higher than 40 mIU/mL indicates primary ovarian failure. POF resulting in secondary amenorrhea can be due to genetic cause such as XO/XX mosaicism and 47XXX. Carriers of fragile X permutation are at an increased risk to develop POF, with a reported prevalence of 10–20%. Therefore, patients with secondary amenorrhea and high gonadotropin levels

Table 54–4. Differential diagnosis of galactorrhea-hyperprolactinemia.

Pituitary tumors secreting prolactin
  Macroadenomas (>10 mm)
  Microadenomas (<10 mm)

Hypothyroidism
Idiopathic hyperprolactinemia
Drug-induced hyperprolactinemia
Interruption of normal hypothalamic-pituitary relationship   Pituitary stalk section

Peripheral neural stimulation
  Chest wall stimulation
    Thoracotomy
    Mastectomy
    Thoracoplasty
    Burns
    Herpes zoster
    Bronchogenic tumors
    Bronchiectasis
    Chronic bronchitis
  Nipple stimulation
    Stimulation of nipples
    Chronic nipple irritation
  Spinal cord lesion
  Tabes dorsalis
  Syringomyelia

Central nervous system disease
  Encephalitis
  Craniopharyngioma
  Pineal tumors
  Hypothalamic tumors
  Pseudotumor cerebri

Table 54–5. Differential diagnosis of hypoestrogenic amenorrhea (hypogonadotropic hypogonadism).

Hypothalamic dysfunction
  Kallmann's syndrome
  Tumors of hypothalamus (craniopharyngioma)
  Constitutional delay of puberty
  Severe hypothalamic dysfunction
  Anorexia nervosa
  Severe weight loss
  Severe stress
  Exercise

Pituitary disorder
  Sheehan's syndrome
  Panhypopituitarism
  Isolated gonadotropin deficiency
  Hemosiderosis (primarily from thalassemia major)

should have karyotype analysis and screened for the fragile X mutation. In addition, POF can be due to an autoimmune process, ovarian infectious disease such as mumps oophoritis, or a physical insult such as surgery, irradiation, or chemotherapy.

Patients who bleed in response to the progestin challenge (ie, whose ovaries are secreting estrogen) fit into one of 4 categories: (1) virilized, with or without ambiguous genitalia; (2) hirsute, with polycystic ovaries, hyperthecosis, or mild maturity-onset adrenal hyperplasia; (3) nonhirsute, with hypothalamic dysfunction; or (4) amenorrheic secondary to systemic disease.

Table 54–7 sets forth the differential diagnosis for patients with amenorrhea who respond to progestin challenge test and are considered to have anovulation. Clinical examination, transvaginal ultrasound, and hormonal profile (FSH, LH, androgens, insulin) may be helpful in establishing the diagnosis of PCOS.

Complications

The complications of amenorrhea can be numerous, including infertility and psychosocial developmental delays with lack of normal physical sexual development. Hypoestrogenic patients can develop severe osteoporosis and fractures, the most hazardous to life being femoral neck fracture (see Chapter 59). The complications associated with amenorrhea in patients who respond to progestin challenge are endometrial hyperplasia and carcinoma (see Chapter 59) resulting from unopposed estrogen stimulation.

Treatment

A. Management of Patients Desiring Pregnancy—Ovulation Induction

1. Ovulation induction in patients with amenorrhea-galactorrhea with pituitary macroadenoma—Dopamine agonist drugs such as cabergoline and bromocriptine remain the first-line treatment of hyperprolactinemia of any cause, including macroadenomas. These drugs can decrease prolactin secretion and tumor size. Surgical therapy—transsphenoidal or frontal removal of the pituitary adenoma or the entire gland—may be required if tumor size or secretion are resistant to dopamine agonists, the lesion is rapidly enlarging or causing symptoms such as visual changes or headaches, or in women with giant adenomas (>3 cm) who wish to discontinue agonist treatment for conception and the duration of pregnancy. Approximately half of surgically treated patients will menstruate normally after this procedure.

2. Ovulation induction in patients with amenorrhea-galactorrhea without macroadenoma (including patients with microadenomas)—These patients ovulate readily in response to dopamine agonist treatment, with dose titrated until serum prolactin is normal. Patients are maintained on the lowest dose necessary to maintain normal

Table 54–6. Progesterone and estrogen/progesterone challenge test methods.

Progesterone challenge		
Medication	**Duration**	**Estrogen/Progesterone Challenge**
Medroxyprogesterone acetate (Provera) 5 mg bid, orally	5-7 days	Conjugate equine estrogen 1.25 mg bid or estradiol 2 mg bid on days 1 to 21 followed by a progestational agent for 7-10 days (doses at left)
Norethindrone acetate (Aygestin), 5 mg bid, orally	5-7 days	
Progesterone in oil (Gestin), 100 mg, intramuscular	Single dose	
Micronized progesterone (Prometrium), 100 mg tid, orally	5-7 days	
Micronized progesterone vaginal tablets (Endometrin) 100 mg bid or Micronized progesterone vaginal gel 8% (Crinone) Once daily	7 days 7 days	

bid, twice a day; tid, three times a day.

prolactin levels. Once pregnancy has been achieved, the agent can be discontinued. Patients with macroadenomas may need to continue therapy throughout pregnancy to avoid further growth of the lesion.

Patients taking drugs that raise the prolactin level should discontinue them if possible, but continued use of such drugs is not a contraindication to therapy.

3. Ovulation induction in patients with hypothyroidism—Amenorrheic patients with hypothyroidism frequently respond to thyroid replacement therapy.

Table 54–7. Differential diagnosis of eugonadotropic eugonadism (progestin-challenge positive).

Mild hypothalamic dysfunction
Emotional stress
Psychologic disorder
Weight loss
Obesity
Exercise induced
Idiopathic
Hirsutism-virilism
Polycystic ovary syndrome (Stein-Leventhal syndrome)
Ovarian tumor
Adrenal tumor
Cushing's syndrome
Congenital and maturity-onset adrenal hyperplasia
Systemic disease
Hypothyroidism
Hyperthyroidism
Addison's disease
Cushing's syndrome
Chronic renal failure
Many others

4. Ovulation induction in patients with primary ovarian failure—According to Rebar and associates, patients with primary ovarian failure can be made to ovulate only under very rare circumstances. Patients with reversible ovarian failure include those with autoimmune oophoritis, who can be successfully treated with corticosteroids. Otherwise, almost all patients with primary ovarian failure fall into the category of idiopathic premature ovarian failure and cannot be made to ovulate. In vitro fertilization (IVF) with donor oocytes is the only way they can have children.

Any patient with a Y chromosome should undergo oophorectomy to prevent tumor development.

5. Ovulation induction in patients with hypoestrogenic hypothalamic amenorrhea (progestin-challenge negative)—In these patients with low estrogen levels, the pituitary does not release high quantities of LH and FSH (as would be expected with an intact, normally functioning, negative feedback mechanism). Therefore, even though clomiphene citrate (an antiestrogen) is unlikely to stimulate gonadotropin release, many reproductive endocrinologists treat such patients successfully with a single course of clomiphene citrate, 150 or 250 mg daily for 5 days, on the chance that ovulation will occur.

Injections of exogenous gonadotropins (human recombinant follicle-stimulating hormone combined with human recombinant luteinizing hormone or human menopausal gonadotropin [hMG]) is usually first-line therapy. Patients showing some ovarian stimulation by clomiphene can be treated with a combination of clomiphene and hMG—the advantage being a reduction in the amount of hMG required and thus a substantial cost savings. Ovulation induction with gonadotropins must be carefully monitored with serial ultrasound and estradiol determinations to avoid hyperstimulation. Hyperstimulation is the stimulation of too many follicles, with associated ovarian enlargement and ascites, as well as other systemic abnormalities.

If a specific and potentially reversible cause of amenorrhea can be identified (eg, marked weight loss), it should be corrected.

6. Ovulation induction in patients who bleed in response to progestin challenge—Virtually all of these patients respond to clomiphene citrate. The starting dose is 50 mg orally daily for 5 days. This can be increased to a maximum of 250 mg orally daily in 50-mg increments until ovulation is induced. Efficacy of clomiphene, however, plateaus at 100 mg/d. This medication is approved by the US Food and Drug Administration for use up to 150 mg/d. Ovulation occurs 5–10 days after the last dose. Patients with elevated androgens who do not respond to clomiphene citrate may respond to combined treatment with an oral hypoglycemic agent and clomiphene. If clomiphene therapy with or without oral hypoglycemic agents is ineffective, gonadotropin therapy may be attempted. Care must be taken in using FSH in these patients, as they are likely to become hyperstimulated.

Laparoscopic ovarian drilling (LOD) is a surgical method of ovulation induction in PCOS patients. LOD involves electrocautery or laser drilling of the ovarian cortex, with the goal of creating foci of laser or thermal damage in the cortex and ovarian stroma. In general, at least 6 puncture sites 2–4 mm in depth are made in the ovary away from the hilum. The mechanism of action is unknown, but may involve destruction of androgen-producing stromal cells, a sudden drop in ovarian androgen levels, improved follicular microenvironment, or increased gonadotropin secretion. This procedure may cause postoperative pelvic adhesions, resulting in tubal compromise.

B. Management of Patients Not Desiring Pregnancy

Patients who are hypoestrogenic must be treated with a combination of estrogen and progesterone to maintain bone density and prevent genital atrophy. The dose of estrogen varies with the age of the patient. Oral contraceptives are good replacement therapy for most women. Combinations of 0.625–1.25 mg of conjugated estrogens orally daily on days 1 through 25 of the cycle with 5–10 mg of medroxyprogesterone acetate on days 16 through 25 are a suitable alternative. Calcium intake should be adjusted to 1–1.5 g of elemental calcium daily.

Patients who respond to the progestin challenge require occasional progestin administration to prevent the development of endometrial hyperplasia and carcinoma. Oral contraceptive pills may be used to regulate the menstrual cycle. Oral contraceptives also help with management of hirsutism. Alternatively, progestational medication in a dose detailed in Table 54–6 for 10–13 days every month or every other month is sufficient to induce withdrawal bleeding and to prevent the development of endometrial hyperplasia. Patients with hyper-prolactinemia need periodic prolactin measurements and radiographic cone views of the sella turcica to rule out the development of macroadenoma.

Prognosis

The prognosis for amenorrhea is good. It is not usually a life-threatening clinical event, as with proper evaluation, tumors can be recognized and treated. Many patients with hypothalamic amenorrhea will spontaneously recover normal menstrual cycles.

Virtually all amenorrheic women who do not have premature ovarian failure can be made to ovulate with a dopamine agonist, clomiphene citrate, insulin-sensitizing agents, and gonadotropins.

Abrahamson MJ, Snyder PJ. Treatment of hyperprolactinemia due to lactotroph adenoma and other causes. *UpToDate Online* 2005;13.1. Available at www.uptodate.com.

Practice Committee of American Society for Reproductive Medicine. Current evaluation of amenorrhea. *Fertil Steril* 2008; 90(Suppl 5): S219–S225. PMID: 19007635.

Diamanti-Kandarakis E. Polycystic ovarian syndrome: pathophysiology, molecular aspects and clinical implications. *Expert Rev Mol Med* 2008;10:e3. PMID: 18230193.

Heiman DL. Amenorrhea. *Prim Care* 2009; 36:1–17, vii. PMID: 19231599.

Master-Hunter T, Heiman DL. Amenorrhea: evaluation and treatment. *Am Fam Physician* 2006; 73:1374–1382.

Rebar RW. Premature ovarian failure. *Obstet Gynecol* 2009;113:1355–1363. PMID: 19461434.

Rebar RW. Premature ovarian "failure" in the adolescent. *Ann N Y Acad Sci* 2008;1135:138–145. PMID: 18574219.

Rothman MS, Wierman ME. Female hypogonadism: evaluation of the hypothalamic-pituitary-ovarian axis. *Pituitary* 2008;11:163–169. PMID: 18404388.

The Rotterdam ESHRE/ASRM-Sponsored PCOS Consensus Workshop Group. Revised 2003 consensus on diagnostic criteria and long-term health risks related to polycystic ovary syndrome. *Fertil Steril* 2004;81:19–25. PMID: 14711538.

Torre DL, Falorni A. Pharmacological causes of hyperprolactinemia. *Ther Clin Risk Manag* 2007; 3:929–951. PMID: 18473017.

55 Hirsutism

Ariel Revel, MD

ESSENTIALS OF DIAGNOSIS

- Excess coarse body hair in sex hormone–dependent areas
- Only in women and children
- Ferriman–Gallwey score ≥8 (Fig. 55–1)
- Adult male distribution pattern
- Testing for elevated androgens is not recommended in mild cases.
- Main causes are polycystic ovary syndrome, idiopathic, congenital adrenal hyperplasia, androgen-secreting tumors, Cushing syndrome, acromegaly, drugs.
- Topical and/or systemic treatments control hirsutism in most cases.
- Allow 4–6 months for any treatment to be effective.

Hirsutism, unwanted hair growth, is a common and distressing condition that, although often thought to be a cosmetic problem, significantly affects psychologic well-being. In Western society, excessive facial or body hair in women is unacceptable. Women who do not conform to a prevailing feminine ideal of physical appearance because of hirsutism may feel unattractive and suffer from low self-esteem, and such women may find social interactions difficult. Hirsutism is however, more than a cosmetic problem because it usually represents a hormonal imbalance, resulting from a subtle excess of androgens that may be of ovarian origin, adrenal origin, or both. The underlying cause of hirsutism is usually polycystic ovary syndrome (PCOS). It is important to differentiate idiopathic hirsutism from other causes. Physicians should be familiar with therapies for these conditions.

Pathogenesis

A. Hair Growth Cycle

The hair growth cycle comprises 3 phases: anagen (growth phase), catagen (involution phase), and telogen (rest phase). Hormonal regulation plays an important role in the hair growth cycle in a site-specific pattern. Androgens increase hair follicle size, hair fiber diameter, and the proportion of time terminal hairs spent in the anagen phase. Androgen excess in women leads to increased hair growth in most androgen sensitive sites, but will manifest with loss of hair in the scalp region, in part by reducing the time scalp hairs spends in the anagen phase.

B. The Sebaceous Glands

The sebaceous glands are microscopic glands in the skin that secrete an oily/waxy matter, called sebum, to lubricate the skin and hair. They are found in greatest abundance on the face and scalp, though they are distributed throughout all skin sites except the palms and soles.

C. Types of Hair

Hair can be categorized as either vellus (fine, soft, and not pigmented) or terminal (long, coarse, and pigmented). Follicle size and type of hair can change in response to numerous factors, particularly androgens. Nonetheless, the number of hair follicles does not change over an individual's lifetime.

D. The Role of Androgens

Androgens are necessary for terminal hair and sebaceous gland development and mediate differentiation of pilosebaceous units into either a terminal hair follicle or a sebaceous gland. In the former case, androgens transform the vellus hair into a terminal hair; in the latter, the sebaceous component proliferates and the hair remains vellus.

D. Male-Pattern Hair Growth

Male-pattern hair growth occurs in sites where relatively high levels of androgen are necessary for pilosebaceous unit differentiation. Although androgen underlies most cases of hirsutism, there is only a modest correlation between the quantity of hair growth and androgen levels. This is

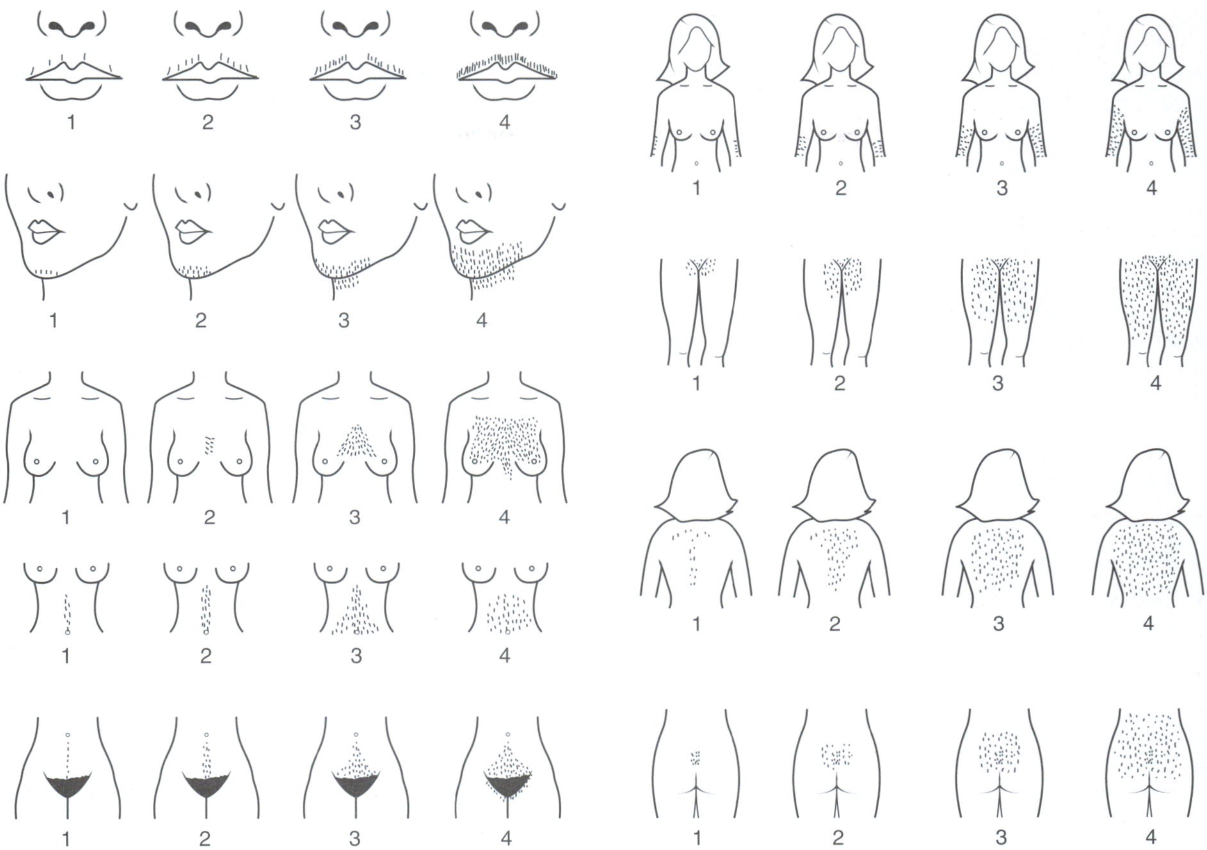

▲ **Figure 55–1.** Ferriman–Gallwey hirsutism scoring system. Each of the 9 body areas most sensitive to androgen is assigned a score from 0 (no hair) to 4 (frankly virile), and these separate scores are summed to provide a hormonal hirsutism score. (Reproduced, with permission, from Hatch R, et al. *Am J Obstet Gynecol* 1981; 140:850–830. [Fig. 5]. © Elsevier.)

thought to result from the fact that stimulation of hair growth from the follicle does not depend solely on circulating androgen concentrations, but also depends on local factors and variability in end-organ sensitivity to circulating androgens

E. Physiology of Androgens

Androgens are steroids that stimulate the development of male secondary sex characteristics and consequently promote the growth of sexual hair. The major androgens are testosterone, dihydrotestosterone, androstenedione, dehydroepiandrosterone (DHEA), and dehydroepiandrosterone sulfate adrenocorticotropic hormone (DHEAS). In order to comprehend the role played by elevated levels of androgens in the development of hirsutism, one must understand the sources of androgens, their metabolic pathways and sites of action, and their interrelationship with other steroid hormones such as estrogens and corticosteroids.

1. Production—All steroid hormone production begins with the 2-stage rate-limiting step of cholesterol conversion to pregnenolone, which is regulated by trophic hormones. In the nonpregnant woman, androgens are produced by both the ovaries and the adrenals, as well as by peripheral conversion. The rate-limiting step in androgen formation is the regulation of P450c17 gene expression, which is dependent on the concentrations of luteinizing hormone (LH) in the ovary and adrenocorticotropic hormone (ACTH) in the adrenal cortex.

2. Ovarian production of androgens—Androgens are produced by the normal ovary as precursors in the synthesis of estrogens. When gonadotropin-releasing hormone (GnRH) is secreted in a pulsatile fashion, thecal cells are stimulated to secrete and bind LH. In response to ligand binding, the theca cells of the preantral follicle produce androstenedione, DHEA, and testosterone. In the normal female, follicle-stimulating hormone (FSH) secreted from granulosa cells stimulates the granulosa cells to aromatize these androgens to the estrogens, estrone and estradiol. This relationship produces a system of androgen anabolism and catabolism balanced and coordinated to meet the needs of the follicular cycle.

3. Adrenal production of androgens—Stimulation of the adrenal gland by ACTH results in androgen production in the zona reticularis and zona fasciculata of the adrenal cortex. The main androgen manufactured is DHEAS, with smaller amounts of DHEA and androstenedione. A phenomenon called adrenarche occurs and is usually chronologically timed before menarche in females. During this period, the adrenal cortex has a significant increase in adrenal hormone production, as a result of increased responsiveness of androgens and their precursors to the circulating levels of ACTH. This results in adrenocortical secretion of DHEAS at a level similar to that of cortisol secretion. Controversy remains regarding the causative factors.

4. Circulation

A. TESTOSTERONE—Testosterone, by virtue of its plasma concentration and its potency, is one of the major androgens. It is the second most potent androgen after dihydrotestosterone, and circulating levels are 20–80 ng/dL in adult women. The ovary and the adrenals contribute equally to testosterone production, with each supplying approximately 25% of the total circulating level. The other 50% of circulating testosterone is derived from peripheral conversion of androstenedione, although the ovarian contribution to testosterone levels may increase during the periovulatory portion of the menstrual cycle. Peripheral levels of testosterone display a slight diurnal variation that parallels that of cortisol. In normal women, 99% of testosterone is protein-bound, of which 80% is bound to sex hormone-binding globulin (SHBG) and 19% is loosely bound to albumin. The remaining 1% is free and unbound. The free and albumin-bound testosterone are the biologically active forms of circulating testosterone.

B. DIHYDROTESTOSTERONE—Circulating levels of dihydrotestosterone, the most potent androgen, are 2–8 ng/dL or one-tenth those of testosterone. Although both the ovary and the adrenal gland secrete it, most dihydrotestosterone is produced by peripheral conversion of testosterone by 5α-reductase.

C. ANDROSTENEDIONE—Androstenedione, one of the 17-ketosteroids, is not very potent, with only 20% of the effectiveness of testosterone. Synthesis and secretion occur mostly in the ovaries and adrenals in equal amounts, with the remaining 10% being produced peripherally. Androstenedione levels display a diurnal variation paralleling that of cortisol and may simultaneously increase by as much as 50% when cortisol levels rise. Moreover, periovulatory increases in androstenedione levels can also be observed. In contrast to testosterone, androstenedione is bound mainly to albumin and secondarily to SHBG.

D. DHEA AND DHEAS—DHEA and DHEAS, both weak androgens, have approximately 3% of the effectiveness of testosterone and are the other major precursors of 17-ketosteroids. DHEA is primarily produced by the adrenals (60–70%), with ovarian production and hydrolysis of DHEAS accounting for the remainder. DHEA has a large diurnal variation similar to that of cortisol. Conversely, DHEAS is derived almost entirely from the adrenal, has only slight diurnal variation, and circulates in high concentrations. The DHEAS level may provide a good clinical assessment of adrenal function.

5. Action—The skin and hair follicles are androgen-responsive and thus have the capacity to metabolize androgens. DHEA, androstenedione, and testosterone enter the target cell and are reduced to dihydrotestosterone by 5α-reductase. Dihydrotestosterone is then bound to a cytoplasmic receptor protein that transports the androgen into the cell nucleus, where it is bound to chromatin and initiates transcription of stored genetic information. In the hair follicle, this promotes hair growth, leading to increased hair growth and initiating the conversion of vellus to terminal hair.

In females a certain amount of androgenic stimulation is expected, with the greatest levels noted at puberty, when these increased levels result in the clinical appearance of pubic hair and axillary hair. Similarly, androgens stimulate the facial pilosebaceous glands, resulting in the pubertal development of acne.

Metabolic conversion of androgens to dihydrotestosterone may be accelerated. This results in irreversible conversion of vellus hair to terminal hair in areas of androgen-sensitive skin. Thus, in excess androgens are pathologic, and the clinical signs and symptoms of hirsutism and virilization result.

Hirsutism results from an interaction between the plasma androgens and the apparent sensitivity of the hair follicle to androgen. The sensitivity of the hair follicle is determined in part by the local metabolism of androgens, particularly by conversion of testosterone to dihydrotestosterone by 5α-reductase, and subsequent binding of these molecules to the androgen receptor. Some women have hirsutism without hyperandrogenemia (idiopathic hirsutism). Most women with a 2-fold or greater elevation of androgen levels have some degree of hirsutism or an alternative pilosebaceous response, such as acne vulgaris, seborrhea, or pattern alopecia.

F. Definition of Hirsutism & Hypertrichosis

Hirsutism is defined as the development of androgen-dependent terminal body hair in a woman in places in which terminal hair is normally not found.

Hirsutism usually represents androgen overproduction or enhanced androgen metabolism in the skin. This is most often manifested as increased "midline hair" on the upper lip, chin, ears, cheeks, lower abdomen, back, chest, and proximal limbs. Most women with a two-fold or greater elevation of androgen levels have some degree of hirsutism or an alternative pilosebaceous response, such as acne vulgaris, seborrhea, or pattern alopecia. Nevertheless, some women have hirsutism without hyperandrogenemia ("idiopathic hirsutism").

Hypertrichosis is a generalized excessive hair overgrowth occurring on the trunk and hands and *not* localized to the androgen-dependent areas of the skin. Although the mechanisms of hypertrichosis are poorly defined, it is not thought to be an androgen-dependent process. There are 2 distinct types of hypertrichosis: generalized hypertrichosis, which occurs over the entire body, and localized hypertrichosis, which is restricted to a certain locations, such as on the extremities, the head, and the back. Hypertrichosis may also be either congenital or, more commonly, acquired later in life. Congenital forms of hypertrichosis are X-linked dominant traits. Causes of acquired hypertrichosis include cancer metabolic disorders, anorexia, thyroid disorders, and most commonly drugs or chemicals such as oral phenytoin, diazoxide, minoxidil, and cyclosporine. Acquired generalized hypertrichosis can be obtained through cancer. The hair that grows due to this condition is known as malignant down.

G. Etiology

The goal of working up selected hirsute women is to attempt to determine the specific etiology and to provide a baseline in case it becomes necessary to reassess the patient because of progression of the disorder. Table 55–1 details the ovarian, adrenal, and iatrogenic causes of hirsutism, whereas Table 55–2 details the etiology of hypertrichosis.

Prevention

Hirsutism is generally not a preventable condition; thus most causes of hirsutism are beyond a woman's control. Patients should be advised to avoid unnecessary medicines known to cause hirsutism, control obesity, and prevent insulin resistance.

Clinical Findings & Diagnosis

It is important to define the age of onset and to correlate it to puberty. Important aspects of history of hirsute patients are detailed in Table 55–3.

A. Symptoms & Signs

Examination should assess the distribution of excess hair. Weight and height are measured to calculate body mass index (BMI). Physical examination should search for acanthosis nigricans, representing insulin resistance. Signs of virilization, such as clitoromegaly, male pattern balding, deepening voice, or decreased breast size, should be assessed. The Ferriman–Gallwey grading system (Fig. 55–1) system provides a subjective determination of severity of hirsutism. It is especially useful to determine treatment effectiveness and for research purposes. Hair growth is rated from 0 (no growth of terminal hair) to 4 (complete and heavy cover) in 9 locations, giving a maximum score of 36. The 9 locations measured are the upper lip, chin, chest, upper back, lower back, upper abdomen, lower abdomen, the upper arms, and the thighs. In white women, a score of 8 or higher is regarded as indicative of androgen excess. With other ethnic groups, the amount of hair expected for that race should be considered.

This rating scale has since been modified by the American Association of Clinical Endocrinologists to include a total of 19 locations, with the 10 extra locations being sideburns, neck, buttocks, inguinal area, perianal area, forearm, leg, foot, toes, and fingers. Each area has its own specified definition of the 4-point scale.

Table 55–1. Differential diagnosis of hirsutism.

Ovarian nonneoplastic causes
Polycystic ovary syndrome
Stromal hyperplasia
Stromal hyperthecosis
Hyperandrogenism, insulin resistance, acanthosis nigricans (HAIR-AN)
Ovarian neoplastic causes
Sertoli-Leydig cell tumors
Hilar cell tumors
Germ cell tumors
Gynandroblastomas
Granulosa cell tumors
Gonadoblastomas
Ovarian tumors with functional stroma
Pregnancy-related causes
Theca lutein cysts
Luteoma of pregnancy
Adrenal causes
Congenital adrenal hyperplasia
Adrenal tumors
Cushing's syndrome
Hyperprolactinemia
Iatrogenic causes
Methyltestosterone
Danazol
Anabolic steroids
19-Nortestosterones
Idiopathic hirsutism

Table 55–2. Etiology of hypertrichosis.

Cancer
Dermatomyositis
General systemic illness
Hypothyroidism
Other endocrine disorders
Malnutrition
Porphyria cutanea tarda

B. Psychologic Dysfunction

Cystic acne, hirsutism, and alopecia can have a devastating psychosocial effect in young girls and women of reproductive age. These manifestations may be associated with severe anxiety and depression. The occurrence of obesity in conjunction with hyperandrogenism can have a further negative effect on self-esteem and self-image. The fear of social rejection can make some women reclusive and may retard development of their social skills and confidence. Correction of the underlying pathophysiologic condition can help ameliorate the psychologic dysfunction.

C. Laboratory Findings

Measurement of serum testosterone concentrations helps identify the occasional case of severe androgen excess that needs further investigation, but it is not essential in women with a clearly benign presentation, especially as testosterone assays perform poorly in the female range. According to current guidelines, testosterone measurement is needed only for women with moderate to severe hirsutism, when other symptoms of polycystic ovary syndrome (PCOS) are present, or when there is rapid progression of hirsutism or other signs of virilization. Obese women with PCOS, particularly those with a family history of type 2 diabetes, should be assessed for metabolic syndrome with an oral glucose tolerance test and cholesterol profile. The value of laboratory tests for mild to moderate hirsutism is not proven. The investigation of severe cases should include free and total testosterone levels, prolactin, LH, and FSH. Obese patients with PCOS could benefit from glucose tolerance tests and cholesterol levels.

Table 55–3. Important aspects of the patient history.

How quickly has the hair growth progressed?
What measures have been used to control excess hair?
Do you have any other features of androgen excess (acne or alopecia)?
What is the pattern of menstruation?
Has her weight changed recently?
What is the history of use of the oral contraceptive pill?
Is there a family history of type 2 diabetes?

D. Imaging Studies

Sonographic scan of the ovaries is important in the evaluation of PCOS. Computerized tomography (CT) of the adrenal glands should be performed only when a high index of suspicion of tumor exists, especially when hair growth is sudden and heavy.

Differential Diagnosis of Excessive Hair Growth

Because some excess hair results from medical disorders, it is important to distinguish excess hair that is the result of an underlying medical problem from hair growth that is simply a cosmetic concern. Underlying medical problems of hirsutism and hypertrichosis are detailed in Tables 55–1 and 55–2, respectively.

Excessive growth of sexual hair may be due to excessive androgen production, increased sensitivity of the hair follicle to androgens, or increased conversion of weak androgens to potent androgens. Potential sources of increased androgens include the ovaries, the adrenal glands, exogenous hormones, and other medications.

Figure 55–2 provides an approach to the workup for hyperandrogenism that depends on both assessing the degree of hirsutism and elucidating risk factors for PCOS, virilizing disorders, androgenic medications, and other endocrinopathies.

A. Ovarian Neoplastic Disorders Causing Hirsutism

Androgen-secreting ovarian neoplasms usually present with rapidly developing hirsutism, amenorrhea, and virilization and are rare causes of hirsutism. The most common androgen secreted by these tumors is testosterone, with serum testosterone levels usually in excess of 200 ng/dL. Most hormone-secreting neoplasms are palpable on pelvic examination and are unilateral.

1. Sertoli-leydig cell tumors and hilar (leydig) cell tumors—These are ovarian neoplasms typically associated with hirsutism and virilization. Sertoli-Leydig cell tumors constitute <0.5% of all ovarian tumors and occur mainly in young, menstruating females. Hilar cell tumors are rare neoplasms and are usually encountered in older women. Their presentation is often more indolent and less dramatic than that of Sertoli-Leydig cell tumors. Other ovarian neoplasms that may be associated with hirsutism are the gynandroblastomas, germ cell tumors, granulosa cell tumors, and gonadoblastomas. The latter occur mainly in male patients, with gonadal dysgenesis and resultant female phenotypes.

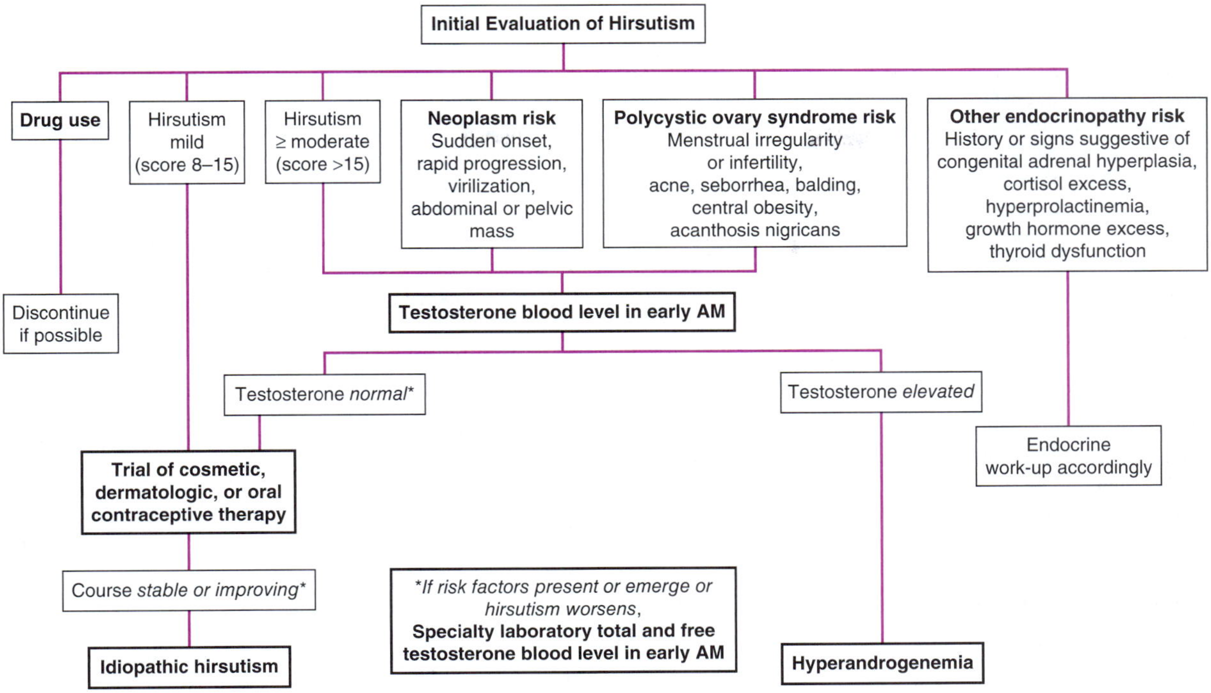

▲ **Figure 55–2.** Suggested algorithm for the initial evaluation of hirsute women for hyperandrogenism. Risk assessment includes more than the degree of hirsutism. Medications that cause hirsutism include anabolic or androgenic steroids (consider in athletes and patients with endometriosis or sexual disfunction) and valproic acid (consider in neurologic disorders). If hirsutism is moderate or severe or if mild hirsutism is accompanied by features that suggest an underlying disorder, elevated androgen levels should be ruled out. Disorders to be considered, as shown, include neoplasm and various endocrinopathies, of which polycystic ovarian syndrome (PCOS) is the most common. Plasma testosterone should be rechecked in the early morning on day 4–10 of the menstrual cycle in regularly cycling women, the time for which norms are standardized. Plasma total testosterone should be rechecked along with free testosterone in a reliable laboratory if the plasma total testosterone is normal in the presence of risk factors or progression of hirsutism on therapy. Simultaneous assay of 17-hydroxyprogesterone may be indicated in subjects at high risk for congenital adrenal hyperplasia. A small minority of women initially diagnosed with idiopathic hirsutism by this algorithm will later be found to have otherwise asymptomatic idiopathic hyperandrogenism or previously unsuspected infertility as their only noncutaneous manifestation of PCOS. (Data from Rosenfeld RL. *N Engl J Med* 2005; 353:2578–2588.)

2. Ovarian tumors with functional stroma—Ovarian tumors with functional stroma are categorized as germ cell tumors containing syncytiotrophoblast cells and idiopathic and pregnancy-related tumors. In these tumors, the neoplastic cells do not secrete steroid hormones directly, but stimulate secretion by the ovarian stroma either within or immediately adjacent to the tumor. These tumors have been described in essentially all tumors that occur in the ovary, whether benign or malignant, metastatic or primary.

B. Ovarian Nonneoplastic Disorders Causing Hirsutism

PCOS, the most common cause of hirsutism, is typically associated with menstrual irregularities, infertility, and obesity. Histologic changes seen in PCOS include a thickened ovarian capsule and numerous follicular cysts surrounded by a hyperplastic, luteinized theca interna. The pathophysiology of this disease is not fully understood; proposed causes include ovarian dysregulation, a disturbance of the hypothalamic–pituitary axis, adrenal androgen excess, and increased insulin resistance. Regardless of the underlying defect, the degree of hyperandrogenism and the individual's sensitivity to androgens may result in the complaint of hirsutism in 80% of these patients.

Other nonneoplastic ovarian disorders associated with hirsutism include stromal hyperplasia and stromal hyperthecosis. Stromal hyperplasia results in the hypersecretion of androgens from hypertrophic ovaries. It has a peak incidence between 60 and 70 years of age and is usually associated with uniform enlargement of both ovaries. Stromal hyperthecosis is a proliferation of stroma with foci of luteinized thecal cells and also results in bilateral ovarian involvement. It frequently results in the clinical manifestations of virilism, obesity, hypertension, and disturbances of glucose metabolism, with most patients showing histologic evidence of concurrent stromal hyperplasia. A syndrome known as hyperandrogenism, insulin resistance, acanthosis nigricans (HAIR-AN) has also been described; however, this is thought to most likely represent a variation of one of the nonneoplastic disorders, rather than denoting a separate disease entity.

C. Pregnancy-Related Disorders

During pregnancy, elevated androgen levels that lead to severe hirsutism and virilization may be due to any of the previously mentioned conditions; however, pregnancy-specific disorders also exist.

1. Theca lutein cysts (Hyperreactio Luteinalis)—These are benign neoplasms that can cause bilateral ovarian enlargement, hirsutism, and, infrequently, virilization. These cysts occur almost exclusively in pregnancy and have an increased incidence in pregnancies complicated by gestational trophoblastic disease. Ovarian biopsy reveals cysts lined mostly with luteinized theca cells, but luteinized granulosa cells may also be present. Typically, resolution of the cysts occurs after pregnancy.

2. Luteoma of pregnancy—Is a benign human chorionic gonadotropin (hCG)–dependent ovarian tumor that may develop during pregnancy. High levels of testosterone and androstenedione are present, and virilization may occur in up to 25% of affected mothers and 65% of female fetuses. In most patients, spontaneous regression of the neoplasm and return of androgen levels to normal occur in the postpartum period.

D. Adrenal Disorders Causing Hirsutism

1. Enzyme deficiencies—Enzyme deficiencies affecting adrenal and ovarian steroidogenesis represent the second most common cause of hyperandrogenism in postmenarchal females, and congenital adrenal hyperplasia (CAH) represents the most common disorder in this group. CAH is inherited as an autosomal recessive trait, and is present in 1–5% of women who complain of hirsutism. It results from mutations in enzymes required for adrenal steroidogenesis. The most common form of CAH is characterized by a deficiency of 21-hydroxylase, with case reports of similar occurrences in patients with 3β-hydroxysteroid dehydrogenase and 11β-hydroxylase deficiencies. These defects prohibit cortisol synthesis from its precursor 17β-hydroxyprogesterone. The expectant decrease in serum cortisol stimulates pituitary secretion of ACTH in an effort to normalize cortisol levels. Higher levels of ACTH stimulate adrenal production of intermediates in the biosynthetic pathway of cortisol. Consequently, these intermediates cannot be used for cortisol production because of enzyme defects and are instead shunted into the biosynthetic pathways for androgens, with resultant increases in testosterone and androstenedione. Classical CAH is usually diagnosed in females during the neonatal period because of androgen-induced ambiguous genitalia (pseudohermaphroditism); however, a minor enzyme deficiency termed acquired, adult-onset CAH may go unrecognized until puberty, when hirsutism, amenorrhea, and virilization may occur. CAH causes severe hirsutism if adherence to glucocorticoids is poor. Late-onset CAH is important to exclude in hirsute women wishing to conceive. Glucocorticoids are the treatment of first choice during periconception.

2. Adrenal neoplastic disorders—Adrenal tumors are a rare cause of hirsutism, although when present, symptoms may be acute and quite severe. The main androgen produced by adrenal neoplasms is DHEAS, with serum levels usually >700–800 μg/dL. Rarely, adrenal neoplasms may secrete testosterone; when this occurs, testosterone values are usually higher than 200 ng/dL.

3. Cushing's syndrome—Cushing's syndrome and the associated overproduction of cortisol may increase androgen levels and cause hirsutism. The syndrome has 3 known etiologies: (1) adrenal tumor, (2) ectopic production of ACTH by a nonpituitary tumor, or (3) excess production of ACTH by the pituitary (Cushing's disease). Because androgens are formed from intermediates in the synthesis of cortisol, increased serum and tissue levels of cortisol and its intermediates may result in hyperandrogenism and clinically present as hirsutism, regardless of the underlying cause of this syndrome.

4. Other causes—Hyperprolactinemia has been shown to produce mild hirsutism. Several investigators have reported increased DHEAS levels with hyperprolactinemia. This likely results from adrenal stimulation after prolactin binds to its numerous receptors on the adrenal gland. Despite increased androgen secretion, clinical manifestations are mild or absent, due to the inhibitory effects of prolactin on the conversion of testosterone to dihydrotestosterone (DHT) and its metabolites.

The adrenal gland may be the source of excess androgen production in the absence of an identifiable cause. The cause of this adrenal hyperactivity is not clear, but mild enzyme deficiencies, stress, and hyper-functioning of the entire adrenal gland have been postulated as probable causes.

E. Iatrogenic Mechanisms Causing Hirsutism

Exogenous sources of androgens should also be considered as possible causes of hirsutism. Methyltestosterone, danazol, and anabolic steroids such as oxandrolone may lead to excessive hair growth. The 19-nortestosterones in low-dose oral contraceptives rarely cause hirsutism or acne.

1. Idiopathic hirsutism—Hirsutism that occurs without adrenal or ovarian dysfunction, in patients with normal menstrual cycles and in the absence of any exogenous source of steroid hormones is termed idiopathic hirsutism. The term idiopathic hirsutism is thought to be a misnomer, since a likely cause has been elucidated. When normal levels of testosterone, unbound testosterone, DHEAS, dihydrotestosterone, and androstenedione are present, increased 5α-reductase enzyme activity appears to be the major mechanism of action. This enzyme converts testosterone to the more potent dihydrotestosterone in the hair follicle. Many patients with idiopathic hirsutism have an elevated level of plasma 3α-androstanediol glucuronide, a metabolite of dihydrotestosterone, thought to reflect the increased peripheral androgen metabolism, which is responsible for the clinical manifestation of hirsutism.

In summary, hirsutism may result from an ovarian disorder, an adrenal disease, an iatrogenic cause, or an increase in peripheral androgen metabolism. Rarely, other endocrinologic disturbances such as hypothyroidism or acromegaly may be associated with excessive hair growth. An important clinical correlation is that hirsutism may be accompanied by infertility as a result of the underlying abnormality. Because infertility may be the inciting factor triggering a patient to seek medical care, questions regarding a history of hirsutism should be a part of any infertility workup.

Treatment

The overall quality of primary evidence of the relative efficacy of treatments for hirsutism is weak and is based on small studies of short duration that lack quality-of-life outcomes. Recently, however, systematic reviews have amalgamated this evidence, and new guidelines are now available (Table 55–4). It should be explained that hair grows in cycles. Thus it can take months for an individual hair follicle to proceed through catagen, anagen, and telogen phases.

Table 55–4. Treatment of hirsutism.

Nonsystemic treatments
Shaving
Threading
Waxing
Depilatory creams
Electrolysis
Laser epilation
Photoepilation
Lifestyle changes
Local
Eflornithine
Systemic treatment
Oral contraceptive pills
Gonadotropin-releasing hormone agonists
Androgen receptor antagonists
Cyproterone acetate
Spironolactone
Flutamide
Finasteride
Glucocorticoids
Dopamine
Insulin-lowering drugs
Cimetidine
Ketoconazole

A. Lifestyle Changes

Lifestyle changes that promote weight loss through diet and physical exercise are useful in obese patients. Obesity is present in 60% of patients with PCOS, the most common form of hirsutism and hyperandrogenism. Weight loss in patients with hyperandrogenism, with or without the clinical presence of PCOS, should be the first therapeutic option because it decreases androgen levels, increases SHBG, and may restore ovulation. As little as a 7% reduction in body weight can restore fertility, decrease hirsutism, and improve the response to induction of ovulation. Lifestyle measures that promote weight loss through diet and exercise are of paramount importance because obesity has an adverse effect on the outcome of all systemic treatments.

B. Medical

1. Local—Eflornithine, a topical agent, is an irreversible inhibitor of ornithine decarboxylase, an enzyme that catalyzes the rate-limiting step for follicular polyamine synthesis, which is necessary for hair growth. Eflornithine hydrochloride cream 13.9% (Vaniqa) is approved in many countries for the treatment of unwanted facial hair in women. Eflornithine does not remove hair but acts to reduce the rate of hair growth.

A large sponsored randomized trial showed a 26% reduction in facial hair after 24 weeks of treatment, with most of the benefit achieved in 8 weeks. Nevertheless, Endocrine Society Clinical Practice Guideline recommends against the use of topical antiandrogen therapy.

2. Systemic treatment—Systemic treatment reduces stimulation of the anagen growth phase by testosterone. Thus enough follicles have to pass through anagen before a clinical effect is observed. The goal of treatment is to find the lowest effective dose of treatment that maintains the benefit gained in the first phase of treatment. For all pharmacologic therapies for hirsutism a trial of at least 6 months should be conducted before making changes in dose, changing medication, or adding medication. Medical suppression of hirsutism is detailed in Table 55–5.

3. Oral contraceptive pills—The primary driver of ovarian androgen secretion is LH, which can be suppressed using a combined oral contraceptive pill. The effectiveness of oral contraceptives in suppressing hirsutism will depend on the content of ethinylestradiol (20–35 μg) and on the nature of the progestogen. Pills containing progestogens with antiandrogenic properties, such as cyproterone acetate and drospirenone found in Diana and Yasmin, respectively, are effective in hirsutism. Pills containing levonorgestrel and norethisterone are more androgenic and could potentially exacerbate hirsutism. Third-generation progestogens such as desogestrel or gestodene have relatively neutral androgenic effects, and oral contraceptives containing these compounds can usefully be combined with an antiandrogen such as spironolactone. Only 1 small randomized controlled trial has compared different oral contraceptive pills, and current guidelines do not recommend one specific pill for treating hirsutism.

4. Gonadotropin-releasing hormone agonists—Severe hirsutism of ovarian origin can sometimes be treated by gonadotropin-releasing hormone (GnRH) analogues. GnRH analogs inhibit the secretion of gonadotropins from the pituitary gland, thereby inhibiting the secretion of androgens and estrogens from the ovary. Although GnRH agonists acutely stimulate ovarian production of androgens and estrogens, continued therapy causes a sustained decrease in ovarian steroid production compared with pretreatment levels. This suppression continues for the duration of GnRH agonist therapy. Significant decreases in serum levels of estradiol, testosterone, and androstenedione occur during treatment, although adrenal androgens are usually unaffected.

As a result of the hypoestrogenism associated with ongoing GnRH therapy, a potential risk of osteoporosis and menopausal symptoms exists with long-term therapy. However, concomitant use of estrogen and progesterone replacement therapy may counteract the adverse effects. Newer studies suggest that spironolactone may also simulate this effect.

Most studies have shown greater improvement of hirsutism with the use of GnRH agonists alone or in combination with oral contraceptives as compared with combination oral contraceptives alone; however, some studies show comparable efficacy. Endocrine society guidelines suggest against using GnRH agonists except in women with severe forms of hyperandrogenemia, such as ovarian hyperthecosis, who have a suboptimal response to oral contraceptive pills and antiandrogens.

Table 55–5. Suppression of hirsutism over baseline over 6 months compared with placebo.

Metformin	19.1%
Finasteride	20.3%
Oral contraceptive pills	27%
Thiazolidinediones	31.5%
Combination cyproterone acetate & ethinylestradiol	36%
Spironolactone	38.4%
Flutamide	41.3%

5. Androgen receptor antagonists—In a proportion of women, ovarian suppression alone may not be sufficient, and antiandrogens will need to be added. Patient-important hirsutism that remains despite ≥6 months of monotherapy with an oral contraceptive justify combination therapy by adding an antiandrogen.

Antiandrogens are efficacious for treating hirsutism. There are 4 androgen receptor antagonists currently being used for the treatment of hirsutism. Despite proven efficacy in numerous clinical trials, none of these drugs has been approved by the US Food and Drug Administration for this indication. Additionally, similar reported efficacy has been reported with all of these medications. Hence the agent of choice should be dictated by the individual's response, reported side effects, and known contraindications. All antiandrogens, and particularly finasteride, are potentially teratogenic, so some clinicians prescribe them only to women using reliable contraception.

A. Cyproterone acetate—This potent agent was the first androgen receptor antagonist used to treat hirsutism and is widely prescribed in Europe to treat hirsutism. Antiandrogenic effects result from competitive displacement of dihydrotestosterone from its receptor and reduction of 5α-reductase activity in the skin. Progestational activity results in gonadotropin suppression with subsequent suppression of ovarian testosterone secretion. Cyclical administration of 50–100 mg on days 1–10 of the menstrual cycle combined with oral estrogen on days 1–21 produces therapeutic levels. More prolonged use tends to induce amenorrhoea because of its progestogenic properties. This method counters hypoestrogenism and irregular bleeding and prevents pregnancy and the potential teratogenic complications that may result. Although effective in 50–75% of hirsute women, significant side effects include decreased libido, mental depression, and hepatotoxicity, which is rarely seen when cyclic administration is performed. Clinical studies have shown efficacy equivalent to that of spironolactone, with the latter showing fewer side effects (see next section). Currently, cyproterone acetate is not available in the United States.

B. Spironolactone—Spironolactone, an aldosterone antagonist traditionally used as a diuretic in the treatment of hypertension, is also used to treat hirsutism. Cochrane review showed that spironolactone can effectively suppress hirsutism. It possesses antiandrogenic properties and exerts its peripheral antiandrogenic effects in the hair follicle by competing for androgenic receptors and displacing dihydrotestosterone at both nuclear and cytosol receptors. It also lowers testosterone levels by inhibiting the cytochrome P450 monooxygenases that are required for biosynthesis of androgens in gonadal and adrenal steroid-producing cells. Serum levels of SHBG, DHEAS, and DHEA are unaltered by treatment with spironolactone. The dosage used for treatment of hirsutism is between 50 and 200 mg/d. Serum androgen levels will drop within a few days of the start of treatment, and a clinical response can usually be seen within 2–5 months. Side effects include fatigue, transient diuresis, polydipsia, menorrhagia or unscheduled menstrual bleeding, gastro-intestinal bleeding and breast tenderness, but no long-term problems have been encountered. Its anti-mineralocorticoid and diuretic properties are rarely prominent in young women. Because spironolactone is a potent antiandrogen, all women using it should use effective contraception. Nevertheless, women taking spironolactone should be sent for periodic screening of potassium level to identify hyperkalemia.

c. Flutamide—Flutamide is a potent, highly specific, nonsteroidal antiandrogen with no intrinsic hormonal or antigonadotropin activity. Although the exact mechanism of action is unknown, it competitively inhibits target tissue androgen receptor sites. Recent studies suggest that 250 mg 1–3 times daily is a highly effective treatment for moderate to severe hirsutism. Side effects include decreased appetite, amenorrhea, decreased libido, or dry skin. A rare but serious reported side effect is hepatotoxicity. Consequently, flutamide is usually reserved for resistant cases of hirsutism, and liver enzymes should be checked regularly in patients who are taking the drug. Additionally, because of possible teratogenic effects, contraception must be used with this therapy. Endocrine Society Clinical Practice Guideline recommends against flutamide for the treatment of hirsutism.

d. Finasteride—If additional treatment is needed, then finasteride would be a sensible option because it has a different mode of action. Finasteride is the newest antiandrogenic agent used for hirsutism. It is a selective type 2 5α-reductase inhibitor that blocks the conversion of testosterone to dihydrotestosterone. It has proven efficacy in up to 86% of patients with a subjective improvement rate of 21–45% when 5 mg is administered orally over 3 months to 1 year. Side effects at this dosage are usually mild or absent and include headaches, transient gastrointestinal upset, and an unexplained increase in total testosterone.

6. Glucocorticoids—Dexamethasone is used mainly to treat hirsutism in patients with hyperandrogenism of adrenal origin. Chronic low-dose dexamethasone, 0.5–1 mg orally taken at bedtime, will provide adequate adrenal androgen suppression. Diminution of hair growth is reported in 16–70% of patients. Glucocorticoid therapy has fallen out of favor due to frequent side effects, potential for adrenal suppression, and evidence that these agents are less effective than antiandrogens, even when there is a clear adrenal cause of hyperandrogenism. However, their use may be justified in some patients, as recent data suggest that concomitant use of glucocorticoids with GnRH agonists may prolong the disease-free interval when therapy is discontinued. Moreover, glucocorticoids are the treatment of choice to decrease ACTH levels and thereby decrease formation of androgenic precursors of cortisol for patients with CAH.

7. Dopamine—Dopamine is a centrally acting inhibitor of prolactin secretion and is frequently used in the treatment of hyperprolactinemia. Recently, hirsutism scores were shown to decrease significantly during dopamine treatment of hyperandrogenic women with hyperprolactinemia.

8. Insulin-Lowering Drugs—Insulin, which acts as a co-gonadotrophin and amplifies LH-induced testosterone production, is a secondary driver of ovarian androgen secretion. Troglitazone, an insulin-sensitizing agent of the thiazolidinedione class, results in a decrease in androgen level in patients with polycystic ovarian syndrome. Additionally, it has been shown that the administration of 600 mg/d results in improvement of hirsutism in this population. Endocrine Society Clinical Practice Guideline recommends against the use of insulin-lowering drugs for the treatment of hirsutism.

Conveniently, women for whom suppression of LH is not possible (eg, obese women who should not take the oral contraceptive pill because of the risk of thrombosis) are often the very women for whom suppression of insulin is most effective. Nevertheless, insulin sensitizers are of limited use as sole treatment for hirsutism.

9. Cimetidine—Cimetidine, an H2-receptor antagonist, has weak antiandrogenic properties. Recent studies show minimal or no beneficial effect in hirsutism.

10. Ketoconazole—Ketoconazole is a synthetic imidazole derivative that blocks adrenal and gonadal steroidogenesis; it has been advocated by some as a treatment for hirsutism. However, serious side effects result in poor compliance and preclude long-term use. Its use should be avoided because safer therapeutic regimens exist.

C. Mechanical Therapy

The goal of mechanical therapy is to limit new hair growth without affecting existing hair. For this reason, mechanical depilators such as lasers, electrolysis devices, creams, and waxes are often used as supplemental therapy (Table 55–4). Recent technology has made this procedure faster, easier, less painful, and generally free of any serious adverse effects. Many women will be familiar with routine methods of hair removal such as shaving, threading, waxing, and using depilatory creams and can be reassured that these methods do not exacerbate hair growth. Electrolysis and laser epilation or photoepilation are also widely available. A review of 11 trials of laser and light-assisted hair removal in 444 patients showed a 50% reduction in hair over 6 months but noted that the long-term efficacy of these treatments is not well established. Laser treatment is less effective in darker skin because a contrast is needed between skin and hair pigments, but some types of photoepilation can be of benefit patients with for darker skin.

D. Surgical Treatment

In the minority of hirsute patients in whom a specific cause can be identified, therapy should be directed toward the underlying disorder. For example, ovarian and adrenal tumors should be surgically excised. Additionally, women with Cushing's disease are treated with transsphenoidal pituitary microsurgery. Alternatively, when Cushing's syndrome is caused by an adrenal tumor, simple adrenalectomy is sufficient. Finally, acromegaly can be treated by transsphenoidal hypophysectomy. For persistent disease, bilateral adrenalectomy or pituitary irradiation is appropriate.

Similarly, a minority of older women may fail to respond to medical management for hyperthecosis despite good compliance. For these women, bilateral oophorectomy may be justified as definitive therapy.

Although wedge resection of the ovary has been successfully used to induce ovulation, it is not recommended for the treatment of hirsutism. This surgical procedure exposes patients to the risks of both anesthesia and possible formation of adhesions. More importantly, this procedure results in only a transient decrease in androgen levels and has successfully reduced the rate of hair growth in only 16% of patients. Wedge resection should not be used as a treatment for hirsutism.

Prognosis

Prognosis for women with hirsutism, hypertrichosis, and precocious sexual hair development depends on the underlying conditions leading to these physical findings, early appropriate evaluation, and appropriate treatment.

A. Follow-up

The success of treatment is usually based on subjective assessment, and clinicians should not contribute to unrealistic expectations of effectiveness. Patient expectations should be discussed, as even compliant patients should expect no more than 25% reduction in hair growth using systemic treatment. Some patients see no benefit, and some are resistant to any systemic treatment.

Women with mild hirsutism may not notice much benefit, and some women will prove resistant to all treatments. Psychologic interventions may be useful for women with unsatisfactory outcomes, but no trials have assessed the effectiveness of such interventions specifically for hirsutism. Testosterone measurements can be misleading because oral contraceptives cause a rise in SHBG, which results in an increase in the total blood testosterone concentration. No specific guidelines exist for monitoring long-term treatments, but it seems logical to measure liver function in users of cyproterone acetate; plasma potassium, liver function, and renal function in users of spironolactone; and vitamin B_{12} concentrations in users of metformin (which is associated with low concentrations of this vitamin).

In conclusion, hirsutism is a common problem, the effect of which is often underestimated. Various treatment options are available, which—when used in logical combinations and tailored to the individual's clinical profile—can achieve good results in most cases.

Azziz R, Carmina E, Sawaya ME. Idiopathic hirsutism. *Endocr Rev* 2000;21:347–362. PMID: 10950156.

Paus R, Cotsarelis G. The biology of hair follicles. *N Engl J Med* 1999;341:491–497. PMID: 10441606.

Deplewski D, Rosenfield RL. Role of hormones in pilosebaceous unit development. *Endocr Rev* 2000;21:363–392. PMID: 10950157.

Ferriman DM, Gallwey JD. Clinical assessment of body hair growth in women. *J Clin Endocrinol* 1961:21:1440–1447.

Goodman N, Bledsoe M, Cobin R, et al. American Association of Clinical Endocrinologists medical guidelines for the clinical practice for the diagnosis and treatment of hyperandrogenic disorders. *Endocrine Pract* 2001;7:120–134. PMID: 12940239

Koulouri O, Conway GS. A systematic review of commonly used medical treatments for hirsutism in women. *Clin Endocrinol* 2008;68:800–805. PMID: 17980017.

Martin KA. Evaluation and treatment of hirsutism in premenopausal women: an endocrine society clinical practice guideline. *J Clin Endocrinol Metab* 2008;93:1105–1120. PMID: 18252793.

Yildiz BO. Assessment, diagnosis and treatment of a patient with hirsutism. *Nat Clin Pract Endocrinol Metab* 2008; 4:294–300. PMID: 18332896.

Endometriosis

56

Susan Sarajari, MD, PhD
Kenneth N. Muse, Jr., MD
Michael D. Fox, MD

ESSENTIALS OF DIAGNOSIS

- Endometriosis is a disorder in which abnormal growths of tissue, histologically resembling the endometrium, are present in locations other than the uterine lining.
- Although endometriosis can occur very rarely in post-menopausal women, it is found almost exclusively in women of reproductive age.
- All other manifestations of endometriosis exhibit a wide spectrum of expression.
- The lesions are usually found on the peritoneal surfaces of the reproductive organs and adjacent structures of the pelvis, but they can occur anywhere in the body (Fig. 56–1).
- The size of the individual lesions varies from microscopic to large invasive masses that erode into underlying organs and cause extensive adhesion formation.
- Similarly, women with endometriosis can be completely asymptomatic or may be crippled by pelvic pain and infertility.

Epidemiology

Endometriosis is a common and important health problem of women. Its exact prevalence is unknown because surgery is required for its diagnosis, but it is estimated to be present in 6–10% of women in the reproductive age group and 25–35% of infertile women. It is seen in 1–2% of women undergoing sterilization or sterilization reversal, in 10% of hysterectomy surgeries, in 16–31% of laparoscopies, and in 53% of adolescents with pelvic pain severe enough to warrant surgical evaluation. Endometriosis is the commonest single gynecologic diagnosis responsible for hospitalization of women aged 15–44, being found in more than 6% of patients.

Cramer DW. Epidemiology of endometriosis. In: Wilson EA (ed): *Endometriosis*. New York, NY: Alan R. Liss; 1987, p. 5.

Gruppos Italiano per lo Studio Dell'Endometriosi. Prevalence and anatomical distribution of endometriosis in women with selected gynaecological conditions: results from a multicentric Italian study. *Hum Reprod* 1994;9:1158–1162. PMID: 7962393.

Olive DL, Schwartz LB. Endometriosis. *N Engl J Med* 1993; 328:1759–1769. PMID: 8110213.

Wheeler JM. Epidemiology and prevalence of endometriosis. *Infertil Reprod Med Clin North Am* 1992;3:545.

Zhao SZ, Wong JM, Davis MB, et al. The cost of inpatient endometriosis treatment: an analysis based on the Healthcare Cost and Utilization Project Nationwide Inpatient Sample. *Am J Manag Care* 1998;4:1127–1134. PMID: 10182888.

Pathogenesis

The cause of endometriosis is complex, and the leading theories include retrograde menstruation with transport of endometrial cells, metaplasia of coelomic epithelium, hematogenous or lymphatic spread, and direct transplantation of endometrial cells. A combination of these theories is likely to be responsible.

A theory of retrograde menstruation was proposed during the 1920s. It was postulated that endometriosis occurred because viable fragments of endometrium were shed at the time of menstruation and passed through the fallopian tubes. Once in the pelvic cavity, the tissue became implanted on peritoneal surfaces and grew into endometriotic lesions. Subsequent observations have confirmed that some degree of retrograde menstruation normally occurs in women with patent tubes, that outflow tract obstructions (cervical stenosis, transverse vaginal septa) increase the incidence of endometriosis, and that intentional deposition of endometrium onto peritoneum can initiate endometriosis. Also, the risk of developing the disease is higher in women with prolonged menstrual flow and in those with short menstrual cycle lengths (more menses per year). This theory is simple, attractive, and easily explains why endometriosis is most

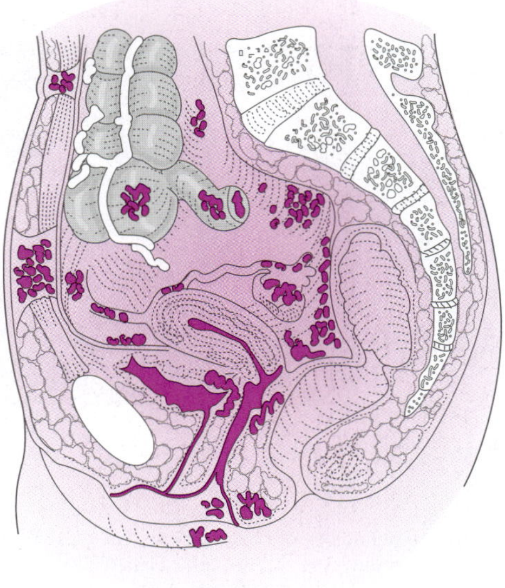

▲ **Figure 56–1.** Common sites of endometrial implants (endometriosis). (Reproduced, with permission, from Way LW (ed). *Current Surgical Diagnosis & Treatment.* 7th ed. Los Altos, CA: Lange; 1985.)

commonly found on the peritoneal surfaces of the ovaries, cul-de-sac, and bladder and why lesions may develop in episiotomies and other incisions. However, it does not explain why all women do not develop endometriosis, nor does it explain the rare cases of endometriosis in the lung, brain, or other soft tissues or in nonmenstruating subjects (women with Turner's syndrome or with absent uteri).

There is evidence that altered humoral and cell-mediated immunity plays a role in the pathogenesis of endometriosis. The activity of natural killer cells may be reduced, and deficient cellular immunity may cause an inability to recognize endometrial tissue in abnormal locations. Endometriosis may occur when the deficiency in cellular immunity allows menstrual tissue to implant and grow on the peritoneum.

Genetic influences in the development of endometriosis have also been described. Studies have found that 7–9% of endometriosis patients' first-degree female relatives are diagnosed with the disease—significantly greater than the control rate of 1–2%. Further investigation has revealed a possible role for the HLA-B7 allele. The expression of HLA-B7 has been shown to inhibit the cytotoxic activity of natural killer-like T lymphocytes, suggesting that the growth of ectopic endometrial cells might be under genetic control.

American College of Obstetricians and Gynecologists: Endometriosis. ACOG Technical Bulletin No. 114. Washington, DC: ACOG; July 2010.

Coxhead D, Thomas EJ. Familial inheritance of endometriosis in a British population: A case control study. *J Obstet Gynaecol* 1993;13:42.

Ho HN, Wu MY, Yang YS. Peritoneal cellular immunity and endometriosis. *Am J Reprod Immunol* 1997;38:400–412. PMID: 9412723.

Oosterlynck DJ, Meuleman C, Waer M, Koninckx PR, Vandeputte M. Immunosuppressive activity of peritoneal fluid in women with endometriosis. *Obstet Gynecol* 1993;82:206–212. PMID: 8336865.

Ramey JW, Archer DF. Peritoneal fluid: Its relevance to the development of endometriosis. *Fertil Steril* 1993;60:1–14. PMID: 8513924.

Schenken RS. Pathogenesis, clinical features, and diagnosis of endometriosis. Up To Date 2005.

Semino C, Semino A, Pietra G, et al. Role of major histocompatibility complex class I expression and natural killer-like T cells in the genetic control of endometriosis. *Fertil Steril* 1995;64:909–916. PMID: 7589633.

Pathology

The gross appearance of endometriosis at operation is usually quite characteristic and, to an experienced surgeon, is sufficient for diagnosis. The smallest (and presumably earliest) implants are red, petechial lesions on the peritoneal surface. With further growth, menstrual-like detritus accumulates within the lesion, giving it a cystic, dark brown, dark blue, or black appearance. The surrounding peritoneal surface becomes thickened and scarred. These "powder burn" implants typically attain a size of 5–10 mm in diameter. With progression of disease, the number and size of lesions increase, and extensive adhesions may develop. When present on the ovary, cysts may enlarge to several centimeters in size and are called **endometriomas** or "chocolate cysts." Severe disease can erode into underlying tissues and distort the remaining organs with extensive adhesions. In addition to these traditional presentations, endometriosis lesions can have a variety of nonclassical appearances: clear vesicles, white or yellow spots or nodules, circular folds of peritoneum ("pockets"), and visually normal peritoneum (lesions so small they can only be detected microscopically).

The distribution of lesions also exhibits a characteristic pattern. Solitary lesions are possible, but multiple implantations are the rule. The most common site of disease is the ovary (approximately half of all cases), followed by the uterine cul-de-sac, posterior broad ligament, uterosacral ligaments, uterus, fallopian tubes, sigmoid colon, appendix, and round ligaments. Implants may occur over the bowel, bladder, and ureters; rarely, they may erode into underlying tissue and cause blood in the stool or urine, or their associated adhesions may result in stricture and obstruction of these organs. Implants can occur deep in tissue, especially on the cervix, posterior vaginal fornix, or within wounds contaminated by endometrial tissue. Very rarely, endometriosis is found distant from the pelvis, in such sites as the lung, brain, and kidney. Pleural implantations are associated with recurrent right pneumothoraces at the time of menses, termed **catamenial pneumothorax** . Similarly, lesions in the central nervous system can cause catamenial seizures.

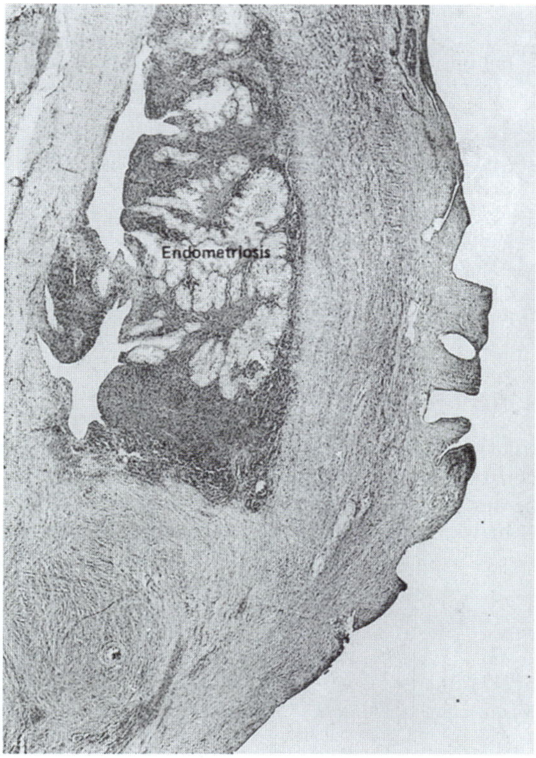

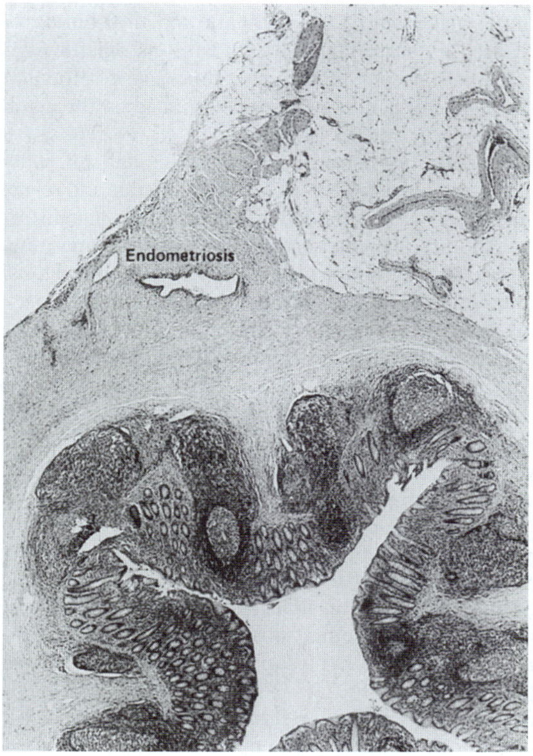

▲ **Figure 56–2.** Histologic appearance of endometriosis. **Left:** Endometriosis of ovary. **Right:** Endometriosis of cervix.

The microscopic finding that these lesions are composed of tissue histologically resembling endometrial glands and stroma gives endometriosis its name (Fig. 56–2). The normal endometrial appearance is best seen in small, early lesions; with advanced disease, cyst formation, and fibrosis, the wall of the implant is lined by a monolayer of cells, if at all. Blood is present inside the cyst, and hemosiderin-laden macrophages are found in the cyst wall.

Bergqvist A, Ferno M. Estrogen and progesterone receptors in endometriotic tissue and endometrium: Comparison according to localization and recurrence. *Fertil Steril* 1993;60:63–68. PMID: 8513960.

Murphy AA, Green WR, Bobbie D, dela Cruz ZC, Rock JA. Unsuspected endometriosis documented by scanning electron microscopy in visually normal peritoneum. *Fertil Steril* 1986;46:522–524. PMID: 3743803.

Schenken RS. Pathogenesis, clinical features, and diagnosis of endometriosis. Up To Date 2005.

Pathologic Physiology

Overproduction of prostaglandins by an increase in cyclooxygenase-2 activity as well as overproduction of estrogen by increased aromatase activity are considered key factors in the development of endometriosis. Progesterone resistance is also seen, which weakens the antiestrogenic effect of progesterone. This can lead to a chronic inflammatory response, and the most commonly found inflammatory cytokines are interleukin 1,6, and 8, and tumor necrosis factor α.

It is generally agreed that pelvic pain occurs premenstrually in endometriosis patients. Because of this, pain from endometriosis is thought to be due to stimulation from estrogen and progesterone during the menstrual cycle; the tissue of the implant is stimulated to grow in much the same way as is the endometrium. The implants enlarge and may undergo secretory change and bleeding; however, the fibrotic tissues surrounding the implants prevent the expansion and escape of hemorrhagic fluid that occurs in the uterus. With subsequent cycles, this process repeats itself. Pain is produced by pressure and inflammation within and around the lesion, by traction on adhesions associated with the lesions, by the number of implants and their proximity to nerves and other sensitive structures, and by the mass effect of large lesions. Although this sequence of events explains why premenstrual pelvic pain can occur in endometriosis, it is incomplete, because many patients with extensive endometriosis have no pain. It is a common observation that the occurrence and severity of pain from endometriosis bear little relationship to the amount and distribution of the disease. Severe pain in patients with endometriosis is associated with deeply infiltrating lesions, and it is thought that the degree of pain is perhaps determined by the depth of invasion.

The relationship between endometriosis and infertility has been more extensively investigated. Moderate and severe endometriosis is associated with pelvic adhesions that distort pelvic anatomy, prevent normal tubo-ovarian apposition, and encase the ovary. Implants can destroy ovarian and tubal tissue, although occlusion of fallopian tubes is rare.

It is not difficult to understand how advanced disease can result in infertility, but minimal or mild endometriosis, in which pelvic anatomy is entirely normal except for a few peritoneal surface lesions, can also cause infertility. The mechanism by which this occurs is unknown. Various theories have been proposed to explain this phenomenon.

Several investigators have examined peritoneal fluid abnormalities. The peritoneal fluid is an ultrafiltrate of plasma, with <5 mL normally present in the pelvis. After ovulation, a transient rise to approximately 20 mL occurs. The volume of peritoneal fluid and the concentrations of various hormones and other substances in it affect the processes of ovulation, ovum pickup, tubal function, and sperm function.

A marker for ovarian reserve, antimüllerian hormone, has also been found to be decreased in early-stage endometriosis.

Bedaiwy MA, Falcone T, Sharma RK, et al. Prediction of endometriosis with serum and peritoneal fluid markers: a prospective controlled trial. *Hum Reprod* 2002;17:426–431. PMID: 11821289.

Bulun SE. Endometriosis. *N Engl J Med* 2009;360:268–279. PMID: 19144942.

Koninckx PR, Meuleman C, Demeyere S, Lesaffre E, Cornillie FJ. Suggestive evidence that pelvic endometriosis is a progressive disease, whereas deeply infiltrating endometriosis is associated with pelvic pain. *Fertil Steril* 1991;55:759–765. PMID: 2010001.

Lemos NA, Arbo E, Scalco R, Weiler E, Rosa V, Cunha-Filho JS. Decreased anti-Mullerian hormone and altered ovarian follicular cohort in infertile patients with mild/minimal endometriosis. *Fertil Steril* 2008;89:1064–1068. PMID: 17624337.

Mansour G, Aziz N, Sharma R, Falcone T, Goldberg J, Agarwal A. The impact of peritoneal fluid from healthy women and from women with endometriosis on sperm DNA and its relationship to the sperm deformity index. *Fertil Steril* 2009;92:61–67. PMID: 19409553.

Pittaway DE, Ellington CP, Klimek M. Preclinical abortions and endometriosis. *Fertil Steril* 1988;49:221–223. PMID: 2448170.

Rodriguez-Escudero FJ, Neyro JL, Corcostegui B, Benito JA. Does minimal endometriosis reduce fecundity? *Fertil Steril* 1988;50:522–524. PMID: 3410104.

Steele RW, Dmowski WP, Marmer DJ. Deficient cellular immunity in endometriosis. *Am J Reprod Immunol* 1984;6:33–36. PMID: 6476182.

Said TM, Agarwal A, Falcone T, Sharma RK, Bedaiwy MA, Li L. Infliximab may reverse the toxic effects induced by tumor necrosis factor alpha in human spermatozoa: an in vitro model. *Fertil Steril* 2005;83:1665–1673. PMID: 15950634.

Switchenko AC, Kauffman RS, Becker A. Are there endometrial antibodies in sera of women with endometriosis? *Fertil Steril* 1991;56:235–241. PMID: 2070852.

Syrop CH, Halme J. Peritoneal fluid environment and infertility. *Fertil Steril* 1987;48:1–9. PMID: 3109960.

Vercellini P, Trespidi L, De Giorgi O, Cortesi I, Parazzini F, Crosignani PG. Endometriosis and pelvic pain: relation to disease stage and localization. *Fertil Steril* 1996;65:299–304.

Risk Factors

Risk factors for endometriosis include family history, early menarche, long duration of menstrual flow, heavy bleeding during menses, and shorter cycles. Regular exercise of >4 hr/wk, higher parity, and longer duration of lactation were all associated with a decreased risk for endometriosis.

Cramer DW, Missmer SA. The epidemiology of endometriosis. *Ann N Y Acad Sci* 2002;955:11–22; discussion 34–6, 396. PMID: 11949940.

Missmer SA, Hankinson SE, Spiegelman D, et al. Reproductive history and endometriosis among premenopausal women. *Obstet Gynecol* 2004;104:965–974. PMID: 15516386.

Signorello LB, Harlow BL, Cramer DW, Spiegelman D, Hill JA. Epidemiologic determinants of endometriosis: a hospital-based case-control study. *Ann Epidemiol* 1997;7:267–741. PMID: 9177109.

Prevention

Prevention of endometriosis is not currently possible. Traditionally, women with relatives affected by endometriosis—or in whom the diagnosis has recently been made—are advised not to postpone childbearing. The merits of this advice have not been proved. A more thorough understanding of the pathophysiology of endometriosis is required before preventive strategies can be devised.

Clinical Findings

Endometriosis is common among women of reproductive age, and its prevalence increases to 30–40% among infertile women. Clinical findings vary greatly depending on the number, size, and extent of the lesions and on the patient population being examined.

The diagnosis of endometriosis is often strongly suspected from a patient's initial history. Infertility, dysmenorrhea, and dyspareunia are the main presenting complaints. Most patients complain of constant pelvic pain or a low sacral backache that occurs premenstrually and subsides after menses begins. Dyspareunia is often present, particularly with deep penetration. Lesions involving the urinary tract or bowel may result in bloody urine or stool in the perimenstrual interval. Implantations on or near the external surfaces of the cervix, vagina, vulva, rectum, or urethra may cause pain or bleeding with defecation, urination, or intercourse at any time in the menstrual cycle. Adhesions from endometriosis may cause discomfort at any time during the cycle, and a sensation of pelvic pressure may result if large masses are present. Premenstrual spotting may occur and is more likely to be associated with endometriosis than with luteal phase inadequacy. It must be emphasized, however, that many patients either have no symptoms or have infertility as their only symptom and that the extent of disease often has little correlation with the severity of symptoms.

The physical examination may also be helpful in discerning whether endometriosis is present. Classically, pelvic examination reveals tender nodules in the posterior vaginal fornix and pain upon uterine motion. The uterus may be fixed and retroverted due to cul-de-sac adhesions, and tender adnexal masses may be felt because of the presence of endometriomas. Careful inspection may reveal implants in healed wounds, especially episiotomy and caesarean section incisions, in the vaginal fornix, or on the cervix. Biopsy may be required to prove that the lesions are due to endometriosis. However, many patients have no abnormal findings on physical examination.

For the vast majority of patients, endometriosis is included in the differential diagnosis of infertility or pelvic pain. Endometriosis should be suspected in any patient of reproductive age complaining of pain or infertility. Medical treatment can be given for pelvic pain thought to be due to endometriosis, but the specific diagnosis of endometriosis should not be made unless documented by direct visualization. The final diagnosis of endometriosis can only be made at laparoscopy or laparotomy, by direct observation of the implants. Occasionally, an isolated endometrioma is removed, and the diagnosis must be made histologically by the demonstration of "endometrial" glands and stroma or of hemosiderin-laden macrophages in the cyst wall.

Except for special circumstances, such as urography or sigmoidoscopy for suspected bowel or urinary involvement, ancillary diagnostic studies (ultrasound, x-rays, computed tomography scans) are of little help in diagnosis. CA-125 is often elevated in women with endometriosis; however, it has been shown that this marker is elevated in many other pelvic diseases and therefore has little specificity in the diagnosis of endometriosis. However, an elevated CA-125 that returns to normal levels after medical or surgical treatment can be helpful in the evaluation for recurrences.

American College of Obstetricians and Gynecologists. Endometriosis. ACOG Technical Bulletin No. 114. Washington, DC: ACOG; July 2010.

Fauconnier A, Chapron C, Dubuisson JB, Vieira M, Dousset B, Breart G. Relation between pain symptoms and the anatomic location of deep infiltrating endometriosis. *Fertil Steril* 2002; 78:719–726.

Vlahos N, Fortner KB. Emerging issues in endometriosis. *Postgrad Obstet Gynecol* 2005;25:1–9.

Differential Diagnosis

The varied presentations of endometriosis mandate that it be considered in the differential diagnosis of virtually all pelvic disease. In particular, the pain, infertility, and adhesions associated with endometriosis must be distinguished from similar symptoms accompanying pelvic inflammatory disease and pelvic tumors. Usually this will require operative evaluation. A patient with a persistent adnexal mass >5 cm should never be presumed to have an endometrioma even if endometriosis has been diagnosed previously. Such masses require surgical diagnosis.

Complications

True complications of endometriosis are few. Implants over the bowel or ureters may cause obstruction and silent impairment of renal function. The erosive nature of the lesions in advanced aggressive disease can cause a myriad of symptoms, depending on the tissue damaged. Endometriomas can cause ovarian torsion or can rupture and spill their irritating contents into the peritoneal cavity, resulting in a chemical peritonitis. Excision of endometriosis causing catamenial seizures or pneumothorax may be necessary.

Schorlemmer GR, Battaglini JW. Pneumothorax in menstruating females. *Contemp Surg* 1982;20:53.

Zwas FR, Lyon DT. Endometriosis: An important condition in clinical gastroenterology. *Dig Dis Sci* 1991;36:353–364. PMID: 1995273.

Classification

Several classification schemes to assist in describing the anatomic location and severity of endometriosis at operation have been created. Although none is entirely satisfactory, the scoring systems are useful for reporting operative findings and for comparing the results of various treatment protocols. The revised American Fertility Society classification is the most commonly used system and is given in Table 56–1 and Figure 56–3. It should be noted that this system does not correlate well with the symptoms of pain, dyspareunia, or infertility, but is mainly designed for uniform recording of operative findings.

American College of Obstetricians and Gynecologists. Endometriosis. ACOG Technical Bulletin No. 114. Washington, DC: ACOG; July 2010.

Table 56–1. American Society for Reproductive Medicine revised classification of endometriosis.

	Endometriosis	<1 cm	1–3 cm	>3 cm
Peritoneum	Superficial	1	2	4
	Deep	2	4	6
Ovary	R Superficial	1	2	4
	Deep	4	16	20
	L Superficial	1	2	4
	Deep	4	16	20
	Posterior Cul-de-sac Obliteration	Partial	Complete	
		4	40	
	Adhesions	<1/3 Enclosure	1/3–2/3 Enclosure	>2/3 Enclosure
Ovary	R Filmy	1	2	4
	Dense	4	8	16
	L Filmy	1	2	4
	Dense	4	8	16
Tube	R Filmy	1	2	4
	Dense	4[1]	8[1]	16
	L Filmy	1	2	4
	Dense	4[1]	8[1]	16

[1]If the fimbriated end of the fallopian tube is completely enclosed, change the point assignment to 16. Staging: Stage I (minimal): 1–5; stage II (mild): 6–15; stage III (moderate): 16–40; stage IV (severe): > 40. (Reproduced, with permission, from American Society for Reproductive Medicine. Revised ASRM classification of endometriosis: 1996. *Fertil Steril* 1997; 67:819.)

Treatment

Treatment options are dictated by the patient's desire for future fertility, her symptoms, the stage of her disease, and to some extent her age. It must be emphasized that therapy for endometriosis requires operative inspection of the lesions for correct diagnosis and staging and to be sure that the patient's symptoms are attributable to endometriosis only.

A. Expectant Management

In asymptomatic patients, those with mild discomfort, or infertile women with minimal or mild endometriosis, expectant management may be appropriate. Although endometriosis is generally felt to be a progressive disease, there is no evidence that treating an asymptomatic patient will prevent or ameliorate the onset of symptoms later. Many reports have found expectant management of infertile women with minimal or mild endometriosis to be as successful as medical or surgical therapies.

B. Analgesic Therapy

Analgesic treatments include nonsteroidal anti-inflammatory agents and prostaglandin synthetase-inhibiting drugs. These drugs are appropriate sole therapy for endometriosis when the patient has mild premenstrual pain from minimal endometriosis, no abnormalities on pelvic examination, and no desire for immediate fertility.

C. Hormonal Therapy

The goal of treatment with hormonal therapy is to interrupt the cycles of stimulation and bleeding of endometriotic tissue. This can be achieved with various agents.

1. Oral contraceptive pills (OCPs)—OCPs are a good choice for patients with minimal or mild symptoms. Generally monophasic products are used, which are prescribed either cyclically or continuously for 6–12 months. The continuous exposure to combination oral contraceptive

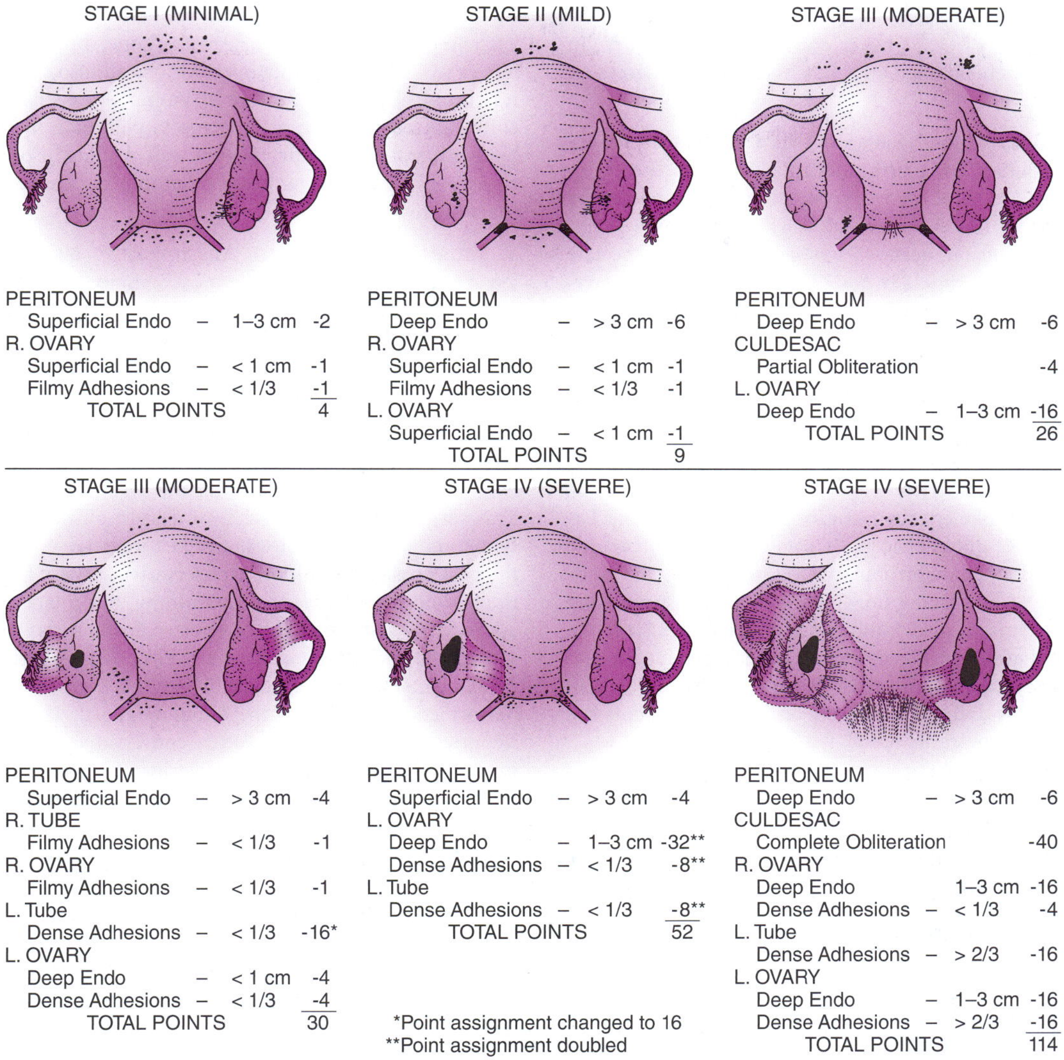

▲ **Figure 56–3.** Staging of endometriosis. Determination of the stage or degree of endometrial involvement is based on a weighted point system (see Table 56–1 for point values). Distribution of points has been arbitrarily determined and may require further revision or refinement as knowledge of the disease increases. To ensure complete evaluation, inspection of the pelvis in a clockwise or counterclockwise fashion is encouraged. Number, size, and location of endometrial implants, plaques, endometriomas, and/or adhesions are noted. For example, 5 separate 0.5-cm superficial implants on the peritoneum (2.5 cm total) would be assigned 2 points. (The surface of the uterus should be considered peritoneum.) The severity of the endometriosis or adhesions should be assigned the highest score only for peritoneum, ovary, tube, or cul-de-sac. For example, a 4-cm superficial and a 2-cm deep implant of the peritoneum should be given a score of 6 (not 8). A 4-cm deep endometrioma of the ovary associated with more than 3 cm of superficial disease should be scored 20 (not 24). In patients with only 1 set of adnexa, points applied to disease of the remaining tube and ovary should be multiplied by 2. Points assigned may be circled and totaled. Aggregation of points indicates stage of disease (minimal, mild, moderate, or severe). The presence of endometriosis of the bowel, urinary tract, fallopian tube, vagina, cervix, skin, and so forth should be documented under "additional endometriosis." Other pathology such as tubal occlusion, leiomyomata, uterine anomaly, and so forth should be documented under "additional pathology." All pathology should be depicted as specifically as possible on the sketch of pelvic organs, and means of observation (laparoscopy or laparotomy) should be noted.(Reproduced, with permission, from American Society for Reproductive Medicine. Revised ASRM classification for endometriosis: 1996. *Fertil Steril* 1997;67:820.)

pills results in decidual changes in the endometrial glands. Continuous use of OCPs has been shown to be effective in decreasing dysmenorrhea and may also retard progression of endometriosis.

2. Progestins—These agents work via a mechanism similar to that of the OCPs, causing decidualization in the endometriotic tissue. Oral medroxyprogesterone acetate can be prescribed as a 10–30-mg dosage daily. An alternative regimen is norethindrone acetate 5 mg daily or megestrol acetate prescribed as a 40-mg daily dose. Depot medroxyprogesterone acetate 150 mg administered intramuscularly can also be given as a single injection every 3 months.

The levonorgestrel-releasing intrauterine device has also been shown to relief dysmenorrheal and pelvic pain. Eighty percent of women treated with progestins have a partial or complete relief of pain.

3. Danazol—Danazol is a 19-nortestosterone derivative with progestin-like effects. Danazol acts via several mechanisms to treat endometriosis. It acts at the hypothalamic level to inhibit gonadotropin release, inhibiting the midcycle surge of luteinizing hormone and follicle-stimulating hormone. Danazol also inhibits steroidogenic enzymes in the ovary that are responsible for estrogen production. As a result, a hypoestrogenic environment is created. This, in addition to the androgenic effects of danazol, prevents the growth of endometriotic tissue.

The dosage of danazol is 400 to 800 mg/d in divided doses for 6 months. Side effects of danazol include acne, oily skin, deepening of the voice, weight gain, edema, and adverse plasma lipoprotein changes. Most changes are reversible upon cessation of therapy, but some (such as deepening of the voice) may not be.

Pain relief is achieved in up to 90% of patients taking danazol.

4. GnRH agonists—Gonadotropin-releasing hormone (GnRH) agonists are analogues of the 10-amino-acid peptide hormone GnRH. With the continuous administration of GnRH analogues, suppression of gonadotropin secretion occurs, resulting in elimination of ovarian steroidogenesis and suppression of endometrial implants. Pain related to endometriosis is relieved in most cases by the second or third month of therapy. GnRH agonists can be administered intramuscularly as leuprolide acetate 3.75 mg once a month, intranasally as nafarelin 400 to 800 μg daily, or subcutaneously as goserelin 3.6 mg once a month.

The use of these agents is generally limited to 6 months because of the adverse effects associated with a hypoestrogenic state, particularly loss of bone mineral density. Other side effects include vasomotor symptoms, vaginal dryness, and mood changes.

Many side effects can be minimized by providing add-back therapy in addition to the GnRH agonists in the treatment of endometriosis. The addition of 2.5 mg of norethindrone or 0.625 mg of conjugated estrogens with 5 mg/d of medroxyprogesterone acetate seems to provide relief of vasomotor symptoms and decrease bone mineral density loss in a 6-month treatment period. The addition of 5 mg of norethindrone acetate alone or in conjunction with low-dose conjugated equine estrogen seems to eliminate the loss of bone mineral density effectively as well. Adding bisphosphonates, parathyroid hormone, or calcitonin can also minimize the bone loss.

5. Aromatase inhibitors—Anastrozole (1 mg daily) and letrozole (2.5 mg daily) are the most commonly used aromatase inhibitors. They act by inhibiting the enzyme aromatase, which functions in the conversion of androgens to estrogens. They can be used as an adjuvant treatment combined with other agents such as GnRH analogs.

6. Surgical treatment—In women who want to preserve fertility, who have severe disease, or who have adhesions, conservative surgical therapy is the treatment of choice. This surgery attempts to excise or destroy all endometriotic tissue, remove all adhesions, and restore pelvic anatomy to the best possible condition. Conservative surgery has traditionally been performed at laparotomy, but a laparoscopic approach is associated with a shorter hospital stay and less morbidity, and it is more cost effective. This is particularly true in contemporary practice, where this therapy is usually performed at the time of the initial diagnostic laparoscopy. Reported pregnancy rates after conservative surgery are inversely proportional to the severity of disease and vary greatly. In counseling patients, approximate pregnancy rates of 75% for mild disease, 50–60% for moderate disease, and 30–40% for severe disease should be quoted; however, individualization of therapy is stressed.

Presacral neurectomy to relieve pain should be performed only in selected cases, such as women with recurrent endometriosis, severe incapacitating dysmenorrhea, or disease that did not respond to initial treatment, as efficacy of this treatment is controversial.

If the patient does not desire future childbearing and has severe disease or symptoms, definitive surgery is appropriate and often curative. This entails total abdominal hysterectomy, bilateral salpingo-oophorectomy, and excision of remaining adhesions or implants. If endometriosis remains after excision, postoperative medical therapy may be indicated. After this or after complete excision, hormone replacement therapy is indicated. Estrogen-progestin therapy may be used without reactivating the endometriosis, but individualization of therapy is required.

7. Assisted Reproduction—Infertile women with endometriosis who are older, or who have failed other therapies for infertility, can undergo assisted reproduction, such as ovulation induction with intrauterine insemination or in vitro fertilization (IVF). However, it was found that women with endometriosis undergoing IVF have significantly lower pregnancy rates, fertilization rates, implantation rates, mean number of oocytes retrieved, and peak estradiol concentrations as compared with women with tubal factor infertility. The need to treat women surgically or medically before starting an IVF cycle remains unclear.

American College of Obstetricians and Gynecologists. Endometriosis. ACOG Technical Bulletin No. 114. Washington, DC: ACOG; July 2010.

Barbieri RL. Hormonal treatment of endometriosis: The estrogen threshold hypothesis. *Am J Obstet Gynecol* 1992;166:740–745. PMID: 1536260.

Barbieri RL, Ryan KJ. Danazol: Endocrine pharmacology and therapeutic applications. *Am J Obstet Gynecol* 1981;141: 453–463. PMID: 7025640.

Cook AS, Rock JA. The role of laparoscopy in the treatment of endometriosis. *Fertil Steril* 1991;55:663–680. PMID: 1826275.

Dlugi AM, Miller JD, Knittle J. Lupron depot (leuprolide acetate for depot suspension) in the treatment of endometriosis: A randomized placebo-controlled, double-blind study. *Fertil Steril* 1990;54:419–427. PMID: 2118858.

Krasnow JS, Berga SL. Endometriosis and gamete intrafallopian transfer. *Assisted Reprod Rev* 1993;3:121.

Luciano AA, Turksoy RN, Carleo J. Evaluation of oral medroxyprogesterone acetate in the treatment of endometriosis. *Obstet Gynecol* 1988;72:323–327. PMID: 2970029.

Maouris P. Asymptomatic mild endometriosis in infertile women: The case for expectant management. *Obstet Gynecol Surv* 1991;46:548–551. PMID: 1832214.

Marcoux S, Maheux R, Bérubé S. Laparoscopic surgery in infertile women with minimal or mild endometriosis. *N Engl J Med* 1997;337:217–222. PMID: 9227926.

Speroff L, Glass RH, Kase NG. *Clinical Gynecologic Endocrinology and Infertility*. 6th ed. Philadelphia, PA: Lippincott Williams & Wilkins; 1999, p. 1063.

Schenken RS. Classification and treatment of endometriosis. Up To Date 2005.

Surrey ES, Add-Back Consensus Working Group. Add-back therapy and gonadotropin hormone agonists in the treatment of patients with endometriosis: can a consensus be reached? *Fertil Steril* 1999;71:420–424. PMID: 10065775.

Surrey ES, Gambone JC, Lu JK, Judd HL. The effects of combining norethindrone with a gonadotropin-releasing hormone agonist in the treatment of symptomatic endometriosis. *Fertil Steril* 1990;53:620–626. PMID: 2108056.

Vlahos N, Fortner KB. Emerging issues in endometriosis. *Postgrad Obstet Gynecol* 2005;25:1–9.

Yates M, Vlahos N. Endometriosis and in vitro fertilization. *Postgrad Obstet Gynecol* 2003;23.

Prognosis

Proper counseling of patients with endometriosis requires attention to several aspects of the disorder. Of primary importance is the initial operative staging of the disease to obtain adequate information on which to base future decisions about therapy. The patient's symptoms and desire for childbearing dictate appropriate therapy. Most patients can be told that they will be able to obtain significant relief from pelvic pain and that treatment will assist them in achieving pregnancy.

Long-term concerns must be more guarded in that all current therapies offer relief but not cure. Even after definitive surgery, endometriosis may recur, but the risk is very low (approximately 3%). The risk of recurrence is not significantly increased by estrogen replacement therapy. After conservative surgery, reported recurrence rates vary greatly but usually exceed 10% in 3 years and 35% in 5 years. Pregnancy delays but does not preclude recurrence. Recurrence rates after medical treatment also vary and are similar to or higher than those reported after surgical treatment.

Although many patients are concerned that endometriosis will progress inexorably, experience has been that conservative surgery avoids the necessity for hysterectomy in the great majority of cases. The course of endometriosis in any individual is impossible to predict at present, and future treatment options should greatly improve what can now be offered.

57 Assisted Reproductive Technologies: In Vitro Fertilization & Related Techniques

Konstantinos G. Michalakis, MD, PhD
Alan H. DeCherney, MD
Alan S. Penzias, MD

In vitro fertilization (IVF) is a process by which egg cells are fertilized in vitro, that is, by sperm outside of the womb. IVF is a major treatment in infertility when other methods of assisted reproductive technology have failed. Assisted reproductive technologies (ART) include multiple techniques that allow gamete manipulation outside the body and have evolved greatly over the past 2 decades.

IN VITRO FERTILIZATION

IVF involves egg retrieval from the ovary, fertilization in the laboratory (fluid medium), and replacement of the zygote in the patient's uterus. The first live birth resulting from this technique occurred in June 1978. Since then, over 1 million children have been born throughout the world with the use of assisted reproduction.

Assisted reproductive techniques have been used for more than 20 years, reporting an increasing number of cycles treated, an increasing pregnancy rate, and an increase in live births per cycle (from 6.6% in 1985 to 27% in 2006) for IVF. In 2003 there were 122,872 ART cycles (99.4% were IVF cycles), whereas in 2006, 41,343 live-birth deliveries were reported; approximately <1.0% were gamete intrafallopian transfer for fertilization (GIFT) and <1.0 % accounted for zygote intrafallopian transfer (ZIFT) cycles. In approximately half of the ART cycles (53%), intracytoplasmic sperm injection (ICSI) is used.

One of the most important prognostic predictors for pregnancy is the age of the female partner. Whereas for women younger than 35 years, live birth rate/cycle varies from 30 to 35%, women older than 40 years face live birth rates <6%, down to 2.4%. Table 57–1 presents data according to the National Summary and fertility reports of the US Department of Health and Human Services.

Approximately 39% of patients who undergo egg retrieval will become pregnant with sonographic documentation of an intrauterine pregnancy (clinical pregnancy); 82% of these patients will carry to term. Many "biochemical pregnancies" occur, but these should not be included in pregnancy statistics. A biochemical pregnancy is one in which serum levels of human chorionic gonadotropin (hCG) rise and then fall before sonographic detection of pregnancy is possible. Eggs are almost always obtained by aspiration, and under ordinary circumstances, approximately 75% of eggs will fertilize and cleave. The clinical pregnancy rate of approximately 34% per embryo transfer per IVF cycle (women <35 years old) is > 20–25% pregnancy rate per cycle observed in spontaneous conceptions in the general population.

The success rate with ART has been augmented by replacing more than 1 embryo, but doing so results in one of the major complications of ART treatment: the development of multiple gestations. In 2002, the European Society of Human Reproduction and Embryology (ESHRE) reported a multiple gestation incidence between 26.3 and 29.1%, whereas in the United States, among pregnancies from fresh donor cycles, 57.3% were singletons, 37.1% were twins, and 5.6% were triplets or more. Although multiple gestations are often welcomed by the infertility couples, they are riskier pregnancies that may result in preterm births.

Indications

The basic concept of IVF–embryo transfer (IVF-ET) initially was to bypass the potential mechanical obstacles of the female reproductive tract. It was first developed for patients with severe tubal disease, for patients with bilateral salpingectomy, or for women whose tubes are so badly damaged that they cannot function. As expertise increased, the variations of IVF and ICSI applied to a wider spectrum of other infertility problems. Indications for ART now include the following:

1. Male factor infertility
2. Tubal disease (tubal and pelvic adhesions)
3. Absent or damaged fallopian tubes
4. Endometriosis
5. Preimplantation genetic diagnosis (PGD)
6. Need for third-party reproduction/donor eggs or gestational surrogate

Table 57–1. In vitro fertilization.

Cycles performed in relation to age groups				
	<35 y	35–37 y	38–40 y	>40 y
Number of cycles performed	54,386	31,127	25,933	26,752
Outcomes according to age groups				
	<35 y	35–37 y	38–40 y	41–42 y
% cycles resulting in pregnancy	45.2	37.7	23.5	19.0
% cycles resulting in live births	37.4	31.1	20.6	
Average number of embryos transferred	2.0	2.5	3.8	2.9
% of twin gestation	38.5	12.5		
% of cancellations	12.2	6.6	13.2	

7. Unexplained infertility
8. Age-related infertility
9. Decreased ovarian reserve
10. Recurrent intrauterine insemination failure

When the probability of conception by ART exceeds that of conception by conventional therapy, ART appears to be the procedure of choice. Because of an increased incidence of infertility in our modern society, the timing of reproduction tends to move to the right of the female reproductive curve, as career-women work earlier and conceive later. Thus there is an increased awareness and availability of ART, and the application of such alternatives has expanded.

Although IVF is successful in treating many infertility problems, its success hinges on entry of sperm into the egg. It was initially hoped that routine IVF could be used to compensate for severe oligospermia (<5 million sperm/mL). However, early results were often poor. Modern microsurgical techniques with ICSI are now used in several cases, attempting placement of sperm directly into the cytoplasm of the oocyte. This is discussed in detail later. In addition to male factor issues, another barrier to success with IVF is hydrosalpinx (fluid collection in the fallopian tube). This condition may interfere with implantation, and additional surgery may be needed so that implantation and pregnancy rates improve.

Technique

IVF consists of the following steps:

1. Ovarian stimulation
2. Oocyte retrieval
3. Fertilization with capacitated sperm and ICSI
4. Embryo culture
5. Embryo transfer

A. Ovarian Stimulation—Superovulation

Multiple eggs increase the possibilities of producing multiple embryos, which adds to the likelihood of successful conception. Apart from that, multiple eggs are desired because some eggs will not develop or fertilize after retrieval. By using fertility medication, the ovaries are stimulated to produce several high-quality eggs, and timing for aspiration is better controlled.

Almost all ART programs use superovulation. The type of ovulation-induction therapy varies from group to group. The following methods are used alone or in combination:

1. Combination of gonadotropins and gonadotropin-releasing hormone (GnRH) analogues
2. Combination of gonadotropins and GnRH antagonist
3. Follicle-stimulating hormone (FSH) products—urinary or recombinant
4. Human menopausal gonadotropins—urinary or recombinant
5. Luteinizing hormone (LH) agonists
6. Clomiphene citrate (rarely)

In order to monitor the number and growth of follicles, as well as the uterine lining, superovulation is carefully monitored with ultrasound. To assess the function of the follicles, serial serum estradiol levels are drawn. At least 2 or 3 follicles should be developing before proceeding with egg aspiration; otherwise, the cycle is usually abandoned, and an alternative stimulation regimen is selected for a subsequent cycle. Serum estradiol levels are complementary to ultrasonography in evaluating the maturation and growth of the developing follicles (200 pg/mL per mature follicle is expected). There is evidence that the pattern of serum estradiol may predict the cycles most likely to result in pregnancy. When the mature follicles have reached at least 17 mm in diameter and the amount of estradiol reaches approximately 500 pg/mL, 10,000 IU of hCG (either urinary or recombinant) are usually administered to induce ovulation. Ovulation and subsequent retrieval usually occurs 36 hours after hCG injection.

The introduction of GnRH agonists or antagonists to superovulation regimens has drastically reduced the likelihood of a premature LH surge; consequently, they are used in the majority of IVF patients in the United States. There are many ways to add an agonist in the whole procedure: commonly the GnRH agonists are administered on day 21 or the previous cycle (long protocol) or at the beginning of menses, along with the addition of gonadotropins (short protocol), and they are continued until the day of hCG. When GnRH antagonists are used, treatment with antagonists begins after 5–6 days of gonadotropins or when the lead follicle is 13 mm, whereas recent data allow the antagonist initiation even with a 16–17 mm leading follicle. The antagonists have the advantage of requiring fewer injections; however, there may not be a difference in pregnancy rates between the agonists or the antagonists.

B. Oocyte Retrieval

Aspiration of the preovulatory follicles is performed approximately 34–36 hours after the hCG injection. Egg aspiration is performed using either of 2 methods. Laparoscopy was the first method to be used and is rarely used today. The current method uses ultrasonography to direct transvaginal aspiration (occasionally, egg collection is performed through the abdominal wall under ultrasound guidance, in cases in which the ovaries are abnormally placed). In transvaginal aspiration, a needle is passed through the posterior vaginal fornix using a vaginal ultrasound probe and directed into the ovary. Fluid from the follicles is drawn into a test tube to retrieve the eggs. The advantage of ultrasound aspiration is that it can be performed on an outpatient basis (approximately 30-minute procedure), it is simpler, less invasive, and less expensive.

C. Fertilization With Capacitated Sperm and ICSI

Freshly ejaculated sperm cannot fertilize an egg; the sperm must be capacitated. Fortunately, capacitation is a very simple process in humans and involves only a short incubation period in a culture medium, soon after the collection procedure.

Because of the nature of the superovulatory process, eggs will be in different stages of maturation. Once the eggs have been identified, the embryologist classifies them as either mature (preovulatory) or immature. Mature eggs have an expanded cumulus oophorus , have undergone the first meiotic division (and so the first polar body is visible), and are usually fertilized 5 hours after aspiration, whereas immature eggs have a very compact cumulus, have not undergone the first meiotic division. and can be incubated in the laboratory for up to 36 hours before fertilization. If sperm and eggs are mixed too early, fertilization and cleavage will not take place. Between 50,000 and 150,000 motile sperm are placed with each egg.

Male infertility has been considered a major contributory factor to infertility. In order to face and eventually bypass male factor, microassisted fertilization techniques, principally ICSI, were developed. In the context of assisted conception, they seem to have revolutionized the management of couples with so-called male factor infertility. The causes of spermatogenetic failure found in most cases of male infertility remain largely idiopathic, however, and unfortunately, there is no effective treatment to improve spermatogenesis for idiopathic male infertility patients. For male factor infertility (<5 million total normal motile sperm/mL), ICSI has resulted in higher fertilization rates and expanded possibilities for cryopreservation. In this procedure, 1 normal motile sperm is selected per oocyte and injected through the intact zona pellucida directly into the cytoplasm away from the polar body. Other indications for ICSI include surgically retrieved sperm (for men with azoospermia who need testicular or epididymal biopsy), cryopreserved oocytes, or cases in which PGD is performed for single gene disorders. For couples with borderline quality semen, ICSI results in higher fertilization rates than IVF, and couples with very poor semen will have better fertilization outcomes with ICSI than with subzonal insemination or additional IVF. In 2005, approximately 60% of all ART cycles in the United States involved intracytoplasmic sperm injection, whereas in 2006, it was used in 1 in 2 cycles.

D. Embryo Culture

Embryos are incubated in an atmosphere of ≤5% carbon dioxide and 37°C temperature, close to the temperature of the fallopian tubes. Various culture media are used and are often supplemented with either the patient's serum or synthetic albumin as well as essential and nonessential amino acids and sugars. At various intervals after the attempted fertilization, the embryos are examined in order to identify pronuclei, which confirm fertilization (genetic material from both partners), as well as the stage of cleavage.

After pronuclei identification, the embryos will develop for another 24 hours. At this point, embryos are usually monitored for cell division and should have evolved to 2- or 4-cell embryos.

Embryos can be cultured for various days, mostly relevant to the reproductive obstacles the parents were facing. Embryos can be cultured for:

- **2 Days**—This type of culture is used for couples who have a low number of embryos available for transfer or who have embryos that are slowly developing. Those embryos are transferred at the 2- or 4-cell stage.
- **3 Days**—Embryos cultured for 3 days are checked for gene activations and cleavage, thus increasing the potential of transferring a viable embryo. These embryos are usually transferred at the 6- to 8-cell stage.
- **5 Days**—These embryos reach the blastocyst stage. Blastocysts consist of 12 to 16 cells and are ready for implantation into the uterus.

E. Embryo Transfer

After 3–5 days of laboratory culture, the embryos are replaced into the patient's uterus, a procedure termed **embryo transfer**. Before transfer, the embryos are graded from A to D depending on their appearance and on the degree of fragmentation. Embryos that are not transferred at this time can be cryopreserved and stored in liquid nitrogen use in later IVF cycles, if necessary. If day 5 or 6 transfers are performed, the embryos are at the blastocyst stage, as mentioned earlier. There are 2 types of embryo transfers:

- Day 3 embryo transfer, which is performed 72 hours after egg retrieval
- Blastocyst transfer, which is the transfer of blastocysts and, as mentioned, raises the possibilities of transferring a healthy embryo

The decision of how many embryos to transfer is made by the patient in conjunction with the physician and the embryologist in accord with the American Society for Reproductive Medicine (ASRM) recommendations based on the patient's age (Table 57–2). The exact number of embryos transferred depends on the number of embryos produced, the health of the embryos, the risk level for multiple pregnancy, and the woman's age.

Most embryo transfers are performed under direct visualization with 2-dimensional (2-D) or 3-dimensional (3-D) ultrasounds. Before the embryo transfer is performed, the patient is usually asked to drink water to fill the bladder. A full bladder helps straighten the uterus as well as improve visualization by ultrasound during the transfer. The embryologist prepares the best embryos by aspirating them into a small catheter with some media, and after the physician cleans the cervix with culture media and aspirates the extra cervical mucous, the catheter is passed transcervically into the uterus, and the embryos are injected into the uterine cavity under direct visualization, usually in the space at the top of the uterus. The probability of pregnancy after embryo transfer can be affected by the patient's age, the cause of infertility, the endometrial thickness, and the average embryo grade.

In some patients, assisted hatching or an opening in the zona is performed in order to improve implantation. This is thought to be beneficial in older patients (age 38 years and older) who have harder zonae; however, it is not routinely performed in all IVF centers.

Retrospectively, the decision to establish such recommendations indeed helped the number of multiple births decrease substantially, although the absolute number did not ultimately increase because of the increase in total IVF births.

Table 57–2. Recommended number of embryos to transfer.

Age (years)	Number
<35	2 (consider 1 if previous successful IVF cycle, great embryos, first IVF)
35–37	2–3
38–40	3–4
>40	5
Age independent	In some cases, such as previous failed IVF cycles or unfavorable prognosis, OK to transfer more

F. Luteal Phase Support

In order to avoid a short period of luteal phase, after embryo transfer is performed, progesterone supplementation is usually recommended by most physicians until approximately 7 weeks' gestation. Progesterone administration tends to correct the ratio of estradiol to progesterone and as a result provide a secretory endometrium, which is needed for the implantation. Progesterone is usually administered by an intramuscular injection or by a vaginal suppository or gel.

Complications

Few risks are associated with ART. The risks of ART can be considered in 5 major areas:

A. Risks Associated with Drugs Used to Stimulate Egg Production

1. Ovarian hyperstimulation syndrome—This syndrome is characterized by ovarian enlargement, ascites, and hemoconcentration, whereas the clinical manifestations are abdominal distention, abdominal discomfort, and nausea. Its incidence reaches 5%. Risk factors include polycystic ovary syndrome, multiple follicles, and high estradiol levels. The prognosis is usually worse in patients who get pregnant and have this syndrome. Patients with this syndrome may be at risk for blood clots. In 0.5–1.0% of all IVF cycles, admission is required, with fluid drainage and replacement of albumin. This situation resolves in 1–2 weeks.

2. Cancer—Two studies suggested that the use of the drug clomiphene increases the risk of ovarian cancer, although this has not been reported in other studies. Uterine, cervical, or breast cancer incidence does not increase with IVF.

B. Surgical Risks Associated with IVF

- General anesthetic and intravenous sedation: similar risk to any other surgery.
- Damage to other structures: 1 in 2500 retrievals.
- Pelvic infection: This could occur as a result of the needle insertion and manipulations and requires antibiotic treatment and, rarely, abscess drainage.

C. Risks Associated with Pregnancy

1. Multiple gestations—The likelihood of a twin pregnancy is 10% (0.5% for triplets) with the use of clomiphene, 20–30% after IVF with 2 embryos (increased incidence of triplets in 3 embryo replacement), and 10–20% after intrauterine implantation treatment (1–2%). The complications of multiple pregnancy are increased risk of miscarriage, increased risk of premature labor, increased risk for hemorrhage and high blood pressure, increased requirement for caesarian section, increased loss of an infant, and increased risk of an abnormal infant with a physical or learning disability. Transferring more embryos does not necessarily lead to a greater IVF success rate.

2. Ectopic and heterotopic pregnancies—Patients who undergo an ART procedure are at twice the risk for having an ectopic pregnancy as the general population (1–3% of all pregnancies from embryo transfer). Heterotopic pregnancies, which are rare but seen more commonly with ART, involve cases in which there is an intrauterine pregnancy and an ectopic pregnancy (usually in the fallopian tube) in the same patient.

3. Miscarriage—No difference has been reported in relation to naturally conceived pregnancies.

4. Preterm birth and low-birth-weight infants—These are higher in patients undergoing IVF.

D. Risk of an Abnormal Baby

The risk of congenital abnormalities may be slightly higher in patients who use ART; however, this concept is still controversial (2.6% risk of an abnormal baby with IVF, 2.0% with natural conception). In patients who use ICSI, the risk of imprinting disorders, such as Angelman's syndrome and Beckwith-Wiedemann syndrome, may be increased.

Intellectual impairment seems to occur more often in offsprings of fathers who had to go through ICSI or surgical extraction of sperm.

Babies born after replacement of thawed embryos do not show any increased incidence of abnormalities.

E. Cost

Currently only a few states allow health insurance to cover infertility treatment, which leaves many couples with tremendous expenses (the estimated cost per delivery is $66,667).

OTHER TECHNIQUES RELATED TO IVF-ET

Ovum Donation

Embryos have been donated from one woman to another with many resultant live births. Women who receive donated embryos include those with ovarian failure (premature, autoimmune) or absence (eg, gonadal dysgenesis), diminished ovarian reserve, or genetically transmitted disorders.

Ovum donation can occur under either of 2 circumstances. One circumstance is the infertile patient who produces a large number of oocytes during her own IVF or GIFT cycle and elects to donate some of them to another woman who is otherwise incapable of producing eggs. The other, more common circumstance involves the recruitment of a woman who undergoes superovulation and oocyte retrieval purely for the purpose of donating her oocytes. The donor may be known to the patient (a family member or friend) or, more commonly, may be anonymous. Although the genetics of the resulting pregnancy are derived from the husband and the donor, the infertile woman incapable of producing her own eggs goes through the pregnancy. In these cases, the endometrium of the recipient must be primed with estrogen and progesterone before transfer of the donated embryos, and progesterone and estrogen supplementation must be maintained for at least 10 weeks. The number of embryos transferred is decided based on the age of the donor, not the age of the recipient.

Gestational Surrogacy

A surrogate mother is a woman who is pregnant with a child but who does not intend to raise it after birth. The intended parent(s) is an individual or couple who intends to raise the child after its birth. In traditional surrogacy the surrogate is pregnant with her own biological child, but this child was conceived with the intention of relinquishing the child to be raised by others.

In gestational surrogacy the surrogate becomes pregnant via embryo transfer with a child of which she is not the biological mother. In altruistic surrogacy, the surrogate receives no financial reward for her pregnancy, whereas in commercial surrogacy, the gestational carrier is paid to carry out the pregnancy by the infertile couple. This procedure is legal in several countries.

Gamete Intrafallopian Tube Transfer (GIFT)

GIFT is an alternative to IVF but is used infrequently, typically for women with unexplained infertility or with normal tubal function plus endometriosis. Live birth rates per cycle are approximately 25–35% at most infertility centers. However, with the improved pregnancy rates in IVF, GIFT procedures are rarely done now. Usual indications for GIFT nowadays include patients who have moral or religious objections to IVF and want to have fertilization in vivo rather than in vitro. As with IVF, superovulation is induced, and the follicles are aspirated vaginally under ultrasound guidance. The eggs are then identified in the laboratory. Thereafter, sperm is collected and capacitated, and laparoscopy is performed. Sperm are then mixed with the eggs and drawn up into a catheter. The sperm and eggs can also be separated by an air bubble in the catheter, after which they are transferred into one of the fallopian tubes, permitting in vivo fertilization and cleavage.

Obviously, GIFT is useful only in patients who have normal tube function and are not of advanced age. It has been argued that the requirement of normal tubal function renders the direct comparison of IVF-ET and GIFT results impossible. Among proponents of each technique, there is vigorous ongoing debate regarding the advantages of GIFT over IVF-ET.

In unexplained infertility, IVF-ET will differentiate the etiology of fertilization problems between egg and sperm; GIFT will not. Additionally, GIFT exposes patients to the risks of general anesthesia and laparoscopy. GIFT is now rarely used.

Zygote Intrafallopian Transfer (ZIFT)

Zygote intrafallopian transfer (ZIFT) is used to treat infertility that is caused by a blockage in the fallopian tubes that prevents the normal binding of sperm to the egg. ZIFT is a procedure that combines IVF and GIFT. Ovulation is induced and the oocytes are removed and fertilized in vitro. Soon thereafter, the zygotes are placed into the fallopian tubes by laparoscopy, similar to GIFT, and the embryo travels to the uterine cavity. ZIFT has a success rate of 64.8% in all cases, but is now rarely used.

Preimplantation Genetic Diagnosis (PGD)

PGD is a technology that has been around since early 1990. It allows many genetically heritable diseases to be identified using a variety of molecular biologic techniques. These techniques include but are not limited to polymerase chain reaction and fluorescent in situ hybridization. Currently, there are mainly 2 groups of patients for which PGD is indicated.

1. Couples with a high risk of transmitting an inherited condition that is either a monogenic disorder (autosomal recessive, autosomal dominant, or X-linked disorders) or a chromosomal structural abnormality/translocation.
2. Couples whose embryos are screened for chromosome aneuploidies in the context of IVF procedures. The technique mostly used for screening is actually referred to as preimplantation genetic screening (PGS) and is used to increase the chances of an ongoing pregnancy. The main reasons for this procedure are advanced maternal age or history of recurrent miscarriages. Patients with nonobstructive azoospermia are also candidates for PGD.

Recent advances in embryo manipulation have made possible the removal of 1 or 2 cells, or blastomeres, from a developing 8-cell human embryo without harm to the embryo. Biopsy of the first and/or second polar bodies can also be done for several single-gene defects. In patients at risk of passing along a heritable genetic disease, PGD has made possible the identification of normal embryos (those with no risk of passing the heritable disease). PGD is available for a large number of monogenic disorders; the most frequently diagnosed autosomal recessive disorders are β-thalassemia, sickle cell disease, cystic fibrosis, and spinal muscular atrophy type 1. These normal embryos are then transferred back to the patient. More than 1000 live births have been reported after application of these techniques. PGD is also performed for patients with recurrent miscarriages, previous failed IVF cycles, aneuploidy diagnosis for patients with advanced maternal age, and for sex selection, but these indications are still controversial.

Cryopreservation

Cryopreservation is a process by which cells or whole tissues are preserved by cooling to low subzero temperatures, such as (typically) 77 K or −196° C (the boiling point of liquid nitrogen). At these low temperatures, all biologic activities, including cell death, are stopped.

As expected, the combination of cryopreservation and IVF means that embryos or eggs are frozen to be used at a later time after thawing (unfreezing). Cryopreservation of embryos is very successful and has greatly improved since the first case in 1983. Survival rates of frozen embryos have been reported to be between 50 and 90%. Before implanting thawed embryos, the patient's cycle is usually synchronized so that embryo transfer occurs during the implantation window of the uterus. Consequently, pretreatment with estrogen and progesterone is recommended. In 2003, the live birth rate per transfer of frozen embryos was 27%.

Cryopreservation of oocytes has been gaining attention and has improved over the past few years. In the fall of 2004, the American Society for Reproductive Medicine (ASRM) issued an opinion on oocyte cryopreservation concluding that the science was "promising" because recent laboratory modifications have resulted in improved oocyte survival, fertilization, and pregnancy rates from frozen-thawed oocytes in IVF. The ASRM noted that from the limited research performed to date, there does not appear to be an increase in chromosomal abnormalities, birth defects, or developmental deficits in the children born from cryopreserved oocyes. Pending further research, oocyte cryopreservation should be introduced into clinical practice only on an investigational basis and under the guidance of an institutional review board.

Cryopreservation of ovarian tissue is of interest to women who want to preserve their reproductive function beyond the natural limit or whose reproductive potential is threatened by cancer therapy. Research on this issue is promising; autologous transplantation is the process by which the ovary is removed and transferred to a different location, such as the forearm or abdomen.

Allen VM, Wilson RD, Cheung A; Genetics Committee of the Society of Obstetricians and Gynaecologists of Canada (SOGC); Reproductive Endocrinology Infertility Committee of the Society of Obstetricians and Gynaecologists of Canada (SOGC). Pregnancy outcomes after assisted reproductive technology. *J Obstet Gynaecol Can* 2006;28:220–250. PMID: 16650361.

Althuis MD, Moghissi KS, Westhoff CL, et al. Uterine cancer after use of clomiphene citrate to induce ovulation. *Am J Epidemiol* 2005;161:607–615. PMID: 15781949.

American Society for Reproductive Medicine. *Guidelines on Number of Embryos Transferred*. Birmingham, AL: ASRM; 2004.

American Society for Reproductive Medicine, Society for Assisted Reproductive Technology. 2005: *Assisted Reproductive Technology Success Rates: National Summary and Fertility Clinic Reports*. Atlanta, GA: Centers for Disease Control and Prevention; 2007.

Andersen AN, Goossens V, Ferraretti AP, et al. Assisted reproductive technology in Europe, 2004: results generated from European registers by ESHRE. *Hum Reprod* 2008;23:756–771. PMID: 18281243.

Andersen AN, Goossens V, Bhattacharya S, Ferraretti AP, Kupka MS, de Mouzon J, Nygren KG; and The European IVF-monitoring (EIM) Consortium, for the European Society of Human Reproduction and Embryology (ESHRE). Assisted reproductive technology and intrauterine inseminations in Europe, 2005: Results generated from European registers by ESHRE: The European IVF Monitoring Programme (EIM), for the European Society of Human Reproduction and Embryology (ESHRE). *Hum Reprod* 2009; 24:1267–1287.

British Fertility Society. Factsheet: Risks and complications of assisted conception. http://www.fertility.org.uk. Accessed March 13, 2012.

Byk C. Preimplantation genetic diagnosis: an ambiguous legal status for an ambiguous medical and social practice. *J Int Bioethique* 2008;19:87–104, 125. PMID: 19244944.

Centers for Disease Control and Prevention. CDC Report 2005. National Summary and Fertility Clinic Report. http://www.cdc.gov/ART/ART/ART2005. Accessed March 13, 2012.

Dickey RP. The relative contribution of assisted reproductive technologies and ovulation induction to multiple births in the United States 5 years after the Society for Assisted Reproductive Technology/American Society for Reproductive Medicine recommendation to limit the number of embryos transferred. *Fertil Steril* 2007;88:1554–1561. PMID: 17481621.

Elizur SE, Lerner-Geva L, Levron J, Shulman A, Bider D, Dor J. Cumulative live birth rate following in vitro fertilization: study of 5,310 cycles. *Gynecol Endocrinol* 2006;22:25–30. PMID: 16522530.

The ESHRE Capri Workshop Group. Multiple gestation pregnancy. *Hum Reprod* 2000;15:1856–1864. PMID: 10920117.

The Practice Committee of the American Society for Reproductive Medicine. Ovarian tissue and oocyte cryopreservation. *Fertil Steril* 2004;82:993–998. PMID: 15482797.

Fawole AO, Oladapo OT. An evaluation of embryo, zygote and oocyte cryopreservation in assisted reproductive technology. *Afr J Med Med Sci* 2007;36:325–334. PMID: 18564648.

Guidelines on number of embryos transferred. *Fertil Steril* 2006;86:5(Suppl):S51–S52. PMID: 17055845.

Jensen A, Sharif H, Frederiksen K, et al. Use of fertility drugs and risk of ovarian cancer: Danish population based cohort study. *BMJ* 2009;338:b249. PMID: 19196744.

Jensen A, Sharif H, Olsen JH, Kjaer SK. Risk of breast cancer and gynecologic cancers in a large population of nearly 50,000 infertile Danish women. *Am J Epidemiol* 2008;168:49–57. PMID: 18448441.

Jensen A, Sharif H, Svare EI, Frederiksen K, Kjaer SK. Risk of breast cancer after exposure to fertility drugs: results from a large Danish cohort study. *Cancer Epidemiol Biomarkers Prev* 2007;16:1400–1407. PMID: 17585058.

JOINT SOGC-CFAS. Guidelines for the number of embryos to transfer following in vitro fertilization No 182, September 2006. *Int J Gynaecol Obstet* 2008;102:203–216. PMID: 18773532.

Kashyap S, Moher D, Fung MF, Rosenwaks Z. Assisted reproductive technology and the incidence of ovarian cancer: a meta-analysis. *Obstet Gynecol* 2004;103:785–794. PMID: 15051576.

Kojima Y, Kurokawa S, Mizuno K, et al. Gene transfer to sperm and testis: future prospects of gene therapy for male infertility. *Curr Gene Ther* 2008;8:121–134. PMID: 18393832.

Lintsen AM, Eijkemans MJ, Hunault CC, et al. Predicting ongoing pregnancy chances after IVF and ICSI: a national prospective study. *Hum Reprod* 2007;22:2455–2462. PMID: 17636281.

Mahutte NG, Arici A. Role of gonadotropin-releasing hormone antagonists in poor responders. *Fertil Steril* 2007;87:241–249. PMID: 17113088.

Malizia B, Hacker M, Penzias A. Cumulative live-birth rates after in vitro fertilization. *N Engl J Med* 2009; 360:236–243. PMID: 19144939.

Muasher SJ, Abdallah RT, Hubayter ZR. Optimal stimulation protocols for in vitro fertilization. *Fertil Steril* 2006;86:267–273. PMID: 16753157.

Myers ER, McCrory DC, Mills AA, et al. Effectiveness of assisted reproductive technology (ART). *Evid Rep Technol Assess* 2008:1–195. PMID: 18620469.

National summary and fertility clinic reports: Assisted reproductive technology success rates. U.S. Department of Health and Human Services, Centers for Disease control and prevention, http://www.cdc.gov/ART/ART2006/508PDF/2006ART.pdf. Accessed March 13, 2012.

Olivennes F, Cunha-Filho JS, Fanchin R, Bouchard P, Frydman R. The use of GnRH antagonists in ovarian stimulation. *Hum Reprod Update* 2002;8:279–290. PMID: 12078838.

Ombelet W, De Sutter P, Van der Elst J, Martens G. Multiple gestation and infertility treatment: registration, reflection and reaction-the Belgian project. *Hum Reprod Update* 2005;11: 3–14. PMID: 15528214.

Palermo G, Jons H, Devroey P, Van Steirteghem AC. Pregnancies after intracytoplasmic injection of single spermatozoon into an oocyte. *Lancet* 1992;340:17–18. PMID: 1351601.

Pandian Z, Bhattacharya S, Vale L, Templeton A. In vitro fertilisation for unexplained subfertility. *Cochrane Database Syst Rev* 2005:CD003357. PMID: 15846658.

Pandian Z, Templeton A, Serour G, Bhattacharya S. Number of embryos for transfer after IVF and ICSI: a Cochrane review. *Hum Reprod* 2005;20:2681–2687. PMID: 16183994.

Pantos K, Stefanidis K, Pappas K, et al. Cryopreservation of embryos, blastocysts, and pregnancy rates of blastocysts derived from frozen-thawed embryos and frozen-thawed blastocysts. *J Assist Reprod Genet* 2001;18:579–582. PMID: 11804424.

Pelinck MJ, Vogel NE, Hoek A, et al. Cumulative pregnancy rates after three cycles of minimal stimulation IVF and results according to subfertility diagnosis: a multicentre cohort study. *Hum Reprod* 2006;21:2375–2383. PMID: 16751647.

Practice Committee of American Society for Reproductive Medicine. Repetitive oocyte donation. *Fertil Steril* 2008;90(Suppl):S194–S195. PMID: 19007628.

Seif MM, Edi-Osagie EC, Farquhar C, Hooper L, Blake D, McGinlay P. Assisted hatching on assisted conception (IVF & ICSI). *Cochrane Database Syst Rev* 2006:CD001894. PMID: 16437437.

Sharlip ID, Jarow JP, Belker AM, et al. Best practice policies for male infertility. *Fertil Steril* 2002;77:873–882. PMID: 12009338.

Sills ES, Healy CM. Building Irish families through surrogacy: medical and judicial issues for the advanced reproductive technologies. *Reprod Health* 2008 4;5:9. PMID: 18983640.

Sills ES, Walsh DJ, Walsh AP. Results from the advanced reproductive technologies: fresh vs. frozen? *Ir Med J* 2008;101:288; author reply 289. PMID: 19051622.

Society for Assisted Reproductive Technology; American Society for Reproductive Medicine. Assisted reproductive technology in the United States: 2001 results generated from the American Society for Reproductive Medicine/Society for Assisted Reproductive Technology registry. *Fertil Steril* 2007;87:1253–1266. Erratum in: *Fertil Steril* 2007;88:1020. PMID: 17276436.

Speroff L, Fritz MA. *Clinical Gynecologic Endocrinology and Infertility*. 7th ed. Philadelphia, PA: Lippincott Williams & Wilkins; 2005.

Stephenson EL, Mason C, Braude PR. Preimplantation genetic diagnosis as a source of human embryonic stem cells for disease research and drug discovery. *BJOG* 2009;116:158–165. PMID: 19076947.

Steptoe PC, Edwards RG. Birth after the reimplantation of a human embryo. *Lancet* 1978;2:366.

Stern JE, Cedars MI, Jain T, et al. Assisted reproductive technology practice patterns and the impact of embryo transfer guidelines in the United States. *Fertil Steril* 2007;88:275–282.

Tarlatzis BC, Bili H. Intracytoplasmic sperm injection. Survey of world results. *Ann N Y Acad Sci* 2000;900:336. PMID: 79723.

Thornhill AR, deDie-Smulders CE, Geraedts JP, et al. Best practice guidelines for clinical preimplantation diagnosis (PGD) and preimplantation genetic screening (PGS). *Hum Reprod* 2005;20:35–48. PMID: 15539444.

Vahratian A, Schieve LA, Reynolds MA, Jeng G. Live-birth rates and multiple-birth risk of assisted reproductive technology pregnancies conceived using thawed embryos, USA 1999–2000. *Hum Reprod* 2003;18:1442–1448. PMID: 12832370.

Verlinsky Y, Cohen J, Munne S, et al. Over a decade of experience with preimplantation genetic diagnosis: a multicenter report. *Fertil Steril* 2004;82:292–294. PMID: 15302270.

Vyjayanthi S, Tang T, Fattah A, Deivanayagam M, Bardis N, Balen AH. Elective cryopreservation of embryos at the pronucleate stage in women at risk of ovarian hyperstimulation syndrome may affect the overall pregnancy rate. *Fertil Steril* 2006;86:1773–1775. PMID: 17011557.

Witsenburg C, Dieben S, Van der Westerlaken L, Verburg H, Naaktgeboren N. Cumulative live birth rates in cohorts of patients treated with in vitro fertilization or intracytoplasmic sperm injection. *Fertil Steril* 2005;84:99–107. PMID: 16009164.

58 Contraception & Family Planning

Ronald T. Burkman, MD
Amnon Brzezinski, MD

CONTRACEPTION

Decision making concerning fertility control is, for many people, a deeply personal and sensitive issue, often involving religious or philosophical convictions. Thus it is important for the clinician to approach the subject with particular sensitivity, empathy, maturity, and nonjudgmental behavior.

Despite the introduction of modern contraceptives, unintended or unplanned pregnancies continue to be a major problem in the United States and worldwide. According to the 2009 National Survey of Family Growth, there were a total of 6,408,000 pregnancies in the United States, of which 49.2% were unintended. Among the unintended pregnancies, nearly half result in a pregnancy termination and more than 10% in spontaneous abortion, a substantial degree of pregnancy wastage. Unintended and unplanned pregnancies have social and economic ramifications; they also have a significant impact on public health. Approximately 40% of unintended pregnancies occur among women who do not desire pregnancy yet do not use a method of contraception. Approximately 60% of unintended pregnancies occur among women using some form of birth control. Such data suggest that many women and couples are inadequately motivated to use contraception, that side effects may be problematic for some, that access may be an issue for others, or that some methods may be difficult for women to use correctly. However, encouraging is the latest report of the National Survey of Family Growth (2009) that the teenage pregnancy rate dropped 40% from 1990 to 2005, reaching an historic low of 70.6 per 1000 women aged 15–19 years. Rates fell much more for younger than for older teenagers.

Individual Indications for Birth Control

Contraception is practiced by most couples for personal reasons. Many couples use contraception to space their children or to limit their family size. Others desire to avoid childbearing because of the effects of preexisting illness on the pregnancy, such as severe diabetes or heart disease. For all of these types of decisions, clinicians must provide accurate information about the benefits and risks of both pregnancy and contraception. However, medical conditions that may substantially increase the risk of using some form of contraception usually increase the risks associated with pregnancy to an even greater extent. As a matter of public policy, some countries, especially those that are less developed, promote contraception in an effort to curb undesired population growth.

Legal Aspects of Contraception

Contraceptives are prescribed, demonstrated, and sold throughout most of the United States without restriction.

Despite high rates of unprotected intercourse and unintended pregnancy, the pros and cons of providing contraceptive information and materials to teenagers have been vigorously debated. Most states either have legislation that permits access to contraception for persons under 18 years or have not addressed the issue legislatively. There is a general consensus among physicians that teenagers should be given contraceptive advice and prescriptions within the limits of the law. Physicians must be careful to avoid imposing their own religious or moral views on their patients.

Health care providers are obliged to provide all persons requesting contraception with detailed information about use of the method(s) and its benefits, risks, and side effects so that the patient can make an informed choice relative to a particular method. Not only is the provision of this information of ethical and legal importance, but such counseling is likely to increase the likelihood that the method will be used appropriately with overall improved compliance. Documentation of the discussion with the patient and her understanding of what has been said is important both clinically and legally. In particular, when using methods that require instrumentation or surgery and that also may require intervention by a health care professional for discontinuation (eg, intrauterine contraceptive device [IUD], injectable progestin, or sterilization), signed consent forms that outline the information discussed and the patient's understanding of it may reduce potential legal issues should a problem occur. If needed, the signed consent form serves as evidence that the patient was given counseling about use of a particular birth control method, that she appeared competent to understand what was said to her, and that she consented to receive contraceptive management in the manner specified.

METHODS OF CONTRACEPTION

The available methods of contraception can be classified in many ways. For this discussion, traditional or folk methods are coitus interruptus, postcoital douche, lactational amenorrhea, and periodic abstinence (rhythm or natural family planning). Barrier methods include condoms (male and female), diaphragm, cervical cap, vaginal sponge, and spermicides. Hormonal methods encompass oral contraceptives and injectable or implantable long-acting progestins. In addition, the IUD and sterilization (tubal ligation or vasectomy) are part of the contraceptive armamentarium. Sterilization is discussed in Chapter 46.

COITUS INTERRUPTUS

One of the oldest contraceptive methods is withdrawal of the penis before ejaculation. This process results in deposition of the semen outside the female genital tract. It has the disadvantage of demanding sufficient self-control by the man so that withdrawal precedes ejaculation. Although the failure rate probably is higher than that of most methods, reliable statistics are not available. Failure may result from escape of semen before orgasm or the deposition of semen on the external female genitalia near the vagina.

POSTCOITAL DOUCHE

Plain water, vinegar, and a number of "feminine hygiene" products are widely used as postcoital douches. Theoretically, the douche flushes the semen out of the vagina, and the additives to the water may possess some spermicidal properties. Nevertheless, sperm have been found within the cervical mucus within 90 seconds after ejaculation. Hence the method is ineffective and unreliable.

LACTATIONAL AMENORRHEA

The lactational amenorrhea method can be a highly efficient method for breastfeeding women to use physiology to space births. Suckling results in a reduction in the release of gonadotropin-releasing hormone, luteinizing hormone (LH), and follicle-stimulating hormone (FSH). β-Endorphins induced by suckling also induce a decline in the secretion of dopamine, which normally suppresses the release of prolactin. This results in a condition of amenorrhea and anovulation. During the first 6 months, if breastfeeding is exclusive, menses are mostly anovulatory and fertility remains low. A recent World Health Organization (WHO) study on lactational amenorrhea revealed that during the first 6 months of nursing, cumulative pregnancy rates ranged from 0.9 to 1.2%. However, at 12 months, pregnancy rates rose as high as 7.4%. When using lactation as a method of birth control, the mother must provide breastfeeding as the only form of infant nutrition. Supplemental feedings may alter both the pattern of lactation and the intensity of infant suckling, which secondarily may affect suppression of ovulation. Second, amenorrhea must be maintained. Finally, the method should be practiced as the only form of birth control for a maximum of 6 months after birth. If another pregnancy is undesired, most practitioners advise lactating women to use a reliable contraceptive method starting 3 months after delivery.

Van der Wijden C, Kleijnen J, Van den Berk T. Lactational amenorrhea for family planning. *Cochrane Database Syst Rev* 2003:CD001329. PMID: 14583931.

MALE CONDOM

The condom, or contraceptive sheath, serves as a cover for the penis during coitus and prevents the deposition of semen in the vagina. The most common material used for male condom manufacture is latex, although available condoms are also made from polyurethane material and lamb ceca. The advantages of the condom are that it provides highly effective and inexpensive contraception as well as protection against sexually transmitted infections (STIs). Some condoms now contain a spermicide, which may offer further protection against failure, particularly if the condom breaks. Given the concern about STIs, including HIV, condom use should be recommended for all couples except those in a mutually monogamous relationship.

The condom probably is the most widely used mechanical contraceptive in the world today. Condoms made of latex or polyurethane are impervious to both sperm and most bacterial and viral organisms that cause STIs or HIV infection. However, the less commonly used lamb's cecum condom is not impermeable to such organisms. The failure of all condoms results from imperfections of manufacture (approximately 3 in 1000); errors of technique, such as applying the condom after some semen has escaped into the vagina; and escape of semen from the condom as a result of failure to withdraw before detumescence. In typical use, failure rates with condoms range from 10 to 30% in the first year of use.

When greater contraceptive effectiveness is desired, a second method such as contraceptive vaginal jelly or foam should be used in conjunction with the condom. This combination significantly reduces the chances for condom failure due to mechanical or technical deficiencies. No association has been established between the use of vaginal contraceptives (spermicides) and the occurrence of congenital malformations if a pregnancy occurs.

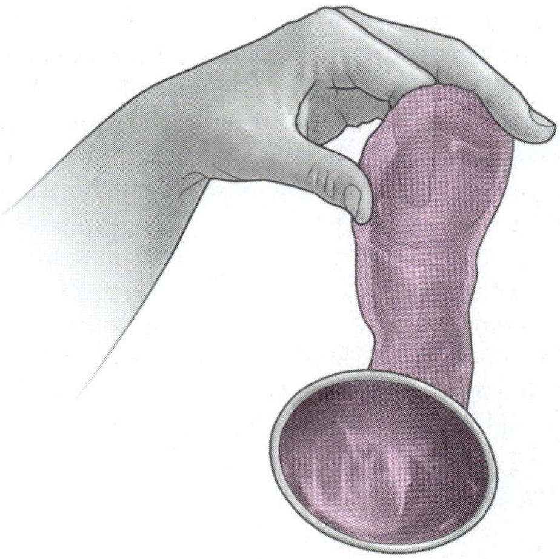

▲ **Figure 58–1.** The female condom.

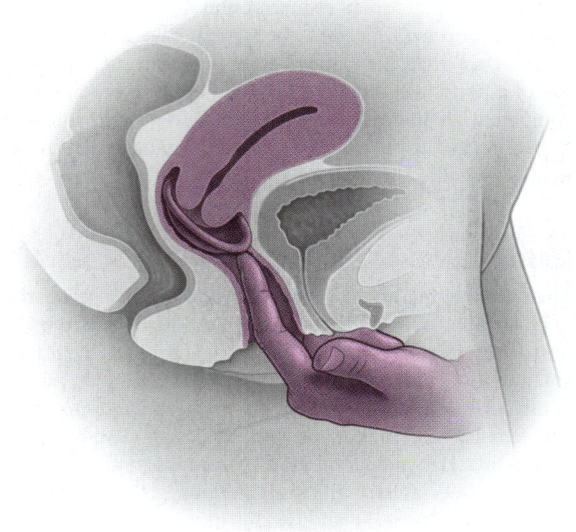

▲ **Figure 58–2.** The diaphragm.

FEMALE CONDOM

The female condom (Fig. 58–1) is made of thin polyurethane material with 2 flexible rings at each end. One ring fits into the depth of the vagina, and the other ring sits outside the vagina near the introitus. Female condoms have the advantage of being under the control of the female partner and of offering some protection against STDs. Significant disadvantages may be their cost and overall bulkiness. Comparisons of the female condom with other female barrier methods such as the diaphragm and cervical cap indicate that typical use failure rates are comparable. The 6-month probability of failure during perfect use of the condom is 2.6%, which is much lower than the initial prediction of 15%. Perfect use of the female condom may reduce the annual risk of acquiring HIV by more than 90%.

Bounds W. Female condoms. *Eur J Contracept Reprod Health Care* 1997;2:113–116. PMID: 9678099.

Gilliam ML, Derman RJ. Barrier methods of contraception. *Obstet Gynecol Clin North Am* 2000;27:841–858. PMID: 11091990.

Kulig J. Condoms: the basics and beyond. *Adolesc Med* 2003; 14:633–645. PMID: 15122165.

VAGINAL DIAPHRAGM

The diaphragm (Fig. 58–2) is a mechanical barrier between the vagina and the cervical canal. Diaphragms are circular rings ranging from 50–105 mm in diameter. They are designed to fit in the vaginal cul-de-sac and cover the cervix. Although the designs vary, the arcing spring version probably is the easiest for most women to use. A contraceptive jelly or cream should be placed on the cervical side of the diaphragm before insertion because the device is ineffective without it. This medication also serves as a lubricant for insertion of the device. Additional jelly should be introduced into the vagina on and around the diaphragm after it is securely in place. The diaphragm can be inserted up to 6 hours before intercourse and should be left in place for at least 6–24 hours after intercourse. When the diaphragm is of proper size (as determined by pelvic examination and trial with fitting rings) and is used according to directions, its failure rate is as low as 6 pregnancies per 100 women per year of exposure. With typical use, however, the pregnancy rate is 15–20 pregnancies per 100 woman-years. The diaphragm has the disadvantages of requiring fitting by a physician or a trained paramedical person and the necessity for anticipating the need for contraception. Weight alterations and deliveries might change the vaginal diameter. Therefore, the fit of the diaphragm to the user must be assessed yearly during the routine pelvic examination. Failures may result from improper fitting or placement and dislodgment of the diaphragm during intercourse. It cannot be used effectively by women with significant pelvic relaxation, a sharply retroverted or anteverted uterus, or a shortened vagina. As with condoms, diaphragms offer some protection against STIs. The only side effects are vaginal wall irritation, usually with initial use or if the device fits too tightly, and an increased risk of urinary tract infections due to pressure of the rim against the urethra and alterations in the composition of the vaginal flora.

Allen RE. Diaphragm fitting. *Am Fam Physician* 2004;69:97–100. PMID: 14727824.

CERVICAL CAP

Cervical caps (Fig. 58–3) are small, cuplike diaphragms placed over the cervix that are held in place by suction. To provide a successful barrier against sperm, they must fit tightly over the

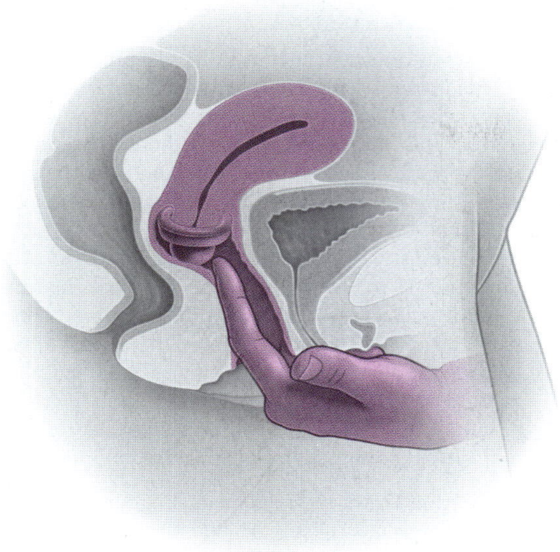

▲ **Figure 58–3.** Cervical caps.

cervix. Because of variability in cervical size, individualization is essential. Tailoring the cap to fit each cervix is difficult, greatly limiting the practical usefulness of the method. In addition, many women are unable to feel their own cervix and thus have great difficulty in placing the cap correctly over the cervix. Because of these problems, the cervical cap has few advantages over the traditional vaginal diaphragm. Although some advocates of the cervical cap recommend that it remain in place for 1 or 2 days at a time, a foul discharge often develops after approximately 1 day of use. With proper use, the efficacy of the cervical cap is similar to that of the diaphragm, with dislodgment being the most frequently cited cause of failure in most reports. The cap should be left in place for 8–48 hours after intercourse, and its proper placement over the cervix should be confirmed by digital self-examination after each sexual act.

SPERMICIDAL PREPARATIONS

Spermicidal vaginal jellies, creams, gels, suppositories, vaginal sponge, and foams, in addition to their toxic effect on sperm, act as a mechanical barrier to entry of sperm into the cervical canal. The only spermicide available in the United States contains nonoxynol 9, which is a long-chain surfactant that is toxic to spermatozoa. Spermicides can be used alone or in conjunction with a diaphragm or condom. Some foam tablets and suppositories require a few minutes for adequate dispersion throughout the vagina, and failures may result if dispersion is not allowed to occur. In general, when used alone, spermicides have a failure rate of approximately 15% per year with perfect use but double that rate with typical use. These chemical agents may irritate the vaginal mucosa and external genitalia. Recent evidence indicates that spermicides containing nonoxynol 9 are not effective in preventing cervical gonorrhea, chlamydia, or HIV infection. In addition, frequent use of spermicides containing nonoxynol 9 without a barrier has been associated with genital lesions that may be linked to increased risk of HIV transmission.

Raymond EG, Chen PL, Luoto J. Contraceptive effectiveness and safety of five nonoxynol-9 spermicides: a randomized trial. *Obstet Gynecol* 2004;103:430–439. PMID: 14990402.

Richardson BA. Nonoxynol-9 as a vaginal microbicide for prevention of sexually transmitted infections. *JAMA* 2002;287:1171–1172. PMID: 11879115.

PERIODIC ABSTINENCE

It has long been known that women are fertile for only a few days of the menstrual cycle. The periodic abstinence (rhythm or natural family planning) method of contraception requires that coitus be avoided during the time of the cycle when a fertilizable ovum and motile sperm could meet in the oviduct. Fertilization takes place within the tube, and the ovum remains in the tube for approximately 1–3 days after ovulation; hence the fertile period is from the time of ovulation to 2–3 days thereafter.

Accurate prediction or indication of ovulation is essential to the success of the periodic abstinence method. Data from surveys in developed and developing countries performed during the past decade indicate the use of natural family planning methods varies from 0 to 11%. Pregnancy rates vary, but most reliable studies report 1-year life-table pregnancy rates between 10 and 25 per 100 woman-years.

1. The **calendar method** predicts the day of ovulation by means of a formula based on the menstrual pattern recorded over a period of several months. Ovulation ordinarily occurs 14 days before the first day of the next menstrual period. The fertile interval should be assumed to extend from at least 2 days before ovulation to no less than 2 days after ovulation. An overlap of 1–2 days of abstinence either way increases the likelihood of success. Successful use of this approach is based on the knowledge that the luteal phase of a menstrual cycle is relatively constant at 14 days for normal women. Furthermore, for this approach to be successful as the only form of contraception requires regular menstrual cycles so that the various timing schedules retain validity. Although this is the most commonly used method of periodic abstinence, it is also the least reliable, with failure rates as high as 35% in 1 year's use.
2. A somewhat more efficacious approach to periodic abstinence is the **temperature method,** as more reliable evidence of ovulation can be obtained by recording the basal body temperature (BBT). The vaginal or rectal temperature must be recorded upon awakening in the

morning before any physical activity is undertaken. Although it is often missed, a slight drop in temperature occurs 24–36 hours after ovulation. The temperature then rises abruptly approximately 0.3–0.4°C (0.5–0.7°F) and remains at this plateau for the remainder of the cycle. The third day after the onset of elevated temperature is considered the end of the fertile period. For reliability, care must be taken by the woman to ensure that true BBTs are recorded (ie, that temperature elevations due to other causes such as fever do not provide misleading information). A distinct limitation of this technique is that prediction of timing of ovulation in any given cycle is retrospective, making it difficult to predict the onset of the fertile period.

3. The **combined temperature and calendar method** uses features of the 2 methods to more accurately predict the time of ovulation. Failure rates of only 5 pregnancies per 100 couples per year have been reported in studies of well-motivated couples.
4. The **cervical mucus (Billings) method** uses changes in cervical mucus secretions as affected by menstrual cycle hormonal alterations to predict ovulation. Starting several days before and until just after ovulation, the mucus becomes thin and watery, whereas at other times the mucus is thick and opaque. Women using this approach are trained to evaluate their mucus on a daily basis. Success rates are similar to those described for the combined temperature and calendar method. Advantages of this approach include relative simplicity and lack of a requirement for charting. Disadvantages include difficulty in evaluating mucus in the presence of vaginal infection and the reluctance of some women to evaluate such secretions.
5. The **symptothermal method,** if used properly, probably is the most effective of all the periodic abstinence approaches. It combines features of both the cervical mucus and the temperature methods. In addition, symptoms that may occur just prior to ovulation, such as bloating and vulvar swelling, are used as adjuncts to ovulation.

The most accurate method of determining ovulation time is to demonstrate the LH peak in serum specimens. Because of the cost and the time required for serial measurements of LH level that are essential to indicate the abrupt rise, this method is impractical as a method of birth control. It is valuable in the treatment of infertility, however, when the optimal time for coitus or artificial insemination is of great importance.

Figure 58–4 shows the relationships among ovulation, BBT, serum levels of LH and FSH, and menses. At least 20% of fertile women have enough variation in their cycles that reliable prediction of the fertile period is impossible.

Epidemiologic studies of women using periodic abstinence have suggested an increased incidence of congenital anomalies, such as anencephaly and Down syndrome, among children resulting from unplanned pregnancies. Animal experiments have shown delayed fertilization results in an increased incidence of aneuploidy and polyploidy in offspring, thus suggesting a possible explanation for similar human fetal anomalies. However, despite a theoretical explanation for the occurrence of such birth defects, it is important to recognize that much of the data are subject to bias, and

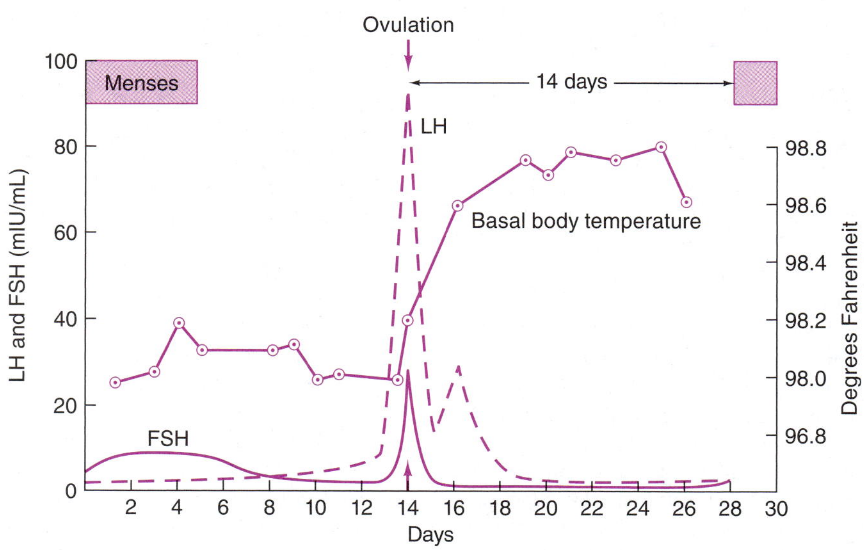

▲ **Figure 58–4.** Relationships among ovulation, basal body temperature, and luteinizing hormone (LH) and follicle-stimulating hormone (FSH) surges in the normal menstrual cycle.

concluding that such associations have been conclusively proved would be inappropriate.

ORAL HORMONAL CONTRACEPTIVES

Oral contraceptives, when placed in general use in 1960, heralded the modern era of contraception. Oral contraceptives provide an estrogen, ethinyl estradiol, and a progestin. The most commonly used progestins in the United States are the estranes: norethindrone and norethindrone acetate; the gonanes: levonorgestrel, desogestrel, and norgestimate; and the spironolactone analogue drospirenone. When first developed, the 2 principal regimens of oral contraception were combined and sequential. The sequential method has been abandoned in the United States because several studies showed a higher than normal incidence of endometrial cancer in women using this method of contraception. In the most commonly used combined method, pills containing both estrogen and progestin are taken each day for 21 days, followed by 7 days of placebo pills, during which time most women experience withdrawal bleeding. Over the past several decades the estrogen content has been reduced by a factor of 3-fold to 4-fold, such that the current dose of ethinyl estradiol ranges between 15 and 35 μg. Similarly, the progestin content has been substantially reduced. In general use, the combined regimen is started either with the onset of the menstrual cycle or on the Sunday closest to the start of menses. Because most oral contraceptive preparations are packaged in 28-day regimens, the Sunday start approach may be easier to follow for some women. However, a good practice is to recommend use of an additional form of contraception during the first week of the cycle to maximize efficacy. Recently, some practitioners have initiated an approach in which birth control pills are started on the day of the office visit if pregnancy is unlikely. It appears this approach may reduce unwanted pregnancies. However, backup contraception is required for at least 7 days after initiation of the method. With standard oral contraceptive preparations, withdrawal bleeding can be expected within 3–5 days after completion of the 21-day regimen of active pills.

The newest approach with combined oral contraceptives is to administer active pills for a prolonged period of time, causing extended periods of amenorrhea (extended-use regimen). A preparation of 84 days active pills followed by 7 days free of was approved by the US Food and Drug Administration (FDA) in 2003. The continuous use of a 30-μg ethinylestradiol and 3-mg drospirenone formulation over 126 days was reportedly safe, efficacious, and well accepted by the users. Although this approach is designed to reduce the number of withdrawal bleeding episodes to 3–4 per year, a significant number of women experience irregular bleeding, especially during the first few cycles of use. In 2007 the FDA approved for use an extended-use oral contraceptive (ethinylestradiol/levonorgestrel 20 μg/90 μg) that is designed for 365 days of continuous use. The pregnancy rate attributable to method failure in a large noncomparative trial of healthy, sexually active women during treatment for 12 months was 15 per 2134 women (adjusted Pearl Index 1.26 per 100 women-years of use). There were no differences in pregnancy rates over 12 months between of continuous-use and cyclical use in a small, randomized, unblinded trial. In small trials, hormonal and ultrasound changes indicative of reinstated ovulation occurred within a month of discontinuation of the drug, and menstruation began again in most women within 90 days. The incidence of adverse effects was similar in continuous-use and cyclical regimens.

The serum levels of FSH and LH throughout the normal menstrual cycle are shown in Figure 58–5A. During a typical cycle under the combined oral contraceptive regimen (Fig. 58–5B), there is no rise during the first half of the cycle; thus the growth of the dominant follicle and ovulation do not occur, and there are no midcycle alterations of FSH and LH levels. Oral contraceptives change the consistency of cervical mucus, resulting in less sperm penetration; make the endometrial lining less receptive to implantation; and alter tubal transport of both sperm and oocytes. During the sequential oral contraceptive regimen (Fig. 58–5C), the estrogen stimulates LH secretion in an irregular manner. There is no concomitant early rise in FSH level when progestin is added, and another LH surge usually is produced. When a progestin-only regimen (Fig. 58–5D) is followed (see Progestin-Only Pill), there are multiple LH surges but no significant changes in FSH levels.

A comprehensive survey of reported data indicates that the return of fertility in former oral contraceptive users (both cyclic and extended/continuous regimens) in women who stop use in order to conceive is comparable to that observed with other contraceptive methods.

Advantages

Benefits that are reasonably established include reduction in risk of ovarian and endometrial cancer, ectopic pregnancy, pelvic inflammatory disease (PID), menstrual disorders, benign breast disease, and acne. Emerging benefits include protection against bone mineral density loss, development of colorectal cancer, and progression of rheumatoid arthritis. Multiple observational studies have documented that combination oral contraceptives decrease the risk of ovarian cancer by 40–80% and endometrial cancer by approximately 50%. These effects take place after 1 year of use, and protection persists for a significant period after oral contraceptive use is discontinued. Oral contraceptives also reduce the risk of ectopic pregnancy by approximately 90% and the risk of acute salpingitis by as much as 50–80% in some studies, although other studies suggest the protection occurs to a lesser extent. However, birth control pills do not offer protection against lower tract infections such as gonorrhea or chlamydia. Oral contraceptives reduce menstrual blood loss as well as dysmenorrhea. There is a 30–50% overall decrease in benign fibrocystic conditions of the breast. Randomized placebo-controlled trials have demonstrated a reduction in acne lesions with some oral contraceptive preparations.

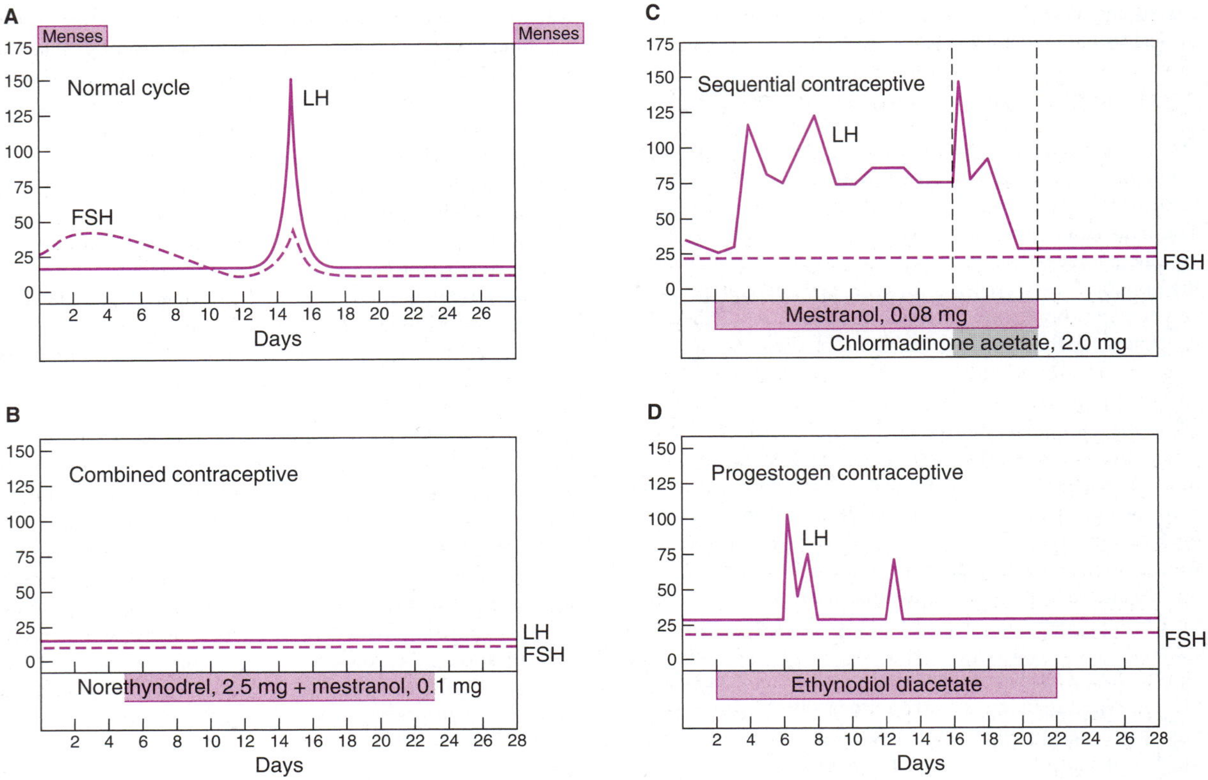

▲ **Figure 58–5.** Serum levels (in mIU/mL) of follicle-stimulating hormone (FSH) and luteinizing hormone (LH) during the menstrual cycle, with and without oral contraception. **A:** During a normal cycle without medication. **B:** During a typical cycle with combined medication (see text). **C:** During a typical cycle with sequential medication (see text). **D:** During progestin-only medication. (Reproduced, with permission, from Odell WD, Moyer DL. *Physiology of Reproduction*. St. Louis, MO: Mosby; 1971.)

Disadvantages & Side Effects

Much attention has been paid to a possible relationship between the use of oral contraceptives and the incidence of thromboembolic disease, including pulmonary embolism. Use of most current combination oral contraceptives roughly triples a user's risk of venous thromboembolism (VTE) from approximately 3 to 9 events per 100,000 users annually, although some studies of formulations containing desogestrel suggest that the risk could climb as high as 7-fold. However, it is important to recognize that even with the worst-case scenarios, the attributable risk annually is approximately 18 additional events per 100,000 users compared with nonusers of combination oral contraceptives. VTE risk is enhanced by risk factors such as recent leg trauma, pelvic surgery, stasis (but not varicose veins), and the presence of the mutation known as factor V Leiden. Although the presence of this latter clotting abnormality markedly elevates a user's risk of VTE, the absolute risk is still low such that routine screening for the disorder among all potential oral contraceptive users would not be cost effective.

Myocardial infarction (MI) is a rare condition that occurs among combination oral contraceptive users only in the presence of risk factors such as hypertension, diabetes, severe dyslipidemia, and, in particular, cigarette smoking. Age above 35 years and smoking also act synergistically to increase risk; thus prescribing combination oral contraceptives to women over 35 years who smoke is not recommended. However, even with a 20- to 30-fold relative risk of MI among smoking combination oral contraceptive users, this risk equates to only a maximum of 500–600 events per million woman-years. However, unlike VTE, in which the case fatality rate in the reproductive age group is <1%, the case fatality rate for MI is approximately 50%.

Stroke is a rare condition among women in the reproductive age group, with hemorrhagic stroke somewhat more common than ischemic stroke. Among nonsmoking women, the rates range from 6–46 events per million woman-years; combination oral contraceptive use increases that risk only if risk factors such as age, cigarette smoking, migraine headaches (for ischemic but not hemorrhagic stroke), and especially hypertension are present. Overall, the relative risk of stroke varies between 2-fold and 10-fold, depending on the number of risk factors present.

Although cancer of the cervix among users of oral contraceptives has been a matter of concern, a major problem with many studies attempting to examine this relationship is confounding factors such as multiple sexual partners, age at first intercourse, and frequency of sexual activity and the concomitant use of barrier contraceptive methods. A recent meta-analysis determined that the risk of cervical cancer among oral contraceptive users compared with nonusers increased with duration of use, reaching a relative risk of approximately 4 after 10 years. For several decades, concern has been expressed regarding the possible association between oral contraceptive use and breast cancer. In 1996, a collaborative project representing a reanalysis of 54 studies demonstrated that for current users of oral contraceptives, the relative risk of breast cancer for users compared with women who had never used oral contraceptives was 1.24. This small increase in risk persisted for approximately 10 years after discontinuation of oral contraceptive use, with the risk essentially disappearing after that time. In addition, there was no overall effect of oral contraceptive use by dosage, specific formulation, duration of use, age at first use, age at time of cancer diagnosis, or family history of breast cancer. The pattern of disappearance of risk after 10 years coupled with a tendency toward localized disease suggests that the overall effect may represent detection bias or perhaps a promotional effect. Another recent, large population-based case-control study showed that neither current nor past use of any type of oral contraceptive increased the risk of breast cancer compared with population-based controls. Further, the results did not vary according to potential risk factors such as estrogen dose, duration of use, family history of breast cancer, or age at initiation of use. Other infrequent problems occasionally noted with oral contraceptive use include hypertension, cholelithiasis, and benign liver tumors. However, none of these problems occurs frequently enough to be of significant concern to most users.

Because the current formulations are associated with significant reductions in risk of serious sequelae, side-effect control will be of greater importance to most users in the future. Furthermore, studies have shown that compliance is affected by occurrence of side effects and that such "minor" problems, particularly spotting and breakthrough bleeding, account for approximately 40% of the discontinuations. Approximately 10–20% of women experience intermenstrual bleeding, including breakthrough bleeding and spotting, in the first few months of use. With today's formulations, such problems stabilize after approximately 6 months and are seen in only approximately 5% of users. Missed menstrual periods or amenorrhea are relatively infrequent and of little clinical significance, except that these problems can raise concern as regarding contraceptive failure. Nausea may be seen in up to 10% of users; as with intermenstrual bleeding, this is a duration effect that declines rapidly after several months of use. Significant headaches and weight gain are far less frequent than reported with higher-dose preparations.

Contraindications for use of oral contraceptives include pregnancy; undiagnosed vaginal bleeding; prior history of VTE, MI, or stroke; women at increased risk for cardiovascular sequelae, such as active systemic lupus erythematosus, uncontrolled diabetes, or hypertension, and cigarette smokers over age 35 years; current or prior breast cancer; and active liver disease.

Because compliance and a clear understanding of how to take oral contraceptives are important to their successful use, health care providers should take the time at the initial visit to explain the packaging of the brand being prescribed, discuss the side effects, review how to start the first cycle, and discuss what to do when pills are missed. It should be emphasized that the patient package insert provides useful information on these topics. In addition, users should be encouraged to contact their provider or someone in the office or clinic who is familiar with oral contraceptive health care if problems occur. Finally, users should be advised to use alternate forms of contraception if oral contraceptive use is interrupted because of forgotten pills or the occurrence of side effects.

Table 58–1 lists the currently available oral contraceptives and their contents.

Progestin-Only Pill (Minipill)

Several studies have demonstrated that a small daily quantity of a progestin alone, usually norethindrone or levonorgestrel, provides reasonably good protection against pregnancy without suppressing ovulation. The method has several advantages: the side effects attributable to the estrogen component of conventional oral contraceptives are eliminated because no estrogen is given, and no special sequence of pill-taking is necessary because the minipill is taken every day. Although the mechanism of action of progestin-only pills is not known, it has been postulated that the cervical mucus becomes less permeable to sperm and that endometrial activity goes out of phase so that nidation is thwarted even if fertilization does occur. In clinical trials, progestin-only oral contraceptives result in a pregnancy rate of approximately 2–7 pregnancies per 100 woman-years. Unlike combined oral contraceptives, which permit a certain margin of patient error and forgetfulness, minipill progestin agents must be taken each day promptly. Even a delay of 2–3 hours diminishes the contraceptive effectiveness for the coming 48 hours. Progestins given alone are associated with side effects, particularly irregular bleeding. Progestin-only contraceptives are ideal for women for whom estrogen is contraindicated. Ideal candidates include older women who smoke; women with sickle cell anemia, mental retardation, migraine headache, hypertension, or systemic lupus erythematosus; or women who are breastfeeding.

Table 58–1. Oral contraceptive agents in use.

	Estrogen (mg)	Progestin (mg)	
Combination tablets			
Loestrin 1/20	Ethinyl estradiol 0.02	Norethindrone acetate	1
Loestrin 1.5/30	Ethinyl estradiol 0.03	Norethindrone acetate	1.5
Ovcon-35	Ethinyl estradiol 0.035	Norethindrone	0.4
Brevicon	Ethinyl estradiol 0.035	Norethindrone	0.5
Modicon			
Nordette	Ethinyl estradiol 0.03	L-Norgestrel	0.15
Ortho-Cept, Desogen	Ethinyl estradiol 0.30	Desogestrel	0.15
Ortho-Cyclen	Ethinyl estradiol 0.35	Norgestimate	0.25
Lo/Ovral	Ethinyl estradiol 0.03	DL-Norgestrel	0.3
Ovral	Ethinyl estradiol 0.05	DL-Norgestrel	0.5
Demulen 1/50	Ethinyl estradiol 0.05	Ethynodiol diacetate	1
Demulen 1/35	Ethinyl estradiol 0.35	Ethynodiol diacetate	1
Ovcon 50	Ethinyl estradiol 0.05	Norethindrone	1
Ovcon 35	Ethinyl estradiol 0.35	Norethindrone	0.4
Norinyl 1/50	Mestranol 0.05	Norethindrone	1
Norinyl 1/35	Ethinyl estradiol 0.35	Norethindrone	1
Ortho-Novum1/50			
Ortho-Novum 1/35	Ethinyl estradiol 0.35	Norethindrone	0.4
Alesse	Ethinyl estradiol 0.20	Levonorgestrel	0.1
Levlite	Ethinyl estradiol 0.20	Levonorgestrel	0.1
Levlen	Ethinyl estradiol 0.30	Levonorgestrel	0.15
Nordette	Ethinyl estradiol 0.30	Levonorgestrel	0.15
Yasmin	Ethinyl estradiol 0.30	Drospirenone	3
Yaz	Ethinyl estradiol 0.20	Drospirenone	3*
Combination tablets—multidose			
Biphasic			
Ortho-Novum 10/11			
Day 1–10	Ethinyl estradiol 0.035	Norethindrone	0.5
Day 11–21	Ethinyl estradiol 0.035	Norethindrone	1
Jenest-28			
Day 1–7	Ethinyl estradiol 0.35	Norethindrone	0.5
Day 8–21	Ethinyl estradiol 0.35	Norethindrone	1

(Continued)

Table 58–1. Oral contraceptive agents in use. (Continued)

	Estrogen (mg)	Progestin (mg)	
Mircette			
Day 1–21	Ethinyl estradiol 0.20	Desogestrel	0.15
Day 22–26	Ethinyl estradiol 0.10	None	
Triphasic			
Tri-Norinyl			
Day 1–7	Ethinyl estradiol 0.035	Norethindrone	0.5
Day 8–16	Ethinyl estradiol 0.035	Norethindrone	1
Day 17–21	Ethinyl estradiol 0.035	Norethindrone	0.5
Day 22–28		Placebo	
Triphasil, Tri-Levlen			
Day 1–6	Ethinyl estradiol 0.030	Levonorgestrel	0.05
Day 7–11	Ethinyl estradiol 0.040	Levonorgestrel	0.075
Day 12–21	Ethinyl estradiol 0.030	Levonorgestrel	0.125
Day 22–28		Placebo	
Ortho-Novum 7/7/7			
Day 1–7	Ethinyl estradiol 0.035	Norethindrone	0.5
Day 8–14	Ethinyl estradiol 0.035	Norethindrone	0.75
Day 15–21	Ethinyl estradiol 0.035	Norethindrone	1
Day 22–28		Placebo	
Ortho-Tri-Cyclen			
Day 1–7	Ethinyl estradiol 0.35	Norgestimate	0.180
Day 8–14	Ethinyl estradiol 0.35	Norgestimate	0.215
Day 15–21	Ethinyl estradiol 0.35	Norgestimate	0.250
Multiphasic			
Estrostep Fe			
Day 1–5	Ethinyl estradiol 0.20	Norethindrone	1
Day 6–12	Ethinyl estradiol 0.30	Norethindrone	1
Day 13–21	Ethinyl estradiol 0.35	Norethindrone	1
Natazia (Qlaira)			
Days 2	Estradiol Valerate 3	Dienogest	
Days 5	Estradiol Valerate 2	Dienogest	2
Days 17	Estradiol Valerate 2	Dienogest	3
Days 2	Estradiol Valerate 1	Dienogest	
Days 2	Placebo	Dienogest	

(*Continued*)

Table 58–1. Oral contraceptive agents in use. (Continued)

	Estrogen (mg)	Progestin (mg)	
Daily progestin tablets			
Micronor	. . .	Norethindrone	0.35
Nor-QD	. . .	Norethindrone	0.35
Ovrette	. . .	DL-Norgestrel	0.075
Extended-regimen			
Seasonale **(84 days)**	Ethinyl estradiol 0.03	Norgestrel	0.15
Seasonique (91 days)	Ethinyl estradiol 0.03Ethinyl estradiol 0.01	Norgestrel	0.15
Lybrel (365 days)	Ethinyl estradiol 0.20	Levonorgestrel	0.09

Note: The estrogen-containing compounds are arranged in order of increasing content of estrogen (ethinyl estradiol and mestranol have similar potencies).Some of the above oral contraceptives are available as generic formulations.
*Active pills take 24 of 28 days.

Emergency Contraception

Postcoital or emergency contraception is a therapy used to prevent unwanted pregnancy after unprotected intercourse or after a failure to use a contraceptive method appropriately. The major methods used for emergency contraception include combination oral contraceptives containing the progestin levonorgestrel (also known as the Yuzpe method), levonorgestrel tablets given alone, or the copper T 380A IUD. The hormonal methods prevent pregnancy by delaying or inhibiting ovulation or by disrupting the function of the corpus luteum. The usual combination hormonal formulation consists of 100 μg ethinyl estradiol and 500–600 μg levonorgestrel in several tablets administered twice, 12 hours apart. Under current recommendations, the first dose is administered within 72 hours of intercourse. The levonorgestrel-alone formulation requires administration of 750 μg of the progestin twice, also 12 hours apart. Many authorities currently recommend initial dosing within 72 hours, although data suggest this approach may be effective as long as 5 days after intercourse. Furthermore, data suggest that a single dose of 1500 μg levonorgestrel may be as effective as the 2-dose regimen. The IUD may inhibit implantation or possibly interfere with sperm function. The T 380A is inserted within 7 days from the time of unprotected intercourse.

Nausea occurs in approximately 50% and vomiting in 20% of the combination hormonal emergency contraception users. Administration of an antiemetic (eg, meclizine) 1 hour before may reduce this effect. The levonorgestrel-only approach is associated with rates of nausea and vomiting that are 50 and 70% lower than the rates experienced by combination emergency contraception users, respectively.

LONG-ACTING HORMONAL CONTRACEPTION

Depot medroxyprogesterone acetate (DMPA), an aqueous suspension of 17-acetoxy-6-methyl progesterone, has been used as a contraceptive in the United States for at least 4 decades. The usual dose is 150 mg administered intramuscularly into the gluteus maximus or deltoid every 3 months. The mechanisms of action include suppression of ovulation by suppressing the surge of gonadotropins, thickening cervical mucus to impede ascent of sperm, and thinning of the endometrium such that implantation of a blastocyst is less likely. Although labeled as effective for up to 13 weeks, the contraceptive activity actually persists for approximately 4 months after an injection, allowing some leeway for providers to schedule follow-up injections. During 1 year of use, the perfect use failure rate is 0.3 pregnancies per 100 woman-years, whereas the failure rate with typical use is 3 pregnancies per 100 woman-years.

Use of DMPA is associated with several health benefits. The risk of ectopic pregnancy is significantly lower among users compared to women who do not use contraception. The risk of endometrial cancer is reduced by as much as 80%, an effect that is long term and increases with duration of use. Studies have shown as much as a 70% reduction in the frequency of sickle cell crises; the mechanism for this effect is not known. Some women with endometriosis have improvement of symptoms with use of DMPA.

Use of DMPA does not increase the risk for arterial or venous disease. The most significant potential risk associated with DMPA use is a reduction in bone mineral density. Overall, prospective studies of at least 1 year's duration have shown a maximum reduction of 1.5–2.3% in bone mineral density. No studies have shown any increase in fracture risk. Finally, retrospective studies have shown improvement in bone mineral density when DMPA was discontinued. Until further data become available, adequate calcium intake should be encouraged for DMPA users, particularly young patients and longer term users. Irregular bleeding and prolonged menstrual flow are not uncommon during the first 6 months of use. However, with continued use, many women become amenorrheic, and up to 70% of users experience no menses after 1 year. Mood change and depression have been reported in association with DMPA use. However, most studies are uncontrolled. Although earlier studies suggested DMPA users gained an average of 5 lb after 1 year of use, a recent randomized clinical trial demonstrated that DMPA was not associated with significant weight gain or changes in variables that might lead to weight gain. Finally, when DMPA users stop injections in an effort to achieve pregnancy, the return to baseline fertility may take an average of 10 months.

Implants

Although no implantable contraceptives currently are available in the United States, clinical trials of a single-rod implant 4 cm long and 2 mm in diameter have been completed. This system releases etonogestrel, the major metabolite of desogestrel, and maintains its efficacy for up to 3 years. The rod usually is inserted in the upper arm, using a trocar. Removal is easier than with other implants because it is a single-rod system. The likely mechanism of action is similar to that of DMPA. Overall efficacy is extremely high, with no reported pregnancies in more than 70,000 cycles of use. No major complications have been reported to date. Side effects include menstrual abnormalities and weight gain.

Vaginal Ring

The vaginal ring (Fig. 58–6) is approximately 5 cm in diameter and 4 mm thick. The ring is flexible. It releases ethinyl estradiol and etonogestrel at fairly constant rates. The ring is worn for 3 weeks per month, although the ring's reservoir contains enough contraceptive steroid for approximately 14 more days. The ring maintains its efficacy even if it is removed for up to 3 hours, although it is designed to be left in place even during intercourse. Users are instructed to insert the ring high into the vagina; fitting by a health professional is not required. The overall pregnancy rate over 1 year of use is 0.65 pregnancies per 100 woman-years.

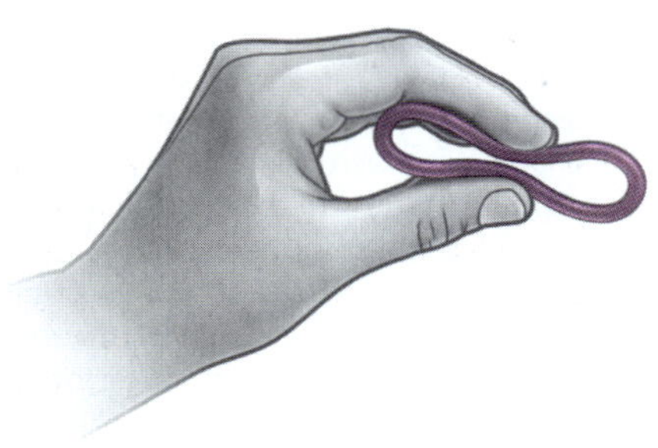

▲ Figure 58–6. The vaginal ring.

No published data indicate the rates of major side effects or potential noncontraceptive benefits. However, because the vaginal ring contains steroids that are used in combination oral contraceptives, rates of serious side effects may be similar, and some of the noncontraceptive benefits may accrue to users of this method. Minor side effects are similar to those seen in users of combination oral contraceptives, although the frequency of breakthrough bleeding and spotting appears lower. Approximately 10–15% of users report vaginal-related symptoms, such as slight discomfort, a sensation of a foreign body, leukorrhea, vaginitis, or coital problems. There are reports that the ring might be used in an extended regimen, although this regimen was not yet approved by regulatory institutions.

Transdermal Patch

The transdermal contraceptive patch is 20 cm^2, roughly the size of a small adhesive-back (Post-It) pad consisting of 3 layers. The transdermal contraceptive patch is designed to deliver norelgestromin, the active metabolite of norgestimate, and ethinyl estradiol daily for a 7-day period. After 7 days, the patch is removed and a new patch is applied to another skin site. Three consecutive 7-day patches are applied in a typical cycle, followed by a 7-day patch-free period to allow withdrawal bleeding. Application sites include the buttocks, lower abdomen, upper outer arm, and upper torso, except for the breasts. Because this is a combination steroid preparation, the same contraindications noted for combination oral contraceptives use apply.

The transdermal contraceptive patch has a method use rate of 0.70 and a typical use rate of 0.88 pregnancies per 100 woman-years. These rates are comparable to pregnancy rates achieved with current oral contraceptives. However, a failure rate approaching the typical use failure rate seen with combination oral contraceptive users was noted for women weighing over 198 pounds who used the patch.

Although few reports have documented the rates of serious adverse events, one should assume that the events and risks will be similar to those noted for combination oral contraceptives. To date, 1 published study has indicated that the risk of venous thromboembolism is similar to that of an oral contraceptive. Similarly, no data on noncontraceptive benefits are available. The frequency of side effects such as headache and nausea are similar to that seen among users of combination oral contraceptives, although contraceptive patch users have application site reactions, more breast symptoms (only during the first 2 cycles), and more dysmenorrhea than combination oral contraceptive users. The pattern of breakthrough bleeding and spotting with the transdermal contraceptive patch is similar to that seen with oral contraceptive users. No evidence indicates that use of the patch influences body weight. Among users, 1.8% of women required replacement for complete detachment and 2.9% became partially detached. Detachment rates were similar for women living in warm, humid climates and for women who were subjected to vigorous exercise, swimming, and sauna use compared with other users. When patches do become detached, users should attempt to reattach them if possible, without using ancillary adhesives or tape. If detachment has occurred for 24 hours or less, the cycle continues as usual, with the patch changed on the previously determined change day. If detachment has occurred for more than 24 hours, a new patch should be applied, backup contraception should be used for 1 week, and the day that the new patch is applied now becomes the patch change day.

Anderson FD, Hait H. A multicenter, randomized study of an extended cycle oral contraceptive. *Contraception* 2003;68: 89–96. PMID: 12954519.

Audet M, Moreau M, Koltun WD, et al. Evaluation of contraceptive efficacy and cycle control of a transdermal contraceptive patch vs an oral contraceptive. *JAMA* 2001;285:2347–2354. PMID: 11343482.

Barreiros FA, Guazzelli CA, de Araújo FF, Barbosa R. Bleeding patterns of women using extended regimens of the contraceptive vaginal ring. *Contraception* 2007;75:204–208. PMID: 17303490.

Barnhart KT, Schreiber CA. Return to fertility following discontinuation of oral contraceptives. *Fertil Steril* 2009;91:659–663. PMID: 19268187.

Burkman RT. Cardiovascular issues with oral contraceptives: evidenced-based medicine. *Int J Fertil Womens Med* 2000;45: 166–174. PMID: 10831186.

Burkman RT. The transdermal contraceptive system. *Am J Obstet Gynecol* 2004;190:S49.

Burkman R, Schlesselman JJ, Zieman M. Safety concerns and health benefits associated with oral contraception. *Am J Obstet Gynecol* 2004;190:S5–S53. PMID: 15105798.

Croxatto HB. Clinical profile of Implanon: a single-rod etonogestrel contraceptive implant. *Eur J Contracept Reprod Health Care* 2000;5(suppl 2):21–28. PMID: 11246604.

Darney PD. Implantable contraception. *Eur J Contracept Reprod Health Care* 2000;5(suppl 2):2–11. PMID: 11246603.

Dunn S, Guilbert E, Lefebvre G, et al. Emergency contraception. *J Obstet Gynaecol Can* 2003;25:673–687. PMID: 12908020.

Foidart JM, Sulak PJ, Schellschmidt I, Zimmermann D; Yasmin Extended Regimen Study Group. The use of an oral contraceptive containing ethinylestradiol and drospirenone in an extended regimen over 126 days. *Contraception* 2006;73:34–40. PMID: 16371292.

Harrison-Woolrych M, Hill R. Unintended pregnancies with etonogestrel implant (Implanon): a case series from postmarketing experience in Australia. *Contraception* 2005;71:306–308. PMID: 15792651.

Kaunitz AM. Current concepts regarding use of DMPA. *J Reprod Med* 2002;47:785–789. PMID: 12380407.

Jick SS, Kay JA, Russmann S, Jick H. Risk of nonfatal venous thromboembolism in women using a contraceptive transdermal patch and oral contraceptives containing norgestimate and 35 microg of ethinyl estradiol. *Contraception* 2006; 73:223–228. PMID: 16472560.

Kuohung W, Borgatta L, Stubblefield P. Low-dose oral contraceptives and bone mineral density: an evidence-based analysis. *Contraception* 2000;61:77–82. PMID: 10802271.

Lara-Torre E. "Quick Start," an innovative approach to the combination oral contraceptive pill in adolescents. Is it time to make the switch? *J Pediatr Adolesc Gynecol* 2004;17:65–67. PMID: 15010044.

Le J, Tsourounis C. Implanon: a critical review. *Ann Pharmacother* 2001;35:329–336. PMID: 11261531.

Marchbanks PA, McDonald JA, Wilson HG, et al. Oral contraceptives and the risk of breast cancer. *N Engl J Med* 2002;346: 2025–2032. PMID: 12087137.

Meckstroth KR, Darney PD. Implant contraception. *Semin Reprod Med* 2001;19:339–354. PMID: 11727176.

Moreno V, Bosch FX, Muñoz N, et al. Effect of oral contraceptives on risk of cervical cancer in women with human papillomavirus infection: the IARC multicentric case-control study. *Lancet* 2002;359:1085–1092. PMID: 11943255.

Mulders TMT, Dieben TO. Use of the novel combined contraceptive vaginal ring NuvaRing for ovulation inhibition. *Fertil Steril* 2001;75:865–870. PMID: 11334895.

Parsey KS, Pong A. An open-label, multicenter study to evaluate Yasmin, a low-dose combination of oral contraceptive containing drospirenone, a new progestogen. *Contraception* 2000;6:105–111. PMID: 10802275.

Rosenberg MJ, Burnhill MS, Waugh MS, Grimes DA, Hillard PJ. Compliance and oral contraceptives: a review. *Contraception* 1995;52:137–141. PMID: 7587184.

Roumen FJ, Apter D, Mulders TM, Dieben TO. Efficacy, tolerability and acceptability of a novel contraceptive vaginal ring releasing etonogestrel and ethinyl oestradiol. *Hum Reprod* 2001;16:469–475. PMID: 11228213.

Sanchez-Guerrero J, Uribe AG, Jimenez-Santana L, et al. A trial of contraceptive methods in women with systemic lupus erythematosus. *N Engl J Med* 2005;353:2539–2549. PMID: 16354890.

Wagstaff AJ. Continuous-use ethinylestradiol/levonorgestrel 20microg/90microg: as an oral contraceptive. *Drugs* 2007;67:2473–2479. PMID: 17983260.

Webb AM. Emergency contraception. *BMJ* 2003;326:775–776. PMID: 12689951.

Westhoff C. Clinical practice. Emergency contraception. *N Engl J Med* 2003;349:1830–1835. PMID: 14602882.

INTRAUTERINE CONTRACEPTIVE DEVICES

Two types of IUDs are available in the United States: the copper T 380A device and a levonorgestrel-releasing device (Fig. 58–7). The T 380A is a T-shaped device approximately 36 mm in length and 32 mm in diameter that contains 380 mm^2 of copper on its vertical and side arms. Two monofilament strings are attached to the vertical arm to ascertain placement in the uterus over the course of use. This IUD has a useful lifespan of at least 10 years. The exact mechanism of action is unknown, although current theories include spermicidal activity, interference with either normal development of ova or the fertilization of ova, and activity on the endometrium that may promote phagocytosis of sperm and that may impede sperm migration or capacitance. No data

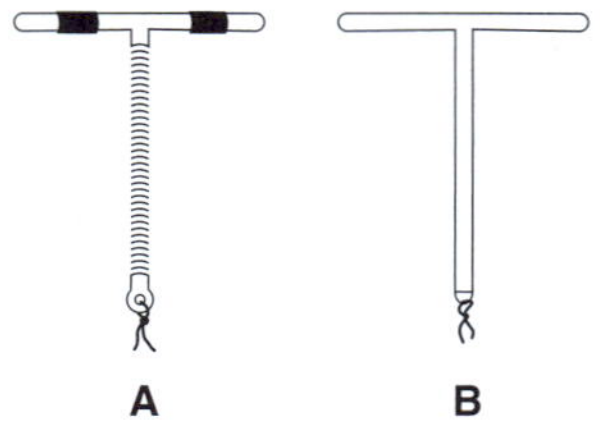

▲ **Figure 58–7.** Intrauterine contraceptive devices currently available in the United States. **A**: The copper T 380A device; **B**: the levonorgestrel device.

support this or other IUDs as abortifacients. The perfect use failure rate with the T 380A is 0.6 pregnancies per 100 woman-years and approximately 0.8 for typical use. In the past, IUDs were associated with an increased risk for PID around the time of insertion. However, by restricting use to mutually monogamous couples and couples currently at low risk of STIs, the absolute risk of PID in association with IUD use is almost negligible. PID appears to be associated primarily with the insertion of the device (Fig. 58–8) and not with its duration of use. Currently, with appropriately selected users, the rate of PID is approximately 1 case per 1000 insertions. Women at risk for HIV infection or who are already infected are not believed to be candidates for use of this device. Other ideal candidates are women in whom combination hormonal contraception is contraindicated. The other major risks reported in association with use of this IUD include ectopic pregnancy, spontaneous abortion, uterine perforation, and expulsion. Although 5–8% of pregnancies that occur with use of this IUD are ectopic, overall, because of the high effectiveness of this device, the absolute risk of ectopic pregnancy in users is substantially less than that experienced by nonusers of contraception. In addition, if a user becomes pregnant with the device in place, the risk of a spontaneous abortion is approximately 50%. Removing the device when the strings can be readily identified will reduce this risk by approximately 50%. If the pregnancy continues with the IUD in place, users should be apprised of an increased risk for premature rupture of the membranes and preterm delivery. Uterine perforation, which occurs at the time of insertion, has been reported at a rate of 1–2 events

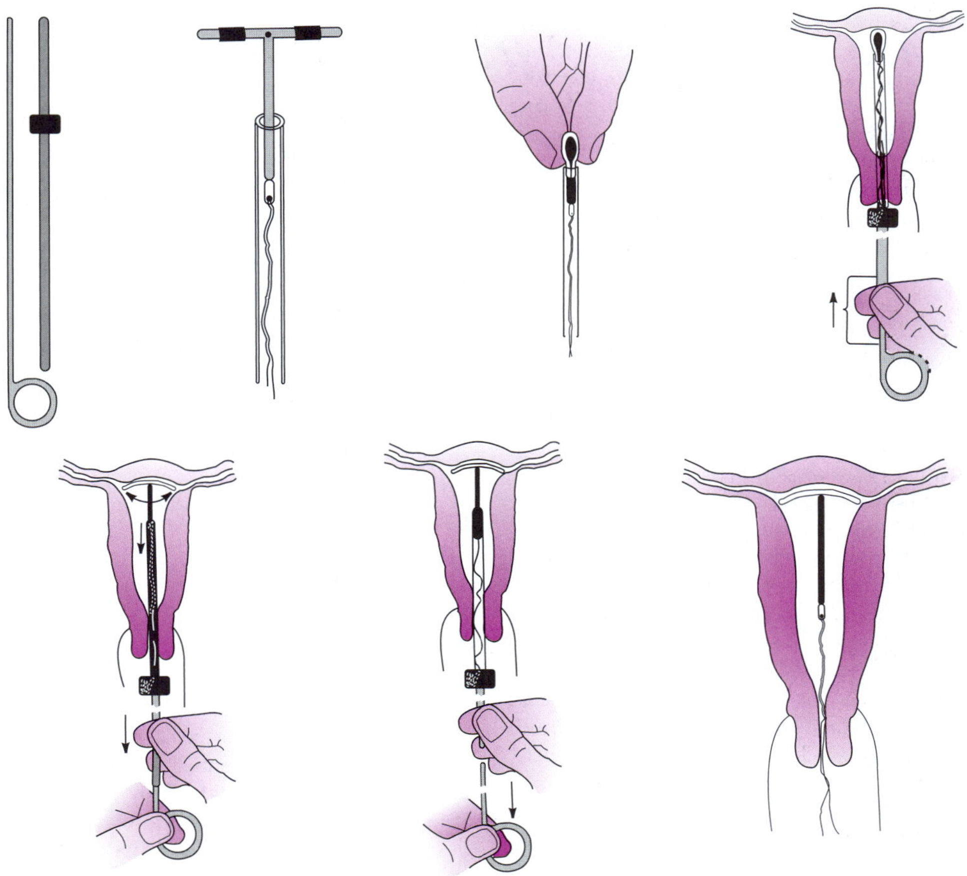

▲ **Figure 58–8.** Insertion of the ParaGard T 380A intrauterine copper contraceptive device.

per 1000 insertions. This risk is minimized by performing a preinsertion pelvic examination to determine the position of the uterus and by using a tenaculum to straighten the uterine axis during insertion. Expulsions of the device are more common in the first few weeks of use, with rates of approximately 5%. Minor side effects include abnormal bleeding and cramping. Use of nonsteroidal anti-inflammatory drugs often will reduce the overall amount of flow as well as reduce cramping.

The levonorgestrel-releasing intrauterine device (LNG-20 IUD) has a T-shaped frame with a reservoir on the vertical arm that releases the progestin levonorgestrel daily. Two monofilament strings are attached to the vertical arm. Blood levels of levonorgestrel among users are approximately 25% the levels seen among users of oral contraceptives containing this progestin. In contrast to the copper T 380A device, the LNG-20 IUD has a life span of 5 years in clinical trials. The primary mechanisms of action of the LNG-20 IUD are thickening the cervical mucus to impede ascent of sperm and altering the uterotubal fluid to also interfere with sperm migration. This IUD causes anovulation in approximately 10–15% of cycles and changes the characteristics of the endometrium to reduce the likelihood of implantation. Candidates for use of this IUD fit the same profile as those who would consider use of the T 380A. The perfect and typical use pregnancy rates are 0.1 pregnancies per 100 woman-years after 1 year of use, and the cumulative pregnancy rate over 5 years is 0.7 pregnancies per 100 woman-years. Approximately 50% of the pregnancies that occur are ectopic. However, as with the T 380A device, the absolute risk of ectopic pregnancy still is substantially lower than that experienced by nonusers of contraception. Because the LNG-20 IUD releases a potent progestin at the endometrial level, the bleeding pattern is substantially different from that seen with the T 380A. During the initial 3–4 months of use, some women experience irregular bleeding that may be heavy at times. However, after a few months of use, most women experience a significant decrease in menstrual flow by as much as 70%. In some studies, 20–25% of users become amenorrheic in the second year of use. In addition, dysmenorrhea tends to improve with use of this device. Because of the effectiveness of the LNG-20 IUD in reducing menstrual blood flow, it has been used for treatment of menorrhagia, a significant noncontraceptive benefit. Major risks with this IUD are similar to those noted for the copper T 380A, except that PID has not been associated with use of this device. The minor side effects of bleeding and cramping are less frequent with this device, except for irregular bleeding patterns during the first few months of use. Some women have reported headache, acne, or mastalgia, which could be related to the systemic effects of the progestin.

A not infrequent issue with IUD use is the management of missing strings. First, the patient should be encouraged to use a backup contraceptive method until she is evaluated. If the IUD strings cannot be seen even with gentle probing of the endocervical canal, one should perform a pregnancy test if indicated and consider ordering a transvaginal ultrasound to determine whether the IUD is intrauterine, intraperitoneal, or likely has undergone expulsion. If the patient is pregnant, an ectopic pregnancy must be excluded. If the IUD is determined to be intraperitoneal in location, removal usually is indicated because of likely peritoneal irritation by the device.

Backman T, Rauramo I, Huhtala S, Koskenvuo M. Pregnancy during the use of levonorgestrel intrauterine system. *Am J Obstet Gynecol* 2004;190:50–54. PMID: 14749634.

Rose S, Chaudhari A, Peterson CM. Mirena® (Levonorgestrel intrauterine system): a successful novel drug delivery option in contraception. *Adv Drug Deliv Rev* 2009;61:808–812. PMID: 19445984.

MALE CONTRACEPTION

The development of contraceptive methods for men poses a different challenge because men are continuously producing sperm and therefore are continuously fertile, unlike women who have a limited number of fertile days each month. Recent surveys have shown that men want to be more involved in contraception decisions, and women trust their male partners to take an active role in this area. The current research is focused on developing contraceptive injections, implants, or vaccines that will reduce a male's sperm count low enough to levels unlikely to cause pregnancy, but without damaging lifetime sperm production. Tests are currently being conducted overseas, and the information in this field will continue to be expanded. Nonsurgical steroidal methods comprising various derivatives of the androgens and their receptors are in various phases of clinical trials in men. The ideal male contraceptive should be coital-independent, nonsurgical, reversible, effective, and should not alter androgen levels or libido. Several nonsteroidal molecules and vaccines are being investigated in animal models for male contraception.

Naz RK, Rowan S. Update on male contraception. *Curr Opin Obstet Gynecol* 2009;21:265–269. PMID: 19469045.

CONTRACEPTION OVER 40

The majority of women 40–49 years of age need an effective method of contraception because the decline in fertility with age is an insufficient protection against unwanted pregnancy. Although pregnancy is less likely after the age of 40 years, the clinical and social consequences of an unexpected pregnancy are potentially detrimental. No contraceptive method is contraindicated by advanced reproductive age alone; thus there is a need to discuss the effectiveness, risks, and noncontraceptive benefits of all family planning methods for women in this age group. A review of the literature demonstrated that decline in fecundity in the fifth decade is insufficient for contraceptive purposes; thus a family planning method is needed. Sterilization is by far the most common method in several countries. Copper IUDs and hormone intrauterine systems have similar effectiveness, with fewer than 1% failures in the first year of typical use. Special considerations in this age group include the frequency of menstrual irregularity, sexual problems, and the possibility of menopausal symptoms, all of which may respond to hormonal methods of contraception.

The ESHRE Capri Workshop Group. Female contraception over 40. *Hum Reprod Update* 2009;15:599–612. PMID: 19458038.

INDUCED ABORTION

Induced abortion is the deliberate termination of pregnancy in a manner that ensures that the embryo or fetus will not survive. Societal attitudes toward elective abortion have changed markedly in the past few decades. In some situations the need for abortion is accepted by most people, but political and medical attitudes regarding induced abortion have continued to lag behind changing attitudes. Certain religious objections continue to prevail, resulting in personal, medical, and political conflicts.

Approximately one-third of the world's population lives in nations with nonrestrictive laws governing abortion. Another third live in countries with moderately restrictive abortion laws (ie, in countries where unwanted pregnancies may not be terminated as a matter of right or personal decision but only on broadly interpreted medical, psychologic, and sociologic indications). The remainder live in countries where abortion is illegal without qualification or is allowed only when the woman's life or health would be severely threatened if the pregnancy were allowed to continue.

An estimated 1 of every 4 pregnancies in the world is terminated by induced abortion, making it perhaps the most common method of reproduction limitation. In the United States, estimates of the number of criminal abortions performed before legalization of the procedure ranged from 0.25–1.25 million per year. The number of legal abortions now being performed in the United States approximates 1 abortion per 4 live births. In 1997, there were 1.33 million induced abortions compared with 3.88 million live births.

The procedures being used in the United States for legally induced abortions during the first trimester are relatively safe. Table 58–2 shows that first-trimester legal abortions are consistently safer for the woman than if she used no birth control method and gave birth. Table 58–2 also shows that although the number of maternal deaths related to births steadily increased from 5.6 to 22.6 per 100,000 women as age increased, the age-related increase in number of deaths per 100,000 women per year from legal abortions was insignificant.

Table 58–2. Pregnancy-related deaths per 100,000 women per year in developed countries compared with deaths resulting from legal abortion as a means of contraception.

	Age Groups (Years)					
Type of Birth Control	15-19	20-24	25-29	30-34	35-39	40-44
No birth control; birth related	5.6	6.1	7.4	13.9	20.8	22.6
First-trimester abortion only; method related	1.2	1.6	1.8	1.7	1.9	1.2

(Adapted from Tietze C. Induced abortion: 1977 supplement, Table 11. *Rep Popul Fam Plann* 1977; 14[2nd ed. Suppl]:16.)

In general, the risk of death from legal abortion is lowest when it is performed at 8 menstrual weeks or sooner. During 1988–1997, the overall death rate for women obtaining legally induced abortions was 0.7 per 100,000 legal induced abortions. The risk of death increased exponentially by 38% for each additional week of gestation. Compared with women whose abortions were performed at or before 8 weeks of gestation, women whose abortions were performed in the second trimester were significantly more likely to die of abortion-related causes. The relative risk (unadjusted) of abortion-related mortality was 14.7 at 13–15 weeks of gestation (95% confidence interval [CI] 6.2, 34.7), 29.5 at 16–20 weeks (95% CI 12.9, 67.4), and 76.6 at or after 21 weeks (95% CI 32.5, 180.8). Up to 87% of deaths in women who chose to terminate their pregnancies after 8 weeks of gestation may have been avoidable if these women had accessed abortion services before 8 weeks of gestation.

Legal Aspects of Induced Abortion in the United States

The United States Supreme Court ruled in 1973 that the restrictive abortion laws in the United States were invalid, largely because these laws invaded the individual's right to privacy, and that an abortion could not be denied to a woman in the first 3 months of pregnancy. The Court indicated that after 3 months a state may "regulate the abortion procedure in ways that are reasonably related to maternal health" and that after the fetus reaches the stage of viability (approximately 24 weeks) the states may refuse the right to terminate the pregnancy except when necessary for the preservation of the life or health of the mother. Still, much opposition is raised by various "right-to-life" groups and religious groups. In spite of this opposition, more than 1 million procedures are still performed annually in the United States, with approximately one-third performed on teenaged women. The patient must be informed regarding the nature of the procedure and its risks, including possible infertility or even continuation of pregnancy. The rights of the spouse, parents, or guardian also must be considered and permission obtained when indicated (until the individual woman's rights are clearly established). State laws must be obeyed with special reference to residence, duration of pregnancy, indications for abortion, consent, and consultations required.

Evaluation of Patients Requesting Induced Abortion

Patients give varied reasons for requesting abortion. Because in some cases the request is made at the urging of the woman's parents, in-laws, husband, or peers, every effort should be made to ascertain that the patient herself desires abortion for her own reasons. In addition, one should be certain that the patient knows she is free to choose from among other methods of solving the problem of unplanned pregnancy, such as adoption or single-parent rearing.

Although the majority of abortions are performed as elective procedures (ie, because of social or economic reasons as opposed to medical reasons), some women still request such services for medical or surgical indications. For example, continuation of pregnancy may pose a threat to the life of women with certain medical conditions, such as Eisenmenger's syndrome and cystic fibrosis. Other indications are pregnancy resulting from a rape or pregnancy with a fetus affected with a major disorder, such as trisomy 13. In any event, the ultimate decision rests with the pregnant woman. Help from social agencies should be made available as necessary. A complete social history, medical history, and physical examination are required. Particular attention must be given to uterine size and position; the importance of accurate calculation of the duration of pregnancy (within 2 weeks but preferably within 1 week) cannot be overstated. With uncertainty, pelvic sonography should be used liberally. Routine laboratory tests should include pregnancy tests, urinalysis, hematocrit level, Rh typing, serologic tests for syphilis, culture for gonorrhea, and Pap smear.

Methods of Induced Abortion

Numerous methods are used to induce an abortion: suction or surgical curettage; medical abortion (performed with mifepristone alone, or with a combination of mifepristone and misoprostol or other prostaglandins), induction of labor by means of intraovular or extraovular injection of a hypertonic solution or other oxytocic agent; dilatation and evacuation; extraovular placement of devices such as catheters, bougies, or bags; hysterotomy—abdominal or vaginal; hysterectomy—abdominal or vaginal; and menstrual regulation.

The method of abortion used is determined primarily by the duration of pregnancy, with consideration for the patient's health, the experience of the physician, and the available physical facilities. The risk of repeat abortion is associated with various sociodemographic characteristics, but apparently the method of abortion used is not a risk factor for repeat termination of pregnancy.

Suction curettage on an outpatient basis performed under local or light general anesthesia can be accomplished with a high degree of safety. The safety of outpatient abortion and the shortage of hospital beds have led to the development of single-function, "freestanding" abortion clinics. In addition to providing more efficient counseling and social services, these clinics have effectively reduced the cost of abortion. Many hospitals have "short-stay units," which match the efficiency of outpatient clinics but also offer the backup facilities of the general hospital.

A. Suction Curettage

Suction curettage is the safest and most effective method for terminating pregnancies of 12 weeks' duration or less. This technique has gained rapid worldwide acceptance, and more than 90% of induced abortions in the United States are now performed by this method. The procedure involves dilatation of the cervix by instruments or by hydrophilic *Laminaria* tent (see Induction of Labor by Intra-Amniotic Instillation), followed by insertion of a suction cannula of the appropriate diameter into the uterine cavity (Fig. 58–9). Most procedures are performed using a paracervical block with local anesthesia with or without additional medication for sedation. Standard negative pressures used range from 30–50 mm Hg. Many physicians follow aspiration with light instrumental curettage of the uterine cavity.

The advantages of suction over surgical curettage are that suction curettage empties the uterus more rapidly, minimizes blood loss, and reduces the likelihood of perforation of the uterus. However, failure to recognize perforation of the uterus with a cannula may result in serious damage to other organs. Knowledge of the size and position of the uterus and the volume of the contents is mandatory for safe suction curettage. Moreover, extreme care and slow minimal dilatation of the cervix, with special consideration for the integrity of the internal os, should prevent injury to the cervix or uterus. Attention to the decrease in uterine size that occurs with rapid evacuation helps to avoid uterine injury.

When performed in early pregnancy by properly trained physicians, suction curettage should be associated with a very low failure rate. The complication rate should be <1% for infection, approximately 2% for excessive bleeding, and <1% for uterine perforation. The risk of major complications, such as persistent fever, hemorrhage requiring transfusion, and unintended major surgery, ranges between 0.2 and 0.6% and is proportional to pregnancy duration. The incidence of mortality for suction curettage is approximately 1 in 100,000 patients.

B. Surgical Curettage

Surgical ("sharp") curettage has been used for first-trimester abortion in the absence of suction curettage equipment.

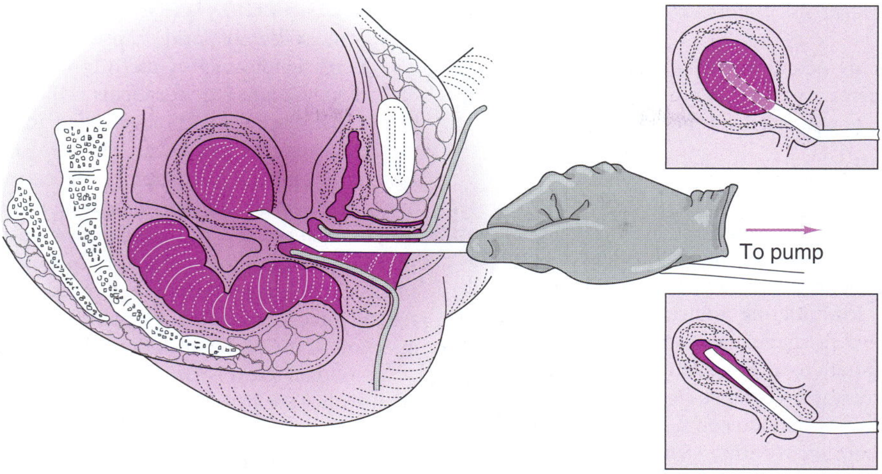

▲ **Figure 58–9.** Suction method for induced abortion.

This procedure is performed as a standard dilatation and curettage, such as for the diagnosis of abnormal uterine bleeding or for the removal of endometrial polyps. The blood loss, duration of surgery, and likelihood of damage to the cervix or uterus are greatly increased when surgical curettage is used. In addition, the risk of uterine synechiae or Asherman's syndrome is increased with this approach. Accordingly, suction curettage is generally preferred over sharp curettage for first-trimester termination procedures.

Bartz D, Goldberg A. Medication abortion. *Clin Obstet Gynecol* 2009;52:140–150. PMID: 19407520.

Bartlett LA, Berg CJ, Shulman HB, et al. Risk factors for legal induced abortion-related mortality in the United States. *Obstet Gynecol* 2004;103:729–737. PMID: 15051566.

Creinin MD. Randomized comparison of efficacy, acceptability and cost of medical versus surgical abortion. *Contraception* 2000;62:117–124. PMID: 11124358.

Grimes DA, Creinin MD. Induced abortion: an overview for internists. *Ann Intern Med* 2004;140:620–626. PMID: 15096333.

Haimov-Kochman R, Arbel R, Sciaky-Tamir Y, Brzezinski A, Laufer N, Yagel S. Risk factors for unsuccessful medical abortion with mifepristone and misoprostol. *Acta Obstet Gynecol Scand* 2007;86:462–466. PMID: 17486469.

Hubacher D, Grimes DA. Noncontraceptive health benefits of intrauterine devices: a systematic review. *Obstet Gynecol Survey* 2002;57:120–128. PMID: 11832788.

Niinimäki M, Pouta A, Bloigu A, et al. Frequency and risk factors for repeat abortions after surgical compared with medical termination of pregnancy. *Obstet Gynecol* 2009;113:845–852. PMID: 19305329.

Vargas J, Diedrich J. Second-trimester induction of labor. *Clin Obstet Gynecol* 2009;52:188–197. PMID: 19407525.

C. Medical Abortion

Medical methods for pregnancy termination in early gestation offer women an alternative to surgical evacuation and have the potential to improve access globally to safe abortion. Several drug regimens are used with varying efficacy, including mifepristone plus misoprostol, misoprostol alone, and methotrexate plus misoprostol. Where available, a mifepristone plus misoprostol regimen is most frequently used and is highly effective for early abortion. Overall, women who choose medical abortion report high levels of satisfaction.

Women with first-trimester pregnancies <49 days from their first day of the last menstrual period may be eligible for medical abortion. An alternative method of medical abortion consists of the administration of an oral antiprogestin (RU-486 [mifepristone]) followed by oral misoprostol 48 hours later. The reported success rate of this method is >90%, provided the protocol is started before 7 weeks from the last menstrual period. Complications include cramping, bleeding due to incomplete abortion, and failure to evacuate the uterus necessitating completion by suction curettage. With one of the more common protocols, 50 mg methotrexate is administered orally, followed by 800 mg misoprostol per vagina (by the patient at home) 3–7 days later using the same tablets as those used for oral dosing. The patient is seen at least 24 hours after the misoprostol administration; a vaginal ultrasound is performed to determine whether there has been passage of the gestational sac. If abortion has not occurred, the misoprostol dose is repeated. The patient is then followed up in 4 weeks; if abortion has not occurred by this time, a suction curettage is typically performed. If fetal cardiac activity is noted on ultrasound, office follow-up is more frequent. Efficacy with this method is up to 98% for pregnancies up to 49 days' gestation; complete abortion rates are inversely proportional to duration of gestation. Nausea is the most frequently reported side effect. Older age, previous spontaneous abortions, and multigravidity are apparently independent risk factors for unsuccessful medical abortion.

Contraindications include active liver disease, active renal disease, severe anemia, acute inflammatory bowel disease and coagulopathy, or anticoagulant therapy.

D. Induction of Labor by Intra-Amniotic Instillation

The Japanese developed this technique for induced abortion after the first trimester. Currently, the technique is used almost exclusively for initiating midtrimester abortion. The original procedure consisted of amniocentesis, aspiration of as much fluid as possible, and instillation into the amniotic sac of 200 mL hypertonic (20%) sodium chloride solution. In most (80–90%) cases, spontaneous labor and expulsion of the fetus and placenta occur within 48 hours. This technique has been modified, primarily to reduce the injection–abortion interval, and as a result of the development of other agents that initiate labor when instilled intra-amniotically.

Because of the problems associated with hypertonic sodium chloride, many clinicians have used intra-amniotic hyperosmolar (59.7%) urea, usually with oxytocin or prostaglandin or intra-amniotic prostaglandin alone. These approaches result in injection–abortion intervals of 16–17 hours for urea and 19–22 hours for prostaglandin. The urea is instilled in a fashion similar to that described for hypertonic sodium chloride. The prostaglandin, most frequently prostaglandin F_{2a} (PGF_{2a}), usually is instilled as a single dose of 40–50 mg or as 2 doses of 25 mg instilled 6 hours apart. When oxytocin is used to augment these agents, doses as high as 332 mU/min are required to produce uterine contractions because of the relative insensitivity of the myometrium to oxytocin at this stage of pregnancy. To avoid water intoxication, the oxytocin is made up in highly concentrated solutions and given at slow rates.

It is advantageous to soften the unripe cervix with *Laminaria* tents placed in the cervix a few hours before amniocentesis is performed. Such an approach markedly reduces the risk of cervical injury.

Midtrimester abortion induced by this method must be accomplished with scrupulous aseptic surgical technique, and the patient must be monitored until the fetus and placenta are delivered and postabortion bleeding is under control. The complication rate is high—up to 20% in some institutions—and the mortality rate is comparable to that of term parturition. Fortunately, because first-trimester abortion is now more readily available, more women are consulting their physicians early and thus availing themselves of the much safer suction curettage.

Several types of complications are associated with the use of instillation agents. Retained placenta is the most common problem; rates ranging from 13 to 46% have been reported. The placenta usually can be removed without difficulty using ring forceps and large curettes with the patient under local anesthesia. Hemorrhage may be caused by retained products or atony; coagulopathy is seen in up to 1% of patients in whom hypertonic sodium chloride is used. Infection can occur but is reduced significantly by use of prophylactic antibiotics in high-risk situations (eg, in patients with early ruptured membranes and during injection–abortion intervals >24 hours). Cervical laceration can occur but is reduced by the use of *Laminaria* tents. Hypernatremia can occur with the use of hypertonic sodium chloride if the drug is absorbed rapidly by the placental bed or if it is given intravascularly by mistake.

Failure of labor to expel the products of conception necessitates either a repetition of the procedure if the membranes are still intact or oxytocin stimulation, usually by intravenous injection or use of the dilatation and evacuation technique.

Emotional stress is an important factor for many women because they are awake at the time of the expulsion of the fetus and the fetus is well formed. (The emotional stress is also a factor for hospital personnel—a problem impossible to avoid.)

E. Induction of Labor with Vaginal Prostaglandins

Second-trimester abortions are most commonly performed in the United States via dilation and evacuation; however, there are instances in which the use of systemic abortifacients is necessary. Lack of trained staff to perform late abortion procedures, fetal anomalies, and patient preference are important considerations when selecting the method of termination. Second-trimester abortions with misoprostol-only protocols require higher doses, side effects are more common, and the time to complete the abortion is longer in comparison with mifepristone-misoprostol combinations. Feticidal agents are recommended to avoid transient fetal survival. Prostaglandin E_2 given intravaginally can be used to induce midtrimester abortion. Vaginal suppositories containing 20 mg are used every 3–4 hours until abortion occurs; the presence or absence of labor determines whether the prostaglandin E_2 should be stopped. Misoprostol, a synthetic prostaglandin E_1 analogue, is also used. Treatment–abortion intervals, rates of incomplete abortion, and complications are similar to those described for instillation agents. The major disadvantages are significant gastrointestinal side effects, a higher incidence of live abortion, and a more frequent occurrence of fever.

F. Dilatation & Evacuation

This technique for inducing midtrimester abortion is essentially a modification of suction curettage. Because fetal parts are larger at this stage of pregnancy, most operators use serial placement of *Laminaria* tents to effect cervical dilatation with less likelihood of injury. Larger suction cannulas and specially designed forceps are used to extract tissue. In most instances, the operation can be performed in the outpatient setting using paracervical block anesthesia and intravenous sedation on patients with pregnancies up to 18 weeks' gestation. Complications include hemorrhage (usually due to atony or laceration), perforation, and rarely infection. Retained tissue is uncommon, especially when tissue is carefully inspected for completion at the end of each procedure. Compared with instillation techniques or vaginal prostaglandin, the overall incidence of complications (in pregnancies up to 18 weeks' gestation) is less with dilatation and evacuation. In addition, most patients prefer the technique because it is an outpatient procedure and the woman does not undergo labor.

G. Hysterotomy & Hysterectomy

The use of hysterotomy and hysterectomy is currently reserved for special circumstances such as the failure to complete a midtrimester abortion due to cervical stenosis or the management of other complications. Both approaches, compared with other techniques discussed, have unacceptably high rates of morbidity and mortality, and neither should be used as a primary method.

H. Menstrual Regulation

Menstrual regulation consists of aspiration of the endometrium within 14 days after a missed menstrual cycle or within 42 days after the beginning of the last menstrual period by means of a small cannula attached to a source of low-pressure suction, such as a syringe or other suction machine. This is a simple and safe procedure that can be readily performed in the office or outpatient clinic, usually without any anesthetic, although paracervical block can be used if necessary. Menstrual regulation was used extensively in the 1970s and 1980s before reliable, inexpensive, and sensitive urine pregnancy tests became available. It offered a safe early approach to pregnancy termination; however, approximately 40% of women were not pregnant at the time of the procedure. With the advent of urine pregnancy tests that have the ability to document pregnancy even before a missed menstrual period, standard first-trimester suction curettage probably is more widely used. Complications are similar to those described for suction curettage except that persistent pregnancy is more common, particularly when very early menstrual regulation procedures are performed.

I. RU-486

RU-486 (mifepristone) is a synthetic drug, developed by French pharmacologists, that acts at least partially as an antiprogestational agent. When given orally in conjunction with a prostaglandin such as misoprostol, it effects first-trimester abortion. Complications include failure to terminate a pregnancy, incomplete abortion, and significant uterine cramping.

Follow-Up of Patients After Induced Abortion

Follow-up care after all procedures must be ensured. After abortion by all methods, human Rho (D) immune globulin (RhoGAM) should be administered promptly if the patient is Rh-negative, unless the male partner is known to be Rh-negative. The patient should take her temperature several times daily and report fever or unusual bleeding at once. She should avoid intercourse or the use of tampons or douches for at least 2 weeks. The physician should discuss with the patient the possibility that emotional depression, similar to that after term pregnancy and delivery, may occur after induced abortion. Follow-up care should include pelvic examination to rule out endometritis and parametritis, salpingitis, failure of involution, or continued uterine growth. Finally, effective contraception should be made available according to the patient's needs and desires.

Long-Term Sequelae of Induced Abortion

Many studies during the past 2 decades have examined the possible long-term sequelae of elective induced abortion. Most of the attention has focused on subsequent reproductive function; unfortunately, many of the studies had inherent biases and serious methodologic flaws. Despite these problems, enough information is available to provide relative estimates of potential risks. Data from some studies suggest that midtrimester pregnancy loss is more common in women who have undergone 2 or more induced or spontaneous abortions. However, women who have undergone 1 procedure have essentially the same risk as women who have experienced a single term pregnancy. Regarding low birthweight, only women who have undergone a first-trimester procedure by sharp curettage under general anesthesia appear to have increased risks. The reason for this association might be related to the method of dilatation used. Finally, studies that have examined both ectopic pregnancy and infertility have failed to show any consistent association between these adverse events and prior induced abortion.

Burkman RT. Clinical pearls: factors affecting reported contraceptive efficacy rates in clinical studies. *Int J Fertil Womens Med* 2002;47:153–161.PMID: 12199411.

Chandra A, Martinez GM, Mosher WD, Abma JC, Jones J. Fertility, family planning, and reproductive health of US women: data from the 2002 National Survey of Family Growth. National Center for Health Statistics. *Vital Health Stat* 2005;23:1–160. PMID: 16532609.

Dailard C, Gold RB. *Fulfilling the Promise: Public Policy and U.S. Family Planning Clinics.* New York: The Alan Guttmacher Institute; 2002.

Kubba A, Guillebaud J, Anderson RA, MacGregor EA. Contraception. *Lancet* 2000;356:1913–1919. PMID: 11130398.

Ventura MA, Abma JC, Mosher WD, Henshaw SK. Estimated pregnancy rates for the United States, 1990–2005: an update by Stephanie J. Centers for Disease Control and Prevention National Center for Health Statistics National Vital Statistics System. *Natl Vital Stat Rep* 2009;58:1-14. PMID: 20121003.

59

Menopause & Postmenopause

Lauren Nathan, MD

ESSENTIALS OF DIAGNOSIS

- Natural menopause diagnosed after 12 months of amenorrhea with no obvious pathologic cause
- Average age 51 years
- Estradiol <20 pg/mL and follicle-stimulation hormone level 21–100 mU/mL helpful in establishing the diagnosis
- Induced menopause is defined as permanent cessation of menstruation after bilateral oophorectomy or ablation of ovarian function (ie, by chemotherapy or radiation)
- Premature menopause defined as menopause reached at or before age 40 and can be natural or induced
- Perimenopause/menopause transition defined by menstrual cycle and hormonal changes that occur a few years before and 12 months after the final menstrual period resulting from natural menopause
- May be associated with vasomotor symptoms, sleep disturbance, and vaginal/urinary symptoms

General Considerations

According to the 2010 US census, of the 155 million women in this country, 41 million were 55 years of age or older. Most of these women had or shortly would have their last menstrual period, thus becoming postmenopausal. As a woman at age 55 years can expect to live another 28 years, a large portion of the female population is without ovarian function and lives about one-third of their lives after this function ceases. Consequently, physicians caring for women must understand the hormonal and metabolic changes associated with the menopause, or "change of life," and the potential benefits and risks of hormone therapy (HT).

According to the Comite des Nomenclatures de la Federation Internationale de Gynecologie et d'Obstetrique, the **climacteric** is the phase of the aging process during which a woman passes from the reproductive to the nonreproductive stage. The signals that this period of life has been reached are referred to as "climacteric symptoms" or, if more serious, as "climacteric complaints." **Perimenopause,** or **menopausal transition,** refers to the part of the climacteric before the menopause occurs when the menstrual cycle is likely to be irregular and when other climacteric symptoms or complaints may be experienced. The **menopause** is the final menstruation, which occurs during the climacteric. **Postmenopause** refers to the phase of life that comes after the menopause.

To develop a more functional staging system of reproductive aging, the Stages of Reproductive Aging Workshop (STRAW) was held in 2001 and again 10 years later in another workshop called "STRAW +10". The specific goals of the workshop were to (a) develop a useful staging system for reproductive aging, (b) revise nomenclature, and (c) identify knowledge gaps that should be addressed by the research community. STRAW + 10 also added more supportive criteria using endocrinologic parameters (Follicle Stimulation Hormone [FSH], anti-mullerian hormone [AMH], Inhibin B) and Antral Follicle count [AMC]). According to STRAW +10, reproductive aging is divided into 7 stages (−5 to +2), with −5 beginning with menarche and +2 being defined as the late menopause. This staging system is not applicable to women who have undergone hysterectomy or endometrial ablation, who have chronic menstrual irregularity such as polycystic ovarian syndrome (PCO), or who have chronic illness and undergoing chemotherapy. STRAW +10 may also not be applicable to women with other chronic illnesses such as HIV-AIDs but further research into this population needs to be carried out in order to better characterize ovarian function across time in this group of patients.

The **menopausal transition,** or **perimenopause,** is divided into 2 stages—early (−2) and late (−1) and encompasses a wide age range. Both stages vary in length and both are characterized by an elevation in early follicular phase follicle-stimulating hormone (FSH). In stage −2, the menstrual cycles remain regular, but the cycle length changes by 7 days or more (ie, cycle length becomes 24 days instead of 31). FSH may be elevated but levels are variable. AMH,

Inhibin B and AMC are all low. Duration is variable. Stage −1 (late menopausal transition) is characterized by an interval of amenorrhea of ≥60 days and is typically characterized by increased variability in cycle length. FSH is usually >25 IU/L during this stage. AMH, Inhibin B and AMC are low. Many women begin to experience symptoms during this time which may include vasomotor symptoms, and sleep disturbance. The duration is typically 1-3 years. The early postmenopausal period (stage +1) is divided into +1a, +1b and +1c and includes the first 6 years following the final menstrual period. +1a begins 12 months following the last menstrual period and marks the end of the menopausal transition or "perimenopause". During stage +1, FSH remains elevated while AMH, Inhibin B and AMC drop further and become very low. The late postmenopausal period (stage +2) begins 6 years after the final menstrual period and continues until death.

Harlow SD, Gass M, Hall JE, et al. Executive Summary of the Stages of Reproductive Aging Workshop + 10: Addressing the Unfinished Agenda of Staging Reproductive Aging. *J Clin Endocrinol Metab*, 2012;97:1159–1168. PMID: 22344196.

U.S. Census Bureau. Age and Sex Composition: 2010. www.census.govprod/cen2010

Pathogenesis

A. Perimenopausal State

The decades of mature reproductive life are characterized by generally regular menses and a slow, steady decrease in cycle length. Mean cycle length at age 15 years is 35 days, at age 25 years it is 30 days, and at age 35 years it is 28 days. This decrease is a result of shortening of the follicular phase of the cycle, with the luteal phase length remaining constant. After age 45 years, altered function of the aging ovary is detectable in regularly menstruating women (Fig. 59–1). The mean cycle length is significantly shorter than in younger women and is attributable to a shortened follicular phase. The luteal phase is of similar length, and progesterone levels are no different from those observed in younger women. Estradiol levels are lower during portions of the cycle, including active follicular maturation, the midcycle peak, and the luteal phase. Concentrations of FSH are strikingly elevated during the early follicular phase and fall as estradiol increases during follicular maturation. FSH levels at the midcycle peak and late in the luteal phase are also consistently higher than those found in younger women and decrease during the midluteal phase. Luteinizing hormone (LH) concentrations are indistinguishable from those observed in younger women. The mechanism responsible for this early rise of FSH is probably related to inhibin. **Inhibin** is a polypeptide hormone that is synthesized and secreted by granulosa cells. It causes negative feedback on FSH release by the pituitary. As the oocyte number decreases, inhibin levels fall, resulting in a rise in FSH levels.

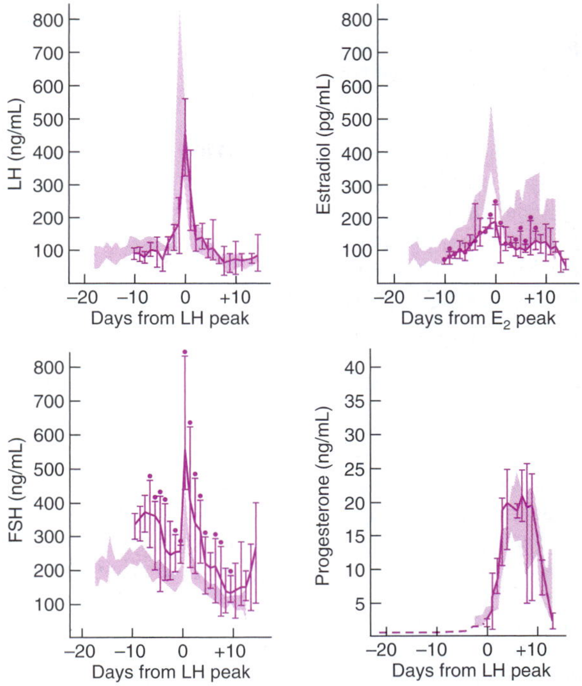

▲ **Figure 59–1.** Mean and range of LH, FSH, estradiol (E_2), and progesterone levels in women over age 45 with regular menstrual cycles. Shaded area represents the mean (±2 SEM) in cycles found in young women. (Reproduced, with permission, from Sherman BM, Korenman SG. Hormonal characteristics of the human menstrual cycle throughout reproductive life. *J Clin Invest* 1975;55:699.)

The transition from regular cycle intervals to the permanent amenorrhea of menopause is characterized by a phase of marked menstrual irregularity. The duration of this transition varies greatly among women. Those experiencing the menopause at an early age have a relatively short duration of cycle variability before amenorrhea ensues. Those experiencing it at a later age usually have a phase of menstrual irregularity characterized by unusually long and short intermenstrual intervals and an overall increase of mean cycle length and variance.

The hormonal characteristics of this transitional phase are of special interest and importance. The irregular episodes of vaginal bleeding in premenopausal women represent the irregular maturation of ovarian follicles with or without hormonal evidence of ovulation. The potential for hormone secretion by these remaining follicles is diminished and variable. Menses are sometimes preceded by maturation of a follicle with limited secretion of both estradiol and progesterone. Vaginal bleeding also happens after a rise and fall of estradiol without a measurable increase in progesterone, such as is seen during anovulatory menses.

From these findings, it is clear that the transitional phase of menstrual irregularity is not one of marked estrogen deficiency. During the menopausal transition, high levels of FSH appear to stimulate residual follicles to secrete bursts of estradiol. Occasionally, estradiol levels will rise to concentrations 2 or 3 times higher than is normally seen, probably reflecting the recruitment of more than 1 follicle for ovulation. This may be followed by corpus luteum formation, often with limited secretion of progesterone. Because the episodes of follicular maturation and vaginal bleeding are widely spaced, premenopausal women may be exposed to persistent estrogen stimulation of the endometrium in the absence of regular cyclic progesterone secretion.

B. Menopausal State

The 2 types of menopause are classified according to cause.

1. Physiologic menopause—In the human embryo, oogenesis begins in the ovary around the third week of gestation. Primordial germ cells appear in the yolk sac, migrate to the germinal ridge, and undergo cellular divisions. It is estimated that the fetal ovaries contain approximately 7 million oogonia at 20 weeks' gestation. After 7 months' gestation, no new oocytes are formed. At birth, there are approximately 1–2 million oocytes, and by puberty this number is reduced to 300,000–500,000. Continued reduction of oocyte numbers occurs during the reproductive years through ovulation and atresia. Nearly all oocytes vanish by atresia, with only 400–500 actually being ovulated. Very little is known about oocyte atresia. Animal studies show that estrogens prevent the atretic process, whereas androgens enhance it.

Menopause apparently occurs in the human female because of 2 processes. First, oocytes responsive to gonadotropins disappear from the ovary, and second, the few remaining oocytes do not respond to gonadotropins. Isolated oocytes can be found in postmenopausal ovaries on very careful histologic inspection. Some of them show a limited degree of development, but most reveal no sign of development in the presence of excess endogenous gonadotropins.

The average age at menopause in the United States is 50–51 years. There does not appear to be any consistent relationship between age at menarche and age at menopause. Marriage, childbearing, height, weight, and prolonged use of oral contraceptives do not appear to influence the age of menopause. Smoking, however, is associated with early menopause.

Spontaneous cessation of menses before age 40 years is called **premature menopause,** or **premature ovarian failure.** It appears that approximately 0.9% of women in the United States may experience this early cessation of function. Cessation of menstruation and the development of climacteric symptoms and complaints can occur as early as a few years after menarche. The reasons for premature ovarian failure are unknown.

Disease processes, especially severe infections or tumors of the reproductive tract, can occasionally damage the ovarian follicular structures so severely as to precipitate the menopause. The menopause can also be hastened by excessive exposure to ionizing radiation; chemotherapeutic drugs, particularly alkylating agents; and surgical procedures that impair ovarian blood supply. The possibility of associated endocrine or chromosomal abnormalities should also be considered.

2. Artificial menopause—The permanent cessation of ovarian function brought about by surgical removal of the ovaries or by radiation therapy is called an artificial menopause. Irradiation to ablate ovarian function is rarely used today. Artificial menopause is used as a treatment for endometriosis and rarely may be used to treat estrogen-sensitive neoplasms of the breast and endometrium. More frequently, artificial menopause is a side effect of treatment of intra-abdominal disease (eg, ovaries are removed in premenopausal women because the gonads have been damaged by infection or neoplasia). When laparotomy is being performed for intra-abdominal or pelvic disease (ie, hysterectomy for leiomyomata), elective bilateral oophorectomy is sometimes used to prevent ovarian cancer. In some women who are genetically predisposed to ovarian cancer, elective laparoscopic oophorectomy is also performed.

C. Changes in Hormone Metabolism Associated with the Menopause

After the menopause, there are major changes in androgen, estrogen, progesterone, and gonadotropin secretion, much of which occurs because of cessation of ovarian follicular activity (Fig. 59–2).

1. Androgens—During reproductive life, the primary ovarian androgen is androstenedione, the major secretory product of developing follicles. In postmenopausal women, there is a reduction of circulating androstenedione to approximately 50% of the concentration found in young women, reflecting the absence of follicular activity. In the year following the last menstrual period, the levels of this hormone are steady. In older women, there is a circadian variation of androstenedione, with peak concentration between 8:00 AM and 12 noon, and the nadir occurring between 3:00 PM and 4:00 AM. This rhythm reflects adrenal activity. The clearance rate of androstenedione is similar in pre- and postmenopausal women; therefore, the change in levels of circulating hormone reflects changes in production. Thus the average production rate of androstenedione is approximately 1.5 mg/24 h in older women, a rate that is 50% of the rate found in premenopausal women. The source of most of this circulating androstenedione appears to be the adrenal glands, but continued secretion by the postmenopausal ovary accounts for approximately 20%.

For testosterone, the level found in postmenopausal women is only minimally lower than that found in premenopausal women before oophorectomy and is distinctly higher than the level observed in ovariectomized young women. There is also a prominent circadian variation of this androgen, with the highest levels occurring at 8:00 AM and the nadir at

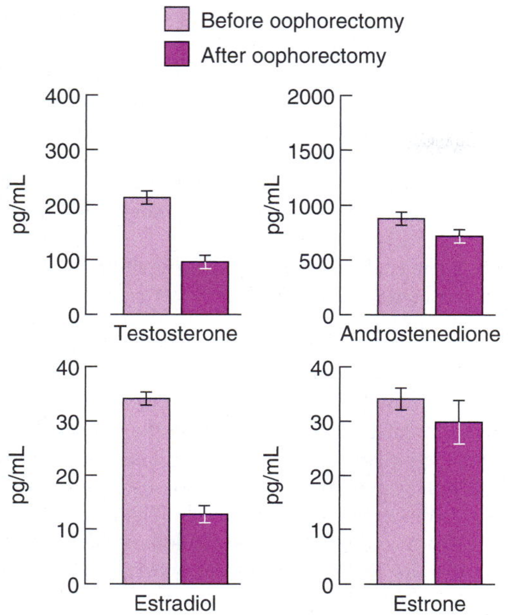

▲ **Figure 59–2. Serum androgen and estrogen levels in 16 postmenopausal women with endometrial cancer before and after oophorectomy.** (Reproduced, with permission, from Judd HL. Hormonal dynamics associated with the menopause. *Clin Obstet Gynecol* 1976; 1:775.)

4:00 PM. There is no difference in the clearance rate of testosterone before and after the menopause. Thus the production rate in older women is approximately 150 μg/24 h, a rate that is only one-third lower than the rate seen in young women.

The source of circulating testosterone is more complex than that of androstenedione. Oophorectomy after menopause is associated with a nearly 60% decrease in testosterone. There is no change in the metabolic clearance rate of the androgen with oophorectomy; therefore, the fall in the circulating level reflects alterations of its production rate. Approximately 15% of circulating androstenedione is converted to testosterone. The small simultaneous fall of androstenedione after oophorectomy can only account for a small portion of the total decrease of testosterone. The remainder of the loss presumably represents loss from direct ovarian secretion of testosterone. Direct ovarian secretion in the postmenopausal ovary is larger than the amount secreted directly by the premenopausal ovary. Large increments in testosterone have been found in the ovarian compared with the peripheral veins of postmenopausal women. These increments are greater than those observed in premenopausal women, supporting the hypothesis that the postmenopausal ovary secretes more testosterone directly than the premenopausal ovary. Hilar cells and luteinized stromal cells (hyperthecosis) are present in most postmenopausal ovaries and have been shown to produce testosterone in premenopausal women. Presumably, these cells could do the same in postmenopausal subjects.

A proposed mechanism for increased ovarian testosterone production by postmenopausal ovaries is the stimulation of gonadal cells still capable of androgen production by excess endogenous gonadotropins, which, in turn, are increased because of reduced estrogen production by the ovaries. This increased ovarian testosterone secretion, coupled with a reduction of estrogen production, and decrease in sex hormone-binding globulin (SHBG) may partly explain the development of symptoms of defeminization, hirsutism, and even virilism occasionally seen in older women.

Levels of the adrenal androgens dehydroepiandrosterone (DHEA) and dehydroepiandrosterone sulfate (DHEAS) are reduced by 60% and 80%, respectively, with age. Whether these reductions are related to the menopause or to aging has not been determined. Again, a marked circadian variation of DHEA has been observed. Whether a similar rhythm is present for DHEAS is unknown. As with younger subjects, the primary source of these 2 androgens is thought to be the adrenal glands, with the ovary contributing <15%. Thus the marked decreases of DHEA and DHEAS reflect altered adrenal androgen secretion, and this phenomenon has been called the *adrenopause*. The mechanism responsible for it is unknown.

In premenopausal women, plasma androstenedione is approximately 1.5 ng/mL. Plasma testosterone is approximately 0.3 ng/mL. Mean DHEA and DHEAS levels are approximately 4 ng/mL and 1600 ng/mL, respectively, in samples drawn at 8:00 AM.

In postmenopausal women, the mean plasma androstenedione concentration is reduced by at least 50%, to approximately 0.6 ng/mL. Plasma testosterone levels are only slightly reduced (to approximately 0.25 ng/mL). Plasma DHEA and DHEAS levels are decreased to mean levels of 1.8 ng/mL and 300 ng/mL in women in their sixties and seventies.

2. Estrogens—After a woman has passed the menopause, there is good clinical evidence of reduced endogenous estrogen production in most subjects. When circulating levels have been assessed, the greatest decrease is in estradiol. Its concentration is distinctly lower than that found in young women during any phase of their menstrual cycle and is similar to the level seen in premenopausal women after oophorectomy. A decrease of this estrogen occurs up to 1 year after the last menstrual period. There does not appear to be a circadian variation of the circulating concentration of estradiol after the menopause. The metabolic clearance rate of estradiol is reduced by 30%. The average production rate is 12 μg/24 h.

The source of the small amount of estradiol found in older women has been established. Direct ovarian secretion contributes minimally, but the adrenal glands are the major source. Investigators who have examined the concentrations of estradiol in adrenal veins have reported minimal increments, arguing against direct adrenal secretion being a major contributor. Although both estrone and testosterone are converted in peripheral tissues to estradiol, it is conversion from estrone that accounts for most estradiol in older women.

After the menopause, the circulating level of estrone decreases—not as much as that of estradiol—and overlaps with values seen in premenopausal women during the early follicular phase in menstrual cycles. There is a circadian variation of circulating estrone, with the peak in the morning and the nadir in late afternoon or early evening. This variation is not as prominent as that observed for the androgens. In postmenopausal women, there is a 20% reduction of estrone clearance, and the average production rate is approximately 55 μg/24 h.

The adrenal gland is the major source of estrone. Direct adrenal or ovarian secretion is minimal. Most estrone results from the peripheral aromatization of androstenedione. The average percent conversion is double that found in ovulatory women and can account for the total daily production of this estrogen. Aromatization of androstenedione occurs in fat, muscle, liver, bone marrow, brain, fibroblasts, and hair roots. Other tissues may also contribute but have not been evaluated. To what extent each cell type contributes to total conversion has not been determined, but fat cells and muscle may be responsible for only 30–40%. This conversion correlates with body size, with heavy women having higher conversion rates and circulating estrogen levels than slender women.

During normal menstrual life, the mean plasma estradiol fluctuates from 50–350 pg/mL and estrone from 30–110 pg/mL. In postmenopausal women, the mean estradiol level is approximately 12 pg/mL, with a range of 5–25 pg/mL. The mean estrone level is approximately 30 pg/mL, with a range of 20–70 pg/mL. Estradiol levels in normal young women do not overlap with those observed in postmenopausal subjects. The finding of estradiol levels below 21 pg/mL can be helpful in establishing the diagnosis of menopause, as the fall of this estrogen is the last hormonal change associated with loss of ovarian function. There is substantial overlap of estrone levels in younger and older women. Measurement of this estrogen is not helpful in determining the ovarian status of a patient.

3. Progesterone—In young women, the major source of progesterone is the ovarian corpus luteum after ovulation. During the follicular phase of the cycle, progesterone levels are low. With ovulation the levels rise greatly, reflecting the secretory activity of the corpus luteum. In postmenopausal women, the levels of progesterone are only 30% of the concentrations seen in young women during the follicular phase. Because postmenopausal ovaries do not contain functional follicles, ovulation does not occur and progesterone levels remain low. The source of the small amount of progesterone present in older women is felt to be caused by adrenal secretion, as dexamethasone suppresses its level, adrenocorticotropic hormone (ACTH) increases its level, and human chorionic gonadotropin (hCG) administration has no effect.

In young menstruating women, the mean progesterone level is approximately 0.4 ng/mL during the follicular phase of the cycle, with a range of 0.2–0.7 ng/mL. During the luteal phase, progesterone levels rise and fall, reflecting corpus luteum function; the mean level is approximately 11 ng/mL, with a range of 3–21 ng/mL. In postmenopausal women, the mean progesterone level is 0.17 ng/mL. To date, no clinical use has been established for the measurement of progesterone in postmenopausal women.

4. Gonadotropins—With the menopause, both LH and FSH levels rise substantially, with FSH usually higher than LH. This is thought to reflect the slower clearance of FSH from the circulation. The reason for the marked increase in circulating gonadotropins is the absence of the negative feedback of ovarian steroids and inhibin on gonadotropin release. As in young women, the levels of both gonadotropins are not steady, but instead show random oscillations. These oscillations are thought to represent pulsatile secretion by the pituitary. In older women, these pulsatile bursts occur every 1–2 hours, a frequency similar to that seen during the follicular phase of premenopausal subjects. Although the frequency is similar, the amplitude is much greater. This increased amplitude is secondary to increased release by the hypothalamic hormone gonadotropin-releasing hormone (GnRH) and enhanced responsiveness of the pituitary to GnRH because of low estrogen levels. Studies with rhesus monkeys suggest that the site governing pulsatile GnRH release is in the arcuate nucleus of the hypothalamus. The large pulses of gonadotropin in the peripheral circulation are believed to maintain the high levels of the hormones found in postmenopausal women.

During reproductive life, the levels of both FSH and LH range from 4–30 mU/mL, except during the preovulatory surge, when they may exceed 50 mU/mL and 100 mU/mL, respectively. After the menopause, both rise to levels above 100 mU/mL, with FSH rising earlier and to higher levels than LH.

When contradictory or uncertain clinical findings make the diagnosis of the postmenopausal state questionable, measurement of plasma FSH, LH, and estradiol levels may be helpful. This situation occurs frequently in women after hysterectomy without oophorectomy. The findings of plasma estradiol below 20 pg/mL and elevated FSH and LH levels are consistent with cessation of ovarian function. In practical terms, it is not necessary to measure LH.

D. Physical Changes Associated with the Menopause

1. Reproductive tract—Because estrogen functions as the major growth factor of the female reproductive tract, there are substantial changes in the appearance of all the reproductive organs. Most postmenopausal women experience varying degrees of atrophic changes of the vaginal epithelium. The vaginal rugae progressively flatten and the epithelium thins. This may lead to symptomatic atrophic vaginitis (see Atrophic Vaginitis).

There are also atrophic changes of the cervix. It usually decreases in size, and the canal may become stenotic. There is a reduction of secretion of cervical mucous. This may contribute to excessive vaginal dryness, which may cause dyspareunia.

Atrophy of the uterus is also seen, with shrinkage of both the endometrium and myometrium. This shrinkage can be beneficial to women who enter the climacteric with uterine myomas. Reduction in size and elimination of symptoms frequently prevent the necessity for surgical treatment. The same applies to adenomyosis and endometriosis, both of which usually become asymptomatic after the menopause. Palpable and symptomatic areas of endometriosis generally become progressively smaller and less troublesome. With cessation of follicular activity, hormonal stimulation of the endometrium usually ceases. Endometrial biopsy may reveal anything from a very scanty, atrophic endometrium to one that is moderately proliferative. Spontaneous postmenopausal bleeding may occur in the presence of any of these patterns. Endometrial tissue revealing glandular hyperplasia (with or without uterine bleeding) is an indication of enhanced estrogenic stimulation from either endogenous estrogen production (eg, increased conversion of androgen) or from exogenous intake of estrogen.

The oviducts and ovaries also decrease in size postmenopausally. Although this produces no symptoms, the small size of the ovaries makes them difficult to palpate during pelvic examination. A palpable ovary in a postmenopausal woman must be viewed with suspicion, and the presence of an ovarian neoplasm must be considered.

The supporting structures of the reproductive organs suffer loss of tone as estrogen levels decline. Postmenopausal estrogen deficiency may be associated with symptomatic progressive pelvic relaxation.

2. Urinary tract—Estrogen plays an important role in maintaining the epithelium of the bladder and urethra. Marked estrogen deficiency may produce atrophic changes in these organs similar to those that occur in the vaginal epithelium. This may give rise to atrophic cystitis, characterized by urinary urgency, frequency, incontinence, and dysuria. Recurrent urinary tract infection may also develop in the setting of estrogen deficiency. Loss of urethral tone, with pouting of the meatus and thinning of the epithelium, favors the formation of a urethral caruncle with resultant dysuria, meatal tenderness, and occasionally hematuria. Treatment of symptomatic women involves topical vaginal estrogen (see Estrogen Therapy).

3. Mammary glands—Regression of breast size during and after menopause is psychologically distressing to some women. For those who have been bothered by cyclic symptoms of breast pain and cyst formation, the disappearance of these symptoms postmenopausally is a great relief.

Erickson GF. Normal ovarian function. *Clin Obstet Gynecol* 1978;21:31–52. PMID: 343955.

Judd HL. Hormonal dynamics associated with the menopause. *Clin Obstet Gynecol* 1976;19:775–788. PMID: 791558.

Judd HL, Judd GE, Lucas WE, Yen SS. Endocrine function of the postmenopausal ovary: concentrations of androgens and estrogens in ovarian and peripheral vein blood. *J Clin Endocrinol Metab* 1974;39:1020–1024. PMID: 4430702.

Judd HL, Shamonki IM, Frumar AM, Lagasse LD. Origin of serum estradiol in postmenopausal women. *Obstet Gynecol* 1982;59:680–686. PMID: 7078905.

Judd HL, Davidson BJ, Frumar AM, Shamonki IM, Lagasse LD, Ballon SC. Serum androgens and estrogens in postmenopausal women with and without endometrial cancer. *Am J Obstet Gynecol* 1980;136:859–871. PMID: 7361834.

Prevention of Menopause

Nothing can prevent the physiologic menopause (ie, ovarian function cannot be prolonged indefinitely), and nothing can be done to postpone its onset or slow its progress. However, artificial menopause can often be prevented. When ionizing radiation is used for the treatment of intra-abdominal disease, incidental ablation of ovarian function often cannot be avoided. In such cases, if an operation will serve equally well to treat intra-abdominal disease, it should be used in preference to radiation therapy in order to preserve the ovaries.

Elective removal of the ovaries to prevent ovarian cancer is frequently performed at laparotomy or laparoscopy in premenopausal women, with deliberate acceptance of artificial menopause. This form of therapy is increasingly used in women with genetic predisposition to breast and ovarian cancer. However, in low-risk women this remains controversial.

Clinical Conditions Associated with Menopause

A. Atrophic Vaginitis

1. Pathogenesis—As the epithelium thins after menopause, the capillary bed shines through as a diffuse or patchy reddening. Rupture of surface capillaries produces irregularly scattered petechiae, and a brownish discharge may be noted. Further atrophy of the vaginal epithelium renders its capillary bed increasingly sparse, so that the hyperemic appearance gives way to a smooth, shiny, pale epithelial surface. The epithelium lacks glycogen, which leads to a reduction in lactic acid production and an increase in the vaginal pH to 5.0–7.0. This is associated with disappearance of lactobacilli. Early in the process, local bacterial invasion may initiate vaginal pruritus and leukorrhea. Vaginal burning, soreness, dyspareunia, and a thin watery or serosanguineous discharge may also occur. Minimal trauma with examinations or coitus may result in slight vaginal bleeding. Urinary complaints, including urinary frequency, urgency, dysuria, and urge incontinence, have also been described in association with atrophic vaginitis.

2. Diagnosis—There is no specific test that reliably quantifies the degree of atrophy. Clinical decision making is therefore generally based on patient symptomatology and findings on physical examination. However, vaginal cytology has been used to assist in the diagnosis of atrophic vaginitis. The degree of maturation of exfoliated vaginal epithelial cells, as revealed by stained vaginal smears, is an index of estrogenic activity. Among the various methods of assessing the smears, the following are most commonly used: the **maturation index** consists of a differential count of 3 types of squamous cells—parabasal cells, intermediate cells, and superficial cells, in that order—expressed as percentages (eg, 10/85/5); a greater percentage of parabasal cells reflects a greater degree of atrophy. The **cornification count** is the percentage of precornified and cornified cells among total squamous cells counted. This is actually a simplified maturation index, because this percentage is essentially the same as that of the superficial cells.

The assessment of exfoliated vaginal epithelial cells is influenced not only by the level of estrogenic activity, but also by other hormones (particularly progesterone and testosterone), local vaginal inflammation, local medication, vaginal bleeding, the presence of genital cancer, the location of the vaginal area sampled, and variations in end-organ (epithelial) responses to estrogenic influence. Thus women with identical levels of circulating estrogens may have quite different cytograms.

The great variation in cytologic findings leads to the following conclusions regarding the use of smears in the clinical management of postmenopausal women: (1) the smear is only a rough measure of estrogenic status, and it may sometimes be grossly misleading. (2) The vaginal cytogram cannot predict whether or not an individual woman is experiencing menopausal signs and symptoms. (3) The smear cannot be used as the sole guide to steroid supplementation therapy; clinical signs and symptoms are more dependable for this purpose.

3. Treatment—Symptomatic atrophic vaginitis may be managed with water-soluble lubricants and/or topical vaginal estrogens, which are available in the form of creams, tablets, or estradiol-releasing rings (see Estrogen Therapy). Systemic estrogens are also effective in the treatment of atrophic vaginitis, but vaginal preparations are preferred when estrogen therapy is being used solely for the treatment of vulvovaginal atrophy.

B. Hot Flushes

1. General considerations—The most common and characteristic symptom of the climacteric is an episodic disturbance consisting of sudden flushing and perspiration, referred to as a **hot flash** or **flush.** It is observed in approximately 75% of women who go through the physiologic menopause or have a bilateral ovariectomy. Of those having flushes, 82% experience the disturbance for more than 1 year, and 25–50% complain of the symptom for more than 5 years. Most women indicate that hot flushes begin with a sensation of pressure in the head, much like a headache. This increases in intensity until the physiologic flush occurs. Palpitations may also be experienced. The actual flush is characterized as a feeling of heat or burning in the face, neck, and chest, followed immediately by an outbreak of sweating that affects the entire body but is particularly prominent over the head, neck, upper chest, and back. Less common symptoms include weakness, fatigue, faintness, and vertigo. The duration of the whole episode varies from momentary to as long as 10 minutes; the average length is 4 minutes. The frequency varies from 1–2 per hour to 1–2 per week. In women with severe flushes, the mean frequency is 54 minutes.

Investigators have characterized the physiologic changes associated with hot flushes and have shown that the symptoms result from true alterations in cutaneous vasodilation, perspiration, reductions of core temperature, and elevations of pulse rate. Fluctuations in electrocardiographic data probably reflect changes in skin conductance. Changes in heart rhythm and blood pressure have not been observed.

The patient's awareness of symptoms does not correspond exactly with physiologic changes. Women become conscious of symptoms approximately 1 minute after the onset of measurable cutaneous vasodilation, and discomfort persists for an average of 4 minutes, whereas physical changes persist for several minutes longer.

2. Pathogenesis—The exact mechanism responsible for hot flushes is unknown, but physiologic and behavioral data indicate that symptoms result from a defect in central thermoregulatory function. Several observations support this conclusion: (1) the 2 major physiologic changes associated with hot flushes—perspiration and cutaneous vasodilation—are the result of different peripheral sympathetic functions. Excitation of sweat glands results from sympathetic cholinergic fibers, and cutaneous vasodilation is under the control of tonic α-adrenergic fibers. It seems unlikely that any peripheral event could cause both cholinergic excitation of sweat glands and α-adrenergic blockade of cutaneous vessels, and it is well recognized that these are the 2 basic functions triggered by central thermoregulatory mechanisms that lower the central temperature. (2) During a hot flush, the central temperature decreases because of cutaneous vasodilation and perspiration. If hot flushes were the result of some peripheral event, the body's regulatory mechanisms would be expected to prevent such a decrease. (3) There is also a change in behavior associated with hot flushes. Women feel warm and have a conscious desire to cool themselves by throwing off the bedcovers, standing by open windows or doors, fanning themselves, or by other means. This behavior is observed even in the presence of a steady or decreasing central temperature.

Most investigators believe the core temperature of the body is maintained near a central set point that is controlled by central thermoregulatory centers, particularly those in the rostral hypothalamus. This central set point temperature is analogous to a thermostat setting. Hot flushes appear to result from a narrowing of the thermoregulatory set point such that smaller than normal increases in core body temperature activate heat loss responses. As a consequence, heat loss mechanisms, both physiologic and behavioral, are activated so that the core temperature will be brought in line with the new set point; this results in a fall of central temperature.

Because hot flushes occur after the spontaneous cessation of ovarian function or following oophorectomy, it is presumed that the underlying mechanism is initiated through endocrinologic changes related primarily to ovarian estrogen withdrawal. Low estrogen levels alone do not appear to trigger hot flushes; prepubertal children and patients with gonadal dysgenesis have low estrogen levels but not flushing. Patients with gonadal dysgenesis do experience symptoms if they are given estrogens that are later withdrawn. Thus it appears that estrogen must be present and then withdrawn for hot flushes to be experienced.

Changes in central nervous system (CNS) concentrations of norepinephrine (NE) and serotonin likely play an important role in the development of hot flushes. Animal and human studies indicate that NE plays an important role in the etiology of hot flushes. Increased levels of NE have been correlated with a narrowing of the thermoneutral zone, and it has been demonstrated that plasma levels of metabolites of NE increase after a hot flush. In addition, use of pharmacologic agents that alter central noradrenergic activity (ie, clonidine, serotonin and norepinephrine reuptake inhibitors [SNRIs]) have been shown to lessen the severity and/or frequency of vasomotor symptoms.

Studies also suggest a role for serotonin in the development of vasomotor symptoms. Serotonin is thought to be important in thermoregulation, as studies have shown an increase in stimulation of serotonin receptors after a thermostimulus, which then results in sensation of a hot flush. In addition, an association between serotonin levels and severity of vasomotor symptoms in menopausal women has been demonstrated. Finally, the selective serotonin reuptake inhibitors (SSRI) class of drugs has been shown to be effective in the management of vasomotor symptoms in postmenopausal women.

A close temporal association between the occurrence of flushes and the pulsatile release of LH has been demonstrated. However, the observation that flushes occur after hypophysectomy suggests that they are not directly caused by LH release. The appearance of hot flushes in women with defects in GnRH release or synthesis (Kallmann's syndrome) also suggests GnRH itself is not involved in the flushing mechanism. The absence of hot flushes in women with hypothalamic amenorrhea and hypoestrogenemia is intriguing. These women have defects in neurotransmitter or neurochemical input to their GnRH neurons. In particular, excessive endogenous opioid and dopamine input to GnRH neurons may account for chronic suppression of GnRH release, leading to hypothalamic amenorrhea. The absence of hot flushes in these women suggests that altered afferent input of neurotransmitters or neurochemicals to the GnRH neuron that is secondary to hypogonadism leads to hot flushes.

Hot flushes are a greater annoyance than most physicians recognize. Patients frequently complain of night sweats and insomnia. There is a close temporal relationship between the occurrence of hot flushes and nighttime awakening. Women with frequent flushes may experience flushes and awakening episodes hourly, which may cause a profound sleep disturbance that may, in turn, cause cognitive (memory) and affective (anxiety) disorders in some women.

3. Treatment—Estrogens are the principal medications used to relieve hot flushes. Estrogens block both the perceived symptoms and the physiologic changes. Their use also relieves some aspects of the sleeping disorder. Estrogen administration has been shown to enhance hypothalamic opioid activity in postmenopausal women. This increase of hypothalamic opiates may be involved in the relief of hot flushes with estrogen administration.

Progestins also block hot flushes and represent a reasonable form of substitutional therapy in women who cannot take estrogens. However, because addition of progestins to hormone therapy has been associated with an increased risk of breast cancer, a progestogen would not be the ideal alternative to estrogen for women who are seeking to avoid effects on breast disease. **Clonidine,** a centrally acting alpha agonist, is more effective than a placebo but is associated with side effects. More recently, certain **SSRIs and SNRIs** have been shown to be effective in the treatment of hot flashes. Their side effects may limit their overall benefit, but they are one of the first alternative choices in women who are not taking estrogen. Certain SSRIs may also affect the metabolism of tamoxifen to its active metabolite through the enzyme, CYP2D6, a member of the cytochrome P450 oxidase enzyme system. SSRIs such as paroxetine and fluoxetine have been associated with increased breast cancer recurrence and/or death amongst women using tamoxifen. Therefore, until further studies are available, caution must be used when using SSRIs, particularly paroxetine and fluoxetine, in women receiving tamoxifen. **Black cohosh** may have modest effects in decreasing hot flashes, but concerns remain regarding its potential to stimulate breast and uterine tissue. **Gabapentin** also decreases hot flashes by 50–80% and is therefore comparable to estrogen according to certain studies. However, sedation is a major side effect that limits its acceptability for many women. Small doses at night may be useful for women suffering from night-time awakening due to vasomotor symptoms. **Tibolone** is a synthetic steroid with estrogenic, progestogenic, and androgenic properties that alleviates menopausal symptoms and has been used in other countries for this purpose, as well as to preserve bone mineral density. However, its long-term safety profile with regard to breast and endometrial cancer remains controversial. Its mechanism of action would suggest that it is unlikely to increase the risk of breast cancer. However, the Million Women Study reported an increased risk of breast cancer among participants using tibolone as compared with controls. In addition, tibolone was associated with an increased risk of breast cancer recurrence in a randomized trial of breast cancer patient using tibolone for relief of vasomotor symptoms. Tibolone's action on the endometrium also suggests that it is unlikely to cause endometrial proliferation. This is supported by findings from studies demonstrating a low incidence of vaginal bleeding and an absence of endometrial hyperplasia on histology. However, rates of endometrial cancer were also increased in the Million Women Study. Further study is required to ascertain whether tibolone can be used long term without increased risks for breast and endometrial cancer. Tibolone's potential to modify risk for cardiovascular disease is also unknown. However, a study evaluating the effect of tibolone on myocardial blood flow demonstrated that tibolone improved myocardial blood flow in women with ischemic heart disease. Vitamins E and K, mineral supplements, and phytoestrogens have all been tried to alleviate menopausal symptoms, but have not been proven beneficial. Many women express a preference for **bioidentical hormones (BHT)**, with the expectation that they are safer, with comparable efficacy. The term may be used to describe varying formulations and therefore is not used consistently amongst patients or practitioners. For some, the term refers to hormones that are chemically identical to those produced by humans and includes formulations that are well-tested, US Food and Drug Administration (FDA)–approved brand names. For the majority of others, the term refers to custom-made hormone formulations that provide different doses and routes of administration of estrogens and progestogens. These compounded formulations are not subject to the same regulatory approval process as brand name formulations, and therefore safety, efficacy, and consistency are in no way assured. Cost to the patient can also be greater for these compounded formulations because they are often not covered by third-party payers. The FDA has declared that claims of compounding pharmacies stating that BHT drugs avoid the risks of FDA-approved treatments and these drugs reduce the risk of serious illness such as heart disease, stroke, or breast cancer are not supported by credible scientific evidence. They further state that safety and efficacy of estriol in these formulations has not been proven. Therefore, incorporation of estriol into these formulations may not occur without an investigational new drug authorization. According to the 2010 North American Menopause Society position statement: "Filled prescriptions for BHT should include a patient package insert identical to that required for products that have regulatory-agency approval. In the absence of efficacy and safety data for any specific prescription, the generalized benefit-risk ratio data of commercially available HT products should apply equally to BHT."

C. Osteoporosis

1. General considerations—Osteoporosis is defined as a systemic skeletal disorder characterized by low bone mass and microarchitectural deterioration of bone tissue, with a consequent increase in fragility of bone and susceptibility to risk of fracture. Although gradual bone loss occurs in all humans with aging, this loss is accelerated in women after cessation of ovarian function. After attainment of peak bone mass by age 25–30 years, bone loss begins, accelerates in women at menopause, and then slows again but continues into advanced years at a rate of 1–2% per year (Fig. 59–3). Women can lose up to 20% of their bone mass in the 5–7 years after menopause.

Osteoporosis affects an estimated 10 million Americans 50 years of age or older, 80% of whom are women. Of Americans 50 years of age or older, 34 million are estimated to have low bone mass at the hip, placing them at increased risk for osteoporosis. Osteoporosis is most severe in women who have had early oophorectomy or premature ovarian failure, and in those with gonadal dysgenesis. Osteoporosis occurs most often in whites, followed by Asians, Hispanics, and African Americans.

Bone loss produces minimal symptoms, but leads to reduced skeletal strength. Thus osteoporotic bones are more susceptible to fractures. The most common sites of fracture are in the vertebral body, proximal femur, and distal forearm/wrist. Recent figures from the National Osteoporosis Foundation show that osteoporosis is responsible for more than 1.5 million fractures per year. Due to the

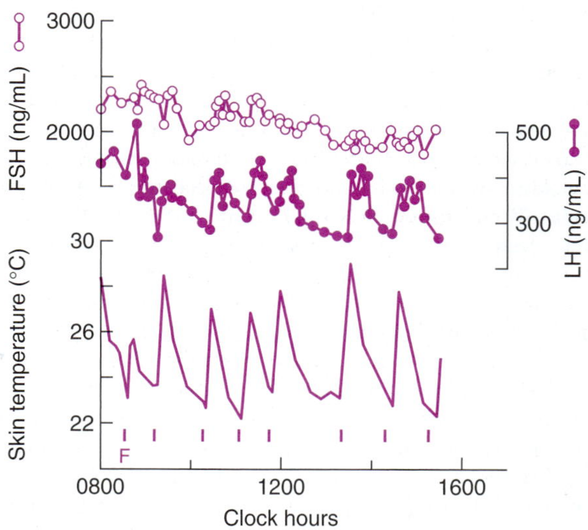

▲ **Figure 59–3.** Changes in metacarpal cortical width, as determined by sequential measurements in pre- and postmenopausal women, age range 30–50 years. Note bone loss in postmenopausal women. (Reproduced, with permission, from Nordin BEC, et al. Postmenopausal osteopenia and osteoporosis. *Front Horm Res* 1975; 3:131.)

aging population, the prevalence of osteoporosis is expected to increase such that by 2020, 1 in 2 Americans is expected to have or be at risk for osteoporosis of the hip. Approximately 1 in 2 women older than the age of 50 years will have an osteoporosis-related fracture in her remaining lifetime. The incidence of hip fractures in women is 2–3 times that in men. The mortality rate associated with hip fractures is between 10 and 20% within 12 months after the injury. Of survivors, 15–25% are permanently disabled. The estimated cost for osteoporosis-related fractures in the United States totals more than $17 billion per year. According to the Surgeon General, these costs could double or triple by the year 2040.

Risk factors include certain lifestyle choices (ie, increased caffeine intake, smoking, excessive alcohol intake, lack of exercise, lifetime of low calcium intake), hormonal factors (ie, estrogen deficiency from menopause, eating disorders), genetic factors (ie, family history, cystic fibrosis, Ehlers Danlos), endocrinologic disorders (hyperparathyroidism, adrenal insufficiency, hyperthyroidism), medical disorders (ie, lupus, malabsorption syndromes, lymphoma), medication use (ie, corticosteroids, chemotherapy, excess thyroid supplementation), vitamin D deficiency, slender body size, and advanced age.

2. Pathogenesis—Bone loss occurs because bone resorption is excessive, bone formation is decreased, peak bone mass is low, or a combination of all 3 factors. Bone remodeling is regulated by many factors, including systemic hormones, local cytokines, prostaglandins, and local growth factors. Of the systemic hormones, sex steroids, parathyroid hormones, glucocorticoids, thyroid hormones, and growth hormone/insulinlike growth factors likely play a role.

Ovarian estrogen and estrogen administered postmenopausally are protective against osteoporosis. The exact mechanisms by which estrogen regulates bone remodeling are incompletely understood. Estrogens likely modulate osteoclast and osteoblast function possibly via effects on cytokines and growth factors such as transforming growth factor-β and tumor necrosis factor-α (TNF-α). Estrogens may decrease the depth of erosion of osteoclasts.

Interleukin-1 (IL-1) and TNF-α derived from bone marrow macrophages stimulate bone resorption and may inhibit bone formation. There is evidence to suggest they may be regulated by estrogen, as IL-1 activity in bone increases immediately after the menopause or oophorectomy. Furthermore, it has been shown in animal models that inhibition of IL-1 and TNF-α after ovariectomy attenuates bone loss. IL-6 and prostaglandins, especially prostaglandin E_2, are also involved in bone remodeling and are regulated by sex steroids. Other factors, such as insulin-like growth factor and fibroblast growth factor, also likely play a role in the pathogenesis of osteoporosis and may be regulated by sex steroids.

Androgens play a role in bone remodeling as androgen deficiency is associated with increased bone loss. The precise mechanism by which androgens alter bone remodeling is unknown but may involve conversion to estrogen. For example, men with aromatase deficiency have an elevated risk of developing osteoporosis, possibly due to decreased conversion of androgen to estrogen.

Progestogens may affect bone remodeling in a similar way to estrogens and androgens, but the mechanisms underlying these effects are not well understood. It is possible that they work through glucocorticoid receptors.

Parathyroid hormone (PTH) also plays a role in bone remodeling. PTH stimulates bone resorption, and absence of this hormone inhibits development of osteoporosis in animal and human studies. Thus far, it does not appear that PTH is elevated in most women with osteoporosis or that the sensitivity of bone to PTH is enhanced. It is interesting that the amino-terminus of PTH (1-34) inhibits bone resorption.

Thyroid hormones increase bone resorption. The exact mechanism is not fully understood, but possibly involves accelerated osteoclast function and altered calcium metabolism.

Growth hormone stimulates bone remodeling; however, studies evaluating the effect of exogenous growth hormone administration on established osteoporosis are inconclusive. Recently, new factors were discovered that are involved with the regulation of bone remodeling: osteoprotegerin, a naturally occurring protein, and RANKL (receptor activator of nuclear factor kappa beta ligand) both regulate osteoclastogenesis and bone resorption.

Genetic factors may also affect risk for osteoporosis. Variants in the estrogen receptors α and β expressed in bone are associated with altered risk for osteoporosis and fracture. Variants in the vitamin D receptor gene and bone morphogenetic protein 2 may also play a role in the pathogenesis of osteoporosis.

3. Diagnosis & monitoring—Although much has been done to study urinary and serum factors as predictors of osteoporosis, the most predictive test remains bone densitometry with dual-energy x-ray absorptiometry (DXA). Results are given in grams or g/cm^2. In 1994, the World Health Organization created a clinically useful definition of osteoporosis. Bone mineral density (BMD) results are reported using T and Z scores. The T score is the number of standard deviations (SD) above or below the mean bone mineral density for sex-matched young normal controls. The Z score compares the patient with an age- and sex-matched population. Normal bone density is defined as a T score > −1.0 SD at the spine, hip or forearm. Osteopenic patients have T scores between −1.0 and −2.5, whereas osteoporotic patients have T scores below −2.5. In most studies, a decrease by 1 SD in mass increases the risk of fracture 2–3-fold. In postmenopausal women, the WHO T-score criteria should be applied. In premenopausal women, WHO BMD criteria should not be applied and other criteria should be used (ie, ethnic or race adjusted Z-scores, with −2.0 indicating low bone density for chronologic age).

Assessment of risk factors has not been nearly as predictive of fracture risk as density measurement. Similarly, assessment of biochemical markers of bone turnover have not been shown to be useful for diagnosing osteoporosis but may give some indication of future risk for fracture and/or be useful for monitoring response to antiresorptive therapy. Markers of bone formation include serum bone-specific alkaline phosphatase and osteocalcin. Markers of bone resorption include serum C-telopeptide (CTX) and urinary N-telopeptide (NTX).

National Osteoporosis Foundation has created a set of guidelines for the use and interpretation of measurement of bone mineral density. Measurements of bone mineral density are recommended for the following groups: (1) all postmenopausal patients younger than age 65 years who have ≥1 additional risk factors for osteoporosis (other than being white, postmenopausal, and female); (2) all women age 65 years and older regardless of additional risk factors; (3) postmenopausal women who present with fractures; (4) women considering therapy for osteoporosis if testing would facilitate the decision; (5) women who have been on hormone replacement therapy for prolonged periods; (6) women who have been on treatment to monitor the treatment effect; and (7) women considering discontinuation of treatment.

Another tool to assess risk and guide treatment is the Fracture Risk Algorithm (FRAX). This tool incorporates BMD, as well as other factors, to assess 10-year probability of hip fracture and 10-year probability of major osteoporotic fracture. It is most useful in patients with low hip BMD as opposed to low spine BMD. Special consideration needs to be taken into account for patients with normal hip BMD but low spine BMD, as FRAX incorporates hip BMD measurements. It is also intended for postmenopausal women, not for younger women. Therapy can be considered in patients with a 10-year probability of hip fracture of ≥3% and 10-year probability of major osteoporosis-related fracture of ≥20%. The FRAX calculator can be accessed at http://www.shef.ac.uk/FRAX/tool.jsp?locationValue=9.

4. Prevention and treatment—All individuals at risk for or who have been diagnosed with osteoporosis should be advised to consume adequate **calcium** (minimum of 1200 mg elemental calcium per day). The National Osteoporosis Foundation recommends **vitamin D** (800–1000 IU/d). Smoking cessation, avoidance of excessive alcohol intake, and participation in regular weight-bearing and muscle strengthening exercise should be encouraged. Pharmacologic therapy should be strongly considered in women with a hip or vertebral fracture, in women with BMD scores below −2.5 with no risk factors, and in women with BMD T-scores below −1.0 with a 10-year probability of hip fracture of ≥3% or a 10-year probability of major osteoporotic fracture of ≥20%. Current pharmacologic therapy for osteopenia/osteoporosis, listed in alphabetical order, includes (1) **bisphosphonates**, (2) **calcitonin**, (3) **estrogens** (with or without progestogens), (4) **parathyroid hormone**, (5) **raloxifene**, and (6) **denosumab**.

Bisphosphonates are excellent choices for prevention and treatment of osteoporosis. They are potent antiresorptive agents that bind to hydroxyapatite crystals on the surface of bones, enter osteoclasts, and decrease resorptive actions by reducing the production of hydrogen ions and lysosomal enzymes. In addition, they have indirect effects, causing osteoblasts to produce substances that inhibit osteoclasts. They increase bone mineral density at the spine, wrist, and hip in a dose-dependent manner and decrease the risk of vertebral fractures by 30–50%. In addition, they reduce the risk of subsequent nonvertebral fractures in women with osteoporosis. There are 4 bisphosphonates currently available for oral administration. **Alendronate** is approved by the FDA for the prevention of osteoporosis (5 mg daily and 35 mg weekly) and for the treatment of established osteoporosis (10 mg daily or 70 mg weekly). **Risedronate** is approved by the FDA for prevention and treatment of postmenopausal osteoporosis. The recommended daily dose is 5 mg daily or 35 mg weekly. **Ibandronate** is approved for both prevention and treatment of postmenopausal osteoporosis. It has the advantage of being available in an oral daily (2.5 mg) and oral monthly (150 mg) dosing regimen, as well as an intravenous regimen of 3 mg given every 3 months. The 2.5-mg daily and 150-mg monthly oral doses are approved for prevention and treatment of osteoporosis. The 3-mg intravenous dose is approved for treatment of osteoporosis. **Zoledronic acid** is approved for prevention and treatment of osteoporosis in postmenopausal women. It is given as 5-mg intravenous infusion over 15 minutes once yearly for treatment or once every 2 years for prevention. Intestinal absorption of bisphosphonates is poor, and therefore these medications should be taken in the morning with 8 ounces of water, before consumption of any food or beverage. Nothing else should be taken by mouth for at least 30–60 minutes after oral dosing. The patient should also remain upright for 30 minutes after administration. The most common side effects of bisphosphonates are gastrointestinal. Pain in the joints, bone, and muscle may also occur. Risks include gastric and esophageal ulceration and, rarely, osteonecrosis of the jaw. Most cases of osteonecrosis of the jaw have been described in cancer patients being treated with intravenous bisphosphonates, but some cases have occurred in patients being managed for postmenopausal osteoporosis. Some studies suggest an increased risk of esophageal cancer following bisphosphonate use, but others do not. Further study is needed to assess whether there is a direct link between use of bisphophonates and esophageal cancer. More recently, an increase in the risk of atypical fracture of the femur has been reported in women using bisphosphonates for >5 years. The risk is probably small, but should be discussed with patients who are considering use of this class of drug, or who have been using these drugs for prolonged periods of time. The FDA has required a labeling change of bisphosphonates to reflect this risk and will continue to monitor these outcomes closely. Clinicians and patients should be aware that diagnosis of these atypical fractures has been preceded by new onset thigh or groin pain.

Calcitonin is a peptide hormone that inhibits osteoclast activity and therefore inhibits bone resorption. It demonstrates positive effects on bone mineral density at the lumbar spine, although less effectively than estrogen or bisphosphonates. Salmon calcitonin is the most potent form and is available for intranasal administration or as a subcutaneous injection. Calcitonin 100 IU is given subcutaneously daily or every other day; the intranasal calcitonin dose is 200 IU daily. The most frequent side effect with the intranasal route is rhinitis. Other antiresorptive therapies, such as bisphosphonates, are preferred over calcitonin, as they produce greater increases in bone mineral density. However, because of calcitonin's analgesic properties, calcitonin is the preferred therapy in patients with pain from vertebral fracture.

Until recently, **estrogen** was the mainstay of therapy for prevention and treatment of postmenopausal osteoporosis. However, with the findings from the Women's Health Initiative (WHI) trial demonstrating overall greater health risks than benefits from hormone therapy, it is no longer first-line therapy for prevention of osteoporosis. Osteoporosis prevention does remain an FDA-approved indication for estrogen therapy, however. It is best used in women who would otherwise use estrogen/hormone therapy for management of menopausal symptoms, or in women who cannot tolerate alternate antiresorptive therapies.

In observational studies, estrogen decreases the risk of hip fractures by 25–50%, of vertebral fractures by approximately 50%, and reduces the risk of other fractures. Daily dosages of 0.3–0.625 mg of conjugated estrogens, 0.5–1 mg of micronized estradiol, 1.25 mg of piperazine estrone sulfate, 0.025–0.05 mg of transdermal estradiol, and a new low dose (0.014 mg) of transdermal estradiol all are appropriate for the prevention of osteoporosis. The lower doses (ie, 0.3 mg of conjugated equine estrogens) are not as effective as higher doses but do prevent bone loss. For best results, therapy should begin soon after the menopause.

Parathyroid hormone, teriparatide (PTH [1-34]) has been approved by the FDA for use in women and men who are at high risk for fracture, including those with previous fracture, multiple risk factors for fracture, and previous failed treatment. Despite its potential deleterious effect on bone, intermittent administration of recombinant PTH stimulates bone formation, and clinical trials support its use in the treatment of osteoporosis. It should only be used in high-risk patients because of its high cost, the need for daily injection, and a possible risk for osteosarcoma.

Selective estrogen receptor modulators (SERMs) are nonhormonal agents that bind to estrogen receptors and may exhibit either estrogen agonist or antagonist activity. Currently, there are 3 SERMs approved for use in humans (tamoxifen, toremifene, and raloxifene); however, raloxifene is the only SERM approved for the prevention and treatment of osteoporosis. It exhibits estrogen agonist properties in the bone (inhibits osteoclast function) and the liver (decreases low-density lipoprotein cholesterol) and acts as an antagonist in the breast and uterus. Raloxifene 60 mg daily for 24 months is associated with a 1–2% increase in lumbar spine and hip bone density.

Combination Therapy has been evaluated in the prevention and/or treatment of osteoporosis. This typically takes the form of a bisphosphonate (ie, alendronate) and systemic estrogen. Small increases in BMD have been seen with combination therapy, but the effect on fracture risk is unknown.

Other therapies have been proposed for osteoporosis treatment and prevention, some without proven benefit. **Progestins** decrease biochemical markers of bone resorption and preserve bone density. When used as monotherapy for osteoporosis, they may be more effective at preserving bone in the wrist than in the spine.

Fluoride has been used in Europe and the United States and is associated with a marked increase in trabecular bone, but did not improve fracture rates, and in some studies fracture rates were increased. This may be a result of a lack of increase in cortical bone. Sodium fluoride is generally not recommended for the treatment of osteoporosis.

Phytoestrogens are plant-derived compounds that have weak estrogen-like effects. Although some animal studies are promising, no effects on the incidence of fractures in humans have been shown.

Tibolone (see Hot Flushes) also increases lumbar spine and femoral neck bone density. Its effects on bone are comparable to those of estrogens. As discussed previously, however, issues regarding long-term safety are currently being evaluated.

D. Sexual Dysfunction

The determinants of sexual behavior are complex and interrelated. Sexual function is believed to be regulated by 3 general components: the individual's motivation (also called desire or libido), endocrine competence, and sociocultural beliefs. Decreased libido is reported with increasing age. However, the relative contributions of the primary decrease in desire, anatomic limitations to sexual function, or beliefs that sexual behavior is inappropriate in older women to this decreased libido are unknown.

The hypoestrogenemic state leads to atrophy of the internal genitalia. Although dyspareunia is the most obvious symptom of vaginal atrophy, suboptimal sexual functioning can occur without frank dyspareunia. Diminished genital sensation (and therefore decreased sensory output in the arousal phase), lessened glandular secretions, less vasocongestion, and decreased vaginal expansion may not be perceived as discrete symptoms by the postmenopausal female, but may influence her perception that she is less responsive.

Genital atrophy, one cause of postmenopausal sexual dysfunction, responds to estrogen therapy. The specific impact of estrogen on libido has been difficult to determine. Improved anatomy may also have a positive psychologic impact and may indirectly encourage sexual motivation.

The role of androgen therapy in female sexual dysfunction is an active area of investigation. Despite the fact that the postmenopausal ovary continues to be a major source of androgens for several years after menopause, androgen levels overall are decreased, and this may contribute to the decrease in libido seen during menopause. Furthermore, the addition of testosterone to hormone therapy has been shown to improve sexual function in women in randomized, placebo controlled trials. However, improvements in sexual function have been modest at best. In addition, long-term safety has not been established. Some studies have suggested an increased risk of breast cancer amongst women using androgens. Therefore, its use remains controversial.

Campisi R, Camilletti J, Mele A, Erriest J, Pedroni P, Guiglioni A. Tibolone improves myocardial perfusion in post-menopausal women with ischemic heart disease: an open-label exploratory pilot study. *J Am Coll Cardiol* 2006;47:559–564. PMID: 16458136.

Dimitrakakis C, Keramopoulos D, Vourli G, Gaki V, Bredakis N, Keramopoulos A. Clinical effects of tibolone in postmenopausal women after five years of tamoxifen therapy for breast cancer. *Climacteric* 2005;8:342–351. PMID: 16390769.

Gambone J, Meldrum DR, Laufer L, Chang RJ, Lu JK, Judd HL. Further delineation of hypothalamic dysfunction responsible for menopausal hot flashes. *J Clin Endocrinol Metab* 1985;59:1097–1102. PMID: 6436285.

Kenemans P, Bundred NJ, Foidart JM, et al. Safety and efficacy of tibolone in breast cancer patients with vasomotor symptoms: A double blind, randomized, non-inferiority trial. *Lancet Oncol* 2009; 10:135–146. PMID: 19167925.

Krapf JM, Simon JA. The role of testosterone in the management of hypoactive sexual desire disorder in postmenopausal women. *Maturitas* 2009; 63:213–219. PMID: 19487090.

National Osteoporosis Foundation. *Physician's Guide To Prevention and Treatment of Osteoporosis.* Washington, DC: National Osteoporosis Foundation; 2010.

Ness RB, Albano JD, McTiernan A, Cauley JA. Influence of estrogen plus testosterone supplementation on breast cancer. *Arch Intern Med* 2009;169:41–46. PMID: 19139322.

North American Menopause Society. Estrogen and progestogen use in postmenopausal women: 2010 position statement of the North American Menopause Society. *Menopause* 2010;17: 242–255. PMID: 20154637.

Panay N, Al-Azzawi F, Bouchard C, et al. Testosterone treatment of HSDD in naturally menopausal women with the ADORE study. *Climacteric* 2010; 13:121–131. PMID: 20166859.

Rapkin AJ. Vasomotor symptoms in menopause: physiologic condition and central nervous system approaches to treatment. *Am J Obst Gynecol* 2007; 196:97–106. PMID: 17306645.

Schwenkhagen A, Studd J. Role of testosterone in the treatment of hypoactive sexual desire disorder. *Maturitas* 2009; 63:152–159. PMID: 19359109.

US Food and Drug Administration. Pharmacy Compounding/ Compounding of Bio-Identical Hormone Replacement Therapies, 2009. www.fda.gov/News/Events/Testimony/ucm154031.htm

World Health Organization. Assessment of fracture risk and its application to screening for postmenopausal osteoporosis. Report of a WHO Study Group. *World Health Organ Tech Rep Ser* 1994;843:1. PMID: 7941614.

Differential Diagnosis of Common Signs and Symptoms During Menopause

Signs and symptoms similar to those of the climacteric can be caused by a variety of other diseases. In general, seeing the entire clinical picture is helpful in establishing the proper diagnosis. The absence of evidence of other disease points to cessation of ovarian function, whereas the presence of prominent features of other conditions, in the absence of other climacteric symptoms, suggests a nonclimacteric origin.

A. Amenorrhea

By definition, the primary symptom of the menopause is the absence of menstruation for 12 months. Amenorrhea can occur for many reasons, of which physiologic menopause is only one. Cessation of ovarian function is by far the most common reason for amenorrhea to occur in women in their forties or early fifties. Persistent amenorrhea in younger women may be a result of premature cessation of ovarian function, but must be differentiated from other causes. Obvious features of specific disease often suggest the proper diagnosis (ie, extreme weight loss in anorexia nervosa, galactorrhea in hyperprolactinemia, hirsutism and obesity in polycystic ovarian disease).

B. Hot Flashes

Several diseases can produce sensations of flushing that may be misinterpreted as menopausal vasomotor symptoms. Notable are hyperthyroidism, pheochromocytoma, carcinoid syndrome, diabetes mellitus, tuberculosis, and other chronic infections. None of these disorders produces the specific symptoms associated with the climacteric (ie, short duration and specific body distribution). Moreover, the absence of other signs or symptoms of the climacteric suggest some other cause of the flushes should be sought.

C. Abnormal Vaginal Bleeding

Before the menopause, irregular vaginal bleeding is expected and does not necessitate a diagnostic workup in many cases. However, organic disease can occur at this time, and some patients require evaluation. If a woman is in her forties or fifties and experiences an increase in cycle length and a decrease in the quantity of bleeding, menopausal involution can be presumed, and endometrial sampling is usually not necessary. However, if menses become more frequent and heavier, spotting between menses occurs, or any pattern of irregular bleeding persists, assessment of the endometrium should be performed. The usual procedure is an endometrial biopsy or dilatation and curettage (D&C) to rule out endometrial hyperplasia or cancer. The disadvantage of the former is that entry into the endometrial cavity may not be accomplished in the setting of a stenotic os, and the drawbacks of the latter are greater expense, risk and need for anesthesia.

It is most unusual for a woman to experience vaginal bleeding because of ovarian activity by 6 months after the menopause. Thus postmenopausal bleeding is much more ominous and necessitates evaluation each time it occurs. The only exception to this rule is the uterine bleeding associated with estrogen replacement therapy. Other guidelines are recommended for this type of bleeding (see Estrogen Therapy).

Organic disease is commonly associated with postmenopausal bleeding. Endometrial polyps may be found, which can be resected via the hysteroscope. Endometrial hyperplasia may be discovered, frequently in obese women. This can be treated by the periodic administration of progestin or by hysterectomy. If hyperplasia develops in a woman taking estrogens, the addition of progestins should be considered. If hyperplasia develops unrelated to hormone replacement, surgery should be considered if the patient is a good surgical risk or is not reliable in taking progestins. The finding of endometrial cancer necessitates appropriate therapy depending on the stage and grade of the tumor.

D. Vulvovaginitis

Many specific vulvar and vaginal diseases (ie, trichomoniasis and candidiasis) may mimic the atrophic vulvovaginitis of estrogen deficiency. Their special clinical characteristics usually suggest more specific diagnostic testing. When pruritus and thinning of the vaginal epithelium or the vulvar skin are the only manifestations, therapeutic testing with local applications of estrogen may help to establish the diagnosis of vulvovaginitis. When any whitening, thickening, or cracking of vulvar tissues is present, biopsy to rule out carcinoma is mandatory. Raised or erosive lesions should also be sampled. Biopsy to rule out carcinoma is also necessary for suspicious looking vaginal or cervical lesions.

E. Back Pain

Occasionally, the pain of vertebral compression from osteoporosis may mimic that of gastric ulcer, renal colic, pyelonephritis, pancreatitis, spondylolisthesis, acute back strain, or herniated intervertebral disk.

Common Clinical Conditions of the Aged, Postmenopausal Woman: Controversial Role of Estrogens

A. Coronary Heart Disease (CHD)

Heart disease affects approximately 8 million women in the United States. Deaths caused by CHD in women number more than 230,000 per year. The incidence of death from CHD increases with age in all populations and both sexes. Substantially more heart disease is seen in younger men, with the onset of cardiovascular problems occurring an average of 10 years later in women. Before the age of menopause, very few women die of a heart attack. After the menopause, a woman's risk increases progressively such that CHD rates in women after menopause are 2–3 times those of women of the same age before menopause. Statistics such as these, indicating a role for both sex and menopause on the development of CHD, have led to the suggestion that estrogen deficiency that occurs after menopause is at least partially responsible for the increased risk of CHD in postmenopausal women.

The first attempts at ascertaining whether cessation of ovarian function is associated with an increased incidence of heart disease came from large epidemiologic studies. The Framingham study, in which nearly 3000 women were examined biennially, revealed that after the menopause, there is indeed an increased incidence of heart disease that is not just age-related. In the Nurses' Health Study cohort of 121,700 women, after controlling for age and cigarette smoking, women who had a natural menopause had no appreciable increase in risk compared with that of premenopausal women. However, women who underwent a bilateral oophorectomy and no estrogen replacement had an increased risk (relative risk = 2.2) compared with that seen in premenopausal women.

Case-control studies were also performed comparing the degree of CHD or the incidence of myocardial infarction in women who had undergone early oophorectomy with age-matched premenopausal controls. Most of these studies revealed an increased risk of cardiovascular disease after ovarian excision. All these reports have been criticized because of patient selection bias, particularly of the controls.

Numerous case-control and large-cohort studies have also since been carried out to assess the role of exogenous estrogens administered during menopause on morbidity and mortality from CHD. Most have shown a beneficial impact of exogenous estrogens on morbidity and mortality from CHD. Although the magnitude of change and the consistency of results appear compelling, it must be recognized that all these studies are observational and that the choice of controls has been questioned. In particular, women who take estrogens are more health conscious and must see a doctor regularly to receive their medication, whereas women who do not take estrogens may or may not receive regular medical checkups. Thus some or all of the apparent benefits of estrogens on heart disease may have been a consequence of these other considerations.

Based on these observational/case-controlled studies suggesting a beneficial effect of estrogens, numerous experimental studies were performed attempting to elucidate the mechanism(s) by which estrogens could prevent CHD. Evidence for both an indirect effect on circulating lipids and a direct action on the vascular system was found. Orally administered estrogens influence hepatic lipid metabolism and raise high-density lipoprotein (HDL) cholesterol and triglycerides and lower low-density lipoprotein (LDL) cholesterol. The impact of nonorally administered estrogens is of lesser magnitude and takes longer to become apparent.

Numerous studies have shown that estrogen and progesterone receptors are present in the heart and aorta. Thus the subcellular components necessary for direct hormonal action exist in these tissues. Endothelial cells of the arteries produce factors in response to estrogen. One of the most potent of these is believed to be nitric oxide (NO). NO exerts several effects on the arterial wall. It increases intracellular cyclic guanosine monophosphate in the arterial smooth muscle, which results in vasodilation. It also inhibits platelet adhesion and aggregation, as well as monocyte adherence to the arterial endothelium. Estrogen appears to increase NO production, and this may be important in preventing coronary vasospasm and thrombus formation. Estrogen has been shown in animals to prevent atherosclerosis. It has also been shown in a rabbit model to prevent 2 of the earliest steps in the atherogenic process—adhesion and migration of monocytes. This likely occurs through an NO-mediated mechanism. Estrogens also likely have adverse effects on the vessel wall. Estrogens lead to a hypercoagulable state which may increase the risk of coronary events. Although these mechanisms are only partially understood, they emphasize the importance of studying the direct effects of estrogen on the vascular system.

Interestingly, use of estrogen had been widespread for many years, yet it was not until recently that large-scale, prospective, randomized, placebo-controlled studies evaluating the effect of hormone therapy on relevant clinical end points in humans were performed. One of the first of these studies was the Heart and Estrogen/Progestin Replacement Study (HERS), which studied the use of estrogen and progestin in the secondary prevention of coronary events in women with known CHD. HERS showed that treatment with oral conjugated equine estrogen (CEE) plus medroxyprogesterone acetate (MPA) did not reduce the overall rate of CHD events in postmenopausal women with established heart disease. Furthermore, there was an early increased risk of CHD events within the first year of starting HT. In addition, the ERA (Estrogen Replacement and Atherosclerosis) Trial, which was the first randomized angiographic end point trial to test the effect of HT on the progression of atherosclerosis in postmenopausal women with documented coronary stenosis, showed no benefit of CEE either alone, or in combination with MPA, on angiographic progression of disease. Consequently, it is suggested that physicians not prescribe estrogen therapy (ET)/HT for the sole purpose of *secondary* prevention of coronary events.

The *primary* prevention of CHD by HT also had not been evaluated in a prospective, randomized fashion until recently. The WHI, a large, multicenter, prospective, randomized, placebo-controlled trial of primarily healthy postmenopausal women, was initiated to assess the effects of a specific regimen of CEE alone or in combination with MPA on several health-related outcomes, including CHD. The combined estrogen/progestin portion of the study was stopped after 5.2 years as overall health risks exceeded benefits. The increased risks included a greater number of cardiovascular events. The estrogen-only arm of the study was continued for approximately 7 years. This arm of the study was stopped early because of an increased risk of stroke. Overall, there was no reduction in the risk of coronary events. Interestingly, there appeared to be a trend toward a decreased risk of coronary events in the younger subset of postmenopausal women. This finding was confirmed in a subanalysis of the data for the 50–59-year-old age group where the investigators reported a lower relative risk for the combined end points of myocardial infarction, coronary death, coronary revascularization, and confirmed angina among women ages 50–59 years using estrogen alone. In addition, in the subset of women who were 50–59 years of age who were placed on the estrogen-alone arm, lower levels of coronary artery calcium were observed, suggesting that in this group of recently postmenopausal women that estrogen alone slows the development of calcified coronary atherosclerotic plaque.

There were several limitations of the WHI study. It did not assess different dosages, types of estrogens and progestogens, nor different routes of administration (ie, transdermal vs. oral). Finally, many of the subjects had become menopausal several years before entry into the study. Consequently, it was not possible to precisely ascertain whether starting HT with the onset of menopause, when initiation or more rapid acceleration of atherosclerosis may take place, is beneficial. Because estrogen has been shown in experimental models to prevent the very earliest steps in atherogenesis, but to raise cardiovascular risk in the setting of established atherosclerosis (possibly via increases in clotting factors), it is possible that the adverse cardiovascular effects seen in this study may have been because many women started HT following the onset of menopause when subclinical atherosclerotic changes and irreversible endothelial damage may have already set in. In order to evaluate the possible role of age and/or years since menopause in the development of CHD, WHI investigators performed additional analyses in various subgroups of women. These additional analyses suggested no effect of age (i.e. 50-50 vs. 70-79 year of age). However, there were was a suggestion that greater numbers of years since menopause was associated with greater risk. Women starting within 10 years of menopause had fewer CHD events than those starting >20 years since menopause. However, statistical analyses of the combined WHI trials did not demonstrate that time since menopause altered CHD risk overall. This emphasizes the importance of continuing to study the effects of estrogen, particularly in younger, recently postmenopausal women. Additional studies are currently underway to assess whether estrogen administration to younger, healthy, recently postmenopausal women is safe from a cardiovascular standpoint.

The decision to use HT should be based primarily on the proven benefits of ET/HT on other systems, the potential risks of therapy, and patient preference. It should not be prescribed for prevention of CHD. Short-term use of HT for relief of postmenopausal symptoms is still an option for women without contraindications.

B. Diabetes Mellitus

Hormone therapy may decrease the risk of developing diabetes in postmenopausal women. In the HERS trial, the incidence of diabetes was significantly lower in women receiving HT as compared to women receiving placebo. The WHI trial revealed similar results whereby the incidence of diabetes was less in the HT group as compared with the placebo group. The differences between groups in both studies persisted after adjusting for body mass index and waist circumference. These results provide some reassurance regarding the effects of HT on glucose tolerance in women. However, HT should not be prescribed to postmenopausal women for prevention of diabetes.

C. Mood Disorders

Studies assessing the effects of estrogen on depression and other mood disorders are conflicting. Although some studies suggest beneficial effects of estrogen, others, including the recent WHI, do not. Early cross-sectional surveys of community or large, general, medical practice–based populations attempted to measure the temporal association of depression and irritability to the cessation of menses. Some reports indicated an increased incidence of minor symptoms such as irritability, dysphoria, and nervousness early in the menopausal transition.

Reports from community-based cohort studies have refined knowledge in the area of mood, mentation, and menopause. The initial longitudinal report of the US cohort found an increase in overall nonspecific symptom reporting at the menopause. Depression for more than 2 interviews was noted in 26% of the cohort. Perceived health, rather than menopause or coincident life stresses, was most related to depression in this study. These findings are consistent with the concept of variability in a woman's response to the menopause; individual characteristics and self-perceptions appear to be important determinants of each woman's experience of the climacteric.

Hypotheses regarding the etiology of the affective complaints at the menopause also include a primary biologic cause (eg, an alteration in brain amines). Studies using the opioid antagonist naloxone have demonstrated that estrogen deficiency is associated with low levels of endogenous opioid activity and that estrogen supplementation increases opioid activity. These findings suggest that central neurotransmitters may contribute to the etiology of affective and cognitive complaints. Sociologic factors postulated to cause psychologic symptoms, such as negative cultural values attached to aging, may also promote a negative climacteric experience.

Double-blind studies have found improvements in self-reported irritability, mild anxiety, and dysphoria in women treated with estrogen alone or when combined with progestin. Improvement of the Beck depression score in women without hot flushes indicates that estrogens likely have direct effects on brain function.

Depression and other quality-of-life outcomes were studied in the WHI trial. Overall, CEE alone, or in combination with medroxyprogesterone acetate, did not improve depressive symptoms among postmenopausal women ages 50–79 years after 1 and 3 years. In a subgroup analysis of 50–54-year-old women experiencing hot flashes, estrogen plus progestin improved hot flashes and sleep disturbance, but no other quality-of-life outcomes. In the estrogen-alone group, there was a slight improvement in sleep disturbance and social functioning, but no other quality-of-life outcomes measured. Therefore, a role for HT/ET in improving depressive symptoms after the menopause remains unproven.

D. Cognitive Decline

As life expectancy in women has risen, there has been more research regarding the effects of estrogen on cognitive functioning in postmenopausal women. Research indicates that estrogen influences areas of the brain known to be important for memory. However, recent data from the WHI suggests that estrogen alone or in combination with progestin does not decrease, and in fact may increase, the risk of cognitive decline in women older than 65 years of age.

E. Skin & Hair Changes

With aging, noticeable changes occur in the skin. There is generalized thinning and an accompanying loss of elasticity, resulting in wrinkling. These changes are particularly prominent in the areas exposed to light (ie, the face, neck, and hands). "Purse-string" wrinkling around the mouth and "crow's feet" around the eyes are characteristic. Skin changes on the dorsum of the hands are particularly noticeable. In this area, the skin may be so thin as to become almost transparent, with details of the underlying veins easily visible.

Histologically, the epidermis is thinned, and the basal layers become inactive with age. Dehydration is typical. Reduction in the number of blood vessels to the skin is also seen. Degeneration of elastic and collagenous fibers in the dermis also appears to be part of the aging process.

These skin changes are of cosmetic importance and are of great concern to many women. It is unclear whether these changes are primarily caused by the menopause, aging, or a combination of both factors. It is commonly stated that women undergoing estrogen replacement look younger, and the cosmetic industry has been putting estrogens in skin creams for years for precisely this reason.

The possibility that estrogens may have effects on skin was suggested by the demonstration of estrogen receptors in skin. The number of receptors is highest in facial skin, followed by skin of the breasts and thighs. This gives credence to the hypothesis that estrogens affect the skin.

Skin circulation is decreased in women after oophorectomy. Radiolabeled thymidine incorporation (an index of new DNA metabolism) is reported to decrease during the several months after oophorectomy. In some animal studies, estrogens increase the mitotic rate (a reflection of growth) of skin. Estrogens may alter the vascularization of skin. They also change the collagen content of the dermis, as reflected by mucopolysaccharide incorporation, hydroxyproline turnover, and alterations of the ground substance. In addition, dermal synthesis of hyaluronic acid and dermal water content are enhanced.

Skin collagen content and thickness have been studied in postmenopausal women. Decreases of both have been observed at a rate of 1–2% per year. The losses correlated with the number of years since the menopause, but not with chronologic age. Estrogen replacement prevents these losses or restores both parameters to premenopausal values. The greatest recovery is observed in women who began with low values. These data were interpreted to indicate that estrogen can prevent loss in women with high skin collagen levels, whereas it can restore content as well as prevent further loss in women with low collagen levels. Although these results are promising, it remains unclear whether they are clinically relevant. Estrogen should not be prescribed to improve the appearance of skin.

After the menopause, most women note some change in patterns of body hair. Usually there is a variable loss of pubic and axillary hair. Often there is loss of lanugo hair on the upper lip, chin, and cheeks, together with increased growth of coarse terminal hairs; a slight moustache may become noticeable. Hair on the body and extremities may either increase or decrease. Slight balding is seen occasionally. All of these changes may be partly a result of reduced levels of estrogen in the face of fairly well-maintained levels of testosterone.

F. Miscellaneous Symptoms

Many other symptoms are attributed to the endocrine changes of the postmenopausal state, but a direct cause-and-effect relationship has not been established for them. Some of these so-called climacteric symptoms are so common that they deserve brief mention.

Symptoms possibly related to specific autonomic nervous system instability—but equally attributable to anxiety or other emotional disturbances—are paresthesia (pricking, itching, formication), dizziness, tinnitus, fainting, scotomas, and dyspnea. Symptoms clearly not of endocrine origin are weakness, fatigue, nausea, vomiting, flatulence, anorexia, constipation, diarrhea, arthralgia, and myalgia.

Many women erroneously believe that the endocrine changes accompanying menopause will produce a steady weight gain. Women and men do tend to gain weight at this time of life, but the cause is usually a combination of decreased exercise and possibly increased caloric intake. There may be some redistribution of body weight occasioned by the deposition of fat over the hips and abdomen. Perhaps this is partly an endocrine effect, but more likely it is the result of decreased physical activity, reduced muscle tone, and other effects of aging.

Many of the previously mentioned symptoms occasionally respond promptly to administration of estrogen. This should not mislead physicians into assuming a specific endocrine action for what is actually a placebo effect.

Anderson GL, Limacher M, Assaf AR, et al; The Women's Health Initiative Steering Committee. Effects of conjugated equine estrogen in postmenopausal women with hysterectomy. *JAMA* 2004;291:1701. PMID: 15082697.

Ding EL, Song Y, Malik VS, Liu S. Sex differences of endogenous sex hormones and risk of type 2 diabetes: a systematic review and meta-analysis. *JAMA* 2006;295:1288–1299. PMID: 16537739.

Espeland MA, Rapp SR, Shumaker SA, et al. Conjugated equine estrogens and global cognitive function in postmenopausal women: the Women's Health Initiative Memory Study. *JAMA* 2004;291:2959–2968. PMID: 15213207.

Hulley S, Grady D, Bush T, et al. Randomized trial of estrogen plus progestin for secondary prevention of coronary heart disease in postmenopausal women. Heart and Estrogen/Progestin Replacement Study research group. *JAMA* 1998;280:605–613. PMID: 9718051.

Kanaya AM, Herrington D, Vittinghoff E, et al. Glylcemic effects of postmenopausal hormone therapy: the Heart and Estrogen/progestin Replacement Study. A randomized, double-blind, placebo-controlled trial. *Ann Intern Med* 2003;138:1–9. PMID: 12513038.

Manson JE, Hsia J, Johnson KC, et al. Estrogen plus progestin and the risk of coronary heart disease. *N Engl J Med* 2003;349:523–534. PMID: 12904517.

Manson JE, Allison MA, Rossouw JE, et al. Estrogen therapy and coronary artery calcium. *N Engl J Med* 2007;356:2591–2602. PMID: 17582069.

Margolis KL, Bonds ED, Rodabough RJ, et al. Effect of oestrogen plus progestin on the incidence of diabetes in postmenopausal women: results from the Women's Health Initiative Hormone Trial. *Diabetologia* 2004;47:1175–1187. PMID: 15252707.

Nathan L, Stackhouse J, Goulandris N, Snowling MJ. Estradiol inhibits leukocyte adhesion and transendothelial migration in vivo: possible mechanisms for gender differences in atherosclerosis. *Circ Res* 1999; 85:377–385. PMID: 10455066.

Prentice RL, Manson JE, Langer RD, et al. Benefits and Risks of postmenopausal hormone therapy when it is initiated soon after menopause. *Am J Epidemiol* 2009;170:12–23. PMID: 19468079.

Rapp SR, Espeland MA, Shumaker SA, et al. Effect of estrogen plus progestin on global cognitive function in postmenopausal women: the Women's Health Initiative Study: a randomized trial. *JAMA* 2003;289:2663–2672. PMID: 12771113.

Estrogen Therapy

Every woman with menopausal symptoms deserves an adequate explanation of the physiologic event she is experiencing to dispel her fears and address symptoms such as hot flashes and sleep disturbance. Reassurance should be emphasized. Specific reassurance about continued sexual activity is important.

As long as ovarian function is sufficient to maintain some uterine bleeding, no treatment is usually required. Occasionally, women complain of hot flushes while menstrual function is still present. Treatment with low-dose oral contraceptive pills, if no contraindications exist, will relieve these symptoms and help to regulate menstrual cycles during the menopausal transition.

A. Indications

Estrogen therapy has been used for many years for a variety of symptoms and conditions seen in the aged female population. However, despite suggestions from observational and experimental studies that estrogens prevent many common conditions of aging, such as Alzheimer's disease and CHD, estrogen therapy has only been proven to be effective in the prevention of osteoporosis, treatment of vasomotor symptoms, and treatment of vulvovaginal atrophy. Results from the WHI further call into question the degree to which estrogen can act as a "cure-all" for the common conditions of aging, particularly those affecting the brain and heart. Benefits beyond those already established are still possible, but await proof in large-scale studies in humans. Therefore, use of estrogens should be limited to the currently FDA-approved indications: prevention of osteoporosis, treatment of vasomotor symptoms, and treatment of vulvovaginal atrophy (see D. Management Guidelines for Estrogen Therapy).

B. Complications

Before discussing the management of estrogen replacement, it is necessary to review the complications of and contraindications to this type of therapy. These play an important role in the ultimate decision regarding treatment for all patients.

1. Endometrial cancer—The role of estrogen therapy in the development of endometrial cancer is one of the most highly charged issues related to the menopause. Current concerns are based on several lines of investigation. The scope of investigative efforts lead to the conclusion that estrogen stimulation of the endometrium, unopposed by progesterone, causes endometrial proliferation, hyperplasia, and, finally, neoplasia. In most studies, a strong association has been found, with 2- to 8-fold overall risk ratios. High dosage and prolonged treatment increase the risk. Disease is local in most cases, although more widespread invasive tumors have been reported. Consequently, it is recommended that a progestogen be added to ET to reduce the risk of endometrial hyperplasia or carcinoma. Some women may experience adverse side effects from progestogen therapy. In addition, increasing concerns about the role of progestogens in increasing risk of breast carcinoma amongst women using estrogen–progestogen therapy (EPT) have led to further efforts to find alternatives to progestogens to counteract the effects of estrogen on the endometrium. Agents with estrogen agonist/antagonist activity are currently being investigated as such possible alternatives.

2. Breast cancer—Early age at menarche and older age at menopause are known risk factors for breast cancer, and early oophorectomy is known to give protection against this disease. Ovarian activity is an important determinant of risk, thus estrogen may play a role in the development of breast cancer. Studies in rodents support that view. More than 30 epidemiologic studies have been published since 1974 to determine the possible link between postmenopausal estrogen use and breast cancer. In general, the later studies have had better design, quality, and analytic strategies. The number of subjects in more recent studies has also been larger. These results have not always agreed. The recent prospective, randomized WHI trial also addressed this issue. In this study there was an increased risk of invasive breast cancer in the estrogen/progestin arm. However, in the estrogen-alone arm, the risk of breast cancer was not increased compared with controls.

Despite this inconsistency in studies, some trends have been observed: (1) Long-term use (ie, 4–10 years) has been associated with mild increased risk in some of the meta-analyses and the WHI. (2) The addition of a progestin does not appear to decrease risk and may increase risk. (3) Finally, risk does not vary in strata of family history of breast cancer or with benign breast disease.

It must be remembered that all women are at risk for breast cancer. Thus instructions for breast self-examination, a careful breast assessment, and routine screening mammography should be a part of the medical care of all older women.

3. Thromboembolic disease—Use of oral contraceptives increases the risk of overt venous thromboembolic disease and subclinical disease extensive enough to be detected by laboratory procedures such as ^{125}I fibrinogen uptake and plasma fibrinogen chromatography. The risk of venous thromboembolic disease was also increased among users of ET/EPT in the WHI, as well as among users of HT in the HERS trial.

The effects of estrogen on the clotting mechanism may contribute to or be responsible for a generalized hypercoagulable state. Oral estrogens affect synthesis of coagulation factors through a first-pass effect in the liver, an effect associated with an increased risk of thromboembolic disease. The risk for thromboembolic events with use of ET/EPT is also likely further increased amongst patients with inherited thrombophilias.

Use of transdermal estrogens is probably associated with a lowered risk for thromboembolic events as compared with use of oral estrogens. However, randomized trials are needed to better characterize the effects of transdermal estrogens on risk for clinical thromboembolic events.

4. Stroke—Several recent studies suggest that HT is associated with an increased risk of stroke. In the EPT arm of the WHI, there was an increased risk of ischemic stroke among those using EPT when compared with the placebo. In the estrogen-alone arm of the WHI, there was also a statistically significant increased risk of stroke after approximately 7 years of follow-up, and this outcome led to the trial being terminated.

5. Uterine bleeding—If patients are given sequential estrogen and progestins, the majority will experience some uterine bleeding, particularly soon after initiation of therapy. This bleeding can occur during the treatment-free interval (scheduled bleeding) or while the medications are being administered (unscheduled bleeding). Hyperplastic endometrium can develop with this type of therapy. If the bleeding is heavy or prolonged, a biopsy should be performed. In women using a combined continuous regimen of estrogen and progestin, bleeding is common in the first several months of therapy and usually doesn't indicate endometrial pathology. However, if bleeding persists in these patients, or is prolonged or heavy at any time, endometrial sampling should be performed. If endometrial hyperplasia is present, the medications can be discontinued, progestin dose can be increased, or a progestin can be given each day of estrogen administration. Whichever approach is adopted, a repeat biopsy should be performed to make certain that the hyperplastic endometrium has resolved. The cost-effectiveness ratio for periodic biopsy in women who do not bleed or bleed only during the medication-free interval is poor and indicates that such biopsy is probably unnecessary.

In women taking estrogen only, the incidence of endometrial hyperplasia can be as high as 25% after only 12 months of therapy. Hyperplasia occurs in women who do not experience vaginal bleeding, bleed only during the medication-free interval, or bleed during drug administration. Thus a pretreatment biopsy and yearly endometrial biopsies are necessary in all women receiving estrogens alone to assess for the presence of hyperplasia. Again, estrogen withdrawal or combined EPT may be used to treat the hyperplasia. The incidence of endometrial cancer will likely be reduced if the programs discussed previously are instituted.

6. Gallbladder disease—An increased incidence of gallbladder disease has been reported after estrogen replacement therapy. Estrogens cause increased amounts of cholesterol to collect in bile. Two primary bile salts, cholate and chenodeoxycholate, are produced by liver cells. In women taking estrogen, decreased levels of chenodeoxycholate and increased levels of cholate are found in bile. Chenodeoxycholate inhibits activity of the enzyme β-hydroxy-β-methylglutaryl-CoA reductase, which regulates cholesterol synthesis, and a decrease in chenodeoxycholate may therefore cause increased activity of β-hydroxy-β-methylglutaryl-CoA reductase, leading to increased synthesis of cholesterol. Bile normally has a 75–90% saturation in cholesterol, and even small increases of this substance can initiate cholesterol precipitation and stone formation. Three-fourths of gallstones are composed predominantly of cholesterol.

7. Lipid metabolism—Estrogen replacement also has an impact on circulating lipids. As discussed earlier, many of these effects are favorable. However, others may pose increased risk. Most lipids are bound to proteins in the blood, and the concentrations of the various types of lipoproteins are associated with varying risks of heart disease. Lower levels of HDL cholesterol and higher concentrations of total cholesterol, LDL cholesterol, very-low-density lipoprotein cholesterol, and triglycerides are associated with increased risk of atherosclerosis and coronary artery disease. Estrogen replacement decreases LDL cholesterol and increases HDL cholesterol and triglycerides. Use of conjugated estrogens, 0.625 mg/d or less, causes approximately a 10% increase in HDL cholesterol. Much attention has been focused on the impact of estrogens on lipoproteins to explain what appeared to be a beneficial effect of HT on heart disease in earlier observational studies of younger postmenopausal women. The impact of estrogen-induced increases in triglycerides on cardiovascular risk is unclear. In patients with familial defects of lipoprotein metabolism, estrogen replacement therapy is associated with massive elevations of plasma triglycerides, leading to pancreatitis and other complications. However, this is a very unusual complication of estrogen replacement. Transdermal estrogens are probably less likely to raise triglyceride levels and thus are preferred in women with an elevation in triglyceride levels.

8. Miscellaneous—Other side effects of estrogen therapy include uterine bleeding, generalized edema, mastodynia and breast enlargement, abdominal bloating, signs and symptoms resembling those of premenstrual tension, headaches (particularly of a "menstrual migraine" type), and excessive cervical mucous. These side effects may be dose related or idiosyncratic, and are managed by lowering the dosage, by use of another agent, or by discontinuation of the medication.

C. Contraindications to Estrogen Replacement Therapy

Contraindications to ET are as follows: (1) Undiagnosed abnormal vaginal bleeding; (2) known, suspected, or history of cancer of the breast; (3) known or suspected estrogen-dependent neoplasia; (4) active deep vein thrombosis, pulmonary embolism, or a history of these conditions; (5) arterial thromboembolic disease (myocardial infarction, stroke); and (6) liver dysfunction or disease. In general, ET should be avoided in patients with a diagnosis of endometrial cancer. ET may stimulate growth of malignant cells remaining after treatment of breast or endometrial carcinoma and may thus hasten the recurrence of cancer. Therefore, it is prudent to avoid systemic ET in breast cancer patients and most endometrial cancer patients. Recently, it was suggested that women with early (stage 1) and well-differentiated (grade 1) endometrial cancer can be administered estrogens after primary treatment of the cancer. Care must be exercised in following this recommendation until it has been properly studied. Any decision to use ET/EPT after a diagnosis of endometrial cancer should be made in consultation with the patient's oncologist. Patients who have had estrogen receptor–positive malignant tumors of the breast probably should not receive systemic estrogen supplements. Topical vaginal estrogens to treat symptoms of urogenital atrophy in breast/endometrial cancer patients might be acceptable, but should first be discussed with the patient's oncologist. A history of treated carcinoma of the cervix or ovary is not a contraindication to ET. Estrogens may have undesirable effects on some patients with preexisting seizures, hypertension, fibrocystic disease of the breast, uterine leiomyoma, collagen disease, familial hyperlipidemia, migraine headaches, chronic thrombophlebitis, and gallbladder disease. At the low dosages recommended for replacement therapy, increased growth of uterine myomas, endometriosis, or chronic cystic mastitis is rarely a concern.

D. Management Guidelines for Estrogen Therapy

1. General—Only general guidelines can be offered, because risks and benefits must be evaluated for each patient. Numerous formulations of estrogen and estrogen plus progestin are available (Table 59–1). Current indications for ET are relief of menopausal symptoms (including hot flushes and vaginal atrophy) and prevention of osteoporosis. Caution should be exercised in providing therapy for other conditions until more definitive studies have been performed. If symptoms of hot flushes and vaginal atrophy are moderate to severe, therapy may be used for the shortest duration possible; minimal or no symptoms may not require hormones.

In women who require pharmacologic intervention for prevention of **osteoporosis,** estrogen may be used. However, ET for osteoporosis prevention is generally reserved for those women who are otherwise using estrogen for menopausal symptoms and/or who cannot tolerate other antiresorptive therapies. Lower dosages of estrogen are being increasingly used for prevention of osteoporosis to minimize the risks of estrogen therapy. There are several options available for use of estrogen or estrogen plus progestin for prevention of osteoporosis (Table 59–1). In the past, standard doses included 0.625 mg of conjugated equine estrogens, 0.05 mg of transdermal estradiol, and 1 mg of micronized estradiol. However, 0.3 mg of conjugated equine estrogens, 0.5 mg of micronized estradiol, and 0.025-mg transdermal

Table 59–1. Preparations of estrogens and progestogens available in the United States for hormone therapy.

Agent	How Supplied	Special Features
Oral estrogens for management of vasomotor and genitourinary symptoms; strongly consider progestogen for women with intact uterus		
Conjugated equine estrogens	0.3 mg, 0.45 mg, 0.625 mg, 0.9 mg, 1.25 mg tablets	Well studied, well tolerated; approved for prevention of osteoporosis, 0.625 mg dose used in WHI study
Estradiol	0.5 mg, 1 mg, 2 mg tablets	Well tolerated; approved for prevention of osteoporosis
Piperazine estrone (estropipate)	0.75 mg, 1.5 mg, 3 mg tablets	
Synthetic conjugated estrogens	0.3 mg, 0.45 mg, 0.625 mg, 0.9 mg, 1.25 mg tablets	Not approved for prevention of osteoporosis
Transdermal estrogens for management of vasomotor symptoms and genitourinary atrophy; strongly consider progestogen for women with intact uterus		
Estradiol patch (mg/day)	0.025 mg, 0.0375 mg, 0.05 mg, 0.06 mg, 0.075 mg, 0.1 mg patches	Well tolerated, 10% skin rash, available in weekly and biweekly formulations; approved for prevention of osteoporosis
Estradiol gel	0.06% gel; 0.75 mg estradiol per pump	Not approved for prevention of osteoporosis
Estradiol spray	1.5 mg/spray	Not approved for prevention of osteoporosis
Transdermal estrogen for prevention of osteoporosis		
Estradiol patch (low dose)	0.014 mg	Only approved for prevention of osteoporosis; not approved for prevention of vasomotor symptoms or genitourinary atrophy
Intravaginal ring for treatment of vasomotor symptoms and genitourinary atrophy; strongly consider progestogen for women with intact uterus		
Estradiol acetate	0.05 mg/day and 0.1 mg/day over 3 months	Remains in place for 3 months; not approved for prevention of osteoporosis

(*Continued*)

Table 59–1. Preparations of estrogens and progestogens available in the United States for hormone therapy. (Continued)

Agent	How Supplied	Special Features
Vaginal estrogens for treatment of genitourinary atrophy (doses inadequate to treat vasomotor symptoms)		
Creams		
Conjugated equine estrogens	0.625 mg/g cream	Not approved for prevention of osteoporosis or vasomotor symptoms
Estradiol	0.1 mg/g cream	Not approved for prevention of osteoporosis or vasomotor symptoms
Tablets		
Estradiol	0.010 mg tablet	Not approved for prevention of osteoporosis or vasomotor symptoms
Rings		
Estradiol	0.0075 mg/day released over 3 months	Remains in place for 3 months; not approved for prevention of osteoporosis or vasomotor symptoms
Oral Progestogens		
Medroxyprogesterone acetate	2.5 mg, 5 mg, 10 mg tablets	Well tolerated, well studied
Micronized progesterone	100 mg, 200 mg capsules	Well tolerated, possible somnolence
Megestrol acetate	20 mg, 40 mg scored tablets	Not used routinely for postmenopausal hormone therapy
Norethindrone	0.35 mg tablets	Available as contraceptive "minipill"
Norethindrone acetate	5 mg scored tablets	Dosage probably too large for routine hormone therapy
Intrauterine Progestin		
Levonorgestrel releasing IUD	20 μg/day	Not routinely used for postmenopausal hormone therapy, approved for use as contraceptive and heavy menstrual bleeding; remains in place for 5 years; may prevent endometrial hyperplasia with fewer side effects but not approved for this use.
Estrogen/Progestogen combination formulas indicated for treatment of menopausal symptoms in women with a uterus		
Oral		
Conjugated equine estrogens (CEE)/medroxyprogesterone acetate (MPA)	0.3 mg CEE/1.5 mg MPA; 0.45 mg CEE/1.5 mg MPA; 0.625 mg CEE/2.5 mg MPA; 0.625 mg CEE/5 mg MPA; 0.625 mg CEE days 1–14, then 0.625 mg CEE/5 mg MPA days 15–28	Well tolerated, well studied, approved for prevention of osteoporosis, 0.625 mg/2.5 mg preparation used in WHI study
Estradiol/norethindrone acetate	1 mg estradiol/0.5 mg norethindrone	Approved for prevention of osteoporosis
Estradiol/norgestimate	1 mg estradiol × 3 days, alternating with 1 mg estradiol/0.09 mg norgestimate × 3 days	Intermittent progestin; approved for prevention of osteoporosis
Ethinyl estradiol/norethindrone acetate	2.5 μg ethinyl estradiol/ 0.5 mg norethindrone; 5 μg ethinyl estradiol/ 1 mg norethindrone	Approved for prevention of osteoporosis
Estradiol/drospirenone	1 mg estradiol/5 mg drospirenone	Not approved for prevention of osteoporosis
Transdermal patches		
Estradiol/norethindrone acetate	0.05 mg estradiol/0.14 mg norethindrone per day; 0.05 mg estradiol/0.025 mg norethindrone per day	Not approved for prevention of osteoporosis
Estradiol/levonorgestrel	0.045 mg estradiol/0.015 mg levonorgestrel per day	Approved for prevention of osteoporosis

patches also prevent bone loss, although not as well as higher doses. A new **low-dose** (0.014 mg/d) transdermal formulation of estradiol was recently FDA approved for prevention of osteoporosis. Early commencement of prophylaxis after cessation of ovarian function will maintain the highest bone density. Initiation of HT well after the menopause will stop bone loss, but will not return bone density to that which was present at the time of the menopause.

For women with **hot flashes,** a standard dosage of estrogen, such as 0.3–0.625 mg of conjugated equine estrogens, 0.025 mg transdermal estradiol, or 0.5 mg oral estradiol should be given daily (Table 59–1). Higher doses may be necessary to relieve hot flashes. Progressive reduction of dosage should be attempted as soon as feasible. Additional formulations containing estradiol, synthetic estrogens, and estrogens plus progestins are also available (Table 59–1).

In women who are suffering from **atrophic vaginitis,** vaginal preparations can be used and are preferred over systemic estrogens. These preparations are available in the form of creams (ie, CEEs or estradiol 0.25–2 g given nightly for 2 weeks, followed by twice weekly), tablets (10 μg estradiol given nightly for 2 weeks, followed by twice weekly), and rings (estradiol releasing rings, which remain in place for 3 months at a time) (Table 59–1). With the tablets, rings, and lowest dose creams, endometrial proliferation is rare. However, higher doses, presence of vaginal bleeding, or other risk factors may necessitate periodic endometrial biopsy or ultrasound to assess the endometrial thickness. Progestogens may be necessary to prevent endometrial proliferation in some cases.

2. Progestogen–estrogen therapy—One of the most serious concerns about estrogen replacement is the occurrence of endometrial hyperplasia or cancer. Progestogens oppose the action of estrogen on the endometrium. Progestogens reduce the number of estrogen receptors in glandular and stromal cells of the endometrium. These agents also block estrogen-induced synthesis of DNA, and they induce the intracellular enzymes estradiol dehydrogenase and estrogen sulfotransferase. The former reduces estradiol to the much less potent estrone, whereas the latter converts estrogen to estrogen sulfates for rapid elimination from endometrial cells. In addition, full secretory transformation occurs if the progestogen is given at a large enough dosage for a sufficient length of time.

Progestogens reduce the occurrence of endometrial cancer. Epidemiologic studies show significant reduction of the occurrence of endometrial cancer with estrogen plus progestogen compared with estrogen alone. One study indicated use of the progestogen for more than 10 days a month reduced the occurrence more than use for a shorter interval. In treating women with hormones, a more practical concern is the prevention of endometrial hyperplasia. Initially, British investigators showed that high-dose estrogens (1.25 mg or greater of CEEs) resulted in 32% hyperplasia, whereas low doses (0.625 mg or less) stimulated 16% hyperplasias in women followed up for 15 months. In women given estrogen plus progestins, the occurrence of hyperplasia was 6% and 3%, respectively. In comparing length of therapy, 7 days of progestogen reduced the occurrence of hyperplasia to 4%, 10 days reduced it to 2%, and 12 days eliminated hyperplasia. Direct comparisons in drug trials have also shown reductions of hyperplasia in women given estrogens and progestogens compared with those given estrogen alone. It should be pointed out that the majority of endometrial lesions observed in women in these trials were either cystic or simple hyperplasias, which could be reversed by giving a progestogen or discontinuing the estrogen.

One option is to administer a progestogen such as medroxyprogesterone acetate at a dosage of 5–10 mg/d for 12–14 days each month (see Table 59–1). If this is accomplished, 80–90% of women will experience some vaginal bleeding monthly toward the end of or after the progestogen is administered. An alternative is to prescribe a lower dosage, 2.5 mg, continuously. Many newer formulations of hormone therapy contain both estrogen and progestin (Table 59–1). The combined, continuous administration of estrogen plus progestogen is the most common mode of administration today. This regimen promotes endometrial atrophy and results in amenorrhea in 70–90% of women who use continuous therapy for more than 1 year. The remainder will bleed occasionally, with the bleeding usually being less frequent, shorter, and lighter than with sequential therapy.

Administration of progestogens can be associated with other uncomfortable side effects including fatigue, depression, breast tenderness, bloating, menstrual cramps, and headaches. It is also important to keep in mind that it was a progestogen-containing regimen that was used in the WHI trial that was discontinued largely because of a trend toward an increased risk of **breast cancer**. In the estrogen-only arm, breast cancer rates were not increased over control levels. This raises concerns about the potential role of progestogens in increasing breast cancer risk. This concern combined with potential progestogen side effects may lead to elimination of or nonstandard progestogen administration. If lower dosages or shorter duration of progestogens are used, endometrial sampling to diagnose the development of hyperplasia or cancer should be performed. Use of locally administered progestogens through the use of the levonorgestrel intrauterine device is also being considered as an alternative strategy to minimize systemic side effects and risks while maintaining endometrial protection.

Chlebowski RT, Anderson GL, Gass M, et al. Estrogen plus progestin and breast cancer incidence and mortality in postmenopausal women. *JAMA* 2010; 304:1684–1692. PMID: 20959578.

Beral V, Bull D, Reeves G; Million Women Study Collaborators. Endometrial cancer and hormone-replacement therapy in the Million Women Study. *Lancet* 2005;365:1543–1551. PMID: 15866308.

Prentice RL, Chlebowski RT, Stefanick ML, et al. Conjugated equine estrogens and breast cancer risk in the Women's Health Initiative clinical trial and observational study. *Am J Epidemiol* 2008; 167:1407–1415. PMID: 18448442.

Rossouw JE, Anderson GL, Prentice RL, et al; Writing Group for the Women's Health Initiative. Risks and benefits of estrogen plus progestin in healthy postmenopausal women: Principal results from the Women's Health Initiative randomized controlled trial. *JAMA* 2002;288:321–333. PMID: 12117397.

Prognosis

The prognosis for the postmenopausal woman who does not develop clinically manifest estrogen deficiency includes only the ordinary hazards of disease and aging. For the woman who does develop signs of estrogen deficiency, hormone therapy can correct physical symptoms and signs and prevent the development of osteoporosis. Correction of minor distressing symptoms and signs can improve the general well-being of the postmenopausal woman and help her to pursue a vigorous life. However, HT for the postmenopausal woman who does not need it serves no purpose and can cause unpleasant side effects and impose unnecessary risks to her health.

Domestic Violence & Sexual Assault

60

Michael C. Lu, MD, MPH
Jessica S. Lu, MPH
Vivian P. Halfin, MD

For many victims of domestic violence and sexual assault, the first contact with the health care system is with the obstetrician-gynecologist or primary care doctor. Consequently, it is critical that these physicians be knowledgeable in the identification, evaluation, and treatment of such patients.

DOMESTIC VIOLENCE

ESSENTIALS OF DIAGNOSIS

- Chronic pelvic pain
- Sexual dysfunctions, such as decreased interest or arousal, dyspareunia, or anorgasmia
- Chronic or recurrent vaginitis
- Anxiety or tears before or during the pelvic examination
- Persistent multiple bodily complaints, such as chronic headaches, palpitations, abdominal complaints, or sleep and appetite disturbances
- Eating disorders
- Somatoform disorder
- Depressed or suicidal
- Anxiety or sleep disorders
- May self-medicate with alcohol or other substances
- Posttraumatic stress disorder
- Personality disorders characterized by maladaptive character traits
- Multiple personality disorder

Although the home is often thought of as a safe haven, it is the site of the most common manifestations of violence in our society today. Domestic or intimate partner violence typically refers to violence perpetrated against adolescent and adult females within the context of family or intimate relationships. Although victims of domestic violence may be male or female, 90–95% of the victims are women. Domestic violence is characterized by a behavior pattern manifested in physical and sexual attacks, as well as psychologic and economic coercion.

The abuser uses the behavior in order to establish and maintain domination and control over the victim. Because abuse is usually accompanied by shame and guilt, the victim often does not report the abuse. As a result of significant underreporting, it is difficult to compile exact data on the incidence of domestic violence. Every year, approximately 4–5 million women are believed to be battered by their intimate partners. Violence by an intimate partner accounts for approximately 21% of all the violent crime experienced by women. More than 40% of all female murder victims are murdered by their husbands, boyfriends, or ex-partners. It is estimated that at least one-fifth of all American women will be physically assaulted by a partner or ex-partner during their lifetime.

Violent acts may include threats, throwing objects, pushing, kicking, hitting, beating, sexual assault, and threatening with or using a weapon. Domestic violence frequently includes verbal abuse, intimidation, progressive social isolation, and deprivation of things such as food, money, transportation, or access to health care. The violence typically occurs in a predictable, progressive cycle. The tension-building phase is characterized by arguing and blaming as anger intensifies. This leads to the battering phase that may involve verbal threats, sexual abuse, physical battering, and use of weapons. The battering phase is followed by a honeymoon phase during which the abuser may deny the violence, make excuses for battering, apologize, buy gifts, and promise never to do it again, until the next cycle begins. Although unemployment, poverty, and alcohol and substance abuse increase the likelihood of abuse, domestic violence cuts across all racial, ethnic, religious, educational, and socioeconomic lines. Domestic violence often occurs within a framework of family violence that can include child abuse, elder abuse, or abuse of adults who are disabled. It is estimated that child abuse occurs in 33–77% of families where adults are abused.

Prevention

If the violence has escalated to the point where the patient is afraid for her safety or that of her children, she should be offered shelter. An important step in addressing ongoing violence is to help the victim establish a safety plan. The American College of Obstetricians and Gynecologists (www.acog.org) distributes pocket cards with suggested steps for making an exit plan. These cards can be handed to the patient or left in patient restrooms where a woman can pick it up without concern of being seen by an accompanying partner.

Providing educational materials about domestic violence and its consequences can sometimes help victims take action toward ending the violence. These materials demonstrate to women that their physicians' offices are both a resource and a safe place should they decide to take action. A list of referral resources should be readily available in medical offices. The list should include telephone numbers for police departments, emergency departments, shelters for battered women, rape crisis centers, counseling services, self-help programs, and advocacy agencies that can provide legal, financial, and emotional support.

Clinical Findings

Survivors of domestic violence or sexual abuse may present to health care professionals in a variety of clinical settings. The prevalence of domestic violence among patients in ambulatory care settings is estimated to be between 20 and 30%.

Such patients commonly report chronic pelvic pain to their gynecologists. A history of sexual abuse is found in significantly more women with chronic pelvic pain as compared with other gynecologic conditions. Others may complain of sexual dysfunctions such as decreased interest or arousal, dyspareunia, or anorgasmia. Incest victims have a very high rate of sexual dysfunction and may avoid sex or seek it out compulsively. Still others may present with chronic or recurrent vaginitis. Some women may present for a routine gynecologic appointment but become anxious and tearful before or during the pelvic examination.

Some women present to their primary care physicians with persistent multiple bodily complaints, such as chronic headaches, palpitations, abdominal complaints, or sleep and appetite disturbances. Eating disorders may be more common among abuse victims. Others may have a somatoform disorder. This condition is characterized by physical symptoms suggesting a physical condition for which there are no demonstrable organic findings or physiologic mechanisms. In the face of a negative workup, there may be evidence of or a presumption that the symptoms are linked to psychologic factors or conflicts. Women who meet the criteria for somatoform disorder often have a history of abuse.

In a mental health setting, victims of domestic violence or sexual assault may note feeling depressed or suicidal. They may have anxiety or sleep disorders that they may self-medicate with alcohol or other substances. Most commonly, these women may have posttraumatic stress disorder (PTSD), which occurs in individuals who have experienced a psychologically distressing event that is outside the range of usual human experience. Symptoms of PTSD include re-experiencing the traumatic event through intrusive memories, dreams, flashbacks, or exposure to events symbolic of the trauma. Patients with PTSD also exhibit a "psychic numbing," that is, they are detached from other people and have difficulty feeling emotions, especially those associated with intimacy or sexuality. Other clinical syndromes include personality disorders characterized by maladaptive character traits. In very extreme cases, patients may have multiple personality disorder, characterized by having ≥2 distinct personalities existing within them. This disorder is marked by a disturbance in the normally integrated functions of identity, memory, and consciousness as the result of dissociation from traumatic experiences.

The problem of domestic violence in pregnancy merits special mention because it is a threat to both the mother and her developing fetus. Estimates of prevalence of domestic violence in pregnancy are in the range of 1–20%, with most studies identifying rates between 4 and 8%. These estimates suggest that violence is a more common problem for pregnant women than preeclampsia, gestational diabetes, and placenta previa, conditions for which pregnant women are routinely screened and evaluated. Some evidence suggests that violence may escalate during pregnancy, especially in the postpartum period. Abuse is associated with increased physical and psychological stress, inadequate prenatal care utilization, poor nutrition and weight gain, and increased maternal behavioral risks (cigarette, alcohol, and substance abuse). These may lead to problems with fetal growth and development. Physical trauma can cause abruptio placentae, preterm labor, preterm premature rupture of membranes, and maternal and fetal injuries and demise.

Differential Diagnosis

Although battered women seek medical care frequently, as few as 1 in 20 are correctly identified by the practitioner to whom they turn for help. Barriers to diagnosis include the practitioner's lack of knowledge or training, lack of recognition of the widespread prevalence of the problem, time constraints, fear of offending the patient, and a feeling of powerlessness in the area of treatment. Research suggests that the use of abuse assessment questions on standard medical records may increase screening and documentation. In addition, because many women will not voluntarily disclose abuse, asking each patient directly about prior or ongoing victimization increases the likelihood of disclosure.

The screening assessment should be prefaced with a statement to establish that screening is universal, such as,

"I would like to ask you a few questions about physical, sexual, and emotional trauma because we know that these are common and affect women's health." Direct questioning using behaviorally specific phrasing should follow:

- Has anyone close to you ever threatened to hurt you?
- Has anyone ever hit, kicked, choked, or hurt you physically?
- Has anyone, including your partner, ever forced you to have sex?
- Are you ever afraid of your partner?

Disclosure rates will be higher when the questions are asked face to face by the health care provider rather than through a questionnaire and when behaviorally specific descriptions rather than the terms "abuse," "domestic violence," or "rape" are used. Abuse victims are often accompanied to health care appointments by the perpetrator, who may appear overprotective or overbearing, and may answer questions directed toward the woman. It is important to ask the patient questions in private, apart from the male partner. It is also important to ask the patient questions apart from children, family, or friends and to avoid using them as interpreters when asking questions about violence.

In the office setting, the most effective and efficient strategy for providing assistance to a woman who has disclosed abuse involves acknowledging and documenting the trauma, assessing immediate safety and establishing a safety plan, and providing patient education and referrals to community support services. An essential first step is to acknowledge the trauma. It is important to reinforce to the victim that she is not to blame, as many victims have trouble believing that they are not responsible for the abuse.

Documenting domestic violence is no different from documenting other patient interactions, but such documentation may provide important supportive evidence in the courtroom to put an end to the violence. Direct quotations of the patient's explanation of her injuries should be recorded. Photographs may be taken after consent is granted. Every effort should be made to maintain confidentiality to avoid retaliation by the perpetrators when they suspect disclosure of abuse. The physician or health care professional may be required by state law to report actual or suspected domestic violence.

Once domestic violence is acknowledged and documented, the next step is to assess immediate safety and to establish a safety plan. Lethality of the violence should be assessed by asking questions such as:

- Has your partner ever threatened to kill you or your children?
- Are there weapons in the house?
- Does your partner abuse alcohol or use drugs?
- Is it safe for you to go home?
- Are the children (or other dependents) safe?

Treatment

Given the high rate of psychiatric symptomatology in this population, referral for psychiatric screening and counseling can be useful. Patients who are experiencing posttraumatic stress disorder can benefit from psychotherapy and possibly medication as well. Those with depression, substance abuse, or anxiety, personality, or dissociative disorders will also require ongoing treatment. Psychiatrists or other mental health professionals can serve to coordinate a variety of treatment modalities for the victims: individual, couples, and family therapy; detoxification and substance abuse treatment; and advocacy groups.

Despite the best efforts of physicians and other health care professionals, some women may initially be unable to extirpate themselves from victimization. For such women, an encounter with a health care system that they experience as nonblaming, accessible, and supportive will help to maximize the chances of their making a positive life change at some future point.

Campbell JC. Health consequences of intimate partner violence. *Lancet* 2002;359:1331–1336. PMID: 11965295.

Chambliss LR. Intimate partner violence and its implication for pregnancy. *Clin Obstet Gynecol* 2008;51:385–397. PMID: 18463468.

Rabin RF, Jennings JM, Campbell JC, Bair-Merritt MH. Intimate partner violence screening tools: a systematic review. *Am J Prev Med* 2009;36:439–445.e4. PMID: 19362697.

Rhodes KV, Levinson W. Interventions for intimate partner violence against women: Clinical applications. *JAMA* 2003;289: 601–605. PMID: 12578493.

Sarkar NN. The impact of intimate partner violence on women's reproductive health and pregnancy outcome. *J Obstet Gynaecol* 2008;28:266–271. PMID: 18569465.

United States Preventive Services Task Force. Screening for family and intimate partner violence: Recommendation statement. *Ann Fam Med* 2004;2:156–160. PMID: 15083857.

Wathen CN, MacMillan HL. Interventions for violence against women: Scientific review. *JAMA* 2003;289:589–600.

SEXUAL ASSAULT

ESSENTIALS OF DIAGNOSIS

- Complaints of having been mugged
- Concerns about acquired immune deficiency syndrome (AIDS) or other sexually transmitted diseases
- Psychiatric symptoms include depression, anxiety, or a suicide attempt
- PTSD
- Somatic symptoms include disturbed sleeping and eating patterns, gastrointestinal irritability (with nausea predominating), musculoskeletal soreness, fatigue, tension headaches, and intense startle reactions

- Symptoms of vaginal irritation occur in more than 50% of victims
- Rectal pain and bleeding are frequent in patients subjected to anal penetration
- Gynecologic trauma
- Escape through the use of alcohol and drugs

Sexual assault is any sexual act performed by one person on another without the person's consent. Sexual assault includes genital, oral, or anal penetration by a part of the accused's body or by an object. It may result from force, the threat of force either on the victim or another person, or the victim's inability to give appropriate consent. Many states have now adopted the gender-neutral legal term *sexual assault* in favor of *rape*, which traditionally referred to forced vaginal penetration of a woman by a male assailant.

An estimated 700,000 to 1,000,000 American women are sexually assaulted every year. These estimates are higher than official crime reports because the majority of cases go unreported. According to one estimate, only 30% of rapes are reported to the police, and 50% of rape victims tell no one. At least 20% of adult women, 15% of college-age women, and 12% of adolescent girls have experienced sexual abuse and assault during their lifetime. Sexual assault occurs in all age, racial-ethnic, and socioeconomic groups, but its incidence may be higher for African American women and for adolescent females. In several studies, approximately one-fourth to one-half of the victims of sexual assault were younger than the age of 18 years. The very young, the elderly, and the physically or developmentally disabled may be particularly vulnerable to sexual assault.

Several variants of sexual assault deserve special mention. **Marital rape** is defined as forced coitus or related sexual acts within a marital relationship without the consent of a partner. **Acquaintance rape** refers to those sexual assaults committed by someone known to the victim. More than 75% of adolescent rapes are committed by an acquaintance of the victim. When the acquaintance is a family member, including step-relatives and parental figures living in the home, the sexual assault is referred to as **incest.** When the forced or unwanted sexual activity occurs in the context of a dating relationship, it is referred to as **date rape.** In this situation, the woman may voluntarily participate in sexual play but coitus occurs, often forcibly, without her consent. Alcohol use is frequently associated with date rape. "Date rape drugs" such as flunitrazepam (Rohypnol) and gamma-hydroxybutyrate (GHB) have also been used to diminish a woman's ability to consent or to remember the assault.

Statutory rape refers to sexual intercourse with a female under an age specified by state law (ranging from 14–18 years of age); the consent of an adolescent younger than this age is legally irrelevant because she is defined as being incapable of consenting. **Child sexual abuse** is defined as contact or interaction between a child and an adult when the child is being used for the sexual stimulation of that adult or another person. All 50 states and the District of Columbia mandate reporting of child abuse, including child sexual abuse. Nearly half of the states also require physicians to report statutory rape. Physicians should be familiar with the laws in their states; failure to report sexual assault against children may subject the physicians to fines and incarceration for up to 1 year.

Our society has many misperceptions about sexual assault. The victims are often blamed for having encouraged the assault by their behavior or dress, for not sufficiently resisting the assault, for being promiscuous, or for having ulterior motives for pressing charges. This misplaced culpability is often internalized by the victims, which (in addition to fear of retribution) may explain their reluctance to report the violent crime to the authorities. Another common misperception is that rape is an impulsive or aggressive extension of normal sex drive on the part of the rapist. The motivation for most sexual assault, however, seems not to be sexual gratification but rather degradation, terrorization, and humiliation of the victim. The assault is often a demonstration of power (power rape), anger (anger rape), or sadism manifested in ritualized torture or mutilation of the victim (sadistic rape) on the part of the rapist.

Prevention

Much of this chapter addresses the role and responsibilities of the health care professional in caring for victims of domestic violence and sexual assault after they have occurred. One of the greatest challenges for health care and public health professionals working to improve women's health continues to be the epidemic of violence against women in our society and around the world. A great deal remains to be learned and done about the primary prevention of violence.

Clinical Findings

The majority of rape victims who come to emergency rooms do not openly admit to having been sexually assaulted. Instead, they may complain of having been mugged or may voice concerns about acquired immune deficiency syndrome (AIDS) or other sexually transmitted diseases. Others may present with psychiatric symptoms including depression, anxiety, or a suicide attempt. Unless the primary care physician, obstetrician-gynecologist, or psychiatrist obtains a sexual history, assault victims will remain unidentified as such and will be inadequately treated.

A "rape-trauma" syndrome often occurs after a sexual assault. The initial response (acute phase) may last for hours or days and is characterized by a distortion or paralysis of the individual's coping mechanisms. The initial outward responses vary from complete loss of emotional control (crying, uncontrolled anger) to an unnatural calm and detachment (although some physical signs such as shaking or lowered skin temperature are usually present). The latter behavior represents the victim's need to reestablish control over herself and her environment while simultaneously abandoning the defense mechanism of denial and allowing the renewed invasion of privacy represented by the questioning and examination. The initial reactions of shock, numbness, withdrawal, and denial typically abate after the first 2 weeks. However, studies suggest there is a period, occurring from 2 weeks to several months postassault, in which symptomatology returns and may intensify. It is at this time that the victim may begin to seek help for her symptoms, often without telling the health care provider of the sexual assault that precipitated these symptoms.

The next phase (delayed phase) may occur months or years after the sexual assault and is characterized by chronic anxiety, feelings of vulnerability, loss of control, and self-blame. Long-term reactions include anxiety, nightmares, flashbacks, catastrophic fantasies, feelings of alienation and isolation, sexual dysfunction, psychologic distress, mistrust of others, phobias, depression, hostility, and somatic symptoms. More than half of rape victims experience substantial difficulty in reestablishing sexual and emotional relationships with spouses or boyfriends. Thirty-three percent to 50% of victims report suicidal ideation; suicide attempts have been reported in nearly 1 in 5 rape victims who do not seek treatment.

PTSD is a common long-term sequela of sexual assault, characterized by psychic numbing, intrusive re-experiencing of the trauma, avoidance of stimuli associated with the trauma, and intense psychologic distress. Women with prior victimization histories often have more severe sequela. Women assaulted sexually by family members or dates experience as severe levels of distress as women assaulted by acquaintances or strangers.

Up to 40% of victims who are sexually assaulted sustain injuries. Although most injuries are minor, approximately 1% of the injuries require hospitalization and major operative repair, and 0.1% are fatal. Somatic symptoms are common during the acute phase and include disturbed sleeping and eating patterns, gastrointestinal irritability (with nausea predominating), musculoskeletal soreness, fatigue, tension headaches, and intense startle reactions. Symptoms of vaginal irritation occur in more than 50% of victims, and rectal pain and bleeding are frequent in patients subjected to anal penetration. Ongoing health concerns include gynecologic trauma, risk of pregnancy, and the potential for contracting infections or sexually transmitted diseases, including HIV. Victims may also seek to escape the pain of rape's effects through the use of alcohol and drugs.

Rape victims appear to be frequent users of medical services in the months and years after the assault. In one study, visits to physicians increased 18% in the year of the assault, 56% in the following year, and 31% in the year after, compared with previctimization levels. Reintegration of the self after sexual assault is a slow process that may take months to years as the victim works through the trauma and the loss of the event and replaces it with other life experiences. The prognosis for complete recovery is improved if health care professionals responsible for the victim's care have a supportive, nonjudgmental approach and a well-developed understanding and competent treatment of the emotional, as well as physical, consequences of sexual assault.

Differential Diagnosis

The physician evaluating the victim has both medical and legal responsibilities and should be aware of state statutory requirements. Such requirements may involve the use of sexual assault assessment kits, which list the steps necessary and the items to be obtained for forensic purposes. If personnel trained in collecting samples and information are available, it is appropriate to request their assistance.

Informed consent must be obtained before examining a sexual assault victim. A careful history and physical examination should be performed in the presence of a chaperon or victim advocate. The patient should be asked to state in her own words what happened and to identify or describe her attacker, if possible. The history should include inquiry about last menstrual period, contraceptive use, preexisting pregnancy and infection, and last consensual intercourse before the assault. The patient's activities in the interval between the assault and the examination—whether the patient has eaten, drunk, bathed, douched, voided, or defecated—might affect findings on physical examination; such activities must be recorded.

A careful physical examination of the entire body should be performed. The physician should search for bruises, abrasions, or lacerations about the neck, back, buttocks, and extremities. Bite marks should be noted, particularly about the genitalia and breasts. Injuries to the mouth and pharynx may result from oral penetration. Injuries should be documented with photographs or drawings in the medical record. *Rape* and *physical assault* are legal terms that should not be used in medical records. Instead, the physician should report findings as "consistent with the use of force."

A pelvic examination should be performed. Injuries to the vulva, hymen, vagina, urethra, and rectum should be noted. Occasionally, foreign objects may be found in the orifices. The speculum must be moistened only with saline. Two milliliters of normal saline are injected into the vaginal vault. Nonabsorbent cotton swabs should be used to sample fluid from this vaginal pool and should then be placed in sterile glass tubes and refrigerated. Air-dried, nonfixed smears of this same fluid should be placed on glass slides. A Papanicolaou (Pap) test may also be obtained. Evidence of coitus will be present in the vagina for as long as 48 hours after the attack. Motile sperms may be noted in the vagina for up to 8 hours after intercourse, but may be present in the cervical mucous for as long as 2–3 days. Nonmotile sperm may be noted in the vagina for up to 24 hours and in the cervix for up to 17 days. Acid phosphatase is an enzyme found in high concentrations in the seminal fluid. Evidence of acid phosphatase should be sought by swabbing the vaginal secretions, even in the absence of sperm because the attacker may have had a vasectomy. DNA evaluation may also be performed from the vaginal swab. Nonmotile sperm may be found in the rectum for up to 24 hours after the assault, and acid phosphatase can also be detected in the rectum.

A wet mount or vaginal swab should be obtained to detect *Trichomonas vaginalis.* Testing for *Neisseria gonorrhoeae* and *Chlamydia trachomatis* should be performed from specimens from any sites of penetration or attempted penetration. A serum sample should be collected for subsequent serologic analysis if test results are positive. The risk of acquiring gonorrhea from sexual assault is estimated to be between 6 and 12%. Baseline serologic tests for hepatitis B virus, HIV, and syphilis should also be offered. The risk of acquiring syphilis from sexual assault is estimated to be 3%; the risk of acquiring HIV is undetermined.

An important part of the physician's legal responsibilities is to collect samples for forensic purposes. Pubic hair combings should be collected to look for pubic hair from the assailant. Fingernail scrapings should be obtained to look for skin or blood of the attacker. Skin washings and clothing should be investigated for the presence of blood or semen. A Wood light may be helpful because dried semen will fluoresce under its light. Saliva should be collected from the victim. Because seminal fluid is rapidly destroyed by salivary enzymes, identification of seminal fluid in the mouth after a few hours is difficult. Consequently, victims should be encouraged to come to a medical facility immediately after an assault, where they can be evaluated before they bathe, urinate, defecate, wash out their mouths, or clean their fingernails.

Proper processing and labeling of collected specimens is crucial. All collected specimens are placed in a larger sealed container and processed in a "chain of evidence" fashion. The person who collects the specimens verifies their completeness by signature on the sealed master container. The individual to whom they are transferred must verify by signature that all specimens were received in an untampered state. Thus each individual who has "custody" of the specimens during processing must verify that they were transmitted without alteration until they are turned over to the responsible law enforcement agency. The name of the law enforcement agent who receives the specimens should be noted in the medical record.

Treatment

Treatment of physical injuries sustained at the time of assault should be initiated immediately; prophylactic medical treatment may be indicated for prevention of sexually transmitted infections and pregnancy. For prophylaxis against sexually transmitted infections, empiric recommended antimicrobial therapy for chlamydial, gonococcal, and trichomonal infections may be given. One such regimen consists of the following:

- Ceftriaxone 125 mg intramuscularly in a single dose, plus
- Metronidazole 2 g orally in a single dose, plus
- Doxycycline 100 mg orally 2 times a day for 7 days

Alternative treatment may be given as recommended by the US Centers for Disease Control and Prevention. In addition, it is recommended that hepatitis B immunoglobulin be administered intramuscularly as soon as possible, but certainly within 14 days of exposure. It should be followed by the standard 3-dose active immunization series with hepatitis B vaccine at 0, 1, and 6 months, beginning at the time of passive immunization. Prophylaxis against HIV is controversial.

Emergency contraception can be offered as prophylaxis against pregnancy. The risk of pregnancy after sexual assault has been estimated to be 2–4% in victims who were not using some form of contraception at the time of the assault. A serum pregnancy test should be obtained before administration of emergency contraception to evaluate for preexisting pregnancy. Emergency contraception should be given within 72 hours of the assault, although it can still be effective up to 120 hours later. There are several different methods of emergency contraception. For many years, the most common method (Yuzpe method) involved the use of high-dose combined oral contraceptives within 72 hours of unprotected coitus, repeated 12 hours after the first dose. More recently, use of a progestin-only method has become popular. This method involves the use of levonorgestrel 0.75 mg, in 2 doses 12 hours apart, or a 1-time dose of 1.5 mg within 72 hours of unprotected coitus. A randomized study showed that this is more effective and better tolerated than the Yuzpe method. Levonorgestrel prevented 85% of pregnancies that would have occurred without treatment.

As most patients suffer significant psychologic trauma as a consequence of sexual assault, the physician must be prepared to provide access to counseling. It is preferable that follow-up psychologic counseling be provided by individuals who have extensive experience in the management of crisis response to rape. Even if the victim appears to be in control emotionally, she will probably experience aspects of rape-trauma syndrome at some time in the future. She should be made aware of the symptoms that she may experience and advised to seek help if and when these symptoms occur. No patient should be released from the facility until specific follow-up plans are made and agreed upon by the patient, physician, and counselor.

A follow-up visit should be scheduled approximately 2 weeks after the assault for repeat physical examination and collection of additional specimens. Testing for *N gonorrhoeae, C trachomatis*, and *T vaginalis* should be repeated unless prophylactic antimicrobials have been provided. Follow-up counseling should be discussed again at the second visit. Additional visits may be scheduled according to the victim's needs; an additional follow-up visit approximately 12 weeks after the sexual assault is advisable to collect sera for detection of antibodies against *T pallidum*, hepatitis B virus (unless vaccine was given), and HIV (repeat test at 6 months). During each of these visits, assessment of the patient's psychologic symptoms should be performed, and referrals for further counseling are made as indicated.

American College of Obstetricians and Gynecologists. Psychosocial risk factors: perinatal screening and intervention. ACOG Committee Opinion No. 343. Washington, DC: ACOG; 2006.

American College of Obstetricians and Gynecologists. Emergency oral contraception. ACOG Practice Bulletin No. 25. Washington, DC: ACOG; 2001.

Centers for Disease Control and Prevention. 2006 Sexually transmitted disease treatment guidelines. http://origin.cdc.gov/STD/treatment/default.htm. Accessed March 17, 2010.

Jina R, Jewkes R, Munjanja SP, Mariscal JD, Dartnall E, Gebrehiwot Y. Report of the FIGO Working Group on Sexual Violence/HIV: Guidelines for the management of female survivors of sexual assault. *Int J Gynaecol Obstet* 2010;109:85–92. PMID: 20206349.

Jones RF 3rd, Horan DL. The American College of Obstetricians and Gynecologists: Responding to violence against women. *Int J Gynaecol Obstet* 2002;78:S75–S77. PMID: 12429443.

Kaplan DW et al. Care of the adolescent sexual assault victim. *Pediatrics* 2001;107:1476–1479. PMID: 11389281.

Patel M, Minshell L. Management of sexual assault. *Emerg Med Clin North Am* 2001;19:817–831. PMID: 11554289.

Welch J, Mason F. Rape and sexual assault. *BMJ* 2007;334:1154–1158. PMID: 17540944.

Index

NOTE: A *t* following a page number indicates tabular material, and *f* following a page number indicates a figure.

D

P